GUIDE TO DRUG PROTOTYPES   CONTINUED

NURSING
Pharmacology

Norma L. Pinnell, MSN, RN

College of Nursing
Southern Illinois University at Edwardsville
Edwardsville, Illinois

College of Nursing
Deaconess Health System
St. Louis, Missouri

W.B. SAUNDERS COMPANY
A Division of Harcourt Brace & Company
Philadelphia   London   Toronto   Montreal   Sydney   Tokyo

W.B. SAUNDERS COMPANY

A Division of Harcourt Brace & Company

The Curtis Center
Independence Square West
Philadelphia, Pennsylvania 19106

NOTICE

Pharmacology is an ever-changing field. Standard safety precautions must be followed, but as new research and clinical experience broaden our knowledge, changes in treatment and drug therapy become necessary or appropriate. The authors of this work have carefully checked the generic and trade drug names and verified drug dosages to ensure that the dosage information in this work is accurate and in accord with the standards accepted at the time of publication. Readers are advised, however, to check the product information currently provided by the manufacturer of each drug to be administered to be certain that changes have not been made in the recommended dose or in the contraindications for administration. This is of particular importance in regard to new or infrequently used drugs. It is the responsibility of the treating physician or health care provider, relying on experience and knowledge of the client, to determine dosages and the best treatment for the client. The authors cannot be responsible for misuse or misapplication of the material in this work.

THE PUBLISHER

Library of Congress Cataloging–in–Publication Data

Nursing pharmacology/[edited by] Norma L. Pinnell.
     p.   cm.
    ISBN 0–7216–6482–2
    1. Pharmacology.   2. Nursing   I. Pinnell, Norma Nolan.
    [DNLM: 1. Pharmacology—nurses' instruction.   2. Drug Therapy–
–nurses' instruction.   3. Drugs—nurses' instruction. QV 18 N9745
1995]
RM300.N885 1996
615'.1—dc20
DNLM/DLC
for Library of Congress   94-20441
                                                       CIP

NURSING PHARMACOLOGY   ISBN 0–7216–6482–2

Printed in the United States of America

Last digit is the print number: 9 8 7 6 5 4 3 2 1

To my husband,
Tom,
for his constant love, support,
and encouragement.

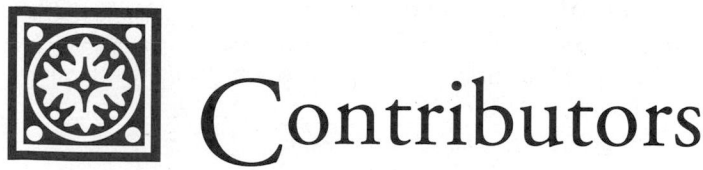

Contributors

Dottye Akerson, MSN, RN
Associate Clinical Professor, Barnes College of Nursing, University of Missouri–St. Louis, St. Louis, Missouri
Antimycobacterial Drugs

Lasca Beck, MS, RN
Nursing Liaison, Arizona State University West, and Faculty Associate, Arizona State University, Tempe, Arizona
Drugs Used in Ocular Disorders

Elizabeth A. Buck, PhD, RN
Professor, Jewish Hospital College of Nursing and Allied Health, St. Louis, Missouri
Drugs Affecting Plasma Lipids and Coagulation Factors; Overview of the Renal System

Ellen J. Burge, MSN, RNC
Formerly Assistant Professor, Community Health, DePauw University School of Nursing, Indianapolis, Indiana; presently Maternal-Infant Clinical Nursing Instructor, King Fahad National Guard Hospital, Riyadh, Kingdom of Saudi Arabia
Drugs Used to Manage Poisoning

Jeanne E. Catanzaro, MSN, RN
Instructor, Jewish Hospital College of Nursing and Allied Health, St. Louis, Missouri
Diuretics

Jacquelyn M. Clement, PhD, RN
Associate Professor, Southern Illinois University at Edwardsville School of Nursing, Edwardsville, Illinois
Drugs Affecting Plasma Lipids and Coagulation Factors

Elizabeth Ann Coleman, PhD, RNP
Associate Professor, College of Nursing, and Program Leader, Women's Oncology, Arkansas Cancer Research Center, University of Arkansas for Medical Sciences, Little Rock, Arkansas
Overview of Normal and Neoplastic Cell Growth

Rhonda W. Comrie, MSN, RN
Lecturer, Southern Illinois University at Edwardsville School of Nursing, Edwardsville, Illinois
Opioid and Nonopioid Analgesics

Sandra L. Forney, MS, RNC
Edwardsville, Illinois
Drug Therapy in Childbearing and Breastfeeding Clients

Sandy Forrest, PhD, RN
Department Chair and Professor, Department of Nursing and Radiologic Sciences, Mesa State College, Grand Junction, Colorado
Psychotherapeutic Drugs

William R. Gerber, MD
Assistant Professor of Obstetrics and Gynecology, St. Louis University School of Medicine; Active Staff, St. Louis University Health Sciences Center, St. Mary's Health Center, and Deaconess Hospital, St. Louis, Missouri
Overview of Female and Male Reproductive Systems; Drugs Affecting the Female Reproductive System; Local Anesthesia

Susan Grinslade, MSN, RN
Associate Professor, Jewish Hospital College of Nursing and Allied Health, St. Louis, Missouri
Antiviral Drugs

Gail Estock Haller, MS, RN
Assistant Professor, Division of Nursing, McKendree College, Lebanon, Illinois
Drug Therapy in the Elderly Client; Antiseptics, Disinfectants, and Sterilants

Rhoda Headley, MSN, RN
Staff Nurse, Neuroradiology, Barnes Hospital, St. Louis, Missouri
Overview of the Central Nervous System; Drugs Used to Treat Parkinson's Disease

Judith K. Hedrick-Thompson, MSN, RN
Formerly Clinical Specialist—Enterostomal Therapist, presently Collaborative Care/Carepath Coordinator, St. John's Mercy Medical Center, St. Louis Missouri
Overview of the Digestive System

Donna Henry, MSN, RN
Instructor of Nursing, Illinois Eastern Community Colleges, Olney, Illinois
Antihypertensive Drugs; Drugs Affecting the Upper Gastrointestinal Tract

June Hertell, MSN, RN
Clinical Assistant Professor, Barnes College of Nursing, University of Missouri–St. Louis, St. Louis, Missouri
Antiparasitic Drugs

Barbara B. Hodgson, RN
Drug Research Coordinator, Diabetes Center, University of South Florida, Tampa, Florida
Nasal Decongestants, Antitussives, and Mucolytics

Alan W. Hopefl, PharmD
Clinical Coordinator, AmeriNet, St. Louis, Missouri
HIV Therapy

V. Lynn Horning, MSN, RN
HIV Nurse Educator, 18th MEDCOM, United States Army, Republic of Korea
Drugs Used to Treat Dermatologic Conditions

Sonja Howard, MS, RN, CCRN
Patient Care Manager, BJC Health System, St. Louis, Missouri
Drugs that Affect Vascular Tone

Pamela E. Hugie, MSN, RN
Assistant Professor, Weber State University, Ogden, Utah
Drugs Affecting Hypothalamic and Pituitary Functions; Drugs Affecting Thyroid and Parathyroid Function

Joyce M. Hunter, MSN, RN
Clinical Professor, Barnes College of Nursing, University of Missouri–St. Louis; Staff Nurse PRN, Acute Psychiatric Unit, Barnes Hospital, St. Louis, Missouri
Substance Abuse and Addiction

Karen C. Johnson-Brennan, EdD, RN
Professor of Nursing and Associate Director, School of Nursing, San Francisco State University, San Francisco, California
Hyperuricemic Drugs

Kathy M. Ketchum, MS, RN
Doctoral Student and Research Assistant, St. Louis University, St. Louis, Missouri
Antifungal Drugs

Robert J. Kizior, BS, RPh
Educational Coordinator, Department of Pharmacy, Alexian Brothers Medical Center, Elk Grove Village, Illinois
Antiarrhythmic Drugs; Antibiotics; Drugs Used to Treat Dermatologic Conditions; Drugs Used to Manage Poisoning

Joan M. Kulpa, EdD, MSN, RN
Associate Professor, Nursing, Bradley University, Peoria, Illinois
Overview of the Endocrine System

Pamala D. Larsen, PhD, RN
Associate Professor, School of Nursing, University of Northern Colorado, Greeley, Colorado; Administrative Supervisor, Poudre Valley Hospital, Fort Collins, Colorado
Drugs Affecting the Male Reproductive System

Sharon Jones Layton, BSN, RN
Formerly Director of Educational Services, presently Nursing Administration, Staff Nurse, Citizens Memorial Hospital, Bolivar, Missouri
Drugs Used for Diagnostic Procedures

Sandra Lindquist, MEd, MSN, RN
Associate Professor, Barnes College of Nursing, University of Missouri–St. Louis, St. Louis, Missouri
Overview of the Autonomic Nervous System

Kim Litwack, PhD, RN
Associate Professor, College of Nursing, University of New Mexico, Albuquerque, New Mexico
Antiarrythmic Drugs

Judy Malkiewicz, PhD, RN
Associate Professor, School of Nursing, University of Northern Colorado, Greeley, Colorado
Immunosuppressant and Immunostimulant Drugs; Ear Preparations

Jan Hoot Martin, PhD, RN, GNP
Associate Professor, School of Nursing, University of Northern Colorado, Greeley, Colorado
Immunosuppressant and Immunostimulant Drugs; Ear Preparations

Mary Mirch, MS, RN
Associate Professor, Glendale Community College, Glendale, California
Nonsteroidal, Anti-inflammatory Drugs

Karen Muench, MSN, MSEd, RN
Nursing Instructor, Division of Nursing, McKendree College, Lebanon, Illinois
Adrenal Corticoids

Jean Nelson, MEd, MSN, RN
Clinical Assistant Professor, Barnes College of Nursing, University of Missouri–St. Louis, St. Louis, Missouri
Drugs Affecting the Lower Gastrointestinal Tract

Marguerite Newton, PhD, RN
Assistant Professor, Southern Illinois University at Edwardsville School of Nursing, Edwardsville, Illinois
Legal Foundations of Pharmacologic Practice; Overview of Biologic Defense Mechanisms

Pamela Mohler Pickens, PharmD, BCNSP
Clinical Pharmacist I: Oncology/Nutrition, St. Agnes Medical Center, Fresno, California
Fat-Soluble Vitamins; Water-Soluble Vitamins; Minerals

Janet D. Pierce, DSN, RN, CCRN
Assistant Professor, University of Kansas School of Nursing, Kansas City, Kansas
Overview of the Cardiovascular System

Julia Ann Raithel, MSN, RN

Assistant Professor, Deaconess College of Nursing, St. Louis, Missouri

Drugs Used to Regulate Blood Glucose Levels; Overview of the Respiratory System

Robyn Rice, MS, RN

Associate Clinical Professor, Barnes College of Nursing, University of Missouri–St. Louis; Medical-Surgical Clinical Nurse Specialist, Family Services and Visiting Nurse Association, Alton, Illinois

Substance Abuse and Addiction; Overview of the Automonic Nervous System; Overview of Biologic Defense Mechanisms; HIV Therapy

David J. Ritchie, PharmD

Assistant Professor of Pharmacy Practice, St. Louis College of Pharmacy; Clinical Pharmacist, Infectious Diseases, Barnes-Jewish Hospitals, St. Louis, Missouri

Antifungal Drugs

Bernadette Roche, MS, CRNA

Adjunct Professor, DePaul University; Instructor and Program Director, Ravenswood Hospital Medical Center School of Anesthesia; Manager, Anesthesia Services, Department of Anesthesia, Ravenswood Hospital Medical Center, Chicago, Illinois

Anesthetic Agents

Angela M. Rossington, MSN, RN

Health Educator and Adjunct Associate Professor in Women's Health, Alfred University; formerly Assistant Professor of Nursing, Alfred University College of Nursing, Alfred, New York

Principles of Antimicrobial Therapy; Antibiotics

Linda Ruholl, MS, RNC

Nursing Instructor and Pharmacology Instructor, Lake Land College, Mattoon, Illinois

Skeletal Muscle Relaxants; Urinary Tract Antiseptics

Janice Rumfelt, EdD, MSN, RNC

Assistant Professor, Southern Illinois University at Edwardsville School of Nursing, Edwardsville, Illinois

Drug Therapy in the Neonate and Pediatric Client

Terry L. Seaton, PharmD, BCPS

Assistant Professor, St. Louis College of Pharmacy; Clinical Pharmacist, Department of Family Medicine, St. John's Mercy Medical Center, St. Louis, Missouri

Central Nervous System Stimulants

Martha A. Spies, MSN, RN

Assistant Professor, Deaconess College of Nursing, St. Louis, Missouri

Fluid, Electrolyte, and Nutritional Balance; Agents Affecting the Volume and Ion Content of Body Fluids; Enteral and Parenteral Nutritional Therapy

Cynthia Mills Spiro, MSN, RN

Instructor, Medical-Surgical Nursing, Barnes College of Nursing, University of Missouri–St. Louis; Cardiology Clinical Nurse Specialist, Private Cardiology Practice, St. Louis, Missouri

HIV Therapy

Janet L. Melnik Stewart, MNEd, RN

Nursing Instructor, The Western Pennsylvania Hospital School of Nursing, Pittsburgh, Pennsylvania

Histamine-Receptor Agonists and Antagonists

Michael F. Thomure, MD

Instructor, Division of Reproductive Endocrinology and Infertility, Department of Obstetrics and Gynecology, St. Louis University School of Medicine; Active Staff, St. Mary's Health Care Center, Deaconess Hospital, and St. Louis University Health Sciences Center, St. Louis, Missouri

Drugs Affecting the Female Reproductive System

Patricia Ugo, MSN, RN

Enterostomal Therapist and Nutrition Support Nurse, St. John's Mercy Medical Center, St. Louis, Missouri

Fat-Soluble Vitamins; Water-Soluble Vitamins; Minerals

Carol M. Viamontes, MSN, RN

Clinical Nurse Specialist, Maternal-fetal Medicine, St. Mary's Health Center, St. Louis, Missouri

Overview of Female and Male Reproductive Systems; Drugs Affecting the Female Reproductive System; Local Anesthesia

Myrna Brenner Wacker, MS, RNC

Instructor of Nursing, Southern Illinois University at Edwardsville School of Nursing, Edwardsville, Illinois

Cultural Influence on Drug Therapy; Nurse's Role in Drug Therapy in the Home

Joan Domigan Wentz, MSN, RN

Assistant Professor, Jewish Hospital College of Nursing and Allied Health, St. Louis, Missouri

Drugs Affecting the Parasympathetic Nervous System; Drugs Affecting the Sympathetic Nervous System

Sharee A. Wiggins, MSN, RN, CRNI

Clinical Assistant Professor, Critical Care, University of Kansas School of Nursing, Kansas City, Kansas

Overview of the Cardiovascular System

Barbara J. Wirick, MSN, CEN

Assistant Professor of Nursing, Weber State University; Staff Nurse, Emergency Department, McKay Dee Hospital, Ogden, Utah

Antiepileptic Drugs; Bronchodilating Drugs and Related Agents

Linda Nattkemper York, MSN, RN

Instructor, Barnes College of Nursing, University of Missouri–St. Louis, and Consultant, Independence Center, St. Louis, Missouri

Central Nervous System Stimulants

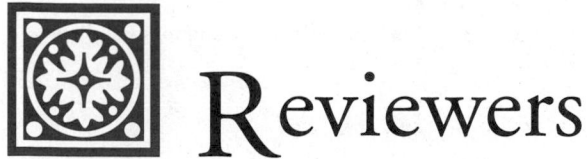

Reviewers

Gerald Banet, MSN, RN
Department of Neurology, St. Louis University Health Sciences
Center, St. Louis, Missouri

George Battaglia, PhD
Department of Pharmacology, Stritch School of Medicine, Loyola
University Chicago, Maywood, Illinois

Sheryl Lee Buck, PhD
Loyola University Medical Center, Maywood, Illinois

Kathleen Blais, EdD, RN
School of Nursing, Florida International University, Miami, Florida

Gloria M. Blatti, EdD, MA, RN, FNP
Adelphi University, Garden City, New York

Karna Bramble, PhD, RNC, GNP
College of Nursing, California State University, Long Beach, Long
Beach, California

Constance F. Buran, DNS, RN
College of Nursing, University of Indianapolis, Indianapolis, Indiana

Jessie M. Clemmons, MNSc
American Nurses Association, Arkansas Nurses Association,
National League of Nurses, Arkansas National League of Nurses,
Pine Bluff, Arkansas

Barbara A. Cline, MSN, RN
School of Nursing, Kent State University, Kent, Ohio

Charles Robert Craig, PhD
Professor of Pharmacology and Toxicology, Department of
Pharmacology and Toxicology, West Virginia University Health
Sciences Center, Morgantown, West Virginia

Janet D. Dionne, MSN, RN
Assistant Professor, Community College of Denver, Denver, Colorodo

Leonard A. Fahien, AB, MD
Department of Pharmacology, University of Wisconsin Medical
School, Madison, Wisconsin

Janet M. Farahmand, EdD, MSN, CRN
Associate Professor and Project Director—Graduate Program,
School of Nursing and Health Sciences, Neumann College,
Aston, Pennsylvania

Elizabeth Anne Farren, PhD, RN
College of Nursing, Baylor University, Dallas, Texas

Sister Catherine Feuerstein, OSF, MSN
Neumann College, Aston, Pennsylvania

Jacqueline L. Gaddy, MSN, RN, CDE
School of Nursing, Southern Illinois University, Edwardsville,
Illinois

Susan L. Gatto, MSN, RNP
College of Nursing, University of Central Arkansas, Conway, Arkansas

Elizabeth Gloss, EdD, RN
College of Nursing, State University of New York, Health Science
Center Brooklyn, New York, New York

Barbara Eunice Gould, MEd, BScPhm
School of Health Sciences, Seneca College of Applied Arts and
Technology, Willowdale, Ontario, Canada

Pauline M. Green, PhD, RN
College of Nursing, Howard University, Washington, DC

Patricia A. Higham, MEd, BSN, RN
Instructor, St. John's Hospital School of Nursing,
Springfield, Missouri

Doris Hoerdeman, MSN, RN
School of Nursing, Methodist Medical Center of Illinois,
Peoria, Illinois

Barbara Dawn Horton, MS, RN
School of Nursing, Arnot Ogden Medical Center, Elmira, New York

Brenda P. Johnson, MSN, RN
Instructor, College of Nursing, Southeast Missouri State University,
Cape Girardeau, Missouri

Jodell Kuzneski, MNEd, RN
Chairperson, Department of Nursing/Allied Health, Indiana
University of Pennsylvania, Indiana, Pennsylvania

Vicky M. Lagle, MSN, RN, ARNP(C)
Assistant Professor, College of Nursing, Spalding University,
Louisville, Kentucky

Nada Light, MA, BSN, RN
Capital Community Technical College, Hartford, Connecticut

Lola Gayle McKay, MS, CRNA
Associate Program Director, School of Anesthesia, Abbott
Northwestern Hospital, and Adjunct Faculty, St. Mary's College,
Minneapolis, Minnesota

Janet Lynn Melnick, MNEd, BSN, RN
School of Nursing, The Western Pennsylvania Hospital,
Pittsburgh, Pennsylvania

Dorothy M. Obester, PhD, MSN, BSNEduc, RN
Professor, Higher Education, School of Nursing, St. Francis College,
Loretto, Pennsylvania

Nancy O'Donnell, MSN, RN
Associate Professor, Department of Nursing, J. Sargeant Reynolds
Community College, Richmond, Virginia

Keith M. Olsen, PharmD
Associate Professor of Pharmacy, Pharmacy Practice, University of
Arkansas for Medical Sciences, Little Rock, Arkansas

Sue Ann Pflum, BSN, RN, CARN
Past President, National Nurses Society on Addictions, Chicago, Illinois

Susan Quatre, BSN, RN
Instructor, School of Nursing, Gavilan College, Gilroy, California

Margaret Anne Reilly, PhD
Research Scientist, Nathan Kline Research Institute, Orangeburg,
New York; Adjunct Assistant Professor, Concordia College,
Bronxville, New York; Instructor in Pharmacology, Phillips–Beth
Israel School of Nursing, New York, New York

Kenneth W. Renton, PhD
Department of Pharmacology, Dalhousie University, Halifax, Nova
Scotia, Canada

Rosemary Ricks-Saulsby, MSN, MA, RN
Christian Nurses Association, Department of Nursing, Trinity
Christian College, Palos Heights, Illinois

Robin William Rockhold, PhD
Department of Pharmacology and Toxicology, The University of
Mississippi Medical Center, Jackson, Mississippi

Carol E. Roe, MSN, RN
Department of Nursing, Kalamazoo Valley Community College,
Kalamazoo, Michigan

Sharon P. Shipton, MSN, RN, AS
Associate Professor, College of Nursing, Youngstown State
University, Youngstown, Ohio

Ann S. Syfrett, MN, RN
Division Chair, Associate Degree of Nursing Faculty of Health
Science, Gulf Coast Community College, Panama City, Florida

Gopi A. Tejwani, PhD
Department of Pharmacology, Ohio State University College of
Medicine, Columbus, Ohio

Joan Kay Ulloth, MSN, RN
Associate Professor, School of Nursing, Kettering College of
Medical Arts, Kettering, Ohio

Paula J. Vehlow, MS, RN
Lincoln Land Community College, Springfield, Illinois

Michael J. A. Walker, PhD
Department of Pharmacology and Therapeutics, University of
British Columbia, Vancouver, British Columbia, Canada

Kay L. Wold, MS, RN
Associate Professor and Chair, Department of Nursing, Minnesota
Intercollegiate Nursing Consortium, Gustavus Adolphus College,
St. Peter, Minnesota

Bruce H. Woolley, PharmD
Professor, Pharmacology and Nutrition, Brigham Young University,
Provo, Utah

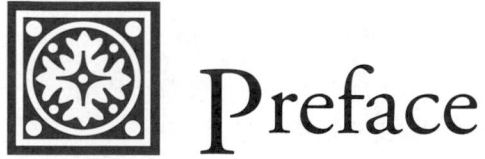

Preface

Professional nurses need to be knowledgeable about pharmacology. They need to understand the overall therapeutic plan of care and the role of drug therapy. In addition, nurses must be aware of the responsiblities that develop as a consequence of the drug regimen. This text, *Nursing Pharmacology*, addresses these responsibilities and blends in-depth pharmacology with clear, consistent nursing considerations.

Nursing Pharmacology is divided into two parts, with each part subdivided into units and chapters. Chapters in Part One discuss the basic concepts of pharmacology, including basic terms, legal foundations of pharmacologic practice, drug preparations and formulations, and general principles of drug action. Biopsychosocial aspects, life-span and cultural influences, self-treatment, drug therapy in the home, and over-the-counter drugs are also discussed.

Part Two addresses the clinical aspects of pharmacology. Units in this part are organized according to body systems. Each chapter within a unit discusses drugs or drug categories that affect that particular body system. This approach enables students to associate specific drug groups with specific body systems. Thus as students acquire essential knowledge of pharmacology, they retain it more easily by making a connection to what they already know. For each body system, normal anatomy and physiology are reviewed and various pathologic conditions discussed.

Within each drug group or category, usually one drug that typifies the features of all members of the group can be identified. This drug is viewed as a prototype. Since other drugs in the category are similar to the prototype, to understand the prototype is to understand the basic properties of all group members. *Nursing Pharmacology* uses this prototype approach to teach pharmacology. Within each chapter a prototype for each drug group or category is presented in depth. Pharmacotherapeutic, pharmacodynamic, pharmacokinetic, and pharmaceutic data are provided for each prototype. In addition, undesired clinical responses; contraindications and precautions; life-span considerations; drug-drug, drug-nutrient, and drug-environment interactions; and specific drug-related nursing considerations are discussed. Examples of other drugs in the category are briefly discussed or presented in table format.

Clinical chapters have many useful features. Each chapter begins with objectives that are integrated into an easy-to-follow outline of key concepts and terms to review. Concept Review boxes that summarize key points made in the text are placed throughout each chapter. A consistent, easy-to-scan format is used for drug tables. These tables present drugs by their generic names and describe how the drugs are supplied as well as their dosages, routes of administration, and key nursing considerations. Most chapters contain standardized body system illustrations that clearly indicate common undesired clinical responses associated with specific drugs or drug categories. Life-span considerations address the effects of drugs on clients of all ages—particularly children, the elderly, adults, and pregnant and lactating women.

Another distinguishing feature within each chapter is the consistent use of the nursing process. The nursing process is viewed as one component that helps to distinguish nursing from other health care professions. Using the nursing process format to present nursing care related to drug therapy reinforces the student's prior learning and facilitates the learning of new content. To assist students to identify with the importance of nursing research, research boxes are presented throughout this book. These boxes contain summaries of nursing research and suggest student activities related to the research topic.

Ancillary materials that are available include the *Instructor's Manual, Student Study Guide, and ExaMaster.* The *Instructor's Manual* for *Nursing Pharmacology* contains learning objectives and teaching and learning strategies. Included are suggestions for the instructor, class assignments, focus points for lecture or discussion, clinical site experiences, group activities, and suggestions for guest speakers. The manual also contains transparency masters for use in the classroom and a testbank of multiple-choice questions that correspond with the chapters in the textbook. The *Student Study Guide* contains a variety of activities, including study questions, sample multiple-choice questions, crossword puzzles, and critical-thinking exercises. These activities are meant to help students retain what they have learned and to identify areas that remain unclear. The *EXAMaster* is an easy to use computerized testbank.

NORMA L. PINNELL

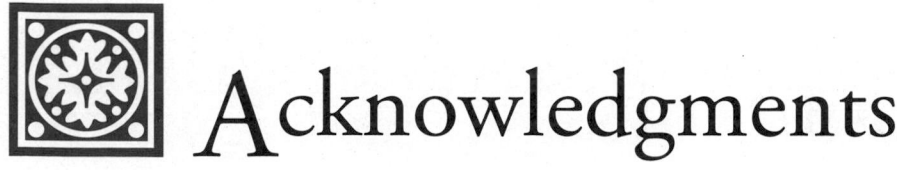

Acknowledgments

Many people helped to make this book a reality. To these individuals I offer my thanks.

To Thomas H. Pinnell, my husband, who made many sacrifices to assure completion of this project. Without his assistance and encouragement this book would not exist.

To Daniel T. Ruth, former editor at W.B. Saunders, who supervised the acquisition and production of the text and gave this project unfailing support.

To Rachel Bedard, developmental editor, who helped design and release the final manuscript to production.

To Susan Bielitsky, former editorial assistant at W.B. Saunders, who provided support and encouragement during manuscript preparation.

To Thomas Eoyang, Vice President & Editor-in-Chief, Nursing Books, who provided guidance during the final stages of production.

To the many contributors, who shared their expertise and knowledge.

To the many reviewers, who enhanced this book with their comments and corrections.

To Robert Kizior, BS, RPh, who reviewed chapters for current and essential information.

To Diane Crowder, RPh, Mark Krinski, RPh, and Ted Thalmann, RPh, who shared their expertise in clinical pharmacology.

To Lynn Crammond, BS, RPh, Adjunct Professor, Southern Illinois University, Edwardsville, School of Dental Medicine, Alton, Illinois, who critiqued the original content outline and shared her resources.

To Guy W. Aton, MD, who shared his expertise and resources.

NORMA L. PINNELL

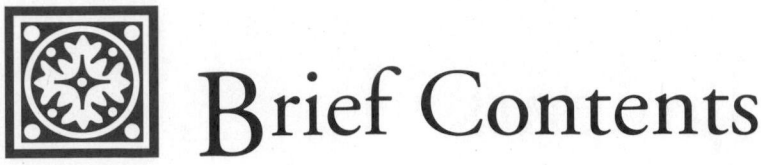

Brief Contents

Detailed Contents

PART TWO
CLINICAL ASPECTS OF PHARMACOLOGY

UNIT V
Drugs Affecting the Central Nervous System

UNIT VIII
Drugs Affecting the Renal System

UNIT IX
Drugs Affecting the Endocrine System

UNIT XIII
Antimicrobial Drugs

PART one

BASIC CONCEPTS OF
Pharmacology

Orientation to Pharmacology

CHAPTER 1

Introduction to Pharmacology

NORMA L. PINNELL

⊛ **Historic Perspective**
LEARNING OBJECTIVE: Describe the historic development of the science of pharmacology.
KEY TERM: Pharmacopeia

⊛ **Basic Terms**
LEARNING OBJECTIVE: Define selected terms associated with pharmacology.
KEY TERMS:
Drug, over-the-counter (OTC) drugs, pharmacodynamics, pharmacognosy, pharmacokinetics, pharmacology, pharmacotherapeutics, pharmacy, prescription drug, toxicology

⊛ **Drug Classification**
LEARNING OBJECTIVE: Discuss three methods for classifying drugs.
KEY TERM: Prototype

⊛ **Drug Nomenclature**
LEARNING OBJECTIVE: Describe the nomenclature used in assigning names to drugs.
KEY TERMS:
Bioequivalent, chemical name, generic name or nonproprietary name, official name, proprietary name or trade name

⊛ **Sources of Drug Information**
LEARNING OBJECTIVE: List two official sources and two unofficial sources of drug information.

*P*harmacology is a young science, dating from the middle of the nineteenth century. It draws on physiology and biochemistry and provides a foundation for clinical medicine.

HISTORIC PERSPECTIVE

The use of chemicals to produce biologic effects on living organisms comprises an ancient branch of human knowledge. Potent natural chemicals were discovered as people foraged for food. Through a slow system of trial and error humans learned that some fruits, roots, berries, and barks were safe to eat but that others produced discomforting effects on the body. Knowledge about natural chemicals was acquired and transmitted from generation to generation through folklore and cultural beliefs.[1,2]

Primitive Era

Probably the first natural product used internally for medical purposes was the cathartic. Laxative chemicals were frequently found in nature in the form of purgative plants and mineral salts. These purgative substances were used for mystical or magic purposes, that is, cleansing the body of evil spirits thought to exist in the sick person.

Ancient and Middle Ages

Pharmacologically active substances were used traditionally in many ancient cultures, including those of the Chinese, Egyptians, Hebrews, Greeks, and Arabs. Ancient Egypt is considered the "cradle" of pharmacology. The *Ebers Medical Papyrus,* an Egyptian compilation of drug lore dating from approximately 1550 BC, refers to the use of opium and castor oil. Such documents also describe preservative substances used to prevent decay of the body after death. These papers were probably the earliest documents devoted entirely to medicine.

The Greco-Roman civilization also used many drugs in its medical practice. Although Hippocrates, often called the Father of Medicine, used few drug preparations in the treatment of disease, his fifth century BC writings mentioned more than 400 drugs. Another Greek physician, Dioscorides, described approximately 600 drugs in his encyclopedic work on medical material. Many of these drugs are still listed in current sources of drug information.

Additional early collections of information about drugs were found in China. Near 2700 BC, a book of mixtures for medicinal use and a textbook of medicine existed. Substances such as rhubarb, senna, and ginseng were favorite remedies.

During the Middle Ages medical practice in Europe returned to a primitive philosophy, and natural remedies were the primary source of drugs. Herbs, including belladonna, were cultivated in the gardens of medieval monasteries for their medicinal properties. Isolated centers of learning preserved some older drug knowledge, but few new remedies were developed. One source of new remedies was Galen (AD 131 to 210), who developed many preparations of plant drugs.

During the eighth century AD Arabs swept throughout Asia Minor and Northern Africa and into Spain. The Arabs absorbed the teaching of Hippocrates and Galen and advanced the science of medicine and pharmacy in many ways. They contributed many new plant drugs and used mineral substances to treat disease. In addition, the Arabs compiled the first **pharmacopeia** (an authoritative essay on drugs and their preparations).

Medicine During the Renaissance

During the Renaissance, plants and herbs were classified, and the relationship of dose to toxicity was recognized. The use of pure chemical agents as drugs also was fostered by the beginnings of empirical chemistry. During the sixteenth century the Swiss physician Paracelsus introduced mercury for treatment of syphilis. He advocated the use of single drugs, instead of mixtures, to treat diseases. For his contributions, Paracelsus is often considered the "father of pharmacology."

By the mid-sixteenth century New World natives were using cocoa, chili, balsam, castor oil, sassafras, sarsaparilla, and tobacco for medicinal purposes. Many of these products were exported to Europe. Native Americans also used mushrooms, peyote, and morning glory as hallucinogens.

Nineteenth Century Medicine

Knowledge of chemistry played a major role in the advancement of drug knowledge during the nineteenth century. Investigation centered on the site and mode of actions of drugs. It became possible to extract the active ingredients of medicines for study, and some chemicals became available in their pure form. As the sciences of chemistry and biology developed, a modern science of pharmacology emerged.

Among the discoveries of this period were anesthetics, injection techniques, and antipyretic analgesics such as aspirin. Medical therapy was characterized by measures designed to force the body to resume normal functions; violent purges, sweating, emetics, and bloodletting were favorite treatments.

Modern Medicine

Pharmacology has evolved into a complex science since the beginning of the twentieth century. Now purified chemicals are prepared from all conceivable natural materials, including minerals, plant and animal tissues, and microbial cultures. In addition, drugs are developed and modified through chemical synthesis. Chemicals can enhance, suppress, or manipulate every body function.

With the availability of chemicals with powerful effects on the body, the problem of drug abuse has surfaced on a worldwide level. In addition, a multitude of chemical substances for use by industry and agriculture permeates the environment and influences the health of each individual.

BASIC TERMS

The science of pharmacology has a language of its own.[3-5] You should know the meaning of the terms used in drug therapy.

Pharmacology

Pharmacology is the study of the history, sources, and physical and chemical properties of drugs. Pharmacology also includes the study of the effects of drugs on living systems.

Pharmacy

Pharmacy is the branch of health science that deals with the preparation and dispensing of drugs. The term describes the process of compounding, dispensing, and selling drugs.

Pharmacotherapeutics

Pharmacotherapeutics is the branch of pharmacology that deals with drugs or chemicals used in medicine for the treatment, prevention, and diagnosis of disease. It sometimes is used synonymously with the term *clinical pharmacology*.

Pharmacokinetics

Pharmacokinetics is the study of the movement of drugs in the body. It includes the processes of absorption, distribution, biotransformation (metabolism), and excretion of drugs.

Pharmacodynamics

Pharmacodynamics is the experimental science that deals with interactions between chemical components of living tissues or systems and foreign chemicals. These interactions are studied by using techniques from physiology and biochemistry.

Pharmacognosy

Pharmacognosy is the study of drugs that come from natural sources such as plants, animals, or minerals and their products. Pharmacognosy has recently emerged as an important pharmaceutical science.

Toxicology

Toxicology is the study of poisons—chemical substances harmful to health or that damage life. The study of the adverse effects of drugs on living organisms also is included.

Drug

Any chemical substance that influences living systems could be considered a **drug.** The term frequently is used synonymously with the word *medication* to mean a pharmacologic agent that interacts with living organisms to produce biologic effects. Although drugs are used to some extent for diagnosis, their chief value lies in the prevention, treatment, and symptomatic relief of disease.

Prescription Drugs

Prescription drugs cannot be sold to the consumer without a prescription and must be labeled with the legend, "CAUTION: Federal Law Prohibits Dispensing Without Prescription." Physicians, dentists, veterinarians, and other legally authorized health practitioners write prescriptions as part of their specific practice. Most prescriptions are written on printed forms and usually contain the following information:
- Client information (e.g., name, address, age)
- Date prescribed
- The R_x symbol
- Name and dosage of the prescribed medication
- Quantity to dispense
- Directions for the client
- Refill and/or labeling instructions
- Prescriber's name
- Prescriber's signature

If the prescribed drug is a controlled substance, the following information also is needed:
- Address of client
- Prescriber's address
- Drug Enforcement Administration (DEA) number of the prescriber

Federal law allows a nurse to prepare prescription orders (including controlled substances) for the signature of the licensed prescriber. The Durham-Humphrey Amendment to the Federal Food, Drug and Cosmetic Act specifies that refill instructions may be given orally by the licensed prescriber or a legally authorized representative. The legally authorized representative of the physician is usually a nurse.[5] See Chapter 8 for additional information on labeling.

Nonprescription or Over-the-Counter Drugs

Nonprescription or **over-the-counter (OTC) drugs** can be acquired legally by the client without a prescription order. Chapter 11 contains additional information about OTC drugs, including their risks and benefits and the nurse's role in consumer education.

DRUG CLASSIFICATION

Since there are thousands of drugs, similar drugs are grouped together for the purpose of study and for ease of prescribing. Usually drugs are grouped or classified according to chemical, pharmacologic, and/or therapeutic classification. In **chemical classification,** drugs of like chemical structure are grouped together, regardless of differences in source or pharmacologic activity. In **pharmacologic classification,** drugs are grouped ac-

cording to their physiologic activities and mechanisms of action. **Therapeutic classification** organizes drugs according to similar therapeutic indications or uses.

Studying drugs according to classifications, groups, or categories helps you develop an orderly and systematic approach to the science of pharmacology. For this reason pharmacologic classifications or groupings provide the organizing framework in the clinical chapters of this text.

Another method of systematizing your study is to concentrate on the best-established and most important drug or drugs in each group or category. Individual drugs that represent groups of drugs are called **prototypes.** Once the prototype of each group is thoroughly understood, other drugs in that category or group can be studied more easily.

CONCEPT REVIEW

Chemical, pharmacologic, and therapeutic classifications organize drugs into groups.

Prototypes are individual drugs that represent groups of drugs.

DRUG NOMENCLATURE

One reason pharmacology appears complex to students is that individual drugs may have more than one name. A single drug may have a chemical, generic or nonproprietary, official, and trade (brand) or proprietary name. Different names identify the drug and its function for different groups of people (i.e., manufacturers, health professionals, and consumers).[6-9]

Chemical Name

During the early stages of drug development a drug is assigned a **chemical name.** This is a systematically derived name that clearly and precisely identifies the chemical structure of the drug. Chemical names are quite complex and are not capitalized. For example, the chemical name for ibuprofen is ($\pm$)-2-(p-isobutylphenyl) propionic acid. To facilitate the dispensing of drugs, each drug substance is also given a generic name.

Generic or Nonproprietary Name

The **generic name** is related to the official name of a drug and is **nonproprietary** (independent of any particular manufacturer). This name is either handed down from antiquity, acquired from biochemistry, or assigned by the United States Adopted Names (USAN) Council.

Generic names are not capitalized, and they reflect important pharmacologic or chemical characteristics of the drug. For example, the generic name of ($\pm$-2-(p-isobutylphenyl) propionic acid is ibuprofen.

A drug manufacturer can patent a generic name with the United States Patent Office for 17 years. Once the drug is patented, the original drug manufacturer can license other companies to produce or sell the drug. Once a manufacturer's

DRUG NOMENCLATURE

Chemical name	$(\pm\text{-}2\text{-}(p\text{-isobutylphenyl})$ propionic acid
Generic or non-proprietary name	ibuprofen
Official name	ibuprofen
Trademark (brand) or proprietary name	Advil, Ibuprofen, Medipren, Motrin, Nuprin

patent for the generic drug has expired, other companies are free to market the drug under their own trademarked name or under the generic name.

What maintains the quality of generic drugs? What determines that generic drugs are chemically the same and therefore interchangeable (i.e., **bioequivalent**)? In 1984 the Drug Price Competition and Patent Term Restoration Act established the Food and Drug Administration's (FDA) approval process for generic drugs. This act requires that generic drugs be chemically equivalent to the previously approved product. However, a manufacturer need only prove that a drug is bioequivalent, not clinically or therapeutically equivalent.

Three general criteria must be met to obtain FDA approval for a generic drug:

1. The generic product must contain the same amount of active ingredients in the same dosage form and with the same route of administration as the previously approved product. The generic product does not have to contain the same fillers and additives as the approved product.
2. Equivalent manufacturing standards must be followed.
3. The generic drug must be bioequivalent to the approved product.

Since the nonactive ingredients in generic preparations differ, the therapeutic effect of the drug and response of the client to the drug are influenced. This is a major concern when substituting generic products for approved products.[10]

Trade (Brand) Name or Proprietary Name

When a drug is ready for commercial distribution, the drug manufacturer may decide not to use the generic name and instead assign the drug a trademarked or brand name. The FDA must approve all trademarked or brand names.

The trademarked or brand name is usually short and easy to recall. If the name is registered, it is followed with the superscript R and is considered a **proprietary** or **trade name** owned by the drug manufacturer. Only the company that initiated the registration process can use the registered trademarked or brand name. When the drug is manufactured by more than one company, each company may market its product under its own trademarked or brand name.

Unlike the chemical or generic name, a trademarked or brand name begins with a capital letter. Some of the trade-

marked or brand names for ibuprofen are Motrin, Advil, Medipren, Nuprin, and Ibuprofen.

Official Name

In 1962 the federal government mandated the use of **official names.** The official name is usually the same as the generic name and is listed in an official pharmacopeia or formulary. For a preparation to qualify as an official drug, it must conform to standards cited in the *United States Pharmacopeia (USP).* Once these standards are met, the letters *USP* are placed after the drug's name.

SOURCES OF DRUG INFORMATION

Health care professionals who prescribe, dispense, or administer medication require reliable and current drug information. This information is available through both official and nonofficial sources.

Official Sources in the United States

In the United States official sources of information are the *USP,* the *United States Pharmacopoeia Dispensing Information (USP-DI),* and the *National Formulary.*

The *USP* was first published in 1820 and was adopted as an official source of drug data and standards in 1906 by the United States Congress. The *USP* is published every 5 years; supplements are published as needed. The Committee of Revision of the United States Pharmacopeial Convention is responsible for updating the *USP.* This committee consists of consumers and a group of experts from a variety of fields.

The *USP* contains information on single drugs of proven therapeutic value and low toxicity, which are listed according to official names. Chemical, physical, and biologic properties and standards for identity, strength, and purity are presented for each drug. In addition, information on method of storage and on dosage range for therapeutic use is included.

In 1888 the American Pharmaceutical Association established the *National Formulary.* At that time the formulary contained drug data and standards. Between 1906 and 1974 it was considered an official source for drug standards by the United States government. In 1975 the last edition of the *National Formulary* was published, and standards from the formulary were combined with those in the *USP.* The *USP* is now the only official book of drug standards in the United States.

The *USP-DI* is a compilation of dispensing information for a wide variety of drugs. It also contains information appropriate for clients receiving the listed drugs and is frequently used as a teaching guide. The *USP-DI* is issued annually; supplements are published throughout the year.

Official Sources in Great Britain and Canada

Standards for drugs vary from country to country. For Great Britain and Canada there are several references available, including the *British Pharmacopoeia (BP),* the *British*

SOURCES OF DRUG INFORMATION

Official Sources

The *United States Pharmacopeia (USP)*
The United States Pharmacopeial Convention, Inc.
Mack Printing Company
Easton, PA

Compendium of Pharmaceuticals and Specialties (CPS)
Canadian Pharmaceutical Association
Ottawa, Ontario
Canada

The *British Pharmacopoeia (BP)*
Office of the British Pharmacopoeia Commission
London, England

British Pharmaceutical Codex (BPC)

European Pharmacopoeia (EP)
Pharmaceutical Press
London, England

Unofficial Sources
American Drug Index
J.B. Lippincott
Philadelphia, PA

American Hospital Formulary Services (AHFS) Drug Information
American Hospital Formulary Services
American Society of Hospital Pharmacists
Bethesda, MD

AMA Drug Evaluations
American Medical Association
Chicago, IL

Bioavailability of Drug Products
American Pharmaceutical Association
Washington, DC

Drugs Available Abroad
Gale Research, Inc.
Detroit, MI

Drug Facts and Comparisons
Facts & Comparisons/J.B. Lippincott Co.
St. Louis, MO

Index Nominum: International Drug Directory
Swiss Pharmaceutical Society
Medpharm Scientific Publishers
Stuttgart, Germany

Martindale: The Extra Pharmacopoeia
The Pharmaceutical Press
London, England

Merck Index
Merck & Co., Inc.
Rahway, NJ

Physicians' Desk Reference (PDR)
Medical Economics Data
Montvale, NJ

Physicians' Desk Reference for Nonprescription Drugs
Medical Economics Data
Montvale, NJ

The United States Pharmacopeia Dispensing Information (USPDI)
The United States Pharmacopoeial Convention, Inc.
Mack Printing Company
Easton, PA

POISONDEX
Mircromedex Inc.
Denver, CO

Pharmaceutical Codex (BPC), the *Canadian Formulary,* the *European Pharmacopoeia,* and the *British National Formulary.*

The *BP* is published every 5 years and is similar to the *USP.* Drugs listed in this book are considered official and are subject to legal control. The *British National Formulary* contains detailed descriptions of the properties, actions, and therapeutic uses of most drugs in current use. This book is prepared by a committee of the British Medical Association and the Pharmaceutical Society of Great Britain.

Unofficial Sources of Information

There are many unofficial sources of information. Some of them are *Physicians' Desk Reference (PDR), Physicians' Desk Reference for Nonprescription Drugs, American Hospital Formulary Service (AHFS) Drug Information* book, *Drug Facts and Comparisons,* the *Internist's Compendium of Drug Therapy, POISONDEX,* and *TOXLINE.*

The *PDR* is an annual publication intended primarily for use by prescribers. Drugs are listed by generic name, brand name, and manufacturer. The product information section contains complete information not unlike that found in the package insert that accompanies a drug.

The *PDR* also contains a section with color photographs of more than 1000 commercially available drugs. This is an excellent source for use in identifying unknown drug products by their appearance. The *PDR* does not contain implications for drug administration nor nursing data. Thus this source is less useful for the individual dispensing the drug directly to the client.

The *Physicians' Desk Reference for Nonprescription Drugs,* also published annually, is meant as a companion volume to the *PDR* and is organized in a similar manner. The volume is divided into the Manufacturers' Index, Product Name Index, Product Category Index, and Active Ingredients Index. There is also a Product Identification Section.

The American Society of Hospital Pharmacists issues the *AHFS Drug Information* book. It contains a comprehensive, evaluative approach to individual drugs and serves as a good resource for physicians and pharmacists.

Drug Facts and Comparisons contains actions, indications, warnings, interactions, contraindications, precautions, adverse reactions, dosage, and prescribing and patenting information for each drug. Information about related or competing drugs is also available. This reference is published annually in a bound book, in a loose-leaf notebook, and in a microfiche version. The loose-leaf and microfiche versions are updated monthly.

The *Internist's Compendium of Drug Therapy* is published annually and is used primarily by prescribers. It is organized according to therapeutic classification. In some larger categories drugs are arranged into groups with similar physiologic actions. The book contains approximately 2000 prescription and OTC drugs. One section of the book contains color photographs of more than 1800 products. Comprehensive clinical pharmacokinetic data on commonly used drugs are available as are drug information resources.

The most current sources of drug information are electronically accessed databases. Two extensive computer-accessible toxicology databases are *POISONDEX* and *TOXLINE*. The National Library of Medicine produces *TOXLINE*. This source contains more than 850,000 citations from 1965 to the present date. Both databases are available directly from poison control centers and cover medicinal, commercial, industrial, and botanical sources of poison.

CONCEPT REVIEW

A single drug may have a chemical, generic or nonproprietary, official, and trade (brand) or proprietary name. Different names identify the drug and its function for different groups of people (i.e., manufacturers, health professionals, and consumers).

Drug information is available through official and nonofficial sources.

SUMMARY

Knowledge of the science of pharmacology should be built on an understanding of its history. Pharmacology has an interdisciplinary basis. For example, nutrition, chemistry, geology, botany, microbiology, and animal and human physiology contribute to the process of drug development. Thus you must possess some knowledge in all these areas. In addition, to help you fulfill your role in drug therapy, you must learn new terminology and use new sources of information.

REFERENCES

1. Leake, C.D. (1975). *An historical account of pharmacology to the twentieth century.* Springfield, IL: Charles C Thomas.
2. Weatherall, M. (1990). *In search of a cure: A history of pharmaceutical discovery.* New York: Oxford University Press.
3. Cordell, G.A. (1990). Pharmacognosy—High tech pharmaceutical science. *Pharmacia-Journal of Turkish Pharmacists' Association, 30*(3), 169-181.
4. Goodman, R., Gilman, E.W., Rall, T., Nies, A., & Taylor, P. (Eds.). (1990). *Goodman and Gilman's: The pharmacological basis of therapeutics* (8th ed.). New York: Pergamon Press.
5. Smith, C.M., & Reynard, A.M. (1992). *Textbook of pharmacology.* Philadelphia: W.B. Saunders.
6. Bruch, M.K., & Larson, E. (1989). An early historical perspective on the FDA regulation of OTC drugs. *Infection Control & Hospital Epidemiology, 10,* 527-528.
7. Fleeger, C.A. (Ed.). (1991). *USAN and the U.S.P. dictionary of drug names.* Rockville, MD: United States Pharmacopeial Convention.
8. Jacox, A., & Kolassa, M. (1992). Cost and regulation of drugs. *Nursing Economics, 10*(1), 66-69.
9. Sanborn, M., Godwin, H., & Pessetto, J. (1991). FDA drug classification system. *American Journal of Hospital Pharmacy, 48,* 2659-2662.
10. Huntington, A.G. (1990). Generic drugs reexamined. *Physician Assistant,* January, 13, 17.

BIBLIOGRAPHY

Anonymous. (1992). Exhibit to explore history of pharmacy. *Indiana Medicine, 86*(2), 1, 3.

Hayes, L. (1992). Ancient remedies provide clues in search for 'new' medicines. *Chemecology, 21*(5), 10-11.

Labreche, D.G. (1989). The rise and fall of the apothecary: Will history repeat itself? *Pharmacotherapy, 9*(2), 105-111.

Lehne, R.A. (1994). *Pharmacology for nursing care* (2nd ed.). Philadelphia: W.B. Saunders.

Morin, L. (1990). Tips for generic substitution. *Montana Pharmacist, 13,* 14-15.

Navarra, T. (1990). The history of a love affair. *American Journal of Nursing, 90,* 91, 93-96, 98.

Svedmyr, N. (1991). Clinical advantages of the aerosol route of drug administration. *Respiratory Care, 36,* 922-930.

CHAPTER 2

Legal Foundations of Pharmacologic Practice

MARGUERITE NEWTON

⊛ United States Drug Legislation

LEARNING OBJECTIVE: Summarize major legislation that influenced drug development in the United States.

KEY TERMS:

Legend, nonprescription, prescription

⊛ Canadian Drug Legislation

LEARNING OBJECTIVE: Summarize major legislation that influenced drug development in Canada.

⊛ International Drug Control

LEARNING OBJECTIVE: Describe attempts at international drug control.

⊛ Standardization of Drugs

LEARNING OBJECTIVES:

Identify official publications for the United States, Great Britain, and Canada.

Discuss the over-the-counter drug review process.

⊛ Development of New Drugs

LEARNING OBJECTIVE: Describe the developmental process for new drugs.

⊛ Investigational and Orphan Drugs

LEARNING OBJECTIVES:

Explain the meaning of the term *orphan drug*.

Define the term *investigational drug*.

KEY TERMS:

Investigational drug, orphan drug

⊛ Impact on Role of Nurse

LEARNING OBJECTIVE: Discuss the impact of state and federal legislation on the role of the nurse.

CONCEPTS AND TERMS TO REVIEW

Review the section in Chapter 1 that describes the *USP* and *National Formulary*.

Read the section in Chapter 5 on therapeutic index.

---

*D*uring the past 20 years, dramatic changes have occurred in the development of new drugs and new drug delivery systems. Intense research has produced major biomedical breakthroughs (e.g., drugs for the treatment of acquired immunodeficiency syndrome [AIDs]) and has provided modification of older drugs to increase their effectiveness.

The current trend is toward more involvement of the general population in their health care. As the client becomes more knowledgeable and involved in health care, the nurse's responsibilities also expand. The nurse has the most contact with the client and thus has a major role in educating the client

and monitoring him or her for therapeutic and undesired clinical responses. This role can be performed only if the nurse has a comprehensive understanding of pharmacology.

This chapter traces the history of drug legislation in the United States and Canada. The legal and regulatory processes involved in drug development, testing, and administration are also presented. In addition, the legal aspects of the nurse's role in drug administration are addressed.

UNITED STATES DRUG LEGISLATION

Before the twentieth century, minimal legislation existed to regulate drug production, efficacy, purity, and distribution. In the 1800s, patent medicines prevailed. Extravagant claims declaring cures for all manner of ailments and diseases from cancer and asthma to malaria, gonorrhea, and gallstones were made for these medicines. Products included Lydia E. Pinkham's Tonic, Kick-A-Poo Sagwa, Dr. Johnson's Mild Combination Treatment for Cancer, and Dr. Shreve's Anti-Gallstone Remedy. Such products did not have to prove their claims or list their active ingredients, which ranged from alcohol or opium to morphine in teething medicine for babies.[1]

Early Federal Legislation

It became apparent that laws were necessary to control the development and distribution of medicinal products. The first attempt by the U.S. government to regulate the quality of drugs, the **Import Drugs Act,** was passed in 1848. This act provided for inspection of imported drugs at the port of entry into the United States. Any impure drugs could be destroyed or sent back to the country of origin.

Another major step occurred in 1902 when the **Biologics Control Act** was passed. This act gave the U.S. Public Health Service control over licensing of biologics laboratories and their products. This act was precipitated by the death of 12 children from tetanus contamination of a diphtheria antitoxin.[1] After the passage of this act, activists promoted legislation to regulate drugs further and to control food purity. Opposition to further legislation came principally from the manufacturers of patent medicines.[1]

In 1906 the **Federal Pure Food and Drugs Act** was passed. Unfortunately, this law provided no standards for safety and efficacy of drugs. Further, the law did not regulate the labeling and therapeutic claims made for products by the pharmaceutical manufacturers. The Sherley Amendment, which regulated labeling, was added to the act in 1912. In 1931 reorganization in the federal government led to formation of the Food and Drug Administration (FDA).[1]

Federal Food, Drug, and Cosmetic Act

The issue of drug safety gained national attention in 1937 when the antibiotic sulfanilamide was introduced as a cherry elixir for children. This drug was marketed without prior testing on animal or human subjects. Unfortunately, diethylene glycol was one of its ingredients. This powerful nephrotoxin, an ingredient in antifreeze, killed more than 100 people. This tragic event provided the impetus for the passage of the **Federal Food, Drug, and Cosmetic Act** in 1938. This act stipulated that a drug's safety must be proved before marketing. It also set more stringent labeling requirements and allowed the FDA to inspect pharmaceutical factories.[1] In 1952 the **Durham-Humphrey Amendment** to the act established two categories of drugs: **prescription** or **legend drugs** and **nonprescription** or **over-the-counter (OTC) drugs.** This act specified that habit-forming drugs and drugs not safe for use except under the supervision of a licensed practitioner were prescription drugs. Legend or prescription drugs must bear the legend "Caution: Federal Law Prohibits Dispensing Without Prescription."

Further major amendments to the Food, Drug, and Cosmetic Act were introduced in 1962. These amendments **(Kefauver-Harris amendments)** required proof of efficacy and safety before marketing of a drug. The precipitating factor that motivated passage of the amendments was the thalidomide tragedy in late 1961. Thalidomide, a sedative, was used widely by pregnant women in Europe. Many women who

TABLE 2–1
Summary of Major Legislation in the United States

Date	Drug Legislation	Restrictions
1906	Pure Food and Drugs Act	Restricted sale and manufacture of drugs. Marketed drugs had to meet strength and purity standards. *United States Pharmacopeia* and *National Formulary* adopted as drug standards.
1912	Sherley Amendment	Prohibited fraudulent therapeutic claims.
1914	Harrison Narcotic Act	Attempted to control narcotics and the resultant addiction and dependence.
		Defined *narcotic* as a legal term.
1938	Federal Food, Drug, and Cosmetic Act	Set labeling requirements.
		Required drug toxicity studies before FDA approval.
		Gave FDA enforcement power to recall drugs deemed unsafe.
1952	Durham-Humphrey Amendment	Established over-the-counter (OTC) as a category for drugs sold without a prescription.
		Designated prescription category as *legend drugs.*
1962	Kefauver-Harris Amendment	Set safety and efficacy standards for drug approval. All drugs from 1938 to 1962 were tested for efficacy and safety.
1970	Controlled Substances Act	Mandated research for drug dependence and abuse prevention and treatment.
		Established five schedules for controlled drugs and set prescriptive limits.
		Encouraged more support for law enforcement efforts.
1978	Drug Regulation and Reform Act	Shortened drug investigation time.
1984	Drug Price and Competition and Patent Term Restoration	Established that generic drugs could be marketed on basis of bioequivalence.

took the drug delivered babies with a rare birth defect, phocomelia, which is characterized by gross malformation or complete absence of arms and legs. Thalidomide was not a problem in the United States since the FDA had prevented its import. The Kefauver-Harris amendments also required that all drugs introduced between 1932 and 1962 undergo testing for effectiveness. In addition, the amendments established rigorous procedures for testing new drugs[1,2] (see the section "Development of New Drugs" and Table 2–1).

Controlled Substance Legislation

The first legislation to address drug addiction and dependence was the **Harrison Narcotic Act** of 1914. This act attempted to regulate importation and marketing of narcotic drugs by imposing taxes. As a result of this act, *narcotic* became a legal term.

In 1970 the Federal Comprehensive Drug Abuse Prevention and Control Act was enacted. A section of this act is the **Controlled Substances Act (CSA)** The CSA is implemented by the Drug Enforcement Administration (DEA), an agency established within the Department of Justice in 1973. This act strengthened the role of law enforcement in the control of drug abuse and established a system of drug classification for controlled substances. The schedule classifies substances according to their abuse potential. Table 2–2 summarizes the five categories and provides examples of drugs in each category.[1]

Procedures designed to meet federal and state regulations for use of controlled substances must be addressed by all health care facilities. The pharmacy determines the documentation procedure. Some agencies use computers to record and validate use of controlled substances. The computer program records the name of the client, prescriber, and individual administering the drug, in addition to dose, time of administration, and amount of drug remaining in stock. A manual count of controlled drugs remaining in stock is done periodically. Agencies without computer systems have similar procedures but do all of the recording manually.

CANADIAN DRUG LEGISLATION

Canadian drug legislation history echoes that of the United States. The first law that addressed the purity of food, drink, and drugs was approved in 1875. The **Canadian Food and Drug Act** was enacted in 1953 and is enforced by the Health Protection Branch (HPB) of the Department of National Health and Welfare. This act controls drug research and development, drug advertising, and product information and monitors the safety of all drug products. The distribution of all potentially addictive drugs is also controlled by this act.

Legislation in Canada classifies drugs as *nonprescription, prescription,* or *restricted.* Nonprescription drugs are further classified as *proprietary* or *OTC.* Prescription drugs include Schedule F drugs and Schedule G drugs. **Schedule F drugs** can be sold and refilled only by prescription. Drugs listed in Schedule F include antibiotics, hormones, and tranquilizers. Labels for these drugs must be clearly marked with "Pr," prescription required. **Schedule G drugs** are controlled drugs (e.g., amphetamines and barbiturates). Controlled drugs must be identified by "C" on the label. Restricted drugs are listed in **Schedule H** and are available only to institutions for research.

TABLE 2–2
United States Controlled Drug Schedule

Schedule	Definition	Examples of Drugs
I	Drugs are available only for research and have no legal use. Special permission for use must be obtained from FDA. Only exception is peyote use by Native Americans	Peyote LSD (lysergic acid diethylamide) Mescaline Heroin Psilocybin
II	Drugs have therapeutic use but also have high abuse potential. Prescriptions for these drugs must be rewritten; no refills are allowed. Federal law provides for an emergency telephone prescription order.	Amphetamine Morphine Cocaine Opium
III	Drugs have lower abuse potential but can be abused. Prescriptions must be rewritten after five refills. Refills must be made within 6 months of date of issue.	Stimulants not covered in other schedules Products containing amobarbital, pentobarbital, secobarbital Paregoric Anabolic steroids
IV	Drugs have a lower potential of abuse relative to drugs in schedule III. Potential for psychologic dependence exists.	Phenobarbital Pentazocine (Talwin) Chlordiazepoxide (Librium) Diazepam (Valium)
V	Drugs have a low abuse potential. State-to-state requirements vary. Prescription may not be required in some states. In some states, pharmacy must dispense only limited amounts and must keep a record of purchases.	Terpin hydrate with codeine Triaminic expectorant with codeine Diphenoxylate hydrochloride with atropine sulfate (Lomotil) Robitussin A-C

Hallucinogenic drugs and lysergic acid diethylamide (LSD) are included in this group.

The **Canadian Narcotic Control Act** was originally passed in 1961; it has been amended several times since that date. This act governs the possession, sale, manufacture, production, and distribution of narcotics. Narcotics (e.g., cocaine, codeine, morphine, and opium) are drugs used primarily for relief of pain, but they also possess significant psychotropic activity. Labels for these drugs must include the proprietary and common names of the drug, names of the manufacturer and the distributor, and the symbol "N."[3]

INTERNATIONAL DRUG CONTROL

The first efforts to achieve international drug control occurred in 1912 at the "Opium Conference" at The Hague, Netherlands. Governments represented at the conference developed treaties that limited the manufacture of opium for medicinal and scientific purposes and controlled production and distribution of raw opium. In 1964 all existing treaties were combined into one act directed at controlling narcotics. This act prohibited narcotic production, manufacture, and trade for nonmedicinal purposes. It established a system for international control of opium transactions by countries that produce opium, and it required import certificates and export authorization. At the same time, the International Narcotic Control Board was established to enforce these laws.

CONCEPT REVIEW

Legislation to protect the consumer from unsafe or ineffective drugs was slow to develop.

Currently the United States, Canada, and other countries are attempting to control the development and distribution of prescription and nonprescription drugs.

STANDARDIZATION OF DRUGS

A standard is something established as a rule or basis of comparison in measuring, for example, quantity and quality. Drug standardization is an attempt to have all drugs meet minimal expectations for purity, safety, and effectiveness.

Drug Standards in the United States

In the United States, standardization of drugs was slow to develop. Physicians outraged by the presence of substandard and contaminated drugs led the movement to develop a national pharmacopeia *(United States Pharmacopeia [USP]).* This book contains only drugs that meet stringent criteria for quality, purity, and strength.

Drug Standards in Great Britain and Canada

In Great Britain the *British Pharmacopoeia (BP)* serves the same function as the *USP* in the United States. Drugs listed in the *BP* must meet established standards. The British Pharmacopoeia Commission prepares and reviews this publication. In Canada the *Canadian Formulary* contains formulas for preparations commonly used in that country. The Canadian Food and Drug Act recognizes this as an official publication.

Over-the-Counter Drug Review

The OTC drug review does not evaluate each product. Instead, the review focuses on each ingredient in the product and the proposed therapeutic category (e.g., antacid, antifungal, digestive aids). Its purpose is to determine if the ingredients are safe and effective for use in self-treatment. The process also reviews claims and recommends appropriate labeling.

Many OTC drugs originally are marketed as legend or prescription drugs. However, if FDA regulations are met, drugs can be reclassified from prescription to OTC marketing status. Examples of reclassified drugs include hydrocortisone, ibuprofen, and promethazine.[4]

DEVELOPMENT OF NEW DRUGS

Development and testing of new drugs is an expensive, lengthy process lasting 6 to 12 years and costing millions of dollars. Drug development follows a prescribed five-step sequence mandated by the FDA.

Initially researchers conduct animal studies to determine toxicity, therapeutic effects, therapeutic index, median effective dose, and pharmacokinetics of the agent. Dosage form also is determined at this time. After the preclinical tests, which may take 1 to 3 years, the drug developer may apply to the FDA for permission to begin clinical testing. If approval is received, the drug is granted **Investigational New Drug status,** and clinical testing begins.

Clinical testing is divided into four phases and may take 5 to 9 years to complete. Early **phase I** testing usually involves 75 to 150 human volunteers. Results of a complete blood analysis, urine chemistries, electrocardiogram, and physical examination must be obtained for each volunteer before he or she may participate in the studies. These test results serve as baseline data; the tests are repeated at predetermined intervals during the studies.

In **phase II** researchers investigate the drug's therapeutic effectiveness for a particular disease. Therefore drugs are tested on individuals with the disease. These tests are conducted under extremely controlled conditions and may involve as many as 500 to 1000 subjects. Dosage range is also studied during phase II. In **phase III** double-blind, controlled studies are conducted, again using individuals with the disease. Studies may involve 1500 to 5000 subjects and often include the use of placebos.

Upon completion of the clinical and preclinical testing, the data are submitted to the FDA for review. Safe and effective drugs are granted **New Drug Application (NDA) status.** When this occurs, **phase IV** or postmarketing surveillance begins. During the early portion of the phase the new drug is released for marketing on a limited basis. All clients receiving the drug are monitored. In the late stage of phase IV the drug is released for general marketing. Reporting of drug response is not required at this point.

There are severe limitations to the present testing procedure. Little drug testing is done in women. In fact, almost all women of child-bearing potential are excluded from clinical trials. Therefore limited information is available about how women respond to drugs. Minimal drug testing is done on different ethnic groups. Therefore information is not available, for example, on how the response of African-Americans to a particular drug varies from the response of a Korean.[1,5-9]

INVESTIGATIONAL AND ORPHAN DRUGS

Some drugs are approved for use by the FDA without completing the long five-step sequence.

Investigational Drugs

As indicated previously, new drug testing takes 6 to 12 years. During this time deaths or disabilities occur that could be prevented if the new drug were available. Consumer groups, concerned about the delay in drug development, lobbied for changes in the research or testing process. As a result, in 1987 the FDA established the **Treatment Investigational New Drug Exemption.** It allows drugs that have passed phase II to be prescribed for treatment purposes. However, use of investigational drugs is limited to closely monitored situations in which the prescriber is extremely knowledgeable about the disease and therapy.

Orphan Drugs

In an attempt to promote research on drugs for rare diseases that afflict a small percent of the population, the **Orphan Drug Act** was passed in 1983. Pharmaceutical companies receive a tax credit and a 7-year patent extension for any drug developed to treat a disease identified in this legislation. Based on data from FDA documents, 33 orphan drugs were developed and approved from 1983 through 1989. Products were intended for a wide range of rare diseases, including growth failure, porphyria, cytomegalovirus retinitis, and anemia associated with end-stage renal failure. To a degree, the act has been successful. However, unresolved issues exist that must be examined as changes in technology and third-party payer coverage evolve.[10]

CONCEPT REVIEW

New drug development is a long and expensive process. The process consists of preclinical and clinical testing and postmarketing surveillance.

In an attempt to meet the needs of the consumer, the FDA has shortened the developmental process for special categories of drugs, investigational drugs and orphan drugs.

IMPACT ON ROLE OF NURSE

A nurse must be familiar with the legal foundations of drug administration. He or she must know what drugs are controlled substances and what drugs can be administered only with a prescription. A nurse must know the regulations established by the state nurse practice act and understand the procedures at his or her agency.

In addition, if involved in drug research, the nurse must know his or her legal and ethical responsibilities. Any client involved in research must provide informed consent. This means that the client has been told about the research and agrees to participate. The client must be provided information about the procedure and his or her role, expected risks and benefits, and expected effects. The researcher is responsible for conveying the information, but the nurse is responsible for assessing the client's understanding. The nurse should also have a thorough knowledge of the drug being studied and the study protocol.

SUMMARY

Legislation has helped to standardize drugs. In the United States the FDA enforces the Federal Food, Drug, and Cosmetic Act, which stipulates that a drug's safety must be proved before marketing. This act also identifies two categories of drugs: prescription and nonprescription. The Controlled Substances Act, which is implemented by the DEA, describes a schedule of drug classification for controlled substances. The schedule classifies substances according to their abuse potential. In addition, the FDA has established a five-step drug development process that involves preclinical and clinical testing and postmarketing surveillance.

REFERENCES

1. Cocchetto, D., & Nardi, R. (1992). *Managing the clinical drug development process.* New York: Marcell Dekker.
2. Lehne, R.A. (1994). *Pharmacology for nursing care* (2nd ed.). Philadelphia: W.B. Saunders
3. Krogh, C. (1993). *Compendium of pharmaceuticals and specialties: The Canadian reference for health professionals* (28th ed.). Ottawa, Ontario: Canadian Pharmaceutical Association.
4. American Pharmaceutical Association (1990). *Handbook of nonprescription drugs* (9th ed.). Washington, DC: National Professional Society of Pharmacists.
5. Beer, D. (1988). *Generic drugs: A guide to FDA approval requirements.* Clifton, NJ: Prentice Hall Law & Business.
6. Carroll, P., & Maher, V. (1990). Legal issues in experimental investigations of medications. *Advancing Clinical Care, 5*(3), 6.
7. Jenkins, J., & Hubbard, S. (1991). History of clinical trials. *Seminars in Oncology Nursing, 7,* 228-234.
8. Smith, C. (1992). *The process of new drug discovery and development.* Boca Raton, FL: CRC Press.
9. Lee. C. (1993). *Development and evaluation of drugs: From laboratory through licensure to market.* Boca Raton, FL: CRC Press.
10. Asbury, C. (1991). The Orphan Drug Act. *JAMA, 265,* 893-897.

BIBLIOGRAPHY

Canha, B. (1990). Research or treatment: What is the FDA's role? *AIDS—Patient Care, 4,*(6), 3-5.

Cassidy, J., & MacFarlane, D. (1991). The role of the nurse in clinical cancer research. *Cancer Nursing, 14*(3), 124-131.

Cheson, B.O. (1991). Clinical trials programs. *Seminars in Oncology Nursing, 7,* 235-242.

FDA recommendations regarding latex products. (1992). *Images, 11*(1), 12-13.

Hodges, L.C., Patterson, R., & Rapp, C.G. (1990). Clinical trials: The role of the neuroscience nurse. *Journal of Neuroscience Nursing, 22*(3), 195-198.

How each state stands on legislative issues affecting advanced nursing practice. (1990). *Nurse Practitioner: American Journal of Primary Health Care, 15*(1), 11-18.

Joranson, D. (1990). A new drug for the states: An opportunity to affirm the role of opioids in cancer pain relief. *Journal of Pain and Symptom Management, 5,* 333-336.

Office of the Federal Register, National Archives and Records Administration. (1993). *Code of federal regulation: Food and drugs.* Washington, DC: U.S. Government Printing Office.

Rodman, M. (1992). New FDA approvals: How to use them, when to suggest them. *RN Magazine, 55*(3), 58-65.

General Principles of Pharmacology

CHAPTER 3

Pharmaceutic Phase

NORMA L. PINNELL

⊛ **Sources of Drugs**

LEARNING OBJECTIVE: Describe four sources from which drugs are derived.

KEY TERMS:

Alkaloids, glycosides, gums, oils, pharmaceutic phase, resins

⊛ **Excipients Used in Drugs**

LEARNING OBJECTIVES:

Define the term *excipient*.

Name four types of excipients found in drugs.

KEY TERMS:

Disintegration, dissolution, active ingredient, excipient

⊛ **Drug Routes**

LEARNING OBJECTIVE: Describe three major drug administration routes.

KEY TERMS:

Enteral, hypodermic, implants, intraarterial, intraarticular, intracutaneous, intradermal, intramuscular, intraspinal, intrathecal, intravenous, parenteral, subcutaneous, sublingual, topical, transmucosal

⊛ **Dosage Forms and Preparations**

LEARNING OBJECTIVES:

Define the term *dosage form*.

Describe four dosage forms for each of the three major drug administration routes.

KEY TERMS:

Ampule, cartridges, dosage forms, emulsion, enteric coated, patches, semisolids, solids, solution, suspensions, sustained release, troches (lozenges), vials

⊛ **Drug Stability and Storage**

LEARNING OBJECTIVE: Discuss three factors that affect the stability of drugs.

K nowledge of the general principles of pharmacology provides a basis for understanding how drugs produce therapeutic and adverse effects. These general principles usually are organized according to the pharmaceutic, pharmacokinetic, pharmacodynamic, and pharmacotherapeutic phases. The pharmaceutic phase is discussed in this chapter.

The **pharmaceutic phase** includes information on sources of drugs, constituents of drug products, and formulation of drugs into effective **dosage forms** (preparations or delivery systems). Also included in this phase are routes of administration, drug stability, and drug storage.

SOURCES OF DRUGS

Various sources provide the active ingredients (components responsible for producing the action) of a drug: plants, animals, minerals, and organic and inorganic chemicals.[1-3]

Plant Sources

Leaves, roots, seeds, and other parts of plants are processed for use as drugs. Products that result from this initial processing of plant parts are known as *crude drugs*. When the pharmacologically active constituents are separated from these crude preparations, the resulting products are more potent and usually more reliable than the crude drug. Pharmacologically active substances produced from plants include alkaloids, glycosides, gums, resins, and oils.

Alkaloids Alkaloids are among the most important naturally derived drugs. These alkaline-organic-chemical compounds are composed of carbon, hydrogen, nitrogen, and oxygen and are usually specific to a given plant species. Alkaloids taste bitter and are poorly soluble in water. When combined chemically with acids, alkaloids form water-soluble salts. Examples of alkaloids are atropine, scopolamine, cocaine, quinine, morphine, and codeine.

PHARMACOLOGICALLY ACTIVE SUBSTANCES FROM PLANTS

Alkaloids
Alkaline-organic-chemical compounds
Composed of carbon, hydrogen, nitrogen, and oxygen
Bitter tasting
Poorly soluble in water
Combined with acids, form water-soluble salts

Glycosides
Compounds of sugar units and a nonsugar component
Sugar probably increases solubility, absorption, permeability, and cellular distribution of the glycosides

Gums
Plant exudates
Polysaccharides

Resins
Complex substances
Semisolid or solid plant exudates
Amorphous in structure
Insoluble in water

Oils
Highly viscous liquids
Liquid form of lipids
VOLATILE OILS
  Evaporate easily
  Pleasant odor and taste
FIXED OILS
  Greasy
  Do not evaporate easily

Glycosides Glycosides are compounds composed of sugar units, usually glucose, and a nonsugar component. Actions of the glycosides are not dependent on the presence of the sugar. However, the sugar probably increases solubility, absorption, permeability, and cellular distribution of the glycosides. Common glycosides are mustard, vanilla, wild cherry, and licorice. Some glycoside drugs are the cardiac glycosides and the anticoagulants, coumarin and dicumarol.

Gums Gums are plant exudates that are polysaccharides. Some of these exudates swell and form gelatinous masses when water is added. Other gums remain unchanged and form translucent, hydrophilic (water-attracting) colloidal masses. Gums are in bulk laxatives, binders for tablets, and dental adhesives. Some gums sooth irritated skin and mucous membranes.

Resins Resins are complex substances of plant origin. They are semisolid or solid plant exudates that are amorphous (indistinct) in structure and insoluble in water. Benzoin, an antiseptic, is a commonly used resin.

Oils Oils are highly viscous liquids—the liquid form of lipids. Oils generally are classified as volatile or fixed. **Volatile**

oils evaporate easily and have a pleasant, pungent odor and taste. These oils (e.g., peppermint, spearmint, menthol, cinnamon, lemon, camphor, and wintergreen) are used as aromatics and as flavoring agents. **Fixed oils** are greasy and do not evaporate easily. Some fixed oils (e.g., castor oil) are laxatives. Others are emollients in cosmetics (e.g., almond oil), solvents for injections (e.g., corn oil, peanut oil, and sesame oil), bases for suppositories (e.g., cocoa butter), or substitutes for butter (e.g., safflower oil).

Animal Sources

Body fluids or glands of animals can be sources of drugs. Drugs obtained from animal sources include hormones extracted from animal endocrine glands (e.g., insulin), oils and fats (e.g., cod-liver oil), and enzymes (e.g., pepsin and pancreatin).

Mineral Sources

Metallic and nonmetallic minerals provide various inorganic materials not present in plants and animals. Mineral sources may be in their natural state or combined with other ingredients to form acids, bases, or salts. Examples of drugs from mineral sources are iron and potassium preparations.

Chemical Sources

Most drugs currently in use today are produced in laboratories by researchers. These drugs are from organic (animal or plant life forms) or inorganic substances or a combination of the two. Man-made drugs are classified as synthetic or semisynthetic. **Synthetic drugs** are artificially produced in the laboratory and have greater purity than naturally derived drugs. Chemical modification of natural substances produces **semisynthetic drugs.**

EXCIPIENTS USED IN DRUGS

Besides the **active ingredient,** several inert substances called **excipients** form the bases of drugs. Drugs may contain diluents, fillers, binders, disintegrators, and dissolution enhancers and retardants. In addition, some drugs contain lubricants, wetting agents, antiadherants, antioxidants, preservatives, pH stabilizers, coatings, flavorings, and colorings. These excipients influence the disintegration, dissolution, and rate of absorption of the active ingredient. (**Disintegration** is the actual breakdown of a dosage form in the aqueous contents of the digestive tract. Once the dosage form disintegrates, it is free to enter a solution as solute particles; this is called **dissolution.**) Most excipients must pass Federal Food and Drug Administration (FDA) approval.[4-6]

CONCEPT REVIEW

Drugs are derived from animal, plant, mineral, and chemical sources.

Besides an active ingredient, inert substances called *excipients* comprise most drugs.

EXCIPIENTS USED IN DRUGS

Color Additives
D & C red No. 22
D & C yellow No. 10
FD & C blue No. 1, 2, 3
FD & C red No. 40
Anthocyanin (grape skin extract)
Betacyanin (beet extract)

Flavoring Agents
Cinnamon
Ethanol
Orange oil
Tincture of orange peel

Binders
Cornstarch
Potato starch
Wheat starch
Cellulose

Coating Agents
Shellac
Sucrose
Wax
Cellulose
Acrylic acid
Paraffin

Fillers
Cellulose
Lactose
Polyvinylpyrrolidone
Water
Ethanol
Gelatin solutions
Glucose syrups
Sucrose derivatives

Sweetening Agents
Aspartame
Saccharin
Sorbitol
Dextrose
Lactose
Mannitol

Preservatives
Benzalkonium chloride
Benzoic acid
Benzyl alcohol
Chlorobutanol
Phenol

Disintegrators
Cellulose
Cornstarch

Diluents
Lactase
Sucrose

Lubricants
Polyethylene glycol
Magnesium stearate
Sodium benzoate
Zinc stearate
Stearic acid
Talc
Paraffins
Waxes

DRUG ROUTES

Drugs have either a local or a systemic effect. In a local effect the drug effects are confined to one area of the body. For systemic effects to occur, drug absorption and delivery to the body tissues by way of the lymphatic or vascular system must occur. The major route of administration for local effect is topical; the major routes for systemic effect are oral, enteral, and parenteral. Some topically administered drugs produce both local and systemic effects.[4,7-10]

Oral Route

Drugs given orally are administered by mouth. Oral drug administration is the most commonly used route. This route is usually safe, simple, convenient, and inexpensive. However, it is not necessarily the best route in every case. Both drug and client variables influence the effectiveness of orally adminis-

tered drugs. (These variables are discussed in Chapters 4, 5, 7, 9, 10, and 13 through 15.)

Enteral Route

With the enteral route, the agent is administered directly into the stomach or small intestine. This route is usually associated with the administration of essential nutrients and fluids. (Dosage forms and preparations for this route are discussed in Chapter 75.)

Parenteral Routes

Parenteral refers to any route other than the gastrointestinal tract by which a drug is injected or infused. Intradermal or intracutaneous, subcutaneous (**hypodermic**), intramuscular, intravenous, intraarterial, intrathecal or intraspinal, and intraarticular are all parenteral routes.

Intradermal or **intracutaneous** administration involves injection of a drug into or just under the skin layer. This route frequently is used during skin testing for allergies. With the **subcutaneous (SC, SQ, sub-Q)** route, drugs are injected into the layer of fat that lies immediately under the skin. Many sites are available for subcutaneous injections. With the **intramuscular (IM)** route, drugs are injected directly into a muscle mass. The principal sites for IM injections are the gluteal, deltoid, and vastus lateralis muscles.

Intravenous (IV) medication is injected directly into a vein. This route of administration provides the most rapid, predictable drug delivery. Drugs administered intravenously are given in concentrated or diluted preparations. Administration of these drugs is by continuous IV drip or infusion over a period of seconds, minutes, or hours. The IV infusion of large volumes of fluids (**venoclysis**) uses products known as large-volume parenterals. Venoclysis supplies electrolytes and nutrients, restores blood volume, and replaces body fluid. (See Chapters 71 and 72 for more information on fluid and elec-

---

PARENTERAL ROUTES

subcutaneous (hypodermic) Injection of a solution into layer of fat immediately under skin (abbreviated SC, SQ, or sub-Q)

intramuscular Injection of a solution into striated muscle fibers beneath subcutaneous layer of tissue (abbreviated IM)

intravenous Infusion of medication or fluids directly into vascular system (abbreviated IV)

intradermal or intracutaneous Injection of a drug into space just under surface of skin; used most commonly in skin testing for allergies

intrathecal Infusion or injection of a drug within either subarachnoid or subdural space, directly into cerebrospinal fluid

intraspinal Infusion or injection of a drug within vertebral canal or spinal cord

intraarticular Injection of a drug into a joint

trolyte replacement.) The **intraarterial** route involves injecting a drug directly into an artery. Drugs given in this manner are administered slowly since the drug effect cannot be neutralized.

The **intrathecal** route administers drugs directly into either the subarachnoid or subdural space. This route is used when it is not possible to achieve sufficient plasma levels for diffusion into the cerebrospinal fluid. Drugs can also be injected within the vertebral canal or spinal cord **(intraspinal)**. Parenteral products administered by the intrathecal or intraspinal routes must be of the highest purity. The **intraarticular** route administers drugs directly into a joint. Solutions of anti-inflammatory and local anesthetic drugs routinely are administered by this route.

Topical Route

Drugs are administered topically to any externally accessible tissue. Topical preparations are applied to the skin, cornea, or mucous membranes of the eye, mouth, oropharynx, nose, rectum, vagina, or urethra. These preparations have astringent, antiseptic, bacteriostatic, cleansing, anesthetic, emollient, antibiotic, anti-inflammatory, and fungicidal effects. Although most topically applied drugs exert their effects on local tissues, some drugs administered topically diffuse through the skin **(transdermal)** or the mucous membranes **(transmucosal)** into the bloodstream and produce systemic effects.[11]

The **sublingual** method of drug administration produces systemic responses. Sublingual drugs are placed under the tongue where they dissolve. The active ingredient of the drug is absorbed by the blood vessels on the underside of the tongue and is circulated through the body.

With **buccal** administration, a drug is held against the mucous membranes of the cheek until dissolved. The active ingredient of the drug acts locally on the mucous membranes of the mouth or systemically when absorbed by the mucosa or swallowed in the saliva. Buccal and sublingual routes are similar. However, buccal tablets usually dissolve slowly to give prolonged effects, whereas sublingual tablets disintegrate or dissolve rapidly, giving a rapid drug response. These methods are not interchangeable. Therefore read the prescription order carefully to avoid errors.

Instillation involves the placement of a drug into a body cavity or orifice such as the urinary bladder, rectum, vagina, nose, ears, or conjunctival sac of the eyes. Solid, semisolid, and liquid dosage forms are used for instillation purposes. The active drug ingredient in these products produces local and/or systemic responses.

Currently, some anticonvulsants, nonnarcotic and narcotic analgesics, bronchodilators, antiemetic agents, and antibacterial agents are administered by rectal instillation. With rectal administration the rate and extent of drug absorption is usually lower than with oral absorption. However, studies show that serum levels for some drugs administered rectally exceed serum levels after oral administration. Local irritation is one problem associated with repeated rectal drug instillation. Therefore you must carefully assess the client's tolerance to this method of drug administration.[12]

Finely dispersed, nebulized, or aerosolized drug particles are administered by the **inhalation** method. These drug particles produce direct effects on the respiratory tract. The active drug ingredient in some drugs also produces systemic responses.

Intradermal Implants

Some drugs such as male hormones and female contraceptive agents are administered via intradermal implants. During a minor surgical procedure the drugs are implanted in dermal pockets. The active ingredients of these drugs are released slowly over months or years.

DOSAGE FORMS AND PREPARATIONS

Drugs are transported or delivered into the human body in a variety of ways. Seldom are they administered in their pure chemical form; instead, drugs are prepared in a dosage form that maximizes the stability and usefulness of the medication.[4,7,8,13,14]

Preparations for Oral Use

Drugs for oral administration are prepared as liquids or solids. **Solid** drug preparations can be tablets, capsules, Caplets (trademark for capsule-shaped tablet), Spansules (trademark for sustained release capsule), troches, powders, and granules. Liquid drug preparations are usually solutions, suspensions, or emulsions.

A **solution** is a clear liquid preparation that contains at least one solvent, usually water, and one or more dissolved solutes. Solutions are usually flavored and colored to mask the taste and/or appearance of the solute. They are easy to administer and absorb rapidly. Solutions frequently are used for pediatric and geriatric clients or individuals who have difficulty swal-

---

EFFECTS FROM TOPICAL PREPARATIONS

▸ *Astringents* cause vasoconstriction and tissue contraction, which decrease or stop secretions. Astringents will toughen tissue.

▸ *Antispetic* and *bacteriostatic agents* inhibit the growth or multiplication of bacteria on skin or mucous membrane.

▸ *Cleansing agents,* when applied topically, remove dirt, crusts, secretions, and debris.

▸ *Anesthetics* produce a loss of feeling or sensation on the surface of the skin or mucous membrane.

▸ *Emollients* soothe and soften the skin.

▸ *Antibiotics* and/or *bactericidal agents* are antagonistic to other forms of life.

▸ *Anti-inflammatory agents* reduce or counteract inflammation.

▸ *Fungicidal agents* destroy fungi on the surface of the skin or mucous membrane.

DOSAGE FORMS AND PREPARATIONS

Oral

SOLIDS
Tablets
Caplets
Capsules
Troches (lozenges)

LIQUIDS
Solutions
Syrups
Elixirs
Tinctures
Suspensions
Emulsions

Topical (Skin and/or Mucous Membrane)

Aerosols
Baths
Creams
Foams
Gels
Liniments
Lotions
Nebulizers

Ointments
Pastes
Patches
Powders
Soaks
Sprays
Suppositories
Tinctures

Parenteral
Ampules
Vials
Cartridges
Intravenous infusion fluids

Implants
Capsules
Pellets

---

lowing solid dosage forms. If solutions are not prepared, packaged, or stored properly, they are subject to contamination by bacteria, molds, and dust. In addition, if solutions are not stored in containers with tight-fitting caps, the solvent evaporates and produces a more concentrated drug solution.

Syrups are solutions that contain a high concentration of dissolved sugar. Syrups are frequently used to disguise unpleasant-tasting drugs. **Elixirs** are also solutions, but the solvent is a sweetened and aromatic mixture of alcohol and water. Elixirs are often used with drugs that do not dissolve in water alone. A **tincture** is an alcoholic or hydroalcoholic solution in which alcohol is the primary solvent. An example of a tincture is iodine tincture, a mixture of iodine and sodium iodide in alcohol and water.

Suspensions are liquid dosage forms that contain solid drug particles suspended in a liquid medium. In aqueous suspensions the liquid carrier is water. Some suspensions have a greater concentration of drug than a solution. All suspensions must be thoroughly mixed immediately before administration to assure uniformity of dosage.

When fine droplets of oil are dispersed in water or when droplets of water are dispersed in oil, an **emulsion** is formed. The unpleasant taste and odor of medicinal oils (e.g., castor oil or mineral oil) are masked when they are dispersed in water containing a flavoring agent.

Many solid dosage forms exist; **tablets** are probably the most common. Most tablets are formed by compressing a mixture containing the pure drug and inactive components into a

solid form. These solid dosage forms contain an ingredient that disintegrates on contact with fluid in the stomach. The tablet then breaks into smaller particles that dissolve and release the active drug. Tablets are not stable in all environments. Some deteriorate, especially in humid weather, whereas other tablets harden.

Some tablets are **scored** to facilitate convenient division into halves or quarters. In some instances a **coating** is applied to tablets. The coating alters the rate of disintegration, improves the appearance or taste of the drug, and/or improves the stability of the active ingredient. An **enteric coating** prevents tablets from dissolving in the stomach. Instead, the drug dissolves in the neutral or alkaline pH environment of the small intestine. Drugs that irritate the stomach or are destroyed by the acid environment of the stomach are usually enteric coated. Since the enteric coating is present to ensure safe, effective drug administration, crushing the tablet to ease swallowing is not recommended.[15-18]

Certain tablets are **layered.** The layers represent different drugs or separate doses of the same drug. Tablets containing separate doses of the same drug are called **sustained-release tablets.** (The layers are released at different times in the gastrointestinal tract, thus prolonging the action of the drug.) These tablets should not be crushed. Crushing sustained-release tablets allows absorption of too much of the drug at one time and could shorten the duration of the drug's action.

Effervescent and **chewable tablets** are also available. A variety of products, including antacids, analgesics, denture cleaners, and potassium and nutritional supplements, are available in compressed effervescent tablets. These tablets supply premeasured amounts of drugs or chemicals in a convenient, rapidly dissolving form. Effervescent tablets are completely dissolved in a liquid, usually water, immediately before administering.

Chewable tablets are crushed in the mouth before swallowing. These tablets frequently contain large amounts of drugs intended for absorption or local effect in the gastrointestinal tract. Chewable forms of antacids, vitamins, and antibiotics are available.

Recently drug manufacturers have developed **Caplets.** These drugs are in tablet form but are coated with a gelatin shell to make swallowing easier and to decrease the chance of drug tampering.

Capsules are a powder, liquid, or oil form of a drug enclosed in either a hard or soft soluble gelatin shell. **Hard gelatin capsules** consist of two parts that slide together to enclose the medicinal content. (To decrease the incidence of tampering, hard gelatin capsules are being manufactured so that separation of the two parts is impossible.) **Soft gelatin capsules** encapsulate medicinal liquids. These capsules are completely sealed. Both hard and soft gelatin capsules are administered intact; the shell is not removed before administration.

Some capsule products contain small drug-impregnated beads that slowly release the active drug at different times, thus producing a sustained-action effect. These **sustained-release capsules,** or **Spansules,** are useful for drugs that are metabolized or excreted rapidly. As with sustained-release tablets, these capsules should not be opened. Removal of the gelatin shell could allow absorption of a large quantity of the drug in a short time, resulting in a shortened duration of action and an increased potential for adverse reactions.[19]

Troches, or **lozenges,** are solid dosage forms that are dissolved slowly in the mouth. As they dissolve, drugs that produce an antiseptic or anesthetic effect on the tissues of the buccal cavity or throat are released.

Preparations for Parenteral Use

Parenteral drugs are prepared, packaged, and administered in a way that maintains sterility. Parenteral drugs are supplied in ampules, single-dose and multiple-dose vials, cartridges, and large-volume containers for IV infusion fluids.

Ampules are molded glass containers; the tops of ampules are broken off to allow insertion of a needle and withdrawal of the medication. Once the ampule is opened, any remaining medication is discarded because the solution is no longer sterile. One problem associated with the use of ampules is contamination of the drug solution with glass particles.[20]

❧ NURSING RESEARCH

Giambrone, A.J. (1991). Two methods of single-dose ampule opening and their influence upon glass particulate contamination. *Journal of the American Association of Nurse Anesthetists, 59,* 225-228.

One of the hazards of opening glass ampules is particulate contamination. Studies have shown that intravenous administration of these fragments of glass can cause injury to the brain, lungs, spleen, kidneys, liver, and venous systems of laboratory animals. In an attempt to determine the safest method of opening glass ampules, the researcher compared two methods: snapping by hand and using a commercial ampule opener.

Once the ampules were opened, the contents were aspirated, using a nonfilter needle. The contents were then filtered and examined under a microscope for glass fragments. Size and number of glass fragments were recorded.

The study found no difference in glass contaminants in the two groups. Since particulate contamination is a potential hazard, use of filtering devices (placed within the intravenous fluid line or contained within the needle used to aspirate the ampule content) is recommended.

STUDENT ACTIVITIES

- Talk with a nurse anesthetist in your agency and determine what techniques are used to prevent aspiration of glass particles.
- Share these research findings with the nurse anesthetist in your agency.

Vials are closed glass or plastic containers with rubber stoppers. Vials contain a single dose or multiple doses of liquid or powdered drugs. When the medication is supplied in a powdered dosage form, a diluent is injected through the stopper. Before withdrawing the medication, air equivalent to the dosage volume must be added to the vial. Multiple-dose vials usually contain a preservative and are used more than once if sterility is maintained.[21]

Cartridges are single-dose units of parenteral solution that are supplied in a glass tube or cylinder. A cartridge may or may not have a needle attached. Cartridges are inserted into specially designed metal or plastic holders and are used like other needle-syringe units.

Intravenous infusion fluids come in glass or plastic containers that hold 150, 250, 500, or 1000 ml of fluids. Large-volume infusion containers for drugs requiring large amounts of diluents, for total parenteral nutrition, or for drugs administered by continuous infusion rates are available.

Preparations for Topical Use

An enormous variety of dosage forms is available for topical therapy, including solutions, emulsions, powders, suspensions, clear and opaque gels, oils, and semisolid creams, ointments, and pastes.[4,12,22,23] **Creams** typically are **semisolid,** nongreasy, water-soluble emulsions. Creams contain lipids and other moisturizers and are applied by rubbing the preparation into the skin. Moisturizers and most hand lotions are classified as creams.

Ointments differ from creams because they are oily or fatty suspensions of drugs. These preparations have bases with low solubility in water and are not easily washed off by water or perspiration. The most commonly used ointment bases are petrolatum and lanolin. Ointments that are thick and viscous and do not soften substantially from body heat are called ***pastes.*** Pastes contain a high percentage of insoluble solids. They are good protective barriers because they form an unbroken, water-impermeable film on the skin surface. Pastes can also absorb harmful chemicals before the chemicals reach the skin.

Liniments are thinner than ointments and consist of fluid mixtures of drugs and water, oil, soap, and other ingredients. Liniments are applied by rubbing. A **gel,** or jelly, is a clear or translucent semisolid that liquefies when applied. Gels are frequently used as lubricants and as carriers for spermicidal agents. Aqueous suspensions, solutions, or emulsions of drugs are **lotions.** Lotions are not rubbed into the skin but are dabbed onto the surface.

Additional liquid or semisolid preparations used on the skin and mucous membranes are tinctures, aerosols, sprays, foams, baths, and soaks. Alcoholic or water-soluble solutions of drugs (tinctures) are often applied to the skin for protective and/or anti-infective purposes. Iodine tincture and benzoin tincture compound are examples of topically applied tinctures. **Aerosols** are solid or liquid particles suspended in a gas under pressure. They are a major component of respiratory therapy. **Nebulization** is also a method for administering drugs via the respiratory route. Through a nebulizer, the client inhales a fine mist or powdered drug preparation. **Foams** are aerated, semisolid drug preparations under pressure. These preparations are sprayed directly on the skin or mucous membrane. **Baths** and **soaks** provide direct contact between the skin and a drug preparation. Bran, starch, or gelatin baths for pruritus and magnesium sulfate soaks for local inflammation are examples of these topical preparations.

Plasters, powders, and patches are solid dosage forms applied to the skin. **Plasters** usually have an adhesive mixture as their base. They soften in response to body heat and adhere to the skin. **Powders,** fine particles obtained by grinding or crushing a solid, are applied by light dusting of the skin. Powders absorb moistures from the skin. With **patches,** a gradual transdermal or transmucosal absorption of a drug preparation occurs. The total amount of drug on the patch is typically larger than the amount absorbed.

Suppositories and nebulizers are topical preparations used only on mucous membranes. **Suppositories** are administered rectally and vaginally. The drug preparation is mixed with a solid base such as cocoa butter, glycerin, or polyethylene glycol that melts at body temperature. Suppositories can produce local (anti-infective) and systemic (antipyretic and antiemetic) responses. Most suppositories are bullet shaped and approximately 2.5 cm long. Because they melt at body temperature, suppositories usually require refrigeration.

Preparations for Intradermal Implants

Most implantable drugs are relatively insoluble in water. These drugs are prepared in high molecular compounds. The compounds are then placed in capsules or pellets. Small amounts of drug are continuously released from the capsule or pellet.[24]

CONCEPT REVIEW

The three major drug administration routes are oral, parenteral, and topical.

Drugs are transported into the human body in a variety of ways.

The dosage form used for a particular drug affects its stability and usefulness.

DRUG STABILITY AND STORAGE

Both the potency and effect of a drug are influenced by the way in which the drug is handled and stored. As soon as drugs or chemical compounds are produced, they begin to deteriorate and decompose. This process gradually continues and may eventually result in altered effectiveness or toxicity once the drug is administered.

Many drugs change composition when exposed to incorrect external temperatures. Not all drugs are stored at room temperature. Some drugs must be refrigerated (2° to 15° C); some must be stored in a freezer (0° C); and others must be stored at temperatures no higher than 40° C. Guidelines for storage are established by the *United States Pharmacopeia.*

Some drugs are sensitive to light or moisture. Light-sensitive drugs are stored in amber-colored containers to prevent deterioration. In liquid dosage forms, color change, precipitation, or gas formation suggests deterioration. With solid or semisolid dosage forms, a change in color or appearance can denote deterioration. If changes are noted, the drug is not used. Moisture can cause drugs to disintegrate before being administered. To prevent deterioration or alteration caused by moisture, a device containing a moisture absorbent silica gel is packaged with some drugs. In addition, the mouth of the container is vacuum sealed with paper or foil.

At some point after production, a drug reaches a period when its effectiveness decreases. Because of this fact, pharmaceutical companies establish expiration dates and print them on the label or package insert of each drug. These expiration dates are estimates. Thus a drug is not instantly rendered useless or harmful on a specific date. However, to avoid the danger of diminished effectiveness or increased toxicity, do not use drugs after their expiration date.[25-27]

SUMMARY

The pharmaceutic phase is concerned with sources of drugs and excipients used in drug products. In addition, routes of administration, drug stability and storage, and formulation of drugs into effective dosage forms or preparations are part of the pharmaceutic phase.

Most drugs are man-made and are classified as semisynthetic or synthetic. In addition to man-made drugs, plants, animals, and minerals are sources of drug products. The primary dosage forms are solids, semisolids, and liquids. These dosage forms are administered to the body through a variety of routes. The majority of drugs are administered through the gastrointestinal tract—oral, buccal, sublingual, and rectal. Parenteral drugs commonly are administered through intradermal, subcutaneous, intramuscular, and intravenous routes.

All drugs must be handled and stored in a manner that prevents deterioration and decomposition. Improper handling and storage can decrease drug effectiveness or increase drug toxicity.

REFERENCES

1. Arena, J.M. (1989). Plants that poison. *Emergency Medicine, 21*(1), 20-21, 31-32, 34-35, 37-38, 48-51, 58-62, 64.
2. Hayes, L. (Ed.). (1992). Ancient remedies provide clues in search for 'new' medicines. *Chemecology, 21*(5), 10-11.
3. Wagner, D.T. (1989). The pharmacist's role in rain-forest conservation. *American Pharmacy, NS29*(9), 39-40.
4. Banker, G., & Rhodes, C. (1989). *Modern pharmaceutics* (2nd ed.). New York: Marcel Dekker.
5. Cohen, J.L., Hubert, B.B., Leeson, L.J., et al. (1990). Development of U.S.P. dissolution and drug release standards. *Pharmaceutical Research, 7,* 983-987.
6. Smolinske, S.C. (1992). *Handbook of food, drug, and cosmetic excipients.* Boca Raton, FL: CRC Press.
7. Ansel, H., & Popovich, N. (1990). *Pharmaceutical dosage forms and drug delivery systems* (5th ed.). Philadelphia: Lea & Febiger.
8. Avis, K.E., Lieberman, H., & Lachman, L. (1992). *Pharmaceutical dosage forms, parenteral medications* (2nd ed.). New York: Marcel Dekker.

9. Druce, H. (1991). The nasal route for drug administration. *Hospital Practice, 26*(3A), 19-20, 22-23.

10. Williams, D.B., & Johnson, C. (1991). Dosage forms and routes of administration. *Georgia Journal of Hospital Pharmacy, 5*(2), 25-27.

11. Cleary, G.W. (1991). Transdermal drug delivery. *Cosmetics & Toiletries, 106,* 97-104, 106-109.

12. Van Hoogdalem, E.J., De Boer, A.G., & Breimer, D.D. (1991). Pharmacokinetics of rectal drug administration. Pt I. General considerations and clinical applications of centrally acting drugs. *Clinical Pharmacokinetics, 21*(1), 11-26.

13. Chien, Y.W. (1992). *Novel drug delivery systems* (2nd ed.). New York: Marcel Dekker.

14. Madan, P.L. (1990). Sustained release dosage forms. *U.S. Pharmacist, 15,* 39-43, 47-51.

15. Lehmann, S., & Barber, J.R. (1991). Giving medications by feeding tube: How to avoid problems. *Nursing '91, 21*(11), 58-61.

16. Mitchell, J.F., & Pawlicki, K.S. (1990). Oral dosage forms that should not be crushed: 1990 revision. *Hospital Pharmacy, 25,* 329-335.

17. Parks-Veal, P.M. (1991). Oral dosage forms that should not be crushed. *Georgia Journal of Hospital Pharmacy, 5*(1), 28.

18. Williams, P.J. (1989). How do you keep medicines from clogging feeding tubes? *American Journal of Nursing, 89,* 181-182.

19. Wordell, D.C. (1988). Should you crush that tablet? *Nursing '88, 18*(1), 48-49.

20. Giambrone, A.J. (1991). Two methods of single-dose ampule opening and their influence upon glass particulate contamination. *Journal of the American Association of Nurse Anesthetists, 59,* 225-228.

21. Arrington, M.E., Gabbert, K.C., Mazgaj, P.W., & Wolf, M.T. (1990). Multidose vial contamination in anesthesia. *AANA-Journal, 58,* 462-465.

22. Henderson, M.L. (1991). Physiology of the body's largest organ. *U.S. Pharmacist, 16,* 4, 6, 8-9.

23. Dolovich, M. (1991). Clinical aspects of aerosol physics. *Respiratory Care, 36,* 931-938.

24. Waldman, S.D. (1990). Implantable drug delivery systems: Practical considerations. *Journal of Pain and Symptom Management, 5*(3), 169-174.

25. Dalton-Bunnow, M.F., & Halvachs, F.J. (1990). Update on room-temperature stability of drug products labeled for refrigerated storage. *American Journal of Hospital Pharmacy, 47,* 2522-2524.

26. Thoma, K., & Klimek, R. (1991). Photostabilization of drugs in dosage forms without protection from packaging materials. *International Journal of Pharmaceutics, 67,* 169-175.

27. Treloar, A. (1989). Are the drugs in your bag effective? *Practitioner, 233,* 1435-1436.

BIBLIOGRAPHY

Biddle, C., & Gilliland, C. (1992). Transdermal and transmucosal administration of pain-relieving and anxiolytic drugs: A primer for the critical care practitioner. *Heart and Lung: Journal of Critical Care, 21*(2), 115-124.

Bindler, R., & Bayne, T. (1991). Medication calculation ability of registered nurses. *IMAGE: Journal of Nursing Scholarship, 23,* 221-224.

Colaizzi, J.L. (1990). Basic pharmaceutics of oral dosage forms. *U.S. Pharmacist, 15,* 24-31.

Kottke, M.K., Stetsko, G., Rosenbaum, S.E., & Rhodes, C.T. (1990). Problems encountered by the elderly in the use of conventional dosage forms. *Journal of Geriatric Drug Therapy, 5*(2), 77-92.

McQuay, H.J. (1990). The logic of alternative routes. *Journal of Pain and Symptom Management, 5*(2), 75-77.

Murphy, J.I. (1990). Tube feeding problems and solutions. *Advanced Clinical Care, 5*(2), 7-11.

Paice, J.A., & Magolan, J.M. (1991). Intraspinal drug therapy. *Nursing Clinics of North America, 26,* 477-498.

Powers, J.E., & Cascella, P.J. (1990). Comparison of methods used to prepare tablets for nasogastric tube administration. *Journal of Pharmacy Technology, 6,* 60-62.

Ranade, V.V. (1990). Drug delivery systems. Pt 4. Implants in drug delivery. *Journal of Clinical Pharmacology, 30,* 871-889.

Ripamonti, C., & Bruera, E. (1991). Rectal, buccal, and sublingual narcotics for the management of cancer pain. *Journal of Palliative Care, 7*(1), 30-35.

Svedmyr, N. (1991). Clinical advantages of the aerosol route of drug administration. *Respiratory Care, 36,* 922-930.

Technique with multidose vials leads to pseudomonad infections. (1990). *Hospital Infection Control, 17*(6), 73-74.

CHAPTER 4

Pharmacokinetic Phase

NORMA L. PINNELL

⊛ Factors Affecting the Pharmacokinetic Processes

LEARNING OBJECTIVES:
Define the four pharmacokinetic processes.
Discuss two factors that affect all pharmacokinetic processes.
KEY TERM: Pharmacokinetic phase

⊛ Absorption of Drug Molecules

LEARNING OBJECTIVES:
Describe the impact of drug solubility on drug absorption.
Explain four ways drugs cross cell membranes.
Discuss five factors that affect absorption of drug molecules.
KEY TERMS:
Absorption, active transport, bioavailability, filtration, passive diffusion, pinocytosis, solubility

⊛ Distribution of Drug Molecules

LEARNING OBJECTIVE: Describe three factors that influence the distribution of drug molecules.
KEY TERMS:
Affinity, blood-brain barrier, competitive binding, distribution, nonspecific binding, placental barrier, plasma-protein binding

⊛ Biotransformation of Drug Molecules

LEARNING OBJECTIVE: Explain three factors that alter the biotransformation process.
KEY TERMS:
Biotransformation, first-pass phenomenon, metabolites, pharmacoanthropology

⊛ Excretion of Drug Molecules and Metabolites

LEARNING OBJECTIVE: Describe renal excretion of drug molecules.
KEY TERMS:
Clearance, enterohepatic recycling, excretion

⊛ Pharmacokinetic Effects on Plasma Levels

LEARNING OBJECTIVE: Explain pharmacokinetic effects on plasma levels.
KEY TERMS:
Loading dose, maintenance dose, plasma half-life, plateau principle, therapeutic index

---

CONCEPTS AND TERMS TO REVIEW

Review the following physiologic functions: passive diffusion, active transport, filtration, and pinocytosis.
Review the chemical processes of hydrolysis, oxidation, reduction, and synthesis.
Review glomerular filtration and active tubular secretion mechanisms of the renal system.
Review description of routes of administration and dosage forms in Chapter 3.

The **pharmacokinetic phase** includes the processes of drug absorption, distribution, biotransformation, and excretion (Fig. 4–1). These processes determine the intensity and duration of a drug's action. The manner in which a drug produces its effects occurs during the pharmacodynamic phase, which is discussed in Chapter 5.

FACTORS AFFECTING THE PHARMACOKINETIC PROCESSES

Why is it necessary to administer some drugs more frequently than other drugs? Why do some drugs produce unexpected responses in individuals? Drug absorption, distribution, biotransformation, and excretion determine the number of drug molecules to reach action sites, the intensity of drug action, and the duration of drug action.

ABSORPTION OF DRUG MOLECULES

Absorption is the process by which a drug passes from the site of administration into venous or lymphatic circulation. All drugs, except those administered directly into venous circula-

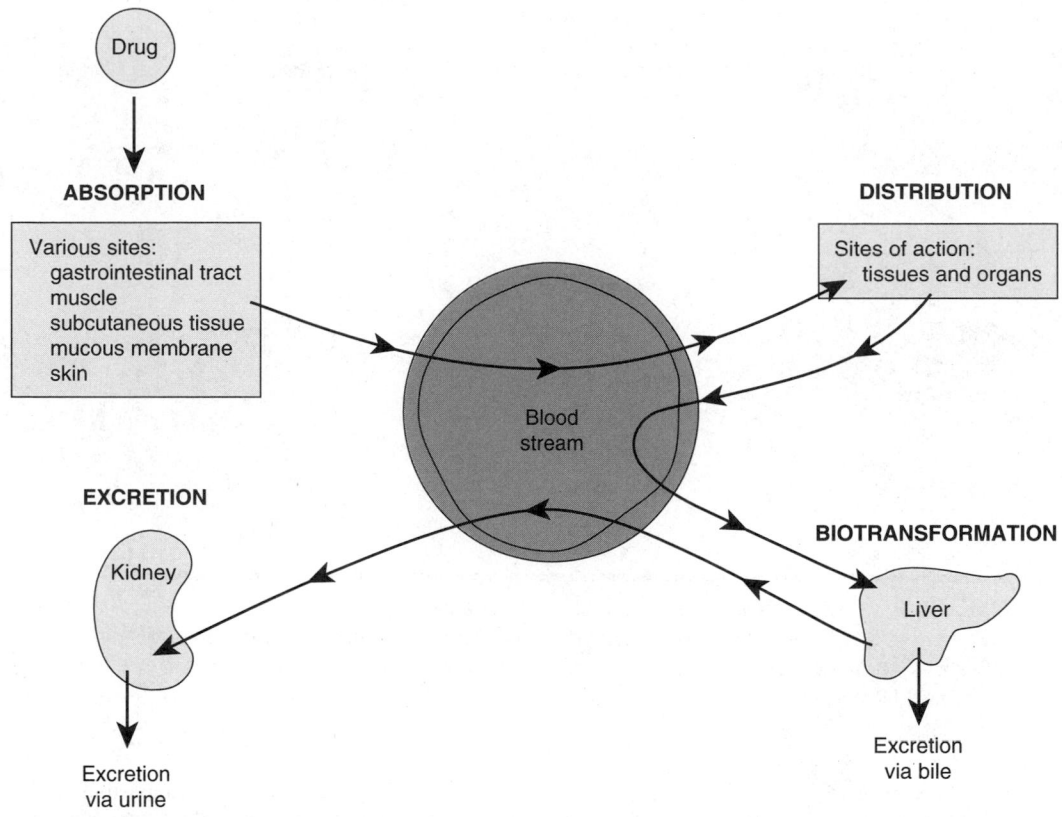

FIGURE 4–1   Pharmacokinetic processes. Drug molecules are absorbed into the bloodstream and distributed to action sites. After biotransformation, which usually occurs in the liver, most drug molecules are excreted by either the liver or kidneys.

tion or applied topically, must be absorbed before they can produce actions in the body. In most instances the total amount administered is ultimately not available to produce pharmacologic effects; some drug molecules are lost during the processes of absorption and distribution. **Bioavailability** is the term used to describe the proportion of the administered drug available to produce effects.[1-5]

Many factors influence the absorption of drugs. Two of the most important factors are drug solubility and ability of the drug to pass through cell membranes.

Drug Solubility

For absorption to occur, drugs must be in a solution form. Solids, semisolids, and liquids are the most common forms of drug preparations. Solid and semisolid dosage forms such as tablets, capsules, troches, powders, and granules must initially disintegrate in body fluids. Particles produced by the disintegration process move into liquids and form solutions or suspensions that can be absorbed. **Solubility** denotes the ability of a drug to dissolve and form a solution. Liquid dosage forms (e.g., solutions, suspensions, and emulsions) bypass the disintegration and dissolution process.

Excipients (inert substances used as fillers and binders) used to produce and stabilize the drug can affect solubility. For ex-

ample, alcohol-based products have enhanced solubility and absorption, whereas oil-based products have delayed solubility and absorption. To facilitate disintegration and dissolution of drugs, excipients that act as disintegrators are added to some drug products.[6-8]

Since cell membranes contain lipids, drugs must be both water and fat soluble. Solubility in fat (lipid) is essential for diffusion of drug molecules across lipid-rich cell membranes.

Movement Across Cell Membranes

Cell membranes are composed of proteins, lipids, and carbohydrates; they help regulate the composition of the intracellular environment. During absorption, drug molecules cross cell membranes by passive diffusion, active transport, filtration, and/or pinocytosis (Fig. 4–2). **Passive diffusion** is the most common process by which drugs cross membranes. Diffusion is the random movement of drug molecules from the place of highest drug concentration to the place of lowest concentration. Diffusion is usually more rapid if a higher drug dose is administered because it produces a greater concentration gradient. In other words, the drug moves from the drug-rich extracellular environment to the drugfree intracellular environment. In addition to diffusing across cell membranes, some drug molecules diffuse between adjacent cells. The

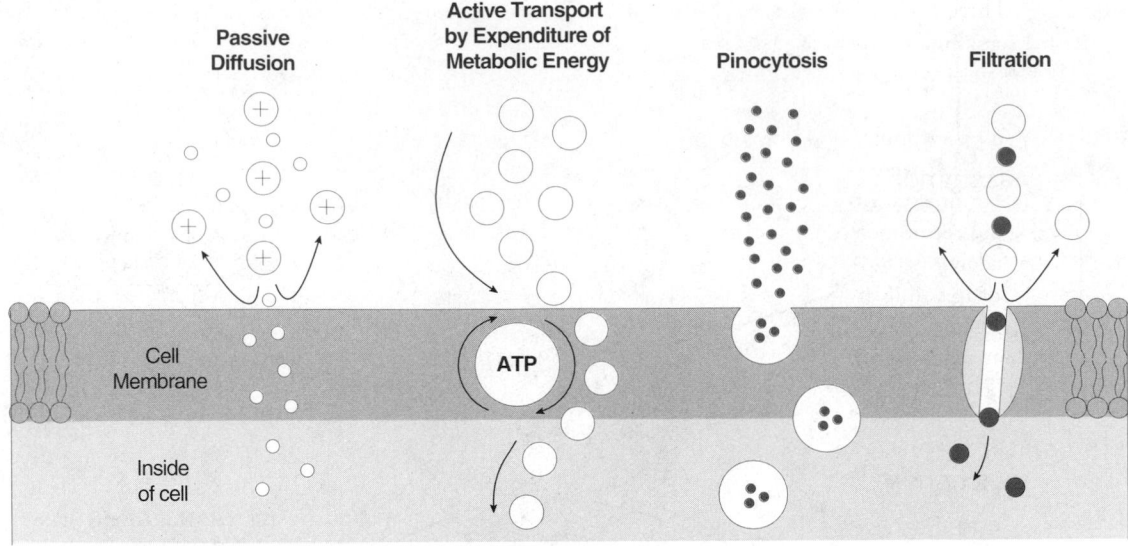

FIGURE 4–2   Movement of drug molecules across cell membranes. Molecules from most drugs cross cell membranes by passive diffusion. Only nonionized lipid-soluble drug molecules diffuse easily. Movement of drug molecules also occurs by active transport, pinocytosis, and filtration.

process of diffusion also regulates the movement of drug particles out of the bloodstream into target cells.

Active transport is the movement of molecules across a cell membrane against a concentration gradient. This process requires the expenditure of metabolic energy. Active transport is also an essential component in the excretion of drugs by the kidneys. In **filtration,** drug molecules pass through membrane pores from an area of highest concentration to an area of lowest concentration. This process is driven by a pressure gradient, either osmotic or hydrostatic. Filtration, like active transport, does not have a major role in drug absorption but is essential in the excretion process. A few drugs cross cell membranes by **pinocytosis.** During pinocytosis the cell membrane surrounds and engulfs a substance on its outer surface and carries the substance inside the cell.[9-11]

Several other factors influence absorption. They include route of administration, dosage form, drug concentration, condition of absorptive surface, ionization of drug solution, and size of drug molecule.

Route of Administration

The route of administration affects the absorption process significantly. Therefore this factor must be considered when determining dosages and monitoring for drug effects, adverse reactions, and side effects.

Oral route   The oral route is the slowest route to produce effects, primarily because of the rate of absorption. Drugs administered orally are absorbed into the venous and lymphatic circulation through the mucosal membranes that line the entire length of the gastrointestinal tract.

Few drugs are absorbed in the mouth, even though the lining of the oral cavity is thin and has a rich blood supply. However, drugs that dissolve rapidly in the salivary secretion of the mouth (e.g., oxytocin and nitroglycerin) are absorbed.

These drugs enter general circulation directly, thus avoiding destruction from gastrointestinal fluids and the liver.

The absorption rate of drugs from the stomach is variable and depends on gastric motility, emptying time, and pH. In addition, the presence or absence of food and the amount and composition of gastric secretions influence drug absorption. Generally, drugs ingested with food are absorbed more slowly than drugs taken on an empty stomach. The normal gastric emptying time of 4 hours is prolonged by factors such as vigorous exercise, pain, emotional stress, drugs, and gastric surgery. In addition, ingestion of bulky or fatty foods, carbohydrates, hot foods, or foods with high viscosity prolongs the rate of gastric emptying. Mild exercise, hunger, cold foods, and ingestion of dilute liquids hasten gastric emptying time.

Some drugs and food form complexes that cannot pass through the mucosal lining of the gastrointestinal tract. For example, the antibiotic tetracycline combines with calcium and other polyvalent cations (e.g., Ca^{2+} and Mg^{2+}) to form complexes that are excreted unabsorbed in the feces. In addition, some drugs are destroyed by the high acidity and peptic activity of gastric contents. Achlorhydria (absence of hydrochloric acid in the stomach) promotes absorption of weak acids and inhibits absorption of weak bases.[12]

NURSING RESEARCH

Strong, A., Wolff, H., Kinder, S., & Lubischer, A. (1991). Drug administration in relation to meals in the institutional setting. *Heart & Lung, 20*(1), 39-44.

A study was conducted on 183 adult clients in two short-term and two long-term care settings. The purpose of the study was to investigate adherence to literature recommendations for the administration of five cardiovascular drugs. Three of the drugs were to be administered in the fed state, one in the fasting state, and one in either state but with consistence of administration maintained.

Findings showed that timing recommendations for dosing in relation to meals were not considered in these institutions. Drug administration schedules were arbitrarily established, and recommendations from the literature were not considered.

Use of standard drug administration schedules established by hospital policy could have serious consequences. Medication schedules need to be designed to achieve the greatest drug bioavailability.

STUDENT ACTIVITIES

- Review the agency's policy and procedure manual to determine established drug administration schedules.

- Select three clients at random and determine if their drugs are being administered as recommended by literature.

Most drugs administered orally are absorbed from the small intestine. The convoluted lining of the duodenum contains millions of small capillaries that absorb drug molecules directly into the systemic circulation. Intestinal motility, amount and composition of intestinal fluids, gastrointestinal flora, blood flow to the intestines, and the physiologic status of the gut influence drug absorption from this site.

Increased intestinal motility enhances or diminishes the absorption of drugs. The disintegration of solid and semisolid drugs is accelerated by increased intestinal motility, thus enhancing the absorption of drugs. However, the increased motility also hastens the passage of drugs through the intestines, reducing the time of contact between the drug and mucosal surface and decreasing drug absorption.

The pH of the intestines is approximately 4.0 to 5.0 in the duodenum, and it becomes progressively more alkaline in the small intestine (6.0 to 7.5). Therefore basic drugs are better absorbed farther along the intestinal tract. Certain drugs are metabolized by enzymes located in the mucosal membrane of the intestines. Other drugs are significantly destroyed within the small intestine before the drugs reach systemic circulation.

Parenteral route   The most common parenteral routes used by nurses are intradermal, subcutaneous, intramuscular, and intravenous. Drugs administered via the intradermal route diffuse slowly from the injection site into the local microcapillary system. Drugs administered subcutaneously are usually in aqueous solutions. To reach systemic circulation, these drug molecules must cross the extracellular compartment, reach a capillary, and diffuse across the blood vessel membrane. Although absorption is slow from subcutaneous sites, the rate is still faster than with intradermal injections.

As with subcutaneous injections, drugs administered intramuscularly must reach a capillary and diffuse through the vessel wall. Since muscle tissue is more richly supplied with blood vessels, absorption is more rapid than with the subcutaneous route.

Drug absorption from subcutaneous and intramuscular sites is influenced by the condition of the injection site and the blood perfusion at the site. For example, clients in shock have diminished tissue perfusion. Drugs administered subcutaneously or intramuscularly to these individuals are absorbed slowly. Some muscles normally have greater blood supply than other muscles. For example, drugs administered intramuscularly in the deltoid muscle are absorbed faster than drugs administered in the larger gluteal muscle because of greater blood flow. Massaging or applying heat to subcutaneous or intramuscular injection sites accelerates blood flow and enhances absorption. Absorption can be slowed by constricting or occluding blood perfusion in the area. Techniques used to slow absorption include application of cold to the injection site or local injection of a vasoconstrictor.

Intravenous administration of drugs provides the most rapid and accurate drug action. Since intravenous drugs are administered directly into the circulatory system, the intravenous route bypasses the absorption process. Drugs injected by the intravenous route pose the greatest potential for adverse and toxic effects.[8,13-15]

Topical route   Less absorption occurs through topical application to the skin and mucous membranes than with oral and parenteral routes. Most drugs applied topically to the skin are meant for local effect only. The epidermis of the intact skin acts as a lipid barrier, allowing absorption of only lipid-soluble substances. However, absorption through the skin is enhanced if the area is covered with an occlusive dressing or if the skin is broken.

As noted in Chapter 3, mucous membranes commonly used for the administration of drugs include the sublingual, buccal, nasal, conjunctival, vaginal, and rectal mucosa. When drugs are applied to mucous membranes with vascular beds close to the surface (e.g., sublingual and rectal), absorption is rapid. A benefit to topical drug administration is that drugs quickly enter the vascular system and are not destroyed by gastrointestinal secretions. In addition, some topical routes are beneficial because they bypass the first-pass phenomenon of the liver. (This phenomenon is discussed later in the chapter.)

Drugs instilled into the ears usually result in negligible absorption. Absorption from ophthalmic instillation depends on the type of preparations or dosage form (i.e., solutions or ointments) used. Drugs administered via nasal instillation can cause local or systemic effects. In addition, the large alveolar-capillary network of the lungs provides an excellent location for drug absorption. Inhaled drug molecules diffuse rapidly from the alveolar space to the bloodstream.[8,13-15]

Dosage Form

Drugs administered in a liquid dosage form are already in solution and thus are immediately available for absorption. Drugs administered in a solid or semisolid form must first disintegrate and go into a solution.

Oral preparations   The soluble gelatin shell of most capsules dissolves in the stomach within 10 to 20 minutes. Thus the drug becomes available for dissolution and absorption at a rate almost equal to that for liquid dosage forms. Since tablets must disintegrate first, they are absorbed more slowly.

If capsules and tablets are enteric coated, disintegration is delayed. Enteric-coated drug products are designed to disintegrate in the alkaline environment of the small intestines. Because the disintegration process is delayed with this dosage form, it is difficult to project the onset of action. If the enteric coating disintegrates in the stomach, poor absorption may result. In addition, when gastric emptying is prolonged, enteric-coated tablets or capsules remain inactive in the stomach for hours. Absorption is also delayed if the enteric coating does not dissolve promptly when the dosage form reaches the intestines. In some cases individuals eliminate the dosage form intact in their stool.

Theoretically, the active ingredient in sustained-release capsules is absorbed slowly over an 8- to 12-hour period. However, most solid and semisolid drug preparations reach the end of the small intestine within 3 to 4 hours after oral administration. Thus a substantial amount of the drug contained in the sustained-released preparation may be excreted in the stool without being absorbed.[16,17]

Parenteral preparation   Drugs administered intramuscularly are usually in solutions, suspensions, or emulsions. Some of these preparations are formulated to be absorbed slowly **(depot preparations).** With delayed drug absorption, drug activity is prolonged and frequency of injections decreased. This technique usually is not used with subcutaneous injections because of the potential for tissue damage. Instead, drug preparations for subcutaneous injections are usually aqueous solutions.

In general, only aqueous solutions are administered intravenously. These solutions produce an immediate rise in the plasma concentration level and thus reduce the onset-of-action time to a minimum. Some fat emulsions are administered intravenously during parenteral feeding (hyperalimentation).[7,13,18-20] (See Chapter 75 for further discussion of hyperalimentation.)

Drug Concentration

The concentration of free-unbound drug influences the rate at which a drug enters circulation. High concentrations of free drug accelerate absorption; high plasma levels of protein-bound drugs lower free drug concentrations and slow absorption.

Condition of Absorptive Surface

Whether the drug is administered orally, parenterally, or topically, the condition of the absorptive surface influences the rate of absorption. Damaged, impaired, or surgically removed absorptive surfaces decrease the amount of drug absorbed into the body.

Essentially, the larger the surface area, the faster the absorption. One of the largest surface areas for drug absorption is the small intestines. However, the amount of absorptive surface area can be significantly decreased by gastrointestinal surgery (e.g., jejunoileal bypass and gastrectomy). In addition, gastrointestinal diseases such as inflammatory bowel disease and celiac disease decrease the amount of normal surface area available.[21]

The absorptive area for parenteral injections can also be compromised. Bruised or inflamed tissue caused by frequent injections or failure to rotate injection sites diminishes absorption. Inflammation and extravasation (leaking) at intravenous sites can also impair absorption of drugs. In addition, circulation to the absorptive surface influences the rate of absorption. Basically, the rate of absorption is proportional to the rate of blood flow.

Drug Ionization

A drug in solution is ionized (electrically charged) or nonionized. Ionized drugs do not diffuse easily across lipid membranes and therefore are absorbed poorly. Nonionized drug molecules are soluble in lipids and easily diffuse through lipid membranes. Few drugs are all ionized or all nonionized; they are usually a balance between the two.

The pH of the drug environment largely determines if drug molecules will be ionized or nonionized. For example, in the stomach, a strongly acidic environment (pH, 1.0 to 2.0), acid drugs remain nonionized and are therefore more rapidly absorbed.

Size of Drug Molecule

The size of a drug molecule is also a factor in absorption. Small molecules penetrate cell membranes more quickly. Drugs with molecular weights of less than 60,000 usually pass through capillary walls easily. This is true even if the drugs are ionized and have low lipid solubility. Capillaries of the central nervous system are an exception (see discussion of blood-brain barrier, below).[8]

CONCEPT REVIEW

Absorption represents the stage from the time the drug enters the body until it enters the venous or lymphatic circulation.

Many factors influence the absorption of drugs, including drug solubility, ability of the drug to pass through cell membranes, route of administration, dosage form, drug concentration, condition of absorptive surface, ionization of drug solution, and size of drug molecule.

DISTRIBUTION OF DRUG MOLECULES

Distribution describes the process by which drug molecules are transported by body fluids to sites of action. Once absorbed into circulation, drug molecules must still reach reactive tissues—sites that respond to the drug. In the process of being distributed to reactive tissues, drug molecules are also distributed to tissues sites where no effects are produced (storage sites) and to sites where inactivation occurs.

Unless a drug is administered for its direct effects on the components of the blood, drug molecules must cross capillary membranes to reach their sites of action. Because of the concentration gradient, the movement of drug molecules out of the blood is quicker than absorption. Although drug distribution can occur by active transport, pinocytosis, and filtration through pores, the process primarily involves diffusion. Several factors influence the distribution of drugs, including cardiac output, regional blood flow, plasma protein binding, drug concentration, physiologic barriers, and reservoir and/or storage sites.

Cardiac Output and Regional Blood Flow

Cardiac output and regional blood flow affect the initial phase of drug distribution. The quantity of drug that enters the tissue is proportional to the rate of blood flow through that tissue.

Plasma-Protein Binding

Within the vascular compartment, a drug is either bound to plasma proteins, usually albumin, or circulates in a free or unbound state. Only those drug molecules not bound to plasma proteins are able to produce pharmacologic effects and be metabolized and/or excreted. **Plasma-protein binding** renders drug molecules pharmacologically inactive (Fig. 4–3).

The percentage of drug molecules bound to plasma proteins depends, in part, on the chemical structure of the drug.

This structure also influences the intensity of the interaction between the binding sites and the drug molecules.

Binding of a drug to plasma protein is generally reversible, nonspecific, and competitive. Reversible binding indicates that the interaction between the binding site and the drug molecule is not permanent. A drug that binds tightly to plasma proteins is said to have a high **affinity;** the proportion of free or unbound drug will be low. For example, generally in excess of 90% of most antipsychotic drugs bind to plasma proteins. Conversely, a drug with low affinity for plasma proteins will have a higher percentage of free drug. An example of a drug that binds poorly is aminoglycoside, an antibacterial drug. Less than 10% of it is bound by plasma protein. The same proportion of bound and free drug is maintained in the blood at all times. Thus when free drug molecules leave the plasma, drug molecules are released from plasma protein to reestablish the proper ratio between bound and free molecules. (See Chapter 5 for additional discussion of affinity.)

Nonspecific binding indicates the plasma proteins will bind with many different drugs. **Competitive binding** means molecules of different drugs compete for binding sites. In situations in which the drugs have differing affinity levels, the drug that binds more strongly will be more extensively bound. Competitive binding is the basis for many drug interactions.

If the individual has a disease such as hypoalbuminemia that causes a low level of plasma protein, drug molecules will have diminished binding sites, resulting in higher-than-normal plasma levels of the free drug. This situation can cause overdose or toxicity.

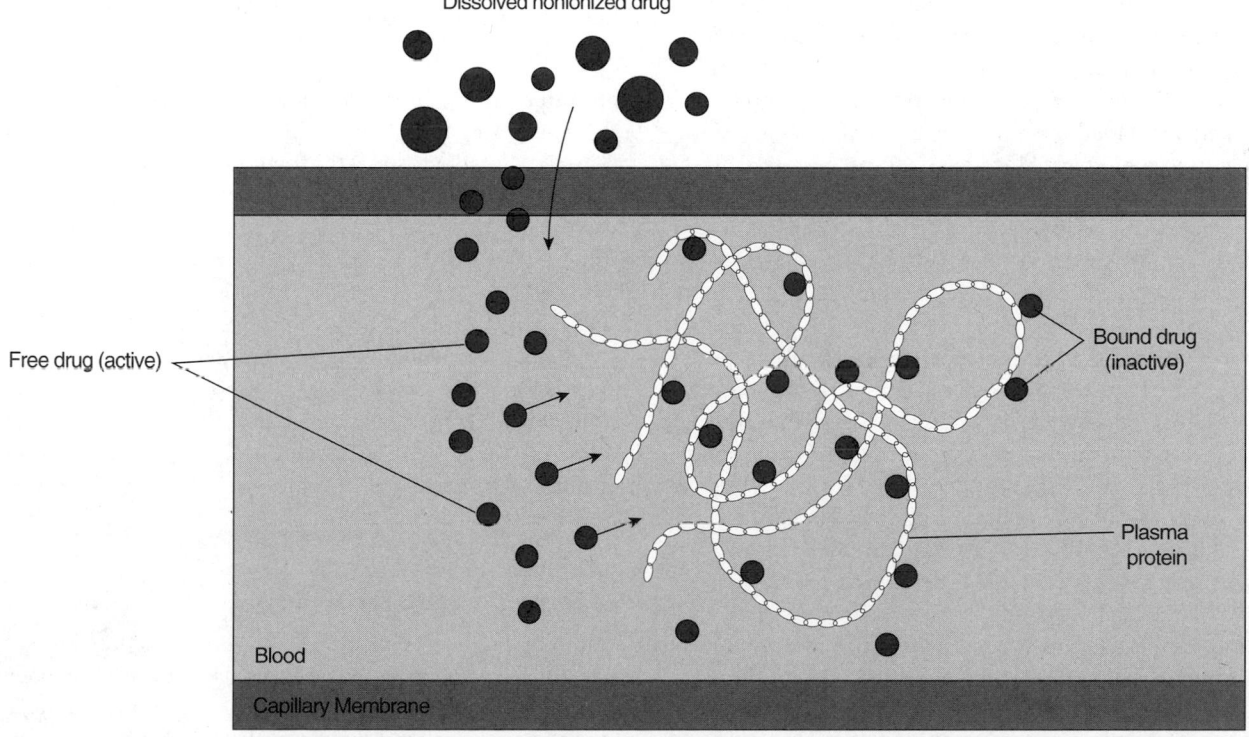

Dissolved nonionized drug

Free drug (active)

Bound drug (inactive)

Plasma protein

Blood

Capillary Membrane

Figure 4–3   Plasma protein-bound drug molecules versus free drug molecules. Once absorbed, drug molecules bind to plasma proteins. The percentage of bound drug molecules depends on the drug and the availability of protein-binding sites. Only drug molecules that are not bound to plasma proteins (free-drug molecules) are able to produce pharmacologic effects.

Drug Concentration

The rate at which a drug leaves the circulation is proportional to the concentration gradient of unbound drug from plasma to extracellular water. If the plasma level of unbound drug is high, the drug will quickly move into the extracellular water. In some instances the initial dose of a drug is increased to raise the plasma-drug concentration level.

Physiologic Barriers

Capillary networks in some organs prevent certain drugs from crossing cell membranes, thus establishing a physiologic barrier. The two most important barriers are the blood-brain barrier and the placental barrier.

Capillaries in the central nervous system differ from all other capillaries—a morphologic difference called the **blood-brain barrier.** In a few areas of the brain (i.e., lateral nuclei of the hypothalamus, pineal body, posterior lobe of the hypophysis, and areas of the fourth ventricle) the barrier is absent. Consequently, these areas of the brain are able to respond to changes in the chemical composition of blood.

The blood-brain barrier prevents entrance into the central nervous system of drugs poorly soluble in lipids. Because of the barrier, some drugs have little or no effect on the functioning of the central nervous system, even if they are present in the blood in large amounts. Newborns are more sensitive to lipid-soluble drugs than older children and adults because the blood-brain barrier is not fully developed at birth. (See Chapter 17 for additional information on the blood-brain barrier.)

The **placental barrier** is produced by the membranes of the placenta. It is not an absolute barrier to the passage of drugs. Lipid-soluble, nonionized compounds readily pass from the maternal bloodstream into the blood of the fetus. (See Chapter 13 for more information.) Note that both the placental barrier and the blood-brain barrier allow the passage of lipid-soluble drug molecules. Since many drugs are at least to some degree lipid soluble (nonionized) at physiologic pH, they can cause some central nervous system side effects and are potential risks to the fetus.[9,11]

Drug Reservoirs

Drug reservoirs, or storage sites, include fat, bone, teeth, and kidneys. Fatty, or adipose, tissues serve as a depot for lipid-soluble drugs such as barbiturates and anticoagulants. Since the blood flow in fat is slow, accumulated drugs remain for long periods of time. These drugs may not be released into the bloodstream until after drug administration has stopped. If an individual loses weight quickly, the amount of body fat decreases, and large amounts of stored drugs can be released into the blood.

Structures composed primarily of calcium such as bone and teeth can accumulate or store drugs that bind with calcium. Radioactive elements such as radium and environmental pollutants such as lead and arsenic are stored in bone. The antibiotic tetracycline is stored in teeth and bone. This drug can interfere with the growth of bones when it crosses the placental barrier and accumulates in skeletal tissue of the fetus. Tetracycline can also cause a brownish discoloration of permanent teeth if administered during the prenatal period or early childhood.

Since a large quantity of blood flows through the kidneys, these organs are exposed to a large amount of drugs. Although few therapeutic drugs accumulate in kidney tissues, metals such as lead and mercury can reach high concentration levels.

CONCEPT REVIEW

Distribution is the process of transporting drug solutions in body fluids to various sites.

Within the vascular compartment, a drug is either bound to plasma proteins or circulates in a free or unbound state.

Only those drug molecules not bound to plasma proteins are able to produce pharmacologic effects and be metabolized and/or excreted.

Physiologic barriers (i.e., blood-brain barrier and placental barrier) are capillary networks that prevent certain drugs from crossing cell membranes.

Within the body are reservoirs and/or storage sites where drugs accumulate.

Equilibrium between bound and free drug molecules assures that all molecules eventually will be freed and able to leave the circulatory system.

BIOTRANSFORMATION OF DRUG MOLECULES

Biotransformation, or metabolism, is the process by which the body modifies or alters the chemical structure of the drug. This process usually reduces the amount of active drug in the body. However, not all drugs are metabolized to the same extent or by the same mechanisms. Some drugs are not metabolized; they pass through the body and are excreted in an unchanged form.

During biotransformation most drugs are converted to **metabolites.** Qualities of metabolites differ from those of the original drug. For example, some metabolites are more active pharmacologically or more water soluble than the parent drug. In some instances active metabolites prolong the duration of drug action. Drugs may also be converted to inactive metabolites that are ready for excretion.

Biotransformation Sites

Although the site of most drug metabolism is the liver, enzymes capable of breaking down drugs are present in all body tissues. Drugs can be metabolized in the placenta, kidneys, lungs, blood plasma, and intestinal mucosa. Enzymes at biotransformation sites alter drugs through hydrolysis, oxidation, reduction, and synthesis.

Hepatic Metabolism

Within the liver, the microsomal enzyme system is responsible for metabolizing drugs. Several types of chemical transformation occur, but the hepatic enzyme system usually creates water-soluble compounds that are more easily excreted by the kidneys. Enzymes within this system are nonspecific; in other words, many drugs are metabolized by the same enzyme. More enzymes are produced by the liver if drug concentrations are extremely high, thus allowing the microsomal enzyme system to metabolize drugs more quickly.

Several factors such as age, nutritional status, and liver disease can modify, inhibit, or accelerate hepatic drug metabolism. Some substances suppress hepatic drug metabolism by diminishing the ability of hepatocytes to function properly. Drugs also compete for the same hepatic enzyme system; thus one drug inhibits the metabolism of another drug. In some instances the client may receive drugs that stimulate the liver's ability to metabolize other drugs.

Another important concept associated with biotransformation is the **first-pass effect** or **phenomenon.** Drugs taken orally and absorbed from the small intestine are transported by portal circulation directly to the liver before entering general circulation. Hepatic metabolism may inactivate or activate a fraction of the absorbed drug or have no effect. The bioavailability of a drug is reduced if the drug is inactivated. If metabolism of the drug by the liver is highly efficient, the amount of drug to reach systemic circulation will be substantially lowered. When the capacity of the liver to metabolize a particular drug is extremely high, the drug can be completely inactivated on its first pass through the liver (Fig. 4–4).

Factors Altering Biotransformation

Drugs disappear from the blood and site of action at a rate proportional to the concentration at any given moment. In an individual with cardiovascular, hepatic, or renal disease, drug metabolism is usually prolonged. When the metabolism of drugs is delayed for any reason, cumulative drug effects occur. These effects are manifested as excessive or prolonged responses to ordinary doses of drugs. Stimulation of drug metabolism or biotransformation usually produces a state of apparent drug tolerance.

Interethnic differences account for individual variations in drug responsiveness. Research in this area is increasing, giving rise to a new field called **pharmacoanthropology.** Studies have shown that the interethnic differences include genetic inability to metabolize a drug in the expected manner and structural variations in the binding sites in the body. One significant genetic difference concerns the ability of different races to achieve acetylation of certain drugs. (Acetylation is the biotransformation of drugs in the liver by acyl transferase enzymes.) Some ethnic groups are classified as fast acetylators and others as slow acetylators. Ethnic groups that are slow acetylators are more prone to toxic effects. In addition to physiologic differences among ethnic groups, coinciding environmental conditions (e.g., poverty and nutritional status) affect the absorption, distribution, biotransformation, and excretion of drugs.[22,23]

An example of this variation occurs with the use of alcohol and caffeine. Alcohol is metabolized by the liver enzyme alcohol dehydrogenase in Caucasians. In Asians the enzyme aldehyde dehydrogenase metabolizes alcohol. This enzyme works faster. As a result, unpleasant effects such as facial flushing and palpitations occur. Caffeine is excreted faster by Caucasians than by Asians as a result of liver-enzyme differences.

Note that the liver enzyme system of the very young and the elderly may not metabolize drugs efficiently. In the young the liver enzyme system is not fully developed, whereas in the older adult the function of the system may be diminished. (See Chapters 14 and 15 for further discussions of this topic.) These individuals must be monitored carefully for possible toxic effects.

CONCEPT REVIEW

Biotransformation or metabolism is the process by which the body modifies or alters the chemical structure of the drug.

During biotransformation most drugs are converted to active metabolites.

The microsomal enzyme system of the liver is responsible for metabolizing most drugs.

Drugs administered orally and absorbed from the small intestine are transported by portal circulation directly to the liver. Hepatic metabolism may immediately inactivate all of the absorbed drug; this is called the *first-pass effect* or *phenomenon.*

Many factors, including age, disease state, and ethnic differences, influence the biotransformation process.

EXCRETION OF DRUG AND METABOLITES

Excretion describes the movement of drugs or drug metabolites from the tissues into circulation and from circulation into the organs of excretion. The rate of removal of drug molecules from the body is termed **clearance.** Routes of excretion include the renal system, gastrointestinal tract, pulmonary system, skin, saliva, perspiration, tears, and breast milk.

Renal Excretion

Most drugs are excreted through the renal system. However, before lipid-soluble drugs are excreted from the kidneys, some form of biotransformation must convert them to water-soluble metabolites. Excretion of drugs and metabolites through the kidneys involves two processes: glomerular filtration and active tubular secretion (Fig. 4–5). In filtration small drug molecules move by passive diffusion from the blood vessels in the kidneys into the tubule. In active secretion drug

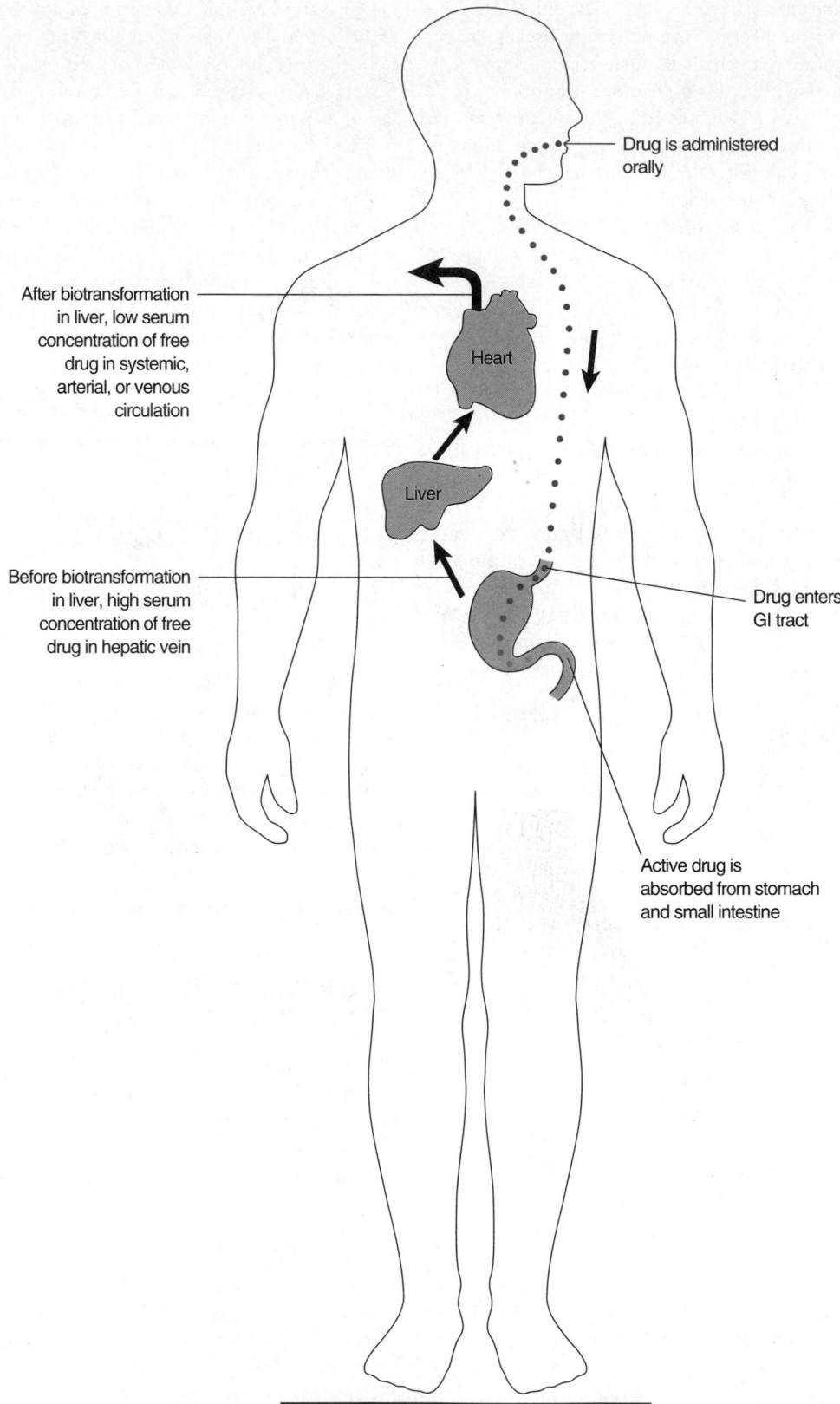

Drug is administered orally

After biotransformation in liver, low serum concentration of free drug in systemic, arterial, or venous circulation

Heart

Liver

Drug enters GI tract

Before biotransformation in liver, high serum concentration of free drug in hepatic vein

Active drug is absorbed from stomach and small intestine

FIGURE 4–4 First-pass phenomenon.

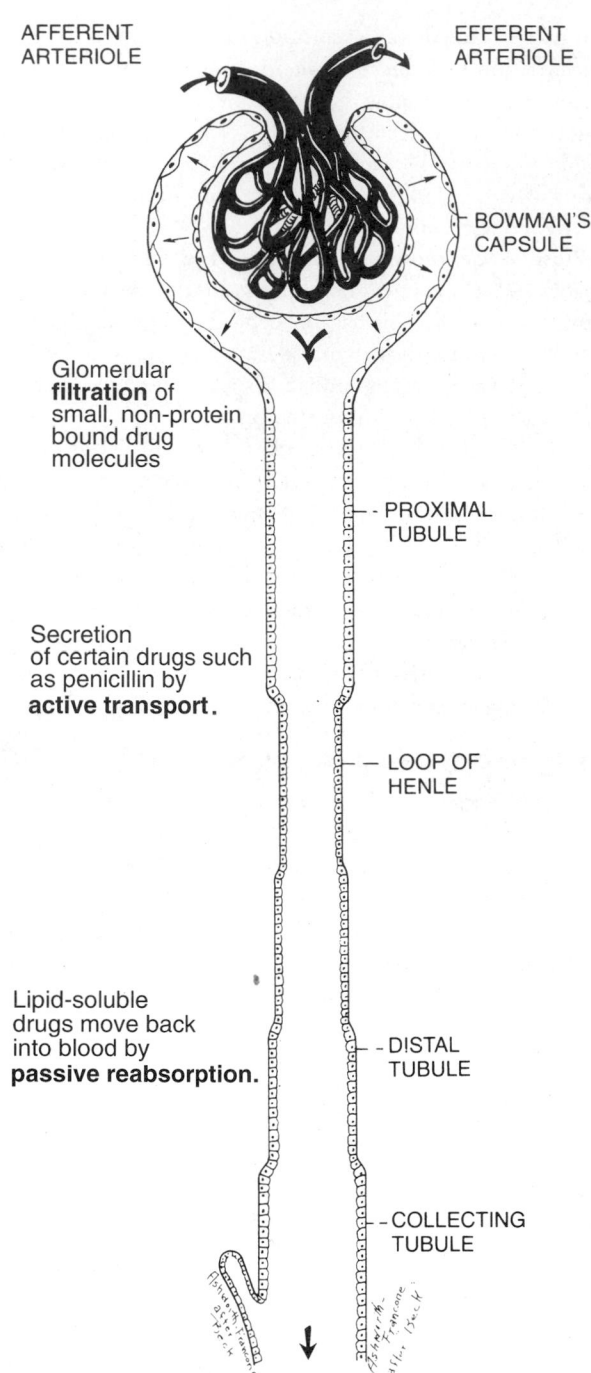

AFFERENT ARTERIOLE

EFFERENT ARTERIOLE

BOWMAN'S CAPSULE

Glomerular **filtration** of small, non-protein bound drug molecules

PROXIMAL TUBULE

Secretion of certain drugs such as penicillin by **active transport.**

LOOP OF HENLE

Lipid-soluble drugs move back into blood by **passive reabsorption.**

DISTAL TUBULE

COLLECTING TUBULE

FIGURE 4–5 Urinary excretion of drugs. (From Jacob, S., & Francone, C.A. [1989]. *Elements of anatomy and physiology* [2nd ed.]. Philadelphia: W.B. Saunders.)

Several factors affect the rate of drug excretion from the kidneys, including the concentration of the drug in plasma, urinary pH, molecular weight of the drug, maturity of the kidney, kidney function (absence or presence of disease), and renal blood flow. Altering urinary pH can enhance or delay excretion of some drugs. For example, acidic urine reduces the excretion of weak acid drugs; alkaline urine delays the excretion of weak bases. Loss of kidney function allows drugs to accumulate in the body. Clients with kidney disease usually require reduced drug dosages to compensate for reduced excretion ability.

Hepatic Excretion

Some drugs or drug metabolites are released by the liver into the bile and are eliminated in feces. Approximately 600 to 1000 ml of bile are formed each day. Thus this method of excretion can dispose of significant amounts of drug.

After their excretion into bile and their return to the intestine, some drug molecules are reabsorbed into the bloodstream. These drug molecules are returned to the liver and secreted again into bile. This process is called **enterohepatic recycling.** Enterohepatic recycling affects mainly basic drugs because they are nonionized in alkaline intestinal pH.[5,7]

Pulmonary Excretion

Pulmonary excretion occurs primarily with gaseous substances or vapors such as those used to produce anesthesia. The pulmonary system also excretes limited amounts of alcohol through exhaled air.

Miscellaneous Routes of Excretion

The skin eliminates a comparatively small amount of drugs. Although it is theoretically possible, excretion of drugs in perspiration, saliva, and tears is relatively unimportant. In lactating women certain drugs are also excreted in breast milk.

CONCEPT REVIEW

Drug excretion describes the movement of drugs or drug metabolites from the tissues into circulation and from circulation into the organs of excretion.

Clearance is the rate of removal of drug molecules from the body.

Routes of excretion include the renal system, gastrointestinal tract, pulmonary system, skin, saliva, perspiration, tears, and breast milk.

---

molecules are transferred from the blood to the tubule by a mechanism requiring energy.

The renal excretory mechanisms have the net effect of removing the free drug brought to the kidneys by the renal artery blood. Some drugs are totally excreted on the first pass through the kidneys. Other drugs require several passes through the kidneys before total excretion occurs.

PHARMACOKINETIC EFFECTS ON PLASMA LEVELS

Measurement of serum concentration levels of a drug provides an indication of the extent of disintegration, dissolution, and absorption. Serum levels also reflect the influence of drug distribution, metabolism, and excretion. For most drugs, low

plasma concentration levels are ineffective, whereas excessively high concentration levels can be toxic.

Determining plasma levels is particularly useful with drugs that have a narrow range between a lethal and a therapeutic dose **(therapeutic index).** Plasma levels are also used to monitor the client's compliance with the drug therapy. In instances in which drugs are administered prophylactically, plasma levels help determine if plasma concentration levels are in a therapeutically effective range.[3,5,20]

Single-Dose Administration

Single-dose administration of drugs facilitates study of the time course or time response of a drug. The time-response aspect of drugs varies significantly with the route of administration.

Onset of action   Once a drug is administered and absorption begins, blood levels begin to rise. However, there is no measurable response until a minimally effective concentration is reached. The phrase *onset of action* describes the length of time needed for a drug to reach the minimally effective concentration level.

Peak serum level   The term *peak serum level* reflects the maximum concentration that a drug can reach. It does not reflect the intensity of the drug action.

Time to peak action   Once the initial response begins, the intensity of the response increases, usually paralleling the rise of blood concentration. The time from drug administration to the development of maximum effect is called *time to peak action.*

Duration of action   As soon as a drug begins to circulate in the blood, metabolism and excretion begin. Eventually drug elimination exceeds the absorption rate, and the peak serum concentration and effect begin to decline. When the blood concentration falls below the level needed to produce an effect, drug action ceases, even though drug molecules remain in the blood. Therefore the *duration of action* represents the time during which blood levels of a drug are above the minimum effective concentration (Fig. 4–6).

Plasma, or biologic, half-life of drugs   Biotransformation and excretion determine the drug's **plasma,** or **biologic, half-life.** Biologic half-life of a drug is the length of time required to reduce the original plasma concentration by 50%. This figure varies among individuals and is used to determine the frequency of drug administration.

The drug's half-life does not change with drug dosage. The body still takes the same amount of time to eliminate one half of the drug present in the body. For example, if a 500-mg dose of a drug with a half-life of 4 hours is administered, 250 mg of the drug remain in the plasma after 4 hours. If a 1000-mg dose of the same drug is administered, 500 mg remain in the plasma after 4 hours. In the example of the 1000-mg dose, plasma concentration continues to decrease by 50% every 4 hours (i.e., 250 mg after 8 hours; 125 mg after 12 hours).

Repeated Drug Administration

Although there are instances in which a drug is administered only once, it is more common to give a drug repeatedly. Since the duration of action of most drugs is relatively short in relation to the length of time the effects are needed, repeated drug administration is used. When a drug is administered more than once, loading doses, maintenance doses, and plateau levels must be considered.

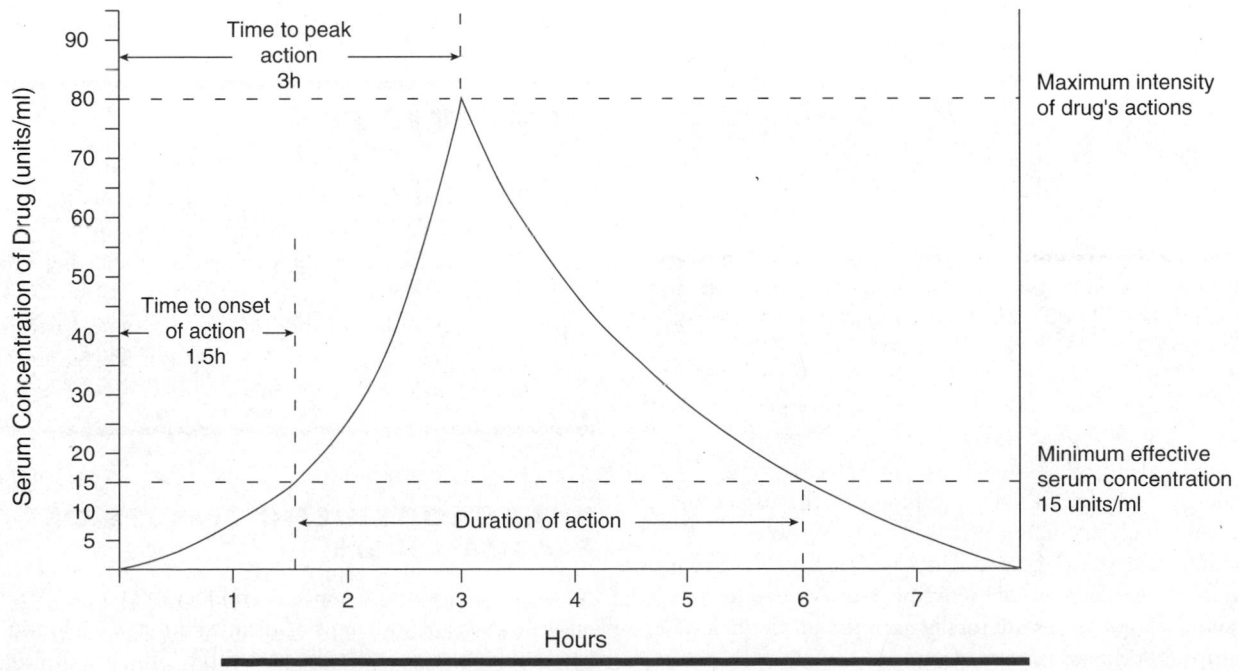

FIGURE 4–6   Time-response aspect of single-dose administration of drug.

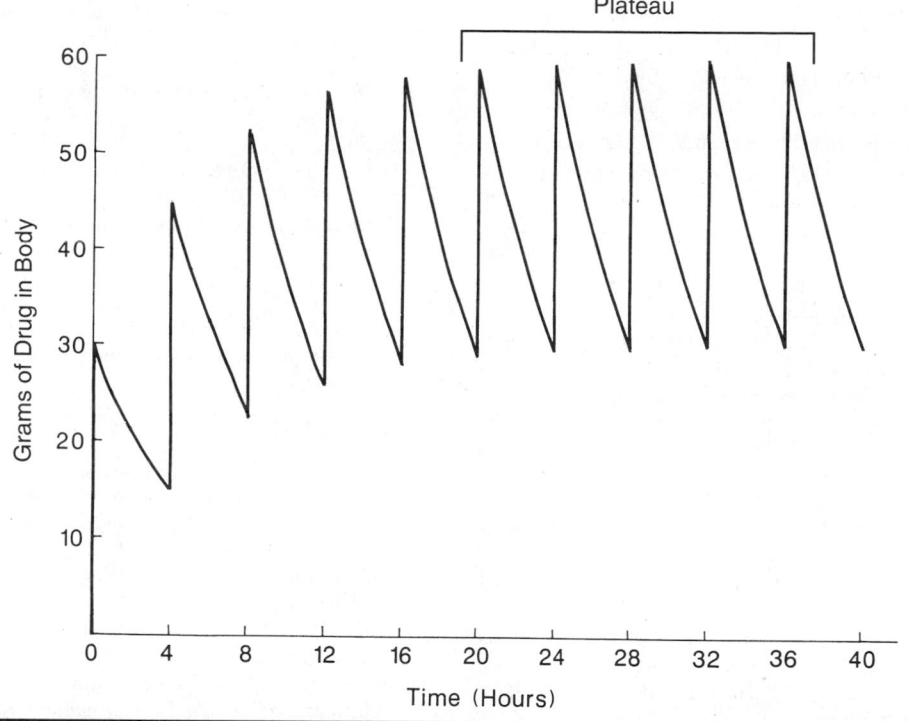

FIGURE 4–7   Plateau principle. (From Smith, C.M., & Reynard, A.M. [1992]. *Textbook of pharmacology*. Philadelphia: W.B. Saunders.)

Plateau principle   When a consistent dose of a drug is repeatedly administered at regular intervals, the concentration of the drug in the blood eventually will reach a constant level **(plateau).** As long as the drug is administered in the same manner (i.e., same dose and frequency), the blood concentration level remains within a limited range. However, the serum concentration level will still reflect peaks and troughs unless the drug is administered by continuous intravenous infusion (Fig. 4–7).

CONCEPT REVIEW

The blood or serum concentration level of a drug can be correlated with anticipated therapeutic response.

The time course or time response of a drug includes the onset of action, peak serum level, peak action, and duration of action times.

When a consistent dose of a drug is administered repeatedly at regular intervals, the concentration of the drug in the blood will eventually reach a plateau.

Loading doses of a drug are administered to achieve rapid therapeutic serum levels.

Loading dose   At times an effective blood level of a drug must be reached quickly. To achieve this goal, a larger-than-usual first dose is administered. This initial dose is the **loading dose.**

Maintenance doses   Once the desired blood concentration level is achieved, the usual recommended dose is administered. The subsequent doses administered to maintain a relatively constant effect are **maintenance doses.**

SUMMARY

This chapter discussed the four pharmacokinetic processes that influence drug action: absorption, distribution, biotransformation, and excretion. Absorption represents the stage from the time the drug enters the body until it enters the venous or lymphatic circulation. Distribution describes the process by which drug solutions are transported by body fluids to sites of action. Biotransformation, or metabolism, is the process by which the body modifies or alters the chemical structure of the drug. This process usually reduces the amount of active drug in the body. During biotransformation most drugs are converted to inactive metabolites. Drug excretion describes the movement of drugs or drug metabolites from the tissues into circulation and from circulation into the organs of excretion. Together these processes regulate plasma levels of drugs and determine the intensity and length of pharmacologic action.

The chapter also discussed a variety of factors that affect the four pharmacokinetic processes. However, you should remember that the most important factor is the individual client. All aspects (e.g., genetic background, physiologic status, psychologic status, and environmental elements) associated with a client can alter the pharmacologic action of drugs and produce a wide variation in clinical response.

REFERENCES

1. Clark, W., Brater, D.G., & Johnson, A.R. (1992). *Goth's medical pharmacology.* St. Louis: Mosby–Year Book.
2. DiPalma, J.R., & DiGregorio, J. (Eds). (1990). *Basic pharmacology in medicine.* New York: McGraw-Hill.
3. Gibaldi, M. (1990). *Biopharmaceutics and clinical pharmacokinetics.* Philadelphia: Lea & Febiger.
4. Goodman, R., Gilman, E., Rall, T., Nies, A., & Taylor, P. (Eds.). (1990). *Goodman and Gilman's: The pharmacological basis of therapeutics* (8th ed.). New York: Pergamon Press.
5. Grymonpre, R., & Zhanel, G. (1990). Pharmacokinetics made easy. *Canadian Pharmaceutical Journal, 123,* 322-325.
6. Katzung, B. (Eds.). (1992). *Basic and clinical pharmacology.* Norwalk, CT: Appleton & Lange.
7. Schwertz, D.W. (1991). Basic principles of pharmacologic action. *Nursing Clinics of North America, 26,* 245-261.
8. Smith, C., & Reynard, A. (1992). *Textbook of pharmacology.* Philadelphia: W.B. Saunders.
9. Hole, J.W. (1993). *Human anatomy and physiology* (6th ed.). Dubuque: Wm. C. Brown.
10. Seeley, R., Stephens, T., & Tate, P. (1992). *Anatomy and physiology* (2nd ed.). St. Louis: Mosby–Year Book.
11. Tortora, G.J., & Grabowski, S.R. (1993). *Principles of anatomy and physiology* (7th ed.). New York: Harper Collins.
12. Gugler, R., & Allgayer, H. (1990). Effects of antacids on the clinical pharmacokinetic of drugs: Update. *Clinical Pharmacokinetics, 18,* 210-219.
13. Nahata, M.C. (1993). Intravenous infusion conditions: Implications for pharmacokinetic monitoring. *Clinical Pharmacokinetics, 24,* 221-229.
14. Strong, A., Wolff, H., Kinder, S., & Lubischer, A. (1991). Drug administration in relation to meals in the institutional setting. *Heart & Lung, 20*(1), 39-44.
15. Van Hoogdalem, E., de Boer, A., & Breimer, D. (1991). Pharmacokinetics of rectal drug administration: Pt 1. *Clinical Pharmacokinetics, 21*(1), 11-26.
16. Madan, P.L. (1990). Sustained release dosage forms. *U.S. Pharmacist, 15,* 39-43, 47-51.
17. Melia, C.O., & Davis, S. (1989). Review article: Mechanisms of drug release from tablets and capsules. Dissolution. *Alimentary Pharmacology and Therapeutics, 3,* 513-525.
18. Ansel, H., & Popovich, N. (1990). *Pharmaceutical dosage forms and drug delivery systems* (5th ed.). Philadelphia: Lea & Febiger.
19. Avis, K.E., Lieberman, H., & Lachman, L. (1992). *Pharmaceutical dosage forms, parenteral medications* (2nd ed.). New York: Marcel Dekker.
20. Williams, R.L. (1992). Dosage regimen design: Pharmacodynamic considerations. *Journal of Clinical Pharmacology, 32,* 597-602.
21. Gubbins, P.O., & Bertch, K.E. (1991). Drug absorption in gastrointestinal disease and surgery: Clinical pharmacokinetic and therapeutic implications. *Clinical Pharmacokinetics, 21,* 431-437.
22. Goddard, H. (1990). Treating differences: How race affects drug therapy. *Canadian Pharmaceutical Journal, 123,* 314-315.
23. Wood, A.J., & Zhou, H.H. (1991). Ethnic differences in drug disposition and responsiveness. *Clinical Pharmacokinetics, 20,* 350-373.

BIBLIOGRAPHY

Amidon, G., DeBrincat, G., & Najib, N. (1991). Effects of gravity on gastric emptying, intestinal transit, and drug absorption. *Journal of Clinical Pharmacology, 31,* 968-973.

Biddle, C., & Gilliland, C. (1992). Transdermal and transmucosal administration of pain-relieving and anxiolytic drugs: A primer for the critical care practitioner. *Heart & Lung, 21*(2), 115-124.

Caralis, P. (1991). How ethnicity affects disease and therapy. *Consultant, 31*(7), 49-56.

Durnas, C., Loi, C.M., & Cusack, B.J. (1990). Hepatic drug metabolism and aging. *Clinical Pharmacokinetics, 19,* 359-389.

Guyon, G. (1989). Pharmacokinetic considerations in neonatal drug therapy. *Neonatal Network: Journal of Neonatal Nursing, 7*(5), 9-12, 27-30.

Gwilt, P.R., Nahhas, R.R., & Tracewell, W.G. (1991). The effects of diabetes mellitus on pharmacokinetics and pharmacodynamics in humans. *Clinical Pharmacokinetics, 20,* 477-490.

Kauffman, R.E., & Kearns, G.L. (1992). Pharmacokinetic studies in paediatric patients. Clinical and ethical considerations. *Clinical Pharmacokinetics, 23*(1), 10-29.

Korth-Bradley, J.M. (1991). A pharmacokinetic primer for intravenous nurses. *Journal of Intravenous Nursing, 14*(1), 16-26.

Kudzma, E. (1992). Drug response: All bodies are not created equal. *American Journal of Nursing, 92*(12), 48-50.

McLeod, H.L., & Evans, W.E. (1992). Pediatric pharmacokinetics and therapeutic drug monitoring. *Pediatrics in Review, 13,* 413-421.

Swan, S.K., & Bennett, W.M. (1992). Drug dosing guidelines in patients with renal failure. *Western Journal of Medicine, 156,* 633-638.

Threlkeld, J.A. (1992). Nursing implications in kinetic modeling. *ANNA Journal, 19*(2), 178-181.

Yuen, G.J. (1990). Altered pharmacokinetics in the elderly. *Clinics in Geriatric Medicine, 6,* 257-267.

CHAPTER 5

Pharmacodynamic Phase

NORMA L. PINNELL

Theories of Drug Action

LEARNING OBJECTIVES:

Describe two structurally nonspecific drug actions produced by physical modification of the cell's environment.

Describe two structurally nonspecific drug actions produced by chemical modification of the cell's environment.

Explain the drug-receptor theory of drug action.

Discuss the drug-enzyme theory of drug action.

KEY TERMS:

Agonist, antagonist, antimetabolites, competitive antagonist, drug action, drug effects, drug-enzyme interaction, drug-receptor interaction, non-competitive antagonist, receptor, structurally nonspecific, structurally specific

Factors Affecting Pharmacodynamics

LEARNING OBJECTIVE: Summarize three factors that affect pharmacodynamics.

KEY TERMS:

Circadian rhythms, drug potency, efficacy

Dose-Response Relationship

LEARNING OBJECTIVE: Diagram the dose-response curve for two drugs.

KEY TERM: Dose-response curve

Therapeutic Index

LEARNING OBJECTIVE: Explain the importance of the therapeutic index.

KEY TERM: Therapeutic index

CONCEPTS AND TERMS TO REVIEW

Review the biochemical interaction between enzymes and substrates.

Review content in Chapter 4 on plasma level profile.

Review content in Chapter 4 on the influence of ethnic background on the pharmacokinetic process.

*P*harmacodynamics is the process by which cell physiology is altered by a drug. The process involves a series of events produced by the presence of a chemical compound in a living organism. To initiate this series of events, an appropriate concentration level of the chemical compound must exist in the body. This means that the molecules of the compound must move from their point of entry into the body to the vicinity of the tissues with which they react. An interaction between drug molecules and cellular components of the target organ occurs when sufficient drug molecules are available at effector or target sites.

THEORIES OF DRUG ACTION

Before discussing theories of drug action, the difference between drug effect and drug action must be clarified. The **drug action** is the interaction between a drug and the target organ. Body responses that result from the drug action represent **drug effects.** Drug effects are dose related. (Information on the effects of drugs on the body—therapeutic effects, adverse effects, side effects, and toxic effects—are presented in Chapter 6.)

Drugs act by manipulating the body's own natural processes; they do not produce new functions. Drugs inhibit or activate biochemical or physiologic processes or replace elements needed to initiate or enhance a process. Many drug actions are produced by chemical or physical alteration of the cell's external or internal environment. These drugs do not combine with specific biologic receptors. Drugs that produce their action in this manner are considered **structurally non-specific.** Some drugs produce their effects by interacting with enzymes. Most drugs, however, produce their effects by combining with receptors. The group of drugs that produce effects

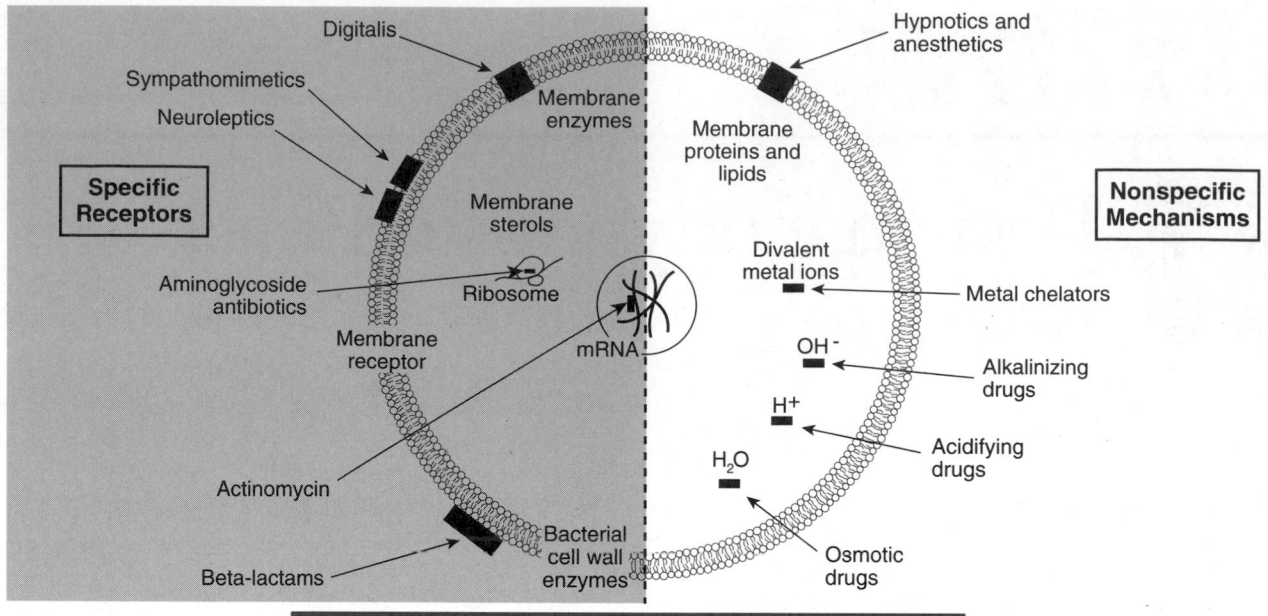

FIGURE 5–1   Specific and nonspecific structural mechanisms.

through enzyme interactions or combination with receptors is considered **structurally specific**[1,2] (Fig. 5–1).

Structurally Nonspecific Drugs

Drugs that demonstrate no structural specificity and act by more general effects on cell membranes and cellular processes do so by physiochemical means. These drugs alter the external environment of the cell or penetrate cell membranes, thus interfering with some cell function or metabolic process.

Physical modification   Drugs that physically modify the cell's environment do not change specific cellular or enzyme functions. Instead, they modify the environment by producing a protective barrier, reducing surface tension, or altering the characteristics of the fluid in the membrane. For example, petroleum jelly and sunscreen produce protective barriers. Petroleum jelly applied to the skin repels liquids; application of a sunscreen prevents penetration of ultraviolet rays. The effectiveness of many stool softeners is based on their ability to reduce the surface tension of fecal material, allowing absorption of water.

Chemical modification   Although structurally nonspecific drugs do not alter or modify specific cellular functions, chemical modification of the cell's environment can create specific changes in cellular function. Some drug categories that act by altering the chemistry of the cell's environment are antacids, osmotic diuretics, antiseptics, and electrolyte replacements. For example, active ingredients in antacids (e.g., sodium bicarbonate, aluminum hydroxide gel, magnesium hydroxide, magnesium trisilicate, magnesium oxide, and calcium carbonate) alter the pH of body fluids. Osmotic diuretics such as mannitol (Osmitrol) alter the composition of the body fluid. These drugs elevate the osmolarity of plasma, glomeru-

lar filtrate, and tubular fluid. This in turn decreases the reabsorption of fluid and electrolytes.

Structurally Specific Drugs

Typically, structurally specific drugs alter cell function through facilitation or depression of membrane transport or by enhancing or inhibiting energy metabolism. Modification of cell function can be caused by drug-receptor interaction or drug-enzyme interactions.

Drug-receptor interactions   The action of many drugs is produced by the interaction of the drug with a specialized region of a cell called a **receptor.** Receptors are found on the surface of the cell or within the target cell. Most receptors are cellular proteins or nucleic acids. However, they can also be lipids, enzymes, or carbohydrate residues. The number of receptors available for binding and the attraction of the receptors for the drug affect the final response. Some receptors are less selective of the drugs with which they interact. In many cases similar chemical compounds can occupy the same receptor.

The molecular structure of protein allows each specific receptor to assume a different shape. These differing shapes among receptors support the structural-specific theory of the relationship between the receptor and the drug. This structure-specific relationship has often been likened to that between a lock and key (Fig. 5–2); that is, a reciprocal or complementary configuration exists between the chemical structure of the drug molecule and the receptor.

The ability to bind to the receptor and the ability to stimulate an action by the receptor are two different aspects of drug action. **Affinity** is the term used to describe the propensity of a drug to be at a given receptor site. Drugs with high affinities have a high attraction to a receptor site. When receptors are

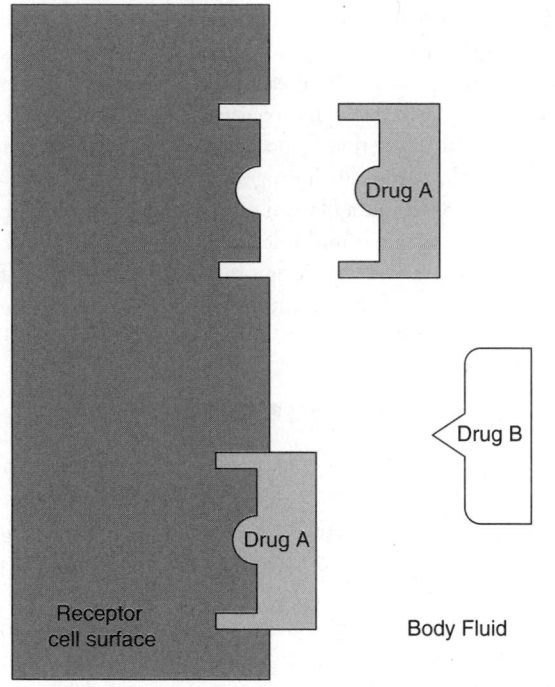

FIGURE 5–2   Receptor site and drug molecule.

highly specific and have high affinities for the compound that binds to them, very low concentrations can initiate biologic activity.

An **agonist** is a drug that has affinity for a receptor and the ability to initiate the desired therapeutic effect (efficacy). An **antagonist** is a drug that has affinity for the receptor but is unable to produce biologic effects. In other words, antagonists have affinity for a receptor but no efficacy. Antagonists are also called receptor blockers. A **competitive antagonist** has an affinity for the same receptor sites as an agonist. The competition with the agonist for the receptor site inhibits the action of the agonist. In this case the drug action is determined by the drug (agonist or antagonist) that occupies the most receptor sites. **Noncompetitive antagonists** combine with different parts of the receptor mechanism and inactivate the receptor so that the agonist cannot be effective.

The interaction between an agonist and its receptor is only temporary. In most instances the drug and receptor form a reversible complex. During the time that the complex exists, cellular properties are changed, and a response is produced.

Drug-enzyme interaction   Many drugs are thought to produce their effects by combining with enzymes. Drug-enzyme interactions can stimulate or inhibit cellular function.

An enzyme is a protein that acts as a catalyst to produce or increase the rate of a chemical reaction. Enzymes react with a substance (substrate) to produce their effects. Some drugs have a structural resemblance to an enzyme's substrate molecule, causing the enzyme to interact with the drug. Drugs resembling substrates are called **antimetabolites.** Antimetabolites can either block normal enzymatic action or promote the production of other substrates.[1-5]

CONCEPT REVIEW

Structurally nonspecific drugs act by producing chemical or physical alteration of cellular fluids or cell membranes.

Structurally specific drugs act through specific receptors or enzyme interactions.

Structurally specific drugs alter cell function by facilitating or depressing membrane transport or by enhancing or inhibiting energy metabolism.

Modification of cell function can be caused by drug-receptor interaction or drug-enzyme interaction.

FACTORS AFFECTING PHARMACODYNAMICS

Numerous factors affect pharmacodynamics.[1,6] These factors include drug efficacy, drug potency, circadian rhythms, and interethnic factors.

Drug Efficacy

Efficacy is the term used to describe the drug's ability to initiate a biologic activity. Whereas the term *affinity* describes the capacity of a drug to engage in binding, efficacy is the capacity of the drug to initiate activation. It also describes the drug's maximum therapeutic ability.

Drug Potency

Drug potency differs from drug efficacy. The term **drug potency** refers to the relative amount of a drug required to produce the desired response. The drug potency of one drug can be compared with another drug to establish the more potent drug. For example, morphine sulfate, a narcotic analgesic, frequently is used to evaluate the potency of other narcotics. An intramuscular 10-mg dose of morphine sulfate provides the pain relief associated with an intramuscular dose of 100 mg of meperidine (Demerol).

Circadian Rhythms

The term *circadian* denotes a period of approximately 24 hours. **Circadian rhythm** describes a regular recurrence of certain activities within that 24-hour period. Daily body rhythms such as those for hormone levels, renal function, blood pressure levels, and body temperature can alter the pharmacodynamic of drugs. For example, aspirin administered at 7:00 AM remains in the body for 22 hours; aspirin administered at 7:00 PM lasts only 17 hours. This delay in the pharmacokinetic process of aspirin is probably due to altered renal function and influences the serum concentration level and the clinical response.

Circadian rhythms are also important factors in determining safe versus toxic drug doses. A distinct 24-hour rhythm of vulnerability or resistance to drugs has been identified. However, federal research guidelines do not consider the circadian rhythms of the animals or humans being tested.

One extensively studied area of **chronopharmacology** (study of cellular rhythms in relationship to drug therapy) is the relationship of adrenocortical function and corticosteroid drug administration. The secretion of corticosteroids by the adrenal cortex has a 24-hour rhythm, with the highest concentration expected after the usual time of awakening. When corticosteroids are administered either daily or on alternate days, adrenal suppression can be minimized by timing administration with the circadian crest in adrenocortical function.[7-10]

Interethnic Influences

As indicated in Chapter 4, interethnic differences affect the pharmacokinetic process. They also influence the pharmacodynamic process. For example, Asian clients are at risk for unusually high plasma concentrations of psychotropic drugs. Awareness of this risk may help you to detect and prevent serious adverse drug effects.[11]

CONCEPT REVIEW

Several factors, including drug efficacy, drug potency, pathologic states, circadian rhythms, and interethnic influences, affect the pharmacodynamic phase.

DOSE-RESPONSE RELATIONSHIP

The biologic response to a drug usually increases as drug concentration increases. The intensity of a response to a drug is related to the number of activated receptors or the rate of activation.

Dose-response curve The relationship between the drug dose administered and the response generated is an S-shaped curve called the **dose-response curve.** This curve is obtained by plotting the observed response against the dose of a drug used to elicit that response. Several important properties about the drug, including a threshold for each drug-induced response and a plateau response, are illustrated by the curve. Drugs produce multiple predictable biologic effects—for each effect a dose response curve may be drawn. Dose-response curves help determine the relative safety of a drug[1,12-14] (Fig. 5-3).

THERAPEUTIC INDEX

Once an investigational dose range has been established, a therapeutic dose range must be determined. The therapeutic dose range reflects the dose that provides therapeutic efficacy while producing minimum adverse effects. This range is called the **therapeutic index.** Since many drugs have more than one therapeutic effect, drugs usually have several therapeutic indices. Therapeutic indices are determined through animal studies during investigational testing.

A therapeutic index (TI) reflects the ratio of the drug dose that is lethal in 50% of the tested animals (LD_{50}) to the dose that is therapeutically effective in 50% of tested animals (ED_{50}). Therefore the formula for the therapeutic index is $TI = LD_{50}/ED_{50}$. For a drug that induces sleep in 50% of the tested population at a dose of 2.5 mg/kg and is lethal at a dose of 2500 mg/kg, the ratio is 2500 to 2.5. The drug is said to have a therapeutic index of 1000. This therapeutic index would mean that the amount of drug required to produce a

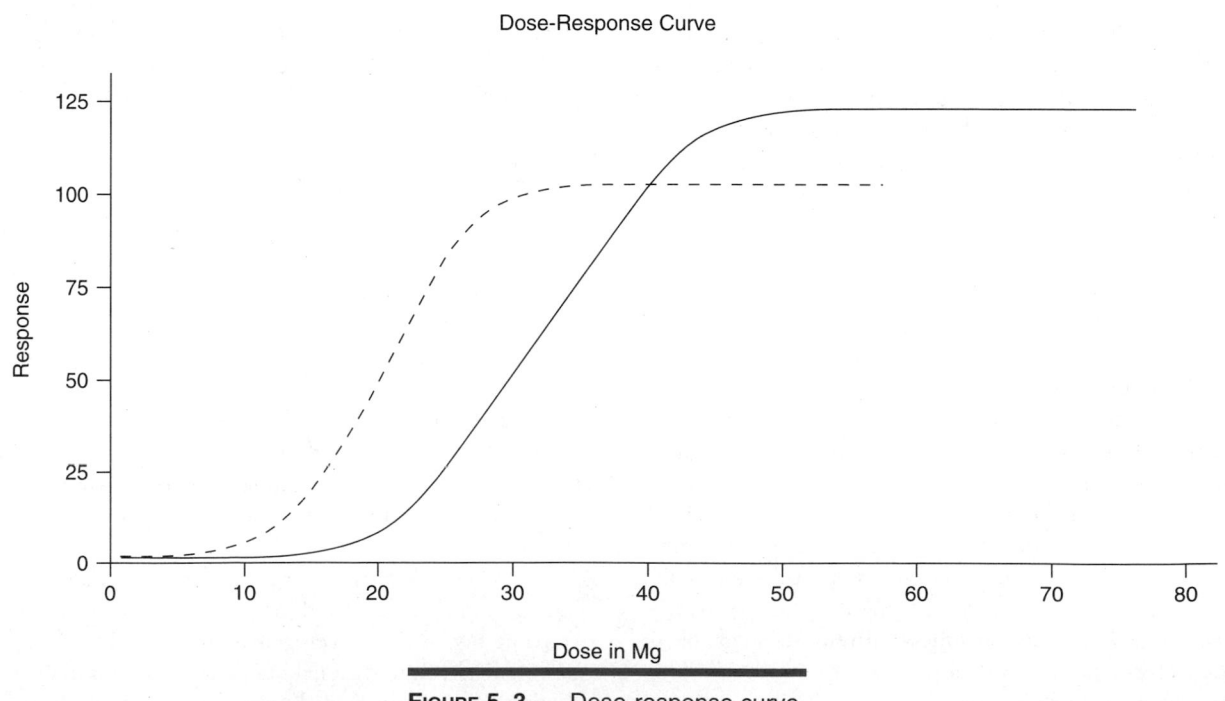

Dose-Response Curve

FIGURE 5-3   Dose-response curve.

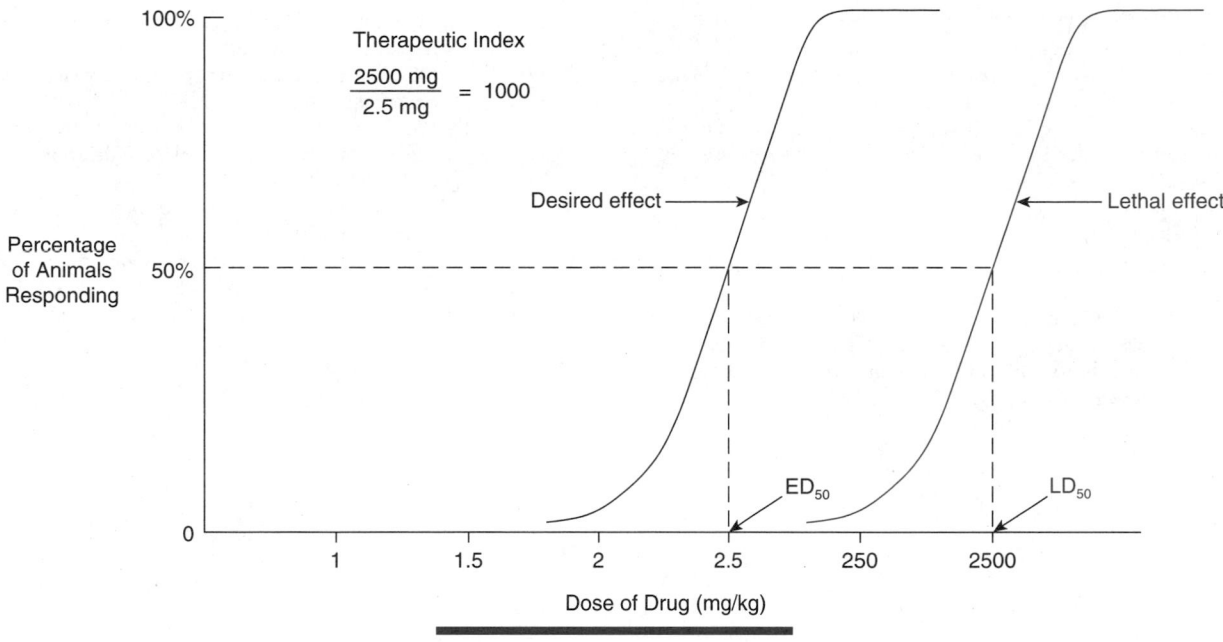

FIGURE 5–4   Therapeutic index.

lethal effect in 50% of the animals would be 1000 times that required to produce a therapeutic effect in 50% of animals tested.

A large therapeutic index is preferred. If the difference between the two doses is small, the drug has a narrow therapeutic index, and use in humans may not be indicated. During drug testing involving humans, the therapeutic index usually represents the ratio between the minimum effective dose for 50% of the clients and the dose that elicits adverse reactions in 50% of the clients[1,12,13] (Fig. 5–4).

CONCEPT REVIEW

The dose-response curve illustrates a threshold for each drug-induced response and a plateau response.

The therapeutic-dose range reflects the dose that provides therapeutic efficacy while producing minimum adverse effects.

SUMMARY

This chapter discussed theories of drug action, factors affecting pharmacodynamics, dose-response relationship, and therapeutic index. Drug actions are produced by either structurally nonspecific or structurally specific methods. Drug actions produced by chemical or physical alteration of cellular fluids or cell membranes are considered structurally nonspecific. Drugs that produce their action through specific interaction with enzymes or in combination with biologic receptors are considered structurally specific.

The pharmacodynamics of a drug are affected by circadian rhythms and interethnic influences. In addition, the drug's affinity, efficacy, and potency affect the dose-response curve.

The dose-response curve illustrates several important properties about the drug, including a threshold for each drug-induced response and a plateau response. This curve is determined for each predictable biologic effect of the drug.

In addition to the dose-response curve, a therapeutic dose range must be determined for each drug. This range reflects the dose that provides therapeutic efficacy while producing minimum adverse effects. This range is called the *therapeutic index.*

REFERENCES

1. Clark, W., Brater, D.G., & Johnson, A.R. (1992). *Goth's medical pharmacology.* St. Louis: Mosby–Year Book.
2. Goodman, R., Gilman, E., Rall, T., Nies, A., & Taylor, P. (Eds.). (1990). *Goodman and Gilman's: The pharmacological basis of therapeutics* (8th ed.). New York: Pergamon Press.
3. Levine, R. (1990). *Pharmacology: Drug actions and reactions* (4th ed.). Boston: Little, Brown.
4. Schwertz, D.W. (1991). Basic principles of pharmacologic action. *Nursing Clinics of North American, 26,* 245-262.
5. Smith, C.M., & Reynard, A.M. (1992). *Textbook of pharmacology.* Philadelphia: W.B. Saunders.
6. Gwilt, P.R., Nahhas, R.R., & Tracewell, W.G. (1991). The effects of diabetes mellitus on pharmacokinetics and pharmacodynamics in humans. *Clinical Pharmacokinetics, 20,* 477-490.
7. Aronson, J.K. (1990). Chronopharmacology: Reflection on time and a new text. *Lancet, 335,* 1515-1516.
8. Fehm, H.L., & Born, J. (1991). Evidence for intrainment of nocturnal cortisol secretion to sleep process in human beings. *Neuroendocrinology, 53,* 171-176.
9. Von-Roemeling, R. (1991). The therapeutic index of cytotoxic chemotherapy depends upon circadian drug timing. *Annual of New York Academic Science, 618,* 292-311.
10. Willis, J. (1990). Keeping time to circadian rhythms. *FDA Consumer, 24*(6), 18-21.
11. Kudzma, E. (1992). Drug response: All bodies are not created equal. *American Journal of Nursing, 92*(12), 48-50.

12. Cocchetto, D., & Nardi, R. (1992). *Managing the clinical drug development process.* New York: Marcell Dekker.

13. Smith, C. (1992). *The process of new drug discovery and development.* Boca Raton, FL: CRC Press.

14. Williams, R.L. (1992). Dosage regimen design: Pharmacodynamic considerations. *Journal of Clinical Pharmacology, 32,* 597-602.

BIBLIOGRAPHY

Bower, B. (1991). Got no rhythm: Stalling biological clocks. *Science News, 139,* 150.

Coy, K.M., Imperi, G., & Lambert, C.R. (1990). Application of time series analysis to circadian rhythms: Effect of beta-adrenergic blockade upon heart rate and transient myocardial ischemia. *American Journal of Cardiology, 66,* 226-246.

DiPalma, G., & DiGregorio, J. (Eds). (1990). *Basic pharmacology in medicine.* New York: McGraw-Hill.

Greener, M. (1990). Towards the magic bullet: Improving specificity in drugs. *Professional Nurse, 6*(3), 171-172, 174.

Kauffman, R.E., & Kearns, G.L. (1992). Pharmacokinetic studies in paediatric patients. Clinical and ethical considerations. *Clinical Pharmacokinetic, 23*(1), 10-29.

Lehne, R.A. (1994). *Pharmacology for nursing care.* (2nd ed.). Philadelphia: W.B. Saunders.

Reville, B., & Almadrones, L. (1989). Continuous infusion chemotherapy in the ambulatory setting: The nurses' role in patient selection and education. *Oncology Nursing Forum, 16,* 529-535.

Schwertz, D.W., & Buschmann, M.T. (1989). Pharmacogeriatrics. *Critical Care Nursing Quarterly, 12*(1), 26-37.

CHAPTER 6

 Individual Variation
in Drug Response

NORMA L. PINNELL

⊛ Desired Clinical Response to Drugs

LEARNING OBJECTIVES:

Discuss how desired clinical responses are determined.
Describe five factors that affect individual clinical
responses.

KEY TERM: Pharmacogenetics

⊛ Undesired Clinical Response to Drugs

LEARNING OBJECTIVES:

Define the terms *side effects, toxic effects,* and *adverse
reactions.*

Differentiate predictable from unpredictable adverse
responses.

KEY TERMS:

Adverse reactions, predictable adverse reactions, side
effects, toxic effects

⊛ Responses to Single Drug Administration

LEARNING OBJECTIVE: Describe four adverse responses to
single drug administration.

KEY TERMS:

Allergy, cellular tolerance, cross-tolerance, cumulative
effect, dependence, idiosyncratic response,
intolerance, metabolic tolerance, tolerance

⊛ Responses to Drug Combinations

LEARNING OBJECTIVE: Describe four responses to a
combination of drugs.

KEY TERMS:

Additive response, antagonism, interaction,
potentiation, summation, synergism

⊛ Iatrogenic Responses

LEARNING OBJECTIVES:

Define the term *iatrogenic.*
Explain five iatrogenic responses to drug therapy.

KEY TERMS:

Blood dyscrasias, carcinogenesis, mutagenesis,
teratogenesis

⊛ Nursing Considerations

LEARNING OBJECTIVE: Describe the role of the nurse
regarding individual variation in drug response

CONCEPTS AND TERMS TO REVIEW

Review section in Chapter 2 on stages of new drug development.
Review sections in Chapters 3 and 4 on factors affecting
the pharmacokinetic and pharmacodynamic phases.

---

*I*n Chapter 2 information on how new drugs are developed
and tested was presented. Criteria for new drug development are established by the Food and Drug Administration
(FDA) with the hope of promoting desired clinical responses
and minimizing untoward reactions. However, because each
individual is different, body responses that result from the action of a drug vary among individuals. This chapter provides
an overview of some of the factors that affect individual clinical responses and undesired and iatrogenic responses. In addition, responses produced by single drug administration or
drug combinations are discussed.

DESIRED CLINICAL RESPONSE
TO DRUGS

How does a primary care provider know what response to expect from a drug? Does the desired clinical response occur with
all individuals?

Determination of Desired Response

It is not until the late phases of clinical testing that a new
drug is administered to an individual with the disease. Until

that time testing is conducted on animals and healthy individuals. This testing in healthy volunteers evaluates the drug's metabolism in and biologic effects on humans.

When the new drug is tested in a client, therapeutic effects, dosage range, and safety are determined. However, even this phase of clinical testing may exclude many individuals. For example, in the past only Caucasian males were used to test new drugs. It is possible that complete information about the clinical response to a drug is not known until postmarketing studies are completed.

Factors Affecting Individual Clinical Responses

Factors such as drug dose, dosage form, route and time of administration, and circadian rhythms are discussed in Chapters 4 and 5. These factors affect the pharmacokinetic and pharmacodynamic phases and therefore affect the clinical response to drugs. Other aspects also affect the clinical response to drug therapy.

Body size and weight   Body size or mass influences drug concentration, distribution, and action and affects the clinical response to the drug. As the body size of the client increases, drug concentration decreases. Conversely, as the body size decreases, drug concentration increases. In a client with a large body mass, drug molecules may never reach a concentration that elicits a clinical response, but a client with a small body mass is at increased risk for toxic effects. Therefore the drug dosage must be adjusted according to the client's body size or mass. When possible, drug dosage should be based on **body surface area.** Body surface area considers the client's weight and amount of muscle and adipose tissue.

Gender   Differences related to the gender of the individual are associated with skeletal frame, hormone and metabolic levels, and the proportion of adipose tissue, water, and muscle mass. Bones of the male are generally larger and heavier than those of the female; thus body surface area in the male is greater, diminishing drug concentration. In addition, because men have proportionately more muscle tissue and less adipose tissue than women, they have a greater basal metabolic rate (BMR) than females. However, during pregnancy, a female's BMR may increase 20% because of the metabolic activity of the fetus.[1] An increased rate of metabolism produces faster drug biotransformation.

Age   Drug sensitivity varies with age. Neonates have immature body systems, incomplete excretory mechanisms, and decreased body mass (e.g., the liver of the newborn lacks many of the metabolizing enzymes needed for biotransformation of drugs). These factors increase to normal during the first few weeks or months of life. However, until maturity of the body systems occurs and body mass increases, dosage adjustment is necessary. (See Chapter 14 for additional discussion of this topic.)

Elderly individuals have decreased muscle mass, increased adipose tissue, and deteriorating metabolic and excretory mechanisms. With the change in body mass, drug concentrations are altered. In addition, excessive drug storage in adipose tissue can occur. These individuals are also at higher risk for toxic effects caused by deteriorating hepatic and renal function. Elderly clients may also have concomitant physical conditions that alter drug effect. (See Chapter 15 for additional discussion of this topic.)

Genetic factors   Genetic (inherited) differences can significantly alter the response of individuals to drugs. The field of **pharmacogenetics** (study of genetic influence on pharmacokinetic and pharmacodynamic processes) addresses individual responses to drug therapy that may have a genetic link.

In some instances the differences arise from genetic deficiencies in drug metabolism or receptor sensitivity. For example, because of genetic insufficiency, some individuals are unable to metabolize succinylcholine (a muscle relaxant). If this drug is administered to these individuals, prolonged muscle paralysis occurs. Other drugs whose rate of metabolism is genetically determined include isoniazid, a drug used to treat tuberculosis, and procainamide, an antiarrhythmic drug.[2]

Ethnic differences   Ethnic differences are important factors, accounting for individual variations in drug responsiveness. For example, several studies have shown a difference in the response of Afro-Americans, Chinese, and Caucasians to antihypertensive drugs. Chinese clients are sensitive to the beta-blocking and hypotensive actions of propranolol (Inderal). In clinical practice these individuals require lower doses of this drug. Afro-Americans also demonstrate altered sensitivity to the drug. In these individuals the sensitivity is due to the ethnic group's increased parasympathetic tone.[2]

These differences in drug response are a relatively neglected area of investigation. Drug doses should not be prescribed to different ethnic populations without consideration of ethnic pharmacokinetic and pharmacodynamic variation.

Pathophysiologic factors   Many pathologic conditions alter drug response. Renal, hepatic, gastrointestinal (GI), and cardiovascular diseases are capable of producing pharmacokinetic changes and altering drug response. For example, clients with GI diseases may not be able to absorb drugs administered orally. Some cardiovascular diseases produce decreased cardiac output. This decrease in circulating blood volume alters drug distribution. Diminished hepatic function slows biotransformation of most drugs, and renal dysfunction alters excretion of drugs and drug metabolites.

Psychosocial factors   The client's belief in the effectiveness of drugs influences clinical response. In many instances a strong belief in the power of drugs potentiates the drug effects. Conversely, hostility and mistrust of medicine and health care personnel can diminish drug effects. (See Chapter 10 for additional information on psychosocial factors affecting drug therapy.)

Nutritional factors   Diet composition, eating habits, and nutritional diseases alter clinical response. For example, a high-protein, low-carbohydrate diet promotes rapid metabolism of drugs, whereas a high-protein or high-fat diet decreases biliary excretion of some drugs. In these situations drug response can be either enhanced or diminished. In addition, malnutrition alters drug response. Protein, mineral, and vitamin deficiencies alter enzyme activity, affecting drug metabolism and drug activity.

Environmental factors   Studies have shown that smoking, high altitudes, and environmental temperatures are capable of modifying drug response. Smoking alters the plasma concentration of some drugs, and oxygen deprivation created by high altitudes increases an individual's sensitivity to various drugs. In addition, summer temperatures cause certain drugs to have dangerous side effects that do not occur during the winter. For example, a number of drugs drastically impair the body's ability to release heat, making the individual highly susceptible to heat stroke.

CONCEPT REVIEW

Determination of desired clinical response is established early in the development of a new drug. However, complete information about clinical response to the drug may not be determined until the postmarketing period.

Many factors, including gender, age, nutrition, body size, disease states, and cultural, ethnic, genetic, psychosocial, and environmental factors, affect individual clinical responses to drugs.

UNDESIRED CLINICAL RESPONSE TO DRUG THERAPY

Undesired clinical response to drugs occurs regardless of careful testing and monitoring. Within this text undesired clinical responses are classified as side effects, toxic effects, or adverse reactions.

Side Effects

Drugs do not produce one single effect; instead they produce multiple or secondary effects. **Side effects** are responses, other than the expected clinical response, that occur at normal, therapeutic doses. Some side effects are beneficial; other side effects are undesirable. In some instances drugs are administered to exploit their side effects. For example, diphenhydramine hydrochloride (Benadryl) is classified as an antihistamine. However, it is frequently used to promote sleep and/or decrease restlessness because of its side effect of sedation.

Toxic Effects

Toxic effects usually result from high doses or increased sensitivity to normal doses of a drug. Toxicity is inversely related to the therapeutic index of a substance. If a drug has a wide therapeutic margin of safety, the potential for toxic effects is usually low. Conversely, if a drug has a narrow therapeutic index, the potential for toxic effects is high. In some drugs the therapeutic index is extremely narrow; these drugs are considered dangerous even in therapeutic doses. Digoxin, a cardiac glycoside, and lithium, a drug for manic-depression, are examples of drugs with narrow therapeutic indices.

Adverse Reactions

An **adverse reaction** or **response** is an unwanted, undesired, and possibly harmful side effect of a drug. Adverse responses to drugs can occur immediately or can take days, weeks, or months to develop. In some situations adverse reactions are **predictable**—the reaction is anticipated. For example, barbiturates are central nervous system (CNS) depressants. However, a predictable response that occurs with some clients is CNS excitation.

RESPONSES TO SINGLE DRUG ADMINISTRATION

Even with careful monitoring, no drug is completely safe and free of adverse effects. Common adverse responses associated with single drug administration include intolerance, drug allergy, idiosyncratic responses, tolerance, cumulation, and dependence.

Intolerance

Intolerance is the occurrence of side effects or adverse reactions to the normal pharmacologic doses of a drug. For example, some clients experience severe respiratory depression after receiving the usual analgesic dose of morphine.

Allergy

A **drug allergy** is the reaction of the body's immune system to the presence of drug molecules. The body perceives the drug as a foreign substance—an antigen. Six to 10% of all adverse responses are allergic reactions.

Drug allergy, or hypersensitivity, is divided into two types: immediate and delayed. **Immediate hypersensitivity** occurs within a period of minutes to hours after exposure. These reactions are due to immunoglobulin E (IgE) antibodies that have been produced through prior exposure to the allergen. Immediate hypersensitivity reactions are frequently associated with the administration of antibiotics, intravenous (IV) contrast material (x-ray dye), horse serum, antitoxin, vaccines, local anesthetics, narcotics, and aspirin and related drugs.

These reactions are manifested in many forms. A mild reaction usually consists of urticaria (hives), pruritus, rhinitis, wheezing, rashes, photosensitivity, angioedema, and GI symptoms. *Anaphylaxis* and *anaphylactic shock* are the terms used for severe, potentially life-threatening allergic reactions. Clinical features of anaphylaxis include wheezing, coughing, laryngeal edema, shortness of breath, altered level of consciousness, shock, hypotension, and arrhythmias. The client may also experience nausea, vomiting, abdominal pain, diarrhea, tearing, and feelings of impending doom.[3,4]

Delayed hypersensitivity reactions are sometimes called *cell-mediated hypersensitivity*. These reactions are mediated by T lymphocytes and normally require 36 to 48 hours to develop.

One type of delayed hypersensitivity is a response called *serum sickness* in which the client experiences urticaria, fever, joint pain, and swollen lymph nodes (lymphadenopathy). This reaction is frequently caused by antibiotics and iodides.[4,5]

Idiosyncratic Responses

Idiosyncratic responses are unusual or abnormal responses to a drug, responses different from those normally expected of a specific drug or dose. This term is used most often to describe a state of altered drug metabolism. The cause of an idiosyncratic response is usually genetic.[2,6]

Tolerance

Tolerance represents a decreased response to a drug as a consequence of prior exposure. This decreased response may be divided into two categories: metabolic or pharmacokinetic tolerance and cellular or pharmacodynamic tolerance. If tolerance is caused by a reduction in drug concentration at receptor sites, it is classified as **metabolic tolerance.** Metabolic tolerance is usually due to an increased rate of biotransformation of the drug. Drug tolerance caused by adaptive changes that take place at the receptor or in systems closely connected with the drug's action sites is called **cellular tolerance.**[4] In either situation diminished effectiveness of the drug occurs unless the dose is increased.

With some drugs, **cross-tolerance** develops; that is, tolerance to one drug confers tolerance to another. It is not unusual for drugs of a given class or category to display cross-tolerance. For example, individuals tolerant to one barbiturate are usually tolerant to all barbiturates.

Cumulative Effects

With **cumulative effects,** the body is unable to metabolize and excrete one dose of a drug before the next dose is administered; that is, the drug accumulates in the body. Accumulation of drug molecules in the body is influenced by many factors, including pathologic conditions, malnutrition, and developmental stage of the client. To prevent the occurrence of cumulative effects, serum levels are used to monitor many drugs.

Dependence

Dependence can be divided into physical and psychologic dependency. In either situation it occurs as a consequence of prior exposure to a drug. In **physical dependency** the drug is required for normal function—nerve cells require the drug's presence. Physical dependence is defined in terms of the signs and symptoms displayed after termination of the drug. These signs and symptoms are called *withdrawal* or *abstinence syndrome.*

In **psychologic dependency** the individual has a craving for the effect or response that the drug produces. For example, the individual may use the drug to obtain relief from tension and emotional discomfort. (See Chapter 12 for additional information on substance misuse, abuse, and addiction.)

RESPONSE TO COMBINATIONS OF DRUGS

The incidence of adverse reactions increases as the total number of drugs prescribed for an individual client increases. Common adverse responses associated with combinations of drugs include addition or summation, synergism, potentiation, antagonism, and interaction.

Additive Response or Summation

Summation or **additive response** occurs when the combined effect of two drugs is equal to the sum of the effects of each drug administered alone. For example, drug *A* has X effect; drug *B* has Z effect. When taken together, the combination produces X + Z effects. Combining acetaminophen with codeine sulfate is an example of a beneficial additive effect. Summation or additive effects can only occur when drugs do not interact.[4]

Synergism

A **synergistic effect** occurs when the addition of a second drug yields a combined effect greater than the sum of the effects of the two drugs administered alone. In this instance synergism can be viewed mathematically. For example, drug *A* has the effect of 1 and drug *B* has the effect of 1. The combined effects of the drugs equal 3 instead of 2. The prolonged hypnotic effect of alcohol combined with a hypnotic drug is an example of synergism.

Potentiation

Potentiation is a particular form of synergism. In potentiation only one in a pair of drugs produces a particular effect, with the second drug intensifying or prolonging the effect of the active agent. For example, hydroxyzine (Vistaril) is frequently administered with meperidine (Demerol) to enhance the analgesic effect of meperidine.

Antagonism

An **antagonistic effect** is the opposite of synergism. The combined effect of two drugs is less than that of either one of the drugs alone. Addition of the second drug diminishes or eliminates the effect of the first drug. Any antidote may be regarded an antagonist. For example, gastric absorption of most toxins is diminished when activated charcoal is administered. The activated charcoal forms a stable complex with the poison, preventing its systemic absorption.

When an effect of a drug is diminished at a common receptor site, the term **pharmacologic antagonism** is used. For example, for a client experiencing signs and symptoms of morphine toxicity, naloxone (Narcan) is administered. This narcotic antagonist competes for the same receptor sites as the morphine and prohibits the effects produced by the morphine.

A drug that produces a pharmacologically opposite effect but at a different site is also called an *antagonist.* For example, norepinephrine and acetylcholine are mutually antagonistic in regard to the heart rate. But they affect different sites in the sinoatrial node. The term *physiologic antagonism* is used to describe opposing effects at distinct sites.[4,7]

Interaction

An **interaction** is the process of two or more things acting on each other. In drug therapy drug-drug, drug-nutrient, and drug-environment interactions occur.[8] Interactions are discussed in more depth in Chapter 7.

IATROGENIC RESPONSES

The term *iatrogenic* refers to responses produced unintentionally during the treatment of a client. The most common iatrogenic responses associated with drug therapy are dermatologic responses, hematologic responses, hepatic toxicity, ocular toxicity, ototoxicity, nephrotoxicity, and teratogenic effects. In addition, drug therapy can produce sexual dysfunction (decreased libido and impotence) and pulmonary changes (pulmonary fibrosis and pneumonitis).

Dermatologic Responses

The skin is the most commonly affected organ in the body. Acne, psoriasis, eczema, and maculopapular rashes are mild dermatologic responses associated with certain drugs. Severe responses include exfoliative dermatitis (skin becomes scaly) and erythema multiforme exudativium (Stevens-Johnson syndrome).[7,9]

Hematologic Responses

Drugs can affect the formed elements of the blood (erythrocytes, leukocytes, and platelets). These effects by drugs can produce conditions such as leukopenia, thrombocytopenia, hemolytic or aplastic anemia, and bone marrow depression. Hematologic responses or **blood dyscrasias** are serious and can result in death. The client should report any generalized weakness, fatigue, infection, or bruising that occurs after drug therapy has been initiated.[9]

Nephrotoxicity

Nephrotoxicity is associated with a number of drugs. The kidneys are at risk because they have the highest blood supply and oxygen consumption per gram of tissue of any tissue in the body. Drugs excreted by the kidneys or carried by the blood through the kidneys can damage these organs. It is believed that toxic effects are produced in part by drug molecules binding with brush border receptors in the renal proximal convoluted tubules.[10]

Two pathologic conditions produced by drugs are interstitial nephritis and toxic nephropathy. When potentially nephrotoxic drugs are prescribed for an individual, baseline blood urea nitrogen and creatinine levels should be determined before therapy and periodically during therapy.[11]

Hepatic Toxicity

The liver is the first organ to receive the drug once it is absorbed from the intestine. Drug damage to the liver usually involves the hepatocytes (functional cells of the liver) and bile channel injury. This damage results in biliary obstruction, hepatitis-like syndromes, and hepatic necrosis. Liver function studies are obtained before starting these drugs and are repeated periodically for clients receiving long-term therapy.

Ocular Toxicity

Eyes are subject to direct and indirect injury by drugs. Direct injury results from contact with a drug (e.g., inadvertent administration of otic solution instead of ocular solution). Indirect injury results from systemic absorption of a drug.

Some systemic drugs produce mild symptoms such as blurring of vision and disturbance of color vision. These changes are usually reversible and disappear when the drug is discontinued. For example, digoxin (Lanoxin) produces blurred or yellow vision that disappears once drug clearance occurs. Other systemic drugs produce major changes in the cornea, lens, retina, or optic nerves. These changes are usually not reversible. It is recommended that a complete eye examination be performed before beginning drugs that can produce these effects.

Ototoxicity

The factors that produce ototoxicity are not fully understood. Researchers believe that damage results from primary or secondary effects of drugs. Primary effects are produced when drugs bind to the plasma membrane of the outer hair cells of the cochlea and vestibular apparatus. Secondary effects occur when drugs affect the vestibular and auditory branches of the eighth cranial nerve. Damage to this nerve produces dizziness, balance difficulties, and hearing loss. Some antibiotics and chemotherapeutic drugs are capable of inducing ototoxicity.[10]

Teratogenesis

Teratogenesis describes the production of physical defects in the developing embryo. These changes occur as a result of placental transfer of drugs and/or harmful substances. Since many drugs cross the placental barrier, all drugs are contraindicated in pregnant and possibly pregnant women unless prescribed by the primary care provider.

The response to a teratogenic drug depends on the timing of the exposure. The embryo is at greatest risk during the first trimester (day 1 through 56) of pregnancy. Exposure during the first trimester can lead to obvious anatomic malformations since the form of the internal organs is being established. Birth defects that result from exposure to teratogens in later pregnancy are different. Exposure during the second and third trimester can injure the nervous, endocrine, and immune systems and the developing teeth.[12]

In an attempt to limit teratogenesis and to facilitate decisions about drug therapy during pregnancy, the FDA has categorized drugs according to the potential harm to the fetus.

Drugs are classified according to five pregnancy categories: A, B, C, D, and X. Drugs in category A are the least dangerous to the fetus. In contrast, drugs classified in category X are the most dangerous. These drugs cause harm to the human fetus, and their risks outweigh any therapeutic benefit. Occasionally a drug is classified as *NA* to indicate that controlled studies have not been done on the drug. Chapter 13 contains additional information on drugs and the pregnant client.

FDA PREGNANCY CATEGORIES

A No risk to the fetus has been detected, based on acceptable and controlled studies in pregnant women.

B No evidence of risk to humans has been detected, based on either positive findings in animals but negative findings in human studies or negative findings in animal studies and the absence of adequate data from human trials.

C Potential risk is present either because there are no data from human studies and animal studies show adverse effects or no studies have been conducted. Drugs with a Pregnancy Category C rating may be used when potential benefits outweigh potential risks to the fetus.

D There is evidence of fetal harm, based on data either obtained from investigational studies or collected after the drug was approved and used in pregnant women. Category D drugs may be used during pregnancy if there is a favorable benefit-to-risk ratio.

X The drug is contraindicated during pregnancy; the potential risks clearly outweigh any real or anticipated benefits.

Mutagenesis

Mutagenesis means the induction of genetic mutation. Some drugs produce chromosomal changes that result in permanent alteration of genetic structure.

Carcinogenesis

Carcinogenesis indicates that a substance has the ability to induce cancer or predispose an individual to the disease. Highly carcinogenic drugs are not released for use. However, it is possible that carcinogenic drugs may not be identified until after years of clinical use.

CONCEPT REVIEW

Iatrogenic responses are produced unintentionally during the treatment of a client. The most common iatrogenic responses associated with drug therapy are dermatologic responses, hematologic responses, hepatic toxicity, ocular toxicity, ototoxicity, nephrotoxicity, and teratogenic effects.

⊞ NURSING CONSIDERATIONS

The primary focus of your care is constant close observation of the client. Protecting your client is your top priority, for you are with the client more than any other health care provider. Therefore you are in the best position to prevent undesired reactions by early recognition and intervention.

Your first responsibility is to know which drugs are more likely to produce undesired reactions, what type of response is expected, and how to recognize the reaction as soon as possible. Any drug can cause undesired reactions; however, certain drugs cause the vast majority of reported undesired clinical responses. Anticoagulants, antimicrobials, bronchodilators, cardiac drugs, CNS drugs, hormones, and diagnostic agents are especially prone to producing adverse reactions.[13]

Most health care agencies have drug reference books available for the care providers. Additional sources of information are package inserts and the agency's pharmacist. Use these resources to help you know what type of response to expect.

🦎 NURSING RESEARCH

Fahs, P. S., & Kinney, M. (1991). The abdomen, thigh, and arm as sites for subcutaneous sodium heparin injections. *Nursing Research, 40,* 204-207

The purpose of this study was to evaluate the effectiveness of three subcutaneous injection sites. The 101 subjects, ranging in age from 20 to 94 years, were randomly placed in one of three groups. Group A received injections in the abdomen, group B in the thigh, and group C in the arm. Each subject received three injections at one site. Activated partial thromboplastin time (APTT) was measured before initiation of heparin and 4 hours after the first injection. Bruising was measured at 48, 60, and 72 hours after injection.

There were no statistically significant differences among the groups for changes in APTT or bruising at 60 and 72 hours after injection. Therefore the clinical practice of using the abdomen as the primary site for subcutaneous heparin injections was not supported.

Future studies in this area should consider the subject's weight, size, proportion of adipose tissue, gender, and ethnic background. All these factors influence the response to subcutaneous injections.

STUDENT ACTIVITIES

• Read the procedure for low-dose heparin therapy at your assigned agency.
• Request permission to monitor several clients receiving subcutaneous heparin therapy. Check the charts of these clients and record their age, weight, and ethnic background. Monitor and record dosage, site of injection, and degree of bruising. Determine if any differences exist.

• Interview a client receiving low-dose heparin therapy injections in the abdomen. Determine the client's psychologic response to these injections, i. e., any fears or discomfort.

If you assess an undesired reaction, contact the primary care provider immediately. If the reaction is an allergic response, do not administer the next dose. If the drug is being administered intravenously, stop the infusion. The drug may be discontinued permanently or the dose altered to limit the signs and symptoms of the reaction. In some cases it will be necessary for you to administer an antidote.

All caregivers should be informed that the client has experienced an undesired reaction to a drug. Note the name of the drug clearly on the outside of the medical record. Within the record, record the signs and symptoms of the reaction. Tell the client which drug caused the reaction, and suggest that the client carry a card or wear a bracelet that contains the name of the drug.

Drug manufacturers monitor adverse reactions and report them to the FDA. The FDA also welcomes reports from nurses whose clients have experienced serious reactions, especially with drugs that have been on the market 3 years or less. According to the FDA, the following constitute serious reactions: response is life threatening; causes death; leads to hospitalization or prolongs hospitalizations, or results in permanent or severe disability.[9]

The Joint Commission on Accreditation of Healthcare Organizations (JCAHO) requires that hospitals have an adverse drug reaction reporting program in place. JCAHO also requires that all significant reactions be reviewed to assure quality care. According to JCAHO, a significant reaction is one in which the drug must be discontinued; the client requires treatment with another drug to diminish the reaction, or the length of the hospitalization is prolonged.[9]

SUMMARY

The desired clinical response to a drug is determined after years of animal and human studies and trials. Even after an extensive test period, undesired clinical responses may still occur. Consideration of causative factors such as age, gender, body surface area, ethnic background, and physical state can prevent some undesired clinical responses. The role of the nurse is to know factors that may precipitate undesired responses and early manifestations of the responses.

REFERENCES

1. Seeley, R., Stephens, T., & Tate, P. (1992). *Anatomy and physiology* (2nd ed.). St. Louis: Mosby–Year Book.
2. Wood, A.J., & Zhou, H.H. (1991). Ethnic differences in drug disposition and responsiveness. *Clinical Pharmacokinetics, 20,* 350-373.
3. Roth, R. (1990). Allergic response. *Emergency, 22*(6), 28-32.
4. Smith, C., & Reynard, A. (1992). *Textbook of pharmacology.* Philadelphia: W.B. Saunders.
5. Goodman, R., Gilman, E., Rall, T., Nies, A., & Taylor, P. (Eds.). (1990). *Goodman and Gilman's: The pharmacological basis of therapeutics* (8th ed.). New York: Pergamon Press.
6. Kudzma, E. (1992). Drug response: All bodies are not created equal. *American Journal of Nursing, 92*(12), 48-50.
7. Levine, R. (1990). *Pharmacology: Drug actions and reactions.* Boston: Little, Brown.
8. Mathewson, M.K. (1989). Drug interactions. *Critical Care Nurse, 9*(4), 84-92.
9. O'Donnell, J. (1992). Understanding adverse drug reactions. *Nursing '92, 22*(8), 34-40.
10. Walker, E.M., Fazekas-May, M.A., & Bowen, W.R. (1990). Nephrotoxic and ototoxic agents. *Clinics in Laboratory Medicine, 10,* 323-354.
11. Garfinkel, H., Porter, G., & Whelton, A. (1988). Renal failure: Are drugs the cause? *Patient Care, 22*(14), 71-74, 77, 80.
12. Lehne, R.A. (1994). *Pharmacology for nursing care* (2nd ed.). Philadelphia: W.B. Saunders.
13. Heenan, A. (1989). Side effects of drugs: Monitoring adverse reactions. *Nursing Times, 85*(39), 25-27, 29.

BIBLIOGRAPHY

Acute drug reactions in the elderly (1989). *Emergency Medicine, 21*(4), 50, 55-56.
Carruth, A., & Boss, B. (1990). More than they bargained for: Adverse drug effects. *Journal of Gerontological Nursing, 16*(7), 27-30.
DeHart, R.L. (1990). Medication and the work environment. *Journal of Occupational Medicine, 32,* 310-312.
Greener, M. (1990). Towards the magic bullet: Improving specificity in drugs. *Professional Nurse, 6,* 171-174.
Jahns, B.E., & Levy, D.B. (1991). Common drug reactions and interactions. *Emergency, 23*(11), 22-26, 29-31.
Orfan, N., & Patterson, R. (1992). Anaphylaxis management update. *Physician Assistant, 16*(4), 67-70, 73, 76.
Santo-Novak, D., & Edwards, R.M. (1989). Rx: Take caution with drugs for elders. *Geriatric Nursing, 10*(2), 72-75.
Snow, B. (1989). SEDBASE: On-line for drug side effects and interactions. *Database, 12*(1), 85-94.

CHAPTER 7

Drug Interactions

NORMA L. PINNELL

⊛ **Drug-Drug Interactions**

LEARNING OBJECTIVES:

Describe two mechanisms involved in pharmacokinetic interactions.

Explain one mechanism involved in pharmacodynamic interactions.

KEY TERM: Drug-drug interaction

⊛ **Drug-Nutrient Interactions**

LEARNING OBJECTIVES:

Summarize three effects of drugs on nutritional status.

Discuss the pharmacologic effects of food.

Describe the effect of nutrients on drugs.

KEY TERM: Drug-nutrient interaction

⊛ **Drug-Environment Interactions**

LEARNING OBJECTIVE: Describe two examples of drug-environment interactions.

KEY TERM: Drug-environment interaction

⊛ **Clinical Implications of Drug Interactions**

LEARNING OBJECTIVES:

Discuss the clinical implications of drug interactions.

Describe the role of the nurse in the prevention of interactions.

CONCEPTS AND TERMS TO REVIEW

Review section on the oral route of administration in Chapter 4.

Examine the meaning of the concepts *affinity* and *competitive binding* in Chapter 4.

Review the section on drug-receptor interactions in Chapter 5.

---

*E*very day the number of possible drug-drug, drug-nutrient, and drug-environment interactions increases. There are two practical approaches to this problem: (1) understand the main types and mechanisms of drug interactions and (2) have available resources that list all known interactions.

This chapter provides an overview of the main types and mechanisms of drug interactions. General information on drug-drug, drug-nutrient, and drug-environment interactions is presented. Examples of specific drug interactions are discussed in each of the clinical chapters in Part II of the book.

DRUG-DRUG INTERACTIONS

A **drug-drug interaction** occurs whenever the action of a drug is modified by another pharmacologically active chemical substance. The interaction can be physical, chemical, or biologic.[1]

Direct Physical or Chemical Interactions

In a direct drug-drug interaction each drug is modified (e.g., using protamine sulfate to neutralize the effects of circulating heparin or digoxin immune Fab (Digibind) to decrease the level of circulating digoxin).[2,3]

Direct interactions also occur when certain parenteral drug solutions are combined. In some situations the interaction causes the formation of a precipitate. If a precipitate appears, the solution must be discarded. However, not all direct interactions between parenteral drug solutions are visibly evident; therefore it is important to determine drug-drug compatibility before mixing the solutions.

This same form of direct interaction can occur when two or more liquid-oral dosage forms are combined. Again, determine drug-drug compatibility if liquid drug solutions are being mixed to facilitate oral or enteral administration.

NURSING RESEARCH

Collins, J.L., & Lutz, R. (1991). In vitro study of simultaneous infusion of incompatible drugs in multilumen catheters. *Heart & Lung, 20,* 271-277.

Multilumen catheters are commonly used to administer incompatible drugs simultaneously to critically ill clients. Limited information is available about the safety and efficacy of this practice.

This study used an in vitro model flow system to examine the physicochemical phenomena that occur when two incompatible drugs (phenytoin [Dilantin] and total parenteral nutrition) are simultaneously administered through multilumen catheters. Video recordings were made of the drug interactions, and assays of phenytoin concentration were performed on samples of the circulating fluid.

Recordings revealed white clouds of phenytoin precipitation near the tip of the double-lumen catheter but not the triple-lumen catheter. There was also an average 6% loss of phenytoin to precipitate with the double-lumen catheter. In some instances millimeter-sized fragments of phenytoin precipitate were seen dislodging from the tip of the double-lumen catheter.

Clinical significance of the study has not been assessed. However, possible complications such as pulmonary emboli, thrombophlebitis, and catheter occlusion are a concern. In addition, the reduced bioavailability of a drug may significantly reduce desired clinical response.

STUDENT ACTIVITIES

- Review the procedure manual in your assigned agency and determine the protocol for administering drugs through multilumen catheters.
- Study four drugs commonly administered through multilumen catheters. Focus your attention on possible drug-drug interactions.
- Determine if any attempt is made in your agency to separate incompatible drugs (i.e., different times of administration).

Pharmacokinetic Interactions

Pharmacokinetic interactions occur when the absorption, distribution, biotransformation, or excretion of one drug is affected by another drug.

Alteration in oral drug absorption　Oral drugs can combine to form complexes that are not absorbed in the stomach. For example, antacids can form complexes with many drugs, decreasing the second drug's effectiveness. Antacids also elevate gastric pH. This action decreases the ionization of basic drugs in the stomach and increases the ability of the body to absorb these drugs. Conversely, antacids have the opposite effect on the absorption of weak acids. Gastric antacids also accelerate the dissolution rates of some drugs; for example, antacids dissolve the coating of bisacodyl (Dulcolax), an action that enhances gastric absorption of bisacodyl. Drugs such as morphine and codeine decrease gastric motility. This lengthens the time that other drugs are in contact with the gastrointestinal (GI) mucosa and increases the amount of drug absorbed.[3,5-7]

Alterations in distribution　The most common interactions affecting drug distribution involve one drug's displacing another drug from plasma proteins. The diuretic ethacrynic acid (Edecrin) displaces oral hypoglycemic drugs such as tolbutamide (Orinase) from plasma protein. This may produce higher-than-anticipated circulating levels of tolbutamide, resulting in hypoglycemia. Another example occurs with the anticoagulant warfarin (Coumadin). Warfarin can be displaced by the anti-inflammatory drug phenylbutazone (Butazolidin), causing elevated prothrombin times due to excess free warfarin.[3,6,7] Some drugs interfere with the storage of other drugs. For example, quinidine decreases the binding of digoxin in peripheral tissues. As a result, serum digoxin levels increase.[6]

Inhibition of drug biotransformation　Drugs can modify the metabolism or biotransformation of other drugs. Disulfiram (Antabuse) is used to treat alcohol addiction. Disulfiram inhibits the hepatic metabolism of ethanol, causing serum acetaldehyde levels to rise. As a result, the individual experiences a variety of unpleasant and undesirable symptoms.[6]

Phenobarbital, a barbiturate, increases the metabolism of some drugs by stimulating the action of hepatic enzymes. Concurrent administration of phenobarbital increases the metabolism of drugs such as anticoagulants, steroids, and digitoxin and may result in inadequate drug effect as a result of lowered serum concentrations.[3,6,7]

Alteration of excretion　Excretion of drugs can be altered by changes in the urinary pH. Therefore any drug that alters the urinary pH potentially can increase or decrease the excretion of other drugs. Usually acidic drugs such as phenobarbital are excreted faster in alkaline urine. Basic drugs (e.g., meperidine [Demerol], imipramine [Tofranil]) are excreted more quickly in acidic urine.[3,6,7]

Pharmacodynamic Interactions

Pharmacodynamic interactions result from the combined action of drugs at receptor sites. The interaction of two drugs at the same receptor site usually results in an inhibitory effect on both drugs. However, as noted in the previous chapter, pharmacodynamic drug-drug interactions may be beneficial, as in the case of some additive, synergistic, and potentiating effects.

CONCEPT REVIEW

Drug-drug interactions involve the modification of a drug's action by another pharmacologically active substance.

In direct physical or chemical drug-drug interactions, each drug is modified.

Pharmacokinetic drug-drug interactions alter the absorption, distribution, biotransformation, and excretion processes.

Pharmacodynamic interactions result from the combined action of drugs at receptor sites.

DRUG-NUTRIENT INTERACTIONS

Drug-nutrient interactions are a commonly overlooked aspect of drug therapy. However, over the past few years increased attention has been given to the interaction of drugs with certain nutrients. Drugs can affect the nutritional status of the client by altering nutrient absorption, metabolism, utilization, and excretion. Conversely, the client's nutritional status can affect the action of drugs by altering absorption, distribution, biotransformation, and excretion. In addition, some foods and beverages contain pharmacologic substances capable of producing undesirable effects in the body.

Effect of Drugs on Nutritional Status

Drugs that affect gastric and/or intestinal motility can decrease absorption of glucose, protein, sodium, potassium, and some vitamins. Mineral oil acts as a physical barrier to and solvent for fat-soluble vitamins. Drugs that reduce cholesterol (bile acid sequestrants) decrease absorption of vitamin B_{12}, iron, fat-soluble vitamins, glucose, and electrolytes. Surface-active agents (stool softeners) also alter absorption of nutrients; and broad-spectrum antibiotics destroy intestinal flora that synthesize vitamin K.[8,9]

Drugs can affect nutrition by decreasing taste sensitivity, producing unpleasant tastes in the mouth, or yielding an aftertaste. These changes can cause anorexia in the client. Other drugs such as antipsychotic agents stimulate appetite, and some drugs specifically depress the appetite.

Drugs can alter nutrient metabolism and utilization. For example, anticonvulsants such as phenytoin, phenobarbital, and primidone (Mysoline) cause accelerated metabolism of vitamin D. Since vitamin D is essential for calcium absorption, a decrease in vitamin D can lead to decreased calcium absorption. These same anticonvulsants utilize folic acid, which can lead to clinical manifestations of folate deficiency states.[8–10]

Excretion of nutrients is also altered by drugs. Loop and thiazide diuretics cause an increased excretion of sodium, potassium, and magnesium. Diuretics also influence calcium excretion; loop diuretics increase urinary excretion of calcium, and thiazide diuretics decrease excretion of calcium. Clients given chronic high-dose aspirin therapy are subject to increased ascorbic acid excretion and potassium depletion. Fluid and electrolyte imbalances are common side effects of steroids, nonsteroidal anti-inflammatory drugs, and some antihypertensive agents.[8,9,11]

Effect of Nutrients on Drugs

Studies have shown that nutritional status is an important determinant of drug response. Dietary modifications are essential for clients who are at nutritional risk (i.e., less than ideal weight or with a low serum albumin level, low lymphocyte count, or unintentional, rapid weight loss). In addition, since food, beverages, and mineral or vitamin supplements can alter the pharmacokinetics of a drug, the client's intake must be monitored closely.

Foods decrease, delay, or increase the absorption of drugs. Inactive complexes can result from drugs that bind to nutrients, rendering both the drug and nutrient unavailable for absorption. For example, when given with milk, dairy products, or antacids, tetracycline (an antibiotic) binds with the cations present in these products to form an inactive complex. Food delays the absorption of many drugs, including acetaminophen, aspirin, and potassium. Absorption of some drugs (e.g., phenobarbital, ampicillin, penicillin G, and tetracycline) is decreased when administered with food or too close to mealtime. Acidic beverages can interfere with absorption of penicillin and erythromycin, both antibiotic drugs. Increased absorption of drugs can be caused by foods that decrease first-pass metabolism or decrease gastric emptying time. Fatty foods can increase the absorption of some drugs (e.g., griseofulvin [Fulvicin, Grifulvin V, and Grisactin], an antifungal agent, and hydrochlorothiazide with triamterene [Dyazide], a diuretic).[9–11]

Some drugs (e.g., Sudafed syrup, Feosol elixir, potassium chloride liquid, phenytoin suspension, and digoxin elixir) may not be well absorbed when given during continuous enteral feeding. The mixture of feeding and drug may cause gel formation, tube clogging, and drug precipitation. With clients receiving continuous enteral feeding, it is recommended that drugs be given as a single-bolus dose 1 hour or more after the formula flow has been temporarily discontinued and the feeding tube has been rinsed with water.[11]

Food and drugs can also be antagonists, altering the usual action of the drug. For example, the oral anticoagulant warfarin and vitamin K are antagonists. If clients receiving warfarin consume excessive amounts of foods rich in vitamin K such as broccoli, brussels sprouts, cabbage, kale, spinach, asparagus, lettuce, or liver their prothrombin time may decrease.

Another example of antagonistic action occurs between levodopa and pyridoxine. Clients receiving levodopa for Parkinson's disease must limit their intake of pyridoxine, which is found in large amounts in meat, fish, and poultry. Pyridoxine is a cofactor in the peripheral decarboxylation of levodopa to dopamine. Since dopamine cannot cross the blood-brain barrier, clinical manifestations of parkinsonism may be exacerbated in clients receiving levodopa and ingesting large amounts of these foods. In addition, certain amino acids in protein inhibit the absorption of levodopa and reduce the amount of the drug that crosses the blood-brain barrier. Restricting the protein intake of clients receiving levodopa improves the client's response to drug therapy.[10,12]

The use of alcohol with drugs can result in clinically significant interactions. Drug metabolism is affected by both acute and chronic use of alcohol. Chronic use of alcohol results in enzyme reduction, which causes decreased metabolism of drugs. Large amounts of alcohol over a short period of time or small amounts in an individual who seldom drinks can cause an additive or synergistic effect with central nervous system depressants.

Many fermented foods such as wine, beer, and aged cheese contain tyramine. Tyramine is also present in bread or crackers containing cheese, homemade yeast bread, beef and chicken livers, summer sausage, smoked, dried, or pickled fish, and broad bean pods. With monoamine oxidase (MAO) inhibitors, tyramine triggers the release of norepinephrine from sympathetic nerve endings and epinephrine from adrenal glands. The release of these substances can result in a hypertensive reaction or crises. Headaches, palpitations, nausea, and vomiting are frequent clinical manifestations of this interaction. MAO inhibitors include certain antidepressants and antihypertensive drugs. In addition, the chemotherapeutic drug procarbazine hydrochloride (Matulane) has MAO inhibitory properties. Clients taking these drugs should follow a tyramine-restricted diet.[9-11]

Natural licorice or licorice extracts containing glycyrrhizinic acid can complicate hypertension and digitalis therapy. Glycyrrhizinic acid is a sweet compound in licorice roots that has mineralocorticoid activity. It can cause sodium retention and potassium excretion. Most domestic licorice is made with a synthetic licorice flavor and presents no problem.[8-10,13]

Pharmacologic Effects of Food

Pharmacologic substances found in some food and beverages can affect the health of individuals. For example, hydroxytryptamine exists in pineapples and bananas; dihydroxyphenylalanine (DOPA) is present in broad beans, and oxalates are present in some foods. In addition, selenium, potassium, calcium, magnesium, and sodium are present in grains and other foods.

Pesticides and heavy metal residues have been detected in several species of edible fish. Food additives such as preservatives, antioxidants, bleaching and maturing agents, surface-active agents, acidulates, buffers, special dietary sweeteners, and flavors are used in processing food. Water, soft drinks, and alcoholic beverages may contain various metals, xanthines, and histamines.[14,15]

CONCEPT REVIEW

Drugs can affect the nutritional status of the client by altering nutrient absorption, metabolism, utilization, and excretion.

The client's nutritional status can also affect the action of drugs by altering absorption, distribution, biotransformation, and excretion.

Some foods and beverages contain pharmacologic substances capable of producing undesirable effects in the body.

DRUG-ENVIRONMENT INTERACTIONS

Drug-environment interactions involve several aspects, including storage of the drug and impact of the environment on the drug's pharmacokinetic and pharmacodynamic processes. Most drugs are sensitive to the environment. Excessive heat, light, or moisture or sudden temperature changes can affect the stability of the drug. Therefore it is important to follow the manufacturer's recommendations about storage. This information is found in package inserts. It is also available in official sources of information such as the *United States Pharmacopoeia (USP)*, the *United States Pharmacopoeia Dispensing Information (USP-DI)*, the *National Formulary*, the *British Pharmacopoeia (BP)*, the *British Pharmaceutical Codex (BPC)*, the *Canadian Formulary*, the *European Pharmacopoeia*, and the *British National Formulary*. Failure to follow these guidelines can alter the drug's action and the clinical response.

It is also important to monitor the client's environment while he or she is receiving certain drugs. Some drugs (e.g., amitriptyline, imipramine, and tolbutamide) can cause photosensitivity. These drugs make the skin extremely sensitive to sunlight. Even brief exposure can cause a bad sunburn, hives, or skin rash. Other drugs (e.g., atropine, belladonna alkaloids [Donnatal], benztropine [Cogentin]) reduce the body's tolerance to heat and/or inhibit the body's ability to reduce body temperature. Either one of these effects can lead to heat stroke in hot weather or during exercise.

CLINICAL IMPLICATIONS OF DRUG INTERACTIONS

Drug interactions potentially can significantly alter the outcome of drug therapy. As a result of interactions, the intensity of drug responses may be increased or reduced. Interactions that increase the intensity of a drug response also increase the potential for adverse reactions and toxic effects.

The more drugs a client receives, the greater is the risk of an interaction. Therefore the total number of drugs must be kept to a minimum. If the client's condition warrants multiple-drug therapy, close observation of the client is essential.

Effective, safe use of drugs requires cooperation and collaboration of all individuals involved—the client, primary care provider, pharmacist, and nurse. Your role in drug therapy is based on a thorough assessment of the client and on an understanding of the drug to be administered. Obtain a drug history before administering any drug. Determine if the client has received the prescribed drug previously. If so, ask the client to describe the past response to the drug. Assess the appropriateness of the prescribed drug. Ask yourself: "What is the expected response to the drug?" "Is the prescribed dose within recommended, safe limits?" "Is the prescribed route compatible with the client's condition?" "Is the drug compatible with other drugs being administered to the client?" "Is the drug compatible with the client's dietary patterns?" Make certain you know the action of the drug and possible side effects and interactions. Only after these aspects have been addressed should you administer the prescribed drug.

SUMMARY

Three types of drug interactions can occur: drug-drug, drug-nutrient, and drug-environment. Drug-drug interactions occur whenever the action of a drug is modified by another pharmacologically active chemical substance. This type of interaction may involve the pharmacokinetic or pharmacodynamic processes or a direct drug-drug interaction.

The importance of drug-nutrient interactions has become an item of concern in recent years. Drugs can affect the nutritional status of the client; conversely, the client's nutritional status can affect the action of the drug. In addition, some foods and beverages contain pharmacologic substances capable of producing undesirable effects in the body.

Minimum research has been done about drug-environment interactions. However, this area is just as important as drug-drug and drug-nutrient interactions. Care must be taken that drugs are stored properly and that the client is educated about environmental restrictions.

All health care providers have an important role in preventing drug interactions. Before any drug therapy is initiated, a thorough assessment of the client must be completed. This assessment should include a drug and diet history. Once drug therapy has been established, close observation of the client for unusual signs and symptoms is imperative.

REFERENCES

1. Mathewson, M.K. (1989). Drug interactions. *Critical Care Nurse, 9*(4), 84-91.
2. Jahns, B.E., & Levy, D.B. (1991). Common drug reactions and interactions. *Emergency, 23*(11), 22-26, 29-31.
3. Porterfield, L.M. (1989). Drug interactions. *Advancing Clinical Care, 4*(6), 15-16.
4. Collins, J., & Lutz, R. (1991). In vitro study of simultaneous infusion of incompatible drugs in multilumen catheters. *Heart & Lung, 20,* 271-277.
5. Lehne, R.A. (1994). *Pharmacology for nursing care* (2nd ed.). Philadelphia: W.B. Saunders.
6. Cunningham, R., & Smith, C. (1992). Interactions: Drug allergy; Drug-drug; Drug-food. In C. Smith, & A. Reynard (Eds.), *Textbook of pharmacology* (pp. 1090-1102). Philadelphia: W.B. Saunders.
7. Tatro, D.S. (Ed.). (1990). *Drug interaction facts.* St. Louis: Facts and Comparisons Division, J.B. Lippincott.
8. Roe, D.A. (1988). *Diet and drug interactions.* New York: Van Nostrand Reinhold.
9. Trovato, A., Nuhlicek, D.N., & Midtling, J.E. (1991). Drug-nutrient interactions. *American Family Physician, 44*(5), 1651-1658.
10. Graedon Enterprise. (1991). *Drug & food interactions.* Durham, NC: King Features.
11. McPherson, M.L. (1989). Drug and dietary interactions: Guidelines for counseling the home health care patient. *Home Health Care Practice, 1*(4), 27-37.
12. Cerrato, P.L. (1991). Nutrition support: Diet therapy helps this drug work better. *RN, 54*(2), 71-72, 74.
13. Litteral, J. (1990). What are the clinical important drug-nutrient interactions? *Pediatric Nursing, 16,* 594-596.
14. Food additives: What they do. (1992). *Chemecology, 21*(2), 4-5.
15. Murray, J., & Healy, M. (1991). Drug-mineral interactions: A new responsibility for the hospital dietitian. *Journal of the American Dietetic Association, 91*(1), 66-70, 73.

BIBLIOGRAPHY

Cerrato, P. (1992). The patient's eating—Why is he losing weight? *RN, 55*(4), 77-80.

De Hart, R. (1990). Medication and the work environment. *Journal of Occupational Medicine, 32,* 310-312.

Food and drug interactions. (1991). *Health & You, 7*(2), 43-45.

Garabedian-Ruffalo, S. (1990). Drug compatibility chart. *Critical Care Nurse, 10*(3), 28-29.

Gora, M.L., Tschampel, M.M., & Visconti, J.A. (1989). Considerations of drug therapy in patients receiving enteral nutrition. *Nutrition in Clinical Practice, 4*(3), 105-110.

Grauer, K. (1991). Problems of polypharmacy and intercurrent disease. *Hospital Practice Symposium, Suppl 26*(2), 20-25.

Hones, C.M., & Reddick, J.E. (1989). Drug-nutrient interaction counseling programs in upper Midwestern hospitals: 1986 survey results. *Journal of the American Dietetic Association, 89,* 243-245.

Kumpf, V. (1992). Pharmacists help identify, treat drug-related malnutrition. *Provider, 18*(1), 41.

Lamy, P.P. (1990). Most common drug interactions are predictable, avoidable. *Provider, 16*(7), 35-36.

Miller, C. (1990). When medication harms as well as helps. *Geriatric Nursing, 11,* 301-302.

Moha, M., Watson, R., & Leonard-Green, T. (1990). Nutritional effects of marijuana, heroin, cocaine, and nicotine. *Journal of the American Dietetic Association, 90,* 1281-1287.

Snow, B. (1989). SEDBASE: Online for drug side effects and interactions. *Database, 12*(1), 85-94.

Strong, A., Wolff, H., Kinder, S., & Lubischer, A. (1991). Drug administration in relation to meals in institutional setting. *Heart & Lung, 20,* 39-44.

Drug Therapy and the Nurse

CHAPTER 8
Drug Therapy and the Nursing Process

DRUG THERAPY AND THE
Nursing Process

NORMA L. PINNELL

CONCEPTS AND TERMS TO REVIEW

Review section, "Impact on Role of Nurse," in Chapter 2.
Review information about dosage forms and routes of administration in Chapter 3.
Review section, "Role of Nurse," in Chapter 6.

*T*he term *process* denotes the act of moving forward continuously, proceeding from one point to another on the way to a goal. Process is a method used to produce, accomplish, or attain a specific result. The nursing process is just such a dynamic process. It is the structure or framework around which a nurse organizes his or her care. It represents an organized, systematic method for examining the client's health status, identifying the client's needs, and determining appropriate solutions to meet these needs.

OVERVIEW OF THE NURSING PROCESS

The nursing process, which is composed of five phases or steps, is flexible and adaptable to any practice setting. These phases, **assessing, diagnosing, planning, implementing,** and **evaluating,** are interrelated; completion of one phase automatically leads into the next phase (Fig. 8–1).

During the assessing phase the nurse is responsible for completing a database on the client. This database may consist of an assessment interview, nursing health history, wellness assessment, cultural assessment, spiritual assessment, developmental assessment, nutritional assessment, and physical assessment. Depending on the situation, one or all of these assessment measures are used.

Although theoretically the database is never complete, the nurse must at some point decide he or she has enough information to provide safe, individualized care. At this point the

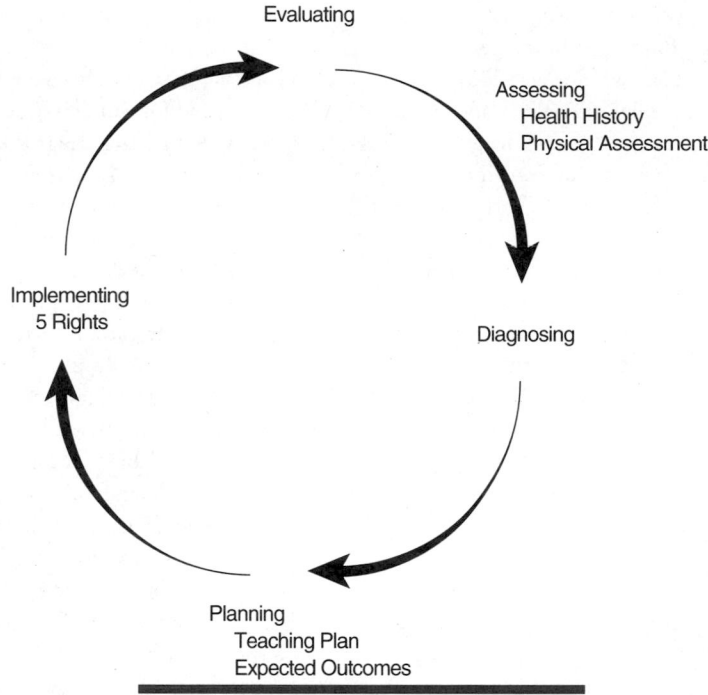

FIGURE 8–1   Nursing process in action.

data are analyzed, and nursing diagnoses are formulated. If several diagnoses exist, they should be placed in order of priority.

The actual plan of care varies from practice setting to practice setting. The plan includes goals, objectives, expected outcomes, and interventions for each diagnosis. Since the goals and objectives should be individualized for each client based on the assessed data, this textbook considers only expected outcomes and interventions. Once the plan of care has been developed, it is implemented and the outcomes of care evaluated.

ASSESSING THE CLIENT

Nonadherence to drug therapy is a major public health problem. Approximately 25% to 50% of the population in the United States does not follow drug regimens properly. Prevention of this problem begins with a thorough assessment of clients and their needs.

Health History

The **health history** is gathered during the assessment interview. This is an information-gathering interview in which therapeutic communication is used to obtain subjective data from the client. The health history does *not* contain objective data or inferences. Depending on the situation, the health history may include an extensive wellness assessment, dietary history, developmental assessment, cultural assessment, and spiritual assessment.

During the health history you, as the nurse, must gather a complete drug history. Determine drugs, both prescription and nonprescription, currently taken. (In soliciting a nonpre-

scription drug history, it helps to proceed according to drug class [i.e., cough or cold medication, analgesics, antacids].) Question the client about dosage, route, and frequency of administration for each drug. Ask about therapeutic and undesired clinical responses to each drug.

Ask the client if there are any known allergies; if the client has a drug allergy or has experienced a previous hypersensitivity reaction, flag the medical record. Many drugs are compounds of two or more drugs; in such a situation, determine the ingredients of these products. Also determine if the client has experienced sensitivity to drugs similar in chemical structure to new ones being prescribed.

Determine how much the client knows about the condition for which each drug was prescribed. Does the client believe a need for the drug still exists? Or was the drug prescribed years ago and no one has discontinued it? Determine why the client takes over-the-counter (OTC) drugs. Did he or she see them advertised? Did a friend or relative recommend that he or she take them? Did a health professional suggest they be taken?

You must identify ethnic, psychologic, and socioeconomic factors that may influence health decisions and medicine use. (See Chapters 9 and 10 for more discussion of these topics.) Lack of social support or a mistrust of drugs by family members can affect drug use. Determine if the client is self-medicating with herbs, roots, or ethnic remedies. (See Chapter 11 for discussion of self-medication practices.)

Assess the use of caffeine, nicotine, alcoholic beverages, or street drugs. Determine how long and how much the client has smoked, for smoking influences the metabolism of some drugs (e.g., smoking increases the metabolism of theophylline). When caffeine is ingested in amounts of 200 mg or more, it is considered a pharmacologic agent. Therefore quantify the client's use of caffeine-containing foods and beverages such as coffee, tea, soft drinks, and chocolate. Caffeine acts as a central nervous system (CNS) and myocardial stimulant and a diuretic. It may have a synergistic effect with some drugs.[1]

When talking to the client, assess his or her learning needs. Include an assessment of the client's literacy level and language most easily understood. This information is important when planning verbal and written instructions. Evaluate the mental status of the client to establish a baseline if confusion or cognitive changes develop after a new drug is administered. Also determine the client's compliance history. Has the client decided to discontinue previously prescribed drugs? What influenced the client's actions?

Physical Assessment

The **physical assessment** is an evaluation of the client's health status through the use of observation, auscultation, percussion, and palpation. This database contains objective data—data that is verifiable or confirmed by other assessment means.

A complete physical assessment has four major parts: general survey or initial observation of the client's general appearance and behavior; vital signs measurement; assessment of height and weight; and physical examination or assessment of all structures, organs, and body systems. In some settings you do not have the opportunity to perform a complete assessment. In these situations conduct a modified assessment based on knowledge of the client's history and complaints.

This text does not describe the techniques used during the physical assessment; thus you must study references that focus on this topic and have supervised practice to perfect physical assessment skills.

CONCEPT REVIEW

The nursing process is composed of five phases: assessing, diagnosing, planning, implementing, and evaluating.

During assessing you collect a health history, which consists of subjective data. This is information the client must tell you.

You also perform a physical assessment. It provides objective data—data that can be verified or validated.

FORMULATING NURSING DIAGNOSES

Before reaching a conclusion about nursing diagnoses, you must analyze the database. Ask yourself: Does the client have a history of noncompliance with drug therapy? Does the client have a history of undesired clinical responses from drugs? Are the dose, route of administration, and time schedule for each prescribed drug appropriate? Do any of the client's drugs have the potential to interact? Is there a risk of drug-nutrient or drug-environment interactions? Are any of the drugs a dupli-

cation in therapy? Is the client taking the same drug under two different names?

Once the data have been analyzed and the decision reached about the need for nursing intervention, nursing diagnoses are developed. A **nursing diagnosis** is a two-part statement that reflects the client's response and the etiologies or causative factors for that response. In some instances the nursing diagnosis reflects a response the client is at risk for developing if appropriate actions by health care professionals are not taken.

The first part of the diagnostic statement consists of a diagnostic label and the second part consists of the causes. The two parts are joined by the phrase *related to.* Although the North American Nursing Diagnosis Association (NANDA) has developed a list of diagnostic labels (see box), you are free to use other diagnostic labels. For example, if you are unable to find an appropriate diagnostic label on the list, develop one that is specific for the client. REMEMBER: NANDA's list of approved diagnostic labels was originated by nurses who developed them based on their client's specific data.

Examples of nursing diagnoses related to drug therapy include the following:

- High risk for injury related to side effects of drug such as dizziness and drowsiness.
- Altered thought processes related to effects of drugs on central nervous system.
- Knowledge deficit regarding drug action, administration techniques, and undesired clinical responses related to language difficulties.
- Altered nutrition: less than body requirement related to side effects from drug (nausea, vomiting, anorexia).
- Noncompliance with drug therapy related to lack of funds to purchase drugs.
- Self-esteem disturbance related to need for long-term drug therapy.

DEVELOPING THE PLAN OF CARE

The plan of care includes teaching or discharge preparations and expected outcomes. To reduce drug error and enhance drug compliance, develop the teaching plan and begin your teaching as soon as possible. Make certain you have the most current information about the drugs. If in doubt, check a recent pharmacology reference or consult with the pharmacist. Tailor the plan to meet the client's interests and level of understanding. Review of the assessment data should provide clues about these aspects. In addition, ask yourself: "What does the client need to know?" "What psychomotor skills does the client need to maintain health?" and "What environmental barriers might prevent the client's performing desired behaviors?"

Learning requires motivation. **Motivation** describes what directs the individual's actions. If this aspect was not assessed previously, you must assess the client's motivation to learn before continuing with the teaching plan. Many environmental and personal factors affect the client's behavior and therefore learning (Fig. 8–2). Also assess the client's **developmental**

NANDA-APPROVED NURSING DIAGNOSTIC LABELS

Activity intolerance

Activity intolerance, high risk for

Adjustment, impaired

Airway clearance, ineffective

Alcohol drinking patterns, dysfunctional*

Anxiety

Aspiration, high risk for

Body image disturbance

Body temperature, high risk for altered

Breastfeeding, effective

Breastfeeding, ineffective

Breastfeeding, interrupted

Breathing pattern, ineffective

Caregiver role strain

Caregiver role strain, high risk for

Communication, impaired verbal

Community coping, ineffective*

Community coping, potential for enhanced*

Confusion, acute*

Constipation

Constipation, colonic

Constipation, perceived

Decisional conflict (specify)

Decreased cardiac output

Defensive coping

Denial, ineffective

Diarrhea

Disuse syndrome, high risk for

Diversional activity deficit

Dysfunctional ventilatory weaning response

Dysreflexia

Environmental interpretation syndrome, impaired*

Family coping: compromised, ineffective

Family coping: disabling, ineffective

Family coping: potential for growth

Family processes, altered

Family processes: addictive behavior (individual and family), altered*

Fatigue

Fear

Fluid volume deficit

Fluid volume deficit, high risk for

Fluid volume excess

Gas exchange, impaired

Grieving, anticipatory

Grieving, dysfunctional

Growth and development, altered

Health maintenance, altered

Health seeking behaviors (specify)

Home maintenance management, impaired

Hopelessness

Hyperthermia

Hypothermia

Incontinence, bowel

Incontinence, functional

Incontinence, idiopathic fecal*

Incontinence, reflex

Incontinence, stress

Incontinence, total

Incontinence, urge

Individual coping, ineffective

Infant behavior, disorganized*

Infant behavior, high risk for disorganized*

Infant behavior, potential for enhanced organized*

Infant feeding pattern, ineffective

Infection, high risk for

Injury, high risk for

Knowledge deficit (specify)

Loneliness, high risk for*

Management of therapeutic regimen (individuals), ineffective

Management of therapeutic regimen (families), ineffective*

Noncompliance (specify)

Nutrition: less than body requirements, altered

Nutrition: more than body requirements, altered

Nutrition: potential for more than body requirements, altered

Oral mucous membrane, altered

Pain

Pain, chronic

Pain, labor*

Continued on following page.

NANDA-APPROVED NURSING DIAGNOSTIC LABELS CONTINUED

Parental role conflict

Parent/infant attachment, altered*

Parenting, altered

Parenting, high risk for altered

Peripheral neurovascular dysfunction, high risk for

Personal identity disturbance

Physical mobility, impaired

Poisoning, high risk for

Post-trauma response

Powerlessness

Preservation/quality of life, alteration in*

Protection, altered

Rape-trauma syndrome

Rape-trauma syndrome: compound reaction

Rape-trauma syndrome: silent reaction

Relocation stress syndrome

Role performance, altered

Self-care deficit

    Bathing/hygiene

    Dressing/grooming

    Feeding

    Medication administration*

    Toileting

Self-esteem, chronic low

Self-esteem, situational low

Self-esteem, disturbance

Sensory/perceptual alterations (specify) (visual, auditory, kinesthetic, gustatory, tactile, olfactory)

Self-mutilation, high risk for

Sexual dysfunction

Sexuality patterns, altered

Skin integrity, impaired

Skin integrity, high risk for impaired

Skin integrity: pressure ulcer, high risk for impaired*

Sleep pattern disturbance

Social interaction, impaired

Social isolation

Spasticity*

Spiritual distress

Spiritual well being, opportunity for enhanced*

Suffocation, high risk for

Sustain spontaneous ventilation, inability to

Swallowing, impaired

Terminal illness response*

Thermoregulation, ineffective

Thought processes, altered

Tissue integrity, impaired

Tissue perfusion, altered (specify type) (renal, cerebral, cardiopulmonary, gastrointestinal, peripheral)

Trauma, high risk for

Unilateral neglect

Urinary elimination, altered

Urinary filtration syndrome, impaired*

Urinary retention

Violence, high risk for: self-directed or directed at others

From *NANDA Nursing Diagnoses and Classification* 1992–1993. Philadelphia: North American Nursing Diagnosis Association.
*1994 diagnoses in progress.

level since it influences readiness to learn, and readiness to learn depends on maturation. Therefore knowledge of the client's state of development enables you to develop a relevant and individualized teaching plan. A number of theoretic frameworks are available for assessing development. For example, Erikson's eight stages of man present the developmental tasks for each age group, which include normal expectations in the areas of motor control, cognitive functions, and expression of feelings. Piaget's theory can help in evaluating the client's cognitive development. This theory affects how you teach since thinking changes according to chronologic age.

Basic information that belongs in the **teaching plan** includes the following[2,3]:

- Brand and generic name of drug
- Desired actions and therapeutic effects
- Drug dose and time schedule for administration
- Administration techniques (e.g., take drug with food; take drug on an empty stomach)
- Appropriate actions if drug dose is missed
- Effects on body (e.g., change in color of stool or urine)
- Undesired clinical responses
- Appropriate actions if undesired responses occur

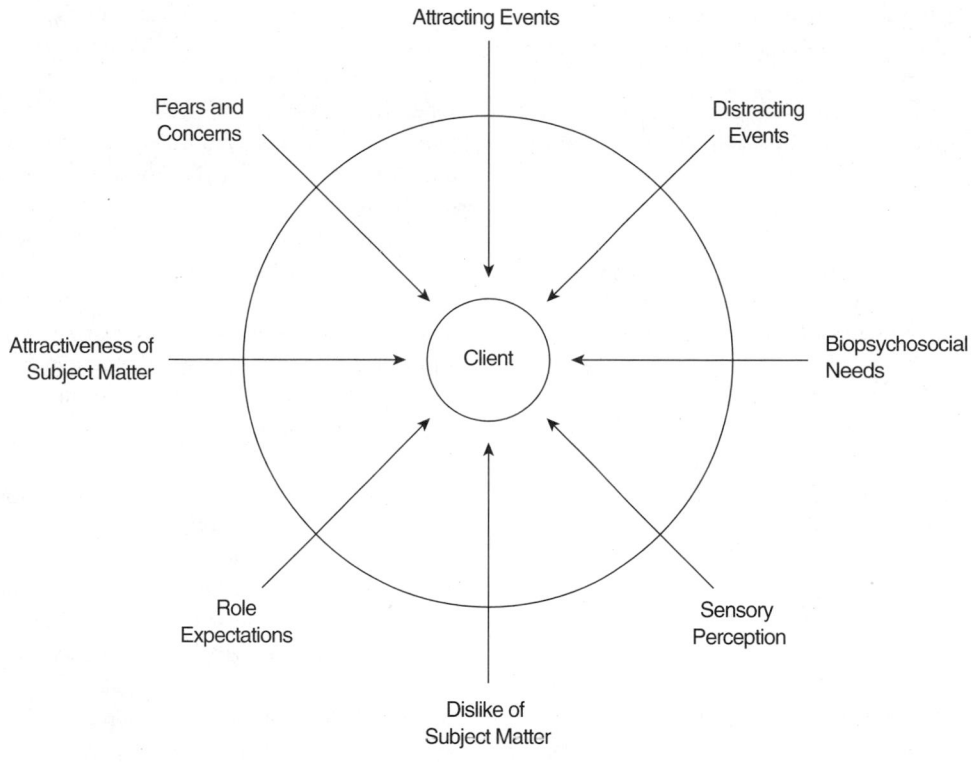

FIGURE 8–2   Environmental and personal factors affecting learning behavior.

- Anticipated length of drug therapy
- Activities to avoid (e.g., do not drive or operate machinery)
- Potential drug-drug, drug-nutrient, and drug-environment interactions

Include information about the impact of OTC drugs such as vitamins, laxatives, and minor analgesics and the need to contact the primary care provider or pharmacist before taking any new drug. Incorporate into the plan safety reminders and information on proper drug storage:

- Keep all drugs in original labeled containers
- Discard drugs no longer being used (i.e., old prescription drugs) or OTC drugs inappropriate in the current situation
- Protect drugs from excessive heat, light, and moisture (e.g., do not store drugs above a stove or sink or in a window)
- Store drugs out of reach of children and pets
- Store drugs for other family members in a separate place to prevent inadvertently taking the wrong drug
- Develop a list of drugs being taken
- Distribute the drug list to all health care providers to decrease the risk of drug-drug interactions

The plan of care must also address the issue of client **compliance.** Compliance begins with the client's being able to read and understand the instructions on the drug container. Data that appear on the original prescription are transferred to the label on the container (Fig. 8–3). The pharmacist also places on the container stickers that provide specific administration directions (e.g., "Drink at least one glass of water with each dose"). Teaching the client how to interpret this information increases drug therapy compliance.

Having a realistic schedule for drug administration increases the likelihood of compliance with drug therapy. (Before suggesting adjustments in the drug schedule, consult with the primary care provider or pharmacist.) Sometimes more drugs can be administered at the same time. For example, drugs taken once daily could be administered at one time in the morning instead of at different times throughout the day. Normal client mealtimes, bedtime, and waking time are important considerations. Do not arbitrarily schedule a drug for 8 AM if the client does not usually awaken until 10 AM. Drugs may also be scheduled according to times that are significant to the client and easy for him or her to remember. For example, if the client has an establshed daily pattern (i.e., awaken at 6 AM, drive to work at 7:30 AM, take a break at 10:30 AM), schedule drug administration to fit that schedule.

NURSING RESEARCH

Conn, V., Taylor, S., & Kelley, S. (1991). Medication regimen complexity and adherence among older adults. *IMAGE: Journal of Nursing Scholarship, 23,* 231-235.

The purpose of this study was to examine the relationship between medication regimen complexity and adherence among older adults recently discharged from hospitals (N = 178) and those not recently hospitalized (N = 98). Medication regimen complexity was measured using the Medication Complexity Index, which measures number, frequency, and types of activities required to execute the drug regimen. Adherence to the regimen was based on pill count and verbal self-report by the subjects.

The negative correlations between drug regimen complexity and adherence were in the predicted direction but did not achieve statistical significance. Relatively high adherence scores were reported by these subjects compared to those in some other reported research. Researchers suggest that future research should investigate the relationship between medication regimen complexity and other aspects of drug management.

STUDENT ACTIVITIES

- Conduct a ministudy on medication regimen complexity and adherence. Interview 10 nonhospitalized subjects over the age of 65 years. Determine their current drug usage and identify factors that they perceive complicate the drug regimen. Determine if these individuals ever fail to comply with their drug regimen. If so, question them about the reasons for not complying.
- Using these same individuals, determine the amount and type of teaching that each client had before beginning the current drug regimen.

Administration systems also facilitate compliance. The system is developed specifically for the client, based on his or her individual situation. It should be accessible, inexpensive, and easy to use. Commercial pill containers with individual compartments for drugs are available. These compartments are la-

beled with times of day and days of the week. Egg cartons or envelopes are less expensive versions of this system; these containers can also be labeled by times of day and days of the week. (Disadvantage of all these methods is that they require removing the drugs from the original container.) Other methods include charts that list the drugs and the times to take them. The charts may be color coded to facilitate remembering and may have a place to check off doses as they are taken.

Recognition of the client's basic needs also contributes to compliance. If the client has unmet needs for food, clothing, or shelter, he or she may not see a particular drug regimen as a priority. You may need to connect the family with resources to meet these needs before the client or family can move on to complying with the drug treatment.

Once you know what you need to teach and the client's willingness and ability to learn, decide on appropriate **teaching techniques** or **strategies.** Include in the teaching plan a variety of instructional techniques to facilitate learning and enhance the retention of information. Schedule teaching sessions when the client is most receptive to learning. In some situations it may be necessary to involve a family member or friend in the sessions. Learning is usually more effective when the client is active rather than passive in the teaching-learning process. Demonstrations, practice sessions, and return demonstrations give the client the opportunity to be an active learner. Providing the client immediate feedback and making him or her aware of progress encourages him or her and facilitates learning. Always allow time for questions and discussions of concerns.

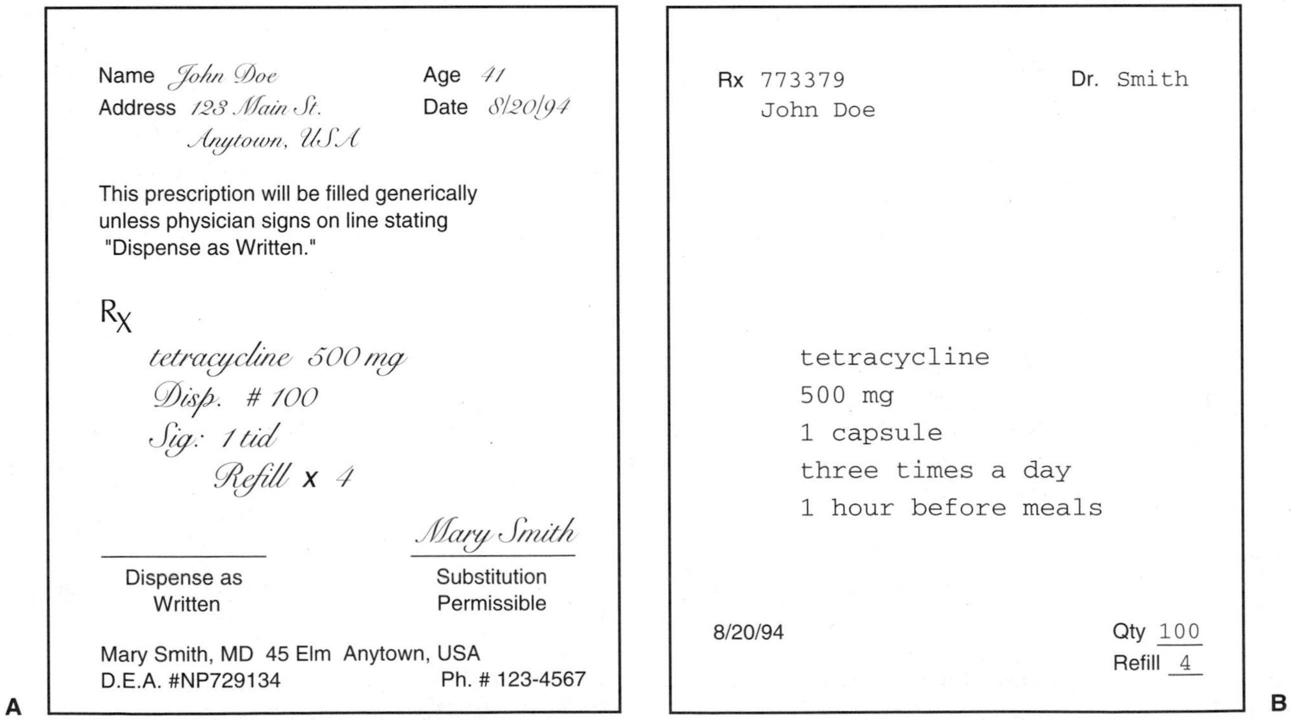

FIGURE 8–3   Information from the prescription **(A)** written by the primary care provider is transferred to the drug container label **(B).**

The use of literature to supplement and reinforce verbal teaching is recommended. Information is available from a variety of professional, consumer, and government groups. For example, the National Council on Patient Information and Education, a nonprofit organization, is an excellent source for both literature and referrals.[4]

Always review literature for accuracy and appropriateness before dispensing to the client. When reviewing the material, consider the reading level required to understand the material.[5]

Drug cards are helpful when teaching the client about drug therapy. These cards are tailored to meet the needs of the client and might include the name of the drug, the reason for taking the drug, the dose to be taken, the time of day to take the drug, and the possible side effects of the drug. Also consider including hints on administering the drug (e.g., do not crush the tablet; take with an 8-ounce glass of water).

Before the plan of care is complete, identify **expected outcomes** for the teaching. What behavior must the client display to validate that learning has occurred? What is the desired response to the nursing intervention (teaching)? Expected outcomes usually contain the following:

- A description of the change, specific behavior, or response that must be evident as a result of the nursing action
- A statement defining the limits of acceptable behavior or performance

---

CONCEPT REVIEW

After the database is complete, the data are analyzed and nursing diagnoses developed. A nursing diagnosis is a two-part statement that describes the client's response and the contributing factors for that response.

During the planning phase a plan of care is developed. It provides a guide for the actual care that is to follow. The plan includes information on the teaching needs of the client and expected outcomes.

IMPLEMENTING THE PLAN OF CARE

This phase of the nursing process includes the nursing activity necessary to implement the nursing and medical plans of care. If you are the nurse administering the drug, your first responsibility is to determine if the prescribed drug is accurate as to route, dose, dosage form, and frequency of administration. If you do not know this information, check a reference before preparing the drug. In addition, you are responsible for knowing the pharmacologic action, desired clinical response, contraindications and precautions, and undesired clinical responses of all drugs you administer. Possible drug interactions and allergies of the client must also be considered before the drug is administered.

Preparing the Drug

Once you have determined that the various parameters of the drug prescription are correct, prepare the drug for administration. A general guide to use in drug administration is the "five rights": right drug, right dose, right client, right time, and right route of administration.[6]

Right drug   Always read the label three times: when selecting the drug (container or unit-dose pack), when removing the drug from the container, and when returning the container to its storage place or before discarding the unit-dose packaging. Never use a drug from a container that is unlabeled. Use special care when administering drugs with similar names (e.g., Coumadin, coumarin). If the drug is in a unit-dose pack, keep the dose packaged until immediately before administering it.

Right dose   Determining the correct dose of a drug is sometimes difficult because three systems of measurement are used in prescribing drugs: metric, apothecary, and household. Although the metric system is gradually replacing the apothecary system in the United States, you must be familiar with all three systems and be able to convert from one system to another.

Usually drugs are supplied in the required dosage, making dose calculation unnecessary. However, if dosage calculation is needed, several calculation methods are available. Perhaps the most popular and most basic formula is:

$$\frac{D}{H} \times V = \text{Amount to give}$$

D symbolizes the desired dose (the dose prescribed by the primary care provider); V is the vehicle or form and amount in which the drug is supplied (e.g., tablet, capsule); and H, or on-hand dose, is the drug dose on the label container.

Basic Formula

Order: tetracycline, 1000 g PO
Available: tetracycline, 250-mg capsule

$$\text{Formula: } \frac{1000}{250} \times 1 \text{ capsule} = 4$$

Another method for calculating drug doses is ratio and proportion:

$$\text{H:V::D:X.}$$

The H and V on the left side of the equation are the known quantities, dose on-hand and vehicle. D and X on the right side of the equation are the desired dose and the unknown amount to give. To determine X, multiply the means (V and D) and the extremes (H and X).

Ratio and Proportion

Order: tetracycline, 1000 g PO
Available: tetracycline, 250-mg capsule
Formula: 250:1::1000:X
250X = 1000
X = 4 capsules

Drug doses for pediatric and elderly clients are frequently provided in official sources of drug information. In Chapter 14, *Drug Therapy in the Neonate and Pediatric Client,* formulas for calculating doses according to body surface area and weight are explained. These dosage guidelines should be available at all nursing stations, crash carts, outpatient clinics, and emergency departments.

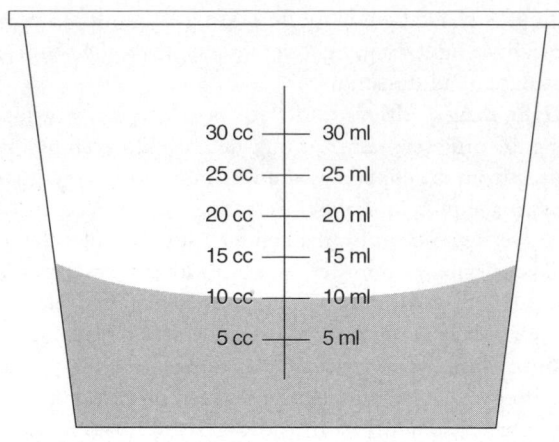

FIGURE 8–4   Measuring liquids. Always measure the volume of a liquid at the lowest point of the meniscus. This medicine glass or cup contains 10 ml of liquid.

Once the dose is calculated, it must be correctly measured. Depending on the dose, liquid dosage forms for oral administration are measured with medicine glasses or cups, droppers, and syringes. Most medicine glasses have measurements for all three systems of measurement. Select the proper measurement system and pour the medication. Always measure the volume of a liquid medicine at the lowest point of the meniscus (Fig. 8–4). Some drugs are measured with a calibrated dropper. To ensure the proper dosage, hold the dropper vertically while squeezing the bulb. Insert the tip of the dropper in the liquid and slowly release the bulb; the liquid is drawn up into the dropper. In some instances, small oral doses are also measured in calibrated needleless syringes.

Sterile needles and syringes are used to measure and administer drugs for parenteral injections. Different types of syringes are available (e.g., tuberculin, insulin, general purpose). These syringes vary in size (e.g., 1, 3, 5, 20, and 50 ml) and in calibrations, minims (0.01 ml), units, and milliliters. Parenteral drugs for injections are supplied in multiple- and single-dose vials and ampules.

🌿 NURSING RESEARCH

Bindler, R., & Bayne, T. (1991). Medication calculation ability of registered nurses. *IMAGE: Journal of Nursing Scholarship, 23,* 221-224.

The purpose of this study was to investigate errors in drug calculation that contribute to medication errors. A convenience sample of 110 registered nurses in four western states completed a demographic questionnaire and a 20-item drug calculation test. The test assessed mathematical calculating ability rather than clinical decision making. A short conversion table was attached to the examination.

Test scores ranged from 20% to 100% correct. The modal score was 80%. Eighty-one percent of the sub-

jects were unable to calculate doses correctly 90% of the time, and 43.6% of the subjects' test scores were below 70% accuracy.

STUDENT ACTIVITIES

• Determine if drug calculation tests are administered to new employees at your assigned agency.
• Interview a nurse from the quality assurance or risk management department to learn if drug calculation affects medication errors at this agency.
• Request permission to administer a drug calculation test to nurses at your assigned agency.   🌿

Right client   Once the drug is properly prepared, the next step is to administer it to the right client. Use every means of identification available. Call the individual by name, and check the client's wrist identification band. If the client is in bed, check the identification tag on the bed. If the client is physically able, ask him or her to state his or her name. If you are caring for a child and the parent or caregiver is present, ask the parent or caregiver to tell you the child's name. Explain to the client what you are doing. If the client questions the appearance, dosage, time, or method of drug administration, always recheck the order before administering the dose.

Right time   The written order for the drug specifies the number of times per day to administer the drug. In some instances the order may state the exact hours of administration or give general guidelines such as "administer before meals" or "administer 1 hour after meals." If the exact time is not indicated, drug administration usually follows a schedule established by the agency.

To be most effective, drug schedules should be based on knowledge of the desired effect of the drug, characteristics of the drug, possible interactions with other drugs, and the client's daily schedule. Once a schedule is established, it is important to adhere to it. As a rule, administer drugs within ½ hour of the scheduled time. This is especially important for drugs such as antimicrobial agents that must maintain a constant serum concentration level.

Right route of administration   Be certain you know the prescribed route for the drug and that the route is compatible with the drug's properties. The individual writing the prescription should indicate the desired route of administration. If a route is not specified, check with the prescriber for clarification.

As discussed in Chapter 3, numerous routes are used for drug administration: oral, enteral, parenteral, and topical. Some drugs can be administered by only one route. However, many drugs are available in a variety of dosage forms, permitting administration by more than one route.

Drugs administered orally must be followed with sufficient fluids to ensure that the drug enters the stomach. In general, it is recommended that the client drink at least 100 ml of liquid with oral tablets or capsules. These fluids also enhance the drug's absorption and effectiveness. In addition, it is recommended that everyone drink at least 2 L of water daily to replace lost body water. In some situations properties of the drug require that the client drink additional quantities of water. Therefore specific directions such as "drink 10 to 12 glasses of water daily" must be followed carefully.

To enhance absorption or prevent gastric upset, constipation, or diarrhea, some oral drugs are best administered with food. Other drugs must be given on an empty stomach. You may need to mix liquid dosage forms with fruit juices to mask unpleasant tastes or to prevent harming or staining the teeth. (As you progress through the text, specific nursing measures related to administration of each prototype drug or drug category are presented.)

Parenteral drug administration techniques vary according to site of injection or infusion, properties of the drug, and characteristics of the client. Two aspects that must be considered are selection of appropriate needle and syringe and determination of proper injection site. Needles are available in various gauges and lengths. The term **needle gauge** refers to the diameter of the lumen; larger gauge numbers indicate smaller lumen diameters. The usual range of needle gauges is from 18 to 27. **Needle lengths** usually vary from $\frac{3}{8}$ to 2 inches. Table 8–1 lists needle lengths and gauges for subcutaneous, intramuscular, and intradermal injections.

Type of injection, drug properties, and characteristics of the client also determine injection site and angle and volume of drug administered. **Intradermal injections** are usually administered in the inner aspect of the forearm. Care must be taken that the drug is *not* inadvertently administered into the subcutaneous tissue. The needle is inserted at a 10- to 15-degree angle with the bevel upward. Usually only 0.01 to 0.1 ml of isotonic drug solution is injected. **Subcutaneous injections** are administered into fat pads on the abdomen, upper hips, upper back, lateral upper arms, and lateral thighs (Fig. 8–5). The needle is inserted at a 45-, 60-, and 90-degree angle (Fig. 8–6). Usual volume of drug injected is 0.5 to 2 ml in each injection site. **Intramuscular injections** are administered into the ventrogluteal, dorsogluteal, deltoid, and vastus lateralis muscles (Fig. 8–7). The needle is injected into the skin at a 90-degree angle. Usual drug volume administered per injection site is 0.5 to 5 ml, based on the injection site and size of the client (see Fig. 8–6).[8,9]

The **intravenous (IV) route of administration** is used to administer drugs and infuse large volumes of nutrients or replacement fluids. Methods used are IV push, IV piggyback, or IV infusion. All of these methods use a peripheral or central IV line or implanted port. **IV push** or **bolus** involves rapid ad-

ministration of 0.1 to 10 ml of undiluted drug in 30 seconds to 5 minutes. **IV piggyback,** or intermittent infusion, involves infusion of 25 to 100 ml of diluted drugs or 5 to 20 ml of more concentrated drugs in 15 to 60 minutes. Constant and variable-rate infusions involve administering 0.2 to 1000 ml/hour. This method is used for drugs that must be highly diluted, for high-volume hydration and nutrition, and for keep-open vein infusions.[10–12]

Before mixing drugs in the same syringe or administering drugs through existing IV lines, you must determine the compatibility of the agents involved. Several general rules should be kept in mind when assessing the compatibility and stability of two agents:

- Check the pH values of each drug. Drugs with the same pH value are usually compatible.
- Usually if one member of a chemical group is incompatible with another agent, other members of that group will also be incompatible.
- Because of the danger of salts and precipitate formation, minerals such as calcium, magnesium, phosphorus, and bicarbonate should not be mixed or piggybacked to another IV admixture.
- If no information exists about compatibility, separate syringes or IV lines should be used.

Topical drug preparations are applied to the skin, cornea, or mucous membranes of the mouth, oropharynx, nose, rectum, vagina, urethra, or conjunctiva. Administration techniques for most of these routes are discussed in later chapters: rectum (Chapter 14), metered dose inhaler (Chapter 45), cornea and conjunctiva (Chapter 64), and ear (Chapter 65).

Documentation

Documentation, sometimes considered the "sixth right" of drug administration, validates every aspect of your actions from client teaching to administration of the drug. Document your actions immediately. If your actions involved client teaching, record what was taught, methods used in the teaching session, and client response. If you administered a drug, record the name of the drug, dose, route, time, and date and your initials or signature. For injections, note the injection site used. With some drugs (e.g., analgesics, antiemetics, sedatives), you must record the client's response. To assist in accurate recording of drugs administered, most health care agencies use a graphic format. Each setting adapts the graphic to meet its needs.

TABLE 8–1

Needle Length and Gauge Based on Injection Site

Type of Injection	Needle Gauge	Needle Length (Inches)
Intradermal	25, 26, 27	3/8, 1/2, 5/8
Subcutaneous	25, 26, 27 (most common, 25)	3/8, 1/2, 5/8, 7/8 (usually 5/8)
Intramuscular	19, 20, 21, 22 (most common, 20 and 21)	5/8, 1, 1½, 2 (most common, 1½)

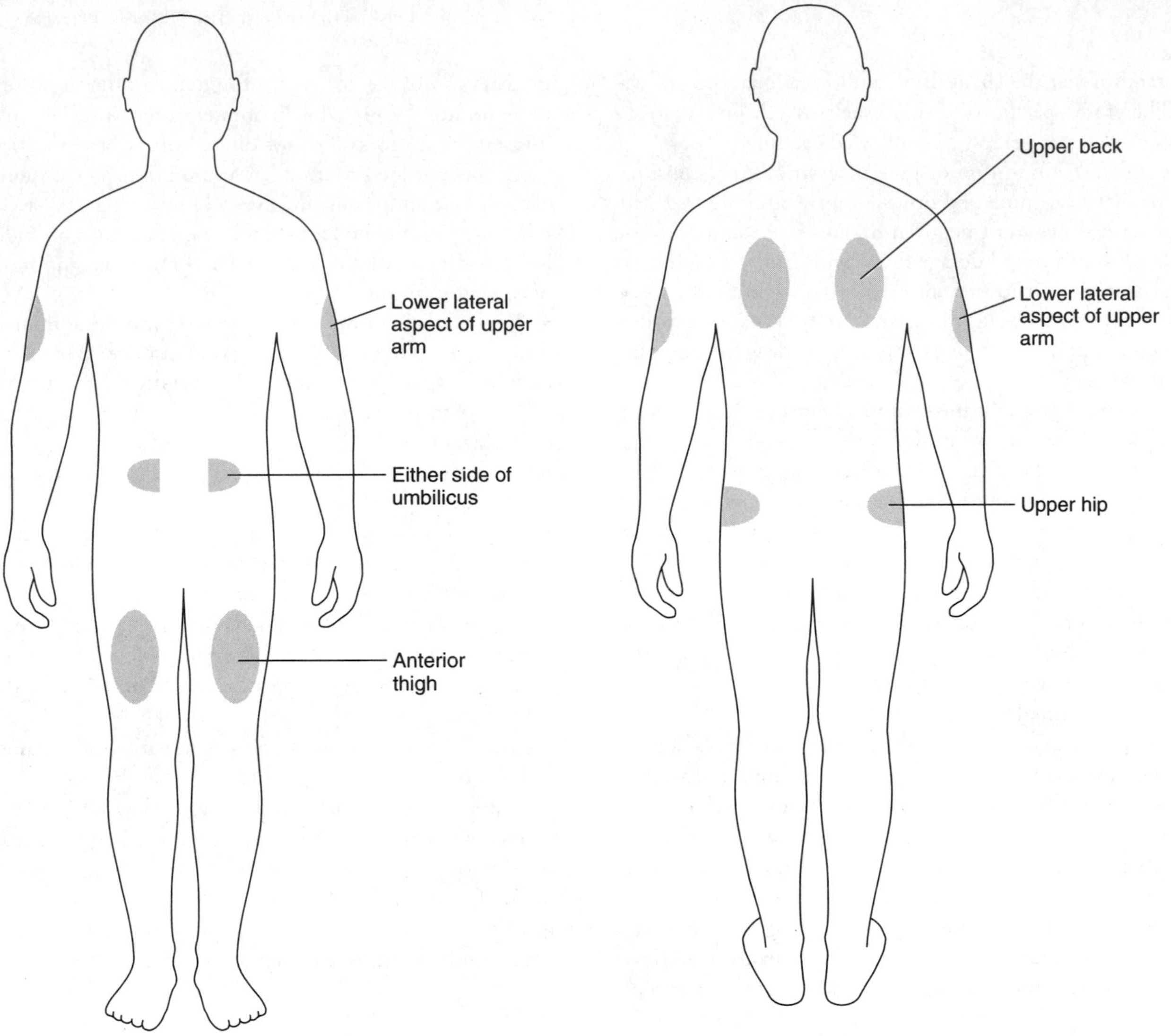

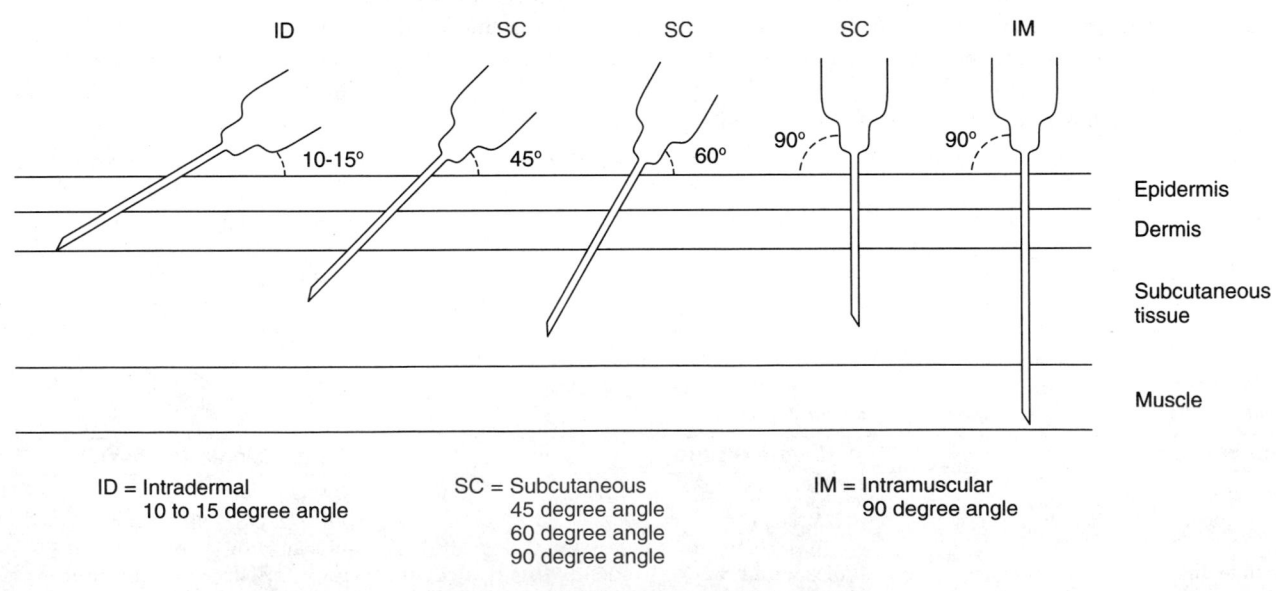

Lower lateral
aspect of upper
arm

Either side of
umbilicus

Anterior
thigh

Upper back

Lower lateral
aspect of upper
arm

Upper hip

FIGURE 8–5   Subcutaneous injection sites.

ID   SC   SC   SC   IM

10-15°   45°   60°   90°   90°

Epidermis

Dermis

Subcutaneous
tissue

Muscle

ID = Intradermal
    10 to 15 degree angle

SC = Subcutaneous
    45 degree angle
    60 degree angle
    90 degree angle

IM = Intramuscular
    90 degree angle

FIGURE 8–6   Angles for injections.

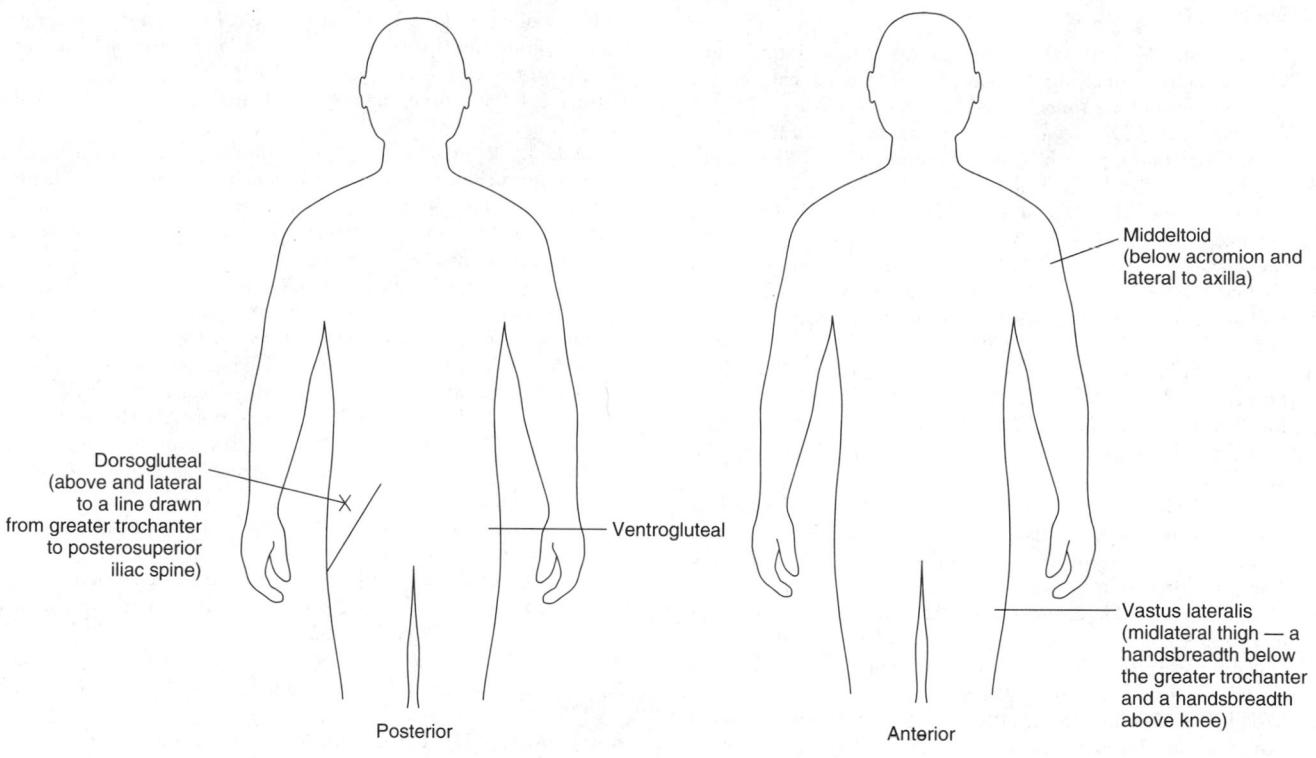

Posterior

Anterior

Dorsogluteal
(above and lateral
to a line drawn
from greater trochanter
to posterosuperior
iliac spine)

Ventrogluteal

Middeltoid
(below acromion and
lateral to axilla)

Vastus lateralis
(midlateral thigh — a
handsbreadth below
the greater trochanter
and a handsbreadth
above knee)

FIGURE 8–7   Intramuscular injection sites.

EVALUATING EFFECTIVENESS OF PLAN OF CARE

In the evaluating phase of the nursing process you assess the client's response to the nursing and medical interventions. Note the client's response to the drug. Is there a change in behavior? Has the blood pressure decreased? Is the pulse rate more regular? Have the signs and symptoms of infection diminished?

You may also request that serum levels be determined for drugs with an established therapeutic or toxic range. Monitor diagnostic studies to determine toxic effect on the liver and kidneys. Toxicity is usually reflected in altered laboratory values such as blood urea nitrogen, serum creatinine, and liver enzyme levels.

Review the plan of care. Are changes needed? Are there additional assessment data that alter the original plan? Are the nursing diagnoses appropriate, or must they be altered? Review expected outcomes for the plan of care. Were they accomplished? Discuss outcomes with the client, and decide if additional time for achievement is needed or if outcomes are not realistic.

CONCEPT REVIEW

The fourth phase is implementing. In this phase you execute the plan of care. This is the action phase of the nursing process. For a client receiving drug therapy, implementing focuses on the five rights.

The last phase is evaluating—you determine the effectiveness of the plan of care and document the client's response. Evaluation may lead to redefining the nursing diagnoses and redevelopment of the plan of care.

SUMMARY

The nursing process, which consists of five steps or phases—assessing, diagnosing, planning, implementing, and evaluating—is flexible and adaptable. It provides an organized, systematic method for examining the client's health status, identifying the client's needs, and determining appropriate solutions to meet these needs.

REFERENCES

1. McPherson, M. (1989). Drugs and dietary interactions: Guidelines for counseling the home health care patient. *Journal of Home Health Care Practice, 1*(4), 27-37.
2. Azzarello, J. (1989). Reviewing your patient's medication regimen: A systemic approach. *Home Healthcare Nurse, 7*(6), 24-26.
3. Conn, V., Taylor, S., & Kelley, S. (1991). Medication regimen complexity and adherence among older adults. *IMAGE: Journal of Nursing Scholarship, 23,* 231-235.
4. Merkatz, R., & Couig, M.P. (1992). Helping America take its medicine. *American Journal of Nursing, 92*(6), 56-60, 62.
5. McLaughlin, G. (1969). SMOG grading: A new readability formula. *Journal of Reading, 12,* 639-646.
6. Sullivan, G.H. (1991). Five "rights" equal 0 errors . . . medication errors. *RN, 54*(6), 65-66, 68.
7. Bindler, R., & Bayne, T. (1991). Medication calculation ability of registered nurses. *IMAGE: Journal of Nursing Scholarship, 23,* 221-224.
8. Kee, J., & Marshall, S. (1992). *Clinical calculations with applications to general and specialty areas.* Philadelphia: W.B. Saunders.
9. Newton, M., Newton, D., & Fudin, J. (1992). Reviewing the "big three" injection routes. *Nursing '92, 22*(2), 34-41.
10. Dick, M., Maree, S., & Gray, J. (1992). How to boost the odds of a painless IV start. *American Journal of Nursing, 92*(6), 49-51.
11. Millam, D. (1993). How to teach good venipuncture technique. *American Journal of Nursing, 93*(7), 38-41.
12. Wood, L.S., & Gullo, S.M. (1993). IV vesicants: How to avoid extravasation. *American Journal of Nursing, 93*(4), 42-46.

BIBLIOGRAPHY

Blais, K., & Bath, J.B. (1992). Drug calculation errors of baccalaureate nursing students. *Nurse Educator, 17*(1), 12-14.
Cohen, M.R. (1992). Even night drug cabinet can cause problems. *Nursing '92, 22*(7), 9.
Collins-Colon, T. (1990). Do it yourself: Medication management for community based clients. *Journal of Psychosocial Nursing & Mental Health Services, 28*(6), 25-29, 34-35.
Gibson, J. (1989). A new approach to better medication compliance. *Nursing, 19*(4), 49-51.
Hanisak, J., & Shaw, H.L. (1991). Similar packaging for heparin, potassium chloride, and 1% lidocaine by one drug manufacturer causes concern. *Journal of Emergency Nursing, 17,* 367-368.
Heath, S., & McArthur, J. (1991). Risk management: Reducing the incidence of medication errors. *The Provider, 16,* 30-35.
Lee, L., Wellman, G.S., Birdwell, S.W., & Sherrin, T.P. (1992). Use of an automated medication storage and distribution system. *American Journal of Hospital Pharmacy, 49,* 851-855.
Lehman, S., & Barber, J.R. (1991). Giving medication by feeding tube: How to avoid problems. *Nursing '91, 21*(11), 58-61.
Ludwig-Beymer, P., Czurylo, K.T., Gattuso, M.C., Hennessy, K.A., & Ryan, C.J. (1990). The effect of testing on the reported incidence of medication errors in a medical center. *Journal of Continuing Education in Nursing, 21*(1), 11-17.
Murphy, J. (1991). Reducing the pain of intramuscular (IM) injections. *Advancing Clinical Care, 6*(4), 35.
Powers, J.E., & Cascella, P.J. (1990). Comparison of methods used to prepare tablets for nasogastric tube administration. *Journal of Pharmacy Technology, 6,* 60-62.
Rein, A., Tiburzi, T., & Parks, V. (1992). Comparison of technologies in medication administration. *Nursing Economics, 10,* 233-235.
Ross, F.M. (1989). Doctor, nurse and patient knowledge of prescribed medication in primary care. *Public Health, 103,* 131-137.
Smith, L.S. (1990). Those medication error dilemmas! *Advancing Clinical Care, 5*(5), 50-51.
Walters, J.A., Puetz, C., Sala, S.M., Hanson, K., et al. (1992). Developing and implanting a tool to measure severity of medication errors. *Journal of Nursing Care Quality, 6*(4), 33-43.
Wilkinson, R. (1991). The challenge of intravenous therapy. *Nursing Standard, 5*(28), 24-27.

The Individual and Drug Therapy

CHAPTER 9

 Cultural Influence on Drug Therapy

MYRNA BRENNER WACKER

❋ Concepts Relevant to Culture

LEARNING OBJECTIVES:
Define terms relevant to culture.
Explain the concepts culture shock, acculturation, and ethnocentrism.
Differentiate between the terms *culture* and *ethnicity*.
KEY TERMS:
Acculturation, culture, culture shock, ethnicity, ethnocentrism, stereotyping, transcultural nursing

❋ Cultural and Ethnic Implications Related to Drug Therapy

LEARNING OBJECTIVES:
Describe the influence of culture on drug therapy.
Discuss the influence of ethnicity on drug therapy.

❋ Role of the Nurse

LEARNING OBJECTIVE: Incorporate culturally appropriate nursing measures into a client's drug therapy program.

❋ Specific Cultural Variations Affecting Drug Therapy

LEARNING OBJECTIVE: Identify specific cultural variations that affect drug therapy.

CONCEPTS AND TERMS TO REVIEW

Review content on self-medication in Chapter 11.
Review content on the effects of ethnic background on pharmacokinetics, pharmacodynamics, and individual response to drugs (Chapters 4–6).

---

*I*mmigration into the United States is on the rise, and each ethnic group brings with it a unique set of values that influences health practices and beliefs. This influx of immigrants, along with the current pluralistic society, makes it essential for nurses to understand and adapt culturally sensitive approaches to clinical care. In an attempt to address this aspect of nursing, Leininger[1] developed the concept of **transcultural nursing.** Transcultural nursing is a formal area of study and practice focused on the cultural beliefs, values, and lifeways of diverse cultures. It also includes the use of this knowledge to provide culturally specific or culturally universal care to individuals, families, and groups of particular cultures.

This chapter presents some of the cultural and ethnic factors that influence drug therapy. The role of the nurse is described and specific cultural and ethnic variations summarized. It is always important not to stereotype when considering groups of individuals. Not everyone within a group may accept or follow all of the practices of that group. Therefore use the information in this chapter as a guide for planning individualized nursing care.

CONCEPTS RELEVANT TO CULTURE

Culture describes nonphysical characteristics such as beliefs, customs, values, norms, behavioral patterns, and lifestyle practices shared by a group. These characteristics, which guide the members of the group in their thinking and actions, are socially transmitted from one generation to the next. Although some individuals interchange the words *ethnicity* and *culture,* they are not synonymous. **Ethnicity** describes common biologic and/or physical characteristics of a group of people. Ethnic differences include skin color, hair color, shape of eyes, race, language, and dialect.[2] An individual is born into an ethnic group but may adopt characteristics from other ethnic groups' culture.

Culture Shock

When an individual encounters a new culture, feelings of bewilderment, confusion, disorganization, and frustration are common. The individual may feel unable to adapt to differences in language, word meanings, activities, time, and customs that are part of the new culture. This experience is called **culture shock.**[3]

Acculturation

The process of changing one's cultural patterns to those of the host society is called **acculturation.**[4] The degree or amount of individual acculturation is a crucial factor in the study of culture. Some individuals are absorbed more rapidly into the mainstream of the dominant culture. Other individuals never assimilate components of the dominant culture. Factors that influence acculturation are social class, length of time in the dominant culture, degree of identity with either culture, value orientation, and contact with cultural transmitters such as the elderly or media.

Ethnocentrism of Nurses

As previously indicated, nurses must meet the challenge of providing nursing care that is culturally sensitive and appropriate. Too often nurses are ethnocentric in their approach to health care delivery. (**Ethnocentrism** is the belief that one's own cultural practices and beliefs are superior to others.[5]) When care is approached in this manner, nurses may attempt to impose their cultural beliefs on the clients. In addition, the personal value system of the nurse may put him or her in conflict with cultures that do not reflect that system.

Some nurses do not feel confident in caring for the culturally diverse. Schools of nursing, facing the need to provide large quantities of technical information, may not adequately prepare students to give care to clients from different cultures. Decreased confidence and lack of knowledge may cause the nurse to stereotype individuals from different cultural or ethnic groups. **Stereotyping** prevents recognition of individual differences, and everyone from a particular culture is viewed as the same.

CULTURAL AND ETHNIC FACTORS INFLUENCING DRUG THERAPY

All aspects of an individual's cultural and ethnic background influence drug therapy. However, for purposes of this discussion, five areas are considered: biologic characteristics, health/illness values and beliefs, self-treatment, dietary patterns, and response to service.

Biologic Characteristics

Previous chapters noted that the pharmacokinetic and pharmacodynamic phases were influenced by an individual's ethnic origin. (See Chapters 4 through 6 for additional information on the influence of ethnicity on drug therapy.) In addition, susceptibility to disease varies among ethnic groups. For example, African-Americans and Native Americans are especially susceptible to tuberculosis; Hispanics and Native Americans are especially susceptible to diabetes; and individuals from Asia Minor, India, the Mediterranean, and the Caribbean and African-Americans are especially susceptible to sickle cell anemia.[2,6]

Health and Illness Values and Beliefs

Since culture is the frame of reference or design by which individuals live their lives, it has an eminent effect on how health and illness are perceived. These perceptions, based on cultural values and beliefs, result in actions. For example, definitions of health vary between the United States and Third World countries. Individuals considered healthy in a Third World country may be considered ill in the United States.

Beliefs about disease prevention and health promotion also vary among countries. These beliefs influence whether or not an individual believes these activities are valuable. Values and beliefs also influence drug treatment. For example, the general belief in the United States is that people should not have to endure pain. This belief leads to the use of over-the-counter (OTC) drugs for minor discomfort that may be ignored in other cultures.

Self-treatment

In some cultures the beliefs about prevention and treatment of illness are outside the realm of modern scientific medicine. For example, many Hispanics believe in the hot-and-cold theory. This theory categorizes diseases and treatments as "hot" or "cold." The treatment goal is a balance of the two states. For example, penicillin, a hot drug, would be inappropriate for a hot condition such as a fever. However, acetylsalicylic acid, aspirin, a hot drug, could be used for the treatment of arthritis, a cold condition. Adherence to these and similar beliefs may lead to noncompliance with prescribed drug therapy.

Natural folk medicine is widely practiced in the United States. This form of prevention or treatment includes remedies that have been passed down for generations. The remedies use herbs, plants, minerals, or other natural substances. For example, extensive use of natural substances such as ginseng (a perennial plant with a thick, aromatic root) occurs in Chinese cultures. Eating raw garlic or wearing garlic on the body to prevent illness is another example of natural folk medicine. (See Chapter 11 for more information on self-medication and self-treatment.)

Self-treatment also includes the use of healers, healing ceremonies, or protective objects. Many cultures have individuals in their communities who are designated as healers. These individuals perform ceremonies meant to correct different health problems. For example, the medicine man is the traditional healer of Native Americans. In some cultures protective objectives such as religious medals, charms, and trinkets are worn or hung in the home to prevent illness and harm.

Dietary Patterns

Dietary patterns are another facet of culture that can affect drug therapy. Interaction of food and drugs can either alter the effect of the drug or alter the nutritional effect of the food. (See Chapter 7 for more information on drug-nutrient interactions.) For example, diets high in sodium chloride such as the diets of African-Americans or the Japanese can adversely affect individuals receiving drug therapy for hypertension.

Response to Service

Beliefs about communication, time orientation, space, privacy, locus of control, and family influence the individual's response to the nurse and health care system. **Communication** is the key to the therapeutic nurse-client relationship. Verbal and nonverbal communication techniques such as language, touch, gestures, facial expressions, and eye contact differ considerably among cultures. Inappropriate use of these techniques diminishes the effectiveness of the nurse-client relationship and ultimately affects adherence to drug therapy.

Personal space involves an individual's feelings toward the space around himself or herself. These feelings are influenced by culture. In fact, different cultural or ethnic groups have varying norms and definitions associated with the space. Being sensitive to the client's attitudes toward personal space is important. In addition, some cultures are much more modest than others about parts of their bodies and body function. This need for **privacy** can interfere with drug treatments and assessments, particularly in a hospital setting.

Time orientation also varies among cultures. The concept of absolute time with reliance on a clock is foreign to many cultures. In some cultures punctuality is not valued. This creates a problem when specific timing of drug dosages is essential. Time orientation difference may also become important in long-term planning of health care.

Clients whose culture generally demonstrates an external **locus of control** may have problems exhibiting self-care behaviors. These individuals are not experienced in decision making, and they may lack the confidence to administer and monitor their drug regimen. Finally, the **family role** varies significantly among cultures. In some cultures, care cannot proceed without the approval of the dominant group or member.

CONCEPT REVIEW

The nurse must learn to avoid ethnocentrism in relating to clients.

In assessing the client, the nurse must consider biologic characteristics, health and illness values and beliefs, self-treatment, dietary patterns, and response to service.

▦ NURSING CONSIDERATIONS

To function effectively as a nurse, it is crucial that you develop a trusting relationship with the client and family. To do this, you must understand your own values and beliefs and be willing to learn about other cultures.

Assessing   An accurate, comprehensive assessment is essential for determining effective nursing interventions. Several cultural assessment tools or guides are available (Fig. 9–1). References for some of these tools are listed at the end of the chapter.[2,7–9]

HEALTH HISTORY   Communication often creates the most insurmountable problems for the nurse caring for clients from diverse cultural backgrounds. Yet effective communication is the key to gathering a thorough health history. You must consider the client's communication style before initiating the formal interview process.

In some cultures written words are more powerful than spoken words. In other cultures verbal communication dominates. This information affects the type of health history format you use: formal versus informal; written versus verbal. Do individuals in this cultural group use silence as a mode of communication? Does their normal communication pattern include talking in a low volume? a loud volume? Is touch an appropriate vehicle for conveying feelings? Is the use of gestures and eye behavior a part of their communication style?[2]

For clients with English as a second language, translators may be needed. These translators should be the same gender as the client and should understand medical concepts and terminology. Even clients who understand English may have difficulties understanding medical and scientific terminology. Ask the clients if they understand the terms being used. Demonstrate patience and respect for their language. Do not rush their response to your questions. Speak slowly and distinctly and use simple language.

How questions are asked is also important. Open-ended questions or declarative statements are usually the most productive. Questions such as, "What do you think caused your problem?" "What does your sickness do to you?" "What type of treatment do you think you should receive?" and "What results do you hope to receive from this treatment?" will gather information about the health problem and the expectations of the client. Since some clients are reluctant to admit to folk beliefs, avoid asking questions specifically directed at this area such as, "Do you use folk healers in your culture?"

Clients from diverse cultural backgrounds may not display the same symptoms or necessarily describe the same symptoms for a particular health problem. The words and manner used by the client to present health concerns follows a culturally determined pattern. In some situations, symptoms or illnesses that exist in one culture do not exist in others. For example, such cultural conditions as ghost sickness, fallen fontanel, high or low blood, and arctic hysteria are not discussed in most annals of Western medicine.[10]

PHYSICAL ASSESSMENT   During the physical assessment, you need to address the **biologic characteristics** of your client. Consider the client's features, skin color, and body size.

Determining a baseline skin color is essential. The assessment should be made in the daylight or under at least a 60-watt bulb. Observe skin surfaces having the least pigmentation such as the palms of the hands, soles of the feet, the abdomen, and buttocks. Look for the underlying red tones typical of all skin. If a dark-skinned client has pallor, the red tone is absent.[2]

Another category of difference between cultures is susceptibility to disease. The increased or decreased incidence of a particular disease may be genetically induced, environmental, or a combination of the two. For example, some Native Americans have a tuberculosis rate 7 to 15 times higher than non–Native Americans. The tuberculosis rate in African-Americans is three times higher than in white Americans. In this case the susceptibility to tuberculosis may be genetic or environmental. Jews of Eastern European ancestry are genetically at risk for Tay-Sachs disease; African-Americans are genetically at risk for sickle cell disease. Knowledge of the client's disease susceptibility should help focus your assessment and direct diagnostic testing.[2,8]

Diagnosing   The list of diagnostic labels developed by the North American Nursing Diagnosis Association (NANDA) is focused on the dominant Western health care model and does not meet the needs of culturally diverse clients.[12] However, if you analyze the data base from a cultural viewpoint, the labels retain their usefulness. For example, you can expect a Japanese client who usually eats a traditional diet to have problems adjusting to a low-sodium diet. Therefore the diagnosis "Altered nutrition: less than body requirements related to dislike of low-sodium food" is appropriate.

Planning   Care should be planned based on the client's needs as identified by the client and nurse together. Integrating cultural factors into the plan allows you to acknowledge the importance of the client as a unique individual. This also makes the care more acceptable to the client. For example, Native American healing ceremonies may be used in conjunction with scientific medical treatment. Plans also should address the areas of cultural conflicts. For instance, if a folk remedy is known to interfere with a medication, you must decide how to approach the client to resolve this conflict effectively.

Another important part of the planning phase is collaboration with other health professionals. Sharing of information by all those caring for the client allows joint problem solving and consistent interventions.

Implementing   Incorporation of cultural beliefs into practice can be done in a variety of ways. One method is altering screening tests to fit the need of the cultural group. For example, some items on the Denver Developmental Screening Test are not universally known to all children. In some areas pavement, lakes, hedges, or curtains do not exist. Substituting familiar words (e.g., road, ocean, or palm trees) will help you

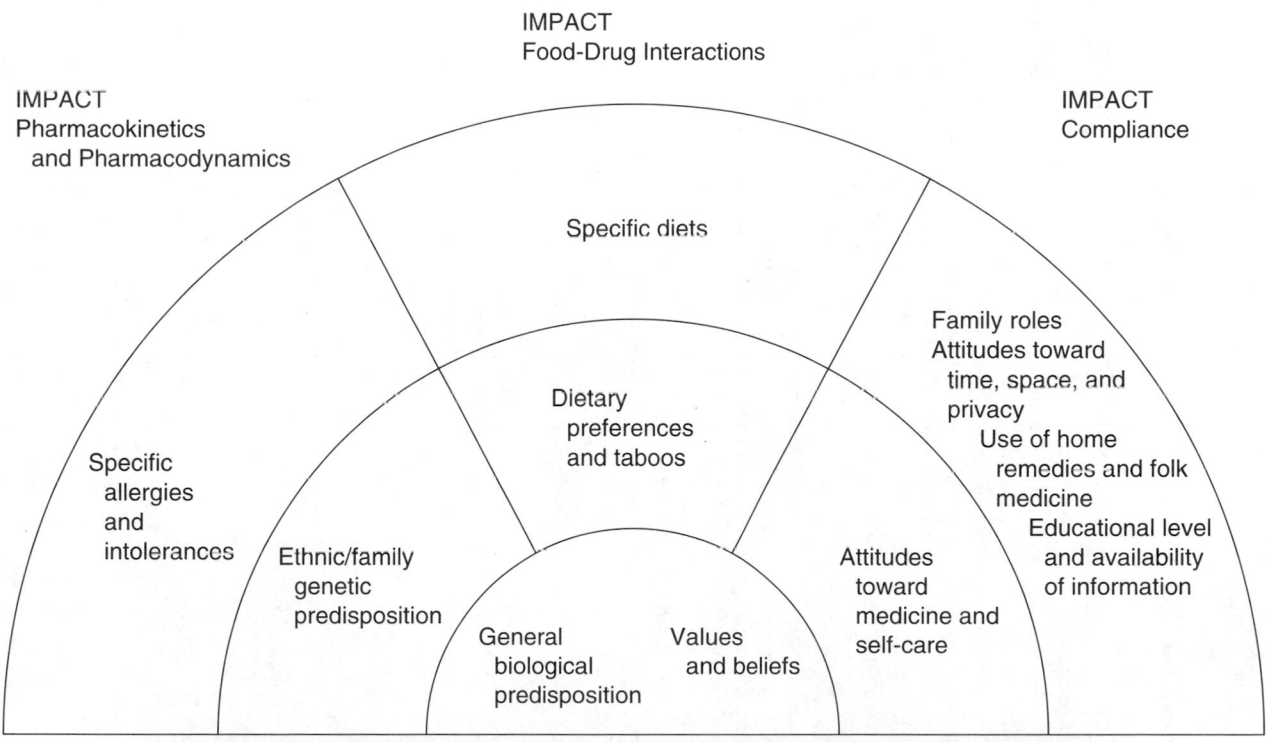

FIGURE 9–1   Facets of cultural assessment. This figure illustrates some of the areas of cultural assessment that may affect drug therapy for clients. The areas in the center are the most general and difficult to assess. The outer areas are more specific and easier to assess.

TABLE 9–1

Specific Cultural and Ethnic Variations Affecting Drug Therapy

Biologic Characteristics	Health and Illness Values and Beliefs	Self-Medication	Dietary Patterns	Response to Service
Hispanic Americans				
Individuals of Puerto Rican, Cuban, Mexican, and Central and South American descent	Blend of Indian, European, and Spanish Catholic influences	Herbs and plants used both for prevention and curative effects	Diets high in carbohydrates, low in animal protein	**COMMUNICATION**
Skin tones from light to dark brown	People viewed holistically	Amulets (charms, talismans, trinkets, etc.) and medals used for prevention and healing	Deficiencies in vitamin A, iron, and calcium common	Spanish language predominant
Susceptible to diabetes, heart disease, hypertension, cerebrovascular accidents, pernicious anemia, cancer, melanomas, communicable diseases (AIDS, respiratory tract infections, and tuberculosis), diarrhea, parasitic infections, complications of pregnancy, nutritional deficiencies, obesity, and substance abuse	Health a result of balance and harmony with natural and supernatural environments	Folk healers, *curanderos*, use rituals to heal the sick	Beans, flour and corn tortillas, vegetables such as chiles and corn, and fruits such as bananas usual menu items	Dialects and accents differ according to land of origin
	Health associated with the ability to work and fulfill roles	Other folk healers such as herbalists and witches also used		Native language retained because of pride in language and culture
	Conventional disease prevention measures not highly valued	Mistrust of "outside" health care providers		Usually not fluent in second language
	Illness a part of life to be endured (God's will)			Out of respect, may feign agreement with what is being said
	Male value on being tough; illness seen as a weakness			Reluctant to discuss personal matters with strangers
	Diseases classified as hot or cold			Small talk expected before business
	Treatment for disease designed to bring a balance to body through use of the opposite temperature treatment (e.g., hot foods, beverages, herbs, and plants used to treat cold disease)			Indirect communication techniques common
	Disease caused by external factors such as sinning, "evil or bad eye" (*mal ojo*), fright (*mal de susto*), witches (*mal puesto*), food (*empacho*), or dislocation of body parts (*caída de la mollera*)			Sensitive to criticism
				TIME
				Present oriented
				Reluctant to consider the future: delay of gratification not an important value
				Punctuality not an important value
				SPACE
				Comfortable with close interpersonal distance
				Touch acceptable form of expression, especially among family members
				Value physical presence such as that of family
				PRIVACY
				Body modesty valued
				Strong social value that women do not expose their bodies to men or other women
				LOCUS OF CONTROL
				External locus of control
				Fatalistic about their control over what happens to them
				FAMILY
				Turn to family first to meet needs; do not like to seek help outside family
				View themselves as family members first, individuals second
				Paternalistic role for the men
				Men minimally involved in child care
				When people are ill decided by women
				What to do when people are ill decided by men
				Religion and family priest important in decision making

Asian Americans

Americans of Chinese, Taiwanese, Japanese, Korean, Vietnamese, Cambodian, Laotian, and Far Eastern descent Exhibit the epicanthic fold, giving the slanted eye appearance Yellow to tan skin Mongolian spots, dark bluish pigmentation areas, in the sacral and gluteal regions of babies Short stature Susceptible to glucose-6-phosphate dehydrogenase deficiency, a hemoglobin abnormality characterized by red blood cell destruction and anemia when exposed to certain drugs such as analgesics, sulfonamides, antimalarials, antibacterials, vitamin K, probenecid and quinidine Susceptible to thalassemia, tuberculosis, parasitic infections, malaria, malnutrition, anemia, hepatitis, and cancers of nasopharynx, esophagus, stomach, liver, and cervix Japanese sensitive to alcohol	Chinese medicine from religious philosophies of Taoism: Health seen as a state of spiritual and physical harmony with nature Yin and Yang forces of energy: yin is female, negative, dark, and cold; yang is male, positive, warm and bright Illness occurs with imbalance of yin and yang Treatment of illness aimed at restoring balance Blood drawing seen as dangerous; blood is source of life for the body Chinese theory of energy conduits and sensitive points: Conduits called *acupoints;* form basis for acupuncture and acupressure Acupuncture and acupressure restore energy flow and proper rhythm. Disease or illness prevention important Japanese health practices closely tied to Shinto religion; emphasis on physical fitness Other Asian cultures have various beliefs (e.g., cosmic forces influence behavior; balance in humors prevents and treats illness) May be fatalistic about disease	Medicinal herbs used widely (e.g., herbal teas, ginseng, turtle shells, sea horses) Remedies restore the yin and yang balance Herbs available in special shops Cambodians apply ointment and rub a coin over affected area; use cupping (placing a hot cup over affected area); pinch affected areas Eastern Asian families have cultural healers Some Eastern cultures use amulets to prevent evil spirits	Milk and milk products often avoided because of lactose intolerance Do not like icy drinks; prefer warm or hot beverages Iron avoided during pregnancy because it is believed to harden bones in the body Prefer lightly cooked vegetables; small amounts of meat or fish Rice main carbohydrate; noodles also eaten in some cuisines High intake of sodium chloride in diet (MSG and soy sauce) Low dietary intake of cholesterol and fat	**COMMUNICATION** Linguistic diversity, even among groups in one country Silence valued Nonverbal communication and context important Touch during conversation not considered polite Emotional outbursts and expression of pain discouraged Minimum eye contact Self-expression discouraged Harmony, respect, formal approach valued Disagreements not verbalized Direct confrontation and conflict avoided **TIME** Time considered a process, not an absolute Planning for future, calmness, and time for daily ceremony valued Present important; past considered priceless **SPACE** Noncontact people More comfortable side by side than face to face **PRIVACY** Avoid calling attention to self; value humility Expect individuals to knock before entering their room Showing the bottom of the shoe, pointing the foot, touching an individual's head considered impolite **LOCUS OF CONTROL** Self-control and stoicism important **FAMILY ROLE** Extended family valued Female subservient to male who is dominant member Respect elders, duty, and obligation to parents Obligation to sick more important than individual rights

Table continued on following page.

TABLE 9–1 Continued

Specific Cultural and Ethnic Variations Affecting Drug Therapy

Biologic Characteristics	Health and Illness Values and Beliefs	Self-Medication	Dietary Patterns	Response to Service
Native Americans More than 200 tribal groupings exist in the United States, each with its own particular language, customs, and belief system Tan to dark tan skin Mongolian spots on buttocks and backs of children common Life expectancy at birth lower than norm High risk for many health problems, especially those influenced by socioeconomic conditions Increased rates of obesity, hypertension, heart disease, diabetes, end-stage renal disease, tuberculosis, arthritis, diseases of spine and connective tissue, chronic obstructive pulmonary disease, neoplasms, cerebrovascular hemorrhage, parasitic infections, pneumonia, and kidney infection Increased mortality rate from infectious diseases—meningitis, hepatitis—and sexually transmitted diseases Metabolize alcohol differently; higher rates of alcoholism and fetal alcohol syndrome Many are lactose intolerant	Health viewed holistically and supernaturally as a life cycle of birth, life, and death Death part of life; essential component of natural harmony Religion integral part of life and health Nature works in harmony with itself Humans interdependent with nature Violation of harmony creates illness Other causes of illness are witchcraft, sorcery, spirits, violation of taboos, and loss of soul Minor aches and pains a part of life; do not need treatment Treating the body with respect important	Religion, medicine, and magic go together May use folk and modern scientific systems together Concept of medicine looks beyond scientific medicine; not always directed toward a cure for illness Variety of folk health practitioners Variety of healing techniques such as meditation, ceremonies, interpretation of dreams, chanting, singing, massage, herbs, bone pressing, and belly rubbing Disease prevention and healing addressed Disease prevention accomplished through herbal teas, charms, and fetishes to ward off evil Medicine men do both psychologic and physical healing Herbalists have knowledge of use of herbs in healing (e.g., herbs used in sweat baths to draw out evil; pinon tree sap to treat leg ulcers, and goldenrod for colds, sore throat, and cough)	Diet high in fat and carbohydrates, low in fresh fruits and vegetables Deficiencies in calcium, phosphorus, iron, and vitamin A Favorite foods, especially in the Southwest, fried bread, beans, corn, and squash Meat and blue cornmeal believed to give strength to the Navajo Decreased consumption of dairy products if lactose intolerance exists Food has social value Some foods such as corn and squash have sacred symbolism and are used in tribal ceremonies	**COMMUNICATION** Different language spoken by each tribe Complexity of languages makes difficult to translate into English; medical terminology especially difficult Exhibit little self-disclosure May remain silent rather than speak in unpredictable situations Do not like interruptions, direct questions, or hurried conversations Little eye contact given Nonverbal communication watched closely Pointing, firm handshakes, and note taking considered impolite Converse in a low tone of voice; expect listener to listen closely **TIME** Present oriented Not clock conscious View time on a continuum with no beginning and no end Events begin when everyone agrees it is time to begin Place a high value on the past **SPACE** May have specific traditional beliefs about personal space Sharing important value **LOCUS OF CONTROL** External locus of control **FAMILY** Strong commitment to family and tribe Family extremely important, including both the nuclear and extended family Family important in care of sick Staying with hospitalized individuals is important Elderly revered for wisdom and experience Family roles flexible In some tribes descent is matrilineal—women have power; maternal grandmother's permission may be necessary for health care for family members In other tribes individual considered independent—no one has the right to speak or make decisions for another; children, for example, allowed to make decisions about whether they will take prescribed medication

African-Americans

Majority descendants of slaves brought from Africa

Many intermarried with other ethnic and racial groups to produce a heterogeneous group

Cultural differences are influenced strongly by social class

Various shades of brown and black pigmented skin

Shorter life expectancy than Caucasians

Mature earlier; larger physiques

Mongolian spots on sacral and buttock areas of children

Skin problems: keloids, pseudofolliculitis, and hyper- and hypo-pigmentation

Increased rate of cardiovascular disease, hypertension, cancer, accidents, influenza, pneumonia, periodontal problems, substance abuse, malnutrition, AIDS, and obesity, especially in women

High infant mortality rate

Sickle cell anemia, a genetically inherited disorder, occurs only in African-Americans

Increased incidence of glucose-6-phosphate dehydrogenase deficiency as a result of certain drug therapies or stressful conditions

---

Life viewed as a process

All things, living and dead, influence each other

Nature of an individual is energy, not matter

Health seen as harmony with nature

No separation of mind, body, and spirit

Illness attributed to disharmony, demons, and evil spirits

Goal of treatment is to remove demons and evil spirits from the body

Everything has an opposite (i.e., for every birth there must be a death)

Illness may be seen as a punishment

Wide variety of beliefs:

Practice of Voodoo from West Africa—voodoo entails many rituals and procedures, including white harmless magic and black dangerous magic; may view illness as resulting from a hex

Traditional healers—usually older women, "Granny"; use herbs and roots for treatment of illness

Spiritualists

Objects such as copper or silver bracelets to prevent illness, poultices, oils, powders, rituals, and ceremonies

Prayer

Pica—ingesting nonfood material such as clay or starch

Salt pork, greens such as collard and mustard greens, chard, and kale, chicken, pork, and black-eyed peas are favored foods

Food preparation by boiling and frying

Problem digesting dairy products if lactose intolerance is present

Deficiencies in calcium, iron, and niacin

COMMUNICATION

Variety of dialects—difference in pronunciation, grammar, and syntax; may be related to education and socioeconomic level

Use of body movement such as facial gestures, hand and arm movements, expressive stances, handshakes, and hand signals

TIME

Present oriented

Do not value punctuality

Time flexible and elastic; events begin when they arrive

SPACE

Closer personal space than norm

PRIVACY

Privacy not valued

Higher involvement ratio with others

LOCUS OF CONTROL

External locus of control

FAMILY

Matriarchal—assist family members in illness and advise when to seek help

Large supportive kin and non-kin networks

Respect for elders

Religion and ministers important

Uniqueness, individuality, and assertiveness valued

Data from Giger and Davidhizar;[2] Murray and Zentner;[3] and Spector[4] were used in compiling this table.

assess word comprehension. However, you must remember that an altered tool cannot be used to document a child's performance specifically.[8]

You can also incorporate cultural beliefs into many of the technical procedures that are performed. For example, there are strict rules about the roles of men and women concerning modesty. Men from many cultures, including African-Americans, Hispanic Americans, and Mediterranean groups, may feel uncomfortable about receiving certain aspects of care from a female (e.g., an intramuscular injection in the buttock). If this is the problem, either arrange for a male to perform the care or provide as much privacy as possible.

Teaching also requires special effort, especially for those whose comprehension of English is limited. Visual aids are helpful and can increase understanding. In instances of cultural conflict, explain to the client the problems that commonly occur if advice is not followed. Attempts to shame the client or force compliance are usually counterproductive.

You also have important roles as a client advocate, whether with a physician, a particular health care agency, or the health care system in general. You are often in the position to have the best knowledge of the client and his or her needs and are the most adept at communicating this knowledge to others.

NURSING RESEARCH

Frye, B. (1991). Cultural themes in health-care decision making among Cambodian refugee women. *Journal of Community Health Nursing, 8*(1), 33-44.

This research study focused on perceptual differences between Cambodian refugee women and health care providers. The study investigated the areas of types and causes of diseases, illness behaviors, treatment modalities, and patterns of health-care decision making and accessing care.

According to the cultural group studied, disease is caused by disequilibrium that results in a state of internal "bad wind." The bad wind can be released through coin rubbing or oppositional treatment (hot or cold). A primary concern for the refugees when accessing and selecting care providers was the need for help with the language and cultural comfort.

Implications for the study were the need to combine traditional healing practices with scientific ones and the need for health care providers to use knowledge of specific cultural beliefs when planning and implementing care.

STUDENT ACTIVITIES

• Interview five clients. Identify their cultural and ethnic groups. Ask the clients to share with you information on the areas investigated in this study: areas of types and causes of diseases, illness behaviors, treat-

ment modalities, and patterns of health-care decision making and accessing care.
• Compare these findings with those reported in the study.

Evaluating   Evaluate both the process (what care is being given) and the outcome (what happens to the client as a result of the care). If the client is not adhering to medical therapy, examine the actions of the client and the reasons for the behavior. In addition, examine the actions of the health care providers—why was the care by the health care professionals ineffective?

VARIATIONS AFFECTING DRUG THERAPY IN SPECIFIC CULTURES

To provide you with a basis for culturally sensitive health care, cultural and ethnic information about four different cultural groups is summarized in Table 9–1. These statements are generalizations; the degree to which a given individual meets these generalizations is individually determined.

SUMMARY

The United States is a culturally and ethnically diverse nation. This diversity influences health, health care, and the response to health care. It is your responsibility as a nurse to provide culturally sensitive nursing care. To do this, you must overcome your own ethnocentrism.

Culturally appropriate care is based on a cultural assessment. When performing this assessment, consider the following six areas: communication style, dietary patterns, response to service, self-treatment practices, health and illness values and beliefs, and biologic characteristics. Assessment findings in these areas vary with the cultural group being assessed. Once the data base has been established, incorporate the client's culture into the plan of care as much as possible.

REFERENCES

1. Leininger, M. (1989). The transcultural nurse specialist: Imperative in today's world. *Nursing & Health Care, 10,* 251-256.
2. Giger, J., & Davidhizar, R. (1991). *Transcultural nursing.* St. Louis: Mosby–Year Book.
3. Murray, R., & Zentner, J. (1993). *Nursing assessment and health promotion strategies through the lifespan* (5th ed.). Norwalk, CT: Appleton & Lange.
4. Spector, R. (1991). *Cultural diversity in health and illness* (3rd ed.). Norwalk, CT: Appleton & Lange.
5. Ross, B., & Cobb, K. (1990). *Family nursing: A nursing process approach.* Redwood City, CA: Addison-Wesley.
6. Kudzma, E. (1992). Drug response: All bodies are not created equal. *American Journal of Nursing, 92*(12), 48-50.
7. Bloch, B. (1983). Bloch's assessment guide for ethnic/cultural variations. In Orque, M., Bloch, B., & Monroy, L. *Ethnic nursing care: A multicultural approach.* St. Louis: C.V. Mosby.
8. Niederhauser, V. (1989). Health care of immigrant children: Incorporating culture into practice. *Pediatric Nursing, 15,* 569-574, 584-585.

9. Rosenbaum, J. (1991). A cultural assessment guide. *Canadian Nurse, 87*(4), 32-33.

10. Hoeman, S. (1989). Cultural assessment in rehabilitation nursing practice. *Nursing Clinics of North America, 24,* 277-289.

11. Geissler, E. (1991). Transcultural nursing and nursing diagnoses. *Nursing and Health Care, 12,* 190-203.

12. Frye, B. (1991). Cultural themes in health-care decision making among Cambodian refugee women. *Journal of Community Health Nursing, 8*(1), 33-44.

BIBLIOGRAPHY

Barney, K. (1991). From Ellis Island to assisted living: Meeting the needs of older adults from diverse cultures. *American Journal of Occupational Therapy, 45,* 593.

Budd, J. (1991). The Plains Indians: Cultural considerations in use of apnea monitors. *Neonatal Network—Journal of Neonatal Nursing, 9*(6), 55-57.

Caralis, P. (1991). Hypertension in Hispanic-Americans: How ethnicity affects disease and therapy. *Consultant, 31*(7), 49-51, 54-56.

Henkel, J., & Kennerly, S. (1990). Cultural diversity: A resource in planning and implementing nursing care. *Public Health Nursing, 7*(3), 145-149.

Kelly, J., & Frisch, N. (1990). Use of selected nursing diagnoses: A transcultural comparison between Mexican and American Nurses. *Journal of Transcultural Nursing, 2*(1), 16-21.

Leininger, M. (1990). Issues, questions, and concerns related to the nursing diagnosis cultural movement from a transcultural nursing perspective. *Journal of Transcultural Nursing, 2*(1), 23-32.

Lile, J.L., & Hoffman, R. (1991). Medication taking by the frail elderly in two ethnic groups. *Nursing Forum, 26*(4), 19-24.

Lopez, J., & Hendrickson, S. (1991). Family visits and different cultures. *AXON, 12*(3), 59-62.

Martin, M., & Henry, M. (1989). Cultural relativity and poverty. *Public Health Nursing, 6*(1), 28-34.

Nicholle, P.H. (1990). Cultural considerations in teaching the Saudi Arabian renal transplant recipient. *ANNA Journal, 17,* 377-380.

Rairdan, B., & Higgs, Z.R. (1992). When your patient is a Hmong refugee. *American Journal of Nursing, 92*(3), 52-55.

Uhl, J. (1991). Health promotion—A cultural affair. *Journal of Professional Nursing, 7*(5), 267.

CHAPTER 10

Psychosocial Factors Affecting Drug Therapy

NORMA L. PINNELL

CONCEPTS AND TERMS TO REVIEW

Reexamine cultural aspects that influence drug therapy. Review Chapters 4 and 5 for physiologic factors that affect the pharmacokinetic and pharmacodynamic phases of drug therapy.

---

*I*n previous chapters the impact of physiologic and cultural factors on drug therapy is discussed. However, drug therapy is also influenced by psychosocial factors. These factors can alter the client's response to and compliance with drug therapy.

HEALTH BEHAVIORS

Behavior is an observable response to environmental stimuli and includes verbal reports about emotional state, perceptions, and thoughts. The primary purpose of behavior is to meet the needs of the individual or group.[1] **Health behaviors** usually result from health beliefs and can positively or negatively affect health. Positive health behaviors are activities that enhance health, prevent illness, or detect illness.[2] Positive health behaviors are also known as health-seeking or health-protective behaviors.[3]

Health behaviors are also influenced by the individual's perception of health. Health is perceived uniquely by each individual. The individual's perception of health varies from day to day and is influenced by culture, socioeconomic status, age, knowledge, and preexisting state of health or illness.

HEALTH PROMOTION AND ILLNESS PREVENTION MODELS

Paradigms and models have been developed to explain the concepts of health, illness, and health behaviors. These models can provide a basis for predicting client compliance with and response to drug therapy.

Health Belief Model

Rosenstock's Health Belief Model was developed in the early 1950s. This model is used to explain why some individuals take actions to avoid illness while others fail to do so. If the individual is to take action, the individual must perceive that (1) he or she is susceptible to an illness, (2) the illness is serious enough to warrant action, and (3) the action will be of benefit. Variables (e.g., age, gender, ethnicity, personality, social class, peer and reference group pressure, and prior contact with an illness) influence the individual's perception of the benefits and barriers of preventive action.[4]

The model also provides a way of understanding how clients will comply with health care therapies. For example, drug immunization programs are used to prevent infectious diseases such as pneumonia, diphtheria, pertussis, tetanus, measles, mumps, and influenza. Other drugs are also administered prophylactically to prevent diseases. The Health Belief Model can predict the client's behavior in relation to these prevention activities.

Human Ecologic Model

The Human Ecologic Model uses a biopsychosocial approach to explain the client's health-wellness status. According to this model, factors that affect health and health-seeking activities include lifestyle, stress management, affiliation with others, cultural norms, social support, and personality. All biopsychosocial components are interrelated and interdependent.[5]

Resource Model of Preventive Health Behavior

The Resource Model of Preventive Health Behavior considers the social and health resources available to the individual since these resources affect the individual's preventive health behaviors. Health resources include health status, concern about health, social and personal support systems, feelings about independence in caring for self, and general psychologic well-being.[6,7]

🌺 NURSING RESEARCH

Pender, N.J., Walker, S.N., Sechrist, K.R., & Frank-Stromborg, M. (1990). Predicting health-promoting lifestyles in the workplace. *Nursing Research, 39,* 326-332.

A model proposed as explanatory and predictive of health-promoting lifestyles was evaluated in a sample of 589 employees enrolled in employer-sponsored health-promotion programs. Employees who reported more health-promoting lifestyles perceived themselves as competent in handling life situations, defined health as high-level wellness, evaluated their health positively, and perceived their health as affected by significant others.

STUDENT ACTIVITIES

- Develop a brief tool for assessing health-promoting activities.
- Using the tool, interview at least 10 individuals to determine their health-promoting behaviors. Identify any behaviors that might affect drug therapy. 🌿

PSYCHOSOCIAL FACTORS AFFECTING DRUG THERAPY

In the preceding section several psychosocial factors that influence health-seeking or health-protective behaviors (e.g., psychologic response, personality, attitudes and beliefs, and support systems) were identified. These factors also affect drug therapy. In addition, compliance with and response to therapy are influenced by locus of control, client participation in treatment, client–health-care provider relationship, and the symbolic meaning of drugs to the client.

Psychologic Response

The term **illness behavior** describes the response of an individual to an illness. Five stages of illness behavior have been identified: symptom experience, assumption of the sick role, medical care contact, dependent client role, and recovery and rehabilitation.[9] During the first stage, symptom experience, the individual may try self-treatment strategies such as using home remedies or over-the-counter drugs. During the first, second, and third stages, *denial* of symptoms may occur. If this happens, the individual may delay seeking health care. If denial of the medical diagnosis occurs, the individual may consult a variety of health-care providers in an attempt to find someone who will say what he or she wants to hear. The individual using denial may forget to take prescribed drugs or continue to use self-treatment strategies.

Other psychologic responses associated with drug therapy include anxiety, anger, shame, fear, and powerlessness. These responses can enhance or negate drug action. *Anxiety,* a feeling of uneasiness, apprehension, and/or dread, is a common response to drug therapy. With anxiety, the client usually has difficulty identifying the specific cause of the apprehension. However, *fear* is a feeling of dread related to an identifiable source. Clients may fear the adverse reactions associated with specific drugs (e.g., alopecia with chemotherapeutic agents or impotence with antihypertensive drugs). Other clients may be afraid that the desired response to the drug will not occur. Many clients fear dependence on or addiction to sedative, hypnotic, or analgesic drugs. If these fears are not addressed, the client may decrease the dosage of the drug or discontinue the drug before the course of therapy is complete.

Some clients may experience *anger.* The anger may be expressed directly or indirectly toward significant others or health-care providers or both. These feelings of anger may prevent the client from adhering to the treatment plan. In some situations the client uses the sick role to gain attention or to control others. Effective drug therapy prevents the client from benefitting from the illness; this may produce feelings of anger in the client. The family may also be angry if drug therapy is successful since family roles and relationships will be changed.

Individuals who believe that their illness (e.g., tuberculosis, lice infestation, or a sexually transmitted disease) is socially unacceptable may experience *shame*. These feelings may prevent the client from seeking health care or complying with drug therapy. Illness may also lead to a perceived loss of control over one's body or life. This feeling is termed *powerlessness*. Powerlessness can affect the individual's participation in health-care activities and decisions.

Attitudes and Beliefs

An *attitude* is a point of view or a way of thinking or feeling. *Beliefs* are ideas, convictions, or opinions. Attitudes and beliefs are acquired through social experiences—with family, the culture, education, religion, socioeconomic status, and health. Attitudes and beliefs can have a positive or negative effect on drug action. For example, the client's past conditioning to drugs, the illness, health-care system, and health-care providers determines the client's response to drug therapy.

In addition, *expectations* of the client often affect drug response. For example, therapy is usually more effective when the client has a positive attitude about the drug being used. Positive expectations of the client are enhanced if health-care providers consistently assure the individual of the benefits of the drug. If the client does not expect positive results, the drug is less likely to be effective. This is especially true in relationship to analgesic, sedative, and hypnotic drugs.

Placebos (inert substances such as distilled water, normal saline, lactose, or sugar solutions) are used during experimental drug studies or to produce desired responses in the absence of chemical activities. Therapeutic use of placebos depends on positive expectations of the client. When placebos are prescribed, health-care providers administering the placebos must encourage positive expectations. If the client believes a drug has been administered and anticipates a positive response, the desired effect may be achieved. Placebos have been effective in alleviating pain, anxiety, and sleeplessness.

Expectations of the client can also produce undesired clinical responses to drugs. For example, if the client has experienced adverse reactions to an antibiotic in the past, these reactions may occur again with other antibiotic drugs. Or if the client had nausea and vomiting with a general inhalation anesthetic, this reaction may occur with all future anesthetics. The client may also experience symptoms similar to those experienced by a friend or relative receiving the same drug. In some situations the client experiences undesired clinical responses to a drug after being educated about the drug's adverse reactions and side effects. This is especially true if the client has a high level of suggestibility.

Support System

A client with a strong support system of family members or significant others usually maintains high self-esteem. High self-esteem produces positive drug responses and promotes compliance.

Locus of Control

Clients with an internal locus of control believe they control their own lives. These individuals are more prone to seek medical care and follow treatment plans. However, they also usually have their own ideas about taking drugs. They may compare their knowledge about drugs and illness with the prescribed drug and the actions of the health-care provider. In some instances the individuals with a strong internal locus of control alter treatment plans in an attempt to maintain control of their own health care. On the other hand, an individual with an external locus of control believes fate and external forces control his or her life. Therefore he or she may not question the proposed treatment plan or verbalize negative and positive responses to the drug therapy.[10]

Symbolic Meaning of Drugs

Drugs have symbolic meanings such as danger, dependency, help, or protection for most individuals. Some individuals gain a feeling of security or well-being from drugs. These individuals view drugs as helpful. If drugs are viewed as symbols of danger, the client may be hesitant to take prescribed drugs or may interpret cure as a threat to the emotional security of illness. Drug therapy may also disturb an individual's self-image of independence (Fig. 10–1).

CONCEPT REVIEW

Several psychosocial factors influence the client's compliance with and response to drug therapy. These factors vary from client to client and even from day to day with the same client.

▨ NURSING CONSIDERATIONS

Consideration must be given to physiologic, psychosocial, and cultural factors that affect drug therapy.

Assessing   During the initial assessment, determine the client's attitudes and beliefs about drug therapy. Ask the client about previous experiences with this specific illness. Determine if this particular drug has been prescribed in the past. If so, ask the client if the desired response was achieved. Determine what current expectations the client has concerning drug therapy. If possible, identify specific meanings that drugs have for the client.

Diagnosing   After analysis of the collected data, identify appropriate diagnostic labels. Possible diagnostic labels include the following

Anxiety	Ineffective denial
Altered health maintenance	Noncompliance
Body image disturbance	Powerlessness
Fear	Self-esteem disturbance
Health-seeking behaviors	

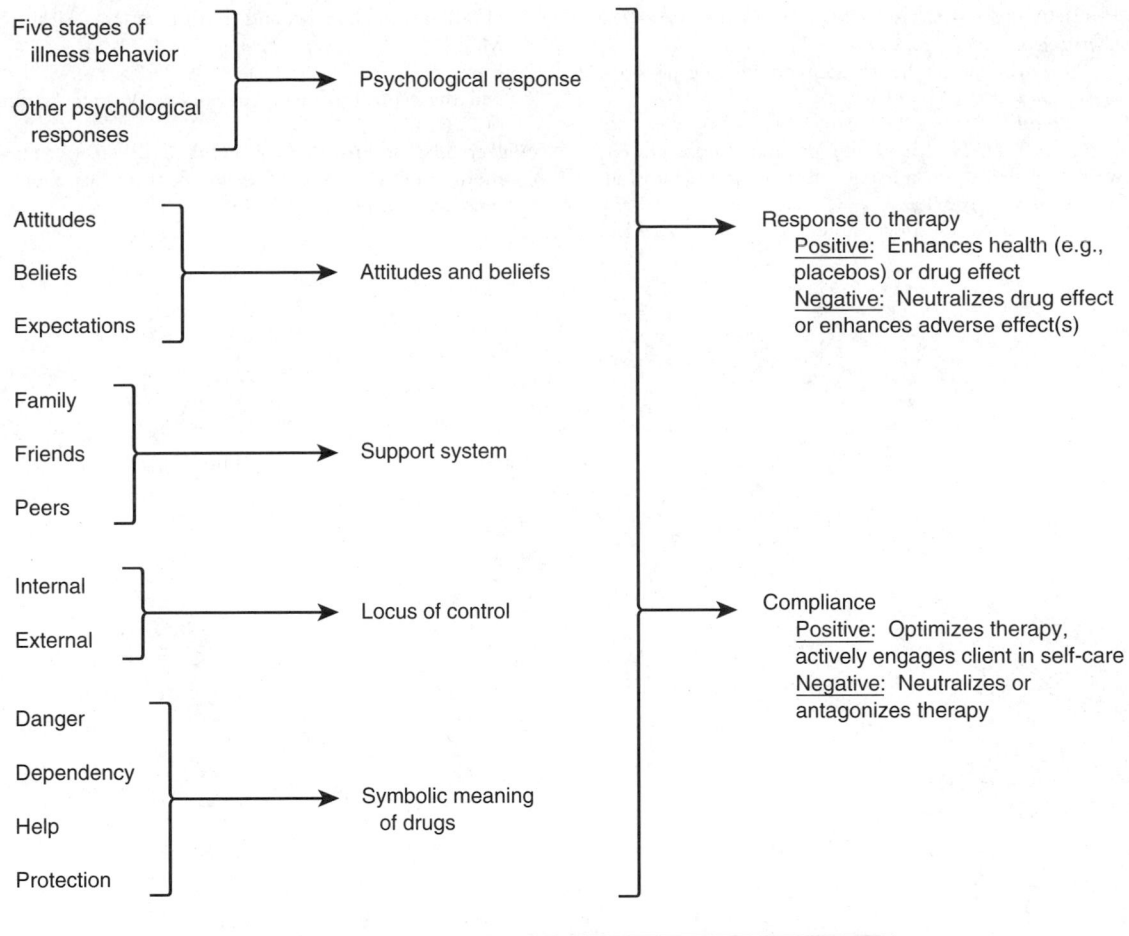

FIGURE 10–1   Psychosocial factors affecting drug therapy.

Planning   Develop a plan of care that is specific for the client's needs. Expected outcomes should address improved compliance and response to drug therapy.

Implementing   Interventions should include increased client participation in therapy and increased contact with health-care providers. Include the client in decision making. These factors usually have a positive impact on compliance and drug response. In addition, help the client to explore feelings about drugs and drug therapy actively.

Evaluating   Evaluate the client's response to the drug and determine his or her participation in the treatment plan. Determine if expected outcomes have been met and what revisions are necessary in the initial plan of care.

SUMMARY

When administering drugs, address all aspects that affect drug response, including physiologic, cultural, and psychologic factors. Since psychologic factors are difficult to evaluate, they are frequently overlooked. To prevent this from occurring, develop an assessment plan that incorporates these factors.

REFERENCES

1. Murray, R.B., & Zentner, J.P. (1993). *Nursing assessment and health promotion: Strategies through the life span* (5th ed.). Norwalk, CT: Appleton Lange.
2. Pender, N.J. (1987). *Health promotion in nursing practice* (2nd ed.). Norwalk, CT: Appleton Lange.
3. Bigbee, J., & Jansa, N. (1991). Strategies for promoting health promotion. *Nursing Clinics of North America, 26,* 895-913.
4. Rosenstock, I.M., Strecher, V.J., & Becker, M.H. (1988). Social learning theory and the health belief model. *Health Education Quarterly, 15,* 175-183.
5. Shaver, J. (1985). A biopsychosocial view of human health. *Nursing Outlook, 33*(4), 186-191.
6. Kulbok, P.P. (1985). Social resources, health resources, and preventive health behavior: Patterns and predictions. *Public Health Nursing, 2*(2), 67-81.
7. Kulbok, P., & Baldwin, J.H. (1992). From preventive health behavior to health promotion: Advancing a positive construct of health. *Advances in Nursing Science, 14*(4), 50-64.
8. Pender, N.J., Walker, S.N., Sechrist, K.R., & Frank-Stromborg, M. (1990). Predicting health-promoting lifestyles in the workplace. *Nursing Research, 39,* 326-332.
9. Suchman, E. (1965). Stages of illness and medical care. *Journal of Health Human Behavior, 6,* 114.
10. Brady, T.J. (1990). Point: Patient control of treatment is essential. *Arthritis Care and Research, 3*(3), 163-166.

BIBLIOGRAPHY

Blair, J.E. (1993). Social learning theory: Strategies for health promotion. *AAOHN Journal, 41,* 245-249.
Frank-Stromborg, M., Pender, N.J., Walker, S.N., & Sechrist, K.R. (1990). Determinants of health-promotion lifestyle in ambulatory cancer patients. *Social Science and Medicine, 31,* 1159-1168.

Lauver, D. (1992). A theory of care-seeking behavior. *Image—The Journal of Nursing Scholarship, 24,* 281-287.

Pender, N.J. (1990). Expressing health through lifestyle patterns. *Nursing Science Quarterly, 3*(3), 115-122.

Pender, N.J., Barkauskas, V.H., Hayman, L.L., Rice, V.H., & Anderson, E.T. (1992). Health promotion and disease prevention: Toward excellence in nursing practice and education. *Nursing Outlook, 40*(3), 106-112.

Pender, N.J., Walker, S.N., Sechrist, K.R., & Stromborg, M.F. (1988). Development and testing of the Health Promotion Model. *Cardiovascular Nursing, 24*(6), 41-43.

Polifroni, E.C., & Storrs, C.T. (1993). Psychological determinism and the evolving nursing paradigm. *Nursing Science Quarterly, 6*(2), 63-68.

Walker, S.N., Sechrist, K.R., & Pender, N.J. (1987). The health-promoting lifestyle profile: Development and psychometric characteristics. *Nursing Research, 36,* 76-81.

CHAPTER 11

Self-treatment

NORMA L. PINNELL

⊛ **Self-care**

LEARNING OBJECTIVE: Discuss factors that influence the self-care movement that exists in the United States.

⊛ **Self-treatment**

LEARNING OBJECTIVE: Define important terms associated with self-treatment.

KEY TERMS:
Self-administration, self-medication, self-treatment

⊛ **Self-treatment Using Over-the-Counter Drugs**

LEARNING OBJECTIVES:
Describe factors that influence the use of OTC drugs.
Summarize hazards associated with the use of OTC drugs.

⊛ **Miscellaneous Self-treatment Practices**

LEARNING OBJECTIVE: Describe several self-treatment measures.

KEY TERMS:
Acupressure, acupuncture, herbalism, homeopathy

⊛ **Nurse's Role in Consumer Education**

LEARNING OBJECTIVE: Discuss the nurse's role in consumer education.

> ### CONCEPTS AND TERMS TO REVIEW
>
> Review section on the self-care movement in a basic nursing textbook.
> Review section on nonprescription drugs in Chapter 2.

*S*elf-treatment is increasing. As availability of self-treatment resources and products increases and health care costs escalate, more and more individuals are assuming control over their own health care. Within the United States, self-treatment is part of the self-care movement.

SELF-CARE

Self-care is a process by which individuals function effectively on their own behalf in health promotion, health decision making, and disease prevention, detection, and treatment. Self-care emphasizes that the individual is the *subject* of health care decision action, not an *object* of it. Self-care practices include anything that individuals do on their own behalf to promote or improve their health status. They can include traditional and nontraditional medical practices, folk or popular remedies, and care of self during periods of illness.

Most individuals are more comfortable with health promotion and disease prevention and detection practices than disease treatment practices. However, in today's health care system the client frequently is required to provide self-care during periods of illness. The frequency and length of hospital admission have significantly decreased. In addition, more treatments, surgeries, and procedures are being done without hospitalization. All of these factors force the client to assume an active role in this aspect of self-care.

SELF-TREATMENT

For purposes of this text, the term **self-treatment** describes the practice of treating oneself with over-the-counter (OTC) drugs or folk, home, or popular remedies. Self-medication is a part of self-treatment. **Self-medication** is viewed as the act of properly and responsibly treating oneself with nonprescription drugs. When done properly, self-medication is a desirable and important component of primary health care. Although self-medication is a self-care practice, not all self-care involves self-medication.

The term *self-medication* has a different meaning in most institutional settings. In these settings (e.g., hospitals, extended care facilities, rehabilitation units), self-medication usually describes the procedure of allowing clients to administer their own prescription drugs. This is used as a teaching tool in an attempt to ready the client for discharge and to involve the client in self-care.[1,2]

Another aspect of self-treatment is self-administration. **Self-administration** refers to the use of prescribed drugs for other than prescribed purposes. For example, the client saves prescription drugs from one illness episode and self-prescribes them when similar signs and symptoms occur, or a wife shares her prescribed antimicrobial agents with her husband because his symptoms are similar to hers.

CONCEPT REVIEW

The idea of self-treatment may have started with the self-care movement. This movement encouraged health care consumers to become responsible for their health care. As they assumed more responsibility, consumers also became more active in the care process.

SELF-TREATMENT USING OVER-THE-COUNTER DRUGS

OTC drugs are sold without medical supervision or prescription. The high incidence of self-medication is a major concern of health professionals.

Factors Influencing OTC Drug Use

Many factors affect self-medication. For example, attitudes, beliefs, values, education, age, and gender influence the pattern and extent of self-medication. Frequently self-medication is due to the inconvenience and cost of seeking professional guidance.

Age often determines the type of OTC drugs used and the frequency of use. Younger individuals, under the age of 55 years, are more prone to use OTC drugs to relieve the discomforts associated with minor cuts and scratches, colds, sinus problems, acne, and headaches. OTC drug use for individuals over 55 years of age focuses on the relief of constipation, sleeping problems, arthritis, and other age-related discomforts.[3,4] Some studies indicate that use of OTC drugs declines in the very elderly (i.e., individuals over the age of 85). In addition, the total number of different types of OTC drugs is lower in this age group.[3,5]

🐾 NURSING RESEARCH

Conn, V.S. (1992). Self-management of over-the-counter medications in older adults. *Public Health Nursing, 9*(1), 29-36.

A sample of 186 adults age 65 years and over was interviewed and asked to describe their use of 16 OTC substances. Most of the interviewees reported using specific OTC preparations often. Few subjects acknowledged being influenced by advertisements. Health care providers were common but not exclusive sources of information about the products used. Some overuse of laxatives was noted, as was continuation of antacid administration for excessive lengths of time for persisting symptoms. Few subjects were aware of precautions associated with the OTC drugs being used. The results of the study indicate the need for educational programs for older adults.

STUDENT ACTIVITIES

• Develop a brief tool for assessing OTC drug use in older adults.
• Interview 10 individuals between the ages of 60 and 70 years and 10 individuals between the ages of 71 and 81 years. Ask each individual to complete your assessment tool. Compare the results of the two groups for differences and similarities in OTC drug use. 🌿

Men and women report different reasons for using OTC drugs. Women are more likely to seek relief from anxiety, obesity, indigestion, headaches, fatigue, sleeping problems, and skin problems. Men use OTC drugs to relieve muscle aches and pains, colds, and minor cuts and scratches.[3,4]

Another factor influencing the selection of OTC drug is the pharmacist. The pharmacist has an enormously expanded role in providing information, advice, and counseling. In one study a typical pharmacist made an average of 320 recommendations a month within the 33 OTC product categories included in the study. Findings also show that most pharmacists recommend specific products for the treatment of adult cough and cold, diarrhea, athlete's foot, jock itch, children's cough, allergies, vaginal fungus infections, throat discomfort, and hemorrhoids.[7]

Existing signs and symptoms of health problems affect the choice and use of OTC drugs. For example, one study analyzed self-care practices of independently living older adults with joint problems. Most subjects took nonprescription drugs for relief. One quarter of these individuals did not seek assistance in making the drug choice but used a trial-and-error approach.[8] Another study analyzed the self-medication practices of individuals with spinal cord injury. The focus of the study was on practices aimed at managing chronic pain. Many of the subjects used alcohol to achieve pain relief. In addition, the use of OTC analgesic drugs significantly increased.[9]

Problems Associated With OTC Drug Use

Even though many consumers are well informed, other individuals harbor misinformation and inaccurate beliefs about drugs. Consumers tend to gather bits and pieces of information from health professionals, advertisements, friends, relatives, and media. Even the *Physicians' Desk Reference,* which is published for use by prescribers of drugs, is available in most major bookstores, offering the consumer another source of information. However, access to information only provides a means of informing the consumer; it does not ensure understanding of the material. Information or knowledge without understanding leads to poor self-medication decisions.

Unclaimed prescriptions are another problem that occurs with increased accessibility of OTC drugs. In some instances the client is diagnosed by a primary care provider, and a prescription drug is ordered; but the prescription is never claimed by the client. One study indicated that cost (63%), forgetfulness (33.6%), and improved condition (31.8%) were major reasons for not claiming prescriptions. However, factors such as client did not want medicine (24.1%), lack of communication (17.3%), and client disagrees with physician (2.6%) also contributed to the high number of unclaimed prescriptions.[10] In many instances these individuals, once diagnosed, turn to OTC drugs and home remedies for symptom relief.

Numerous other risks are involved in using OTC drugs. For example, a large percent of the general population does not consider these products drugs. Individuals may not realize that many of the OTC drugs were prescription drugs before being switched to the nonprescription category. This lack of concern about OTC products makes the individual vulnerable to drug-drug, drug-nutrient, and drug-environment interactions, overdose, and toxic effects.

In some instances the individual does not understand or cannot accurately diagnose the seriousness of the signs and symptoms. In addition, OTC drugs may mask the actual problem while relieving signs and symptoms. Many OTC drugs contain ingredients that may be harmful to the client (e.g., alcohol, caffeine). Since some individuals do not or cannot read the label (i.e., small print, lack of ability) on the container, they remain unaware of these ingredients until problems develop.

MISCELLANEOUS SELF-TREATMENT PRACTICES

A variety of self-treatment practices exist (e.g., herbalism, homeopathy, traditional medicine, acupressure, and acupuncture). **Herbalism** is the use of leaves, flowers, stems, or roots of plants to treat illness. Use of herbal remedies increased significantly as warnings about food additives and preservatives increased. At present, health food stores and stores that sell natural organic vitamins, cosmetics, and vegetables abound. However, not all herbal remedies are harmless. For example, chamomile, which is used as an appetite stimulant, can produce skin rash and severe hypersensitivity reactions in individuals allergic to ragweed.

Homeopathy is a system of therapeutics founded by Samuel Hahnemann (1755-1843). In this system of healing, diseases are treated by drugs capable of producing in healthy individuals the same symptoms as the disease being treated. Homeopathic drugs are administered in small amounts.

Traditional health care includes folk beliefs and practices that have been passed down through tradition. Many of these beliefs and practices are used today as an alternative to, or in addition to, practices of the modern health care system. Traditional health practices include using home remedies and reliance on cultural and spiritual healers. These healers may use herbs, magical, or religious remedies.

Acupressure is a noninvasive technique. Pressure from the practitioner's fingers is applied to acupuncture sites to cure or treat diseases. **Acupuncture** requires the insertion of needles into specific points in the body to relieve discomfort. Neither acupressure nor acupuncture requires the use of drugs.

CONCEPT REVIEW

Self-treatment involves the use of OTC drugs or folk, home, or traditional remedies to treat oneself.

The number and variety of OTC drugs have drastically increased in recent years. Use of these drugs offers the consumer certain benefits but also poses a threat to the individual's health status.

As health care technology increases, more individuals are selecting alternative health care practices. This trend is expected to continue in the future.

NURSE'S ROLE IN CONSUMER EDUCATION

Health care providers must be alert for self-treatment practices in clients. Often the client does not volunteer information about self-treatment. Since the practice of self-treatment is widespread, you must educate the client to reduce the negative consequences of this practice. One important point to make with all clients is the need to select one pharmacy and get to know the pharmacist. That pharmacist is a resource for an appropriate OTC drug choice.

SUMMARY

Self-treatment involves both self-medication and self-administration practices. These practices produce a threat to the safety and health of the consumer. Self-treatment also includes the use of alternative health care practices such as herbalism, traditional remedies, and healers. Health care professionals must be alert to the possibility of such practices and assess these areas during the health history.

REFERENCES

1. Coudreaut-Quinn, E., Emmons, M., & McMorrow, M. (1992). Self-medication during inpatient psychiatric treatment. *Journal of Psychosocial Nursing, 30*(12), 32-36.
2. Johns, C. (1990). Steps to self-medication. *Nursing Times, 86*(11), 40-41.
3. American Pharmaceutical Association. (1990). *Handbook of nonprescription drugs* (9th ed.). Washington, DC: Author.
4. Campbell, R.K., White, J., & Hansten, P. (1992). Prescription and over-the-counter drugs: The ins and outs. *Diabetes Forecast, 45*(2), 35-39.
5. Conn, V.S. (1991). Older adults: Factors that predict the use of

over-the-counter medication. *Journal of Advanced Nursing, 16,* 1190-1196.

6. Conn, V.S. (1992). Self-management of over-the-counter medications by older adults. *Public Health Nursing, 9*(1), 29-36.

7. Gannon, K. (1991). Hot, hot, hot: New switches to brighten OTC market. *Drug Topics, 135*(15), 32-34, 41-42, 45-46, 50, 52, 55.

8. Conn, V. (1990). Joint self-care by older adults. *Rehabilitation Nursing, 15,* 182-186.

9. Radwanski, M. (1992). Self-medicating practices for managing chronic pain after spinal cord injury. *Rehabilitation Nursing, 17,* 312-318.

10. McCaffrey, D., Smith, M., & Banahan, B. (1993). Why prescriptions go unclaimed. *Pharmacist,* (August), 58, 60, 62, 64-65.

BIBLIOGRAPHY

Brehm, B. (1993). *Essays on wellness.* New York: Harper Collins College Publishers.

Bruch, M.K., & Larson, E. (1989). An early historical perspective on the FDA's regulation of OTC drugs. *Infection Control & Hospital Epidemiology, 10,* 527-528.

Pesznecker, B., Patsdaughter, C., Moody, K., Albert, M., et al. (1990). Medication regimens and the home care client: A challenge for health care providers. *Home Healthcare Services Quarterly, 11*(1/2), 9.

Sidel, V., Beizer, J., Lisi-Fazio, D., et al. (1990). Controlled study of the impact of educational home visits by pharmacists to high-risk older patients. *Journal of Community Health, 15*(3), 163-174.

CHAPTER 12

Substance Abuse and Addiction

ROBYN RICE • JOYCE M. HUNTER • NORMA L. PINNELL

⊛ Substance Abuse

LEARNING OBJECTIVES:
Define the term *substance abuse.*
Describe the progressive phases of substance abuse.
KEY TERMS:
Circumstantial use, experimental phase, intensified use, social-recreational phase, substance abuse

⊛ Addiction

LEARNING OBJECTIVES:
Define the term *addiction.*
Differentiate between substance abuse and addiction.
KEY TERMS:
Addiction, compulsive phase, dependence

⊛ Theories of Substance Abuse and Addiction

LEARNING OBJECTIVE: Summarize two theories of substance abuse.

⊛ Biopsychosocial Manifestations of Substance Abuse

LEARNING OBJECTIVES:
Identify major physical manifestations of long-term substance abuse and addiction.
Describe the psychosocial impact of substance abuse and addiction on the client.

⊛ Nursing Process

LEARNING OBJECTIVES:
Identify appropriate assessment parameters for the individual who is a substance abuser.
List two nursing diagnoses appropriate for the individual who is a substance abuser.
Outline a plan of care for a client with a substance abuse problem.

⊛ Commonly Abused Drugs

LEARNING OBJECTIVE: Summarize essential information about alcohol, cocaine, and marijuana.
KEY TERMS:
Acetaldehyde, hash, hash oil, hallucinogens

CONCEPTS AND TERMS TO REVIEW

Review physiology of the central nervous system.
Review section in Chapter 4 on the distribution of drug molecules.

Why does the 17-year-old high school student become an alcoholic? What causes the 26-year-old nurse to start freebasing cocaine? These behaviors are based on many factors. For example, the individual's physical status, self-con-

cept, and interactions with family and friends influence behavioral responses. Perceptions of pain, illness, and health and personal health beliefs also affect the behavior of the individual.

The use of mind- or mood-altering substances is not new; it is probably as old as the human race. Drugs to relieve pain or anxiety, to promote sleep, or to suppress one's appetite are routinely prescribed. In addition, home remedies and over-the-counter (OTC) drugs are used to promote a sense of well-being. However, abuse of or addiction to a substance is an illness. Treatment of this illness requires a comprehensive plan that includes pharmacologic and behavioral therapy.

SUBSTANCE ABUSE

Substance abuse refers to excessive use of mind- or mood-altering substances. Currently the most frequently abused substances are caffeine, alcohol, nicotine, cocaine, and marijuana. Studies have shown that the selection of these substances usually follows a pattern. The progression starts with wine or beer, progresses to cigarettes, then to hard liquor, to marijuana, and finally to other illicit drugs such as cocaine.

In addition, the actual pattern of usage is progressive. Initially the substance abuse is short term and nonpatterned; this occurs during the **experimental phase.** During the next phase, **social-recreational,** the individual begins to use drugs at social gatherings. No longer is experimentation the intent— the individual wants to experience the mood-altering effects along with others. **Circumstantial** or **situational use** occurs next. In this phase the individual uses the drug to help him or her accomplish a particular task. Drug usage of this nature may have little impact on the individual or can result in spontaneous death from overdose. From situational use the individual progresses to **intensified use** in which the substance abuse is long term and patterned. The last phase is **compulsive use.**[1,2]

ADDICTION

According to the American Nurses' Association (ANA), **addiction** is "an illness characterized by compulsion, loss of control, and continued patterns of abuse despite perceived negative consequences."[3] Addiction represents the **compulsive phase** of substance abuse. In this phase there is a high frequency of substance use and physical and psychologic dependency. With **dependence,** the individual has signs and symptoms of withdrawal if the drug intake is interrupted.

With addiction, there are changes in emotional and cognitive states that are due to the continuous presence of one or more drugs in an individual's system. Progressive deterioration of the individual and disintegration of the family unity occur. Typically the individual experiences decreased coping abilities, loss of support systems, and financial instability.

THEORIES OF SUBSTANCE ABUSE AND ADDICTION

There are several theories or models of substance abuse and addiction, including disease model, interactive model, sociocultural model, learning theory model, behavioral model, family systems theory, and genetic theory. Three of these models are described in the following sections.

Disease Model

The disease model of addiction was originally developed by Jellinek to describe alcoholism; it is now applied to addiction in general. According to this model, addiction is a progressive disease that has both physiologic and psychologic aspects. The physical components include biologic factors such as genetic predisposition to addiction and chemically altered brain function. The psychologic components of addiction include an obsession with the use of the substance.[2,4]

Learning Theory Model

The learning theory model views substance abuse as a learned response to tension. Tension occurs within the individual, and a desire for alleviation of the tension is created. The individual uses substances that reduce the tension to a more tolerable level. Repeated achievement of this tension-reduction effect establishes a cycle of psychologic and behavior reinforcement.

Sociocultural Model

The sociocultural model suggests that substance abuse is conveyed through the socialization process. Verbal and nonverbal behaviors convey that substance use is appropriate. Usage of a drug, particularly by parents, is often perceived by children as a pattern to emulate. Group influence and peer pressure are especially important to the adolescent. Therefore adolescent acceptance or rejection of drugs may be associated with peer usage.[5,6]

CONCEPT REVIEW

Substance abuse is not a new phenomenon. It is the excessive use of substances for mood-altering effects.

Addiction occurs when the individual is physically and psychologically dependent on a substance. Addiction depends on the compulsion to use the substance, not on the quantity of the substance or on the frequency of use.

BIOPSYCHOSOCIAL MANIFESTATIONS OF SUBSTANCE ABUSE

Biopsychosocial manifestations of substance abuse depend on the type of substance, method of administration, frequency of drug use, and the individual's overall health status. The longer substance abuse persists, the more body systems involved. Most of the physical manifestations illustrated in Figure 12–1 represent changes that occur with long-term use.

In addition to physical manifestations, cognitive and psychosocial changes occur. Cognitively, the abuser develops impaired judgment, recall, and problem-solving abilities. Psychosocial manifestations include anger, denial, withdrawal, and loss of self-control. Feelings of anxiety, paranoia, depression, apathy, shame, and failure arise. The individual may experience a sense of powerlessness and destructiveness toward self and family. Excessive use of defense mechanisms, including denial, rationalization, and projection, occurs. In addition, guilt, isolation, and antisocial behaviors occur.[3,7,8]

As substance abuse continues, interpersonal relationships, particularly those with the family, are impaired and disrupted.

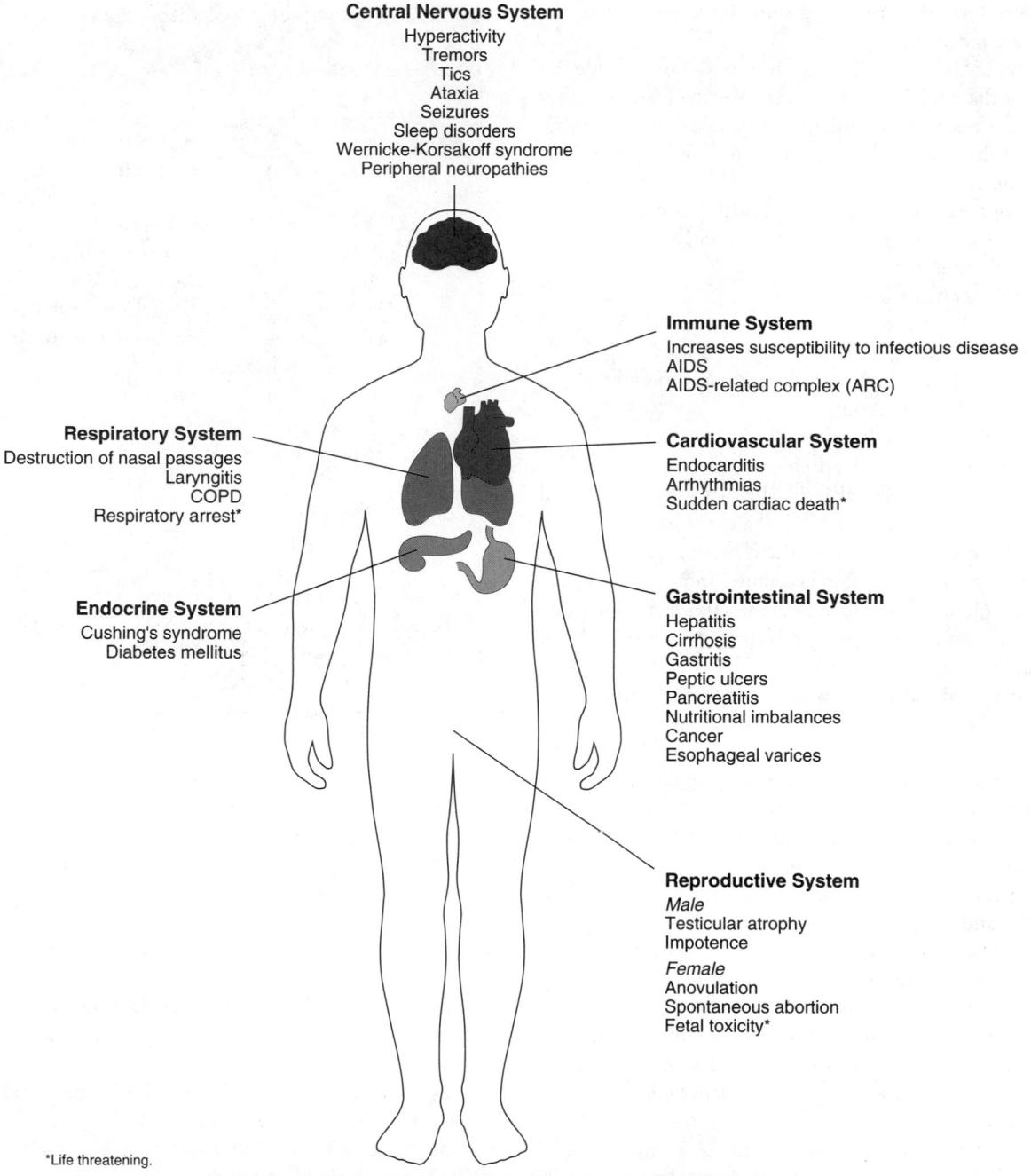

Central Nervous System
Hyperactivity
Tremors
Tics
Ataxia
Seizures
Sleep disorders
Wernicke-Korsakoff syndrome
Peripheral neuropathies

Immune System
Increases susceptibility to infectious disease
AIDS
AIDS-related complex (ARC)

Respiratory System
Destruction of nasal passages
Laryngitis
COPD
Respiratory arrest*

Cardiovascular System
Endocarditis
Arrhythmias
Sudden cardiac death*

Endocrine System
Cushing's syndrome
Diabetes mellitus

Gastrointestinal System
Hepatitis
Cirrhosis
Gastritis
Peptic ulcers
Pancreatitis
Nutritional imbalances
Cancer
Esophageal varices

Reproductive System
Male
Testicular atrophy
Impotence

Female
Anovulation
Spontaneous abortion
Fetal toxicity*

*Life threatening.

FIGURE 12–1   Physical manifestations of substance abuse.[3,7,8]

Communication, role performance, and sexual interactions become distorted. Concerned family or friends may show signs of co-dependence or coping strategies that contribute to the progression of the illness. For example, they may provide the abuser with money for living expenses that the abuser uses for drug purchases. Family and friends feeling guilt over the abuser's illness or remorse for past events may compensate in unhealthy ways. To protect the user, the family may act as if nothing is wrong or may terminate outside friendships and community visibility. The response by children in the family to abuse may take the form of rigid, compulsive roles and emo-tional distancing. Children of addicted parent(s) usually do poorly in school and show withdrawal, anger, or aggressive behaviors.

NURSING CONSIDERATIONS

Clients who are substance abusers are seen in a variety of health care settings (e.g., emergency departments, psychiatric units, general medical-surgical units, and home-health situations). Therefore all nurses need some understanding of the care of these individuals.

The intent of the following section is to provide an overview of the nurse's role in the care of a client who is either a substance abuser or an addict. It is not possible within the structure of this textbook to address such a complex-client situation completely.

Assessing As with any client, a **health history** should be gathered as soon as possible. Questions such as the following provide important data:

• When did you first use drugs?
• What drugs do you use?
• When you use a drug, in what setting is it used?
• How frequently do you use it (daily, weekly, monthly)?
• How do you take the drug(s)?
• What was the last drug(s) you took?
• When did you last take the drug?

Learn how the individual feels when they use a drug and what behavior changes occur. Ask if the client has experienced withdrawal symptoms. Question the client about hospitalizations or arrests related to substance abuse. Inquire if client has experienced blackouts (periods of amnesia). Determine if the client thinks that drug use is a problem and if the client ever tried to control the use of drugs.[1,2]

During the **physical assessment** observe the general appearance of the client. Does the client have an unsteady gait? Are the client's eyes red or glassy in appearance? When the client answers your questions, is there slurring of speech? Note if the client is underweight or overweight. Observe the client's hygiene and clothing. Record inappropriate affect, confusion, or agitation.

During the cardiac assessment assess for the presence of tachycardia and arrhythmias. Measure the client's blood pressure carefully since hypertension occurs as a complication of long-term substance abuse. Assess the client's respiratory status for hyperventilation, cough, or abnormal breath sounds. During the neurologic assessment examine pupil size and reaction; note dilated or unequal pupils. Test deep-tendon reflexes. Ask the client questions that evaluate long- and short-term memory.

Examine the client's nose and throat. Is the nose red and bulbous with broken blood vessels? (This condition is usually associated with prolonged, excessive alcohol intake.) Is there erythema of the nasal mucosa and pharynx; swelling of the nasal turbinates; or necrosis, perforation, or bleeding of the nasal septum? (These physical changes are usually associated with cocaine snorting—inhalation of the powder through a straw or rolled currency.) Inspect the skin for tracks or lesions over veins. They are commonly found on forearms, in the antecubital fossa, on legs, or between toes. Observe for bruising, hair loss, jaundice, or pale skin associated with hepatic or nutritional disorders.

Diagnosing The diagnosis phase for this client serves two purposes: to determine if the client meets the diagnostic criteria for a substance abuse disorder and to develop an appropriate nursing diagnosis.

DIAGNOSTIC CRITERIA FOR SUBSTANCE ABUSE DISORDER

Substance Dependence

A. Client meets at least three of the following criteria:
1. Client needs to increase amount of substance to achieve desired effect, or diminished effects result from continued use of same amount.
2. Substance often is used in larger amounts or over a longer period than client intended.
3. Client has persistent desire for substance or has made at least one unsuccessful attempt to diminish or control substance use.
4. Substantial time is spent in securing, using, and recovering from effects of substance.
5. Frequent intoxication or withdrawal symptoms prevent fulfillment or major obligations.
6. Major social, occupational, or recreational activities are reduced.
7. Client continues substance abuse despite knowledge of negative consequences.
B. Some symptoms have persisted for at least 1 month or have occurred repeatedly over a longer period.

Adapted from American Psychiatric Association (1987). *Diagnostic and statistical manual of mental disorders* (3rd ed., rev.). Washington, DC: Author

Data analysis follows the assessment of your client. The American Psychiatric Association has developed criteria to assist in diagnosing substance abuse disorders. These criteria are listed in the box. As you analyze your data, compare your findings with the criteria. If your client meets at least three of the seven criteria listed, a diagnosis of substance abuse disorder is appropriate.

Next develop nursing diagnoses. Appropriate nursing diagnoses for the client who is a substance abuser include the following:

• High risk for injury related to client's limited adaptive resources.
• Social isolation related to unaccepted social behaviors.
• Self-care deficit related to cognitive impairment.
• Disturbed body image related to physical changes caused by substance abuse.
• Impaired verbal communication related to substance abuse.

Planning Planning must be comprehensive in nature. It includes both the client and family or significant other in the formation of realistic long- and short-term goals. The goals must recognize the realities of the client's lifestyle and habits and the degree of commitment of everyone involved. Coordination of health services and therapies and multidisciplinary referrals are a part of this process. See box for some resources.

Based on the nursing diagnoses used in the plan of care, appropriate expected outcomes include the following:

• Client demonstrates lifestyle changes to protect self from injury.

- Client identifies causes of social isolation.
- Client performs self-care activities within level of own ability.
- Client verbalizes understanding of body changes.
- Client demonstrates suitable verbal communication skills.

Implementing   Education, along with support and encouragement regarding positive changes in lifestyle, plays a significant part in the client's plan of care. Responsibility for recovery and optimal health is placed on the client once physiologic and psychologic stability has been established. This is often a long-term process and involves the attainment of client self-awareness and acceptance. Coping styles and needs of those involved with the client should be periodically reinforced.

Community health nurses have an important role in the development and implementation of programs that foster the health of local residents. Interventions include public education about illicit drug and alcohol abuse and identification of signs and symptoms of substance abuse. Public education about the deleterious effects of substance abuse is the best prevention.

Evaluating   Evaluation of interventions involves the client's, family's, or significant other's response to the plan of care. Continually assess the client's progression to goal achievement and accomplishment of expected outcomes.

COMMONLY ABUSED DRUGS

In the United States today there are three main categories of abused chemicals: sedatives, stimulants, and hallucinogens. Individuals who are anxious people tend to abuse sedatives, alcohol, or marijuana. Individuals with affective (manic-depressive) disorders and attention deficit disorders are more predisposed to abuse stimulants.[9]

As previously mentioned, the most frequently abused substances include caffeine, alcohol, nicotine, cocaine, and marijuana. Caffeine and nicotine are discussed in Chapter 22. Alcohol, cocaine, and marijuana are described in this chapter.

Central Nervous System Depressants

Central nervous system (CNS) depressants are pharmacologic agents that have a depressive effect on the brain and spinal cord.

CNS DEPRESSANT PROTOTYPE
ETHANOL

The *National Household Survey on Drug Abuse: Population Estimates 1991* reported approximately 68% of the total population in the United States consumed alcohol (ethanol) during 1991. Other studies indicate that there are more than 18 million alcoholics in the United States. In addition, alcohol abuse contributes to approximately 50% of all traffic accidents, suicides, and homicides.[7,11,12]

Types of Alcohol Consumed   Alcohol is available in many forms (e.g., beer, wine, dessert wine, distilled liquor). Each form contains different amounts of alcohol. For example, dessert wines usually have an alcohol content of 20%, whereas distilled liquor has an alcohol content of 40%. The alcoholic content produces the pharmacologic effect.[13]

Other products that contain alcohol may also be abused. Alcohol is a solvent in many medicinal compounds and an ingredient in shaving lotions and mouthwashes. When alcohol is not available, individuals may resort to drinking these substances.

Pharmacokinetics   After ingestion, alcohol is rapidly absorbed from the stomach and the small intestine. As the gastric alcohol concentration increases, the rate of absorption increases and then decreases as the alcohol restricts the blood supply to the stomach. The ingestion of food or milk also slows gastric absorption of alcohol. Complete absorption of alcohol usually takes 2 to 6 hours. After absorption, alcohol is uniformly distributed throughout body tissue and fluids.[13]

The body metabolizes approximately 90% to 98% of ingested alcohol. The small amount that is not oxidized is excreted in the urine or exhaled by the lungs. Most ingested alcohol is metabolized in the liver.[13]

Pharmacodynamics   Alcohol's exact mechanism of action is unclear. Some research has demonstrated that alcohol affects the brain by interacting with specific protein constituents of the brain cell membranes. Other studies suggest that alcohol increases blood levels of norepinephrine. In addition, alcoholics have increased urinary levels of catecholamines during periods of ingestion and withdrawal.[12,13]

There has been research on alcohol's interactions with γ-aminobutyric acid (GABA), the major inhibitory neurotransmitter of the mammalian brain. The GABA receptor has recognition sites for GABA, barbiturates, and benzodiazepines that produce effects similar to those of alcohol. Studies indicate that alcohol may also affect these sites.[14]

Additional research suggests that another neurotransmitter-receptor system, the glutamate system and its *N*-methyl-D-aspartate (NMDA) receptor, may mediate many of the acute effects of alcohol. The activity of glutamate, an amino acid that appears to be the main excitatory neurotransmitter of the mammalian brain, is affected by alcohol.[15,16]

Physiologic Effects Alcohol produces a general dose-dependent depression of the CNS. Many of the initial behavioral changes that follow alcohol ingestion are caused by the effects of alcohol on the reticular formation. The reticular formation, which extends through the middle portion of the brain stem upward to the thalamus, initiates diffuse activation of the cerebral cortex. The cortex is susceptible to the depressant effects of alcohol.[13]

Undesired Clinical Responses Alcohol affects almost every organ system in the body, either directly or indirectly. The liver, the primary site of alcohol metabolism, can be severely affected by excess alcohol ingestion. In the liver alcohol is converted to **acetaldehyde.** It is then oxidized to acetate and excreted as carbon dioxide and water. This metabolic conversion of alcohol is critical because acetaldehyde is highly toxic to the liver and other organs.

Chronic alcoholism is associated with elevated levels of acetaldehyde. As the alcoholic drinks, acetaldehyde levels rise, impairing liver function and further increasing the levels of acetaldehyde. Liver damage may take the form of steatosis (fatty liver), alcoholic hepatitis, and cirrhosis. Liver damage is characterized by jaundice, an enlarged liver, abdominal pain, fever, portal hypertension, kidney failure, gastrointestinal (GI) bleeding, esophageal varices, and abnormal accumulation of fluid in the abdomen (ascites).[12,13]

Regular alcohol consumption may precipitate inflammation of the esophagus and exacerbate existing peptic ulcers. The risk of esophageal cancer and chronic atrophic gastritis is higher in alcohol abusers. Heavy alcohol consumption is the principal cause of chronic pancreatitis and is a common cause of acute pancreatitis.[12] Malnutrition resulting from poor eating habits can arise from reduced overall food intake and from deficiencies of specific nutrients. Results of nutritional deficiencies include anemia, neuropathy, Wernicke's disease, and depressed cellular and hormonal functions. Alcohol also affects carbohydrate, lipid, and protein metabolism.[12]

Alcohol can affect the heart muscle itself, producing cardiomyopathy and cardiac arrhythmias. Chronic alcohol consumption is associated with a significant increase in hypertension and may contribute to ischemic heart disease. Alcohol may alter circulatory functions by affecting the release and actions of hormones and related substances.[12,13,17] CNS complications of alcoholism include delirium tremors, Korsakoff's psychosis, dementia, seizures, ataxia, paresthesia, and peripheral neuropathies.[12,13]

Pharmacologic Agent Used to Treat Alcohol Abuse Disulfiram (Antabuse) is one of several aldehyde dehydrogenase inhibitors that raise the plasma level of acetaldehyde after ethanol ingestion. Ingesting alcohol while disulfiram is in the body produces blurred vision, nausea, vertigo, anxiety, and cardiovascular effects such as hypotension, palpitations, tachycardia, and flushing of the face and neck. Symptoms begin within 15 minutes of the alcohol ingestion and may last for several hours. Thus the usual pleasant reaction to ethanol is changed to an unpleasant reaction resulting from the body's reaction to the acetaldehyde.[4,18]

Like any drug, disulfiram has side effects. Drowsiness and fatigue are common complaints during the early phase of treatment. These responses can be managed by administering the disulfiram at bedtime. Garliclike breath also occurs in individuals receiving disulfiram.[4]

NURSING RESEARCH

Trinkoff, A., Eaton, W., & Anthony, J. (1991). The prevalence of substance abuse among registered nurses. *Nursing Research, 40*(3), 172-175.

The purpose of this research was to estimate the prevalence of substance abuse and depression among a population-based sample of registered nurses. A comparison was made between nurses and other employed individuals.

Subjects were obtained from a probability sample of households that were part of the National Institute of Mental Health Epidemiologic Catchment Area Program. Of the adults interviewed in the project, 143 were less than age 65 years and were currently working as registered nurses. These nurses were matched by neighborhood of residence and gender to a comparison group of non-nurses.

Estimates of the odds of substance use and depression among the nurses (n = 143) and nonnurses (n = 1410) were calculated. Nurses were no more likely to have engaged in illicit drug use than nonnurses. Nurses were also less likely to have experienced problems with alcohol abuse than nonnurses.

STUDENT ACTIVITIES

- Complete a 1980-to-1990 literature search of this topic.
- Compare the findings of this research study with findings in two additional studies.

CONCEPT REVIEW

Alcohol is the most socially accepted, widely used drug. Alcohol abuse is extremely destructive to the human body. Changes occur in the heart, pancreas, liver, stomach, esophagus, intestines, and skeletal muscle. Metabolic changes induced by alcohol consumption can cause variations in blood glucose levels, increases in uric acid levels, and deposition of fat in the liver.

Central Nervous System Stimulants

CNS stimulants are pharmacologic agents that can increase cortical alertness and electrical activity throughout the brain

TABLE 12–1

Generic and Street Names of Commonly Abused CNS Stimulants[1,8,20]

Generic Name	Street Name(s)
Cocaine hydrochloride	Dope, coke, snow, lady, gold dust
Cocaine freebase	Crack
Racemic amphetamine	Uppers, bennies
Methamphetamine	Speed, meth, crystal, whites
Methamphetamine freebase	Ice
Amphetamine complex	Black beauty, black Cadillacs

and spinal cord. Included in this category are amphetamines, cocaine, synthetic amphetamine-like drugs, caffeine, and nicotine. Generic and street names for some of the commonly used stimulants are included in Table 12–1.

CNS STIMULANT PROTOTYPE
COCAINE

Before 1980, cocaine abuse was considered a minor drug abuse problem. However, during the 1980s, cocaine use increased dramatically. Cocaine is a white crystalline powder. It is self-administered by almost any route, but the preferred method is snorting or inhalation for absorption through the nasal mucosa. In addition, cocaine is absorbed well through the buccal membranes and may be injected intravenously.[20]

Pharmacokinetics Compared to other CNS stimulants, cocaine has a very short half-life. After intranasal or buccal absorption, effects usually last 5 to 15 minutes. Once in the bloodstream, cocaine is rapidly metabolized to benzoylecgonine by the liver. It is excreted by the kidneys. Cocaine may be detected in the urine for 24 to 36 hours after use. To maintain CNS stimulation over long periods, cocaine must be inhaled or injected every 15 to 30 minutes.[20]

Pharmacodynamics Cocaine is an alkaloid found in the leaves of the plant *Erythroxylon coca*. Its effects have been linked to a direct effect on cortical cells and to an alteration of central catecholamine levels. Cocaine is known to inhibit the reuptake of norepinephrine at adrenergic synapses, which may account for some of its central and peripheral effects.[20,21]

Undesired Clinical Responses Intravenous (IV) injection or smoking cocaine can cause sudden death as a result of ventricular fibrillation, myocardial infarction, cerebrovascular accident, or respiratory arrest.[7] Signs of circulatory collapse caused by excessive adrenergic stimulation, hyperventilation, and irregular pulse may occur. In addition, hyperactive psychomotor reflexes and agitation, including facial tics or twitching muscles, have been reported. In the individual who snorts cocaine powder, perforation and bleeding of the nasal septum occur. Pulmonary effects include rhonchi and wheezes.[22]

Pharmacologic Agents Used to Treat Cocaine Abuse Several compounds are used in the treatment of cocaine abusers. Cocaine users frequently develop depression after cocaine use is discontinued. For these individuals, antidepressant therapy has been helpful. One antidepressant prescribed is **desipramine hydrochlo-**

ride (Norpramin, Pertofrane), a tricyclic antidepressant. Desipramine HCl restores normal levels of neurotransmitters in the CNS. **Bromocriptine mesylate** (Parlodel), a dopamine receptor agonist that facilitates binding of dopamine to postsynaptic receptors, has been used successfully in suppression of withdrawal symptoms. Another dopamine agonist, **amantadine hydrochloride** (Symmetrel), has also been used to suppress withdrawal symptoms and craving.[21,22]

CONCEPT REVIEW

The abuse of stimulant drugs is a major problem in the United States. The ability of these drugs to stimulate the cortex and alleviate fatigue make them perfect choices for casual and hard-core abuse.

Stimulants can produce behavior patterns that resemble psychosis and paranoid states. In toxic doses stimulants can produce death caused by cardiovascular collapse or CNS depression.

Hallucinogens

Naturally occurring mood-altering substances have been used for centuries in some cultures. Most of these substances have been replaced by more potent and usually more toxic synthetic agents. Several terms are used to describe these drugs: *hallucinogens, psychotogens,* and *psychedelics.* For purposes of this text they are called *hallucinogens.*

Hallucinogens alter the normal functioning of the peripheral nervous system and CNS. These drugs are grouped according to their chemical composition. Group I contains substances having an indole nucleus. This group includes lysergic acid diethylamide (LSD), psilocybin, dimethyltryptamine (DMT), and diethyltryptamine (DET). Group II includes substances containing β-phenethylamines or substituted phenyl alkylamines such as mescaline and amphetamine-like drugs. Group III contains cannabis (marijuana) and phencyclidine (PCP), which are not related structurally to each other

TABLE 12–2

Generic and Street Names of Commonly Abused Hallucinogens[1,2,8,23]

Hallucinogen	Street Name(s)
Cannabis (marijuana)	Acapulco gold, ace, ashes, baby, broccoli, grass, hemp, jive, joint, Mary Jane, pot, THC, weed
Hash, hashish	Black hash (hashish containing opium), black Russian (potent, dark hashish)
Lysergic acid diethylamide (LSD)	Acid, battery acid, Berkeley blood, big D, chief, HCP, sugar, sunshine, window pane
Mescaline	Bad seed, big chief, cactus, peyote, pink wedge, white light
Phencyclidine (PCP)	Angel dust, flying saucers, hair hog, mist, peace pill

or to the compounds in group I or II.[23] Generic and street names for some of the commonly used hallucinogens are included in Table 12–2.

HALLUCINOGEN PROTOTYPE
MARIJUANA

Marijuana is a complex psychoactive substance containing more than 400 chemicals; 61 of them are cannabinoids. The primary psychoactive constituent is tetrahydrocannabinol (THC), which is concentrated in the resin in the flowering tops and leaves of marijuana plants.[7,10] Potency of any marijuana preparation depends on the amount of resin it contains and the potency of the resin.

Three types of cannabis preparations are available on the "street": marijuana, hash, and hash oil. Marijuana is the most prevalent; it is composed of dried leaves, stems, and flowers of the plant. Marijuana is smoked or added to food items. **Hash,** or hashish, is a potent concentrate of the resin derived from the flowering tops of plants. **Hash oil** is very concentrated THC made by boiling hashish.[23]

Pharmacokinetics Ingested marijuana is metabolized in the liver, whereas marijuana inhaled by smoking is metabolized to some extent in the lungs. Since different enzyme systems are involved in these sites, different metabolites are possible.

THC absorbed into systemic circulation leaves the bloodstream rapidly. It is stored in various body compartments, with highest concentrations in fatty tissues. It is also taken up quickly by tissues well supplied by blood (e.g., liver, spleen, lungs, kidneys, testes, and ovaries). From the fatty tissues, THC is slowly released back into systemic circulation. Measurable levels of THC in the blood of chronic users can be detected for 6 days after the last marijuana cigarette was smoked. In frequent users the plasma half-life is approximately 19 hours. Metabolites of THC are eliminated through the feces and in small amounts through the urine. These metabolites may be found for weeks after the last drug use.[23]

Pharmacodynamics The mechanisms by which THC and its metabolites produce behavioral and physiologic effects are currently not well understood. It is known that these compounds affect brain amine levels, produce ultrastructural changes in some neurons, and cross biologic membranes.[8,22,23]

Undesired Clinical Responses Effects on the respiratory system are due in part to the direct effects of marijuana. Laryngitis, bronchitis, and asthmalike conditions, including obstructive airway disease, have been observed. Hoarseness, rhonchi, or wheezing may be present. CNS manifestations include dilated or glassy pupils, ataxia, and panic reactions. Effects on the cardiovascular system include tachycardia and orthostatic hypotension. Reproductive disorders include decreased sperm production and testosterone levels, testicular atrophy, and altered menstruation. If marijuana is used during pregnancy, fetal toxicity and organ malformation may occur.[7,8,23]

CONCEPT REVIEW

Hallucinogens comprise a diverse group of synthetic and naturally occurring chemicals considered highly toxic.

These substances can alter reality and judgment and produce delusions and hallucinations.

SUMMARY

Substance abuse is a major health care problem in the United States. The cause of drug abuse is complex, varying over time, across geographic regions, by drug, and by characteristics of drug users. Peer pressure, curiosity, depression, attempts to increase or improve performance, and many other reasons have been offered to explain why people use and abuse mood-altering substances.

Nurses in every area come in contact with clients who abuse substances. Although the identifying characteristics and treatment approaches differ, substance abuse may exist in clients of all ages, from adolescents to the elderly. Therefore all nurses should address this topic during their initial assessment of the client.

REFERENCES

1. McFarland, G., & Thomas, M. (1991). *Psychiatric mental health nursing: Application of the nursing process.* Philadelphia: J.B. Lippincott.
2. Haber, J., McMahon, A., Price-Hoskins, P., & Sideleau, B. (1992). *Comprehensive psychiatric nursing* (4th ed.). St. Louis: Mosby–Year Book.
3. American Nurses' Association. (1987). *The care of client with addictions: Dimensions of nursing practice.* Kansas City, MO: Author.
4. Bennett, G., & Woolf, D. (1991). *Substance abuse: Pharmacologic, developmental, and clinical perspectives* (2nd ed.). Albany, NY: Delmar Publishers.
5. Hahn, E. (1993). Parental alcohol and other drug (ADD) use and health beliefs about parent involvement in ADD prevention. *Issues in Mental Health Nursing, 14,* 237-247.
6. Vega, W.A., Zimmerman, R.S., Warheit, G.J., Apospori, E., & Gil, A.G. (1993). Risk factors for early adolescent drug use in four ethnic and racial groups. *American Journal of Public Health, 83*(2), 185-189.
7. Bartholomew, S. (1990). Chemical dependence: Recognition and intervention. *Physician Assistant, 7,* 15-28.
8. Lowinson, J.H., Ruiz, P., & Millman, R. (Eds.). (1992). *Substance abuse: A comprehensive textbook.* Baltimore: Williams & Wilkins.
9. Compton, P. (1989). Drug abuse: A self-care deficit. *Journal of Psychosocial Nursing and Mental Health Services, 27*(3), 22-26.
10. American Psychiatric Association. (1987). *Diagnostic statistical manual of mental disorders* (3rd ed., rev.). Washington, DC: Author.
11. National Institute on Drug Abuse. (1991). *National household survey on drug abuse: Population estimates 1991.* Rockville, MD: U.S. Department of Health and Human Services.

12. U.S. Department of Health and Human Services. (1990). *Alcohol and health.* Rockville, MD: Author.
13. Woolf, D. (1991). CNS depressants: Alcohol. In G. Bennett and D. Woolf, *Substance abuse* (2nd ed., pp. 13-29). Albany, NY: Delmar Publishers.
14. Glowa, J., Crawley, J., Suzdak, P., & Paul, D. (1989). Ethanol and the GABA receptor complex: Studies with partial inverse benzodiazepine receptor agonist Ro 15-4513. *Pharmacological Biochemistry and Behavior, 31,* 767-772.
15. Hoffman, P., Rabe, C., Moses, F., & Tabakoff, B. (1989). *N*-methyl-*D*-aspartate receptors and ethanol: Inhibition of calcium flux and cyclic GMP production. *Journal of Neurochemistry, 52* 1937-1940.
16. Lovinger, D., White, G., & Weight, F. (1989). Ethanol inhibits NMDA-activated ion current in hippocampal neurons. *Science, 243,* 1721-1724.
17. Urbnuo-Marquex, A., et al. (1989). The effects of alcoholism on skeletal and cardiac muscle. *New England Journal of Medicine, 320,* 409-415.
18. Petersen, E. (1992). The pharmacology and toxicology of disulfiram and its metabolites. *Acta Psychiatrica Scandinavica Suppl, 369,* 7-13.
19. Trinkoff, A., Eaton, W., & Anthony, J. (1991). The prevalence of substance abuse among registered nurses. *Nursing Research, 40*(3), 172-175.
20. Holbrook, J. (1991). CNS stimulants. In G. Bennett and D. Woolf, *Substance abuse* (2nd ed., pp. 44-54). Albany, NY: Delmar Publishers.
21. Johnson, D., & Vocci, F. (1993). Medications development at the National Institute on Drug Abuse: Focus on cocaine. In F. Tims and C. Leukerfeld (Eds). *Cocaine treatment: Research and clinical perspectives* (pp. 61-65). Rockwell, MD: National Institute on Drug Abuse.
22. Tims, F., & Leukefeld, C. (Eds.) (1993). *Cocaine treatment: Research and clinical perspectives.* Rockville, MD: National Institute on Drug Abuse.
23. Holbrook, J. (1991). Hallucinogens. In G. Bennett and D. Woolf, *Substance abuse* (2nd ed., pp. 68-80). Albany, NY: Delmar Publishers.

BIBLIOGRAPHY

Holmstrom, C. (1990). Substance abuse in the elderly. *Psychiatric Nursing, 31*(1), 6-8.

Hunt, C. (1991). Understanding symptoms eases drug withdrawal process. *Provider, 17*(11), 39.

Kaufman, E., & McNaul, J.P. (1992). Recent developments in understanding and treating drug abuse and dependence. *Hospital and Community Psychiatry, 43,* 223-236.

McCaffery, M., Ferrell, B., O'Neil-Page, E., & Lester, M. (1990). Nurses' knowledge of opioid analgesic drugs and psychological dependence. *Cancer Nursing, 13*(1), 21-27.

McCaffery, M., & Vourakis, C. (1992). Assessment and relief of pain in chemically dependent patients. *Orthopaedic Nursing, 11*(2), 13-27.

Mohs, M., Watson, R., & Leonard-Grer, T. (1990). Nutritional effects of marijuana, heroin, cocaine, and nicotine. *Journal of the American Dietetic Association, 90,* 1261-1267.

Shuttleworth, A. (1990). Let nurses be an effective weapon against drug abuse. *Professional Nurse, 5,* 226.

Solari-Twadell, P.A. (1991). Recreational drugs: Societal and professional issues. *Nursing Clinics of North America, 26,* 499-509.

Tucker, C. (1990). Acute pain and substance abuse in surgical patients. *Journal of Neuroscience Nursing, 22,* 339-350.

CHAPTER 13

DRUG THERAPY IN
Childbearing and Breastfeeding Clients

SANDRA L. FORNEY

◉ Drug Therapy in the Childbearing Client

LEARNING OBJECTIVES:

Explain physiologic factors affecting drug response in childbearing clients.

Identify appropriate nursing considerations related to the administration of drugs to childbearing clients.

Discuss general guidelines to use in teaching women about drug therapy during pregnancy.

Identify drugs belonging to each of the Food and Drug Administration Pregnancy Categories.

Describe the effects of drugs on the newborn.

KEY TERMS:

Cell differentiation, embryonic period, fetal period, organogenesis, ovum, teratogen

◉ Drug Therapy in the Breast-Feeding Client

LEARNING OBJECTIVES:

Describe physiologic factors affecting drug response in breast-feeding clients.

List appropriate nursing considerations related to the administration of drugs to breast-feeding clients.

Discuss general guidelines to use in teaching women about drug therapy during lactation.

KEY TERMS:

Colostrum, lactation, myoepithelial cells, oxytocin, prolactin

---

CONCEPTS AND TERMS TO REVIEW

Review Chapter 4, which describes the pharmacokinetic processes of absorption, distribution, biotransformation, and excretion.

Review the processes of simple diffusion, pinocytosis, and active transport.

Reexamine fetal development in an anatomy and physiology book.

Drug therapy in childbearing and breast-feeding clients requires special considerations. Any drug or chemical substance taken by the client has the potential to cross into the embryo, fetus, or nursing newborn or infant.

Recent studies indicate that 75% of women use 3 to 10 different prescription or over-the-counter (OTC) drugs per pregnancy. (OTC drug use occurs at a rate four times that of prescribed drugs.) Drugs most frequently ingested are dietary supplements, antiemetics, antacids, antihistamines, analgesics, antibiotics, tranquilizers, hypnotics, and diuretics. These drugs reach the breast-feeding newborn or infant by crossing the blood-milk barrier. They reach the embryo or fetus through the maternal-placental-fetal circulation. When this occurs, the blood level of drug in the fetus can reach 50% to 100% of the maternal blood level. If fetal exposure to the drug produces a permanent alteration in form or function, the substance is labeled a **teratogen.**[1]

Nursing care of childbearing and/or breast-feeding clients requires knowledge of the physiologic changes that occur during pregnancy and lactation. This chapter reviews these changes and provides information on the mechanisms involved in drug transfer to the fetus or nursing newborn or infant. In addition, guidelines are provided for the development of care plans for the pregnant or nursing client and for client teaching.

DRUG THERAPY IN THE CHILDBEARING CLIENT

Few drugs are considered safe; thus all drugs should be avoided by the childbearing client when possible. However, for some pregnant clients, drug therapy is a necessity. For example, drugs are used (1) to treat chronic diseases such as asthma, epilepsy, diabetes mellitus, and cardiac problems; (2) to treat pregnancy-induced problems such as premature labor and hypertension; (3) for therapeutic effect in the fetus (e.g., cardiac glycosides or glucocorticoid); and (4) during labor (e.g., analgesics or anesthetics). In these cases the timing and dose of the drug are critical with regard to the period of embryonic or fetal development.

Fetal Growth During Pregnancy

Growth during pregnancy is divided into three developmental time periods: ovum, embryonic period, and fetal period. The **ovum** comprises the period from fertilization of the egg to the implantation of the products of conception into the uterus. This is a time of cell multiplication, not **cell differentiation.** Drugs taken during this time can damage most or all of the cells. If this damage occurs, the ovum can not survive.[1,2] If the drugs damage only a few cells, the ovum continues without developing deficits. Thus, the drugs have an all-or-nothing effect.

The **embryonic period** lasts from the second to the eighth week of development, which includes most of the first trimester. During this time, **organogenesis** occurs. The cells grow in number and differentiate into specialized cells to form organs and tissues. Placental function begins near the fifth week of embryonic life. Placental integrity is essential in transporting maternal substances for embryonic growth.[1,3,4]

Unintentional exposure of the embryo to teratogenic substances may occur at the beginning of the embryonic period if the client does not know that she is pregnant. However, since placental function does not begin immediately at the time of conception, the growing fetus is provided some natural protection during this time. Even so, if a teratogenic substance reaches the embryo in sufficient amounts, large numbers of cells are destroyed, and the embryo cannot survive. If fewer cells are destroyed, malformations and fetal anomalies occur.[5]

The **fetal period** lasts from week 8 until birth. This period is characterized by cell growth, further cell differentiation, and cell migration. Normal human anatomy was laid down during the embryonic period. Now these structures grow in size and develop physiologic function. The completed organ system is more resistant to teratogenic insult than the embryo. Drugs administered during the fetal period usually do not produce structural changes; instead, the drugs alter future growth or functional development.[1,3,6] For example, diethylstilbestrol (DES) exposure in the pregnant woman can cause defects in the fetus that are not evident until the reproductive age. At that time, female offspring may have müllerian anomalies and vaginal adenosis and carcinoma. Male offspring may have reproductive tract abnormalities such as epididymis cysts, hypotrophic testes, capsular induration, and pathologic semen.[4]

Tetracycline administered during pregnancy is associated with staining of the teeth in children and retarded limb growth in premature infants. Sulfonamides administered in the last weeks of pregnancy compete with bilirubin attachment of protein-binding sites, resulting in neonatal jaundice.[7] (NOTE: Through the remainder of this chapter, the terms *fetal* and *fetus* will be used, although the fetus may actually be in the embryonic period of development.)

Physiologic Changes That Influence the Pharmacokinetic Processes

Physiologic changes associated with pregnancy influence the pharmacokinetic properties of drugs (Fig. 13–1). The following section examines the effects of pregnancy on each process.

ABSORPTION

Changes associated with pregnancy influence the absorption of orally, topically, and parenterally administered drugs. Factors that alter absorption of **orally** administered drugs include nausea, vomiting, decreased gastrointestinal (GI) tone and motility, and altered gastric and intestinal pH levels. Some clients experience heartburn, nausea, and vomiting during the first trimester. These symptoms usually alter the eating habits of the client and may ultimately reduce the amount of drug available for absorption. High levels of circulating progesterone in pregnancy produce a decrease in GI tone and motility. Thus drugs remain in the stomach longer, allowing more absorption to occur. For drugs absorbed from the small intestine, the delay in the stomach delays peak concentration levels in maternal circulation. If the drug undergoes biotransformation in the stomach, the lengthened time in the stomach allows for greater metabolism, decreasing the amount of drug available for absorption in the small intestine. Some drugs pass through the stomach unaltered. For these drugs, lengthened exposure to the mucous membranes in the small intestine increases the amount absorbed. In addition, the amount of hydrochloric acid secretion is reduced during the first two trimesters and is increased during the third trimester. Drugs administered during the first two trimesters that require an acid environment are absorbed more slowly, thus delaying peak serum concentration levels.[7,8]

Altered blood flow to the skin and mucous membranes during pregnancy affects **topically** administered drugs. Blood flow to the hands increases to six times normal, and twice the normal blood flow occurs in the feet. Only small increases occur in the forearms and legs. Therefore absorption of topical or transdermal drugs varies according to the site of the drug's application. Pulmonary function also changes with pregnancy. Although the respiratory rate remains unchanged, the amount of air inhaled per minute increases. In addition, the blood supply to the lungs increases. The combination of increased ventilatory rate and blood flow enhances drug absorption. General anesthetic gases and other drugs administered via the inhalation route produce a more rapid effect.[19] **Parenterally** admin-

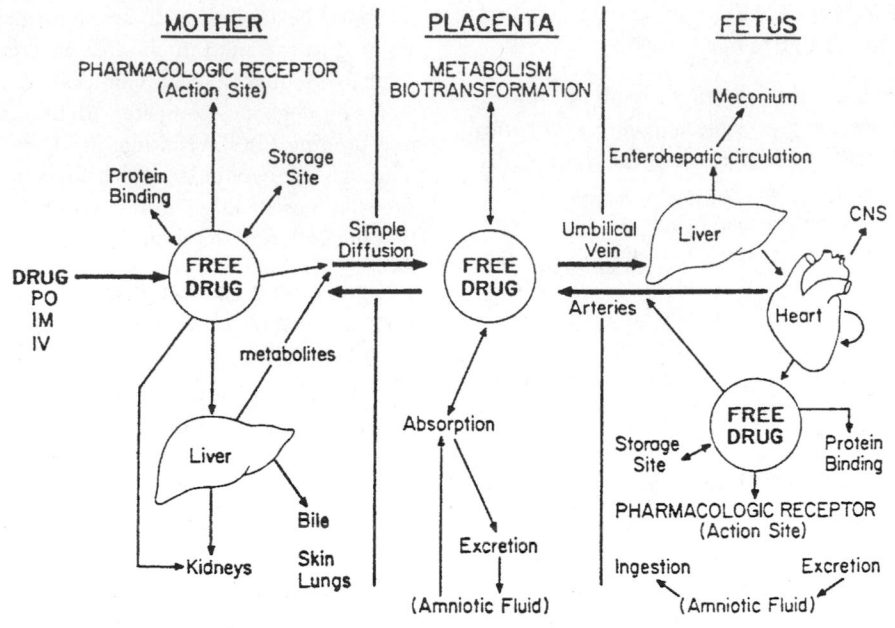

FIGURE 13–1   Drug pathways within maternal, placental, and fetal units. (From Rayburn, W.F., Zuspan, F.P. (1992). *Drug Therapy in Obstetrics and Gynecology.* Norwalk, CT: Appleton & Lange.)

istered drugs are also affected. Circulating blood flow is faster; blood volume and cardiac output are increased, and renal clearance is faster.

DISTRIBUTION

Several physiologic changes occur in the mother, placenta, and fetus that affect the distribution of drugs. By the middle of the second trimester, the cardiac output increases approximately 50%. It remains elevated throughout the rest of the pregnancy. Maternal total body water, extracellular volume, and plasma volume increase. The increase in extracellular fluid volume produces a decrease in drug concentration levels late in pregnancy. The rate of albumin production increases, but there is an overall decrease in serum albumin level because of the expansion in plasma volume.[8] The number of available receptor or binding sites decreases. These sites are occupied by other hormones or endogenous substances that increase during pregnancy. For example, there is an increase in estrogen and progesterone. These hormones are strongly protein bound. In addition, there is an increase in the metabolism of fatty acids, which are carried in the plasma attached to proteins. Since fewer sites are available for binding drugs, more free, unbound drug is distributed throughout the body. The weight gain that occurs during pregnancy also affects drug distribution. The additional weight results in an increase in maternal body fat. As a result, drugs distributed to fatty tissues remain in the body longer and are more slowly released into the bloodstream. This longer retention time may later affect the delivery of drugs to the breast-feeding newborn.[10]

The **placenta** varies in function and structure according to the stage of gestation. Changes that occur late in gestation make it easier for drugs to transfer to the fetus. These changes include (1) increased uteroplacental blood flow; (2) increased placental surface area; (3) decreased thickness of the semipermeable lipid membranes between the placental capillaries; (4) greater physical disruption of placental membranes; and (5) more acidic fetal circulation to "trap" basic drugs.[8,9]

Most drugs cross the placenta by simple diffusion, but transport also occurs by facilitated diffusion, active transport, and pinocytosis. The actual amount of drug to reach the fetus depends on the drug's molecular weight, lipid solubility, degree of ionization, and extent of protein binding. **Lipid-soluble drugs** are easily transported between the mother and the fetus. Water-soluble drugs transfer into the fetus easily but do not return as easily to the mother. These drugs accumulate in the amniotic fluid around the fetus. Most drugs have a **molecular weight** of less than 500. Drugs with a molecular weight less than 600 readily cross the placenta. Those with molecular weights greater than 1000 such as heparin rarely cross the placenta. Since stronger **ionized drugs** have a greater affinity for protein binding, they replace weaker ionized drugs, increasing the level of the weaker drug in circulation.[8,9]

Besides characteristics of the drug, placental transport is also affected by the placental blood flow, pH gradient between mother and fetus, and the placental metabolism. Some drugs affect placental enzyme activity. Others reduce placental blood flow or interfere with normal transport functions of the placenta. These factors not only alter drug distribution but influence the development of the fetus.[8,9]

Drug level within the **fetus** is determined by cardiac output, tissue affinity and binding, drug metabolism, renal excretion, recirculating amniotic fluid, and permeability of specialized membranes. Drug molecules enter the fetus by traveling through the umbilical vein to the portal vein and into the liver.

In the liver drugs are either metabolized or shunted through the ductus venosus into the right side of the heart. The heart distributes the blood and the drug molecules to essential organs, following the pathway of least resistance. Since the fetus has lower levels of plasma proteins and fewer protein-binding capacities than the mother, more free, unbound drug is available. These free, unbound drug molecules easily enter the brain since the blood-brain barrier is poorly developed. Drug molecules in the fetal circulation also compete with other drugs or compounds for protein-binding sites. Eventually, more than half of the cardiac output is returned through the umbilical arteries to the placental and maternal circulation.[6,8]

BIOTRANSFORMATION

Blood flow through the **maternal** liver remains unchanged during pregnancy with only minimal stasis occurring. However, maternal metabolism of drugs by the liver is diminished by the increase of circulating steroid hormones. These hormones compete for plasma protein-binding sites.[8]

Metabolism of drug molecules in the **fetus** occurs primarily in the fetal liver. The hepatic microsomal enzymes produce oxidation and conjugation reactions. Some drugs such as phenobarbital or alcohol stimulate further enzyme activity. Prolonged narcotic, phenobarbital, or alcohol exposure conjugates bilirubin in the neonate. Metabolism of drugs by the **placenta** occurs but is not well understood. The placenta is capable of reduction, conjugation, and hydrolysis.[8]

EXCRETION

Since there is increased cardiac output during pregnancy, a corresponding increase in renal perfusion and glomerular filtration occurs. Renal blood flow increases 25% to 50%, and glomerular filtration increases 50%. These changes increase the excretion of drugs by the kidneys. Late in pregnancy, the size and weight of the uterus increase. As a result, when the client lies on her back, renal blood flow is decreased. This results in decreased excretion and prolonged effects of drugs excreted by the kidneys.[8]

Excretion of drugs is slower and less efficient in the fetus because of the immature development of the kidneys. The primary routes of elimination are the placenta and the fetal urine. Urine is excreted into the amniotic fluid. Swallowing of the urine by the fetus results in recirculation of some drugs.[8]

CONCEPT REVIEW

Physiologic factors affect drug response in childbearing clients.

Maternal Factors
- Reduced tone and motility of the GI tract
- Altered secretion of hydrochloric acid
- Increased weight gain
- Increased intercellular and extracellular volume
- Increased blood volume
- Increased plasma protein production
- Greater competition for plasma protein binding sites

Fetal Factors
- Placental metabolism and integrity
- Umbilical blood flow
- Immature blood-brain barrier
- Immature hepatic and renal systems
- Reduced plasma protein binding sites
- High proportion of water-to-body mass

NURSING CONSIDERATIONS

Nurses who have contact with the childbearing client must assess the client carefully and intervene in a manner helpful to both the mother and fetus.

Assessing   A baseline health history and drug history must be collected on each client. Using a holistic approach is essential. The **health history** should include physiologic, social, psychologic, cultural, and economic information. Include the client's perception of her current health status. Ask the client to describe her health promotion and protection patterns. Explore the client's nutritional intake (e.g., ask if there are pica practices that expose the fetus to drugs or chemicals). Ask questions that will help investigate the client's social support systems, cultural and religious aspects, and self-concept. Include questions about feelings toward and about drugs, coping mechanisms, level of stress, and locus of control.

Ask questions about the client's place of employment to determine if she is exposed to teratogenic substances. Determine if the client is exposed to pesticides, solvents, anesthetic gases, heavy metals, and/or radiation. Hobbies should be explored for environmental hazards such as lead solder use in making jewelry or working with stained glass. The client's history should also identify cultural practices that put women at risk for chemical or drug exposure. For example, Islamic and Hindu women use certain cosmetics (kohl and surma) that contain lead. Certain Asian and Mexican folk remedies also contain lead.[11,12]

While obtaining the **drug history,** ask the client about the use of social drugs such as tobacco, caffeine, alcohol, and street drugs. Determine if the client is currently taking any OTC or prescription drugs. To help identify drug use, ask how the client copes with the general discomforts of pregnancy or if chronic health problems exist. Determine if the client uses any ethnic or folk remedies. Also ask about allergies and past adverse reactions. Determine the client's knowledge level about each drug being taken. Can the client describe the drug, provide information about the dose and frequency of administration, explain what the drug does, and describe the adverse reactions associated with the drug?

Diagnosing   After obtaining a thorough history, data analysis determines appropriate nursing diagnoses. These diagnoses include the following:
- High risk of injury to fetus related to maternal ingestion of drugs.
- High risk of altered nutrition: less than body requirements related to pica practices.

- High risk of injury to fetus related to work place teratogens.
- Noncompliance related to maternal desire for continued ingestion of illicit drugs.

Planning   The plan of care must take into consideration the well-being of both the fetus and the mother. Client education is a major part of the plan. The client should be taught healthful lifestyle practices such as proper diet, rest, exercise, and avoidance of alcohol, caffeine, and tobacco. Teach the client that any drug can reach the fetus and interfere with growth and development. Provide her with information about nondrug measures for relief of common health problems and discomforts of pregnancy. Instruct the client to contact the primary health care provider before taking any drugs.

Develop expected outcomes with the client. These outcomes should reflect the nursing diagnoses appropriate for the client. Possible expected outcomes include the following:

- Client verbalizes factors that contribute to possible injury of fetus.
- Client demonstrates lifestyle changes to reduce injury to the fetus.
- Client identifies lifestyle and cultural factors that predispose to inadequate nutrition during pregnancy.
- Client participates in development of a plan to eliminate use of illicit drugs.

Implementating   If drug use is indicated during pregnancy, the prescriber should select a drug that is unlikely to cause teratogenic effects. Newer drugs should be avoided; instead, drugs that have been thoroughly studied should be used. Because of slower absorption, the oral route is recommended.

TABLE 13–1
FDA Pregnancy Categories

Category	Examples of Drugs in Categories
A	Prenatal vitamins
	Multivitamins
B	Penicillin
	Cephalosporins
	Immune globulins for hepatitis B
C	Antivirals
	Cholinergics
	Anticholinergics
	Tranquilizers
	Laxatives
	Cardiac drugs
	Select vaccines
D	Anticonvulsants
	Tetracyclines
	Progesterones
	Anticoagulants except heparin
	Antithyroids except sodium iodide
	Many diuretics
	Most antineoplastics
X	Estrogens
	Vaccines for rubella, smallpox, measles, mumps
	Sodium iodide

In addition, the smallest dose should be given for the shortest time possible.

As indicated in Chapter 2, the Food and Drug Administration (FDA) has assigned five categories to prescription drugs (Table 13–1) that indicate a drug's potential for causing birth defects. These range from A (remote possibility of teratogenic effects) to X (risk of teratogenic effect outweighs any therapeutic benefits—use contraindicated). In later chapters the FDA pregnancy category is identified for most drugs described.

Evaluating   To determine whether the interventions were appropriate, examine the continued drug practices during pregnancy. If a drug has been discontinued, has the client actually quit taking the drug? If a drug has been changed, has the client followed through with the change? Examination of the newborn at birth gives an indication of the effects of drugs during pregnancy. However, some effects are not visible for days, months, or even years.

🌿 NURSING RESEARCH

Butters, L., & Howie, C. (1990). Awareness among pregnant women of the effect on the fetus of commonly used drugs. *Midwifery, 6*(3), 146-154.

Studies have shown that pregnant women continue to take substantial quantities of drugs, particularly OTC drugs. Awareness of the effects on the fetus of commonly used drugs, cigarettes, and alcohol among 514 women in the postnatal wards of two maternity units in Glasgow, Scotland, was assessed by self-completion questionnaire.

Most of the subjects recognized that the fetus is most at risk of being harmed by drugs during the first 3 months of pregnancy. The majority of the subjects felt it was safest not to smoke and were aware of the adverse effects of smoking on fetal growth. More than half thought that alcohol should be avoided altogether during pregnancy and considered alcohol harmful to breastfed babies. A generally high level of awareness of commonly used drugs was demonstrated by these subjects, but areas requiring further health education were noted.

STUDENT ACTIVITIES

- Visit a prenatal clinic and determine what information is given to pregnant clients about the use of drugs.
- Request permission to audit the chart of 10 postpartum women. After reading the health history, record information about their use of drugs during pregnancy. Compare your findings with the Apgar score for the infants. 🌿

Effects of Drugs on Neonates

Some of the problems associated with drug use and the neonate are low birth weight, fetal alcohol syndrome, and crack (cocaine-exposed) babies.

LOW BIRTH WEIGHT

Studies suggest that caffeine, tobacco, and alcohol contribute to low birth weights. The half-life of caffeine triples during the third trimester of pregnancy because caffeine clearance decreases, thus increasing the exposure of the fetus. In addition, caffeine consumption by the mother increases the levels of circulating catecholamines, which cause vasoconstriction in uteroplacental circulation and reduce the blood flow to the fetus. This can affect fetal growth and cause fetal hypoxia.[13,14] Smoking is a contributing factor in 20% to 40% of the cases of low-birth-weight infants in the United States. Smoking is usually associated with a 150- to 200-g reduction in infant birth weight. Women who consume alcohol during pregnancy have more stillbirths, low-birth-weight infants, and lower placental weights than women who do not. Alcohol probably contributes to intrauterine growth retardation.[14]

FETAL ALCOHOL SYNDROME

The most serious adverse effect associated with alcohol is fetal alcohol syndrome. Fetal alcohol syndrome is not associated with single drinking binges but occurs when the pregnant woman consistently drinks more than 80 to 100 g of alcohol daily. The most severe abnormalities seen with this syndrome are facial dysmorphology, prenatal and postnatal growth deficiencies, and central nervous system (CNS) involvement. Facial abnormalities involve the eyes, nose, and the mouth. CNS involvement includes microcephaly, hypotonia, irritability in infancy, and hyperactivity in childhood.[14,15]

COCAINE-EXPOSED INFANTS

In women who use cocaine during pregnancy there is a significant incidence of abruptio placentae, prematurity, and growth retardation. Drug-exposed infants are significantly smaller at birth. During the first week of life these infants generally show such neurobehavioral symptoms as tremulousness, irritability, hypertonia, poor sucking and feeding, regurgitation, yawning, and sneezing.[16,17]

DRUG THERAPY IN THE BREAST-FEEDING CLIENT

With the delivery of the fetus, the client experiences a reversal in the physiologic changes created in her body by the pregnancy. If the client chooses to breast-feed, she must continue to monitor her drug or chemical use since anything she ingests potentially can cross into the breast milk for ingestion by the newborn. The following section reviews the production of breast milk, the transfer of drug molecules into the breast milk, and the pharmacokinetic properties of the newborn.

Production of Milk

The term **lactation** refers to the secretion and ejection of milk by the mammary glands. **Prolactin** from the anterior pituitary gland is the principal hormone that promotes lactation.

Even though prolactin levels increase as the pregnancy progresses, no milk is secreted because estrogens and progesterone inhibit the effectiveness of the prolactin. After delivery, the levels of these hormones in the mother's blood decrease, and the inhibition is removed. Breast milk is a suspension of fat in a protein-mineral-carbohydrate solution. It is produced in the **myoepithelial cells** of the alveoli of the breast. Substances that comprise breast milk originate in the maternal circulation.

After delivery, the client planning to breast-feed begins nursing her child. Sucking by the infant stimulates **oxytocin** release. Oxytocin induces myoepithelial cells surrounding the outer walls of the alveoli to contract, thereby compressing the alveoli and ejecting the milk. This process is called **milk ejection** or **let-down.** The removal of the milk from the breast stimulates further milk production. If the sucking stimulation ceases, the prolactin secretion diminishes and reduces the amount of breast milk produced. Maternal nutrition and state of health also affect the amount of breast milk produced.

For the first 3 to 4 days, the newborn receives **colostrum.** Colostrum is more viscous, higher in proteins and minerals, and lower in fat and carbohydrate than breast milk. Changes in fat and carbohydrate content gradually take place as the milk changes into transitional milk and then into the whole breast milk. Initially the newborn takes approximately 7 to 14 ml of milk at each feeding. By the end of the first week, the newborn is receiving approximately 500 ml of milk in the same 24-hour period. Later the newborn ingests an average of 800 ml in 24 hours.[18]

Lactation and Drugs

Plasma drug concentration levels and mammary blood flow determine the amount of drug distributed to the breast for possible metabolism and delivery to the newborn in breast milk. Mammary blood flow is influenced by the metabolic activity in the mammary gland and the release of lactogenic hormones in response to infant suckling. Blood flow is also affected by the decrease in intramammary pressure from removal of milk from the breast and the use of certain drugs.[8]

The ability of the drug molecule to pass into the breast milk also influences the amount of drug exposure to the fetus. Some of the same factors that influenced passage of drug molecules across the placental barrier are important in determining what drugs pass into breast milk. In general, drugs cross the cell membrane by passive diffusion. However, some drug molecules are moved by pinocytosis, facilitated diffusion, or active transport. Unbound, nonionized, lipid-soluble drugs of low molecular weight pass more easily and in greater amounts into the breast milk. Large drug molecules enter the breast milk in limited quantities unless the molecules have a high lipid content. Drugs that are tightly bound to plasma proteins typically do not enter breast milk. However, drugs are transported into the milk bound to milk proteins or on the surface of the lipid component of the milk fat globule. Drugs also pass more easily into colostrum than into transitional or whole breast milk.[19,20]

The amount of milk produced alters the amount of drug available to the newborn. Heavy smoking decreases milk supply, as do drugs with sympathomimetic activity. Some drugs act on the hypothalamus to increase or decrease the release of prolactin inhibiting factor (PIF). Drugs that increase the output of PIF include monoamine oxidase (MAO) inhibitors, pyridoxine hydrochloride, levodopa (L-Dopa), and bromocriptine mesylate (Parlodel). Drugs that suppress prolactin inhibiting factor include phenothiazines, cimetidine (Tagamet), and certain antihypertensives such as reserpine and methyldopa (Aldomet). Metoclopramide hydrochloride (e.g., Reglan) is a potent stimulator of prolactin release and is used in women with dereased milk flow.[8]

Effects of Drugs on Newborn

The effect of a drug on a nursing infant depends on newborn's maturity; both gestational age and chronologic age are important. The younger, less mature newborn usually ingests smaller amounts of milk and handles drug exposure poorly. In addition, the milk composition and the changing physiologic characteristics of the newborn influence the pharmacokinetic properties of the drug.

ABSORPTION

The amount of drug absorbed from the breast milk is influenced by the functional readiness of the GI tract, which includes the infant's gastric acidity and gastric emptying time. **Gastric acid secretion** is variable and depends on both birth weight and newborn gestational age. Presence of gastric acid is rarely seen in newborns less than 32 weeks' gestation. In the full-term newborn the gastric acid secretion increases for the first 10 days. It drops between the tenth and thirtieth days and gradually reaches the lower limits of adult values by the third month.

Gastric emptying is variable and is influenced by several factors, including prematurity, peristaltic rate, presence of bacterial flora, type of feeding, and presence of disease. For the first 6 to 8 months, the newborn has irregular peristalsis; then gradually regular peristalsis is established. Although little is known about GI flora colonization and flora metabolic activity, it is known that colonization is affected by postnatal age, type of delivery, type of feeding, and presence of drugs. Disease states may prolong or decrease gastric emptying. For example, with steatorrhea or diarrhea, the drug passes through the GI tract more quickly, decreasing the amount of absorption. The type of newborn diet also influences gastric emptying. Breast-fed newborns have a faster emptying time than formula-fed newborns. Feeding of long-chain fatty acids or those with higher caloric density slows gastric emptying.[21]

DISTRIBUTION

Distribution in the newborn is influenced by body water content, fat content, protein binding, and regional blood flow. Newborns have a greater total water content and a greater ratio of extracellular-to-intracellular fluid volume. This distribution dilutes the extracellular drug concentration. Fat content, protein quantity, and the ability of protein to bind drugs are lower in newborns. Plasma protein drug binding depends on several age-related variables such as amount of protein avail-

able, available binding sites, and the presence of endogenous substances that compete for binding sites. During the first week of life, bilirubin levels are often elevated because of increased red cell destruction and limited liver conjugation capacity. At birth the binding affinity of bilirubin is much less than in the adult. When drugs compete with bilirubin for the same binding sites, the end result can be excessively high levels of unconjugated bilirubin (neonatal jaundice) or high levels of drugs yielding toxic effects.[21]

BIOTRANSFORMATION

The primary organ for drug metabolism in the newborn is the liver. The kidneys, intestines, skin, adrenal glands, and mammary epithelium are also capable of biotransformation.

The liver is capable of the following enzyme activities: oxidation, reduction, hydrolysis, and conjugation. At birth the infant has low concentrations of some hepatic microsomal enzymes. **Oxidation enzymes** are present in the fetal liver at levels comparable to those of the adult liver. Unfortunately, the activity of the oxidizing enzyme system is greatly reduced in the neonate. **Hydrolytic enzyme** levels are also reduced during the neonatal period, resulting in highly erratic and variable rates of activity. **Conjugation enzymatic reactions** are primarily responsible for synthesis of water-soluble compounds. **Detoxifying** includes the ability to combine harmful materials with glucuronic acid. Low levels of glucuronyl transferase and uridine diphosphate glucuronide dehydrogenase are present. Since drugs are unable to conjugate with glucuronic acid, they remain in the body longer. This system does not become functional until 1 to 2 weeks of age.[21]

Postnatal age, pathology, and previous exposure to enzyme inducers such as phenobarbital influence the rate of hepatic maturation. The initially slow enzyme activity is followed by a period of rapid enzyme activity that even surpasses adult metabolic capacity.

EXCRETION

Most drugs are excreted from the body by the kidneys. Renal excretion is influenced by the rate of glomerular filtration, tubular secretion, and tubular reabsorption. The amount of drug filtered by the glomerulus depends on the functional capacity of the glomerulus, the integrity of the renal blood flow, and the extent of drug-protein binding. **Renal blood flow** increases as a result of functional maturation, cardiac output, and a reduction in peripheral vascular resistance. At birth the renal blood flow averages 12 ml. Adult levels are reached at 5 to 12 months of age.[21]

Before 34 weeks of gestation, the **glomerular filtration rate** is minimal. Maturation occurs in the nephrons between weeks 34 and 36. The glomerular filtration rate in the newborn is approximately 2 to 4 ml per minute. This rate doubles in 2 weeks and reaches adult values (125 ml/min) by 5 months of age.[21]

Tubular secretory function is the slowest developing function—much slower than glomerular filtration. Tubular function approaches adult levels at approximately 7 months of life.[21]

CONCEPT REVIEW

Physiologic factors affect drug response in breast-feeding
   clients

Maternal Factors
- Mammary epithelial metabolism capability
- Mammary blood flow
- Level of drug in mother's body

Fetal Factors
- Immature digestive system
- Immature renal and hepatic system
- Immature enzyme activity
- Few plasma proteins
- Amount of newborn fat and water content
- Type of feeding
- Concentration of drug in milk
- Duration of feeding
- Volume of milk ingested
- Timing of feeding in relation to drug ingestion by
  mother

✷ NURSING CONSIDERATIONS

As with the pregnant client, care follows the steps in the nursing process.

Assessing   The decision to breast-feed is usually made before delivery. Therefore the nurse in the hospital or delivery center must reenforce instructions previously given to the client. However, if the decision to breast-feed has not been made, the nurse's role changes.

Initially, collect a complete health history that focuses on drug usage and nutritional patterns of the mother. Review the client's past and present lifestyle practices for drug and chemical use. Ask specific questions about drugs routinely taken by the client. Ask questions such as the following: "Do you take any prescription or OTC medications? If so, what is the purpose, starting date, dose, and frequency of each?" "How much per day do you consume of the following beverages: coffee, tea, cola, cocoa?" "Do you drink alcoholic beverages?"

Diagnosing   After obtaining a thorough history, analyze the data to determine the areas in which nursing interventions are needed. The following nursing diagnoses may be appropriate for the breast-feeding mother:
- Interrupted breast-feeding related to neonatal physiologic jaundice.
- High risk for injury to newborn related to maternal ingestion of drugs.
- High risk for altered nutrition: less than body requirements related to increased demands of breast-feeding.
- Anxiety related to prescribed drug regimen during breast-feeding.

Planning   In addition to addressing the specific nursing diagnoses appropriate for the client, client education must be provided. Encourage healthful lifestyle measures such as a nu-

tritious diet, exercise, plenty of rest, and avoidance of caffeine, alcohol or tobacco. Tell the client to use nondrug measures for common health problems and preventive measures such as handwashing and cleansing nipples before breast-feeding to avoid health problems. Teach the client about the lactation process and how substances are converted into breast milk. Emphasize that any OTC, prescribed, or illicit drug can reach the newborn. Remind the client to tell all health care providers that she is breast-feeding. If prescribed drugs are necessary, provide the client with information on the drug's potential for crossing into the milk.

Implementing   If drug use is indicated during breast-feeding, a drug is selected that is least likely to cause an effect in the newborn. Newer drugs should be avoided; those selected should be well-known, with studies identifying expected effects. Use of long-acting drugs should be avoided. In addition, the smallest dose needed should be prescribed for the shortest time possible. The drug should be administered after breast-feeding or before the newborn's long sleeping periods to lessen the amount of the drug in the breast milk. During the early period of breast-feeding, use of lipid drugs should be avoided since they cross into the milk faster if the milk is colostrum or early transitional milk. Because of the immature liver in a neonate, use of drugs detoxified in the liver should also be avoided.

TABLE 13–2

Examples of Drugs to Avoid and Drugs to Use with Caution During Breast-Feeding

Drug/Drug Category	Possible Response in Newborn
DRUGS TO AVOID	
Cocaine	Signs of withdrawal, seizures, behavioral developmental problems
Lithium citrate (Cibalith-S, Lithobid/Cibalith)	Central nervous system disturbance, impaired cardiovascular function
Methotrexate sodium (Folex, Mexate)	Immune suppression
Bromocriptine mesylate (Parlodel)	Suppressed lactation
Cyclosporine (Sandimmune)	Potential nephrotoxicity, possible immune suppression
Ergotamine tartrate	Vomiting, diarrhea, suppressed lactation
Alcohol	Large doses: drowsiness, diaphoresis, growth retardation, Cushing's syndrome
Marijuana	Drowsiness
DRUGS TO USE WITH CAUTION	
Estrogen	Feminization
Diazepam (Valium)	Sedation, cumulative effect in infant
Phenobarbital	Sedation, decreased responsiveness
Tetracycline	Possible staining of developing teeth
Sulfonamides	Increased risk for kernicterus, neonatal jaundice
Aluminum antacids	Developmental retardation
Phenytoin (Dilantin)	Methemoglobinemia

Options should be discussed with the client on whether or not to continue breast-feeding while receiving drug therapy. If drug therapy is indicated, the expected adverse effects to the mother and her newborn should be explained and information provided on what to do if they occur. If using drugs harmful to the newborn cannot be avoided, it may be necessary to interrupt breast-feeding temporarily.

The American Academy of Pediatrics has developed a list of drugs and chemicals that transfer into human milk.[22] The drugs are divided into five groups:

1. Drugs not to administer to any breast-feeding client
2. Drugs to administer with caution
3. Drugs whose effects are unknown
4. Drugs requiring temporary discontinuation of breast-feeding
5. Drugs that are safe

Use this resource when caring for a mother who is breast-feeding (Table 13–2).

Evaluating To determine if the interventions were appropriate, examine the continued drug practices during breast-feeding and determine if breast-feeding continued successfully. Examine the health status of the newborn, including its growth and feeding patterns, sleep and wake cycles, behavior, responsiveness, and comfort levels. Examine the health status of the mother, including comfort and coping levels. Evaluate the maternal-newborn unit for bonding behaviors.

SUMMARY

In conclusion, any drug has the potential to reach the fetus or the breast-feeding newborn. Serum drug levels of 50% to 100% of the mother's blood concentration level have been detected in fetuses. In the newborn who is breast-feeding, serum drug levels of 1% to 2% have been detected. When drug therapy is necessary, health care providers should review the categories identified by the FDA indicating a drug's potential for causing birth defects and the American Academy of Pediatrics' list of drugs and chemicals transferred into human milk. The drug therapy chosen should take into consideration the development of the fetus or newborn and seek to avoid potential harm.

REFERENCES

1. Cunningham, F.G., MacDonald, P.C., Gant, N.F., Leveno, K.J., & Gilstrap, L.C. (1993). *Williams obstetrics* (19th ed.). Norwalk, CT: Appleton & Lange.
2. Kuller, J.M. (1990). Effects on the fetus and newborn of medications commonly used during pregnancy. *Journal of Perinatal and Neonatal Nursing, 3*(4), 73-87.
3. Gilstrap, L.C., & Little, B.B. (1992). *Drugs and pregnancy*. New York: Elsevier.
4. Briggs, G.G., Freeman, R.K., & Yaffe, S.J. (1990). *Drugs in pregnancy and lactation: A reference guide to fetal and neonatal risk* (3rd ed.). Baltimore: Williams & Wilkins.
5. Ives, T.J., & Tepper, R.S. (1990). Drug use in pregnancy and lactation. *Primary Care, 17*, 623-645.
6. Verklan, M.T. (1989). Safe in the womb? Drug and chemical effects on the fetus and neonate. *Neonatal Network, 8*(1), 59-65.
7. Olds, S.B., London, M.L., & Ladewig, P.A. (1992). *Maternal-newborn nursing: A family-centered approach* (4th ed.). Menlo Park, CA: Addison-Wesley.
8. Rayburn, W.F., & Zuspan, F.P. (1992). *Drug therapy in obstetrics and gynecology* (3rd ed.). Norwalk, CT: Appleton-Century-Crofts.
9. Reece, E.A., Hobbins, J.C., Mahoney, M.J., & Petrie, R.H. (1992). *Medicine of the fetus and mother*. Philadelphia: J.B. Lippincott.
10. Mattison, D.R. (1990). Transdermal drug absorption during pregnancy. *Clinical Obstetrics and Gynecology, 33*, 718-727.
11. Lidstrom, I. (1990). Pregnant women in the workplace. *Seminars in Perinatology, 14*, 329-333.
12. Brown, M.J., Bellinger, D., & Matthews, J. (1990). In utero lead exposure. *American Journal of Maternal Child Nursing, 15*(2), 94-96.
13. McKim, E.M. (1991). Caffeine and its effects on pregnancy and the neonate. *Journal of Nurse-Midwifery, 36*, 229-231.
14. Aaronson, L.S., & Macnee, C. (1989). Tobacco, alcohol, and caffeine use during pregnancy. *JOGNN, July/August*, 279-285.
15. Butters, L., & Howie, C. (1990). Awareness among pregnant women of the effect on the fetus of commonly used drugs. *Midwifery, 6*(3), 146-154.
16. Jhaveri, M.K., Schechter, C., Gertner, M., & Holzman, I. (1993). Perinatal cocaine/crack exposure in infants: A different perspective. *Neonatal Intensive Care, 5*(3), 18-19.
17. Saylor, C., Lippa, B., & Lee, G. (1991). Drug-exposed infants at home: Strategies and supports. *Public Health Nursing, 8*(1), 33-38.
18. Riordan, J., & Auerbach, K.G. (1993). *Breastfeeding and human lactation*. Boston: Jones & Bartlett.
19. O'Dea, R.F. (1992). Medication use in the breastfeeding mother. *NAACOG's Clinical Issues in Perinatal and Woman's Health Nursing, 3*, 598-604.
20. Lawrence, R.A. (1989). Breastfeeding and medical disease. *Medical Clinics of North America, 73*, 583-603.
21. Reed, M.D., & Besunder, J.B. (1989). Developmental pharmacology: Ontogenic basis of drug disposition. *Pediatric Clinics of North America, 36*, 1053-1074.
22. Committee on Drugs, American Academy of Pediatrics (1989). Transfer of drugs and other chemicals into human milk. *Pediatrics, 84*, 924-936.

BIBLIOGRAPHY

Anderson, P.O. (1991). Drug use during breast-feeding. *Clinical Pharmacy, 10*, 594-624.

Dattell, B.J. (1990). Substance abuse in pregnancy. *Seminars in Perinatology, 14*(2), 179-187.

Kacew, S. (1993). Adverse effects of drugs and chemicals in breast milk on the nursing infant. *Journal of Clinical Pharmacology, 33*, 213-221.

Knott, C., & Reynolds, F. (1990). Therapeutic drug monitoring in pregnancy: Rationale and current status. *Clinical Pharmacokinetics, 19*, 425-433.

Krauer, B., & Dayer, P. (1991). Fetal drug metabolism and its possible clinical implications. *Clinical Pharmacokinetics, 21*, 70-80.

Miller, R.K. (1991). Fetal drug therapy: Principles and issues. *Clinical Obstetrics and Gynecology, 34*, 241-249.

Niebyl, J.R. (1991). Drugs with little or no potential fetal toxicity. *Contemporary OB/GYN, 36*(5), 71-80.

Niebyl, J.R. (1991). Drugs with potential fetal toxicity. *Contemporary OB/GYN, 36*(4), 68-78.

Notarianni, J.J. (1990). Plasma protein binding of drugs in pregnancy and in neonates. *Clinical Pharmacokinetics, 18*, 20-36.

Ito, S., Blajchman, A., Stephenson, M., Eliopoulos, C., & Koren, G.

(1993). Prospective follow-up of adverse reactions in breast-fed infants exposed to maternal medication. *American Journal of Obstetrics and Gynecology, 168,* 1393-1399.

Peters, H., & Theorell, C.J. (1991). Fetal and neonatal effects of cocaine use. *Journal of Obstetric, Gynecologic, and Neonatal Nursing, 20*(2), 121-126.

Rurak, D.W., Wright, M.R., & Axelson, J.E. (1991). Drug disposition and effects in the fetus. *Journal of Developmental Physiology, 15*(1), 33-44.

Weiss, J., & Hansell, M.J. (1992). Substance abuse during pregnancy: Legal and health policy issues. *Nursing and Health Care, 13,* 472-479.

CHAPTER 14

DRUG THERAPY IN THE
Neonate and Pediatric Client

JANICE RUMFELT

⚜ Physiologic Factors Affecting Drug Response

LEARNING OBJECTIVES:

Describe three physiologic factors that affect drug response in the neonate and pediatric client.

Define terms used to describe pediatric clients.

KEY TERMS:

Adolescent, infant, neonate, newborn, preschooler, school-age, toddler

⚜ Pharmacokinetic Differences in Children of Various Ages

LEARNING OBJECTIVES:

Explain three factors affecting absorption of drugs in pediatric clients.

Summarize two factors affecting distribution of drugs in pediatric clients.

Discuss age-related alterations in drug metabolism.

Identify age-related alterations in drug excretion.

⚜ Preparing for Drug Administration

LEARNING OBJECTIVES:

List factors that must be assessed before administering drugs to a child.

Develop appropriate nursing diagnoses for the pediatric client.

Summarize important developmental changes that influence drug therapy for the pediatric client.

⚜ Administering Drug Preparations

LEARNING OBJECTIVE: Describe age-related modifications needed for administering drugs to pediatric clients.

KEY TERMS:

Body surface area, Clark's rule, Fried's rule, nomogram, Young's rule

⚜ Unique Response of Children to Drugs

LEARNING OBJECTIVES:

Discuss drug efficacy in the pediatric client.

Summarize major points associated with age-related drug toxicity.

CONCEPTS AND TERMS TO REVIEW

Reexamine processes in the pharmacokinetic phase from Chapter 4.

Review content on individual variation in drug response in Chapter 6.

Review normal growth and development from the neonate through the adolescent.

Giving drugs to children goes far beyond the "five rights" of correct drug, dose, route, time, and child. Although the primary care provider writes the order for the precise amount of a particular drug to be given by a specific route at a specified frequency, it is the nurse who administers the drug. This gives the nurse the legal responsibility for verifying that the drug dosage is within recommended limits and that the drug and route are appropriate for the child's age and condition. Nurses are expected to know anticipated actions, possible undesired clinical responses, and signs of drug toxicity in children, just as in adults.

Successful administration of drugs to children requires that you, the nurse, possess skillful techniques for drug administration and knowledge of normal growth and developmental patterns. This chapter includes information on how the child's age and condition affect the action of drugs in the body, the safe calculation of pediatric dosages, and age-related developmental considerations. It does not include information about the psychomotor skills required for preparing and administering drugs (see a pediatric nursing text for this information).

PHYSIOLOGIC FACTORS AFFECTING DRUG RESPONSE

Knowledge of how the growth and development process affects the disposition of drugs in the body has greatly expanded during the past 20 years. The immaturity of body organs and systems is known to create unique responses to drugs.[1-3]

Height, Weight, and Body Surface Area

Between birth and physical maturity the individual's height increases approximately three and one half times, and the weight increases approximately 20 times. Body surface area, measured by the relationship of height and weight, increases approximately seven times.

TERMS USED TO DESCRIBE PEDIATRIC CLIENTS

newborn a human offspring from the time of birth through the twenty-eighth day of life

neonate a newborn

infant a young child from the end of the first month of life to the end of the first year of life

toddler a child between the ages of 12 and 36 months

preschooler a child between 3 and 6 years of age

school-age a child between 6 years of age and puberty

adolescent a child between the onset of puberty and the cessation of physical growth (approximately 11 to 19 years of

---

Integumentary System

The relatively larger body surface area in children results in proportionately more skin. Children's skin has a thin epidermis and dermis. Since children also have a greater proportion of body fluid, the skin is well hydrated. Increased vascularization and the development of exocrine and apocrine glands and the corneal strata layer are other maturational changes of the skin that affect percutaneous absorption.

Muscle-Fat Composition

The body's composition of fat varies considerably across the life span. Body fat represents approximately 16% of the neonate's body weight, 23% of a 1-year-old child's weight, 8% to 12% of a preschooler's weight, and 15% of an adult's weight.

The percentage of muscle per body weight rises with age. Neonates, infants, and young children have a relatively small skeletal muscle mass. During infancy the average is 25% as compared to 40% in adulthood.[4]

Central Nervous System: Blood-Brain Barrier

The blood-brain barrier in the hypothalamus is immature in neonates.

Renal System and Body Fluids

Both glomerular filtration and renal blood flow are diminished in the neonate, infant, and young child. Both factors are approximately one third of the adult rate. The glomerular filtration rate of the full-term neonate is approximately 38 ml per minute. This rate doubles around 2 months, reaches 110 ml per minute by 6 months of age, and achieves adult levels (115 to 125 ml per minute) by 2 to 3 years of age. In addition, tubular secretion and reabsorption rates are greatly reduced in neonates. These rates do not reach adult levels until approximately 7 months of age. The urinary pH is also more acidic in the neonate.

The percentage of body weight consisting of body fluid is greatest at birth and gradually decreases: 85% in premature neonates; 70% to 80% in term neonates, and 50% to 60% in adults. The extracellular proportion of body fluid in infants is approximately 45% and in adults, 15%. A lesser proportion of body fluid is intracellular in the infant (35%) than in the adult (40%). This greater proportion of extracellular fluid makes infants prone to dehydration. (Table 14–1 depicts the percentage of body weight composition of water, muscle, and fat in the fetus through adulthood.[5])

Gastrointestinal System

Gastric emptying time is prolonged until the infant reaches 6 months of age, and peristalsis may be irregular and unpredictable for several weeks after birth. The pH of gastric contents in the premature neonate is very elevated (alkaline) because of the immature secretion of gastric acid. Full-term neonates and children less than 3 years old also have less acidity than the average adult. Duodenal fluids have decreased en-

TABLE 14–1

Percentage of Body Weight Composed of Water, Muscle, and Fat

Age	Muscle	Fat	Total Body Water	Extra-cellular Water	Intra-cellular Water
Fetus	*	*	94	*	*
Premature infant	*	1	85-86	50	*
Birth	25	16	70-80	45-47	32-35
12 mo	*	22-24	58-60	25-27	41
4 y	*	12	60	24	41
10-11 y	40	18-20	60	17	41
Adult	50	15	50-60	15-19	40

Adapted from Bindler, R.M., Howry, L.B. (1991). *Pediatric drugs and nursing implications.* Norwalk, CT: Appleton & Lange.
* Not determined.

zymatic activity until the infant is approximately 4 months of age. In addition, the liver accounts for 5% of body weight in the neonate and only 2% of adult body weight.

PHARMACOKINETIC DIFFERENCES IN CHILDREN OF VARIOUS AGES

The study of movement of drugs throughout the body focuses on the processes of absorption, distribution, biotransformation, and excretion. These processes are different in premature neonates, full-term neonates, infants, and older children.[6-9]

Absorption Phase

The rate at which drugs move from the site of administration into the vascular system depends on the method of administration, pharmacokinetic qualities of the drug, and specific characteristics of the child.

ORAL ROUTE

In neonates, infants, and young children, absorption of oral drugs is affected by the altered gastric pH, prolonged gastric emptying time, and diminished enzymatic activities of the small intestines. Some drugs respond favorably to the alkaline conditions of the stomach in these individuals; other drugs that are acid-labile may not be adequately absorbed. The prolonged emptying time of the stomach causes drugs to remain in the stomach longer. This extended exposure to the gastric environment may cause more complete absorption of some drugs. However, if the drug normally is absorbed in the small intestine, the delay in the stomach reduces the drug's absorption rate. An altered absorption rate delays or accelerates the attainment of peak serum concentrations and may cause ineffective drug therapy or lead to drug toxicity or overdose.

Neonates have both low lipase concentrations and reduced intraluminal concentrations of bile acid. These factors may prevent the absorption of lipid-soluble drugs. Drug absorption in the duodenal fluids of young infants (1 to 4 months) may also be altered by the low activity of amylase and other duodenal enzymes. For example, the inactive prodrug chloramphenicol palmitate requires pancreatic enzymes for hydrolysis to the active chloramphenicol base.[9]

PARENTERAL ROUTE

Drug absorption from the intramuscular and subcutaneous sites depends primarily on the relative blood flow to muscles. Neonates, infants, and children experience irregular absorption of drugs administered through these routes. Because muscle mass is poorly developed in the sick neonate, this route is rarely used for neonates.

TOPICAL ROUTE

Drugs applied topically usually act locally. However, the thinness of the skin and its high water content results in enhanced percutaneous absorption in neonates and infants. The use of topical drugs avoids the unpredictability of oral and intramuscular absorption and the difficulties of intravenous drug therapy in tiny infants. However, studies have documented that the increased permeability also results in toxic effects after the use of substances such as hexachlorophene soap and steroid creams.

Drugs often are administered rectally to pediatric clients who are unable to or should not take them orally. The rate of absorption for this route appears to vary with the drug.

Distribution Phase

Several factors affect the distribution of drugs in the infant and young child: total body water, body fat, plasma protein binding of the drug, and modification of physiologic functions.

TOTAL BODY WATER

Total body water varies greatly with the age of the individual, with neonates having the greatest amount of body water. As intracellular and extracellular fluid volumes increase or decrease, drug concentration levels respond accordingly. Since young children have greater fluid volume levels, they require high dosages (mg/kg) of water-soluble drugs.

BODY FAT

Lipid-soluble drugs (e.g., barbiturates) are dependent on the amount of fat tissue in the body. Blood levels of these drugs do not rise until the drug has saturated the fatty tissue. Thus the distribution of these drugs is more limited in neonates, infants, and young children than in older children (10 to 12 years of age) and most adults.

PROTEIN-BOUND DRUGS

Binding of drugs to serum proteins is decreased in neonates because of decreased plasma protein concentration, competition for certain binding sites by endogenous compounds such as bilirubin, and differences in the ability of the neonate's albumin to bind with drugs.[10] The decrease in plasma protein binding of drugs can increase their distribution at the cellular level. Thus premature neonates require a higher loading dose to reach a therapeutic serum concentration.

BLOOD-BRAIN BARRIER

Since the blood-brain barrier is not fully effective at birth, the actions of drugs given for their central nervous system (CNS) effect are usually intensified. In addition, drugs given for their effects on other organ systems may have an exaggerated effect on the CNS. Since drug binding to plasma protein does not reach adult levels until the infant is approximately 6 months of age, drug molecules are usually small enough to enter the CNS.[10]

Biotransformation Phase

The biotransformation of drugs is substantially slower in infants than in older children and adults. Maturation of various liver enzyme systems responsible for the biotransformation of drugs proceeds in an uneven manner. For example, the glucuronidation pathway is not completely developed at birth. This can result in prolonged serum concentration of some drugs, leading to toxicity.

An example of this is seen with theophylline, a bronchodilator. The pharmacologic and toxicologic properties of theophylline are similar to those of caffeine. Neonates have extremely slow clearance rates of theophylline as compared to older infants and children. In premature neonates the decreased clearance is related to oxidative pathways. The slowed clearance can lead to toxic effects, with CNS irritation and convulsions.[11–13]

Although biotransformation of drugs is initially slow at birth, this process may exceed adult levels in early childhood because the young child's liver is proportionately larger than that of the adult. Because of the accelerated metabolic rate, the child may require a significantly higher dose of some drugs than the adult.

Excretion Phase

Kidneys are immature in the neonate and young infant. Thus diminished glomerular filtration rate and renal blood flow contribute to the delay in eliminating drugs from the body. Since tubular secretion is also less efficient, drugs primarily eliminated by tubular secretion remain in the body longer.[14]

Tubular reabsorption, which results in reabsorption of substances from the filtrate back into the bloodstream, is affected by the urinary pH. The acidic urine of the neonate promotes nonionization of acidic drugs, causing greater reabsorption of weakly acidic drugs. This increased reabsorption could cause drugs to remain in the body, leading to drug toxicity or overdose. Drugs having narrow therapeutic indexes may require greater intervals between doses.[9,10]

An additional problem is caused by the underdeveloped metabolic pathways of the liver. The liver may not adequately inactivate drugs into water-soluble substances that can be excreted through the kidneys. See box for physiologic factors affecting disposition of drugs in the pediatric client.

CONCEPT REVIEW

Numerous physiologic factors affect drug response in the pediatric client.

Physiologic changes that occur with the normal growth and development process have an impact on all of the pharmacokinetic processes.

Aspects of importance include the body surface area, total body water, and muscle-fat composition of the body.

NURSING CONSIDERATIONS

Children often perceive that the major role of the nurse is to give medicine. In addition, much of the fear that children experience during an illness is associated with receiving medicine, especially when needles are involved.

PHYSIOLOGIC FACTORS AFFECTING DRUG DISPOSITION IN CHILDREN

Absorption
ORAL ROUTE
  Less acidic gastric pH
  Prolonged gastric emptying time
  Irregular peristalsis
  Low enzyme activity
PARENTAL ROUTE
  Variable blood flow
  Decreased skeletal muscle mass
TOPICAL ROUTE
  Thinness of skin
  Hydration of skin

Distribution
Effect of body fluid on concentration and perfusion
Decreased binding of drugs to serum protein
Immature blood-brain barrier
Varied distribution of lipid-soluble drugs based on proportion of body fat

Biotransformation
Immature enzyme systems
Reduced metabolism of drugs
Variable rates of metabolism

Excretion
Immature renal function prolongs drug elimination
Immature hepatic function prolongs drug elimination

Assessing

Before administering any drug, make a quick assessment. When possible, the parent or caregiver should be encouraged to contribute to the assessment data.

During the **health history**, gather the following data:
- Does the child have any allergies?
- How does the child usually respond to taking medicine?
- How is medicine administered at home, or how has it been given by other nurses (i.e., equipment used, child's position, drug mixed with food or juice)?
- Is the child currently receiving any over-the-counter (OTC) drugs?
- Can the child swallow tablets or capsules, or is a liquid dosage form needed?
- Is a parent or caregiver available to be with the child? (Leave the option open for him or her not to stay if that is his or her wish.)
- Is the child, parent, or caregiver familiar with the action, purpose, and potential undesired responses to the drug?

During the **physical assessment**, assess the developmental level of the child, including the child's psychosocial and cognitive development. To help collect data in this area, observe the child's interactions with others and if possible his or her play behaviors. A review of a growth-and-development or a nursing-of-children textbook for characteristics of each developmental stage may be helpful.[1,3,15,16]

Obtain the child's height, weight, and vital signs. Plot the height and weight on a growth grid to facilitate future drug dosage calculations. Record the vital signs carefully; they provide baseline data for parameters after drug administration. Also assess the condition of muscular and subcutaneous tissue. This information helps determine the most appropriate needle size for the child's body build. In addition, assess specific areas related to the client's concern (e.g., pain level, nausea, respiratory status in the asthmatic child, urinary output in the child with pyelonephritis, cardiac status in the child with congestive heart failure).

🌺 NURSING RESEARCH

Curley, M., McDermott, B., Berry, P., et al. (1992). Nurses' decision making regarding the use of sedatives and analgesics in pediatric ICU. *Heart and Lung: Journal of Critical Care, 21,* 296.

The purpose of this study was to identify factors that pediatric critical care nurses consider when administering sedatives or analgesics. The Multidisciplinary ICU: Sedation and Pain Assessment Tool was developed to facilitate data collection. This tool contains client demographic information and 30 items identified in literature as assessment parameters related to pain or agitation in critically ill infants and children.

Pediatric intensive care unit (PICU) nurses were asked to complete the tool anytime they administered a sedative or analgesic and then identify the assessment parameters in the situation. Heart rate and blood pressure ranked high in all categories. The results help describe the constructs of pain and agitation in the PICU population.

STUDENT ACTIVITIES

- Interview six PICU nurses and determine assessment parameters used to diagnose pain and agitation.
- Investigate this subject in nursing literature and determine the basis for administering drugs for pain and agitation.
- Interview five pediatric nurses and determine their views on pain levels of pediatric clients. 🌺

Diagnosing

After the initial assessment data have been collected and examined, cluster the information and identify appropriate nursing diagnoses. Common nursing diagnoses related to administration of drugs to the pediatric client follow:

- Anxiety related to mobility limitation in preparation for drug administration.
- Fear related to anticipated discomfort of receiving medicine.

- Ineffective individual coping related to unwillingness or inability to cooperate due to fear of body harm.
- Noncompliance of parent or caregiver in drug therapy related to inability to use resources to obtain drug. (or) overwhelming nature of child's care. (or) lack of understanding regarding necessity of drug. (or) excessive family demands.
- Powerlessness related to inability to refuse drug or need to be immobilized during administration procedure.
- High risk for poisoning related to inappropriate storage of drugs in the home.
- Impaired tissue integrity related to inappropriate home administration of drug (e.g., inappropriate drug concentration, drug dosage, site selection, or needle length).
- High risk for injury related to inappropriate administration or storage of drugs in the home.

Planning

Your assessment and formulation of nursing diagnoses set the stage for development of a plan that will direct the child's care.

LEGAL CONSENT FOR DRUG ADMINISTRATION

Before administering any drug or treatment, consider the legal aspects of the situation. Because the pediatric client is legally considered a minor, the primary care provider is under legal duty to obtain an informed consent from the parent or legal guardian. When the pediatric client is admitted to a hospital, the parent or legal guardian is asked to sign a form allowing treatment of the child, including the administration of drugs. If adolescents are emancipated minors, they may consent to treatment without parental or guardian permission. In some instances the judiciary system intervenes and provides consent for treatment of a child.

CONSIDERATION OF DEVELOPMENTAL STAGE

Infants develop a sense of trust in the caregiver during the first 6 months of life. By 12 months of age, they have become strongly attached to their primary caregiver and begin to recognize and fear strangers. To diminish this fear, approach infants in a calm and gentle manner and talk to them in quiet, soothing tones.

Toddlers are developing their sense of autonomy as they become masters of their own bodies. Their developing independence is evident as they begin to feed, dress, and undress themselves, walk, talk, and control their urine and feces.

Following rituals and routines helps toddlers learn to master their environment and brings them a sense of security. The toddler is often resistive, says "No!" and has temper tantrums in an effort to assert further autonomy. The major fear of the child continues to be separation from the primary caregiver. Cognitively the toddler begins to display very simple reasoning and enjoys imitating adult behavior.

Preschoolers are busy developing a sense of initiative. They use imagination freely and enjoy fantasizing about people and things in both the real and make-believe world. Preschoolers become aware of their own vulnerability and often exhibit a variety of fears, most of which are related to fear of bodily harm. They do not like anything that intrudes on or invades their body. Preschoolers rapidly develop their vocabulary and often enjoy sharing. Their cognitive abilities demonstrate their developing reasoning skills; yet they lack the logic of the older child.

School-age children have begun to develop a sense of industry and seek recognition for what they are able to do. Their self-esteem grows as their achievements increase. They enjoy learning and take pride in sharing their knowledge and abilities with their friends, families, and nurses. Cognitively they are able to think logically and understand causality. They can verbalize their fears and reason about events that are occurring. They are learning the mental processes of classification and serialization and enjoy collections of all types.

Having learned to take care of their own bodies, school-age children are reluctant to allow others to assume these responsibilities. They readily listen to why they need to take medications and rarely object to doing so. However, do not take this positive attitude for granted; instead give the child verbal recognition for cooperating.

Adolescence is a difficult time for hospitalization. The confinement of hospitalization infringes on the independence that adolescents have just begun to enjoy. There are hospital rules to follow and separation from peers to endure. Adolescents struggling to develop their identity may have that development temporarily interrupted by acute illness or permanently affected by chronic or terminal illness. Cognitively the adolescent has developed the abilities to think abstractly, to hypothesize, and to be both rational and reflective. Adolescents are quite aware of the numerous physical changes occurring in their bodies and are self-conscious and concerned about their body image.[15,16]

Provide privacy for the adolescent during any drug administration that requires exposure of the body (i.e., injections and suppositories). Since adolescents have high expectations of themselves, they want to appear brave. Nevertheless, some move or cry during painful experiences such as injections. Offer the adolescent a hand to hold and an accepting attitude for support. You also must be aware that adolescents who receive drugs that alter the appearance of the body may become anxious and need help to develop appropriate coping skills.

TEACHING PLAN

During this step in the nursing process you develop your teaching plans. Base these plans on the assessed data and the existing knowledge of the child or caregiver. Review the information about the drug therapy supplied by the primary care provider. Was information about the frequency of drug administration, common undesired clinical responses, and anticipated length of drug therapy given to the child or caregiver? If not, this information must be included in the plan. For example, when administering an iron supplement to an infant, tell the caregiver that the infant's stools will become greenish black and that some children experience constipation but others develop loose stools. Also base the teaching plan on what the child or caregiver *wants* to know. Some caregivers want de-

tailed information about the drugs, but others are content to know the basic action.

You are responsible for preparing the child and caregiver for self-administration of drugs in the home. Teaching begins as soon as the decision is made that drug therapy will continue after discharge. Two topics to include in the plan are measurement of the drug dosage and development of a drug schedule that assures the child receives each of the prescribed drugs at the appropriate times.

Provide the caregiver with a few of the small disposable plastic measuring cups or needleless syringes for use at home. These devices can be washed and reused. If the drug is ordered in teaspoons, teach the caregiver either to measure 5 ml in the plastic cup or to use a household measuring teaspoon. Provide the child or caregiver or both the opportunity to prepare and administer the drugs during hospitalization.

Teach the caregiver to establish a daily drug schedule. The schedule should take into account if the drugs will be given with meals or on an empty stomach. If drugs will be administered three or four times a day, tell the caregiver if they should be administered throughout the 24-hour period or only during normal waking hours. After a schedule is developed, help the caregiver develop a system for monitoring and recording drug administration. A cardboard or plastic egg carton or a muffin tin can be used, with the individual cups representing the different hours of administration. Another important teaching point is that the drugs, both in their original containers and in the day's allotment, must be kept out of the reach of younger children.

EXPECTED OUTCOMES

Expected outcomes of the plan of care include the following:
- Child receives accurate doses of the correct drug at appropriate time.
- Child or caregiver discusses the purpose, undesired clinical responses, and administration technique of prescribed drugs.
- Child or caregiver uses resources or support systems effectively.
- Child or caregiver identifies ineffective coping behaviors and consequences.
- Child or caregiver participates in drug treatment plan.
- Child makes choices related to and is involved in drug therapy.
- Caregiver correctly stores drugs in home environment to prevent accidental poisoning of younger children.

CONCEPT REVIEW

Assessment of the child is critical before any drug is administered. When possible, include the parent or caregiver in the assessment process.

The child's developmental level influences all aspects of drug therapy. Therefore knowledge of developmental stages, tasks, and crises is important.

ADMINISTERING DRUG PREPARATIONS

Drug administration to children requires the use of unique skills. You must combine your knowledge of drugs, growth, and development with your communication and psychomotor skills.

Implementing

The first step in the administration of drugs to the pediatric client is to determine if the drug and dose are appropriate for the child.

CALCULATION OF PEDIATRIC DRUG DOSAGES

Recommended pediatric dosages are available for many drugs, but other dosages must be estimated using the adult dosage. See box for four methods for calculating pediatric drug dosages. The first three methods are based on modification of adult dosages. The fourth method uses the body surface area (BSA). None of these methods provides an exact individualized dosage since age, weight, and BSA are only a few of the factors that influence drug response.[18]

Dose calculation according to **body surface area** is the most accurate since it is not based on the assumption that the child is average in size. To use this method the following information is needed:

- Drug order with drug name, dosage, and time frequency
- Child's height and weight in kilograms

FORMULAS FOR CALCULATING PEDIATRIC DOSAGES FROM ADULT DOSAGES

Clark's Rule

$$\frac{\text{Child's weight in pounds}}{150} \times \text{Adult dose} = \text{Child's dose}$$

Fried's Rule

$$\frac{\text{Age in months}}{150} \times \text{Adult dose} = \text{Infant's dose}$$

Young's Rule

$$\frac{\text{Child's age in years}}{\text{Age in years} + 12} \times \text{Adult dose} = \text{Child's dose}$$

Body Surface Area Rule

$$\frac{\text{Child's surface area (m}^2)}{1.73 \text{ m}^2} \times \text{Adult dose} = \text{Child's dose}$$

- BSA nomogram for children
- Recommended adult drug dosage

The **nomogram** developed by West for estimation of BSA uses a child's height and weight to determine the specific BSA (Fig. 14–1). This information is then applied to the BSA formula to obtain a drug dosage for a specific child.

Fried's rule and Young's rule determine pediatric drug doses based on the child's age. **Fried's rule** is primarily used for children less than 1 year of age, whereas **Young's rule** is for children between 2 and 12 years. Since the maturational development of infants and children is variable, age is not an accurate basis for drug dosing. Therefore these rules are not frequently used.

Calculating the **drug dosage according to body weight** is appropriate when the child is of usual stature. (See box for formula and example of dosage calculation based on body weight.) Most drug references give recommendations for milligrams per kilograms of body weight dosages for children of different ages. The following information is needed to calculate this dose:

- Drug order with drug name, dosage, and time frequency
- Child's weight in kilograms (1 kg equals 2.2 lb)
- Pediatric dosage as listed by the manufacturer or hospital formulary
- Information on how the drug is supplied.

Clark's rule determines a pediatric dosage based on the child's weight in pounds and the average adult weight of 150 pounds. Since the average adult weight has increased in recent years, the fixed constant of 150 pounds can lead to underdos-

---

DOSAGE CALCULATION BASED ON BODY WEIGHT

Example

A 3-week old, 8-lb neonate is to receive 120 mg of cefotaxime (Claforan) q8h.

Formula

1. Determine the child's weight in kilograms.
   The infant's weight is 8 lbs, or 3.62 kg.

2. Use a drug reference to determine recommended milligrams per kilograms of body weight per 24 hours (note if dosage recommendation varies with age or specific pathology).

3. Determine dose parameters by multiplying the child's weight by the minimum and maximum daily dose of the drug.

   50 mg/kg/d × 3.62 kg = 181 mg
   150 mg/kg/d × 3.62 kg = 543 mg

   Safe range of this drug is 181 to 543 mg/kg/d.

4. Determine total amount of drug to administer per day.

   120 mg/kg × 3 doses (q8h) = 360 mg

   NOTE: If drug reference recommends dosage as mg/kg dose, omit step 4.

5. Compare drug dosage ordered with calculated safe range; 360 mg is within the safe dosage range of 181 to 543 mg/24 h.

6. If drug dosage varies from safe-dose range, consult with primary care provider.

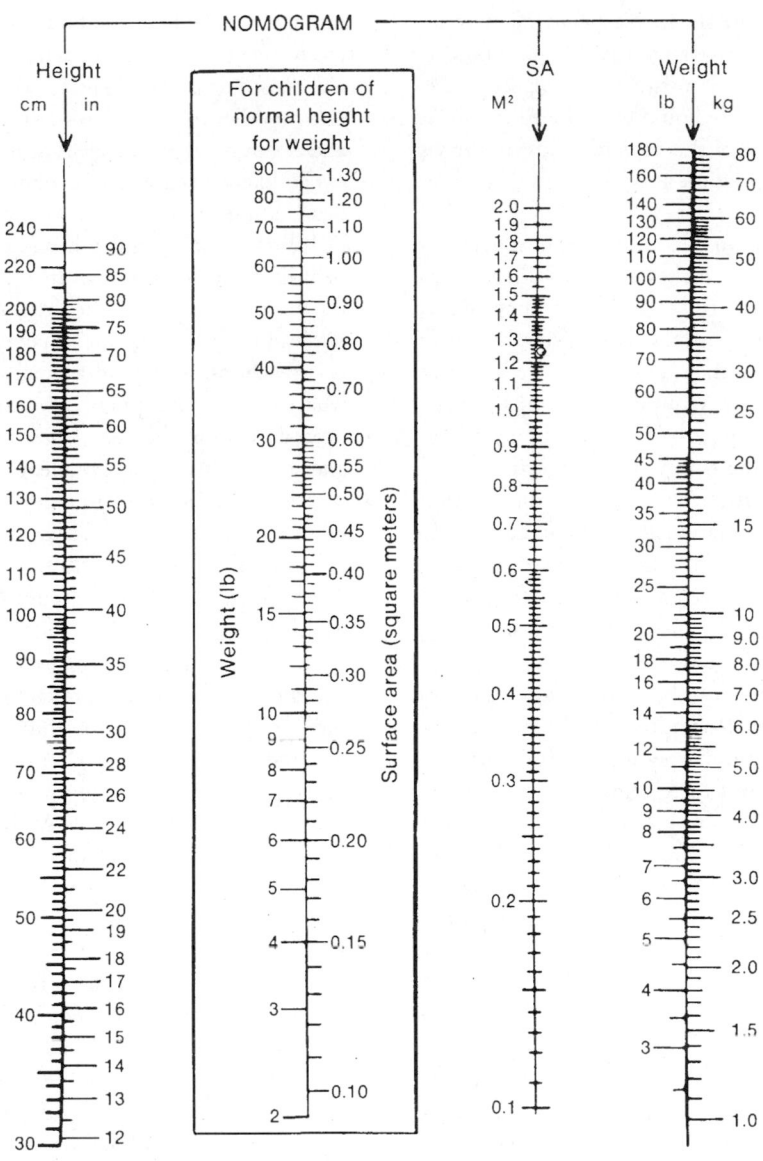

FIGURE 14-1   West nomogram for infants and children.

ing infants and children. Therefore using Clark's rule is not recommended.

DRUG ADMINISTRATION THROUGH THE ORAL ROUTE

Giving drugs by mouth is the preferred route for children because it is less threatening and causes less discomfort than other routes. Most drugs can be dissolved, suspended in liquid preparations, or chewed.

Infants usually receive liquid dosage forms. If the drug is not supplied in a liquid form, determine if the tablet can be crushed or the capsule opened. Tablets are easily crushed with a mortar and pestle. Since the crushed drug often clings to the side of the container, take special care to get all of the medicine. After each use, wash the mortar and pestle and dry them immediately to prevent mixing remnants of the crushed drug with the next drug that is crushed for a different client. If a

mortar and pestle are not available, place the tablet between two small paper soufflé cups and crush it. Mix the crushed drug particles with a small amount (½ teaspoon) of liquid, jelly, syrup, or strained baby food (e.g., applesauce). Honey should not be used because of the risk of botulism. Mixing drugs with essential foods such as formula, milk, juice, or cereal is also not recommended because the child may develop a dislike for that food and refuse to eat it.

If the drug dosage is less than one tablet, additional preparation is needed. If the tablet is scored, break the tablet on the scored line. (Special devices for splitting tablets are available but may not be accurate.) You can also crush the tablet finely and dissolve it in 2 ml of water in a syringe. If, for example, one fourth tablet is the required dose, administer 0.5 ml of the solution (0.25 × 2 ml = 0.5 ml).

When measuring liquid dosage forms, use a small plastic needleless syringe to measure amounts less than 5 ml. Measure amounts greater than 5 ml in small, plastic medicine cups. When drugs are ordered in teaspoons, the dosage should be converted to milliliters to assure consistency. Some drugs (e.g., vitamin and iron preparations) in liquid form are administered with a dropper. Since the size of the drop depends on the viscosity of the liquid, the dropper used for these drugs contains milliliter markings.

Physically, the young infant has poor head control and sucks readily on anything that makes contact with the lips. Therefore a nipple, needleless syringe, or dropper may be used to administer oral drugs. If possible, administer the drugs when the infant is hungry and the sucking response to objects placed near the mouth is strong. Hold the infant in a partially upright position or have the upper body elevated on a pillow.

If a nipple is used, place the empty nipple into the infant's mouth and fill the inner portion with the drug preparation. Gradually add more drug preparation as the infant empties the nipple with sucking. If a syringe or dropper is used, place the drug preparation on the side or back of his or her tongue. This prevents the normal thrusting of the tongue during sucking from pushing the drug out of the mouth.

A small plastic cup or spoon can be used to administer oral drugs to older infants. This techique allows you to collect drooled medicine with the cup or spoon and readminister it. Drooling is reduced if you wait for the infant to swallow between deposits of the drug. Various methods are used to elicit a swallow reflex in an infant. Blowing a small puff of air into the face of infants less than 11 months old frequently elicits a swallow reflex.[19] Another approach is using a thumb to pull the infant's chin gently up and stroking the infant's neck.

As the infant becomes older, gentle restraint of the arms is often needed. Place the infant's near arm behind your own body and hold the infant's other arm. This leaves you a free hand to hold and administer the medicine. You can also "mummy" the infant with a baby blanket or sheet. If a second individual is present, ask him or her to restrain gently or "busy" the infant's hands with toys. The other individual can also distract the infant by talking, singing or making noises with the mouth while you place the medicine into the infant's mouth. The infant should be encouraged and comforted during and after the procedure. Hugging, stroking, and rocking of the infant result in the association of pleasant sensations with the giving of medicine.

Toddlers present a different challenge for the nurse. It is important to establish a relationship with the toddler before attempting to gain his or her cooperation in taking medicine. Simple explanations may not be understood but often promote the toddler's trust. Use an attitude which conveys that you expect the child to take the medicine willingly. Do not ask the toddler, "Will you take this medicine for me?" That approach provides the toddler with the opportunity to be negative both verbally and in action.

Since toddlers like the security provided by routines, they accept medicine more easily if administration methods are similar to those used at home. You still should crush solid dosages forms. However, if possible, you can prepare the drug

mixture according to methods used at home. Also ask the parent or caregiver if a cup or spoon is the most appropriate vehicle. Most nurses prefer the small plastic cup since it allows the older toddler to assert autonomy by holding the medicine cup and it can be used to collect drooled medicine.

Toddlers need positive reinforcement on completion of drug administration. Use of verbal praise, hugs, clapping of hands, stickers, and other positive actions for cooperative behaviors usually results in future cooperation when it is time for the child to receive the drug again. Force and restraint often lead to more resistant behaviors.

Preschoolers require a positive approach. Briefly explain what is going to happen; allow the child some choice in the procedure if possible (e.g., cup or spoon for oral dosage forms) and then administer the drug. It is not unusual for the preschooler to attempt to delay taking the drug by asking to perform other tasks such as going to the bathroom. Allow one delay and then proceed with the administration process. Make it clear to the child that the medicine is not a form of punishment.

When needleless syringes are used to measure small amounts of oral drugs, preschoolers often like to show that they can push the plunger and squirt the medicine into their own mouth. Just like the older toddler, preschoolers enjoy dramatic play and often enjoy pretending they are giving medicine to a doll or stuffed toy. Many preschoolers respond positively to the challenge of showing how quickly they can make the medicine disappear into their tummies. They often look forward to the positive verbal rewards and attention they receive for being "good medicine takers." An excellent reward for preschoolers is a chart of stickers or stars showing how many times they cooperated. The child can show the chart to parents and relatives and take it home to show their siblings and friends.

To familiarize yourself with the actual taste of a drug, take a very small taste. This helps you describe the taste to the child. Most manufacturers attempt to camouflage any offensive smell or taste of oral drugs. However, a number of strategies make oral dosage forms more palatable. For example, before giving the drug, allow the child to suck on a Popsicle or small ice cube to numb the tongue. If not contraindicated, ask the child if he or she would like to mix the medicine with a small amount of sweet-tasting substance such as syrup, pureed fruit, jam or jelly, or chocolate sauce. If possible, allow the child to select a "chaser" such as water, juice, cracker, or Popsicle to take after the medicine. If the child is nauseated, have him or her drink a carbonated beverage poured over finely crushed ice either immediately before or after taking the drug.

School-agers are generally cooperative. Learning is an important part of their life, and they are eager for explanations about their drugs. Later they may share this information with other nurses and family members. This serves as a form of achievement for the child and helps to build self-esteem.

If several drugs are being administered, allow school-agers to choose which drug to take first or what fluid to drink with their medicine. Many children like to save and collect the medicine cups and syringes that were used. You may also give school-agers the responsibility for recording the amount of water they drink when taking their drugs or for returning to their room to receive a specific drug at a specific time.

The early school years are an appropriate time for the child to learn to swallow capsules, pills, and tablets. Children may be anxious but at the same time eager to develop this ability. Capsules are usually the easiest to learn to swallow since they do not begin to dissolve in the mouth and thus do not cause an unpleasant taste. To help the school-ager learn, have the child swallow very small pieces of candy such as a red hot; then progressively increase the size of the pieces. Success with each piece gives the child confidence to progress to larger size pieces.

Adolescents should be given as much information about their drugs as they request. If the adolescent does not ask questions, assess what information they already have about the drugs and provide further opportunities for them to ask questions.

Most adolescents have learned to swallow pills. However, some may reluctant to do so; offer these individuals the choice of liquid dosage forms. Adolescents can also be given the responsibility for determining when they need as-needed drugs and for taking certain drugs at prescribed times.

DRUG ADMINISTRATION THROUGH THE PARENTERAL ROUTE

A great deal of anxiety is associated with receiving injections, particularly in children. Whether the injection is intradermal, intramuscular, subcutaneous, or intravenous, a needle is involved, and the idea of having it puncture the skin results in fear.

Determining the site for **intramuscular injections** is based on the size of the muscles, tissue integrity, presence of major nerves and vessels, and amount of solution to be injected. Permanent disability has been reported when drugs have been injected too close to the sciatic or other large nerves. In addition, repeated use of the same site is avoided since that has been associated with reduced absorption of drug, fibrosis of the muscle, and subsequent muscle contractures.

Four major sites are recommended for intramuscular injections in children: gluteal or dorsogluteal, vastus lateralis, ventrogluteal, and deltoid muscles. Since the **gluteus maximus** or **dorsogluteal muscle** is not well developed until the child has walked for at least 1 year, this site is not recommended in children from birth to 2 years of age. In addition, the sciatic nerve runs through the medial portion of the muscle mass and may not assume its mature position until after 2 years of age. The **vastus lateralis,** a large muscle mass that is free of major nerves and vessels, is the preferred site for most age groups. The **ventrogluteal site** is not generally recommended for children less than 3 years of age.[18] However, Beecroft and Redick[20] recently challenged this recommendation and suggested that the site is safe even before children walk, for the ventrogluteal site is relatively free of major nerves and vessels. It has minimal subcutaneous tissue and well-defined landmarks and is easily acces-

sible.[20] The **deltoid muscle,** which is located approximately 1 to 1½ inches below the acromion process of the shoulder, is not recommended for children less than 2 years of age. However, this site is sometimes used for immunizations with children as young as 18 months. Less pain and fewer side effects are associated with immunizations injected in the deltoid muscle than with those in the vastus lateralis muscle.[21]

Selection of needle size depends on the size of the child and the quantity of drug to be injected. To help determine the proper needle length, grasp the vastus lateralis or deltoid muscle between the thumb and forefinger and choose a needle that is approximately half of that length. Use the same technique for the other two injection sites but select a needle length that is slightly more than half the distance of the bunched tissue. To minimize discomfort, use the smallest gauge needle possible (25 to 30). The amount of solution injected into a particular site with each dose depends on the size of the muscle and tissue integrity. Table 14–2 provides guidelines for intramuscular injections.

Subcutaneous injections are usually administered in the back of the arm, midway between the elbow and shoulder. The abdomen is also a preferred site, especially for insulin injections.

The approach to use when giving injections is based on the age and size of the child. You should administer injections in a manner that decreases both the physical and psychologic trauma experienced by the child.

If the caregiver or parent are present, explain the reason for the injection, and discuss with them how they can participate in the procedure. Little resistance is offered by the neonate and young infant. However, older infants offer resistance as soon as they perceive their movement is being restricted. After the injection, spend time comforting and distracting the infant with rocking, talking, cuddling, and stroking.

Sight of the syringe often provokes fear and crying in toddlers since they may recall previous painful experiences with immunizations. Consequently, it is best that they do not see the syringe until just before receiving the injection. Your approach to the toddler is essentially the same as with the older infant, except that the toddler is stronger and reacts more vigorously to the painful stimuli. Since there is danger of the child's moving and the needle's breaking apart from the hub, never attempt to give a toddler an injection without the assistance of at least one other individual.

It is best not to tell preschool children they are to receive an injection until you are prepared to give it. Their anxiety about painful procedures escalates rapidly. Give a simple, honest explanation. Assist the child to assume the proper position and have another individual available to comfort and hold the child during the injection. Afterward assure the child you are sorry if you caused any discomfort and praise the child for any positive behaviors exhibited.

School-agers usually still have some fear about receiving injections, but most want to cooperate and be perceived by others as "brave." Give the child the opportunity to cleanse the skin site personally and to open the Band-aid while the skin

TABLE 14–2
*Pediatric Guidelines for Intramuscular Injections**

Age	Muscle Group				
	Rectus Femorus	Vastus Lateralis	Gluteus Maximus	Ventrogluteal	Deltoid
Birth to 2 y	0.5-1 ml	0.5-1 ml	Not safe	Not safe	Not safe
2-3	1 ml	1 ml	1 ml	1 ml	0.5 ml
3-7	1.5 ml	1.5 ml	1.5 ml	1.5 ml	0.5 ml
7-16	1.5-2 ml	1.5-2 ml	1.5-2 ml	1.5-2 ml	0.5-1 ml
16-adult	2-2.5 ml	2-2.5 ml	2-3 ml	2-3 ml	1-2 ml

From Kee, J.L., & Marshall, S.M. (1992). *Clinical calculations* (2nd ed., p. 149). Philadelphia: W.B. Saunders.
*The safe use of all sites is based on normal muscle development and size of the child.

dries. Ask if the child wants to hold the hand of a parent or nurse. (If you do not know from previous experience if the child is able to cooperate, have a second adult at the bedside who can assist the child to hold still.) Afterward thank the child for cooperating.

With adolescents, privacy is a major concern. Many adolescents resist thigh injections because they believe they are more painful and dorsogluteal injections because they invade their sense of privacy. Adolescents continue to find injections unpleasant but want to seem unconcerned. Talking often distracts them and helps them relax.

The **intravenous route** is frequently preferred for the administration of drugs to children. However, starting and maintaining an infusion line and administering intravenous drugs in children is beyond the scope of this chapter. See a pediatric nursing text for such information.

DRUG ADMINISTRATION THROUGH THE TOPICAL ROUTE

The primary topical routes used in children are nasal, inhalation, opthalmic, otic, dermatologic, and rectal. With the exception of rectally administered drugs, these routes are discussed in future chapters (Chapter 44, "Nasal Decongestants, Antitussives, and Mucokinetic Drugs"; Chapter 64, "Drugs Used in Ocular Disorders"; Chapter 65, "Otic Preparations"; and Chapter 67, "Dermatologic Agents").

The **rectal route** of drug administration is usually reserved for the child not allowed to take drugs by mouth or unable to tolerate anything orally. Drugs most frequently given by this route are used to control fever or vomiting and to induce sedation and defecation. A major concern related to rectal administration of drugs is that the drug may be expelled before total absorption has occurred. Also if stool is present in the rectal ampulla, absorption of the drug may be delayed.

Make certain that the suppository is firm before you attempt to insert it into the rectum. Placing the wrapped suppository in cold water or in the refrigerator quickly firms it. If the suppository must be divided to obtain the desired dose, divide it lengthwise. (Even then, there is no guarantee that the drug is equally dispersed throughout the petrolatum base.)

Wear a glove when inserting the suppository. Although a small amount of lubricant can be used, the suppository is usu-

ally more manageable if it is slightly moistened with water. Insert the suppository beyond both rectal sphincters to enhance its retention. The urge to expel the suppository lasts 5 to 10 minutes, and the suppository usually requires approximately ½ hour to dissolve.

CONCEPT REVIEW

Throughout the drug administration process, the child's age and developmental status must be considered. All techniques for administering drugs are modified according to these two factors.

One of the primary safety factors involved in drug administration to the pediatric client is accurate dose calculation. Although several formulas are available for determining the correct dose for the child, the most accurate dosages are those provided by the drug manufacturer or those based on body surface area.

UNIQUE RESPONSE OF THE PEDIATRIC CLIENT TO DRUGS

Once the drug is delivered to the target cells, it begins its biochemical action. Results sometimes vary between the child and the adult client because of unique pathophysiologic changes of the tissues and cells.

Drug Efficacy

Drug efficacy is altered by disease states in infants and children. For example, infants between the ages of 1 and 6 months with congestive heart failure require larger doses of digoxin for maintenance therapy than adults. These individuals have an increased binding of digoxin to protein within the myocardium. In addition, the neonatal erythrocytes have more digoxin-binding sites than do adult erythrocytes. This decreases the bioavailability of the drug for binding with the receptors in the myocardium and is responsible for the higher dosage requirement.

Most studies on the influence of liver disease on dosage requirements have been carried out in adults and may not apply uniformly to children. Since the liver is the primary site of drug metabolism, clients with hepatic disease usually have a decreased drug clearance. For example, theophylline clearance may decrease by 45% in a child with viral hepatitis. Children with liver disease must be closely monitored for signs of toxicity.[22]

Since most drugs are excreted by the kidneys, renal failure decreases the dosage requirement of those drugs. Few studies have been done on dosage requirements of children in renal failure, so most dosage adjustments are based on data from adult studies. For drugs with narrow therapeutic ranges, serum concentrations should be measured frequently. The rate of elimination of these drugs is directly proportional to the glomerular filtration rate as measured by the creatinine clearance test. Dosage adjustment for drugs with a wide therapeutic range is necessary only for clients with moderate-to-severe renal failure.[21] Another example of how pathology affects drug efficacy is found in children with cystic fibrosis. These children require increased doses of specific drugs such as aminoglycosides and penicillins.[22]

Drug Toxicity

Toxicity to drugs is a major concern with infants and children. However, do not assume that *all* drugs are more toxic to infants than to adults. Surprisingly, certain drugs are less toxic. This is true for aminoglycosides for which toxicity in adults appears to be related to both peripheral compartment accumulation and the adult client's inherent sensitivity to tissue concentrations.[22]

Two examples of drugs that are more toxic in children include propylene glycol and benzyl alcohol. Propylene glycol, which is added to many injectable drugs to increase their stability, can result in hyperosmolarity in infants. In the past the chemical benzyl alcohol was routinely added to the sterile water used to dilute intravenous drugs. A syndrome of metabolic acidosis, seizures, neurologic deterioration, gasping respirations, hepatic and renal abnormalities, cardiovascular collapse, and death of premature infants was linked to its use. After its elimination from the sterile diluent, a study showed a decline in both mortality rate and the incidence of major intraventricular hemorrhage in low-birth-weight infants. Today, diluents that contain benzyl alcohol are labeled "Not for use in neonates."[22]

SUMMARY

Effective pharmacologic treatment of children is complex— from the calculation of the pediatric dose to the administration of the drug. Understanding the effects of the child's age and physical development on pharmacokinetics and pharmacodynamics is important, but you are not expected to memorize all this specific content. You are expected to be aware that these differences exist and to use reliable drug references as a guide to administering appropriate drugs and dosages to children. It is your legal responsibility to administer the correct drug, in the correct amount, and at the correct time. It is also your responsibility to administer the drug in a manner safe and appropriate for the developmental and individual needs of the child.

REFERENCES

1. Dworetzsky, J., & Davis, N. (1989). *Human development: A lifespan approach.* St. Paul, MN: West Publishing.
2. Stewart, C., & Hampton, E. (1987). Therapy review: Effect of maturation on drug disposition in pediatric patients. *Clinical Pharmacy, 6,* 548-562.
3. Turner, J., & Helms, D. (1991). *Lifespan development* (3rd ed.). New York: Harcourt & Brace.
4. Wu, Y., Nielsen, D., Cassady, S., et al. (1993). Cross-validation of bioelectrical impedance analysis of body composition in children and adolescents. *Physical Therapy, 73,* 320-328.
5. Bindler, R., & Howry, L.B. (1991). *Pediatric drugs and nursing implications.* Norwalk, CT: Appleton & Lange.
6. Dionne, R., & McManus, C. (1993). Pediatric clinical care pharmacodynamics. *Critical Care Nursing Clinics of North America, 5,* 367-379.
7. McLeod, H.L., & Evans, W.E. (1992). Pediatric pharmacokinetics and therapeutic drug monitoring. *Pediatric Review, 13,* 413-421.
8. Nahata, M.C. (1992). Variability in clinical pharmacology of drugs in children. *Journal of Clinical Pharmacy and Therapeutics, 17,* 365-368.
9. Smith, C.M., & Reynard, A.M. (Eds.). (1992). *Textbook of pharmacology.* Philadelphia: W.B. Saunders.
10. Wink, D.M. (1991). Giving infants and children drugs: Precision + caution = safety. *American Journal of Maternal/Child Nursing, 16,* 317-321.
11. Koren, G. (1993). Medications which can kill a toddler with one tablet or teaspoonful. *Journal of Toxicology, Clinical Toxicology, 31,* 407-413.
12. Theophylline and behavioral changes in children. (1992). *Nurses' Drug Alert, 16*(7), 55.
13. Data Pharmaceutica, Inc. (1993). *1993 physicians' genRx.* Smithtown, NY: Author.
14. Guyon, G. (1989). Pharmacokinetic considerations in neonatal drug therapy. Neonatal network. *Journal of Neonatal Nursing, 7*(5), 9-12, 27-30.
15. Murray, R., & Zentner, J. (1993). *Nursing assessment and health promotion: Strategies through the life span* (5th ed.). Norwalk, CT: Appleton & Lange.
16. Newman, B., & Newman, P. (1991). *Development through life: A psychosocial approach* (5th ed.). Pacific Grove, CA: Brooks/Cole.
17. Curley, M., McDermott, B., Berry, P., et al. (1992). Nurses' decision making regarding the use of sedatives and analgesics in pediatric ICU. *Heart and Lung: Journal of Critical Care, 21,* 296.
18. Kee, J.L., & Marshall, S.M. (1992). *Clinical calculations with applications to general and specialty areas* (2nd ed.). Philadelphia: W.B. Saunders.
19. Orenstein, S., et al. (1988). The santmyer swallow: A new and useful infant reflex. *Lancet, 1,* 345-346.
20. Beecroft, P., & Redick, S. (1990). Intramuscular injection practices of pediatric nurses: Site selection. *Nurse Educator, 15*(4), 23-28.
21. Ipp, M.M., et al. (1989). Adverse reactions to diphtheria, tetanus, pertussis-polio vaccination at 18 months of age: Effect of injection site and needle length. *Pediatrics, 83,* 679-682.
22. Nahata, M.C. (1989). Pediatrics. In J.T. DiPiro, et al. (Eds.). *Pharmacotherapy: A pathophysiological approach* (pp. 35-41). New York: Elsevier Science.

BIBLIOGRAPHY

Beecroft, P.C., & Redick, S. (1989). Possible complications of intra-muscular injections on the pediatric unit. *Pediatric Nursing, 15,* 333-336, 376.

Byington, K.C. (1991). Your guide to pediatric drug administration. *Nursing 1991, 21*(8), 82, 84, 86.

Erl, B., & Robbins, P. (1990). Hand-held nebulization therapy. *Journal of Pediatric Nursing: Nursing Care of Children and Families, 5,* 408-409.

Gorman, K., & Poilitt, E. (1992). Relationship between weight and body proportionality at birth, growth during the first year of life, and cognitive development at 38, 48, and 60 months. *Infant Behavior and Development, 15,* 279-296.

Henry, J., & Giordano, B. (1992). Assessment of growth in infants and children: Normal and abnormal patterns. *Journal of Pediatric Health Care, 8,* 289.

Lehne, R.A. (1994). *Pharmacology for nursing care* (2nd ed.). Philadelphia: W.B. Saunders.

Messmer, P., Meehan, R., Gilliam, N., et al. (1993). Teaching infant CPR to mothers of cocaine-positive infants. *Journal of Continuing Education in Nursing, 24,* 217-220.

Morrelli, J. (1993). Pediatric poisonings: The 10 most toxic prescription drugs. *American Journal of Nursing, 93*(7), 27-29.

Rudy, C. (1992). A drop or a dropper: The risk of overdose. *Journal of Pediatric Health Care, 6*(1), 40, 51-52.

CHAPTER 15

DRUG THERAPY IN THE
Elderly Client

GAIL ESTOCK HALLER

⊛ **Common Physiologic Changes Associated With Aging**

LEARNING OBJECTIVE: Describe physiologic changes associated with aging.

⊛ **Alterations in Pharmaceutic, Pharmacokinetic, and Pharmacodynamic Phases**

LEARNING OBJECTIVES:

Summarize effects of aging process on the pharmaceutic phase of the drug therapy.

Explain effects of aging process on pharmacokinetic phase of drug therapy.

Describe effects of aging process on pharmacodynamic phase of drug therapy.

⊛ **Pharmacotherapeutic Problems in the Elderly**

LEARNING OBJECTIVE: Discuss problems associated with drug therapy in the elderly.

KEY TERM: Polypharmacy

⊛ **Role of the Nurse**

LEARNING OBJECTIVE: Describe the role of the nurse in providing drug therapy for the elderly.

*A*n observable change in the demographic structure of the population in the Western world has occurred. Both the number and proportion of the population aged 65 and over have grown. This growth is predicted to continue in the future, with the most rapid increase expected between the years 2010 and 2030 when the "baby boom" generation reaches age 65. Further predictions suggest that the number of the very elderly (85+) will show the greatest growth.

This increase in the number of elderly individuals has raised the average age of clients within the health care system. These clients need individualized, age-related nursing care. The purpose of this chapter is to familiarize you with age-related alterations in the pharmaceutic, pharmacokinetic, and pharmacodynamic phases of drug therapy. Specific pharmacotherapeutic problems associated with the elderly are discussed, and the nursing responsibilities and functions associated with drug therapy in the elderly are addressed.

TERMS RELEVANT TO ELDERLY CLIENTS

elderly Individuals 60 to 85 years old

geriatrics Study and treatment of diseases of the elderly

gerontology Study of all the issues and problems associated with aging, including physiologic, pathologic, psychologic, economic, and sociologic ones

senescence Biologic aging; mental and physical decline associated with the aging process

very elderly Individuals over the age of 85 years

COMMON PHYSIOLOGIC CHANGES ASSOCIATED WITH AGING

From the day of birth, humans begin to age. For each individual the rapidity and manifestations of aging depend on a variety of factors, including heredity, past illness, lifestyle, patterns of eating and exercise, presence of chronic disease, and level of lifetime stress. However, some generalized physiologic changes occur in all individuals; these changes include decreased rate of cell mitosis, deterioration of specialized nondividing cells, increased rigidity and loss of elasticity in connective tissue, and loss of reserve functional capacity. Figure 15–1 summarizes some of the common changes seen in the elderly.[1-3]

ALTERATIONS IN PHARMACEUTIC, PHARMACOKINETIC, AND PHARMACODYNAMIC PHASES

Since the aging process affects the functioning of all body systems, it also affects the pharmaceutic, pharmacokinetic, and pharmacodynamic phases of drug therapy. The nurse must be aware of these effects, both when administering drugs to the elderly client and when observing the client for adverse drug reactions.

Pharmaceutic Phase

In the pharmaceutic phase age-associated sensory and cognitive losses and decreased manual dexterity must be considered. In addition, dermatologic and gastrointestinal (GI) changes can affect drug absorption and distribution. These factors have an impact on selected dosage forms, medication schedules, administration techniques, and storage of drugs (Table 15–1).

Visual changes such as **presbyopia** and having cataracts and glaucoma cause difficulty in reading labels and instructions, distinguishing colors, differentiating among capsules, caplets, and tablets, and preparing dosage forms. Decreased perception to touch and decreased manual dexterity create problems in opening bottles, isolating tiny pills, breaking tablets, and handling and administering parenteral dosage forms. **Presbycusis** (hearing loss) may compromise the client's ability to hear and understand oral instructions completely. Short-term memory loss and alteration in thought processing may result in difficulty in retaining and interpreting instructions.

Pharmacokinetic Phase

The aging process affects absorption, distribution, biotransformation, and excretion of drugs. These changes often influence the dosage requirements, dosage form, and route of administration (Table 15–2).

Absorption Absorption is affected by several changes that occur in the aging process. As the body ages, gastric juice secretion, hydrochloric acid production, GI and esophageal motility, mesenteric blood flow, and size of absorptive surface decrease. Reduction in hydrochloric acid production causes reduced gastric acidity and a rise in pH levels. Consequently orally administered drugs that rely on gastric acid for absorption may be less effective in the elderly. Because decreased GI

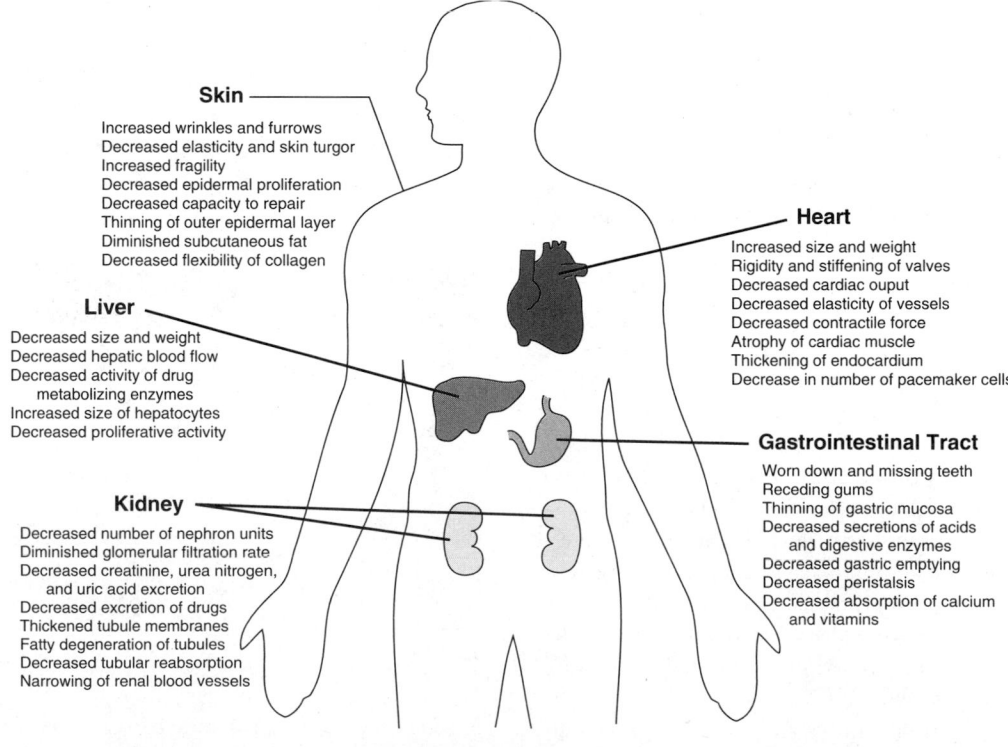

Skin
Increased wrinkles and furrows
Decreased elasticity and skin turgor
Increased fragility
Decreased epidermal proliferation
Decreased capacity to repair
Thinning of outer epidermal layer
Diminished subcutaneous fat
Decreased flexibility of collagen

Heart
Increased size and weight
Rigidity and stiffening of valves
Decreased cardiac ouput
Decreased elasticity of vessels
Decreased contractile force
Atrophy of cardiac muscle
Thickening of endocardium
Decrease in number of pacemaker cells

Liver
Decreased size and weight
Decreased hepatic blood flow
Decreased activity of drug
    metabolizing enzymes
Increased size of hepatocytes
Decreased proliferative activity

Gastrointestinal Tract
Worn down and missing teeth
Receding gums
Thinning of gastric mucosa
Decreased secretions of acids
    and digestive enzymes
Decreased gastric emptying
Decreased peristalsis
Decreased absorption of calcium
    and vitamins

Kidney
Decreased number of nephron units
Diminished glomerular filtration rate
Decreased creatinine, urea nitrogen,
    and uric acid excretion
Decreased excretion of drugs
Thickened tubule membranes
Fatty degeneration of tubules
Decreased tubular reabsorption
Narrowing of renal blood vessels

FIGURE 15–1   Common physiologic changes associated with the aging process.

TABLE 15–1
Aging Factors Affecting the Pharmaceutic Phase

Physiologic Changes	Associated Problems
Sensory Changes	
VISION	
Diminished	Difficulty distinguishing among capsules and tablets, in preparing oral and parenteral dosage forms, and in reading labels
Difficulty in color discrimination	
Presbyopia	Dependency on caregiver
TOUCH	
Decreased dexterity	Difficulty opening bottles, isolating tiny tablets, breaking tablets, and handling and administering oral and parenteral dosage forms
HEARING	
Loss of hearing and sound discrimination	Difficulty understanding verbal instructions
	Loss of self-esteem
Cognitive Changes	
Short-term memory loss	Difficulty in comprehending and retaining verbal and written instructions
Alterations in thought processing	

TABLE 15–2
Physiologic Changes Affecting the Pharmacokinetic Phase

Physiologic Changes in Pharmacokinetic Process	Possible Effects
Absorption	
Decreased gastric acidity	Decreased drug solubility
Reduced gastrointestinal motility	Ineffective absorption of some drugs
Reduced mesenteric blood flow	
Delayed gastric emptying	Extended exposure of drug to gastric mucosa
Diminished absorptive surface	
Impaired epithelial membrane transport	
Distribution	
Reduced muscle mass	
Decreased cardiac output	Delayed circulation of drugs to action sites
Diminished blood flow to tissues	
Decreased levels of serum albumin	Increased availability of protein-bound drugs
Reduction in total body water	Increased sensitivity to water-soluble drugs
Altered tissue permeability	
Increased body fat	Delayed onset of action of fat-soluble drugs
Altered neurotransmitter activity	
Biotransformation	
Decreased liver size and weight	Altered first-pass extraction
Diminished splanchnic blood flow	Prolonged drug half-life
Reduced activity of microsomal drug metabolizing enzymes	Increased plasma concentration
	Increased tissue concentration
Excretion	
Diminished renal blood flow	
Decreased number of glomeruli	Decreased renal drug clearance
Reduced glomerular filtration rate	Prolonged half-life of drugs
Thickened tubular membranes	Elevated plasma levels of drugs
Decreased tubular transport	
Reduced urea and creatinine clearance	
Decreased urine-concentrating capacity	

motility allows the GI mucosa lengthened exposure to orally administered drugs, increased absorption may occur. Other GI changes in the elderly may cause incomplete absorption of some drugs. For example, decreased absorption of calcium and vitamin D is frequently associated with age-related changes in the digestive epithelium.

Additional age-related characteristics of the elderly that affect drug absorption are the decline in cardiac output and regional blood flow. These factors affect absorption of intramuscular, subcutaneous, and topically applied drugs. If the elderly client is bedridden, absorption of drugs administered in the buttock will slow even more because of further reduction of regional blood flow.

Some drugs frequently used by the elderly (e.g., laxatives and antacids) alter the absorption of other medications. For example, since laxatives increase gastric motility, drugs given concurrently will have shortened exposure to GI mucosa. Antacids are absorbents and buffers. They alter absorption of many drugs by altering the pH of the environment. On the other hand, absorption of some orally administered drugs is unaffected by age-related changes. Two drugs that show little change in their absorption rate are acetaminophen and aspirin—drugs frequently used by the elderly for pain.[1,4–6]

Distribution Distribution of drugs in the body is affected by age-related changes such as decreased cardiac output, body muscle mass, total body fluid, and serum albumin; slowed active transport systems; increased adipose tissue; and increased sensitivity to central nervous system drugs. Some of these changes result in slower circulation of drugs to action sites, thus altering the drug's onset and duration of action. Other changes affect the concentration and solubility of drugs in the body.[4,6]

Alterations in body composition (e.g., an increase in body fat) result in retention of lipid-soluble drugs, causing a delayed onset of action. Reduced levels of total-body fluids cause concentration of water-soluble drugs, thus increasing the potential for toxicity. With lower serum albumin levels, drug-binding capacity is inhibited, allowing a greater percentage of free active drug to circulate. Even though the overall serum levels remain normal, the increase in unbound or free drug can produce toxicity and/or drug interactions.

Biotransformation Biotransformation primarily occurs in the liver. As the body ages, the size and weight of the liver generally decrease, splanchnic blood flow diminishes, and activity of microsomal drug-metabolizing enzymes decreases. With the shrinking of the liver, fewer hepatic cells are present to break down drugs. As hepatic function declines, drugs may be metabolized more slowly, resulting in an altered first-pass extraction of orally administered drugs. (Remember that first-pass extraction refers to the amount of a drug that is removed from the bloodstream during the first circulation through the liver after intestinal absorption.) Altered first-pass extraction leads to increased plasma and tissue concentration of some drugs and can result in drug toxicity. Impaired liver function also results in elevated levels of active metabolites of drugs.[1,4]

Excretion   Excretion of drugs is altered by age-related changes in renal physiology. These changes may necessitate adjustments in administration schedules and dosage strength. Most drugs are eliminated from the body by the kidneys after they are metabolized. Excretion rate of drugs depends on renal blood flow, glomerular filtration rate, and urea and creatinine clearance. All these functions are diminished during the aging process.

In many of the elderly these renal changes may be further complicated by other medical problems such as infections, nephrosclerosis, congestive heart failure, diabetic neuropathy, and dehydration. Many of the drugs commonly used in the treatment of geriatric clients (e.g., certain cardiac drugs, diuretics, and antipsychotic drugs) can further diminish renal function.[1,4,6,7]

Pharmacodynamic Phase

All of the previously described age-related physiologic changes also influence the pharmacodynamic phase of drug therapy. In addition, alteration in homeostatic mechanisms, changes in receptor site response, and variation in the permeability of the blood-brain barrier alter a drug's mechanism of action.

In the elderly the action of drugs at **receptor sites** is highly variable. This variability is caused by a change in the number, function, or sensitivity of receptor sites. Receptor-site sensitivity usually increases with age, causing an increase in the effects of a drug. As a result, usual adult dosages should be used with caution to decrease the possibility of toxic reactions. With some drugs (e.g., β-adrenergic agonists such as isoproterenol hydrochloride [Isuprel] and β-adrenergic antagonists such as propranolol hydrochloride [Inderal]), decreased receptor-site sensitivity occurs. To obtain a therapeutic response to these drugs, the usual adult dosage must be increased.[4,6]

The **homeostatic reserves** of the renal, cardiovascular, endocrine, respiratory, and central nervous systems diminish with age. Homeostatic and autonomic mechanisms involved in blood glucose control and bladder function are easily affected by the action of certain drugs. In addition, baroreceptor function declines, making the client more prone to orthostatic hypotension. Since temperature regulation declines with age, the elderly client is sensitive to the effects of drugs that affect thermoregulation. Elderly clients who receive drugs that lower the body temperature are at risk of hypothermia. Some elderly individuals have shown an increase in the permeability of the **blood-brain barrier.** These individuals may have more pronounced cognitive side effects from certain drugs.[4,6]

CONCEPT REVIEW

The aging process influences the pharmaceutic, pharmacokinetic, and pharmacodynamic phases. Dosage form, route of administration, and dosage may require alteration based on the condition of the elderly client.

Physiologic changes in the elderly influence all aspects of the pharmacokinetic phase. These changes may include altered absorption rate of drugs, diminished drug distribution, accelerated drug metabolism, and slowed drug excretion.

Pharmacodynamic changes in the elderly may include altered actions at receptor sites, increased permeability of the blood-brain barrier, and decreased stability of homeostatic mechanisms. As a result of these changes, a clinically significant change in drug effects may result.

PHARMACOTHERAPEUTIC PROBLEMS IN THE ELDERLY

One of the most challenging aspects of working with elderly clients is the identification of specific drug-related problems. Some of the problems associated with this age group are increased incidence of adverse reactions and interactions, polypharmacy, noncompliance with drug regimen, and substance misuse, abuse, and addiction.

Adverse Reactions and Interactions

Many of the adverse reactions and interactions seen in the elderly can be explained by changes produced by aging (e.g., decreased hepatic metabolism, reduced glomerular filtration rate, altered actions at receptor sites, and increased permeability of the blood-brain barrier). Awareness of these changes and their potential harm can help you prevent or minimize problems for this age group.

Adverse reactions are particularly problematic in elderly clients. Statistics indicate that 20% to 25% of hospital admissions in individuals over the age of 65 years are the result of adverse drug reactions. These reactions threaten the quality of life and reduce the client's independence.[6,8,9] Most of the adverse reactions seen in this population group can be attributed to inadequate clinical assessment, excessive prescription of drugs, inadequate supervision, altered pharmacokinetic and pharmacodynamic phases, and lack of compliance.[10] Studies also demonstrate that adverse reactions increase significantly when more than one drug is taken concurrently. Some of the most commonly encountered reactions are mental confusion, constipation, orthostatic hypotension, drowsiness, unsteady gait, depression, agitation, and euphoria.[11,12]

Drug-drug, drug-nutrient, and drug-environment interac-

DRUGS THAT CAN CAUSE CONFUSION IN THE ELDERLY

Drugs Affecting the Central Nervous System
Sedatives
Hypnotics
Anxiolytics
Narcotic analgesics
Psychotherapeutic drugs
Antiparkinsonian agents

Drugs Affecting the Autonomic Nervous System
Anticholinergics

Drugs Affecting the Cardiovascular System
Antiarrhythmics
Antihypertensives

Drugs Affecting the Renal System
Diuretics

Drugs Affecting the Body's Defense System
Histamine blockers

Drugs Affecting the Respiratory System
Antihistamines

---

tions occur in this population just as they do in other age groups. **Drug-drug interactions** in the elderly are usually related to polypharmacy, self-treatment, and self-administration (discussed later in this chapter). An additional cause for drug-drug interactions in this age group is the decrease in serum albumin levels. The reduced levels cause drugs to compete with one another for available receptor sites. One drug might displace another drug, causing more of one drug to be free to interact with other freed drugs.

Drug-nutrient interactions occur more frequently in individuals who change or alter preexisting dietary patterns. Dietary patterns of the elderly are altered for a variety of reasons: anorexia associated with diminished sensations of taste and smell; loss of natural teeth; difficulty chewing meats and fresh fruits and vegetables; and insufficient funds to purchase food. In addition, the elderly are receptive to advertisements about food cures (e.g., they may consume large quantities of one type of food in an attempt to relieve signs and symptoms they are experiencing).

Drug-environment interactions also must be considered. Elderly clients who participate in outdoor activities (gardening, walking for fitness, golf, tennis, etc.) must be assessed carefully for drugs that produce photosensitivity reactions. In addition, since many drugs lose their potency when exposed to air and/or sunlight, it is important to determine where the client's drugs are stored. Some individuals do not leave their drugs in the original containers. If this is the client's pattern of behavior, determine if the prescribed drugs are affected by light or air and teach the client appropriate storage methods.

Polypharmacy

Polypharmacy, the use of multiple medications concurrently, is a concern for health care providers responsible for care of the elderly individual. Studies indicate that the elderly, who represent approximately 12% of the population, take 25% to 31% of all prescription medications.[9,13–16]

The reasons for polypharmacy are many and varied. Even though people are currently living longer and healthier lives than earlier generations, the elderly population remains at risk for numerous health problems. In fact, the majority of the elderly have at least one chronic disease, and many have two or more. The presence of these diseases usually necessitates medical care.

In recent years the focus of medical care for the aged has changed from caring to curing. The aging population wants a cure for the aging process—something that will halt the changes occurring in their bodies. All too frequently, medications are viewed as that cure. Society's expectations may force physicians into prescribing drugs for age-related problems as well as disease states. If not completely satisfied with the results of therapy or if a coexisting illness requires a specialist, the elderly client may seek care from another physician. If this physician does not determine the current drug usage by the client, additional prescriptions may be written. The result is that the client is taking multiple medications concurrently.

NURSING RESEARCH

Pinnell, N., Haller, G., & Wacker, M. (1992). Medication usage in the elderly. Unpublished research study.

This descriptive study used a convenience sample of 190 subjects residing primarily in the Midwest area of the United States. The subjects were noninstitutionalized males and females, 60 years of age and older. Their level of wellness did not exclude them from the study.

Within the survey population, a total of 78% of the subjects took prescription drugs, and 86% took nonprescription drugs. Further analysis revealed that 76% of the males and 79% of the females took prescription drugs, and 73% of the males and 91% of the females took nonprescription drugs. In addition, 61% of the males took both prescription and nonprescription drugs, and 73% of the females took both prescription and nonprescription drugs.

The six drug categories most frequently prescribed were antihypertensives, vasodilators, diuretics, anti-inflammatory agents, electrolyte replacement (potassium), and sedatives/hypnotics/antianxiety agents. The six nonprescription drug categories most frequently used by this group were vitamin/mineral supplements, analgesics, laxatives/stool softeners, antiplatelet agent (aspirin), anti-inflammatory agents, and antacids.

STUDENT ACTIVITIES

- Interview five elderly noninstitutionalized individuals. Determine how many drugs each individual is taking.

Also determine the number of different health care providers being seen. Be certain to ask about prescription and nonprescription drugs.

- Check the records of five institutionalized (i.e., hospital or nursing home) individuals. Determine the number of prescribed drugs being administered. Determine if any drug-drug incompatibilities exist. 🌾

Another reason for the occurrence of polypharmacy is the mobility of the current elderly population. Because they are more mobile than in the past, the elderly rarely use the "corner drugstore" where the "family" pharmacist monitored drug usage. Elderly clients may have prescriptions filled in two or more pharmacies, limiting the pharmacist's ability to check for multiple prescriptions for the same drug or to instruct about potential interactions.

Noncompliance With Drug Regimen

Noncompliance or nonadherence to drug regimen may include taking drugs at the wrong time, increasing the frequency of dosage, discontinuing drugs before treatment is completed, and failing to have prescriptions filled. Studies have shown that compliance with drug therapy drops sharply when more than three drugs are prescribed. Other reasons contributing to noncompliance include limited economic resources, lack of transportation methods, inadequate medication instruction, complicated dosage schedules and packaging methods, and poor labeling practices. Memory impairment, lack of trust in the caregiver, self-medication, and disbelief in the value of the therapy may also contribute to noncompliance. In addition, control of drug usage and observation of drug response are difficult with the increasing numbers of elderly living alone or receiving care in their own homes.[17,18]

🌿 NURSING RESEARCH

Conn, V., Taylor, S.G., & Stineman, A. (1992). Medication management by recently hospitalized older adults. *Journal of Community Health Nursing, 9*(1), 1-11.

The purpose of this study was to describe prescriptive medication management by older adults who had recently been discharged from hospitals. The sample (N = 179) included adults 65 to 101 years of age. These subjects managed a total of 950 prescriptive drugs.

Overall, the subjects reported high confidence in their ability to manage the drugs. The lowest confidence level was reported in the area of ability to recognize unwanted side effects of the drugs.

The most commonly given reason for missed doses was "forgetting"; one fourth of the subjects indicated deliberate omission of drug doses. Almost a half of the subjects received assistance from others with their drug administration.

STUDENT ACTIVITIES

- Interview five elderly individuals in your community who are each receiving at least four prescription drugs. Ask them to describe the frequency of administration for each drug. Determine whether they ever omit doses and what actions they take if they do.
- Ask these same individuals to describe the teaching that accompanied the prescribing of these drugs. 🌾

Self-Medication

Self-medication is common with the elderly individual. As described in Chapter 11, self-medication has two components: self-treatment and self-administration. Self-treatment includes the use of over-the-counter (OTC) drugs and home remedies. In the United States there has been a significant increase in the use of OTC drugs. It has been estimated that over 70% of the elderly population take OTC drugs on a daily basis.[9,16]

A common misuse of self-treatment involves OTC laxatives. Elderly clients frequently rely on laxatives to improve their bowel function. However, using laxatives while taking diuretics or cardiovascular drugs or with decreased fluid intake potentiates the risk of electrolyte imbalance or drug toxicity.

Home remedies also produce problems for the elderly. For example, elderly clients frequently use sodium bicarbonate to relieve symptoms of gastric distress; but intake of large amounts of sodium bicarbonate can lead to metabolic alkalosis. In addition, the increased amount of sodium can be harmful since the elderly have diminished excretory capacity in the kidneys.

Self-administration refers to the use of a prescribed medicine for other than prescribed purposes. Many elderly clients terminate drug regimens early and hoard the remaining drugs for possible future use. Another common practice among the elderly is the sharing of medications with friends and relatives.

Substance Misuse, Abuse, and Addiction

Numerous psychologic and sociologic changes occur with the aging process such as changes in independence, self-esteem, and personality. Emotions may become more labile, and response to stressors may increase. In addition, interest levels in eating, preparing meals, and/or socializing may decrease, and social support systems may diminish. All of these factors may cause substance misuse, abuse, and addiction.

Alcohol abuse is increasingly diagnosed among the elderly population. Some estimates suggest that 10% of independently residing elderly have a problem with alcohol. This problem may be as high as 21% in high-risk groups such as single men and veterans. In many instances alcohol abuse can go unnoticed because the elderly individual exhibits behaviors commonly associated with aging: unsteadiness, missing meals, oversleeping, blackouts, personality changes, accidents, and falls.[19–22]

Since alcohol is a central nervous system (CNS) depressant, oversedation and/or increased CNS depression can occur when the individual combines alcohol with some drugs (e.g., narcotic analgesics, psychotherapeutics, and antihistamines). In addition, alcohol can interfere with the action of other drugs such as antibiotics. (See Chapter 12 for additional information on substance misuse, abuse, and addiction.)

CONCEPT REVIEW

Some of the pharmacotherapeutic problems associated with this age group are increased incidence of adverse reactions and interactions; polypharmacy; noncompliance with drug regimen; and substance misuse, abuse, and addiction.

⊞ NURSING CONSIDERATIONS

It is well-documented that nurses are the health care professionals with whom the elderly client has the most contact. This means that the nurse has the greatest opportunity to monitor the client's response to drug therapy and to discover problems arising from drug usage.

Assessing A holistic approach is essential when assessing the elderly client. A baseline health history, drug history, and physical assessment must be collected on each client. The **health history** should include physiologic, social, psychologic, cultural, and economic information. Ask the client questions about the function of each body system. If the client indicates a problem or health concern, ask more direct questions to help the client describe the problem fully. Include in the health history the client's perception of his or her current health status. Ask the client to describe his or her health promotion and protection patterns. Ask questions that help you investigate the client's social support systems, cultural and religious aspects, and self-concept. Include questions about feelings toward and about drugs, coping mechanisms, level of stress, and locus of control.

Before starting the **drug history,** decide which term you will use when asking questions—drugs, medicines, or medications. The term *drug* may have a different connotation to the older individual. He or she may associate the term only with illegal or street drugs. On the other hand, the term *medication* may exclude frequently used OTC drugs the client does not consider as important since they were purchased without a prescription. Examine the client's responses closely. This information may give you clues to the client's perception of the terms. If not, ask the client to give you his or her interpretation and adjust your questions accordingly.

During the drug history, use open-ended questions as much as possible. This type of question elicits more information than if the client merely has to answer with a one- or two-word response. Make your questions clear; use simple, nontechnical terms. Since processing of information is slowed in some elderly individuals, do not rush the client's response.

In gathering the drug history, consider the following: Is the elderly client currently taking any drugs? Has the individual taken drugs in the past? How frequently does the client taking prescription drugs see a physician? When refills are needed, are requests for refills acquired by telephone, or is an office visit required? Does the client use any ethnic or folk remedies?

Remember it is not uncommon for elderly clients to forget that which is familiar. For example, the "water pill" that has been taken for several years may be overlooked when the client is asked to list current drugs. Be certain to remind the client that you want information on nonprescription drugs also. In addition, ask the client about the use of social drugs such as nicotine, caffeine, alcohol, and street drugs. Include in your drug history questions that will elicit information about allergies and past adverse reactions.

Determine the client's knowledge level about each drug being taken. Can the client describe the drug, provide information about the dose and frequency of administration, explain what the drug does, and describe the adverse reactions associated with the drug? Ask questions that will determine how the client stores drugs. Establish how medications are taken and if special techniques are used to help the client remember when to take the medications.

Ask the client if a prescription drug has ever been discontinued. If it has, determine the reason for the discontinuance (e.g., following medical advice; on advice of family, friends, or media; inability to refill prescription). Ask specifically if the client has ever taken drugs prescribed for a friend or family member or shared medications with anyone. You should determine what pharmacy or pharmacies are used for prescriptions and OTC drug purchases. Ask the client if a drug profile is on file at the pharmacy. Also verify the client's method of paying for drugs.

Hospitalized clients should be asked to have all their drugs brought to the hospital for review by the physician and/or nurse. In the home setting the nurse should ask to see all drugs currently in use. (This review of drugs must include prescription drugs, commonly used OTC drugs, social drugs, and home remedies.)

A system-by-system **physical assessment** of the client is the next step. Some physiologic changes associated with aging have specific implications for drug use. For example, loss of visual acuity may hamper the client's ability to read labels and discriminate between drugs. When you assess the client's motor skills, determine his or her ability to open various types of drug packages. Child-resistant bottles and blister and bubble packages pose problems for many clients. Assess the client's assets and liabilities in sensory perception. Decreases in the senses of smell and taste can lead to diminished appetite and decreased thirst sensation. These changes can lead to increased side effects and decreased benefits from drug regimen. Assess the client's thought processing and integration. This information will provide the basis for an effective teaching plan.

Diagnosing Once the assessment data have been compiled, they must be analyzed and nursing diagnoses established. Many nursing diagnoses are related to drug therapy and the elderly. They may include the following:

- Knowledge deficit regarding drug regimen related to sensory deficits.
- Alteration in comfort: nausea and vomiting related to drug side effects.
- Noncompliance related to lack of knowledge, economic factors, cognitive factors, and/or complexity of drug regimen.

DRUG HISTORY FORM

If clients are not receptive to the term *drugs,* use terms *medicine* or *medication* when asking the client questions.

General Questions About Prescription Drugs

1. What prescription medications do you currently take?
2. Why do you take the medication (e.g., arthritis, pain)?
3. When do you take your medications (frequency and time of day)?
4. What do you do if you miss a dose?
5. Do you take any medications differently from the instructions on the label?
6. Do you have trouble reading the instructions on the label? Removing the cap on the bottle? Opening blister or bubble packs? Preparing the medicine? Swallowing any of your medications?
7. How do you pay for your medications?
8. Have you ever omitted medications because they were too expensive?
9. Where do you store your medications?
10. Do you complete the medication regimen as prescribed?
11. If you do not take all of your prescribed medications, what do you do with the remaining medications?
12. Have you ever taken medication prescribed for another individual?
13. Have your medications been prescribed by more than one health care provider?
14. Where do you get your prescriptions filled?
15. Do you purchase your medications in large quantities?

Questions About Over-the-Counter (OTC) Drugs

1. Do you take OTC medications for any of the following conditions: pain, insomnia, constipation, diarrhea, hayfever, sinus problems, allergies, upset stomach, "nerves"?
2. If you take OTC medications for any of these conditions, what are the names of the medicines?
3. How frequently do you use these medicines?
4. Is your physician aware that you are taking these OTC medications?
5. Have you discussed these OTC medications with your pharmacist?
6. Do you take any vitamins or minerals?
7. Do you use any home remedies?
8. Do you take any medicine to "thin your blood"? If so, was this medication suggested by your physician?

Questions to Determine Potential for Drug-Nutrient Interactions

1. Do you take any health food preparations?
2. How much caffeine do you consume daily? (Determine amount of coffee, tea, chocolate, or caffeinated soda consumed in a 24-hour period.)
3. Do you drink any alcoholic beverages? If so, how much do you drink in 1 day?

Questions About Adverse or Allergic Responses to Medications

1. Have you ever had an allergic reaction to a medication? If so, what was the name of the medication?
2. Can you describe how the medication affected you?
3. What actions were taken when you had your allergic reaction?
4. Have any of your medications ever produced adverse reactions or side effects? What medication was responsible for these effects? What actions were taken when you had these responses?

- High risk for injury related to drowsiness, unsteady gait, and/or confusion associated with drug therapy.
- Self-care deficit related to impaired dexterity associated with drug therapy.
- Alteration in sexual patterns related to drug-induced impotency.
- Alterations in thought process related to fluid and electrolyte imbalance associated with drug regimen.
- Anxiety related to complex medication regimen.
- Alteration in self-image: decreased self-esteem related to dependence on drug therapy.
- High risk for alteration in nutrition: less than body requirement related to side effects of drugs.

Planning   Planning flows from the nursing diagnoses and should involve the client and family if possible. Nurses have a major responsibility for educating clients about drugs. Teaching plans should be developed and shared with the client and his or her significant other.

To enhance assimilation of material, information should be given verbally and in writing. Include in your teaching plan the name, dosage, dose schedule, and therapeutic action of each prescribed drug. In addition, you should include a description of the appearance of the drug, refill information, and approximate duration of therapy. Teach the client about expected adverse reactions and possible drug interactions. Emphasize what actions to take if adverse reactions or drug interactions occur. You should stress the dangers of self-medication and the hazards of noncompliance. Recommend that the client has his or her physician review prescriptions at least every 6 months.

Have the client prepare a list of all prescribed and OTC drugs being taken. This list should be carried by the client at all times. In addition, tell the client to attach a copy of the list to the front of the refrigerator. Suggest to the client that medicine cabinets be cleaned out. Drugs past their expiration date or no longer being taken should be thrown away.

For all OTC drugs currently being used, teach the client to read the labels carefully. Are the drugs being stored properly? Are the drugs being taken as directed on the label? If the small print on the OTC drugs is a problem, suggest that the client use a magnifying glass.

To decrease the incidence of drug-drug interactions, encourage the client always to use the same pharmacy. Teach the client to check with the pharmacist before buying any OTC drug. The pharmacist can tell the client if the OTC drug interacts with prescribed drugs. Instruct the client to read the directions printed on prescription drug containers before leaving the pharmacy; if the client has problems reading the information, the label can be replaced with one using larger type.

As a follow-up to client teaching, you can compile drug information cards. Include on the card information such as drug dose, frequency of administration, and adverse reactions. To help in identifying the drug, tape a tablet or capsule on the card. The medication card can help the client comply with drug regimen and is invaluable if an emergency arises.

Expected outcomes that can be discussed with the elderly client include the following:

- Client will demonstrate appropriate knowledge of prescription drugs.
- Client will develop a list of prescribed and OTC drugs being used.
- Client will demonstrate compliance with drug therapy.
- Client will remain injury free.
- Client will have diminished levels of anxiety.

Implementing   The implementation phase includes administering drugs to older adults in the hospital or home, monitoring response and compliance to drug therapy, and implementing the previously developed teaching plan. For all of these actions, using competent decision making and judgment is essential. In some circumstances it may be necessary to withhold a drug until you communicate with the physician. Based on your observation of the client, you may need to discuss a reduction in drug dosage with the physician. Your assessment might indicate the need for a different dosage route or form (e.g., liquids instead of tablets if swallowing difficulties exist or solid dosage forms if the client has difficulty pouring the liquid form). You may suggest that consideration be given to size, shape, and color of each drug to minimize client confusion. Investigate nonmedical methods of treating common client problems such as constipation and indigestion. Many of these treatment methods are within the nurse's role and may preclude the need for further prescription or OTC drugs.

Before administering a new drug or a drug prescribed on an as-needed basis, review the physiologic status of the client.

Determine if age- or disease-related factors could alter the pharmacodynamic or pharmacokinetic phases of the drug. Ask yourself the following questions: Does the drug have a narrow therapeutic index? What are the adverse or toxic effects of the drug? Could this drug potentiate or inhibit the action of other drugs the client is receiving? Only after you have given consideration to these factors should you administer the drug.

Several aspects of drug administration differ for the elderly client. Since the circulation in the extremities decreases with aging, topical and transdermal dosage forms should be applied to the torso of the elderly client to ensure optimum absorption. In addition, since some elderly clients experience difficulty swallowing, always position the client in an upright position before giving oral drugs.

Hospitalized clients should be supervised as they learn to take their medications before discharge. Have the client start self-administering the least toxic drugs (e.g., vitamins, stool softeners, nonnarcotic analgesics). Leave specified amounts of each drug at the bedside with directions for the client to follow. Each shift of nurses should check the amount of drugs left and reinforce any needed teaching. As the client is ready, add more drugs to the self-administration schedule.

Some nursing homes and chronic care facilities are using drug holidays as an appropriate way to assess the effects of polypharmacy. Drug holidays call for the discontinuation, for a given period of time, of all drugs that the client currently receives. (Exceptions to this rule include the need to substitute regular insulin for the longer-acting insulins.) After a trial drug holiday, it has been found that some drugs can be discontinued or given at a lowered dosage.[4]

For hospitalized clients, you must begin your teaching well before discharge. Teaching should be done slowly to allow time for absorption of the information and for the client to ask questions. You should provide only general information in group sessions. Specific drug information should be given on an individual basis. These teaching sessions should be kept short—15 to 20 minutes at a time. Make certain you speak in a clear, distinct voice and use words meaningful to the individual. Carefully consider the appropriateness of medical terminology.

The decline in motor skills seen in many elderly individuals may require altered self-administration techniques. You should demonstrate the needed skill in simple steps. During the session make certain you have adequate lighting free from glare. Have the client practice the technique and then perform a return demonstration. Ask the client to verbalize each step and provide the rationale involved in the skill along with the return demonstration. This step allows you to assess knowledge and technique. If needed, encourage the client to use adaptive devices such as hearing aids and glasses.

In addition to teaching the client about his or her particular drug regimen, assist the client to establish a system that will facilitate compliance. Simplification of the drug schedule is the first step. Collaborate with the physician to decrease the number of times per day the client must take drugs. Help the client to establish a drug schedule compatible with the prescribed drugs (e.g., drugs to take with meals, drugs to take 2 hours after meals, etc.). As much as possible, arrange the drug schedule so that doses are associated with routine events in the client's life (e.g., mealtimes, favorite television show, bedtime). Suggest that the client set an alarm or timer to help him or her remember when a drug dose is due. Inform the client that there are commercial pill timers he or she can carry with him or her. Prefilled insulin syringes can be used for a diabetic client with diminished vision. The use of individual prefilled envelopes or containers labeled with the name of the drug, day of the week, and time of administration is helpful. A muffin tin, egg carton, or ice cube tray may also be used. In addition, commercially prepared medicine boxes or containers are available.

Evaluating   Part of the evaluation phase includes evaluating the effectiveness of the medications. In addition, the elderly client requires special monitoring for side effects. Adverse reactions are frequently reported with antidepressants, diuretics, antipsychotics, and nonsteroidal anti-inflammatory drugs. Some reactions for which to assess include changes in ambulation and self-care, dry mouth, urinary retention, orthostatic hypotension, restlessness, nausea, vomiting, constipation, and diarrhea.

To evaluate the effectiveness of the plan of care, review the expected outcomes previously developed with the client. In addition, you must evaluate the teaching plan and provide follow-up teaching when necessary.

SUMMARY

This chapter focused on the special needs of the elderly client. Since all phases of drug therapy—pharmacodynamic, pharmacokinetic, and pharmaceutic—are affected by the aging process, nursing care of this age group requires knowledge of the physiology of aging. Aging causes different absorption, distribution, metabolism, and excretion of drugs. Therefore the client may react or respond differently to certain drugs. In some situations the dosage form and route must be altered to meet the special needs of the aging client.

Only with careful, planned nursing care can you prevent the miracles of modern drug therapy from turning into a menace for the elderly. You must look at the client holistically, not focus solely on drug therapy. Improvement in nutrition, use of alternative therapies when possible, and promotion of general health and fitness may result in reduced medication requirements.

REFERENCES

1. Blair, K.A. (1990). Aging: Physiological aspects and clinical implications. *Nurse Practitioner, 15*(2), 14-28.
2. Hogstel, M.O. (1992). *Clinical manual of gerontological nursing.* St. Louis: Mosby–Year Book.
3. Murray, R., & Zentner, J. (1993). *Nursing assessment and health promotion strategies through the lifespan* (5th ed.). Norwalk, CT: Appleton & Lange.
4. Gray, M. (1990). Polypharmacy in the elderly. *Orthopaedic Nursing, 9*(6), 49-54.
5. Levy, D. (1991). Drug therapy and the elderly. *Emergency, 23*(2), 44-49.
6. Tideiksaar, R. (1990). Principles of drug therapy in the elderly. *Physician Assistant, 14*(2), 29-52.
7. Mallet, L. (1991). Age related changes in renal function and clinical implications for drug therapy. *Journal of Geriatric Drug Therapy, 5*(3), 5-29.
8. Brawn, L.A., & Caseleden, C.M. (1990). Adverse drug reactions: Overview of special considerations in the management of the elderly patient. *Drug Safety, 5,* 421-435.
9. Falvo, D.R., Holland, B., Brenner, J., & Benshoff, J. (1990). Medication use practices in the ambulatory elderly. *Health Values, 14*(3), 10-16.
10. Schwertz, D., & Buschmann, M. (1989). Pharmacogeriatrics. *Critical Care Nursing Quarterly, 12*(1), 26-37.
11. Palmieri, D. (1991). Clearing up the confusion: Adverse effects of medications in the elderly. *Journal of Gerontological Nursing, 17*(10), 32-35.
12. Westfall, L., & Pavlis, R. (1987). Why the elderly are so vulnerable to drug reactions. *RN Magazine, 50*(11), 39-43.
13. American Association of Retired Persons and Administration on Aging (1990). *A profile of older Americans.* Washington, DC: U.S. Department of Health and Human Services.
14. Grauer, K. (1991). Problems of polypharmacy and intercurrent disease. *Hospital Practice Symposium Supplement, 26*(2), 20-25.
15. LeSage, J. (1991). Polypharmacy in geriatric patients. *Nursing Clinics of North America, 26*(2), 273-287.
16. Pinnell, N., Haller, G., & Wacker, M. (1992). *Medication usage in the elderly.* Unpublished research study.
17. Cargill, J.M. (1992). Medication compliance in elderly people: Influencing variables and interventions. *Journal of Advanced Nursing, 17,* 422-426.
18. Conn, V., Taylor, S.G., & Stineman, A. (1991). Medication management by recently hospitalized older adults. *Journal of Community Health Nursing, 9*(1), 1-11.
19. Adams, W., Yuan, Z., Barboriak, J., & Rimm, A. (1993). Alcohol-related hospitalizations of elderly people. *Journal of the American Medical Association, 270,* 1222-1225.
20. Chenitz, W., Salisbury, S., & Stone, J. (1990). Drug misuse and abuse in the elderly. *Issues in Mental Health Nursing, 11*(1), 1-16.
21. Holmstrom, C. (1990). Substance abuse in the elderly. *Psychiatric Nursing, 31*(1), 6-8.
22. Sheahan, S.L., Hendricks, J., & Coons, S.J. (1989). Drug misuse among the elderly: A covert problem. *Health Values, 13*(3), 22-29.

BIBLIOGRAPHY

Bender, P. (1992). Deceptive distress in the elderly. *American Journal of Nursing, 92*(10), 29-32.

Carruth, A., & Boss, B. (1990). More than they bargained for: Adverse drug effects. *Journal of Gerontological Nursing, 16*(7), 27-30.

Colt, H., & Shapiro, A. (1989). Drug-induced illness as a cause for admission to a community hospital. *Journal of American Geriatrics Society, 37,* 323-326.

Eng, K., & Emlet, C.A. (1990). Using education to prevent geriatric medication misuse. *Journal of Applied Gerontology, 9,* 185-193.

Feibus, B. (1989). Use and abuse of drugs in the elderly. *Advancing Clinical Care, 4*(4), 21-22.

Gawlinski, A., & Jensen, G. (1991). The complications of cardiovascular aging. *American Journal of Nursing, 91*(11), 26-30.

Gurwitz, J.H., & Avorn, J. (1991). The ambiguous relation between aging and adverse drug reactions. *Annals of Internal Medicine, 114,* 956-966.

Hawe, P., & Higgins, G. (1990). Can medication education improve the drug compliance of the elderly? *Patient Education and Counseling, 16,* 151-160.

Kottke, M.K., Stetsko, G., Rosenbaum, S.E., & Rhodes, C.T. (1990). Problems encountered by the elderly in the use of conventional dosage forms. *Journal of Geriatric Drug Therapy, 5*(2), 77-92.

MacIssac, A.M., & Adamson, C.B. (1989). Multiple medications: Is your elderly patient caught in the storm? *Nursing 89, 19*(7), 60-64.

Quilligan, S. (1990). Tablets to take away: Why some elderly people fail to comply with their medication. *Professional Nurse, 5,* 566-568.

Quilligan, S. (1990). When should you take your tablets? Teaching elderly people about their medication. *Professional Nurse, 5,* 639-640.

Roxe, D. (1989). Renal function, aging, and drug therapy. *Comprehensive Therapy, 15*(8), 13-18.

Short, L., Burnett, M., Egbert, A., & Parks, L. (1990). Medicating the postoperative elderly: How do nurses make their decisions? *Journal of Gerontological Nursing, 16*(7), 12-17.

Stolley, J.M., Buckwalter, K.C., Fjordbak, B., & Bush, S. (1991). Iatrogenesis in the elderly. *Journal of Gerontological Nursing, 17*(9), 12-16.

Taira, F. (1991). Teaching independently living older adults about managing their medications. *Rehabilitation Nursing, 16,* 322-326.

Tesfa, A. (1989). Drug therapy in elderly patients: Diagnosis of drug-related problems. *Recent Advances in Nursing, 23,* 45-52.

CHAPTER 16

NURSE'S ROLE IN
Drug Therapy in the Home

MYRNA BRENNER WACKER

⚛ **Role of the Nurse in the Home Setting**

LEARNING OBJECTIVE: Describe the role of the nurse in managing drug therapy in the home.

⚛ **Application of the Nursing Process**

LEARNING OBJECTIVES:

Apply the nursing process to the management of drug therapy in the home.

Describe major ethical dilemmas related to drug therapy management in the home.

Identify important legal issues affecting drug therapy in home settings.

KEY TERMS:

Compliance, interdisciplinary collaboration, noncompliance, priorities

⚛ **Parenteral Drug Therapy in the Home**

LEARNING OBJECTIVES:

Identify four types of parenteral drug therapy used in the home setting.

Identify specific nursing concerns in the management of parenteral drug therapy in the home.

Describe specific considerations in the administration of controlled substances in the home.

Discuss the administration of chemotherapy at home.

⚛ **Oral Drug Therapy in the Home**

LEARNING OBJECTIVE: Describe specific nursing concerns in the management of oral drug therapy in the home.

CONCEPTS AND TERMS TO REVIEW

Review Chapter 8 for a complete discussion of the role of the nurse in drug therapy.

Review sections in a medical-surgical textbook or procedure manual that describe the care of the client receiving parenteral therapy.

---

*B*ecause of the increase in outpatient treatment and shortened hospital stays, the current trend is toward providing more nursing care in the home. Clients receiving care in the home are more seriously ill and require more intense therapy than those seen in the past. This trend has dramatically changed the role of the nurse who cares for these individuals.

In many instances sophisticated, complex drug delivery systems are being used. Thus the nurse must know how to operate the various systems and have the ability to teach the client or caregiver to do so. This chapter provides an overview of some of the essential points to consider when administering or monitoring drug therapy in the home.

ROLE OF THE NURSE IN THE HOME SETTING

There is a variety of nurses in the community who oversee drug therapy in the home. The primary role of the **community health nurse** is to promote compliance with the drug regimen in the home setting, a setting much less controlled than that of a hospital or long-term care facility. The nurse in this role requires special skills to function effectively, including extensive knowledge of pharmacology and competence in client teaching. The community health nurse also requires skill in motivating the client and caregiver to assume responsibility for self-care.

The **home health nurse** most often cares for the client and caregiver immediately after discharge. This individual establishes drug and treatment regimens and continues to supervise the client during the period of drug therapy. The home health nurse must be capable of managing complex delivery systems for drug administration (e.g., central venous access lines, infusion pumps).

Hospice programs provide care for the terminally ill in their

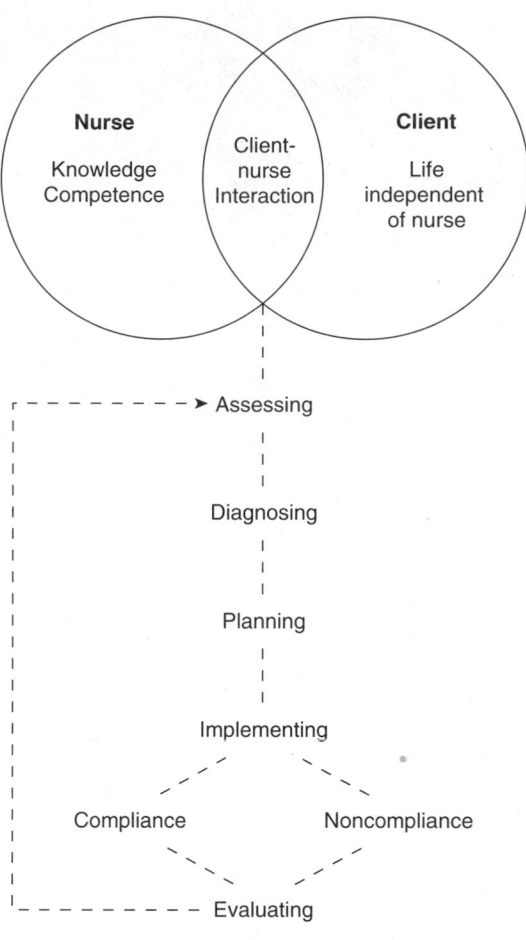

FIGURE 16–1   Drug Therapy Compliance Model.

homes. One important aspect of hospice care is pain management through palliative drugs. The **hospice nurse** works not only with the complexities of pain control but also with the legal issues involved with the use of controlled substances in the home. This nurse must manage complex drug delivery systems and toxic chemotherapy administration in the home.

The **public health nurse,** who works in official health agencies such as health departments, often participates in programs targeted at high-risk populations across the life span. This nurse also receives referrals from the health care system for clients with a variety of health problems such as the deinstitutionalized mentally ill, at-risk prenatal and postpartum clients, infants and children with health problems, and elderly chronically ill clients who need supervision. Many of these high-risk or referred clients are receiving drug therapy.

▨ NURSING CONSIDERATIONS

Regardless of the functions of the nurse in the home setting, nursing care follows the steps in the nursing process. The model in Figure 16–1 illustrates the nursing process as it relates to management of drug therapy in the home. The interlocking circles show the partnership of the client, caregiver, and nurse as they progress through the process. The nurse and client or caregiver have areas of the circles that are open and autonomous. For the nurse, the independent area is professional knowledge and competence. For the client or caregiver, the separate area is the client's life independent from the nurse.

The overlapping portion depicts the essential interaction between the client or caregiver and nurse to form a team, with the goal successful adherence to a drug regimen.

Assessing

The key to an accurate assessment is skillful communication. If the client or caregiver does not trust the nurse, needed information will be missed. It is crucial that the assessment be holistic and examine the myriad of factors such as culture and age that affect the client and determine his or her ability to comply.

During the **health history** a review of all current prescription and nonprescription drugs and previously prescribed drugs is completed. Looking at the total drug regimen alerts the nurse to any drug interactions, duplications, and inappropriateness of drugs or dosages. The client must be asked about previous undesired clinical responses and the names of all primary care providers being seen.

A comprehensive checklist such as illustrated in the box is a valuable resource for the nurse. Use of the checklist provides

HOME MEDICATION ASSESSMENT CHECKLIST	Strength	Barrier
Sociocultural Assessment		
Values and beliefs about health and illness		
Personal long- and short-term health goals		
Communication or language		
Spirituality or religion		
Folk medicine and home remedies		
OTC drugs		
Previous illness experiences		
Response to pain		
Capacity for self-care		
Nutrition and diet		
Hygiene		
Privacy needs		
Time needs		
Support systems and family roles		
Psychologic Assessment		
Learning ability or cognition		
Knowledge base		
Developmental task achievement		
Coping and problem solving		
Physical Assessment		
Systems function		
Sensory function		
Activities of daily living		
Side effects of therapy		
Interactions with therapy		
Environmental Assessment		
Home safety		
Home convenience		
Financial status		
Transportation		
Accessibility of primary care provider		
Accessibility of pharmacist		
Availability of community resources		
COMMENTS:		

needed data for planning effective care with the client or caregiver. If possible, most of the information on the checklist should be solicited during the initial assessment. Elaboration about specific items can be written in the comments space. Information from the checklist can also be used to help resolve barriers to compliance.

Diagnosing

Analyzing the sociocultural, psychologic, physical, and environmental assessment data allows for the development of accurate, meaningful nursing diagnoses. Nursing diagnoses appropriate for the client receiving drug therapy in the home follow:
- Altered body temperature, high risk for, related to side effect of vasoconstrictive medication.
- Cardiac output, decreased, related to failure to take drugs as prescribed.
- Constipation related to side effect of drugs, inadequate fiber and fluids in diet, and inadequate exercise.
- Family coping, compromised, related to inadequate understanding of demands of disease process on client.
- Family coping, disabling, related to exhaustion of caregiver and lack of resources.
- Family processes, altered, related to situational crisis of client's diagnosis.
- Fatigue related to effects of drug therapy.
- Fluid volume excess related to excessive sodium intake.
- Health maintenance, altered, related to priorities, lack of finances, lack of transportation.
- Pain related to reluctance to take adequate dosage of pain medication.
- Poisoning, high risk for, related to unsafe storage of drugs.

Planning

Once the client or caregiver and nurse have identified the important assessment data, including barriers to compliance, joint planning to meet these needs is undertaken. Determining *priorities* must be done with client or caregiver input to ensure client or caregiver ownership and cooperation. One method used to assist in this process is contracting, or a written agreement between nurse and client outlining their mutual goals.

The nurse and the client or caregiver may find they have entirely different priorities. Immediately addressing the priorities of the client or caregiver may remove barriers and allow the nurse to pursue nursing priorities. However, this must be done without placing the client in jeopardy. For example, if a client perceives side effects of the drug as the main problem, this conflict must be resolved, or compliance to the drug therapy may be jeopardized.

Since drug therapy in the home involves situations that are life threatening, safety of the client and caregiver is a high priority of the nurse. For example, in households with small children, safe storage of drugs to prevent poisoning is essential.

Planning also involves determining what resources beyond the nurse are required to meet the client's needs. Working with other disciplines, **interdisciplinary collaboration**, is a significant part of practice when working with clients in the home. For example, close collaboration with the client's primary care provider for aspects of treatment such as dosage adjustments is essential.

This phase also involves developing plans to overcome barriers to compliance. For example, if the barrier is impaired vision, plans can be made to minimize the impact of this problem. Providing information in larger print, use of color coding, or involvement of another family member would be possible alternatives.

Expected outcomes for the plan of care are mutually developed between client or caregiver and nurse. Based on the nursing diagnoses, the following are appropriate outcomes:

- Client avoids over-the-counter (OTC) drugs that interact with current drug regimen.
- Client participates in prescribed drug therapy.
- Client verbalizes the dangers of OTC drugs.
- Client consumes a nutritionally adequate diet, excluding foods that interact with drug therapy.
- Family verbalizes knowledge of client's illness and treatment plan.
- Family participates positively in care of client.

Implementing

Regardless of the situation, there are some general guidelines that should be followed when administering or monitoring drug therapy in the home.

GENERAL GUIDELINES

Conscientious use of *community health standards of practice* provides the basis for quality care.[1] In addition, successful therapy for the client frequently depends on the nurse's ability to establish a situation that allows client or family **compliance,** which means to follow the treatment regimen properly. (**Noncompliance** denotes a client's informed decision not to adhere to a therapeutic recommendation.)

Important factors to consider in assisting the client to achieve compliance are communication and the effective therapeutic relationship. The client's relationship with the care provider is often cited as the most important factor in compliance. In addition, since client self-responsibility is the goal in home care, the client or caregiver must be encouraged to participate in the entire process of care. This participation gives the client or caregiver ownership of the situation and increases the likelihood of compliance. He or she is less likely to follow drug regimens that require significant changes in behavior. However, reinforcement of behaviors by significant others or reference groups such as support groups encourages compliance. In addition, adequate knowledge promotes adherence to therapy.[2] Finally, the nurse working in the home situation must recognize the limitations of that setting. Ultimately the client or caregiver makes the decision to comply or not to comply.

An integral part of managing drug therapy in the home setting is client teaching. Teaching is based on the assessed data and is specific to the client or caregiver situation. The client or caregiver is taught the actions of the prescribed drug, its de-

sired therapeutic effects, and undesired clinical responses. Information on drug-drug, drug-nutrient, and drug-environment interactions is also needed. During the teaching process remember that clients and caregivers are lay individuals and consider the educational preparation that the nurse received to administer the same therapies.

Teaching should include actions to take in case things go wrong and the client is alone. Concise, clearly written instructions are helpful and can serve as a support to the client. Checklists for troubleshooting are also helpful. The nurse should never leave a situation without assurance that the client or caregiver has a very clear idea of what to do in case problems occur and what constitutes serious problems in that particular situation.

REFERRALS

Referral to community resources is also important in the home care setting. Before a referral is made, it must be deemed appropriate, accessible, and acceptable to the client. If these criteria are not met, use of the resource may not occur. Often the nurse must make personal contact with agencies or resources to facilitate the process. With the use of complex resources, keeping a calendar of appointments and home visits for the client is appropriate.

ETHICAL ISSUES

The complexity of care given in the home raises difficult ethical issues. For example, when the client decides not to comply with recommended therapy, what is the correct action for the nurse? Other ethical dilemmas involve termination of care, caregiver issues, reimbursement-driven documentation and care, quality of care, and rationing of health care.

Community health agencies respond to these conflicts in a variety of ways. Agency-based case conferences are vehicles for discussing and resolving conflicts with input from other staff and administrative personnel. Ethics committees provide another possible means of resolving some issues. Other strategies include peer consultation and use of bioethical models and codes of ethics.[3]

LEGAL ISSUES

The current societal trend toward litigation has not escaped this segment of health care. Early hospital discharge of more acutely ill clients with complex treatments compounds the problem for the autonomously functioning community health nurse (see box on p. 138). In addition, managing drug therapy in the home is considered one of the high-risk areas for litigation.[4-6]

Nursing assessment is especially critical in issues of professional negligence. The nurse who fails to complete a comprehensive assessment does not have the necessary information to plan safe, appropriate care. Communication with the client and family, the primary care provider, and other health team members is another critical component in the prevention of litigation problems. Timely reporting of status changes and potential problems is essential for the client's welfare. Accurate documentation of assessments, teaching, and care provides

---

DRUG THERAPY IN SCHOOL SETTINGS

One of the current dilemmas in child health care is drug administration in the school setting. Children with a variety of acute and chronic conditions attend school and require drug administration. Although laws vary from state to state, usually the nurse is the only person in the school setting with legal authorization to administer prescribed drugs. Many schools do not have school nurses or have nurses who are responsible for more than one school. When a nurse is not available, administrators, teachers, or staff members administer drugs. The authorization of lay persons to administer drugs in the school setting is often cited as "in loco parentis" or "in place of the parents." Currently state nurse-licensing boards, state boards of health, and boards of education are debating this issue. In addition to legal issues, there are concerns about possible errors in drug administration, lack of monitoring for side effects, and inappropriate storage of the drugs.

In addition to administering drugs and supervising lay persons who administer drugs, the school nurse has other related responsibilities. Included in these responsibilities are the development of written policies regarding drug administration and documentation and communication with teachers, primary care providers, and families.

---

continuity of care and verification of nursing actions. Copies of instructions given to the client or caregiver confirm the information provided. Documentation giving details of mistakes or potential problems provides protection for both the nurse and agency.

Evaluating

Evaluation includes a review of the client or caregiver's progress toward achievement of expected outcomes. Verbalization and demonstration of a procedure are effective methods of evaluation. However, during the evaluation process the nurse must combine a nonthreatening attitude with a conscientious commitment to correct administration of therapy. The client or caregiver may be dealing with procedures that cause a great deal of fear of failure. The nurse must balance the real need for competent care with the client or caregiver's need for support.

CONCEPT REVIEW

The role of the nurse in the community has changed dramatically in recent years.

Nurses giving direct care to clients in the home need skill in parenteral and oral drug administration tech-

niques. In addition, they must be able to teach the client or caregiver about the prescribed drug regimen and be able to monitor the client for undesired clinical responses.

PARENTERAL DRUG THERAPY IN THE HOME

Emergence of the use of high technology in the home involves the use of diverse methods of parenteral drug therapy.

Specific Nursing Considerations

Thorough and careful assessment is needed before reaching the decision to administer parenteral therapy in the home. Benefits versus disadvantages of each system must be considered. Selection criteria should consider physical condition, motivation, and cognitive ability of client and caregiver, environmental appropriateness, reimbursement sources, and resources.

The nurse must be knowledgeable about the parenteral delivery system and able to provide appropriate supervision of the client or caregiver. Communication between client or caregiver and nurse is a crucial factor. The client or caregiver must have a realistic idea of what the therapy entails from the very beginning. On the other hand, the nurse must be alert to the condition of the caregiver to prevent burnout or exhaustion. The caregiver must be aware of the location of resources and should have continous backup support available.

The complexity of information needed by the client or caregiver presents a challenge to the nurse. A teaching plan prevents omission of important information. A written checklist of information to learn can also be developed. On the checklist, the nurse can document that the client or caregiver demonstrated competence in performing the procedures. The checklist also provides a basis for teaching since it is a record of what has been accomplished, what needs reinforcement, and what remains to be taught.

Working with equipment in the home setting is a special challenge for the nurse. Initially the nurse must determine that the home environment is appropriate for safe and proper operation of the equipment. Then the nurse, client, and caregiver must become comfortable with the machinery. At first all individuals involved may be intimidated by the machine. However, a level of comfort and competence must be achieved through knowledge and practice. Communication among the caregiver, primary care provider, pharmacy, and medical supply company must also be established. In addition, the caregiver and nurse must be skilled in routine maintenance of the machine and in troubleshooting problems as they occur. Keeping spare parts or supplies such as batteries on hand is a helpful practice.

The danger of anaphylaxis from parenteral drug therapy necessitates special planning. Since anaphylaxis is a life-threatening complication, having procedures in place for prompt recognition and treatment of this crisis is critical. Preparation

Teaching Plan for Clients and Caregiver Administering Parenteral Drugs in the Home

Teaching should include information in the following areas:

1. Safety needs
   - Events that constitute an emergency
   - Actions to take immediately
   - Individuals to contact
2. Psychosocial needs
   - What is involved in caring for the client
   - Measures to prevent caregiver burnout
   - Measures to prevent onset of exhaustion in caregiver
   - Feelings that caregiver may experience
3. Environmental needs
   - Home modifications for safety and accessibility
4. Resource needs
   - Availability of financial resources
   - Where to obtain equipment, supplies, and drugs
   - Actions to take if drugs run out
   - Actions to take if equipment fails to function properly
   - Accessibility of primary care provider
   - How to contact primary care provider
   - Accessibility of nurses
   - How to contact a nurse
5. Illness
   - Prognosis for client
   - What to expect during course of the condition
   - Signs and symptoms of complications
   - Actions to take if complications occur
   - When to contact the primary care provider or nurse

6. Drugs
   - Name and dose of each prescribed drug
   - Expected therapeutic effects of each drug
   - Undesired clinical responses associated with each drug
   - Actions to take if these responses occur
   - Special considerations related to use of each drug (e.g., legal restraints with narcotics, disposal of neoplastic agents)
   - Method to maintain drug count
7. Administration procedures
   - Care of tubing and catheters
   - Care of infusion site
   - Supplies needed for dressing changes and other procedures
   - Handling and disposal of soiled supplies such as dressings and needles
   - Indications of complications at infusion site
   - Actions to take if complications occur
8. Machinery or pump
   - Basic parts of infusion pump
   - How the infusion pump operates
   - How to know if machine is functioning properly
   - How alarm system functions
   - Actions to take if alarm activates
   - General maintenance of machine
   - Supplies or spare parts to have available
9. Documentation system
   - Method to document drug treatment and results
   - Monitoring record for routine assessment of client and equipment
   - Method to record undesired clinical responses

for the possibility of anaphylaxis includes determining how to access the local emergency system (e.g., availability of a 911 system), learning about emergency drugs, preparing emergency kits, and developing preestablished protocols and a plan of action.

There are additional considerations when administering home chemotherapy. The Occupational Safety and Health Administration (OSHA) and the Oncology Nursing Society have specific guidelines for handling toxic substances, including recommendations and procedures for spill kits. In addition, a booklet, "Safe Management of Chemotherapy at Home," is available to assist with client and caregiver education.[7,8]

Some form of documentation of care is essential. A form that provides a list of drugs and treatments and the scheduled time of administration is helpful (see box). The caregiver ini-

tials or places a check to indicate that the drug or treatment was administered. Recording the client's response to the therapy and routine client assessment is also important. In addition, a space may be provided for the caregiver to document

Caregiver Drug and Treatment Schedule

	Date Time	Date Time	Date Time	Date Time
Treatments				
Drugs				

contact with the nurse, primary care provider, pharmacist, or medical supply company. Other important information to record includes maintenance of the infusion site and machine. Documentation assists the caregiver in remembering important aspects of care and assists the nurse to evaluate the quality of that care.

Modalities of Parenteral Drug Therapy

Systems used in the home include continuous subcutaneous infusion, peripheral intravenous infusion, central venous access, ambulatory infusion pump, and intraspinal infusion. These different drug delivery systems are discussed briefly in the following section. For information about the actual care of the client and equipment, refer to a medical-surgical textbook or a procedure manual.

Continuous subcutaneous infusion Continuous subcutaneous infusion of narcotics is effective in controlling pain associated with cancer. The advantages are simplicity, safety, and effectiveness. Clients or caregiver can usually accomplish this procedure at home, learning to start the infusion, rotate sites, and operate the infusion pump. This method is especially useful for clients unable to use the oral or rectal dosage form. It is also used for clients needing continuous analgesia or those with no central venous access.[9,10]

Peripheral intravenous infusion Peripheral intravenous infusion is used for clients with short-term therapy or for whom central venous access is a risk or unavailable. Problems associated with use in the home include the need for multiple venipunctures, rotation of intravenous site, pain, sclerosis of the veins, and clotting at site of insertion.

Central venous access Because of the problems associated with peripheral intravenous therapy in the home, central venous access devices are used for long-term home therapy. Usually external devices are used for continuous therapy, and implantable access devices are used for intermittent therapy. Since a wide variety of devices is available, the nurse needs a broad knowledge base. Problems associated with these devices include the potential for infection and catheter occlusion. Thromboocclusion and extravasation are also problems. The client or caregiver must become skilled in aseptic technique to manage care of the catheter and site.[11]

Ambulatory infusion pumps Client-controlled ambulatory infusion pumps provide an effective method of delivering drugs that have few side effects. This drug delivery system frequently is used to administer analgesics. This method lessens the client's anxiety and depression, decreases sedation, increases mobility, and increases the client's feeling of control. A disadvantage is that trained individuals must be available to work with the equipment. Also, adjusting the dosage of the drug to achieve optimal pain control requires skill and teamwork.[12,13]

Intraspinal infusion Intraspinal infusion is used in clients whose pain cannot be controlled by systemic narcotics or who have significant side effects from other regimens. Intraspinal infusion is either epidural or intrathecal. **Epidural infusion** takes place next to the spinal cord and through the dura. Problems encountered are nausea and vomiting and pump failure. Other problems are pruritus, respiratory problems, infection, tolerance, and catheter displacement. The nurse working with this system needs specialized knowledge of spinal drug metabolism. **Intrathecal infusions** do not cross the dura and are given into the subarachnoid space next to the spinal cord. As with epidural infusion, catheters, implantable ports, and pumps can be used. Problems and benefits are similar to those associated with the epidural infusion.[14–16]

Parenteral Narcotic Drug in the Home

With the evolution of home hospice care for clients with cancer, the nurse now provides pain control measures in the home setting. Control of severe cancer pain is usually accomplished through the use of narcotic analgesics. Narcotics are classified as controlled substances. As a result, special precautions must be observed; this is especially true in the unstructured setting of the home.

Controlled substances in the home must be stored and administered in compliance with the Federal Controlled Substance Act and applicable state laws. These drugs must be secured under lock and key, and only the nurse and caregiver should have access. In addition, accurate documentation of use is essential to meet legal requirements. Missing narcotics must be reported and investigated.

When narcotics are used in the home, additional teaching of the client or caregiver is needed. Information on legal constraints, recommended methods of administration, storage, and disposal must be provided. The client or caregiver must be taught how to assess pain levels and effectiveness of treatment and how to manage undesired clinical responses. Sometimes these individuals must learn to deal with conflicting values and beliefs about pain control.[9,17]

☙ NURSING RESEARCH

Dobratz, M., Wade, R., Herbst, L., & Ryndes, R. (1991). Pain efficacy in home hospice patients. *Cancer Nursing, 14*(1), 20-26.

Logan, M., & Bourbonnais, F. (1990). Continuous subcutaneous infusion of narcotics: An exploratory study of patient, family, and nursing concerns. *The Hospice Journal, 6*(1), 60-77.

The purpose of these two studies was to determine what the nurse, client, and family perceived as important in regard to parenteral at-home analgesic therapy. The Dobratz research was a longitudinal study on pain intensity involving 30 home hospice clients. The study suggests that frequent skilled nursing and physician interventions are needed to achieve pain control in the home. It also identified family support and adherence to treatment protocols as variables modifying effective pain control.

The Logan research studied client, family, and nursing concerns associated with continuous subcutaneous infusion of narcotics. Nurses, clients, and caregivers were interviewed when the pump was started, when preparations for home discharge were made, and when the client was at home. Clients and caregiver perceived frequent checks of the equipment and client by the nurse as important. Before caring for the client at home, they wanted information on the pump, infusion site, drugs, and available community resources. Identified nursing concerns were the variety of pumps available and the variations in protocols.

STUDENT ACTIVITIES

- Interview a home health nurse to determine concerns associated with parenteral narcotic therapy in the home setting.
- Seek permission to accompany a home health nurse on two visits to clients receiving parenteral narcotic therapy in their home. Request permission to interview the client and caregiver to determine their concerns about this therapy.

Parenteral Chemotherapy in the Home

Recent trends in this area include the administration of complex chemotherapy through central venous access devices and computerized infusion pumps in the home. This therapy is usually managed by a team that consists of primary care providers, pharmacists, and specially skilled nurses from outpatient oncology clinics and home health care settings. Often programs use an oncology clinical nurse specialist to teach the client or caregiver the complex skills required for maintenance of the therapy.

Benefits of chemotherapy in the home include decreased hospitalizations, decreased morbidity, and increased quality of life. Additional benefits are the independence and control it gives the client. Disadvantages of home chemotherapy are the possibility of serious complications such as anaphylaxis and the high level of skill needed by the client or caregiver to handle drug administration and undesired clinical responses.

The client or caregiver must learn to manage symptoms such as nausea, vomiting, neutropenia, infection, anorexia, stomatitis, and dehydration. Since both the equipment and drug are considered toxic, the client or caregiver must learn the proper handling and disposal of any waste. In addition, the client's excreta such as vomitus, urine, and stool are potentially toxic for a 48-hour period after therapy.[7,8,18-20]

Parenteral Antimicrobial Therapy in the Home

Parenteral drug therapy also extends to intravenous antimicrobial therapy for infections in conditions such as cystic fibrosis, leukemia, human immunodeficiency virus (HIV), brain abscess, and osteomyelitis. As with other home parenteral therapy, this treatment is used as a cost-effective means of providing care while maintaining quality of life. Effectiveness of treatment is comparable to that of the hospitalized treatment plan.

Preferred methods of administration are an implantable port device or a percutaneous catheter. Advantages of the implantable port are ease of care and decreased risk of infection. However, this method is costly, and each dose requires the client to withstand the discomfort of a needle puncture. Percutaneous catheters are also easy to use but require dressing changes, daily heparin flushes, and increased risk of infection or occlusion. Drugs are administered through intravenous push or, more often, an infusion pump.[21-23]

CONCEPT REVIEW

Many drugs are administered through the parenteral drug route.

Several different parenteral delivery systems are used in the home: continuous subcutaneous infusion, peripheral intravenous infusion, central venous access, ambulatory infusion pump, and intraspinal infusion.

Teaching the client or caregiver how to administer drugs through these different systems is an important function of the nurse.

ORAL DRUG THERAPY IN THE HOME

Various oral drugs are used in the home. Successful drug therapy is contingent on the client or caregiver's knowledge of the drug regimen. To help prevent errors in drug administration, the nurse should review the drug label with the client and determine if the instructions are understood. The client should have a written schedule of drugs and dosages that is checked each nursing visit. An understanding of dosages and the dangers of overdose may help prevent self-prescribed dosage adjustments by the client or caregiver.

A drug monitoring system also helps the nurse. This system allows the nurse to record current drugs, dosages, compliance status, client knowledge level, client assessment of effectiveness, nurse assessment of effectiveness, and undesired clinical responses. Information contained in this record should be used to revise and update the plan of care.

SUMMARY

Management of drug therapy is an important function of the nurse who provides care in the home setting. The nurse must know how to administer and monitor a variety of parenteral and oral drug regimens. In addition, special legal and ethical issues must be addressed by the nurse.

Use of the nursing process gives the nurse a framework for providing individualized, quality care. The overall goal of the nurse is to assist the client or caregiver to become competent in self-care. To assure achievement of the goal, the nurse must use effective communication and teaching skills. In addition, the nurse must have a broad knowledge of pharmacology.

REFERENCES

1. American Nurses' Association. (1986). *Standards of community health nursing practice.* Kansas City, MO: Author.
2. Kontz, M. (1989). Compliance redefined and implications for home care. *Holistic Nursing Practice, 3*(2), 54-64.
3. Lanik, G. (1989). Ethical decision making for community health nurses. *Journal of Community Health Nursing, 6*(2), 95-102.
4. Brent, N. (1989). Administering controlled substances in the home: Minimizing the risk of potential diversion. *Home Healthcare Nurse, 7*(4), 6-7.
5. Brent, N. (1993). Criminal law and the home health care nurse. *Home Healthcare Nurse, 11*(1), 11-12.
6. Perdew, S. (1989). Liability issues. In C. Malloy and J. Hartshorn (Eds.). *Acute care nursing in the home: a holistic approach.* Philadelphia: J.B. Lippincott.
7. Blecke, C. (1989). Home chemotherapy safety procedures. *Oncology Nursing Forum, 16,* 719-721.
8. Sansivero, G., & Murray, S. (1989). Safe management of chemotherapy at home. *Oncology Nursing Forum, 16,* 711-713.
9. Logan, M., & Bourbonnais, F. (1990). Continuous subcutaneous infusion of narcotics: An exploratory study of patient, family, and nursing concerns. *The Hospice Journal, 6*(1), 79-77.
10. Murphy, D. (1990). Home pain management: Continuous infusion of narcotics. *Journal of Intravenous Nursing, 13,* 355-359.
11. Wickham, R. (1990). Advances in venous access devices and nursing management strategies. *Nursing Clinics of North America, 25,* 345-361.
12. Peplin, N. (1989). Intractable pain management with intravenous narcotic administration at home. *Journal of Intravenous Nursing, 12,* 228-232.
13. Swanson, G., Smith, J., Bulich, R., New, P., & Shiffman, R. (1989). Patient-controlled analgesia for chronic cancer pain in the ambulatory setting: A report of 117 patients. *Journal of Clinical Oncology, 7,* 1903-1908.
14. Blue, C., & Purath, J. (1989). Home care of the epidural analgesia patient: The nurse's role. *Home Healthcare Nurse, 7*(4), 23-30.
15. St. Marie, B. (1989). Administration of intraspinal analgesia in the home care setting. *Journal of Intravenous Nursing, 12*(3), 164-168.
16. Williams, A., Beaulaurier, K., & Seal, D. (1990). Chronic cancer pain management with the Du Pen epidural catheter. *Cancer Nursing, 13,* 176-182.
17. Dobratz, M., Wade, R., Herbst, L., & Ryndes, T. (1991). Pain efficacy in home hospice patients. *Cancer Nursing, 14*(1), 20-26.
18. Cawley, M. (1990). Recent advances in chemotherapy. *Nursing Clinics of North America, 25,* 377-391.
19. Palmer, P., & Meyers, F. (1990). An outpatient approach to the delivery of intensive consolidation chemotherapy to adults with acute lymphoblastic leukemia. *Oncology Nursing Forum, 17,* 553-558.
20. Wandel, J., Sullivan, D., Gramm, R., & Hetzer, P. (1990). Ambulatory care for patients with acute leukemia: An alternative to frequent hospitalization. *Journal of Professional Nursing, 6,* 300-309.
21. Chattopadhyay, R., Catania, P., & Mergener, M. (1990). Therapeutic outcome of elderly and nonelderly patients receiving home intravenous antimicrobial therapy. *American Journal of Hospital Pharmacy, 47,* 335-339.
22. Hammond, L., Caldwell, S., & Campbell, P. (1991). Cystic fibrosis, intravenous antibiotics, and home therapy. *Journal of Pediatric Health Care, 5*(1), 24-30.
23. Hinkle, J. (1990). Home antibiotic therapy for brain abscesses. *Journal of Intravenous Nursing, 13*(3), 172-176.

BIBLIOGRAPHY

Brown, R. (1991). Selection and training of patients for outpatient intravenous antibiotic therapy. *Review of Infectious Diseases, 13*(2), 147-151.

Carr, P. (1990). The medication maze. *Home Healthcare Nurse, 8*(1), 55-56.

Collins-Colon, T. (1990). Do it yourself medication management for community based clients. *Journal of Psychosocial Nursing, 28*(6), 25-29.

Cowan, M. (1993). Home care of the pregnant woman using terbutaline. *MCN, 18*(2), 99-103.

Graveley, E., & Dseasohn, C. (1991). Multiple drug regimens: Medication compliance among veterans 85 years and older. *Research of Nursing and Health, 14*(1), 51-58.

Haddad, A., Keefer, K., & Stein, J. (1993). Teamwork in home infusion therapy: The relationship between nursing and pharmacy. *Home Healthcare Nurse, 11*(1), 40-46.

Jaffe, M. (1993). *Nursing procedures for home care.* Albany, NY: Delmar Publishers.

Klimas, S. (1992). Home healthcare dilemma: The client at risk. *Home Healthcare Nurse, 10*(2), 13-14.

Moeser, L. (1991). Anaphylaxis a preventable complication of home infusion therapy. *Journal of Intravenous Nursing, 14*(2), 108-112.

Stuck, A.E., & Tamai, I.Y. (1991). Medication management in the home. *Clinics of Geriatric Medicine, 7,* 733-748.

PART
two

CLINICAL ASPECTS OF
Pharmacology

Drugs Affecting the Central Nervous System

CHAPTER 17

OVERVIEW OF THE
Central Nervous System

RHODA HEADLEY

*T*he central nervous system (CNS) is a complex network that directs body systems and controls movement, sensation, and thought. Through this network interactions with the external environment and changes in the internal environment occur. This chapter provides a brief review of the anatomy and physiology of the CNS. Knowledge of this information will help you understand the relationship between functional disturbances and the pharmacologic basis of treatment. In addition, it will help you understand the impact drug therapy has on the CNS.

NERVOUS TISSUE

The neuroglia and the neuron are the two types of cells that comprise the nervous system. The **neuroglia cells** supply nutrients to the neuron, help maintain the electric potential of the neuron, and phagocytize waste products from injured neurons. They also help produce cerebrospinal fluid (CSF) and form the protective myelin sheath for axons of the CNS. **Neurons** perform the essential work of the nervous system; that is, they conduct impulses.

NEURON STRUCTURE AND FUNCTION

Neurons react to physical and chemical changes occurring in their surroundings. They also conduct nerve impulses to other neurons and to cells outside the nervous system.

Cell Body, Dendrites, Axon

A neuron consists of a cell body, one long axon, and one or more shorter dendrites (Fig. 17–1). Axons carry impulses away from the cell body, whereas dendrites conduct impulses to the cell body. Cell bodies of neurons form the gray matter of the brain, brain stem, and spinal cord, and axons form the white matter.[1–3]

Cell Membrane Potential

Neuron cells are surrounded by a cell membrane that usually is polarized. The outer surface of a polarized nerve cell membrane is positively charged and the inner surface negatively charged. This **polarization** is caused by an unequal distribution of ions on either side of the membrane. The three most important ions in neuronal function are sodium, potassium, and chloride.

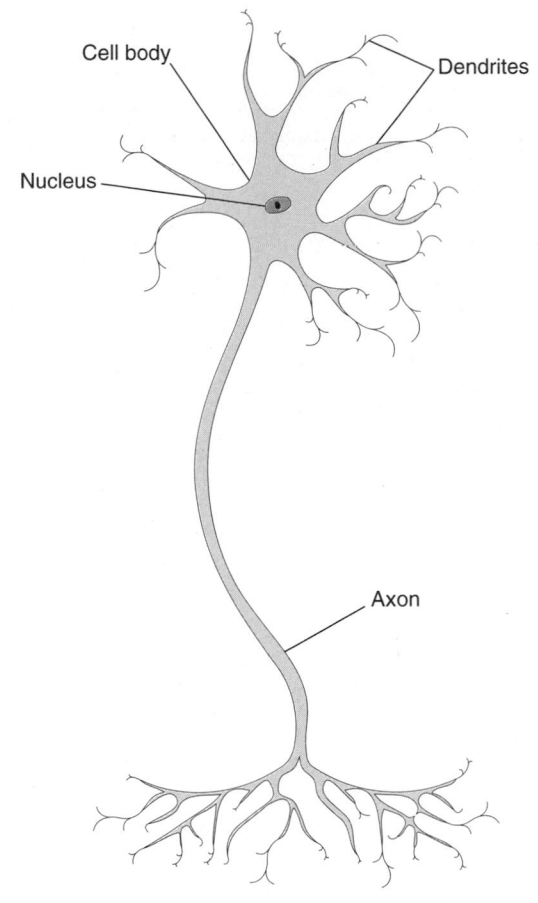

FIGURE 17–1 Neuron: basic functional unit of the nervous system.

Resting potential When neuron cells are at rest (not conducting an impulse), there is a greater concentration of sodium ions outside the membrane and a greater concentration of potassium ions inside the membrane. The difference in electric charge between the two locations is the **resting potential.** While the nerve cell membrane is undisturbed, the membrane remains in this state.

Impulse conduction If the neuron cell in a resting state is stimulated, the membrane's resting potential becomes less negative. If repeated stimuli occur, a level called the **threshold potential** is reached. Once the threshold potential is reached, the membrane's permeability changes. Sodium ions rush into the cell as potassium ions diffuse outward. As a result, the membrane loses its electric charge and becomes depolarized. This rapid sequence of changes involving **depolarization** and repolarization is called an **action potential.** When an action potential occurs at one point in a nerve cell membrane, it triggers other action potentials. These action potentials cause the nerve fiber to fire a **nerve impulse.**[4,5]

Synapse

A **synapse** is the junction between the processes of neurons or between a neuron and an effector organ. Most synapses are axodendritic (from axon to dendrite), axosomatic (from axon to soma), or axoaxonic (from axon to axon). The narrow gap that separates the axon terminal of one nerve cell from another nerve cell or effector organ is the synaptic cleft.

Synaptic transmission There are two types of synapses—chemical and electric; these synapses have structural and functional differences. Almost all nerve impulses within the CNS are chemically transmitted. The **presynaptic neuron** secretes a chemical substance, a **neurotransmitter,** into the synaptic cleft. This neurotransmitter acts on receptor proteins in the membrane of the **postsynaptic neuron** to excite, inhibit, or modify its sensitivity. Chemical synapses always transmit signals in one direction—from the presynaptic neuron to the postsynaptic neuron.

The role of electric synapses in the CNS is not clearly understood. Electric synapses have direct channels called *gap junctions.* These junctions conduct electricity from one cell to the next by allowing the free movement of ions from the interior of one cell to the next. Gap junctions are common in visceral smooth muscle, cardiac muscle, and developing embryos. Only a few gap junctions are present in the CNS.

Neurotransmitter substances More than 40 different chemical substances are believed to function as synaptic transmitters. Both excitatory and inhibitory neurotransmitter substances exist. These neurotransmitters are divided into small-molecule–rapid-acting transmitters and large-molecule–slow-acting transmitters.

The small-molecule–rapid-acting transmitters produce most of the acute responses of the nervous system. Excitatory neurotransmitters in this group include aspartic acid and glutamate. The inhibitory neurotransmitters in the group are γ-aminobutyric acid (GABA) and glycine. Monoamine neurotransmitters (norepinephrine, epinephrine, dopamine, and serotonin) are excitatory at some synapses and inhibitory at others. Acetylcholine is an excitatory neurotransmitter at the neuromuscular junction but has an inhibitory effect at other synapses.

The large-molecule–slow-acting neurotransmitters are called *neuropeptides.* Neuropeptides usually cause prolonged effects that last for days or even months. Some of the important neuropeptides include the endorphins, enkephalins, and

---

CONCEPT REVIEW

Nervous tissue within the CNS consists of neurons and neuroglia. Neurons are responsible for initiating and conducting impulses.

When neurons are not conducting an impulse, the concentration of ions between the intracellular and extracellular environments is unequal.

When a neuron in a resting state is stimulated, sodium ions move inward and potassium ions diffuse outward, producing an action potential.

An action potential or impulse travels along nerve fibers from one neuron to another.

Electric and/or chemical factors assist in the transmission of an impulse across the junction.

TABLE 17–1

Location and Effect of Major Neurotransmitters

Substance	Location	Effect
Acetylcholine	Secreted by neurons in pyramidal cells of the motor cortex, neurons in the basal ganglia, motor neurons in the skeletal muscles, presynaptic neurons in the autonomic nervous system (ANS), and postsynaptic neurons of the sympathetic nervous system	Excitatory or inhibitory
Monoamines		
Norepinephrine	Secreted by neurons located in the brain stem and hypothalamus and in some ANS synapses	Excitatory or inhibitory
Serotonin	Secreted by neurons in the brain stem	Generally inhibitory
Dopamine	Secreted by neurons in the substantia nigra of the basal ganglia and some ANS synapses	Generally excitatory
Histamine	Secreted by neurons in the hypothalamus	Generally inhibitory
Amino Acids		
Glycine	Secreted primarily by neurons in the spinal cord	Most postsynaptic inhibition in the spinal cord
γ-Aminobutyric acid	Secreted by neurons in the spinal cord, cerebellum, basal ganglia, and other areas of the cerebral cortex	Postsynaptic inhibition in the brain; some presynaptic inhibition in the spinal cord
Glutamate and aspartate	Secreted by presynaptic terminals in the sensory pathways and in many areas of the cerebral cortex	Excitatory
Neuropeptides		
Endorphins and enkephalins	Widely distributed in the CNS and peripheral nervous system	Generally inhibitory
Substance P	Neurons in the spinal cord, brain, and sensory neurons associated with pain	Generally excitatory

substance P. Some neuropeptides also function as hormones.[1,4,5] See Table 17–1 for a summary of the location and effects of major neurotransmitters.

STRUCTURES AND FUNCTIONS OF THE CNS

Anatomically, the human body is composed of the CNS and the peripheral nervous system (PNS). The CNS consists of the brain and spinal cord. Spinal nerves, peripheral nerves, and the autonomic nervous system (ANS) comprise the PNS. The **afferent** division of the PNS transmits action potentials to the CNS. Action potentials are carried away from the CNS by the **efferent** division of the PNS.

Protection and Coverings

Structures in the CNS are protected by bones, meninges, and CSF. Without these protective mechanisms, the structures would be vulnerable to trauma.

Bones   The skull is the bony framework of the head. It is composed of the eight bones of the cranium and the 14 bones of the face. The cranium is the part of the skull that encloses the brain and provides the protective vault for brain tissues. A series of bones (vertebrae), stacked one on another to support the head and trunk, forms the vertebral column. Vertebrae also help protect the spinal column from direct trauma.

Meninges   Three layers of meninges cover the brain and spinal cord: the dura mater, arachnoid mater, and pia mater. The dura mater is a tough double-layered fibrous membrane that lines the interior of the skull and vertebral column. An ex-

tremely thin and delicate layer of meninges, the arachnoid mater, loosely encloses the brain and spinal cord. A space, the subdural space, separates the dura and the arachnoid mater. The innermost layer of meninges is the pia mater. It is a mesh-like vascular membrane that covers the entire surface of the brain and spinal cord. The pia mater of the cord is thicker and less vascular than that of the brain.

Cerebrospinal fluid   CSF normally is a clear, colorless, odorless liquid that fills the ventricles of the brain and the subarachnoid space of the brain and spinal cord. This fluid acts as a shock absorber to cushion CNS structures from injury. CSF is composed of water, a small amount of protein, oxygen, carbon dioxide, electrolytes (sodium, potassium, chloride), and glucose.

Blood-Brain Barrier

The term *blood-brain barrier* refers to the barrier that separates the blood from the parenchyma. Capillaries of the brain are the most likely location of the blood-brain barrier. Brain capillaries have tighter junctions between endothelial cells than capillaries in other parts of the body, thus limiting their permeability. Brain capillaries also do not contain fenestrae (pores) and have very few pinocytotic vesicles.

Recent research has shown that the blood-brain barrier does not exist in all parts of the brain. Certain small areas around the floor of the third and fourth ventricles (near the pituitary gland and hypothalamus) apparently do not have a blood-brain barrier. Studies also reveal that mechanical injury to the brain, exposure to certain toxins, irradiation, and CNS tumors alter the blood-brain barrier.[6]

The blood-brain barrier is permeable to water, oxygen, carbon dioxide, nonionic solutes such as glucose, and lipid-soluble substances such as alcohol and general anesthetics. It is slightly permeable to electrolytes and other ionic substances and almost impermeable to plasma proteins and large organic molecules in certain drugs and other exogenously administered chemicals.

Although the significance of the blood-brain barrier is unclear, it is unlikely that it developed only to protect the brain from potentially toxic drugs or other exogenous material that might enter through the systemic circulation. The blood-brain barrier probably serves to maintain the internal environment of the brain and prevent a sudden increase in concentration of water-soluble ionized substances, including neurotransmitters.

CONCEPT REVIEW

The brain and spinal cord are protected by bones, meninges, and CSF.

The blood-brain barrier helps maintain the internal environment of the brain and prevent a sudden increase in concentration of water-soluble ionized substances.

Brain

The major regions of the adult brain are the cerebrum, diencephalon (thalamus and hypothalamus), midbrain (mesencephalon), pons, medulla oblongata, and cerebellum (Fig. 17–2). The medulla oblongata, pons, and midbrain constitute the brain stem.[1,2,4,7,8]

Cerebrum   The cerebrum is the largest part of the mature brain. The outermost portion of the cerebrum consists of a thin layer of gray matter called the **cerebral cortex.** It is estimated that the cerebral cortex contains nearly 75% of all the neuron cell bodies in the nervous system. Beneath the cerebral cortex is a mass of white matter that comprises the bulk of the cerebrum. This mass contains bundles of myelinated nerve fibers that connect neuron cell bodies of the cortex with other parts of the nervous system.

The cerebrum is divided into two large masses called **cerebral hemispheres.** Each hemisphere contains four major lobes: frontal, parietal, occipital, and temporal. Primary functions of the **frontal lobe** are related to motor activity, including the motor aspects of speech, expressions of emotions and behavior, and abstract reasoning. Processing sensory input in the primary sensory cortex, located directly behind the primary motor cortex, is the principal function of the **parietal lobe.** The parietal lobe functions to recognize spatial relation-

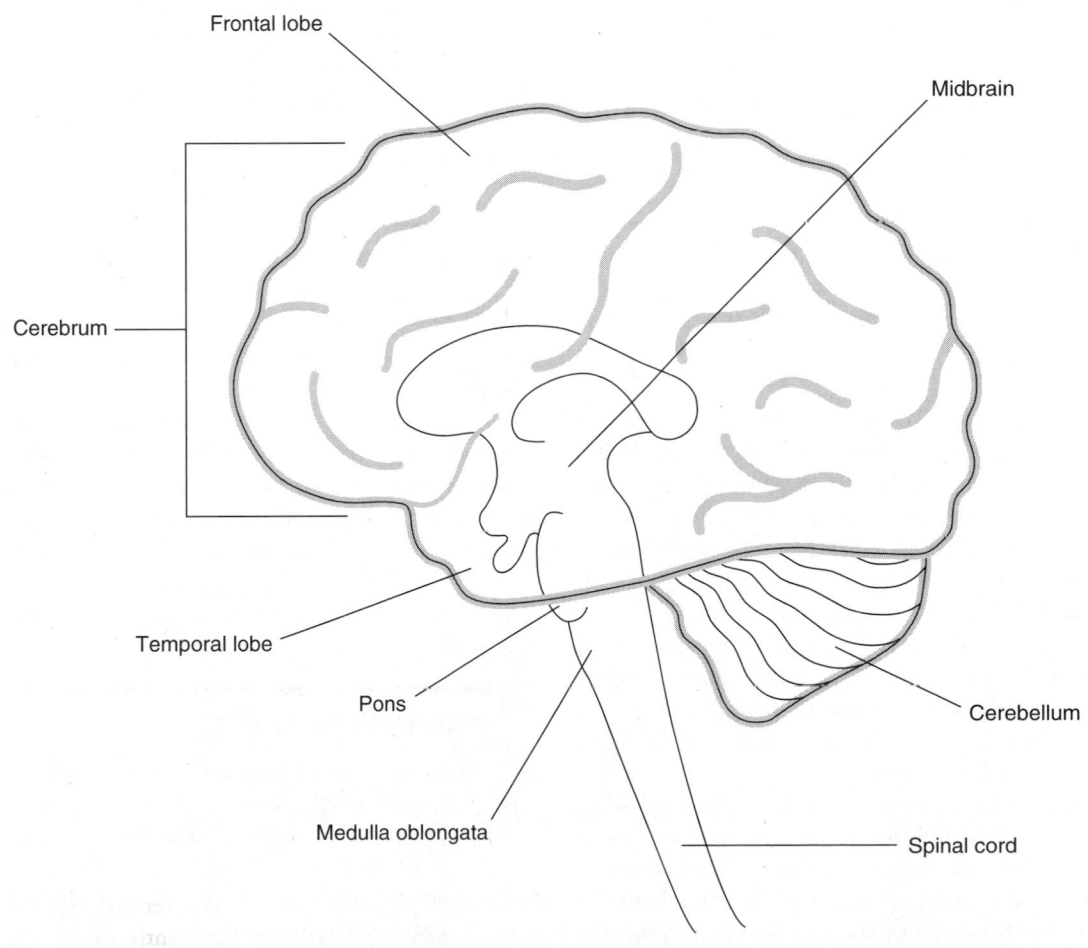

Frontal lobe

Midbrain

Cerebrum

Temporal lobe

Pons

Cerebellum

Medulla oblongata

Spinal cord

FIGURE 17–2   Structures of the central nervous system. The brain, brain stem, and spinal cord function together to control movement, sensation, thought, and emotion.

ships such as size, shape, and texture and to comprehend written communication. Interpretation of sensations related to hearing, taste, smell, and balance is a function of the **temporal lobe.** The anterior portion of the temporal lobe is also involved in memory, behavior, emotion, and personality. The **occipital lobe** contains the primary visual cortex and visual associative areas.

Located deep within the cerebral hemispheres are the **basal ganglia.** The precise function of these structures is not completely understood. Neuron cell bodies contained in the basal ganglia are known to serve as relay stations for motor impulses originating in the cerebral cortex and passing into the brain stem and spinal cord. Also, most of the inhibitory neurotransmitter dopamine is produced in the basal ganglia.

Brain stem   The region of the brain that connects the cerebrum to the spinal cord is called the **brain stem.** It consists of the diencephalon, midbrain, pons, and medulla oblongata. Ten of the 12 cranial nerves originate in the brain stem.

The **diencephalon,** which includes the thalamus and hypothalamus, lies between the cerebral hemispheres and above the midbrain. Located on either side of the third ventricle, the **thalamus** functions as a central relay station for sensory impulses ascending from other parts of the nervous system to the cerebral cortex. All sensory pathways, except the olfactory, have connections to thalamic nuclei. In addition, the thalamus has numerous connections to other areas of the brain. These connections are important in the integration of cerebral, cerebellar, and brain stem activity.

The **hypothalamus** lies below the thalamic nuclei and forms the lower walls and floor of the third ventricles. The hypothalamus plays a key role in maintaining homeostasis by regulating a variety of visceral activities and linking the nervous and endocrine systems. Among the many important functions of the hypothalamus are the following:

1. Regulation and maintenance of body temperature
2. Regulation of heart rate and arterial blood pressure
3. Regulation of water and electrolyte balance
4. Regulation of thirst and hunger
5. Regulation of sleep and wakefulness

Structures in the general region of the diencephalon also play an important role in emotional responses. These structures form a complex called the **limbic system.** The limbic system works with the cerebral cortex, brain stem, and hypothalamus to normalize the expression of emotions such as anger, fear, anxiety, sexual feelings, pleasure, and sorrow.

The **midbrain** is located between the diencephalon and the pons. It contains bundles of myelinated nerve fibers that join lower parts of the brain stem and spinal cord with higher parts of the brain. The midbrain also includes several masses of gray matter that serve as reflex centers.

The **pons** lies on the underside of the brain stem and separates the midbrain from the medulla oblongata. Impulses to and from the medulla oblongata and the cerebrum are transmitted by the dorsal portion of the pons. The ventral portion transmits impulses from the cerebrum to centers within the cerebellum. Regulation of respiration and activation of the reticular formation (see below) are achieved by neurons located in the pons. In addition, the nuclei for the fifth (trigem-

inal), sixth (abducens), seventh (facial), and eighth (acoustic) cranial nerves are located in the pons.

The **medulla oblongata** is continuous with the pons above and the spinal cord below. Nuclei within the medulla oblongata function as control centers for vital visceral activities. These centers include the cardiac center, vasomotor center, and respiratory center. Other nuclei within the medulla oblongata function as centers for reflexes associated with coughing, sneezing, swallowing, vomiting, and hiccoughing. In addition, the nuclei for the ninth (glossopharyngeal), tenth (vagus), eleventh (spinal accessory), and twelfth (hypoglossal) cranial nerves are located in the medulla.

Scattered throughout the medulla oblongata, pons, and midbrain is a complex network of nerve fibers called the **reticular formation.** The reticular formation has both sensory and motor functions. It receives input from higher brain regions that control skeletal muscles. It also alerts the cortex to incoming sensory signals. The reticular formation also has an influence on auditory sense, equilibrium, and pain sensation.

The portion of the reticular formation responsible for alerting the cortex to incoming sensory signals is called the **reticular activating system (RAS).** The RAS is also responsible for maintaining consciousness and for awakening from sleep.

Cerebellum   The cerebellum is the second largest portion of the brain and occupies the inferior and posterior aspects of the cranial cavity. Coordinating and refining muscle activity, especially rapid, repetitive movements, are important functions of the cerebellum. The cerebellum also plays an important role in equilibrium and proprioception.

Spinal Cord

The spinal cord is a slender nerve column that passes downward from the brain into the vertebral canal. The cord tapers to a point and terminates near the intervertebral disc that separates the first and second lumbar vertebrae. The spinal cord has 31 segments; each segment gives rise to a pair of spinal nerves. These nerves branch out to various body parts and connect with the CNS.

The spinal cord has two major functions: conducting nerve impulses and serving as a center for spinal reflexes. Nerve tracts of the spinal cord provide a two-way communication system between the brain and body parts. Tracts that conduct impulses from the body and carry sensory information to the brain are called *ascending tracts.* Tracts that conduct motor impulses from the brain to muscles and glands are called *descending tracts.*[4,5]

CONCEPT REVIEW

The brain is the largest and most complex part of the nervous system.

The major regions of the adult brain are the cerebrum, diencephalon (thalamus and hypothalamus), midbrain (mesencephalon), pons, medulla oblongata, and cerebellum.

The medulla oblongata, pons, and midbrain comprise the brain stem.

EFFECTS OF DRUGS ON CNS

The effects of drugs on the CNS are produced by selective (specific) or nonselective (nonspecific) actions. Most drugs exhibit selective or specific actions.[8,9]

Drugs With Nonselective Actions

Drugs with nonselective actions modify neurotransmitters by increasing the amount of the neurotransmitter at the synapse or by causing a decrease in the physiologic response to the neurotransmitter. These responses are achieved in the following ways:

1. Altering the rate of synthesis of a neurotransmitter substance
2. Altering the rate of release of the substance
3. Altering the length of time that the neurotransmitter substance is in the synapse
4. Altering the rate of enzymatic breakdown of the neurotransmitter substance

CNS depressants and stimulants are examples of drugs with apparently nonspecific mechanisms of action. CNS depressants include the anesthetic gases (e.g., nitrous oxide, ethylene, halothane), alcohol, and some hypnotic sedatives (e.g., barbiturates). These pharmacologic agents depress excitable tissue at all levels of the CNS by stabilizing neuronal membranes, resulting in a decrease in the amount of neurotransmitter released by the nerve impulse. Depression of postsynaptic responsiveness and ion movement also result.

CNS stimulants can excite the CNS by blocking the inhibition of a neurotransmitter, increasing the release of a neurotransmitter, prolonging neurotransmitter action, or a decreasing synaptic recovery time. General CNS stimulants include the methylxanthines (caffeine and theophylline).

Drugs With Selective Actions

Drugs that selectively modify CNS function can either depress or excite neuron function or can produce both effects simultaneously on different parts of the CNS. The principal classes of selective CNS drugs are anticonvulsants, antiparkinsonian agents, opioid and nonopioid analgesics, antiemetics, analgesic antipyretics, antidepressants, and antipsychotic agents.

Although selectivity of action is a desired effect, these drugs usually influence several CNS functions to varying degrees. When only one response is desired in a therapeutic situation, other responses are regarded as limitations of the drug.

SUMMARY

The CNS consists of the brain and spinal cord. These structures process, integrate, store, and respond to information from the PNS. The afferent division of the PNS transmits action potentials to the CNS. Action potentials are carried away from the CNS by the efferent division of the PNS.

Cells of the nervous system are the neuroglia and neurons. Neuroglia cells support and aid the neurons of the CNS. Neurons receive stimuli and transmit action potentials. An action potential is produced by an unequal distribution of ions on each side of the cell membrane of the neuron. Once produced, the action potential moves along the nerve fiber. When the action potential arrives at the presynaptic terminal, a neurotransmitter is released. This substance diffuses across the synaptic cleft and binds with the receptors of the postsynaptic terminal to produce a response in the effector cell or organ.

Drugs produce effects in the CNS by selective (specific) or nonselective (nonspecific) actions. Drugs that produce a response by nonselective actions affect the neurotransmitters. If the drug acts directly on specific structures and/or functions in the CNS, it is classified as having selective actions.

REFERENCES

1. Guyton, A. (1991). *Basic neuroscience: Anatomy and physiology* (2nd ed.). Philadelphia: W.B. Saunders.
2. Guyton, A. (1991). *Textbook of medical physiology* (8th ed.). Philadelphia: W.B. Saunders.
3. Tortora, G., & Grabowski, S. (1993). *Principles of anatomy and physiology* (7th ed.). New York: Harper-Collins.
4. Hole, J. (1993). *Human anatomy and physiology* (6th ed.). Dubuque, IA: Wm. D. Brown.
5. Seeley, R., Stephens, T., & Tate, P. (1992). *Anatomy and physiology* (2nd ed.). St. Louis: Mosby–Year Book.
6. Craig, C. (1990). Introduction to central nervous system pharmacology. In Craig, C., & Stitzel, R. (Eds.). *Modern Pharmacology* (3rd ed.) (pp. 389-400). Boston: Little, Brown.
7. Carey, J. (Ed.). (1992). *Brain concepts: Brain development.* Washington, DC: Society for Neuroscience.
8. Carey, J. (Ed.). (1992). *Brain concepts: How the brain ages.* Washington, DC: Society for Neuroscience.
9. Moline, K. (1992). Cognitive-enhancing drugs. *Headlines,* May/June, 22-23.

BIBLIOGRAPHY

Carey, J. (Ed.). (1992). *Brain concepts: Drugs and the brain.* Washington, DC: Society for Neuroscience.
Carey, J. (Ed.). (1990). *Brain facts.* Washington, DC: Society for Neuroscience.
Hickey, J. (1992). *Clinical Practice of Neurological and Neurosurgical Nursing* (3rd ed.) (pp. 10-45). Philadelphia: J.B. Lippincott.

CHAPTER 18

Sedatives, Hypnotics, and Anxiolytics

NORMA L. PINNELL

⊛ **Sedatives, Hypnotics, and Anxiolytics**

LEARNING OBJECTIVES:

Summarize general characteristics of drugs in this category.

Plan care for a client receiving a sedative, hypnotic, or anxiolytic drug.

KEY TERMS:

Anxiolytic drugs, hypnotic drugs, sedative drugs

⊛ **Barbiturates**

LEARNING OBJECTIVES:

Summarize general characteristics of barbiturates.

Differentiate among long-acting, short-acting, and ultra-short-acting barbiturates.

Summarize essential information about phenobarbital, the prototype for this category.

Identify other drugs in this particular category.

KEY TERM: γ-Aminobutyric acid (GABA)

⊛ **Benzodiazepines**

LEARNING OBJECTIVES:

Summarize general characteristics of benzodiazepines.

Distinguish between benzodiazepines used as anxiolytic drugs and those used as hypnotics.

Summarize essential information about diazepam, the prototype for this category.

Explain the action of flumazenil, a benzodiazepine antagonist.

⊛ **Azapirones**

LEARNING OBJECTIVE: Summarize essential information about buspirone hydrochloride, the prototype for this category.

⊛ **Imidazopyridines**

LEARNING OBJECTIVE: Summarize essential information about zolpidem, the prototype for this category.

⊛ **Miscellaneous Drugs Used as Sedatives, Hypnotics, and Anxiolytics**

LEARNING OBJECTIVE: Describe at least two other categories of drugs used as sedatives or hypnotics.

⊛ **OTC Preparations for Sleep**

LEARNING OBJECTIVE: Discuss the significance of OTC sleep aids.

CONCEPTS AND TERMS TO REVIEW

Review anatomy and physiology of the central nervous system.

Review content on substance abuse, tolerance, and physical and psychologic dependence in earlier chapters.

*A*nxiety, fatigue, and insomnia are among the most common symptoms for which drug therapy is prescribed. The history of the development of sedatives or hypnotics and anx-

iolytics is long and complicated. Alcohol, the oldest known sedative, was used both medically and nonmedically for generations. Eventually a variety of other, presumably safer drugs was developed.

The development of barbiturates in the early 1900s was initially seen as a potentially safe and effective medical advance. However, it was not long until numerous undesired clinical responses, including the potential for addiction, were recognized. The next major advance after the barbiturates was the development of meprobamate in the mid-1950s. After meprobamate, the first benzodiazepine appeared on the market in 1961. As experience with meprobamate and benzodiazepine drugs was gained, it became apparent that drug dependency developed with these drugs also.[1,2] The search for safe, effective drugs that produce sedation or reduce anxiety or both still continues.

This chapter focuses on barbiturates and benzodiazepines. In addition, information on new compounds, azapirones and imidazopyridines, is presented. Other drug groups used as sedatives, hypnotics, and anxiolytics are briefly mentioned, as are over-the-counter (OTC) sleep aids.

SEDATIVES, HYPNOTICS, AND ANXIOLYTICS

Some drugs are specifically developed to promote sedation, produce sleep, or reduce anxiety. In other instances drugs are administered for their predictable adverse effects (i.e., sedation or drowsiness).

Pharmacotherapeutics

Drugs discussed in this chapter are used to promote rest and sleep and to reduce anxiety. **Sleep** is a naturally occurring state of unconsciousness during which the cerebrum rests and from which an individual can be aroused by external stimuli. The sleep-wake cycle is one of the body's circadian rhythms. It follows an approximate 24-hour cycle that is linked to light and dark.

Sleep can be divided in two phases: rapid eye movement (REM) and non–rapid eye movement (NREM) sleep. Transition from the awake state to the NREM phase is marked by decreased concentrations of serotonin, norepinephrine, and acetylcholine. The transition to REM phase is marked by increased acetylcholine levels and further decline in serotonin and norepinephrine levels. Sleep is also divided into four stages. Stages 1 and 2 are periods of light sleep, whereas stages 3 and 4 are periods of deep sleep.[3,4]

Large portions of the adult population in the United States are dissatisfied with the quality of their sleep. Problems with sleep are more common in clients with chronic illness. Disruptions in sleep patterns act as an additional stressor and further compromise the condition of these clients.

In addition, 40% to 50% of clients over 50 years of age report insomnia. Sleep efficiency declines in these individuals. Nighttime sleep is shorter, lighter, and more fragmented. Although elderly clients may actually be in bed for longer periods of time, they spend less time sleeping. Sleep stages in the older adult also change. REM, stage 3, and stage 4 sleep decrease, and stages 1 and 2 increase.[4–6]

Adults dissatisfied with their sleeping patterns frequently seek solutions from primary care providers in the health care system. One therapeutic option in the treatment of poor sleep is the prescription of sedative, hypnotic, or anxiolytic drugs. One study reports that the use of hypnotic drugs increases with age, from 3.6% of clients aged 65 to 69 years to 6.6% of those aged 80 to 84 years.[5,7]

Anxiety is a state in which an individual experiences feelings of uneasiness, dread, and inadequacy. Anxiety is usually accompanied by a variety of autonomic nervous system manifestations, including tachycardia, palpitations, irregular heart rhythm, dizziness, tremor, excessive sweating, dry mouth, abdominal pain, and headache.

Many anxiety disorders have been identified, including generalized anxiety disorder, panic disorder, agoraphobia, social phobia, posttraumatic stress syndrome, and obsessive-compulsive disorders. Anxiety is also a common occurrence with many organic diseases such as hypoglycemia, anemia, hyperthyroidism, and mitral valve prolapse. Anxiety is an important symptom in clients with other psychiatric conditions (e.g., mood disorders, schizophrenia).[8]

General Characteristics

Sedative drugs produce a calming or depressant effect on the central nervous system (CNS). The degree of sedation is based on subjective data from the client or observation of the client's behavior. (Currently sedation is also used in some references to describe the reduction of anxiety produced by anxiolytic drugs.) **Hypnotic drugs** produce or promote sleep by depressing the CNS.

Although the actual action of sedatives and hypnotics is not clear, it is hypothesized that they interfere with nerve impulse transmission in the reticular activating system. This area of the brain is responsible for sleep and arousal mechanisms. Some drugs are capable of promoting relaxation *and* inducing sleep. Low doses of these drugs usually produce relaxation and enable the client to rest, and higher doses actually induce sleep.

Anxiolytic drugs antagonize and relieve anxiety. Most of these drugs depress the CNS. Anxiolytic drugs must be used in conjunction with other therapy such as behavior modification or anxiety-reduction training.

▨ NURSING CONSIDERATIONS

Care of the client receiving sedative, hypnotic, or anxiolytic drug therapy is based on the steps in the nursing process.

Assessing During the **health history** ask the client to describe his or her usual sleep and rest patterns. You may want to collect a complete sleep or rest history. Questions such as the following are important:

• What time do you usually go to bed?
• What time do you usually wake up in the morning?
• Do you fall asleep easily?
• Do you usually sleep all night without waking up?
• If awakened, do you fall asleep again quickly?

Ask the client about prebedtime activities such as reading, drinking warm milk, or exercising. Determine the client's usual sleeping environment (e.g., type of bed, number of pillows used, number of blankets used, and amount of light, noise, and ventilation).

It may be beneficial to have the client keep a sleep log. Ask clients to document daily the time they go to bed, time they fall asleep, awakenings during the night, time of awakening in the morning, and time they get out of bed. Ask them to describe their feelings on awakening (e.g, rested, tired, groggy).

Also ask them to document the time, duration, and frequency of naps.

Since stress and anxiety affect rest and sleep, both aspects must be assessed. Establish how the individual perceives stress, and determine what produces stress for the client. Ask the client to describe symptoms that develop when a stressful situation occurs. Discuss with the client techniques used for stress reduction and the effectiveness of these techniques. Also ask the client about the availability of a support system.

Since numerous drugs contribute to sleep disturbance, gather a drug history. Prescription drugs such as thyroid hormones, theophylline, phenytoin, levodopa (Dopar, Larodopa), methyldopa (Aldomet), steroids, and epinephrine can impair sleep onset or reduce the depth of sleep. Beta-blocking drugs and quinidine-related antiarrhythmic drugs can produce nightmares.[6]

Determine if the client has existing health problems that might prevent the use of sedatives or anxiolytic drugs (e.g., glaucoma, hypertension, chronic obstructive pulmonary disease). Ask the client specific questions about past and existing substance use, suicide attempts, caffeine, tobacco, and alcohol intake, and use of street or illicit drugs.

During the **physical assessment,** observe for disorientation, listlessness, or restlessness. Physical signs such as mild, fleeting nystagmus, ptosis of eyelids, slight hand tremor, dark circles under eyes, changes in posture, and frequent yawning are characteristics of sleep pattern disturbance.

Diagnosing A thorough assessment of the client provides a basis for nursing diagnoses. The following are examples of nursing diagnoses appropriate for the client receiving anxiolytics, sedatives, or hypnotics:

• High risk for injury related to impaired judgment, impaired motor skills, dizziness, and drowsiness associated with drug therapy.
• Sleep pattern disturbance related to rebound insomnia associated with sedative or hypnotic therapy.
• Sensory or perceptual alterations related to photosensitivity associated with drug therapy.
• Social isolation related to alterations in mental status.
• Impaired gas exchange related to respiratory depression associated with drug therapy.
• Fatigue related to altered body chemistry (e.g., drug withdrawal).

Planning Planning for the client receiving sedatives, hypnotics, and anxiolytics involves a variety of activities. Before sedative or hypnotic drugs are prescribed, an effort should be made to remove or reverse factors contributing to sleep disturbance. Plan to review the assessment data with the client and assist the client to recognize factors contributing to insomnia. Teach the client about the normal sleep-wake cycle and ways to improve sleep habits. Other points to include in the teaching plan are listed in the box.

With some clients, progressive muscle relaxation is a successful therapy for reducing stress and promoting relaxation and sleep. With progressive muscle relaxation the client is taught to focus on a muscle group and to tense that group for

5 to 7 seconds. The client then relaxes that muscle group for 30 to 40 seconds, and the cycle is repeated. Another technique that can be taught is guided imagery. Guided imagery or visualization involves imaging a pleasant scene or image that blocks other mental activity and reduces stress.[9]

Plan to teach measures to reduce stress and anxiety to clients scheduled to receive anxiolytic drugs. Include information on drug tolerance and dependence and the need for follow-up care. Caution the client not to drive or engage in other potentially hazardous activities until clinical response to the drug is determined.

Incorporate into the teaching plan information on drugs to avoid (e.g., alcohol, other CNS depressants). Inform the client to consult with a primary care provider before using OTC drugs and caution him or her against abruptly discontinuing any of these drugs after long-term use. Teach the client that sedative, hypnotic, and anxiolytic drugs do not provide pain relief.

With the client, develop expected outcomes based on the selected nursing diagnoses. Appropriate outcomes include the following:
• Client remains injury free.
• Client reports improvement in sleep and rest patterns.
• Client verbalizes factors associated with sensory or perceptual alterations.
• Client participates in activities at level of personal ability.
• Client demonstrates improved ventilation.
• Client reports improved sense of energy.

Implementing Document the client's mental status before administering any of these drugs and closely monitor the client's activity after each administration. With hypnotics and some sedatives, appropriate measures must be used to ensure the client's safety (e.g., side rails up, call signal within reach, no unsupervised smoking). Also make the environment conducive to rest by decreasing noises, lowering the room lights, and offering the client reading materials. Use relaxation techniques also (e.g., mental imagery, soft music, reading, back rub, warm bath, warm milk).

METHODS OF IMPROVING SLEEP HABITS

Teach the client to
▶ Establish a regular rising time in the morning.
▶ Avoid taking naps during the day.
▶ Incorporate daily exercise into personal schedule.
▶ Avoid heavy evening meals.
▶ Avoid alcohol, coffee, cola, tea, and chocolate after the evening meal.
▶ Perform quiet activities (e.g., reading, taking warm bath) before going to bed.
▶ Perform relaxing or productive activities when unable to sleep; do not lie in bed if unable to sleep.

Ensure that oral doses are swallowed and not hoarded. Also monitor the client for signs of overdose (e.g., slurred speech, continued somnolence, respiratory depression, confusion) and tolerance, increased anxiety, or wakefulness. These responses should be carefully documented and reported to the primary care provider.

Evaluating   The therapeutic goal of the drug therapy is to promote relaxation, sleep, or decrease anxiety. Observe the client's behavior and collect subjective data from the client about, for example, energy level and stamina. Review the expected outcomes with the client to determine if they are met. Monitor serum concentration levels of drugs when possible.

CONCEPT REVIEW

Sedative, hypnotic, and anxiolytic drugs are used to promote rest and sleep and to reduce anxiety. These drugs are not meant for long-term therapy. Other forms of treatment (e.g., behavior modification, guided imagery) are required in addition to drug therapy.

Care of clients receiving these drugs requires careful assessment and planning. Focus of the care plan is on teaching since drug therapy usually continues after discharge.

BARBITURATES

With the development of safer and more effective drug compounds the use of barbiturates has decreased.

General Characteristics

Resources frequently divide barbiturates into short-, intermediate-, and long-acting drugs. All barbiturates have the potential to produce a similar pharmacologic effect: nonselective depression of CNS function. Barbiturates do not have selective analgesic effects. In fact, sedative (low) doses may increase the sensation of pain (hyperalgesic effect). Barbiturates have similar side effects, adverse reactions, contraindications, and precautions.

Pharmacodynamic effects are not clear. Barbiturates depress the sensory cortex and motor activity and alter cerebellar function. One possible explanation involves aminobutyric acid. **γ-Aminobutyric acid (GABA)** is a naturally occurring inhibitory neurotransmitter. Low doses of barbiturates exert a GABA-like action or enhance the effects of GABA.[10] Barbiturates may also selectively abolish noradrenergic excitation and can decrease the release and turnover of acetylcholine.[1]

Barbiturates are rapidly distributed to all tissues and fluids in the body. The drugs are bound to plasma and tissue protein in varying degrees, depending on the dosage form and preparation. The drugs also have varying degree of lipid solubility. High concentrations of them are found in the brain, liver, and kidneys. Barbiturates do not impair normal hepatic function; in fact, they enhance liver microsomal enzymes. All barbiturates can produce respiratory depression. The degree of depression depends on the dose.[11,12]

BARBITURATE PROTOTYPE
PHENOBARBITAL, PHENOBARBITAL SODIUM

Phenobarbital (Barbita, Luminal, Luminal Sodium), a long-acting barbiturate, is classified as a controlled substance Schedule IV.

Pharmacotherapeutics Uses   In the past phenobarbital was used as a long-acting sedative or hypnotic. Although it is still used for these purposes, its primary use is treatment of all forms of epilepsy, status epilepticus, and febrile seizures in children. This aspect of the drug is discussed in Chapter 21.

Pharmacokinetics   The drug is absorbed in varying degrees based on the route of administration. Seventy to ninety percent of an oral dose is absorbed. Onset of action occurs in approximately 60 minutes; peak action occurs in 8 to 12 hours and peak brain levels in 10 to 15 hours. Duration of action of the oral dose is 10 to 12 hours. Intramuscularly administered phenobarbital has a slightly faster onset than an orally administered preparation. When administered intravenously, onset of action occurs within 5 minutes and maximal CNS depression within 15 minutes.

Phenobarbital has the lowest lipid solubility, plasma binding capacity, and brain-protein binding of all the barbiturates. The drug is metabolized in the liver and has a half-life of 53 to 118 hours. The half-life of the drug is increased to 60 to 180 hours in children and newborns. With repeated administration, phenobarbital stimulates the liver cells to synthesize more of the enzymes responsible for metabolizing the drug. This effect can lower blood levels of metabolized drugs and shorten their plasma half-lives. Phenobarbital is excreted by the kidneys; 25% to 50% of the drug is eliminated unchanged in the urine.[13]

Pharmacodynamics   As previously indicated, the exact mechanism of action is not clear.

Pharmaceutics   Phenobarbital is manufactured by numerous drug companies. It can be administered orally, intramuscularly, and intravenously. The drug is available in capsules, tablets, and parenteral solutions and as an elixir. The oral dosage forms of phenobarbital are in a free acid state. Sodium salts are present in the injectable dosage forms.

Undesired Clinical Responses   The major adverse responses to phenobarbital are apparent in the CNS. The drug can produce stimulation, delirium, depression, drowsiness, lethargy, hangover headache, flushing, and hallucinations. Common gastrointestinal (GI) reactions are nausea and vomiting. The integumentary system also exhibits adverse reactions to phenobarbital. These reactions include rashes, urticaria, Stevens-Johnson syndrome, and angioedema. Local pain, swelling, tissue necrosis, and thrombophlebitis can result from parenteral doses.[11,13]

Phenobarbital, like all barbiturates, can be habit forming. Tolerance and psychologic and physical dependence

TABLE 18–1
Barbiturate Prototype and Major Drugs in Category

Drug and Available Dosage Forms	Dosage and Route of Administration	Nursing Considerations

PHENOBARBITAL, PHENOBARBITAL SODIUM
 	
(Barbital, Luminal, Luminal Sodium)
HOW SUPPLIED
  Capsules: 16 mg
  Elixir: 15 or 20 mg/5 ml
  Tablets: 30 or 60 mg
  IM, IV: 30, 60, 65, or 130 mg/ml
  Cartridge needle unit: 30, 60, or
    130 mg
	Sedation
	ADULTS
	Oral: 30-120 mg/d in two to three divided doses
	CHILDREN
	Oral: 6 mg/kg/d in three divided doses
	Insomnia
	ADULTS
	PO, IM: 100-130 mg
	CHILDREN
	PO, IM: 3-6 mg/kg
	Preoperative Sedation
	ADULTS
	IM: 100-200 mg 1-1½ h before surgery
	CHILDREN
	IM: 16-100 mg 1-1½ h before surgery
		Assess
		Review nursing health history and assessment.
		Assess for preexisting conditions that would contraindicate use of barbiturates (e.g., hepatic disease, lactation, respiratory disease).
		Interventions
		Do not use parenteral solution if discolored or contains a precipitate.
		Do not mix with other parenteral solutions.
		Limit total IM volume to 5 ml.
		Administer IM medication in a large muscle to avoid tissue irritation.
		Check IV infusion site frequently; extravascular infusion may cause local tissue damage and necrosis.
		Monitor
		Monitor mental status: mood, sensorium, affect, long- and short-term memory.
		Monitor indications of respiratory distress or depression or both.
		Evaluate
		Evaluate results from blood studies, liver function tests during long-term treatment.
		Evaluate for therapeutic serum level, 15-40 μg/ml

Secobarbital, Secobarbital Sodium
 	
(Seconal, Seconal Sodium, Secogen Sodium)
HOW SUPPLIED
  Capsule: 50 or 100 mg
  IM, IV: 50 mg/ml
	Insomnia
	ADULTS
	PO, IM: 100-200 mg hs
	CHILDREN
	IM: 3-5 mg/kg, not to exceed 100 mg
	Preoperative Sedation
	ADULTS
	Oral: 200-300 mg 1-3 h preoperatively
	CHILDREN
	Oral: 50-100 mg 1-2 h preoperatively
		See phenobarbital with following additions or exceptions.
		Implement
		Do not administer more than 5 ml in one site.
		Monitor
		Monitor for toxic serum level: 3-40 μg/ml.
		Evaluate
		Evaluate for therapeutic serum level: 2-5 μg/ml.

Pentobarbital, Pentobarbital Sodium
 	
(Nembutal Sodium)
HOW SUPPLIED
  Capsule: 50 or 100 mg
  Elixir: 20 mg/5 ml
  IM, IV: 50 mg/ml
  Rectal suppository: 30, 60, 120, and 200 mg
	Insomnia
	ADULTS
	Oral: 100 mg hs
	IM: 150–200 mg
	IV: 100 mg
	CHILDREN
	Based on individual age and weight
	Preoperative Sedation
	ADULTS
	Oral: 100 mg
	IM: 150–200 mg
	CHILDREN
	PO, IM: 2-6 mg/kg; maximum: 100 mg
		See phenobarbital with following additions or exceptions.
		Assess
		Determine if client is allergic to tartrazine (FD&C, yellow dye no. 5), which has caused reactions in susceptible individuals.
		Implement
		Store below 30° C (86° F).
		Monitor
		Monitor for toxic serum level: >10 μg/ml
		Evaluate
		Evaluate for therapeutic serum level: 1-5 μg/ml.

*Food, Drug and Cosmetic (Act).

may occur with continued use. As tolerance develops, the amount of drug needed to maintain the same level of effectiveness is increased.

Contraindications and Precautions Phenobarbital should not be administered to individuals with hypersensitivity to barbiturates, hepatic disease, respiratory disease, or a history of addiction. The drug is also not recommended for use in the elderly individual or the lactating female. Precaution is needed when phenobarbital is administered in the presence of anemia, pain, or fever.

Drug-Drug Interactions Phenobarbital lowers the plasma levels of the anticoagulant warfarin and causes a decrease in anticoagulant activity. It also enhances the metabolism of exogenous corticosteroids. Absorption of orally administered griseofulvin is decreased by phenobarbital, thus decreasing serum concentration levels.

Other relevant drug interactions include interactions with other CNS depressants, rifampin, and valproic acid (Depakene, Depakote). All of these interactions increase the barbiturate effect.[14]

Life-Span Considerations Phenobarbital is classified as a Pregnancy Category D drug. In addition, caution should be used when phenobarbital is administered to a nursing woman since small amounts of it are excreted in the milk.

Children and elderly clients usually require lower doses of phenobarbital. Drug effects may take longer to wear off, and there is more risk of hepatotoxicity. Elderly clients may react with marked excitement, depression, and confusion when administered phenobarbital.

Specific Drug-Related Nursing Considerations Prepare parenteral solutions of phenobarbital in a separate syringe since it is not compatible with all drugs. For example, it is not compatible with diazepam, meperidine, morphine, chlorpromazine, or promethazine.[15]

Anticipate periodic laboratory evaluation of organ systems, including hematopoietic, renal, and hepatic systems, for clients receiving long-term therapy. Monitor serum concentration levels; therapeutic level is 15 to 40 μg/ml.

MISCELLANEOUS RELATED DRUGS

Secobarbital or **secobarbital sodium** (Seconal) is a short-acting barbiturate. It is classified as a Schedule G drug in Canada and as a Controlled Substance Schedule II drug in the United States. Secobarbital selectively depresses neurons in the posterior hypothalamus and limbic structures. The drug is used as a mild sedative and a hypnotic. When administered orally, it has a rapid onset of action (within 10 to 15 minutes) and has its peak effect within 3 to 4 hours. Its average half-life is 25 hours.

Butabarbital sodium (Butisol, Buticaps) is used for mild daytime sedation, preoperative sedation, and short-term treatment for insomnia. This barbiturate is classified as a Schedule III drug. When administered by mouth, it has an onset of action of 45 to 60 minutes. Peak action occurs within 3 to 4 hours. Butabarbital has a short duration of action; its average half-life is 20 to 50 hours.

Pentobarbital or **pentobarbital sodium** (Nembutal Sodium) depresses activity of brain cells. It is used for short-

TABLE 18–2
Serum Levels of Barbiturates

Serum Levels	Therapeutic (μg/ml)	Toxic (μg/ml)
Amobarbital	1-5	10-30
Butabarbital	1-2	10-40
Pentobarbital	1-5	> 10
(therapeutic coma)		20-50
Phenobarbital	15-40	35-80
Secobarbital	2-5	3-40

Data from Chernecky, C., Krech, R., & Berger, B. (1993). *Laboratory tests and diagnostic procedures.* Philadelphia: W.B. Saunders.

term treatment of insomnia, as a daytime sedative, for preoperative sedation, and in an emergency to control seizures. For treatment of insomnia, therapy should be limited to 2 weeks. In the United States, pentobarbital is classified as a Controlled Substance Schedule II; in Canada it is a Schedule G drug. Pentobarbital is administered orally and rectally. When administered orally its onset of action occurs with 15 to 30 minutes, and the duration of action lasts 4 to 6 hours. If the drug is administered rectally, onset of action is slow (4 to 6 hours), and the half-life of the drug is 15 to 48 hours. Table 18–1 summarizes information about barbiturates. Table 18–2 shows serum levels of barbiturates.

Thiopental, methohexital, and **thiamylal** are classified as ultrashort-acting barbiturates and are used intravenously for surgical induction or sedation. These drugs are discussed in Chapter 24.

CONCEPT REVIEW

Pharmacodynamic effects of barbiturates are not clear. These drugs depress the sensory cortex, decrease motor activity, alter cerebral function, and produce drowsiness, sedation, and hypnosis.
Phenobarbital is used primarily to treat seizures.

BENZODIAZEPINES

The majority of prescriptions for benzodiazepines are written by primary care providers who treat anxiety or insomnia in an attempt to control other disease processes (e.g., hypertension). The selection of the most appropriate benzodiazepine is made on the basis of the pharmacokinetic and adverse-reaction profiles of the drugs.

General Characteristics

Benzodiazepines have anxiolytic, amnesic, sedative, and anticonvulsant properties. Some benzodiazepines produce musculoskeletal relaxation; others have hypnotic qualities. Benzodiazepines have many dose-related actions, which are the result of selective effects on the CNS.

Benzodiazepines affect a large number of CNS sites, including hypothalamic areas involved in stress response. Mood-altering and emotional effects of benzodiazepines are due to decreased neuronal activity in limbic systems (hippocampus and amygdala). Recent research indicates that benzodiazepines enhance the inhibitory action of GABA in the CNS; and specific benzodiazepine receptors have been identified in the limbic system on GABA receptors. Stimulation of these sites by benzodiazepine produces cell membranes that are less susceptible to depolarization by excitatory neurotransmitters—the anxiolytic effect.[2,17] Mental confusion and amnesia associated with benzodiazepines are related to effects on the hippocampus and cortical association areas. Sleep-promoting properties of benzodiazepine arise from cortical effects or effects on sleep-wakefulness clocks. Effects of benzodiazepine on muscle function and motor control are due to their actions on supraspinal, reticular, and cerebellar systems.[8]

These drugs are well absorbed and widely distributed in body tissues. Benzodiazepines usually are very lipid soluble. Therefore they remain longer in an obese individual or in individuals whose fat-to-lean body mass is increased, such as the elderly. Benzodiazepines have long half-lives and most produce pharmacologically active metabolites. Half-life and duration of pharmacologic action depend on whether a single dose is administered or multiple doses are administered throughout the day over a period of several days or weeks. These drugs are metabolized in the liver and excreted primarily in urine. Reduced renal or hepatic function related to disease or aging also extends the duration of drug effect.[1]

Benzodiazepines should be administered in the smallest possible dose, as infrequently as possible, over the shortest period of time. Long-term use may produce habituation and rebound insomnia with discontinuation.[3,18]

Short-acting anxiolytics are oxazepam (Serax), midazolam (Versed), alprazolam (Xanax), and lorazepam (Ativan). Their half-lives are 1 to 26 hours. Long-acting benzodiazepines are diazepam (Valium), clorazepate (Tranxene), chlordiazepoxide (Librium), and prazepam (Centrax). Half-lives for this group are much longer, 20 to 200 hours.[19] Flurazepam (Dalmane), temazepam (Restoril), and triazolam (Halcion) are currently marketed as hypnotics in the United States. However, benzodiazepines that do not have Food and Drug Administration (FDA) approval as hypnotics are often used as such. Most benzodiazepines are classified as Controlled Substances Act IV drugs.

The therapeutic uses of benzodiazepines include:
- Generalized anxiety disorder
- Atypical anxiety disorder
- Panic disorder
- Posttraumatic stress disorder
- Somatization disorder
- Major depression
- Anxiety related to stressful life events
- Preoperative anxiety
- Chronic disease to relieve the uneasiness

BENZODIAZEPINE PROTOTYPE
DIAZEPAM

Chlordiazepoxide was the first benzodiazepine developed. However, diazepam most typifies the drug category.

Pharmacotherapeutics Primary uses of diazepam include promotion of sedation, relaxation, and muscle relaxation. Although not officially classified as a hypnotic drug, it does promote sleep. It may be useful for short-duration treatment of symptomatic anxiety and is effective in reducing acute ethanol withdrawal symptoms. At low doses it is administered for anxiolytic and sedative effects in the immediate preoperative period and during surgical procedures performed with the client under local or regional anesthesia. Higher doses are used for induction of general anesthesia. However, it does not have any analgesic effect and does not enhance the analgesic effects of narcotics.

Pharmacokinetics Rate of absorption after oral administration varies considerably among benzodiazepine compounds; diazepam is one of the most rapidly absorbed. It is 80% to 90% protein bound. Diazepam is a highly lipid-soluble drug that easily penetrates the CNS. Within the brain, there is selective localization first in gray matter and then white matter. From the brain the redistribution is from highly perfuse tissues to adipose tissue.[8]

Onset of action and duration of action differ among clients. In addition, there is a discrepancy between observed and perceived effects of this drug and serum and brain levels. Generally onset of action after oral administration occurs within 15 to 45 minutes and diminishes in 3 to 4 hours. Peak serum level occurs after 1 to 2 hours; blood level remains elevated for 6 or more hours. Diazepam is metabolized by liver microsomal systems; it undergoes oxidation and conjugation. It has two active metabolites, which may contribute to its long half-life (20 to 100 hours) and prolonged effect. Metabolites of diazepam are excreted by the kidneys.[3,8,13]

Pharmacodynamics Actions of diazepam are produced by the same mechanisms previously described in this section.

Physiologic Effects Diazepam produces many physiologic effects. The main system affected by diazepam is the CNS. CNS effects of diazepam include sedation, calming, drowsiness, hypnosis, anterograde amnesia, and impaired cognitive functioning. Diazepam decreases cerebral blood flow and oxygen consumption. Clients appear relaxed; some clients experience slurred speech, muscle incoordination, and ataxia.

Diazepam produces some effects on the **cardiovascular system.** At low doses there are insignificant reductions in cardiac output and blood pressure. At higher doses there is a decrease in systemic vascular resistance. Hypotension is more likely in hypovolemic or debilitated clients or with the concurrent use of narcotics.

Effects on the **respiratory system** are dose related. Tidal volume and respiratory rate are reduced with low doses. Significant respiratory depression occurs only with doses that exceed those needed for relief of anxiety or promotion of sleep. Respiratory response is more evident in elderly clients or clients with chronic obstructive pulmonary disease.

Within the **renal system,** diazepam decreases renal blood flow and glomerular filtration rate. **Musculoskeletal system** changes are produced by an effect on supraspinal, reticular, and cerebellar systems. Diazepam also produces muscle relaxation by increasing presynaptic inhibition. In addition to the direct effects on motor control systems, relaxation of tense skeletal muscles is one of the consequences of the supraspinal antianxiety ef-

fects.[3,8] Figure 18–1 presents a summary of the physiologic effects of diazepam.

Pharmaceutics Diazepam is available in a variety of dosage forms for oral, intramuscular, and intravenous administration. If administered orally, usually the lowest available dose is administered two to three times daily. Although the long duration of action permits once-a-day dosing, doses are divided to decrease sedation. The dose

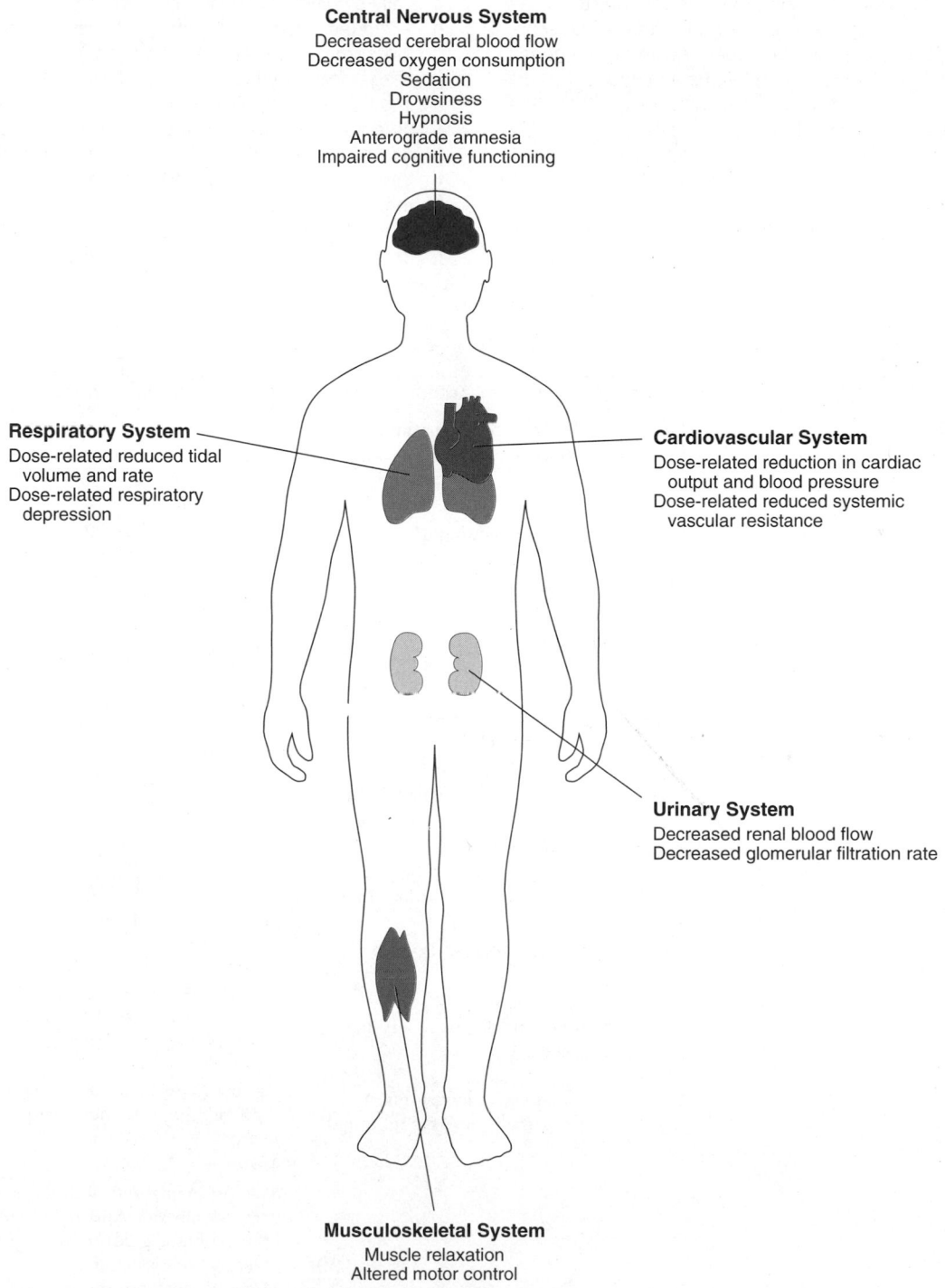

Central Nervous System
Decreased cerebral blood flow
Decreased oxygen consumption
Sedation
Drowsiness
Hypnosis
Anterograde amnesia
Impaired cognitive functioning

Respiratory System
Dose-related reduced tidal
  volume and rate
Dose-related respiratory
  depression

Cardiovascular System
Dose-related reduction in cardiac
  output and blood pressure
Dose-related reduced systemic
  vascular resistance

Urinary System
Decreased renal blood flow
Decreased glomerular filtration rate

Musculoskeletal System
Muscle relaxation
Altered motor control

FIGURE 18–1   Physiologic effects of the benzodiazepine diazepam.

is then titrated to a level that controls the anxiety but does not cause anxiety or other undesired clinical responses.[2]

Undesired Clinical Responses Psychomotor impairment occurs with all benzodiazepines at therapeutic doses. Drowsiness, mental confusion, and incoordination may occur, particularly in elderly clients. These effects are dose related and are potentiated by other depressants such as alcohol, barbiturates, or narcotics.[2]

Tolerance readily develops to the sedative effects of benzodiazepine but develops slowly or not at all to the antianxiety effects. Depression, insomnia, anterograde amnesia, and paradoxical agitation occur with abrupt cessation.[14] A small percentage of individuals taking a benzodiazepine at therapeutic doses has withdrawal symptoms. Appearance of withdrawal symptoms may occur within 1 to 2 days after withdrawal of a benzodiazepine with a short half-life or within 3 to 4 days with the longer half-life drugs.

Contraindications and Precautions Use of antianxiety agents must be evaluated in light of the fact that non-prescription substances (e.g., alcohol) are readily available and widely used. This introduces the possibility of toxicity and addiction and increases the risk of poor nutrition, obesity, and organ damage (e.g., liver, pancreas, brain). Sedative effect produced by diazepam may also limit its use in individuals who must remain mentally alert. In addition, these drugs are used with caution in clients with renal or hepatic failure and in clients with glaucoma.

Drug-Drug and Drug-Nutrient Interactions Clinically significant drug interactions may occur with benzodiazepines. Alcohol and other CNS depressants potentiate the sedative effects of diazepam. In addition, cimetidine (Tagamet), erythromycin, and oral contraceptives may impair the metabolism of diazepam and increase its pharmacologic effects.[2] Excessive coffee intake or concurrent use of an appetite suppressant may negate the desired therapeutic effects of diazepam.[3] Taking diazepam with magnesium–aluminum hydroxide antacids decreases its rate but not extent of GI absorption. Antacids containing only aluminum increase diazepam's absorption.[20]

TABLE 18–3
Benzodiazepine Prototype

Drug Name	Dosage and Route of Administration	Nursing Considerations

DIAZEPAM
 	
(Valium)
HOW SUPPLIED
  Uncoated tablet: 2, 5, and 10 mg
  Sustained-action capsule: 15 mg
  Oral solution: 5 mg/ml, 5 mg/5 ml, 10 mg/10 ml
  IM, IV: 5 mg/ml, 10 mg/2 ml
	Dosage is individualized for maximum beneficial effect.
	
	Anxiety
	ADULTS
	Oral tablet: 2-10 mg bid to qid
	Oral capsule: 15-30 mg/d
	Moderate Anxiety
	IM, IV: 2-5 mg; repeat in 3-4 h if needed
	Severe Anxiety
	IM, IV: 5-10 mg; repeat in 3-4 h if needed
	Symptomatic Relief in Acute Alcohol Withdrawal
	ADULTS
	Oral: 10 mg tid or qid during first 24 h; reduce to 5 mg tid or qid
	Acute Alcohol Withdrawal
	ADULTS
	IM, IV: 10 mg initially, then reduce to 5-10 mg in 3-4 h as needed
	Relief of Skeletal Muscle Spasm
	ADULTS
	Oral: 2-10 mg tid or qid
	IM, IV: 5-10 mg initially, then 5-10 mg in 3-4 h if needed
	CHILDREN
	Start initial therapy with lowest dose and increase as required; 1-2.5 mg tid or qid
		Assess
		Review nursing health history and assessment.
		Assess for preexisting conditions that would contraindicate use of diazepam (e.g., hepatic disease, lactation).
		Review results of hepatic studies: AST, ALT, LDH, alkaline phosphatase.
		
		Interventions
		Assess blood pressure (lying and standing); if BP drops 20 mm Hg, hold drug and notify primary care provider.
		Administer IV solution into large vein to decrease chance of extravasation.
		Do not use parenteral solution if discolored or contains a precipitate.
		Crush tablet if client unable to swallow whole.
		Administer oral preparation on empty stomach unless GI symptoms occur; then administer with food or milk.
		Administer IM in a large muscle to avoid tissue irritation.
		Assist with ambulation during initial therapy since drowsiness and dizziness occur.
		Teach client to rise slowly to avoid syncope.
		Teach client not to discontinue drug abruptly.
		Instruct client to avoid OTC preparations, alcohol ingestion, and other psychotropic drugs.
		
		Monitor
		Monitor mental status: mood, sensorium, affect, long- and short-term memory.
		Monitor blood studies: CBC during long-term therapy.
		Monitor hepatic studies.
		
		Evaluate
		Evaluate therapeutic response: decreased anxiety, restlessness, insomnia.

Ethnic Differences in Drug Disposition and Responsiveness Doses used in Chinese clients are lower than those prescribed for Caucasians. Concentrations of diazepam and its metabolite dimethyl-diazepam are higher in Orientals, as reflected by a significantly lower clearance level.[21]

Life-Span Considerations Diazepam should be avoided in the first trimester of pregnancy because of an increased incidence of cleft lip and palate associated with its use. It is classified as a Pregnancy Category D drug.

Specific Drug-Related Nursing Considerations Monitor the client for paradoxical excitement and mood and affect changes. Instruct the client to avoid using diazepam with alcohol or other CNS depressants. Inform the client that food and antacids decrease absorption. Instruct the client to separate the intake of antacids and diazepam by at least 1 hour.

Caution the client that coordination and reflexes may be impaired; therefore driving or operating dangerous equipment may be injurious. Inform the client that the drug can produce significant anterograde amnesia. Often the client cannot recall conversations with health care providers. If daytime sedation is excessive, direct the client to take the largest dose in the evening hours.

If given parenterally, the drug should not be mixed with other drugs. In addition, parenteral diazepam is in a propylene glycol and ethanol solution, which causes pain during injection and may lead to phlebitis. Monitor vital signs, specifically blood pressure, before and after parenteral administration. Table 18–3 summarizes information about diazepam.

MISCELLANEOUS RELATED DRUGS

As indicated previously, numerous benzodiazepines are on the market. These drugs have pharmacotherapeutic and pharmacodynamic properties similar to those of diazepam. Onset of action, half-life, and dosage range for several benzodiazepines are summarized in Table 18–4.

Several benzodiazepines are routinely prescribed for the elderly client. They include temazepam, triazolam, and flurazepam. These drugs can produce postural hypotension,

TABLE 18–4

*Benzodiazepines: Onset of Action, Half-Life, Dosage Range of Oral Adult Doses**

Benzodiazepines	Onset of Action (min)	Half-Life (h)	Daily Dosage Range (mg)
Alprazolam (Xanax)	30-45	6.3-26	0.15-1.5
Chlordiazepoxide HCl (Librium)	15-45	24-48	5-80
Clorazepate dipotassium (Tranxene)	15-45	24-48	15-30
Diazepam (Valium)	15-45	20-100	4-40
Flurazepam (Dalmane)	15-45	24-100	15-30
Lorazepam (Ativan)	30-55	12-18	2-6
Oxazepam (Serax)	45-90	5.7-10.9	30-60
Temazepam (Restoril)	45-90	9.5-12.4	15-30
Triazolam (Halcion)	2-30	1.5-5.5	0.125-0.50

*Data from references 1, 5, 6, 13, and 28.

dizziness, and depression in this age group. For the elderly, immediate- or short-acting benzodiazepines that contain inactive metabolites such as alprazolam, lorazepam, oxazepam, temazepam, and triazolam are suggested.

Benzodiazepine-Receptor Antagonist

Flumazenil, released in early 1992, is a specific benzodiazepine-receptor antagonist that is structurally related to midazolam. It blocks the CNS effects of benzodiazepine by competitively binding to benzodiazepine receptors. Onset of action is rapid (clinically apparent arousal occurs within 1 to 5 minutes), and duration of action is approximately 3 hours. The dosage range is 0.1 to 1.0 mg IV, with an average dose of 0.4 mg. Flumazenil does not possess clinically significant intrinsic pharmacologic activity. In other words, it is not administered for effects other than blocking the actions of benzodiazepine. It is not effective with other nonbenzodiazepine sedatives and anesthetics, with the possible exception of zolpidem.[22,23]

CONCEPT REVIEW

Benzodiazepines have a broad spectrum of actions, varying with the compound, dosage, and client sensitivity.

Benzodiazepine receptors are widely distributed in the CNS. Many of these receptors are connected with GABA-receptor systems and chloride channels.

When administered alone, benzodiazepines have a large therapeutic index. Tolerance, habitation, and physical dependence can occur with therapeutic and higher doses.

AZAPIRONES

The drug in this group is not chemically or pharmacologically related to the benzodiazepines, barbiturates, or other sedative/anxiolytic drugs.

AZAPIRONE PROTOTYPE
BUSPIRONE HYDROCHLORIDE

Buspirone hydrochloride (BuSpar), approved by the FDA in 1986, was the first azapirone introduced. This drug does not cause any appreciable sedation or interfere with psychomotor performance. It has no potential for abuse and does not produce physical dependence; therefore it is not a controlled substance.

Pharmacotherapeutics Buspirone is used in the treatment of anxiety disorders or for the short-term relief of symptoms of anxiety.

Pharmacokinetics Buspirone is rapidly absorbed and undergoes extensive first-pass metabolism. Peak serum levels are achieved in 40 to 90 minutes. Approximately 95% of buspirone is plasma-protein bound. The drug is metabolized primarily by oxidation, producing several pharmacologically active metabolites. Buspirone is excreted in the urine and feces. The average elimination half-life of unchanged drug is approximately 2 to 3 hours.[13]

Pharmacodynamics Mechanism of action is unknown. Azapirones do not affect GABA. They appear to exert their anxiolytic effect by modulating the activity of the neurotransmitter serotonin. Buspirone does not produce an immediate anxiolytic effect. It takes at least 1 week before any significant improvement in the symptoms is seen, and it takes a full 4 weeks before maximal response is produced.[24-26]

Pharmaceutics Buspirone is supplied in 5- and 10-mg tablets for oral administration. The usual dosage is 5 mg three times a day.

Undesired Clinical Responses Buspirone has been associated with nausea, dizziness, insomnia, and headaches. Weight gain has been reported, and nervousness and excitement occasionally occur.

Contraindications and Precautions Since buspirone HCL is metabolized by the liver and excreted by the kidneys, its administration to clients with severe hepatic or renal impairment is not recommended.

Drug-Drug Interactions Buspirone interacts with monoamine oxidase (MAO) inhibitors, so this combination should be avoided. Its use with psychotropic drugs has not been studied to any extent; therefore concomitant administration of these drugs should be approached with caution.

Life-Span Considerations Buspirone is classified as a Pregnancy Category B drug. The extent of its excretion in human milk is not known; therefore use in nursing mothers should be avoided. Safety and effectiveness with clients below 18 years of age have not been determined.[13]

IMIDAZOPYRIDINES

Imidazopyridines represent a new class of compounds.

IMIDAZOPYRIDINE PROTOTYPE
ZOLPIDEM

Zolpidem (Ambien) is structurally unrelated to benzodiazepines and binds more selectively to neuronal receptors involved in inducing sleep. It apparently does not have significant antianxiety, anticonvulsant, or muscle-relaxing actions. Zolpidem is classified under Schedule IV of the Controlled Substances Act.

Pharmacotherapeutics Zolpidem is a new sedative-hypnotic approved for short-term (7 to 10 days) treatment of insomnia. It apparently does not suppress Stages 3 and 4 of the sleep cycle and produces little or no rebound insomnia when therapy is discontinued.

Pharmacokinetics Zolpidem is rapidly absorbed; serum concentration peaks are reached in 1.6 hours. Absorption is slowed when the drug is taken with food. The drug is metabolized by the liver; its elimination half-life is approximately 2½ hours. Only the inactive metabolites of the drug are excreted in the urine, so doses are not reduced for individuals with renal disease.

Pharmacodynamics Zopidem binds to the same neuronal receptors as the benzodiazepines: the GABA receptor–chloride channel complex.

Pharmaceutics It is available as tablets for oral administration. In most adults 10 mg at bedtime is adequate. In the elderly and clients with impaired liver function, treatment should start with a 5-mg dose.

Undesired Clinical Responses Undesired responses are dose related. With short-term use, daytime drowsiness, dizziness, and diarrhea have been reported. With long-term use (28 to 35 days), dizziness and drug hangover occur.

Contraindications and Precautions Zolpidem should be used with caution in clients with hepatic dysfunction, diseases that affect metabolism or hemodynamics, or compromised respiratory function. It should also be used with care in depressed individuals because of the risk of intentional overdose.

Drug-Drug Interactions Other drugs with CNS activity may enhance zolpidem's depressive effects. Flumazenil reverses the sedation and hypnotic effects of the drug.

Life-Span Considerations In elderly clients the drug reaches higher serum concentrations and is cleared more slowly. Dosage adjustments are needed.

Specific Drug-Related Nursing Considerations Carefully evaluate the client for underlying physical or psychiatric disorders. Elderly or debilitated clients should be closely monitored for cognitive or behavioral abnormalities. Counsel clients not to take the drug with alcohol. Also instruct the client on adverse effects, memory problems, tolerance, dependence, and withdrawal.[27]

CONCEPT REVIEW

Buspirone is a relatively new compound used to treat anxiety. It is not chemically or pharmacologically related to the benzodiazepines, barbiturates, or other sedative or anxiolytic drugs.

Buspirone does not cause any appreciable sedation or interfere with psychomotor performance. Since it has no potential for abuse and does not produce physical dependence, it is not a controlled substance.

Zolpidem is a new sedative-hypnotic approved for short-term (7 to 10 days) treatment of insomnia. It is classified under Schedule IV of the Controlled Substances Act.

MISCELLANEOUS DRUGS USED AS SEDATIVES, HYPNOTICS, AND ANXIOLYTICS

A variety of other drugs is used as sedatives, hypnotics, and anxiolytis. Selection of these drugs is based on desired clinical response.

Chloral Hydrate

Chloral hydrate (Noctec) is a chloral derivative. It is a CNS depressant with properties similar to those of the barbiturates and is used to induce sleep. Rapid metabolism of chloral hydrate forms the metabolite trichloroethanol, which produces sedation. Trichloroethanol has a half-life of 4 to 12 hours.

Chloral hydrate is available in several dosage forms: capsules, syrup, and suppositories. Recommended dose is 0.5 to 1 g 30 minutes before bedtime. Chloral hydrate is subject to abuse and is classified as a Schedule IV drug. As a result of its high therapeutic index, chloral hydrate addicts may ingest extremely large amounts of the drug.[29]

🌿 NURSING RESEARCH

Klein, E.R. (1992). Premedicating children for painful invasive procedures. *Journal of Pediatric Oncology Nursing, 9*(4), 170-179.

Children with cancer experience anxiety about their treatment and invasive tests. Responses of pain, fear, and anxiety are well documented in other studies. These responses may cause developmental delay, sleeping and eating disorders, nausea and vomiting, nightmares, and depression.

Previous studies reported that only a small percentage of children receive premedications and that no clear standard for either drugs or dosages existed. This study explored the attitudes and perceptions of physicians and nurses about medicating children before procedures. Findings showed that most pediatric oncology specialists medicate their clients before invasive procedures. The most common premedications are midazolam, meperidine, promethazine hydrochloride, chlorpromazine hydrochloride, chloral hydrate, lorazepam, and fentanyl.

STUDENT ACTIVITIES

- Develop a questionnaire regarding attitudes and perceptions of health care providers about premedicating children for invasive techniques.
- Distribute the questionnaire to at least six nurses and primary care providers who care for children who require painful, invasive procedures.
- Compare your findings with those described in this research article. 🌿

Carbamates

Meprobamate (Equanil, Miltown) is a carbamate derivative that affects numerous sites in the CNS, including the thalamus and limbic system. Although newer, more effective drugs are available, meprobamate is still used in the treatment of anxiety disorders. The usual adult dose for anxiety is 1.2 to 1.6 g per day in divided doses. Meprobamate is classified as a Schedule IV drug.

Sedating Antihistamines

A common clinical response to antihistamines (H_1-blocking agents) is drowsiness, sedation, and sleep. **Diphenhydramine** (Benadryl) is widely used by prescription and OTC as a sleep aid. The degree of sleep quality and duration produced by diphenhydramine are dose dependent. Other antihistamines such as **hydroxyzine hydrochloride** (Atarax) and **hydroxyzine pamoate** (Vistaril) have been used as anxiolytic drugs. (Antihistamines are discussed in Chapter 50.)

Neuroleptic Drugs

Low doses of antipsychotic drugs have been used in the treatment of anxiety, especially in the elderly. A major limitation in their use is the potential for the client to develop extrapyramidal syndromes or tardive dyskinesia. Neuroleptic drugs are not recommended for nonpsychotic clients with sleep disorders. (Neuroleptic drugs are discussed in Chapter 20.)

OTC Preparations for Sleep

OTC preparations marketed as sleep-inducing drugs contain agents approved by the FDA. At present, diphenhydramine hydrochloride and diphenhydramine citrate are approved as active ingredients in these sleep aids. In addition, products containing doxylamine succinate are being marketed under approved New Drug Applications (NDAs). Both diphenhydramine and doxylamine belong to the ethanolamine class of antihistamines.

SUMMARY

A large portion of the population seeks treatment for anxiety or insomnia or both. Anxiolytic, sedative, or hypnotic drugs are frequently prescribed for these individuals. The major group of drugs prescribed today is the benzodiazepines. These drugs are safer and more effective than previous drugs used (e.g., barbiturates, carbamates, antihistamines).

Dangers with most drugs in these categories are the potential for abuse and the occurrence of psychologic and physical dependence. Sedatives, hypnotics, and anxiolytics should be used in combination with behavioral modification therapy and relaxation training.

REFERENCES

1. Berstein, J.G. (1988). *Handbook of drug therapy in psychiatry* (2nd ed.). Littleton, MA: PSG Publishing.
2. Steiner, J. (1991). Anxiety an update on pharmacologic therapy. *Journal of the American Academy of Physician Assistants, 4,* 421-426.
3. Hollister, L., & Csernansky, J. (1990). *Clinical pharmacology of psychotherapeutic drugs* (3rd ed.). New York: Churchill Livingstone.
4. Murray, R., Zentner, J. (1993). *Nursing assessment and health promotion: Strategies through the life span* (5th ed.). Norwalk, CT: Appleton & Lange.
5. Conrad, K. (1990). Sedative hypnotic drug use in the elderly. *Physician Assistant, 14*(8), 59-60.
6. Nakra, B., Grossberg, G., & Peck, B. (1992). Insomnia in the elderly. *American Family Physician, 43,* 477-483.
7. Fillingim, J. (1992). Insomnia: Diagnosis and treatment in general practice. *Physician Assistant, 16*(4), 47-50.
8. Smith, C., & Reynard, A. (Eds.). (1992). *Textbook of pharmacology.* Philadelphia: W.B. Saunders.
9. Weinberger, R. (1991). Teaching the elderly stress reduction. *Journal of Gerontological Nursing, 17*(10), 23-27.
10. Baldessarini, R.J. (1990). Drugs and the treatment of psychiatric disorders. In A.G. Goodman, T.W. Rall, A.S. Nies, & T. Palmer (Eds.), *Goodman and Gilman's the pharmacological basis of therapeutics* (8th ed., pp. 383-435). New York: Pergamon Press.
11. Katzung, B. (Ed.). (1992). *Basic and clinical pharmacology.* Norwalk, CT: Appleton & Lange.
12. DiPalma, J., & DiGregorio, J. (Eds.). (1990). *Basic pharmacology in medicine.* New York: McGraw-Hill.
13. U.S. Pharmacopeial Convention. (1990). *The United States pharmacopeia* (22nd rev.). Rockville, MD: Author.

14. Levy, D.B. (1991). Common drug reactions and interactions. *Emergency, 23*(11), 22-26, 29-31.

15. Tatro, D.S. (Ed.). (1990). *Drug interaction facts* (2nd ed.). St. Louis: Facts and Comparisons Division, J.B. Lippincott.

16. Chernecky, C., Krech, R., & Berger, B. (1993). *Laboratory tests and diagnostic procedures*. Philadelphia: W.B. Saunders.

17. Biggio, G., & Costa, E. (Eds.). (1990). *GABA and benzodiazepine receptor subtypes: Molecular biology, pharmacology, and clinical aspects*. New York: Raven Press.

18. Shorr, R., & Bauwens, S. (1992). Diagnosis and treatment of outpatient insomnia by psychiatric and nonpsychiatric physicians. *American Journal of Medicine, 93*, 78-82.

19. Porterfield, L.M. (1991). Update on anxiolytics. *Advancing Clinical Care, 6*(5), 14-15.

20. Chase, S. (1993). OTC interactions: Antacids. *RN*, pp. 46-50.

21. Wood, A.J., & Zhou, H.H. (1991). Ethnic differences in drug disposition and responsiveness. *Clinical Pharmacokinetics, 20,* 350-373.

22. Kasson, B. (1992). Flumazenil: A specific benzodiazepine antagonist. *AANA Journal, 60,* 474-476.

23. Spiess, B. (1990). Two new pharmacological agents for the 1990s: Flumazenil and propofol. *Journal of Post Anesthesia Nursing, 5*(3), 186-189.

24. Feighner, J.P., & Cohn, J.B. (1989). Analysis of individual symptoms in generalized anxiety—A pooled multistudy, double-blinded evaluation of buspirone. *Neuropsychobiology, 3,* 124-130.

25. Rakel, R.E. (1990). Long-term buspirone therapy for chronic anxiety: A multicenter international study to determine safety. *Southern Medical Journal, 83,* 194-198.

26. Yocca, F.D. (1990). Neurochemistry and neurophysiology of buspirone and gepirone: Interaction of presynaptic and postsynaptic 5-HT$_{1A}$ receptors. *Journal of Clinical Psychopharmacology, 10,* 6S-12S.

27. Meyer, C. (1993). New drugs: In the realm of the brain. *American Journal of Nursing, 93*(8), 58, 60-61.

28. Biddle, C., & Gilliland, C. (1992). Transdermal and transmucosal administration of pain-relieving and anxiolytic drugs: A primer for the critical care practitioner. *Heart and Lung: Journal of Critical Care, 21*(2), 115-124.

29. Buck, M.L. (1992). Chloral hydrate use during infancy. *Neonatal Pharmacology Quarterly, 1*(1), 31-37.

30. Klein, E.R. (1992). Premedicating children for painful invasive procedures. *Journal of Pediatric Oncology Nursing, 9*(4), 170-179.

BIBLIOGRAPHY

Aker, J. (1990). Review of current research on midazolam and diazepam for endoscopic premedication. *Gastroenterology Nursing, 13*(Res Suppl 2), 24S-28S.

Balter, M., & Uhlenhuth, E. (1991). The beneficial and adverse effects of hypnotics. *Journal of Clinical Psychiatry*, (Suppl 52), 16-23.

Burch, E.A. (1990). Use and misuse of benzodiazepines in the elderly. *Psychiatric Medicine, 8,* 97-105.

Carey, J. (Ed.). (1991). *Sleep and Dreaming*. Washington, DC: Society for Neuroscience.

Charney, D.S., Jrystal, J.H., Delgado, P.L., & Heninger, G.R. (1990). Serotonin-specific drugs for anxiety and depressive disorders. *Annual Review of Medicine, 41,* 437-446.

Gold, C. (1992). Xanax: Pros and cons. *Journal of Psychosocial Nursing, 30*(6), 36-37.

Johnson, L.C., et al. (1990). Daytime sleepiness, performance, mood, nocturnal sleep: The effect of benzodiazepine and caffeine on their relationship. *Sleep, 13*(2), 121-135.

Tiller, J.W.G., & Schweitzer, I. (1992). Benzodiazepines: Depressants or antidepressants? *Drugs, 44*(2), 165-169.

Walsh, J.K., & Mahowald, M. (1991). Avoiding the blanket approach to insomnia: Targeted therapy for specific causes. *Postgraduate Medicine, 90,* 211-214, 217-219, 223-224.

CHAPTER 19

Opioid and Nonopioid Analgesics

RHONDA W. COMRIE

⊛ Pain

LEARNING OBJECTIVES:

Describe the pathway from nociceptors to the brain.
Name three major biochemical mediators.
Explain the function of biochemical mediators.
Discuss methods of classifying the sensation of pain.

KEY TERMS:

Acute pain, biochemical mediator, chronic pain, endorphin, neuromodulator, nociceptor, mild pain, moderate pain, pain, pain pathway, psychogenic, severe pain, somatogenic

⊛ General Characteristics of Opioid and Nonopioid Analgesics

LEARNING OBJECTIVE: Differentiate between the terms *narcotic* and *opioid*.

KEY TERMS:

Analgesia, analgesic, narcotic, opioid

⊛ Nursing Considerations

LEARNING OBJECTIVE: Plan care for the client receiving analgesic therapy.

KEY TERMS:

Continuous subcutaneous infusion, epidural infusion, patient-controlled analgesia

⊛ Nonopioid Analgesics

LEARNING OBJECTIVE: Describe the action of acetylsalicylic acid on the central nervous system.

KEY TERMS:

Hyperalgesia, para-aminophenol derivative

⊛ Opioid Analgesics

LEARNING OBJECTIVES:

Explain the pharmacodynamic properties of opioid analgesics.
Describe the effects of morphine on at least four body systems.
Summarize essential information about the opioid analgesic prototype morphine.
Describe essential information about meperidine and codeine.

KEY TERMS:

Agonist-antagonist, delta receptor, kappa receptor, mu receptor, sigma receptor, opioid agonist, opioid poisoning, opium

⊛ Mixed Opioid Agonist-Antagonists

LEARNING OBJECTIVE: Summarize essential information about pentazocine, the prototype for mixed opioid agonist-antagonist drugs.

⊛ Opioid Antagonists

LEARNING OBJECTIVES:

Summarize essential information about naloxone, the prototype for opioid antagonists.
Identify pharmacotherapeutic uses for naloxone.

CONCEPTS AND TERMS TO REVIEW

Review anatomy and physiology of the central nervous system in Chapter 17.
Reexamine the meaning of the terms *agonist* and *antagonist*.
Review material on epidural and intrathecal routes of administration in Chapter 3.

---

*P*ain relief is a primary concern of health care professionals. Yet in a society in which substance use and abuse are a major problem, these same individuals are often uncertain about how to alleviate pain *and* prevent the negative responses to analgesics.

Pain is a complex phenomenon composed of sensory, motivational, and cognitive experiences and responses. Sensory aspects of pain include strength, intensity, and spatial interpretations. These sensations are mediated through afferent nerve fibers, the spinal cord, the brain stem, and higher brain centers. The result is immediate withdrawal from the painful stimulus. Motivational and cognitive aspects determine the individual's learned approach and avoidance behavior to pain. Motivational behaviors are mediated through the interaction of the reticular formation, limbic system, and brain stem. The individual's cognitive interpretation of appropriate pain behavior is learned through male and female roles, cultural preferences, and past experiences. Cognition may block, moderate, or enhance the perception of pain.

Pain is a subjective experience and cannot be described by anyone other than the individual experiencing it. Therefore careful attention to the type of pain the individual is experiencing, the meaning of pain to that individual, and the individual's response to pain control measures are important. It is also important to remember that you, the nurse, bring a variety of experiences to each individual's report of discomfort. To manage all of these factors, providing pain relief must be approached with a sound knowledge base.

Information in this chapter provides a basis for well-informed decision making regarding pain relief. Pain mediators, pain pathways, and pain modulators are discussed. An overview of nursing care for the individual receiving opioid or nonopioid analgesics is provided as is general information about these drugs. In addition, guidelines are provided to aid in the selection of nonopioid versus opioid drugs for pain relief.

PAIN

Pain is an unpleasant sensory and emotional experience. It is caused by stimulation of specialized nerve endings and is associated with actual or potential tissue damage.

Physiology of Pain

The physiology of pain is complex and is influenced by psychologic or emotional reactions of the individual. Portions of the nervous system responsible for the sensation and perception of pain include afferent pathways, central nervous system (CNS), and efferent pathways.

NEUROANATOMY OF PAIN

Pain results when an unpleasant or noxious substance stimulates mechanical, chemical, or thermal receptors (**nociceptors**) in the body. The distribution of nociceptors throughout the body varies. Areas with a high distribution include subcutaneous tissue, periosteum, deep fascia, ligaments, joint capsules, and the cornea of the eye. Skeletal muscles, bone, and cartilage possess relatively few pain receptors.[1]

Nociceptors excite primary afferent fibers that carry pain messages to the spinal cord. Of the afferent fibers, larger A-delta fibers conduct the pain impulse most quickly. Small C-fibers are the slowest conductors, and B-fibers are intermediate in size and speed of conduction. Afferent fibers are located in peripheral tissues and enter the CNS through the dorsal horn of the spinal cord. Biochemical mediators, released from the afferent neuron to the neurons in the dorsal horn, influence how the impulse is transmitted to the brain.[1,2]

From the dorsal horn the impulse is transmitted primarily to the spinothalamic tract neurons. This tract connects to the brain stem where the thalamus and other control centers are located. When the pain message reaches the thalamus, the sensation of pain arrives at consciousness. From there the stimulus is disseminated to both cerebral hemispheres. Fibers in the somesthetic (sensory) and associative areas of the parietal lobe discriminate between the locality and intensity of the pain. Fibers in the frontal lobe stimulate the limbic system, which probably determines how each individual responds to the pain episode.[1] Figure 19–1 illustrates the **pain pathway** from nociceptor to brain.

BIOCHEMICAL MEDIATORS

As mentioned previously, **biochemical mediators** such as neurotransmitters and neuromodulators are key elements in the transmission of pain impulses to the CNS. **Neuromodulators** such as substance P, prostaglandins, potassium, bradykinins, histamines, and lymphokines exist in tissues and are released when nociceptors are traumatized. All neuromodulators do not function in the same manner. For example, release of substance P occurs at more than one site. When released by nociceptors, substance P causes vasodilation and edema in peripheral tissues. Once substance P is released at the dorsal horn, it binds to the secondary neuron and elicits the action potential that transmits the pain impulse to the spinal cord. Substance P and other neurotransmitters contribute to the modulation of pain in both the afferent and efferent fibers of the spinal cord.[2]

The neuromodulators prostaglandins, bradykinins, and histamines are also released as a result of damage to cell membranes. They depolarize adjacent nociceptors producing pain. *Potassium* release occurs through the process of transduction as ion channels of the primary afferent fibers open and allow the influx of sodium. The result is an action potential by which pain impulses are transmitted. Gamma-aminobutyric acid (GABA) is released at the dorsal horn of the spinal cord. It has a role in spinal regulation of pain.

Endorphins (enkephalin, dynorphin, and β-lipotropin) are neuropeptides that inhibit transmission of pain impulses in the spinal cord and brain. All endorphins act by attaching to opiate receptors on the plasma membrane of the afferent neuron. The combination of opiate receptors and endorphins blocks the release of excitatory neurotransmitters such as substance P.[1,2]

Substances released in the upper CNS also assist in pain regulation. For example, the modulatory or descending pain system releases substances such as serotonin and norepinephrine that inhibit the transmission of pain in the dorsal horn. One area in the midbrain, the nucleus raphe magnus, sends descending projections to the dorsal horn of the spinal cord. This mechanism causes the release of serotonin, which inhibits nociceptive transmission. In addition, neurons from the pons

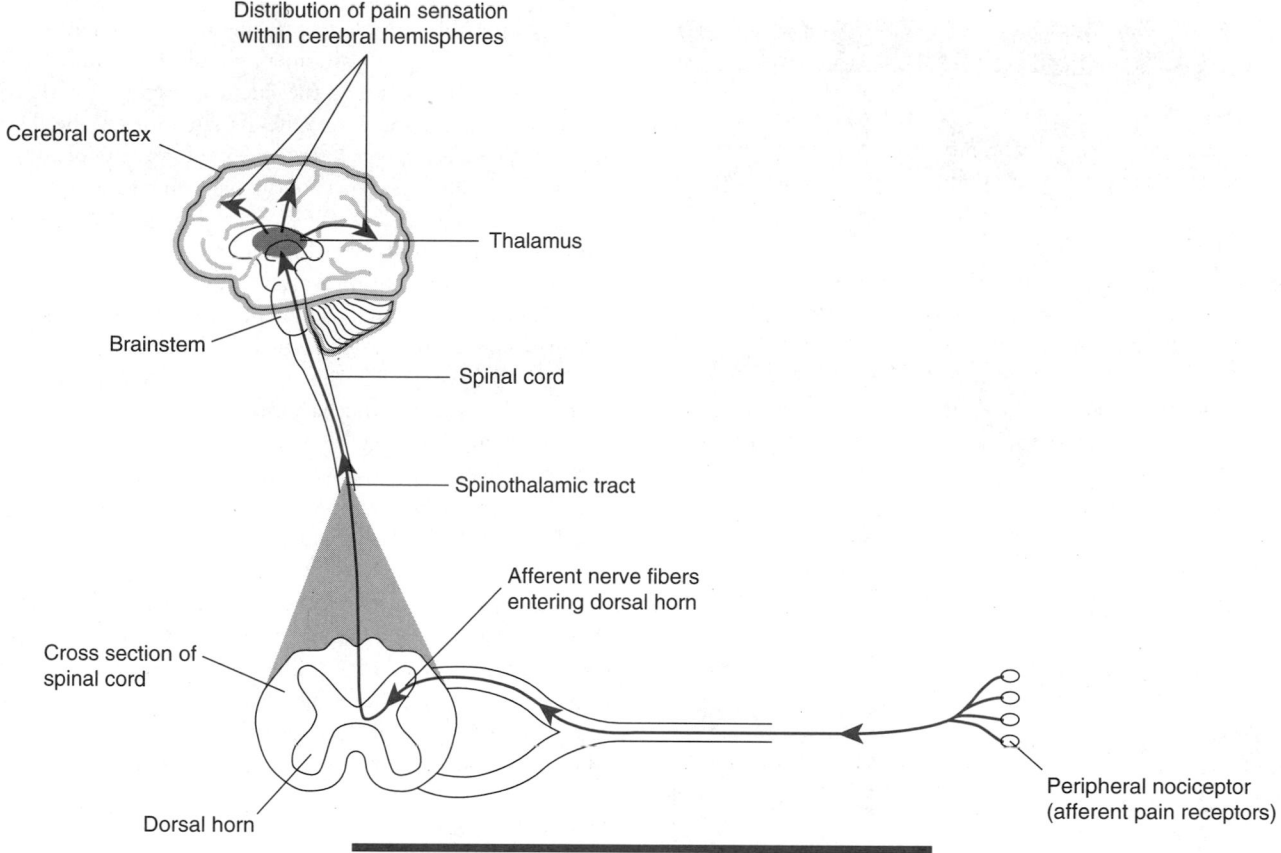

Distribution of pain sensation within cerebral hemispheres

Cerebral cortex

Thalamus

Brainstem

Spinal cord

Spinothalamic tract

Afferent nerve fibers entering dorsal horn

Cross section of spinal cord

Peripheral nociceptor (afferent pain receptors)

Dorsal horn

FIGURE 19–1   Pain pathway from nociceptor to brain.

release noradrenergic substances that inhibit nociceptive transmission within the dorsal horn itself.[1,2]

Classification of Pain

Several methods of pain classification exist (e.g., origin of pain, duration of discomfort, level of discomfort). The term **somatogenic** means originating in the body. Somatogenic pain such as the discomfort associated with appendicitis has a cause that originates in the body. In contrast, the term **psychogenic** means that there is an emotional or psychologic origin. With psychogenic pain, there is no known physical cause. However, psychogenic pain is not imaginary; it may be just as intense as somatogenic pain.

Pain is also classified as acute or chronic. **Acute pain** is a protective mechanism that alerts the individual of injury or harm to the body. Onset of acute pain is usually sudden and is relieved after the biochemical mediator is removed. **Chronic pain** is persistent, lasting at least 6 months. With chronic pain, the cause is frequently unknown. Onset of chronic pain may be sudden or insidious; usually chronic pain does not respond to therapy.[3]

Level of pain is another method of classification. Pain is considered mild, moderate, or severe. **Mild pain** often refers to levels of discomfort that do not interfere with daily activities. **Moderate pain** is more distracting, and activity is somewhat limited. Extreme limitation of activity or immobilization occurs with **severe pain.**

GENERAL CHARACTERISTICS OF OPIOID AND NONOPIOID ANALGESICS

The term **analgesic** describes drugs that are used to produce **analgesia,** the absence of sensibility to pain. Nonopioid, weak opioid, and strong opioid drugs are available. In addition, adjuvant drug therapies, drugs not normally identified for analgesia, are used for specific types of pain. (See box on p. 168 for examples of adjuvant drug therapies.) Nondrug pain therapies such as biofeedback, relaxation training, or hypnotherapy are also used in combination with drug therapies to ensure more comprehensive pain management. Selection of pain therapy is based on a full assessment of each client. Factors that influence the treatment plan include the client's mood, client's pain interpretation, severity of pain episode, and length of pain experience.[3,4]

Since opioid drugs are habit forming, they are regulated under the United States Controlled Substance Act. According to this act, addictive or habit-forming drugs are labeled **narcotics.** Therefore opioid drugs are legally considered narcotics. However, for our purpose the term **opioid** is more accurate than the term *narcotic* since opioid specifically refers to drugs that bind to opioid receptors. *Narcotics* is a general term that has several meanings. For example, it is used in literature to describe agents that induce narcosis. It also refers to any substance that produces dependence, whether it is a listed drug or produced on the street.[5]

ANALGESIC ADJUVANTS

Some drugs not classified as analgesics are effective against certain types of pain. These drugs may enhance the effect of analgesics, have their own analgesic activity, or counteract the side effects of analgesics. Most of these drugs are used for adults and children.

▶ **Tricyclic antidepressants** such as amitriptyline, imipramine, or desipramine are used to treat neuropathy and posttherapeutic neuralgia. These drugs also decrease depression associated with the pain experience.

▶ Some **antihistamines** such as hydroxyzine administered intramuscularly possess analgesic, antiemetic, and mild sedative qualities.

▶ **Benzodiazepines** such as diazepam and lorazepam are used to treat acute anxiety or muscle spasm associated with acute pain.

▶ **Caffeine** increases analgesia when given with aspirin-like drugs for uterine cramping, dental pain, headaches, or episiotomy pain. Other pain syndromes may also respond to caffeine.

▶ **Dextroamphetamine** produces additive analgesia when combined with opioids in the postoperative period.

▶ **Steroids** may cause lysis of some tumors and relieve painful nerve or spinal cord compression by acting to decrease the edema in the tumor and nerve tissue. Pain may be exacerbated by rapid withdrawal of steroid.

Data from American Pain Society. (1992). *Principles of analgesic use in the treatment of acute pain and cancer pain* (3rd ed.). Skokie, IL: Author.

CONCEPT REVIEW

The sensation of pain is an individualized experience. No one can describe the feeling except the individual experiencing the pain.

Once nociceptors are stimulated, the pain sensation follows a pathway to the brain. This pathway involves afferent nerve fibers, the central nervous system, and efferent nerve fibers. Biochemical mediators, neurotransmitters and neuromodulators, influence the transmission of the pain impulse.

⊞ NURSING CONSIDERATIONS

Pain is not a singular entity but a composite of many events. In addition, most adults have learned a response to pain that is culturally acceptable. This leads some clients to voice pain loudly, whereas other clients have been taught that expressing pain is a sign of weakness.

Assessing Regardless of the situation, always begin with an assessment. During the assessment remain as open and objective as possible. Listen to the client carefully and observe behavioral cues. A pain assessment should be included in the initial **health history.** For the client currently experiencing acute, severe pain, abbreviate the assessment. Ask the following: (1) Where is the pain? (2) Is the pain in the same location as before? (3) How do you rate the pain on a scale of 0 to 10, with zero as the least severe? (4) What drug have you taken to reduce the pain, and how did it work?[6]

If the client's condition warrants, expand your assessment. Begin by asking, "What is the meaning of pain for you?" Clients who view pain as a spiritual challenge may be less likely to request pain relief than those who view pain as a physiologic problem. Individuals who have not experienced total pain relief for a long time may not recall what it means to be pain free. Their requests for pain relief may be grounded in a belief that they cannot be pain free. Other clients jump to negative conclusions when pain is present, believing that the presence of pain indicates a fatal disease or malignant growth.[7]

Determine the specific location of the pain. Use drawings that depict all sides of the human body to help the client localize pain sites (Fig. 19–2). Determine when the client first experienced the pain (onset of pain) and if the pain sensation has changed since that time. Ask how long the pain lingers (duration of pain) and if it recurs under the same circumstances.

Ask the client to describe the intensity, severity, and quality of the pain. Encourage clients who are able to provide a self-report of pain to use descriptive words to express the level of pain. Record the client's exact words (e.g., throbbing, sharp, knifelike, dull, ache). Clients with difficulty describing pain intensity present a challenge. For them the use of pain scales may be helpful. As indicated previously, you may ask the client to rank pain on a **numeric scale** between 0 and 10, with 0 equal to no pain and 10 equal to worst possible pain. A numeric scale can be developed into a **visual analog** for clients with difficulty with verbal communication. **Descriptive scales** may also be used. With descriptive scales, phrases are used to describe the pain experience (e.g., no pain, medium pain, or most severe pain possible). Figure 19–3 depicts a combination of a visual analog and a descriptive scale. Note that a vertical scale is used. Studies have suggested that vertical scales are easier to use than horizontal scales.[8] Clients unable to use numeric or descriptive scales can use the Wong-Baker Faces Pain Rating Scale. This scale uses a series of six faces with expressions that range from smiling to crying. The client points to the face that best correlates to the level of pain intensity experienced.[3,5]

Even when assessment tools are used, the client's self-report remains the most reliable description of pain intensity. This is true even if behavioral cues do not correlate with the pain level described. Objective signs such as grimacing or tachycardia may be absent in the client with chronic pain.[3] In addition, the use of sedatives, hypnotics, or other CNS depressants can dull affect.

Determine what, if any, pain-relief therapies have been used by the client. List what treatments, home remedies, or professional therapies have been tried. Include the results of

LOCATION: Client or nurse marks drawing to indicate pain site(s).

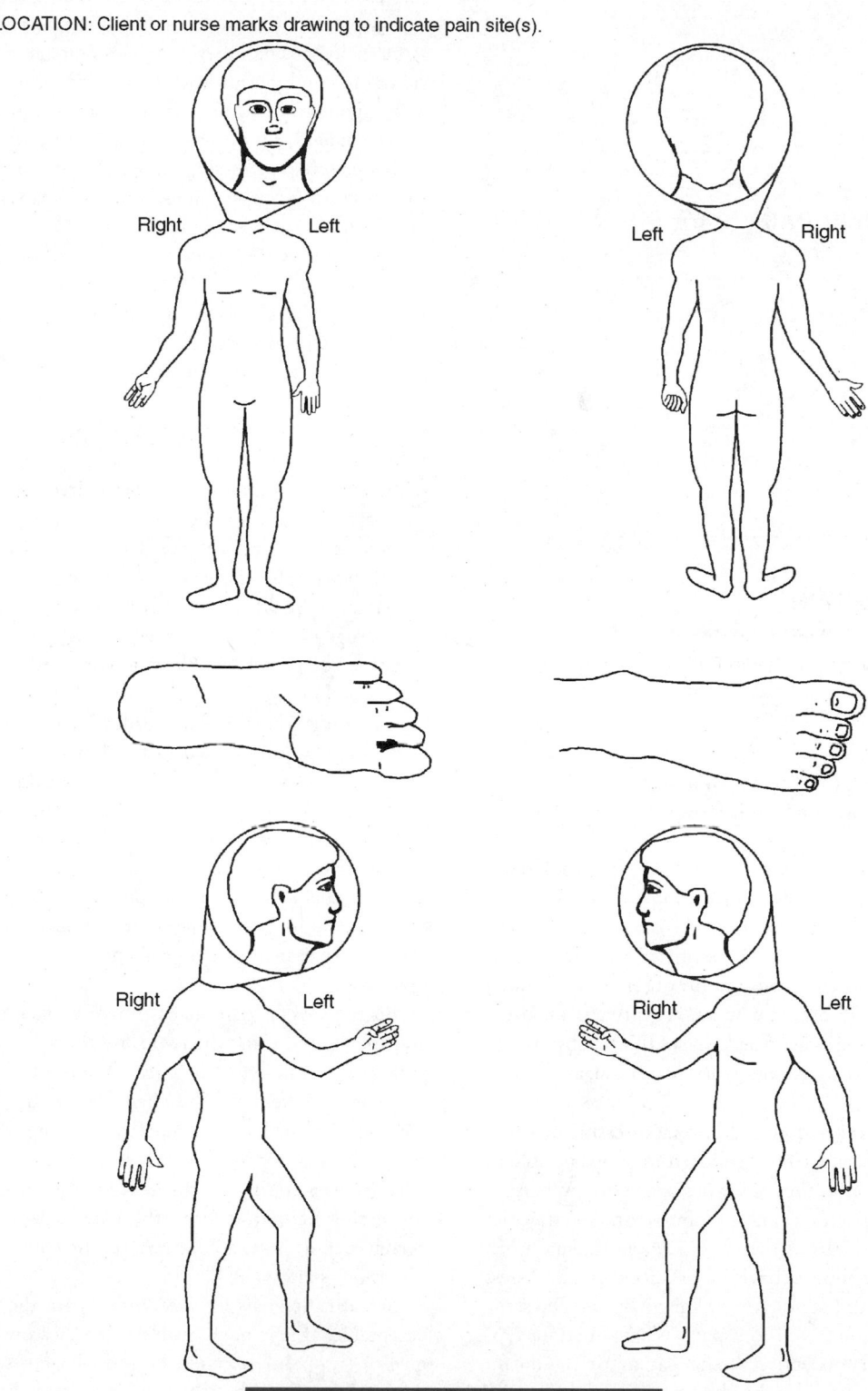

FIGURE 19–2   Human pain site locations.

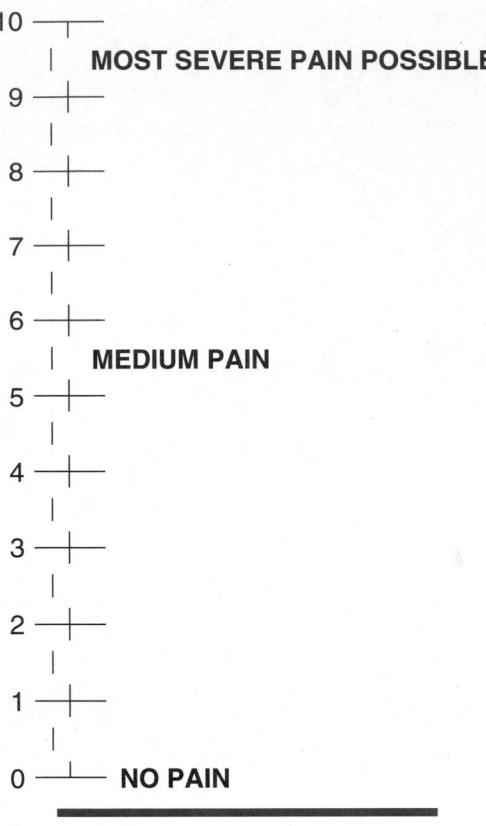

10 ── ┬
    | **MOST SEVERE PAIN POSSIBLE**
9 ─── ┼
    |
8 ─── ┼
    |
7 ─── ┼
    |
6 ─── ┼
    | **MEDIUM PAIN**
5 ─── ┼
    |
4 ─── ┼
    |
3 ─── ┼
    |
2 ─── ┼
    |
1 ─── ┼
    |
0 ── ┴ **NO PAIN**

FIGURE 19–3   Visual pain analog.

each treatment. Pay close attention to which therapies have been successful. Assess also for previous negative experiences with analgesics (i.e., undesired clinical responses or withdrawal from other opioids).[4]

Obtain **physical assessment** data to complete your database. Observe the client at rest and during routine activities such as ambulation, turning in bed, or morning care. Although vital sign changes are not specific or sensitive indicators of pain, these parameters can support observations. Watch for behavioral cues from clients who are cognitively impaired, psychotic, or emotionally disturbed. In addition, observe infants, children, elderly, or clients who do not speak English carefully.

Infants and **children** require additional assessment strategies. Although infants and young children may not be able to express pain levels clearly, they do experience pain. When assessing pain in this age group, tailor your assessment strategies to the individual child. Assess the child's developmental level, and determine if the child's behavior is age appropriate. Assess the child's language skills and use of imagination. Does the child have a long or short attention span? What situations typically cause the child anxiety? Ask the parent or significant other to provide terms used by the child to describe pain (e.g., owie, boo-boo, hurt). Obtain a description of how the child demonstrates pain. Does the child become restless, fussy, or agitated? Does the child cry or hold the involved body part? Some children experiencing pain cannot sleep, play, or participate in conversation.

Studies show that infants and neonates demonstrate physiologic changes when experiencing pain. For example, fluctuations in transcutaneous partial oxygen pressure occur during surgical procedures in this age group. Changes in heart rate and respiratory parameters may also appear in the child with acute pain. (Remember that physiologic changes must be viewed in combination with other data.) Children, like adults, who experience chronic pain may not demonstrate any physiologic changes if they have adapted to the stressful situation.[9]

Diagnosing   Nursing diagnoses for the client receiving analgesics are based on analysis of the database. Possible nursing diagnoses include the following:

- Pain (acute) related to ineffectiveness of opioid or nonopioid drug therapy.
- Chronic pain related to misconceptions about the use of opioids or other forms of pain relief.
- Anxiety related to undesired clinical response to drug therapy.
- Constipation related to decreased peristalsis associated with opioid drugs.
- High risk for injury related to impaired neurologic responses associated with opioid drugs.
- High risk for fluid volume deficit related to nausea, vomiting, and diarrhea associated with drug therapy.
- Ineffective breathing pattern related to effects of mu receptor drugs.
- Sensory or perceptual alterations related to drowsiness and mental clouding from opioid drugs.

Planning   Health care professionals often fear that the client will develop physical or psychologic dependence on opioids.[10] However, statistics do not support this concern. Opioid tolerance and dependence occur less than 1% of the time in clients who receive opioids for short-term postoperative use.[2] Psychologic dependence and addiction are unlikely events unless the client has experienced prior drug abuse.[4] Consequently, you must consider your own attitudes and beliefs before you try to plan care for a client who is scheduled to receive opioids.

Begin plans for pain management by determining what you and the client mean when you use the word *pain*. Establish a pain rating scale with the client; choose the scale that works best for the client. If the client can recall previous painful episodes, ask the client to practice by using the rating scale for those episodes. Determine if relaxation, distraction, or imagery is useful as a coping mechanism for the client. If so, practice the useful techniques with the client. Planning for physical agents such as heat, cold, massage, movement, rest, or immobilization is also valuable.

Set realistic goals for how much pain the client believes is acceptable. If it is not possible to eradicate the pain totally, a goal of "no pain" may not be realistic. For some clients pain relief might mean that the level is decreased to a more tolerable level or that the client may be able to engage in activities of daily living.

Managing pain among known or suspected substance-abuser clients is a major concern. Guidelines established by the American Pain Society are useful when dealing with this issue.

(Recommendations from these guidelines are summarized in the box.) As with any client, review the goals of treatment with these individuals. Emphasize what medical, ethical, and legal consequences will occur if drug abuse behaviors are identified.[4]

Ask these clients to agree to specific treatment guidelines. Provide clear instructions, preferably in writing, to help ensure client cooperation. Asking the client to sign or otherwise acknowledge the guidelines also aids cooperation—no assumptions are "left hanging." For the client receiving pain therapy in a clinical setting, tampering with drug infusion delivery systems, hoarding oral doses of opioid analgesics, or using nonprescribed narcotics (e.g., cocaine) must result in clearly stated consequences. Indicate to the client that drug toxicology screening will be used to confirm independent drug use. For the client in the community setting, include in the guidelines information about doses and frequency of administration. State how many days the drug will be used, and indicate how long the prescription should last. State in the guidelines that random urinary checks may be conducted. Specify that all opioid drug prescriptions must be obtained through one primary care provider. Attempts to falsify prescriptions or obtain them from another source are not allowed. If the client claims that the drug was stolen, make certain a police report with that information documented is available.[4]

The final aspect of planning is the establishment of expected outcomes. Expected outcomes for use of analgesics that affect the CNS include the following:
• Client reports acute pain is relieved.
• Client verbalizes control of chronic pain.
• Client reports that anxiety is reduced to a manageable level.
• Client returns to normal patterns of bowel elimination.
• Client remains free of injury.
• Client's fluid volume is maintained at a functional level as evidenced by adequate urinary output, moist mucous membranes, and good skin turgor.
• Client establishes an effective respiratory pattern.
• Client maintains usual level of consciousness.

Implementing Nonopioids and opioids are usually administered orally or parenterally. However, other routes are also used such as continuous intravenous (IV), subcutaneous (SC), or epidural infusion, drug implant systems, or intranasal administration. Regardless of the dosage form used or the route of administration, a team approach to pain management is most effective.

Nurse-administered analgesia The traditional method of treating pain is by nurse-administered analgesia. With this method pain medication is administered on a schedule or on an as-needed basis. The role of the nurse is to assess the client and decide the following:
• If the client is in pain
• The level or intensity of the pain
• Whether to provide analgesia
• How much to medicate
• If other adjuvant interventions are appropriate
Decisions made by the nurse should be based on verbal complaints from the client, behavior exhibited by the client, and the pathophysiology that exists.

USE OF OPIOIDS IN CHEMICALLY DEPENDENT CLIENTS

▶ Localize the cause of the pain. Is there an infectious process present? Is tissue ischemia causing higher pain levels? Has there been an adverse sequela to the treatment?

▶ Determine if substance abuse is current or from the past. Clients currently abusing a substance may require dosages higher than the usual recommended levels to achieve pain relief.

▶ Use the same guidelines for use of an opioid as used for a nonabusing client. Do not combine agonist-antagonist drugs with methadone; withdrawal may be precipitated. Titrate loading doses to achieve pain relief. Keep in mind that the client may be tolerant to opioids.

▶ Regular practices of offering nonopioid drugs for mild pain should be continued. Appropriate use of nonopioid drugs reduces the dosage requirement for opioid analgesia.

▶ Establish specific guidelines in the practice setting when opioid analgesics are used.

▶ Abide by the guidelines that have been set. Do not allow the drug abuser to manipulate the rules. For example, once tapering of the opioid doses has begun, avoid renegotiation unless other complications are present.

▶ Consult with other pain management team members for further assessment data and personal support.

Data from Agency for Health Care Policy and Research. (1992). *Acute pain management: Operative or medical procedures and trauma.* DHHS Pub. No. AHCPR 93-0032.

Nurse-administered analgesia frequently leads to undertreatment of the pain episode. Clients may minimize their pain or wait until the pain becomes unbearable before requesting pain relief to avoid receiving drugs. Some clients fail to verbalize pain needs because of attitudes expressed verbally or nonverbally by nurses. In some instances clients limit their requests for analgesias because of undesired responses to the drugs (e.g., nausea, vomiting, constipation). In addition, the nurse may not adequately assess the pain episode or may lack correct pharmacologic information about the analgesics.[11]

The intermittent dosing that occurs with nurse-administered analgesia causes wide swings in the blood level of the analgesic, resulting in sedation immediately after a dose and unacceptable pain levels preceding the next dose. Consistent, continuous analgesia produces the best pain relief. Controlled studies have shown that providing drugs around the clock in anticipation of pain recurrence actually reduces the amount of pain medication used.[12] However, if an around-the-clock dosage schedule is interrupted, it may cause a resurgence in the level of pain. In addition, it may take longer to regain pain control.[13]

Continuous infusion methods Patient-controlled analgesia (**PCA**) avoids some of the problems associated with nurse-administered analgesia. PCA is a method of drug delivery that permits the client to self-administer a precise dose of opioids as needed. As much as possible, the PCA allows the client to control pain therapy.

PCA is accomplished using a microprocessor-controlled infusion pump. An opioid, usually morphine, meperidine, or hydromorphone, is stored in a tamper-resistant device within the infusion pump. The infuser or infusion pump is attached to an intravenous infusion line.

After the primary care provider prescribes a specific amount of drug to be delivered at timed intervals, the microprocessor is programmed. On most PCA devices the following settings are possible: flow rate (dosage), flow type (continuous or intermittent), milligrams per dose, and time required between doses. Safe upper limits of dosages are programmed according to the total dose and time. Infusion pumps allow either a 1-hour or 4-hour cumulative dose limit. A lockout feature on the infusion pump prevents the client's receiving doses too often. In addition, most PCA devices record the number of injection attempts, the number of injections actually administered, and system problems or errors. Through evaluation of these data, the pain management team determines if the client requires higher dosages.

When the PCA is first started, a loading dose is administered by the nurse. This dose is usually one half of the recommended intramuscular (IM) dose of the drug. The PCA dosage is then titrated upward for satisfactory pain relief. For example, 5 mg of morphine may initially be ordered, then repeated every 5 minutes until the pain is relieved. The client must be instructed to press the hand-held button whenever definite discomfort is felt. If the button is depressed completely and the specified time period has elapsed, the infuser delivers a bolus of the drug. A typical on-demand dose is 1 mg of morphine every 6 minutes.

After a period of time, the client usually receives an oral analgesic. The oral drug should be administered around the clock to make the transition from PCA easier for the client. When the oral drug is started, the PCA doses must be titrated downward to achieve safe drug levels.[11,14]

🌿 NURSING RESEARCH

McKenzie, R., Rudy, T., & Ponter-Hammill, M. (1992). Side effects of morphine patient-controlled analgesia and meperidine patient-controlled analgesia: A follow-up of 500 patients. *AANA Journal, 60,* 282-286.

The purpose of the study was to evaluate pain relief and side effects of morphine sulfate and meperidine hydrochloride to determine their potential differences. Certified Registered Nurse Anesthetists (CRNAs) conducted a structure interview of 500 female patients 24 hours after major gynecologic, urologic, or breast surgery. Patients' responses on a four-point scale of *none, mild, moderate,* and *severe* were collected for pain intensity, degree of nausea, severity of vomiting and itchiness, and degree of sedation experienced since the operation.

No statistically significant differences for pain intensity, degree of nausea, severity and incidence of vomiting, or degree of sedation were found. However, a significant difference was found in the incidence rates of mild itchiness, which occurred more frequently in the morphine PCA group.

STUDENT ACTIVITIES

• Review five charts of clients receiving morphine PCA and five charts of clients receiving meperidine PCA. Note the number of complaints of pain, nausea, vomiting, sedation, and itchiness in each group.
• Interview nurses on surgical units and determine which drug, in their opinion, produces the most undesired responses.

Continuous subcutaneous infusion (CSI) is often used for chronic moderate-to-severe pain. This method of administration uses the technique of hypodermoclysis (introduction of fluids into subcutaneous tissues) to deliver opioid analgesics. Before the subcutaneous fluids are started, assess the client for renal or metabolic problems that might interfere with safe drug administration. If the client is receiving a restricted fluid diet, CSI may not be suitable. You also should assess the client for available subcutaneous sites. If there are inadequate sites, poor absorption and perfusion result.[16,17]

To administer opioids via the CSI route, a 25- to 27-gauge subcutaneous needle is inserted into subcutaneous tissue at a 30- to 45-degree angle. To facilitate assessment of the infusion site, the area is covered with a clear plastic dressing. The tubing is then attached to an infusion pump that provides continuous infusion and intermittent boluses. In addition, the infusion pump should have a lockout safety feature. The infusion pump is programmed so that no more than 1 to 2 ml/h is infused; higher rates usually result in decreased absorption. Infusion sites are rotated every 5 to 7 days. You should monitor the client carefully for respiratory depression when the treatment is first initiated and assess the infusion site for inflammation on a regular basis.[17]

Epidural infusion of opioids is used for acute postoperative pain, chronic pain, and pain associated with labor and delivery (see box). This route is contraindicated for clients with upper extremity or chest pain, pain above the level of T1. It is also not recommended for clients who have bleeding or clotting disorders, are receiving anticoagulant therapy, or have spinal abnormalities.

An epidural catheter is usually inserted by an anesthetist or anesthesiologist. Initially a needle is inserted into the lumbar interspace at the level that requires analgesia or at L4 or L5. A catheter is advanced through the needle to a point approximately 4 cm into the epidural space; the needle is then removed. The catheter is connected to an infusion pump for continuous infusion or capped for intermittent dosing.

Drugs most often used for epidural analgesia are morphine, fentanyl, meperidine, or hydromorphone. These opioids react with pain modulators in the spinothalamic tract and parts of the brain. Common undesired responses associated with epidural administration of opioids include pruritus around the face, head, and neck; nausea and vomiting; hypotension; respiratory depression; urinary retention; weakness; and numbness.

Recommended doses are much smaller than those administered intravenously. Therefore you must use caution when calculating dosages for epidural infusion. Monitor the insertion site for infection, leaking, or bleeding, and assess the client's intake and output for the first 24 hours. Do not administer other opioids or CNS depressants before consulting with the primary care provider. In addition, naloxone, an opioid antagonist, should be kept at the bedside.[3,4,18,19]

Life-span considerations Administration of opioids and nonopioid analgesics to neonates, infants, children, and the elderly requires special consideration. Undermedication of children's pain has resulted from inappropriate beliefs on the part of nurses and primary care providers about the amount of pain children experience.[9] Initial research in this area was conducted in 1968. After this early study, additional research on the undertreatment of pain in children was conducted throughout the 1970s and 1980s. However, these studies had little effect on the health care that professionals provided to children in pain. Finally the United States Congress commissioned a panel of health care experts to develop clinical practice guidelines for pain management across the life span. These guidelines were published in 1992 and provide an outline for effective management of acute pain.[20,21]

Children receiving opioids for an extended time can become tolerant of the dose. If higher doses are required, the drug should be titrated based on the results of the therapy, not necessarily staying within standard dosage parameters. The younger the client, the shorter is the duration of drug action.[5] Therefore recommended starting doses may not be sufficient.

As with adults, when you provide continuous, consistent pain medication, the drugs are more effective. Use the pain medication record, the child's report of pain levels, and the physiologic cause of pain (e.g., surgery, cancer, procedures) to assist with the choice of pain management.[9] If episodes of breakthrough pain (pain between scheduled drug doses) occur, immediate evaluation of the treatment plan is needed.[21]

Some children receiving intramuscular injections for pain may deny discomfort to avoid injections. If you suspect this is true, discuss with the primary care provider the possibility of using a PCA. Children as young as 7 years old are able to use this method successfully. If needed, the parent or nurse may activate the dosing. Use of intravenous, transmucosal, or oral drugs should also be considered.[9] Children who are unable to express pain should not be on an as-needed schedule.[21] These individuals are also candidates for other methods of treatment.

Other nondrug therapies effective with children include play and activity therapy, art, music, distraction, simple relaxation techniques, hypnosis, immobilization, or the use of hot or cold. Infants benefit from pacifiers, swaddling, holding, or rocking. Encourage parents or significnat others to hold, stroke, sing, hum, or read to the child. In addition, ask that the child's favorite toys be made available.[9]

Elderly clients are physiologically more sensitive to analgesics. Since the duration of analgesia from opiates increases with the client's age, these clients are more sensitive to higher peak responses and longer duration of pain relief. These individuals are also at greater risk for gastric and renal toxicity from nonsteroidal anti-inflammatory drugs (NSAIDs).[3,22]

Evaluating   To determine what changes are needed in the plan of care, compare the expected outcomes with current assessment data. Data are collected by direct observation of the client and from review of the client's medical record. All documentation of pain therapy must be consistent and comprehensive. Research has shown that using a pain flow sheet or pain treatment record is one of the most effective methods of achieving high-quality care of clients in pain. Allowing clients to quantify their pain subjectively provides information for selection of further pain relief measures.

NURSING RESEARCH

Faries, J., et al. (1991). Systematic pain records and their impact on pain control: A pilot study. *Cancer Nursing, 14,* 306-313.

The purpose of this pilot study was to examine the impact of using a systematic nursing pain assessment tool and pain flow sheet. Researchers questioned whether or not pain management would improve using standardized forms. Nurses on a hospital medical oncology unit participated in the study, along with a control group of 23 clients and a treatment group of 20 clients.

For the control group, nurses used routine charting of pain in the nurses' narrative notes. For subjects in the treatment group, nurses used standardized pain assessment and documentation forms. Results showed that the subjects in the treatment group reported significantly lower average pain intensity ratings on the third day of follow-up. Additionally, they reported a greater decrease in pain intensity from day 1 to day 3 as compared with the control group. The researchers concluded that systematic documentation is a valuable tool in facilitating effective pain management.

STUDENT ACTIVITIES

- Check the procedure manual in your assigned agency and validate the charting method used for pain assessment and treatment.
- Audit five charts and determine if the procedure for documentation is being followed.
- Interview a nurse who is familiar with the quality assurance program in your agency. Determine if the effectiveness of the current charting method has been studied.

In addition to using pain flow sheets or pain treatment records, use specific parameters when evaluating pain relief measures. If feasible, identify pain levels at specific time intervals (e.g., every hour or every 2 hours). Document the pain assessment, both initially and periodically, and the pain control measures used. Include events such as treatments or procedures that may have contributed to increased pain.[24]

Sedation scales should be a standard feature of pain therapy documentation. These scales reflect how easily or poorly the client is aroused. The client's respiratory rate, pulse, and blood pressure should be assessed at the same time as the level of consciousness. If the client frequently drifts off to sleep during conversation, the opioid's dose should be reduced. If the client is difficult to arouse, the opioid must be discontinued. In addition, if excessive sedation is present, naloxone, an opioid antagonist, may be administered.[4]

CONCEPT REVIEW

Effective pain therapy is a challenge for health care professionals. Many factors influence the client's and the nurse's response to pain episodes. These factors must be assessed and analyzed so that they do not interfere with the treatment plan.

Nonopioid drugs are usually administered orally or topically. Opioid drugs are administered orally, parenterally, and topically. A variety of delivery systems are available for use in pain therapy.

NONOPIOID ANALGESICS

The nonopioid analgesic category includes salicylates, NSAIDs, para-aminophenol derivatives, and anthranilic acids. Salicylates are discussed briefly in this chapter and presented in detail in Chapter 51 with the NSAIDs.

Salicylates

Salicylic acid is the parent derivative of this group of drugs. The prototype is acetylsalicylic acid (aspirin).

SALICYLATE PROTOTYPE
ACETYLSALICYLIC ACID

Acetylsalicylic acid is used alone for relief of mild pain or in combination with opioids for use with moderate-to-severe pain levels. Salicylates do not cause dependence and are used more widely than other categories of analgesics.

Acetylsalicylic acid and most nonopioid drugs inhibit the enzyme cyclooxygenase. Inhibition of this enzyme prevents the biosynthesis and release of prostaglandins. Prostaglandins, which do not normally exist in cells, are synthesized from phospholipids and released when there is trauma to the cell membrane. Prostaglandins in small amounts cause **hyperalgesia,** an increased sensitivity to stimulation that normally does not cause pain. However, increased levels of prostaglandins sensitize nociceptors of C-fibers by lowering their threshold to thermal, mechanical, and chemical stimuli.[1] In the presence of prostaglandins, pain mediators exert a greater effect on pain receptors such as bradykinin, histamine, and substance P. The result is modification of the nociceptive signal.[5]

Acetylsalicylic acid is associated with many undesired clinical responses. The most common responses involve the gastrointestinal (GI) system and include nausea, heartburn, epigastric discomfort, and anorexia. GI bleeding may result from inhibition of the synthesis of prostaglandins, which normally help protect the gastric mucosa. Other reactions include hives, rashes, angioedema, and prolonged bleeding time.[5,25]

DIFLUNISAL Diflunisal (Dolobid) is an analgesic, anti-inflammatory drug that is a derivative of salicylic acid. It is a peripherally acting nonnarcotic analgesic that inhibits prostaglandin synthesis, thus reducing mediators of pain. Although it does not directly affect the CNS, it does prevent the initiation of the nociceptor pain pathway.

Diflunisal is rapidly and completely absorbed after oral administration, with peak plasma concentrations occurring within 2 to 3 hours. The drug provides significant analgesia within 1 hour and maximum analgesia within 2 to 3 hours.[25]

Para-aminophenol Derivatives

The **para-aminophenol derivatives** are aminobenzenes derived from acetanilid. Phenacetin and acetaminophen are structurally similar compounds.[26]

PARA-AMINOPHENOL DERIVATIVE PROTOTYPE
ACETAMINOPHEN

Acetaminophen has been available as a nonprescription drug in the United States since 1955. As a nonprescription drug, it has numerous trade names (e.g., Anacin 3, Panadol, Tempra, Tylenol). In addition, acetaminophen is an ingredient in a variety of prescription drugs (e.g., acetaminophen; butalbital-acetaminophen; chlorzoxazone-acetaminophen; codeine phosphate).

Pharmacotherapeutics Acetaminophen is effective for relief of headache, dysmenorrhea, myalgias, and neuralgias. It is also used to reduce fevers.

Pharmacokinetics After ingestion acetaminophen is rapidly and completely absorbed. Acetaminophen is only slightly bound to protein. It reaches a peak plasma concentration in 30 to 60 minutes and has a plasma half-life of 2 hours. Acetaminophen is extensively metabolized by hepatic microsomal enzymes and is almost entirely excreted by the kidneys within 24 hours.[26]

Pharmacodynamics Acetaminophen is a weak prostaglandin inhibitor. Little is known of the mechanism of its analgesic properties, although its major actions are on the CNS rather than in the periphery.[26]

Pharmaceutics Acetaminophen is available in a variety of oral dosage forms, including tablets, capsules, solutions, effervescent granules, and wafers. It is also available in suppositories.

Undesired Clinical Responses Acetaminophen has few undesired clinical responses when administered for short time durations and at recommended doses. However, when it is taken in massive doses or for prolonged periods (daily or weekly for years), serious hepatic and renal side effects have been reported.[26]

Contraindications and Precautions Acetaminophen should be used with caution in individuals with preexisting renal or hepatic disorders.

Life-Span Considerations Acetaminophen should be used with caution during pregnancy. Although safe for short-term use, high daily dosages have been associated with anemia in the mother and kidney disease in the neonate. To date, no ill effects have been reported in nursing infants.

Table 19–1 contains additional information about nonopioid analgesics.

CONCEPT REVIEW

Nonopioid analgesic drug categories include salicylates, nonsteroidal anti-inflammatory drugs, para-aminophenol derivatives, and anthranilic acids.

Most nonopioid analgesics act by inhibiting the enzyme cyclooxygenase. Inhibition of this enzyme prevents the biosynthesis and release of prostaglandins. When present, prostaglandins sensitize nociceptors of C-fibers by lowering their threshold to thermal, mechanical, and chemical stimuli.

OPIOID ANALGESICS

Writings as far back as the third century BC refer to the use of opium. **Opium,** the Greek name for poppy juice, is obtained from the juice of the *Papaver somniferum* poppy. In 1806 the pure form of morphine was extracted from opium. Now more than 20 distinct alkaloids are known, including codeine and papaverine.[5]

Opioid analgesics interact with four major receptors, mu, kappa, sigma, and delta, that exist both within and outside the CNS. Effects mediated by **mu receptors** include analgesia, respiratory depression, and euphoria. **Kappa** and **delta receptors** also mediate analgesia. In addition kappa receptors mediate respiratory depression, miosis, and sedation. Activation of

sigma receptors produces hallucinations, dysphoria, seizures, and increased irritability.[26,27]

Based on how each opioid analgesic binds with receptors, it is classified as a full agonist, a partial agonist, or a mixed agonist-antagonist. **Full** or **pure opioid agonists,** including morphine and morphinelike preparations, bind to mu receptors to produce analgesia, sedation, constipation, or respiratory depression. **Partial agonists** have affinity for and stimulate physiologic activity at the same cell receptors as opioid agonists but produce only a submaximal body response. Partial agonists also stimulate physiologic activity at sigma receptors. **Mixed agonist-antagonists** block opioid effects at mu receptors. However, these drugs also act to produce effects that are morphinelike on kappa receptors.[4,5]

OPIOID ANALGESIC PROTOTYPE
MORPHINE SULFATE

Morphine sulfate, a Schedule II Drug under the United States Controlled Substance Act, is the principal opium alkaloid. Its use was not controlled until early in the twentieth century when it was noted that its effects led to compulsive drug use and addiction.

Morphine is readily absorbed from the GI tract and subcutaneous and muscle tissue. It is also absorbed through the nasal and lung mucosa and the skin. Additionally, morphine is administered intravenously, epidurally, and intrathecally. Because morphine's action is clinically superior, it is the standard against which new analgesics are measured. Using morphine 10 mg IM or SC and morphine 30 mg orally as the standard, equianalgesic doses are calculated to determine the strength of other opioids (Table 19–2).

Pharmacotherapeutics Morphine sulfate is used primarily to relieve moderate-to-severe pain. If used preoperatively, its effect is to reduce the client's anxiety, assist with induction of anesthesia, and reduce the required dose of anesthesia during surgery. It is considered the drug of choice for clients with pain from myocardial infarction, pulmonary edema, and dyspnea from acute left ventricular failure.[5]

Pharmacokinetics Absorption depends on the route of administration. Morphine ingested orally is generally absorbed in 1½ to 2 hours. After absorption it makes a first pass through the liver before reaching systemic circulation. In the liver extensive drug metabolism occurs. Consequently, oral doses must be larger than parenteral doses to produce equivalent analgesic effects. Oral dosage forms are adjusted to provide steady, long-lasting pain relief. This is the easiest form for long-term use in the home.[5] Absorption after IM or SC injection occurs in 30 to 60 minutes.

Distribution of morphine occurs quickly. After administration morphine rapidly leaves the blood and enters the kidneys, lungs, liver, and spleen. It enters the skeletal muscle in smaller proportions. However, to be effective, morphine must cross the blood-brain barrier and enter the CNS. Since the drug is not very lipid soluble, it does not cross the barrier easily. Therefore only a small fraction of the administered dose of morphine reaches opiate receptor sites.[5,26] Other opioids that are more lipid soluble such as codeine, heroin, and methadone cross at higher rates.[3]

TABLE 19–1
Nonopioid Analgesics

Drug	Dosage and Route of Administration	Nursing Considerations
SALICYLATES: DIFLUNISAL (Dolobid) HOW SUPPLIED Tablets: 250, 500 mg	***Mild-to-Moderate Pain*** ADULTS Initial dose: 1000 mg, then 500 mg q8-12h Maximum dose: 1500 mg/24 h ***Osteoarthritis and Rheumatoid Arthritis*** ADULTS 500-1000 mg in two divided doses	***Assess*** Determine if client is pregnant; diflunisal is classified as a Pregnancy Category C drug. ***Implement*** 500 mg of diflunisal is comparable to 650 mg of acetylsalicylic acid. Initial large dose shortens length of time to onset of action. Administer drug with 250 ml of water or milk or administer with food. Do not crush tablets. Advise client that tablets must not be chewed. Observe for increased plasma levels of acetaminophen, oral anticoagulants, hydrochlorothiazide, or indomethacin when administered concurrently with diflunisal. Assess for peripheral edema in clients with compromised cardiac function. Assess for hemorrhagic states or gastric irritation. ***Monitor*** Monitor bleeding time and liver function studies. Monitor for undesired clinical responses (e.g., nausea, dyspepsia, GI pain, diarrhea, constipation, flatulence). ***Evaluate*** Evaluate for peak effect in 2-3 h. Plasma half-life is 8-12 h.
PARA-AMINOPHENOL DERIVATIVES: ACETAMINOPHEN HOW SUPPLIED Tablets: 160, 325, 500, 650 mg Chewable tablets: 80 mg Capsules: 500 mg Oral solution: 100 mg/ml Oral liquid: 160 mg/5 ml, 500 mg/15ml Elixir: 120–325 mg/5 ml Wafers: 120 mg Effervescent granules: 80 mg Suppositories: 120, 125, 300, 325 650 mg	***Mild-to-Moderate Pain*** ADULTS Oral: 325–650 mg q4-6h or 1g t.i.d. or q.i.d. Maximum dose: 4000 mg/24 h CHILDREN 10-15 mg/kg q4-6h	***Assess*** Assess for pain levels. Assess for hypersensitivity to acetaminophen. ***Implement*** 650 mg of acetaminophen is equianalgesic to 650 mg of acetylsalicylic acid or 30-60 mg of codeine. Minimal toxic dose is 1000 mg or 140 mg/kg. Minimal lethal dose is 1500 mg or 200 mg/kg. Peak hepatotoxicity occurs 72-96 h after overdose. Oral *N*-acetylcysteine is specific antidote for toxicity. ***Monitor*** Monitor for undesired clinical responses. ***Evaluate*** Evaluate for peak effect in 30 min to 1 h. Plasma half-life is 2-3 h.

As indicated previously, onset of action and duration of action depend on the route of administration. Onset of action of orally administered morphine is highly individualized; duration of action is approximately 4 to 12 hours. Onset of action after IM or SC administration occurs in 10 to 30 minutes; duration of action is 4 to 5 hours. Peak action after an IV bolus occurs in 15 to 30 minutes. Intrathecal or epidural administration of opioids produces profound analgesia with very small doses. These effects can last up to 24 hours.[5,25,27]

Biotransformation of morphine occurs in the liver; most **excretion** occurs in the kidneys. Morphine is excreted in the urine in a modified form called *morphine-6-glucuronide*. A small percentage of morphine is excreted in the feces. Only traces of morphine are found in the body after 48 hours.[5]

TABLE 19–1 *Continued*
Nonopioid Analgesics

Drug	Dosage and Route of Administration	Nursing Considerations
ANTHRANILIC ACIDS: MEFENAMIC ACID (Ponstel) **HOW SUPPLIED** Capsules: 250 mg	**Mild-to-Moderate Pain** ADULTS Initial dose: 500 mg, then 250 mg q6h as needed	**Assess** Assess for hypersensitivity to nonsteroidal anti-inflammatory drugs. Determine if client is pregnant; mefenamic acid is classified as Pregnancy Category C drug. Determine age of client. Safety and efficacy in children <14 y have not been established. **Implement** 250 mg of mefenamic acid is equianalgesic to 650 mg of acetylsalicylic acid. Administer with food or milk to decrease gastric distress. **Monitor** Monitor length of time client receives mefenamic acid. In United States use is approved for only 7 d. Monitor for undesired responses (e.g., nausea, vomiting, severe diarrhea, peptic ulceration, CNS disturbances, blood dyscrasia). **Evaluate** Evaluate for peak effect in 2-4 h. Plasma half-life is 2 h.
MECLOFENAMATE SODIUM (Meclomen) **HOW SUPPLIED** Capsules: 50, 100 mg	**Mild-to-Moderate Pain** ADULTS 50 mg q4-6h Maximum dose: 400 mg/24 h	Same as mefenamic acid with the following exceptions and additions. **Monitor** Monitor long-term drug therapy with CBC and renal and hepatic function studies. **Evaluate** Evaluate peak effect in 30 min to 1 h. Plasma half-life is 1-2 h.

Pharmacodynamics Morphine provides analgesia by binding preferentially to the mu and delta receptors. Morphine targets areas involved with regulation of pain perception, respiration, and affective behaviors. Effects of this interaction are analgesia, drowsiness, changes in mood, respiratory depression, decreased GI motility, nausea, vomiting, and alterations on the endocrine and autonomic nervous systems.[5]

Physiologic Effects of Morphine on Various Body Systems Morphine affects several body systems. For example, it depresses respirations by decreasing the body's responsiveness to CO_2. Depression of respiration is considered a serious predictable, dose-related side effect of morphine and all opioid agonists.[28] Morphine also decreases or abolishes the cough reflex. Most opioids, including morphine, cause constriction of the pupil. Pupillary constriction is the result of central effects on the oculomotor nucleus since morphine has minimal direct effects on pupillary muscles. Because of its stimulation of the chemoreceptor trigger zone in the medulla, morphine induces nausea and vomiting in some individuals. Morphine also causes decreased propulsive activity in the small and large intestines. It increases biliary tract tone and pressure and can induce biliary colic.[26,27] Figure 19–4 illustrates some of the effects of morphine on body systems.

Pharmaceutics Morphine is manufactured by a variety of drug companies. It is available in tablet, solution, and elixir for oral administration. Tablets may be administered by rectum, stoma, or vagina. A hydrogel suppository is also available for rectal administration. Sterile parenteral solutions are available for SC, IM, IV, or intraspinal delivery. Drug doses are titrated to effect since a wide range of doses is required.

Undesired Clinical Responses The major side effects of morphine are apparent in the CNS. Morphine produces dizziness, mental clouding, dysphoria, and, in some instances, delirium. Perhaps the most serious undesired response is respiratory depression. The occurrence of respiratory depression varies with the route of administration. After an IV injection, depressant effects begin in approximately 7 minutes; effects begin approximately 30 minutes after an IM injection and up to 90 minutes after a SC injection. With all of these routes, the depressant effect may persist for 4 to 5 hours.

Morphine also causes nausea, vomiting, and constipa-

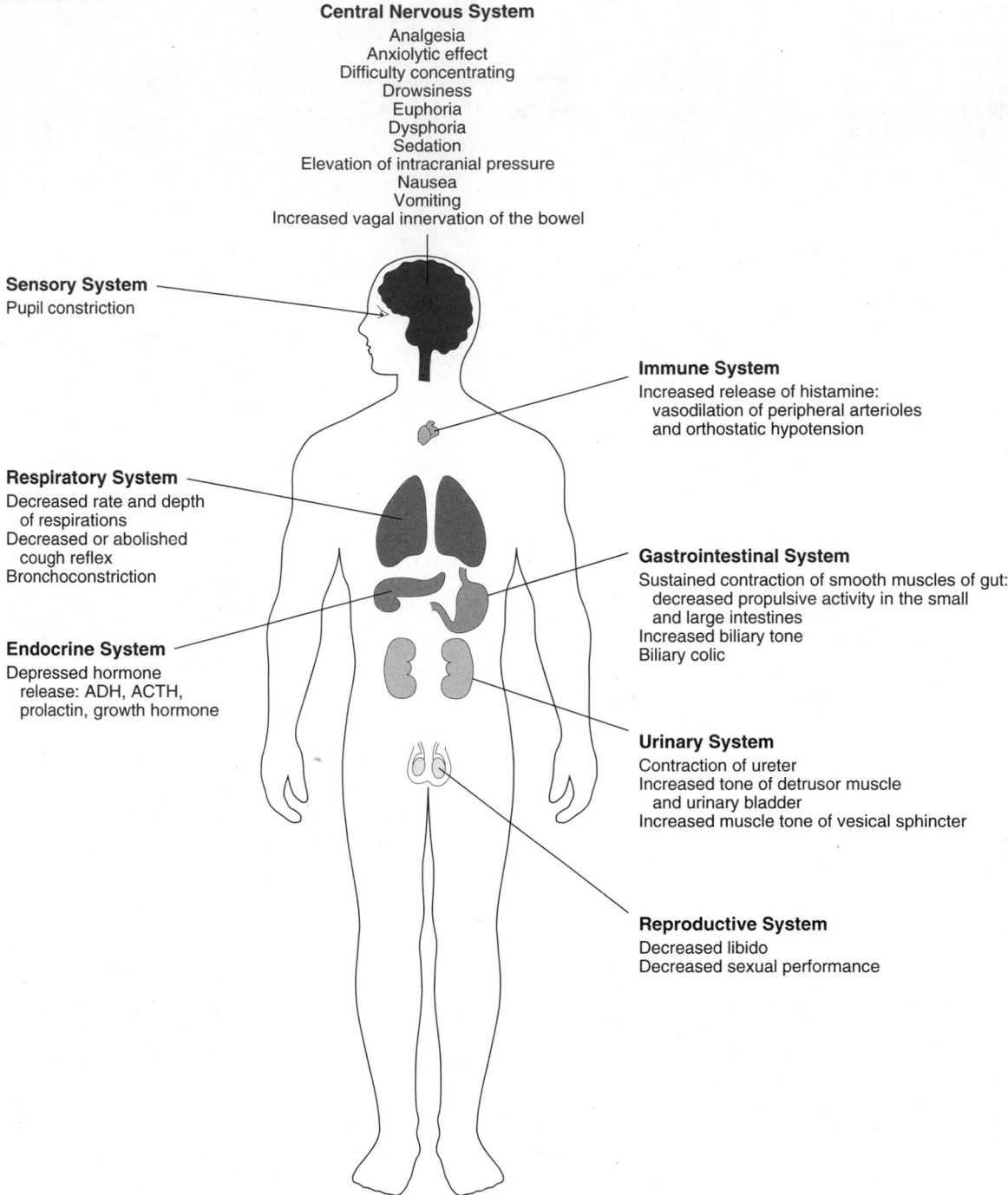

Central Nervous System
Analgesia
Anxiolytic effect
Difficulty concentrating
Drowsiness
Euphoria
Dysphoria
Sedation
Elevation of intracranial pressure
Nausea
Vomiting
Increased vagal innervation of the bowel

Sensory System
Pupil constriction

Immune System
Increased release of histamine:
   vasodilation of peripheral arterioles
   and orthostatic hypotension

Respiratory System
Decreased rate and depth
   of respirations
Decreased or abolished
   cough reflex
Bronchoconstriction

Gastrointestinal System
Sustained contraction of smooth muscles of gut:
   decreased propulsive activity in the small
   and large intestines
Increased biliary tone
Biliary colic

Endocrine System
Depressed hormone
   release: ADH, ACTH,
   prolactin, growth hormone

Urinary System
Contraction of ureter
Increased tone of detrusor muscle
   and urinary bladder
Increased muscle tone of vesical sphincter

Reproductive System
Decreased libido
Decreased sexual performance

FIGURE 19–4   Physiologic effects of morphine on various body systems.

tion. Clients receiving morphine sometimes report an increased sensitivity to pain once the actions of the drug wear off. Uncommon allergic reactions include urticaria and skin rashes. It is possible for health care personnel to develop contact dermatitis.[5]

Other undesired clinical responses to morphine and other opioid analgesics are tolerance and physical and psychologic dependence. *Tolerance* means that the current dose is not adequate to maintain the original effect and usually occurs when opioid analgesics are used for chronic pain treatment. Additionally, the client develops a tolerance to undesired clinical responses associated with

the drug, making it possible to administer a dose that far exceeds standard limits.[3] Morphine also produces a psychologic craving and a physical dependence that may result in addiction. Substance misuse, abuse, and addiction are discussed in more detail in Chapter 12.

Opioid poisoning is also possible. Acute poisoning with morphine and other opioids occurs with overdoses. Signs and symptoms of poisoning are predictable and characteristically include coma, pinpoint pupils, and respiratory depression, which frequently are called *the triad*. Treatment consists of support of respiratory and cardiovascular functions plus the administration of the antagonist naloxone. (Naloxone is discussed in a later section of this chapter.)[26]

Contraindications and Precautions Use of opioid analgesics is contraindicated in individuals with previous episodes of hypersensitivity to opioids and in clients with head injuries or increased intracranial pressure. Because of morphine's pharmacokinetic properties, it should not be used for clients with severe liver and kidney impairment. It also should not be administered to clients with reduced blood volume.

Since morphine causes increased biliary tract tone and can produce biliary colic, it should not be administered to clients after biliary tract surgery. It is also contraindicated for clients after surgical anastomosis of the GI tract.[1,3,25]

Drug-Drug Interactions A mixed agonist-antagonist opioid should never be administered to a client who is currently receiving a pure mu agonist such as morphine. Doing so may precipitate withdrawal-like symptoms. An additive sedative effect occurs when opioids and psychotropic drugs are combined. Alcohol, barbiturates, and other CNS depressants should be avoided.

Administration of morphine and other opioid analgesics concurrently with anticholinergic drugs can intensify drug-induced constipation and urinary retention. Antihypertensive drugs or other drugs that lower the blood pressure can compound the drug-induced hypotension.

Use caution when offering any opioid analgesic to a client with a history of drug abuse. Although it may be done safely, the client must agree to more specific parameters regarding use during acute pain episodes. (See box p. 171.)

Life-Span Considerations Use of morphine during delivery can suppress uterine contractions and produce respiratory depression in the neonate. Morphine should not be administered during labor and delivery of a premature infant. It also should not be administered to the infant after delivery. For the critically ill elderly client, it may be necessary to prescribe 50% of the usual adult dose or extend the dosing interval.

Specific Drug-Related Nursing Considerations Determine the client's respiratory rate before administering morphine or any opioid analgesic. Clients with respiratory diseases are especially sensitive to respiratory depression and must be monitored carefully. Since morphine causes cough suppression, instruct the client to deep-breathe and cough at regular intervals. Also determine the lung status by auscultating for rales routinely.

Teach the client that drowsiness is a common side effect. Instruct the client not to drive or operate heavy machinery after receiving a dose. Inform the client that light-headedness and dizziness are possible indications of orthostatic hypotension. Instruct the client to sit or lie down if these reactions occur. Inform the client to move slowly when changing positions from a supine or seated position to an upright position to minimize the occurrence of hypotension. Hospitalized clients may require assistance with ambulation.

The diet of a client receiving long-term oral opioid therapy should include fiber to counteract the drug's effects on GI function. Help the client choose foods that are tasty and provide necessary nutrients. Monitor bowel function carefully. Note frequency and characteristics of stools, and auscultate bowel sounds at regular intervals. Consult with the primary care provider about need for a stool softener or laxative.

Since morphine can cause urinary hesitancy and retention, tell the client to void every 4 hours. Monitor intake and output and palpate the lower abdomen every 4 hours for bladder distention. Clients with prosthetic hypertrophy require careful monitoring.

MISCELLANEOUS DRUGS IN CATEGORY

Although many new pure opioid analgesics have been developed, none of them is superior to morphine. All of the drugs are essentially equal to morphine in regard to analgesic effect, abuse liability, and potential for undesired clinical responses. Table 19–2 summarizes equianalgesic doses for opioid analgesics.

Meperidine Meperidine is one of the most frequently prescribed opioids for moderate-to-severe pain. It has almost all of the major properties described previously for morphine.

TABLE 19–2
Equianalgesic Doses for Opioids[3,4,13]

Drug	Approximate Equianalgesic Dose (mg), Oral	Approximate Equianalgesic Dose (mg), Parenteral	Conversion Factor: IM, SC, IV to PO
OPIOID AGONISTS			
Morphine	30*	10	3
Hydromorphone	7.5	1.5	5
Levorphanol	4	2	2
Meperidine HCl	300	75	4
Codeine	200(NR)	120	1.6
Oxycodone	30	—	—
Methadone	20	10	2
MIXED AGONIST-ANTAGONIST			
Pentazocine	150	30	2.5

NR = Not recommended.

*Equianalgesic dose may not be suggested initial dose.

INSTRUCTIONS: To convert from one drug to another, determine the equianalgesic dose compared to morphine 10 mg, IM, SC, IV, or 30 mg PO. The new drug is calculated based on how it measures against that standard and compares to the dose that client is currently receiving. For example, to convert from morphine 60 mg PO to hydromorphone parenteral, calculate: $60 = 30x$, $2 = x$, $(2)(1.5) = 3$, the equianalgesic dose of hydromorphone.

Meperidine is approximately one sixth as potent as morphine (e.g., 75 mg IM of meperidine produces analgesia equivalent to 10 mg of morphine). However, in sufficient doses it produces equivalent analgesia. In addition, in equianalgesic doses meperidine is shorter acting, less constipating, and without pupillary constriction and cough suppressant activity.[26]

Undesired clinical responses of meperidine are similar to those of morphine and include respiratory depression, mental clouding, dizziness, nausea, vomiting, dysphoria, and urinary retention. Phenytoin enhances the biotransformation of meperidine, causing faster elimination of the drug and requiring higher meperidine doses for effectiveness. Meperidine may interact with MAO inhibitors to cause blood pressure changes similar to those of malignant hypertension. Additionally, the combination can cause excitation, delirium, hyperpyrexia, and convulsions.

Meperidine is available in tablets and a syrup for oral administration and in sterile solution for parenteral use. Meperidine's duration of action is approximately 2 to 4 hours. It is metabolized in the liver to normeperidine. Normeperidine is twice as toxic as meperidine and has a longer half-life.
With chronic administration, normeperidine can accumulate. Therefore meperidine should not be used for long-term therapy.[26]

Methadone Methadone is a synthetic, strong opioid agonist drug with effects similar to those of morphine. It is used as an analgesic, for treatment of acute withdrawal after termination of opioid therapy, and for long-term management of opioid dependence.

Methadone is available in tablet form for oral administration and as a sterile solution for IM and SC injection. It has a long duration of action and repeated dosing can result in accumulation.[26]

Codeine Codeine is considered a moderate-to-strong opioid agonist. The effects of codeine are similar to those of morphine. Codeine is usually administered orally, although parenteral (IV, IM, or SC) administration is possible.

Oral administration of codeine is used to treat mild-to-moderate pain and as a cough suppressant. Low doses of codeine are frequently combined with acetylsalicylic acid and other nonsteroidal anti-inflammatory compounds for management of pain associated with dental or orthopedic procedures. (Combinations of opioid and nonopioid analgesics are numerous. Some of the more commonly prescribed drug combinations are listed in Table 19–3.) When administered alone, codeine is classified under Schedule II of the Controlled Substance Act. The combination drug preparations are classified under Schedule III. Undesired clinical responses associated with codeine are essentially the same as those described for morphine. With oral doses, the most common complaint is constipation.[5,26]

Propoxyphene Propoxyphene (Darvon, Dolene) has analgesic effects approximately equal to those of acetylsalicylic acid; thus it is used to treat mild-to-moderate pain. It does not have the antitussive quality of some opioid analgesics.

TABLE 19–3

Frequently Prescribed Opioid and Nonopioid Drug Combinations

Drug Combinations	How Supplied
Acetaminophen with codeine*	7.5, 15, 30, or 60 mg codeine with 300 mg acetaminophen
Phenaphen-650 with codeine	30 mg codeine with 650 mg acetaminophen
Aspirin with codeine	15, 30, or 60 mg codeine with 325 mg aspirin
Fiorinal with codeine capsules	7.5, 15, or 30 mg codeine with 325 mg aspirin, 40 mg caffeine, and 50 mg butalbital
Lortab, Lortab 5, Lortab 7 tablets	2.5, 5, or 7 mg hydrocodone bitartrate with 325 mg acetaminophen
Vicodin tablets	5 mg hydrocodone bitartrate with 500 mg acetaminophen
Percodan tablets	4.5 mg oxycodone HCl and 0.38 mg oxycodone terephthalate with 325 mg aspirin
Mepergan Fortis capsules	50 mg meperidine with 25 mg promethazine HCl
Darvocet-N 50 or 100 tablets	50 or 100 mg propoxyphene napsylate with 650 mg acetaminophen
Percocet tablets	5 mg oxycodone HCl and 325 mg acetaminophen

*Various trade names with this combination include Tylenol with codeine, Myapap and codeine, Phenaphen with codeine.

Propoxyphene is commonly administered in combination with acetylsalicylic acid, acetaminophen, and caffeine.

Although frequently considered devoid of serious side effects, propoxyphene has the potential for producing acute and chronic toxicity. In acute overdoses it can be rapidly fatal. It is second only to barbiturates as a prescription drug associated with drug fatalities. Clients must be educated about the potential for abuse and potential drug-drug interactions.[26] Propoxyphene is classifed as a Pregnancy Category B drug; if used at term or for prolonged therapy, it is considered a Category D drug.

Fentanyl, alfentanil, and sufentanil These drugs are strong opioid analgesics used primarily for induction and maintenance of surgical anesthesia. They have rapid onset of action and relatively short duration of action. These drugs are discussed in more detail in Chapter 24.

Miscellaneous opioid analgesics Hydrocodone (e.g., Vicodin) and **oxycodone** (Percodan, Percocet) have analgesic properties similar to those of codeine. Both drugs are administered orally to relieve mild-to-moderate pain. Hydrocodone is available only in combination with aspirin or acetaminophen; it is classified under Schedule III. Oxycodone, whether administered alone or in combination with aspirin or acetaminophen, is classified under Schedule II.[25,26] See Table 19–4 for additional information about opioid analgesics.

TABLE 19–4
Opioid Agonists: Prototype and Major Drugs in Category

Drug	Dosage and Route of Administration	Nursing Considerations

MORPHINE SULFATE
  (Oramorph SR, MS Contin, Roxanol SR, Roxanol 100)
HOW SUPPLIED
Tablets: 15, 30 mg
Sustained-release tablets: 30, 60, 100 mg
Oral solution: 20 mg/ml, 100 mg/5 ml alcohol free
Injectable: 0.5 mg/ml up to 15 mg/ml in syringes, vials, and ampules
	Dosage is highly individualized and based on age, body weight, pain intensity, and vital sign status. Doses listed are standardized beginning doses. Adult doses are referenced for individuals >50 kg of body weight.
	ADULTS
	Oral: 15-30 mg q4h as needed.
	    Sustained-release tablet: 30 mg q8-12h
	SC, IM: 10 mg q3-4h
	IV
	    Bolus—2.5-15 mg in 4-5 ml of water for injection; administer over 4 to 5 min
	    PCA (concentration of 1.0 mg/ml): initial dose, 1.0 mg after loading dose; dose range, 0.5-2.5 mg; lockout range, 5-10 min
	    CSI (concentration of 10-50 mg/ml): dose titrated from 24-h morphine requirement; starting dose, 10 mg/h; infusion rate, 0.70-1.30 ml/h
	Epidural: initial injection of 5 mg; if relief not achieved in 1 h, increment doses of 1-2 mg may be administered. Do not exceed 10 mg during first 24 h; for continuous infusion, 2-4 mg/24 h recommended
	Intrathecal: Usually one-tenth of epidural dose; a single injection of 0.2-1 mg may provide relief for 24 h
	Rectal: 10-20 mg q3-4h
	ELDERLY ADULTS
	Lower dosages are required in the elderly; titrate for pain relief
	CHILDREN
	Oral: 0.3 mg/kg q3-4h
	SC, IM, IV: 0.1-0.2 mg/kg q3-4h
		Assess
		Obtain baseline respiration, pulse, and blood pressure.
		Determine if client is pregnant. During pregnancy drug is classified as a Pregnancy Category B drug. At term morphine is classified as a Pregnancy Category D drug.
		Assess for current status of chemical dependency. Schedule II drugs have high abuse potential.
		
		Implement
		Do not mix parenteral solution with diazepam, meperidine, phenobarbital, sodium bicarbonate, or thiopental.
		If mixed with atropine, chlorpromazine, hydroxyzine, or scopolamine, administer within 15 min.
		Do not crush or allow client to chew sustained-release tablet.
		Have opioid antagonist immediately available, especially with IV use.
		Anticipate that a continuous IV infusion of naloxone may be prescribed for concurrent use with intrathecal therapy.
		To facilitate rectal administration of tablets, place tablets in a soluble medium or capsule.
		
		Monitor
		Monitor respiratory status.
		Monitor urinary output.
		Monitor for undesired clinical responses such as sedation, drowsiness, respiratory depression, euphoria, hypotension, constipation.
		Monitor for opioid poisoning—the triad of coma, pinpoint pupils, and depressed respirations.
		
		Evaluate
		Evaluate for peak effect in 30 min to 1 h.
		Plasma half-life is 2-3 h.
		See "morphine" with the following additions or exceptions.

Codeine (codeine sulfate, codeine phosphate) HOW SUPPLIED Codeine phosphate Soluble tablets: 30, 60 mg Injection: 30-60 mg/ml in syringes and single and multidose vials Codeine sulfate Soluble tablets: 15, 30, 60 mg Tablets: 15, 30, 60 mg	ADULTS Oral: 15–60mg q4–6h IV, SC, IM: 15–60mg q4–6h CHILDREN Oral: 0.5mg/kg q4–6h SC, IM: 0.5mg/kg q4–6h	**Assess** Determine if client is pregnant. Codeine is classified as Pregnancy Category C drug. With prolonged use or at term, codeine is considered a Pregnancy Category D drug. **Implement** 60 mg of codeine is equivalent to 650 mg of acetylsalicylic acid or acetaminophen. Elderly clients have increased sensitivity to drug. **Evaluate** Evaluate for onset of drug in 30 min. Peak effect is in 45-90 min. Plasma half-life is 3-4 h.

Table continued on following page.

TABLE 19–4 *Continued*
Opioid Agonists: Prototype and Major Drugs in Category

Drug	Dosage and Route of Administration	Nursing Considerations
		See morphine with the following additions and exceptions.
Meperidine hydrochloride		**Assess**
(Demerol HCl, Pethadol)	**ADULTS**	Assess clients for renal function, sickle cell disease, or CNS disease. Such clients are at high risk of meperidine-induced toxicity.
HOW SUPPLIED	Oral: not recommended	
Tablets: 50, 100 mg scored and unscored tablets	IM: 50–150 mg q3-4h	Determine if client is pregnant. Meperidine is classified as Pregnancy Category B drug. If use is long term or with high doses at delivery, it is considered a Pregnancy Category D drug.
Syrup: 50 mg/5 ml	IV	
Injection:	PCA (concentration of 10 mg/ml): starting dose, 10 mg after loading dose; dose range, 5-25 mg; usual lockout range, 5-10 min	**Implement**
0 mg/ml in syringes, ampules, and multidose vials		Use IM route in preference over SC since drug is irritating to tissues.
	Epidural: 10-40 mg bolus; infuse at rate of 5-20 mg/h	
	CHILDREN	Do not mix meperidine and barbiturate solutions.
	Oral: not recommended	**Monitor**
	IM, IV, SC: 1–1.5 mg/kg per dose q3–4h; max: 100mg	Drug should be discontinued after 48 h or at doses >600 mg/24 h.
		Evaluate
		Evaluate for onset of pain relief in 10-15 min.
		Peak effect of drug is in 30-60 min.
		Plasma half-life is 3-4 h.
Fentanyl	**ADULTS**	**Assess**
(Sublimaze, Duragesic, Oralet)	Parenteral: 0.05-0.1 mg q1-2h	Assess for hypersensitivity to adhesives if transdermal delivery system is selected.
HOW SUPPLIED	Transdermal: highly individualized; apply 25 μg as initial dose; if client has preexisting opioid tolerance, calculate 24-h morphine dose and initiate fentanyl transdermal using the recommended dose and titrate upward	
Injection: 0.05 mg/ml in ampules and multidose vials		**Implement**
Transdermal system: 25 μg (2.5 mg), 50 μg (5 mg), 75 μg (7.5 mg), 100 μg (10 mg) in sealed patch	Do not increase more frequently than q3d after initial dose	Fentanyl transdermal is not recommended for postoperative pain.
Lozenges (Oralet): 200, 300, 400 μg	Epidural	Fentanyl intrathecal has limited efficacy for postoperative analgesia because of its short duration of action after a single-dose bolus.
	Bolus dose: 50-200 μg	
	Infusion rate: 50-100 μg/h	Transdermal fentanyl is approximately equianalgesic to 30 mg of sustained morphine q8h.
	CHILDREN	Place transdermal patch on portion of upper torso. Select skin that is not irritated.
	Oralet used for preoperative and postoperative pain	Change patch q72h.
		Store unused transdermal systems out of reach of children.
		Discard used systems safely.
		Monitor
		Monitor for fever, which increases rate of transdermal drug absorption.
		Monitor for breakthrough pain with patch.
		Evaluate
		Onset of pain relief for parenteral doses is 10 min.
		Onset of pain relief with oralet is 20-40 min.
		Peak effect of parenteral doses is 20-30 min.
		Plasma half-life of fentanyl is 3-4 h.

CONCEPT REVIEW

Most opioids are potent analgesics. The prototype for this group is morphine. Morphine produces most of its effects by acting on the mu receptors in the CNS. However, morphine produces physiologic effects on many other body systems. These effects are often considered predictable, dose-related side effects.

The most serious undesired clinical response associated with morphine therapy is respiratory depression. When morphine overdose occurs, acute or opiate poisoning develops. This condition produces a triad of signs and symptoms: respiratory depression, pinpoint pupils, and coma.

MIXED OPIOID AGONIST-ANTAGONISTS

There are five agonist-antagonist drugs: pentazocine, nalbuphine, butorphanol, dezocine, and buprenorphine. All of these drugs except buprenorphine act as antagonists at mu receptors and agonists at kappa receptors. These drugs have a low potential for abuse, produce less respiratory depression, and have less powerful analgesic actions. The prototype for the group is pentazocine.

AGONIST-ANTAGONIST PROTOTYPE

PENTAZOCINE LACTATE

Pentazocine (Talwin) was the first widely marketed mixed agonist-antagonist analgesic.

Pharmacotherapeutics Pentazocine is used for the relief of moderate-to-severe pain. It may also be used for postoperative medication and as a supplement to surgical anesthesia.

Pharmacokinetics Pentazocine produces analgesia and drowsiness similar to that produced by morphine. Thirty mg of pentazocine is equivalent to 10 mg of morphine or 80 to 100 mg of meperidine. Pentazocine's duration of action of 3 hours is similar to that of morphine.

Pharmacodynamics Analgesia produced by pentazocine is probably due to an agonistic action at the kappa receptor sites.

Pharmaceutics Pentazocine lactate is available in sterile solution for IV, IM, and SC use. For oral therapy pentazocine is dispensed in tablets that contain naloxone, which is added to prevent abuse.

Undesired Clinical Responses The most common undesired reactions are nausea, vomiting, dizziness or lightheadedness, and euphoria. Some clients receiving pentazocine have experienced hallucinations (usually visual), disorientation, confusion, and seizures. Pentazocine can produce respiratory depression and sedation. Tolerance and dependence can also develop. Additionally, soft-tissue induration and nodules can occur at injection sites.

Contraindications and Precautions Pentazocine should not be administered to clients hypersensitive to it. Special care should be taken when prescribing this drug to emotionally unstable clients and those with a history of drug misuse. Pentazocine should be used with caution for clients with respiratory conditions or impaired renal or hepatic function.

Drug-Drug Interactions Pentazocine should not be administered to a client who is physically dependent on a pure opioid agonist. This can precipitate an abstinence syndrome.

Life-Span Considerations Safe use of pentazocine during pregnancy has not been established. It is classified as a Pregnancy Category B drug; if used at term or for prolonged usage, it is considered a Pregnancy Category D drug. Pentazocine should be used with caution in women delivering premature infants. The use of pentazocine for clients under the age of 12 years is not recommended. Elderly clients have an increased sensitivity to the drug and have more undesired clinical responses than other age groups.

Specific Drug-Related Nursing Considerations Rotate sites of injection to decrease tissue irritation.

MISCELLANEOUS DRUGS IN CATEGORY

Nalbuphine (Nubain) has pharmacologic actions similar to those of pentazocine. It has approximately the same potency and duration of effect as morphine. Nalbuphine has proportionately less respiratory depressant effect than morphine. With prolonged treatment, physical dependence can develop. However, nalbuphine has a low abuse potential and is not regulated under the Controlled Substance Act. It is classified as a Pregnancy Category B drug; if used at term or for prolonged usage, it is considered a Pregnancy Category D drug. Nalbuphine is available in sterile solution for IM, IV, and SC injection.

Butorphanol (Stadol) is a more potent kappa agonist. Its duration of action and undesired clinical responses are similar to those of morphine. However, there is less respiratory depression than with morphine. Butorphanol increases cardiac work and should not be administered to clients with cardiac disorders. It is classified as a Pregnancy Category B drug; if used at term or for prolonged usage, it is considered a Pregnancy Category D drug. Butorphanol has a low abuse potential and is not regulated by the Controlled Substance Act. It is administered parenterally and by nasal spray.

Dezocine (Dalgan) is a new opioid agonist/antagonist. Its analgesic effects are equivalent to those of morphine. It is currently classified as a Pregnancy Category C drug and is not regulated by the Controlled Substance Act. Dezocine is available in sterile solution for IM and IV administration.

Buprenorphine (Buprenex) is a unique opioid. It is a partial agonist at mu receptors and an antagonist at kappa receptors. Buprenorphine is long acting and quite potent. A dose of 0.3 mg IM has analgesic effects equivalent to those of 10 mg of morphine. Peak effects occur in approximately 1 hour, and analgesic action can be sustained for up to 6 hours. Buprenorphine has low potential for abuse and is classified as a Schedule V drug. It is available in sterile solution for IM or slow IV injection.[1,26,29–31] Table 19–5 summarizes information on opioid agonists and opioid agonists-antagonists.

CONCEPT REVIEW

Most mixed opioid agonist-antagonist analgesics act as agonists on kappa receptors and antagonists on mu receptors. Since they have less potential for abuse, some of the drugs are not regulated by the Controlled Substance Act. These drugs produce fewer analgesic actions and less respiratory depression.

OPIOID ANTAGONISTS

Two pure opioid antagonists are available: naloxone and naltrexone. These drugs block the effects of opioid agonists. Naltrexone is used as adjunct therapy in the treatment of opioid addiction.

TABLE 19–5

Opioid Agonists and Agonist-Antagonists: How Supplied, Dosage, Route of Administration, Nursing Considerations

Opioid Agonists and Agonist-Antagonists	Dosage and Route of Administration	Nursing Considerations
Hydromorphone hydrochloride (Dilaudid) **HOW SUPPLIED** 1-10 mg/ml in syringes, ampules, and vials Tablets: 1, 2, 3, 4 mg Suppository: 3 mg	ADULTS Oral: 2–4 mg q4-6h Parenteral SC, IM: 1–2 mg q4-6h PCA (concentration of 0.2 mg/ml): initial dose, 0.2 mg after loading dose; dose range, 0.05-0.4 mg; lockout range, 5-10 min Epidural: Bolus dose, 0.5-3 mg Infusion, 0.15-0.3 mg/h Rectal: 3 mg q6-8h CHILDREN Oral: 0.06 mg/kg q3-4h Parenteral: 0.015 mg/kg q3-4h	Evaluate for onset of pain relief in 30 min. Peak effect of drug is 30-90 min, depending on route of administration. Plasma half-life is 2-4 h.
Levorphanol tartrate (Levo-Dromoran) **HOW SUPPLIED** Tablet: 2 mg Parenteral: 2 mg/ml in 1-ml ampules or 10-ml vials	ADULTS Oral: 2-4 mg q6-8h Parenteral: 2 mg q6-8h CHILDREN Oral: 0.04 mg/kg q6-8h Parenteral: 0.02 mg/kg q6-8h	Instruct client that drug has a bitter taste. Inject IV doses slowly. Protect drug from light. Evaluate for onset of pain relief in 30 min. Peak effect of drug is 60-90 min. Plasma half-life is 10-12 h.
Oxymorphone hydrochloride (Numorphan) **HOW SUPPLIED** 5 mg suppository 1, 1.5 mg/ml in ampules and multidose vials	ADULTS Parenteral: 1–1.5 mg q4–6h Rectal: 5 mg q4-6h CHILDREN Not recommended	Evaluate for onset of pain relief in 10 min. Peak effect of drug in 30-90 min.
Oxycodone (Roxicodone) **HOW SUPPLIED** Tablet: 5 mg Solution: 5 mg/5 ml	ADULTS Oral: 5mg q6h	10 mg oxycodone is equivalent to 90 mg of codeine. Evaluate for onset of pain relief in 15 min. Peak effect occurs in 45-60 min.
Propoxyphene (dextropropoxyphene) *Propoxyphene hydrochloride* (e.g., Darvon Pulvules, Dolene, Doxaphene) *Propoxyphene napsylate* (e.g., Darvon-N) **HOW SUPPLIED** Capsules: 32, 65 mg Tablets: 100 mg Suspension: 10 mg/ml	ADULTS 65 mg q4h CHILDREN Not recommended ADULTS 100 mg q4h	65 mg of propoxyphene HCl or 100 mg of propoxyphene napsylate is equivalent to 32 mg of codeine orally or 650 mg of acetylsalicylic acid or acetaminophen. Evaluate for onset of pain relief in 60 min. Peak effect occurs in 60-90 min. Plasma half-life is 6-12 h.
Methadone hydrochloride (Dolophine HCl) **HOW SUPPLIED** Scored tablets: 5, 10 mg Tablets: 5, 10 mg Oral solution: 5 mg/5ml, 10 mg/5 ml Oral disket tablet: 40 mg 10 mg/ml in 1-ml ampules and 20-ml vials	ADULTS Oral: 5–20 mg q4–8h Parenteral: 2.5–10 mg q3–4h CHILDREN Oral: individualized Parenteral: individualized	Oral form results in longer duration of analgesic effect. Dissolve tablets in orange juice or citrus-flavored drink for use with clients receiving maintenance dose for treatment of substance abuse. Evaluate for onset of pain relief in 15 min. Peak effect occurs in 60-120 min. Plasma half-life is 21-25 h.
Pentazocine lactate (Talwin) **HOW SUPPLIED** 30 mg/ml in ampules, syringes, and vials Talwin NX: 50 mg with 0.5 mg naloxone Talwin compound: 12.5 mg with 325 mg aspirin	ADULTS IM, IV, SC: 30 mg q3-4h Maximum IV dose: 30 mg Maximum IM, SC dose: 60 mg Maximum daily dose: 360 mg Oral: 50 mg q3–4h	50 mg of pentazocine is equivalent to codeine, 60 mg oral. Rotate injection sites; drug is highly irritating to tissues. Use SC route only if necessary. Evaluate for onset of pain relief in 15 min. Peak effect occurs in 30-60 min. Plasma half-life is 2-3 h.
Nalbuphine hydrochloride (Nubain) **HOW SUPPLIED** 10-20 mg/ml in 1- and 10-ml vials, in 1-ml ampules, in 1-ml syringes	ADULTS Parenteral: 10 mg q3–6h	Determine that a drug free interval has occurred when switching from an opioid agonist to nalbuphine. Evaluate for onset of pain relief in 15 min. Peak effect occurs in 45-60 min. Plasma half-life is 4-6 h.

TABLE 19–5 *Continued*

Opioid Agonists and Agonist-Antagonists: How Supplied, Dosage, Route of Administration, Nursing Considerations

Opioid Agonists and Agonist-Antagonists	Dosage and Route of Administration	Nursing Considerations
Butorphanol tartrate (Stadol) **HOW SUPPLIED** 10 mg/ml nasal spray in 2.5-ml metered dose spray pump Injection:1-2 mg/ml in 1-, 2-, and 10-ml vials	**ADULTS** Parenteral: 1–2 mg q3-4h Nasal spray: 1 mg (one spray in one nostril); may be repeated in 60-90 min if pain relief is not achieved; with continued severe pain, repeat two-dose sequence in 3-4 h Initial 2 mg dose (one spray in each nostril) may be used in client who will remain recumbent; may repeat after 3-4 h **CHILDREN** Not recommended	2 mg of butorphanol is equivalent to 10 mg of morphine. Nasal spray produces analgesia equivalent to IM injection. Monitor respiratory rate. Drug causes respiratory depression approximately equal to that of 10 mg of morphine. Ceiling effect of respiratory depression is 30-60 μg/kg. Evaluate for onset of pain relief in 10 min. Peak effect of drug occurs in 30-60 min. Plasma half-life is 2-4 h.
Dezocine (Dalgan) **HOW SUPPLIED** Injection: 5, 10, 15 mg/ml	**ADULTS** IM: 5–20 mg q3-6h IV: 2.5–10mg q2–4h	10 mg of dezocine is equivalent to 10 mg morphine. Evaluate for onset of pain relief in 30 min. Peak effect occurs in 30-150 min.
Buprenorphine hydrochloride (Buprenex) **HOW SUPPLIED** 0.324 mg/ml in 1-ml ampules (equivalent to 0.3 mg)	**ADULTS** IM: 0.3 mg q6h **CHILDREN** Not recommended	0.4 mg of buprenorphine is equivalent to 10 mg of morphine. Evaluate for onset of pain relief in 15 min. Peak effect occurs in 45-60 min. Plasma half-life is 2-3 h.

OPIOID ANTAGONIST PROTOTYPE

NALOXONE HYDROCHLORIDE

Naloxone (Narcan) is a structural analog of morphine.

Pharmacotherapeutics Naloxone HCl is used to treat opioid overdose, postoperative opioid-induced depression, and opioid-induced neonatal respiratory depression. It causes reversal of the effect of opioid agonists, either pure or synthetic.

Pharmacokinetics Effects from naloxone occur almost immediately when administered by IV injection; effects persist for approximately 1 hour. After IM or SC injection, effects begin within 2 to 5 minutes and remain for several hours. Naloxone is rapidly distributed throughout the body. Metabolism occurs in the liver, and excretion of naloxone is through the kidney.

Pharmacodynamics Naloxone is a competitive antagonist for mu, kappa, sigma, and delta opioid receptors. Naloxone does not produce respiratory depression, psychologic dependence, or pupillary constriction. Without the presence of opioids, naloxone has virtually no effects in doses up to 12 mg. At higher doses slight drowsiness may occur.

Pharmaceutics Naloxone HCl is meant for parenteral delivery, and sterile solutions for injection are available.

Undesired Clinical Responses When used with clients who are known or suspected to be physically dependent on opioids, naloxone precipitates acute abstinence or withdrawal syndrome. Symptoms include nausea, vomiting, sweating, tachycardia, elevated blood pressure, and tremors. The syndrome appears within minutes after administration and diminishes in approximately 2 hours. The severity of the syndrome is related to the dose of naloxone and the degree of dependence the client is experiencing. Cardiovascular complications have also been noted with the use of naloxone.[32]

Contraindications and Precautions The major contraindication is hypersensitivity to the drugs. In addition, naloxone is classified as a Pregnancy Category B drug.

Specific Drug-Related Nursing Considerations Beginning with small doses in settings outside of the emergency room allows the opportunity for retention of some analgesic effects of the opioid agonist. In the emergency room larger doses, up to 2 mg, are necessary for rapid reversal of opioid overdose.[33]

MISCELLANEOUS DRUGS IN CATEGORY

Naltrexone (Trexan) is used as adjunct therapy for maintenance of detoxification in formerly opioid-dependent individuals. This drug is available in tablet form for oral administration. It is classified as a Pregnancy Category C drug and produces a variety of undesired clinical responses, which include difficulty sleeping, nervousness, headache, low energy, GI disturbances, joint and muscle pain, delayed ejaculation, decreased sexual potency, and allergic responses. Additional undesired responses include abdominal cramping, nausea, vomiting, itching, skin rash, chills, increased thirst, and changes in liver test values. Naltrexone is contraindicated for use during active opioid dependence states. It should not be administered to clients with acute hepatitis or liver failure.[32,33] Table 19-6 summarizes information on opioid antagonists.

CONCEPT REVIEW

Opioid antagonists bind to opioid receptor sites within the CNS, thus reversing the effects of opioid (narcotic) agents.

Naloxone HCl is a widely used opioid antagonist. It is used primarily to treat opioid overdose or severe respiratory depression produced by opioid agonists.

TABLE 19–6
Opioid Antagonists[1,28,32,33]

Opioid Antagonists	Dosage and Route of Administration	Nursing Considerations
NALOXONE HCl (Narcan) **HOW SUPPLIED** 0.02, 0.4, 1 mg/ml in 1- and 2-ml ampules, syringes, and vials	**Opioid Overdose** **ADULTS** IV: 0.4-2 mg; may repeat at 2- to 3-min intervals **CHILDREN** IV: 0.01 mg/kg; may give 0.1 mg if needed May be administered IM or SC if IV route not available **Opioid Respiratory Depression** **ADULTS** Titrate for response Begin with IV dose of 0.1-0.2 mg at 2- to 3-min intervals **CHILDREN** IV: inject increments of 0.005-0.01 mg at 2- to 3-min intervals	**Assess** Assess for level of sedation, respiratory distress, or pupillary constriction. Obtain vital signs. Attempt to arouse client; use the following sedation scale: 0 = Awake, alert 1 = Occasionally drowsy, easy to arouse 2 = Frequently drowsy, easy to arouse 3 = Somnolent, difficult to arouse (S) = Normal sleep, easy to arouse **Implement** Administer low dosage initially for clients in respiratory distress from opioid depression. Observe for an increase in respiratory rate within 2-3 min if given IV. **Monitor** Duration of the effect after IV dose is 1-4 hr; after SC dose it is 2-5 h. **Evaluate** Be alert for further respiratory depression, especially for an opioid drug with a long half-life or with SC or epidural administration.
Naltrexone HCl (Trexan) **HOW SUPPLIED** Tablets: 50 mg	**ADULT** Initial dose: 25 mg; if no signs of opioid withdrawal, give additional 25 mg Daily maintenance dose: 50 mg	See naloxone HCl Client should be opioid-free before administration.

SUMMARY

Opioid agonists bind to opioid receptor sites in the CNS to reduce pain sensation. In the process sedation and respiratory depression are usually produced. In addition, these drugs produce a wide variation of physiologic effects. Most opioid agonists are regulated under the Controlled Substance Act.

Mixed opioid agonist-antagonist analgesics also relieve pain. However, most of these drugs act on kappa receptor sites instead of mu receptors. Opioid antagonists are used to block the effects of opioid agonists. These drugs are used to treat opioid overdose or severe opioid-induced respiratory depression.

REFERENCES

1. DiGregorio, G.J., Barbieri, G.J., Sterling, G.H., Camp, J.F., & Prout, M.F. (Eds.) (1990). *Handbook of pain management* (3rd ed.). West Chester, PA: Medical Surveillance.
2. Paice, J.A. (1991). Unraveling the mystery of pain. *Oncol Nurs Forum, 18,* 843-849.
3. American Pain Society. (1992). *Principles of analgesic use in the treatment of acute pain and cancer pain* (3rd ed.). Skokie, IL: American Pain Society.
4. Agency for Health Care Policy and Research. (1992). *Acute pain management: Operative or medical procedures and trauma.* DHHS Pub. No. AHCPR 93-0032.
5. Gilman, A.G., et al. (Eds.) (1990). *Goodman and Gilman's: The pharmacological basis of therapeutics* (8th ed.). New York: Macmillan.
6. McCaffery, M., & Beebe, A. (1989). *Pain: Clinical manual for nursing practice.* St. Louis: C.V. Mosby.
7. Burckhardt, C. (1990). Chronic pain. *Nursing Clinics of North America, 25,* 863-870.
8. Walco, G., & Dowite, N. (1991). Vertical versus horizontal visual analogue scales of pain intensity in children. *Journal of Pain and Symptom Management, 6,* 200.
9. Eland, J. (1990). Pain in children. *Nursing Clinics of North America, 25,* 871-884.
10. McCaffery, M., Ferrell, B., O'Neil-Page, E., & Lester, M. (1990). Nurses' knowledge of opioid analgesic drugs and psychological dependence. *Cancer Nursing, 13*(1), 21-27.
11. Slack, J., & Faut-Callahan, M. (1991). Pain management. *Nursing Clinics of North America, 26,* 463-476.
12. Wenrich, J. (1991). Acute pain service in a community hospital. *Journal of Post Anesthesia Nursing, 6,* 324-330.
13. Agency for Health Care Policy and Research. (1992). *Acute pain management in adults: Operative procedures, quick reference guide for clinicians.* DHHS Pub. No. AHCPR 92-0019.
14. Jackson, D. (1989). A study of pain management: Patient controlled analgesia versus intramuscular analgesia. *Journal of Intravenous Nursing, 12*(1), 42-51.
15. McKenzie, R., Rudy, T., & Ponter-Hammill, M. (1992). Side effects of morphine patient-controlled analgesia and meperidine patient-controlled analgesia: A follow-up of 500 patients. *AANA Journal, 60,* 282-286.
16. Bruera, E., Legris, M., Kuehn, N., & Miller, M. (1990). Hypodermoclysis for the administration of fluids and narcotic analgesics in patients with advanced cancer. *Journal of Pain and Symptom Management, 5,* 218-220.

17. Poniatowski, B. (1991). Continuous subcutaneous infusions for pain control. *Journal of Intravenous Nursing, 14*(1), 30-35.
18. McNair, N. (1990). Epidural narcotics for postoperative pain: Nursing implications. *Journal of Neuroscience Nursing, 22,* 275-279.
19. Wild, L., & Coyne, C. (1992). The basics and beyond: Epidural analgesia. *American Journal of Nursing, 92*(4), 26-36.
20. Betz, C.L., Hunsberger, M.M., & Wright, S. (1994). *Family-centered nursing care of children* (2nd ed.). Philadelphia: W.B. Saunders.
21. Agency for Health Care Policy and Research. (1992). *Acute pain management in infants, children, and adolescents: Operative and medical procedures. Quick reference guide for clinicians.* DHHS Pub. No. AHCPR 92-0020.
22. Hughey, J. (1989). Pain medications and the elderly. *Topics in Emergency Medicine, 11*(3), 61-71.
23. Faries, J., Mills, J., Goldsmith, K., Phillips, K., & Orr, J. (1991). Systematic pain records and their impact on pain control: A pilot study. *Cancer Nursing, 14,* 306-313.
24. Lee, D., McPherson, M., & Zuckerman, I. (1992). Quality assurance: Documentation of pain assessment in hospice patients. *American Journal of Hospice & Palliative Care, 9*(1), 38-44.
25. U.S. Pharmacopeial Convention. (1990). *The United States pharmacopeia* (22nd rev.). Rockville, MD: Author.
26. Smith, C., & Reynard, A. (1992). *Textbook of pharmacology.* Philadelphia: W.B. Saunders.
27. Hayes, S.R., & Vogelsang, J. (1991). Opiate receptors and analgesia: An update. *Journal of Post Anesthesia Nursing, 6*(2), 125-128.
28. Pasero, C, & McCaffery, M. (1994). Avoiding opioid-induced respiratory depression. *American Journal of Nursing, 94*(4), 25-30.
29. Data Pharmaceutica, Inc. (1993). *1993 physicians' genRx.* Smithtown, NY: Author.
30. Grass, J. (1992). Fentanyl: Clinical use as postoperative analgesic. *Journal of Pain and Symptom Management, 7,* 419-430.
31. Payne, R. (1992). Transdermal fentanyl: Suggested recommendations for clinical use. *Journal of Pain and Symptom Management, 7,* 540-544.
32. Burke, D., & Dunwoody, C. (1990). Naloxone: A word of caution. *Orthopedic Nursing, 9*(4), 44-46.
33. Goodrich, P. (1990). Naloxone hydrochloride: A review. *AANA Journal, 58*(1), 14-16.

BIBLIOGRAPHY

Biddle, C., & Gilliland, C. (1992). Transdermal and transmucosal administration of pain-relieving and anxiolytic drugs: A primer for the critical care practitioner. *Heart and Lung: Journal of Critical Care, 21*(2), 115-124.

Cavillo, E. (1991). Review of the literature on culture and pain of adults with focus on Mexican-Americans. *Journal of Transcultural Nursing, 2*(2), 16-23.

Ferrell, B., Eberts, M., McCaffery, M., & Grant, M. (1991). Clinical decision making and pain. *Cancer Nursing, 14,* 289-297.

Jacox, A., Ferrell, B., Heidrich, G., Hester, N., & Miaskowski, C. (1992). A guideline for the nation: Managing acute pain. *American Journal of Nursing, 92*(5), 49-55.

Klein, E. (1992). Premedicating children for painful invasive procedures. *Journal of Pediatric Oncology Nursing, 9*(4), 170-179.

Krames, E. (1993). Intrathecal infusional therapies for intractable pain: Patient management guidelines. *Journal of Pain and Symptom Management, 8,* 36-46.

Mooney, N. (1991). Pain management in the orthopedic patient. *Nursing Clinics of North America, 26*(1), 73-87.

Sawaki, Y., Parker, R., & White, P. (1992). Patient and nurse evaluation of patient-controlled analgesia delivery systems for postoperative pain management. *Journal of Pain and Symptom Management, 7,* 443-453.

Timmons, M.E., & Bower, F. (1993). The effect of structured preoperative teaching on patients' use of patient-controlled analgesia (PCA) and their management of pain. *Orthopedic Nursing, 12*(1), 23-31.

Waldman, S. (1990). Implantable drug delivery systems: Practical considerations. *Journal of Pain and Symptom Management, 5,* 169-174.

CHAPTER 20

Psychotherapeutic Drugs

NORMA L. PINNELL • SANDY FORREST

⊛ **Neurotransmitters and the Central Nervous System**

LEARNING OBJECTIVE: Identify the major neurotransmitters involved in behavioral disorders.

⊛ **Psychotherapeutic Drugs**

LEARNING OBJECTIVE: Describe the four major groups of psychotherapeutic drugs.

KEY TERMS:

Antidepressant drugs, bipolar disorders, neuroleptic drugs

⊛ **General Nursing Considerations**

LEARNING OBJECTIVE: Plan care for a client receiving psychotherapeutic drugs.

KEY TERMS:

Drug-free phase, initiation phase, maintenance phase, stabilization phase

⊛ **Neuroleptic Drugs**

LEARNING OBJECTIVES:

Explain the two primary methods of classifying neuroleptic drugs.

Describe three extrapyramidal effects produced by neuroleptic drugs.

Summarize important information about the low-potency neuroleptic prototype drug chlorpromazine.

Discuss essential information about the high-potency neuroleptic prototype drug haloperidol.

Explain why clozapine is considered an atypical neuroleptic drug.

KEY TERMS:

Akathisia, acute dystonia, neuroleptic malignant syndrome, parkinsonism, tardive dyskinesia

⊛ **Antidepressant Drugs**

LEARNING OBJECTIVES:

Summarize important information about the tricyclic antidepressant prototype drug imipramine.

Discuss essential information about the selective serotonin-reuptake inhibitor prototype drug fluoxetine.

Summarize information about monoamine oxidase inhibitors.

KEY TERMS:

First-generation drugs, hypertensive crisis, irreversible inhibition, reversible inhibition, second-generation drugs, secondary amines, tertiary amines

⊛ **Drugs Used to Treat Bipolar Disorder**

LEARNING OBJECTIVE: Summarize information about lithium carbonate.

⊛ **Drugs Used to Treat Anxiety Disorders**

LEARNING OBJECTIVE: Discuss the use of drugs to treat major anxiety disorders.

CONCEPTS AND TERMS TO REVIEW

Review anatomy and physiology of the central nervous system (CNS). Clarify your understanding of the extrapyramidal tract.

Reexamine the functions of neurotransmitters, especially serotonin, norepinephrine, dopamine, and acetylcholine.

Review the use of anxiolytic drugs in the treatment of mild-to-moderate anxiety.

---

*B*efore the advent of modern psychotropic agents, the mentally ill were treated with a variety of somatic therapies: psychoanalysis, seclusion, physical restraints, hydrotherapy, and psychosurgery. Gradually medicinal agents such as insulin, sedatives or stimulants, herbs, and opiates became available and were used to affect moods and emotions or to alleviate distressing mental symptoms. Although these measures provided beneficial effects, they had severe limitations.

In the early 1950s two newly developed drugs, reserpine and chlorpromazine, revolutionized the use of chemical agents in treating mental illness. Mood-elevating effects of monoamine oxidase (MAO) inhibitors were discovered in the late 1950s, and the discovery of the tricyclic compound imipramine came in the 1960s.

Psychopharmacology has grown tremendously in the last several decades. Generally, these drugs have a rapid effect and are often the first treatment of choice for clients with mental illness. These drugs, however, should be viewed as components of a larger treatment plan that includes a comprehensive medical evaluation and continuous assessment of therapeutic interventions and desired goals.

This chapter focuses on the various categories of psychotherapeutic drugs; when appropriate, prototypes are discussed. This information provides knowledge of psychopharmacologic treatment as a guide for nursing care.

NEUROTRANSMITTERS AND THE CENTRAL NERVOUS SYSTEM

All behavior is regulated by the interrelationship of chemical and structural parts of the CNS. Alterations in any part of the system may result in altered behavioral responses. CNS functions are dependent on the action of neurotransmitters, which are amino acids produced by the brain and stored in inactive forms in synaptic vesicles. These substances are necessary for the transmission of messages across nerve synapses, and their formation is kept in homeostatic balance. When the presynaptic neuron is activated, the neurotransmitter is released in an active form and attaches itself to a receptor on the postsynaptic cell, invoking activities characteristic of that cell. Inhibition of neurotransmitter action is due to enzymatic transformation of the neurotransmitter to inactive substances or to reuptake.

Of the numerous neurotransmitters identified, **acetylcholine, dopamine, norepinephrine,** and **serotonin** increase and decrease the rate of neuron stimulation, thereby regulating changes in mood states, thought processes, and psychomotor responses. Psychoactive agents indirectly moderate these changes by depressing the CNS, thus inhibiting the function of the subcortical areas of the brain (hypothalamus, limbic system, and reticular activating system). This results in an excess or deficiency in neurotransmitter formation, release, or reuptake and a corresponding alteration in symptoms.

Acetylcholine

Acetylcholine is secreted by many areas of the brain. Reduction in the amount of acetylcholine secreted causes cognitive changes.

Dopamine

Dopamine is secreted by neurons that originate in the midbrain; sensitivity of receptor sites to dopamine is possibly the cause of psychotic behavior. Drugs that block the transmission of dopamine result in diminished disordered thinking and related signs.

Norepinephrine

Norepinephrine is secreted by cell bodies in the reticular formation system of the brain stem and hypothalamus. This area is associated with feelings of rage and aggression, maintains sleep-wake patterns, and directs the release of chemicals that stimulate responses to emotional stimuli such as increased heart and respiratory rates in panic states. Low norepinephrine-to-epinephrine ratios have been documented in suicidal clients.

Serotonin

Serotonin is secreted by areas of the nuclei of the brain, including the hypothalamus, pineal gland, midbrain, and spinal cord. Alterations in serotonin levels are associated with changes in behaviors and mood states.

PSYCHOTHERAPEUTIC DRUGS

Administered safely and consistently, psychotherapeutic drugs improve the client's accessibility to other therapeutic modalities, thereby assisting them to regain functional and productive lives. Recently these drugs were placed into groups based on their target symptoms. Each group of drugs regulates maladaptive behaviors indirectly when the chemical composition of the drug interacts with cellular chemicals and enzymes.

Neuroleptic (Antipsychotic) Drugs

Neuroleptic drugs, which were called *major tranquilizers,* modify the moods and thoughts of individuals with altered perceptions of reality. They are used to treat psychotic disorders such as schizophrenia, psychotic depression, and drug-induced psychoses. Neuroleptic drugs reduce symptoms such as hallucinations, delusions, disorganized thinking, and withdrawn behavior. Of the currently available neuroleptic drugs in the United States, no single drug is more or less effective in the treatment of symptoms of psychosis.

Antidepressant Drugs

Depressive disorders range from a mildly depressed mood associated with a life event to a cluster of symptoms that suggest major depression. **Antidepressant drugs** are specific for the treatment of depression and reduce symptoms such as feelings of hopelessness and helplessness. All currently available antidepressants are equally effective in treating major depression. However, some drugs are more likely to benefit particular clients.

Drugs Used to Treat Bipolar Disorders

This group of drugs regulates acute manic episodes and is useful in long-term prophylactic treatment of bipolar disorders. (**Bipolar disorders** are affective disorders in which both manic and depressive episodes occur.)

Anxiolytic Drugs

Anxiolytic drugs are called *minor tranquilizers.* These drugs are discussed in Chapter 18 as treatment for mild-to-moderate anxiety. More severe anxiety disorders such as agoraphobia, panic disorder, obsessive-compulsive disorder, and generalized anxiety disorder comprise the largest group of psychiatric disorders.

▓ NURSING CONSIDERATIONS

Even with an increased understanding of the biologic component of psychiatric illness, psychotropic drugs are generally prescribed for the specificity of their therapeutic effect, not according to a specific diagnosis. You, the nurse, are responsible for gathering clinical information that confirms or refutes the efficacy of these drugs. This is best done through direct observation, evaluation, and reporting based on continuous assessment of client behaviors.

Assessing   Gather baseline data from the client, family members, friends, other health team members, medical records, and community agencies. Identify past and present prescription and over-the-counter (OTC) drug use. Determine why each drug was taken and the length of time the drug was used. Assess dosages and frequency of administration and ask the client about undesired clinical responses. If the client has an established psychiatric diagnosis, determine how the drugs affect his or her psychiatric symptoms. Evaluate the client's dietary habits and use of alcohol. Note any aspects that might lead to drug interactions.

Determine the client's potential for therapeutic compliance. Assess the client's insight and comprehension of what is being communicated. Determine his or her ability to communicate directly and accurately. Note myths, fears, and attitudes toward drug therapy. Is the client willing to take prescribed drugs? What is the client's capacity for self-medication? Is there a need for environmental control or family involvement?

Assess the client's mental and emotional status. Evaluate the client's general appearance and type and degree of behavioral dysfunction. Note behavioral patterns such as tremors, restlessness, excitement, and patterns of speech. Assess psychologic processes such as affect, mood, cognition, judgment, memory, thought content and organization, and interpersonal patterns.

Review all diagnostic test results and perform a complete review of body systems, including a genetic history. Consider ethnic variations since they affect drug therapy. For example, Asians, particularly Chinese, appear to require significantly smaller doses of neuroleptics, tricyclic antidepressants, and lithium.[1,2]

Diagnosing   Use the baseline assessment to identify and evaluate findings within and outside the normal limits. Because client response to psychotropic drugs is highly individualized, nursing diagnoses are diverse. Examples of appropriate diagnoses include the following:
- High risk for injury related to inappropriate drug-nutrient, drug-drug, or drug-environment interactions.
- High risk for violence: self-directed related to perceived guilt.
- High risk for noncompliance related to lack of insight.

- Sleep pattern disturbance related to hyperactivity associated with drug therapy.
- Nutrition, altered: more than body requirements related to psychotropic therapy.
- Sensory-perceptual alterations related to exogenous chemical alterations (e.g., mind-altering drugs, CNS depressants).

Planning   Work with the client, caregiver, and other health care team members to establish realistic therapeutic goals. Goals should include maximizing drug effectiveness and minimizing adverse effects. In addition, client or caregiver education is imperative.

Expected outcomes are also established during the planning phase. Outcomes reflect the nursing diagnoses. Appropriate expected outcomes follow:
- Client verbalizes factors that contribute to possible injury.
- Client verbalizes understanding of why behavior occurs.
- Client participates in the development of treatment plan.
- Client reports improvement in sleep patterns.
- Client maintains appropriate eating patterns and exercise program.
- Client uses resources effectively and appropriately.

Implementing   Generally there are four phases (initiation, stabilization, maintenance, drug free) of psychotropic treatment. During each phase observations are made of expected and undesired changes in the presenting symptoms. These observations provide a base for determining appropriate adjustments in the prescribed drug regimen.
- **Initiation phase**   During this phase the dose is initiated at a low level. The dose is then titrated upward until the clients symptoms are controlled. Close observation and assessment of the client's response are essential during this time of dose adjustment.
- **Stabilization phase**   This phase generally occurs within 3 to 6 weeks. During this phase the client's symptoms ideally are eliminated or significantly relieved. Assess carefully for undesired clinical responses and behavior changes.
- **Maintenance phase**   After remission of the client's target symptoms, the drug is slowly reduced to a minimum dose. Again observation and assessment are essential to determine if the reduction in dose alters the client's behavior patterns.
- **Drug-free phase**   Usually in newly diagnosed clients a drug is not discontinued until after 6 to 8 months of treatment. Chronic clients continue taking the drug for an indefinite period of time. However, with these individuals there may be brief periods of discontinuance to allow observation of drug-free behavior.

Once the specific psychotropic drug has been selected, education of the client, family members, and any other significant individuals is essential. Include the following in your teaching:
- Purposes and reasons for administering the drug
- Administration schedule
- Undesired clinical responses and actions to take to minimize them

This education may ensure that the drug is taken as prescribed and safeguard against noncompliance, which is a common cause of recurrence of symptoms and hospitalization.

Throughout drug therapy assess the client carefully for undesired clinical responses. All psychotropic drugs produce side effects and adverse reactions; some of these responses are life threatening.

🌿 NURSING RESEARCH

Garvey, C.A., Gross, D., & Freeman, L. (1991). Assessing psychotropic medication side effects among children: A reliability study. *Journal of Child and Adolescent Psychiatric and Mental Health Nursing, 4*(4), 127-131.

The primary purpose of this pilot study was to determine the effectiveness and consistency of health care providers in assessing psychotropic drug side effects. The tool used was the Dosage Record Treatment Emergent Symptom Scale (DOTES), a rating scale for measuring the presence and intensity of psychotropic drug side effects.

Five nurses were trained in a 1-hour session to use DOTES. After training, three of the raters watched a videotape of a nurse interviewing a 13-year-old child and then completed the DOTES rating scale. A total of 28 symptoms was assessed; there was disagreement on 5 of the 28 items, an 82% agreement rate. The other two raters examined the reasons for disagreement using process tracings.

The study suggests that DOTES is a useful measure for systematic assessment of side effects among children using psychotropic drugs.

STUDENT ACTIVITIES

- Share this article with nurses in the child or adolescent psychiatric unit of your assigned agency.
- Determine if the agency uses any form of rating scale to maintain consistency in monitoring undesired clinical responses.

Evaluating   You are responsible for evaluating all available data related to the established goals and expected outcomes. These data include decreases in primary symptoms, physiologic and behavioral reactions, and signs and symptoms of adverse drug reactions.

CONCEPT REVIEW

There are four major psychotherapeutic drug groups. Each group represents drugs used to relieve specific symptoms (e.g., depression, manic behavior).

Assessment and client education are primary functions of the nurse. These functions begin with initial client contact and continue throughout drug therapy.

NEUROLEPTIC DRUGS

Neuroleptic drugs induce a behavioral state characterized by psychomotor slowing, emotional quieting, and an indifference to external stimuli. These drugs are no longer called *major tranquilizers* or *tranquilizing drugs* because their psychologic effects are seldom pleasant or euphoric. Consequently, neuroleptic drugs are rarely encountered as drugs of abuse.

Classification of Neuroleptic Drugs

Drug selection is based on the drug's potential to decrease symptoms with a minimum of major undesired clinical responses. Neuroleptic drugs can be classified according to potency or chemical structure.

Potency   Although neuroleptic drugs differ in potency, all are essentially equal in ability to relieve symptoms of psychosis. The term *potency* refers to the size of dose needed to elicit a given response; potency does not imply effectiveness of the drug. Thus if drug X has a higher potency than drug Y, the dose of drug X required to produce desired responses is smaller than the required dose of drug Y. Although potency does not affect effectiveness of a drug, it is important in regard to undesired clinical responses—the more potent the drug the more significant the side effects and adverse reactions. Table 20–1 identifies the potency of common neuroleptic drugs.

Chemical structure   Chemically the traditional neuroleptic drugs are organized into five classes: phenothiazines, butyrophenones, dibenoxazepines, dihydroindolones, and thioxanthenes. One of these groups, phenothiazines, is further separated into three subdivisions—aliphatic, piperidine, piperazine. A new class called *dibenzodiazepines* contains clozapine (Clozaril), an "atypical" antipsychotic drug used with a subgroup of schizophrenic clients who cannot tolerate or who do not respond to other drugs.

Pharmacodynamics

The exact mechanism of action of neuroleptic drugs is not known because the etiology of the major psychotic disorders is unknown. However, it is believed that traditional neuroleptic drugs block a variety of receptors within and outside the CNS. These drugs block receptors for dopamine, acetylcholine, histamine, and norepinephrine.

TABLE 20–1
Potency of Common Neuroleptic Drugs

Potency	Drug
Low	Chlorpromazine (Thorazine)
Low	Chlorprothixene (Taractan)
Low	Mesoridazine (Serentil)
Low	Thioridazine (Mellaril)
Medium	Acetophenazine (Tindal)
Medium	Loxapine (Loxitane)
Medium	Molindone (Moban)
Medium	Perphenazine (Trilafon)
Medium	Triflupromazine (Vesprin)
High	Fluphenazine (Prolixin)
High	Haloperidol (Haldol)
High	Thiothixene (Navane)
High	Trifluoperazine (Stelazine)

Antagonism of dopamine neurotransmission appears to underlie both positive and negative effects of these drugs. Dopamine receptors are probably blocked in the limbic and frontal cortical areas, producing therapeutic effects. If centers in the brain stem are affected, an antiemetic effect is produced (see box on p. 195). Negative effects are generated by blockade of dopamine receptors in the extrapyramidal system and the hypothalamic-pituitary axis. When receptor sites in the extrapyramidal system are blocked, motor dysfunctions occur. If the sites are in the hypothalamic-pituitary axis, hormonal alterations occur.

Undesired Clinical Responses

The following section considers undesired responses common to most neuroleptic drugs.

Adverse behavioral symptoms   Long-term treatment with neuroleptic drugs can induce tolerance and physiologic dependence. On withdrawal of the drugs, symptoms may be worse than before treatment. This phenomenon is called **neuroleptic-induced supersensitivity psychosis.**

Extrapyramidal symptoms   Neuroleptic drugs commonly produce extrapyramidal symptoms as undesired clinical responses (Fig. 20–1). These symptoms are caused by dopamine blockade or depletion in the basal ganglia. This lack of dopamine mimics idiopathic pathologies of the extrapyramidal system. Extrapyramidal symptoms include acute dystonia, parkinsonism, akathisia, and tardive dyskinesia. Acute dystonia, parkinsonism, and akathisia occur early in drug therapy and can be controlled with a variety of drugs. Tardive dyskinesia occurs late in therapy and has no satisfactory treatment.[4,5]

Akathisia, characterized by pacing and squirming, is an uncontrollable need for the client to be in constant motion. The syndrome usually develops within the first 2 months of treatment and occurs most frequently with the use of high-potency neuroleptic drugs. It is managed effectively with β-adrenergic blockers, benzodiazepines, and drugs such as diphenhydramine, which has both anticholinergic and sedative properties. Reduction in neuroleptic drug dosage or a switch to a low-potency drug is also effective treatment.[6]

The client experiencing akathisia becomes increasingly agitated, irritable, and unresponsive to limit setting. Frequently these responses are mistaken for worsening of the condition instead of undesired clinical responses to the drug therapy. If more drugs are given in an attempt to control the client's behavior, more severe akathisia develops.

Acute dystonia develops within the first few days of drug therapy. Characteristics include severe spasm of the muscles of the tongue, face, neck, or back. More severe manifestations include involuntary upward deviation of the eyes (**oculogyric crisis**) and tetanic spasms of the back muscles that cause the trunk to arch forward (**opisthotonus**). Acute dystonia occurs most frequently in men and is rare in clients more than 40 years of age. The neuroleptic drug is discontinued as soon as indications of the condition are noted. With the more intense symptoms (i.e., oculogyric crisis and opisthotonus), immediate parenteral infusion of an anticholinergic drug is needed.[4–6]

Symptoms of **parkinsonism**—akinesia, masklike facies, drooling, shuffling gait, cogwheeling, rigidity, stooped posture, and tremor at rest—develop within the first month of therapy and are indistinguishable from those of idiopathic Parkinson's disease. Amantadine (Symmetrel) and some traditional anticholinergic drugs used to treat Parkinson's disease have been used to treat these symptoms.[6]

Tardive dyskinesia occurs after years of drug therapy. Manifestations include repetitive, involuntary, and purposeless movements of a choreoathetoid type involving the mouth, tongue, neck, trunk, and extremities. Movements of the mouth and tongue include sucking, smacking of lips, lateral jaw movements, and fly-catching darting of the tongue. Involuntary movements that involve the tongue and mouth interfere with chewing, swallowing, and speaking. In some clients, symptoms decrease after a dosage reduction. In others, tardive dyskinesia is irreversible.

Tardive dyskinesia occurs more frequently in older clients and is more common in females and those with history of prior brain damage. Researchers have reported no difference in the frequency and severity of tardive dyskinesia among Caucasian, Afro-American, and Hispanic clients.[6–9]

Neuroleptic malignant syndrome   The **neuroleptic malignant syndrome** is due to either an acute decrease in dopaminergic activity or an abrupt increase in cholinergic activity. Manifestations of the syndrome include fluctuating consciousness from lethargy and confusion to stupor or coma; extrapyramidal symptoms manifested by increased muscle tone, skeletal muscle rigidity, akinesia, dysarthria, and dysphagia; extreme hyperthermia in the absence of perspiration; autonomic instability, manifested by blood pressure changes; tachycardia, and tachypnea. In addition, laboratory abnormalities such as increased serum creatine phosphokinase levels, hyperkalemia (associated with muscle damage), and leukocytosis (associated with dehydration and stress) occur.[10,11]

This condition is rare but potentially fatal. All neuroleptic drugs are capable of producing the syndrome, but it is more commonly associated with high-potency drugs administered parenterally. Other factors that contribute to its occurrence include dehydration, agitation, and rate of drug administration. The syndrome lasts 7 to 10 days in uncomplicated cases. Treatment is primarily palliative and consists of reducing the temperature and monitoring for complications. Dantrolene (see Chapter 28), a direct-acting muscle relaxant, and bromocriptine (see Chapter 62), a dopamine-receptor agonist, have also been used.[6,12]

Autonomic nervous system effects   Blurred vision, dry mouth, decreased ability to perspire, difficulty urinating, and constipation are common anticholinergic effects. Sympatholytic actions of neuroleptic drugs may produce orthostatic hypotension or acute hypotensive crises. In addition, certain neuroleptic drugs prevent ejaculation through α-adrenergic receptor blocking actions.[13,14]

Metabolic and endocrine effects   Weight gain resulting from increased appetite and decreased activity may be sub-

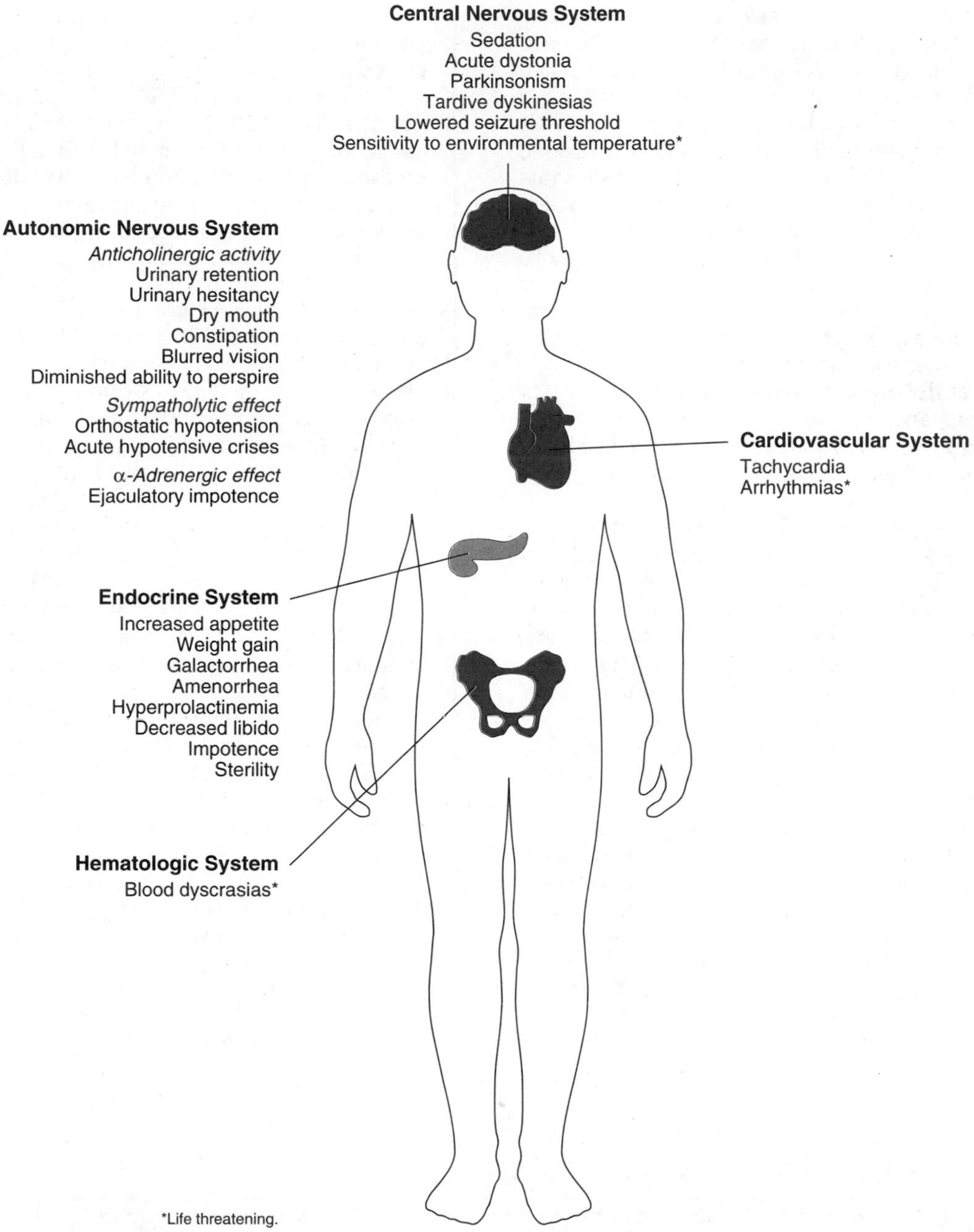

Central Nervous System
Sedation
Acute dystonia
Parkinsonism
Tardive dyskinesias
Lowered seizure threshold
Sensitivity to environmental temperature*

Autonomic Nervous System
Anticholinergic activity
Urinary retention
Urinary hesitancy
Dry mouth
Constipation
Blurred vision
Diminished ability to perspire

Sympatholytic effect
Orthostatic hypotension
Acute hypotensive crises

α-Adrenergic effect
Ejaculatory impotence

Cardiovascular System
Tachycardia
Arrhythmias*

Endocrine System
Increased appetite
Weight gain
Galactorrhea
Amenorrhea
Hyperprolactinemia
Decreased libido
Impotence
Sterility

Hematologic System
Blood dyscrasias*

*Life threatening.

FIGURE 20–1   Undesired clinical responses associated with neuroleptic drugs.

stantial. Galactorrhea, accompanied by amenorrhea, commonly occurs in women because of increased circulating levels of prolactin. The prolactin level increases in response to suppression of release of dopamine blockade, the prolactin-inhibiting factor in the pituitary. Hyperprolactinemia in men is associated with decreased libido, impotence, and sterility.

Low-Potency Neuroleptics

Chlorpromazine, thioridazine, chlorprothixene, and mesoridazine are considered low-potency neuroleptic drugs. Chlorpromazine represents the prototype for this group.

LOW-POTENCY NEUROLEPTIC PROTOTYPE

CHLORPROMAZINE

Chlorpromazine (Thorazine) was the first modern neuroleptic drug. It belongs to the phenothiazine family of compounds.

Pharmacotherapeutics Chlorpromazine is used primarily to treat schizophrenia and other psychotic disorders. It also is used to suppress emesis and to relieve intractable hiccoughs.

Pharmacokinetics Most commonly, chlorpromazine is administered orally but may be given intramuscularly, greatly increasing its effectiveness. It is absorbed erratically and unpredictably from the gastrointestinal (GI) tract. Once in the bloodstream, the drug is rapidly distributed throughout the body, with the highest concentrations in the lungs, liver, adrenal glands, and spleen. It is slowly metabolized in the liver and becomes extensively bound to body tissues, which partially accounts for the slow rate of elimination. Metabolism can be detected for several months after the agent is discontinued, which may contribute to the slow rate of recurrence of psychotic episodes after cessation of drug therapy. Clinical effects of a single dosage can last 24 hours, allowing administration of a daily dose at bedtime to minimize undesirable reactions (e.g., excessive sedation).

Pharmaceutics Chlorpromazine is available in tablet, liquid, syrup, and capsule form for oral administration. It is also available in rectal suppositories and in sterile solution for intramuscular (IM) and intravenous (IV) injection or infusion.

Initial oral dosage for adults is 25 mg three times daily. This dose is gradually increased until symptoms are controlled. Usual maintenance dose is 400 mg per day in divided doses. Parenteral administration is used for clients with more severe symptoms. An initial IM dose of 25 mg is followed in 1 hour by an additional 25 to 50 mg. A daily parenteral dose of 500 mg is usually sufficient to control symptoms.[15]

Undesired Clinical Responses All of the undesired clinical responses previously described can occur with chlorpromazine. Drowsiness during the first or second week of therapy, agranulocytosis, cholestatic jaundice, and granular deposits in the cornea and lens are also associated with chlorpromazine use. In addition, skin rashes may occur, and photosensitivity can lead to severe sunburn, even with a small amount of sun exposure.[15]

Contraindications and Precautions Chlorpromazine should be administered with caution in clients with cardiovascular, liver, or renal disease. Because the drug has a CNS depressant effect, it is used cautiously with clients with chronic respiratory disorders such as asthma and emphysema.[15] Use of this drug is contraindicated in clients with a known history of Parkinson's disease.

Drug-Drug, Drug-Nutrient, Drug-Environment Interactions (Table 20–2) The most important pharmacodynamic interaction of neuroleptics is with other CNS depressants, which induce an additive depressant. Such drugs include conventional sedatives and hypnotics, antihistamine, opiates, and alcohol.[16] Some neuroleptics have an α-adrenergic receptor blocking action that may produce additive orthostatic hypotensive effects when combined with MAO inhibitors. Uptake mechanisms for guanethidine and clonidine are inhibited when administered with chlorpromazine, decreasing their antihypertensive effect. In addition, cigarette smoking increases the metabolism of chlorpromazine and decreases its antipsychotic effect.[17]

Drug-nutrient interactions also occur with chlorpromazine. Chlorpromazine interacts with riboflavin, vitamin B_{12}, and vitamin C, depleting these vitamins. Use of vitamin supplements may be necessary. In addition, high doses of vitamin C may reduce the effectiveness of the neuroleptic drug.

Chlorpromazine-environment interactions include a reduction in the body's tolerance to heat, possibly leading to heat stroke in hot weather or during exercise and photosensitivity.

Life-Span Considerations Most psychotropic agents can be used across the life span, but dosages vary with age. These agents must be used cautiously with the elderly. Age-related changes make elderly clients more susceptible to all of undesired clinical responses previously discussed. For example, neuroleptics are highly protein-bound drugs. When protein levels are low, as is common with the elderly, highly bound drugs circulate freely and can produce toxicity. In addition, with aging, adipose tissue increases in proportion to the total body mass, and total body fluid decreases. As a result, lipid-soluble drugs are retained.[18] Additionally, safety for the use of chlorpromazine during pregnancy has not been es-

TABLE 20–2
Neuroleptic Drugs: Examples of Drug-Drug and Drug-Nutrient Interactions

Drug Involved with Interaction	Effect and Mechanism	Nursing Considerations
Carbamazepine, griseofulvin, rifampin	Increased metabolism with decreased neuroleptic effect	Gather a complete drug history on client. Monitor for response to drug therapy and for decrease in signs and symptoms.
Levodopa	Dopamine blockade causes decreased levodopa effect	Assess for increase in signs and symptoms of Parkinson's disease.
Lithium	Synergistic effect with increased CNS toxicity	Monitor plasma concentration level of lithium: norm, 0.6-1.2 mEq/L.
Phenytoin	Increase or decrease in phenytoin serum levels	Monitor plasma concentration levels of phenytoin: therapeutic range, 10-20 μg/ml; toxic level, 45-112 μg/ml.
Antihypertensive drugs and coronary vasodilators	Peripheral vasodilation causes hypotension	Assess for preexisting cardiovascular disorders. Monitor blood pressure at regular intervals.
Epinephrine	α-Adrenergic blockade and β-adrenergic stimulation cause hypotension	Same as above.
Opiates, sedatives, hypnotics, barbiturates, benzodiazepines, antihistamines	Additive CNS depression causes prolonged somnolence and respiratory depression	Monitor carefully for changes in level of consciousness. Monitor respiratory rate.
Antacids, tea, coffee, milk, fruit juice	Impaired GI absorption decreases phenothiazine effect	Instruct client to avoid ingesting these items.

tablished. There is evidence that chlorpromazine is excreted in the breast milk of nursing mothers.

Specific Drug-Related Nursing Considerations
Instruct clients experiencing orthostatic hypotension to rise carefully from a lying or sitting position, especially in the morning. Caution the client that excessive use of hard candy to relieve the discomfort of a dry mouth may lead to dental cavities.

Weight gain is a significant problem for individuals who already have a diminished sense of self-esteem. Suggest to the client that drinking diet sodas and increasing the amount of daily exercises may help. Talk to the client about calorie-reduction methods.

Teach the client that therapeutic drug effects may not occur for 2 to 3 weeks because of the delay in reaching serum dosage levels. Inform the client that the drug should not be discontinued abruptly; abrupt discontinuance may precipitate symptoms such as gastritis, nausea, vomiting, dizziness, and tremulousness.

MISCELLANEOUS DRUGS IN CATEGORY

Only two other low-potency neuroleptic drugs are discussed in this section, chlorprothixene and thioridazine. **Chlorprothixene** (Taractan) belongs to the thioxanthene class of neuroleptic drugs. Since chlorprothixene is structurally similar to phenothiazines, all precautions and undesired clinical responses previously described should be considered with this drug. The drug is administered orally in tablet or concentrated form. The concentrate contains 100 mg of the drug per 5 ml and may be mixed in milk, water, fruit juice, coffee, or carbonated beverages. A sterile solution for IM injections is available for agitated clients. The initial oral dosage is 25 to 50 mg three or four times daily. Dosage is gradually increased until maximal therapeutic response is achieved. IM dosage is 75 to 200 mg per day in divided doses.[15]

Thioridazine hydrochloride (Mellaril) belongs to the phenothiazine class and the subclass piperidine. It reduces excitement, hypermotility, and agitation. Thioridazine also is used in the treatment of behavioral disorders in clients with epilepsy. Its pharmacologic activity is similar to that of other phenothiazines, including the prototype chlorpromazine. When thioridazine is administered concomitantly with quinidine, it produces an additive myocardial and electrophysiologic effect, which causes cardiac arrhythmias and myocardial depression. If thioridazine is administered concomitantly with propranolol, the plasma level of both drugs is increased, thus increasing the effect of both drugs. Thioridazine is available in tablets and suspensions for oral administration. The initial dosage is 50 to 100 mg three times per day. Dosage is gradually increased until maximal therapeutic effects are achieved; oral dosage should not exceed 800 mg per day.[15]

Medium-Potency Neuroleptic Drugs

Only two medium-potency neuroleptic drugs are discussed in this section. Their contraindications, precautions, and undesired clinical responses are similar to those of other neuroleptic drugs.

Loxapine hydrochloride Loxapine hydrochloride (Loxitane) belongs to the dibenoxazepine class of neuroleptic

---

ANTIEMETIC USE OF PHENOTHIAZINES

Prochlorperazine (Compazine) is one of the most commonly used phenothiazine antiemetics. It is indicated for control of severe nausea and vomiting from various causes. The drug directly affects the chemoreceptor trigger zone by blocking dopamine receptors in this area.

Peak plasma levels of prochlorperazine occur in 2 to 4 hours after oral administration. The intramuscular route provides four to 10 times more active drug than oral doses. Prochlorperazine is 91% to 99% plasma protein bound. It is widely distributed in tissues, with concentrations in the CNS exceeding those in the plasma. The drug is lipophilic; it and its metabolites accumulate in brain, lung, and other lipid tissues. Biotransformation occurs in the liver, resulting in numerous active metabolites. These metabolites persist for prolonged periods, produce undesired clinical responses, and contribute to the biologic activity of the parent drug. After enterohepatic recirculation, metabolites are excreted in the urine and feces.

Oral dosage forms include sustained-release capsules, tablets of various strengths, and a syrup. Rectal suppositories are available in various strengths. For parenteral use the drug is available in ampules, vials, and prefilled syringes.

---

drugs. It is available for oral and IM use. Oral doses of loxapine provide less systemic bioavailability than IM doses do, probably because of first-pass metabolism of the oral dose. The approximate half-life of loxapine after oral administration is 1 to 14 hours; after IM administration, the half-life is approximately 8 to 23 hours. Loxapine is extensively metabolized.[15]

The initial dose of loxapine is 10 mg twice daily. Dosage is then rapidly increased over the next 7 to 10 days until there is effective control of psychotic symptoms. A daily dose higher than 250 mg is not recommended. IM loxapine is used for prompt symptomatic control of acutely agitated clients. The drug is administered IM in doses of 12.5 to 50 mg at intervals of 4 to 6 hours.[15]

Perphenazine Perphenazine (Trilafon) belongs to the phenothiazine class and the subclass piperazine. This drug has actions at all levels of the CNS, particularly the hypothalamus. It is used in the management of manifestations of psychotic disorders and for the control of severe nausea and vomiting in adults.[15]

Perphenazine is available in tablet and liquid concentrate forms for oral administration and in sterile solution for IM or IV injections. The liquid concentrate should be diluted with water, saline solution, milk, carbonated orange drink, or pineapple, apricot, prune, orange, or grapefruit juice. It should *not* be mixed with beverages containing caffeine (coffee, cola), tannics, (tea), or pectinates (apple juice). The initial oral dosage for nonhospitalized clients is 4 to 8 mg three times daily. Once symptoms are controlled, the dosage should be reduced to the lowest effective dosage. For hospitalized psychotic clients the initial oral dosage is 8 to 16 mg two to four times daily. Dosages in excess of 64 mg per day should be avoided. The initial IM dosage is 5 mg every 6 hours. Parenteral dosage should not exceed 15 mg per day in ambulatory clients or 30 mg per day in hospitalized clients. The client should receive oral medication as soon as possible.[15]

High-Potency Neuroleptic Drugs

High-potency neuroleptic drugs are effective in smaller dosages than low- and medium-potency drugs are. However, these drugs produce more significant side effects and adverse reactions.

HIGH-POTENCY NEUROLEPTIC PROTOTYPE

HALOPERIDOL

Although haloperidol (Haldol) belongs to the butyrophenone class of neuroleptic drugs, it still possesses the pharmacologic properties described for the other neuroleptic drugs. Therefore only significant differences are discussed.

Pharmacotherapeutics Haloperidol is used in the management of manifestations of psychotic disorders and to treat tics and vocal utterances of Tourette's disorders in children and adults. Haloperidol has also been used for treatment of severe behavior problems in children.

Pharmacokinetics Haloperidol peaks in 2 to 6 hours, with a duration of action of approximately 72 hours. It is 80% to 90% plasma-protein bound and has a half-life of 12 to 16 hours.

Pharmaceutics Haloperidol is available as tablets and as a concentrate for oral administration. It is also available in a sterile solution for IM injections. Initial oral dosage for adults is 0.5 to 5 mg two or three times daily, depending on the severity of the symptoms. Parenteral administration is used for prompt control of symptoms. A dose of 2 to 5 mg is administered initially, followed by subsequent injections if necessary.[15]

Drug-Drug Interactions When haloperidol and methyldopa are administered concomitantly, dopamine blockade and decreased catecholamine synthesis occur. This mechanism produces signs and symptoms of dementia. In a few individuals the combination of haloperidol and lithium has produced an encephalopathic syndrome that caused irreversible brain damage.[17]

Ethnic Differences in Drug Disposition and Responsiveness Studies suggest that Chinese clients receiving haloperidol maintain a significantly higher plasma level than non-Asians in the United States after IM and oral administration of the drug. Additionally, prolactin concentrations are substantially lower in Caucasians than in Asian clients. The incidence of extrapyramidal reactions after haloperidol use is also increased in Asians. These responses support the need to give Asians clients reduced dosages of the drug.[2,19]

MISCELLANEOUS DRUGS IN CATEGORY

Three additional high-potency drugs are fluphenazine hydrochloride, trifluoperazine, and thiothixene. **Fluphenazine** (Prolixin) belongs to the phenothiazine class and the piperazine subclass. It is used to treat schizophrenia and other psychotic disorders. The drug has activity at all levels of the CNS and on multiple organ systems. Fluphenazine is available in oral and parenteral dosage forms. Oral liquid dosage forms should be shaken gently to disperse the oils and solution. All doses are highly individualized. Adult dosage may range from 2.5 to 10 mg in divided doses every 6 to 8 hours. Generally, the oral dose is two to three times the parenteral dose. Once the symptoms are controlled, oral dosages are reduced to a maintenance dose of 1 to 5 mg per day.[15]

Thiothixene (Navane) belongs to the thioxanthene class and is used in the management of psychotic disorders. Since thiothixene produces antiemetic effects, it is possible that it may mask indications of drug overdose or intestinal disorders. Thiothixene is available both orally and in a sterile solution for IM injections. IM dosages of this drug should be administered deep in a large muscle mass, preferably in the upper outer quadrant of the buttock or the midlateral thigh. It should *not* be administered in the deltoid muscle. In clients with mild conditions an initial dose of 2 mg, three times daily or in clients with more severe conditions an initial dose of 5 mg twice a day is recommended. The usual optimal dose is 20 to 30 mg daily. When more rapid control and treatment are desired, 4 mg of thiothixene IM is administered two to four times daily.[15]

Trifluoperazine (Stelazine) is a member of the phenothiazine class and the subclass of piperazine. It is used in the management of psychotic disorders and for the short-term treatment of generalized nonpsychotic anxiety. Trifluoperazine is available in oral and parenteral dosage forms. Usual initial oral dose is 2 to 5 mg twice a day; optimum therapeutic dosage levels should be reached within 2 to 3 weeks. When the liquid concentrate dosage form is used, it should be added to 60 ml or more of diluent just before administration. Vehicles suggested for dilution include tomato or fruit juice, milk, simple syrup, orange syrup, carbonated beverages, coffee, tea, or water. Semisolid foods such as soup or puddings may also be used. IM injection of 1 to 2 mg is used for prompt control of severe symptoms. The injection solution must be protected from light since exposure causes discoloration.[15]

Atypical Neuroleptic Drugs

Atypical neuroleptic drugs differ from traditional drugs because they produce few extrapyramidal symptoms. Atypical drugs also have a different profile of binding to dopamine receptors, and their effects on various dopamine-mediated behaviors differ from those of traditional neuroleptic drugs.[15]

ATYPICAL NEUROLEPTIC PROTOTYPE

CLOZAPINE

Clozapine (Clozaril) was approved for use in the United States by the Food and Drug Administration (FDA) in 1989.

Pharmacotherapeutics Clozapine is used in the treatment of schizophrenia. Because of the significant risk of agranulocytosis and seizures associated with its use, clozapine should be used only in clients who have not responded to standard neuroleptic drugs.

Pharmacokinetics Clozapine tablets and solution have the same bioavailability. The drug is approximately 95% bound to serum proteins. It is almost completely metabolized before excretion, and only trace amounts of unchanged drug are detected in the urine and feces. The elimination half-life is 4 to 66 hours, depending on single-dose or multiple-dose administration.[15]

Pharmacodynamics Clozapine is a dibenzodiazepine. It acts as an antagonist at adrenergic, cholinergic, histaminergic, and serotonergic receptors. Clozapine interferes with the binding of dopamine at both D_1- and D_2-receptors, yet it does not cause catalepsy or inhibit apomorphine-induced stereotypy. It appears that clozapine is more active at limbic than at striatal dopamine receptors, which may explain the drug's low extrapyramidal profile.[15]

Undesired Clinical Responses Neuroleptic-in-duced agranulocytosis is a potentially fatal side effect associated with clozapine. This condition usually emerges 10 to 90 days after initiation of treatment. Clients being treated with clozapine must have a baseline white blood cell (WBC) count and differential count before therapy begins, a WBC every week during therapy, and a weekly WBC for 4 weeks after discontinuance of the drug. Clients should be advised to report signs of lethargy, weakness, fever, or sore throat.[15,20,21]

Another significant undesired clinical response is seizures. Seizures apparently are dose related; high doses of clozapine produce the greatest risk. Orthostatic hypotension, tachycardia, electrocardiographic (ECG) changes, congestive heart failure, and myocarditis have also been reported.[15]

Contraindications and Precautions Clozapine should be used with caution in clients with cardiovascular, hepatic, or renal disease. It is contraindicated for clients with a history of seizures or myeloproliferative disorders.

SUMMARY OF NURSING CONSIDERATIONS FOR CLIENTS RECEIVING NEUROLEPTIC DRUGS

Assess

▶ Assess client for preexisting conditions that would prevent the use of neuroleptic drugs (e.g., cardiovascular, renal, or hepatic disorders, glaucoma, Parkinson's disease, chronic constipation, prostatic hypertrophy, or pregnancy).

▶ Review pretreatment diagnostic studies (e.g., renal, hepatic, and hematologic studies, ECG).

▶ Question the client about sulfite allergy if parenteral administration is scheduled. (Ampules contain sulfites and are capable of producing hypersensitivity reactions.)

Implement

▶ Read instructions carefully about parenteral injection site and technique.

▶ Check pediatric dosages carefully.

▶ Instruct client not to exceed prescribed dosage and not to discontinue the drug abruptly.

▶ Provide appropriate safety precautions (e.g., use side rails and call light, supervision) if sedative effects occur.

▶ Keep client lying down for at least ½ hour and observe for hypotension after parenteral administration of the drugs.

▶ Teach client to change positions slowly.

▶ Advise client to avoid tasks that require mental alertness.

▶ Instruct client to avoid alcohol and other CNS depressants.

▶ Teach female clients that drugs may give a false-positive urine pregnancy test. (This possibly is caused by drug metabolite that discolors the urine.)

▶ Inform client to avoid excessive heat (e.g., hot showers, sun bathing, saunas, physical activities in heat of the day).

▶ Advise client to wear sunglasses if photophobia is present and to protect skin with sunscreens, long sleeves, and hats with brims if photosensitivity occurs.

▶ Recommend increased intake of oral fluids and fiber to decrease potential for constipation.

▶ Encourage frequent oral hygiene.

▶ Explain to the client and caregiver the rationale for drug therapy.

▶ For nonhospitalized clients, suggest use of a medical identification tag or bracelet.

▶ Provide client and caregiver a list of undesired clinical responses and actions to take if these responses occur.

Monitor

▶ Observe children, the elderly, and debilitated clients closely for undesired clinical responses.

▶ Monitor for tremor, rigidity, inability to sit still, tongue and jaw movements, and decreased motility.

▶ Monitor blood pressure, especially early in therapy, in clients with impaired cardiovascular function and in clients receiving other drugs that depress the CNS.

▶ Observe for signs of hyperreflexia or muscle twitches.

▶ Monitor laboratory studies that would reflect possible undesired clinical responses:
   Hepatic studies: bile in urine; increased serum transaminase, bilirubin, and alkaline phosphatase levels
   Altered plasma cholesterol levels
   Increased serum prolactin levels

Evaluate

▶ Evaluate plasma concentration levels.

▶ Observe for diminished signs and symptoms of psychotic disorder.

Since clozapine has a potent anticholinergic effect, it is not recommended for use in clients with glaucoma or prostatic hypertrophy.[15]

Drug-Drug Interactions Clozapine may potentiate the hypotensive effects of antihypertensive drugs and the anticholinergic effects of atropine-like drugs. In addition, since clozapine is highly bound to plasma protein, it may increase the plasma concentration levels of other concomitantly administered drugs that are also highly protein bound (e.g., digitoxin, warfarin).[15]

Life-Span Considerations Clozapine is classified as a Pregnancy Category B drug. Safety and effectivness in children below the age of 16 years have not been established.

Specific Drug-Related Nursing Considerations Blood test results should be monitored weekly. Teach the client to report immediately the appearance of lethargy, weakness, fever, sore throat, malaise, or mucous membrane ulceration. Instruct the client to notify the primary care provider before taking any prescription or OTC drugs. Female clients should be instructed not to breastfeed while receiving clozapine.

TABLE. 20–3

Properties of Antidepressant Drugs and Their Related Physiologic Responses

Property	Related Physiologic Responses
Reuptake of norepinephrine	Alleviation of depression
	Erectile and ejaculatory dysfunction
	Tachycardia
	Tremors
Reuptake of serotonin	Alleviation of depression
	Anxiety
	GI tract disturbance
Histamine H_1 blockade	Hypotension
	Potentiation of CNS depressants
	Sedation
Anticholinergic blockade	Blurred vision
	Constipation
	Memory dysfunction
	Sinus tachycardia
	Urinary retention
	Xerostomia
α-Adrenergic blockade	Orthostatic hypotension
	Reflex tachycardia
	Priapism

CONCEPT REVIEW

The terms *neuroleptic* and *antipsychotic* are used interchangeably in some resources.

Traditional neuroleptic drugs include the phenothiazines, butyrophenones, dibenoxazepines, dihydroindolones, and thioxanthenes. These classes describe the drugs' chemical structure.

Neuroleptic drugs are also classified as low-, medium-, and high-potency drugs. The potency reflects the dosage required to achieve effective reduction in signs and symptoms.

Extrapyramidal symptoms are the most significant undesired clinical responses associated with the traditional neuroleptic drugs. These symptoms include acute dystonia, akathisia, parkinsonism, and tardive dyskinesia.

Clozapine is considered an atypical neuroleptic drug. Its action and side effect profile differ from those seen with the traditional drugs.

ANTIDEPRESSANT DRUGS

The number of drugs available for treating depression has been growing rapidly. Tricyclic antidepressants, MAO inhibitors, and lithium were among the original drugs and are sometimes referred to as *traditional antidepressants* or **first-generation drugs.** During recent years a number of other drugs, usually chemically and sometimes pharmacologically different from these earlier classes, have been introduced. These drugs are often called **second-generation drugs.** Second-generation drugs have a more rapid onset of action, more tolerable undesired

clinical responses, and greater safety when taken in overdose. Research has shown that all antidepressants block reuptake of neurotransmitters in the synapse and block certain postsynaptic neurotransmitter receptors. Reuptake of synaptic receptors prevents overstimulation of synaptic receptors by taking released neurotransmitters back into the nerve ending.[22]

Antidepressants differ in terms of clinical activity (Table 20–3), safety, tolerability, likelihood of pharmacodynamic and pharmacokinetic interactions with concomitantly prescribed drugs, and ease of administration. Choice of one antidepressant over another is based on biologic theories of depression, drug efficacy, and side effect profiles. Monitoring antidepressant efficacy is essential to successful drug therapy since drug plasma concentration levels reflect appropriate or inappropriate dosing.[23]

Tricyclic and Chemically Related Antidepressants

There are three broad subtypes of tricyclic and chemically related antidepressants: tertiary amines, secondary amines, and nontricyclics (Table 20–4). The **tertiary amines** group includes amitriptyline hydrochloride (HCL), doxepin HCL, trimipramine maleate, and imipramine HCL; these drugs have frequent and severe undesired clinical responses. The **secondary amines** group includes desipramine HCL, nortriptyline HCL, and protriptyline HCL, which have higher selectivity for norepinephrine-reuptake blockade. Other nontricyclics include bupropion HCL and trazodone HCL, which lack lethal overdose potential and are useful for suicidal clients.

TABLE 20–4

Tricyclic and Chemically Related Antidepressants: Bioavailability, Protein Binding, Plasma Half-life

Tricyclic Antidepressants	Bioavailability (%)	Protein Binding (%)	Plasma Half-life (h)
TERTIARY AMINES			
Amitriptyline HCl (Amitril, Elavil)	31-61	82-96	13-36
Doxepin HCl (Adapin, Sinequan)	13-45	—	8-24
Imipramine HCl (Presamine, Tofranil)	29-77	88-93	6-20 or 18-34
Trimipramine maleate (Surmontil)	—	—	7-30
SECONDARY AMINES			
Desipramine HCl (Norpramin, Pertofrane)	—	70-90	12-30
Nortriptyline HCl (Aventyl, Pamelor)	46-79	93	18-28 or 14-79
Protriptyline HCl (Vivactil)	—	92	55-124
NONTRICYCLICS			
Buproprion HCl (Wellbutrin)	—	85	3.9-23.1 or 11-14
Trazodone HCl (Desyrel)	—	73	13-16

Data from references 6, 15, 17, and 22.

TRICYCLIC ANTIDEPRESSANT PROTOTYPE

IMIPRAMINE HYDROCHLORIDE

The first tricyclic drug used clinically was imipramine (e.g., Janimine, Tofranil). Its structure is similar to that of the phenothiazine class of neuroleptic drugs. In fact, imipramine was originally developed for possible use as a neuroleptic drug. However, clinical trials demonstrated it was more effective as a mood elevator than as an antidepressant.

Pharmacotherapeutics Imipramine is appropriate for treating depression after myocardial infarction and for clients with mild hypertension, peptic ulcer disease, Parkinson's disease, and tardive dyskinesia.

Tricyclic antidepressants, including imipramine, have been used in the treatment of certain childhood disorders for more than 20 years. Research supports the use of tricyclics for preadolescent children as adjunctive therapy for major depression, attention deficit hyperactivity disorder, enuresis, tic disorders, anxiety disorders, and eating disorders.[23]

Pharmacokinetics Imipramine is highly lipid soluble and binds tightly to plasma proteins. Because of these two factors the half-life of imipramine is usually in excess of 20 hours. Asian individuals reach peak plasma levels more quickly than Caucasians. Metabolism of imipramine is through the mixed-function oxidase enzyme system. During metabolism, desipramine, an active metabolite, is formed. The amount of this metabolite usually exceeds that of the parent compound.

Pharmacodynamics Tricyclic antidepressants block reuptake of norepinephrine more than that of serotonin. Imipramine blocks the amine pump both for norepinephrine and serotonin. The metabolite desipramine specifically blocks uptake of norepinephrine.

Pharmaceutics Imipramine is available for oral administration in 10-, 25-, and 50-mg tablets. It is also available in sterile solution for IM injections. The initial oral dose for hospitalized clients is 100 mg per day in divided doses. This dose may be gradually increased to 200 mg per day. If no response occurs in 2 to 3 weeks, the dose is increased to 250 to 300 mg per day. Initial IM dose is up to 100 mg per day in divided doses.[15]

Undesired Clinical Responses Blockade of neurotransmitter reuptake is probably responsible for many of the undesired clinical responses seen with use of tricyclic antidepressants. Reactions differ significantly and predictably according to the neurotransmitter being blocked. Use of imipramine is associated with responses such as tremors, tachycardia, and erectile and ejaculatory dysfunction.[22]

Additionally, cardiotoxicity is a chief concern with tricyclic use. These drugs, including imipramine, have a quinidine-like effect on the cardiac conduction system.[24] Conduction defects and arrhythmias may occur. Imipramine can also produce orthostatic hypotension, sedation, delirium, confusion, and cognitive impairment.[25]

Anticholinergic symptoms are especially troubling to clients. They include blurred vision, urinary retention, constipation, and dry mouth. The dry mouth from decreased salivation causes impairment in oral rinsing with subsequent increases in debris, bacterial growth, and oral acids that encourage caries development.[24,25]

Contraindications and Precautions Imipramine use should be avoided in clients with orthostatic hypotension, cardiovascular disease, glaucoma, history of seizure, prostatic hypertrophy, and hyperthyroidism. Its use is also contraindicated during the acute recovery period after a myocardial infarction.[15]

Drug-Drug, Drug-Nutrient, Drug-Environment Interactions Imipramine is a basic drug; it is excreted more quickly in acidic urine, resulting in lowered blood levels. Foods such as bread, bacon, corn, lentils, meat, fish, and fowl acidify urine.[26] In addition, imipramine produces photosensitivity, so clients must avoid direct sunlight.

Imipramine is involved in numerous drug-drug interactions. For example, tobacco smoking produces an enzyme activity that decreases the plasma level of imipramine. Phenothiazines and tricyclic antidepressants interact to decrease the metabolism of both drugs, thus enhancing the effects of both drugs. Several antiarrhythmic drugs (e.g., quinidine, procainamide, lidocaine, propranolol) have an additive quinidine-like effect with imipramine. This effect decreases myocardial contractility and produces arrhythmias.[16]

Ethnic Differences in Drug Disposition and Responsiveness Studies indicate that Asians and Hispanics are less tolerant to tricyclic antidepressants than Caucasians. Both of these groups develop undesired clinical responses at lower doses than Caucasians. In addition, they appear to respond to lower doses and have lower effective concentrations of the drugs than Caucasians.[19]

Life-Span Considerations Tricyclic antidepressants have been used in the treatment of certain childhood disorders for more than 20 years, and indications for their use in the pediatric population are increasing. Research supports the use of these drugs for preadolescent children as adjunctive therapy for major depression, attention deficit hyperactivity disorder, enuresis, tic disorders, anxiety disorders, and eating disorders.[24]

Tricyclic antidepressants are the greatest prescription killers among the pediatric age group. The increase in use of these drugs in the pediatric population provides more opportunities for toxic exposure in children. An early indication of poisoning may be extreme drowsiness. Within minutes, the child may develop seizures and lapse into a coma. Deaths are linked to cardiac disturbances and intractable seizures.[27]

Specific Drug-Related Nursing Considerations Assess the client, especially the elderly individual, for diseases associated with depression: dehydration, acid-base imbalance, anemia, infections, congestive heart failure, cerebrovascular disease, chronic obstructive pulmonary disease, dementia, and Parkinson's disease. In addition, collect and analyze a drug history for drugs that may cause depression.

Anticipate that the client initially will receive approximately one fourth the maximal usual daily dose for adults. (Asian individuals require smaller doses.) This dose is administered for 2 to 3 weeks before a dose increase is considered (Table 20–5).

It usually takes 2 to 4 weeks for the client to experience a clinical response. However, undesired clinical responses may start much sooner and interfere with client compliance. Explain to the client that some discomfort is likely to occur during the first few weeks of therapy.

Be careful when administering the drug; check drug doses closely. An overdose of tricyclic antidepressants is dangerous, for it can cause complete atrial-ventricular dissociation, ventricular arrhythmia, and death. Common clinical features of tricyclic poisoning include dry mouth, blurred vision, dilated pupils, sinus tachycardia, pyramidal neurologic signs, and dizziness. Coma, convulsions, respiratory depression, hypotension, and ECG abnormalities may accompany severe poisoning.[22]

MISCELLANEOUS DRUGS IN CATEGORY

Amitriptyline and doxepin are also tertiary amines. The active metabolite of **amitriptyline HCl** (Elavil) is nortriptyline. Amitriptyline has a selective action of blocking uptake of serotonin; nortriptyline blocks both norepinephrine and serotonin. The end result is predominantly on serotonin. Amitriptyline is especially prone to cause anticholinergic effects. Common undesired clinical responses include xerostomia, urinary retention, constipation, blurred vision, and memory dysfunction, particularly in the elderly individual. Amitriptyline produces photosensitivity. Because of its affinity for histamine H_1 receptors, amitriptyline also has a sedating effect. To decrease GI symptoms, administer amitriptyline with food. **Doxepin HCl** (Sinequan) has strong sedative effects and is used as an anxiolytic and antidepressant drug. It is the most potent histamine H_1 antagonist available in the United States. This drug has a relatively weak blocking action of the amine group.[17,22,25]

Desipramine and nortriptyline are included as secondary amines. Even though **desipramine HCl** (Norpramin, Pertofrane) is a metabolite of imipramine, it is also used as a separate drug entity. Desipramine has fewer sedative, anticholinergic, and α-adrenoreceptor blocking actions than most other tricyclics. Common undesired clinical responses associated with this drug include tachycardia, tremor, and erectile and ejaculatory problems. It interferes with the antihypertensive effects of guanethidine monosulfate (Ismelin) and guanadrel sulfate (Hylorel) and potentiates the pressor effects of sympathomimetic amines. Doses are similar to those of imipramine. **Nortriptyline HCl** (Aventyl), the metabolite of amitriptyline, is also used as a separate drug entity. This drug

TABLE 20–5
Tricyclic Antidepressants: Dosages* and Therapeutic Plasma Concentrations

Tricyclic Antidepressants	Usual Initial Oral Dose (mg)†	Daily Oral Dosage Range (mg)†	Maximum Daily Dose (mg)†	Therapeutic Plasma Concentrations (ng/ml)
Amitriptyline	75	50-200	300	100-250
Buproprion HCl	200	200-300	450	25-100
Desipramine HCl	100	100-200	300	150-300
Doxepin HCl	75	75-150	300	100-200
Imipramine HCl	100	75-300	300	75-250
Nortriptyline HCl	75	50-100	150	50-150
Protriptyline HCl	15	15-40	60	50-150
Trazodone HCl	150	150-400	600	50-250
Trimipramine maleate	75	50-200	250-300	—

Data from references 6, 15, 17, 22, and 28.
*Doses are for adults.
†Divided doses.

is extensively metabolized during the first pass through the liver. Nortriptyline and its metabolites affect noradrenergic, serotonergic, and dopaminergic systems. Since it has fewer toxic symptoms than other antidepressants, it is better tolerated by elderly clients. It is also a preferred drug for clients with congestive heart failure or ischemic disease.[17,22]

Nontricyclic antidepressants include bupropion, trazodone, and amoxapine. These drugs lack lethal overdose potential and are useful for suicidal clients. **Trazodone** (Desyrel) is a phenylpiperazine compound; its pharmacologic action is complex. At some doses the drug acts as a serotonin-receptor antagonist; at other doses it acts both as a serotonin agonist and as an uptake inhibitor. Anticholinergic symptoms are few with trazodone. Major undesired clinical responses include drowsiness, dizziness, headache, nausea, and priapism.[17,25]

Bupropion HCl (Wellbutrin) has a phenethylamine structure. Its exact mode of action is unclear. It has little effect on norepinephrine uptake, no anticholinergic actions, and no inhibiting effects on MAO. Dry mouth is the most common undesired clinical response, although anorexia, mild agitation, difficulty sleeping, and rashes have occurred. More adverse responses occur when bupropion is administered concurrently with levodopa. Bupropion use is contraindicated in clients with a history of head trauma or seizures.[22]

Amoxapine (Asendin) is classified as a dibenzoxazepine but can be considered a tricyclic because of its chemical structure. It is a selective, potent blocker of norepinephrine and is a dopamine-receptor blocker. Amoxapine is a derivative of the neuroleptic drug loxapine. It is further metabolized to hydroxyl metabolites that are three to 10 times as abundant as the parent drug. These metabolites probably account for its antidepressant activity. Amoxapine produces extrapyramidal side effects typical of neuroleptic drugs. It also produces hyperprolactinemia and sexual disturbances in men and amenorrhea-galactorrhea in women.[22,25]

Selective Serotonin-reuptake Inhibitors

As the name indicates, this group contains highly selective serotonin-reuptake blockers.

SELECTIVE SEROTONIN-REUPTAKE INHIBITOR PROTOTYPE

FLUOXETINE HYDROCHLORIDE

Fluoxetine HCl (Prozac) was the first entirely specific serotonin-reuptake inhibitor marketed in the United States for treatment of depression.

Pharmacotherapeutics Fluoxetine is used to treat a variety of depressive states. It is one of the preferred drugs in clients with chronic pain syndrome, organic brain syndrome, angle-closure glaucoma, and hypertension treated with prazosin or clonidine. Fluoxetine is helpful in treating clients with psychomotor retardation.[22]

Pharmacokinetics The capsule and oral solution dosage forms of fluoxetine are bioequivalent. Food delays absorption but does not alter systemic bioavailability. Peak plasma concentrations of fluoxetine of 15 to 55 ng/ml occur after 6 to 8 hours. Approximately 95% of the drug is plasma protein bound. Fluoxetine is extensively metabolized in the liver to norfluoxetine and other metabolites. Norfluoxetine has pharmacologic properties similar to those of fluoxetine. Both fluoxetine and its metabolite have a long elimination half-life, 1 to 3 days for fluoxetine and 7 to 9 days for norfluoxetine. These long elimination half-lives assure that the active drug substances remain in the body for weeks after the drug is discontinued.[15]

Pharmacodynamics The antidepressant action of fluoxetine is presumed linked to its inhibition of CNS neuronal uptake of serotonin. Fluoxetine binds weakly if at all to most postsynaptic receptors. It does not block anticholinergic, histamine H_1, and α_1-adrenergic receptors.[15,22]

TABLE 20–6

Dosages for Selective Serotonin-Reuptake Inhibitors and MAO Inhibitors

Drug	Initial Dose (mg/d)*	Daily Dosage Range (mg/d)*	Maximum Daily Dose (mg/d)*
SELECTIVE SEROTONIN-REUPTAKE INHIBITORS			
Fluoxetine HCl (Prozac)	20	20-40	80†
Fluvoxamine (Luvox)	50	100–300	300
Sertraline (Zoloft)	50	50-200	200
Paroxetine (Paxil)	20	10-50	50
MAO INHIBITORS			
Phenelzine sulfate (Nardil)	45†	15-60†	90†
Tranylcypromine sulfate	30†	30-60‡	60†

*Doses are for adults.
†Divided doses.
Data from U.S. Pharmacopeia (22nd rev.), 1990.

Pharmaceutics Fluoxetine is available in 10-20-mg capsules and a 20 mg/5 ml solution. The initial dosage of fluoxetine is 20 mg per day administered in the morning. Further titration of dosage is unnecessary in most clients. If improvement is not noted after several weeks of therapy, the dosage is gradually increased to a maximum of 80 mg per day[22] (Table 20–6).

Undesired Clinical Responses Fluoxetine lacks many of the anticholinergic, antihistaminic, and hypotensive effects of other antidepressants. Most common undesired clinical responses are nausea, anorexia, diarrhea, anxiety, nervousness, insomnia, and headache.

Contraindications and Precautions Fluoxetine use is contraindicated in clients with known hypersensitivity to the drug. It is used with caution in clients with hepatic or renal dysfunction or both. These individuals usually require lower or less frequent dosages.

Drug-Drug, Drug-Nutrient, Drug-Environment Interactions As indicated previously, food delays absorption of the drug but not bioavailability; therefore it can be administered with food. The drug must be stored at controlled room temperature.

The most dangerous drug-drug interaction is the combination of fluoxetine and MAO inhibitors. This combination has produced serious and sometimes fatal reactions. When fluoxetine is administered concurrently with other antidepressants, the plasma level of the other drug is usually altered.[16]

Life-Span Considerations Fluoxetine is classified as a Pregnancy Category B drug. One study reported that the drug was excreted in human milk; therefore use with nursing mothers is not recommended. Safe and effective use with children has not been established. Fluoxetine is used with caution in the elderly because its activating properties may produce excitement and insomnia in this age group.

Specific Drug-Related Nursing Considerations Some clients develop significant sleeping problems due to drug-induced anxiety or muscle twitching. Therefore you should question the client about sleeping patterns. If sleeping difficulties do not improve, discuss the problem with the primary care provider.

Inform the client that fluoxetine may be taken with meals. Instruct the client to take the drug in the morning. If the dosage exceeds 20 mg per day, advise the client to take a portion of the dose in the morning and the remaining dose later in the day. Caution the client not to discontinue treatment once symptoms improve; relapse may occur.

MISCELLANEOUS DRUGS IN CATEGORY

Sertraline hydrochloride (Zoloft) was approved by the FDA in 1991. Its pharmacologic properties are similar to those of fluoxetine, the prototype for this group. Sertraline is highly protein bound, has an elimination half-life of approximately 26 hours, and undergoes extensive metabolism. It is available in 50- and 100-mg tablets. The initial adult dose is 50 mg once daily. If symptoms do not improve, dose increases at intervals of 1 week are made. The maximum dose is 200 mg per day.[15]

Paroxetine (Paxil) is a new drug used in the treatment of depression. Paroxetine blocks neuronal reuptake of released serotonin, thereby raising concentrations of this neurotransmitter. Administered orally, it is completely absorbed in the GI tract. The plasma concentration peaks in approximately 5 hours. Paroxetine is metabolized by the liver; its metabolites are inactive. The drug is excreted in both the urine and feces; the elimination half-life for paroxetine averages 21 hours.[29]

Common undesired clinical responses include nausea, somnolence, dry mouth, asthenia, dizziness, insomnia, ejaculatory disturbance, and sweating. Most responses are dose related. Paroxetine should not be administered to clients receiving MAO inhibitors. Additionally, at least 14 days should be allowed between discontinuation of the MAO inhibitor and the starting of paroxetine. The drug should also be used with caution in clients with mania or a history of seizures.

The usual adult dose is 20 mg once daily in the morning. The dosage is increased by 10 mg at intervals of 1 week or more until the desired therapeutic response is reached. Maximum dose is 50 mg per day. Approximately 10 days of drug therapy are needed to reach steady-state concentrations.[29]

Monoamine Oxidase Inhibitors

MAO inhibitors were introduced in the 1950s and were the first clinically effective drugs for depression. Only two MAO inhibitors are currently used to any extent: **phenelzine** (Nardil) and **tranylcypromine** (Parnate). These drugs are phenylethylamine derivatives. Since this group does not have a true prototype, pharmacologic properties of the group are discussed.

Pharmacotherapeutics MAO inhibitors are as effective as the tricyclic antidepressants in the treatment of depression. However, because of their undesired clinical responses, they are not the first drugs of choice. However, for clients suffering from atypical depression (i.e., with symptoms of increased sleep and appetite or with depression associated with anxiety) these drugs may be the initial therapy. Additionally, MAO inhibitors are used to treat bulimia, panic disorders, and obsessive-compulsive disorders.[6]

Pharmacodynamics MAO is a cyproprotein enzyme that deaminates monoamines such as serotonin, epinephrine, norepinephrine, dopamine, tyramine, and tryptamine. In nerve terminals, MAO converts monoamine transmitters into inactive substances. MAO in the liver and intestine inactivates biogenic amines present in foods.

MAO inhibitors produce their antidepressant action by increasing brain concentrations of monoamine neurotransmitter substances. This is achieved by blocking MAO-catalyzed metabolism of these substances. This action increases the amount of norepinephrine and serotonin available for release from neurons of the CNS, thus intensifying transmission.

MAO inhibitors produce reversible or irreversible inhibition. Phenelzine and isocarboxazid produce **irreversible inhibition.** Recovery from this form of inhibition requires synthesis of new enzyme, which is a slow process. Thus the effects of these drugs persist for approximately 2 weeks after discontinuation of the drugs. Tranylcypromine produces **reversible inhibition.** This recovery is more rapid, occurring in 3 to 5 days.[6,17,30]

Undesired clinical responses Undesired responses to MAO inhibitors include orthostatic hypotension, impotence, daytime sedation and insomnia, weight gain, muscle cramps, and involuntary muscle jerks. Most of these responses are not dose related.[6]

Drug-drug and drug-nutrient interactions The most severe drug-nutrient interaction associated with these drugs is the **hypertensive crisis** that may occur when tyramine-rich foods or beverages are ingested by the client. (Tyramine, an amino acid, is normally degraded by MAO in the intestine.) While the client is receiving MAO inhibitors, tyramine is not degraded. Once ingested, tyramine promotes release of norepinephrine from sympathetic nerves, leading to symptoms of hypertensive crisis. Symptoms include sudden onset of a severe headache, nausea, sweating, or palpitations. An abrupt and substantial increase in blood pressure occurs, usually within minutes of ingesting the food or beverage. This response, which produces hypertension, headache, nausea, vomiting, and tachycardia, may lead to hyperpyrexia, stroke, coma, or death.[6]

Numerous drug-drug interactions are possible with MAO inhibitors. Vasodilators or phenothiazines administered concurrently with MAO inhibitors can enhance the hypotensive reaction of these antidepressants. When levodopa is administered concurrently with MAO inhibitors, pronounced CNS stimulation and hypertension may occur. CNS depressants, including alcohol, barbiturates, benzodiazepines, chloral hydrate, and opiates, are generally potentiated by MAO inhibitors, producing excessive sedation and CNS depression.[6,16,17]

Specific drug-related nursing considerations Carefully instruct the client about dietary restrictions (see box) and drugs to avoid. Advise the client to limit the daily intake of caffeine-containing beverages to 3 cups or glasses per day. Generally, small quantities of sour cream, yogurt, cottage

cheese, or chocolate may be consumed without ill effects. Instruct the client to avoid the use of nose drops, cold remedies, nasal decongestants, cough syrups, diet pills, and other prescription or OTC drugs that contain vasoconstrictor or stimulant-type drugs.[6,17]

CONCEPT REVIEW

Three major categories of antidepressant drugs are available: tricyclic antidepressants, selective serotonin-reuptake inhibitors, and MAO inhibitors.

Currently the tricyclic antidepressant drugs are the most frequently prescribed. All tricyclic antidepressant drugs possess the same pharmacologic properties. The choice of which tricyclic antidepressant drug to prescribe is usually based on the side effect profile of each drug and the client's physical and psychologic condition.

Selective serotonin-reuptake inhibitors are relatively new to psychopharmacology. Generally, these drugs have fewer undesired clinical responses and contraindications.

MAO inhibitors are not used as frequently as in the past. These drugs can produce a severe hypertensive crisis in clients who do not monitor dietary intake of tyramine.

DRUGS USED TO TREAT BIPOLAR DISORDER

Lithium carbonate is usually the first drug of choice in the treatment of bipolar disorder. Two anticonvulsant drugs, carbamazepine (Tegretol) and valproic acid (Depakote, Depakene), are common second-line drugs used to treat mania and prevent relapse. These drugs are discussed in Chapter 21.

BIPOLAR DISORDER DRUG PROTOTYPE

LITHIUM CARBONATE

Lithium carbonate is a salt of the alkali metal lithium.

Pharmacotherapeutics Lithium is the recommended treatment for bipolar affective disorder. It is also effective in the treatment of recurrent unipolar depression, obsessive-compulsive disorder, aggression, cluster headaches, and alcoholism.[6]

Pharmacokinetics The pharmacokinetic properties of the drug are linked to the physiology of sodium, chloride, potassium, and fluid balance in the individual. Absorption of lithium is rapid after an oral dose and is virtually complete within 6 to 8 hours. Peak plasma levels occur within 30 minutes to 2 hours after the dose. No protein binding occurs. Lithium is distributed in the total body water, shifting slowly into cells. The slow entry into cells may account for the delay of several days before full clinical responses are noted. Exit from cells is also slow.

FOODS AND BEVERAGES THAT INTERACT WITH MAO INHIBITORS

Foods	Beverages
Aged cheese	Red wine (especially Chianti)
Dry sausages	Sherry
Smoked fish	Beer
Fava beans	
Soy sauce	
Sour cream	
Ripe avocado	
Ripe bananas	
Yogurt	
Yeast extract	
Protein dietary supplements	

Lithium levels in the cerebrospinal fluid peak 24 hours later than levels in the extracellular fluid. This concentration is generally 50% of the plasma concentration. Passage into the brain is slow.[17,30] Lithium is not metabolized by the body; it is filtered, reabsorbed, and excreted by the kidneys. Lithium is also excreted in saliva. The ratio of plasma concentration to salivary concentration is fixed.

Pharmacodynamics Lithium alters sodium transport in nerve and muscle cells and effects a shift toward intraneuronal metabolism of catecholamines. However, the specific biochemical mechanism of lithium action in mania is unknown.[15]

Pharmaceutics Lithium carbonate is available in capsule, sustained-action tablet, and uncoated tablet dosage forms for oral administration. The initial dose of lithium is 300 mg twice daily. Dosage is then increased by 300 mg until adequate serum concentration levels are achieved. Optimal client response is usually established and maintained with 1800 mg per day in divided doses. Immediate-release capsules and tablets are usually administered three to four times daily. Doses of controlled-release tablets are administered twice a day.[6,15]

Undesired Clinical Responses Undesired clinical responses include nausea, hand tremor, diarrhea, increased thirst and urination, acne, weight gain, cognitive dulling, and edema. Fatigue, muscular weakness, slurred speech, ataxia, leukocytosis, and nephrogenic diabetic insipidus have also occurred. These responses apparently are dose related.[15]

In addition, lithium interferes with iodine trapping by the thyroid gland and the formation of thyroid hormones. In the course of lithium therapy, clients may develop a goiter or experience hypothyroidism. Studies, including those of triiodothyronine (T_3), thyroxine (T_4), and thyroid-stimulating hormone (TSH), should be obtained before starting lithium therapy and every 1 or 2 years during therapy.[17,30]

Severe and persistent nausea, vomiting, and diarrhea are common early signs of lithium toxicity. Lethargy, weakness, and decreasing levels of consciousness occur next. Tremors, myoclonic movements, increased muscle tonus, increased deep tendon reflexes, and seizures follow. Pulmonary complications and cardiac arrhythmias are the major causes of death.[17]

Contraindications and Precautions Lithium is not recommended for clients with significant renal or cardiovascular disease. In addition, sodium depletion resulting from a salt-restricted diet or the administration of diuretics enhances lithium retention, increasing the serum concentration of lithium. Hypokalemia enhances the toxic potential of lithium.[17]

Drug-Drug Interactions Numerous drugs, when combined with lithium, can increase the serum concentration of lithium. For example, when fluoxetine is administered concurrently with lithium, serum lithium concentration increases, and lithium toxicity is possible. A variety of nonsteroidal anti-inflammatory drugs also increase serum lithium concentrations.[16,17]

Thiazide diuretics and furosemide increase sodium and potassium excretion and lithium reabsorption, leading to increased serum lithium concentration. Potassium-saving diuretics decrease renal clearance of lithium and may also increase lithium serum concentration.[17,30]

Life-Span Considerations Lithium use is not recommended during pregnancy. Since it is excreted in human milk, nursing should not occur during lithium therapy. It is not recommended that lithium be used in children less than 12 years of age. Elderly clients often achieve therapeutic serum levels with lower dosages.[15]

Specific Drug-Related Nursing Considerations Before treatment with lithium is initiated, a complete blood count, urinalysis, thyroid function studies, and a plasma chemistry assay are obtained. Review these results as a part of your initial assessment. Also determine if the client has a history of renal, cardiovascular, or seizure disorders. Additionally, gather a complete drug history and determine if there is a potential for drug-drug interactions.

You must monitor lithium serum concentration levels. The range of therapeutic concentrations is 0.6 to 1.4 mEq/L; maintenance concentration levels are 0.4 to 0.9 mEq/L. Toxic serum levels occur at 2.0 mEq/L.[15,17,28]

CONCEPT REVIEW

Lithium carbonate is the drug of choice in the treatment and prevention of bipolar disorder.

The exact mechanism of action of this drug is not clear. However, its pharmacokinetic properties are closely linked to the sodium, chloride, potassium, and fluid balance of the client.

Monitoring the serum lithium concentration is imperative.

DRUGS USED TO TREAT ANXIETY DISORDERS

In Chapter 18, anxiolytic drugs are discussed from the perspective of treating mild-to-moderate anxiety disorders. However, in some situations, anxiety occurs in a more severe form. Three major categories of anxiety disorders are treated with psychotherapeutic drugs: panic disorder, obsessive-compulsive disorder, and phobias.

Panic disorders respond to tricyclic antidepressants, in particular, imipramine and desipramine. In addition, preliminary data indicate that fluoxetine and phenelzine are effective. Only one drug, phenelzine, has shown any effectiveness in treating phobias. Fluoxetine and trazodone have shown some effectiveness in treating obsessive-compulsive disorders.[31]

SUMMARY

All behavior is regulated by the interrelationship of chemical and structural parts of the CNS. Alterations in any part of the system may result in altered behavioral responses. Psychotherapeutic drugs act to produce a balance in this interrelationship.

REFERENCES

1. Keltner, N., & Folks, D. (1992). Psychopharmacology update. *Perspectives in Psychiatric Care, 28*(1), 33-36.

2. Lin, T. (1986). Multiculturalism and Canadian psychiatry: Opportunities and challenges. *Canadian Journal of Psychiatry, 31,* 681-690.

3. Garvey, C.A., Gross, D., & Freeman, L. (1991). Assessing psychotropic medication side-effects among children: A reliability study. *Journal of Child and Adolescent Psychiatric and Mental Health Nursing, 4*(4), 127-131.

4. Blair, D., & Dauner, A. (1993). Nonneuroleptic etiologies of extrapyramidal symptoms. *Clinical Nurse Specialist, 7,* 225-231.

5. Blair, D., & Dauner, A. (1992). Extrapyramidal symptoms are serious side-effects of antipsychotic and other drugs. *Nurse Practitioner, 17*(11), 56, 62-64, 67.

6. Clod, C. (1991). Psychopharmacology and clinical practice. *Nursing Clinics of North America, 26,* 375-399.

7. Dillon, N.B. (1992). Screening system for tardive dyskinesia: Development and implementation. *Journal of Psychosocial Nursing and Mental Health Services, 30*(10), 3-7, 38-39.

8. Grove, K. (1990). Tardive dyskinesia: A key issue facing the psychiatric/mental health nurse. *Perspectives in Psychiatric Care, 26*(3), 29-32.

9. Sramek, R., Roy, S., Ahrens, T., et al. (1991). Prevalence of tardive dyskinesia among three ethnic groups of chronic psychiatric patients. *Hospital and Community Psychiatry, 42,* 590-592.

10. Ebadi, M., Pfeiffer, R., & Murrin, L. (1990). Pathogenesis and treatment of neuroleptic malignant syndrome. *General Pharmacology, 21,* 367-386.

11. Granner, M., & Wooten, B. (1991). Neuroleptic malignant syndrome or Parkinsonism hyperpyrexia syndrome. *Seminars in Neurology, 11,* 228-235.

12. Caroff, S., & Mann, S. (1993). Neuroleptic malignant syndrome. *Medical Clinics of North America, 77,* 185-200.

13. Sullivan, G., & Lukoff, D. (1990). Sexual side effects of antipsychotic medication: Evaluation and interventions. *Hospital and Community Psychiatry, 41,* 1238-1241.

14. McCarthy, P., & Snyder, J.C. (1992). Orthostatic hypotension: A potential side effect of psychiatric medications. *Journal of Psychosocial Nursing and Mental Health Services, 30*(8), 3-5, 37-38.

15. U.S. Pharmacopcial Convention (1990). *The United States pharmacopeia* (22nd rev.). Rockville, MD: Author.

16. Watsky, E., & Salzman, C. (1991). Psychotropic drug interactions. *Hospital and Community Psychiatry, 42,* 247-256.

17. Berstein, J.G. (1988). *Handbook of drug therapy in psychiatry* (2nd ed.). Littleton, MA: PSG Publishing.

18. Santo-Novak, D., & Edwards, R.C. (1989). Rx: Take caution with drugs for elders. *Geriatric Nursing,* 72-75.

19. Wood, A.J., & Zhou, H.H. (1991). Ethnic differences in drug disposition and responsiveness. *Clinical Pharmacokinetics, 20,* 350-373.

20. Meltzer, H. (1993). New drugs for the treatment of schizophrenia. *Psychiatric Clinics of North America, 16,* 365-385.

21. Safferman, A., Lieberman, J., Kane, J., Szymanski, S., & Kinon, B. (1992). Update on the clinical efficacy and side effects of clozapine. *Innovations and Research, 1*(3), 3-14.

22. Cohn, J., Katon, W., & Richelson, E. (1990). Choosing the right antidepressant. *Patient Care, 24*(12), 88-92, 97-98, 100.

23. Brasfield, K. (1991). Practical psychopharmacologic considerations in depression. *Nursing Clinics of North America, 26,* 651-663.

24. Newcomb, P. (1991). Tricyclic antidepressants and children. *Nurse Practitioner: American Journal of Primary Health Care, 16*(5), 26, 28, 30.

25. Gomez, G., & Gomez, E. (1992). The use of antidepressants with elderly patients. *Journal of Psychosocial Nursing, 30*(11), 21-26.

26. McPherson, A. (1989). Drugs and dietary interactions: Guidelines for counseling the home health care patient. *Journal of Home Health Care Practice, 1*(4), 27-29.

27. Morelli, J. (1993). Pediatric poisonings: The 10 most toxic prescription drugs. *American Journal of Nursing, 93*(7), 27-29.

28. Chernecky, C., Krech, R., & Berger, B. (1993). *Laboratory tests and diagnostic procedures.* Philadelphia: W.B. Saunders.

29. Meyer, C. (1993). New drugs: In the realm of the brain. *American Journal of Nursing, 93*(8), 58, 60-61.

30. Hollister, L., & Csernansky, J. (1990). *Clinical pharmacology of psychotherapeutic drugs* (3rd ed.). New York: Churchill Livingstone.

31. Beeber, L. (1989). Update on medications for the treatment of anxiety. *Journal of Psychosocial Nursing and Mental Health Services, 27*(10), 42-43.

BIBLIOGRAPHY

Farkas, M. (1990). Utilizing the nursing process in the development of a medication group on an inpatient psychiatric unit. *Perspectives in Psychiatric Care, 26*(3), 12-17.

Feltner, D., & Hertzman, M. (1993). Progress in the treatment of tardive dyskinesia: Theory and practice. *Hospital and Community Psychiatry, 44,* 25-34.

Harrington, C., Tompkins, C., Curtis, M., & Grant, L. (1992). Psychotropic drug use in long term care facilities: A review of the literature. *Gerontologist, 32,* 822-833.

Peet, M., & Pratt, J. (1993). Lithium. Current status in psychiatric disorders. *Drugs, 46*(1), 7-17.

Porterfield, L.M. (1990). Today's antidepressants. *Advancing Clinical Care, 5*(3), 7, 21.

Smith, M., & Buckwalter, K.C. (1992). Medication management, antidepressant drugs, and the elderly: An overview. *Journal of Psychosocial Nursing and Mental Health Services, 30*(10), 30-36, 38-39.

Taft, L., & Barkin, R. (1990). Drug abuse: Use and misuse of psychotropic drugs in Alzheimer's care. *Journal of Gerontological Nursing, 16*(8), 4-10, 36-37.

CHAPTER 21

Antiepileptic Drugs

NORMA L. PINNELL • BARBARA J. WIRICK

⚬ Classification of Epileptic Seizures
LEARNING OBJECTIVES:
  Describe the classification of epileptic seizures.
  Define the different types of seizure activities.
KEY TERMS:
  Atonic, clonic, epilepsy, generalized seizures,
    myoclonic, partial seizures, postictal phase, seizure,
    seizure focus, status epilepticus, tonic

⚬ Etiology of Epilepsy
LEARNING OBJECTIVE: Discuss the etiology of epilepsy.

⚬ General Characteristics of Antiepileptic Drugs
LEARNING OBJECTIVE: Discuss general characteristics of
  antiepileptic drugs.

⚬ Nursing Considerations
LEARNING OBJECTIVE: Develop a plan of care for a client
  receiving antiepileptic drugs.
KEY TERM: Aura

⚬ Hydantoins
LEARNING OBJECTIVES:
  Summarize essential information about the
    pharmacokinetic and pharmacodynamic phases of
    phenytoin.
  Describe drug-diet interactions that occur with
    phenytoin.
  Identify five important undesired clinical responses
    associated with phenytoin.

⚬ Barbiturates
LEARNING OBJECTIVE: Describe the action of
  phenobarbital as an antiepileptic drug.

⚬ Deoxybarbiturates
LEARNING OBJECTIVE: Summarize essential information
  about the pharmacokinetic and pharmacodynamic
  phases of primidone.

⚬ Succinimides
LEARNING OBJECTIVE: Identify the primary therapeutic
  use of ethosuximide.

⚬ Oxazolidinediones
LEARNING OBJECTIVE: Identify the primary therapeutic
  use of trimethadione.

⚬ Iminostilbenes
LEARNING OBJECTIVE: Summarize essential information
  about the pharmacokinetic and pharmacodynamic
  phases of carbamazepine.

⚬ Benzodiazepines
LEARNING OBJECTIVE: Identify major benzodiazepines
  used as antiepileptic drugs.

⚬ Miscellaneous Antiepileptic Drugs
LEARNING OBJECTIVE: Summarize essential information
  about the pharmacokinetic and pharmacodynamic
  phases of valproic acid and felbamate.

CONCEPTS AND TERMS TO REVIEW
Review the physiology of the central nervous system.
Read in a medical-surgical textbook about the care of a
  client during a seizure episode.
Review Chapter 18 for additional information on barbi-
  turates and benzodiazepines.

---

*E*pilepsy is not a disease in and of itself. The term *epilepsy*
describes a group of syndromes involving the central nervous system (CNS). These syndromes are characterized by
sudden, transitory, and recurring seizures that involve one or
more of the following systems: motor, sensory, autonomic, or
psychic. Synonyms for the term *epilepsy* are *convulsive disorders*
and *seizure disorders*.[1]

CLASSIFICATION OF EPILEPTIC SEIZURES

Most epileptic seizures are classified as partial or generalized seizures. **Partial seizures** are also known as *focal* or *local seizures.* Simple partial seizures do not impair consciousness. However, impairment of consciousness does occur with complex partial seizures.

A **generalized seizure** may be convulsive or nonconvulsive. These seizures result in impaired or total loss of consciousness and absence, tonic, clonic, tonic-clonic, myoclonic, or atonic seizure activity. (See Table 21–1 for a description of these seizure activities.) The period immediately after a generalized seizure is called the **postictal phase.** During this phase many individuals experience confusion or excessive lethargy or both.

The term **status epilepticus** denotes seizure activity that recurs before recovery from the preceding seizure activity. This condition may become life threatening. The client may experience airway impairment, aspiration, or brain damage.[1,2]

ETIOLOGY OF EPILEPSY

The most prominent features of an epileptic seizure is sustained synchronous neural discharges. The specific mechanism for sustaining the synchronous firing is unknown. It has been suggested that most seizures begin with the synchronous firing of a relatively localized group of neurons, the **seizure focus.** This focus point may remain quiescent over long periods, discharging only intermittently at levels insufficient to produce seizure activity.[1] Traumas, neurologic surgeries, infections, metabolic alterations, congenital anomalies, brain tumors, drug and alcohol abuse, and vascular diseases have all been implicated as causes for seizure disorders.

Other than children under the age of 5 years, the highest incidence of new onset epilepsy occurs in the age group over 65 years of age. In this age group seizure behavior is often confused with other neurologic impairments, thus delaying treatment.[3]

In individuals with seizure disorders numerous factors such as hypoglycemia, fatigue, or lack of sleep, emotional or physical stress, febrile illness, constipation, use of stimulant and depressant drugs, and hyperventilation can precipitate seizures. Some environmental stimuli such as blinking lights, poorly adjusted television screens, loud noises, certain music or odors or simply being startled can also precipitate seizure activity.[2]

GENERAL CHARACTERISTICS OF ANTIEPILEPTIC DRUGS

Since most seizures begin with the synchronous firing of a group of neurons, effective drugs must block or interrupt this process. At present, clinically used antiepileptic drugs decrease membrane excitability by interacting with ion (sodium or calcium) channels or γ-aminobutyric acid (GABA) neurotransmitter receptors.[4,5]

Even though the actions of antiepileptic drugs are similar, their effects on individuals vary considerably. For example, metabolism of antiepileptic drugs generally occurs faster in children. Therefore the half-lives of these drugs are shortest in this age group. In addition, rates of elimination of antiepileptic drugs are slowest in neonates, infants, and children. Thus children require larger dosages, on a milligrams-per-kilogram basis, than adults.[6]

Undesired clinical responses to antiepileptic drugs are more prevalent in the elderly than in other age groups. Many elderly clients have neurologic deficits that render them more vulnerable to the neurotoxic effects (e.g., ataxia and cognitive disturbances) of antiepileptic drugs. In addition, low serum albumin concentrations, frequently associated with the elderly, decrease drug-protein binding. This may mask high serum concentrations of antiepileptic drugs.[6]

Studies suggest that most antiepileptic drugs are teratogenic; therefore their use during pregnancy is not recommended. Despite this recommendation, approximately 1 in every 250 newborns is exposed to antiepileptic drugs in utero. Compared with the general population, this group of newborns has a greater incidence of teratogenic effects. These effects include major malformations, minor anomalies, intrauterine or postnatal growth failure, and psychomotor retardation.[7] Sometimes the use of antiepileptic drugs is essential for the prevention of major seizures and should not be discontinued during pregnancy. In these situations the primary care provider must discuss the potential risks with the female client.[1]

TABLE 21–1
Description of Seizure Activities

Type of Seizure	Activities
Atonic	Sudden loss of muscle tone, leading to head drop or slumping of body
Absence	Sudden, brief impairment of consciousness; may include blank stare, eye movement, and presence or absence of jerking of limbs and body
Clonic	Rhythmic, multiple jerks of all body parts with loss of consciousness
Myoclonic	Brief, single, mild-to-violent jerks of arms or head
Tonic	Rigid, violent muscular contractions; loss of consciousness
Tonic-clonic	Generalized tonic muscle contractions with flexion of the upper extremities and forced extension of the lower extremities; followed by rhythmic contractions of the limbs and loss of consciousness

▓ NURSING CONSIDERATIONS

The goal of antiepileptic therapy is to decrease or eliminate seizure episodes. To achieve this goal, drug therapy and nursing care must be individualized.

Assessing A complete **health history** is one of the most important aspects of the assessment. Inquire about the frequency of seizures. Ask the client or significant other to describe the seizure episode. Determine how long seizure activity lasts and, if applicable, the sequence through which the seizure progresses. Determine if the client has an **aura** before the seizure. (An aura is a subjective sensation [e.g., visual or auditory changes, tingling, numbness, or dizziness] that occurs before the seizure and warns the client of an impending convulsion.) Determine what occurs in the postictal phase. Does the client become drowsy and sleep? Does the client experience confusion, weakness, headache, or muscle ache?

Also gather subjective data about other neurologic aspects. For example, ask the client if he or she experiences any unusually frequent or severe headaches. Determine if the client has a history of head injury. Ask if the client experiences lightheadedness, dizziness, or vertigo or ever has difficulty swallowing or speaking.

If the client is a child, determine if the mother had health problems during pregnancy (e.g., infections, hypertension, diabetes). Determine if there were difficulties during labor and delivery. How long was the labor? Was the baby at term or premature? Did the baby breathe immediately? Ask the mother if the baby's sucking and swallowing seem coordinated. For the older child, determine if he or she has any problems with balance or has demonstrated unexplained falling, clumsiness, unsteady gait, or muscular weakness.[8]

Obtain a current drug history. Ask the client about all antiepileptic drugs and other prescription or over-the-counter drugs. Assess the dosing schedule of all drugs. Establish the client's level of compliance. Does the client take the drug at the times prescribed and in the prescribed dosages? Is the client in the habit of missing doses? Does the client intentionally skip drug doses? If the client does not follow the prescribed schedule, ask why.

Conduct a thorough psychosocial assessment. These data aid in planning long-term care for the client. Pay particular attention to the following: the client's understanding of the disease, the client's adjustment to the diagnosis, the client's manner of coping with the fears and stigma of the diagnosis, and the type of peer and family support available to the client.

After obtaining a health history, perform a **physical assessment,** including a neurologic assessment. This will aid in identifying underlying pathologic changes. During the neurologic assessment test the cranial nerves, inspect and palpate muscles, perform balance tests, and assess coordination and skilled movements. In addition, assess the sensory system and test reflexes.

Diagnosing After analyzing the data collected from the client, formulate appropriate nursing diagnoses. The following are examples of nursing diagnoses for clients receiving antiepileptic drugs:
- Body image disturbance related to dependence on drugs.
- Diarrhea related to undesired response to drug therapy.
- High risk for altered health maintenance related to lack of knowledge about diagnosis, care during seizure episode, drug schedule, and undesired clinical responses associated with drugs.
- High risk for injury related to CNS effects (e.g., drowsiness, visual disturbance, ataxia, unsteadiness, vertigo) produced by drug therapy.
- High risk for altered nutrition: less than body requirements related to discomfort when eating. (Gingival hyperplasia is a problem associated with phenytoin therapy.)
- High risk for altered nutrition: less than body requirements related to nausea and vomiting.
- High risk for altered oral mucous membrane related to phenytoin therapy.
- High risk for social isolation related to fear of seizure activity.

Planning Since epilepsy is a chronic condition, individuals with the disorder must learn to cope with the condition. Therefore the main focus of the planning phase is client education. Major teaching points are summarized in the Teaching/Discharge Plan. In addition, educate the client's family, friends, or significant other about epilepsy and teach what to do during a seizure episode. Teach the client to take the prescribed drugs on a regular basis and caution the client against abrupt reduction of dosage or discontinuance of the drug.

Establish expected outcomes during the planning phase. Appropriate outcomes include the following:
- Client verbalizes acceptance of self.
- Client reestablishes and maintains a normal pattern of bowel elimination.
- Client assumes responsibility for own health care needs.
- Client remains free of injury.
- Client remains free of signs of malnutrition.
- Client demonstrates techniques to restore integrity of oral mucosa.
- Client verbalizes willingness to be involved with others.

Implementing Most antiepileptic drugs are selective for specific seizure disorders. Therefore to control seizures, proper drug selection is essential. The initial medical diagnosis is based on a thorough health history and physical assessment. In addition, diagnostic studies such as electroencephalogram (EEG), computerized tomography (CT), positron emission tomography (PET), and magnetic resonance imaging (MRI) are used. Since additional seizure activity can be precipitated by stress, the client must be prepared emotionally for these studies.

Once drug selection is made, the client must be monitored closely for therapeutic, toxic, and undesired clinical responses to the drugs. Close monitoring of the client is especially important when drug therapy is initiated, when dosages are altered, when drugs are changed, or when other illness occurs. To limit the severity of undesired clinical responses, drug dosages are begun at a low level and are gradually increased until a therapeutic dose is reached.

Since many antiepileptic drugs are CNS depressants, regularly assess mental and neurologic function and behavior. Common gastrointestinal (GI) symptoms that occur with many antiepileptic drugs are nausea, vomiting, and diarrhea.

TEACHING/DISCHARGE PLAN

The following information should be taught to the client and family or significant other:

1. Monitor for and report undesired clinical responses to drugs (drowsiness, ataxia, nausea, vomiting, diarrhea, incoordination) to the primary care provider.
2. Practice proper health measures to reduce seizure activities:
   - Avoid physical or emotional stress.
   - Practice stress management techniques.
   - Eat a well-balanced, nutritious diet with increased amounts of vitamin D.
   - Seek medical care for concurrent illness.
   - Avoid situations that may cause hypoxia, hypoglycemia, sodium and water retention, and exhaustion.
   - Avoid flashing or blinking lights.
   - Avoid alcohol intoxication.
3. Take antiepileptic drug(s) as prescribed:
   - Take drugs regularly at consistent intervals.
   - Take drugs with meals or food to diminish gastric symptoms.
   - Store the drugs out of reach of children.
   - Check with the primary care provider or pharmacist before taking other drugs.
   - Do not reduce dosage abruptly or discontinue drugs without checking with the primary care provider.
4. Wear a medical identification tag or bracelet that indicates you are taking antiepileptic drugs.
5. Use caution when operating a car or other powered machinery.

Gastric symptoms may be reduced by administering the drugs with meals. Once a drug regimen is established, administer doses regularly at consistent intervals.

Control of seizures is an important factor in enhancing the client's self-image and social interaction. Individuals with a seizure disorder often feel embarrassed and humiliated. They may isolate themselves socially because they fear ridicule if a seizure occurs in public. Always treat the individual with respect and acceptance. Provide emotional support and encourage the client to maintain existing social relationships.

Growth and development may be altered throughout all phases of the life span. Developmental tasks of childhood may be delayed. Adolescents may be shunned by peers. Social and job pressures may be placed on adults. All of these factors make it difficult to progress developmentally and socially. Children with seizure disorders may be referred to appropriate professionals. Educate parents to assist the child in overcoming developmental delays that do occur. Community resource referrals for adolescents and adults with epilepsy may be made to assist them in these areas.

Evaluating   Plasma drug levels that produce therapeutic and toxic effects have been established and can be used to evaluate the effectiveness of specific drugs and drug dosages. Plasma drug levels can also help the health care providers monitor compliance and identify causes of toxicity.

Another tool for evaluating the effectiveness of the drug regimen is a seizure-episode record. The record should contain a complete history of all seizure activities. Before discharge, teach the client or significant other how to create and use the record.

During the evaluation phase determine if the client has achieved the expected outcomes developed during the planning phase. If the outcomes were not achieved, determine the reason(s) and revise the plan of care accordingly.

CONCEPT REVIEW

Sustained synchronous discharge of a localized group of neurons precipitates seizure episodes.

Antiepileptic drugs do not cure seizure disorders but do suppress seizure activity.

Antiepileptic drugs should not be discontinued abruptly. Sudden withdrawal of drugs may trigger seizure activity or status epilepticus.

The main focus of nursing care for the individual receiving antiepileptic drugs is client education.

HYDANTOINS

Three hydantoins—phenytoin, mephenytoin, and ethotoin—are available for antiepileptic use. The most commonly prescribed hydantoin is phenytoin.

HYDANTOIN PROTOTYPE

PHENYTOIN

Phenytoin (Dilantin) was introduced as an antiepileptic drug in 1938.

Pharmacotherapeutics   Phenytoin has a broad range of action against many types of seizures. However, it is ineffective against absence seizures. It is indicated for the treatment of grand mal and complex partial seizures and is used frequently to treat and prevent seizures during and after neurosurgic procedures. Intravenous (IV) phenytoin is also effective in controlling tonic-clonic status epilepticus.[1,9,10]

Pharmacokinetics   Since phenytoin is a weak acid, it is insoluble at the pH of gastric juice. Thus orally administered phenytoin is poorly and slowly absorbed in the stomach. Most oral phenytoin absorption occurs in the small intestine. A portion of an oral dose can remain unabsorbed and be eliminated in the feces.[1,11]

Phenytoin is almost 90% bound to plasma protein in adults. After an oral dose the peak blood level is reached in approximately $1\frac{1}{2}$ to 12 hours. The average half-life of phenytoin is 22 hours, but the half-life may range from 7 to 42 hours as a result of absorption and elimination variables in individuals. Several days to weeks of drug therapy may be needed for the client to reach a steady-state plasma level. Phenytoin is metabolized extensively in the liver and is excreted in the urine.[1,9,11]

Pharmacodynamics Phenytoin acts mainly in the motor cortex to normalize abnormal fluxes of sodium across neuron cell membranes during and after depolarization. This reduces the excitability of the nerve and raises the seizure threshold.[5,9]

Pharmaceutics Phenytoin is available in chewable tablets, gelatin capsules, and liquid suspensions for oral administration. Phenytoin sodium is available in a solution for intramuscular (IM) and IV use.[9,10] Table 21–2 summarizes information about phenytoin and other hydantoins.

Undesired Clinical Responses The most common undesired clinical responses encountered with phenytoin therapy involve the CNS. These responses, which are usually dose related, include ataxia, nystagmus, slurred speech, decreased coordination, and mental confusion. Dizziness, insomnia, transient nervousness, muscle twitching, and headaches have also been observed.[10]

Other undesired clinical responses include nausea, vomiting, constipation, toxic hepatitis, and liver damage. Blood dyscrasias such as thrombocytopenia, granulocytopenia, leukopenia, and agranulocytosis have been reported. In addition, phenytoin causes coarsening of facial features, enlargement of the lips, hirsutism, and gingival hyperplasia.[9] Figure 21–1 illustrates undesired clinical responses common to most antiepileptic drugs.

IV phenytoin has additional undesired clinical responses, including hypotension, arrhythmias, cardiovascular collapse, and CNS depression. In addition, local irritation, inflammation, tenderness, necrosis, and tissue sloughing have been reported at the infusion site. Also associated with IV administration of phenytoin is purple-glove syndrome. Although the etiology of purple-glove syndrome is unknown, three stages of the syndrome have been identified: appearance, progression, and resolution.[9,12]

Contraindications and Precautions Administration of parenteral phenytoin is contraindicated for clients with sinus bradycardia, sinoatrial block, second- and third-degree AV block, and Adams-Stokes syndrome. Also phenytoin should not be administered to clients with impaired liver function or clients hypersensitive to hydantoins.[10]

Interference With Laboratory Tests Phenytoin may decrease serum levels of protein-bound iodine (PBI).

Phenytoin may also increase serum levels of glucose, alkaline phosphatase, and γ-glutamyl transpeptidase (GGT).

Drug-Drug and Drug-Nutrient Interactions Concurrent administration of phenytoin with other drugs can result in marked increases or decreases in plasma phenytoin levels. Drugs either inhibit or enhance the metabolism of phenytoin or displace phenytoin from protein-binding sites.[1,13] Phenytoin can also increase or decrease the serum levels of other drugs. Some drugs that interact with phenytoin are listed in the box.

Phenytoin induces microsomal oxidase, leading to accelerated metabolism of vitamin D. Because vitamin D is necessary for the absorption of calcium, a decrease in vitamin D may decrease calcium absorption, causing osteomalacia and rickets. Phenytoin also uses folic acid as a cofactor during enzyme induction. This can produce clinical folate deficiency states. Folic acid supplements may reduce serum levels of phenytoin and decrease the drug's efficacy. The primary care provider should test for folate anemia and prescribe adequate folic acid to prevent the occurrence of anemia. In addition, phenytoin can lower the level of stored vitamin K.[14]

Life-Span Considerations In-utero exposure to phenytoin may produce congenital heart malformations, cleft lip or palate, and fetal hydantoin syndrome. Fetal hydantoin syndrome consists of prenatal growth deficiency, microcephaly, and mental deficiency.[9] In addition, women taking phenytoin should not breast-feed since the drug apparently is secreted in low concentrations in human milk.

The usual dosage of phenytoin in adults is 100 mg tid; children may need a dosage of 4 to 8 mg/kg/d. In the elderly a dosage level of 3 to 4 mg/kg/d may be needed to achieve therapeutic plasma levels.[6]

Specific Drug-Related Nursing Considerations The client's plasma concentration levels must be monitored closely. Plasma concentrations from 10 to 20 µg/ml are therapeutically effective. Concentrations from 30 to 50 µg/ml produce toxicity, and the approximate fatal concentration is 100 µg/ml. Note that the margin between therapeutic and toxic levels is narrow when the drug is administered intravenously.

Since the various preparations of phenytoin exhibit differences in rate and extent of absorption, they are not bioequivalent. Advise the client not to change from one product to another. Also instruct the client to check with the pharmacist when receiving prescription refills to make certain that the same product is supplied each time.

Gingival hyperplasia and softening of the gums are the most common difficulties with phenytoin. These problems can be prevented or controlled in many cases by good oral hygiene. Tell the client to brush his or her teeth at least once daily with a soft toothbrush and to floss daily. If the client is a young child, parents or caregivers should be instructed to brush and floss the child's teeth daily.

DRUG-DRUG INTERACTIONS INVOLVING PHENYTOIN

Increased Phenytoin Effects	Decreased Phenytoin Effects
Amiodarone	Carbamazepine
Cimetidine	Barbiturates
Disulfiram	Ethanol
Isoniazid	Rifampin
Benzodiazepines	Theophylline
Valproic acid	

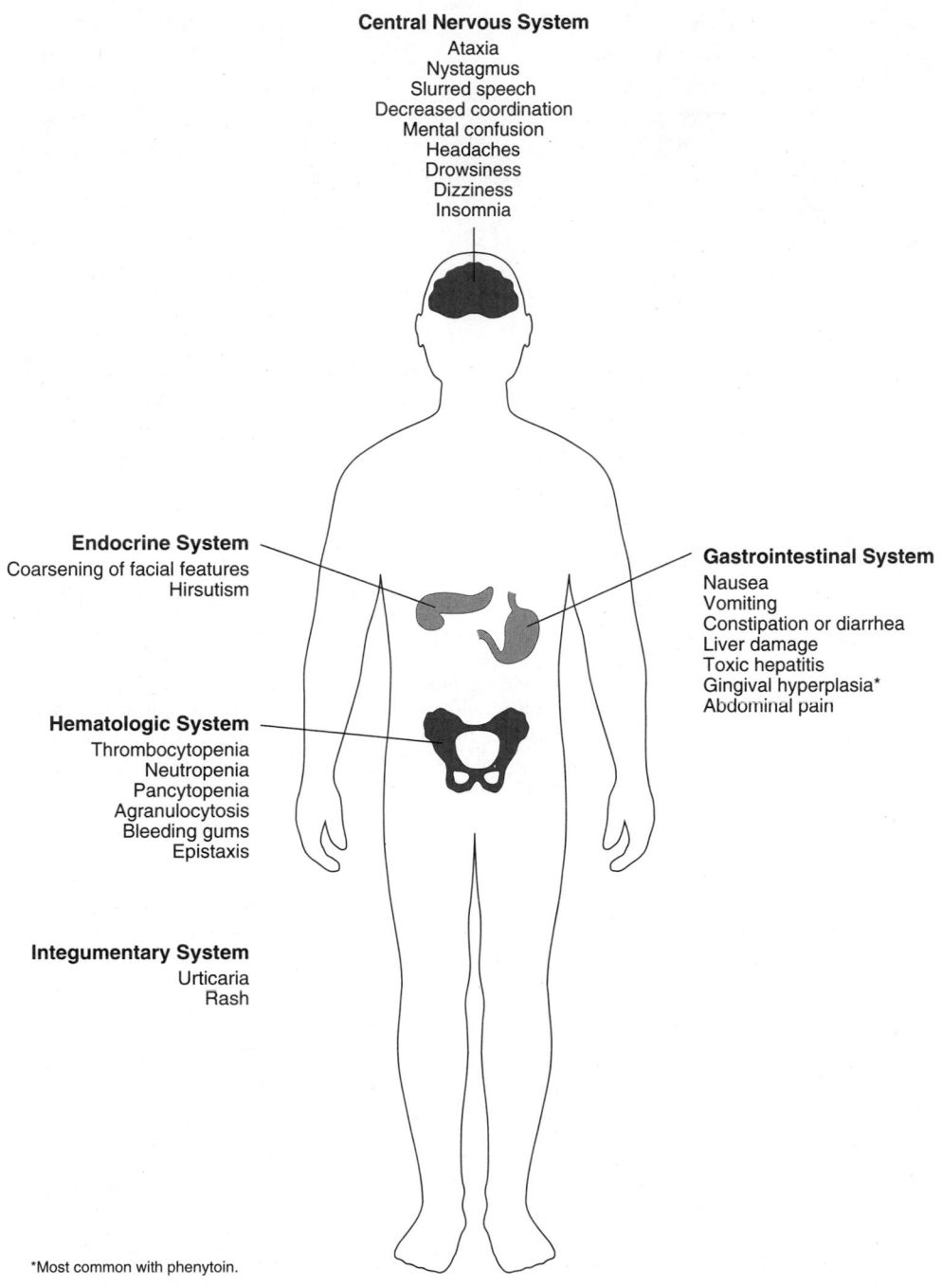

Central Nervous System
Ataxia
Nystagmus
Slurred speech
Decreased coordination
Mental confusion
Headaches
Drowsiness
Dizziness
Insomnia

Endocrine System
Coarsening of facial features
Hirsutism

Gastrointestinal System
Nausea
Vomiting
Constipation or diarrhea
Liver damage
Toxic hepatitis
Gingival hyperplasia*
Abdominal pain

Hematologic System
Thrombocytopenia
Neutropenia
Pancytopenia
Agranulocytosis
Bleeding gums
Epistaxis

Integumentary System
Urticaria
Rash

*Most common with phenytoin.

FIGURE 21-1   Undesired clinical responses common to most antiepileptic drugs.

Phenytoin produces coarsening of facial features and hirsutism in female clients. You may need to provide the client with suggestions for managing these problems. Usually, since shaving of undesirable facial hair leaves a stubble, bleaching is the preferred method of handling hirsutism. Some clients use electrolysis, which destroys hair follicles. The coarsened facial features usually can be altered with careful use of makeup.

When giving phenytoin intravenously, be certain that the solution is clear and not cloudy or precipitated. Because of the possibility of precipitation, do not mix parenteral phenytoin with any IV fluid. The IV dosage of phenytoin should not exceed 50 mg per minute in adults and 1 to 3 mg/kg/min in neonates. Heart rate, rhythm, and blood pressure should be carefully monitored for all clients receiving IV phenytoin. Phenytoin is not recommended for continuous drip infusions.[9,10]

NURSING RESEARCH

Bader, M. (1993). Case study of two methods for enteral phenytoin administration. *Journal of Neuroscience Nursing, 25,* 233-242.

Serum phenytoin levels fall dramatically, often to subtherapeutic levels, when phenytoin is administered enterally. The purpose of this case study was to evaluate the effect of two methods of administering phenytoin suspension in clients concurrently receiving enteral feedings. Effectiveness of each administration technique was based on serum phenytoin levels.

Data revealed that dilution of the suspension and irrigation of the tube produced higher phenytoin levels than the administration of the undiluted suspension. It was suggested that simultaneous administration of other enteral drugs might have interfered with phenytoin absorption in one subject.

STUDENT ACTIVITIES

• Check the procedure manual at your assigned agency and determine the protocol for administering the

drug enterally. Are the drugs diluted? Is the tube irrigated after the administration of the drug?
• Interview a nurse in the quality assurance department of the agency and determine if plasma levels are checked to determine the effectiveness of drugs administered enterally.

MISCELLANEOUS DRUGS IN CATEGORY

Both mephenytoin (Mesantoin) and ethotoin (Peganone) are used to treat seizure disorders. **Mephenytoin** was introduced in 1945 as an antiepileptic drug. Although it is not frequently prescribed today, mephenytoin is approved by the Food and Drug Administration (FDA) for treatment of tonic-clonic, simple partial, and complex partial seizures. Compared to phenytoin, mephenytoin produces more sedation and a

TABLE 21–2
Hydantoins: Prototype and Other Drugs in Category

Drug Name	Dosage and Route of Administration	Nursing Considerations
PHENYTOIN (Dilantin) **HOW SUPPLIED** Chewable tablet: 50 mg Capsule: 30, 100 mg Suspension: 30 or 125 mg/5 ml Injection: 50 mg/ml	**ADULTS** Loading dose (if prescribed): 1 g divided into 400, 300, 300 mg administered at 2-h intervals, followed by usual maintenance dose started 24 h later Oral: with tablets, initial dose, 100 mg tid; usual maintenance dose, 100 mg three or four times a day With suspension, initial dose, 125 mg (1 tsp) tid; can be increased to 125 mg five times a day Parenteral (IV preferred): loading dose, 10-15 mg/kg slowly, not to exceed 50 mg/min; maintenance dose, 100 mg q6-8h **CHILDREN** Oral (tablet or suspension): initial dose, 5 mg/kg/d in two or three equally divided doses; maintenance dose, individualized up to a maximum of 300 mg daily; usual maintenance dose, 4-8 mg/kg/d Parenteral (IV preferred): loading dose, 15-20 mg/kg slowly not to exceed 50 mg/min	**Assess** Collect drug history to detect possible drug-drug interactions. Assess client for preexisting conditions that would contradict use of hydantoins. Collect nutrition history to detect possible drug-nutrient interactions. **Implement** Advise client to wear identification. Instruct client not to change drug brands. Explain that drug may color urine pink, red, or reddish brown. Teach client to brush teeth with a soft toothbrush. Stress the importance of regular visits to the dentist. Do not mix IV solutions with dextrose 5% in water. Do not use cloudy parenteral solution. Begin IV infusion within 1 h of mixing. Discard solution after 4 h. Inject sterile saline solution through same needle or IV catheter after phenytoin sodium injection to avoid venous irritation. Infuse IV solution at rate of 50 mg/min in adults and 1-3 mg/kg/min in neonates. Do not use discolored capsules. Protect drug from light and moisture. Store drug below 30° C. **Monitor** Monitor for undesired clinical responses (e.g., drowsiness, sedation, nausea, vomiting, gingival hyperplasia) Monitor CBC and serum calcium levels q6mo. **Evaluate** Evaluate serum concentration levels. Clinically effective serum level is usually 10-20 μg/ml.

TABLE 21–2 *Continued*
Hydantoins: Prototype and Other Drugs in Category

Drug Name	Dosage and Route of Administration	Nursing Considerations
Mephenytoin (Mesantoin) HOW SUPPLIED Uncoated tablets: 100 mg	ADULTS Initial dose, 50–100 mg/d for the first week, then increase daily dose by 50–100 mg at weekly intervals; average dose, 200–600 mg/d CHILDREN Initial dose, same as for adult; usual required dose, 100–400 mg/d	Same as for phenytoin.
Ethotoin (Peganone) HOW SUPPLIED Uncoated tablets: 250, 500 mg	ADULTS Initial dose, 1 g/d divided into four or six doses taken after meals; usual maintenance dose, 2-3 g/d CHILDREN Initial dose depends on weight, not to exceed 750 mg/d; usual maintenance dose, 500 mg-1 g/d	Same as for phenytoin.

greater risk for serious blood dyscrasias. Because of the toxicity associated with the mephenytoin, the initial dose should be 50 to 100 mg/d for 1 week, with increases of 50 or 100 mg at weekly intervals.[1]

Ethotoin is used to treat tonic-clonic and complex partial seizures. Compared with phenytoin, it is less toxic and has a lower efficacy. It is usually administered in conjunction with other antiepileptic drugs. The half-life of ethotoin is approximately 3 to 9 hours. Its effective plasma concentration level is 15 to 50 µg/ml. To achieve this level, the drug must be administered after meals in four to six divided daily dosages.[1]

CONCEPT REVIEW

Phenytoin has a stabilizing effect on neuronal membranes. It is effective in the treatment of a variety of seizure disorders.

Concurrent administration of phenytoin with other drugs can result in marked increases or decreases in plasma phenytoin levels.

One of the most common undesired clinical responses associated with phenytoin is gingival hyperplasia. In addition, vitamin D, vitamin K, and folate deficiency states are possible with phenytoin therapy.

BARBITURATES

In Chapter 18 the drug category of barbiturates was described. In this chapter the discussion is limited to barbiturates commonly used as antiepileptic drugs.

BARBITURATE PROTOTYPE
PHENOBARBITAL

Phenobarbital was introduced for the treatment of seizures in 1912. Since then it has become one of the most widely used antiepileptic drugs.

Pharmacotherapeutics Phenobarbital is effective against generalized tonic-clonic and simple and complex partial seizures but is not useful in treating absence and myoclonic seizures. Phenobarbital is also used to prevent and treat febrile seizures and alcohol- and drug-withdrawal seizures.[1]

Pharmacodynamics Used as an antiepileptic, phenobarbital may enhance GABA receptor-mediated inactivation. This inhibits abnormal electric brain activity that causes seizures. High concentrations of the drug may also decrease transmitter release and postsynaptic excitation by blocking calcium ion entry into nerve terminals.[1]

Pharmaceutics Phenobarbital is available in oral preparations and sterile solutions for IM or IV administration (see box). Doses of phenobarbital and phenytoin are also combined in a capsule for oral administration.[9,10]

PHENOBARBITAL DOSAGES

Adult Dose
Oral: 60–250 mg/d in divided doses
IM or IV: 100-320 mg; repeat in 6 h if needed to total of 600 mg/d

Pediatric Dose
Oral: 4-6 mg/kg/d in divided doses
IM or IV: 10–20 mg/kg loading dose; then 1–6 mg/kg/d

Specific Drug-Related Nursing Considerations In-utero exposure may produce congenital heart malformations, facial clefts, and other malformations in the neonate. Therefore advise female clients to notify their primary care providers if they believe that they are pregnant.

Like phenytoin, phenobarbital accelerates the metabolism of vitamin D and uses folic acid during enzyme induction. Deficiency states for both of these vitamins are possible. Vitamin B_6 supplements, if prescribed, can reduce the effectiveness of phenobarbital. In addition, food decreases the absorption of phenobarbital. Administer the drug on an empty stomach (i.e., 1 hour before or 2 hours after a meal).[14]

Administer IM injections of phenobarbital sodium deep into large muscles. Do not inject more than 5 ml in one site because of possible tissue irritation. IV infusion is recommended only if the client is unconscious. The rate of IV infusion for adults should not exceed 60 mg/min.[9]

MISCELLANEOUS DRUGS IN CATEGORY

Mephobarbital (Mebaral) is an analog of phenobarbital. It has the same pharmacologic properties, clinical uses, and undesired clinical responses as phenobarbital. During metabolism approximately 75% of a single oral dose of mephobarbital is converted to phenobarbital.[1]

The average dose of mephobarbital for adults is 200 to 600 mg daily. For children under 5 years of age, the desired dose is 16 to 32 mg three to four times daily. Children older than 5 years should receive 32 to 64 mg three to four times daily. Administer mephobarbital at bedtime if seizure activity generally occurs at night. If seizure activities are diurnal, administer the drug during the day.[9]

DEOXYBARBITURATES

Deoxybarbiturates are compounds that contain one less atom of oxygen than barbiturates.

DEOXYBARBITURATE PROTOTYPE

PRIMIDONE

Primidone (Myidone, Mysoline) is nearly identical in structure to phenobarbital. Therefore the pharmacology of the drugs is similar.

Pharmacotherapeutics Primidone is used in the treatment of tonic-clonic and partial seizures. It is not effective against absence seizures. Primidone is also used concurrently with other antiepileptic drugs such as phenytoin and carbamazepine.

Pharmacokinetics Since primidone is not ionized, it is quickly absorbed from the GI tract after oral administration. Primidone is minimally bound to plasma proteins, and plasma concentration levels peak approximately 3 hours after administration. Metabolism of primidone results in two active metabolites—phenobarbital and phenylethylmalonamide (PEMA). The elimination half-life of primidone varies, ranging from 5 to 18 hours. Primidone and PEMA are excreted by the kidneys.[1]

PRIMIDONE DOSAGES

Clients 8 years of age and older who have received no previous treatment for seizure activity are stated on the following regimen:

Days 1-3: 100-125 mg hs
Days 4-6: 100-125 mg bid
Days 7-9: 100-125 mg tid
Day 10 to maintenance: 250 mg tid
Usual maintenance dose: 250 mg tid or qid

Children less than 8 yr old are started on the following regimen:

Days 1-3: 50 mg hs
Days 4-6: 50 mg bid
Days 7-9: 100 mg bid
Day 10 to maintenance: 125-250 mg tid
Usual maintenance dose: 125-250 mg tid or 10-25 mg/kg/d in divided doses

---

Pharmacodynamics Primidone and its two metabolites have antiepileptic actions. However, the exact mechanism of primidone's antiepileptic action is not known.[9]

Pharmaceutics Primidone is available in tablet and suspension preparations for oral administration. The total daily dose of primidone should not exceed 2g (see box).

Undesired Clinical Responses Ataxia and vertigo are the most frequent early undesired clinical responses. These symptoms tend to disappear with continued therapy or reduction of the initial dosage. Nausea, vomiting, anorexia, drowsiness, fatigue, and CNS disturbances have also been reported. In addition, the client may experience the undesired responses that occur with phenobarbital therapy.[1,10]

Contraindications and Precautions Use of primidone is contraindicated in clients hypersensitive to phenobarbital or in clients with porphyria.[9]

Drug-Drug and Drug-Nutrient Interactions Phenytoin and carbamazepine induce the biotransformation of primidone, producing decreased levels of primidone but increased levels of its metabolite phenobarbital. Isoniazid can increase primidone plasma levels.[1]

Like phenytoin, primidone accelerates the metabolism of vitamin D and uses folic acid during enzyme induction. Deficiency states for both of these vitamins are possible. Primidone can also lower the level of stored vitamin K.[14]

Life-Span Considerations Effects of primidone on human pregnancy are unknown. However, studies show an elevated incidence of birth defects in women treated with phenobarbital, the active metabolite of primidone. Studies have also shown that primidone appears in the milk of nursing mothers in substantial quantities.[9]

Specific Drug-Related Nursing Considerations Since therapy with primidone usually extends over prolonged periods, a complete blood count (CBC) should be conducted every 6 months.

SUCCINIMIDES

Three succinimide antiepileptic drugs—ethosuximide, meth-suximide, and phensuximide—are marketed.

SUCCINIMIDE PROTOTYPE
ETHOSUXIMIDE

Ethosuximide (Zarontin) is the most frequently prescribed succinimide antiepileptic drug.

Pharmacotherapeutics Ethosuximide is indicated in the control of absence seizures. It has no clinical efficacy against tonic-clonic and complex partial seizures.

Pharmacokinetics Ethosuximide is absorbed well after oral administration, and peak plasma levels occur within several hours. The drug is water soluble and does not accumulate in fat. Its half-life is 30 hours in children and 60 hours in adults. Most of the drug is metabolized in the liver and excreted in the urine. Approximately 20% to 25% of ethosuximide is excreted unchanged by the kidney. Approximately 40% to 50% is excreted as the inactive hydroxyethyl derivative.[1]

Pharmacodynamics Some studies suggest that etho-suximide depresses the motor cortex, raising the seizure threshold. This action suppresses the brain spike and wave activity, which prevents the lapses of consciousness associated with absence seizures. Other studies suggest that ethosuximide reduces low-threshold calcium current.[5]

Pharmaceutics Ethosuximide is available in capsule and syrup preparations for oral administration. Observation of the client to determine clinical response is the preferred method for establishing dosage.

Undesired Clinical Responses Usually ethosuximide is well tolerated. Minor undesired clinical responses occur in less than 50% of the clients receiving the drug. These responses include nausea, vomiting, anorexia, abdominal pain, diarrhea, weight loss, lethargy, fatigue, and photophobia. Some of these effects may diminish or disappear with continued therapy.[1,10] Other observed undesired clinical responses include hemopoietic complications, drowsiness, headache, irritability, visual disturbance, and urticaria.[9]

Contraindications and Precautions The drug should be used with caution in clients with renal or hepatic dysfunction. It should not be administered to clients allergic to succinimides.

Drug-Drug Interactions Ethosuximide may interact with concurrently administered antiepileptic drugs. For example, the drug increases the lethargy produced by barbiturates and elevates the serum level of phenytoin. When administered with valproic acid, ethosuximide serum levels may increase or decrease.[9,10]

Life-Span Considerations As with most antiepileptic drugs, an elevated incidence of birth defects has been reported in newborns born to women receiving ethosuximide during pregnancy.

Specific Drug-Related Nursing Considerations Caution the client that ethosuximide can cause drowsiness. Advise the client to avoid operating dangerous machinery and motor vehicles while adjusting to the drug. Instruct the client to take the drug with food to reduce GI distress.

Review the results of studies conducted to monitor renal and hepatic function. Even though blood dyscrasias are uncommon, they do occur with ethosuximide. Therefore monitor the client for indications of leukopenia and pancytopenia. In addition, periodic blood serum level results should be obtained, particularly if the client is taking ethosuximide concurrently with other antiepileptics. The therapeutic plasma level is 40 to 100 µg/ml.

CONCEPT REVIEW

Phenobarbital is one of the most widely used antiepileptic drugs. Because phenobarbital has a long half-life, it can be administered once daily to produce relatively constant serum levels.

Mephobarbital is metabolized to phenobarbital. Therefore similar pharmacokinetic and pharmacodynamic properties can be expected.

Primidone also has a chemical structure similar to phenobarbital. The pharmacologic properties of the two drugs are almost identical.

Ethosuximide is the drug of choice for absence seizures.

OXAZOLIDINEDIONES

OXAZOLIDINEDIONE PROTOTYPE
TRIMETHADIONE

Because of its potential to produce fetal malformation and serious undesired clinical responses, trimethadione is not used when other less toxic drugs are effective.

Pharmacotherapeutics Trimethadione was once the drug of choice against absence seizures. It is now used for clients whose absence seizures are not adequately controlled.

Pharmacokinetics Administered orally, trimethadione is rapidly absorbed. Peak serum concentration levels occur in 30 minutes to 2 hours. Metabolism of trimethadione to the active metabolite dimethadione occurs in the hepatic microsomal system. No further metabolism of the drug occurs, and dimethadione is excreted slowly in the urine. The elimination half-life of dimethadione is 10 to 20 days. Therapeutic levels of dimethadione may not be reached for more than 30 days.[1,11]

Pharmacodynamics Mechanism of action for trimethadione is not clearly understood.

Pharmaceutics Trimethadione is available in chewable tablets, capsules, and oral solutions.

Undesired Clinical Responses Both trimethadione and its active metabolite dimethadione are CNS depressants. If administered in high doses, sedation, ataxia, and incoordination can occur. With continued therapy, tolerance to the sedation or drowsiness tends to develop. Other responses associated with this drug are light blindness, dermatologic reactions, and neutropenia.[1] In addition, a myasthenia gravis–like syndrome has been reported.

Contraindications and Precautions Trimethadione should not be administered to a client with a known hypersensitivity to the drug.

Life-Span Considerations Studies suggest that trimethadione has teratogenic effects. The safety of trimethadione during lactation has not been established.[9]

Specific Drug-Related Nursing Considerations Careful medical supervision is required for clients receiving this drug. CBC, liver function tests, and urinalysis should be done before initiating drug therapy and at monthly intervals during therapy. Advise the client to report any skin rash immediately to the primary care provider.

IMINOSTILBENES

IMINOSTILBENE PROTOTYPE

CARBAMAZEPINE

Carbamazepine was first synthesized in the 1950s. It was introduced into clinical practice as an antiepileptic in the United States in the 1960s and early 1970s.

Pharmacotherapeutics Initially carbamazepine was used in the treatment of trigeminal and glossopharyngeal neuralgia. Later it was used as an antiepileptic. As an antiepileptic, carbamazepine is indicated in the treatment of psychomotor and temporal lobe seizures. It is also indicated in the treatment of generalized tonic-clonic seizures, complex partial seizures, and mixed seizures.[1,16]

Since the late 1970s the psychiatric use of carbamazepine has mushroomed. It is used alone or in combination with lithium in the treatment of bipolar affective disorders.[16,17]

Pharmacokinetics Carbamazepine has poor water solubility, and absorption of the drug from the GI tract is slow. Since eating increases the secretion of bile and gastric juice, taking the drug with meals enhances its absorption. Protein binding is approximately 70% to 80%, and attainment of peak serum levels is variable, ranging from 6 to 24 hours. The elimination half-life of carbamazepine ranges from 25 to 65 hours initially and decreases to 12 to 17 hours with repeated dosing. Because of these variabilities, it may take several days to establish a dose that maintains therapeutic serum levels (4 to 12 μg/ml). The drug is metabolized in the liver and excreted by the kidneys; 28% of the drug is excreted in the feces.[11,16]

Pharmacodynamics Carbamazepine is chemically unrelated to other antiepileptics. It may reduce chemically and electrically induced seizures by reducing polysynaptic responses in the CNS and depressing nerve transmission, subsequently preventing seizure activity.[5]

Pharmaceutics Carbamazepine is available in tablet, chewable tablet, and suspension form for oral administration.

Undesired Clinical Responses The most common undesired clinical responses are related to the CNS. These responses (e.g., sedation, nausea, weakness, ataxia, diplopia, and mild nystagmus) are dose dependent and can be avoided by dose reduction. Various types of skin eruptions have been reported with the use of carbamazepine, ranging from urticaria to toxic epidermal necrosis. Drug-induced hyponatremia has been reported in some clients. In addition, blood dyscrasias (aplastic anemia, leukopenia, pancytopenia, and agranulocytosis) and abnormal liver function may arise during treatment with the drug.[16,17]

Carbamazepine overdose is potentially life threatening. The initial symptoms, drowsiness and ataxia, are associated with plasma concentrations of 11 to 15 μg/ml. Combativeness, hallucinations, and choreiform movements may occur at levels between 15 to 25 μg/ml. Severe disturbance of consciousness occurs at levels above 25 μg/ml.[16,18]

Contraindications and Precautions Carbamazepine is not recommended for clients with a history of bone marrow depression, hypersensitivity to the drug, or sensitivity to any of the tricyclic compounds (e.g., amitriptyline, desipramine, imipramine).[9]

Drug-Drug Interactions Numerous drug-drug interactions are possible with carbamazepine. For example, the use of thiazide diuretics or furosemide in combination with carbamazepine may produce severe, symptomatic hyponatremia. Cimetidine, isoniazid, and propoxyphene impair the biotransformation and clearance of carbamazepine, producing increased blood levels and a potential for toxicity. Calcium channel blockers such as verapamil and diltiazem and erythromycin antibiotics decrease hepatic metabolism of carbamazepine.[16]

Life-Span Considerations In-utero exposure to carbamazepine may produce spina bifida and hypospadias.[7] The half-life of carbamazepine is shortest in children and the elderly. In addition, the hyponatremia associated with this drug may be a particular concern in the elderly.[6,19]

Specific Drug-Related Nursing Considerations Review results of baseline CBC and liver function studies before administering the initial dose. Monitor CBC results regularly; the drug usually is discontinued if the white blood count (WBC) drops below 3000. Assess the client for signs of aplastic anemia and agranulocytosis, including a tendency to bruise, sore throat, fever, petechiae, and mouth ulcerations.[17] Clients receiving carbamazepine in conjunction with diuretics should also have periodic serum electrolyte determinations.

Dizziness and drowsiness may occur, and the client should be cautioned against operating dangerous machinery or a motor vehicle. As with other antiepileptics, advise the client not to adjust the drug dosage without consulting with the primary care provider. Tell the client to take the drug with food to minimize GI discomfort and to enhance absorption.

BENZODIAZEPINES

In Chapter 18 the drug category of benzodiazepines was described. In this chapter the discussion is limited to the antiepileptic action of these drugs.

BENZODIAZEPINE PROTOTYPE

DIAZEPAM

Pharmacotherapeutics Diazepam is the drug of choice for status epilepticus. It sometimes is used concurrently with primary antiepileptic drugs to treat infantile spasms and atypical absence, myoclonic, atonic, and photosensitive seizures.[1]

Pharmacodynamics Mechanism of action as an antiepileptic drug is to enhance GABA receptor–mediated inhibition. The effectiveness of diazepam is enhanced during biotransformation; both of its metabolites possess antiepileptic properties.

Pharmaceutics As an antiepileptic drug, diazepam is usually administered intravenously. Since repeated doses of IV diazepam are not recommended, a loading dose of another long-acting antiepileptic drug is usually administered in addition to diazepam.[1]

Specific Drug-Related Nursing Considerations Remember that diazepam potentiates actions of other CNS depressants.

MISCELLANEOUS DRUGS IN CATEGORY

Midazolam hydrochloride (Versed), the first water-soluble benzodiazepine, is used as an antiepileptic drug in adults and children. It has been administered intravenously and intramuscularly to treat status epilepticus and repeated epileptic seizures in adults and children.[20]

Clonazepam (Klonopin) has been approved by the FDA for use alone or as an adjunct antiepileptic drug. It is most effective in the treatment of absence seizures, infantile spasms, and myoclonic and atonic seizures. Clonazepam is rapidly absorbed from the GI tract and is approximately 40% to 50% bound to plasma proteins. The elimination half-life varies between 20 and 40 hours, with peak plasma concentration occurring 1 to 3 hours after an oral dose.

Common undesired clinical responses are drowsiness, ataxia, and behavioral changes. These effects are potentiated by concurrent administration of barbiturates. In addition, when clonazepam is administered concurrently with valproic acid, exacerbation of absence seizures may occur. Bronchial hypersecretion and hypersalivation can cause respiratory problems in children.[1,21]

MISCELLANEOUS ANTIEPILEPTIC DRUGS

Although there are numerous other antiepileptic drugs, including gabapentin, lamotrigine, and vigabatrin, only valproic acid and felbamate are discussed in this section.

Valproic Acid

Valproic acid (Depakene) was first used as an antiepileptic drug in Europe. It gained FDA approval in 1978 and is primarily used in the treatment of absence seizures. Valproic acid is also used as an alternative to lithium in the treatment of acute mania and as prophylaxis for bipolar disorder.[17]

Its mechanism of action as an antiepileptic involves decreasing high-frequency repetitive firing of action potentials in the CNS. This action is enhanced by sodium channel inactivation.

When administered orally, valproic acid is rapidly absorbed. The drug is approximately 90% bound to plasma protein, and peak blood levels occur within 1 to 5 hours. Valproic acid is metabolized to at least five metabolites. The amount of valproic acid metabolized to an active metabolite is less in adults than in children.[6,19] The elimination half-life varies between 6 and 18 hours. There is minimal correlation between serum concentration levels and clinical response.[1]

Most common undesired clinical responses are sedation, GI distress, weight gain, alopecia, stomach cramping, tremor, lethargy, and diarrhea. Some of these effects can be minimized by using enteric-coated tablets or administering the drug after meals. Asymptomatic elevation of hepatic enzymes occurs in approximately 15% to 30% of the clients. This occurs during the first several months of therapy. Hepatotoxicity has also been reported. This response usually involves clients under the age of 15 years and occurs during the first 6 months of therapy. Hematologic and liver function parameters must be established before therapy begins. These same studies should be conducted routinely during therapy. Valproic acid interacts with several other antiepileptic drugs, including phenobarbital, primidone, carbamazepine, and phenytoin. These drug-drug interactions alter the serum concentration levels of the drugs involved.[1] Determining serum concentration levels routinely is essential.

Felbamate

Felbamate (Felbatol) is the first epilepsy drug to be approved in 15 years. The drug may be used alone or in combination with other antiepileptic drugs, including phenytoin, valproic acid, and carbamazepine. Felbamate helps control partial seizures and seizures that become generalized in clients age 14 years or older. It is also used to treat Lennox-Gastaut epilepsy syndrome in children 2 to 14 years of age. Although the drug's exact mechanism of action is unknown, studies suggest that felbamate raises the seizure threshold and reduces seizure spread.

Felbamate is administered orally. More than 90% of the oral dose is absorbed; 40% to 50% of the absorbed drug is excreted unchanged in the urine. Most of the remaining drug is metabolized or converted into inactive substances. The half-life for felbamate is 20 to 23 hours.

Dyspepsia, vomiting, constipation, insomnia, headache, and fatigue are frequent undesired clinical responses associated with felbamate. Significant drug-drug interactions involving felbamate and other antiepileptic drugs have been reported. For example, when administered concurrently with phenytoin, the plasma concentration of phenytoin increases, and the clearance of felbamate doubles. When felbamate is administered concurrently with carbamazepine or valproic acid, carbamazepine concentrations decrease, and concentrations of valproic acid increase. Carbamazepine also increases the clearance of felbamate. Plasma concentration levels of all antiepileptic drugs must be monitored.[5,22–25]

• • •

Antiepileptic prototypes and major drugs are presented in Table 21–3.

TABLE 21–3

Antiepileptic Drugs: Prototypes and Major Drugs

Drug Name	Dosage and Route of Administration
SUCCINIMIDE: ethosuximide (Zarontin) HOW SUPPLIED Capsule: 250 mg Syrup: 250 mg/5 ml	Initial dose: 250-500 mg, depending on age; increase dose slowly to a maximum of 1.5 g/d; usual optimal dose for children, 20 mg/kg/d
OXAZOLIDINEDIONE: trimethadione (Tridione) HOW SUPPLIED Capsule: 300 mg Oral solution: 40 mg/ml Chewable tablet: 150 mg	ADULTS Initial dose: 0.9 g daily; increase by 300 mg at weekly intervals; maintenance dose: 0.9-2.4 g daily in three or four equally divided doses CHILDREN Usual dose: 0.3-0.9 g daily in three or four equally divided doses
IMINOSTILBENE: carbamazepine (Epitol, Tegretol) HOW SUPPLIED Chewable tablet: 100 mg Tablet: 200 mg Suspension: 100 mg/5 ml	6-12 y: initial dose, 100 mg bid, increase at weekly intervals; usual maintenance dose, 400-800 mg/d Over 12 y: initial dose, 200 mg bid, increase at weekly intervals to a maximum dose based on age; usual maintenance dose, 800-1200 mg/d
BENZODIAZEPINE: diazepam (Valium, Zetran) HOW SUPPLIED Injection solution: 5 mg/ml Uncoated tablet: 2, 5, 10 mg Sustained-action capsule: 15 mg Oral solution: 5 mg/5 ml, 10 mg/10 ml	ADULTS IV (preferred) or IM: initial dose, 5-10 mg, repeated if necessary at 5- to 10-min intervals to a maximum dose of 30 mg Oral: usual dose, 2-10 mg, two to four times daily CHILDREN IV (preferred) or IM: 30 d to 5 y—0.2-0.5 mg slowly q2-5min to maximum of 5 mg; >5 y—1 mg slowly q2-5min to maximum of 10 mg; can repeat in 2-4 h if necessary Oral: initial dose, 1 mg three or four times daily; increase up to 2.5 mg three or four times daily; not for use in children <6 mo old
Clonazepam (Klonopin) HOW SUPPLIED Uncoated tablet: 0.5, 1, 2 mg	ADULTS Initial dose: not more than 1.5 mg/d divided into three doses; increase if necessary in increments of 0.5-1 mg q3d to maximum recommended daily dose of 20 mg CHILDREN Up to 10 y or 30 kg: initial dose, 0.01-0.03 mg/kg/d given in two or three divided doses; may increase by 0.25-0.5 mg every third day to a maintenance dose of 0.1-0.2 mg/kg/d given in divided doses

MISCELLANEOUS ANTIEPILEPTIC DRUGS

Valproic Acid (Depakene, Depakote, Myproic Acid) HOW SUPPLIED Capsules: 250, 500 mg Delayed release capsules: 125, 250, 500 mg Suspensions: 250 mg/5 ml	Initial dose: Adults 5–15 mg/kg/d; then increase at 1-wk intervals by 5–10 mg/kg/d to maximum recommended dose of 60 mg/kg/d; daily doses >250 mg should be divided CHILDREN Initial dose: 15–45 mg/kg/d; then increase at weekly intervals by 5–10 mg/kg/d
Felbamate (Felbatol) HOW SUPPLIED Tablets: 400, 600 mg Suspensions: 600 mg/5 ml	ADULTS 14 y and older: 1200 mg/d in three to four doses; maximum dose, 3600 mg/d CHILDREN Ages 2-14 y: 15 mg/kg/d; maximum dose, 45 mg/kg/d
Gabapentin (Neurontin)	ADULTS 900–1800 mg/d CHILDREN Over 12 y: 900–1800 mg/d
Lamotrigine (Lamictal)	ADULTS 100–500 mg/d
Vigatrin (Sabril)	ADULTS 1–4 g/d CHILDREN 50–100 mg/kg/d

TABLE 21–4

Summary of Antiepileptic Drugs: Clinical Uses and Therapeutic Serum Levels

Antiepileptic Drug	Clinical Use	Therapeutic Serum Levels
Phenytoin	Most seizures except absence seizures	10-20 µg/ml
Phenobarbital	Generalized tonic-clonic and partial seizures	Adults: 10-25 µg/ml Infants and children: 15-30 µg/ml
Primidone	Most seizure activities except absence seizures	Adults: 5-12 µg/ml Children: 7-10 µg/ml
Ethosuximide	Absence seizures	40-100 µg/ml
Carbamazepine	Most seizure activities except absence seizures	4-12 µg/ml
Clonazepam	Absence and myoclonic seizures	15-60 µg/ml
Valproic acid	Primarily absence seizures	50-100 µg/ml
Felbamate	Broad spectrum of antiepileptic activities	Probably 20-120 µg/ml

CONCEPT REVIEW

Benzodiazepines are used primarily as sedative-antianxiety drugs. However, diazepam, clonazepam, clorazepate dipotassium, and midazolam are also used as antiepileptic drugs.

Usefulness of trimethadione is limited by its toxic effects. It is usually prescribed for clients whose absence seziures are not well controlled.

Carbamazepine is used to treat complex partial and generalized seizures. Although serious side effects have been reported, they are not common.

Valproic acid is used as an adjunctive drug to treat a variety of seizure activities. It has been approved by the FDA for primary use with absence seizures.

Unlike many drugs used to treat seizures, felbamate was developed for use as an antiepileptic drug. This drug was proved effective in treatment of poorly controlled seizures in adults and children.

SUMMARY

A variety of antiepileptic drugs is available to treat seizure activities. Selection of a drug is based on the client's health history, physical assessment, and diagnostic findings. Collection of assessment data and evaluation of clinical responses are important responsibilities of the nurse.

Table 21–4 provides a summary of frequently prescribed drugs, their clinical use, and their therapeutic serum levels.

REFERENCES

1. Chan, A. (1992). Drugs used in the treatment of epilepsy. 320-339.
2. McCance, K.L., & Huether, S.E. (1990). *Pathophysiology: The biologic basis for disease in adults and children.* St. Louis: C.V. Mosby.
3. Lannon, S. (1993). Epilepsy in the elderly. *Journal of Neuroscience Nursing, 25,* 273-285.
4. Gale, K. (1992). GABA and epilepsy: Basic concepts from preclinical research. *Epilepsia, 33*(Suppl. 5), S3-12.
5. MacDonald, R., & Kelly, K. (1993). Antiepileptic drug mechanisms of action. *Epilepsia, 34*(Supp. 5), S1-8.
6. Leppik, I. (1992). Metabolism of antiepileptic medication: Newborn to elderly. *Epilepsia, 33*(Suppl. 4), S32-40.
7. Lindhout, D., & Omtziqt, J. (1992). Pregnancy and the risk of teratogenicity. *Epilepsia, 33*(Suppl. 4), S41-48.
8. Jarvis, C. (1992). *Physical examination and health assessment.* Philadelphia: W.B. Saunders.
9. Data Pharmaceutica, Inc. (1993). *1993 physicians' genRx.* Smithtown, NY: Author.
10. U.S. Pharmacopeial Convention. (1990). *United States pharmacopeia* (22nd rev.). Rockville, MD: Author.
11. Browne, T., & Szabo, G. (1991). New pharmacokinetic methods for the study of antiepileptic medications of the 1990s. *Epilepsia, 32*(Suppl. 5), S66-73.
12. Hanna, D.R. (1992). Purple glove syndrome: A complication of intravenous phenytoin. *Journal of Neuroscience Nursing, 24,* 340-345.
13. Tatro, D.S. (Ed.). (1990). *Drug interaction facts* (2nd ed.). St. Louis: J.B. Lippincott.
14. Trovato, A., Nuhlicek, D., & Midtling, J. (1991). Drug-nutrient interactions. *American Family Physician, 44,* 1651-1657.
15. Bader, M.K. (1993). Case study of two methods for enteral phenytoin administration. *Journal of Neuroscience Nursing, 25,* 233-242.
16. Bernstein, J.G. (1988). *Handbook of drug therapy in psychiatry* (2nd ed.). Littleton, MA: PSG Publishing.
17. Glod, C.A. (1991). Psychopharmacology and clinical practice. *Nursing Clinics of North America, 26,* 375-399.
18. Hollister, L., & Csernansky, J. (1990). *Clinical pharmacology of psychotherapeutic drugs* (3rd ed.). New York: Churchill Livingstone.
19. Kiker, M. (1991). Antiepileptic drugs for children: Carbamazepine and valproic acid derivatives. *Journal of Neuroscience Nursing, 23,* 130-132.
20. Lahat, E., Aladjem, M., Eshel, G., Bistritzer, T., & Katz, Y. (1992). Midazolam in treatment of epileptic seizures. *Pediatric Neurology, 8,* 215-216.
21. Katzung, B. (Ed.). (1992). *Basic and clinical pharmacology.* Norwalk, CT: Appleton & Lange.
22. Bourqeois, B., et al. (1993). Felbamate: A double-blind controlled trial in patients undergoing presurgical evaluation of partial seizures. *Neurology, 43,* 693-696.
23. Efficacy of felbamate in childhood epileptic encephalopathy (Lennox-Gastaut syndrome). (1993). *New England Journal of Medicine, 328,* 29-33.
24. Felbamate (Felbatol): A new choice for seizure control. (1994). *American Journal of Nursing, 94* (3), 58.
25. Ramsay, R. (1993). Advances in the pharmacotherapy of epilepsy. *Epilepsia, 34*(Suppl. 5), S9-16.

BIBLIOGRAPHY

Bvers, V. (1993). Novel antiepileptic drugs: Nursing implications. *Journal of Neuroscience Nursing, 25,* 375-379.

Cloyd, J., Fischer, J., Kriel, R., & Kraus, D. (1993). Valproic acid pharmacokinetics in children. IV. Effects of age and antiepileptic drugs on protein binding and intrinsic clearance. *Clinical Pharmacol Ther, 53*(1), 22-29.

DiIorio, C., Faherty, B., & Manteuffel, B. (1992). Self-efficacy and social support in self-management of epilepsy. *Western Journal of Nursing Research, 14,* 292-307.

Dupuis, R.E., & Miranda-Massari, J. (1991). Anticonvulsants: Pharmacotherapeutic issues in the critically ill patient. *AACN Clinical Issues in Critical Care Nursing, 2,* 639-656.

Rose, B.A. (1993). Neurologic therapies in critical care. *Critical Care Nursing Clinics of North America, 5,* 237-246.

Tate, E. (1993). The clinical challenge of progressive myoclonus epilepsy. *Nurse Practitioner: American Journal of Primary Health Care, 18*(5), 25-28.

VanValkenburg, C., Kluznik, J., & Merrill, R. (1992). New uses of anticonvulsant drugs in psychosis. *Drugs, 44,* 326-335.

CHAPTER 22

Central Nervous System Stimulants

LINDA NATTKEMPER YORK • TERRY L. SEATON

⊛ **Central Nervous System Stimulants**

LEARNING OBJECTIVE: Outline a teaching plan for a client receiving central nervous system stimulants.

⊛ **Cerebral Stimulant: Amphetamine**

LEARNING OBJECTIVES:
Describe three therapeutic uses for amphetamine.
Explain the rationale for four major undesired clinical responses associated with amphetamine.
Summarize essential information aboutamphetamine.
KEY TERMS:
Attention deficit–hyperactivity disorder, amphetamine, enantiomer, narcolepsy

⊛ **Cerebal Stimulant: Amphetamine-Like Drugs**

LEARNING OBJECTIVE: Describe the pharmacodynamic properties of two amphetamine-like drugs.

⊛ **Cerebral Stimulant: Caffeine**

LEARNING OBJECTIVES:
Describe two therapeutic uses for caffeine.
Explain the rationale for four major undesired clinical responses associated with caffeine.
Summarize essential information about caffeine.
KEY TERM: Caffeine

⊛ **Central Nervous System and Ganglionic Stimulant: Nicotine**

LEARNING OBJECTIVES:
Describe two physiologic responses to nicotine.
Develop a teaching plan for a client who smokes.
KEY TERM: Nicotine

CONCEPTS AND TERMS TO REVIEW

Review the anatomy and physiology of the central nervous system.
Reexamine the role of the blood-brain and placental barriers.
Review the location sites and actions of neurotransmitters.

Central nervous system (CNS) stimulants comprise a heterogenous group of drugs whose subgroups (amphetamines and amphetamine-like substances, caffeine, and nicotine) bear little resemblance to one another. As a group, CNS stimulants have limited therapeutic applications. Amphetamines and amphetamine-like substances are used to treat narcolepsy, attention deficit–hyperactivity disorder (ADHD), and exogenous obesity. Caffeine is found in many over-the-counter (OTC) drugs and as an additive to foods and beverages. It is indicated for a limited number of medical conditions. Nicotine in the form of chewing gum and transdermal patches was recently approved by the Food and Drug Administration (FDA) as adjuncts in the treatment of nicotine addiction. In addition, caffeine and nicotine are self-administered throughout the general population.

A nurse must know the physiologic effects produced by CNS stimulants to have the background to provide knowledgeable and effective teaching about these drugs.

CENTRAL NERVOUS SYSTEM STIMULANTS

CNS stimulants are not equivalent to antidepressants. CNS stimulants cannot elevate the mood of the individual without producing excitation. At therapeutic doses these drugs produce increased mental alertness and a sense of well-being. These characteristics also increase the potential for abuse. Thus individuals may use CNS stimulants to induce prolonged periods of wakefulness, perhaps to the point of sleep deprivation, or to induce a state of euphoria.

▦ NURSING CONSIDERATIONS

Nursing care for clients receiving CNS stimulants is based on the steps in the nursing process.

Assessing During the **health history** interview, assess the client's perception about stimulant use in the overall treatment of the condition. Since drug therapy alone is rarely successful for most conditions treated with CNS stimulants, determine the client's willingness to engage in other forms of treatment such as behavioral modification programs and support or self-help groups.

Assess the client's eating patterns. Ask the individual to recall all food and beverages ingested over the last 24 hours. Ask if that menu is typical of most days. Record the individual's daily intake of caffeine. Determine if the client smokes. If so, ask, "At what age did you start smoking?" "How many packs do you smoke per day?" Assess the client's sleep patterns. Ask the client, "What time do you usually go to bed?" "How long does it take for you to fall asleep?" "Do you use any sleep aids?" Determine if the client uses nonprescription CNS stimulants. Assess the client's past and present use of addictive substances.

If the client is already receiving a prescribed CNS stimulant, determine the name of the drug. Ask the client, "How long have you been taking the drug?" "What dose do you take daily?" "Do you ever alter the dose prescribed?" "When was your last examination by the health care provider who prescribed the drug?" "When was your last dose?" Also collect information on past withdrawal episodes and any history of sensitivity or adverse reactions to CNS stimulants.

While obtaining the past medical history or review of systems, ask about heart disease, hypertension, or diabetes. Note the date of the individual's last electrocardiogram. For females, determine the date of the last menses to rule out the possibility of pregnancy. In addition, a thorough head-to-toe **physical assessment** should be performed.

Diagnosing Once the data have been collected and analyzed, develop the nursing diagnoses. Depending on the data base, specific condition being treated, and the prescribed CNS stimulant, several nursing diagnoses are possible:

• Impaired social interaction related to self-concept disturbance.
• Altered thought processes related to inability to concentrate.
• Sleep pattern disturbance related to drug-induced insomnia.
• Ineffective individual coping related to excessive reliance on chemical substances.
• Altered nutrition: less than body requirements related to decreased food intake.
• High risk for injury related to increased motor activity.
• Altered health maintenance related to knowledge deficit about drug regimen.

Planning A primary focus of the plan of care is education. Include in the plan information about support and self-help groups. Support groups for parents of hyperactive children are usually beneficial. Self-help groups such as Smokers Anonymous and Overeaters Anonymous are patterned after the "Twelve Steps" of Alcoholics Anonymous to assist clients in their treatment programs.

Usually CNS stimulants are ineffective if administered without adjunctive therapies. After conferring with the primary care provider, plan to provide the client and/or significant others with information about adjunctive behavioral and educational programs.

Client outcomes include the following:
• Client demonstrates appropriate method of drug administration.
• Client verbalizes the importance of using prescribed adjunctive therapies in addition to the prescribed drug.
• Client lists the adverse effects of the drug.
• Client describes the potential for abuse or addiction and lists measures to reduce the likelihood of its occurrence.

Implementing Initial nursing interventions are directed toward monitoring the effects of the drug regimen. To assist in determining the effectiveness of CNS stimulants, monitor the client's vital signs, weight, mental status, and activity level.

Review anticipated benefits and possible undesired clinical responses of the drug with the client and significant others. Tell clients to use the drug only as prescribed. If tolerance to the desired effects develops, instruct the client to notify the primary care provider rather than attempt to adjust the drug dosage on his or her own. If the client experiences dry mouth, suggest the use of sugarless hard candy or chewing gum. Instruct the client to consult with the primary care provider before using any OTC drugs.

Evaluating Evaluation of the effectiveness of CNS stimulants depends on the category of drug and the purpose for which it was prescribed. Examples include (1) the child with ADHD develops an increased attention span and more appropriate behavior; (2) the client with narcolepsy is able to stay awake and alert during the day; (3) the client desiring to quit smoking is able to abstain from nicotine, with only minimal physical withdrawal symptoms, while learning to deal with psychologic withdrawal; and (4) the client with obesity loses weight at a safe rate.

Regardless of the specific medical condition for which the stimulant is prescribed, the client should be able to verbalize an understanding of the stimulant's side effects and of the regimen necessary for safe and effective self-administration. In addition, the expected outcomes incorporated into the plan of care must be considered.

CEREBRAL STIMULANT: AMPHETAMINE

Amphetamines were discovered in the 1920s as a result of the search for a synthetic substitute for the drug ephedrine, which was being used as an effective treatment for asthma. Ephedrine was so effective and widely used that concern arose that the supply of this naturally occurring substance would be depleted.

Beginning in 1932, amphetamine was marketed as a nonprescription drug in an inhaler (Benzedrine) for the treatment of asthma. In 1937 the American Medical Association (AMA) approved amphetamine for the treatment of narcolepsy. Soon these clients observed decreased appetite and subsequent weight loss. Thus amphetamine quickly became a popular method of weight reduction. During World War II, soldiers used amphetamine to extend periods of wakefulness when sleep was undesirable. By the 1960s amphetamine had become a drug of abuse.

The amphetamine family consists of amphetamine, dextroamphetamine, and methamphetamine. All are powerful CNS stimulants and have significant actions in the periphery. Amphetamines have a high potential for addiction.[1] As a result, all amphetamines are classified by the FDA as Schedule II drugs of the Controlled Substances Act.

AMPHETAMINE PROTOTYPE
AMPHETAMINE SULFATE

Amphetamine is a noncatecholamine, sympathomimetic amine with CNS stimulant activities. It is not a single compound but a mixture of dextroamphetamine and levamphetamine. These two substances are **enantiomers,** substances whose molecular structures are mirror opposites of each other.[1,2]

Pharmacotherapeutics Amphetamine has several therapeutic and nontherapeutic uses. It is frequently abused by individuals to produce euphoria and to promote wakefulness. Amphetamine and amphetamine-like substances such as methylenedioxymethamphetamine (also called *Ecstasy* or *MDMA*) produce effects similar to those of both stimulants and hallucinogens. In fact, the psychologic effects of amphetamine are practically indistinguishable from those produced by cocaine.[1] (See Chapter 12 for a discussion of the social use of drugs.)

Amphetamine is still prescribed for clients with narcolepsy. **Narcolepsy,** which is characterized by an irresistible urge to sleep, can be profoundly disabling and cause impaired job performance, compromised public safety, a sense of social worthlessness, or depression.[3] Stimulants control excessive somnolence and reduce cataplexy and sleep paralysis by suppressing rapid eye movement (REM) sleep. Although stimulants may greatly enhance one's quality of life, complete control of sleepiness is rare.

Amphetamine is used as an adjunct to psychologic, educational, social, and other remedial measures in the treatment of **ADHD.** ADHD is a disruptive behavior disorder that generally occurs in children. Controversy exists whether ADHD progresses into adulthood.

Pharmacokinetics Amphetamine is absorbed well from the gastrointestinal (GI) tract. It is distributed into most body tissues, particularly the brain and CNS. Pharmacologic effects persist for 4 to 24 hours. Both hepatic metabolism and urinary excretion of unchanged drug account for elimination of amphetamine from the body.[2,4]

Pharmacodynamics Amphetamine's pharmacodynamic properties are similar to those of ephedrine. Effects are produced by the release of biogenic amines (dopamine, serotonin, norepinephrine) from neurons in the CNS and periphery.[1] These substances stimulate the medullary respiratory center and produce other effects of CNS stimulation. In addition, amphetamine may directly stimulate some serotoninergic receptors.

Physiologic effects of amphetamine are widespread. In general, amphetamine causes CNS excitation, which results in increased motor activity, mental alertness, mild euphoria, and a decreased perception of fatigue. Although task performance impaired by fatigue may be slightly improved, nervousness produced by amphet-amine hinders performance in healthy individuals. Respiratory stimulation, which is greater in individuals with preexisting respiratory depression, also occurs. Amphetamine may temporarily improve symptoms of depression. However, this effect depends on drug dose, previous mental state, and personality of the individual.[1,5] When amphetamines are discontinued after long-term use, sleep patterns may take several months to return to normal.

Amphetamine causes a marked increase in urinary bladder sphincter contraction. Uterine tone is usually increased. GI motility is either increased or decreased.

Pharmaceutics Amphetamine is administered exclusively by the oral route. Doses vary and are usually individualized for the client. In general, the lowest effective dose should be used[2] (Table 22–1).

Undesired Clinical Responses Amphetamine produces numerous undesired clinical responses. They primarily affect the CNS, GI system, and cardiovascular system. These responses are summarized in Figure 22–1.

Contraindications and Precautions Amphetamine use is contraindicated in clients with arteriosclerosis, angina or other symptomatic cardiac disease, and hypertension. It should not be administered to individuals with hyperthyroidism, glaucoma, or a known history of drug abuse. Amphetamine use is also contraindicated in individuals in agitated states.[2,4]

Drug-Drug Interactions Numerous drugs interact with amphetamine, increasing or decreasing its effectiveness. Some of the drugs that decrease either the absorption or metabolism of amphetamine are listed in the box on p. 225.

Some drugs enhance the effects of amphetamine. GI alkalinizing agents such as sodium bicarbonate increase the absorption of amphetamine. Urinary alkalinizing agents such as acetazolamide (Diamox) decrease the excretion of the drug. In addition, when administered concurrently with meperidine (Demerol), amphetamine increases the analgesic effects of meperidine.[4] Administering amphetamine with some drugs (e.g., methylphenidate [Ritalin] and phentermine [Ionamin]) produces agitation, bizarre behavior, hallucinations, and paranoia.[6]

Interference with Diagnostic Studies Amphetamine can cause a significant elevation in plasma corticosteroid levels, with the greatest increase in the evening.

Amphetamine may interfere with urinary steroid determinations.

Life-Span Considerations It is not known if amphetamine is excreted in breast milk; therefore it should not be administered to nursing mothers. Amphetamine is classified as a Pregnancy Category C drug; it should be used during pregnancy only if the potential benefits justify the potential risk to the fetus. Women who become pregnant while taking amphetamine should notify their primary care provider immediately.[2]

Specific Drug-Related Nursing Considerations Administer amphetamine at least 6 hours before bedtime to minimize the risk of insomnia. Once the desired dose has been achieved, consult with the primary care provider to determine if the sustained-release dosage form can be used.

TABLE 22-1
CNS Stimulants: Prototype and Major Drugs in Category

Drug Name	Dosage and Route of Administration	Nursing Considerations

AMPHETAMINE SULFATE
HOW SUPPLIED
Coated tablet: 10 mg
Uncoated tablet: 5mg
	Narcolepsy
	Adults and children >12 y
	   5-60 mg/d; usual dose, 10 mg/d; may
	   increase 10 mg at weekly intervals
	ADHD
	Children
	3-5 y: 2.5 mg/d; may increase 2.5 mg at
	   weekly intervals until desired response
	   achieved
	≥6 y: 5-40 mg/d; usual dose, 5 one or
	   two times per day; may increase 5 mg/d
	   at weekly intervals
		Assess
		Determine baseline vital signs and weight for
		   comparison during treatment.
		Assess client for preexisting conditions that
		   would contradict use of amphetamines.
		Implement
		Observe mental status for changes in mood,
		   degree of stimulation, and aggressiveness.
		Weigh client at regular intervals.
		Administer last dose at least 6 h before bed-
		   time.
		Suggest use of sugarless chewing gum or
		   hard candy if dry mouth or unpleasant
		   taste develops.
		Encourage adequate fluid and fiber intake.
		   Observe eating patterns.
		Monitor
		Monitor vital signs regularly.
		Monitor sleeping patterns.
		Evaluate
		Base evaluation on purpose:
		   Evaluate for weight loss.
		   Evaluate for daytime wakefulness.
		   Evaluate for decreased hyperactivity and in-
		   creased level of concentration.

Dextroamphetamine Sulfate
(Dexedrine, Ferndex, Oxydess)
HOW SUPPLIED
Uncoated tablet: 5 and 10 mg
Gelatin sustained-release (SR)
capsules: 5, 10, and 15 mg
	Narcolepsy
	Adults: 5-60 mg/d. Initial dose of 10
	   mg/d; may increase 10 mg at weekly in-
	   tervals
	Children 6-12 y: 5mg/d; may increase
	   5mg at weekly intervals
	ADHD
	Children
	3-5 y: see amphetamine dosage
	≥6 y: see amphetamine dosage
		See amphetamine

Methamphetamine Hydrochloride
(Desoxyn, Methampex)
HOW SUPPLIED
Uncoated tablet: 5 mg
Sustained-release uncoated tablet:
5, 10, and 15 mg
	ADHD
	Children ≥6 y: initial dose 5mg once or
	   twice a day; may increase 5 mg at
	   weekly intervals; usual effective dosage
	   20-25 mg/d
		See amphetamine
		Implement
		Instruct client to swallow SR tablets whole;
		   do not crush or chew

AMPHETAMINE-LIKE DRUGS
Methylphenidate Hydrochloride
(Ritalin)
HOW SUPPLIED
Plain-coated, sustained-release tablet:
20 mg
Uncoated tablets: 5, 10, and 20 mg
	ADHD
	Adults: 10-60 mg/d divided 2 or 3 times
	   per day; administer 30-45 min before
	   meals
	Children ≥6 y: initial dose should be
	   small; daily dosage above 60 mg not
	   recommended
		See amphetamine
		Implement
		Administer before 6 PM if drug interferes with
		   sleeping

Assess the client's mental status for changes in mood, activity level, and degree of stimulation or aggressiveness. Also monitor his or her vital signs. Orally administered amphetamine raises both systolic and diastolic blood pressure. The heart rate is often reflexly lowered.[8] Since the release of biogenic amines raises the blood sugar, serum glucose levels and indications of hyper- glycemia should be monitored more closely in the client with diabetes mellitus. In addition, drug-related changes in diet and activity level may alter insulin or oral hypoglycemic requirements.

For the client being treated for exogenous obesity, monitor nutritional intake and exercise program. Weight loss in these individuals is almost entirely due to de-

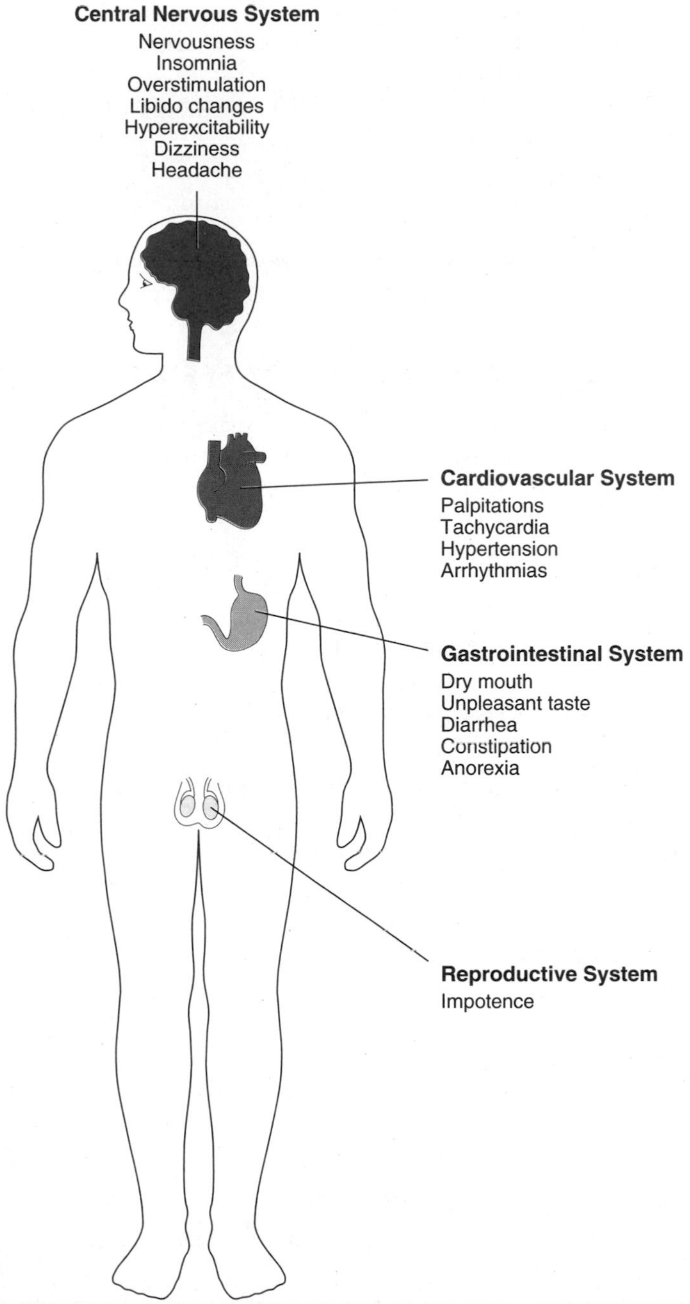

Central Nervous System
Nervousness
Insomnia
Overstimulation
Libido changes
Hyperexcitability
Dizziness
Headache

Cardiovascular System
Palpitations
Tachycardia
Hypertension
Arrhythmias

Gastrointestinal System
Dry mouth
Unpleasant taste
Diarrhea
Constipation
Anorexia

Reproductive System
Impotence

FIGURE 22–1 Undesired clinical responses associated with amphetamines.

SOME DRUGS THAT ALTER EFFECTS OF AMPHETAMINE

Monoamine Oxidase Inhibitors
 Isocarboxazid (Marplan)
 Phenelzine (Nardil)
 Tranylcypromine (Parnate)
Furazolidone (Furoxone)
Phenothiazines
 Haloperidol (Haldol)
 Chlorpromazine (Thorazine)
 Thiothixene (Navane)
 Perphenazine (Trilafon)
Anti-infective Drug
 Methenamine mandelate (Mandelamine)
Antihypertensive Drugs
 Guanethidine (Ismelin)
 Reserpine (Serpasil)
Antimanic Drug
 Lithium carbonate (Lithonate)
Urine Acidifiers
 Ammonium chloride
 Sodium acid phosphate

---

creased food intake and, to a much lesser extent, slightly increased metabolism.[7] In humans, tolerance to the appetite-suppressive effects of amphetamine, probably mediated in the hypothalamic feeding center, develops rapidly. Advise the client that the drug therapy is only for short-term use. Instruct the client to contact the primary care provider if tolerance develops. The client should not independently increase the drug dose.

Counsel families of children with ADHD that amphetamine administration is indicated only after a thorough assessment of the child. The assessment should include observation of behavior at home and school. Explain to the families that drug therapy is not indicated for all children with hyperactivity. Similarly, not all children with hyperactivity benefit from amphetamine use. When drug therapy is initiated, families should be informed that amphetamines will not solve all educational and social problems. Ongoing involvement of the significant other, teachers, and health care providers is necessary. Consult with the primary care provider to determine if children with ADHD can have drug-free periods. These periods, sometimes referred to as "drug holidays," allow assessment of behavior while not receiving the drug.

Educating both the client and significant others is extremely important to maximize effective use of amphetamine and reduce the possibility of abuse. Inform the client and, when appropriate, parents of children not to discontinue the drug abruptly. Abrupt discontinuance of the drug may precipitate a withdrawal episode since dependence can occur. Remind the client to consult with a pharmacist or the primary care provider before taking OTC or other prescription drugs.

MISCELLANEOUS DRUGS IN CATEGORY

Several other amphetamines, including **dextroamphetamine sulfate** (Dexedrine) and **methamphetamine hydrochloride** (Desoxyn, Methampex), are used for the treatment of exogenous obesity and ADHD. As with amphetamine, tolerance to the appetite-suppressant effects of these drugs frequently develops. When tolerance develops, the drug should be discontinued. The dose should not be increased. See Table 22–1 for further information about amphetamines.

CEREBRAL STIMULANT: AMPHETAMINE-LIKE DRUGS

Both methylphenidate hydrochloride and pemoline are structurally dissimilar to the amphetamines. However, their pharmacologic effects are nearly identical.

Methylphenidate Hydrochloride

Methylphenidate hydrochloride (Ritalin) is considered a mild CNS stimulant. Of the various amphetamine-like drugs, it is the best studied and most widely used clinically. However, its mode of action is still not completely understood. Presumably methylphenidate activates the brain-stem arousal system and cortex to produce its stimulant effect. Methylphenidate is used to treat ADHD and narcolepsy. In clients with ADHD, methylphenidate reduces the incidence of inappropriate behaviors and improves learning.[4]

Methylphenidate apparently is readily absorbed from the GI tract. Rate of absorption of extended-release products is slower, but the extent equals that of conventional immediate-release tablets. Hepatic metabolism accounts for the majority of drug removal from the body. Metabolites are excreted almost entirely in the urine, with 80% of the dose eliminated within 24 hours.[2,4,5]

Undesired clinical responses, contraindications, and precautions for methylphenidate are similar to those for amphetamine. As with amphetamine, drug therapy with methylphenidate should be combined with other forms of therapy (i.e., educational programs, support groups).

Pemoline

Pemoline (Cylert) is used to treat ADHD. Although pemoline is a CNS stimulant, it is structurally dissimilar to the amphetamines and methylphenidate. Pemoline's exact mechanism and site of action in humans are not known.[4]

Peak serum concentrations of pemoline after oral absorption occur within 2 to 4 hours. Pharmacologic effects after single-dose administration persist for at least 8 hours. Multiple-dose studies in adults indicate steady-state serum concentrations occur after approximately 3 days. However, when administered to children for treatment of ADHD, pemoline's full therapeutic effects, exhibited by behavioral changes, may not be apparent for 2 to 4 weeks. Pemoline distribution into body tissues is also largely unknown. More than 50% of pemoline is metabolized by the liver; weakly active metabolites do exist. Approximately 75% of an oral dose is excreted in the urine, 43% as unchanged drug, after 24 hours.[2,4]

Pemoline should be administered with caution to clients with impaired renal or hepatic function. Hepatic function studies should be performed before and periodically during therapy. If abnormalities are confirmed or revealed during follow-up studies, use of the drug should be discontinued.[4]

CONCEPT REVIEW

CNS stimulants do not elevate mood but produce increased mental alertness and a sense of well-being.

CNS stimulants can assist with conditions such as attention deficit–hyperactivity disorder, narcolepsy, obesity, and fatigue.

In excessive amounts CNS stimulants can produce euphoria, nervousness, or sleeplessness.

Tolerance to amphetamines and amphetamine-like drugs does develop, and the potential for abuse is high.

CEREBRAL STIMULANT: CAFFEINE

Caffeine belongs to a group of naturally occurring substances known as the methylxanthines. Caffeine is found in chocolate, tea, and coffee. Although caffeine was not identified in coffee until 1820, coffee and the coffee bean have been recognized for centuries as possessing stimulant properties.[9] More recently, caffeine has been added to a variety of products, including soft drinks, OTC analgesics, cold remedies, and appetite suppressants (Table 22–2).

Pharmacotherapeutics

Caffeine has several uses, including CNS stimulation and as an adjunctive therapy with electroconvulsive therapy. It is also used to treat neonatal apnea and headaches.

Widespread social use as a **CNS stimulant** remains the main use of caffeine. Caffeine promotes wakefulness and restores mental alertness in individuals in fatigued conditions. It also is used to offset the sedative effects of antihistamines.

Perhaps the most useful pharmacologic role of caffeine is in the treatment of **neonatal apnea.** In low-birth-weight

TABLE 22-2

Caffeine Content in Common Beverages and OTC Drugs

Item	Range (mg)	Average (mg)
Coffee (5-oz cup)		
Brewed, drip method	60-180	115
Brewed, percolated	40-170	80
Instant	30-120	65
Decaffeinated, brewed	2-5	3
Decaffeinated, instant	1-5	2
Tea (5-oz cup)		
Brewed, major U.S. brands	20-90	40
Brewed, imported brands	25-110	60
Instant	25-50	30
Cola drinks (12 oz)	35-60	40
Cocoa beverage (5 oz)	2-20	4
OTC drugs		
Anacin, Vanquish		32 mg/tab
Excedrin		65 mg/tab
NoDoz		100 mg/tab
Vivarin		200 mg/tab

neonates caffeine citrate has been shown to decrease apneic episodes significantly. Although only theophylline is approved for this condition, caffeine offers several potential advantages and is preferred by some clinicians.[10] These advantages include a larger therapeutic index and fewer peripheral effects such as tachycardia and diuresis.

When combined with either analgesics and/or ergot alkaloids, caffeine is used to abort many types of **headaches,** including vascular, migraine, and cluster headaches. Beneficial effects of these combinations were initially attributed to additive cerebral vasoconstriction, but caffeine also increases absorption of ergotamine. In addition, caffeine appears to possess intrinsic analgesic activity itself.[11] This analgesic activity is independent of improving mood or treating "caffeine-withdrawal headache." The exact mechanism of analgesic effect is not known. Caffeine and sodium benzoate have also been used for treatment of headache associated with spinal puncture.

Caffeine has been safely and successfully used to increase the duration of seizures in clients undergoing **electroconvulsive therapy (ECT)** for severe mental disorders.[12] However, the use of caffeine is generally reserved for clients in whom adequate seizure duration is difficult to achieve.

Caffeine has been used to treat a variety of other conditions. Either alone or in combination with other agents, caffeine has been used for symptomatic relief of tension, fatigue, and fluid retention associated with menstruation. Caffeine restriction has been used to treat breast pain associated with fibrocystic breast disease.[13,14]

❧ Nursing Research

Russell, L.C. (1989). Caffeine restriction as initial treatment for breast pain. *Nurse Practitioner, 14*(2), 36-40.

This study sought to determine the effects of caffeine restriction on breast pain in women with fibrocystic breast changes. A sample of 138 women were surveyed by questionnaire about their past medical history, medication usage, caffeine consumption, and degree of breast pain.

After completing the questionnaire, subjects were examined and counseled about caffeine intake reduction. At the end of 1 year, 81.9% of the subjects had reduced their caffeine intake significantly. Of them, 61% reported a reduction in breast pain. Three percent experienced an increase in breast pain, and 36% reported no change. The author recommends caffeine restriction as a conservative, noninvasive method of managing breast pain associated with fibrocystic breast changes.

STUDENT ACTIVITIES

- Interview as many women as possible with fibrocystic breast changes and assess their caffeine intake.
- Correlate the existence of breast pain and the intake of caffeine for these women.

Pharmacokinetics

Caffeine and caffeine citrate are absorbed well from the GI tract. Peak serum concentrations are reached within 50 to 75 minutes after oral administration of 100 mg of caffeine as coffee. Absorption after intramuscular (IM) administration of caffeine and sodium benzoate apparently is slightly slower than after oral administration. Rectal absorption from suppositories is slow and erratic. Caffeine distributes into all body tissues, including the brain and placenta. Concentrations in human breast milk are approximately 50% of maternal serum concentrations.

Caffeine is rapidly metabolized by the liver. Metabolites and unchanged drug are excreted in the urine. The half-life in adults ranges from 3 to 5 hours. Because of quantitative and qualitative differences in metabolism, the half-life is markedly prolonged (as long as 80 hours) in neonates. This property permits single daily dosing in neonates with apnea.[15]

Pharmacodynamics

Several mechanisms of action have been suggested for caffeine and the other methylxanthines. They include (1) enhancement of calcium permeability in the sarcoplasmic reticulum; (2) reversible blockade of adenosine receptors; and (3) inhibition of cyclic nucleotide phosphodiesterase.[1]

Physiologic effects of caffeine are similar to those produced by other xanthine derivatives. Although these agents predominantly stimulate the cerebral cortex, they probably affect all levels of the CNS. Traditionally caffeine has been considered the most potent CNS stimulant of the methylxanthines, although theophylline (Theo-Dur, Slo-bid) may produce more dangerous CNS stimulation. Clearer and more rapid thought processes and increased wakefulness occur with low to moderate doses of caffeine. With increasing doses, nervousness, tremor, and insomnia may occur. Convulsions may occur at very high doses.

Stimulation of respiratory centers and vasomotor areas results from high doses. It is postulated that caffeine increases the respiratory drive by increasing medullary respiratory sensitivity to carbon dioxide.

Caffeine increases blood pressure in regular consumers of caffeine-containing beverages, probably because of both increased vascular resistance and cardiostimulatory effects. It may also increase blood pressure response to exercise. Caffeine also increases cardiac output and workload by increasing heart rate and force of myocardial contraction. At high doses caffeine may produce tachycardia or supraventricular arrhythmias. In preterm infants caffeine increases cardiac output and possesses pressor effects.[16] In the frail elderly caffeine extends the postprandial fall in blood pressure in individuals with postprandial hypotension.[17]

Human epidemiologic studies are inconclusive in determining the effects of caffeine on fetal growth patterns. Long-term adverse fetal outcomes associated with **moderate** prenatal caffeine exposure have not been consistently identified. (Moderate exposure is defined as less than 300 mg of maternal caffeine consumption per day.) Nonetheless, daily intake of more than 300 mg is generally not recommended for pregnant mothers.[17,18]

Caffeine increases production of urine by enhancing water and electrolyte excretion, probably by increasing glomerular filtration and renal blood flow. Its effects apparently are slightly less than those of theophylline.

Pharmaceutics

Caffeine or caffeine combinations can be administered orally, intramuscularly, or intravenously.

Undesired Clinical Responses

Caffeine produces numerous undesired clinical responses. These responses primarily affect the CNS, GI system, and car-

Central Nervous System
Insomnia
Restlessness
Tremors
Lightheadedness
Tinnitus
Headache
Anxiety neurosis

Cardiovascular System
Tachycardia
Extrasystoles
Palpitations

Gastrointestinal System
Nausea
Vomiting
Diarrhea
Stomach pain

Urinary System
Diuresis

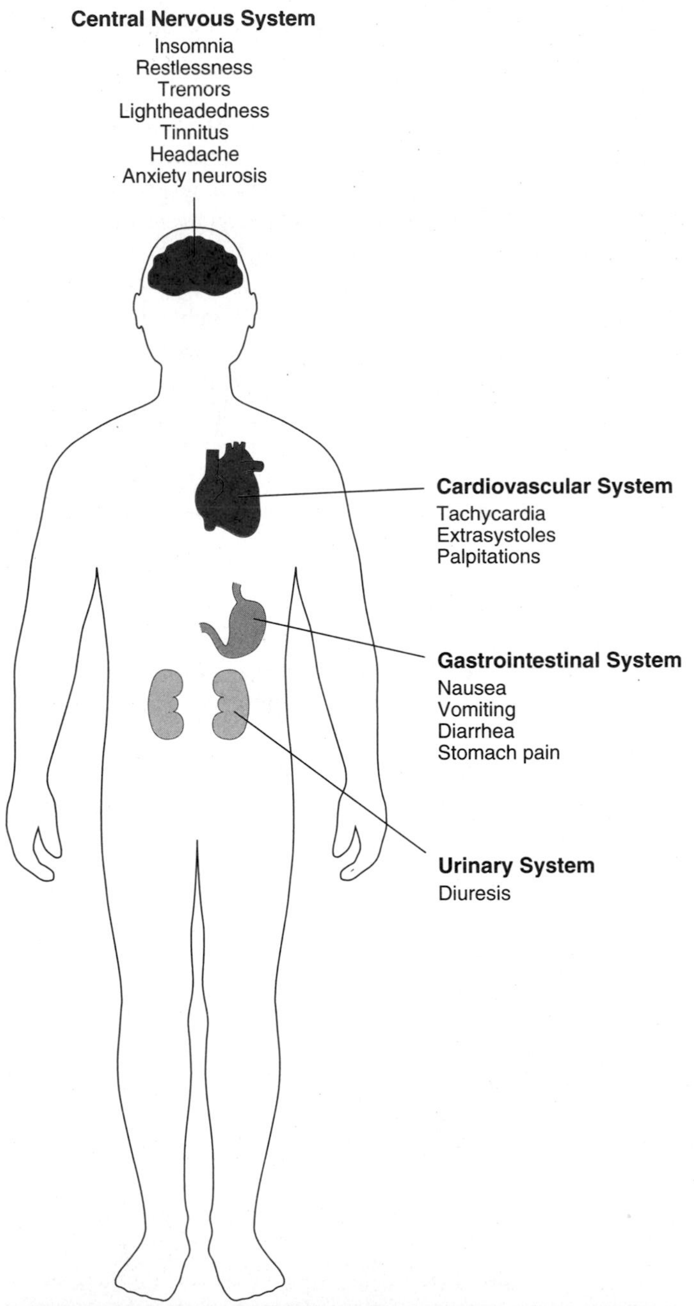

FIGURE 22–2   Undesired clinical responses associated with caffeine.

diovascular system. These responses are presented in Figure 22–2.

Contraindications and Precautions

Because caffeine is a gastric irritant, care should be exercised in administering it to clients with a history of peptic ulcer. Caffeine should also be avoided by clients with symptomatic cardiac arrhythmias and after an acute myocardial infarction.

Drug-Drug and Drug-Nutrient Interactions

Numerous drugs interact with caffeine, increasing or decreasing its effectiveness. Some of the drugs that increase the effects of caffeine are listed in the box below. Some drugs (e.g., phenytoin [Dilantin]) limit or decrease the effects of caffeine. In other situations caffeine decreases or limits the effects of the other drug in the interaction (e.g., adenosine [Adenocard], dipyridamole [Persantine], lorazepam [Ativan], and timolol [Timoptic]).

In addition to caffeine, coffee and tea also contain tannins, which may interfere with absorption of analgesics, antipsychotics, and antihistamines. Therefore clients should be cautioned against taking drugs with coffee or tea.

Specific Drug-Related Nursing Considerations

The nurse's major role in relation to caffeine is client education. Caffeine is usually viewed by the public as an ingredient in a social beverage. It not viewed as a drug. Therefore assessing the level of caffeine intake and educating the client about the physiologic effects of caffeine on the body are important.

It is especially important to assess caffeine consumption in all pregnant or breast-feeding women. Pregnant women should be told about the potential sources of caffeine and counseled to reduce caffeine intake below 300 mg per day.[19]

SOME DRUGS THAT INCREASE EFFECTS OF CAFFEINE

Cimetidine (Tagamet)
Quinoline antibiotics
   Ciprofloxacin (Cipro)
   Enoxacin (Penetrex)
Oral contraceptives
Disulfiram (Antabuse)
Methoxsalen (Oxsoralen)

CONCEPT REVIEW

Caffeine is a cerebral stimulant commonly used to promote wakefulness or to offset the sedative effects of antihistamines.

Caffeine significantly reduces apneic episodes in low-birth-weight neonates, can abort many types of headaches, and is used in electroconvulsive therapy. Negative effects of caffeine include nervousness, tremor, and insomnia; increased blood pressure; tachycardia or supraventricular arrhythmia; and gastric irritation.

CENTRAL NERVOUS SYSTEM AND GANGLIONIC STIMULANT: NICOTINE

Tobacco has played an important role in American and European history. When Columbus arrived in the Western Hemisphere, he discovered Native Americans smoking cigars, something totally unknown in Europe at the time. Later, under British rule, tobacco became the major export and source of income for the colonies. The popularity of tobacco in England inspired efforts to limit or prohibit its use.

Early reports on nicotine suggested a wide range of medical uses, including the treatment of ulcers, headaches, asthma, rheumatism, colds, toothache, and stroke. However, subsequent use and research have shown these reports were not valid.

Unlike amphetamine and caffeine, nicotine is not consumed in its pure form. Raw nicotine is highly toxic. Chewed or smoked tobacco absorbed through the skin generally provides serum nicotine concentrations below a level of acute poisoning. However, young children continue to remain potential victims of nicotine poisoning if they ingest tobacco left within their reach.

Pharmacotherapeutics

Nicotine currently has no therapeutic use. However, recent concerns about tobacco's addictive potential and its well-documented health hazards have prompted pharmaceutical manufacturers to develop nicotine replacement products. These products are marketed as nicotine gum and transdermal nicotine patches. When combined with comprehensive behavioral modification, counseling, and support, nicotine replacement therapy may help individuals quit smoking.

Pharmacokinetics

Because of the extensive lung absorptive surface and absorption from buccal mucosa, nicotine is rapidly absorbed into the systemic arterial circulation after inhalation of tobacco smoke. When nicotine polacrilex (Nicorette Gum) is chewed, nicotine absorption is somewhat slower. After oral ingestion, only minimal amounts of nicotine reach the systemic circulation because of extensive first-pass metabolism. Nicotine is also slowly absorbed through the skin after application of a transdermal system.[2,4]

Distribution of nicotine in human tissues has not been well studied. However, it apparently is readily distributed into brain and placental tissues. It is also excreted in breast milk. Plasma nicotine concentrations vary significantly after either buccal or transdermal administration. Blood levels produced by gum chewing persist as long as the gum is chewed but fall rapidly thereafter. In contrast, after applying a single nicotine patch, plasma nicotine concentrations peak in 3 to 6 hours and persist for at least 16 to 24 hours. After patch removal, plasma concentrations may persist for several hours because a reservoir of nicotine remains in the skin.[2,4]

The primary metabolite of nicotine, cotinine, is not pharmacologically active. The plasma half-life of cotinine is 10 to 40 hours. Nicotine elimination is subject to wide variation, with accumulation occurring in some individuals. Only 10% to 20% of nicotine is excreted as unchanged drug in the urine.[2,4]

Pharmacodynamics

By stimulating ganglionic (nicotinic) cholinergic receptors, nicotine produces many autonomic effects, both centrally and peripherally. Nicotine readily crosses the blood-brain barrier and binds to acetylcholine receptors. As a result, many neurotransmitters such as acetylcholine, norepinephrine, dopamine, serotonin, vasopressin, growth hormone, and adrenocorticotropic hormone (ACTH) are released. CNS stimulation and paradoxical relaxation occur, causing increased alertness, increased ability to concentrate, and a calming effect. These immediate and short-lived effects contribute to development of physical and psychologic dependence. Central effects also include stimulation of the respiratory center and medullary chemoreceptor trigger zone.

Peripherally, nicotine appears to cause catecholamine release that produces dose-dependent increases in heart rate, stroke volume, systolic and diastolic blood pressure, and oxygen consumption. GI effects, mediated largely through cholinergic stimulation, are characterized by increased smooth muscle tone and activity. Nicotine also appears to exhibit mild antidiuretic activity.

Pharmaceutics

As indicated previously, nicotine is available as a gum and in transdermal patches. The gum is available in pieces containing either 2 mg or 4 mg of nicotine. Each piece is chewed several times until the client feels a tingling sensation, which is also described as a "peppery" taste. The gum is then placed between the cheek and gums and held until the sensation goes away. The gum is then chewed several times again, and the process is repeated. Each piece of gum should last approximately 30 minutes. Although treatment is individualized, the average daily use usually is 8 to 16 pieces of gum during the first month. The daily dose should not exceed thirty 2-mg pieces or twenty 4-mg pieces of gum. Use of the gum for longer than 6 months is discouraged and is rarely necessary.[4,20,21]

Transdermal nicotine patches vary. Patches (Nicoderm, Habitrol, Prostep) are available that deliver either 7 mg, 11 mg, 14 mg, 21 mg, or 22 mg per 24 hours. Another patch (Nicotrol) delivers 15 mg; it should be worn only 16 hours per day while the client is awake. Clients who weigh less than 100 pounds, smoke fewer than 10 cigarettes per day, or have cardiovascular disease should begin therapy with a lower strength patch. Generally nicotine replacement should be used for 2 to 4 months to allow the client enough time to develop modified behavior and to manage nicotine abstinence.[4,20,21]

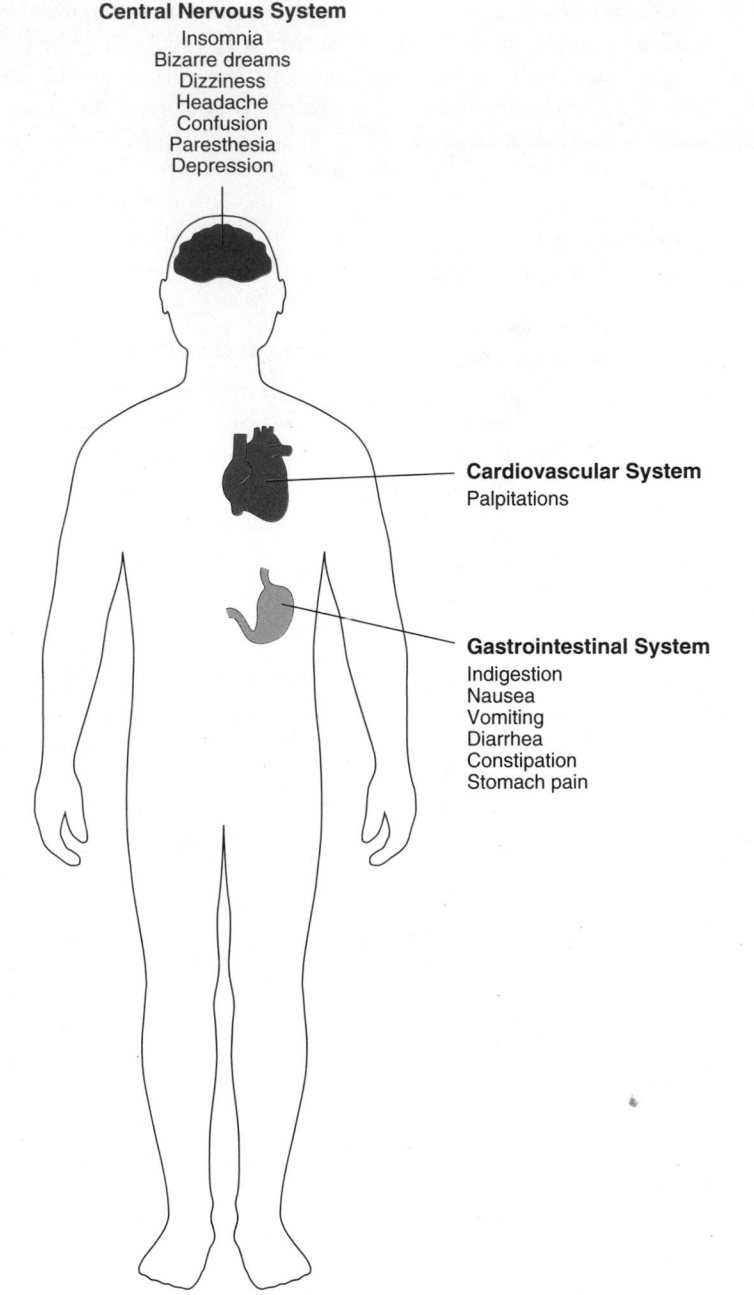

Central Nervous System
Insomnia
Bizarre dreams
Dizziness
Headache
Confusion
Paresthesia
Depression

Cardiovascular System
Palpitations

Gastrointestinal System
Indigestion
Nausea
Vomiting
Diarrhea
Constipation
Stomach pain

F I G U R E 22–3   Undesired clinical responses associated with nicotine.

Undesired Clinical Responses

Nicotine produces numerous undesired clinical responses. They primarily affect the CNS, GI system, and cardiovascular system. These responses are summarized in Figure 22–3. In addition, nicotine gum can cause oral irritation, hoarseness, and jaw pain. The transdermal patches can produce skin rashes.

Contraindications and Precautions

Nicotine use is contraindicated during pregnancy and in clients with active cardiovascular disease (i.e., angina, myocar-

dial infarction). Clients with temporomandibular joint disease should not use the nicotine gum.

Drug-Drug Interactions

A few drug-drug interactions have been established. For example, nicotine increases the effects of adenosine (Adenocard) effects. Cimetidine (Tagamet) increases nicotine's effects.

Specific Drug-Related Nursing Considerations

Most smokers are both physically and psychologically dependent on nicotine. However, when individuals try to quit smoking, those with greater physical dependence appear to have higher abstinence rates when nicotine replacement therapy is used. Physical withdrawal symptoms from nicotine, which include agitation, irritability, anxiety, and nicotine craving, are theoretically reduced by nicotine replacement. By temporarily preventing physical withdrawal, smokers are able to learn to manage psychologic dependence. After incorporating learned coping mechanisms, nicotine replacement therapy is stopped, usually in a tapering fashion.

The nurse's major role is client education. Instruct the client in the proper use of the nicotine replacement system. Teach the client to apply one patch daily to a hairless area of the body and to rotate sites daily to avoid skin irritation. Instruct the client to chew the nicotine gum whenever the urge to smoke occurs. Because many beverages inhibit nicotine absorption, tell the client to avoid drinking 15 minutes before chewing nicotine polacrilex. Inform the client that chewing the gum too rapidly increases the risk for adverse effects and may predispose him or her to transferring the addiction to the gum. Since children are especially vulnerable to the adverse effects of nicotine, advise the client to store the gum and/or patches out of reach of children. Inform the client that if he or she continues to smoke while using either the gum or patches, he or she is at risk for developing toxicity.

CONCEPT REVIEW

Nicotine is a ganglionic stimulant with no current therapeutic use.

Nicotine is readily distributed into brain and placental tissue and is excreted in breast milk.

Nicotine patches and gum allow a gradual withdrawal from tobacco addiction.

SUMMARY

CNS stimulants comprise a heterogenous group of drugs whose subgroups (amphetamine and amphetamine-like substances, caffeine, and nicotine) bear little resemblance to one another. As a group, CNS stimulants have limited therapeutic applications. However, they are used frequently by the general population; thus the nurse's primary role is to provide client education.

REFERENCES

1. Lehne, R.A. (1994). *Pharmacology for nursing care* (2nd ed.). Philadelphia: W.B. Saunders.
2. U.S. Pharmacopeial Convention (1990). *The United States pharmacopeia* (22nd rev.). Rockville, MD: Author.
3. Aldrich, M.S. (1990). Narcolepsy. *New England Journal of Medicine, 324*, 389-393.
4. Data Pharmaceutica, Inc. (1993). *1993 physicians' genRx*. Smithtown, NY: Author.
5. Goodman, R., Gilman, T., Ball, T., Nies, A., & Taylor, P. (Eds.) (1990). *Goodman and Gilman's: The pharmacological basis of therapeutics* (8th ed.). New York: Pergamon Press.
6. Jahns, B.E., & Levy, D.B. (1991). Common drug reaction and interactions. *Emergency, 23*(11), 22-26, 29-31.
7. Foltin, R.W., Kelly, T.H., & Fischman, M.W. (1990). The effects of *d*-amphetamine on food intake of humans living in a residential laboratory. *Appetite, 15*, 33-45.
8. Lynch, J., & House, M.A. (1992). Cardiovascular effects of methamphetamine. *Journal of Cardiovascular Nursing, 6*(2), 12-18.
9. McKim, W.A. (1991). *Drugs and behavior: An introduction to behavioral pharmacology*. Englewood Cliffs, NJ: Prentice-Hall.
10. Fuglsang, G., Nielsen, K., Nielsen, L.K., Jakobsen, P., & Thelle, T. (1989). The effect of caffeine compared with theophylline in the treatment of idiopathic apnea in premature infants. *Acta Paediatrica Scandinavica, 78*, 786-788.
11. Ward, N., Whitney, C., Avery, D., & Dunner, D. (1991). The analgesic effects of caffeine in headache. *Pain, 44*, 151-155.
12. Coffey, C.E., Figiel, G.S., Weiner, R.D., & Saunders, W.B. (1990). Caffeine augmentation of ECT. *American Journal of Psychiatry, 147*, 579-585.
13. Bullough, B. (1990). Methylxanthines and fibrocystic breast disease: A study of correlations. *Nurse Practitioner, 15*(3), 36-44.
14. Russell, L.C. (1989). Caffeine restriction as initial treatment for breast pain. *Nurse Practitioner, 14*(2), 36-40.
15. De Carolis, M.P., Romagnoli, C., Muzii, U., Tortorolo, G., Chiarotti, M., DeGiovanni, N., & Carnevaale, A. (1991). Pharmacokinetic aspects of caffeine in premature infants. *Developmental Pharmacology and Therapeutics, 16*, 117-122.
16. Walther, F.J., Erickson, R.R., & Sims, M.E., (1990). Cardiovascular effects of caffeine therapy in preterm infants. *American Journal of Diseases of Children, 144*, 1164-1166.
17. Barr, H.M., & Streissguth, A.P. (1991). Caffeine use during pregnancy and child outcome: A 7-year prospective study. *Neurotoxicity and Teratology, 13*, 441-448.
18. Mills, J.L., Holmes, L.B., Aarons, J.H., Stupson, J.L., Brown, Z.A., Jovanovic-Peterson, L.G., Conley, M.R., Graubard, B.I., Knapp, R.H., & Metzger, B.E. (1993). Moderate caffeine use and the risk of spontaneous abortion and intrauterine growth retardation. *Journal of American Medical Association, 269*, 593-597.
19. McKim, E.M. (1991). Caffeine and its effects on pregnancy and the neonate. *Journal of Nurse Midwifery, 36*, 226-231.
20. Holdcroft, C. (1992). Efficacy of transdermal nicotine patches for nicotine replacement and smoking cessation. *Nurse Practitioner, 17*(7), 46, 48.
21. Houezec, J.L., & Benowitz, N.L. (1991). Basic and clinical psychopharmacology of nicotine. *Clinics in Chest Medicine, 12*, 681-699.
22. Gora, M.A. (1993). Nicotine transdermal systems. *Annals of Pharmacotherapy, 27*, 742-750.

BIBLIOGRAPHY

Bruera, E., Brenneis, C., Paterson, A.H., & MacDonald, R.N. (1989). Use of methylphenidate as an adjuvant to narcotic analgesics in patients with advanced cancer pain. *Journal of Pain and Symptom Management, 4*, 3-6.

Cerrato, P.L. (1990). Caffeine: How much is too much? *RN Magazine, 53*, 77-80.

Flay, B.R., Ockene, J.K., & Tager, I.B. (1992). Smoking: Epidemiology, cessation, and prevention. *Chest, 102*, 277S-301S.

Franklin, R.A. (1992). Smoking. *Nursing Clinics of North America, 27*, 631-642.

Gulick, E.E., Hayes, J.D., & Kennelly, L.F. (1991). Smoking among women: A life cycle perspective on which to base prevention/cessation interventions. *Oncology Nursing Forum, 18*(1), 91-102.

Heseltine, D., El-Jabri, M., Ahmed, F., & Knox, J. (1991). The effect of caffeine on postprandial blood pressure in the frail elderly. *Postgraduate Medical Journal, 67,* 543-547.

Hollis, J.F., Lichtenstein, E., Vogt, T.M., Stevens, V.J., & Biglan, A. (1993). Nurse-assisted counseling for smokers in primary care. *Annals of Internal Medicine, 118,* 521-525.

Krahn, D.D., Hasse, S., Ray, A., Gosnell, B., & Drenowski, A. (1991). Caffeine consumption in patients with eating disorders. *Hospital and Community Psychiatry, 42,* 313-315.

O'Conner, A.M., et al. (1992). Effectiveness of a pregnancy smoking cessation program. *Journal of Obstetric, Gynecologic, and Neonatal Nursing, 21,* 385-392.

Padula, C.A. (1992). Nurses and smoking: Review and implications. *Journal of Professional Nursing, 8,* 120-132.

Rossignol, A.M., & Bonnlander, H. (1990). Caffeine-containing beverages, total fluid consumption, and premenstrual syndrome. *American Journal of Public Health, 80,* 1106-1110.

CHAPTER 23

DRUGS USED TO TREAT
Parkinson's Disease

RHODA HEADLEY

⊛ Pathophysiology of Parkinson's Disease

LEARNING OBJECTIVE: Describe the pathophysiology of Parkinson's disease.

Key Terms:

Dopamine, dopaminergic cells

⊛ General Characteristics of Drug Group

LEARNING OBJECTIVE: Explain the major pharmacodynamics of the drugs used to treat Parkinson's disease.

⊛ Nursing Process

LEARNING OBJECTIVE: Develop a teaching plan for the client with Parkinson's disease that focuses on drug therapy.

KEY TERMS:

Bradykinesia, akinesia, parkinsonian crisis

⊛ Drugs that Increase Brain Levels of Dopamine

LEARNING OBJECTIVES:

Summarize essential information about levodopa.

Describe one drug-nutrient interaction that alters the effectiveness of levodopa.

Explain the impact of ethnic differences on the effectiveness of levodopa.

Summarize the effect of carbidopa on levodopa administration.

KEY TERMS:

Dyskinesia, on-off phenomenon

⊛ Dopamine-Releasing Drugs

LEARNING OBJECTIVES:

Summarize essential information about amantadine hydrochloride.

Distinguish between the actions of levodopa and amantadine.

⊛ Dopamine Agonists

LEARNING OBJECTIVE: Describe the use of bromocriptine in the treatment of Parkinson's disease.

⊛ Antimuscarinic and Anticholinergic Drugs

LEARNING OBJECTIVES:

Compare the action of antimuscarinic drugs and dopaminergic drugs.

Identify the major adverse reactions of the antimuscarinic drugs used in the treatment of Parkinson's disease.

⊛ Miscellaneous Drugs Used to Treat Parkinson's Disease

LEARNING OBJECTIVES:

Explain the use of diphenhydramine hydrochloride in the treatment of Parkinson's disease.

Describe the action of procyclidine hydrochloride.

CONCEPTS AND TERMS TO REVIEW

Review the anatomy and physiology of the central nervous system.

Review the functions of dopamine and acetylcholine.

Review the section in Chapter 26 that describes antimuscarinic drugs.

---

*P*arkinson's disease, a common disease of the nervous system, was first described in 1817 by James Parkinson. It is a chronic, progressive neurologic disorder characterized by rest tremors, muscle rigidity, bradykinesia, and postural instability. The disease occurs in both men and women of all ethnic backgrounds and almost always develops in clients between the ages of 50 and 70 years.

This chapter provides information on the pathophysiology of Parkinson's disease and the various drugs used to treat the condition. The nurse's role in assessing and planning appropriate care is also presented.

PATHOPHYSIOLOGY OF PARKINSON'S DISEASE

Parkinson's disease is caused by selective and progressive degeneration of dopamine-containing pigmented neurons in the substantia nigra of the midbrain and basal ganglia. **Dopamine** is transmitted to the putamen and caudate nucleus in the basal ganglia. There it inhibits the excitatory signals produced by acetylcholine (ACh), which is produced and secreted by neurons throughout the basal ganglia. ACh-producing neurons transmit excitatory signals throughout the basal ganglia. This stimulation of the basal ganglia results in inhibition of muscle tone throughout the body, thus allowing the refinement of voluntary movement.[1]

The underlying cause of the progressive degeneration of **dopaminergic cells** is unknown. However, research shows that when there is a decrease in dopamine transmitted to the corpus striatum of the basal ganglia, striatal cells under the influence of ACh initiate action potentials more rapidly. This results in progressive muscle rigidity or tremors or both.[2]

Most cases of Parkinson's disease are considered idiopathic in origin. **Idiopathic Parkinson's disease** is believed to be caused by loss of neurons associated with the normal aging process. In the idiopathic form approximately 80% of dopaminergic neurons in the substantia nigra degenerate before the onset of signs and symptoms.[2,3]

Postencephalitic parkinsonism most commonly results from a viral encephalitis infection. Some individuals with this form of the disease develop signs and symptoms within a few weeks of the infection. Others do not develop clinical evidence of the disease for 30 years. **Iatrogenic parkinsonism** is a common side effect of most antipsychotic drugs. Iatrogenic parkinsonism has also been associated with manganese, carbon monoxide, and cyanide toxicity.[3]

GENERAL CHARACTERISTICS OF DRUG GROUP

When dopamine-containing neurons in the substantia nigra degenerate beyond a threshold number, the inhibitory influence of dopamine is decreased, and the excitatory influence of ACh is increased. Therefore the major goal of drug therapy for clients with Parkinson's disease is to restore the balance of cholinergic and dopaminergic activity.

Drugs used in the treatment of Parkinson's disease either increase inhibitory dopamine activity or antagonize excitatory ACh activity. Drugs that increase the amount of dopamine available in the central nervous system (CNS) do so by one of three mechanisms: increasing the amount of dopamine in the brain; releasing dopamine; or acting as dopaminergic agonists. Drugs that antagonize excitatory ACh receptors do so by blunting the excitatory signals from the substantia nigra to the corticospinal motor control system.[4,5]

☒ NURSING CONSIDERATIONS

Most clients with Parkinson's disease are diagnosed and start receiving therapy in a community setting such as a physician's office or clinic. Since there is no known cure, treatment is aimed at controlling symptoms and maintaining the client's functional abilities. This treatment is based on a holistic approach that includes drugs, physical and occupational therapy, counseling, and education.

Assessing   During the **health history** obtain information about the time of onset and progression of the disease. Assess the client's mental status. Question the client about depression and altered thought processes. Assess the social, economic, and emotional impact of the disease on the client. Assess the client's ability for self-care and the ability to perform activities of daily living. Determine if he or she has difficulty starting movements or getting out of chairs. (These subtle changes in movement may be indications of **bradykinesia,** the slowness of purposeful movement.) Other subjective data to gather include presence of fatigue, dysphagia, difficulty with tasks requiring fine movements of the fingers, and heat insensitivity. In addition, ask the client about past and present drug usage. Note the name and dosage of all drugs. Question the client about the effectiveness of the drugs and the presence of undesired clinical responses.

During the **health assessment** observe the client for symptoms of the disease. Check the client's posture and gait (Fig. 23–1). (Usually the posture of a client with Parkinson's disease is stooped, and the client has a characteristic shuffling gait.) Note any muscle rigidity, and determine the client's muscle strength. Observe the client closely for rest tremor. (**Rest tremor** is the easiest symptom of Parkinson's disease to recognize. The tremor usually begins in one hand and often involves all the fingers and thumb.) Assess the client for **akinesia,** the inability to initiate movement. Akinesia causes the masklike facial expression seen in clients with Parkinson's disease. Some symptoms are due to autonomic nervous system dysfunction. They include changes in the pulse rate, orthostatic hypotension, infrequent blinking, heat intolerance, and excessive salivation.[3,6–8]

Diagnosing   Once the database has been established, the data are analyzed and nursing diagnoses developed. Depending on the data analysis, several nursing diagnoses are appropriate for the client receiving drug therapy for Parkinson's disease:

- Self-care deficit related to increase in muscle rigidity.
- Social isolation related to impaired communication.
- High risk for injury related to postural instability.
- Altered health maintenance related to knowledge deficit about drug regimen.
- Anxiety related to change in self-concept, change or threat to health status, threat of death.
- Altered nutrition: less than body requirement related to difficulty swallowing.
- High risk for ineffective coping related to lifestyle changes and dependence on drug therapy.

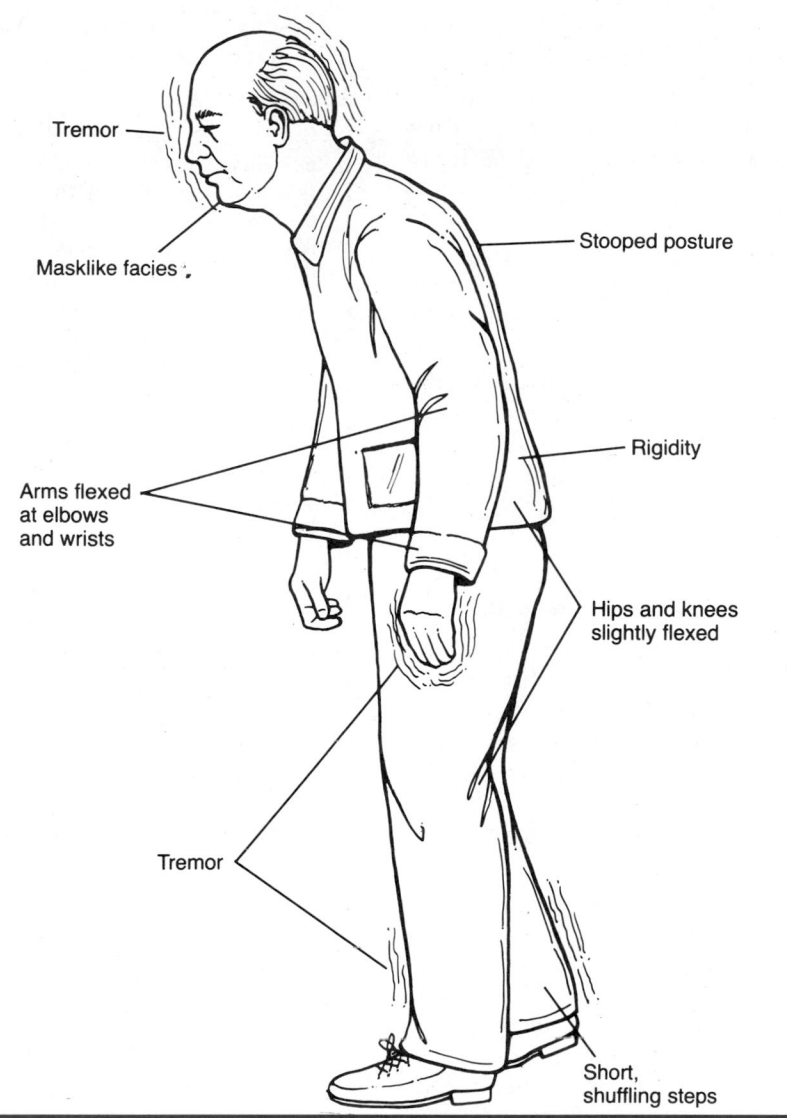

Tremor

Masklike facies

Stooped posture

Arms flexed
at elbows
and wrists

Rigidity

Hips and knees
slightly flexed

Tremor

Short,
shuffling steps

FIGURE 23–1   Clinical manifestations of Parkinsons' disease. (From Monahan, F.D., Drake, T., & Neighbors, M. [1994]. *Nursing Care of Adults.* Philadelphia: W.B. Saunders.

- High risk for altered urinary elimination related to affects of dopaminergic agents or anticholinergics on urinary system.
- High risk for altered bowel elimination: constipation related to affects of anticholinergics.

Planning   The role of the nurse caring for a client with Parkinson's disease includes client and family teaching. Much of the teaching focuses on preparing the client for self-management of the disease. Offer the client information on how to adapt the home environment to minimize the risk of injury. Include teaching on ways to adapt current clothing and personal items (e.g., elastic shoelaces, Velcro patches instead of buttons) so that independence in self-care is facilitated. Plan to teach the client exercises and other measures that will minimize the complications of decreased mobility. Develop a plan for teaching the client about nutrition. For example, tell him or her that semi-solid foods are easier to swallow than liquids or solids.

Instruct the client to decrease intake of vitamin B_6 and high-protein foods since they facilitate the destruction of dopamine. Provide the client information on the planned drug regimen. Include the name and dose of each drug, expected response to the drug, and list of undesired clinical responses.

Expected outcomes that can be discussed with the client include the following:

- Client participates in self-care activities within functional abilities.
- Client remains free from injury.
- Client verbalizes major undesired clinical responses associated with prescribed drugs.
- Client maintains desired body weight.
- Client maintains social interactions with significant others.
- Client establishes regular bowel elimination program.

Implementing Encourage the client to be as physically independent as possible. Focus on the client's functional abilities rather than functional losses. Encourage active participation in self-care activities. Have the client participate in a daily exercise routine that maintains full range of motion in all joints.

Administer drugs as prescribed and evaluate the client's response. Determine the degree of symptom control and the presence of undesired clinical responses. If the client is scheduled for diagnostic tests or surgery, maintain the prescribed dosages of drugs for as long as possible.

Provide the client and family with information about the drug regimen. Discuss symptoms that are expected to improve with each drug, and encourage the client to time activities to correlate with the drug's peak effectiveness. Teach the client and family to recognize fluctuations in response to drugs. Also explain common undesired clinical responses associated with each drug. Tell the client to maintain the prescribed drug regimen to avoid the occurrence of **parkinsonian crisis,** which can be caused by the sudden withdrawal of drugs. This condition is characterized by the abrupt return of marked rigidity, akinesia, tremor, and hyperpyrexia.

Assess both the client's and the family's coping status. Signs of ineffective coping include withdrawal, anger, crying, fatigue, feelings of guilt or worthlessness, decreased ability to concentrate, hypersomnolence, and insomnia. Encourage the client and the family to express their concerns and feelings. If necessary, refer the client to social services or pastoral care personnel.

Evaluating Evaluation of the therapeutic effectiveness of the plan of care involves subjective and objective improvement in the client's response. Evaluate the client's symptoms on a regular basis to determine if there is progression of the disease process. The client's overall functional abilities should be regularly evaluated. In addition, review the expected outcomes to determine if changes in the plan of care are needed.

CONCEPT REVIEW

Drugs used to treat Parkinson's disease primarily increase the dopamine content in the brain, block the neuronal reuptake of dopamine, or directly stimulate the release of dopamine.

The role of the nurse focuses on client teaching and promotion of self-management of the disease process.

DRUGS THAT INCREASE BRAIN LEVELS OF DOPAMINE

The prototype drug currently used to increase brain levels of dopamine is levodopa.

DRUG TO INCREASE DOPAMINE BRAIN LEVELS PROTOTYPE

LEVODOPA

Before 1965, when levodopa (Dopar, Larodopa) was introduced, mortality rates for individuals with Parkinson's disease were almost three times those of the general population. Most pre-levodopa deaths were caused by the effects of progressive immobility, pneumonia, infections, or exhaustion.[3,8]

Pharmacotherapeutics Approximately 75% of clients with Parkinson's disease respond to levodopa therapy. Improvement in rigidity and bradykinesia are usually more dramatic and long lasting than improvement in tremor. Significant improvement usually appears during the second or third week of therapy but may not appear for up to 6 months. Therapeutic effectiveness of levodopa seems to decline after approximately 6 years of treatment.[8]

Levodopa therapy in the long-term management of Parkinson's disease is frequently characterized by wide fluctuations in response within the client. The individual who had normal or near-normal mobility may suddenly develop severe tremors, loss of postural reflexes, and akinesia. These severe symptoms may persist for 30 minutes or up to 4 hours. This condition is called the **on-off phenomenon.** The on-off phenomenon can happen once a day or several times within the day. The condition usually develops after 2 years of levodopa therapy. The exact mechanism causing this phenomenon is unknown but it is believed to be related to an imbalance in physiologic regulatory mechanisms. Some clients seem to have less problem with the on-off phenomenon if the daily dosage of levodopa is divided into smaller, more frequent doses.[9,10]

Pharmacokinetics Levodopa is absorbed from the gastrointestinal (GI) tract by the amino acid transport system. It is rapidly metabolized in the GI tract and liver by l-aromatic amino-acid decarboxylase. In peripheral tissue this enzyme rapidly converts levodopa to dopamine. Since dopamine is not stored at these sites, the amine is further metabolized to 3,4-dihydroxyphenylacetic acid and 3-methoxy-4-hydroxyphenylacetic acid. These products are excreted in the urine unchanged or conjugated with sulfate or glucuronide. A small amount of dopamine is converted to norepinephrine and epinephrine in sympathetic nerve terminals. A significant proportion of dopamine in plasma occurs as the sulfate conjugate.[9,10]

To be effective, levodopa must undergo conversion to dopamine by dopa decarboxylase within the brain. Only about 1% of an oral dose of levodopa actually enters the brain. About 95% of the levodopa absorbed after oral administration is converted to dopamine peripherally. This peripherally produced dopamine cannot penetrate the CNS.[4,9]

Onset of action usually begins in 30 to 45 minutes, with peak plasma concentrations occurring 1 to 3 hours after administration of levodopa. Since levodopa competes with dietary amino acids for absorption from the small intestine and is absorbed by active transport, levodopa absorption is slowed if given with food. Approximately 80% of a dose is excreted in the urine within 24 hours after the dose is administered. A small amount of the drug is excreted in the feces.[4,9,11]

Pharmacodynamics Levodopa is a catecholamine that is the metabolic precursor of dopamine. Dopamine does not cross the blood-brain barrier in sufficient concentrations after systemic administration to be therapeutic. However, levodopa does cross the blood-brain barrier (Fig. 23–2).

The exact mechanism of action of levodopa is unknown. Most of its pharmacologic effects are believed related to newly formed dopamine. The effects of levodopa seem to be mediated by stimulation of both central and peripheral dopamine receptors.[9]

Pharmaceutics Levodopa is available in gelatin capsules and uncoated tablets for oral administration. The dosage of levodopa must be individualized.

Undesired Clinical Responses Undesired clinical responses to levodopa are either early reactions that tend to improve with tolerance to the drug or late-developing symptoms that increase with duration of therapy (Fig. 23–3). The most common early adverse reactions to levodopa include GI symptoms (anorexia, nausea, and vomiting) and orthostatic hypotension. GI symptoms probably are caused by direct stimulation of the chemoreceptor trigger zone in the medulla oblongata by the newly formed dopamine. Orthostatic hypotension probably is caused by the accumulation of dopamine in norepinephrine nerve terminals. Cardiac arrhythmias that occur in some clients are caused by stimulation of β-adrenoceptors in the heart by dopamine. These early symptoms usually subside as tolerance develops over a period of a few weeks. A temporary reduction in the drug dosage also decreases the severity of the symptoms.[4,10]

Reactions to levodopa that tend to increase with the duration of drug therapy probably result from CNS stimulation of dopamine receptors. The most common of these adverse reactions is the development of **dyskinesia.** These abnormal movements of the limbs, hands, trunk, and tongue can be decreased by reducing the dosage of levodopa. However, reduction in the dosage of levodopa causes the symptoms of the disease to become more severe. Many clients prefer to live with the dyskinesia if their overall mobility is improved with levodopa therapy. Other common reactions include dark-colored urine and perspiration, urinary retention or frequency, and hemolytic anemia.

Serious mental disturbances occur in about 15% of clients treated with levodopa. Many individuals receiving long-term levodopa therapy develop severe depression, vivid dreams, delusions, and visual hallucinations.[12] If serious neuropsychiatric disturbances occur, the dosage of levodopa may be decreased or a "drug holiday" started.

Contraindications and Precautions Levodopa should be used with caution in clients with a history of myocardial infarction who have a residual dysrhythmia. The drug is used with caution in clients with bronchial asthma or emphysema who require drug therapy with sympathomimetic drugs. Clients with severe cardiovascular, pulmonary, renal, hepatic, endocrine, or active peptic ulcer disease should also be monitored closely while receiving levodopa. In addition, levodopa is not recommended in clients with wide-angle glaucoma and psychotic disorders.[4,11]

Drug-Drug and Drug-Nutrient Interactions There

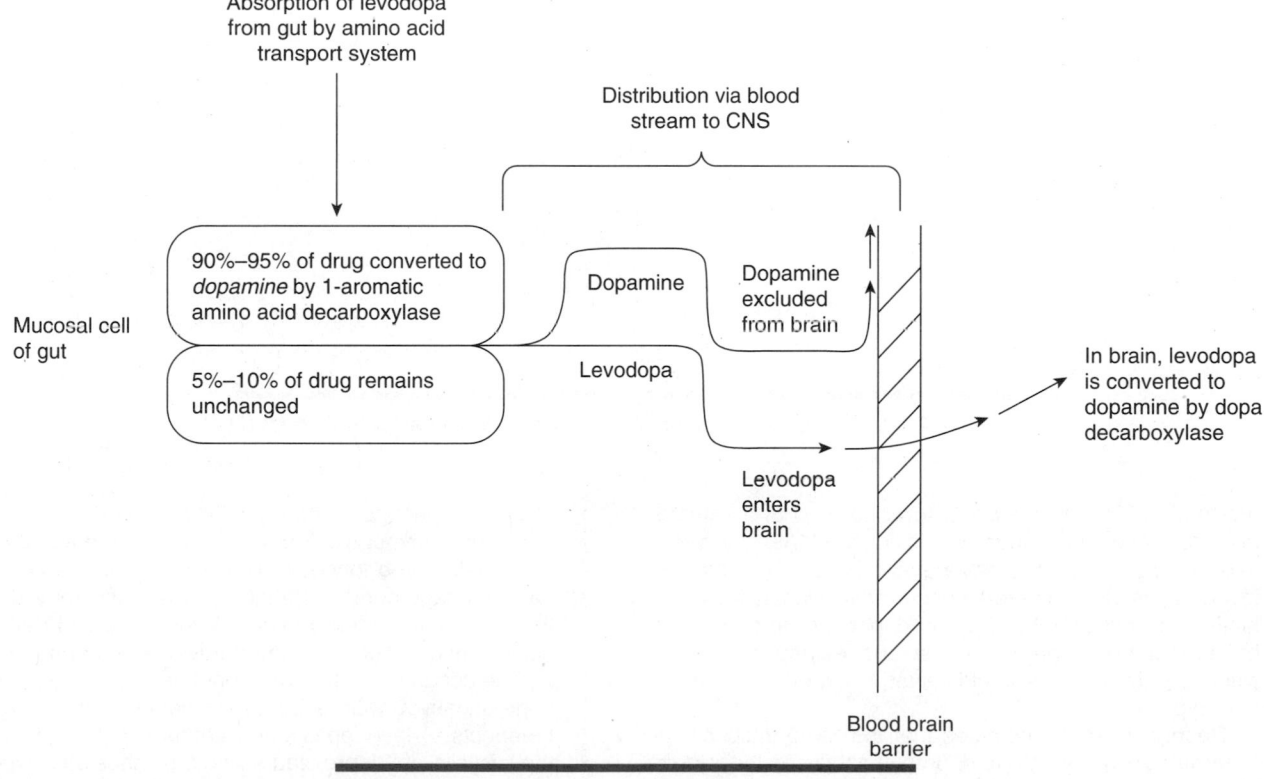

FIGURE 23–2   Distribution of levodopa in the brain.

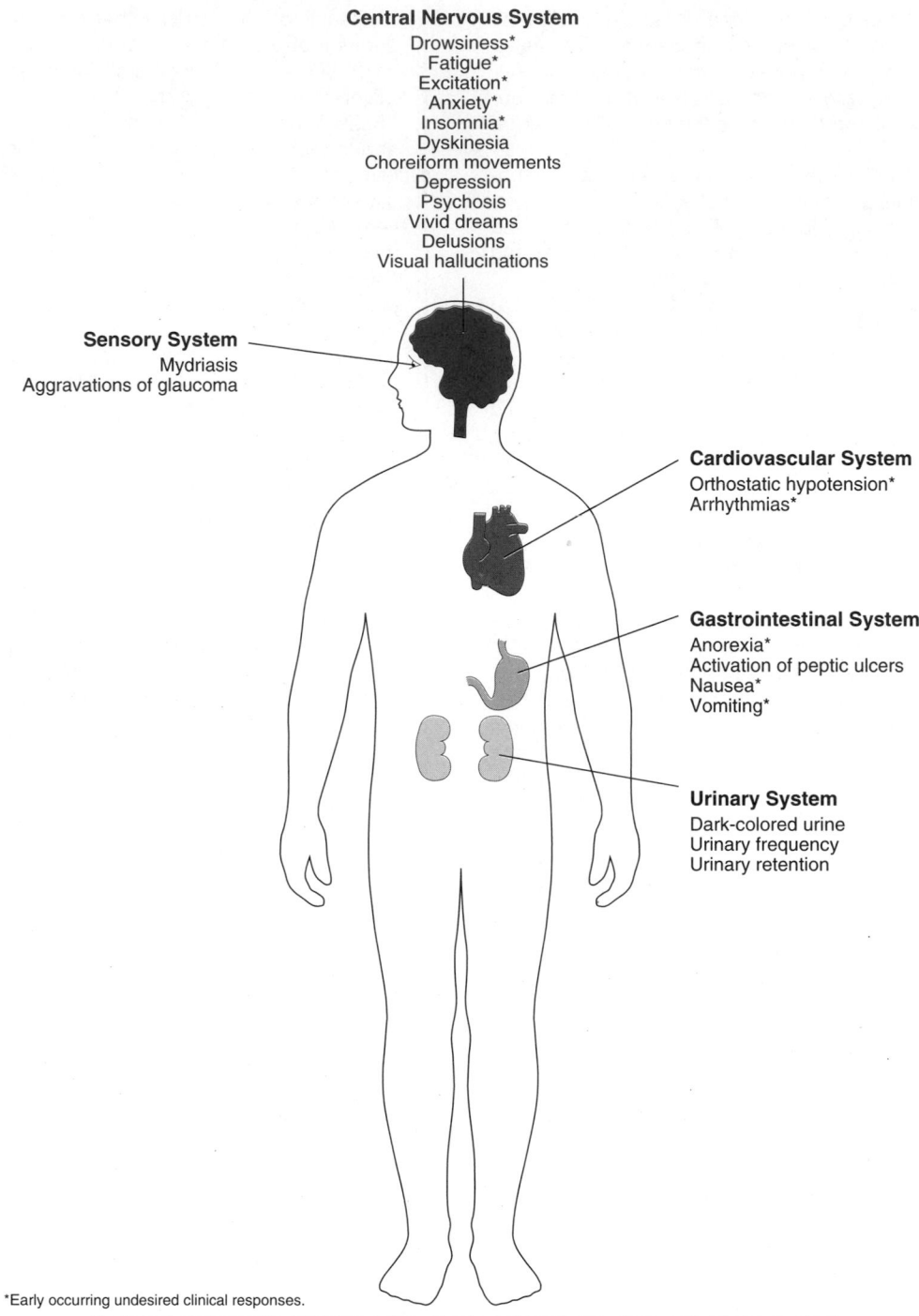

Central Nervous System
Drowsiness*
Fatigue*
Excitation*
Anxiety*
Insomnia*
Dyskinesia
Choreiform movements
Depression
Psychosis
Vivid dreams
Delusions
Visual hallucinations

Sensory System
Mydriasis
Aggravations of glaucoma

Cardiovascular System
Orthostatic hypotension*
Arrhythmias*

Gastrointestinal System
Anorexia*
Activation of peptic ulcers
Nausea*
Vomiting*

Urinary System
Dark-colored urine
Urinary frequency
Urinary retention

*Early occurring undesired clinical responses.

FIGURE 23–3   Undesired clinical responses associated with levodopa.

are numerous **drug-drug interactions.** For example, levodopa and the monoamine oxidase (MAO) inhibitors use common metabolic pathways within the brain. When levodopa is administered concurrently with a MAO inhibitor, a massive buildup of dopamine and a small buildup of both norepinephrine and epinephrine occur within the brain. This could result in hypertensive crisis and hyperpyrexia.[11,12]

Recent research indicates that the MAO inhibitor **selegiline hydrochloride** (L-deprenyl) catalyzes the metab-

olism of dopamine in the brain. This extends the duration of action of levodopa. Studies show that the combination of selegiline and low-dose levodopa administered in the early management of Parkinson's disease may sustain the therapeutic effectiveness of levodopa and delay the appearance of dosage-related adverse reactions.[13,14]

The coadministration of phenothiazine and butyrophenone sedatives with levodopa antagonizes the therapeutic effects of levodopa. Many antidepressants, including the tricyclic antidepressants, cause orthostatic hypotension as an adverse reaction. This could have an additive effect with the orthostatic hypotension of levodopa. Hypotension can be minimized by giving the antidepressant only once a day at bedtime.[11]

Several **drug-nutrient interactions** occur with levodopa therapy. To decrease the GI adverse reactions to levodopa, the drug is frequently given with meals. However, because levodopa competes with dietary amino acids for absorption from the small intestine, food in the stomach slows absorption of the drug. In addition, high-protein foods and pyridoxine interfere with the absorption of levodopa.

Pyridoxine (vitamin B$_6$) is a cofactor in the decarboxylation of levodopa to dopamine. Pyridoxine rapidly reverses the therapeutic effectiveness of levodopa by promoting more rapid peripheral conversion of levodopa to dopamine, thus making less levodopa available for transport to the brain. Clients receiving levodopa should limit their intake of pyrimidine to less than 5 g daily. Dietary sources of pyrimidine include green vegetables, whole grain cereals, wheat germ, legumes, bananas, and meats (especially liver). Since over-the-counter (OTC) multivitamin preparations and fortified cereals contain pyrimidine, their use should be avoided unless approved by the primary care provider.[15,16]

Interference with Diagnostic Studies Levodopa has caused elevated serum and urinary pH levels, false-positive reactions for urinary glucose and ketones, and false elevations of urinary catecholamine results.

Ethnic Differences in Drug Disposition and Responsiveness Levodopa is converted to dopamine by decarboxylation and metabolized to 3-O-methyldopa by catechol-O-methyltransferase (COMT). The metabolite 3-O-methyldopa antagonizes the therapeutic effects of levodopa. Therefore the greater the activity of COMT, the more 3-O-methyldopa produced, diminishing the therapeutic response to levodopa. Orientals (Chinese, Filipinos, and Thais) have increased COMT activity. These individuals require lower doses of levodopa and careful monitoring for dyskinesia.[17]

Specific Drug-Related Nursing Considerations Because levodopa can cause orthostatic hypotension, ideally the client's blood pressure should be monitored every 4 hours during periods of dosage adjustment or when new drugs are added to the drug regimen. If the client is in the home setting, teach the client how to check his or her blood pressure. Tell the client to move slowly from the supine to a standing or sitting position to avoid possible hypotensive episodes. In addition, instruct the family or significant others to report any signs of personality or behavior change that might be related to the drug therapy. Table 23–1 summarizes additional nursing considerations.

TABLE 23-1
Drugs Used to Treat Parkinson's Disease

Drug Name	Dosages and Route of Administration	Nursing Considerations
LEVODOPA (L-dopa, Dopar, Larodopa) **HOW SUPPLIED** Gelatin capsules: 100 mg, 250 mg, 500 mg Uncoated tablets: 100 mg, 250 mg, 500 mg	Dosage must be individualized. Usual initial dosage: 0.5-2 g/d in two or three divided doses Dosage gradually increased by 0.5-0.75 g, q3-7d Maximum dosage, 8 g/d	***Assess*** Determine if client has preexisting conditions (e.g., renal, hepatic, cardiovascular, or pulmonary disease) that would prevent use of levodopa. Gather a complete drug and nutritional history. ***Implement*** Advise client not to take drug with high-protein meals or foods containing pyridoxine. Instruct client to change from recumbent to standing position slowly to avoid dizziness or syncope. Instruct clients with chronic wide-angle glaucoma to have intraocular pressure checked at least yearly. Advise clients with diabetes mellitus that frequent blood sugar monitoring is necessary. Teach client early indications of overdose: muscle twitching and spasmodic winking. ***Monitor*** Monitor for behavioral changes. Monitor vital signs during dosage adjustment and report any alterations. ***Evaluate*** Anticipate significant improvements by second or third week of therapy.

Table continued on following page.

TABLE 23-1 *Continued*
Drugs Used to Treat Parkinson's Disease

Drug Name	Dosages and Route of Administration	Nursing Considerations
Carbidopa-levodopa (Sinemet) HOW SUPPLIED Uncoated tablet: 10 mg/100 mg, 25 mg/100 mg, 25 mg/250 mg Sustained-action tablet: 50 mg/200 mg	If client receiving levodopa, initial dosage: one 25 mg/250 mg tablet tid or qid Dosage increased or decreased by one half to one tablet daily Maximum dosage: eight of the 25 mg/250 mg tablets daily If client not receiving levodopa, initial dosage: one 10 mg/100 mg or 25 mg/100 mg tablet tid Dosage increased by one tablet daily or every other day Maximum dosage: eight tablets daily	Same as levodopa with following exceptions or additions: **Implement** Initial dose usually administered after individual has been without levodopa for a minimum of 8 h. **Monitor** Anticipate that therapeutic and undesired clinical responses occur more rapidly with combination therapy.
Amantadine Hydrochloride (Symadine, Symmetrel) HOW SUPPLIED Capsule: 100 mg Syrup: 50 mg/5 ml	Usual initial dosage: 100 mg once or twice a day	**Assess** Assess for preexisting conditions (e.g., history of seizures, congestive heart failure, peripheral edema, recurrent eczematoid dermatitis) that would contradict use of amantadine. **Implement** Advise client to avoid activities requiring mental alertness until response to drug is determined. Instruct client not to take last daily dose too close to bedtime; insomnia may occur. Teach client to change positions slowly to avoid syncope. Teach client to assess ankles routinely for diffuse, mottled reddening and swelling (livedo reticularis) **Monitor** Monitor for CNS disturbances. Monitor vital signs for at least 3 d after dosage adjustments. **Evaluate** Anticipate lessening of akinesia, rigidity, and excessive salivation within 4-48 h after therapy begins.
Bromocriptine Mesylate (Parlodel) HOW SUPPLIED Gelatin capsule: 5 mg Uncoated tablet: 2.5 mg	**Parkinson's Disease** Initial dosage: one half of 2.5-mg tablet bid with meals Gradual increase q14-28 d by 2.5 mg/d with meals Decrease dosage slowly (2.5-mg increments)	**Assess** Assess baseline blood pressure; therapy should not be started unless vital signs are stable. **Implement** Instruct client to take drug with meals or milk to decrease GI effects. Inform client that mild diuresis may occur in initial phase of drug therapy. Teach client to avoid changing positions too quickly; lightheadedness, dizziness, and syncope can occur. Instruct client to avoid exposure to cold and to report pallor of fingers or toes since digital vasospasm can occur with high dosage. **Monitor** Monitor blood pressure and pulse carefully during first few days of therapy. Monitor hepatic, renal, hematologic, and cardiovascular function periodically. **Evaluate** Anticipate improvements in tremors and rigidity within 2 h of drug administration. Evaluation of response done at least every 2 wk during dosage titration to determine lowest effective dose.

TABLE 23-1 *Continued*
Drugs Used to Treat Parkinson's Disease

Drug Name	Dosages and Route of Administration	Nursing Considerations
Benztropine Mesylate (Cogentin, Glycopyrrolate) HOW SUPPLIED Uncoated tablet: 0.5 mg, 1 mg, 2 mg IM, IV: 1 mg/ml	Usual initial dosage (oral): 1.5 to 1 mg/d Dosage gradually increased to maximum of 6 mg/d Usual maintenance dosage: 2 mg/d	**Assess** Determine if client has preexisting conditions (e.g., narrow-angle glaucoma, myasthenia gravis, obstructive genitourinary disorders) that might contradict therapy with benztropine. **Implement** Administer at bedtime with food or immediately after a meal. Suggest use of mouth rinses, hard candy, or chewing gum to relieve mouth dryness. Auscultate bowel sounds and teach client to monitor elimination pattern since paralytic ileus can occur. Encourage adequate fluid and fiber intake to decrease potential for constipation. Teach client to avoid strenuous activities in hot weather to prevent heat exhaustion or stroke. Be aware of potential for abuse caused by hallucinogenic effects of drug. Teach client about possibility of drowsiness and blurred vision. Advise client to avoid activities requiring mental alertness until response to therapy is determined. Inform client that alcohol and other CNS depressants may increase drowsiness. **Monitor** Monitor status of cardiac function carefully. Monitor individuals with previous history of mental dysfunction for increased symptoms during initial therapy. **Evaluate** Anticipate changes in symptoms in 2 to 3 d.
Trihexphenidyl Hydrochloride (Artane) HOW SUPPLIED Elixir: 2 mg/5 ml Uncoated tablet: 2 mg, 5 mg Gelatin sustained-action capsule: 5 mg Liquid: 2 mg/5 ml	Usual initial dosage: 1 mg/d; dosage increased 2 mg q3-5 d Maximum daily dosage: 10 mg Usual maintenance dosage: 6-10 mg When administered with levodopa, dosage usually decreased	See benztropine mesylate.
Biperiden Hydrochloride (Akineton) HOW SUPPLIED Uncoated tablet: 2 mg IM, IV: 5 mg/ml	**Idiopathic or Drug-Induced Parkinson's Disease** Oral: Initial dosage: 2 mg tid or qid **Acute Drug-Induced Extrapyramidal Symptoms:** IM or IV: 2 mg q30 min up to maximum of 8 mg/24 h	See benztropine mesylate.
Procyclidine Hydrochloride (Kemadrin) HOW SUPPLIED Uncoated tablet: 5 mg	Initial dosage: 2-2.5 mg tid with meals; may be increased to 4-5 mg tid	See benztropine mesylate.
Ethopropazine Hydrochloride (Parsidol) HOW SUPPLIED Uncoated tablet: 10 mg, 50 mg	Initial dosage: 50 mg once or twice a day Maintenance dosage: 100-400 mg/d for mild to moderate symptoms; 500-600 mg/d for severe symptoms	See benztropine mesylate.

Decarboxylase Inhibitors

To decrease peripheral conversion of levodopa to dopamine, decarboxylase inhibitors sometimes are administered concomitantly with levodopa. Addition of decarboxylase inhibitors to levodopa preparations allows administration of lower, less frequent doses of levodopa. In addition, a larger percentage of the administered dosage of levodopa is available for entry into the CNS. The drug combination also promotes therapeutic effectiveness by shortening the onset of drug action and decreasing the peripheral adverse effects of levodopa. However, the development of late-appearing adverse reactions such as the on-off phenomenon does not seem to decrease with the combination therapy.[4,9,10]

DECARBOXYLASE INHIBITOR PROTOTYPE

CARBIDOPA

Carbidopa is administered in combination with levodopa as Sinemet. This fixed-dosage combination is easy for the client to administer. Carbidopa may also be administered as a single agent as Lodosyn. With this approach the primary care provider can individualize the dose of each drug—carbidopa and levodopa. Since carbidopa does not cross the blood-brain barrier, it does not affect the metabolism of levodopa within the brain. When carbidopa is given along with levodopa, levodopa plasma levels and plasma half-life are increased. The amount of levodopa that a client requires is reduced by approximately 75% when carbidopa is added to the drug regimen. Carbidopa also decreases the inhibitory effect of pyridoxine on levodopa.[4]

Carbidopa-levodopa is available as an uncoated oral tablet and in an extended-release dosage form. The dosage of Sinemet or Lodosyn is highly individualized. Precautions for administration and assessment for undesired clinical responses are the same as those for levodopa. See Table 23–1 for a summary of information about dosages and nursing considerations.

CONCEPT REVIEW

Levodopa increases the level of dopamine in the brain. Two major undesired clinical responses associated with levodopa are dyskinesia and mental disturbances. In addition, many drug-drug interactions are possible with levodopa.

Carbidopa decreases or blocks the conversion of levodopa to dopamine in the periphery, allowing more levodopa to cross into the brain. This allows a reduction in the dosage of levodopa.

DOPAMINE-RELEASING DRUGS

The prototype dopamine-releasing drug is amantadine hydrochloride.

DOPAMINE-RELEASING DRUG PROTOTYPE

AMANTADINE HYDROCHLORIDE

Amantadine (Symmetrel) is a synthetic antiviral agent used in the management of influenza A. However, it has been found effective in the treatment of Parkinson's disease.

Pharmacotherapeutics Amantadine is not as effective as levodopa. It produces rapid (sometimes within 2 days) but short-term improvement in approximately two thirds of the clients who receive the drug. Usually akinesia, rigidity, tremor, gait disturbance, and overall functional disability are improved. Optimal results usually occur within 3 months, but tolerance develops within 3 years. Amantadine is usually given along with levodopa therapy or anticholinergic therapy. When amantadine therapy is discontinued, the dosage should be gradually decreased to prevent exacerbations of symptoms.[4,18]

Pharmacokinetics Amantadine is absorbed well from the GI tract. Mean peak blood concentrations occur in 1 to 4 hours. The elimination half-life of amantadine averages 24 hours. The drug is excreted unchanged in urine by glomerular filtration and tubular secretion. The half-life of amantadine is prolonged in clients with impaired renal functioning.

Pharmacodynamics Amantadine's exact mechanism of action is unknown. It is believed that the drug acts by releasing dopamine from the dopaminergic terminals that have not yet degenerated.[4,18]

Pharmaceutics Amantadine hydrochloride is available for oral administration in capsule and syrup dosage forms.

Undesired Clinical Responses The most common undesired responses to amantadine are mild CNS disturbances. These disturbances are reversible, are usually dose related, and appear within a few hours after initiating drug therapy or changing drug dosage. Dizziness, insomnia, nervousness, anxiety, hallucinations, confusion, nightmares, and impaired ability to concentrate are the most frequent CNS disturbances. Nausea is also a common undesired response. In addition, drowsiness, lethargy, and slurred speech have been reported.

Livedo reticularis is a common but not serious clinical response. This condition is characterized by a reddish blue mottle discoloration of the legs and, rarely, the arms. Livedo reticularis probably is caused by local release of catecholamines and abnormal capillary permeability.[4,18]

Contraindications and Precautions Amantadine should be administered cautiously to clients with liver disease, recurrent eczematoid dermatitis, uncontrolled psychosis, or epilepsy and to clients receiving CNS-stimulating drugs. It should also be used with caution in clients with impaired renal functioning, congestive heart failure, peripheral edema, or orthostatic hypotension.[11,12]

Drug-Drug Interactions Concurrent administration of amantadine to clients receiving anticholinergic drugs may increase the undesired clinical responses from the anticholinergic drugs.

Specific Drug-Related Nursing Considerations Advise the client to take the evening dose of amantadine several hours before bedtime if insomnia develops. Teach clients with a history of congestive heart failure to monitor their weight daily. Instruct them to report changes in respiratory status and to check daily for indications of fluid retention in the lower extremities. Because amantadine can cause drowsiness, caution the client to avoid activities requiring mental alertness during periods of dosage adjustment.[18]

DOPAMINE AGONISTS

The prototype dopamine agonist drug is **bromocriptine mesylate** (Parlodel). Bromocriptine is a semisynthetic ergot derivative used primarily for short-term management of amenorrhea or galactorrhea and to prevent postpartum lactation. It has also been approved as adjunctive therapy with levodopa or levodopa-carbidopa in the treatment of Parkinson's disease. The therapeutic efficacy of bromocriptine is considered equal to that of levodopa.

The maintenance dosage of levodopa is usually reduced when bromocriptine is concomitantly administered. This reduction decreases the severity of undesired clinical responses associated with long-term levodopa therapy. However, the combination of levodopa and bromocriptine does not alter the appearance of dyskinesia or the on-off phenomenon. Bromocriptine may be useful in clients who have been treated for several years with levodopa and who are experiencing end-of-dose failure. **End-of-dose failure** or deterioration is a progressive decrease in the duration of therapeutic effects from a dose of levodopa.[14,19] Undesired clinical responses are shown in Figure 23–4.

Recent studies show that **cabergoline,** a long-acting dopamine agonist, could be a suitable drug for providing continuous dopaminergic stimulation. Cabergoline has a high affinity for dopamine receptors. It has an active half-life of more than 60 hours, so the drug may be effective in once-daily doses. The addition of cabergoline to levodopa-carbidopa therapy decreases the severity of the on-off phenomenon.

Pergolide mesylate (Permax), a semisynthetic ergoline derivative, is also a potent dopamine agonist. It is considered approximately 10 times more potent than bromocriptine. In clients with Parkinson's disease, pergolide exerts its therapeutic effect by directly stimulating postsynaptic dopamine receptors in the nigrostriatal system. Pergolide is indicated as an adjunctive treatment to levodopa-carbidopa therapy.[19,21] Table 23–1 provides additional information about dopamine agonists.

CONCEPT REVIEW

Amantadine stimulates the release of dopamine in the brain. Its exact mechanism is not known, and it is not as effective as levodopa.

Dopamine agonists such as bromocriptine and pergolide mesylate stimulate dopamine receptors.

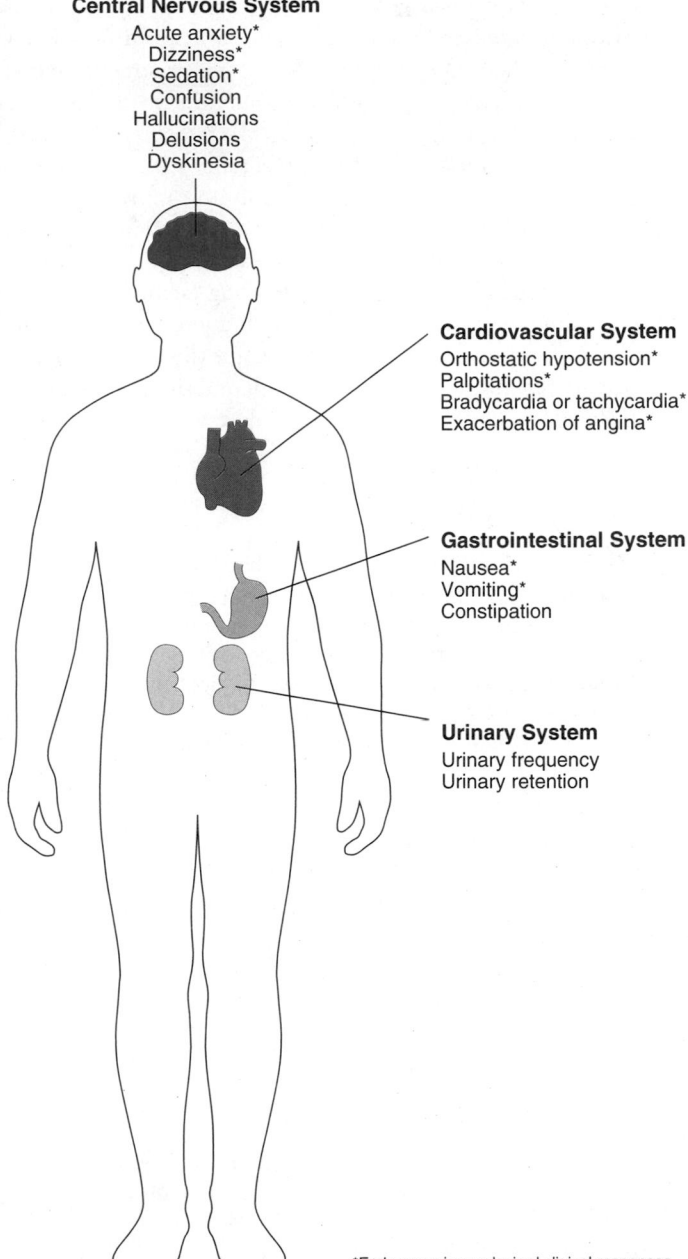

Central Nervous System
Acute anxiety*
Dizziness*
Sedation*
Confusion
Hallucinations
Delusions
Dyskinesia

Cardiovascular System
Orthostatic hypotension*
Palpitations*
Bradycardia or tachycardia*
Exacerbation of angina*

Gastrointestinal System
Nausea*
Vomiting*
Constipation

Urinary System
Urinary frequency
Urinary retention

*Early occurring undesired clinical responses.

Figure 23–4 Undesired clinical responses associated with dopamine agonists.

ANTIMUSCARINIC OR ANTICHOLINERGIC DRUGS

Antimuscarinic drugs are also used to treat Parkinson's disease. Antimuscarinics, also called *anticholinergics* and *parasympatholytics,* antagonize functions controlled primarily by the parasympathetic nervous system. (See Chapter 26 for complete information on anticholinergic drugs.)

Currently, antimuscarinic drugs are used most commonly in the management of mild symptoms in the early stages of the disease process. Antimuscarinic drugs are also used along with levodopa in the management of more severe symptoms as the disease progresses. When used as the primary drug therapy, these drugs are most effective in controlling tremor and rigidity. They are not very effective in the management of akinesia.[10]

Most antimuscarinic drugs maintain their effectiveness with long-term administration. If antimuscarinic drug use is discontinued, the dosage should be reduced gradually. Abrupt withdrawal can result in confusion, exhaustion, and exacerbation of symptoms. The primary limiting factor in the use of these drugs is the appearance of drug-induced (antimuscarinic) adverse reactions. These reactions include dry mouth, dry eyes, urinary retention, and constipation. Confusion, delirium, and hallucinations may occur with high doses.[4,11]

ANTIMUSCARINIC DRUG PROTOTYPE

BENZTROPINE MESYLATE

Benztropine mesylate (Cogentin) is the antimuscarinic drug currently used in the management of Parkinson's disease. Benztropine is a synthetic, centrally acting antimuscarinic that is chemically similar to atropine and diphenhydramine (Benadryl).

Pharmacotherapeutics Benztropine is useful in the treatment of elderly clients who cannot tolerate the CNS-stimulating properties of other antimuscarinic drugs.[10]

Pharmacokinetics After oral administration most antimuscarinic drugs are almost completely absorbed from the GI tract. The exact distribution of these agents is unknown. However, it is believed that they cross the blood-brain barrier since they affect CNS tissue. Onset of action is within 1 hour, and peak concentrations are reached within 4 hours. Duration of action may be as long as 6 hours. The drugs are at least partially metabolized by the liver and excreted as metabolites and unchanged drug in the urine.[4,10,11]

Pharmacodynamics Antimuscarinic drugs block the reuptake of dopamine into presynaptic neurons in the CNS and by suppressing central cholinergic activity. Central cholinergic activity has an excitatory effect on the CNS. An excess of ACh may cause the tremors associated with Parkinson's disease.[10]

Pharmaceutics Benztropine is available in tablet form for oral administration.

Undesired Clinical Responses Common undesired clinical responses include dry mouth, blurred vision, mydriasis, nausea, nervousness, tachycardia, and skin rash. High doses may cause mental confusion, weakness, urinary retention, constipation, paralytic ileus, hyperthermia, and visual hallucinations. Dosage adjustment usually eliminates most of the responses.[4,10]

Contraindications and Precautions Benztropine should be used with caution in clients taking phenothiazines or other drugs with antimuscarinic effects. Use of this drug is not recommended in clients with prostatic hypertrophy, tardive dyskinesia, or episodic tachycardia.[11,12]

Drug-Drug Interactions Concurrent administration of benztropine and other drugs with antimuscarinic effects increases the risk for undesired clinical responses. Concurrent administration of benztropine with pheno-

thiazines or tricyclic antidepressants may cause paralytic ileus, hyperthermia, or heat stroke.[11]

MISCELLANEOUS DRUGS IN CATEGORY

Other antimuscarinic drugs used to treat Parkinson's disease include **ethopropazine hydrochloride** (Parsidol) and **trihexyphenidyl hydrochloride** (Artane). Ethopropazine's specific mode of action in person's with Parkinson's disease is not known. However, most of the symptoms of the disease respond to therapy with this drug. Ethopropazine has been used to treat postencephalitic and idiopathic parkinsonism and drug-induced extrapyramidal symptoms. Trihexyphenidyl exerts a direct inhibitory effect on the parasympathetic nervous system. It is used as an adjunctive treatment of all forms of parkinsonism.[11,12]

MISCELLANEOUS DRUGS USED TO TREAT PARKINSON'S DISEASE

Other drugs used to reduce symptoms of Parkinson's disease include diphenhydramine hydrochloride (Benadryl) and procyclidine hydrochloride (Kemadrin). **Diphenhydramine hydrochloride** is classified as an antihistamine. However, it has significant antimuscarinic activity. (Additional information on diphenhydramine is in Chapter 51.) In clients with Parkinson's disease, diphenhydramine suppresses central cholinergic activity and prolongs the reuptake and storage of dopamine. This drug decreases rigidity and improves voluntary movement and speech. It is especially useful in elderly clients who cannot tolerate more potent CNS-stimulating agents.[12]

Procyclidine hydrochloride (Kemadrin) is a synthetic antispasmodic compound. The drug is a chemical modification of antihistamines. It is used to relieve symptoms of all forms of Parkinson's disease and drug-induced extrapyramidal symptoms. Studies show that procyclidine has an atropine-like action and exerts an antispasmodic effect on smooth muscles. It is a potent mydriatic and inhibits salivation. Procyclidine does not have sympathetic ganglion-blocking activity.[12]

SUMMARY

Parkinson's disease is a chronic, progressive neurologic disorder. At this time symptoms cannot be reversed once the process begins. However, the progression of symptoms can be controlled with pharmacologic agents. Once the diagnosis is confirmed, pharmacologic management is based on the degree of disability caused by the individual's symptoms. If early symptoms do not cause interference with the ability to perform activities of daily living, use of pharmacologic management may be delayed. Most clients eventually are treated with levodopa.

Current research indicates that the initial benefits of levodopa therapy decline after 2 or more years of treatment. For this reason it is beneficial to begin treatment with other drugs. If tremor is the only significant symptom, the client may be treated initially with an antimuscarinic drug. If bradykinesia and rigidity cause difficulty, amantadine alone or in combination with an antimuscarinic drug may be the initial treatment. Once these drugs become ineffective, a dopamine agonist may be used. With this approach, the use of a levodopa-carbidopa combination may be delayed for up to 3 years.

REFERENCES

1. Bradybury, K., & Bauer, M. (1990). Brain graft surgery: A new treatment for Parkinson's disease. *Critical Care Nurse, 10*(8), 15-31.
2. Jellinger, K. (1990). New developments in the pathology of Parkinson's disease. *Advances in Neurology, 53,* 1-13.
3. Vernon, G. (1989). Parkinson's disease. *Journal of Neuroscience Nursing, 21,* 273-282.
4. Cedarbaum, J. (1990). Drugs for Parkinson's disease, spasticity, and acute muscle spasms. In R. Goodman, E. Gilman, T. Rall, A. Nies, & P. Taylor (Eds.), *Goodman and Gilman's: The pharamcological basis of therapeutics* (8th ed., pp. 463-484). New York: Pergamon Press.
5. Hershey, L. (1992). Drugs used in the treatment of Parkinson's disease and other movement disorders. In C. Smith & A. Reynard (Eds.), *Textbook of pharmacology* (pp. 340-357). Philadelphia: W.B. Saunders.
6. Bunting, L., & Fitzsimmons, B. (1991). Depression in Parkinson's disease. *Journal of Neuroscience Nursing, 23,* 158-169.
7. Hughes, A. (1992). What features improve the accuracy of clinical diagnosis in Parkinson's disease: A clinicopathologic study. *Neurology, 42,* 1142-2246.
8. Pleet, A. (1992). Newly diagnosed Parkinson's disease: A therapeutic update. *Geriatrics, 47*(1), 24-29.
9. Juncos, J. (1992). Levodopa: Pharmacology, pharmacokinetics, and pharmacodynamics. *Neurologic Clinics, 10,* 487-509.
10. Rutledge, C. (1990). Drug therapy in parkinsonism and other basal ganglia disorders. In C. Craig & R. Stitzel (Eds.), *Modern Pharmacology* (3rd ed., pp. 500-508). Boston: Little, Brown.
11. U.S. Pharmacopeial Convention (1990). *The United States pharmacopeia* (22nd rev.). Rockville, MD: Author.
12. Data Pharmaceutica, Inc. (1993). *1993 physicians' genRx.* Smithtown, NY: Author.
13. Elizan, T., Moros, D., & Yahr, M. (1991). Early combination of selegiline and low-dose levodopa as initial symptomatic therapy in Parkinson's disease. *Archives of Neurology, 48*(1), 31-34.
14. Le Witt, P. (1992). Treatment strategies for extension of levodopa effect. *Neurologic Clinics, 10,* 511-525.
15. Cerrato, P. (1991). Diet therapy helps this drug work better. *RN Magazine, 54*(2), 71-72, 74.
16. Trovato, A., Nuhlicek, D., & Midtling, A. (1991). Drug-nutrient interactions. *American Family Physician, 44,* 1651-1657.
17. Wood, A., & Zhou, H. (1991). Ethnic differences in drug disposition and responsiveness. *Clinical Pharmacokinetics, 20,* 350-373.
18. Roin, S., & Winters, S. (1990). Amantadine hydrocholoride: Current and new uses. *Journal of Neuroscience Nursing, 22,* 322-325.
19. Collier, D. (1992). Parkinsonism treatment: Part III—Update. *Annals of Pharmacotherapy, 26,* 227-233.
20. Lera, G., et al. (1990). Cabergoline: A long-acting dopamine agonist in Parkinson's disease. *Annals of Neurology, 28,* 593.
21. Goetz, C. (1992). Dopaminergic agonists in the treatment of Parkinson's disease. *Neurologic Clinics, 10,* 527-537.

BIBLIOGRAPHY

Agid, Y., et al. (1990). The efficacy of levodopa treatment declines in the course of Parkinson's disease: Do nondopaminergic lesions play a role? *Advances in Neurology, 53,* 83-95.

Byrd, C. (1993). Neuroleptic malignant syndrome: A dangerous complication of neuroleptic therapy. *Journal of Neuroscience Nursing, 22,* 322-325.

Cedarbaum, J., Gandy, S., & McDowell, F. (1991). "Early" initiation of levodopa treatment does not promote the development of motor response fluctuations, dyskinesias, or dementia in Parkinson's disease. *Neurology, 41,* 622-629.

Gero, E., & Giordano, J. (1990). Ethical considerations in fetal tissue transplantation. *Journal of Neuroscience Nursing, 22,* 9-12.

MacMahon, D., Overstall, P., & Marshall, T. (1991). Simplification of the initiation of bromocriptine in elderly patients with advanced Parkinson's disease. *Age and Aging, 20,* 146-150.

Roos, R., Vredevoogd, C., & van der Velde, E. (1990). Response fluctuations in Parkinson's disease. *Neurology, 40,* 1344-1347.

Waggoner, P. (1992). Case study: Neuroleptic malignant syndrome. *Critical Care Nurse, 12*(7), 22-24.

CHAPTER 24

Anesthetic Agents

BERNADETTE ROCHE

⊛ **General Anesthesia**

LEARNING OBJECTIVE: Describe the three phases of a
general anesthesia.

KEY TERMS:

Autonomic activity, emergence phase, induction phase,
maintenance phase, somatic responses

⊛ **Nursing Considerations: Preoperative**

LEARNING OBJECTIVE: Develop a plan of care for a client
scheduled for surgery.

⊛ **Inhalation Anesthesia**

LEARNING OBJECTIVES:

Explain mechanisms involved in a partial pressure
gradient.

Describe how the blood-gas partition coefficient affects
inhalation anesthesia.

Explain the impact of minimum alveolar concentration
on inhalation anesthesia.

Summarize essential information about each group of
anesthetic gases.

KEY TERMS:

Blood-gas partition coefficient, minimum alveolar
concentration

⊛ **Intravenous Anesthetics**

LEARNING OBJECTIVE: Summarize essential information
about each group of intravenous anesthetics.

⊛ **Nursing Considerations: Postoperative**

LEARNING OBJECTIVE: Discuss the nursing care for a
postoperative client.

CONCEPTS AND TERMS TO REVIEW

Review the physiology of the respiratory system.
Reexamine the principle of partial-pressure gradient.
Read the section on perioperative nursing care in a med-
ical-surgical nursing textbook.

---

*A*nesthesia as it is known today began in the mid-1800s
with the introduction of nitrous oxide (N_2O), diethyl
ether, and chloroform. However, with the exception of N_2O
and the ultrashort-acting barbiturates, the anesthetic agents in
use today are relatively new drugs introduced into clinical
practice within the last 40 years.

General anesthesia can be described as a progressive and reversible depression of the central nervous system (CNS) after
the administration of either inhaled and/or intravenous (IV)
anesthetic agents. It is characterized by unconsciousness, analgesia, muscle relaxation, and decreased activity of the autonomic nervous system (autonomic blockade). None of the

agents in present use safely meets all four of these characteristics. Therefore a combination of IV agents and an inhalation
agent usually is used. Each drug is selected for a specific effect
(i.e., rapid loss of consciousness, analgesia, muscle relaxation,
or autonomic blockade). This is commonly referred to as *balanced anesthesia.*

In the United States the practice of anesthesia is considered
both a medical and nursing specialty. Anesthesiologists (physicians who specialize in anesthesiology) and Certified
Registered Nurse Anesthetists (CRNA) are educated and certified in the specialty of anesthesia.[1] Of the 26 million anesthetics administered yearly in the United States, 65% are administered by CRNAs.

GENERAL ANESTHESIA

General anesthesia can be divided into three separate phases:
induction, maintenance, and emergence.

Induction Phase

Induction of anesthesia begins with the rapid loss of consciousness and onset of analgesia. There is progressive loss of

muscle tone and autonomic activity. Anesthesia during the induction phase is administered intravenously, via mask, intramuscularly, or intranasally. The most common method of induction is IV administration of short-acting drugs such as the ultrashort-acting barbiturates. Potent inhalation agents are also used for inductions by mask. Gas inductions are usually reserved for young children and clients with difficult IV access. The intramuscular (IM) route is used less frequently because of unpredictable results. Intranasal administration of ketamine and midazolam can be used for pediatric inductions.[2]

Maintenance Phase

The **maintenance phase** of general anesthesia lasts as long as necessary for the planned surgical procedure, from skin incision to surgical wound closure. It is characterized by unconsciousness, analgesia, muscle relaxation, obtunded reflexes, and autonomic blockade. During this phase, inhalation anesthetics, IV agents, or a combination of both is administered to maintain an adequate depth of surgical anesthesia. In addition, neuromuscular blocking agents (muscle relaxants) may be administered to provide greater muscle relaxation for the surgeon. Because of surgical stimuli and the large variation in client's anesthetic requirements (i.e., age, state of health, type of illness, drug therapy, and anxiety), the depth of anesthesia must be continually assessed.

The actual depth of anesthesia is monitored by the presence or absence of **somatic responses** (i.e., movement, grimacing, breath holding, phonation) and **autonomic activity** (e.g., tachycardia, hypertension, mydriasis, tearing, and sweating). Since the majority of anesthetized clients are paralyzed with muscle relaxants, somatic responses to surgical stimuli are abolished. Increased autonomic activity indicates "light" anesthesia.

The client's heart rate and rhythm, blood pressure, respiratory rate and depth, oxygenation and ventilation level, and temperature are routinely monitored. Additional monitors (e.g., peripheral nerve stimulators and central IV and intraarterial pressure monitors) are used when the surgery or the physical status of the client dictates their use. Based on the assessed data, the amount of anesthetic agent is adjusted to meet the requirements of the client.

Emergence Phase

During the **emergence phase,** the amount of anesthetic is gradually reduced and eventually terminated as the surgical procedure is completed. As the client emerges from the general anesthesia, autonomic activity, muscle tone, somatic reflexes, and consciousness are regained. During this time, the client requires careful monitoring. In the immediate postoperative period, the client is monitored in the postanesthesia recovery unit (PACU). Emergence and recovery from a general anesthetic depend on type, amount, and duration of anesthetic, client's age, temperature, and status at the completion of surgery, and presence of coexisting disease.

NURSING CONSIDERATIONS: PREOPERATIVE

Preoperative nursing care begins with the first nurse-client contact, whether in the physician's office, the clinic, the emergency room, or the hospital unit.

Assessing A complete client history is part of the preoperative assessment of the surgical client. While taking the **health history,** obtain a history of hospitalizations, medical conditions, and surgical experiences. Determine the client's understanding of the diagnosis, planned surgery, expected outcome of surgery, and sequence of recovery. Specifically ask about allergies, current and past alcohol consumption, caffeine intake, and tobacco or drug use. Determine if the client is taking any drugs, either prescription or nonprescription. It is important to establish the time of the last oral intake and to ascertain the ambulatory surgery client's compliance with any preoperative instructions.

Diagnosing Based on analysis of the data base, several nursing diagnoses are possible for the preoperative client. They include the following:
- Anxiety related to hospitalization, pending surgery, and impact on lifestyle.
- High risk for altered health maintenance related to insufficient knowledge of postoperative activities.
- Knowledge deficit about planned surgery, expected outcomes of surgery, or postoperative routines.

Planning During the preoperative period, the client is prepared for surgery. Preoperative teaching is a major focus of client preparation. To ensure consistent, complete teaching, many agencies have standard teaching plans or check lists for specific topics. Regardless of the method used, the client should be provided information on all preoperative and postoperative activities. Expected outcomes for this phase of the nursing process include the following:
- Client verbalizes realistic expectations of planned surgery and expected outcome.
- Client participates in preoperative preparations.
- Client demonstrates postoperative exercises.

Implementing Drugs prescribed by the nurse anesthetist or anesthesiologist are usually administered to the client before surgery. These drugs are meant to promote sedation, relieve pain, reduce oral secretions, and facilitate a smooth induction of general anesthesia. The preoperative medication consists of a combination of sedatives, analgesics, and antimuscarinic drugs. Common preoperative medications are listed in the box on p. 248. (Sedatives are discussed in Chapter 18, analgesics in Chapter 19, and antimuscarinic drugs in Chapter 26.) After administration of sedatives or narcotics, raise the side rails and instruct the client to remain in bed.

Evaluating The effectiveness of preoperative nursing care is evaluated by comparing the client's status with the expected outcomes. In addition, the effects of the preoperative medications should be evaluated. Evaluation includes assessing the client's level of sedation and a reassessment of vital signs.

COMMON PREOPERATIVE MEDICATIONS

Sedatives	Analgesics
Diazepam (Valium)	Meperidine (Demerol)
Droperidol (Inapsine)	Morphine sulfate
Hydroxyzine hydrochloride	
(Atarax, Vistaril)	
Lorazepam (Ativan)	**Antimuscarinics**
Midazolam hydrochloride	Atropine sulfate
(Versed)	Glycopyrrolate (Robinul)
Pentobarbital sodium	Scopolamine
(Nembutal)	
Promethazine hydrochloride	
(Phenergan)	

CONCEPT REVIEW

General anesthesia consists of three phases: induction, maintenance, and emergence.

In the preoperative period the role of the nurse focuses on preparing the client for surgery. Client education and administration of preoperative medications are a part of this preparation.

Drugs administered during the intraoperative period are administered by specially educated and certified nurses and physicians.

INHALATION ANESTHESIA

Inhalation anesthetics produce a dose-related, reversible depression of the CNS. The degree of CNS depression is directly related to the inhaled concentration of the agent. Absorption, distribution, and elimination of inhalation anesthetics depend on a **partial pressure gradient.** Movement is always from the area with the highest partial pressure to the area with the lowest partial pressure. For example, oxygen diffuses into the blood from the lungs and from the blood into the cells because of a partial pressure gradient between the different areas. Administration of inhalation anesthetics produces a partial pressure gradient at the alveolar-capillary membrane. In response to this gradient, the anesthetic agents diffuse across the alveolar-capillary membrane into the blood. In the blood anesthetic agents also exert a partial pressure that depends on their blood solubility.

Blood-gas partition coefficients are used as a relative index of solubility. The blood-gas coefficient describes the relative affinity of an anesthetic for two different phases: blood and gas. It also describes how the anesthetic will partition itself between the two phases at equilibrium. The larger the blood-gas partition coefficient, the greater the solubility. For example, a blood-gas partition coefficient of 20 indicates that for every part of the anesthetic in the gas phase, 20 parts are dis-

TABLE 24–1
Blood-gas Partition Coefficients for Inhalation Anesthetics

Agent	MW	VP	Bld-gas
Nitrous oxide	44	—	0.47
Isoflurane	184.5	238	1.4
Enflurane	184.5	172	1.9
Halothane	194.4	243	2.3
Desflurane	168	664	0.42
Methoxyflurane	165	23	13.0
Sevoflurane	200	160	0.60

MW = molecular weight; VP = vapor pressure; Bld-gas = blood-gas partition coefficient.

solved in the blood. It is only the part in the gas phase that exerts a partial pressure. The partial pressure gradient between the blood and the brain is the most important factor that determines how fast the drug leaves the blood and diffuses into the brain to exert its anesthetic effects. The more insoluble the drug (i.e., low blood-gas partition coefficient), the greater the partial pressure exerted and the greater the gradient between the two areas. Thus anesthetics with low blood-gas solubility coefficients such as N_2O and desflurane have faster onsets (shorter induction) and recovery periods (faster emergence) than the other inhalation anesthetics. Methyoxyflurane, with a blood-gas partition coefficient of 13, has the longest induction and emergence times. (See Table 24–1 for a summary of the molecular weights, vapor pressure, and blood-gas partition coefficients for various inhalation anesthetics.)

Once in the blood, the drug is distributed throughout the body. Organs that receive the greatest percentage of the cardiac output initially receive the greatest amount of the drug. The body can be divided into four tissue groups: vessel rich, muscle, fat, and vessel poor.[3] (See Table 24–2 for a summary of tissue groups and percent of cardiac output received.) The vessel-rich group, which includes the brain, receives 75% of the drug immediately during administration. All of the inhalation anesthetics are very lipid soluble and diffuse easily into the CNS to exert their effects on neuronal tissue. As mentioned previously, movement of the anesthetic agent from the lungs to the blood and then to the CNS depends on the partial pressure gradient between the three areas. High inspired concentrations of the anesthetic are administered during induction. This creates a

TABLE 24–2
Tissue Groups

Tissue Group	Organs	%Cardiac Output	%Body Weight
Vessel rich	Brain, heart, kidney, splanchnic bed, endocrine glands	75	9
Muscle	Muscle, skin	19	50
Fat	Fat	5	21
Vessel poor	Bone, ligaments, cartilage	1	20

large alveolar-blood partial pressure gradient and encourages the rapid movement of the drug into the blood. The high concentration in the blood creates a second partial pressure gradient between the blood and the CNS. In response to the blood-CNS gradient, the lipid-soluble anesthetic diffuses rapidly into the CNS. During the maintenance phase of the anesthetic, lower concentrations are administered to maintain equilibrium between the lungs and the brain. This results in a constant partial pressure of the anesthetic in the brain. In the emergence phase administration of the inhalation agent is discontinued. As the partial pressure in the blood decreases, the anesthetic agent leaves the brain and reenters the blood for final elimination through the lungs.

Minimum alveolar concentration (MAC) is defined as the amount of an anesthetic that prevents movement in 50% of clients exposed to a noxious stimuli (i.e., skin incision). For example, the MAC of halothane is 0.75. In a group of clients inhaling 0.75% halothane and 99.25% oxygen, 50% will not move during skin incision. The alveolar concentration of the anesthetic is directly related to the concentration in the brain, the site of action of the drug. MAC is a measure of potency and can be used to compare the relative potencies of the different inhalation agents. Generally, 3 to 3.5 times the MAC of any agent is needed for the induction of anesthesia, whereas 1.5 to 2.5 times MAC is necessary to maintain surgical anesthesia.

MAC is influenced by a variety of conditions, including alcohol ingestion (see box). MAC is decreased by acute alcohol ingestion, meaning that less than 0.75% halothane is needed to prevent movement in 50% of surgical clients who are acutely intoxicated. On the other hand, chronic alcohol use increases MAC. Therefore more than 0.75% halothane is needed to prevent movement in clients who ingest alcohol on a regular basis. MACs are also additive; administration of 0.5 MAC of two different agents at the same time is equal in potency to 1.0 MAC of either of the agents.[4–6]

All potent **inhalation anesthetics** produce a dose-related CNS depression. Cortical function is depressed first and medullary and spinal function last. Inhaled anesthetics appear to exert their effects by direct action on the neuronal membrane at a number of sites in the CNS. The exact mechanism by which they interfere with neuronal transmission is unclear. Possible mechanisms include changes in membrane ion permeability, activation of specific membrane receptors, or interference with inhibitory neurotransmitters, specifically γ-aminobutyric acid (GABA).[7]

Inhalational anesthetic agents in use today include desflurane, enflurane, halothane, isoflurane, and N_2O. Methoxyflurane is no longer used in the United States. A new inhalation anesthetic, sevoflurane, is presently undergoing clinical trials in the United States. Inhalation anesthetics are administered through a mask or an endotracheal tube.

With the exception of N_2O, inhalational anesthetics are volatile agents and are liquid at room temperature. Agent-specific vaporizers on the anesthesia machine convert the liquid anesthetics into vapors and control the amount of vapor (concentration) delivered to the client. The client inhales a combination of oxygen and anesthetic vapor.

Nitrous Oxide

N_2O was first prepared by Priestly in 1772 but was not used clinically in the United States until 1844. Because of the euphoric effect observed during inhalation of low concentrations, N_2O was often referred to as *laughing gas*. N_2O is a colorless, odorless gas with a molecular weight of 44. It is stored as a compressed liquid in steel cylinders. Although it is not flammable or explosive, it does support combustion of other flammable agents.

Pharmacotherapeutics N_2O is a potent analgesic. Its use as a sole anesthetic is confined to dental procedures and the second stage of labor. N_2O is a weak anesthetic, with a MAC of 104%; achieving anesthesia is impossible without the danger of hypoxia. When used in combination with other potent inhalation anesthetic agents, 70% N_2O reduces the MAC of those agents by approximately 60%.

Pharmacokinetics With a blood-gas partition coefficient of 0.47, N_2O is a relatively insoluble agent, which accounts for the fast onset and termination of its effects. It is eliminated primarily through the lungs, and approximately 0.004% undergoes metabolism in the gastrointestinal (GI) tract where it is reduced to nitrogen.

Pharmacodynamics N_2O affects most body systems. It is a **CNS** depressant. It increases both cerebral blood flow and intracranial pressure. Unlike the other inhalation agents, it does not decrease cerebral oxygen consumption. N_2O causes centrally mediated stimulation of the **sympathetic nervous system.**

N_2O has several effects on the **cardiovascular system.** When administered alone, it produces a decrease in ventricular function, as evidenced by a decrease in cardiac output, heart rate, and contractility. This depressant action is not always clinically apparent because of the increased sympathetic activity. The sympathetic activity produces an increase in systemic vascular resistance, so there is no overall change in blood pressure.

There are minimal effects on the **respiratory system.** At 50% N_2O, there is normal response to carbon dioxide. Within the **GI system,** N_2O diffuses freely into the bowel. Distention

---

FACTORS THAT INFLUENCE MINIMUM ALVEOLAR CONCENTRATION (MAC)

Decrease MAC	Increase MAC
Hypothermia	Hyperthermia
Pregnancy	Chronic alcohol use
Advanced age	Young age
CNS depressants (opioids, benzodiazepines)	Cocaine
α_2-Agonists (clonidine)	Monoamine oxidase inhibitors
Acute alcohol use	
Hypoxia	

of the bowel may account for the postoperative nausea and vomiting that frequently occurs after its administration. There is no significant change in **renal function,** nor does N$_2$O affect the **skeletal muscle tone.**

Effects on the **reproductive system** vary. There is no effect on uterine tone and contractility when N$_2$O is used during labor and delivery. However, animal studies have shown N$_2$O is teratogenic during early pregnancy. It is thought that the teratogenic effects are due to interference with DNA synthesis. There is also an increased incidence of spontaneous abortion in females exposed to N$_2$O.

Reversible effects on the **hematologic system** occur after prolonged administration (more than 24 hours) of N$_2$O. Extended exposure to N$_2$O depresses hematopoietic function, resulting in anemia, thrombocytopenia, and leukocytopenia. Critically ill patients may be more susceptible and show bone marrow dysfunction with shorter exposure to the drug.

Pharmaceutics   N$_2$O is administered via a mask or endotracheal tube in the following concentrations:
- Analgesia: 30% to 50%
- Balanced general anesthesia: 60% to 70%

Contraindications and precautions   Although N$_2$O has low blood solubility (blood-gas partition coefficient of 0.47), it is 34 times more soluble in blood than nitrogen. N$_2$O diffuses into closed air spaces faster than nitrogen can diffuse out, thus increasing the volume and pressure of the air space. Caution must be used in clients with closed pneumothorax, venous air embolism, bowel obstructions, and middle ear graft procedures. Since N$_2$O also diffuses into air-filled endotracheal tube cuffs, the pressure in the cuff should be closely monitored to avoid tracheal ischemia.[3]

Specific considerations   When N$_2$O administration is discontinued, N$_2$O diffuses rapidly from the blood into the lungs. This dilutes the inspired oxygen concentration to levels of hypoxemia. This "diffusion hypoxia" can be avoided by the administration of 100% oxygen for 5 to 10 minutes when the N$_2$O is discontinued.[3,6]

❧ Nursing Research

Smiley, B., & Paradise, N. (1991). Does the duration of N$_2$O administration affect postoperative nausea and vomiting? *Nurse Anesthesia, 2*(1), 13-18.

Nausea and vomiting are the most frequent postoperative complications in the ambulatory surgical setting. In this study data were gathered from 184 adult, ambulatory cosmetic surgery clients to determine if the use of N$_2$O was associated with the increased incidence of postoperative nausea and vomiting. Anesthesia was induced with thiopental and maintained with an opioid.

Data were analyzed statistically, using the two-way chi-squared test and the Fisher exact test. The major finding was that the incidence of nausea and vomiting was directly related to the duration of the anesthesia in subjects who received N$_2$O. Recommendation based on this study was that N$_2$O use should be avoided in ambulatory cosmetic surgery cases lasting 3 or more hours.

STUDENT ACTIVITIES

- Interview the nurse anesthetist at your assigned agency. Determine the frequency of N$_2$O use and the most frequent postoperative complications associated with this anesthetic gas.
- Interview nurses in the PACU and determine their perception of the most frequently encountered postoperative complications with N$_2$O use.   ❧

Halogenated Hydrocarbons: Halothane

Chloroform was the first halogenated hydrocarbon to gain acceptance as an anesthetic. It is no longer in use as an anesthetic because of associated hepatotoxicity, nephrotoxicity, and cardiac arrhythmias. **Halothane** (Fluothane) is the only halogenated hydrocarbon in use as an anesthetic. It was introduced into clinical practice in 1956, and for a long time it was the most widely used inhalation anesthetic. Halothane is the most potent inhalation anesthetic (MAC, 0.75) in use today with the exception of methoxyflurane, which is rarely used in the United States.

Pharmacotherapeutics   Halothane is a colorless liquid with a sweet, nonirritating odor that makes it an ideal agent for gas induction in children. Because of its potency, halothane can be used alone or as part of a balanced anesthetic.

Pharmacokinetics   Halothane has a molecular weight of 197.39 and is nonexplosive. With a blood-gas partition coefficient of 2.3, halothane is considered a moderately soluble agent. Induction and emergence times with halothane are fairly rapid. Of the inhalation anesthetics in current use, halothane is the one that undergoes the most metabolism. Approximately 80% is eliminated unchanged via the lungs. The remaining 20% undergoes oxidation by the cytochrome P-450 enzymes in the liver.

Pharmacodynamics   Halothane is a **CNS depressant** and produces a dose-dependent reduction in cerebral oxygen consumption. It increases cerebral blood flow, decreases cerebral vascular resistance, and increases intracranial pressure. Halothane also affects the **cardiovascular system.** It is a myocardial depressant and causes a decrease in both heart rate and stroke volume. It sensitizes the heart to the effects of catecholamines, increasing the incidence of ventricular arrhythmias. Halothane decreases systemic vascular resistance.

In the respiratory system a dose-related respiratory depression of the medullary respiratory center and a decreased ventilatory response to carbon dioxide occur. Halothane also affects the **hepatic** and **renal systems.** It has been implicated in postoperative liver enzyme elevation ("halothane hepatitis"). The elevation in liver enzymes is possibly due to abnormal reductive metabolism of halothane in the presence of hepatic hypoxia or an immune-mediated reaction associated with the oxidative pathway.[9] Use of halothane is best avoided in clients with reduced hepatic blood flow or liver disease. There is also a dose-related, reversible decrease in renal blood flow, glomerular filtration rate, and urinary output.

In the **reproductive system** there is a dose-dependent relaxation of uterine tone and contractility during halothane

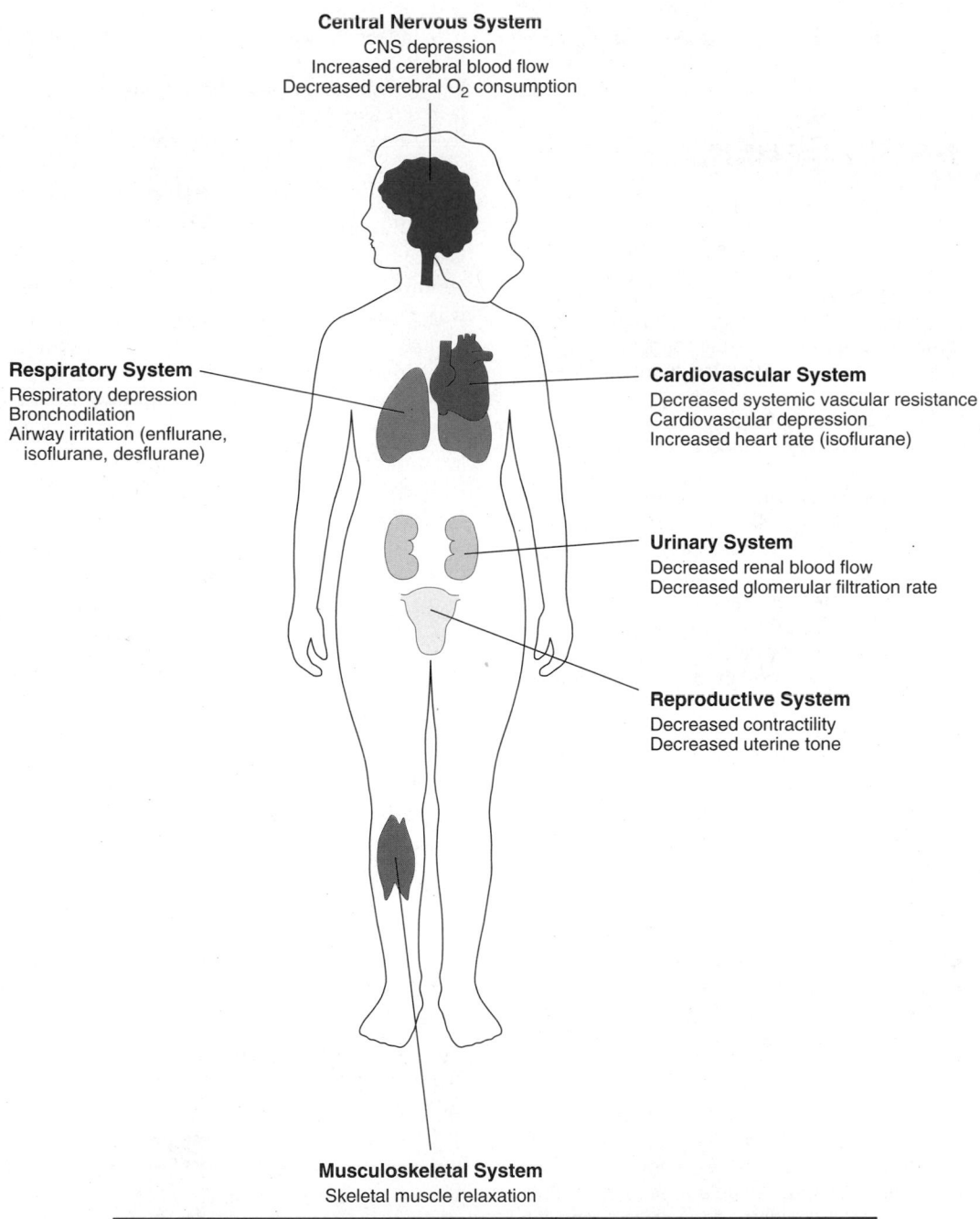

Central Nervous System
CNS depression
Increased cerebral blood flow
Decreased cerebral O_2 consumption

Respiratory System
Respiratory depression
Bronchodilation
Airway irritation (enflurane,
    isoflurane, desflurane)

Cardiovascular System
Decreased systemic vascular resistance
Cardiovascular depression
Increased heart rate (isoflurane)

Urinary System
Decreased renal blood flow
Decreased glomerular filtration rate

Reproductive System
Decreased contractility
Decreased uterine tone

Musculoskeletal System
Skeletal muscle relaxation

FIGURE 24–1   Summary of effects of halogenated hydrocarbons and ethers.

anesthesia. Its effect on the uterus is advantageous for delivery of a retained placenta. In the musculoskeletal system halothane directly relaxes skeletal muscles and potentiates skeletal muscle relaxants used in anesthesia (Fig. 24–1).

Pharmaceutics   Halothane is administered in controlled concentrations (1% to 3%) with a halothane vaporizer. It is administered in combination with 33% to 100% oxygen. N_2O (50% to 60%) often is administered with halothane. This combination has the beneficial effect of reducing the required concentration of halothane.

Halogenated Ethers

Diethyl ether was the first ether used for general anesthesia. Introduced in the mid-1800s, it was used for more than 100

years but gradually fell into disuse. It is highly flammable and explosive, especially in the presence of oxygen. Other disadvantages include prolonged induction and recovery time, unpleasant odor, increased bronchial secretions, and increased activity of the sympathetic nervous system.

Since the 1950s, more stable methyl-ethyl ether anesthetics have been developed. As with the halogenated hydrocarbons, the addition of chlorine and bromine to the ethers increases potency, and the addition of fluorine improves compound stability. Methoxyflurane (1959), enflurane (1972), isoflurane (1981), and desflurane (1992) are the four halogenated ethers available in the United States. Methoxyflurane is rarely, if ever, used. Desflurane, the newest agent, is not yet widely used. Another halogenated ether, sevoflurane, is undergoing clinical trials in the United States. All five agents are nonflammable and nonexplosive.

HALOGENATED ETHER PROTOTYPE

ENFLURANE

Enflurane (Ethrane) was the first of a new series of ether anesthetics: fluorinated methyl-ethyl ethers. It was introduced into clinical practice in 1972 and replaced halothane as the most widely used inhalation anesthetic. With the introduction of its isomer, isoflurane, in 1981, the use of enflurane decreased, although it is still a popular anesthetic.

Pharmacotherapeutics Enflurane is a potent inhalation anesthetic that can be used alone or as part of a balanced anesthetic.

Pharmacokinetics Enflurane is a clear, colorless, sweet-smelling liquid that is nonflammable and nonexplosive. With a blood-gas partition coefficient of 1.91, it is considered a moderately soluble agent with a fairly rapid induction and recovery time. Enflurane is less potent than halothane; its MAC is 1.68. Enflurane undergoes 2% to 8% oxidative metabolism in the liver, but the maximum serum free fluoride ion is not enough to cause renal toxicity.

Pharmacodynamics Like other anesthetic gases, enflurane affects the function of several body systems. Enflurane is a **CNS** depressant; it decreases cerebral oxygen consumption. High concentrations of enflurane may cause "seizurelike" activity to appear on the electroencephalogram (EEG). The incidence of EEG changes is increased in the presence of hypocapnia. Enflurane also causes cerebral vasodilation and increased cerebral blood flow.

On the **cardiovascular system** enflurane causes marked cardiac depression, especially in concentrations greater than 1.5 MAC. It decreases stroke volume, systemic vascular resistance, and blood pressure. Heart rate is increased or remains unchanged. Enflurane has marked effects on the **respiratory system.** Of all the volatile anesthetics, enflurane produces the most respiratory depression. It reduces ventilatory response to hypoxia and hypercarbia and causes bronchodilation. Enflurane's pungent odor may stimulate secretions and elicit coughing and breath holding, especially during induction.

Enflurane's effects on the **hepatic** and **renal systems** are dose related. Enflurane causes a dose-related decrease in liver blood flow but no significant change in hepatic function. It also causes a reversible, dose-related decrease in renal blood flow, glomerular filtration rate, and urinary output. In the **reproductive system** there is a dose-related depression of uterine tone and contractility.

Within the **musculoskeletal system,** enflurane produces skeletal muscle relaxation by interfering with neuromuscular transmission. Like halothane, it potentiates the nondepolarizing muscle relaxants (pancuronium, atracurium, metocurine iodide) used in anesthesia.

Pharmaceutics Induction is achieved using enflurane alone with oxygen or in combination with oxygen–nitrous oxide mixtures. The necessary concentrations for different levels of anesthesia are as follows:

- Induction anesthesia: inspired concentrations of 2.0% to 4.5%
- Maintenance anesthesia: inspired concentrations of 0.5% to 3.0%
- Analgesia: inspired concentrations of 0.25% to 1.0%

MISCELLANEOUS DRUGS IN CATEGORY

Isoflurane (Forane) is an isomer of enflurane. (An isomer is a compound that possesses the same molecular formula as another compound.) Introduced into clinical practice in 1981, it is presently the most widely used volatile anesthetic in the United States.[6] Of all the volatile anesthetics, isoflurane produces the greatest dose-related depression of the CNS; therefore it is used frequently in neurosurgery. Isoflurane also causes cardiovascular and respiratory depression, skeletal muscle relaxation, and decreased uterine tone. Isoflurane undergoes limited hepatic metabolism. It is used at 2% to 3% concentrations for inductions and 1% to 1.5% concentrations for maintenance.

Methoxyflurane (Penthrane) is a highly soluble potent anesthetic that has prolonged induction and recovery times. Of all the volatile anesthetics, methoxyflurane produces the best analgesia. It depresses the CNS and cardiovascular and respiratory systems. Methoxyflurane undergoes extensive metabolism (50%). One of its metabolites, free fluoride ion, is associated with renal toxicity. High-output renal failure is associated with the use of methoxyflurane; therefore it is rarely if ever used in the United States.

Desflurane (Suprane) is the newest volatile anesthetic introduced into clinical practice.[10] Its low blood-gas partition coefficient of 0.42 allows rapid induction and emergence, making it an ideal agent for outpatient surgery. Its effects are similar to those of isoflurane. However, desflurane is more irritating to the airway, which limits its use as an induction agent.[11] With a MAC of 6.0, it is the least potent agent in current use. It undergoes minimal metabolism. Because of its limited use at present, it is too early to predict its fate as an anesthetic.

Sevoflurane was first developed in 1971. It is presently undergoing clinical trials in the United States. It has a blood-gas partition coefficient of 0.68, which results in fast induction and emergence from anesthesia. With a MAC of 1.1, it is a more potent agent than desflurane. Its pharmacodynamic effects are similar to those of the other volatile anesthetics. However, it undergoes significant biotransformation in the liver.[12]

CONCEPT REVIEW

The three major groups of anesthetic gases are N_2O, halogenated hydrocarbons, and halogenated ethers.

The selection of an inhalation anesthetic is based on the anesthetist's preoperative assessment of the client, the planned surgical procedure, and the different properties of the individual agent.

INTRAVENOUS ANESTHETICS

IV anesthetics are used primarily for induction of general anesthesia. Several of the drugs are also used for maintenance of anesthesia in combination with other agents. IV inductions are usually more pleasant for the client. There is a rapid loss of consciousness within 30 to 60 seconds and rapid progression to a surgical depth of anesthesia as other anesthetic agents are administered. When an IV drug is used for maintenance of surgical anesthesia, N_2O and muscle relaxants are usually included as part of the anesthetic. With advances in infusion pump technology and the introduction of more potent IV agents, total IV anesthesia without the use of potent inhalation agents or N_2O may become more common in anesthesia practice.[13]

Ultrashort-Acting Barbiturates

In Chapter 18 the drug category of barbiturates was described. In this chapter the discussion is limited to those barbiturates used for induction of general anesthesia. Three ultrashort-acting barbiturates—thiopental, methohexital, and thiamylal—are used primarily for this purpose.

ULTRASHORT-ACTING BARBITURATE PROTOTYPE

THIOPENTAL

Thiopental (Pentothal), introduced in 1934, is the most popular general anesthesia induction agent.

Pharmacotherapeutics Thiopental is used for IV induction of general anesthesia. It can also be used to treat drug-induced convulsions and to reduce intracranial pressure in clients with severe brain injury. Its antianalgesic effects limit its use as a total anesthetic.

Pharmacokinetics Thiopental is rapidly distributed to the vessel-rich tissue group within 30 to 60 seconds after IV administration. Because of its high lipid solubility, thiopental diffuses rapidly into the CNS. The drug is then distributed to muscles and other tissues, and the plasma concentration of the drug drops. This action accounts for its short distribution half-life of 8.5 minutes. In response to the declining plasma levels, thiopental leaves the CNS and undergoes redistribution to tissues that receive a smaller percentage of cardiac output. This redistribution phase accounts for its short duration of action of 5 to 10 minutes.[14,15]

Thiopental is 75% to 80% protein bound. It is extensively metabolized in the liver where it undergoes oxidation and conjugation by the microsomal enzymes. Its inactive metabolites are excreted by the kidney. Thiopental has the longest elimination half-life, 10 to 12 hours, of the ultrashort-acting barbiturates. Excessive or prolonged administration leads to drug accumulation and excessive drowsiness in the postoperative period.[15]

Pharmacodynamics Thiopental appears to exert its effect by depression of polysynaptic transmission in the CNS. It enhances and possibly mimics the action of GABA, an inhibitory neurotransmitter in the cerebral cortex and reticular activating system. The action of excitatory neurotransmitters such as acetylcholine is also blocked.[14,15]

The **physiologic effects** of thiopental occur primarily in the central nervous, cardiovascular, respiratory, and renal systems. In the CNS, thiopental produces dose-dependent effects that range from mild sedation to unconsciousness. Thiopental does not possess any analgesic effects; in fact, at low doses it causes hyperalgesia. It decreases both cerebral oxygen consumption and cerebral blood flow. Therefore it is beneficial for use in clients with increased intracranial pressure.

With thiopental, there are direct myocardial depression and vasodilation. The medullary vasomotor area is also depressed. Thiopental causes a transient decrease in cardiac output and blood pressure; the heart rate remains the same or slightly increases. In hypovolemic, debilitated, or cardiovascular-compromised clients, an exaggerated response may occur.

There is dose-related respiratory depression due to direct action on the medullary and pontine respiratory centers. Respiratory depression is greater with concurrent administration of narcotics. High doses of thiopental result in apnea. With low doses of thiopental, airway reflexes are increased, and coughing or laryngospasm may occur during induction. Bronchoconstriction in response to an increased parasympathetic tone is not uncommon, especially in susceptible clients such as those with asthma.

Thiopental decreases liver blood flow but does not affect liver function. It also causes reversible decreases in renal blood flow and glomerular filtration rate. When administered to clients with chronic renal failure, the dose should be reduced 50% to 75%.

Pharmaceutics The IV induction dose of thiopental (2% or 2.5% solution) is 3 to 5 mg/kg.

Contraindications and precautions Thiopental is strongly alkaline (pH, 11). Extravascular infiltration causes local tissue damage. In addition, inadvertent intraarterial injection can cause severe vasospasm and tissue necrosis. It is contraindicated in acute intermittent porphyria.

MISCELLANEOUS DRUGS IN CATEGORY

Methohexital sodium (Brevital Sodium) was developed in 1932. It is two to three times more potent than thiopental. Although its actions are similar to those of thiopental, it has a shorter duration of action. With IV administration, the incidence of hiccoughs and myoclonic muscle movements during induction increases. Because of its shorter duration, methohexital is most useful for brief surgical procedures. Induction dose for methohexital 1% is 1 to 2 mg/kg.

Thiamylal sodium (Surital) is used less frequently than the other two ultrashort-acting barbiturates. Its actions and duration of effect are essentially the same as those of thiopental. Induction dose for thiamylal 2.5% is 3 to 5 mg/kg.

Nonbarbiturates

Because of the cardiovascular depression and prolonged recovery associated with the use of barbiturates, the following three unrelated compounds are used as alternative induction agents.

KETAMINE

Ketamine (Ketalar, Ketaject) (1957) is a phencyclidine derivative that produces catalepsy, catatonia, hypertonia, amnesia, and profound analgesia. The client appears to be in a trancelike state, with his or her eyes often remaining open.

Pharmacotherapeutics Ketamine is used for induction and as the sole anesthetic agent for short surgical procedures. It cannot be used alone for visceral surgery. Ketamine is a useful induction agent for children since it can be administered intramuscularly or nasally.

Pharmacokinetics Ketamine is a very lipid-soluble drug, 5 to 10 times more soluble than thiopental. It has a rapid onset of action. Ketamine is 45% to 50% protein bound and has a very short distribution half-life of 10 minutes, which accounts for the 5- to 15-minute duration of action for an IV dose. Ketamine is metabolized in the liver where it undergoes oxidation and conjugation. One of its metabolites has one third the potency of ketamine, which may account for the prolonged CNS effects of the drug. The elimination half-life is 3 hours.

Pharmacodynamics The exact mechanism of action is unknown. It is believed that ketamine antagonizes acetylcholine in the CNS. Ketamine also acts as an agonist at the mu and sigma opioid receptors. This accounts for both its dysphoric effects and its analgesic effects. Ketamine depresses the sensory and motor cortex and the neocorticothalamic system and causes stimulation of the limbic system.

Ketamine has several important **physiologic effects.** After an IV dose of ketamine, loss of consciousness and profound analgesia result. The drug increases cerebral blood flow and cerebral oxygen consumption. It increases intracranial pressure and is best avoided in clients with increased intracranial pressure.

Although ketamine is a direct myocardial depressant, there is an increase in both heart rate and blood pressure secondary to an increase in sympathetic activity. This makes ketamine a useful induction agent for clients in shock. Because of its stimulating effect on the heart, its use should be avoided in clients with coronary and valvular heart disease.

Unlike the barbiturates, protective airway reflexes (pharyngeal and laryngeal) remain active with ketamine. Slight respiratory depression occurs 1 to 2 minutes after IV administration. Respirations return to normal or are slightly increased within a few minutes. Because of its bronchodilator effects, it is useful for induction of the asthmatic client. However, since airway secretions are increased, a preoperative antimuscarinic drug should be administered.

Pharmaceutics Ketamine is available in a sterile solution for parenteral use. The dose varies, based on the desired effects:
• Induction: 1 to 2 mg/kg IV
     5 to 10 mg/kg IM
• Maintenance: 50 to 100 μg/kg per minute (sole agent)
• Maintenance: 15 to 30 μg/kg per minute (in combination with N_2O and narcotics)
• Sedation: 0.1 to 0.3 mg/kg IV

Undesired clinical responses From 5% to 30% of clients who receive ketamine experience nightmares, hallucinations, and emergence delirium. These responses, which may occur 24 hours after administration, are seen more frequently in adults, especially females, and in clients with a history of

personality disorders. Premedication with a benzodiazepine may prevent these responses. Atropine and the sedative droperidol (Inapsine) increase the incidence of emergence delirium, as does excessive sensory stimulation during the recovery phase.

Ketamine also produces a marked increase in oral secretions. Premedication with an antisialagogue is recommended. The antimuscarinic drug glycopyrrolate (Robinul) is preferred.

Contraindications and precautions Ketamine use is avoided in ophthalmologic procedures since it causes nystagmus and increases intraocular pressure. Ketamine is also not recommended for use in clients with a history of psychologic problems.

ETOMIDATE

Etomidate (Amidate) (1973) is an ultrashort-acting sedative-hypnotic approved for use in the United States in the 1980s. It does not possess any analgesic activity. Etomidate is approximately 25 times more potent than thiopental and has a wider margin of safety.

Pharmacotherapeutics Etomidate is used as an induction agent for general anesthesia. Because of its cardiovascular stabilizing effects, it is preferred over thiopental for clients with coronary artery disease. Its short duration and rapid recovery time make it useful in short outpatient surgery.

Pharmacokinetics Etomidate is a highly lipid-soluble compound with an onset of action 30 to 60 seconds after IV administration. Its duration of action is 3 to 5 minutes. Etomidate is approximately 78% protein bound and is 85% metabolized by hydrolysis in the liver and the plasma. Metabolites of etomidate are inactive; approximately 87% are excreted in the urine, with the remainder excreted in the bile. Etomidate has a distribution half-life of 2 minutes and a elimination half-life of 3 hours.

Pharmacodynamics Etomidate depresses the reticular activating system by mimicking or enhancing the action of GABA. It rapidly produces unconsciousness. With etomidate, cerebral blood flow, cerebral oxygen consumption, and intracranial pressure are reduced. Myoclonic muscle movements occur in 30% to 50% of clients; these movements are reduced by premedication with a benzodiazepine or a narcotic.

With a dose of 0.3 mg/kg, there is no significant change in heart rate or cardiac output, and mean arterial blood pressure is slightly decreased. In the respiratory system the tidal volume and minute volume are decreased, but the respiratory rate is increased. Transient apnea may be seen in debilitated clients, and coughing and hiccoughs may be seen on induction. Respiratory depression may be substantial if narcotics are also administered.

Hepatic and renal function are essentially unaltered by etomidate. However, 30% to 40% of the clients experience nausea and vomiting. Although etomidate does not produce muscle relaxation directly, it does potentiate skeletal muscle relaxants. In addition, etomidate suppresses adrenocortical function. Decreased plasma cortisol levels and a decreased response to adrenocorticotropic hormone (ACTH) result 4 to 8 hours after one IV dose. Long-term administration of sedation is not recommended because of the risk of adrenal insufficiency.

Pharmaceutics   Etomidate is available as a sterile solution for injection. The dose for induction purposes is 0.2 to 0.4 mg/kg.

Undesired clinical responses   Etomidate produces pain during IV injection in approximately 30% of clients. This may be prevented by prior injection of lidocaine or fentanyl citrate (Sublimaze). There is a 23% incidence of thrombophlebitis at the infusion site.

PROPOFOL

Although introduced in Europe in 1977, propofol (Diprivan) was not used clinically in the United States until 1989. Propofol is classified as a sedative-hypnotic. It is a highly lipophilic alkyl-phenol derivative.

Pharmacotherapeutics   Because of its ability to produce rapid induction and recovery, propofol is an ideal agent for outpatient surgery, short surgical procedures, electroconvulsive therapy, and endoscopies. It can also be administered as an infusion for maintenance of anesthesia alone or in combination with N_2O and narcotics.

Pharmacokinetics   Propofol has a fast onset of action. Effects of the drug occur within 1 to 2 minutes of IV administration; effects last approximately 4 minutes. The drug is 89% protein bound and is rapidly metabolized in the liver by the microsomal enzymes. Metabolites of propofol are inactive and are excreted in the urine. Propofol has a distribution half-life of 2 to 8 minutes and an elimination half-life of approximately 2 hours.

Pharmacodynamics   The exact mechanism of action for this drug is unknown. There is a dose-related depression of the CNS, ranging from sedation to loss of consciousness. Propofol also decreases intracranial pressure. Recovery from propofol is rapid, and there is no residual sedation or "hang over" effect.

There is also a dose-related depression of the cardiovascular system. Resulting hypotension is greater than that which occurs with thiopental and is worse in clients who are hypovolemic or who have coronary artery disease. Propofol causes profound respiratory depression that is enhanced by prior opioid administration. There is also a dose-related decrease in tidal volume and minute volume. In addition, laryngospasm, coughing, and hiccoughing can occur during induction.

Renal function is not affected. However, prolonged administration of the drug can cause green urine because of the presence of phenols in the urine. Propofol does not effect muscle relaxation directly but does potentiate muscle relaxants used as part of the anesthetic technique.

Pharmaceutics   The dosage of propofol is based on the desired effects:
- Induction: 1.5 to 2.5 mg/kg IV
- Maintenance: 100 to 200 μg/kg per minute (sole agent)
- Sedation: 25 to 75 μg/kg per minute IV

Precautions   Propofol does cause pain during injection. This pain can be avoided by a prior IV injection of lidocaine. Propofol is prepared as an isotonic emulsion of soybean oil, glycerol, and purified egg phosphatide. Because the emulsion can provide an appropriate environment for bacterial growth, it is recommended that the drug be used within 8 hours after the vial is opened.

Benzodiazepine

Benzodiazepines were described in Chapter 18. Only their use as IV anesthetic agents is addressed in this chapter.

Benzodiazepines are used quite frequently during induction and maintenance of general anesthesia:
- Diazepam (Valium) Induction: 0.2 to 0.6 mg/kg IV
  - Sedation: 0.03 to 0.1 mg/kg IV
- Midazolam (Versed) Induction: 0.2 to 0.6 mg/kg IV
  - 2 to 5 μg/kg per minute infusion with narcotics and N_2O
  - Sedation: 0.07 to 0.08 mg/kg IM or IV

Their actions include hypnosis, sedation, anticonvulsant activity, and muscle relaxation. The main action appears to be facilitation of the inhibitory neurotransmitter GABA.[16] The sedation and skeletal muscle relaxation seen with the benzodiazepines are attributed to facilitation of the inhibitory neurotransmitter glycine in the spinal cord and brain stem.

Diazepam has been used in both the preoperative and intraoperative period of anesthesia. However, because of its slow onset and prolonged duration of action, it offers little advantage over thiopental. **Midazolam** is fast replacing diazepam in anesthesia practice because it has greater potency, faster onset of action, and much shorter duration of action.

Opioids

Opioid is a general term used to describe a drug (narcotic analgesic) that binds to the opioid receptor. (Narcotic and nonnarcotic analgesics that affect the CNS are described in Chapter 19.) The opioids used in the practice of anesthesia include the naturally occurring alkaloid morphine and the synthetic compounds fentanyl, sufentanil, and alfentanil. Morphine is a phenanthrene derivative and the oldest narcotic in use at present. It is the standard against which all other narcotics are compared. Fentanyl, alfentanil, and sufentanil are synthetic derivatives; both sufentanil and alfentanil are chemical analogs of fentanyl. Fentanyl is the most commonly used opioid in anesthesia.

OPIOID PROTOTYPE

FENTANYL

Narcotics are used during the induction and maintenance phase of anesthesia.

Pharmacotherapeutics Fentanyl (Sublimaze) is used as a sole agent or in combination with other IV agents, N_2O, or low concentrations of the potent inhalation agents. This balanced technique minimizes doses and side effects while gaining the maximal desired effects of all the drugs.[17]

Pharmacokinetics Fentanyl is 100 times more potent than morphine and 1000 times more potent than meperidine. It is approximately 84% protein bound. Because of its greater lipid solubility, it has a faster onset of action, 4 to 5 minutes, and a shorter duration of action, 30 to 60 minutes, than morphine. The short duration of action is due to redistribution to other tissues. Fentanyl's distribution half-life is 13 minutes; its excretion half-life is 3 hours. Fentanyl is metabolized by hydrolysis in the liver, with 8% excreted unchanged by the kidneys.

Pharmacodynamics The physiologic effects of fentanyl are the same as those of other opioids previously described in Chapter 19. With fentanyl's high lipid solubility, it rapidly gains entrance to the CNS. As a result, analgesia and sedation are produced. With high doses of fentanyl, unconsciousness occurs. However, amnesia may not be present. In fact, one major problem with total narcotic anesthesia is postoperative client recall of intraoperative events.[17]

There is little or no direct myocardial depression seen with fentanyl, a major reason why narcotic anesthesia is commonly used for clients with impaired cardiovascular function. However, when administered with N_2O or a benzodiazepine, a significant decrease in cardiac output and blood pressure occurs.

A dose-related respiratory depression also occurs with fentanyl administration. This is due to direct depression of the medullary respiratory centers and decreased responsiveness of the central and peripheral chemoreceptors. The decrease in respiratory rate, tidal volume, and minute volume can persist into the postoperative period. Narcotic-induced muscle rigidity due to a centrally mediated increase in muscle tone may occur during induction, especially after rapid IV injection of fentanyl. If this occurs, interference with effective ventilation may develop.

Pharmaceutics The actual amount of fentanyl administered depends on a variety of factors, including the client's condition, type and length of surgical procedure, use of other anesthetic agents, and potential need of ventilatory support in the postoperative period:
- Induction and maintenance as sole agent: 50 to 150 μg/kg IV
- Maintenance with other agents: 2 to 10 μg/kg IV

FENTANYL-DROPERIDOL COMBINATION (INNOVAR)

Innovar is a combination of droperidol, a butyrophenone neuroleptic, and fentanyl in a fixed ratio of 50:1. (Each milliliter of Innovar contains 2.5 mg of droperidol and 50 μg of fentanyl.) Innovar, 2 to 4 ml IV, is administered during induction of general anesthesia. Additional fentanyl is titrated during the maintenance period.

Droperidol is a competitive inhibitor of dopamine in the brain, especially in the chemoreceptor trigger zone. Administration of Innovar results in neuroleptic anesthesia, which is characterized by sedation, analgesia, α-adrenergic blockade, catalepsy, and catatonia. Innovar is used as an adjunct to induction of general anesthesia and preoperatively to produce sedation and prevent nausea and vomiting.

Droperidol has minimal cardiovascular and respiratory effects, although it does potentiate the respiratory effects of narcotics. Sedation, antiemetic action, and potentiation of narcotics may persist into the postoperative period. For this reason the doses of all CNS depressants, especially narcotics, must be decreased by one half for 8 hours after the administration

of Innovar. Droperidol is contraindicated in clients with Parkinson's disease because it causes extrapyramidal effects.

MISCELLANEOUS OPIOIDS

Sufentanil (Sufenta) is five to seven times more potent than fentanyl. It is used for major surgery that lasts longer than 2 hours and when ventilatory support may be required in the postoperative period. Sufentanil has a longer redistribution half-life, 18 minutes, and elimination half-life, 2½ hours, than fentanyl. It is 99% metabolized in the liver. As part of a balanced anesthesia technique, sufentanil, 2 to 8 μg/kg IV, is administered in combination with an inhalation agent. For induction and maintenance as a sole agent, 8 to 30 μg/kg is used. Sufentanil in dosages of 1.5 to 4.5 μg/kg can be administered nasally to pediatric clients, with effects occurring in 4 to 10 minutes.[18]

Alfentanil (Alfenta) is a shorter-acting opioid with a potency one fourth to one third that of fentanyl. It is 25 times more potent than morphine. Alfentanil has a much shorter duration of action than fentanyl; it is metabolized in the liver and excreted by the kidney. Alfentanil, 100 to 200 μg/kg IV, is used for induction, and 25 to 150 μg/kg per minute is used for maintenance.

CONCEPT REVIEW

Ultrashort-acting barbiturates, benzodiazepines, opioids, and other drugs are used as IV anesthetics.

These drugs are used as sole agents in the induction and maintenance of an anesthetic or in combination with other IV agents, N_2O, or potent inhalation agents.

IV anesthetic drugs produce CNS depression and have systemic effects on many body systems.

NURSING CONSIDERATIONS: POSTOPERATIVE

After emergence from general anesthesia, the client's condition is considered unstable. The anesthetic drugs continue to affect physiologic functions into the postoperative period. The CNS and cardiovascular and respiratory systems are affected the most.

In the immediate postoperative period, clients recover from anesthesia in the PACU, where they are monitored closely by nurses prepared in this specialty. A detailed preoperative and intraoperative report is provided by the nurse anesthetist before discharge of the client to the care of the PACU nurse.

In the PACU the client is monitored closely for any signs of neurologic impairment, cardiovascular instability, respiratory distress, and pain. All clients recovering from general anesthesia receive 35% to 40% oxygen by aerosol to assure adequate oxygenation. Nevertheless, respiratory distress secondary to narcotic use or prolonged sedation occurs. If sedation is excessive, drugs that reverse the effects of the sedative or narcotic may be necessary. Sedated clients may also exhibit obstructed upper airways because of relaxation of the pharyngeal muscles, including the tongue. In most situations, repositioning the client into a lateral decubitus position is sufficient to resolve the problem.[19,20]

Cardiovascular or hemodynamic instability may occur as a result of prolonged sedation or hypovolemia. Urinary output should be monitored carefully; an output of at least 1 ml/kg per hour is expected. Other causes of cardiovascular instability include myocardial ischemia, pneumothorax, continued surgical bleeding, adrenal insufficiency, or cerebral vascular accident.

Hypertension also occurs in the PACU. Usually it is due to pain, preexisting hypertension, ventilatory distress, or retention of urine. In addition, client agitation may be attributed to pain, full bladder, or cerebral hypoxia. Careful, accurate assessment is mandatory to differentiate the causative factor. Administration of narcotics to a hypoxic client who is incorrectly diagnosed as having pain delays appropriate interventions and may increase existing respiratory distress.[21]

Many surgical clients enter the PACU in a hypothermic state. Hypothermia in these clients is usually the result of cool operating rooms, cold IV and irrigation fluids, and cool anesthetic gases. During major abdominal surgery, heat loss also results from exposure of viscera. In addition, the potent inhalation agents depress the thermoregulatory response; therefore the anesthetized client is unable to compensate for a falling temperature by vasoconstriction and shivering. This hypothermic state slows the recovery from general anesthesia. In addition, the shivering that occurs in response to the lowered body temperature increases the oxygen consumption 200% to 300%. This may have detrimental results in a client with poor cardiovascular reserve. Therefore active rewarming may be necessary in the PACU to return the body temperature to normal.

Specific criteria for discharge from the PACU exist. The client should be easily aroused with verbal stimulation and should be oriented to person, place, and time. (Orientation is relative to preoperative status.) Respiratory and cardiovascular function should be stable. Nausea should be minimal or absent, and the client's temperature should be near normal. In addition, the client must have controlled surgical pain. After discharge from the PACU the client may still be under the effect of the anesthetic drugs administered in the operating room. Continued monitoring by the unit nurse is essential. (Review the section on postoperative care in a medical-surgical textbook.)

SUMMARY

Administration of anesthesia is the responsibility of either a nurse anesthetist or an anesthesiologist, individuals who are educated and certified in the speciality of anesthesia. However, nurses who provide care for clients during the perioperative period must have a basic understanding of the drugs used in the practice of anesthesia. The preoperative and postoperative plan of care for the client should address his or her expectations of anesthesia and the most common anesthesia-related problems encountered in the postoperative period.

REFERENCES

1. Bankert, M. (1989). *Watchful care: A history of America's nurse anesthetists.* New York: Continuum.
2. Walbergh, E.J., & Eckert, J. (1989). Pharmacokinetics of intravenous and intranasal midazolam in children. *Anesthesiology, 71*(Suppl.3A), A1065.
3. Eger, E.I. (1990). Uptake and distribution. In Miller, R.D., (Ed). *Anesthesia* (3rd ed.). New York: Churchill Livingstone.
4. Eger, E.I. (1974). *Anesthetic uptake and action.* Baltimore: Williams & Wilkins.
5. Wood, M., & Wood, A.J. (1990). *Drugs and anesthesia pharmacology for anesthesiologists* (2nd ed.). Baltimore: Williams & Wilkins.
6. Wendell, S.C., & Kingston, H.G. (1992). Inhalation anesthesia. In Barash, P.G., Cullen, B.C., & Stoelting, R.K. *Clinical anesthesia.* Philadelphia: J.B. Lippincott.
7. Stoelting, R.K., & Miller, R.D. (1989). *Basics of anesthesia.* New York: Churchill Livingstone.
8. Smiley, B., & Paradise, N. (1991). Does the duration of N_2O administration affect postoperative nausea and vomiting? *Nurse Anesthesia, 2*(1), 13-18.
9. Brown, B., & Funk, E. (1990). Status of anesthetic hepatotoxicity in the 1990s. *Anesthesiology Review, 17*(6), 15-21.
10. Jones, R.M. (1990). Desflurane and sevoflurane: Inhalation anesthetics for this decade? *British Journal of Anaesthesia, 65,* 527-536.
11. Eger, E.I. (1993). Desflurane: An overview of its properties. *Anesthesiology Review, 20*(3), 87-92.
12. Shiraiski, Y., & Kazuyuki, I. (1990). Uptake and biotransformation of sevoflurane in humans: A comparative study of sevoflurane with halothane, enflurane and isoflurane. *Journal of Clinical Anesthesia, 2,* 381-386.
13. Pace, N., Victory, R., & White, P. (1992). Anesthetic infusion techniques—How to do it. *Journal of Clinical Anesthesia, 4(SI),* 45-52.
14. Olson, R.W. (1988). Barbiturates. *International Anesthesiology Clinics, 26,* 254-261.
15. Fragen, R.J., & Abram, M.J. (1990). Barbiturates. In Miller, R.D. (Ed.). *Anesthesia* (3rd ed.). New York: Churchill Livingstone.
16. Haefely, W.E. (1988). Benzodiazepines. *International Anesthesiology Clinics, 26,* 263-272.
17. Baily, P.T., & Stanley, T.H. (1990). Narcotic anesthesia. In Miller, R.D. (Ed.). *Anesthesia* (3rd ed.). New York: Churchill Livingstone.
18. Estafanous, F.G. (Ed.) (1991). *Opioids in anesthesia II.* Boston: Butterwok-Heinmann.
19. Feeley, T.W. (1990). Assessment and management of patients in the postanesthesia care unit. In Baresh, P. (Ed.). *ASA refresher course, 18* (10).
20. Frost, E.M. (1992). Complications in the post-anesthesia care unit, I. *Current Reviews for Nurse Anesthetists, 15*(12), 97-104.
21. Frost, E.M. (1992). Complications in the post-anesthesia care unit, II. *Current Reviews for Nurse Anesthetists, 15*(13), 105-112.

BIBLIOGRAPHY

Biddle, C. (1991). Transdermal and transmucosal administration of anesthetic drugs. *Journal of American Association of Nurse Anesthetists, 59*(1), 38-45.

Gunn, I.P. (1991). The history of nurse anesthesia education: Highlights and influences. *Journal of American Nurse Anesthetists, 59*(1), 53.

Hanucharurnkui, S., & Vinya-nguag, P. (1991). Effects of promoting patients' participation in self-care on postoperative recovery and satisfaction with care. *Nursing Science Quarterly, 4*(1), 14-20.

Longnecker, D., & Murphy, F.L. (1992). *Introduction to anesthesia* (8th ed.). Philadelphia: W.B. Saunders.

Mansson, M., Fredrikkzon, B., & Rosberg, B. (1992). Comparison of preparation and narcotic-sedative premedication in children undergoing surgery. *Pediatric Nursing, 18,* 337-342, 350-351.

Maree, S.M. (1992). Benzodiazepine and their reversal. *Current Reviews for Nurse Anesthetists, 15*(7), 53-60.

McDonald, D. (1993). Postoperative narcotic analgesic administration. *Applied Nursing Research, 6*(3), 106-110.

Poole, E. (1993). The effects of postanesthesia care unit visits on anxiety in surgical patients. *Journal of Post Anesthesia Nursing, 8,* 386-394.

Thrush, D., Mangar, D., & Alonso, J. (1992). Incidence of arterial oxygen desaturation in cardiac patients premedicated with intramuscular scopolamine and morphine. *Nurse Anesthesia, 3*(2), 53-56.

Drugs Affecting the Autonomic Nervous System

CHAPTER 25

OVERVIEW OF THE
Autonomic Nervous System

SANDRA LINDQUIST • ROBYN RICE

⊛ **Peripheral Nervous System**

LEARNING OBJECTIVE: Describe the components of the peripheral nervous system.

KEY TERMS:

Afferent, efferent, ganglia

⊛ **Autonomic Nerve Fibers**

LEARNING OBJECTIVES:

Differentiate between preganglionic and postganglionic neurons.

Explain autonomic nerve conduction.

KEY TERMS:

Postganglionic fiber, postganglionic neuron, preganglionic fiber, preganglionic neuron

⊛ **Sympathetic and Parasympathetic Functions**

LEARNING OBJECTIVES:

Discuss the effects of neurotransmitter substances in the autonomic nervous system (ANS).

Differentiate between cholinergic and adrenergic fibers.

Differentiate between cholinergic and adrenergic receptors.

Describe the excitatory and inhibitory actions of the ANS.

KEY TERMS:

Acetylcholine, acetylcholinesterase, adrenergic, alpha receptors, autonomic tone, beta receptors, cholinergic, epinephrine, muscarinic receptors, neurotransmitter substances, nicotinic receptors, norepinephrine

⊛ **Drugs Affecting the ANS**

LEARNING OBJECTIVE: Discuss the effects of drugs on the ANS.

CONCEPTS AND TERMS TO REVIEW

Review sections of Chapter 17 for detailed explanations of specific neural structures, impulse conduction, and neurotransmitters.

Review anatomy and physiology for complete discussion of the autonomic nervous system.

---

*T*he autonomic nervous system (ANS), a branch of the peripheral nervous system (PNS), is concerned primarily with involuntary, automatic visceral functions of the body. The ANS innervates tissues such as smooth and cardiac muscle and exocrine and endocrine glands. It regulates a variety of body functions that are usually automatic and not subject to conscious control.[1-3] A primary feature of the ANS is its ca-

pacity to respond almost instantaneously to stressors. For example, in a matter of seconds the blood pressure and heart rate can rise or fall in response to stimulation of the system.

Autonomic signals are transmitted to the body through two major subdivisions: the sympathetic nervous system and the parasympathetic nervous system. The characteristics and functions of these subdivisions are the focus of this chapter. This information will help you understand the relationship between functional disturbances and drug therapy and the impact that drug therapy has on the ANS.

PERIPHERAL NERVOUS SYSTEM

The central nervous system (CNS) and the PNS are subdivisions of the nervous system. The PNS consists of nerves and ganglia.

Nerves and Ganglia

Nerves are bundles of axons and their sheaths that extend from the CNS to peripheral structures. Forty-three pairs of nerves originate from the CNS to form the PNS. Twelve pairs, the **cranial nerves,** originate from the brain. The remaining 31 pairs, the **spinal nerves,** originate from the spinal cord. **Ganglia** are collections or aggregations of nerve cell bodies located outside the CNS.[2-5]

Afferent and Efferent Subdivisions

The PNS is composed of two subdivisions: the afferent (sensory) and the efferent (motor). Action potentials from the sensory organs are transmitted to the CNS by the **afferent** division. The **efferent** division transmits action potentials from the CNS to effector organs (organs that produce an effect) such as muscles and glands. The efferent division of the nervous system is divided into the somatic nervous system and the ANS.

Major sources of stimulation for the ANS originate from centers in the spinal cord, brain stem, and hypothalamus.[3] In addition, some areas of the cerebral cortex such as the limbic system transmit impulses that can influence autonomic activity.

AUTONOMIC NERVE FIBERS

Cell bodies of the efferent nerves of the ANS are located in areas ranging from the midbrain to the sacral region of the spinal cord. Unlike the CNS, the ANS always has at least two neurons involved in the innervation of an effector organ.

The cell body of the **preganglionic** (first) **neuron** is within the CNS. Its myelinated axon, the **preganglionic fiber,** exits the CNS as part of a cranial or spinal nerve. At some point the preganglionic fiber separates from the nerve and extends to an autonomic ganglion. In the autonomic ganglion the preganglionic neuron synapses with a **postganglionic** (second) **neuron.**[3] The postganglionic neuron lies entirely outside of the CNS. Its cell body and dendrites are located in the autonomic ganglion. The axon of a postganglionic neuron, a **postganglionic fiber,** is unmyelinated and terminates in a visceral effector.

Sympathetic Nervous System

Sympathetic nerves originate from T-1 through L-2 segments of the spinal cord and pass into the sympathetic chains of ganglia that lie along the spinal column.[3,4,6] Some sympathetic nerves extend directly from the chains of ganglia to effector organs. Other sympathetic nerves pass through the celiac ganglion or the hypogastric plexus before reaching their effector organs. Because the sympathetic division originates in the thoracic and lumbar segment of the spinal cord, it is also called the *thoracolumbar division.*[3] Fig. 25–1 illustrates the nerve pathways of the sympathetic division.

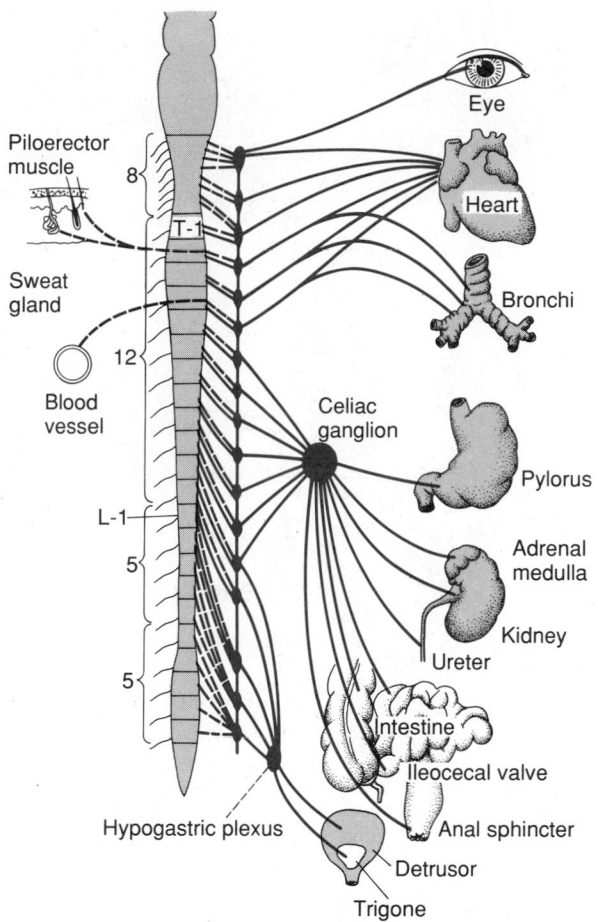

FIGURE 25–1   Sympathetic nervous system. Dashed lines represent postganglionic fibers in the gray rami leading to the spinal nerves or distribution to blood vessels, sweat glands, and piloerector muscles. (From Guyton, A.C. (1991). *Textbook of medical physiology* (8th ed.). Philadelphia: W.B. Saunders.)

Parasympathetic Nervous System

The parasympathetic division originates from preganglionic fibers arising from cells in the brain stem (midbrain, pons, and medulla) and from fibers arising from the second, third, and fourth segments of the sacral spinal cord. Approximately 75% of the parasympathetic nerve fibers involve the tenth cranial nerve, the vagus nerve.[3] Other nerves of the parasympathetic division leave the CNS through cranial nerves III (oculomotor), VII (facial), and IX (glossopharyngeal). Preganglionic fibers of parasympathetic neurons are long; the postganglionic neurons have short axons. Because parasympathetic neurons originate in the brain and the sacral region of the spinal cord, this division is sometimes called the *craniosacral division.*[2,5] Figure 25–2 illustrates the parasympathetic nerve pathways.

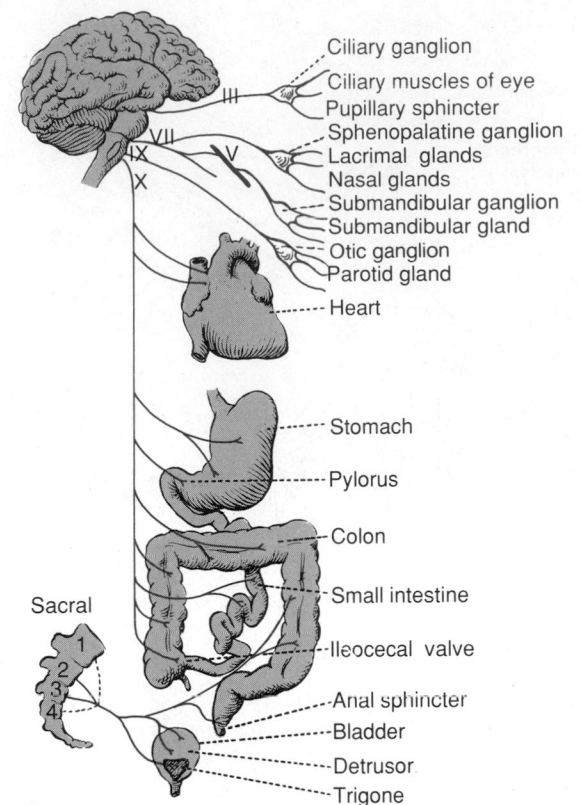

Sacral

Ciliary ganglion
Ciliary muscles of eye
Pupillary sphincter
Sphenopalatine ganglion
Lacrimal glands
Nasal glands
Submandibular ganglion
Submandibular gland
Otic ganglion
Parotid gland
Heart
Stomach
Pylorus
Colon
Small intestine
Ileocecal valve
Anal sphincter
Bladder
Detrusor
Trigone

FIGURE 25–2   Parasympathetic nervous system. (From Guyton, A.C. (1991). *Textbook of medical physiology* (8th ed.). Philadelphia: W.B. Saunders.)

CONCEPT REVIEW

The CNS and the PNS are subdivisions of the nervous system.

The PNS consists of nerves and ganglia.

Autonomic signals are transmitted to the body through two major subdivisions: the sympathetic nervous system and the parasympathetic nervous system.

SYMPATHETIC AND PARASYMPATHETIC FUNCTIONS

Most body structures receive dual innervation; fibers from both the sympathetic and parasympathetic divisions innervate the same structure. Usually the two divisions have opposing effects on an organ, one causing excitation and the other inhibition. This occurs because different neurotransmitters and different neurotransmitter receptors are used.

Neurotransmitters

A neurotransmitter is a chemical synthesized in the nerve cells and stored inside sacs or vesicles of the nerve terminal.[2,7] Because neurotransmitters are chemicals secreted by one cell or

group of cells (preganglionic and postganglionic neurons) and have physiologic control on other cells of the body (i.e., cardiac muscle, smooth muscle, exocrine glands), they are also considered neurohormones by some sources.[3]

Neurons, or nerve cells, use neurotransmitters, or neurohormones, to transmit nerve impulses across synaptic clefts to adjacent neurons. Although the effector organ may have several types of receptors, each receptor recognizes only one specific neurotransmitter. On contact with its specific substance, the receptor site initiates a cellular response. Once the transmitting substance is chemically deactivated by enzymatic activity or moves away from the receptor site to another neuron, the cellular response stops. Acetylcholine, norepinephrine, and epinephrine are the neurotransmitters in the ANS.

Acetylcholine is composed of choline and an acetate molecule and is derived from enzymatic activity by choline acetylase. Once contact with its receptor site is made, acetylcholine is rapidly degraded by the enzyme **acetylcholinesterase** or by nonspecific cholinesterases in blood or tissues.[2] Located in the membranes of cells, acetylcholinesterase degrades acetylcholine back to acetate and choline from which it can again be synthesized into its neurotransmitter form.

Norepinephrine is synthesized in the nerve terminal from the amino acid tyrosine. As the neuron is stimulated by a nerve impulse, norepinephrine is released to act on adjacent cells. Unlike acetylcholine, norepinephrine is not degraded after release but is reabsorbed and stored in the neuronal membrane for future use. Monoamine oxidase (MAO) and catechol-O-methyltransferase (COMT) are two enzymes that degrade norepinephrine in the blood. COMT is found in the liver and the kidneys; MAO is found in many tissues, including the liver and the kidneys.[2,7] Norepinephrine is also stored in the adrenal medulla and is released in response to sympathetic stimulation.

Epinephrine also augments the response of the sympathetic division of the ANS by activating specific receptors for epinephrine and norepinephrine. The adrenal glands secrete epinephrine. When the adrenal glands release epinephrine into the blood, it stimulates cellular activity of effector tissues.

Cholinergic and Adrenergic Fibers

As stated previously, the two synaptic neurotransmitters secreted by sympathetic and parasympathetic fibers are acetylcholine and norepinephrine. Fibers that secrete acetylcholine are called **cholinergic.** **Adrenergic** fibers secrete norepinephrine.

Preganglionic neurons are cholinergic in both the sympathetic and parasympathetic nervous systems. Thus acetylcholine is the preganglionic neurotransmitter for both systems and excites both sympathetic and parasympathetic postganglionic neurons. The postganglionic neurons of the parasympathetic system are all cholinergic. Most of the postganglionic sympathetic neurons are adrenergic.[8]

Because most of the postganglionic neurons in the sympathetic division secrete the adrenergic neurotransmitter norepinephrine, this division is sometimes called the *adrenergic system.* The parasympathetic division is called the *cholinergic system* since its postganglionic neurotransmitter is the cholinergic neurotransmitter acetylcholine.[2,3]

Cholinergic and Adrenergic Receptors

Receptors are proteins located in the membranes of effector cells. When a neurotransmitter combines with a receptor, a response is elicited. There are two types of cholinergic receptors, **muscarinic** and **nicotinic,** and two major structural categories of adrenergic receptors, **alpha** and **beta.** Both α-adrenergic and β-adrenergic receptors can be excitatory or inhibitory. These receptors are further classified into subtypes: alpha 1, alpha 2, beta 1, and beta 2.

Muscarinic receptors Muscarinic receptors are located in the membranes of effector cells at the ends of all postganglionic parasympathetic nerve fibers. Most sweat glands and the smooth muscle in certain blood vessels that receive innervation from cholinergic sympathetic postganglionic fibers also feature muscarinic receptors. Responses from these receptors are excitatory and occur slowly.[4,7–9]

Nicotinic receptors Located on both sympathetic and parasympathetic postganglionic neurons are the nicotinic receptors. They produce rapid, excitatory responses. Nicotinic receptors are also found in the membrane of skeletal muscle fibers at the neuromuscular junction.[4,8]

Alpha receptors Alpha-1 receptors are postsynaptic receptors; they dominate the activity of effector tissues. Activity of the alpha-1 receptors is associated with excitation or stimulatory cellular responses. Alpha-2 receptors are presynaptic autoreceptors and are associated with relaxation or inhibitory cellular responses.[2,9,10]

Beta receptors The exact location of beta-1 and beta-2 receptors is unclear. Most beta-1 receptors are probably located in the heart, whereas beta-2 receptors are found in other tissues. When stimulated, beta-1 receptors increase heart rate and myocardial contractility. They also cause release of renin from the kidney, insulin release from the pancreas, and lipolysis. Beta-2 receptors dilate blood vessels and airways, relax bronchial, ureteral, uterine, and other smooth muscles, and increase glycogenolysis and gluconeogenesis.[2,10]

Excitatory and Inhibitory Actions

Functional characteristics of the ANS distinguish the parasympathetic from the sympathetic nervous system. These characteristics are related to the opposing nature of acetylcholine and norepinephrine on effector tissues. The parasympathetic nervous system works to conserve energy. It dominates more specific regulatory processes of the body such as digestion, cardiac and bladder function, and pupil constriction. The parasympathetic system does not affect the function of apocrine glands, kidneys, systemic arterioles, adrenal medulla, skeletal and piloerector muscles, fat cells, mental activity, and basal metabolism.[2,3,5]

The sympathetic nervous system mobilizes energy in response to stressors or emergency situations. This "fight-or-flight" response has more generalized and widespread effects on the body. For example, sympathetic stimulation causes pupil dilation, increased secretion by the apocrine glands, decreased gastrointestinal peristalsis and tone, and decreased urinary output. When sympathetic neurons of the heart are stimulated, the force of myocardial contraction increases, and the heart rate increases.[2,3,8] Table 25–1 lists the autonomic effects of the sympathetic and parasympathetic systems on various organs of the body.

Sympathetic and Parasympathetic Tone

The sympathetic and parasympathetic systems are continually active. Basic rates of activity are known as **sympathetic tone** and **parasympathetic tone.** The presence of **autonomic tone** means that effector organs are continuously stimulated by minute amounts of neurotransmitter substances. This allows a single nervous system to increase or decrease the activity of a simulated organ.[3]

Each organ or tissue has a dominant transmitting substance, either sympathetic or parasympathetic, that sets its tone. For example, the basal sympathetic tone of arterioles maintains the diameter of the vessel at a midpoint between its minimum and maximum diameter. Activation of the sympathetic system causes the arterioles to constrict. The tone of the gastrointestinal tract is maintained by the parasympathetic nervous system. Motility and secretory functions of the gastrointestinal tract increase when the parasympathetic system is stimulated.[3]

Stimulation: Discrete Versus Mass

In some instances the sympathetic nervous system discharges as a complete unit, that is, mass stimulation. This frequently occurs when the hypothalamus is activated by fear or severe pain. Mass stimulation produces a widespread response throughout the body—the stress or alarm response. At other times, the sympathetic activation occurs in discrete, isolated portions of the system (e.g., the sympathetic control of sweating to regulate body heat).

Control functions of the parasympathetic nervous system are usually highly specific (e.g., parasympathetic cardiovascular reflexes act only on the heart). However, there is a close relationship between some parasympathetic functions. For instance, salivary secretion and gastric secretion can occur independently but often occur together.[3]

CONCEPT REVIEW

Most body structures receive innervation from both the sympathetic and parasympathetic nervous systems.

Acetylcholine, norepinephrine, and epinephrine are the neurotransmitters in the ANS.

Fibers that secrete acetylcholine are called *cholinergic.*

Adrenergic fibers secrete norepinephrine.

The parasympathetic nervous system conserves energy; the sympathetic nervous system mobilizes energy in response to stressors or emergency situations.

TABLE 25–1

Autonomic Effects on Various Organs of the Body

Organ	Effect of Sympathetic Stimulation	Effect of Parasympathetic Stimulation
Eye		
Pupil	Dilated	Constricted
Ciliary muscle	Slight relaxation (far vision)	Constricted (near vision)
Glands	Vasoconstriction and slight secretion	Stimulation of copious secretion (containing many enzymes for enzyme-secreting glands)
Nasal		
Lacrimal		
Parotid		
Submandibular		
Gastric		
Pancreatic		
Sweat glands	Copious sweating (cholinergic)	Sweating on palms of hands
Apocrine glands	Thick, odoriferous secretion	None
Heart		
Muscle	Increased rate	Slowed rate
	Increased force of contraction	Decreased force of contraction (especially of atria)
Coronaries	Dilated (β_2; constricted α)	Dilated
Lungs		
Bronchi	Dilated	Constricted
Blood vessels	Mildly constricted	? Dilated
Gut		
Lumen	Decreased peristalsis and tone	Increased peristalsis and tone
Sphincter	Increased tone (most times)	Relaxed (most times)
Liver	Glucose released	Slight glycogen synthesis
Gallbladder and bile ducts	Relaxed	Contracted
Kidney	Decreased output and renin secretion	None
Bladder		
Detrusor	Relaxed (slight)	Contracted
Trigone	Contracted	Relaxed
Penis	Ejaculation	Erection
Systemic arterioles		
Abdominal viscera	Constricted	None
Muscle	Constricted (adrenergic α)	None
	Dilated (adrenergic β_2)	
	Dilated (cholinergic)	
Skin	Constricted	None
Blood		
Coagulation	Increased	None
Glucose	Increased	None
Lipids	Increased	None
Basal metabolism	Increased up to 100%	None
Adrenal medullary secretion	Increased	None
Mental activity	Increased	None
Piloerector muscles	Contracted	None
Skeletal muscle	Increased glycogenolysis	None
	Increased strength	
Fat cells	Lipolysis	None

From Guyton, A.C. (1991). Textbook of medical physiology (8th ed.). Philadelphia: W.B. Saunders.

DRUGS AFFECTING THE ANS

Drugs can act on the ANS in a variety of ways. For example, they can stimulate or block the action of transmitter substances, promote or decrease impulse transmission, or enhance or diminish the activity of effector organs.

Sympathetic Drugs

Drugs that act on the sympathetic nervous system can be classified as sympathomimetic or sympatholytic. **Sympatho-** **mimetic drugs,** also called *adrenergic,* mimic or act in the same manner as the neurotransmitter substances norepinephrine and epinephrine. These drugs stimulate receptors to activate the sympathetic response of organs and tissues throughout the body. Some sympathomimetic drugs stimulate specific receptor sites, whereas other drugs activate the release of norepinephrine.

Drugs that act on specific receptor sites are classified as **direct-acting sympathomimetic drugs.** For example, isoproterenol (Isuprel) primarily acts on beta receptors. Dobutamine (Dobutrex), a β_1-adrenergic drug, activates cardiac beta-1 receptors to increase the heart rate, improve myocardial contractility, and initiate the release of renin from the kidney. β_2-Adrenergic drugs such as albuterol (Proventil, Ventolin) and metaproterenol (Alupent, Metaprel) selectively stimulate beta-2 receptors to relax bronchiolar and other smooth muscle.[11,12]

Drugs that activate the release of norepinephrine are classified as **indirect-acting sympathomimetic drugs.** These drugs exert their effects only by releasing endogenous catecholamines. Amphetamines are indirect-acting sympathomimetic drugs.

Sympatholytic drugs, also known as *adrenergic blocking agents* or *antiadrenergic drugs,* block or interfere with adrenergic activity at different points in the stimulation process. **Adrenergic neuronal blockers** such as methyldopa (Aldomet), reserpine (Serpasil), and guanethidine (Ismelin) prevent synthesis, storage, or release of norepinephrine in the sympathetic nerve endings.

Drugs such as α-adrenergic or β-adrenergic blockers block alpha- or beta-receptor sites and interfere with activation of sympathetic responses associated with the particular receptor. For example, **α-adrenergic blockers** such as phenoxybenzamine (Dibenzyline) and phentolamine (Regitine) decreases peripheral resistance and lower blood pressure. **β-Adrenergic blockers** such as propranolol (Inderal), nadolol (Corgard), and labetalol (Normodyne, Trandate) can interfere with all beta-receptor activities.[11-13]

Drugs can also block the synaptic transmission of sympathetic impulses from preganglionic to postganglionic neurons. These drugs are called *ganglionic blocking agents.* In blocking sympathetic impulses they reduce peripheral resistance and lower blood pressure. Drugs classified as ganglionic blocking agents include mecamylamine (Inversine) and trimethaphan (Arfonad).[12,13]

Parasympathetic Drugs

Drugs producing typical parasympathetic effects are called *parasympathomimetic drugs.* Parasympathomimetic drugs that stimulate and potentiate the activity of acetylcholine on the parasympathetic system are classified as **cholinergic drugs.** **Muscarinic cholinergic drugs** act directly on the muscarinic receptor sites. These drugs such as bethanechol (Urecholine), carbachol (Miostat), and pilocarpine (Pilocar) stimulate muscarinic receptors. **Nicotinic cholinergic drugs** stimulate nicotinic receptors in synapses between preganglionic and postganglionic neurons in autonomic ganglia. Since nicotinic receptors are located in both sympathetic and parasympathetic postganglionic neurons, these drugs elicit responses from both divisions of the ANS.[3]

Some drugs potentiate the effects of naturally secreted acetylcholine at the parasympathetic nerve endings. These **anticholinesterase drugs** such as edrophonium (Tensilon), physostigmine (Antilirium), neostigmine (Prostigmin), and pyridostigmine (Mestinon) inhibit the enzymatic destruction of acetylcholine by cholinesterase. This action elevates acetylcholine levels and prolongs the action of acetylcholine produced by the body.[12,13]

Parasympatholytic or **anticholinergic drugs** interfere with and block acetylcholine transmission at ganglia, postganglionic parasympathetic receptor sites, and neuromuscular end-plates of skeletal muscle.[12] **Antimuscarinic drugs,** including atropine, oxybutynin (Ditropan), glycopyrrolate (Robinul), and propantheline (Pro-Banthine), inhibit acetylcholine transmission at postganglionic parasympathetic muscarinic receptor sites. **Ganglionic blockers** such as mecamylamine (Inversine) and trimethaphan (Arfonad) interfere with cholingeric transmission at nicotinic receptor sites in the synapses between preganglionic and postganglionic neurons. **Neuromuscular blockers** such as tubocurarine and pancuronium (Pavulon) inhibit acetylcholine transmission at the neuromuscular end-plate of skeletal muscle nicotinic receptor sites.[11-13]

SUMMARY

The ANS is composed of parasympathetic and sympathetic divisions. These divisions interact automatically to maintain a delicate balance within the body's internal environment. The parasympathetic division primarily maintains the ongoing "steady state" of the body, and the sympathetic division mobilizes the body's responses to stressors.

Neurotransmitter substances acetylcholine, norepinephrine, and epinephrine activate tissue receptors throughout the body. Acetylcholine is the neurotransmitter for both parasympathetic and sympathetic preganglionic neurons and parasympathetic (cholinergic) postganglionic neurons. The neurotransmitters for sympathetic (adrenergic) postganglionic neurons are norepinephrine and epinephrine.

Receptors for both divisions of the ANS are located in effector organs and tissues throughout the body. Sympathetic receptors (alpha and beta) and parasympathetic receptors (muscarinic and nicotinic) determine the functional characteristics of the ANS and serve as a basis for neuropharmacologic intervention.

Drugs cause a variety of responses in the ANS. Some drugs have a broad stimulating or inhibiting effect on all receptors within a particular division of the ANS. Other drugs have a selective effect on only one receptor.

REFERENCES

1. Fong, E., Ferris, E., & Shelly, E. (1989). The peripheral and autonomic nervous system. In *Body Structures and Functions* (7th ed.). Albany, NY: Delmar.
2. Guyton, A.C. (1992). *Human physiology and mechanisms of disease* (5th ed.). Philadelphia: W.B. Saunders.
3. Guyton, A.C. (1991). *Textbook of medical physiology* (8th ed.). Philadelphia: W.B. Saunders.
4. Hole, J.E. (1993). *Human anatomy and physiology* (6th ed.). Dubuque, Iowa: Wm. C. Brown.
5. Seeley, R., Stephens, T., & Tate, P. (1992). *Anatomy and physiology* (2nd ed.). St. Louis: Mosby–Year Book.
6. McCance, K., & Huether, S. (1990). Overview of the autonomic system. In *Pathophysiology: The biologic basis for disease in adults and children*. St. Louis: C.V. Mosby.

7. Tortora, G., & Grabowski, S. (1993). *Principles of anatomy and physiology* (7th ed.). New York: Harper Collins.

8. Herlihy, B.L., & Herlihy, J.T. (1991). Cholinergic receptors. *Crticial Care Nurse, 10*(6), 82-83.

9. Manabe, N., Foldes, F.F., Totesik, A., Nagashima, H., Goldiner, P.L., & Vizi, E.S. (1991). Presynaptic interaction between vagal and sympathetic innervation in the heart: Modulation of acetylcholine and noradrenaline release. *Journal of the Autonomic Nervous System, 32,* 233-242.

10. Bennett, B., & Jacob, L. (1987). The autonomic nervous system: Anatomy and effects of stimulation. *Emergency Care Quarterly, 3*(2), 1-9.

11. Lehne, R. (1994). *Pharmacology for nursing care* (2nd ed.). Philadelphia: W.B. Saunders.

12. Smith, C.M., & Reynard, A.M. (1992). *Textbook of pharmacology.* Philadelphia: W.B. Saunders.

13. Goodman, R., Gilman, E., Rall, T., Nies, A., & Taylor, P. (Eds.) (1990). *Goodman and Gilman's: The pharmacological basis of therapeutics* (8th ed.). New York: Pergamon Press.

BIBLIOGRAPHY

Bannister, R. (1990). The diagnosis and treatment of autonomic failure. *Journal of the Autonomic Nervous System, 30,* 19-24.

Claustre, J., Pequignot, J.M., Bui-Xuan, B., Muchada, R., Cottel-Emard, R.M., & Peyrin, L. (1990). Conjugation and deamination of circulating dopamine: Relationship between sulfated and free dopamine in man. *Journal of the Autonomic Nervous System, 29,* 175-182.

Hatch, J.P., Borcherding, S., & German, C. (1992). Cardiac sympathetic activity during self-regulation of heart period. *Biofeedback and Self-Regulation, 17*(2), 89-106.

Johannessen, K.A., Cerqueira, M., Veith, R.C., & Stratton, J.R. (1991). Influence of sympathetic stimulation and parasympathetic withdrawal on Doppler echocardiographic left ventricular diastolic filling velocities in young normal subjects. *American Journal of Cardiology, 67,* 520-526.

Malliani, A., Lombardi, F., Pagani, M., & Cerutti, S. (1990). The neural regulation of circulation explored in the frequency domain. *Journal of the Autonomic Nervous System, 30,* 103-108.

Marley, W.S. (1991). *AANA Journal* course: New technologies in anesthesia: Update for nurse anesthetists—clonidine: An established drug with futuristic indications. *AANA Journal, Anesthetists 59*(2), 161-170.

CHAPTER 26

DRUGS AFFECTING THE

Parasympathetic Nervous System

JOAN DOMIGAN WENTZ

⚙ Neurotransmitters and Receptor Sites

LEARNING OBJECTIVE: Describe the neurotransmitters and receptors found in the parasympathetic nervous system.

KEY TERMS:

Acetylcholine, cholinergic, muscarinic receptors, nicotinic receptors

⚙ Antimuscarinic Drugs

LEARNING OBJECTIVES:

Describe the physiologic response of the body to antimuscarinic drugs.

List four therapeutic uses for these drugs.

Identify two contraindications for the use of antimuscarinic drugs.

Explain the rationale for four major undesired clinical responses associated with these drugs.

Outline a plan of care for a client receiving antimuscarinic drugs.

Summarize essential information about the prototype drug atropine.

KEY TERMS:

Anticholinergic, cycloplegia, impotence, parasympatholytic, xerostomia

⚙ Ganglionic Blockers

LEARNING OBJECTIVE: Discuss the therapeutic uses of ganglionic blockers.

⚙ Parasympathomimetic Drugs

LEARNING OBJECTIVES:

Describe the physiologic response of the body to parasympathomimetic drugs.

List four therapeutic uses for these drugs.

Identify two contraindications for use of parasympathomimetic drugs.

Explain the rationale for four major undesired clinical responses associated with these drugs.

Outline a plan of care for a client receiving parasympathomimetic drugs.

Distinguish between direct-acting and indirect-acting parasympathomimetic drugs.

Summarize essential information about the prototype drug for each subclassification.

KEY TERMS:

Acetylcholinesterase, cholinergic crisis, chronotropic, inotropic, miosis, myasthenia crisis, myopia, pseudocholinesterase

⚙ Ganglionic Stimulants

LEARNING OBJECTIVE: Discuss the therapeutic uses of ganglionic stimulants.

---

*T*his chapter focuses on drugs that affect the parasympathetic branch of the autonomic nervous system (ANS). These drugs are divided into two major groups: drugs that stimulate or mimic the parasympathetic nervous system (PNS) and drugs that suppress or block the PNS. When drugs inhibit the effects of the PNS, the sympathetic nervous system dominates and vice versa.

NEUROTRANSMITTERS AND RECEPTOR SITES

Acetylcholine (ACh) is the preganglionic and postganglionic neurotransmitter for the PNS. Fibers that secrete ACh are called **cholinergic;** therefore the parasympathetic division is called the *cholinergic system.* There are two types of cholinergic receptors, muscarinic and nicotinic.

Muscarinic receptor sites are found mainly on smooth muscle, cardiac muscle, and certain glands (i.e., salivary, mucous, gastric, lacrimal, and sweat). **Nicotinic receptor** sites are found primarily on skeletal muscle. The type of receptor site stimulated, muscarinic or nicotinic, determines the response of the organ.[1] Recently research has identified five subclassifications of muscarinic receptors and two subclassifications of nicotinic receptors.[2] However, these subclassifications are not addressed in this chapter.

Traditionally, drugs that mimic PNS activity have been labeled *parasympathomimetic* or *cholinergic drugs.* Drugs that block parasympathetic activity have been referred to as *parasympatholytic, anticholinergic,* or *cholinergic blockers.* Because knowledge of the ANS is expanding, the classification of autonomic drugs has changed. Currently, drugs that affect ACh are classified as **muscarinic** or **antimuscarinic** and **nicotinic** or **antinicotinic,** according to end-organ response. This classification more clearly and accurately describes the action of the drug, promoting greater understanding of drug uses and adverse reactions.

ANTIMUSCARINIC DRUGS

Antimuscarinic drugs have a relatively specific effect at muscarinic receptors to block the effect of ACh and related agonists. The drugs in this group are sometimes referred to as **parasympatholytic** or **anticholinergic** drugs.

Pharmacotherapeutics

Antimuscarinics have a variety of effects on the body; therefore they are used in the treatment of many disorders. For example, these drugs are used to decrease salivary and mucous secretions before surgery. They are also used to prevent or reduce reflex bradycardia associated with excessive vagal stimulation during the induction stage of anesthesia and tracheal intubation and to reduce laryngospasm during intubation. Anti-muscarinic drugs are used to diminish spasms of the urinary or biliary tract, to reduce the discomfort of colds, allergies, and motion sickness, and to increase the heart rate. They are also used as antidotes for several drug groups (e.g., cholinergics, anticholinesterase drugs, parasympathomimetics, and skeletal muscle relaxants).

Pharmacodynamics

Antimuscarinic drugs compete with ACh for muscarinic receptor sites. In the presence of these drugs, ACh is unable to bind to muscarinic receptor sites and produce an effect. Tissues most sensitive to antimuscarinics are the salivary, bronchial, and sweat glands. Other sites include the gastric parietal cells, the eye, smooth muscle of the gastrointestinal (GI), biliary, and genitourinary (GU) tracts, and cardiac muscle.

As previously noted, antimuscarinic drugs are used to treat a variety of medical disorders. How can one group of drugs affect so many different conditions? A review of other physiologic responses produced by antimuscarinics helps clarify this point. Although some clients experience sedative and general depressant effects from these drugs, most antimuscarinics have no obvious effects on the **central nervous system (CNS).** Antimuscarinics do alter the muscarinic-cholinergic transmissions associated with vestibular disturbances. These conditions such as motion or sea sickness respond well to antimuscarinic drugs. Clients with Parkinson's disease also respond to antimuscarinic drugs. The tremors and rigidity associated with Parkinson's disease probably result from an excess of cholinergic activity and a deficiency of dopamine in the basal ganglia. Thus a combination of an antimuscarinic with a dopamine-like drug usually provides an effective therapeutic approach. Antimuscarinics are also effective for treating organophosphate poisoning. Organophosphate agents (e.g., insecticides) are often muscarinic agonists that increase the amount of ACh at the synapse by inhibiting acetylcholinesterase (AChE).

The effects on the **cardiovascular system** vary. An initial slowing of the heart occurs after small doses or the initial dose of antimuscarinics. The slowing is minor, 4 to 8 beats per minute, and unimportant unless the client already has bradycardia. After the slowing period, blockade of the muscarinic receptors of the heart produces an increase in the heart rate. The increase in rate is more pronounced, 30 to 40 beats per minute, in young adults in whom vagal tone is most marked. Antimuscarinic drugs also increase the conduction velocity between the atria and the ventricles. These drugs have no significant effect on systemic blood pressure since parasympathetic innervation of the resistance and capacitance vessels is lacking.[3]

The **respiratory** and **GU systems** are also affected by these drugs. Antimuscarinics relax bronchial smooth muscle and produce bronchodilation. In addition, they act on bronchial mucous glands to decrease mucous production. In the GU sys-

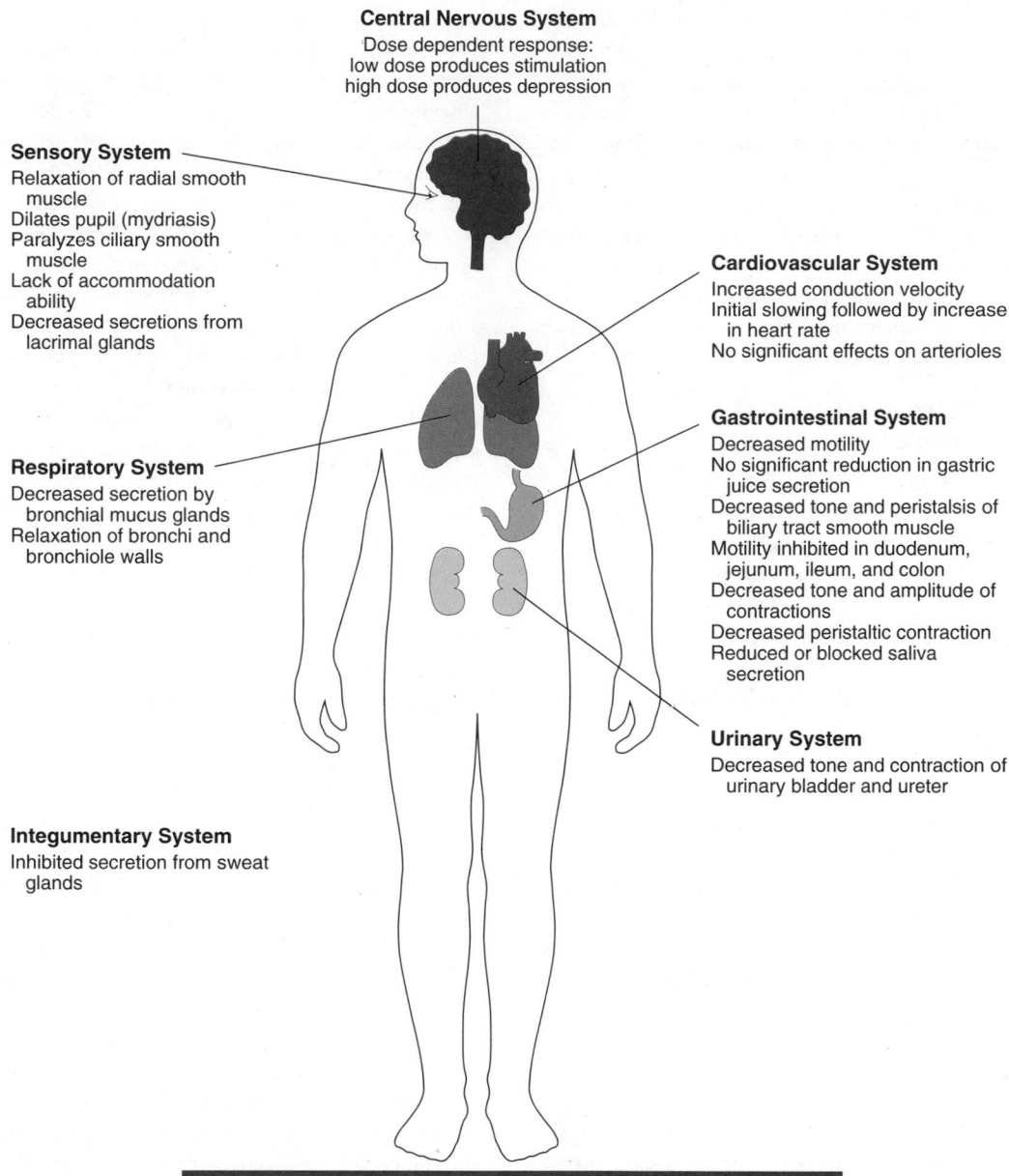

Central Nervous System
Dose dependent response:
low dose produces stimulation
high dose produces depression

Sensory System
Relaxation of radial smooth
  muscle
Dilates pupil (mydriasis)
Paralyzes ciliary smooth
  muscle
Lack of accommodation
  ability
Decreased secretions from
  lacrimal glands

Cardiovascular System
Increased conduction velocity
Initial slowing followed by increase
  in heart rate
No significant effects on arterioles

Respiratory System
Decreased secretion by
  bronchial mucus glands
Relaxation of bronchi and
  bronchiole walls

Gastrointestinal System
Decreased motility
No significant reduction in gastric
  juice secretion
Decreased tone and peristalsis of
  biliary tract smooth muscle
Motility inhibited in duodenum,
  jejunum, ileum, and colon
Decreased tone and amplitude of
  contractions
Decreased peristaltic contraction
Reduced or blocked saliva
  secretion

Urinary System
Decreased tone and contraction of
  urinary bladder and ureter

Integumentary System
Inhibited secretion from sweat
  glands

FIGURE 26–1   Physiologic responses to antimuscarinic drugs.

tem these drugs relax the smooth muscle of the urinary bladder to produce urinary retention. These and other physiologic responses are depicted in Figure 26–1.[2,3]

Contraindications and Precautions

The use of antimuscarinic drugs is contraindicated in clients with hypersensitivity to anticholinergics, obstructed airway, obstructive disease of the GI or GU tract, or myasthenia gravis. They should be used with caution in clients with ulcerative colitis, hyperthyroidism, hepatic or renal disease, prostatic hypertrophy, esophageal reflux, or severe heart disease.[3]

Since antimuscarinics relax the radial and ciliary muscles of the eye, they close the canal of Schlemm. This prevents aqueous humor from flowing out of the anterior chamber, producing increased intraocular pressure. Therefore clients with an-

gle-closure glaucoma should never receive antimuscarinic drugs.

Since the heart rate of the client receiving antimuscarinics usually increases, antimuscarinics are contraindicated in clients with preexisting tachycardia or heart block. In addition, acute myocardial ischemia or infarction should be ruled out before administering these drugs since increasing the heart rate may worsen the ischemia and increase the zone of infarction.[2]

Undesired Clinical Responses

Some of the major side effects associated with antimuscarinic drugs include xerostomia, fever, heatstroke, flushing, thickened mucus, constipation, visual disturbance, urinary retention, and tachycardia. **Xerostomia,** dryness of the mouth, is produced by decreased salivary production. This condition can cause considerable discomfort for the client. Because antimuscarinics diminish the body's ability to perspire and cool itself, individuals receiving these drugs are prone to **heatstroke,** a condition in which the body retains excessive body heat. If this occurs, immediate emergency treatment is required.

Some clients experience depression and/or drowsiness from antimuscarinic drugs. Male clients receiving these drugs may experience **impotence,** the inability to achieve or maintain an erection. This condition usually produces psychologic trauma for the client, and some clients may stop taking the drug in an attempt to correct the situation.[3-6]

Drug-Drug, Drug-Nutrient, Drug-Environment Interactions

Many over-the-counter (OTC) products, particularly antihistamines and antidiarrheal drugs, contain low doses of antimuscarinic agents. Taking prescribed antimuscarinic drugs in conjunction with the OTC drugs can produce undesired clinical responses. Alcohol intake should be reduced while the client is receiving antimuscarinic drugs since it accelerates metabolism of the drugs.

Prescription drugs such as phenobarbital, antacids, antiarrhythmics, digoxin, and monoamine oxidase (MAO) inhibitors also cause problems when administered concurrently with antimuscarinics. MAO inhibitors enhance antimuscarinic effects. These drugs should be discontinued at least 10 days before starting antimuscarinic therapy whenever possible. Phenobarbital stimulates the liver's ability to metabolize drugs; this can lead to significant drug interactions. Antacids block antimuscarinic effects and should be administered 1 hour before or after the antimuscarinic drugs. In addition, antimuscarinics increase the rate and extent of digoxin absorption. If the client is receiving digoxin, monitor the serum digoxin level and assess the client for manifestations of digoxin toxicity.[2]

Food interferes with the absorption of oral antimuscarinics. In addition, many of the synthetic antimuscarinic drugs are prepared in slow-release or extended-action dosage forms. These drugs must not be crushed nor mixed with food or a beverage before administration.

Antimuscarinic drugs also produce drug-environment interactions. These drugs should not be administered to clients exposed to high environmental temperatures. In addition, the drugs must be protected from excessive moisture and light.

Life-Span Considerations

Antimuscarinic drugs must be used with caution in clients over 40 years of age or infants and small children. Doses for these individuals are usually reduced. In the elderly antimuscarinic intoxication causes memory loss and mental confusion.

▦ NURSING CONSIDERATIONS

Since most antimuscarinic drugs produce similar effects, many nursing interventions are also alike. As with any client, care is

administered within the framework of the nursing process.

Assessing   You should begin your care by conducting a thorough health history and physical assessment. During the **assessment interview,** determine if the client has any preexisting conditions such as glaucoma, hyperthyroidism, myasthenia gravis, or prostatic hypertrophy that would contraindicate the use of antimuscarinic drugs. Ask the client if any respiratory disorder exists. Does he or she experience shortness of breath? Does he or she have a cough? If a cough exists, is it productive? Ask the client to describe the color, consistency, and amount of any bronchial secretions. Determine the client's usual bowel and bladder patterns. If constipation exists, it must be corrected before drug therapy is begun.

A drug history is important. Determine what prescribed drugs the client is receiving. Are any of these drugs contraindicated when receiving antimuscarinics? Ask the client to describe methods used to treat cold symptoms. Does he or she use OTC cold remedies?

During the **physical assessment,** focus on the physiologic function of several body systems. As with all assessments, determine the client's blood pressure and pulse. An apical pulse helps you detect preexisting arrhythmias. Assess the client's temperature carefully. Since antimuscarinic drugs limit the body's ability to sweat and reduce elevated body temperatures, the presence of a febrile condition is significant.

In addition to determining the usual respiratory rate, auscultate lung sounds. Note the presence of abnormal breath sounds—crackles, wheezes, gurgles. (Remember that these drugs will decrease and thicken mucous secretion from the bronchial glands.)

If the client is scheduled to receive antimuscarinic drugs for the treatment of Parkinson's disease, determine the client's range of motion and ability to ambulate. To evaluate muscle strength, have the client perform active range-of-motion movements as you apply resistance. Note the strength that the client exerts against resistance.

Assess for the presence of any urinary tract infections. Note the color, odor, and appearance of the urine. Auscultate bowel sounds. Normal peristaltic sounds occur every 5 to 15 seconds. If the client has diminished bowel sound before drug therapy, the probability of constipation increases.

Diagnosing   After data collection, nursing diagnoses are formulated. These diagnoses may include the following:
- Constipation related to decreased bowel tone and motility associated with drug therapy.
- Altered oral mucous membranes related to decreased salivation.
- Impaired swallowing related to decreased salivation.
- Ineffective airway clearance related to thickened tracheobronchial secretions.
- High risk for injury related to altered visual acuity (i.e., photophobia, diminished near vision).
- Ineffective thermoregulation, heatstroke, related to inability to perspire associated with drug therapy.
- Sexual dysfunction related to undesired clinical responses to drugs.
- Noncompliance with medical regimen related to undesired clinical responses to drugs.

Planning The planning phase of the nursing process involves developing individualized teaching and/or discharge plans. When developing your plans, remember the cognitive level of your client. Keep explanations of drug action simple. Most clients will not understand the terms *antimuscarinic* or *neurotransmitter*. Use terms appropriate for the client.

Educate the client about expected clinical responses. Some responses such as dry mouth, constipation, visual disturbances, dry skin, urinary hesitancy, gritty eyes, and drowsiness are expected. Teach the client how to minimize these effects. For example, teach the client to increase fluid and fiber in the diet to relieve constipation; to perform frequent oral hygiene to lessen the dry mouth; and to use skin moisturizers and lotions to ease dry skin.

Teach the client which responses are considered more serious and therefore should not be ignored. Instruct the client to report the following responses immediately to the health care provider:

- Ocular pain after administration of the drug, which could indicate undiagnosed glaucoma
- Major or sudden changes in bowel function, which could suggest a possible bowel obstruction
- Symptoms of heatstroke: initial profuse perspiration followed by insufficient perspiration to maintain temperature within normal limits; hot, dry, flushed skin; dizziness; fainting; and a steady raising of core temperature
- Wheezing or dyspnea, especially in clients with small airway disease—could indicate mucous plugging
- Significant changes in heart rate or rhythm

Drug toxicity is usually avoided by taking the drug as prescribed. If a dose is missed, advise the client to take it as soon as possible. If it is almost time for the next dose, instruct the client not to double the dose but take only the single dose amount. Client should also be instructed to keep antimuscarinic drugs in the original tightly closed, light-resistant container. The drugs should be stored away from moisture and direct light.

Determine if the client is familiar with eyedrop administration. (If teaching in this area is required, follow the procedure described in Chapter 64.) To diminish systemic effects of the drug, teach the client to apply gentle pressure over the lacrimal duct for 1 to 2 minutes immediately after the eyedrops are instilled. This action prevents absorption of the drug by nasal mucosa. Next, instruct the client to close the eyelid gently and roll the eye within the socket to distribute the drug evenly. Eyedrops should be spaced at least 2 to 10 minutes apart to obtain the greatest possible therapeutic effect. Tell the client to begin ophthalmic administration in the evening. If ocular side effects occur, they will not interfere with the days' activities. If eye pain develops after the administration of the eyedrops, instruct the client to notify the health care provider immediately.

Provide the client with a list of OTC drugs or drug categories to avoid while receiving antimuscarinics. Also, suggest alternative drugs to manage colds or allergies. In addition, emphasize the importance of follow-up visits for a client receiving antimuscarinic drug therapy. Often the drug dose will need modification.

During the planning phase, expected outcomes or outcome criteria are established. They reflect the nursing diagnoses and, when possible, are developed with the client. Possible expected outcomes include the following:

- Client maintains airway patency.
- Client maintains normal patterns of bowel functioning.
- Client remains free of injury.
- Client participates in the development of a treatment plan.
- Client reports a decrease in symptoms (dry mouth).
- Client maintains body temperature within normal limits.
- Client verbalizes knowledge of sexual limitations that have occurred.

Implementing Since food interferes with the absorption of oral antimuscarinics, these drugs should be administered 1 hour before meals. Antacids should also be administered 1 hour before or after administering antimuscarinic drugs. A client concurrently receiving antiarrhythmics is at greater risk of developing tachycardia. If the client is receiving digoxin, digoxin toxicity is a possibility. These clients will need frequent cardiac assessments.

Much of the nursing care involved with these drugs is focused on relieving the discomfort associated with drug side effects. Table 26–1 provides a summary of the major undesired clinical responses and related nursing considerations.

If antimuscarinic toxicity develops, anticipate that gastric lavage or induced emesis will be part of the treatment plan. In addition, activated charcoal and saline solution cathartics are administered to inactivate the drug and promote its elimination. To counteract the effects of the antimuscarinic drugs, you may be directed to administer intravenous (IV) physostigmine (Antilirium). Physostigmine is often used when CNS symptoms such as delirium and coma are present. This drug has a short duration of action. It must be administered slowly, or it produces seizures, profound bradycardia, or heart block. Expected responses to physostigmine are the result of increased ACh attaching to muscarinic receptors. These responses include increased salivation and sweating, increased bowel sounds, normalization of heart rate, and improved level of consciousness (LOC).[5]

Evaluating Since there are no laboratory tests that measure therapeutic levels of the drugs, evaluation of antimuscarinic effectiveness depends on the response of the client. You must assess for disappearance of signs and symptoms (e.g., increase in pulse rate). You would also assess for the absence of undesired clinical responses. During the evaluation phase, review the expected outcomes with the client. Determine if the outcomes were met. If they were not, determine what in the plan of care needs changing.

ANTIMUSCARINIC PROTOTYPE
ATROPINE SULFATE

Atropine sulfate is the oldest antimuscarinic and is obtained from the deadly nightshade plant. During the Renaissance period, dilated pupils were considered attractive. To achieve this effect, women chewed the nightshade plant—hence the name *belladonna,* Italian for "beautiful lady."

TABLE 26–1

Antimuscarinic Drugs: Major Undesired Clinical Responses and Related Nursing Considerations

Undesired Clinical Response	Nursing Considerations
Xerostomia (dryness of the mouth from salivary dysfunction)	Provide fluids on a regular basis. Offer ice chips or sugarless, hard candy. Water pic teeth for cleansing purposes. Avoid use of alcohol-based mouthwash. Use lip balm. Use artificial saliva if appropriate.
Fever Heatstroke Flushing	Teach client to: • Avoid prolonged exposure to warm environments. • Wear cottons and wools. • Avoid unnecessary physical exertion, especially in hot weather. • Move slowly. • Stay in the shade when outside. • Wear loose, light clothing. • Stay in air conditioning as much as possible. Offer cool, tepid baths. Monitor body temperature. Provide frequent sponge baths. Provide oscillating fan.
Thickened mucus	Assess for patent airway. Assess lung sounds. Increase oral fluid intake if not contraindicated. Have suction equipment available. Be prepared to administer oxygen.
Diminished near vision Photophobia Lack of pupil reaction to light	Orient client to surroundings. Elevate side rails. Maintain quiet environment. Use low lighting in room. Assist with ambulating activities. Use touch as comfort technique. Teach client to: • Avoid dangerous activities. • Wear sunglasses.
Urinary retention	Assess for voiding pattern. Palpate urinary bladder. Ask client if bladder feels full after voiding. Monitor intake and output. Teach client to: • Assume upright position for voiding. • Perform Credé's maneuver (manual expression of urine from bladder).
Constipation Ileus or failure of appropriate forward movement of bowel contents	Assess for bowel sounds. Determine bowel pattern. Provide high fiber diet (15-40 g/d). Increase oral fluid intake if not contraindicated. Encourage ambulation and/or daily exercise. Offer naturally occurring cathartics (e.g., prunes). Teach client to: • Respond to defecation urge. • Check with primary care provider regarding OTC stool softeners or bulk-forming laxatives.
Tachycardia	Palpate pedal pulses for quality. Palpate skin; should be warm and dry. Report changes in LOC. Report sustained heart rate >20 beats above baseline. Report urinary output <30 ml/h for 2-h period. Minimize activity. Provide quiet environment. Administer oxygen as ordered.
Impotence	Provide privacy during sexual assessment. Determine history of impotence. Allow client opportunity to express feelings. Provide sexual counseling if appropriate. Discuss changing drug with primary care provider.

TABLE 26–1 *Continued*

Antimuscarinic Drugs: Major Undesired Clinical Responses and Related Nursing Considerations

Undesired Clinical Response	Nursing Considerations
Depression	Assess for decreased LOC.
	Observe closely for mood changes.
	Establish trusting relationship.
	Plan for brief, nontask-oriented interactions.
	Use diversionary techniques.
Drowsiness	Raise side rails.
	Assist with ambulation if appropriate.

Atropine is an organic ester of tropic acid and tropine. This alkaloid is isolated from *Atropa belladonna.* Because of the nonspecific action of atropine alkaloids on muscarinic receptors, a large number of synthetic substances have been developed.[3]

Pharmacotherapeutics Atropine has several uses in addition to those discussed in the earlier general section on pharmacotherapeutics. This drug is used to treat **symptomatic sinus bradycardia** and associated frequent **ventricular ectopic beats.** Atropine is also used for treating **ventricular asystole** when there is a possibility of undetected, fine ventricular fibrillation. The drug is particularly useful when **arrhythmias** result from anesthetic, choline ester, or succinylcholine therapy.[4–6]

Atropine is used to produce **mydriasis** (pupil dilation) and **cycloplegia** (paralysis of neural control of ciliary muscle) for examination of the eye and accurate measurement of ocular pressures. In the past atropine was used to treat a wide variety of **GI disorders** such as peptic ulcer disease, irritable bowel syndrome, and spastic colon. In clients with peptic ulcer disease atropine blocks the vagal stimulus, decreasing hydrochloric acid and pepsin secretion. Currently, atropine is used only if the newer drugs are not successful. Atropine is also used as a GI relaxant during diagnostic procedures such as endoscopy.

Atropine is the drug of choice as an antidote to edrophonium chloride (Tensilon), an anticholinesterase drug. During the Tensilon test, which is used to diagnose myasthenia gravis, an IV bolus dose of Tensilon is administered. This causes an increase in the amount of ACh at the synapse. If too much Tensilon is administered, a cholinergic crisis results, and atropine is administered.[3,4]

Pharmacokinetics Atropine is easily absorbed orally, parenterally, and topically from the eye. Protein binding varies and ranges from 2% to 40%. The drug is widely distributed throughout the body, crossing the blood-brain and placental barriers. Most of the drug is metabolized by the liver; the remainder is excreted unchanged by the kidneys.[4–6]

Onset of action occurs 5 to 50 minutes after intramuscular (IM) administration. After oral administration, peak action occurs in 1 to 2 hours. The half-life of the drug is 2 to 6 hours. Duration of therapeutic effect, regardless of route of administration, is 5 hours. However, some therapeutic effects may last up to 1 week.[3,7]

Pharmacodynamics The pharmacodynamics of atropine are the same as those described in the general section on antimuscarinic drugs. One aspect that needs emphasis is the relationship between dosage and responses to antimuscarinics. Not all muscarinic receptors are equally sensitive to blockade by atropine. At some sites, muscarinic receptors are blocked with low doses of antimuscarinic drugs. At other sites, much higher doses are needed to produce blockade.[3,9]

Pharmaceutics Atropine is administered parenterally (IV, IM, and subcutaneous [SC]). It is also administered via aerosol and endotracheal instillation.

Undesired Clinical Responses In addition to the undesired clinical responses discussed in the general section, headache, leukocytosis, restlessness, dizziness, palpitations, and insomnia can occur. Atropine intoxication exhibits a characteristic syndrome. These signs and symptoms are due to an excessive blockade of muscarinic receptors so that normal organ function is disrupted. The manifestations include the following:

1. Extremely dry mouth, dry upper respiratory tract, and dry skin ("dry as a bone")
2. Blushing due to vasodilation of the cutaneous blood vessels in the blush areas of the body ("red as a beet")
3. Diminished visual acuity due to pupil dilation ("blind as a bat")
4. Elevation of body temperature ("hot as a furnace")
5. Hallucinations, bizarre behavior, confusion, delirium, and disturbance of memory ("mad as a hatter")[2,7]

Drug-Drug, Drug-Nutrient, Drug-Environment Interactions Atropine should not be combined in the same syringe with other drugs unless you determine the drugs are compatible. Atropine is not compatible with diazepam (Valium), epinephrine, furosemide (Lasix), heparin, methyldopa (Aldomet), metaraminol (Aramine), or phenytoin (Dilantin).[10]

Life-Span Considerations Since atropine enters breast milk, its use in nursing mothers is controversial. Although not strictly contraindicated, atropine use should be avoided unless absolutely necessary. Infants, children, and elderly clients are especially susceptible to atropine intoxication. Usual dosages are reduced in these individuals.

Specific Drug-Related Nursing Considerations Because of the cardiac effect of atropine, vital signs are monitored frequently with particular attention to the pulse and blood pressure. When atropine is used for eye examinations, instruct the client to wear sunglasses since pupils are unable to constrict fully in response to sunlight. If the examination is done in a primary care setting, advise the client not to drive while the pupil is still dilated. Suggest that a friend or family member provide transportation for the client.

After administration of atropine for GI conditions, monitor the client for frequency of bowel movements. Also, when the GI tract is slowed, there may be en-

TABLE 26–2
Antimuscarinic Drugs: Prototype and Major Drugs in Category

Drug Name	Dosage and Route of Administration	Nursing Considerations
ATROPINE SULFATE (Atrupair, Atropen, Atropine, etc.) HOW SUPPLIED IM, IV, SC: 0.05, 0.1, 0.4, and 1 mg/ml Tablets: 0.4, 0.6 mg	*Preoperative Medication* ADULTS IM: 0.4-0.6 mg, 45-60 min before anesthesia CHILDREN IM: 0.01 mg/kg to a maximum of 0.4 mg 45-60 min before anesthesia *Symptomatic Bradycardia* ADULTS IV or endotracheal: 0.4-1 mg after dilution in 10 ml of normal saline solution; repeat in 5 min; max: 2 mg CHILDREN IV: 0.01 mg/kg to a maximum of 0.4 mg; may repeat q4-6h *Antidote for Anticholinesterase Insecticide Poisoning* ADULTS IV or IM: 2-6 mg; may repeat every hour until symptoms resolved *Treatment of GI disorders* ADULTS Oral: 0.04-0.6 mg q4-6h CHILDREN Oral: 0.01 mg/kg q4-6h; not to exceed 0.4 mg total dose	*Assess* Determine baseline pulse rate. Assess if client is receiving MAO inhibitors, antacids, digoxin, or antiarrhythmic drugs. Assess client for preexisting obstructed airway, myasthenia gravis, intestinal atony, and obstructive disease of GI tract. Assess degree of visual acuity. *Implement* Keep cardiac monitoring equipment, suction equipment, and oxygen available. Keep physostigmine available to treat overdose. Provide ice chips and/or hard, sugarless candy for dry mouth. Obtain order for nonsteroidal analgesic if atropine headache occurs. Provide frequent mouth care. Instruct client to request assistance when ambulating. Advise client to avoid injurious activities. Increase fiber and fluid intake unless contraindicated; if preventive measures do not work, get order for stool softener or laxative. *Monitor* Monitor pulse rate; report rate >20 above baseline. Monitor bowel sounds and bowel elimination pattern. Assess client for undesired clinical responses such as fever, flushing, thickened mucus, constipation, urinary retention, visual disturbances, impotence, depression, and tachycardia. *Evaluate* Observe for desired result of drug administration (e.g., increased strength). See atropine sulfate with the following exceptions: Assess for CNS sedation.
Scopolamine Hydrobromide HOW SUPPLIED IM, IV, SC: 0.3-1 mg/ml	*Preanesthetic sedation* ADULTS Parenteral: 0.3-0.6 mg diluted solution CHILDREN Parenteral: 0.6 µg/kg	See atropine sulfate with the following exceptions: Assess for CNS sedation.
Glycopyrrolate (Robinul) HOW SUPPLIED IM, IV: 0.2 mg/ml Uncoated tablets: 1, 2 mg *Dicyclomine Hydrochloride* (Bentyl, Antispas, Benomine, etc.)	*Preanesthesia* ADULTS 0.004 mg/kg 30-60 min before surgery CHILDREN >2 YEARS OF AGE Same as adult See Chapter 47.	See atropine sulfate with the following exceptions: Instruct client to avoid high environmental temperature. No known major drug interactions.

TABLE 26–2 *Continued*
Antimuscarinic Drugs: Prototype and Major Drugs in Category

Drug Name	Dosage and Route of Administration	Nursing Considerations
Hyoscyamine Sulfate (Anaspaz, Levsin, Cystospaz, Donna-mar, etc.)	See Chapter 47.	
Propantheline Bromide (Pro-Banthine, Probamide)	See Chapter 47.	
Homatropine Hydrobromide (Isopto Homatropine, Homatropine Hbr Ophthalmic, etc.)	See Chapter 64.	
Trihexyphenidyl Hydrochloride (Artane, Trihexane, Trihexidyl Tremen, etc.)	See Chapter 23.	
Benztropine Mesylate (Cogentin, etc.)	See Chapter 23.	

hanced absorption of other drugs because of the prolonged transit time. Clients should be montiored for side effects of those drugs. Table 26–2 includes information on atropine and other drugs in this category.

Miscellaneous Drugs in Category

The other major belladonna alkaloid is **scopolamine hydrobromide.** This drug is an organic ester of tropic acid and scopine and is isolated from *Scopolia carniolica* and *Hyoscyamus niger*.[3] Like atropine, it belongs to the belladonna alkaloid group of muscarinic antagonists.

In most respects the pharmacologic actions of scopolamine are identical to those of atropine. However, these drugs differ in their effects on the CNS. Therapeutic doses of scopolamine produce sedation, whereas therapeutic doses of atropine produce excitation. Scopolamine also acts on the CNS to suppress emesis and motion sickness.[9]

Because of its effects on the CNS, scopolamine is used as a sedative and to treat motion sickness. It is also used as a preanesthetic drug and for obstetric amnesia. Scopolamine is available in sterile solution for injection (IV, IM, and SC). It is also available in an ophthalmic solution.[4]

There are numerous **belladonna alkaloid substitutes**. These newer antimuscarinic drugs, like the belladonna alkaloids, inhibit practically all muscarinic responses. Therefore the actions of these drugs are similar to those of the belladonna alkaloids. Many of these drugs are used to treat peptic disease and are addressed in Chapter 47.

CONCEPT REVIEW

Antimuscarinics act at muscarinic receptors to block the effects of ACh.

Antimuscarinic drugs are used to treat a variety of conditions, including spasms of the urinary and biliary tract, bradycardia, motion sickness, and Parkinson's disease.

Major side effects associated with these drugs include xerostomia, fever, heatstroke, flushing, thickened mucus, urinary retention, and constipation.

Many OTC drugs contain antimuscarinic ingredients.

Antimuscarinic toxicity is an emergency situation.

Treatment for antimuscarinic toxicity may include administration of IV fluids, induced emesis, gastric lavage, and administration of physostigmine.

Atropine sulfate is the prototype drug for this category.

GANGLIONIC BLOCKERS

Because of their lack of selectivity, the ganglionic blocking drugs are of limited clinical use. In the past ganglionic blockers were used to treat essential hypertension. However, since the development of newer, selective antihypertensive drugs, ganglionic blockers are seldom used for this purpose. These drugs are still used in the treatment of hypertensive crisis and the production of controlled hypotension. (Ganglionic blockers are discussed further in Chapter 33.)

PARASYMPATHOMIMETIC (MUSCARINIC AGONIST) DRUGS

Parasympathomimetic drugs mimic or stimulate the PNS. These drugs increase the concentration of ACh at the postganglionic muscarinic receptor sites of the effector organs. Parasympathomimetics usually elicit no response at nicotinic sites. However, when large doses of these drugs are administered, selectivity for muscarinic receptor sites is lost, and nicotinic receptor sites are stimulated.

Parasympathomimetic drugs are divided into direct-acting and indirect-acting subclassifications. Although the physiologic responses produced by these two groups are similar, the modes of action are completely different.

Physiologic Response to Parasympathomimetic Drugs

The presence of ACh at the muscarinic receptor sites produces a variety of physiologic responses. Within the **eye,** ACh stimulation causes contraction of the sphincter of the iris. As a result, **miosis,** or pupil constriction, occurs. Stimulation also contracts the ciliary muscle, causing the lens to thicken. This action permits the eye to focus on near objects more easily (nearsightedness or **myopia**). These changes within the eye stretch the trabecular network of the eye, opening the route to the canal of Schlemm. As a result, aqueous humor escapes from the anterior chamber, and intraocular pressure is reduced.

The major effects on the **cardiovascular system** are a reduction in peripheral vascular resistance and changes in heart activity. ACh decreases the heart rate. This decrease in heart rate is called a negative **chronotropic** effect. It also slows the rate of conduction through the atrioventricular (AV) node and decreases the force of myocardial contraction. The decrease in ventricular force is called a negative **inotropic** effect. In addition, automaticity in the Purkinje fibers is suppressed, decreasing the possibility of ventricular fibrillation.[1,5]

Arteries and veins are **not** innervated by the PNS. Therefore when PNS stimulation occurs, there is no response by these structures. However, there are muscarinic receptors in the arteries and veins that respond to ACh derivatives administered exogenously. When stimulated, these muscarinic receptors cause vasodilation and a decrease in peripheral vascular resistance. With the decrease in peripheral vascular resistance, a chain of events occurs. Initially, hypotension develops. It then stimulates the baroreceptors in the aorta and carotid arteries. The baroreceptors initiate reflex tachycardia to maintain adequate cardiac output.

Within the **respiratory system,** muscarinic receptor site stimulation causes increased bronchial smooth muscle tone and decreased bronchial diameter. In some instances bronchospasms occur. In addition, the stimulation of mucous-producing glands results in the production of excessive thin, watery bronchial secretions.

When muscarinic receptors in the **GI tract** are stimulated, peristaltic activity increases. In addition, various sphincters along the GI tract relax, and GI secretions increase. For example, the parietal cells of the stomach are stimulated to secrete hydrochloric acid. The pancreatic and small intestinal glands are also stimulated but to a lesser extent.

In the **urinary tract** urethral peristalsis increases, the detrusor muscle in the urinary bladder contracts, and the trigone and external sphincter relax. ACh stimulation does not increase urinary production but improves the urinary elimination process. Glands of the **exocrine system** are also affected. Sweat, salivary, and lacrimal secretions are all increased.[2,6,7] These physiologic responses are depicted in Figure 26–2.

Once stimulation of the muscarinic receptor sites is initiated by ACh, what terminates or stops the process? AChE, an enzyme present at synapses, catalyzes the hydrolysis of ACh to choline and acetic acid. Without AChE, ACh would continue to accumulate. An increased concentration of ACh at the muscarinic receptor sites results in exaggeration of the responses produced by the effector organs.

Contraindications and Precautions

Parasympathomimetic drugs are contraindicated in a variety of situations. Clients with asthma or other small airway disease should not receive these drugs since they enhance bronchoconstriction. Since these drugs decrease the heart rate and force of cardiac contraction, they are contraindicated in clients with conditions such as bradycardia, coronary insufficiency, hypotension, or myocardial infarction. They also should not be used with clients with obstructive intestinal or urinary tract disease.

▧ NURSING CONSIDERATIONS

The basis of effective nursing care of clients receiving parasympathomimetic drugs is an understanding of the PNS. The care is built on the five steps of the nursing process: assessment, diagnosis, planning, implementation, and evaluation.

Assessing During the **health history,** assess for any preexisting condition that would contraindicate the use of parasympathomimetic drugs. For example, these drugs are used with caution in individuals with hyperthyroidism, asthma, emphysema, allergies, or a history of seizures.

Determine if the client has a history of coronary insufficiency, heart block, congestive heart failure (CHF), or atherosclerosis. Since parasympathomimetic drugs produce negative chronotropic and inotropic effects, extreme care must be used when administering them to a client with CHF. If the client is receiving cardiac drugs such as quinidine sulfate, particular caution must be exercised. Quinidine prolongs conduction through the AV node. When combined with parasympathomimetic drugs, heart block and/or hypotension can occur.

During the **physical assessment,** carefully assess the client's blood pressure, heart rate and rhythm, and status of peripheral pulses. Since bronchial narrowing occurs with parasympathomimetic drugs, a respiratory assessment is crucial. Auscultate the thorax for breath sounds and note the presence of congestion.

Before administration of parasympathomimetic drugs, assess the GI tract for obstruction. Auscultate the abdomen for bowel sounds. Note the pattern of bowel elimination and the appearance of the stool.

Diagnosing Several nursing diagnoses are appropriate for the client receiving parasympathomimetic drugs. However, you must analyze the client's data base to individualize the diagnoses:

- Sensory/perceptual alteration: visual disturbances related to pupil constriction.
- High risk for injury: physical, related to diminished visual acuity.

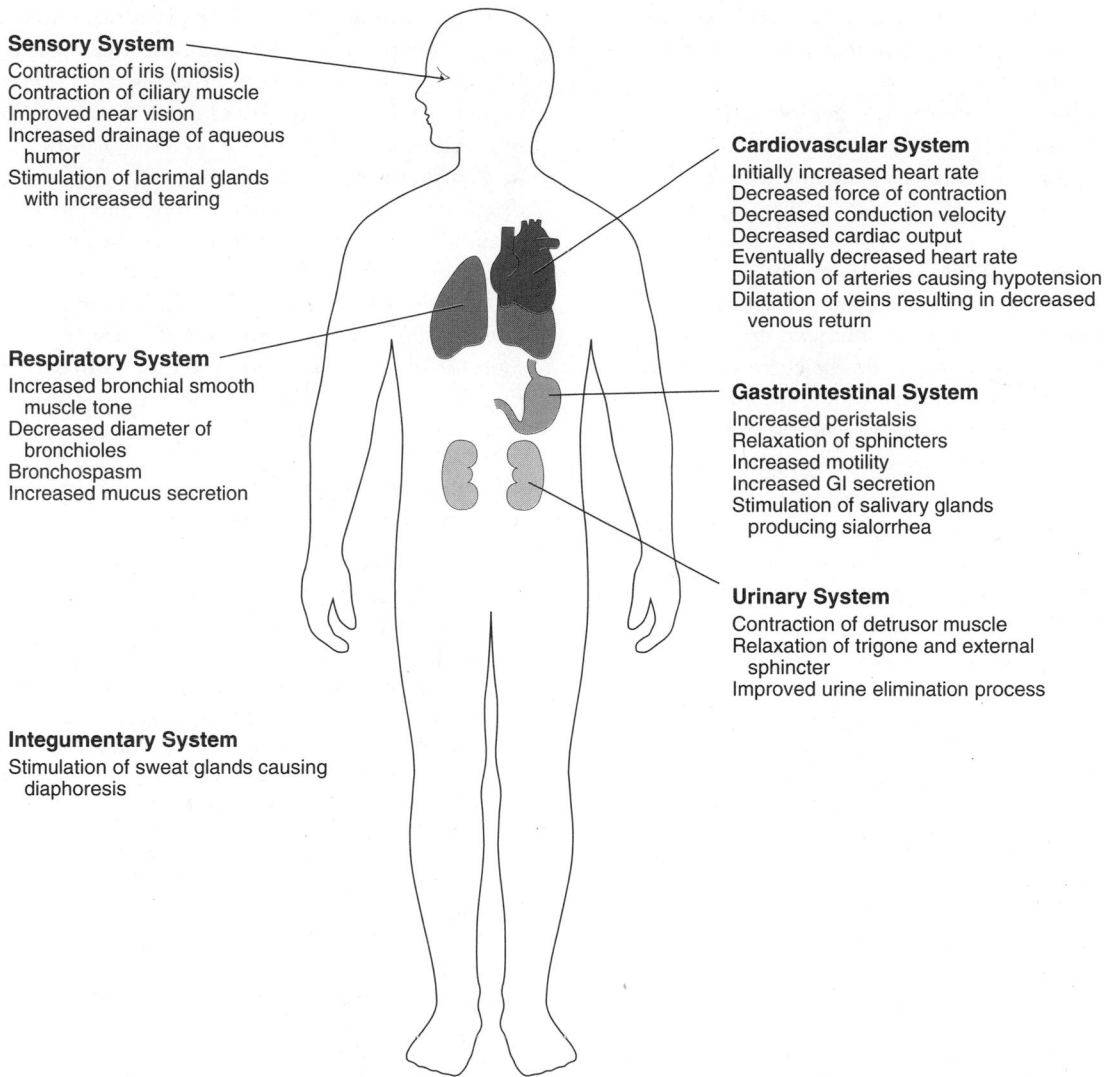

Sensory System
Contraction of iris (miosis)
Contraction of ciliary muscle
Improved near vision
Increased drainage of aqueous
    humor
Stimulation of lacrimal glands
    with increased tearing

Respiratory System
Increased bronchial smooth
    muscle tone
Decreased diameter of
    bronchioles
Bronchospasm
Increased mucus secretion

Integumentary System
Stimulation of sweat glands causing
    diaphoresis

Cardiovascular System
Initially increased heart rate
Decreased force of contraction
Decreased conduction velocity
Decreased cardiac output
Eventually decreased heart rate
Dilatation of arteries causing hypotension
Dilatation of veins resulting in decreased
    venous return

Gastrointestinal System
Increased peristalsis
Relaxation of sphincters
Increased motility
Increased GI secretion
Stimulation of salivary glands
    producing sialorrhea

Urinary System
Contraction of detrusor muscle
Relaxation of trigone and external
    sphincter
Improved urine elimination process

FIGURE 26–2   Physiologic responses associated with parasympathomimetic drugs.

- Impaired gas exchange related to narrowing of airways associated with drug therapy.
- Ineffective breathing patterns related to narrowing of airways and increased bronchial secretions associated with drug therapy.
- Ineffective airway clearance related to increased bronchial secretions associated with drug therapy.

Planning   If the client will be discharged home while taking a parasympathomimetic drug, teach the client about the action of the drug, expected effects, side effects, and dosage regimen. Instruct the client to take the drug on an empty stomach to avoid nausea and vomiting. Tell the client that some annoying side effects are expected, including increased salivation, sweating, abdominal discomfort, and/or flushing. If these symptoms become severe or incapacitating, tell the client to contact the health care provider.[12] Encourage the client to ingest a high-fiber diet to lessen the possibility of constipation.

Symptoms that should be reported immediately are chest pain, dizziness, diarrhea, or headaches, confusion, or seizures. (Headaches and confusion are caused by cerebral artery dilation.) Instruct the client to inform all health care providers that he or she is taking these drugs.[12]

Teach the client the importance of periodic eye examinations, including the measurement of intraocular pressure. Instruct the client to avoid activities that increase intraocular pressure such as straining at the time of defecation, lifting, bending, coughing, or sneezing.

Determine whether the client is familiar with eyedrop administration. If teaching in this area is required, follow the procedure described in the antimuscarinic section of this chapter and in Chapter 64. Inform the client that permanent eye damage is possible if the drugs are not taken as prescribed. Provide the client a list of OTC drugs that may cause pupil dilation. Many of these OTC drugs are used to treat allergies, cold or flu symptoms, or diarrhea and usually contain antihistamines, atropine, or atropine-like compounds.

Before completing your plan of care, discuss expected outcomes with the client. Outcomes that would be appropriate include the following:

- Client establishes an effective respiratory pattern.
- Client remains free of injury.
- Client demonstrates improved ventilation.
- Client demonstrates reduction in congestion with breath sounds clear.

Implementating   While you implement the plan of care, constantly assess for desired and undesired clinical responses. Since high doses of parasympathomimetic drugs can cause a partial or complete AV block, assess the client's cardiac status carefully. Determine the client's blood pressure and apical pulse as indicated by the situation. If the client is hypotensive, communicate with the primary care provider before administering the drug. Since parasympathomimetic drugs can cause a significant decrease in cardiac output, monitor the client's peripheral pulses at least once every 8 hours.

Observe clients for flushing of the skin or diaphoresis, which may signal excessive blood levels of the drug. With excessive levels, the danger of hypotension and/or heart block increases.

Auscultate breath sounds on a regular basis. Assess for indications of bronchoconstriction or an obstructed airway. As the amount of bronchial secretions increase, the client may experience ineffective breathing patterns. Report wheezing or complaints of dyspnea immediately. Have suction equipment and oxygen available. A pulse oximeter for evaluation of oxygen saturation provides a quick, qualitative analysis to support assessed data. In some instances arterial blood gas measurements are obtained. Be prepared to administer epinephrine and/or atropine to reverse the respiratory effects of the parasympathomimetic agent.

For a client who is losing excessive amounts of fluids through diaphoresis, frequent voiding, or diarrhea, fluid and electrolyte management is important. Assess for indications of electrolyte imbalance. Monitor intake and output carefully and record the client's daily weight. Inspect the skin for indications of dehydration.

Evaluating   Evaluation of the effectiveness of the drug is based on the success in obtaining the expected outcomes. Does the client's urinary status improve? Do bowel sounds return? Is there a decrease in abdominal distention? Are secretions diminishing? Is intraocular pressure remaining within normal limits?

Direct-Acting Parasympathomimetic Drugs

Direct-acting parasympathomimetic drugs mimic the effects of endogenous ACh. These drugs are subclassified into two groups: ACh and synthetic choline esters and naturally occurring cholinomimetic alkaloids (i.e., pilocarpine, muscarine, and arecoline). Both drug groups have the muscarinic receptor sites as their principle sites of action. Thus they have similar actions and side effects.

Pharmacotherapeutics   The four main uses of direct-acting parasympathomimetic agents are treatment of glaucoma; treatment of GI tract atony; treatment of urinary retention caused by GU tract atony; and the diagnosis and/or treatment of myasthenia gravis.

Pharmacodynamics   Direct-acting parasympathomimetic drugs are similar in structure and function to endogenous ACh. However, they do not produce the same diffuse effects, nor are they metabolized in the same manner. Endogenous ACh is metabolized by AChE, which is abundant within the bloodstream. Parasympathomimetic drugs are metabolized more slowly by nonspecific **pseudocholinesterases,** permitting an increase in ACh to therapeutic levels.

DIRECT-ACTING PARASYMPATHOMIMETIC PROTOTYPE

ACETYLCHOLINE CHLORIDE

ACh (Miochol) was first produced synthetically by Baeyer in 1867 and is pharmacologically identical to the ACh synthesized in the body.[2]

Therapeutic Uses   ACh has limited therapeutic uses. It is primarily used to manage glaucoma and related eye disorders. In the treatment of glaucoma, the miotic effects of ACh allow aqueous humor to flow from the eye. This reduces intraocular pressure.

Pharmacodynamic Effects   The pharmacodynamic effects of ACh are identical to those caused by stimulation of the PNS. These effects (described in the discussion, Physiologic Response to Parasympathomimetic Drugs, p. 276) are caused by chemical interaction with muscarinic receptor sites. In addition, exogenous ACh can produce unwanted nicotinic responses.

ACh should not be used in individuals with previously shown sensitivity to parasympathomimetic drugs. Adverse reactions or side effects are rare with this drug. However, bradycardia, hypotension, flushing, sweating, and breathing difficulties have been reported.[4]

MISCELLANEOUS DRUGS IN CATEGORY

Other parasympathomimetic drugs that produce prolonged therapeutic actions include carbachol (Miostat, Isopto Carbachol) and bethanechol.

Bethanechol chloride (Duvoid, Urecholine, etc.) is a synthetic ester that is structurally and pharmacologically related to ACh (Table 26–3). It is used primarily to treat urinary retention secondary to surgery or child birth. Bethanechol also is used to treat clients who have suffered a loss in tone in the GI tract.[3]

Bethanechol, as a muscarinic agonist, stimulates the muscarinic receptors of the urinary bladder or GI tract, mimicking the effects of ACh. The parasympathomimetic response increases the tone of the detrusor muscle in the bladder, which results in more complete emptying of the urinary bladder. In addition, there are improved tone and increased contraction of the smooth muscles of the GI tract. This facilitates peristalsis. Increased lower esophageal sphincter tone also occurs, particularly in clients after a vagotomy and antrectomy. Effects pro-

TABLE 26–3
Major Direct-Acting Parasympathomimetic Drugs

Drug Name	Dosage and Route of Administration	Nursing Considerations
BETHANECHOL CHLORIDE (Urecholine, Duvoid) **HOW SUPPLIED** Coated tablet: 10, 25, and 50 mg Uncoated tablet: 5, 10, 25, and 50 mg SC: 5 mg/ml	Dosage and route of administration is individualized **ADULTS** Oral: 10-50 mg, tid or qid SC: Usual dose, 2.5-5 mg	**Assess** Assess baseline blood pressure and heart rate. Determine normal urinary and GI function. Assess client for preexisting GI obstruction, bladder or bowel surgery, peritonitis, or intestinal inflammation. Determine if client is pregnant; bethanechol is classified as a Pregnancy Category C drug. **Implement** Administer tablets on an empty stomach. Administer 2 h after meals if nausea and vomiting occur. Never administer parenteral solution intramuscularly or intravenously. Be aware that effects of oral drug appear within 30-90 min. Effects persist for 60 min. Effects from injection of drug occur in 5-15 min. Notify physician if no urinary output within 30 min after drug administration. Advise client to change positions carefully to avoid dizziness or fainting. Keep epinephrine available for severe cardiovascular or bronchoconstrictor responses. Store tablets in tightly closed container. Avoid storing below temperature of 40° C. Avoid storing injection solution at temperatures below −20° C and above 40° C. **Monitor** Monitor intake and output. Monitor bowel sounds and bowel elimination pattern. Monitor client for undesired clinical responses: abdominal cramps, diarrhea, increased salivation, dyspnea. **Evaluate** Evaluate effectiveness of drug by determining urinary output 1½ h after administration.
Carbachol (Isopto Carbachol, Miostat)	See Chapter 64.	

duced by bethanechol are more prolonged than those seen with ACh since bethanechol is not destroyed by AChE.[13]

Bethanechol is administered only orally or subcutaneously. It has a rapid onset of action. After oral administration, micturition or increased GI motility usually occurs within 30 to 90 minutes. After SC doses, clinical effects are usually observed in 5 to 15 minutes. The IM route of administration must be avoided, for it can result in severe parasympathomimetic symptoms such as hypotension, shock, sudden cardiac arrest, abdominal cramps, and bloody diarrhea.[5]

Bethanechol is contraindicated in the presence of mechanical obstruction of the GU or GI tracts, inflammatory diseases of the GI tract (peptic ulcers), peritonitis, Parkinson's disease, coronary artery disease, hypotension, bradycardia, bronchial asthma, and hyperthyroidism. It should be used with caution in clients already receiving cholinesterase inhibitors, ganglionic blockers, and certain cardiac drugs.[13]

As with most parasympathomimetics, particular caution is advised when giving this drug to children, the elderly, or debilitated clients. Its use is generally discouraged in pregnant women or women who are breastfeeding. In pregnant women the possibility of uterine contractions does exist when parasympathomimetics are administered.[11]

Indirect-Acting Parasympathomimetic Drugs

Drugs that work by blocking AChE are known as *AChE inhibitors, cholinesterase inhibitors, anticholinesterase drugs,* or *indirect-acting parasympathomimetic drugs.* AChE inhibitors are further subclassified into **reversible** or **irreversible drugs.** These terms are somewhat qualitative because all AChE inhibitors are eventually metabolized and eliminated. Their rate of metabolism is what varies. Without intervention, reversible drugs are slowly hydrolyzed, allowing slow regeneration of AChE. Muscarinic effects from these drugs can be interrupted in a few minutes by administering large doses of atropine. The process initiated by irreversible AChE inhibitors take several days or weeks to reverse since new cholinesterase molecules must first be synthesized before cholinesterase enzyme can be produced.

Pharmacotherapeutics   In addition to the therapeutic uses mentioned for direct-acting parasympathomimetic drugs, AChE inhibitors are used to treat myasthenia gravis. Myasthenia gravis is a chronic, autoimmune neuromuscular disease in which the body develops antibodies to the somatic nicotinic receptor sites. As a result, skeletal muscle response is diminished.

Use of an AChE inhibitor in the treatment of myasthenia gravis temporarily increases the amount of ACh at the motor end-plate. Short-acting AChE inhibitors are used to diagnosis myasthenia gravis, and long-acting AChE inhibitors are used for treatment purposes.

The Tensilon test was discussed earlier in the chapter. In this test Tensilon, a short-acting AChE inhibitor, is administered via IV bolus. If the client's muscle weakness dramatically but briefly improves, a diagnosis of myasthenia is made. In clients with known myasthenia gravis, the Tensilon test is also used to differentiate between a **cholinergic crisis,** indicating too much AChE inhibitor, and a **myasthenia crisis,** indicating too little AChE inhibitor. Both crises have similar symptoms. After administration of Tensilon, an improvement in muscle strength points to a myasthenia crisis, whereas no improvement or worsening of symptoms suggests a cholinergic crisis.[14,15]

Pharmacodynamics   When indirect-acting parasympathomimetic drugs inhibit or block the action of cholinesterase, increased concentrations of ACh occur at all receptor sites. There is **not** an increase in the amount of ACh produced, nor is there an increase in the binding capacity of ACh at the receptor site; however, there is an increased concentration or level of ACh and thus an increase in activity of ACh on receptor sites.

Because ACh is produced at a variety of sites, increasing its concentration at these sites produces numerous responses. Unlike muscarinic agonists, which only enhance the effects of ACh at muscarinic receptor sites, AChE inhibitors can enhance the effects of ACh at all autonomic and somatic sites.[2,3]

The enhanced muscarinic responses of AChE inhibitors are the same responses previously described and summarized in Figure 26–2. However, because AChE inhibitors also increase ACh at nicotinic sites and at neuromuscular junctions, additional effects are observed. For example, within the **sympathetic nervous system,** enhanced stimulation of α-, β-, and dopaminergic receptor sites occurs. Increased concentration of ACh in the **adrenal medulla** results in increased release of catecholamines (epinephrine and norepinephrine). Increased availability of ACh at somatic receptor sites results in enhanced skeletal muscle response.[2,8]

The **skeletal muscle response** that occurs is an increase in skeletal muscle contractility, which is the desired response when treating myasthenia gravis. However, high doses of AChE inhibitors eventually produce muscle weakness instead of muscle strength. The continuous skeletal muscle contraction leads to fatigue, fasciculations, and eventually respiratory muscle paralysis.

CNS effects are mainly due to stimulation of the muscarinic receptor sites within the brain. The effects are generally broad in scope and include confusion, slurred speech, decreased reflexes, Cheyne-Stokes respirations, convulsions, and, if untreated, coma. With high doses of AChE inhibitors, CNS depression occurs. It is generally believed that hypoxemia is the cause behind this depressant effect.

A wide range of **cardiovascular effects** can be anticipated when AChE inhibitors are used. The predominant effect is bradycardia, which can lead to a fall in cardiac output. In addition, high doses of AChE inhibitors depress the vasomotor centers of the CNS and cause a fall in blood pressure. These effects can lead to hypoxemia. When hypoxemia occurs, the sympathetic nervous system is stimulated, causing an increase in pulse and blood pressure. In addition, AChE inhibitors stimulate the release of epinephrine from the adrenal medulla, which also increases the pulse and blood pressure.[3,8,9]

Drug-drug, drug-nutrient, drug-environment interactions   In clients with known myasthenia gravis, using a combination of AChE inhibitors and steroids may exacerbate the disorder. To avoid this result, an every-other-day regimen of steroids is recommended.[13] It is also recommended that direct-acting and indirect-acting parasympathomimetic drugs **not** be combined because of possible additive effects.

Organophosphorus compounds used as agricultural insecticides also produce AChE inhibition. With accidental exposure to these agents, drug absorption through the skin, mucous membranes, or by inhalation occurs. Local effects from the drug usually involve the eyes and include marked miosis, ocular pain, hyperemia of the sclera, blurred vision, and a headache over the brow. If the drug is absorbed through the skin, localized sweating and muscular fasciculation at the point of entry occur. Respiratory symptoms include wheezing, rhinorrhea, and increased bronchial secretions. When the AChE inhibitor is ingested, GI symptoms such as nausea, vomiting, abdominal cramps, and diarrhea are the first to appear. With severe drug intoxication, extreme salivation, involuntary defecation and urination, sweating, tearing, bradycardia, and hypotension may occur. Skeletal muscles involuntarily twitch and fasciculate, leading to extreme muscle weakness and eventually paralysis. Death is due to respiratory failure. AChE inhibitors are also used as chemical warfare agents and have been used in suicides. Treatment after contamination with an insecticide or chemical warfare agent consists of administering large doses of atropine for the muscarinic symptoms (i.e., GI, cardiovascular, and respiratory effects). Pralidoxime (Protopam), a cholinesterase reactivator, is used to treat the nicotinic symptoms (skeletal muscle paralysis).[3,8]

INDIRECT-ACTING PARASYMPATHOMIMETIC PROTOTYPE

NEOSTIGMINE

The prototype for indirect-acting parasympathomimetic drugs is neostigmine (Table 26–4). Neostigmine is the oldest member of the AChE inhibitor group and is a member of the reversible inhibitor subgroup. It is available in two forms: *neostigmine bromide* for oral adminis-

TABLE 26–4
Indirect-Acting Parasympathomimetic Drugs: Prototype and Major Drugs in Category

Drug Name	Dosage and Route of Administration	Nursing Considerations
NEOSTIGMINE BROMIDE (Prostigmin, Prostigmin Bromide) HOW SUPPLIED Tablet: 15 mg Uncoated tablet: 15 mg	**Myasthenia Gravis** Varied dosage requirements: 15-375 mg/d Average dose: 150 mg over 24-h period Dosage schedule adjusted for each client	**Assess** Determine normal urinary and GI function. Assess client for preexisting epilepsy, bronchial asthma, bradycardia, hyperthyroidism, cardiac arrhythmias, or peptic ulcer. Assess client for hypersensitivity to bromides. Determine if client is pregnant; neostigmine classified as Pregnancy Category C drug.
NEOSTIGMINE METHYLSULFATE (Prostigmin) HOW SUPPLIED Injection solution 1:4000 (0.25 mg/ml) 1:2000 (0.5 mg/ml) 1:1000 (1 mg/ml)	**Myasthenia Gravis** SC or IM: 1 ml of 1:2000 solution **Urinary Retention** SC or IM: 1 ml of 1:4000 (0.25 mg) to 1:2000 (0.5 mg) solution	**Implement** Administer with milk or food to minimize GI reactions. Administer 30 min before scheduled activities such as eating. Stress importance of taking drugs on time. Keep 1 mg of atropine available as an antidote. Keep suction and life support equipment available. Determine that all cholinergic drugs have been discontinued before administering neostigmine. Teach client responses to report to health care provider. **Monitor** Assess muscle strength ½ h before and 1 h after drug administration. Monitor for excessive acetylcholine effects. Monitor the client for undesired clinical responses: diarrhea, bowel cramps. **Evaluate** Evaluate client for increased muscle strength and/or decreased urinary retention.
Pyridostigmine Bromide (Mestinon, Regonol) HOW SUPPLIED IM, IV: 5 mg/ml Syrup: 60 mg/5 ml Uncoated tablet: 60 mg Sustained-action coated tablet: 180 mg	**Myosthenia Gravis** Dosage adjusted to needs of individual client Average dose: 10 60-mg tablets or 10 5-ml teaspoons daily 1-3 180-mg tablets once or twice daily	See neostigmine with the following exceptions: Safety of drug during pregnancy has not been determined. Administer sustained-release tablets at least 6 h apart.
Edrophonium Chloride (Tensilon) HOW SUPPLIED IM, IV: 10 mg/ml	**Diagnosis of Myasthenia Gravis** ADULTS IV: 2-mg IV push; after 45 s, if no untoward effects, injection of additional 8 mg CHILDREN <34 kg (75 lb) 1 mg initially, followed with 4 mg >34 kg (75 lb) same as adult	See neostigmine with the following exceptions: Observe for increased weakness, fasciculations, respiratory paralysis, bradycardia, and hypotension.

tration and *neostigmine methylsulfate* for parenteral administration.

Pharmacotherapeutics Neostigmine is used for urinary retention and abdominal distention and as an antidote for nondepolarizing neuromuscular junction blockers (tubocurarine, vecuronium, pancuronium, etc.). It is also used in the treatment of myasthenia gravis.

Pharmacokinetics *Neostigmine bromide* is poorly absorbed from the GI tract after oral administration. Because of the poor absorption, 15 mg of neostigmine bromide is equivalent to 0.5 mg of neostigmine methylsulfate parenterally. The extent of absorption of oral doses is approximately 1% to 2% of an ingested 30-mg dose. Peak concentration of neostigmine bromide occurs in 1 to 2 hours. The half-life ranges from 42 to 60 minutes. Protein binding of neostigmine bromide ranges from 15% to 25%. The drug is hydrolyzed by cho-

linesterase and is metabolized by microsomal enzymes in the liver.[4,6]

Neostigmine methylsulfate is administered parenterally. After IM administration, neostigmine methylsulfate is rapidly absorbed and eliminated. In clients with myasthenia gravis, studies indicate the peak plasma levels occur within 30 minutes, and the half-life ranges from 51 to 90 minutes. Approximately 80% of the drug is eliminated in the urine within 24 hours, with approximately 50% unchanged. Clinical effects usually begin within 20 to 30 minutes after the injection and last from 2½ to 4 hours.[4,6,13]

Pharmacodynamics As an anticholinesterase drug, neostigmine blocks the action of cholinesterase at the synapses, preventing breakdown of ACh. This effect allows greater concentration of ACh, with increased muscarinic and nicotinic activity.

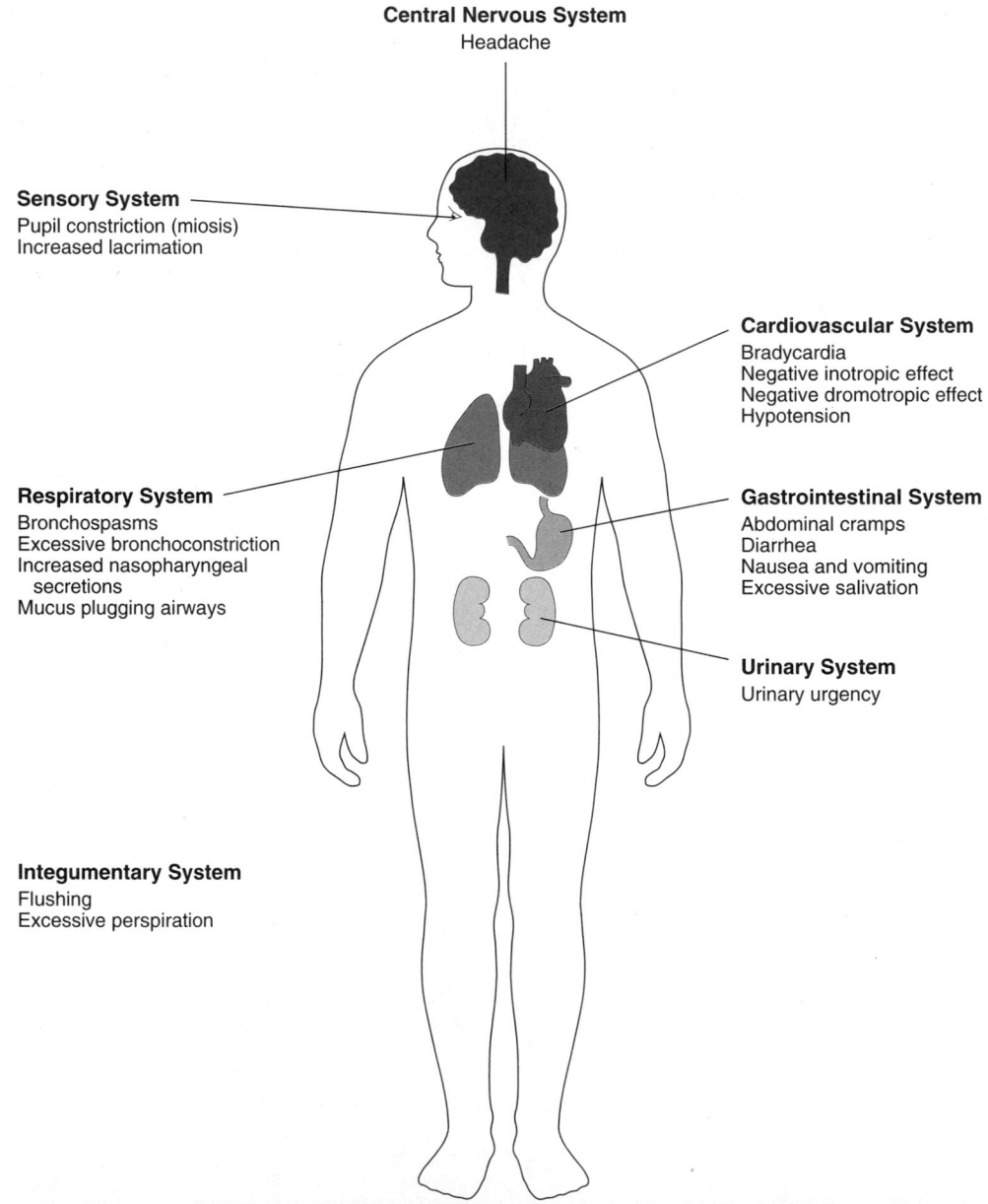

Central Nervous System
Headache

Sensory System
Pupil constriction (miosis)
Increased lacrimation

Cardiovascular System
Bradycardia
Negative inotropic effect
Negative dromotropic effect
Hypotension

Respiratory System
Bronchospasms
Excessive bronchoconstriction
Increased nasopharyngeal
  secretions
Mucus plugging airways

Gastrointestinal System
Abdominal cramps
Diarrhea
Nausea and vomiting
Excessive salivation

Urinary System
Urinary urgency

Integumentary System
Flushing
Excessive perspiration

FIGURE 26–3   Undesired clinical responses associated with parasympathomimetic drugs.

Pharmaceutics As mentioned previously, neostigmine is available for oral and parenteral administration. Neostigmine bromide is prepared in coated and uncoated tablets. Neostigmine methylsulfate is available in sterile solutions for IM, IV, and SC injections.

Undesired Clinical Responses Side effects are usually due to exaggeration of the pharmacologic effects of the drug. Salivation, fasciculation, bowel cramps, and diarrhea are common. Additional undesired clinical responses include headache, dizziness, bradycardia, arrhythmias, increased oral and bronchial secretions, urinary frequency, nausea, and increased peristalsis. See Figure 26–3 for a summary of other undesired clinical responses.

Contraindications and Precautions AChE inhibitors have the same contraindications as other parasympathomimetic drugs. In addition, clients with a diagnosis of pheochromocytoma should not receive AChE inhibitors. Pheochromocytoma is a catecholamine-producing tumor of the adrenal medulla. The catecholamines, epinephrine and norepinephrine, produced by the tumor cause intense vasoconstriction. The vasoconstriction produces extremely high blood pressures (i.e., 300/220). AChE inhibitors can increase epinephrine and norepinephrine release through action of ACh at the nicotinic sites of the adrenal medulla. This potentially can compound the risk for severe hypertension.[12]

Life Span Considerations Neostigmine is classified as a Pregnancy Category C drug. It can also cause uterine irritability and induce premature labor. It is not known if neostigmine is excreted in human milk. Safety and effectiveness in children have not been established.[16]

⊞ NURSING CONSIDERATIONS

The nursing care discussed for clients receiving direct-acting parasympathomimetic agents applies equally to clients receiving AChE inhibitors. This section considers the nursing care associated with the effects of nicotinic receptor stimulation on the skeletal muscle.

Assessing Assessment of these clients includes a thorough history and examination of the musculoskeletal system. You need to determine baseline data on the client's muscle strength, particularly the strength of the intercostal muscles and diaphragm. Is the client becoming weaker? Are there signs of respiratory difficulty?[17]

Since clients receiving long-term AChE inhibitor therapy are at risk for developing cataracts, conduct a careful assessment of the eyes, a step important for early detection and treatment of the cataracts.[2]

Diagnosing Nursing diagnoses associated with the administration of AChE inhibitors are the same as for the direct-acting parasympathomimetic drugs. In addition, the following diagnoses are appropriate because of the somatic influence of the inhibitors:

- High risk for injury related to muscle weakness associated with drug therapy.
- Impaired physical mobility related to muscle weakness associated with drug therapy.
- Fatigue related to muscle weakness associated with drug therapy.

Planning Discharge planning and teaching are essential for clients receiving AChE inhibitors. The client's life may depend on the therapeutic effects of the drug. Therefore teach the client proper drug administration techniques and symptoms of over- and underusage of the inhibitors. Eventually most clients learn to adjust their own drug dose, varying the dose according to the presence of desired therapeutic effects and development of undesirable side effects.

❧ NURSING RESEARCH

Hood, L.J. (1990). Myasthenia gravis: Regimens and regimen-associated problems in adults. *Journal of Neuroscience Nursing, 22,* 358-364.

Two-hundred eighteen persons with myasthenia gravis responded to a mailed survey regarding experiences with their disease. The survey consisted of a 48-item questionnaire that addressed eight key problems encountered in chronic illness. The respondents included 138 females and 80 males, with a mean age of 58.1 years. Most of the subjects (82.1%) received pyridostigmine bromide (Mestinon) as their primary drug. Only 6.9% of the subjects were receiving neostigmine.

One focus of the study was drug side effects and methods used to decrease these effects. The undesired clinical responses reported included diarrhea, frequent urination, abdominal cramps, muscle twitching or fasciculations, inability to sleep well, increased salivation, and muscle spasms. Methods used to decrease the effects of these responses included taking the drug with food, maintaining a strict drug schedule, taking the drug with antacids, avoiding highly spiced foods, and taking prescription or OTC antidiarrheal drugs.

STUDENT ACTIVITIES

- Contact the local support group for the names of individuals with myasthenia gravis and ask to interview some of the members. Determine which drugs they are receiving and what side effects they experience. Ask them to share methods used to control the side effects.
- Compare your findings with those in this study.

Implementing AChE inhibitors given for myasthenia gravis **must** be given on time. They should also be administered on an empty stomach to minimize the potential for nausea and vomiting. In addition, if the drug is taken 30 to 60 minutes before meals, the strength of muscles needed to masticate and swallow is improved.

Since the client may experience urinary urgency, bathrooms should be easily accessible. At night, suggest that the client keep a bedpan, urinal, or bedside commode by the bed. Instruct the client that low lighting in the room, small frequent meals, and frequent mouth care will decrease the discomfort of some of the drug's side effects.

Because myasthenia gravis can worsen without warning, causing extreme muscle weakness, the client needs to plan for alternative methods of summoning help. A touch pad alarm, a small bell that could be knocked to the floor, or heat-sensitive or voice-activated alarms make it easier to summon help.

Teach the client how to monitor for infections. Infections can exacerbate the disease, making an adjustment in the AChE inhibitor dose necessary. Instruct the client to avoid crowds and people with colds or flu. Suggest that the client check with the primary care provider about getting a yearly influenza injection.

In case of a cholinergic crisis, IV atropine sulfate should be readily available for all clients receiving AChE inhibitors. In addition, a resuscitator bag and oral airway should be available. Family members must be taught cardiopulmonary resuscitation in the event of a respiratory arrest from a cholinergic or myasthenic crisis.

Evaluating   The **effectiveness** of treatment depends on the desired outcome. The response of the client is the best criterion to use to evaluate the success of therapy. If AChE inhibitors are administered to treat glaucoma, the intraocular pressure should be maintained below 15 mmHg. Clients receiving the inhibitors for myasthenia gravis should have improved muscle strength. If AChE inhibitors are administered to improve intestinal and/or urinary bladder atony, normal bowel movements and micturition should result. Postoperatively, AChE inhibitors reverse the paralyzing effects of the nondepolarizing muscle relaxants, and muscle strength should improve.

CONCEPT REVIEW

Parasympathomimetic drugs mimic or stimulate the PNS by increasing the concentration of ACh at the postganglionic muscarinic receptor sites of the effector organs.

These drugs are used to treat a variety of conditions, including glaucoma, GI tract atony, urinary retention caused by GU tract atony, and the diagnosis and/or treatment of myasthenia gravis.

Some OTC drugs contain ingredients that enhance the effects of parasympathomimetics.

ACh chloride is the prototype drug for direct-acting parasympathomimetic drugs. Neostigmine is the prototype for indirect-acting parasympathomimetic drugs.

GANGLIONIC STIMULANTS

A complete discussion of parasympathetic drugs must mention ganglionic stimulants. Most ganglionic stimulants have no clinical value (e.g., nicotine is a ganglionic stimulant). Gan-

TABLE 26–5
Physiologic Responses to Antimuscarinic and Parasympathomimetic Drugs

Organ	Antimuscarinics	Muscarinic Agonists
Eye	Contract iris (miosis)	Relax iris (mydriasis)
	Contract ciliary muscle	Relax ciliary muscle
Heart	Decrease pulse rate	Increase pulse rate
	Decrease conduction and contraction	Increase conduction and contraction
Arteries	Dilate	No effect
Veins	Dilate	No effect
Lungs	Increase bronchial smooth muscle tone	Decrease bronchial smooth muscle tone
	Increase mucous production	Decrease mucous production
GI tract	Increase GI smooth muscle tone	Decrease GI smooth muscle tone
GU tract	Increase urinary bladder tone	Decrease urinary bladder tone
Exocrine glands	Increase secretions	Decrease secretions

glionic stimulants also produce CNS stimulation. In this textbook these drugs are discussed in Chapter 22, "Central Nervous System Stimulants."

SUMMARY

As a summary of this chapter, a comparison of the physiologic response to antimuscarinic and parasympathomimetic drugs is provided in Table 26–5. Learn the antimuscarinic effects since these drugs are used more frequently in the clinical setting. The muscarinic agonist effects are the opposite and thus are more easily recalled.

REFERENCES

1. Guyton, A.C. (1991). *Textbook of medical physiology* (8th ed.). Philadelphia: W.B. Saunders.
2. Goodman, A., Gilman, A., Rall, T., Niles, A., & Taylor, P. (Eds.). (1990). *Goodman and Gilman's: The pharmacological basis of therapeutics* (8th ed.). New York: Pergamon Press.
3. Smith, C.M. (1992). Skeletal muscle relaxants. In Smith, C.M., & Reynard, A.M. (Eds.). *Textbook of pharmacology* (pp. 358-366). Philadelphia: W.B. Saunders.
4. Data Pharmaceutica, Inc. (1993). *1993 physicians' genRx.* Smithtown, NY: Author.
5. Kastrup, E.K. (Ed.) (1992). *Facts and comparisons.* St. Louis: J.B. Lippincott.
6. U.S. Pharmacopeial Convention (1990). *The United States pharmacopeia* (22nd rev.). Rockville, MD: Author.
7. Kalant, H., & Roschlau, W. (1989). *Principles of medical pharmacology.* Toronto: Brian C. Decker.
8. Wingard, L., Brady, T., Larner, J., & Schwartz, A. (1991). *Human pharmacology.* St. Louis: Mosby–Year Book.
9. Lehne, R.A. (1990). *Pharmacology for nursing care.* Philadelphia: W.B. Saunders.
10. Garabedian-Ruffalo, S. (1990). Drug compatibility chart. *Critical Care Nurse, 10*(3), 28-29.
11. U.S. Pharmacopeial Convention, Inc. (1991). *USPDI, Drug in-*

formation for the health care professional (Vol. IA) (11th ed.). Rockville, MD.: Author.

12. U.S. Pharmacopeial Convention, Inc. (1991). *USPDI, advice for the patient. Drug information in lay language* (Vol. II). Rockville, MD: Author.

13. Microdex, Inc. (1992). *Drug evaluation monographs* (Vol. 71). Author.

14. Chipps, E. (1991). Myasthenia gravis: The patient in crisis. *Critical Care Nurse, 11*(7). 18-26.

15. Seybold, M. (1991). Update on myasthenia gravis. *Hospital Medicine, 27*(4), 71-72, 77-78.

16. Burke, M.E. (1993). Myasthenia gravis and pregnancy. *Journal of Perinatal and Neonatal Nursing, 7*(1), 11-21.

17. Hickey, J.V. (1991). Myasthenia crisis—Your assessment counts. *RN Magazine, 54*(5), 54-59.

18. Hood, L.J. (1990). Myasthenia gravis: Regimens and regimen-associated problems in adults. *Journal of Neuroscience Nursing, 22,* 358-364.

BIBLIOGRAPHY

Ceron, G., & Rakowski-Reinhardt, A. (1991). Action stat! Autonomic dysreflexia. *Nursing '91, 21*(2), 33.

Goetting, M., & Contreras, E. (1991). Systemic atropine administration during caridac arrest does not cause fixed and dilated pupils. *Annals of Emergency Medicine, 20*(1), 55-57.

Goldblum, K. (1991). Nursing care of the patient with myasthenia gravis. *Insight, 16*(1), 7, 24.

Kelly, B., & Luce, J. (1991). The diagnosis and management of neuromuscular diseases causing respiratory failure. *Chest: The Cardiopulmonary Journal, 99,* 1485-1494.

Mascarella, J., & Hudson, D. (1991). Dysimmune neurologic disorders. *AACN—Clinical Issues in Critical Care Nursing, 2,* 675-684.

Rhynsburger, J. (1989). How to fight MG fatigue . . . myasthenia gravis. *American Journal of Nursing, 89,* 337-340.

Wiseman, E., & Koch, E. (1989). AANA Journal course: Advanced scientific concepts. Update for nurse anesthetists—Anesthesia for patients on anticholinesterase and antiepileptic drugs. *AANA Journal, 57*(1), 78-87.

CHAPTER 27

DRUGS AFFECTING THE
Sympathetic Nervous System

JOAN DOMIGAN WENTZ

⊛ Neurotransmitters and Receptor Sites

LEARNING OBJECTIVES:

Identify the neurotransmitters found in the sympathetic nervous system.

Differentiate between α- and β-receptor sites.

KEY TERMS:

α_1-receptor, β_1-receptor, β_2-receptor, catecholamines

⊛ Sympathomimetic Drugs

LEARNING OBJECTIVES:

Discuss therapeutic uses of sympathomimetic drugs.

Describe general characteristics of all sympathomimetic drugs.

Explain two contraindications for the use of sympathomimetic drugs.

List undesired clinical responses associated with sympathomimetic drugs.

Explain five drug-drug interactions associated with sympathomimetic drugs.

Discuss life span considerations of sympathomimetic drugs.

Outline a plan of care for a client receiving sympathomimetic drugs.

Summarize essential information for each of the seven subcategories of sympathomimetic drugs.

KEY TERMS:

Adrenergic, analeptic effect, anorexigenic effect, direct action, indirect action, mixed action, sympathomimetic

⊛ Sympathomimetics in Over-the-Counter Drugs

LEARNING OBJECTIVES:

Discuss problems associated with the use of OTC drugs that contain sympathomimetics.

Identify three OTC drugs that contain a sympathomimetic ingredient.

⊛ Sympatholytic Drugs

LEARNING OBJECTIVES:

Discuss therapeutic uses of α-blockers.

Describe general characteristics of all adrenergic blockers.

Explain three contraindications for the use of α-blockers.

List undesired clinical responses associated with adrenergic blockers.

Explain five drug-drug interactions associated with α-blockers.

Discuss life span considerations of α-blocker drugs.

Outline a plan of care for a client receiving α-blockers.

Summarize essential information regarding each of the four subcategories of α-blockers discussed in this chapter.

KEY TERMS:

Adrenergic blockers, α-blockers, antiadrenergic, sympatholytic

*T*his chapter focuses on drugs that affect the sympathetic branch of the autonomic nervous system (ANS). Sympathetic drugs either mimic the sympathetic nervous system (sympathomimetic effects) or inhibit the sympathetic nervous system (sympatholytic effects). Drugs that antagonize the effects of the sympathetic nervous system allow the parasympathetic nervous system to predominate and vice versa.

NEUROTRANSMITTERS AND RECEPTOR SITES

Epinephrine, norepinephrine, and dopamine are the neurotransmitters of the sympathetic nervous system. These transmitters are found at target organs and are collectively called **catecholamines.** Sympathetic receptor sites are named *alpha* or *beta*. These sites are further subdivided into alpha 1 (α_1), alpha 2 (α_2), beta 1 (β_1), and beta 2 (β_2) according to end-organ response after stimulation. Recent research shows that more than the α- and β-receptor sites exist.[1] However, in this chapter only drugs affecting α_1, β_1, and β_2-receptor sites are discussed.

α-**Receptors** are concentrated in many areas, including smooth muscles of the arteries and veins, gastrointestinal (GI) tract, endocrine glands, bronchioles, and eye. α-Receptors are not found in the heart. β_2-**Receptors** are located mainly in the bronchioles and blood vessels, and β_1-**receptors** are concentrated in the heart. Epinephrine primarily affects β-receptor sites, whereas norepinephrine primarily affects α-receptor sites.[2]

Alpha stimulation generally opposes beta stimulation. Alpha stimulation constricts blood vessels, contracts sphincters and muscles, and controls secretion—the three *C*'s. Beta stimulation relaxes blood vessels and smooth muscles (dilates), releases renin, and rejuvenates the heart (increases heart rate, conduction, and contractility)—the three *R*'s. An exception to this opposition rule is that both alpha and beta stimulation relax smooth muscle of the GI tract.[3]

SYMPATHOMIMETIC DRUGS

Drugs that mimic the sympathetic nervous system are known as **sympathomimetics, adrenergics,** or adrenergic sympathetic agonists. These drugs are grouped into six subclassifications based on the receptor sites involved and the pharmacodynamics of the drug.

Pharmacotherapeutics

Therapeutic uses of sympathomimetic drugs are based on the pharmacodynamics of the drug. Drugs that stimulate α_1-receptors have two major therapeutic uses: vasoconstriction and mydriasis. The most frequent use is vasoconstriction of vessels in the skin, viscera, and mucous membrane. These drugs promote hemostasis, nasal decongestion, and elevation of systemic blood pressure. In addition, they are routinely used during procedures on the eye since they cause dilation of the pupil (mydriasis). Drugs that stimulate the β_1-receptors in the heart are used to treat cardiac arrest, cardiac failure, atrioventricular heart block, and shock. Stimulation of β_2-receptor sites has limited effect on the uterus and lungs. Drugs that stimulate these receptor sites are used to delay premature labor and to produce bronchodilation.[4–6]

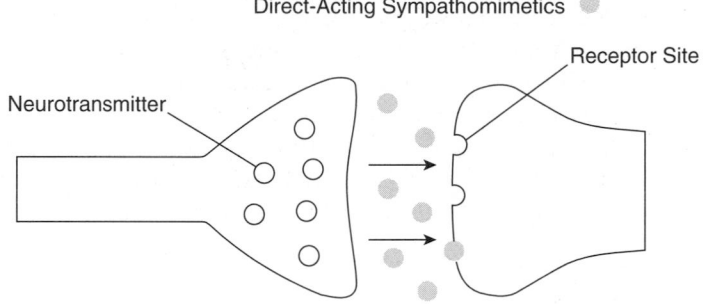

Direct-Acting Sympathomimetics

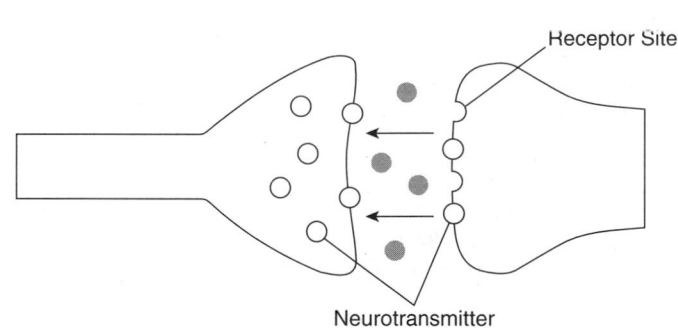

Indirect-Acting Sympathomimetics

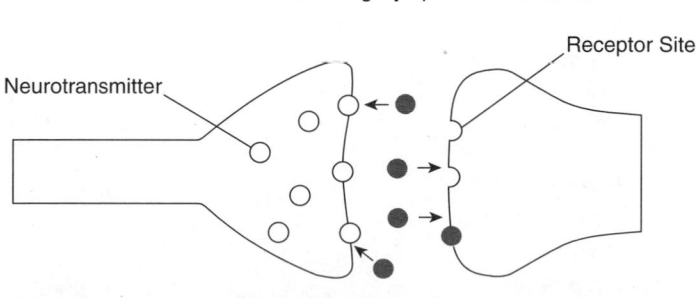

Mixed-Acting Sympathomimetics

FIGURE 27–1   Receptor site stimulation and sympathomimetic drugs.

General Characteristics

Sympathomimetic drugs are naturally occurring or are prepared synthetically. They produce sympathetic responses in several ways. Some sympathomimetic drugs act as neurotransmitters and directly stimulate α- or β-receptor sites (**direct action**) or both. Other drugs stimulate the release of naturally occurring catecholamines (norepinephrine) at the nerve endings. Norepinephrine then stimulates adrenergic receptor sites (**indirect action**). Other indirect actions produced by sympathomimetic drugs involve the blockade of norepinephrine reuptake at the nerve endings or the inhibition of norepinephrine inactivation. Both of these actions increase the amount of transmitter at the nerve ending and thereby increase adrenergic receptor stimulation. For some drugs, the pharmacodynamics involves a mixture or combination of these actions (**mixed action**).[7,8]

Direct-acting sympathomimetic drugs may or may not be selective in receptor site stimulation (Fig. 27–1). For example, some sympathomimetic drugs specifically stimulate **only** α-receptors; others stimulate **only** β_1-receptors, and some stimulate **only** β_2-receptors. Other sympathomimetic drugs stimulate all receptors (α and β). Newer drugs are designed to be more selective, affording them greater use for specific purposes and reducing unwanted side effects. Regardless of the type of action (direct, indirect, or mixed), organ response is similar (Table 27–1).

Contraindications and Precautions

Sympathomimetic drugs must be used with caution in clients with some medical conditions. If these drugs are used to treat elderly clients or clients with cardiovascular and cerebrovascular diseases, hypertension, renal insufficiency, narrow-angle glaucoma, hyperthyroidism, or a history of thyroid hormone therapy, clients must be monitored carefully. Direct-acting sympathomimetic drugs generally constrict blood vessels by alpha stimulation. Administration of these agents to clients with uncontrolled hypertension can exacerbate the hypertension, placing the clients at greater risk for cerebrovascular accidents or myocardial infarctions. Thyroid hormones potentiate the cardiovascular effects of epinephrine. Clients receiving thyroid hormone therapy or who have hyperthyroidism are at risk for tachyarrhythmias when treated concurrently with sympathomimetic drugs. Use of nonselective sympathomimetics is also contraindicated in clients with narrow-angle glaucoma. In fact, direct-acting sympathomimetic drugs can precipitate an attack of acute glaucoma.[3,7]

The use of sympathomimetic drugs is contraindicated in clients with a pheochromocytoma, a catecholamine-producing

TABLE 27–1

Responses of Major Effector Organs to Receptor Site Stimulation

Organ	Receptor Type	Response to Receptor Activation
Cardiovascular System		
Arterioles and large veins	α	Vasoconstriction
	β_2	Dilation
Heart	β_1	Increased heart rate, force of contraction, impulse conduction, and automaticity
Eye		
Iris, dilator muscle	α	Contraction causing mydriasis
Respiratory System		
Bronchial glands	α	Decreased secretion
Bronchial smooth muscle	β_2	Bronchial relaxation
Gastrointestinal Tract		
Motility	α, β_2	Decreased
Sphincters	α	Contracted
Metabolic Effects		
Fat cells	β_1	Increased lipolysis
Skeletal muscle, liver	β_2	Glycogen breakdown
Pancreas	β_2	Increased insulin secretion
Urinary Bladder		
Detrusor	β_2	Relaxation
Trigone sphincter	α	Contraction
		Overall effect—decreased urination
Kidney		
Renin secretion	β_1	Increased secretion
Uterus		
Nonpregnant	β_2	Relaxation
Pregnant	α	Contraction
Male Sex Organs	α	Ejaculation

tumor. When these drugs are used in the presence of a pheochromocytoma, the client is at extreme risk of hypertensive crisis. Caution should also be used when sympathomimetic drugs are administered to clients with diabetes mellitus. Since sympathomimetic drugs increase serum glucose levels, these clients are at greater risk for abnormally high blood sugar levels.[7,8]

Undesired Clinical Responses

Since sympathomimetic drugs affect a variety of receptor sites, a wide range of undesired clinical responses is possible. Most of these responses involve the central nervous system

(CNS), respiratory system, GI system, genitourinary system, endocrine system, eye, and heart. Undesired responses related to stimulation of α_1-receptor sites include hypertension and bradycardia. Parenteral doses of α_1-stimulators produce widespread vasoconstriction and reflex slowing of the heart. In addition, these drugs cause necrosis of local tissue if extravasation of parenteral solutions occurs.

Undesired responses associated with stimulation of β_1-receptor sites include tachycardia, arrthymias, and angina. In addition, these drugs produce an increased oxygen demand in the heart. Stimulation of β_2-receptor sites can produce hypoglycemia[7,8] (Fig. 27–2).

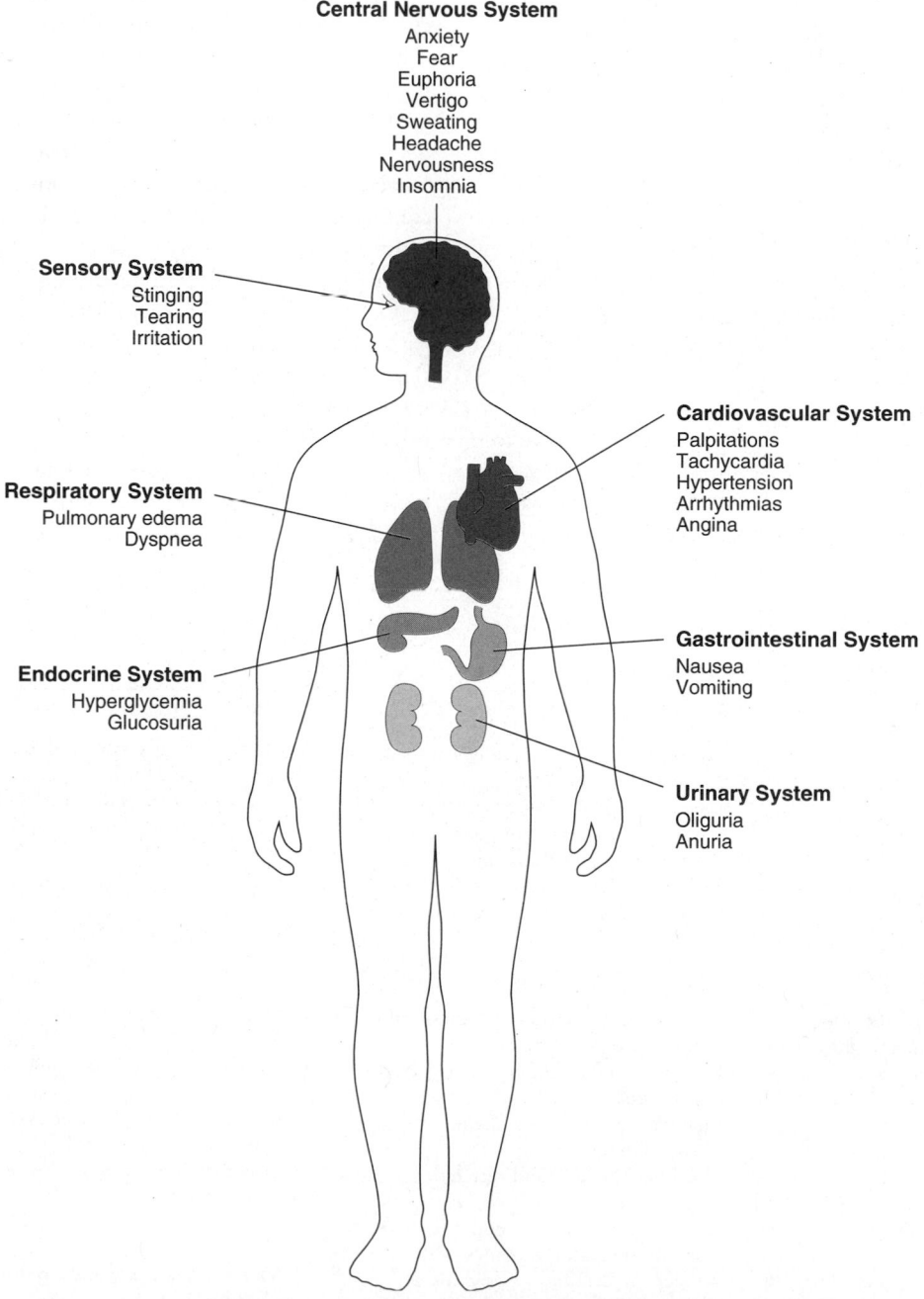

FIGURE 27–2   Undesired clinical responses associated with sympathomimetic drugs.

Drug-Drug, Drug-Nutrient, Drug-Environment Interactions

A variety of **drug-drug interactions** occur with sympathomimetic drugs. Some of the significant interactions involve monoamine oxidase (MAO) inhibitors, tricyclic antidepressants, cardiac glycosides, beta blockers, and cyclopropane or halogen-type general anesthetics. Table 27–2 summarizes information about these interactions. In addition, caution must be used when sympathomimetics are administered concurrently with diuretics, antihistamines, anticholinergics, acidifying agents, and phenytoin (Dilantin).[3,8,9]

Drug-nutrient interactions are more subtle than drug-drug interactions. For example, most sympathomimetics slow peristalsis. When this occurs, the client may experience anorexia and constipation. The most important **drug-environment consideration** is the storage temperature. Most of the injectable solutions must be stored at specific temperatures to prevent deterioration. Specific storage temperatures for some drugs are included in Table 27–4.

Life-Span Considerations

No adequate studies provide evidence for or against the use of sympathomimetic drugs during pregnancy. However, most of these drugs are classified as Pregnancy Category C. They should be used with caution, and the client should be monitored closely.

In addition, children and the elderly are more sensitive to sympathomimetics than are other age groups. Recommended dosages for children have been determined for most sympathomimetic drugs; however, most adult dosages do not reflect the needs of the elderly individual. These individuals require lower doses and closer monitoring of drug effects than young and middle-aged adults.[10]

▨ NURSING CONSIDERATIONS

Nursing care of the client receiving sympathomimetic drugs involves careful assessment, data analysis, planning, and implementation of care. Evaluation of the client's response to nursing care and medical therapy is ongoing, and the plan of care is altered according to the evaluation findings.

Assessing Obtaining a thorough health history and performing a physical assessment are the bases of your care of clients receiving or scheduled to receive sympathomimetic drugs. In some situations the client's condition dictates that the **health history** be gathered at a later time or that data be gathered only from secondary sources. Regardless, you need to determine the presence of preexisting conditions that might prevent the use of these drugs. As indicated previously, these conditions include cardiovascular diseases, hypertension, renal insufficiency, narrow-angle glaucoma, diabetes mellitus, hyperthyroidism, and thyroid hormone therapy.

Collecting a drug history is also important. Although you gather information about all of the client's drugs, your attention should specifically focus on drugs that interact with sympathomimetic drugs. These drug categories include MAO inhibitors, β-blockers, cardiac glycosides, diuretics, antihistamines, anticholinergics, ergot alkaloids, and tricyclic antidepressants.

Since sympathomimetic drugs slow peristalsis, include

TABLE 27–2
Drugs That Interact with Sympathomimetics

Drug Name/Category	Response to Interaction	Nursing Considerations
β-Adrenergic blocker (e.g., propranolol)	Prevents stimulation of β-receptors by sympathomimetic drug Increases activity of α-agonists; can result in severe hypertension, bradycardia, arrhythmias, and heart failure	Monitor cardiac status, blood pressure, and heart rate and rhythm. Assess client for indications of heart failure (e.g., dyspnea, increased weight, edema).
Cardiac glycoside (e.g., digoxin, digitoxin)	May increase ventricular automaticity Increases chance for cardiac arrhythmias	Monitor for signs and symptoms of digoxin toxicity. Assess cardiac rate and rhythm. Monitor electrocardiogram (ECG) for arrhythmias.
Monoamine oxidase (MAO) inhibitor used in the treatment of depression	Prolongs and intensifies effects of sympathomimetic drug Risk of severe or fatal hypertensive crisis and stroke	Usually discontinue administration of MAO inhibitor at least 2 weeks before administration of sympathomimetics.
Tricyclic antidepressant	Blocks uptake of catecholamines by adrenergic neurons Abolishes effects of indirect-acting sympathomimetics Reduces intensity of response to mixed-acting sympathomimetics	If necessary, direct-acting sympathomimetic drugs should be used. Anticipate reduction of dose for the sympathomimetic drug.
General inhalation anesthetics (e.g., Halothane)	Renders myocardium hypersensitive to stimulation by β₂-agonists Can cause development of ventricular arrhythmias and fibrillation	Monitor heart rate and rhythm. Monitor ECG for changes.

questions in the health history about dietary intake, digestion, bowel elimination patterns, and history of GI disorders. Explore all complaints since they may signal preexisting problems that would prevent the use of these drugs. You should also ask questions about the client's urinary elimination patterns. Renal insufficiency is a concern with these drugs. Include in the health history questions such as the following:

• What color is your urine?
• Does your urine appear dark yellow?
• How many times do you urinate daily?
• Have you noticed any change in the frequency of urination?
• Have you noticed any increase or decrease in the amount of urine that you void each time?

During the **physical assessment,** carefully evaluate the client's cardiovascular status. Assess for signs of distress such as dyspnea, restlessness, wheezing, or shallow, labored respirations. Note the client's skin color and degree of capillary refill. Examine the client's tongue and buccal mucosa for indications of central cyanosis; assess lips, earlobes, and nail beds for signs of peripheral cyanosis. Collect baseline blood pressure, pulse, and respiration values.

Carefully assess the client for indications of hypovolemia (e.g., decreased skin turgor, hypotension, dry mucous membranes). The usual sympathetic response to hypovolemia is an increased secretion of **endogenous** epinephrine. Administration of **exogenous** epinephrine could result in either further constriction of blood vessels or no beneficial effect. If additional vasoconstriction occurs, perfusion to the kidneys and heart is compromised.

Examine the client carefully for indications of mechanical obstruction of the bowel. Use the diaphragm of the stethoscope to auscultate the client's abdomen for bowel sounds, and use percussion to detect excessive accumulation of fluid or air in the intestines. Physical assessment of the urinary system should include auscultation of renal arteries in the upper abdominal quadrants. In addition, review the results of laboratory studies used to assess renal function. If the client has diabetes mellitus, establish a baseline blood sugar level before initiation of drug therapy.

Diagnosing Based on analysis of the data base, possible nursing diagnoses for a client receiving sympathomimetic drugs are as follows:

• Constipation related to diminished peristalsis associated with drug actions.
• High risk for impaired tissue integrity related to altered peripheral tissue perfusion.
• Sleep pattern disturbance related to insomnia, nervousness, and restlessness associated with drug therapy.
• Noncompliance related to lack of knowledge about drug regimen.
• Altered nutrition: less than body requirements related to decreased appetite and GI discomfort associated with drug therapy.
• Urinary retention (acute) related to bladder wall relaxation associated with drug actions.

Planning During the planning phase, develop a plan of care and establish expected outcomes based on the plan. Do both of these activities in consultation with the client when possible. Discharge teaching is an important consideration when planning care for individuals receiving sympathomimetic drugs. The teaching-discharge plan focuses on drug administration techniques, desired and undesired clinical responses, actions to take if undesired responses occur, and use of over-the-counter (OTC) drugs.

When sympathomimetic drugs are used to treat open-angle glaucoma, determine if the client is familiar with **eyedrop administration.** (If teaching in this area is required, follow the procedure described in Chapter 64.) If the directions require more than 1 drop of ophthalmic solution, instruct the client to wait 2 to 10 minutes between each drop. This technique allows more complete absorption of the drug, producing a greater therapeutic effect. Also, teach the client not to squeeze the eye shut after instilling the drug; this action causes the drug solution to spill out of the eye. The client receiving a sympathomimetic ophthalmic solution will probably experience photophobia. If this occurs, advise the client to wear sunglasses until the pupils can adapt (constrict) in response to sunlight.

Teach the client to report any eye pain or irritation. If the client experiences systemic side effects (e.g., elevated pulse and blood pressure, restlessness) from ophthalmic administration, teach the individual to occlude the lacrimal duct (at the inner canthus) with an index finger for 2 to 3 minutes after drug administration. This action reduces the concentration of the drug available to the nasal mucosa. The nasal mucosa is highly vascular and can absorb enough drug to cause systemic effects.

Information about systemic effects of the drugs is also important for the client receiving sympathomimetic drugs **intranasally.** Teach the client that systemic effects (e.g., tachycardia, headache, visual changes) may occur. If the client notices any of these responses, the primary care provider should be notified. Nasal administration of sympathomimetic agents should not exceed 3 to 4 days since rebound hyperemia and nasal congestion can occur after discontinuation of the drug.

Sympathomimetic preparations for **inhalation** are available in a nebulizer and in a metered dose inhaler (MDI). Observe the client for proper administration techniques. It is recommended that 3 to 5 minutes elapse between MDI puffs to allow delivery of subsequent drug doses further down the airway. Most inhaled dosage forms are prescribed every 4 hours to minimize side effects. Teach the client that nasal discomfort (stinging) may occur when a nasal sympathomimetic is administered. This discomfort is temporary and should disappear within a few minutes.[10,11] (See Chapter 45 for a detailed description of the proper method of administering inhalation medications.)

Teach the client to count the radial pulse just before using a drug inhaler. Five minutes after inhalation of the drug the client should count the pulse and compare the result to the baseline pulse. If a 20% or greater rise in the pulse rate occurs, the primary care provider should be notified. For example, if the baseline pulse is 74, the pulse rate after inhalation therapy should be less than 89 beats per minute. Elevated posttreatment pulse rates usually indicate adjustments in drug therapy are needed.

Single-dose injection devices that contain a sympathomimetic drug (usually epinephrine) may be prescribed for individuals who are at risk for experiencing an anaphylactic reaction. These clients must be taught when and how to use the self-administration device. Teaching should include indications of an allergic reaction, administration technique, and correct body sites (subcutaneous) for the injection. Teach clients to carry the drug with them at all times. When the drug is stored at home, a cool, dark area is preferred.

In addition to administration techniques, clients must be taught undesired clinical responses and actions to take if these responses occur. For example, since prolonged use of sympathomimetics may produce drug tolerance, teach the client to report any perceived drug ineffectiveness. Administering additional drugs or an increased dosage may be necessary if this occurs.

Instruct the client experiencing CNS effects to rest quietly. In addition, teach the individual to avoid foods or substances high in caffeine or nicotine that could enhance these effects. If these changes persist, the client should notify the primary care provider.

Since sympathomimetic drugs alter bowel and bladder function, instruct the client to report any change in elimination patterns. Difficult or painful urination, abdominal distention, constipation, anorexia, and nausea should be noted. Clients should be taught to monitor their intake and output. If the intake far exceeds the output, the primary care provider should be notified.

Discharged clients who are taking sympathomimetic drugs must thoroughly understand OTC medications. Many OTC drugs used for nasal congestion, colds, and flu have sympathomimetic agents as their main therapeutic ingredient. When they are taken along with prescribed sympathomimetics, serious side effects, especially hypertension, can result. If possible, provide the client a list of commonly used OTC drugs that should be avoided. Some OTC drugs that contain sympathomimetic agents are listed in Table 27–3.

Expected outcomes appropriate for a client receiving sympathomimetic drugs include the following:
• Client returns to normal patterns of bowel functioning.
• Client's skin integrity remains intact.
• Client reports improvement in sleep or rest pattern.
• Client discusses components of the drug therapy plan.

TABLE 27–3
Sympathomimetic Drugs Used in Emergency Situations

Drug	Uses
Epinephrine	anaphylactic shock
	bronchial constriction
	complete heart block
	cardiac arrest
Isoproterenol hydrochloride	status asthmaticus
	Adams-Stokes
	cardiac failure
Methoxamine hydrochloride	hypotensive shock

See Table 27–4 for drug dosages.

• Client maintains adequate nutritional intake.
• Client returns to normal patterns of urinary elimination.

Implementing Before administering any sympathomimetic drug, double-check the label for drug concentration and expiration date. Inspect solutions carefully; fresh solutions are clear and colorless. Since these drug solutions are affected by environmental changes, store them in their original containers, protected from light. Once exposed to light or air, the color of the solution usually changes to pink or brown. These changes indicate oxidation and reduced drug activity.

If the solution must be diluted before administration, check the manufacturer's recommendations. Usually sympathomimetic solutions should not be diluted or mixed with alkaline solutions such as sodium bicarbonate or plain saline. Solutions containing dextrose are preferred since dextrose slows the oxidation process. The drug container should not be opened and the solution not diluted until immediately before administration.

Calculated dosages should be double-checked. Small drug calculation errors can result in major catastrophes, especially with pediatric clients. In addition, using a tuberculin syringe is recommended. If the drug will be administered repeatedly, rotate the injection site to avoid tissue irritation or necrosis due to excessive local vasoconstriction. Massage the injection site to avoid excessive local concentration of the drug.

When administering the drug intravenously, the largest central vein should be used. Veins in the feet and legs should be avoided since these veins frequently contain atherosclerotic plaques. All intravenously administered sympathomimetics must be infused through an infusion pump. During the drug infusion, you should assess the pulse and blood pressure every 2 to 5 minutes or until the blood pressure stabilizes. Direct continuous measurement of arterial and venous pressure is preferred.

Because these drugs have a local vasoconstrictive effect, routinely evaluate pulses distal to the intravenous (IV) site and assess color, warmth, sensitivity, and movement of the distal extremity. Diminished pulse strength or a cool, pale distal extremity could indicate extravasation of drug and should be reported immediately.[1,12]

Hypertension is a serious consequence of any form of sympathomimetic drug therapy. Therefore monitor the client's vital signs carefully and frequently. As indicated previously, assess the heart rate and blood pressure for elevations of 20% or more in relationship to the baseline values. If an elevation occurs, notify the primary care provider. In addition, a combined α- and β-blocking drug such as labetalol (Normodyne, Trandate), oxygen, and other emergency equipment should be available.[1–3]

Since sympathomimetic drugs increase serum glucose levels, periodic evaluation of serum glucose levels with a glucose monitoring device is appropriate. Any persistently elevated blood glucose level must be reported. In some instances a sliding scale of insulin to control blood sugar levels is prescribed.[13]

The overall effect of sympathomimetic activity on the GI smooth muscle is decreased responsiveness. As a result, peristaltic activity is diminished, resulting in constipation and anorexia. Routinely auscultate the client's bowel sounds and assess the elimination pattern. Any change in the bowel sounds or bowel habits should be reported. In addition, if anorexia occurs, offer the client small, frequent meals. If the diminished appetite is prolonged or severe, assess the client's serum albumin, hematocrit, and hemoglobin levels and body weight.

Since excessive sympathomimetic drug usage can decrease renal perfusion through vasoconstriction, assessment of urinary output should be routine. The client should maintain a minimum urinary output of 30 ml/h, indicating adequate renal perfusion. In the event that oliguria or anuria occurs during sympathomimetic therapy, careful evaluation of hydration is indicated.[7,10,12] Urinary retention may also result from improved sphincter contraction. This is especially problematic to clients with benign prostatic hypertrophy.

Evaluating No specific laboratory tests are available to determine the effectiveness of sympathomimetics. The best determination is evaluation of the expected outcomes (e.g., improved blood pressure status, increased cardiac output, return of or increased pulse rate, improved ventilation, decreased bleeding, diminished wheezing, decreased nasal congestion, or decreased intraocular pressure). If these responses are not observed, an adjustment in treatment is indicated.

During evaluation, also review the expected outcomes established earlier with the client. Collect new assessment data and compare the current data with the outcomes. Determine which outcomes were not met and what actions are now required. If possible, discuss the plan with the client before making changes.

🌿 NURSING RESEARCH

Wicks, T.C., Yim, D., Newcomer, T., et al. (1992). Hemostasis and hemodynamics during intranasal surgery: The effects of cocaine, oxymetazoline, and epinephrine. *AANA Journal, 60,* 464-471.

Epinephrine is used frequently as a vasoconstrictor in local anesthetic solutions that are administered with cocaine. In this study, 84 clients presenting for intranasal surgery were randomly assigned to one of four study groups. These clients received either topical cocaine or lidocaine and oxymetazoline. Infiltrative local anesthesia consisted of lidocaine, bupivacaine, and either 1:50,000 or 1:200,000 epinephrine. Findings revealed the epinephrine 1:50,000 offered no greater benefit than epinephrine 1:200,000 based on measures of blood loss and surgeons' satisfaction

STUDENT ACTIVITIES

- Interview a nurse anesthetist at your assigned agency and determine what anesthetic is used for intranasal surgery.
- Determine the reason for this selection of drugs and if other methods have been tried.
- Share the findings of this research study with the anesthetist. 🌿

CONCEPT REVIEW

Drugs that mimic the sympathetic nervous system are known as sympathomimetics, adrenergics, or adrenergic sympathetic agonists.

Drugs that stimulate α_1-receptors have two major therapeutic uses: vasoconstriction and mydriasis.

Drugs that stimulate the β_1-receptors in the heart are used to treat cardiac arrest, cardiac failure, atrioventricular heart block, and shock.

Stimulation of β_2 receptor sites has limited effect on the uterus and lungs.

Sympathomimetic drugs are classified as to type of action: direct acting, indirect acting, and mixed acting.

Careful assessment of each client is essential, since use of these drugs is contraindicated in many situations and can produce life-threatening drug-drug interactions.

DIRECT-ACTING, NONSELECTIVE SYMPATHETIC AGONIST PROTOTYPE

EPINEPHRINE

Epinephrine was one of the first adrenergic agonists used clinically. The drug is identical to the epinephrine synthesized in the adrenal medulla and typifies other sympathomimetic drugs in this category.

Pharmacotherapeutics Epinephrine (Adrenalin, Adrenalin Chloride, Sus-Phrine, etc.) stimulates all four types of adrenergic receptors, α_1, β_1, α_2, and β_2. As a result, epinephrine produces a broad spectrum of beneficial sympathomimetic effects. Epinephrine is used to treat anaphylactic shock, bronchoconstriction, complete heart block, cardiac arrest, and primary open-angle glaucoma (Table 27–3). It is used with local anesthetics to reduce circulation to the surgical site, thus prolonging the action of the anesthetic and minimizing blood loss. The vasoconstriction ability of epinephrine also makes it suitable as a hemostatic agent in the treatment of nosebleeds and tooth extractions. The drug is also useful as a respiratory decongestant, reducing mucous formation.[14-17]

Since epinephrine stimulates both α- and β-receptor sites, it usually is the drug of choice during hypersensitivity reactions. It causes vasoconstriction, an alpha-1 response, and bronchial dilation, a beta-2 response. As a result, blood pressure increases, wheezing (from bronchial constriction) subsides, and vocal cord swelling is minimized, preventing airway obstruction.

A cardiovascular problem for which epinephrine might be prescribed is Stokes-Adams syndrome (Adams-Stokes disease). Clients with Stokes-Adams syndrome have intermittent periods of complete heart block, ventricular standstill, or asystole. **Low** doses of epinephrine increase the time the myocardium spends in diastole. This effect allows greater filling of the heart and improves cardiac output. Because of epinephrine's beta-1 effects, it often improves atrioventricular (AV) conduction. It also sensitizes the myocardium to defibrillation attempts during cardiopulmonary resuscitation by reducing the refractory period of atrial and ventricular muscles (a period when the heart is unable to respond to an electric stimuli) and increasing ventricular automaticity.[1,3,8]

Pharmacokinetics Epinephrine is administered by several routes: intramuscular (IM), IV, subcutaneous (SC), topical, inhalation, and ophthalmic. It is not administered orally since it is destroyed by MAO and catechol-O-methyltransferase (COMT) before it reaches systemic circulation. When epinephrine is administered subcutaneously, absorption is delayed because of local vasoconstriction. IV epinephrine has a 3- to 10-minute onset of action, with a duration of several hours. The duration of action for an IM oil suspension is 4 to 24 hours. Epinephrine is inactivated by uptake into adrenergic nerves and by enzymatic activity and has a short plasma half-life. After enzymatic inactivation or metabolism, it is excreted in the urine.[10,18]

Pharmacodynamics Epinephrine is a direct-acting, nonselective sympathomimetic agent. Although it affects both α- and β-receptor sites, its action is primarily on beta sites.

Physiologic Responses Several body systems and organs respond to the presence of epinephrine. The response of the cardiovascular system and the impact of epinephrine on metabolism are discussed in this section of the chapter. Other physiologic responses are summarized in Figure 27–3.

Epinephrine produces several critical changes within the **cardiovascular system.** Vascular smooth muscles contain two major receptor sites, α and β_2. Epinephrine is a potent vasopressor when it exerts its *alpha effects* on arterioles of the skin, mucosa, kidneys, and veins. This action slightly increases the systolic pressure. Stimulation of β_2-*receptors* in vascular smooth muscle of skeletal muscle, liver, and gut results in relaxation of vessels and a slight fall in diastolic pressure. The overall effect is a moderate increase of mean blood pressure and of the pulse pressure. In addition, the total peripheral resistance, which represents both peripheral vasoconstriction

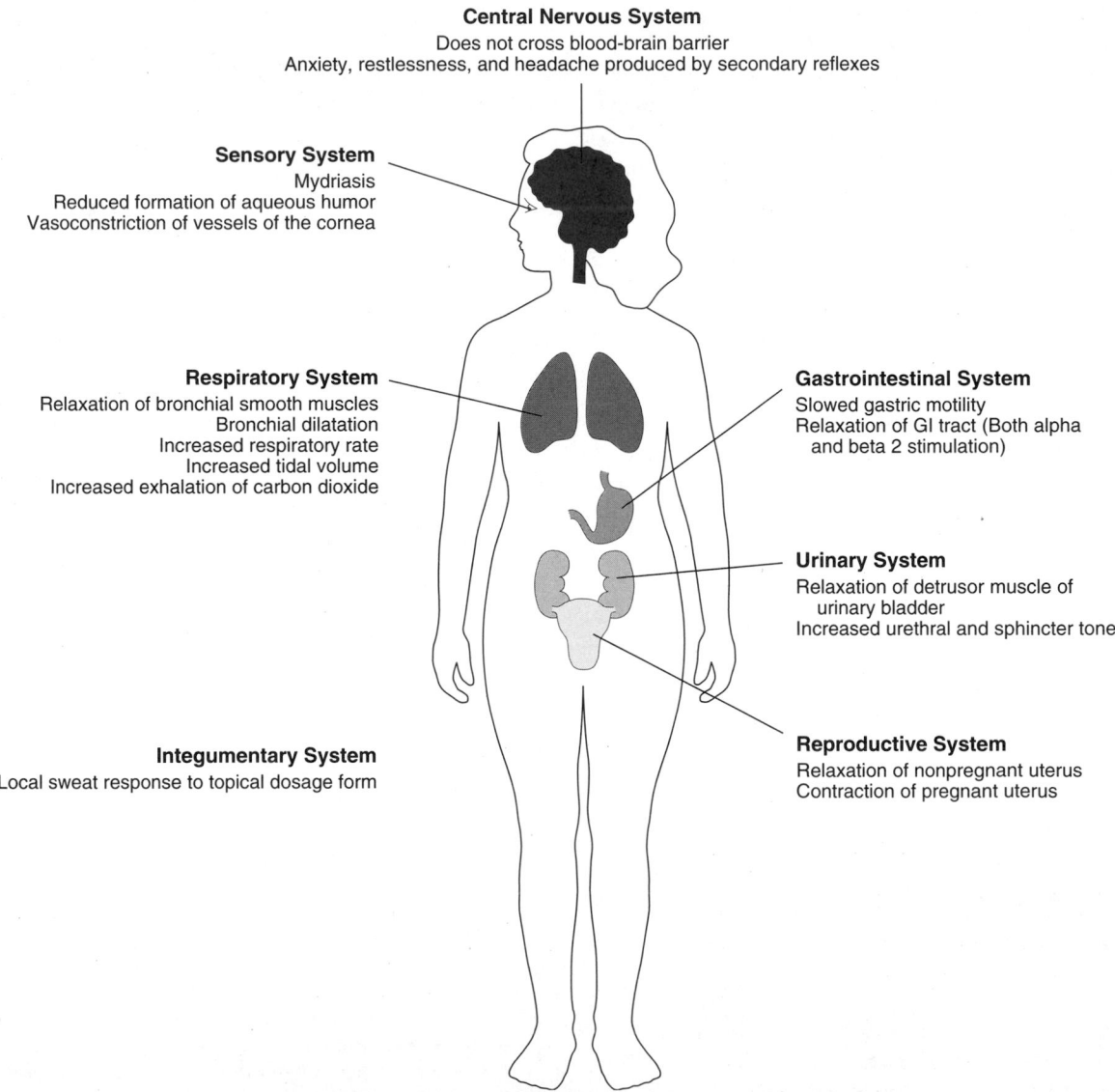

Central Nervous System
Does not cross blood-brain barrier
Anxiety, restlessness, and headache produced by secondary reflexes

Sensory System
Mydriasis
Reduced formation of aqueous humor
Vasoconstriction of vessels of the cornea

Respiratory System
Relaxation of bronchial smooth muscles
Bronchial dilatation
Increased respiratory rate
Increased tidal volume
Increased exhalation of carbon dioxide

Gastrointestinal System
Slowed gastric motility
Relaxation of GI tract (Both alpha and beta 2 stimulation)

Urinary System
Relaxation of detrusor muscle of urinary bladder
Increased urethral and sphincter tone

Integumentary System
Local sweat response to topical dosage form

Reproductive System
Relaxation of nonpregnant uterus
Contraction of pregnant uterus

FIGURE 27–3   Physiologic response to epinephrine.

and vasodilation, falls slightly. These vascular responses are dependent on the dose of epinephrine. At low doses, vasodilation predominates, whereas at higher doses vasoconstriction occurs. The vascular effects of epinephrine and its direct effects on the heart usually increase cardiac output. As a result of this increased cardiac activity, oxygen demand by the cardiac muscles increases.[1,3,18]

Epinephrine also stimulates the β_1-receptors on cells in the kidney's juxtaglomerular apparatus to release renin. Renin release indirectly triggers the release of aldosterone from the adrenal medulla and the formation of angiotensin II. The end result of this action is an elevation in blood pressure.

The effects of epinephrine on **metabolism** are varied and diverse. Epinephrine, through beta-2 stimulation, causes a release of glucagon and inhibition of insulin secretion. It elevates the level of free fatty acids and lactic acids in the blood and causes a 20% to 30% increase in oxygen consumption. Additionally, hypokalemia may result as potassium is taken up by the skeletal muscle cells.[1]

Pharmaceutics Epinephrine is available in a variety of dosage forms and is administered through several different routes. For example, there are different concentrations of sterile solutions for IV, intracardiac, intraspinal, SC, and IM injections. In addition, sterile solutions for instillation into endotracheal tubes and for ophthalmic administration are available. Preparations that can be administered to the respiratory tract include aerosols, sprays, and MDIs. Topical preparations and solutions of epinephrine and lidocaine are also available.

Undesired Clinical Responses Since epinephrine is a direct-acting, nonselective sympathetic agonist, it is capable of producing a wide variation of side effects, adverse effects, and/or toxic effects. The system most affected is the cardiovascular system. Excess alpha-1 stimulation can produce severe vasoconstriction, resulting in hypertensive crisis. Excess stimulation of β_1-receptors in the heart can produce arrhythmias (e.g., tachycardia, premature ventricular contractions, and possibly ventricular fibrillation). In addition, the increased work load and oxygen demand of the heart can cause angina.

Specific Drug-Related Nursing Considerations Any concentration of IV epinephrine solution must be infused slowly through an infusion pump. Also vasodilators such as sodium nitroprusside (Nipride) should be available if reversal of the hypertensive effects of epinephrine is necessary.

Miscellaneous Drugs in Category Dipivefrin hydrochloride (Propine) is a topical ophthalmic drug used only for lowering intraocular pressure in the treatment of open-angle glaucoma. This drug rapidly diffuses into the eye and is metabolized locally to epinephrine. **Norepinephrine bitartrate** (Levophed), which is discussed in Chapter 30, is identical to norepinephrine, the naturally occurring sympathetic neurotransmitter. Unlike epinephrine, the chemical structure of norepinephrine does not contain the methyl group.

DIRECT-ACTING, NONSELECTIVE β-AGONIST PROTOTYPE
ISOPROTERENOL HYDROCHLORIDE

Drugs that stimulate only β-receptors are used mainly to stimulate the heart or to dilate the bronchi. Isoproterenol hydrochloride is the prototype. It stimulates both β_1- and β_2-receptor sites.

Pharmacotherapeutics Isoproterenol (Isuprel, Norisodrine, Vapo-Iso, etc.) is effective in treating acute and chronic asthma and status asthmaticus. It is also used to treat shock, pulmonary hypertension, and symptomatic bradycardia that is resistant to atropine.

Pharmacokinetics Sublingual isoproterenol is poorly absorbed and is rapidly metabolized in the GI tract. It has a half-life of approximately 2 to 5 minutes. The majority of the drug is excreted in its metabolized form by the kidneys. A small portion is excreted in the bile. When administered intravenously, 50% to 70% of the drug is excreted unchanged by the kidney.

Isoproterenol is readily absorbed when given as an aerosol; however, the inhaled form results in an uneven distribution of drug in the bronchioles. Clinical improvement in clients with asthma occurs within 15 to 30 minutes. Further improvements usually occur with repeated inhalation doses. The duration of action of a 1% concentration of inhaled isoproterenol is 2 to 3 hours. The drug is metabolized primarily in the liver and other tissues by COMT.[10,18]

Pharmacodynamics Beta-1 cardiac receptor stimulation by isoproterenol produces positive inotropic (increased force of myocardial contraction) and chronotropic (increased heart rate) effects. This combination results in improved cardiac output. However, this combined effect results in increased myocardial oxygen demand. Isoproterenol also lowers peripheral vascular resistance, causing the diastolic pressure to fall.[19]

Isoproterenol relaxes most smooth muscles. The most pronounced effect is on bronchial and GI smooth muscle. Isoproterenol produces marked relaxation in smaller bronchi and may dilate the trachea and main bronchi.[8]

Pharmaceutics Isoproterenol is available in sublingual tablets, inhalation nebulization solution, inhalation aerosol, and serile solutions for injection (IM, IV, and SC).

Undesired Clinical Responses Side effects from isoproterenol include tremors, headache, dizziness, weakness, nervousness, heart palpitations, nausea, and vomiting. If these responses occur, they should be reported to the primary care provider immediately. In addition, after inhalation therapy the sputum or saliva may appear red or pink tinged; this response is not considered harmful.

Contraindications and Precautions Contraindications to the use of isoproterenol include tachycardia due to digitalis intoxication and preexisting arrhythmias associated with tachycardia. In addition, the drug should be used with caution in clients with coronary insufficiency, diabetes mellitus, hyperthyroidism, hypovolemic shock, or a sensitivity to sympathomimetics. Since deaths have been reported with overuse of inhalation aerosol therapy, the client should be instructed to use the drug only as prescribed.[7,8,10]

Drug-Drug, Drug-Nutrient, Drug-Environment Interactions Epinephrine and isoproterenol should not be administered at the same time since both drugs are direct cardiac stimulants. Their combined effects may induce serious arrhythmias. If desired, they may be alternated if an interval of at least 4 hours elapses.[19]

Clients receiving isoproterenol should not use OTC allergy, cold, or flu medication that contains sympathomimetic ingredients. They should also consult with the primary care provider before self-prescribing any drugs.

Specific Drug-Related Nursing Considerations
Monitor clients receiving IV isoproterenol for cardiac arrhythmias. Individuals with a history of cardiac problems are usually placed on a cardiac monitor while receiving IV drug therapy.

Clients with asthma, bronchitis, or emphysema should be taught that their breathing should improve within 3 to 5 minutes after inhalation or sublingual administration. You may need to review or instruct clients on inhalation techniques. In addition, instruct clients to allow sublingual tablets to dissolve completely under the tongue before they swallow any of the drug. This increases the concentration of the drug and enhances absorption.

Clients should also be instructed to store isoproterenol in the original container, which should be tightly closed and light resistant to avoid exposure to moisture and direct light. Injectable forms of isoproterenol are stable indefinitely when stored in their original container at room temperature.[11]

Miscellaneous Drugs in Category Other drugs in this category include **isoxsuprine hydrochloride** (Vasodilan) and **nylidrin hydrochloride** (Arlidin), which are discussed in Chapter 30.

DIRECT-ACTING, SELECTIVE α-AGONIST PROTOTYPE

PHENYLEPHRINE HYDROCHLORIDE

Phenylephrine hydrochloride is a vasoconstrictor and pressor drug that is chemically related to epinephrine and ephedrine.

Pharmacotherapeutics Phenylephrine hydrochloride (Neo-Synephrine, Mydfrin, Ocu-Phrin, etc.) is used in clients with local ocular disorders for its vasoconstrictor, decongestant, and mydriatic action. It is used during eye examinations when inspection of intraocular structures is desired. It is also used to treat uveitis and postoperative inflammation.

Phenylephrine injections are used to maintain an adequate blood pressure level during spinal and inhalation anesthesia and to treat vascular failure in shock or allergic reactions. In OTC drugs phenylephrine is often the active ingredient used topically to reduce nasal congestion.[10,18,19]

Pharmacokinetics Oral doses of phenylephrine are absorbed poorly; therefore this route of administration is not recommended. Phenylephrine provides vasoconstriction that lasts longer than that of epinephrine and ephedrine. Physiologic responses resulting from IM injections of the drug last approximately 1 to 2 hours. Responses usually last 20 minutes after IV injection and as long as 50 minutes after SC injections. Since phenylephrine is not a catecholamine, it is not metabolized by COMT. MAO activity in the liver is the major metabolic pathway.

The concentration of ophthalmic solutions determines mydriatic effects. Phenylephrine hydrochloride 2.5% and 10% solutions produce maximum mydriasis within 10 to 60 minutes. The mydriasis produced by the 2.5% solution lasts approximately 3 hours, whereas the pupil dilation from the 10% solution lasts 6 hours. Nasal drop or spray decongestion effects last approximately 3 to 6 hours.[12,18,19]

Pharmacodynamics Phenylephrine is a direct-acting, α-receptor sympathetic agonist. The predominant actions of the drug are on the cardiovascular system. Parenteral administration of phenylephrine causes a rise in systolic and diastolic pressures and a marked reflex bradycardia. In addition, phenylephrine considerably increases peripheral vascular resistance.

Pharmaceutics Phenylephrine hydrochloride is available in a variety of dosage forms, including ophthalmic solutions, nasal sprays and drops, and sterile solutions for IM, SC, and IV injections. Ophthalmic solutions are available in 2.5% and 10% concentrations and are usually administered as 1 drop per dose. The lower concentration (2.5%) ophthalmic solution is recommended for elderly clients, since they are frequently more sensitive to the systemic effects of ophthalmic phenylephrine.

As a nasal decongestant, a 0.25% to 1% nasal solution is sprayed or instilled into the nostril every 3 to 4 hours as needed. More frequent use is not recommended because of possible rebound congestion of the mucous membranes. Infants treated for nasal congestion should receive the pediatric strength nose drops, 0.125%, every 2 to 4 hours as needed. Children more than 6 years of age may receive a drop or spray of 0.25% solution every 3 to 4 hours as needed.[3,18]

When phenylephrine is used to treat mild or moderate hypotension, the recommended dose is 2 to 5 mg via SC or IM injection. If the IV route is used, the dose is 0.1 mg to 0.5 mg every 10 to 15 minutes as needed. For children with hypotension, the recommended dose is 0.1 mg/kg by SC or IM injection.[18,19]

Undesired Clinical Responses Usual adverse reactions to phenylephrine injections include headaches, reflex bradycardia, excitability, and restlessness. Occasionally the client experiences arrhythmias. As previously indicated, excessive use of nasal preparations can cause rebound congestion of the mucous membranes of the nostrils. In addition, ophthalmic solutions can produce eye irritation and tearing.

Contraindications and Precautions Clients with a history of a hypersensitivity to sympathomimetic agents or those with narrow-angle glaucoma should not receive phenylephrine hydrochloride. In addition, clients with diabetes mellitus, hyperthyroidism, asthma, and essential orthostatic hypotension should not use phenylephrine. It should be used with caution in clients with coronary artery disease and/or a history of cerebral vascular accident or myocardial infarction.[18]

Specific Drug-Related Nursing Considerations Instruct the client that blurred vision is anticipated with ophthalmic administration of phenylephrine hydrochloride. This reaction should disappear in about 6 hours. Also teach clients to avoid self-medication with OTC drugs, especially those advertised as useful for allergies, colds, or flu, for their use may result in adverse drug-drug interactions.

Miscellaneous Drugs in Category Methoxamine **hydrochloride** (Vasoxyl) is a selective α-agonist that is used only to treat acute hypotension. (See Table 27–4 for additional information on this drug.) Other selective α-agonists used for nasal or ocular problems include **naphazoline, oxymetazoline,** and **tetrahydrozoline.**

Direct-acting, Selective β_1-Agonist Prototype

DOPAMINE

Dobutamine (Dobutrex) and **dopamine** (Intropin) are catecholamines. In therapeutic doses they stimulate β_1-receptors in the heart. This action enhances cardiac contractile force and increases the heart rate. Dilation of some blood vessels, especially those in the mesentery and kidneys, may also occur. The overall physiologic responses to these drugs are increased cardiac output and enhanced peripheral blood flow. These drugs are administered by IV infusion and are used to treat acute heart failure. Dobutamine and dopamine are potent drugs; therefore doses must be double-checked before being administered. Both drugs have a rapid onset of action and a short duration of action. These drugs are discussed more fully in Chapter 30.

Direct-Acting, Selective β_2-Agonist Prototype

ALBUTEROL SULFATE

Albuterol sulfate (Proventil, Ventolin, etc.) was the first selective β_2-agonist approved for use in the United States. Although albuterol sulfate is available in oral, inhaled, and parenteral dosage forms, selective beta-2 stimulating effects occur only when the drug is administered in low doses by inhalation.[12,18]

As a selective β_2-agonist, albuterol sulfate stimulates β_2-receptors located on bronchial smooth muscle, producing bronchodilation. Changes in ventilatory function begin within the first 30 minutes of therapy, and maximum bronchodilation occurs within 1 to 2 hours. The duration of action for albuterol sulfate is 3 to 4 hours. Most of the drug is metabolized by the liver. Albuterol sulfate is excreted by the kidneys, with approximately one fourth excreted unchanged.[18,19] This drug is discussed more fully in Chapter 45.

Indirect-Acting, Nonselective Agonist Prototype

AMPHETAMINE SULFATE

Amphetamines are noncatecholamine, sympathomimetic amines. They produce their effects by stimulating the release of endogenous catecholamines, mainly norepinephrine, from adrenergic nerves. Peripheral actions of these drugs include elevation of systolic and diastolic blood pressure, weak bronchodilation, and respiratory stimulation. Amphetamines also increase or decrease the heart rate. This effect is based on the amount of baroreceptor reflex stimulation that occurs. In addition, amphetamines enter the CNS and produce powerful CNS-stimulating effects.[7,19]

Amphetamines are no longer used for their peripheral sympathomimetic effects. Their indications are related to their effects on the CNS. See Chapter 22 for additional information on this drug category.

Mixed-Acting, Nonselective Agonist Prototype

EPHEDRINE

Ephedrine and other mixed-acting sympathomimetics are not catecholamines. As a group, their chemical structure enables them to enter the CNS much more easily than direct-acting sympathomimetics can.

Pharmacotherapeutics Before the advent of drugs with more beta-2 selectivity and less beta-1 activity, ephedrine was the major drug used for long-term management of asthma. Currently it is rarely used to relieve bronchodilation. It is used to alleviate nasal congestion and to treat acute hypotension. In addition, ephedrine is used as an adjunct to the treatment of myasthenia gravis and to treat mild cases of stress incontinence.[18]

Pharmacokinetics Because ephedrine is not a catecholamine, it is not inactivated by gastric acid and can be administered orally. After oral administration the onset of action is 15 minutes to 1 hour, with a duration of 3 to 5 hours. After an IM injection, the onset of action is 10 to 20 minutes, with a duration of 60 minutes. Ephedrine is relatively resistant to metabolism and is excreted largely unchanged in the urine. The half-life is approximately 3 to 6 hours, depending on urine pH. When the urine is acidic (pH, 5 or less), the half-life is approximately 3 hours. When the urine pH is alkaline (6.3 or above), the half-life is prolonged to approximately 6 hours.[18]

Pharmacodynamics Ephedrine stimulates adrenergic receptors both directly and indirectly. Direct stimulation occurs at both α- and β-receptor sites. Indirect stimulation results from release of norepinephrine from adrenergic nerves.

The clinical response is essentially the same as for nonselective, direct-acting agonists (e.g., epinephrine). The alpha effects result in vasoconstriction, whereas the beta-2 effects result in bronchodilation. Cardiac output and force of myocardial contraction also increase.[3,18]

Systemic administration of ephedrine usually produces mild stimulation of the CNS. This may cause increased wakefulness **(analeptic effect)** and increased resistance to fatigue. In addition, the client's appetite may be suppressed **(anorexigenic effect).**

Pharmaceutics Ephedrine is available in several dosage forms. Sterile solutions for IM, SC, and IV injections are used primarily in the treatment of hypotension. Nasal congestion is treated with oral ephedrine and intranasal spray and gel. Oral tablets are also used in the treatment of asthma.

Undesired Clinical Responses and Contraindications Clients receiving ephedrine are at risk of developing numerous adverse reactions or side effects. The autonomic side effects noted for epinephrine and amphetamine sulfate apply to ephedrine. In addition, CNS reactions such as nervousness, tremors, anxiety, psychosis, hallucinations, depression, paranoia, and seizures occur. Clients receiving ephedrine must also be monitored carefully for physical dependence on the drug.

Ephedrine should not be administered in situations in which vasopressor drugs are contraindicated (e.g., hypovolemic shock). The drug should be used with caution in clients with diabetes mellitus, prostatic hypertrophy, angina pectoris, or chronic heart disease. Chronic use of ephedrine should be avoided since an anxiety reaction may result.[18]

Drug-Drug, Drug-Nutrient, Drug-Environment Interactions In addition to the drugs discussed in the general section on sympathomimetic drugs, others are of major concern with regard to ephedrine. For example, concomitant use of ephedrine and other sympathomimetic agents is not recommended because of the potential for adverse cardiovascular side effects. Ephedrine should not be administered with certain antihypertensive agents (e.g., methyldopa [Aldomet], clonidine [Catapres]). These combinations either diminish the effects of the antihypertensive agent or blunt the expected response of ephedrine.[11,18] In addition, the concurrent administration of theophylline and ephedrine has resulted in increased CNS and GI side effects. Therefore if a client is receiving theophylline and ephedrine is added to the medical management, close assessment of the client for indications of theophylline toxicity is necessary.[18]

Specific Drug-Related Nursing Considerations

TABLE 27–4

Prototype and Major Drugs in Category

Drug Name	Dosage and Route of Administration	Nursing Considerations
DIRECT-ACTING, NONSELECTIVE, SYMPATHETIC AGONIST: EPINEPHRINE (Adrenalin, Adrenalin Chloride, Sus-Phrine) HOW SUPPLIED Injection solution: 1:1000 (1mg/ml), 1:10,000 (0.1 mg/ml), and 1:100,000 (0.01 mg/ml)	Dosage is highly individualized. SC or IM: 0.2 to 1 mg **Cardiac Arrest** ADULTS IV: 0.1-1 mg (1-10 ml of 1:10,000 solution) q5 min CHILDREN IV: 0.01-0.03 mg/kg (0.1-0.3 ml/kg of 1:10,000 solution) q5 min **Local Anesthetic** 1:100,000 (0.01 mg/ml)-1:20,000 (0.05 mg/ml) **Asthma** ADULTS SC: 0.1-0.5 ml of 1:1000 solution; may repeat at 20 min-4 h intervals CHILDREN SC: 0.01 ml/kg of 1:1000 solution; may repeat at 20 min–4h intervals **Endotracheal Tube Administration** 1 mg injected directly into endotracheal tube	**Assess** Obtain baseline heart rate and rhythm and blood pressure values. Assess client for preexisting narrow-angle glaucoma, hypertension, heart disease, hyperthyroidism, diabetes mellitus, or ileus. Determine if client is pregnant; epinephrine is classifed as Pregnancy Category C. Determine baseline blood glucose level. **Implement** Store at 15°-25° C. Protect from light and freezing. Mix solutions thoroughly before administering. Check solutions for particulate matter and discolorations; if present, do not use. Double-check dose before administering. SC is preferred route of administration. IM injection into buttocks should be avoided. Do not prepare epinephrine in same syringe as aminophylline, atropine, diazepam (Valium), lidocaine, isoproterenol (Isuprel), phenytoin (Dilantin), or penicillin G potassium. Follow endotracheal administration with 5 to 10 artificial breaths. Massage injection site to enhance absorption. Teach client how to use single-dose epinephrine devices if necessary. Space administration of ophthalmic solutions at least 10 min apart. **Monitor** Observe parenteral infusion site; infiltration into subcutaneous tissue can cause necrosis of tissue. Monitor urinary output; report anuria or oliguria. Monitor pulse and blood pressure closely for first 3-15 min (or until client stabilizes) after drug administration. Monitor blood glucose levels. Auscultate bowel sounds at least every shift. Monitor for undesired responses: anxiety, headache, fear, and palpitations. **Evaluate** Report significant improvements in client's condition such as improved cardiac output, decreased bleeding, improved ventilation, decreased nasal congestion.
Norepinephrine Bitartrate (Levophed)	See Chapter 30, Table 30–4.	

Stress to the client that many OTC drugs contain ephedrine and that he or she must read the labels on all OTC drugs. Tell the client to consult the primary care provider or local pharmacist about the active ingredient in OTC drugs for asthma, allergies, colds, or flu.

Miscellaneous Drugs in Category Two other mixed-acting sympathomimetic drugs are available for treatment of acute hypotension: **mephentermine** (Wyamine) and **metaraminol** (Aramine). As an α-agonist, metaraminol acts almost exclusively as a vasoconstrictor. Mephentermine constricts more arterioles but, through beta-2 stimulation, dilates others. These drugs are discussed further in Chapter 30.

A summary of sympathomimetic agents, their use, administration, and nursing considerations are in Table 27–4.

CONCEPT REVIEW

Most sympathomimetics are administered through parenteral, nasal, or ophthalmic routes. Few oral preparations are available.

Parenteral doses should be double-checked with another nurse since several solution concentrations are available.

Sympathomimetic drugs should not be administered to individuals with hypertension, cerebrovascular or cardiovascular disease, or diabetes mellitus.

TABLE 27–4 *Continued*
Prototype and Major Drugs in Category

Drug Name	Dosage and Route of Administration	Nursing Considerations
DIRECT-ACTING, NONSELECTIVE β-AGONISTS: ISOPROTERENOL HYDROCHLORIDE (Isuprel, Isuprel Hydrochloride, Isoproterenol Abboject) HOW SUPPLIED Aerosol inhalation solutions: 1:100 and 1:200 (0.5%-1%) Aerosol spray: 0.25% Inhalation solution: 0.5%-5% IM, IV, SC: 0.2-1 mg/ml Tablet, sublingual: 10 and 15 mg	Dosage is highly individualized. **Heart Block, Adams-Stokes Disease, Cardiac Arrest, Cardiac Failure** IV bolus: 0.02-0.06 mg initial dose; 0.01-2 mg subsequent dose range IV infusion: 5 μg/min IM: 0.2 mg initial dose; 0.02-1 mg subsequent dose range SC: 0.2 mg initial dose; 0.15-0.2 mg subsequent dose range Intracardiac: 0.02 mg for cardiac arrest **Intraoperative bronchospasm** IV bolus: 0.001-0.02 mg initial dose; initial dose repeated when necessary **Shock** IV infusion: 0.5-5 μg/min **Chronic Syncope** Sublingual: 10 or 15 mg **Chronic Bronchospasm** ADULTS Sublingual: 10 mg; no more than 60 mg/d CHILDREN Sublingual: 5-10 mg; not to exceed 30 mg/d ADULTS Inhalation: 1 to 2 puffs of metered-dose inhaler; repeat up to six times a day ADULTS OR CHILDREN Hand nebulizer: 5-15 deep inhalations of a 1:100-1:200 solution	**Assess** Assess client for preexisting arrhythmia, coronary insufficiency, diabetes mellitus, or hyperthyroidism. Determine if client is pregnant; isoproterenol is classified as Pregnancy Category C. Obtain baseline heart rate and rhythm and blood pressure. **Implement** Protect solution from light. Store in an opaque container. Store solutions in cool place at 8°-15° C. Store aerosol preparations at 15°-30° C. Do not use if solution is pinkish to brownish in color or contains particulate matter. Dilute solutions in sodium chloride injection, USP, or dextrose injection, USP. Anticipate that usual route of administration is IV infusion or bolus IV injection. Be certain to have oxygen on standby. Be prepared to administer a β-blocker to stop action of isoproterenol. Teach client to use metered-dose inhaler (MDI). Instruct client to allow sublingual tablets to dissolve completely under the tongue before swallowing. Provide frequent mouth care for clients receiving sublingual dosage; sublingual dosage form may damage teeth because of drug acidity. Teach client to avoid OTC drugs containing sympathomimetic drugs. **Monitor** Monitor systemic blood pressure, heart rate, urinary flow, and ECG. Monitor for undesired responses: nervousness, headache, dizziness, irregular heart beat, tachycardia, angina, tremors, weakness, and flushing. **Evaluate** Observe for significant improvements in client's condition.
Isoxsuprine hydrochloride (Vasodilan)	See Chapter 30.	
Nylidrin hydrochloride (Arlidin)	See Chapter 30.	

Table continued on following page.

TABLE 27–4 *Continued*
Prototype and Major Drugs in Category

Drug Name	Dosage and Route of Administration	Nursing Considerations
DIRECT-ACTING, SELECTIVE α AGONIST: PHENYLEPHRINE HYDROCHLORIDE (Neo-Synephrine, Neo-Synephrine Injection) **HOW SUPPLIED** IM, IV, SC: 10 mg/ml	**Mild to Moderate Hypotension** ADULTS SC or IM: 1-10 mg; initial dose not to exceed 5 mg IV: 0.1-0.5 mg; initial dose not to exceed 0.5 mg CHILDREN SC or IM: 0.1 mg/kg **Severe Hypotension and Shock** Continuous IV infusion: 10 mg of drug (1 ml of 1% solution) in 500 ml of dextrose injection, USP, or sodium chloride injection, USP	**Assess** Obtain baseline pulse rate and rhythm and blood pressure values. Determine if client is receiving MAO inhibitors or tricyclic antidepressants. Assess client for preexisting narrow-angle glaucoma, arteriosclerotic cardiovascular disease, cerebrovascular disease, hypertension, bronchial asthma, or hyperthyroidism. Determine if client is pregnant; phenylephrine is classified as Pregnancy Category C. **Implement** Store solutions at 3°-27° C. Protect solutions from light and excessive heat. Check solutions for brownish discoloration; if present, do not use. Do not prepare phenylephrine in same syringe as phenobarbital or phenytoin. Administer IV doses slowly. For IV infusion, be prepared to infiltrate area with phentolamine if extravasation occurs. Administer with caution to elderly clients. Teach client to limit use of OTC nasal solutions to 3-5 days to avoid rebound congestion. **Monitor** Monitor for undesired responses from parenteral doses: headache, reflex, bradycardia, restlessness, and excitability. Monitor vital signs and intake and output. With ophthalmic solutions, monitor client for eye pain and irritation. **Evaluate** Report significant improvements in client's condition.
Methoxamine hydrochloride (Vasoxyl) **HOW SUPPLIED** IM, IV: 20 mg/ml	**Emergency Situation: Hypotensive Shock** IV: 3-5 mg injected slowly IV infusion: 40 mg in 250 ml D_5W to infuse at 5 μg/min IM: 10-15 mg to prolong effect of IV injection **Moderate Hypotension** IM: 5-10 mg **Spinal Hypotension** 3-5 mg slow IV push, followed by 10-15 mg for prolonged effect **Supraventricular Tachycardia** IV: 10 mg by slow push (i.e., 3-5 min)	**Assess** Determine if client has preexisting hypertension, hyperthyroidism, bradycardia, partial heart block, or atherosclerosis. Determine if client is receiving MAO inhibitors, tricyclic antidepressants, an oxytocic agent, or an ergot alkaloid. Determine if client is pregnant; methoxamine is classified as Pregnancy Category C. **Implement** Inspect solution for particulate matter and discoloration. Store solutions at 15°-30° C. Use caution when interpreting cortisol and ACTH plasma levels since this drug influences laboratory test results. **Monitor** Monitor client for undesired responses: nausea, vomiting, hypertension, headache, anxiety, and sweating. Monitor blood pressure. Monitor renal function tests—blood urea nitrogen, creatinine, etc. **Evaluate** Report significant improvements in client's condition.
Clonidine (Catapres, Catapres-TTS)	See Chapter 33.	
Methyldopa (Aldomet)	See Chapter 33.	

TABLE 27–4 *Continued*
Prototype and Major Drugs in Category

Drug Name	Dosage and Route of Administration	Nursing Considerations
DIRECT-ACTING, SELECTIVE β₁-AGONISTS: DOPAMINE HYDROCHLORIDE (Intropin)	See Chapter 30.	
Dobutamine hydrochloride (Dobutrex)	See Chapter 30.	
DIRECT-ACTING, SELECTIVE β₂-AGONIST: ALBUTEROL (Proventil, Ventolin)	See Chapter 45.	
INDIRECT-ACTING, NONSELECTIVE AGONIST: AMPHETAMINE SULFATE HOW SUPPLIED Plain coated tablet: 10 mg Uncoated tablet: 5 mg	***Narcolepsy*** CHILDREN 6-12 y: 5 mg/d; daily dose may be raised by 5-mg increments at weekly intervals ***Attention Deficit Disorder with Hyperactivity*** CHILDREN <3 y: not recommended 3-5 y: 2.5 mg/d; daily dose may be raised by 2.5-mg increments at weekly intervals ≥6 y: 5 mg once or twice daily; daily dose may be raised by 5-mg increments at weekly intervals ***Exogenous Obesity*** ADULTS 5-30 mg/d in divided doses	***Assess*** Assess for history of substance abuse. Assess for use of MAO inhibitors within the last 2 wk. Obtain baseline heart rate and rhythm and blood pressure values. Assess for preexisting hypertension, advanced arteriosclerosis, symptomatic cardiovascular disease, and glaucoma. Determine if client is pregnant; amphetamine is classified as Pregnancy Category C. ***Implement*** Classified under Schedule II of Controlled Substance Act; dispense accordingly. Usually administer first dose when client awakens and then at intervals of 4-6 h. Administer last dose at least 6 h before bedtime. Acidifying the urine shortens effects of drug. Alkaline urine prolongs effects of drug. Drug elevates serum level of growth hormone, changes serum cortisol level, and causes fecal discoloration. Advise client not to discontinue drug abruptly. Teach client to avoid all other drugs unless prescribed by physician. Teach client to avoid caffeine beverages, which may enhance effect of drugs. ***Monitor*** When drug is terminated, assess for withdrawal signs and symptoms; withdrawal develops within 24-48 h. Monitor for undesired responses: palpitations, tachycardia, elevation of blood pressure, restlessness, overstimulation, insomnia, headaches, dryness of mouth, and GI disturbances. ***Evaluate*** Report significant changes in client's condition.

Table continued on following page.

TABLE 27–4 *Continued*
Prototype and Major Drugs in Category

Drug Name	Dosage and Route of Administration	Nursing Considerations
MIXED-ACTING, NONSELECTIVE AGONIST: EPHEDRINE (Ephedrine Sulfate) HOW SUPPLIED Gelatin capsule: 25 and 50 mg IM, IV, SC: 25 and 50 mg/ml Nasal solution: 0.25%-1%	*Relief of Seasonal Allergies* ADULT Oral: 25-50 mg initially; then 25 mg q3-4h; maximum dose in 24 h, 150 mg Intranasal: 2 or 3 drops of 0.25%-1% solution in each nostril qid CHILDREN 6-12 y Oral: 3 mg/kg/d divided into four to six doses or one half of adult dose *Hypotension, Shock* IM, SC: 25-50 mg IV: 10-25 mg injected slowly	*Assess* Assess client for preexisting glaucoma, diabetes mellitus, and hypertension. Determine if client is receiving MAO inhibitors. Obtain baseline blood pressure values and heart rate and rhythm. *Implement* Anticipate that MAO inhibitors should be discontinued at least 2 wk before starting ephedrine. Instruct client not to use intranasal dosage form for more than 4d. Do not administer the drug at night. *Monitor* Monitor intake and output. Monitor client for CNS stimulation: increased wakefulness (analeptic effect), increased resistance to fatigue, and suppressed appetite (anorexigenic effect). *Evaluate* Observe for significant improvements in client's condition.

SYMPATHOMIMETICS IN OVER-THE-COUNTER DRUGS

Sympathomimetics with α-adrenergic agonist activities are found in hundreds of OTC drugs (Table 27–5). These drugs are self-prescribed by individuals for a variety of health problems, including asthma, colds, flu, allergies, nasal congestion, ophthalmic congestion, and cough. Some OTC drugs containing sympathomimetics are used as appetite suppressants. These drugs are intended for short-term relief of minor symptoms. The pharmacodynamics, undesired responses, contraindications, and interactions are similar to the prototypes previously discussed.

Teach the client not to take OTC drugs without checking with the primary care provider or the pharmacist. When purchasing an OTC drug, the client must read the labels carefully. Information such as contraindications, side effects, and possible drug-drug interactions are included on the label or on the package insert. Encourage the clients to purchase all drugs—prescription and OTC—from one pharmacist so that one individual is monitoring their drug usage.

SYMPATHOLYTIC DRUGS

Sympatholytic drugs are also known as **adrenergic blockers** or **antiadrenergic drugs.** These drugs are used to block the effects of the sympathetic nervous system. They inhibit the action of endogenously produced epinephrine and norepinephrine. In addition, they competitively block exogenously administered sympathomimetics. Sympatholytics exert their effects on α_1, α_2, β_1, β_2, and ganglionic receptor sites. α-Adrenergic blocking drugs and nonselective adrenergic blockers are discussed in the following section. Ganglionic blockers are discussed with the parasympathetic drugs in Chapter 26, and β-blockers are discussed in Chapter 30.

Pharmacotherapeutics α-**Blockers** were traditionally used to treat hypertension. An α-antagonist lowers blood pressure by blocking α_1-receptors on arterioles and veins, causing both types of vessels to dilate. However, with the advent of newer, more effective, and safer drugs, α-blockers are now used less frequently for this purpose. Sympatholytic drugs are sometimes used to improve circulation in clients with peripheral vascular conditions such as Raynaud's disease and frostbite. Although α-blockers can relieve symptoms of Raynaud's disease, they are usually ineffective against other peripheral vascular diseases.

α-Blockers are also used to diagnose and temporarily treat pheochromocytoma. With this disease, α-blockers completely block the vasoconstrictive effects of catecholamine and produce a dramatic fall in blood pressure.[8] These drugs are used to reverse the effects of α-agonists or when there is inadvertent infiltration of α-agonists into subcutaneous tissue. Occasionally α-blockers are used in selected clients with urinary obstruction who are poor surgical risks. They provide partial relief from urinary obstruction by relaxing the smooth muscles of the prostate and bladder neck. This same rationale applies to clients with spinal cord injuries who have hypertonic urinary bladder necks. In addition, migraine headaches are sometimes treated with an ergot alkaloid, another α-adrenergic blocking agent. Ergot alkaloids are also used to treat some forms of senility associated with cerebral insufficiency.[3,7,19]

TABLE 27–5
OTC Drugs Containing Sympathomimetic Agents

Product	Dose Form	Sympathomimetic Agent
Actifed	Capsule, tablet, syrup	Pseudoepinephrine hydrochloride, pseudoephedrine hydrochloride
Alka-Seltzer Plus Cold	Tablet	Phenylpropanolamine bitartrate
Allerest	Tablet	Phenylpropanolamine hydrochloride
Benadryl Plus	Tablet	Pseudoephedrine hydrochloride
Bronkaid Mist	Inhaler	Epinephrine
Contac	Timed-release capsule	Phenylpropanolamine hydrochloride
Coricidin D	Tablet	Phenylpropanolamine hydrochloride
Dristan, Advanced Formula	Tablet, caplet	Phenylephrine hydrochloride
Halls Mentho-Lyptus Decongestant	Liquid	Phenylpropanolamine hydrochloride
Novahistine	Elixir	Phenylephrine hydrochloride
Primatene Mist Solution	Inhaler	Epinephrine
Robitussin CF	Syrup	Phenylpropanolamine hydrochloride
Sudafed	Tablet	Pseudoephedrine hydrochloride
Triaminic DM	Timed-release liquid	Phenylpropanolamine hydrochloride

TABLE 27–6
Responses of Major Effector Organs to Alpha or Beta Blockers

Organ	Receptor Type	Response to Receptor Activation
Cardiovascular System		
Arterioles and large veins	α	Dilation
	β_2	Constriction
Heart	β_1	Decreased heart rate, force of contraction, impulse conduction, and automaticity
Eye		
Iris, dilator muscle	α	Miosis
Respiratory System		
Bronchial glands	α	Increased thin secretions
Bronchial smooth muscle	β_2	Bronchial constriction
Gastrointestinal Tract		
Motility	α, β_2	Slightly increased
Sphincters	α	Slightly relaxed
Metabolic Effects		
Fat cells	α, β_1	Decreased lipolysis
Skeletal muscle	α, β_2	Decreased glycogen breakdown
Liver	β_2	Decreased insulin release
Pancreas	α	Increased insulin release

General characteristics α-Blockers have three main methods of action:

1. They can block the synthesis, storage, release, and uptake of norepinephrine by neurons.
2. They can block acetylcholine at the preganglionic synapse.
3. They can competitively or noncompetitively inhibit endogenous catecholamines or exogenous sympathomimetic agents at the receptor site.

α-Blockers are divided into four categories:

1. Noncompetitive, long-acting antagonists.
2. Competitive, short-acting antagonists.
3. Ergot alkaloids.
4. Selective α_1-antagonists.[3,7,19]

Blood vessels contain both α- and β_2-receptor sites. Activation of α-receptors results in vasoconstriction. However, when α-receptors are blocked, β_2-receptors predominate.

TABLE 27–7
Sympatholytic Drug Used in Emergency Situations*

Drug	Uses
Phentolamine mesylate	Hypertensive episodes associated with pheochromocytoma Extravasation of dopamine or norepinephrine infusions

*See Table 27–8 for drug dosages.

Therefore vascular smooth muscles relax with α-blockers, permitting vasodilation, reducing blood pressure, increasing blood flow, and decreasing peripheral vascular resistance (Tables 27–6 and 27–7). Since there are no α-receptors in the heart, there are no cardiac effects from an alpha blockade.[3,7]

Contraindications and precautions The use of α-blockers is contraindicated in individuals with peripheral vascular disease, severe hypertension, cardiovascular disease, or cerebrovascular disease. Since the pharmacokinetics of these drugs involve the liver and kidneys, the drugs should be used with caution when renal or liver disease is present. α-Blockers should also be used with caution in clients who are pregnant.

Undesired clinical responses Several significant adverse reactions or side effects are associated with the use of α-blockers, including orthostatic hypotension, reflex tachycardia, nasal congestion, inhibition of ejaculation, sodium retention, and increased blood volume (Fig. 27–4). The most serious adverse

reaction is orthostatic hypotension. This condition is caused by reduced muscle tone in venous walls. Because of the reduced venous tone, blood accumulates in veins of the lower extremities when the client is erect. As a result, blood return to the heart is reduced; cardiac output is reduced; and the blood pressure falls. Since blood flow to the brain is reduced, the client may experience dizziness, lightheadedness, or syncope.

Reflex tachycardia is caused by triggering the baroreceptor reflex. Vasodilation produced by the α-adrenergic antagonist causes a reduction in the blood pressure. As the blood pressure falls, baroreceptors initiate a reflexive increase in the heart rate through the ANS.[21]

α-Blockers can cause dilation of the blood vessels of the

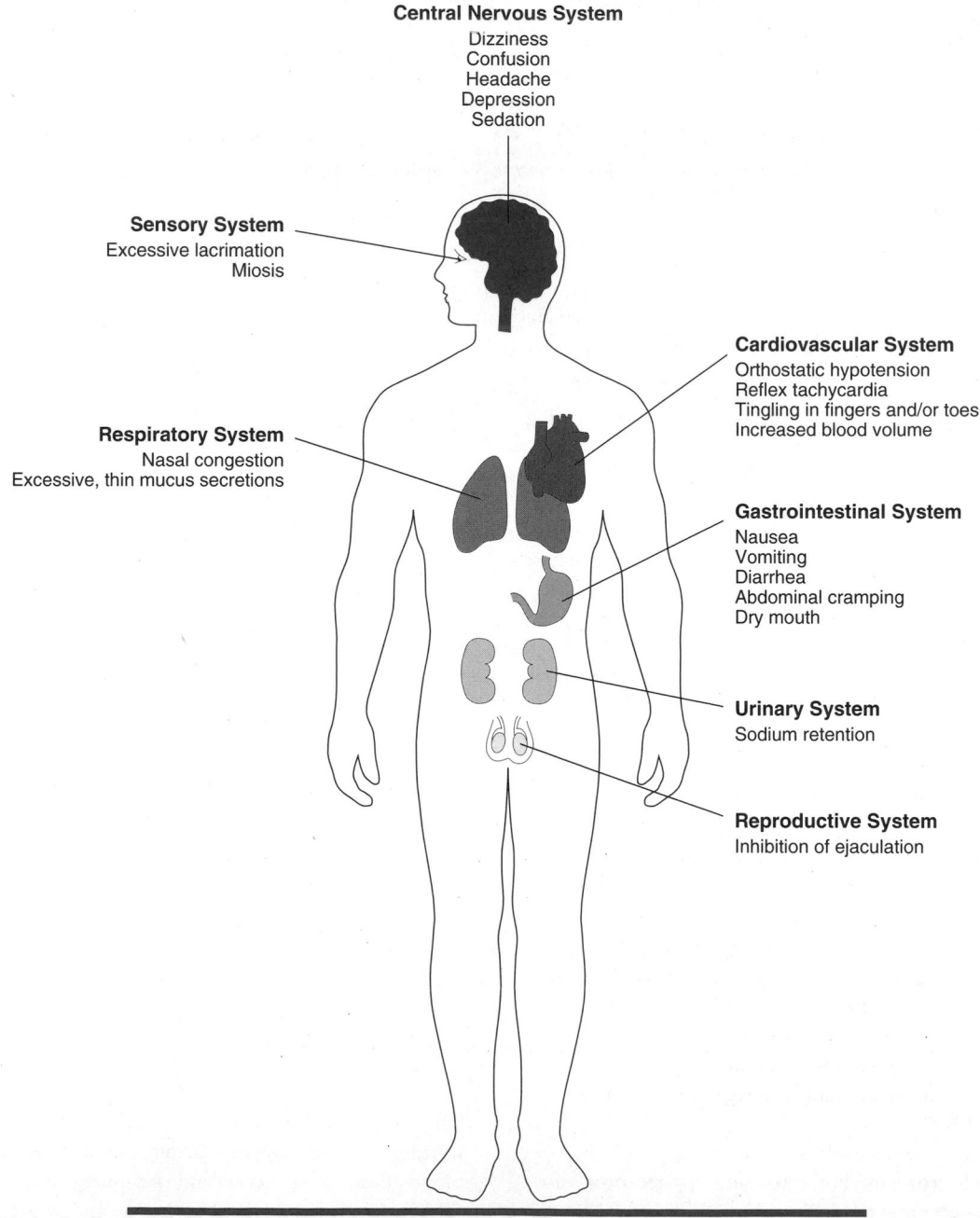

Central Nervous System
Dizziness
Confusion
Headache
Depression
Sedation

Sensory System
Excessive lacrimation
Miosis

Respiratory System
Nasal congestion
Excessive, thin mucus secretions

Cardiovascular System
Orthostatic hypotension
Reflex tachycardia
Tingling in fingers and/or toes
Increased blood volume

Gastrointestinal System
Nausea
Vomiting
Diarrhea
Abdominal cramping
Dry mouth

Urinary System
Sodium retention

Reproductive System
Inhibition of ejaculation

FIGURE 27–4 Undesired clinical responses associated with α-blockers.

nasal mucosa, resulting in nasal congestion. In addition, since stimulation of α_1-receptors is required for ejaculation, blocking of those receptors with an α-adrenergic antagonist can cause reversible impotence. The impotence disappears when use of the α-blocker is discontinued.[7,22]

Clients receiving α-blockers can also experience sodium retention and increased blood volume. By reducing blood pressure, α-blockers can cause retention of sodium and fluid by the kidneys. This increases the circulating blood volume and produces an additional work load on the heart.

Drug-drug, drug-nutrient, drug-environment interactions   Several drugs interact with α-blockers, including sympathomimetic drugs, dopamine, nitroglycerin, anesthetics, and β-blockers. All of these drugs produce hypotension when administered concurrently with sympatholytic drugs. In addition, the drug alcohol should be discouraged during treatment with oral α-blockers. Alcohol consumption precipitates hypotension with reflex tachycardia. Exercise and large meals have the same effect as alcohol, causing vasodilation and potentiation of hypotension and tachycardia.[11] Cigarette smoking should also be discouraged since nicotine stimulates the sympathetic nervous system.

Life span considerations α-Blockers should be administered cautiously to the elderly and to lactating or pregnant women. Safety and effectiveness in children have not been established.

⊞ NURSING CONSIDERATIONS

As with sympathomimetic drugs, nursing care of clients receiving sympatholytic drugs involves careful assessment, data analysis, planning, and implementation of care. Evaluation of the client's response to nursing care and medical therapy is ongoing, and the plan of care is altered based on the findings of the evaluation.

Assessing   As with any client, a thorough health history and physical assessment provide the basis of your care. While obtaining the **health history,** determine if the client has a history of angina pectoris, myocardial infarction, congestive heart failure, or cerebrovascular accident, for the decrease in blood flow and blood pressure from α-blockade could further compromise perfusion to the heart or brain.

Collect a drug history on the client. Focus your questions specifically on drugs that interact with sympatholytics. These drugs include sympathomimetics, β-blockers, and nitroglycerin. Question the client about the use of OTC drugs, particularly antihistamines and drugs used to treat colds, flu, or allergies. In addition, determine if the client has a history of smoking or alcohol consumption.

During the **physical assessment,** carefully evaluate the client's cardiovascular status. Assess for signs of distress such as dyspnea, restlessness, wheezing, or shallow, labored respirations. Note the client's skin color and degree of capillary refill. Collect baseline blood pressure, pulse, and respiration values. Assess for impaired renal function. α-Blockers are excreted through the kidneys and could compromise kidney function.

Diagnosing   Nursing diagnoses related to α-blocker administration include the following:
- Altered nutrition: less than body requirements related to nausea, vomiting, and diminished saliva associated with drug therapy.
- Body image distubance related to sexual dysfunction (inhibition of ejaculation).
- Decreased cardiac output related to diminished venous return associated with drug therapy.
- Altered tissue perfusion, cardiopulmonary, related to decreased venous return.
- High risk for injury related to dizziness, lightheadedness, and syncope associated with drug therapy.
- Fatigue related to decreased cardiac output.
- Fluid volume excess related to increased sodium retention.
- Anxiety related to lack of knowledge about drug regimen.

Planning   Clients scheduled to take an α-blocker at home must be taught the usual drug information: action, side effects, dose, and drug interactions. Teach clients how to count their own pulse. Instruct clients to report a pulse rate of less than 60 or a drop of 20 or more beats per minute from baseline.

Clients should also be taught to monitor their blood pressure. If the blood pressure falls below a set level (based on the client's baseline blood pressure), instruct clients to withhold the drug and contact the primary care provider. Inform clients of the possibility of orthostatic hypotension and teach them to change positions slowly—to rise slowly from a supine to an upright position. If faintness or syncope occurs, teach clients either to lie down or sit down with their head between their knees.

Teach clients that alcohol consumption should be eliminated or decreased and that OTC drugs and other forms of self-medication should be avoided. If a client needs therapy with an OTC drug, drug compatibility should be checked with the pharmacist or primary care provider. Make certain that clients know not to discontinue the α-blocker abruptly; to do so could result in rebound hypertension.

Teach clients what signs and symptoms to report to the primary care provider: increased heart rate, unexplained acute weight gain, swelling of the lower extremities, difficulty breathing, GI upset, dizziness, or lightheadedness. When possible, provide this information to clients in writing, along with a phone number to call with questions.

Expected outcomes that should be discussed with the client include the following:
- Client uses resources and/or support systems effectively.
- Client's fluid volume excess diminishes as evidenced by a decrease in body weight.
- Client reports improved level of energy.
- Client is free of injury.
- Client maintains body weight.
- Client verbalizes understanding of body changes.

Implementing   The blood pressure and heart rate of the client receiving an α-blocker must be monitored carefully. Lying and standing blood pressure should be obtained whenever possible. A fall in blood pressure of 20 mm Hg or more when standing should be reported to the primary care provider.

An infusion pump must be used for administration of IV α-blockers. In addition, clients should be connected to an automatic blood pressure machine or a direct arterial readout to provide continuous monitoring of blood pressure. Clients should be in the supine position during the initial administration of IV α-blockers. For this reason, it is recommended that α-blocker administration begin at night. In addition to monitoring the blood pressure closely, assess the extremities for adequacy of pulses, numbness, coolness, tingling, or weakness. These signs and symptoms could indicate peripheral vascular insufficiency.[3,7,22]

Since there is a danger of orthostatic hypotension, the client should not walk alone during the early stage of drug therapy. Place the call bell within the reach of the client and instruct the client to request assistance before getting out of bed. Allow clients to dangle their legs for 3 to 5 minutes before standing to reduce the risk of hypotensive episodes. In some situations, support stockings are used to diminish venous stasis.

Since α-blockers inhibit salivary flow, possibly contributing to the development of caries, provide clients with frequent mouth care. If drug therapy is long term, encourage clients to see the dentist regularly. α-Blockers also produce dryness of the mouth, so supply clients with ice chips or encourage them to chew sugarless gum.

Evaluating During the evaluation phase, monitor the client to determine the effectiveness of the drug. Is the blood pressure lowered? Are the migraine headaches relieved? Is the client voiding with more ease? In addition, you want to evaluate the presence of undesired clinical responses. Does the presence of adverse reactions or side effects outweigh the effectiveness of the drugs? Finally, review the expected outcomes established during the planning phase. Were these outcomes met by the client? If not, what changes should be made in the plan of care?

CONCEPT REVIEW

- Sympatholytic drugs are also known as *adrenergic blockers* or *antiadrenergic blockers.* These drugs inhibit the action of endogenously produced epinephrine and norepinephrine.
- Vascular smooth muscles relax with α-blockers, permitting vasodilation, reducing blood pressure, increasing blood flow, and decreasing peripheral vascular resistance.
- Several significant adverse reactions or side effects are associated with the use of α-blockers, including orthostatic hypotension, reflex tachycardia, nasal congestion, inhibition of ejaculation, sodium retention, and increased blood volume.
- Careful assessment of each client is essential since these drugs are contraindicated in many situations and can produce life-threatening drug-drug interactions.

NONCOMPETITIVE, LONG-ACTING α-ANTAGONIST PROTOTYPE

PHENOXYBENZAMINE

Individual adrenergic antagonists have a high degree of receptor selectivity. Phenoxybenzamine blocks both α_1- and α_2-receptors.

Pharmacotherapeutics Because phenoxybenzamine is administered orally, it is used for treating chronic disorders such as pheochromocytoma or peripheral vascular disease. In the treatment of pheochromocytoma, it is used before surgical removal of the tumor or during medical management when surgery is too risky. In these clients, adjunctive therapy with β-blockers often is needed to control tachycardia and the increased renin release caused by phenoxybenzamine. In addition, urinary obstruction due to an enlarged prostate has been treated with phenoxybenzamine.[10,19]

Pharmacokinetics Approximately 20% to 30% of phenoxybenzamine is absorbed in its active form in the GI tract. The onset of action is gradual. However, because phenoxybenzamine forms a stable bond with α-receptor sites, the duration of action is prolonged. A single dose can produce an alpha blockade for 3 to 4 days. The drug is highly lipid soluble and can accumulate in adipose tissue. Once the drug is discontinued, it takes several days to reverse the effects of the alpha blockade. Excretion is through the kidneys and biliary system.[18]

Pharmacodynamics Phenoxybenzamine is a long-acting, adrenergic, α-receptor blocking agent. It increases blood flow to the skin, mucosa, and abdominal viscera. The drug also lowers supine and erect blood pressures.[19]

Pharmaceutics Phenoxybenzamine is supplied in 10-mg gelatin capsules. The initial dose is 10 mg twice a day. If necessary, the dosage is increased every other day, usually to 20 to 40 mg two or three times a day.

Drug-Drug, Drug-Nutrient, Drug-Environment Interactions When methyldopa has been administered to clients receiving phenoxybenzamine, total urinary incontinence has occurred. Excessive hypotension and tachycardia result when phenoxybenzamine is administered in combination with other α- and β-agonists. In addition, alcohol enhances the hypotensive effects of phenoxybenzamine.[18]

Life Span Considerations Phenoxybenzamine is classified as a Pregnancy Category C drug. Since the exact effects on the fetus is unknown, the drug should not be administered to pregnant women unless absolutely necessary. It is also not known if this drug is excreted in human milk.[19]

Specific Drug-Related Nursing Considerations Advise the client that it may take several weeks for desired effects to occur. Since long-term therapy can cause GI irritation, the drug should be administered with milk or food. Phenoxybenzamine administration also causes increased gastric acid secretion; therefore if severe GI pain, epigastric distress, or tarry stools occur, the client should notify the primary care provider immediately. If diarrhea develops, the client should try to alleviate the problem with dietary changes instead of OTC drugs.

Assess the client for toxic symptoms of phenoxybenzamine: tachycardia, syncope, vomiting, lethargy, and shock. Inadvertent overdoses are treated with norepinephrine. Epinephrine is not used, since further lowering of the blood pressure could occur because of epinephrine's nonselective action. Since the client will eventually be treated as an outpatient, teach the client the key side effects and what actions to take when they occur.

Instruct the client to not use OTC drugs to reduce the excessive lacrimation and nasal stuffiness produced by phenoxybenzamine. OTC drugs may provide symptomatic relief but can aggravate the side effects associated with α-blockers. Teach the client to expect diminished vision in dim light and to avoid operating a motor vehicle after dark.

COMPETITIVE, SHORT-ACTING α-ANTAGONIST PROTOTYPE

PHENTOLAMINE MESYLATE

Phentolamine mesylate (Regitine) belongs to the group of adrenergic antagonists that produces nonselective alpha blockade. It blocks α_1- and α_2-receptors.

Pharmacotherapeutics Phentolamine is used to control hypertensive episodes in clients with pheochromocytoma. It is also used to prevent dermal necrosis or sloughing after extravasation or IV administration of norepinephrine or dopamine.

Pharmacokinetics Since phentolamine is poorly absorbed from the GI tract, parenteral administration is preferred. If the drug is administered orally, five times the IV dose must be used to achieve the same effect. Onset of action is immediate with IV administration of the drug; however, the duration of α-adrenergic blocking action is short. After IV administration the half-life of phentolamine is approximately 20 minutes. Approximately 13% of a single IV dose appears in the urine in an unchanged state.[10,18,19]

Pharmacodynamics The physiologic effects of phentolamine are similar to those of phenoxybenzamine. In addition, the drug stimulates release of histamine from mast cells, which enhances the secretion of hydrochloric acid and pepsin.[1,3] Pulmonary vascular resistance is also decreased by phentolamine.

Pharmaceutics Phentolamine is available in sterile solutions for IV and IM injections. To reconstitute the drug, dissolve 5 mg in 1 ml of sterile water for injection. The reconstituted solution should be used immediately and not stored.

If the drug is used before surgery in the treatment of pheochromocytoma, 5 mg of phentolamine is administered 1 to 2 hours preoperatively. Phentolamine can also be administered intraoperatively to control blood pressure. Dosage for this purpose is determined by the client's response.

When phentolamine is used to prevent tissue necrosis associated with α-agonist infusion, it is recommended that 10 mg of phentolamine be added to each liter of IV solution containing the agonist. Phentolamine does not alter the pressor effect of the agonist. To treat tissue infiltrated by a sympathomimetic agent, 5 to 10 mg of phentolamine mixed with 10 ml of saline solution is injected into the area of infiltration as soon as possible.[18,23]

Drug-Drug, Drug-Nutrient, Drug-Environment Interactions When secondary cardiac side effects from phentolamine are controlled by β-blockers, decreased cardiac output can result. Phentolamine also antagonizes the vasoconstrictive effects of epinephrine and ephedrine. In addition, combining phentolamine and papaverine in-

tracavernously in the treatment of impotence can induce priapism (persistent abnormal erection of the penis).[18]

Life Span Considerations Because it decreases cardiac output, phentolamine should not be used during pregnancy. Caution is also advised when it is used in the very young and the elderly. Since this drug is hepatotoxic, care should be taken when administering it to elderly clients with reduced liver function.[10,18]

Specific Drug-Related Nursing Considerations While the client is receiving IV phentolamine, monitor the blood pressure continuously. Assess the client carefully for GI problems. Since phentolamine increases the secretion of hydrochloric acid and pepsin, clients with a history of peptic ulcer disease require close monitoring. Assist the client during ambulation and take precautions to protect the client from falls. In addition, have IV phentolamine readily available for any client receiving norepinephrine intravenously in the event of an overdose.

Ergot Alkaloids

Ergot alkaloids are produced by a fungus. Three groups of ergot alkaloids have been isolated: ergotamine, ergonovine, and ergotoxine. The **ergotamine** group (Bellergal, Cafergot, Ergomar, Ergostat, etc.) has potent vasoconstrictive effects and acts as an α-blocker. It is used to manage vascular and migraine headaches. The second group, **ergonovine,** has potent oxytocic (stimulates contractions of myometrium) and vasoconstrictive effects. It does not act as an α-blocker. Drugs in this group (Ergotrate, Methergine, etc.) are used to control uterine hemorrhage. The **ergotoxine** group contains three major alkaloids: ergocornine, ergocristine, and ergocryptine. The ergotoxine drugs (Circanol, Deapril, Hydergine, etc.) are used to treat age-related decline in mental function. This section focuses on the ergotamine group.

ERGOTAMINE GROUP PROTOTYPE

ERGOTAMINE TARTRATE

Pharmacotherapeutics Ergotamine is used to abort or prevent migraine or vascular headaches.

Pharmacokinetics Absorption rates for the drug vary, depending on the specific dosage form used. Once absorbed, ergotamine is widely distributed in the body. It is metabolized in the liver, and 90% of the metabolites are excreted in the bile. The unmetabolized drug is erratically secreted in the saliva, and only traces of the unmetabolized drug appear in the urine and feces. The elimination half-life of ergotamine from the plasma is approximately 2 hours. Some of the drug may be stored in tissues, prolonging therapeutic actions.[19]

Pharmacodynamics Ergotamine constricts peripheral and cranial blood vessels and depresses central vasomotor centers. It works by competitive inhibition, preventing norepinephrine from activating the α-receptors. Ergotamine reduces extracranial blood flow and the amplitude of pain pulsation. Ergotamine constricts arteries and veins yet only slightly increases blood pressure. However, it does increase peripheral resistance and decrease blood flow to various organs.

Pharmaceutics Ergotamine is available in oral and sublingual tablets and suppositories. Therapy should be initiated as soon as possible after the first symptoms of a headache. Dosage should not exceed 6 mg in any 24-hour period.

Undesired Clinical Responses and Contraindications Ergotamine is contraindicated in clients with peripheral vascular disease, coronary artery disease, hypertension, impaired renal or hepatic function, and sepsis. Serious side effects from ergotamine have not been reported; however, transient nausea and vomiting do occur. In addition, sublingual irritation can result with the sublingual dosage form. Assess the client for symptoms of ergotism (chronic poisoning produced by ingestion of ergot): headache, unstable blood pressure, weak, thready pulse, chest pain, decreased circulation to extremities, and CNS symptoms of confusion, excitement, delirium, hallucinations, change in level of consciousness, and convulsions.[18,19]

Specific Drug-Related Nursing Considerations Instruct the client to take ergotamine as soon as an attack begins. In addition, encourage him or her to lie down in a dark room after taking the medication to enhance its effectiveness.

Before administering the drug, determine if the client is pregnant or nursing. If so, do not administer the drug, since it is classified as Pregnancy Category X and can cause fetal harm because of its uterine stimulant actions.

Also do not administer ergotamine to women who may become pregnant. Since ergotamine is secreted into human milk, nursing mothers should not use it. Excessive dosing or prolonged administration of ergotamine can inhibit lactation.[19]

SELECTIVE α_1-BLOCKER PROTOTYPE

PRAZOSIN HYDROCHLORIDE

Prazosin (Minipress) is a selective α-antagonist. It has a greater effect on α_1-receptors than on α_2-receptors. Alpha-1 blockade in the arteries and veins results in a decrease in peripheral vascular resistance and diminished venous return. Consequently, preload is reduced, but cardiac output remains unchanged. Prazosin is usually prescribed to treat hypertension. Although the drug is considered potent, full therapeutic effect from prazosin may not occur for 4 to 8 weeks.[12,18,19] This drug is discussed more completely in Chapter 33.

Miscellaneous α-Blockers

Labetalol (Normodyne, Trandate) is a selective α-blocking and nonselective β-blocking agent used for the treatment of hypertension. It is discussed in more detail in Chapter 33.

TABLE 27–8

Prototype and Major Drugs in Category

Drug Name	Dosage and Route of Administration	Nursing Considerations
NONCOMPETITIVE, LONG-ACTING α-ANTAGONIST: PHENOXYBENZAMINE HYDROCHLORIDE (Dibenzyline) HOW SUPPLIED Gelatin capsule: 10 mg	ADULTS *Loading* 10 mg bid; dosage increased qod if needed *Maintenance* 20-40 mg bid or tid CHILDREN *Loading* 0.2 mg/kg; maximum dosage, 10 mg *Maintenance* 0.4-1.2 mg/kg tid or qid	*Assess* Assess client for preexisting cerebral or coronary arteriosclerosis or renal damage. Obtain baseline heart rate, rhythm, and blood pressure values. Determine if client is pregnant; phenoxybenzamine is classifed as Pregnancy Category C. *Implement* Administer drug with milk or meals. Monitor client's blood pressure and heart rate closely. Stop administering drug and report systolic pressures below 100 and/or heart rates below 60. Teach client to change positions slowly to avoid postural hypotension. If client experiences miosis, use low lighting. Provide consultation for sexual dysfunction if needed. Teach client not to discontinue the drug abruptly. Teach client to avoid consumption of alcohol while taking the drug. Instruct client not to take OTC drugs without checking with physician. *Monitor* Assess for undesired clinical responses: postural hypotension, tachycardia, miosis, nasal congestion, drowsiness, fatigue, GI irritation, and inhibition of ejaculation. *Evaluate* Observe for significant improvements in client's condition.

TABLE 27–8 *Continued*
Prototype and Major Drugs in Category

Drug Name	Dosage and Route of Administration	Nursing Considerations
COMPETITIVE, SHORT-ACTING α-ANTAGONIST: PHENTOLAMINE MESYLATE (Regitine) HOW SUPPLIED IV, IM: 5 mg/ml	**Hypertension Episode Associated With Pheochromocytoma** IV or IM: 5 mg **Extravasation of Norepinephrine** *Prevention* 10 mg to each liter of solution containing norepinephrine *Treatment* 5-10 mg in 10 ml of saline solution injected into area of extravasation within 12 h of incident	**Assess** Obtain baseline heart rate and rhythm. Assess baseline lying and standing blood pressure. Assess client for preexisting myocardial infarction, angina, or coronary insufficiency. Determine if client is pregnant; phentolamine is classified as Pregnancy Category C. **Implement** Use reconstituted solution upon preparation; do not store for later use. Inspect parenteral solutions for particulate matter and discoloration; do not use if present. Be prepared to administer antacids to prevent gastric ulcers from drug-induced increased gastric acid secretion. Watch client closely for orthostatic hypotension. Instruct client to change positions slowly. Teach client to report dizziness or palpitations. **Monitor** Monitor client for undesired clinical responses: prolonged hypotensive episodes, tachycardia, cardiac arrhythmias, weakness, dizziness, nasal stuffiness, nausea, and vomiting. Monitor heart rate and rhythm, blood pressure, skin color, urinary output, and level of consciousness. **Evaluate** Observe client for reduction of hypertension.
α-BLOCKER ERGOTAMINE GROUP: ERGOTAMINE TARTRATE (Ergomar, Ergostat, Wigrettes) HOW SUPPLIED Sublingual tablet: 2 mg	**Migraine or Vascular Headaches** One sublingual tablet at onset of attack; another tablet at ½ h intervals for a total of three tablets Dosage not to exceed 6 mg in 24-h period Weekly dosage limit: 10 mg	**Assess** Assess client for preexisting peripheral vascular disease, coronary heart disease, hypertension, or impaired hepatic or renal functions. Assess for prior substance abuse and/or dependence. Determine if client is pregnant; ergotamine is classified as Pregnancy Category X. **Implement** Do not administer to nursing mothers since drug is secreted into human milk. Teach client to take drug at first indication of migraine. Teach client to notify care provider if nausea, vomiting, irregular heartbeat, numbness or tingling of fingers or toes, or pain or weakness of extremities occurs. Teach client to avoid nicotine and extreme cold for they increase peripheral vasoconstriction. Teach client to take peripheral pulses weekly to detect ergot poisoning. **Monitor** Observe extremities for decreased circulation. Be prepared to administer nitroglycerin, heparin, or low-molecular weight dextran. Monitor the client for undesired responses such as nausea, vomiting, weakness of legs, pain in limb muscles, precardial pain, transient changes in heart rate, and localized edema. **Evaluate** Observe client for decrease in headache symptoms.

Table continued on following page.

TABLE 27–8 *Continued*
Prototype and Major Drugs in Category

Drug Name	Dosage and Route of Administration	Nursing Considerations
α-BLOCKER ERGOTOXINE GROUP: ERGOLOID MESYLATES (Hydergine) HOW SUPPLIED Sublingual tablet: 0.5, 1 mg Uncoated tablet: 1 mg	**Idiopathic Decline in Mental Capacity** 1 mg tid	**Assess** Assess for preexisting acute or chronic psychosis. **Implement** Alleviation of symptoms is gradual; results may not be observed for 3-4 weeks. Administer oral tablets with milk or meals if needed. Store at 15°-30° C. **Monitor** Monitor client for undesired responses such as sublingual irritation, transient nausea, and gastric disturbances. **Evaluate** Observe for improvement in mental status.
SELECTIVE, α₁-BLOCKER: PRAZOSIN (Minipress)	See Chapter 31.	

A summary of sympatholytic agents, their use, administration, and nursing considerations are in Table 27–8.

CONCEPT REVIEW

Most sympatholytic drugs are administered via parenteral or oral routes.

Sympatholytic drugs are used in the treatment of hypertension, pheochromocytoma, migraine or vascular headaches, and infiltration of an α-agonist IV infusion.

SUMMARY

To safely administer drugs that affect the sympathetic nervous system, you must understand the physiologic effects of parasympathetic and sympathetic nervous system stimulation and blockage. If an organ is innervated by both parasympathetic and sympathetic nervous systems, blocking of one system means the other prevails. The physiologic response of the prevailing system is thus observed.

In addition, remember that a variety of names are given to drugs having similar responses (e.g., α-blocker, α-antagonist). Ask yourself if the drug increases or decreases the effects of a specific neurotransmitter. If actions of norepinephrine or epinephrine are increased, the drug mimics the sympathetic nervous system response. If the actions of norepinephrine or epinephrine are diminished, the drug is blocking the sympathetic nervous system response.

REFERENCES

1. Wingard, L., Brady, T., Larner, J., & Schwartz, A. (1991). *Human pharmacology.* St. Louis: Mosby–Year Book.
2. Opie, L. (1992). *Drugs for the heart* (2nd ed.). Orlando, FL: Grune & Stratton.
3. Goodman, A., Gilman, A., Rall, T., Niles, A., & Taylor, P., (Eds.). (1990). *Goodman and Gilman's: The pharmacological basis of therapeutics* (8th ed.). New York: Pergamon Press.
4. Grant, S.A., & Hoffman, R.S. (1992). Use of tetracaine, epinephrine, and cocaine as a topical anesthetic in the emergency department. *Annals of Emergency Medicine, 21,* 987-997.
5. Wicks, T.C., Yim, D., Newcomer, T., et al. (1992). Hemostasis and hemodynamics during intranasal surgery: The effects of cocaine, oxymetazoline, and epinephrine. *AANA Journal, 60,* 464-471.
6. Yamamoto, L.G., et al. (1992). Pulse oximetry and peak flow as indicators of wheezing severity in children and improvement following bronchodilator treatments. *American Journal of Emergency Medicine, 10,* 519-524.
7. Smith, C., & Reynard, A. (1992). *Textbook of pharmacology.* Philadelphia: W.B. Saunders.
8. Kalant, H., & Roschlau, W. (1989). *Principles of medical pharmacology.* Toronto: Brian C. Decker.
9. Miller, C. (1990). When medication harms as well as helps. *Geriatric Nursing,* November/December, 301-302.
10. U.S. Pharmacopeial Convention (1990). *The United States pharmacopeia* (22nd rev.). Rockville, MD.: Author.
11. American Society of Hospital Pharmacists (1991). *Medication teaching manual: A guide for patient counseling* (4th ed.). Bethesda, MD: Author.
12. Capaldo, B., Napoli, R., Di Marino, L., & Sacca, L. (1992). Epinephrine directly antagonizes insulin-mediated activation of glucose uptake and inhibition of free fatty acid release in forearm tissue. *Metabolism, 41,* 1146-1149.
13. *Drug facts and comparisons* (1992). St. Louis: Author.
14. Burns, K.M. (1990). Vasoactive drug therapy in shock. *Critical Care Nursing Clinics of North America, 2,* 167-178.
15. Clements, J.V. (1992). Sympathomimetics, inotropics, and vasodilators, *AACN—Clinical Issues in Critical Care Nursing, 3,* 395-408.
16. Jahns, B.E., Levy, D.B., & Corley, J.R. (1992). ET drug administration. *Emergency, 24*(5), 48-50.
17. Peppers, M.P. (1992). High-dose epinephrine. *Emergency, 24*(2), 23-26.

18. Micromedex. (1993). *Drug evaluation monographs* (Vol. 78). Author.
19. Data Pharmaceutica, Inc. (1993). *1993 Physicians' genRx.* Smithtown, NY: Author.
20. American Pharmaceutical Association (1990). *Handbook of non-prescription drugs* (9th ed.). Washington, DC: Author.
21. Guyton, A.C. (1991). *Textbook of medical physiology* (8th ed.). Philadelphia: W.B. Saunders.
22. Lehne, R.A. (1994). *Pharmacology for nursing care.* (2nd ed.). Philadelphia: W.B. Saunders.
23. Hill, J.M. (1991). Phentolamine mesylate: The antidote for vasopressor extravasation. *Critical Care Nurse, 11*(10), 58-61.

BIBLIOGRAPHY

Bernat, J.L., & Ferrante, J.A. (1992). Helping your patient cope with migraine. *Patient Care, 26*(7), 44-48, 50-54.

Gabai, I.J., & Spierings, E.L. (1990). Diagnosis and management of cluster headaches. *Nurse Practitioner: American Journal of Primary Health Care, 15*(10), 32, 34-36.

Herrmann, S.C., & Feigl, E.D. (1992). Adrenergic blockade blunts adenosine concentration and coronary vasodilation during hypoxia. *Circulatory Research, 70,* 1203-1216.

Oriowo, M.A., Nichols, A.J., & Ruffolo, R.R. (1992). Receptor protection studies with phenoxybenzamine indicate that a single alpha$_1$-adrenoceptor may be coupled to two signal transduction processes in vascular smooth muscle. *Pharmacology, 45*(1), 17-26.

Penn, F., & Mancini, J. (1991). Hemodynamic effects of vasoactive infusions. *AORN Journal, 54,* 613-621.

Peppers, M.P. (1990). Updating epinephrine. *Emergency, 22*(3), 18-23.

Sampson, H.A., Mendelson, L., & Rosen, J. (1992). Fatal and near-fatal anaphylactic reactions to food in children and adolescents. *New England Journal of Medicine, 327,* 380-384.

Viets, J.L., Blades, K.A., Mitchell, N.D., & Perez, W.E. (1990). A review of recent cardioactive and vasoactive drugs in anesthesia. *Nurse Anesthesia, 1*(1), 21-32.

Whipple, J.K., Medicus-Bringa, M.A., Schimel, B.A., et al. (1992). Selected vasoactive drugs: A readily available chart reference. *Critical Care Nurse, 12*(3), 23-29.

Zimmerman, T.J., Sharir, M., Nardin, G., & Fugua, M. (1992). Therapeutic index of epinephrine and dipivefrin with nasolacrimal occlusion. *American Journal of Ophthalmology, 114*(1), 8-13.

Skeletal Muscle Relaxants

LINDA RUHOLL

⊛ Skeletal Muscle Relaxants

LEARNING OBJECTIVE: Identify the different types of skeletal muscle relaxants discussed in this chapter.
KEY TERMS:
Depolarizing, nondepolarizing, peripherally acting

⊛ Skeletal Muscle Contraction

LEARNING OBJECTIVE: Describe the neuromuscular mechanism involved in skeletal muscle contraction.
KEY TERMS:
Acetylcholine, action potential, depolarization, end-plate, muscle tone, repolarization

⊛ Nondepolarizing Neuromuscular Blocking Drugs

LEARNING OBJECTIVES:
Discuss therapeutic uses of nondepolarizing neuromuscular blocking drugs.
Describe two contraindications for the use of nondepolarizing neuromuscular drugs.
List undesired clinical responses associated with nondepolarizing neuromuscular blocking drugs.
Discuss three drug-drug interactions associated with nondepolarizing neuromuscular drugs.
Discuss life span considerations of nondepolarizing neuromuscular drugs.
Summarize essential information about tubocurarine.
KEY TERM: Curare

⊛ Depolarizing Neuromuscular Blocking Drugs

LEARNING OBJECTIVES:
Describe two contraindications for the use of depolarizing neuromuscular drugs.
List undesired clinical responses associated with depolarizing neuromuscular blocking drugs.
Discuss three drug-drug interactions associated with depolarizing neuromuscular drugs.
Discuss life span considerations of depolarizing neuromuscular drugs.
Summarize essential information about succinylcholine.
KEY TERMS:
Malignant hyperthermia, pseudocholinesterase

⊛ Peripherally Acting Skeletal Muscle Relaxants

LEARNING OBJECTIVES:
Discuss therapeutic uses of peripherally acting skeletal muscle relaxants.
Describe two contraindications for the use of peripherally acting skeletal muscle relaxants.
List undesired clinical responses associated with peripherally acting skeletal muscle relaxants.
Discuss three drug-drug interactions associated with peripherally acting skeletal muscle relaxants.
Discuss life span considerations of peripherally acting skeletal muscle relaxants.
Summarize essential information about dantrolene.

CONCEPTS AND TERMS TO REVIEW

Review Chapter 25 for an overview of the autonomic nervous system.
Reexamine the concepts of action potential, polarization, depolarization, and repolarization.

Some muscle-relaxant substances were known to primitive man who used them on arrows and spears when hunting prey. Death of the prey was caused by paralysis of voluntary muscles, specifically the muscles of respiration. Through the years it became apparent that these substances could be of value in medicine. Gradually the more potent substances were refined and used as muscle relaxants during surgery and electroshock therapy. Since the late 1950s less potent skeletal muscle relaxants have been used in the medical management of muscle spasms.

SKELETAL MUSCLE RELAXANTS

Skeletal muscle relaxants are usually classified according to mechanism of action and site of action. Drugs that act at the neuromuscular junction, blocking impulse transmission, are called *neuromuscular blockers.* These drugs fall into two major groups: **nondepolarizing** and **depolarizing neuromuscular blockers.** Other drugs act at sites in or on the muscle. These drugs are called **peripherally acting skeletal muscle relaxants.** Another group of drugs inhibits the function of spinal nerves that control skeletal nerves; they are called **centrally acting skeletal muscle relaxants.** This chapter focuses on neuroblockers and peripherally acting skeletal muscle relaxants. Centrally acting skeletal muscle relaxants are discussed in Chapter 18.

SKELETAL MUSCLE CONTRACTION

Cell bodies of the somatic motor nerves are found in the anterior horn of grey matter in the spinal cord. Motor nerves pass without synapse from the motor neuron in the spinal cord to the muscle fiber. At the muscle fiber the nerves synapse on a specialized area of the muscle, the **end-plate.**

When a command to contract is issued by the brain, a complex series of events is set into motion. Initially an **action potential** sweeps down the motor nerve. When the action potential arrives at the nerve end, the release of the transmitter, **acetylcholine (ACh),** is initiated. ACh binds with nicotinic ACh receptors located on the surface of the end-plate membrane. This combination opens ion channels in the muscle fiber membrane, allowing sodium to enter and potassium to leave the cell and causing a local **depolarization** of the end-plate membrane. If the end-plate potential is strong enough, an action potential is generated on the adjacent muscle and conducted over the muscle membrane to initiate the muscle contraction.[1,2] The depolarization and **repolarization** processes are important for maintaining normal muscle responsiveness to nerve activity. If either process is altered, neuromuscular transmission is affected.

Muscles stay in a state of readiness called **muscle tone.** Depending on the state of the nervous system, normal muscle tone can be increased or decreased. Muscles usually relax after contraction. If not allowed to relax because of nervous system activity, muscles develop spasms, which are caused by the stimulation of entire motor units by a motor neuron. Sustained spasm is called *tetany; spasticity* describes increased muscle tone associated with stiff and awkward movements. Spasms and other sustained contractions are painful and limit function.[1] The exact reason for the pain is unclear. However, since energy demands of the overactive muscle exceed the energy supply, ischemia and accumulation of metabolic wastes result.

NONDEPOLARIZING NEUROMUSCULAR BLOCKING DRUGS

Nondepolarizing blockers are the most widely used group of neuromuscular blocking drugs. These drugs must be administered by skilled clinicians (i.e., nurse anesthetists, anesthesiologists). However, as a nurse, you will care for the client before and after the administration of these drugs. Therefore an understanding of the drugs' actions and their side effects is important.

NONDEPOLARIZING NEUROMUSCULAR BLOCKING PROTOTYPE
TUBOCURARINE HYDROCHLORIDE

Tubocurarine is one of the active ingredients found in arrow poisons used by primitive man. The poisons contained multiple components but were generally called **curare.**

Pharmacotherapeutics Tubocurarine is used in several situations, including endotracheal intubation, as an adjunct to general anesthesia, in ventilator control, as an adjunct to electroshock therapy, and for the diagnosis of myasthenia gravis. When an endotracheal tube is inserted, the client's gag reflexes are triggered. First administering tubocurarine or another nondepolarizing drug prevents these reflexes. Clients with severe psychiatric depression who require electroconvulsive therapy are administered tubocurarine during the therapy to prevent dislocations and fractures of bones during the convulsions. For some clients requiring mechanical ventilation, the natural respiratory drive fights or resists the action of the ventilator. When a neuromuscular blocker is administered, the client's ability to breathe is blocked, and the ventilator assumes complete control.[2-4]

Pharmacokinetics With a single intravenous (IV) dose of tubocurarine to an adult, onset of effects occurs within 1 minute. Maximum paralysis of muscles occurs within 2 to 5 minutes, and duration of effective paralysis lasts 35 to 60 minutes. Full recovery from tubocurarine takes several hours and is dependent on the dose administered. Tubocurarine is eliminated by hepatic metabolic and renal excretion.[2,5] Hepatic or renal disease or hypotension can prolong the action of the drug.[4]

Pharmacodynamics Tubocurarine always carries a positive charge and cannot readily cross membranes. The drug's inability to cross membranes has several implications. First, the drug cannot be administered orally; it must be administered parenterally. Second, since tubocurarine does not cross the blood-brain barrier, it does not effect the central nervous system (CNS). It does not diminish consciousness or the perception of pain. Third, since tubocurarine does not easily cross membranes, it does not readily cross the placental barrier.[3]

Tubocurarine produces its effects by competing with ACh for nicotinic binding sites on the motor end-plate. The drug does not stimulate receptor sites. Muscle groups that are highly innervated are most sensitive to the effects of tubocurarine.[2] Any process that decreases the amount of tubocurarine at the junction reverses muscle relaxation.

Pharmaceutics Tubocurarine is available only in sterile solutions for IV or intramuscular (IM) injection.

Undesired Clinical Responses The most prominent undesired clinical responses from tubocurarine are associated with the respiratory system. The drug can cause excessive paralysis of the muscles of respiration, prolonging respiratory depression and, in some instances, causing respiratory arrest. Some clients experience hypotension. In addition, overdose with tubocurarine can produce prolonged apnea, massive histamine release, and cardiovascular collapse.[2,5]

Contraindications and Precautions Tubocurarine must be used with caution in clients with myasthenia gravis. Electrolyte imbalances also influence the effects of tubocurarine; for example, hypokalemia increases the effects of the drug. Since the drug can cause histamine release, it should not be used in clients with severe allergies or a history of asthma.[2,5,6]

Drug-Drug, Drug-Nutrient, Drug-Environment Interactions Several drugs should not be administered along with tubocurarine, including quinidine sulfate, kanamycin (Kantrex), streptomycin, and gentamicin (Garamycin). These drugs enhance the neuromuscular blockade effect of tubocurarine and cause additional muscle relaxation and respiratory depression. Administering amphotericin B and a thiazide (Diuril, Esidrix, HydroDIURIL) can cause hypokalemia, which enhances the drug's curariform effect.[4,5]

Specific Drug-Related Nursing Considerations Some drugs are physically incompatible with tubocurarine. Therefore it is best to use a separate infusion line for each drug. In addition, do not mix other drugs in the same syringe with tubocurarine.

Make certain that emergency equipment (e.g., oxygen, airway) is available while the client is recovering from the drug's neuromuscular blocking effects. Assess the client's gag reflex and swallowing ability routinely. Do not administer any oral drugs, food, or beverage until the client is able to swallow without difficulty. Also check post-procedural drug orders for potential interactions that could cause the return of curariform effects.

Recovery from tubocurarine neuromuscular blockade can be hastened by the administration of a cholinesterase inhibitor such as neostigmine bromide (Prostigmin), pyridostigmine (Mestinon), or edrophonium (Tensilon). Atropine sulfate frequently is administered before the cholinesterase inhibitor to minimize its muscarinic effects. (See Table 28–2 for additional information about tubocurarine.)

Miscellaneous Drugs in Category

Several neuromuscular blockers are closely related to tubocurarine. These drugs differ primarily in potency and duration of action. **Metocurine iodine** (Metubine), **gallamine triethiodide** (Flaxedil), and **pancuronium** (Pavulon) have a duration of action similar to that of tubocurarine. **Vercuronium** (Norcuron), **atracurium** (Tracrium), and **mivarcurium** (Mavacron) have shorter durations of action when single doses are administered. **Doxacurium** (Nuromax) and **pipecuronium** (Arduan) have the longest duration of action.[2,4,5] Information about the onset of action, peak action, and duration of action for some of these drugs is summarized in Table 28–1.

DEPOLARIZING NEUROMUSCULAR BLOCKING DRUGS

As with nondepolarizing neuromuscular blocking drugs, depolarizing neuromuscular blocking drugs must be administered by skilled clinicians (i.e., nurse anesthetists, anesthesiologists). However, an understanding of the drug actions and side effects is essential for effective client care.

TABLE 28–1

Pharmacokinetic Characteristics of Neuromuscular Blockers

Name and Category	Route of Administration	Time Course*			
		Onset of Effects	Time to Maximum Paralysis (Min)	Duration of Effective Paralysis (Min)	Time to Near Full Recovery
Nondepolarizing Blockers					
Tubocurarine hydrochloride	IV (IM)†	1 min	2-5	35-60	Hours
Atracurium besylate	IV	—	2-5	20-35	60-70 min
Gallamine triethiodide	IV	1-2 min	2-5	15-30	—
Metocurine iodide	IV	1 min	3-5	25-90	Hours
Pancuronium bromide	IV	45 s	3-4	<60	<60 min
Vecuronium bromide	IV	1 min	3-5	25-30	45-65 min
Depolarizing Blocker					
Succinylcholine chloride	IV (IM)†	30 s	1	4-6	—

*Time course of action can vary with dosage and route of administration. The values given are for an average adult dose administered as a single IV injection.
†Usually administered intravenously but may be administered intramuscularly if necessary. (IV = intravenous; IM = intramuscular.)

DEPOLARIZING NEUROMUSCULAR BLOCKING PROTOTYPE

SUCCINYLCHOLINE

Only one depolarizing neuromuscular blocking drug is available in the United States: succinylcholine. Its actions are very different from those of tubocurarine.

Pharmacotherapeutics Like tubocurarine, succinylcholine is given to produce muscle relaxation for clients who receive a general anesthetic or electroshock therapy or require insertion of an endotracheal tube or mechanical ventilation. Succinylcholine (Anectine, Quelicin, Sucostrin) is not used to diagnose myasthenia gravis. It has no effects on the CNS; therefore it does not alter pain perception or level of consciousness.

Pharmacokinetics Succinylcholine has an extremely short duration of action. After an IV injection, onset of action begins in 30 seconds or less. Maximum effects are achieved within 1 minute, and muscle function returns to normal within 4 to 10 minutes. The drug is rapidly degraded by **pseudocholinesterase,** an enzyme in the plasma.[3,4]

Pharmacodynamics Succinylcholine causes muscle relaxation by binding to nicotinic$_2$ (N_2) receptors on the motor end-plate. This binding causes the end-plate to depolarize. The initial response to this depolarization is transient muscle contraction. However, unlike ACh, succinylcholine does not immediately dissociate from the receptor sites. By remaining bound to the receptor sites, succinylcholine prevents repolarization of the end-plate. Thus the end-plate remains in a state of constant depolarization. The drug's ability to maintain depolarization causes the muscle to remain relaxed.[2,4,5]

Pharmaceutics Succinylcholine is available as a premixed sterile solution and as a powder that requires reconstituting. This drug is usually administered intravenously but can be injected intramuscularly.

Undesired Clinical Responses Three major undesired clinical responses are associated with succinylcholine: prolonged paralysis from low pseudocholinesterase activity, malignant hyperthermia, and postoperative muscle pain. In some clients who receive succinylcholine, muscle pain is experienced on recovery from surgery. This pain may be from the muscle contraction that occurs during the initial phase of succinylcholine administration.[2,3,4]

Some individuals have a genetic condition that causes them to produce a form of pseudocholinesterase whose activity is extremely low. If succinylcholine is administered to these individuals, paralysis can last for hours instead of minutes. Clients suspected of having low levels of pseudocholinesterase should be tested before receiving the drug.[3,4]

Malignant hyperthermia develops when succinylcholine is used in combination with certain general anesthetics. This condition is characterized by muscle rigidity and profound elevation of body temperature. (The elevated body temperature is the result of excessive metabolic activity in muscle.) Treatment includes the following: immediate discontinuation of succinylcholine and adjunct anesthetic; cooling of the client; and administration of dantrolene.[3,4,7]

Overdose of succinylcholine produces prolonged apnea. Management of succinylcholine toxicity is purely supportive; there is no specific antidote for succinylcholine toxicity.

Contraindications and Precautions Succinylcholine is contraindicated for individuals with low pseudocholinesterase activity and for clients with a personal or family history of malignant hyperthermia. Since succinylcholine can cause transient increase in intraocular pressure, it should not be used with clients who have acute narrow-angle glaucoma. All neuromuscular blockers should be used with caution in clients with myasthenia gravis.

Drug-Drug, Drug-Nutrient, Drug-Environment Interactions Several drugs cause drug-drug interactions with succinylcholine. The effects of succinylcholine are enhanced or potentiated by antibiotics such as the aminoglycosides and the tetracyclines. Monoamine oxidase (MAO) inhibitors also increase the effects of succinylcholine, and digitalis glycosides enhance the tendency for arrhythmias. When cholinesterase inhibitors are administered to a client receiving succinylcholine, the effects of succinylcholine are intensified. The cholinesterase inhibitors delay succinylcholine deactivation by decreasing the activity of pseudocholinesterase.[2,3,5]

Reconstituted solutions of succinylcholine are unstable and should be used within 24 hours of their preparation. Once opened, premixed solutions are stable for up to 2 weeks. Most solutions must be refrigerated.

Life Span Considerations Succinylcholine is classified as a Pregnancy Category C drug. It is not known if the drug can cause fetal harm when administered to a pregnant woman. Pseudocholinesterase levels are decreased during pregnancy and for several days postpartum. This decrease causes increased sensitivity to succinylcholine in pregnant and postpartum women. Therefore succinylcholine should not be used in this group of clients unless absolutely necessary. Succinylcholine may cause bradycardia in children, especially after a second dose. This effect can be minimized by atropine.[5]

Specific Drug-Related Nursing Considerations As with tubocurarine, make certain that emergency equipment (e.g, oxygen, airway) is available while the client is recovering from the drug's neuromuscular blocking effects. Assess the client's gag reflex and swallowing ability routinely. Do not administer any oral drugs, food, or beverage until the client is able to swallow without difficulty. Also check postprocedural drug orders for potential interactions that could cause the return of curariform effects.

Advise clients who will receive succinylcholine that generalized muscle pain or stiffness may occur in the postoperative period. Be prepared to administer analgesics as necessary. Monitor the postoperative client for indications of malignant hyperthermia when succinylcholine and a general anesthetic were used. Observe the client for muscle rigidity, elevated temperature, and mottling of the skin. Be prepared to administer dantrolene. See Table 28–2 for additional information on succinylcholine.

CONCEPT REVIEW

Tubocurarine produces its effects by competing with ACh for nicotinic binding sites on the motor end-plate.

Recovery from tubocurarine neuromuscular blockade can be hastened by the administration of a cholinesterase inhibitor such as neostigmine bromide, pyridostigmine, or edrophonium.

Several neuromuscular blockers are closely related to tubocurarine. These drugs differ primarily in potency and duration of action.

Succinylcholine causes muscle relaxation by binding to N_2-receptors on the motor end-plate. This binding causes the end-plate to depolarize.

Should an overdose of succinylcholine be administered, the drug does not have an antidote.

TABLE 28–2
Prototypes and Major Drugs in Category.

Drug Name	Dosage and Route of Administration	Nursing Considerations
NONDEPOLARIZING NEUROMUSCULAR BLOCKING DRUGS: TUBOCURARINE CHLORIDE HOW SUPPLIED IM, IV: 3 mg/ml	Dosage is highly individualized. **Surgery** IV: 40-60 U (1 mg = 7 U) administered at time of skin incision; additional 20-30 U in 3-5 min Supplemental doses of 20 U as required Calculate doses based on 0.5 U/lb (1.1 U/kg) **Electroshock Therapy** IV: 0.5 U/lb (1.1 U/kg)	**Assess** Determine baseline laboratory values for factors that may alter response to drug: potassium, calcium, magnesium, blood urea nitrogen (BUN), and creatinine clearance. Determine if client is receiving quinidine sulfate or thiazide diuretic. Determine if client is pregnant. Use of tubocurarine chloride in pregnancy has not been approved. Assess respiratory function before administering drug. Assess for preexisting renal insufficiency, renal disease, or pulmonary disease. **Implement** Do not mix drug with alkaline solution; precipitation will form. Drug must be administered only by a clinician skilled in its use. IV solution should not be administered rapidly. Clients under neuromuscular blockade do not lose consciousness. Maintain professional communication in their presence. Keep a cholinesterase inhibitor (neostigmine or pyridostigmine) available as antidote to toxicity. **Monitor** Monitor respiratory rate since drug causes respiratory depression. Assess client carefully for side effects: tachycardia, hypotension, bronchoconstriction, apnea. Monitor serum electrolyte, especially potassium, levels.
Atracurium Besylate (Tracrium)	ADULTS AND CHILDREN >2 Y IV: 0.4-0.5 mg/kg as bolus; maintain with continuous infusion INFANTS IV: 0.3-0.4 mg/kg as bolus	See tubocurarine chloride.
Metocurine Iodide (Metubine)	Administered as sustained injection over 30-60 s **Endotracheal Intubation** IV: 0.2-0.4 mg/kg **Electroshock Therapy** IV: 1.75-5.5 mg Average dose range: 2-3 mg	See tubocurarine chloride.
Pancuronium Bromide (Pavulon)	IV or IM dosage individualized in each case	See tubocurarine chloride.
Vecuronium Bromide (Norcuron)	*Loading IV Bolus:* 0.08-0.1 mg/kg *Maintenance:* 0.01-0.015 mg/kg during prolonged surgical procedures	See tubocurarine chloride.

TABLE 28–2 *Continued*
Prototypes and Major Drugs in Category

Drug Name	Dosage and Route of Administration	Nursing Considerations
DEPOLARIZING NEUROMUSCULAR BLOCKING DRUGS: SUCCINYLCHOLINE CHLORIDE (Anectine, Quelicin, Sucostrin) HOW SUPPLIED IM, IV: 20 mg/ml	IV and IM dosage individualized in each case	**Assess** Test for serum level of pseudocholinesterase if needed. Determine if client is receiving MAO inhibitor or digitalis glycoside. Assess for genetic disorder of plasma pseudocholinesterase, personal or family history of malignant hyperthermia, myopathies, or acute narrow-angle glaucoma.. Determine if client is pregnant; succinylcholine is classified as Pregnancy Category C. **Implement** Store in refrigerator at 2°-8° C. Multidose vials are stable for 14 days at room temperature. Solutions must be used within 24 h after preparation. Have dantrolene sodium available in case of malignant hyperthermia. **Monitor** If drug is used with inhalation anesthetic, monitor client after surgery for signs of malignant hyperthermia (muscular rigidity, tremor, mottling of skin, elevated temperature). Monitor blood pressure closely.
PERIPHERALLY ACTING SKELETAL MUSCLE RELAXANT: DANTROLENE (Dantrium) HOW SUPPLIED Gelatin capsule 25, 50, and 100 mg IV: 20 mg	**Spasticity** ADULTS Oral: 25 mg/d initially; increase to 25 mg bid to qid; then increase by 25 mg q4-7d; do not exceed 400 mg/d CHILDREN >5 Y Oral: 0.5 mg/kg bid; increase by 0.5 mg/kg up to 3 mg/kg bid to qid **Malignant Hyperthermia** ADULTS AND CHILDREN IV push of 1 mg/kg; may repeat up to total of 10 mg/kg Follow with oral: 4-8 mg/kg/d in divided doses for 1-3 d **Hyperthermia Prophylaxis** ADULTS AND CHILDREN Oral: 4-8 mg/kg/d in three or four divided doses for 1-2 d before	**Assess** Determine if client has preexisting hepatic disease. Determine baseline hepatic function values for client receiving oral preparation. Assess if client is pregnant: safety of drug use in pregnancy has not been determined. **Implement** Administer oral forms with food if GI upset is a problem. If swallowing is a problem, create a suspension by mixing contents of capsule with fruit juice. Administer immediately. For IV infusion, dilute 20 mg in 60 ml sterile water for injection. Shake until solution is clear. Instruct client to avoid CNS depressants and alcohol. Instruct client to avoid driving and using power machinery. Teach client to use sunscreen and protective clothing when outside. **Monitor** Auscultate bowel sounds at each shift. Monitor client for undesired clinical responses: drowsiness, dizziness, insomnia, weakness, and mental confusion. **Evaluate** Evaluate for reduction in muscle spasms.

Table continued on following page.

TABLE 28–2 *Continued*
Prototypes and Major Drugs in Category

Drug Name	Dosage and Route of Administration	Nursing Considerations
Quinine sulfate (Quinite, Quindan, Quinamm, etc.) **HOW SUPPLIED** Gelatin capsules: 200, 300, and 325 mg Plain coated tablet: 260 mg Uncoated tablet: 260 mg	Oral: 1 tablet when retiring; if needed, 1 tablet with evening meal and 1 tablet when retiring	**Assess** Determine if client is pregnant: quinine is classified as Pregnancy Category X. Assess if client is currently taking aluminum-based antacids, digoxin, or product with sodium bicarbonate as an ingredient. **Implement** Quinine can produce an elevated value for urinary 17-ketogenic steroids. **Monitor** Monitor for undesired clinical responses: nausea, vomiting, visual disturbance, tinnitus, and headache. **Evaluate** Evaluate for diminished nocturnal leg cramps.

PERIPHERALLY ACTING SKELETAL MUSCLE RELAXANT

Drugs in this category act directly on skeletal muscle to relieve spasticity. These drugs are used to treat a variety of medical disorders.

▨ NURSING CONSIDERATIONS

The nursing roles associated with peripherally acting skeletal muscle relaxants include assessment, planning, implementation, and evaluation. Because these drugs are used in addition to other forms of therapy, teaching is essential if the client is to receive maximum benefit from the drug.

Assessing   A health history and physical assessment should be completed by the nurse to gather baseline data about the client. Start the **health history** interview by asking the client to describe his or her chief concern—the incident or sensations that led the client to enter the health care system. Ask about events that may have altered bone or muscle function, including falls, trauma, vehicular accidents, and lifting heavy objects. Ask specifically about a past history of muscle spasms, cramping, or stiffness. Note any mention of seizures since some skeletal muscle relaxants can precipitate seizures.

The muscles of the back most likely to exhibit spasms are the paravertebral, the trapezius, and the entire erector group. In the upper arm the deltoid, triceps, or biceps may be involved. In the lower extremities the hamstrings, gluteals, and quadriceps are prone to spasm.

When pain accompanies muscle spasms, a detailed assessment of the client's pain experience is needed. An initial pain assessment includes information about the location, intensity, and quality of the pain. Determine what factors precipitate the onset of pain and what factors relieve or increase the discomfort. A vertical visual analog scale is useful for descriptions of pain intensity. For example, ask the client to rate his or her pain on a scale of 0 to 5, 0 to 10, or 0 to 100. Once the analog scale has been established, all health care team members should use the same numerical scale. (Review Chapter 19 for additional information about pain assessment.)

Ask about other symptoms that often accompany muscle spasms such as loss of appetite, poor concentration, sleeplessness, emotional lability, or disruption of interpersonal relationships. Determine how these alterations have influenced the client's ability to perform activities of daily living, including bathing, dressing, feeding, toileting, and ambulating. Ask questions about work, school, social activities, recreation, household maintenance, and yard work. Inability to work is a major stressor for many adults, whereas missing classes and social activities frustrate children and teenagers.

Collect a drug history. Gather information about prescriptions and over-the-counter (OTC) drugs. Determine if the client has tried any home remedies or self-prescribed treatment methods to relieve the discomfort. If so, assess the effectiveness of these methods.

Determine what the client expects from the drug therapy. At times, clients have unrealistic expectations. Emphasize that skeletal muscle relaxants are useful only when combined with other therapies. To help you develop your teaching plans, also establish the client's level of knowledge.

Physical assessment of the musculoskeletal system begins when you first see the client. If the client is ambulatory, observe the individual's posture and ability to walk. As you assess the client, keep in mind the normal appearance, movement, and function of the various bones, muscles, and joints. Inspect the muscles for symmetry, size, and abnormal movements. Measure and compare the circumference of each arm or leg. A discrepancy of more than 1 cm is considered significant. Assess muscle tone by palpating a muscle at rest and during passive range of motion. Palpation should be gentle to avoid painful pressure on inflamed tissue.[8,9] As you palpate, observe the client for nonverbal indications of pain such as guarding, flinching, or changes in facial expression. Spasms associated with muscle pain are palpable and usually visible.

As you assess the client, move the joints through passive range of motion. There should be even, mild resistance. When spasticity exists, there is increased tone with increasing resistance during muscle lengthening. "Clasp-knife phenomenon" may be apparent in a paralyzed client after a cerebrovascular insult to the corticospinal motor tract. To assess for the phenomenon, gently extend the paralyzed limb. If the phenomenon is present, the limb stiffens with increased resistance to the passive lengthening and then suddenly gives way to full extension, much as a pocketknife blade snaps into the open position. In a client with upper motor neuron disease, spasticity is greater in the flexors of the arms and the extensors of the leg.[8,10]

As with any assessment, obtain baseline vital signs. Baseline bowel function should also be determined because many skeletal muscle relaxants cause constipation or occasionally diarrhea.

Diagnosing Once the database has been established, the data are analyzed and nursing diagnoses developed. Depending on the data analysis, several nursing diagnoses might be appropriate for an individual receiving skeletal muscle relaxants. These diagnoses include the following:

- Impaired physical mobility related to muscle spasms and/or pain.
- Acute or chronic pain related to muscle spasms.
- Fatigue related to long-term efforts to cope with pain and functional disability.
- Anxiety related to a change in health status and/or body image.
- Ineffective individual coping related to inadequate pain management or lack of resources.
- Self-care deficits (bathing, dressing, feeding, toileting) related to decreased mobility.
- Sleep pattern disturbance related to pain.
- Body image disturbance related to changes in physical appearance.
- High risk for altered elimination (constipation) related to decreased intestinal peristalsis associated with some skeletal muscle relaxants.
- High risk for poisoning related to improper storage of drugs in the presence of children.

Planning Include in your teaching plan information about the drug such as drug action, side effects, dosage, and frequency of administration. Instruct clients to take the drug exactly as ordered. (Increasing the dosage does not increase the desired effect but makes side effects more prominent and increases the potential for abuse.) Include what signs and symptoms should be reported to the primary care provider. Also include in the plan any drugs, food, or beverages that should be avoided while skeletal muscle relaxants are being used.

You may also want to include behavioral and cognitive techniques that potentiate the desired effects of skeletal muscle relaxants. For example, guided imagery, distraction, music therapy, and the use of humor are effective among some cooperative clients. Relaxation techniques, including meditation and self-hypnosis, decrease muscle tension and are useful for well-motivated clients.

Since drowsiness and ataxia can occur, instruct the client to avoid driving motor vehicles or operating power machinery such as electric drills, saws, mowers, and household appliances. To avoid dizziness and postural hypotension, the client should be taught to change positions slowly. Since photosensitivity can be a problem for some clients, information about sunglasses and protective clothing is needed.[11]

Before implementing your plan of care, discuss expected outcomes with the client. Some possible outcomes include the following:

- Client attains an optimum level of activity within prescribed restrictions.
- Client rates pain as reduced on the visual analog scale.
- Client establishes and maintains an activity pattern that meets basic needs.
- Client exhibits a relaxed facial expression and easier body movements.
- Client uses appropriate problem-solving skills.
- Client performs targeted self-care activity within physical limitation.
- Client reports improvement in sleep and rest patterns.
- Client verbalizes acceptance of body changes.
- Client returns to normal patterns of bowel functioning.

Implementing Administer peripherally acting skeletal muscle relaxants with food or milk to avoid gastric irritation. If extended-release capsules or tablets are prescribed, they must be swallowed whole; they must not be opened or crushed.

If constipation becomes a problem, unless contraindicated, advise the client to increase bulk and fluid intake. If this increase is ineffective, consult the primary care provider about use of oral stool softeners. Observe the client for signs of unsteadiness or drowsiness. To avoid injury, ambulation and transfer of these clients should be supervised.

Evaluating Compare the client's progress with the outcomes developed during planning. If expected outcomes are not achieved, reassess the client and modify the approaches. Verify that drug information presented earlier is being used by the client and that the drug is actually being taken as prescribed.

🦥 Nursing Research

Davison, L., & Holland, M. (1989). A comparison of vecuronium bromide and atracurium besylate for rapid sequence induction. *Journal of the American Association of Nurse Anesthetists, 57*(1), 37-40.

The purpose of this study was to compare two short-acting, nondepolarizing muscle relaxants, vecuronium and atracurium, with the depolarizing muscle relaxant succinylcholine. Thirty subjects between the ages of 18 and 75 were part of the randomized study. These subjects did meet established criteria, one of which was not having a history of neuromuscular disease.

The subjects were divided into three groups according to the drug used during intubation before general anesthesia was achieved. Conditions at the time of intubation and at the time of 80% to 90% neuromuscular blockade were evaluated. There was statistical significance within all three groups. The final conclusion was that succinylcholine had a significantly faster onset of 80% to 90% neuromuscular blockade.

STUDENT ACTIVITIES

- Interview a nurse anesthetist in your agency and determine what neuromuscular blockers are used during intubation period. Determine the basis for selecting a nondepolarizing or depolarizing drug.
- Share this research article with the nurse anesthetist.

A pain flow sheet is useful to document premedication and postmedication pain levels, vital signs, activity levels, and side effects.[12] Ask the client to rate the pain again on the vertical visual analog scale. Determine if the pain continues to interfere with rest or sleep. Observe the client for improvements in mobility. Ask if the client's overall energy level has increased. Determine the client's progress in carrying out activities of daily living. Repeat assessments are important because surgical intervention sometimes is necessary when conservative therapy has been ineffective.

PERIPHERALLY ACTING SKELETAL MUSCLE RELAXANT PROTOTYPE

DANTROLENE (DANTRIUM)

Peripherally acting, skeletal muscle relaxants have a therapeutic advantage in situations in which the trigger for the muscle spasm is found in the nervous system.

Pharmacotherapeutics Peripherally acting skeletal muscle relaxants help to increase mobility and decrease the pain associated with local trauma and pathologic conditions of the muscles and joints. Conditions that might benefit from skeletal muscle relaxants include fractures, stretch injuries, bone cancer, spasms associated with spinal cord injury, and osteoporosis.[13] In addition, these drugs are used in clients with upper motor neuron diseases such as multiple sclerosis and cerebral palsy that are accompanied by significant spasticity. Dantrolene is also used to reduce the spasticity and mass-reflex movements associated with paraplegic and hemiplegic clients. It is a specific treatment for the management of malignant neuroleptic syndrome and malignant hyperthermia.

Pharmacokinetics The **absorption** of dantrolene is somewhat erratic. Absorption is incomplete (about 70%) after oral administration. Peak blood concentration is reached approximately 5 hours after oral administration. After an IV infusion of dantrolene, the blood concentration level remains at a steady state for approximately 3 hours. More than 1 week may pass before clinical improvement is seen, but if there is no change in 45 days, the drug should be discontinued. The exact **distribution** of dantro-

lene has not been determined. It is known that large amounts of dantrolene are bound to serum albumin. The drug also crosses the placental barrier easily. **Biotransformation** occurs primarily in the liver. Dantrolene is metabolized by the liver into a derivative that is less active than the original form. The plasma half-life of dantrolene is 8.7 hours in adults and 7.3 hours in children. Dantrolene is **excreted** by the kidneys in urine.[2,4,11]

Pharmacodynamics The pharmacodynamics of dantrolene are unique. The drug acts directly on the intracellular space inside skeletal muscle fibers and interrupts the excitation-contraction coupling of the sarcoplasm (the interfibrillary matter of striated muscle) within the intracellular spaces. This action is associated with a reduction of the calcium ions that initiate contraction.[2]

Pharmaceutics Dantrolene is available in gelatin capsules (25, 50, and 100 mg) for oral use. It is also available as a powder for reconstitution as an IV injection.[4]

Undesired Clinical Responses The most frequent undesired responses to dantrolene are drowsiness, dizziness, and muscle weakness. Dantrolene can cause gastrointestinal (GI) disturbances (e.g., diarrhea, nausea, vomiting), mental confusion, myalgia, and abnormal hair growth. Severe liver toxicity and pleural effusion are also possible.[2]

Contraindications and Precautions Dantrolene use is contraindicated in individuals with liver disease. In addition, it may aggravate conditions such as congestive heart failure, asthma, and other obstructive lung disorders. Dantrolene should be used with caution with females and with clients over 35 years of age.[2]

Drug-Drug, Drug-Nutrient, Drug-Environment Interactions Although a definite drug interaction of dantrolene with estrogen therapy has not been established, caution should be taken when the two drugs are given concomitantly. Hepatotoxicity has occurred more frequently in individuals receiving this drug combination. Exposure to sunlight can trigger photosensitivity reactions in clients receiving dantrolene.[4]

Life Span Considerations The safety of dantrolene for women who are or who may become pregnant has not been established. The drug should not be used in nursing mothers. The long-term safety of dantrolene in children less than 5 years old has also not been established.

Extreme caution must be taken if skeletal muscle relaxants are prescribed for elderly clients. Age-related changes make these individuals more vulnerable to undesired clinical reactions to the drugs.

Specific Drug-Related Nursing Considerations If the client has difficulty swallowing, an oral suspension of dantrolene can be created by opening the capsule and mixing the contents with fruit juice. The suspension should be drunk immediately. It is not necessary to give oral dantrolene with food unless gastric upset is a problem. If persistent diarrhea occurs, discontinuation of the drug may be necessary. (However, during long-term use, constipation occurs more commonly than diarrhea.) Since dantrolene capsules contain lactose, lactose-intolerant clients may not be able to use them.

IV dantrolene should be administered carefully to avoid extravasation because the product's high pH is very irritating to tissues. The reconstituted solution must be used within 6 hours of preparation and should be protected from direct sunlight. Since drowsiness and muscle weakness commonly result, keep the client flat for 15 minutes after parenteral administration. Supervise ambulation for the next 2 hours to prevent injury.

If dantrolene is administered on an outpatient basis, follow-up is important. Jaundice, nausea, vomiting, and abdominal pain are signs of liver damage and must be reported to the health care provider at once. Liver function tests should be done before initial administration of dantrolene and periodically during long-term therapy.[11]

Miscellaneous Drugs in Category

Quinine sulfate (Quinite, Quinamm, Quindan, etc.), a cinchona alkaloid, produces skeletal muscle relaxation by three major mechanisms: it increases the refractory period by direct action on the muscle fiber; it decreases the excitability of the motor end-plate; and it affects the distribution of calcium within the muscle fiber. Because of its ability to produce muscle relaxation, quinine is used to prevent and treat nocturnal leg muscle cramps.

Quinine is readily **absorbed** when given orally. Absorption occurs mainly in the upper part of the small intestine. Most of the drug is **metabolized** in the liver and **excreted,** either unchanged or in its metabolized form, in the urine. If the urine is acidic, renal excretion is twice as rapid as with alkaline urine. In addition, small amounts of the metabolized drug appear in the feces, gastric juice, bile, and saliva. Protein binding influences how quinine is **distributed.** Approximately 70% of the plasma quinine is bound to protein. The drug does not readily cross the blood-brain barrier but easily crosses the placental membrane. Peak plasma concentrations of quinine occur within 1 to 3 hours after a single oral dose. The half-life is 4 to 5 hours.

Quinine sulfate should not be administered during pregnancy since it is classified as a Pregnancy Category X drug. Repeated doses or overdose of quinine in some clients can produce a syndrome called **cinchonism.** Manifestations of this syndrome include tinnitus, head-ache, nausea, and altered vision. Symptoms may also involve the GI, nervous, and cardiovascular systems. Adverse reactions to the drug include anginal symptoms, asthmatic symptoms, thrombocytopenic purpura, visual disturbances, allergic reactions, nausea, and vomiting.

Several drug-drug interactions exist. For example, concomitant administration of quinine and digoxin causes increased plasma levels of digoxin. If quinine and aluminum-containing antacids are administered concurrently, the absorption of quinine may be delayed. In addition, if neuromuscular blocking drugs are administered with quinine, respiratory depression may result.[2,4–6] For additional information on peripherally acting skeletal muscle relaxants, see Table 28–2.

CONCEPT REVIEW

Peripherally acting skeletal muscle relaxants are not as potent as the neuromuscular blocking drugs. However, they produce serious adverse reactions and must be administered with caution.

Most peripherally acting relaxants are administered orally.

These drugs are administered most frequently outside of the acute care setting; therefore the role of the nurse must focus on client teaching.

SUMMARY

The three major types of skeletal muscle relaxants discussed in this chapter are nondepolarizing neuromuscular blocking drugs, depolarizing neuromuscular blocking drugs, and peripherally acting skeletal muscle relaxants. The neuromuscular blocking drugs are administered by clinicians with special skills and education. With administration of these drugs, your role primarily involves careful assessment of the client. With the less potent peripherally acting skeletal muscle relaxants, your role includes drug administration and client teaching.

REFERENCES

1. Guyton, A.C. (1991). *Textbook of medical physiology* (8th ed.). Philadelphia: W.B. Saunders.
2. Smith, C.M. (1992). Skeletal muscle relaxants. In Smith, C.M., and Reynard, A.M. (Eds.). *Textbook of pharmacology* (pp. 358-366). Philadelphia: W.B. Saunders.
3. Lehne, R.A. (1994). *Pharmacology for nursing care* (2nd ed.). Philadelphia: W.B. Saunders.
4. Data Pharmaceutica, Inc. (1993). *1993 physicians' genRx.* Smithtown, NY: Author.
5. U.S. Pharmacopeial Convention. (1990). *The United States pharmacopeia* (22nd rev.). Rockville, MD.: Author.
6. Goodman, A., Gilman, A., Rall, T., Niles, A., & Taylor. P. (Eds.) (1990). *Goodman and Gilman's: The pharmacological basis of therapeutics* (8th ed.). New York: Pergamon Press.
7. Ashby, D. (1990). Malignant hyperthermia: A potential crisis in the postanesthesia care unit. *Journal of Post Anesthetic Nursing, 5,* 279-281.
8. Jarvis, C. (1992). *Physical examination and health assessment.* Philadelphia: W.B. Saunders.
9. Grimes, J., & Burns, E. (1992). *Health assessment in nursing practice* (3rd ed.). Boston: Jones & Bartlett.
10. Lombardo, M.C. (1992). Neurologic examination: Evaluation of the neurologic patient. In Price, S.A., and Wilson, L.M. (Eds.). *Pathophysiology: Clinical concepts of disease processes* (4th ed.) (pp. 750-764). St. Louis: C.V. Mosby.
11. McEvoy, G.K. (Ed.) (1991). *AHFS drug information.* Bethesda, MD: American Society of Hospital Pharmacists.
12. Vanderbosch, T.M. (1988). How to use a pain flow sheet effectively. *Nursing '88, 18*(8), 50-51.
13. Hallal, J.C. (1991). Back pain with postmenopausal osteoporosis and vertebral fractures. *Geriatric Nursing, 12,* 285-287.

BIBLIOGRAPHY

Chenitz, W.C., et al. (1991). *Clinical gerontological nursing: A guide to advanced practice.* Philadelphia: W.B. Saunders.

Doege, T.C., & Holinger, P.C. (1990). Understanding and preventing injuries. *American Family Physician, 42,* 680-685.

Dubaybo, B.A., et al. (1991). Use of sedatives and muscle relaxants in acute respiratory failure. *Hospital Formulary, 26,* 278-287.

Elder, N.C. (1991). Abuse of skeletal muscle relaxants. *American Family Physician, 44,* 1223-1226.

Eustace, C. (1991). Back up and wait. *RN, 54*(6), 49-51.

Harvey, S.C. (1990). Skeletal muscle relaxants. In Gennaro, A.R. (Ed.). *Remington's pharmaceutical services* (18th ed.) (pp. 916-923). Easton, PA: Mack Publishing.

Ostgaard, H.C., et al. (1991). Prevalence of back pain in pregnancy. *Spine, 16,* 549-552.

Nasca, R.J. (1990). Back pain in the aging spine. *Topics in Geriatric Rehabilitation, 6*(2), 18-33.

Snyder, M. (1991). *A guide to neurological and neurosurgical nursing* (2nd ed.). Albany, NY: Delmar Publishers.

Drugs Affecting the Cardiovascular System

OVERVIEW OF
The Cardiovascular System

JANET D. PIERCE • SHAREE A. WIGGINS

⊛ **Anatomy of the Cardiovascular System**

LEARNING OBJECTIVES:

Name the microscopic structures of the cardiovascular system.

List macroscopic structures of the cardiovascular system.

KEY TERMS:

Myofibrils, sarcolemma, sarcomere

⊛ **Physiology of the Cardiovascular System**

LEARNING OBJECTIVES:

Describe the conduction system of the cardiovascular system.

Explain the cardiac cycle.

Define the terms associated with cardiac output.

Discuss the regulatory control of cardiovascular function.

KEY TERMS:

Action potential, afterload, contractility, diastole, preload, refractory period, systole

⊛ **Drugs Affecting the Cardiovascular System**

LEARNING OBJECTIVE: Identify four categories of drugs that affect the cardiovascular system.

CONCEPTS AND TERMS TO REVIEW

Review an anatomy and physiology book for a complete discussion of the cardiovascular system.

Review sections in Chapter 17 on resting membrane potential and action potential.

---

*T*he cardiovascular system is responsible for three essential functions: (1) delivery of oxygen and nutrients to the cells of the body; (2) removal of metabolic waste products from the cells; and (3) transportation of other substances from one part of the body to another. A functional cardiovascular system is vital for survival. Without circulation, tissues lack a supply of oxygen and nutrients, and waste substances accumulate.

The cardiovascular system consists of the blood, heart, and blood vessels. Blood is a liquid connective tissue that has three general functions: transportation, regulation, and protection. The heart is the center of the cardiovascular system. It propels blood through thousands of miles of blood vessels. Blood vessels form a closed system of tubes that carry blood away from the heart, transport it to the tissues of the body, and then return it to the heart.

Only the anatomy and physiology of the heart and blood vessels are discussed in this chapter. An overview of the components and functions of blood is presented in Chapter 34. Anatomically the cardiovascular system includes both microscopic and macroscopic structures. Physiologic functions include elements such as the conduction system of the heart, cardiac muscle contraction, and cardiac cycle.

ANATOMY OF THE CARDIOVASCULAR SYSTEM

The anatomy of the cardiovascular system includes microscopic and macroscopic structures. Cardiac fibers and cells are the microscopic structures. The structures of the heart, arterial and venous system, and coronary blood supply are the macroscopic structures.

Microscopic Structure

Based on their appearance in light micrographs, muscle fibers are divided into two types: striated muscle and smooth muscle. Striated muscle is either skeletal or cardiac muscle and is characterized by alternating light and dark bands. In striated muscle there are no defining surface features.[1]

CARDIAC FIBERS AND CARDIAC CELLS

Microscopically, cardiac muscle fibers contain visible striations that appear as a latticework arrangement because the fibers run on a longitudinal axis. The striations are similar in appearance to skeletal muscle except that cells in skeletal muscle are fused. In cardiac muscle the fiber cells, called **myofibrils,** separate, rejoin, and then divide again. Each cardiac muscle cell has only one elongated nucleus. This is in contrast to skeletal muscle cells, which possess many nuclei.[2,3]

Cardiac fibers contain several extraordinary characteristics that enable the heart to contract as a unit. The contracting unit of the myocardium is the **sarcomere.** Its outer covering, the **sarcolemma,** encases the myofibrils. At the end of each sarcomere are separations and branches called **intercalated discs.** These discs are seen microscopically as thick, dark lines across the fibers. They provide the mechanism for rapid conduction of electric impulses across each myofibril. Thus myocardial cells contract simultaneously because depolarization occurs concurrently within each cell. If depolarization begins in any cardiac cell, it quickly spreads throughout the heart; this is why cardiac muscle is called a **functional syncytium.**[3,4]

Myofibrils are thick and thin intracellular filaments (Fig. 29–1). They contain two types of contractile proteins called **actin** and **myosin.** Actin filaments are thin fibers that contain three proteins: actin, tropomyosin, troponin. The myosin filaments are thicker fibrils with overlapping fibers. Actin filaments are attached to **Z**-bands at one end, leaving the opposite end free to interact with the myosin **crossbridges** (small projections from the sides of the myosin filaments). During diastole, the actin and myosin filaments overlap slightly. However, during systole the distance between the **Z**-bands becomes shorter, and the tiny projections on the myosin interact with the actin. Contraction occurs when tropomyosin is moved, exposing the troponin complex to allow the projection from the myosin filament to connect to the actin filament (crossbridging).[1,2,4]

Another important intracellular component related to myocardial contractility is the **sarcoplasmic reticulum (SR).** Both active and passive ion transport occurs within the SR. After depolarization of cardiac muscle, calcium ions stored in the SR are released to bind to troponin. This ionic transport mechanism facilitates actin-myosin filament sliding. Once the sliding movement is complete, the calcium is removed by calcium pumps located within the SR. Removal of calcium allows the actin-myosin filaments to return to a resting position.[4,5]

Within the SR are transverse tubules called T tubules. These tubules penetrate the myofibrils and assist with electric conduction by communicating with the outside of the cell membrane. Action potentials in the T tubules cause a release of calcium from the SR. Electric conduction is achieved not

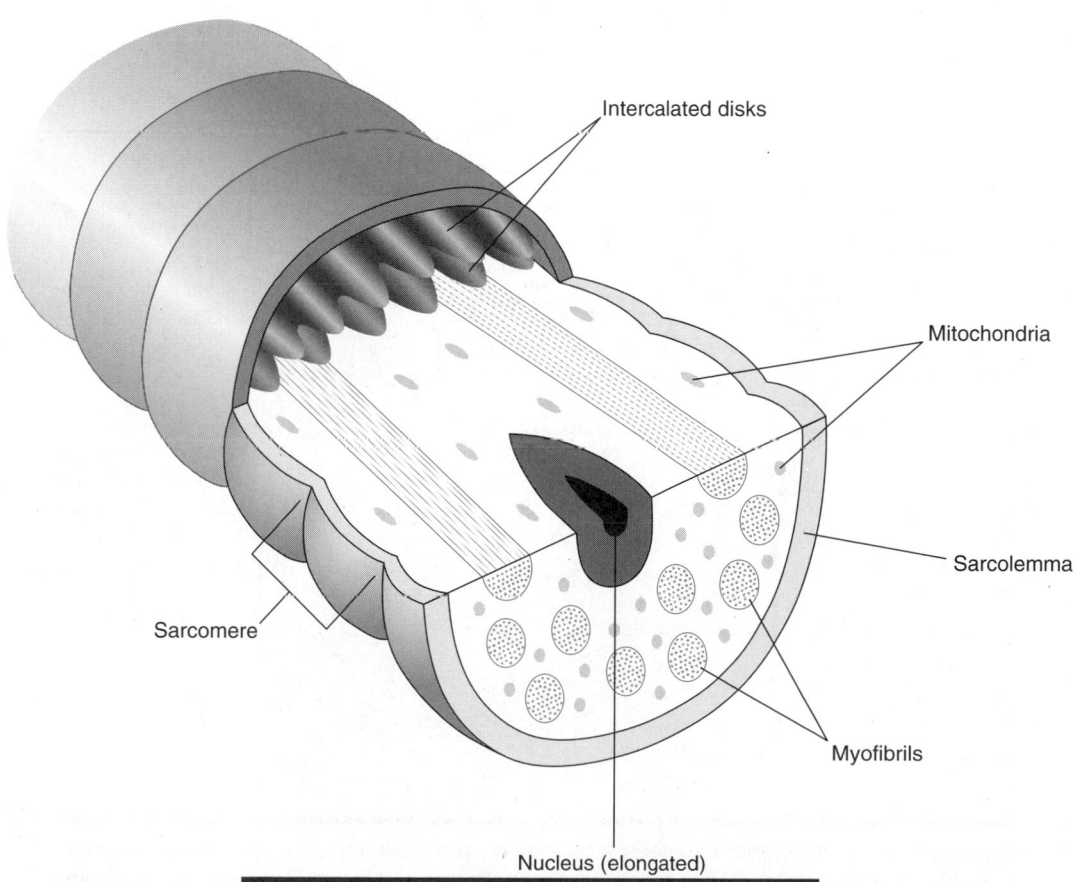

FIGURE 29–1   Components of cardiac muscle fiber.

only by calcium but also by the exchange between sodium and potassium ions.[4-6]

Macroscopic Structures

Important macroscopic structures of the cardiovascular system include the heart, arterial system, and venous system (Fig. 29–2). Coronary blood supply is also considered a macroscopic structure.

HEART

The human heart is a muscular organ that distributes blood throughout the circulatory system. It is located in the mediastinum of the thoracic cavity close to the points of attachment of ribs two through six on the left side. The diaphragm lies below the heart, and the lungs lie on either side. When the heart is viewed anteriorly, it resembles a triangle slanted at a 90-degree angle.

Two atria and two ventricles are the main structures of the heart. The two ventricles form the apex of the heart; the left ventricle forms the anterolateral and posterior surfaces. Usually the apex of the heart is located 9 cm left of the sternal border. It is situated at the midclavicular line of the fifth intercostal space and rests on the central tendon of the di-

aphragm. Two atria constitute the base of the heart, which is parallel to the right edge of the sternal border and extends to the level of the second rib. Arising from the base of the heart are the aortic root, superior vena cava, and pulmonary vessels. Posterior to the heart are the descending aorta, esophagus, trachea, vertebral column, and the inferior vena cava.

The human adult heart is near the size of the individual's clenched fist. It is approximately 10 to 12 cm long and 8 to 10 cm wide. The heart weighs 225 to 255 g in women and 300 to 314 g in men.

A special structure, the **pericardial sac,** encases and protects the heart. This sac is composed of strong, fibrous connective tissues on the outer **(parietal)** surface, whereas epithelial tissue lines the inner **(visceral)** layer. Protection for the heart and a means of attachment to surrounding anatomic structures are provided by the parietal layer. The serous membrane of the visceral layer bathes the heart with fluid and prevents friction during cardiac contractions. To prevent overdistention of the heart during transient periods of volume overload, a strong pericardial sac is essential.[4,7]

Three layers of tissue comprise the heart: epicardium, myocardium, and endocardium. The outer layer, the **epicardium,** is the inner layer of the pericardial sac. The **myocar-**

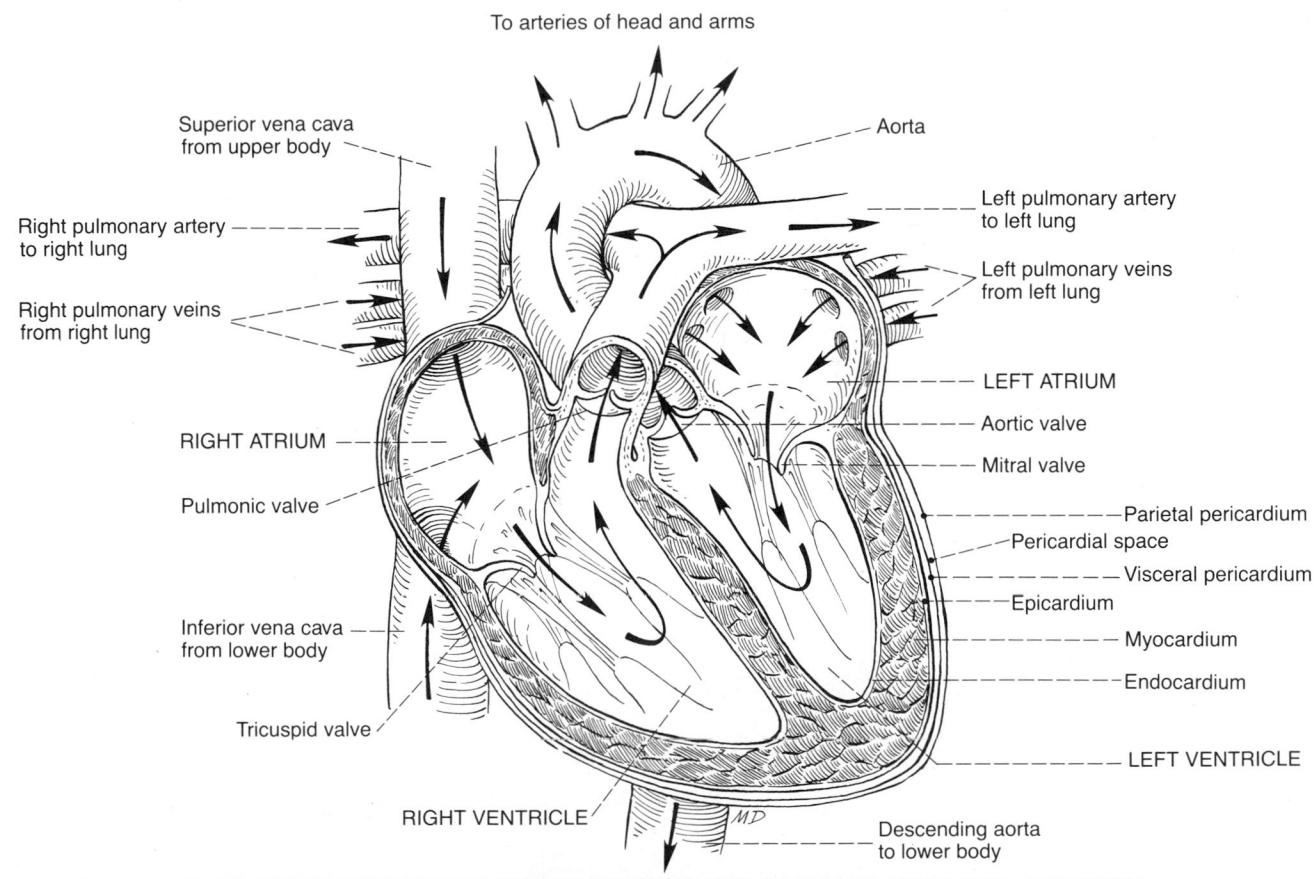

FIGURE 29–2   Anatomic structures of the heart. (From Black, J., & Matassarin-Jacobs, E. [1993]. *Luckmann and Sorensen's medical-surgical nursing: A psychophysiologic approach* [4th ed.]. Philadelphia: W.B. Saunders.)

dium is beneath the epicardium. This thick muscular layer of the heart, the middle layer, is composed of bundles of twisted fibers. It is thinner near the base of the heart and thickens at the apex. The innermost layer, the **endocardium,** is a thin sheet of endothelial tissue that lines the heart chambers.

The atria and ventricles create the four hollow chambers of the heart. Ventricles are more muscular than the atria and are approximately three times thicker. Each side of the heart is divided by a wall called the septum. This partition consists of myocardium covered by endocardium. Two septa separate the heart into separate pumping systems, the right and left sides of the heart.

Four one-way fibrous valves exist within the heart: the atrioventricular (AV) valves and the semilunar valves. Pressure gradients regulate the opening and closing of these valves. **AV valves** lie between the atria and ventricles. Between the right atrium and right ventricle is the **tricuspid valve,** which has three cusps. The left AV valve lies between the left atrium and left ventricle. This valve, the **bicuspid** or **mitral valve,** has two cusps. Attached to the AV valves are four to 10 strong cordlike structures called the **chordae tendineae.** These structures are avascular and arise from the papillary muscles that prevent the valves' opening during systole. **Semilunar valves** prevent blood from flowing backward into the heart. Located in the opening where the pulmonary trunk leaves the right ventricle is the **pulmonary semilunar valve.** Situated at the opening between the left ventricle and aorta is the **aortic semilunar valve.**[1,8–10]

ARTERIAL SYSTEM

The arterial system begins at the aorta and ends at the arterial-capillary interface. **Arteries** are strong, elastic vessels adapted for carrying oxygenated blood away from the heart to the rest of the body. Walls of these blood vessels contain three layers: the tunica intima, tunica media, and tunica adventitia. The **tunica intima,** innermost layer, consists of endothelial cells that form a slippery surface that enhances the flow of arterial blood. A thicker, more powerful layer, the **tunica media,** is next. This layer is composed of smooth muscle cells and elastic tissue. Under the influence of the sympathetic nervous system, smooth muscle of the tunica media changes the diameter of the artery. A strong fibrous connective tissue that supports and protects the artery constitutes the outer layer, the **tunica adventitia.**[2,4,10]

Arterioles, which are microscopic continuations of arteries, give off branches that join capillaries. Although the walls of the larger arterioles have three layers similar to those of the arteries, these walls become thinner and thinner as the arterioles approach the capillaries. **Capillaries** are the smallest blood vessels. They form the connections between the smallest arterioles and the smallest venules.[6]

VENOUS SYSTEM

Veins are blood vessels that carry blood toward the heart. **Venules** are the smallest parts of the venous system; they are formed by the union of several capillaries. Venules rapidly con-

verge to form small veins, which in turn join to form large veins. Gradually the diameters of the vessels increase, ultimately forming the large veins that enter the heart. For the most part, veins remove blood from a particular vascular area by accompanying the arteries that supply the area. The names of the veins are identical to their arterial counterparts.

Veins possess one-way valves that promote the return of blood to the heart. As veins transport partially oxygenated blood to the heart, the size of individual veins increases and the number of veins decreases. Venous blood from the head, neck, and arms is removed by the superior vena cava. Conversely, the inferior vena cava receives blood from the lower body.

Although veins are thinner than arteries, they contain the same three layers (tunica intima, tunica media, and tunica adventitia). The tunica media of veins consists of less muscular and elastic tissue. However, veins contain more fibrous tissue and smooth muscle, which allows for dilation of the veins when large amounts of venous volume are present.[4,11]

Veins are known as the **capacitance vessels** of the circulatory system because of their inherent ability to reserve and distribute large volumes of blood. Veins contain approximately 60% of the circulatory blood volume. The compliance of the venous system is 24 times greater than that of the arterial system. In contrast with the arterial system, large blood volume changes in the venous system generate only small pressure changes within the veins.[4,11]

CORONARY BLOOD SUPPLY

The first two branches of the aorta, the right and left **coronary arteries,** supply blood to the tissues of the heart. The left coronary artery branches into the **circumflex artery** and the **anterior interventricular artery** (or left anterior descending artery). The right coronary artery splits off into two major branches—the **posterior interventricular artery** and the **marginal artery.**[6,7]

Since the heart is constantly working even at rest, the heart aerobically uses most of the oxygen delivered by the coronary blood supply. Therefore any increase in oxygen demand usually results in an increase in coronary blood flow. Normally an individual can increase coronary blood flow five or six times the regular volume if necessary. Many elements, including aortic diastolic blood pressure, pathology, and metabolic, neural, and humoral factors, influence the amount of blood flow to the heart.[12,13]

CONCEPT REVIEW

Cardiac fibers and cells constitute the microscopic structures of the cardiovascular system.

Macroscopic structures of the cardiovascular system include the heart, arterial and venous system, and coronary blood supply.

PHYSIOLOGY OF THE CARDIOVASCULAR SYSTEM

The degree to which the essential functions of the heart are carried out is, for the most part, dependent on normal cardiovascular physiology. The following section discusses electrochemical and electromechanical activities as components of normal cardiovascular physiology.

Conduction System

Cardiac muscle cells have several unique properties that include automaticity, excitability, conductivity, contractility, and rhythmicity. Specialized myocardial cells are responsible for the generation and distribution of electrical cardiac impulses throughout the myocardium. In the healthy individual these electrical impulses originate in the **sinoatrial node (SA).** The SA node, a small, elongated mass of specialized cardiac muscle tissue, is located just beneath the epicardium in the posterior wall of the right atrium (Fig. 29–3).

The SA node is the pacemaker of the heart; it has the highest degree of automaticity (approximately 60 to 100 beats/min). Both the sympathetic and parasympathetic systems innervate the SA node. Sympathetic fibers influence the SA node and increase the rate of impulse generation. Parasympathetic fibers cause the rate of impulse generation in the SA node to decrease.

As a cardiac impulse travels from the SA node into the atrial syncytium, the right and left atria contract almost simultaneously. The cardiac impulse then passes along conducting fibers that lead to another mass of specialized cardiac muscle tissue called the **AV node.** This node is located in the floor of the right atrium near the septum that separates the atria, just beneath the endocardium.

<table>
<tr><td colspan="2">**PROPERTIES OF CARDIAC MUSCLE CELLS**</td></tr>
<tr><td>**Automaticity**</td><td>Ability of cell to depolarize subcutaneously</td></tr>
<tr><td>**Excitability**</td><td>Ability of cell to depolarize in response to a given stimulus</td></tr>
<tr><td>**Conductivity**</td><td>Ability of cardiac cell to transmit a stimulus from cell to cell</td></tr>
<tr><td>**Contractility**</td><td>Ability of cardiac myofibril to shorten in length in response to an electric stimulus</td></tr>
<tr><td>**Refractory state**</td><td>Period during repolarization when cell requires a greater stimulus than normal or cannot depolarize regardless of the intensity of the stimulus</td></tr>
<tr><td>**Rhythmicity**</td><td>Regular rate of automatic electric discharges</td></tr>
</table>

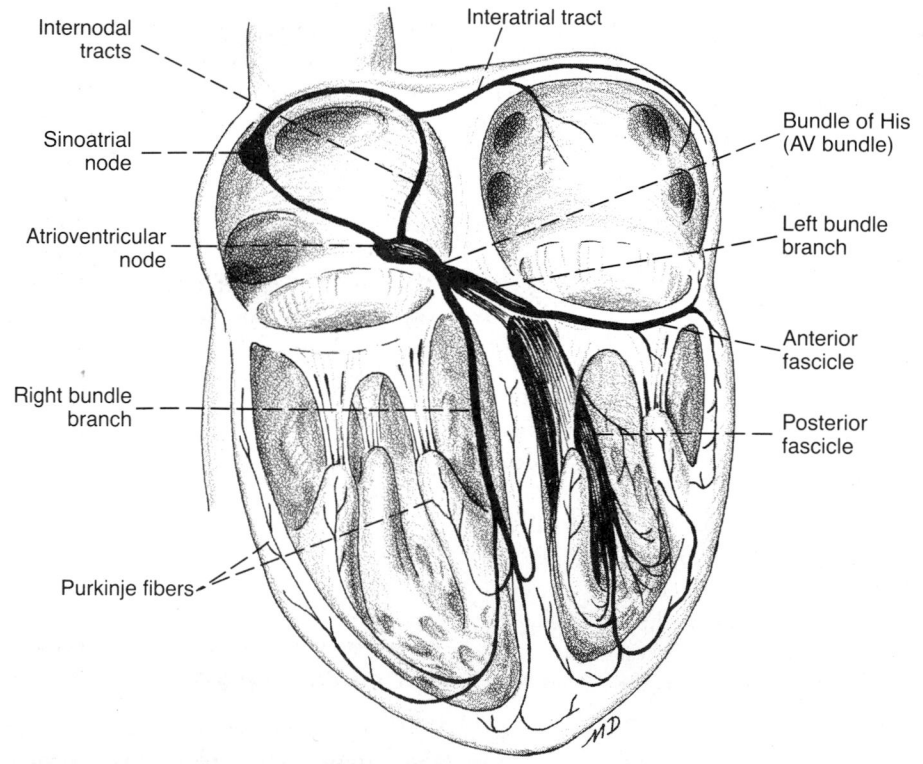

FIGURE 29–3 Conduction system of the heart. (From Black, J., & Matassarin-Jacobs, E. [1993]. *Luckmann and Sorensen's medical-surgical nursing: A psychophysiologic approach* [4th ed.]. Philadelphia: W.B. Saunders.)

Fibers that conduct the cardiac impulse into the AV node slow the impulse velocity. The electrical impulse is delayed still more as it travels through the node; this delay allows time for the atria to empty and the ventricles to fill with blood before ventricular contraction. The inherent automaticity of the AV node is much slower than that of the SA node. If the SA node fails to generate an electrical impulse, the AV node assumes the role of the pacemaker of the heart. However, the pulse rate generated by the AV node is slower, approximately 40 to 60 beats per minute.

From the AV node, the impulse enters the **AV bundle** or **bundle of His,** the only electrical connection between the atria and ventricles. After traveling along the AV bundle, the impulse enters the right and left bundle branches. Finally, large-diameter conduction myofibrils **(Purkinje fibers)** rapidly conduct the impulse into the mass of ventricular muscle tissue. Ventricular cardiac cells also have properties of automaticity, which allow the ventricles to take over as the pacemaker of the heart if higher levels of the conduction system fail to respond. The inherent rate of the ventricles is less than 40 beats/minute.[5–7,9,13,14]

Cardiac Muscle Contraction

Electrically charged ions on either side of the sarcolemma (sodium [Na^+], potassium [K^+], chloride [Cl^-]) begin at equal concentrations. When the sodium-potassium pump in the sarcolemma is activated, potassium is transported inward, causing a higher intracellular potassium concentration. Similarly, more sodium ions transfer out of the cell than diffuse inward. Electrical and concentration gradients are generated by this ionic imbalance, causing ions to move across the semipermeable cell membrane.

An **action potential** is a schematic representation of depolarization and repolarization of cardiac muscle. Action potential in cardiac muscle is caused by fast sodium channels and slow calcium-sodium channels. The slower channels require a longer period to open, but they stay open for approximately 0.7 seconds. This time allows sodium and calcium ions to flow to the interior of the cardiac muscle fiber, causing a prolonged period of depolarization. The plateau in the action potential of cardiac muscle is produced by this prolonged depolarization. The velocity of conduction produced by the action potential is approximately 0.3 to 0.5 m/s.

Cardiac action potential is divided into five phases. During **phase 0,** sodium enters the cardiac cells rapidly, and the interior of the cell becomes positive. As a result, cardiac cells depolarize and begin to contract. **Phase 1** (early rapid repolarization) begins with the abrupt termination of sodium influx into the cardiac cell. As the membrane potential drops, potassium leaves the cell. Soon the cell membrane becomes more permeable to chloride, allowing it to enter the cell.

Phase 2 (plateau) is a prolonged phase of slow repolarization. Potassium continues to leave the cell as sodium enters at a slower rate. During **phase 3** (rapid repolarization), permeability of the cellular membrane to potassium is increased, al-

lowing the interior of the cell to become markedly negative. This is a regenerative process. The membrane potential returns to the resting level, and repolarization is finished.

During **phase 4** (diastole), which is the final phase between action potentials, restoration and initiation of spontaneous diastole occur. The sodium-potassium pump removes sodium that had previously entered the cell during depolarization in exchange for potassium.[2,4,12]

The **refractory period** is the interval during which cardiac cells can be depolarized by electrical stimulation. Two types of refractory periods exist: absolute refractory period (ARP) and relative refractory period (RRP). The **ARP** begins at phase 0 (depolarization) and extends to phase 3. During the ARP, no amount of electrical stimulation generates depolarization of cardiac fibers. The **relative refractory period** extends from the middle of phase 3 to the end of phase 3 and lasts for approximately 0.05 seconds. During this time, a strong stimulus to the cardiac muscle can cause depolarization.[2,4]

Cardiac Cycle

The cardiac cycle refers to the events of a complete mechanical heartbeat (Fig. 29–4). In a normal cardiac cycle the atria contract while the ventricles relax. Then while the ventricles contract, the atria relax. **Systole** refers to the phase of contraction; the phase of relaxation is **diastole.** For healthy adults, the heart completes approximately 72 cardiac cycles per minute; thus the average duration for each cardiac cycle is approximately 0.8 seconds.

Relaxation period   At the end of a heartbeat, all four chambers are in diastole, a period of relaxation. Repolarization of the ventricular muscle fibers initiates relaxation. As the ventricles relax, pressure within the chambers drops, and blood flows into the ventricles.

Ventricular filling   A time of rapid ventricular filling occurs just after the AV valves open. Isovolumic relaxation occurs during rapid filling, and 70% of the blood volume to the ventricles is received passively. (*Isovolumic relaxation* filling occurs between pulmonic and aortic valve closure and tricuspid and mitral valve opening.) The last part of diastole is the slow-filling phase during which the atria contract and force only a small volume of blood into the ventricles. Slow filling is responsible for delivery of 30% of the blood volume received by the ventricles. Through the period of ventricular filling, the AV valves are open, and the semilunar valves are closed.[7,10,11]

Ventricular systole   SA node firing results in atrial depolarization. Near the end of atrial systole, the impulse from the SA node passes through the AV node and into the ventricles. After the spread of electrical activity to the ventricles, myocardial fibers shorten and cause ventricular pressures to rise and exceed atrial pressures. This increase in ventricular pressure forces the tricuspid and mitral valves to close. As the ventricular pressures increase, the intraventricular pressure becomes greater than the aortic and pulmonic pressures, forcing the semilunar valves open. The amount of blood ejected from the ventricles with each contraction is called **stroke volume.**[3,11]

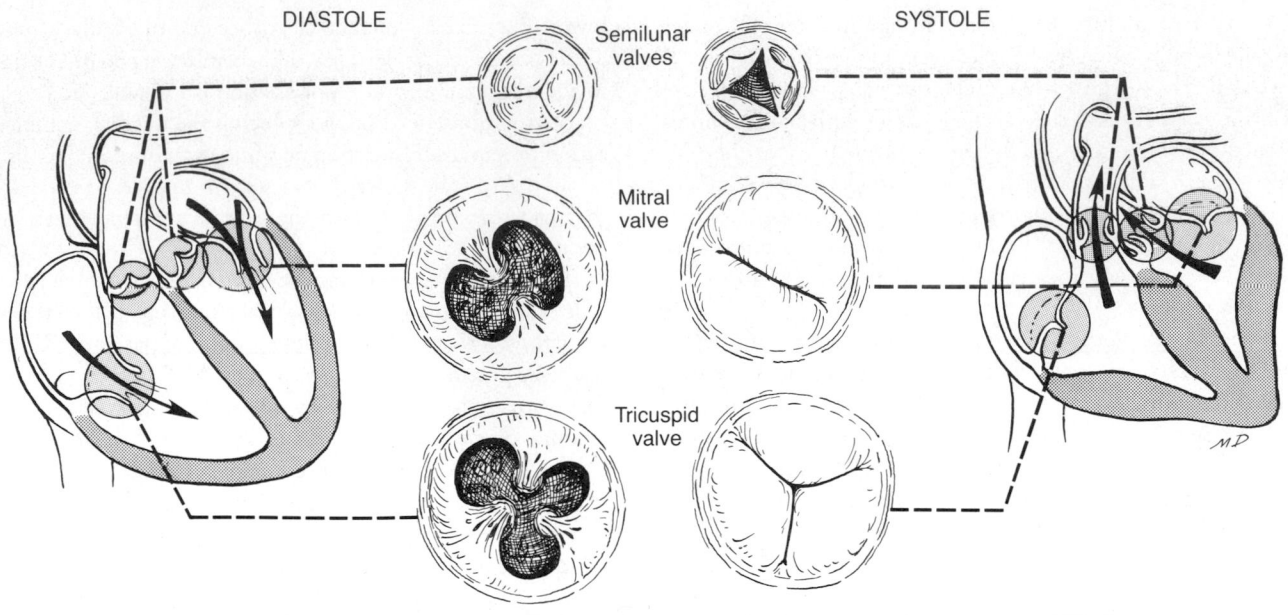

FIGURE 29–4 Heart valve responses during the cardiac cycle. (From Black, J., & Matassarin-Jacobs, E. [1993]. *Luckmann and Sorensen's medical-surgical nursing: A psychophysiologic approach* [4th ed.]. Philadelphia: W.B. Saunders.)

CONCEPT REVIEW

Cardiac muscle cells have the unique properties of automaticity, excitability, conductivity, contractility, and rhythmicity.

Cardiac action potential is divided into five phases.

The cardiac cycle consists of the relaxation period, ventricular filling period, and ventricular systole.

Cardiac Output

The volume of blood pumped out to the body per minute is called **cardiac output.** At rest, the adult heart pumps approximately 4 to 6 L of blood per minute. This amount varies with the actual size of the individual. Stress, exercise, and changes in peripheral or arterial pressure change the cardiac output. Cardiac output is the sum of the stroke volume and heart rate; preload, afterload, and contractility determine the stroke volume.[2-4]

Heart rate The heart rate represents the number of heartbeats per minute. Increasing the heart rate is a primary method of improving cardiac output. However, as the heart rate increases, diastole decreases as does the amount of blood flow to the coronary arteries. A rapid heart rate also increases myocardial oxygen consumption, reducing the amount of energy available for myocardial contractility.

Preload Preload is the end-diastolic stretch on cardiac muscle fiber before contraction. The more the heart is filled during diastole, the greater the force of contraction during systole. This is known as the *Starling law of the heart.* In the body

the preload depends on the volume of blood that fills the ventricles at the end of diastole, the end-diastolic volume (EDV).[2,9,12]

Contractility Contractility is the strength of contraction. *Positive inotropic* factors increase contractility; *negative inotropic* factors decrease contractility. Myocardial contractility can be enhanced by the sympathetic nervous system and the Starling mechanism. In addition, several pharmacologic agents can mimic the sympathetic nervous system, increasing the contractility of the heart.[9,12]

Afterload Afterload is the amount of resistance that the ventricles must overcome to open the semilunar valves and propel blood into the pulmonary and systemic circulatory systems. When the afterload increases, stroke volume decreases, and more blood remains in the ventricles at the end of systole. The primary factor that determines afterload is resistance in the pulmonic and/or systemic vessels.[6,9]

Regulation of Cardiovascular Function

Cardiovascular function is under the control of three regulatory mechanisms: the nervous system, reflexes, and peripheral circulation. These three mechanisms may act independently of each other or in combination.

NERVOUS SYSTEM CONTROL

The sympathetic nervous system is responsible for the "fight-or-flight" phenomenon that occurs under stressful circumstances. Sympathetic nerve fibers in the atria and ventricles have norepinephrine-filled adrenergic nerve endings. The release of norepinephrine can yield two effects—α-adrenergic response or β-adrenergic response. α-Adrenergic response causes arterial vasoconstriction. β-Adrenergic response causes an increase in both heart rate and force of cardiac contraction and dilation in some vascular beds. Anatomically, most sympathetic pathways are near the surface of the heart. These pathways are in close proximity to the coronary arteries and eventually penetrate the myocardium.[4,11]

Parasympathetic nerve fibers originate in the medulla. These fibers control impulses through release of acetylcholine at the vagal endings. Usually acetylcholine stimulates the parasympathetic nervous system (PNS) and depresses myocardial performance. Primarily, the PNS innervates the SA and AV nodes, and the sympathetic nervous system innervates the entire myocardium. When the PNS is stimulated, the heart rate and conduction through the AV node are slowed. In addition, parasympathetic stimulation decreases the peak systolic ventricular pressure and myocardial contractility.[2,4]

CARDIOVASCULAR RECEPTORS AND REFLEXES

Several reflexes also assist with maintaining perfusion to vital organs. **Baroreceptors** located in the carotid sinuses and aortic arch initiate the baroreceptor reflex. Baroreceptors, also called *pressure* or *stretch receptors,* respond to both pressure and volume changes and are essential for the regulation of blood pressure. Baroreceptors are effective when short-term adjustments in blood pressure are needed; they are not effective for long-term regulation of arterial blood pressure. When blood pressure is elevated, baroreceptors respond to the stretch on arterial walls and send an inhibitory impulse to the vasoconstriction center in the medulla. As a result, peripheral vasodilation and bradycardia occur. As arterial blood pressure drops, baroreceptors detect the decrease in vascular stretch and send fewer signals to the medulla. Reduction in the number of impulses increases vasoconstriction and heart rate.[2,4]

Another reflex stimulated by blood pressure variations is the **Bainbridge reflex.** When blood pressure falls, the vagus nerve sends afferent signals to the medulla; efferent signals are returned through the vagus and sympathetic nervous system. The net effect is an increase in heart rate and, hopefully, cardiac output. The increase in heart rate and cardiac output helps prevent damming of blood in the veins, in the pulmonary circulation, and in the atria.[2,4]

Chemoreceptors, located near the bifurcation of the aortic arch and in the carotid sinus, also contribute to control of cardiovascular function. These receptors are mainly responsible for regulating respiration. Chemoreceptors are highly sensitive to low arterial oxygen tension (PaO_2), low pH levels, and high arterial CO_2 tension ($PaCO_2$) levels. These conditions stimulate the chemoreceptors to increase respiratory rate and depth.[2,4]

CONTROL OF PERIPHERAL CIRCULATION

Blood flow is affected by both the resistance and capacitance of vessels. Regulation of peripheral circulation in arteries and veins is under the influence of both intrinsic and extrinsic mechanisms.

Autoregulation is an intrinsic physiologic mechanism that allows each tissue to regulate its own blood flow according to its metabolic needs. There is both acute and chronic local regulation of peripheral circulation. Acute regulation may be due to myogenic or metabolic factors. With myogenic factors, vascular stretch that stimulates vascular smooth muscle dilation is reduced. Vascular smooth muscle contraction occurs when stretch is applied, as is the case with increased arterial blood pressure. With metabolic regulation, the oxygen and nutritional needs of tissues are not met, and vasodilator metabolites are formed and released. Known vasodilator metabolites include prostaglandins, lactic acid, CO_2, phosphates, and adenosine. These metabolites cause dilation of arterial vessels and increase in blood flow. Chronic local regulation of peripheral blood flow is probably due to long-term oxygen deprivation to the tissues. This chronic state causes the formation of collateral blood vessels to meet the metabolic needs of the body.[2,4]

Extrinsic control of peripheral circulation is primarily under the direction of the vasomotor center in the medulla. Two regions in the vasomotor center affect cardiovascular activities: the dorsal lateral medulla *(vasoconstrictor region)* and the ventromedial medulla *(vasodepressor region).* In addition to vascular constriction, the vasoconstrictor region of the medulla increases heart rate and enhances contractility. These actions are produced by the release of norepinephrine. Inhibition of the vasoconstrictor region activates the vasodepressor region, resulting in dilation of the peripheral blood vessels. Emotions and temperature changes also affect peripheral vascular smooth muscle tone.[2,11]

Effects of Ions and Humoral Substances

Hormones and ions can affect circulatory regulation. These substances are found in local anatomic regions or are transported through the vascular system. Humoral substances are classified as vasodilator agents, vasoconstrictor agents, or ionic materials.

There are at least three major vasodilator agents: bradykinin, histamine, and serotonin. **Bradykinin** is a polypeptide that causes arterial dilation and increased capillary permeability. It also regulates blood flow and capillary leakage of fluids in inflamed tissues. When tissues are damaged, mast cells release **histamine,** causing vasodilation. Because of increased capillary permeability produced by the histamines, fluid and plasma proteins leak into the wounded area. **Serotonin** acts as either a vasodilator or a vasoconstrictor. It is believed that serotonin has a local effect rather than a systemic effect.[4,9]

Angiotensin is another potent vasoconstrictive agent. When arterial pressure decreases, the kidneys release renin that activates angiotensin. Angiotensin causes widespread constriction of blood vessels throughout the body. Other vasoconstrictive agents include **epinephrine** and **norepinephrine.** Norepinephrine affects the entire vascular system, but epinephrine does not. **Vasopressin,** antidiuretic hormone (ADH), is also a powerful vasoconstrictor. Vasopressin is produced in the hypothalamus and is secreted into the bloodstream through the pituitary gland. Vasopressin affects water reabsorption in the renal tubules, which helps regulate fluid volume.[4]

Several known ions can either dilate or constrict blood vessels. For instance, potassium causes vasodilation by inhibiting smooth muscle contraction. This is in contrast with calcium, which causes vasoconstriction of smooth muscle. Sodium increases the osmolality of the blood, resulting in arterial dilation. Conversely, if sodium ion concentration is low, osmolality of the blood decreases, and arterial constriction occurs. Chloride exerts vasoconstrictive effects in the renal circulation. However, this effect is not seen elsewhere. Increased concentrations of other substances such as CO_2 and hydrogen ions also cause vasodilation.[3,4]

CONCEPT REVIEW

Cardiac output is based on stroke volume and heart rate. Stroke volume is determined by preload, afterload, and contractility.

Cardiovascular function is under the control of three regulatory mechanisms: the nervous system, reflexes, and peripheral circulation. These three mechanisms may act independently of or in combination with one another.

DRUGS AFFECTING THE CARDIOVASCULAR SYSTEM

Several drug categories are used to treat cardiovascular diseases. In some instances (e.g., in clients with hypertension, congestive heart failure, and coronary artery disease) drugs play an important role in the treatment plan. In clients with other cardiovascular diseases (e.g., valvular diseases, congenital heart diseases, cardiomyopathy) drugs have a minimum impact on the treatment.

Drugs affect the cardiovascular system in a variety of ways. Some act directly on cardiac cells and nerves to produce dromotropic, inotropic, or chronotropic effects. Other drugs alter

the automaticity of cardiac cells, thus correcting life-threatening arrhythmias. Drugs also act on other structures in the cardiovascular system. For example, direct and indirect action on blood vessels by some drugs can produce vasodilation and vasoconstriction. Other drugs act on the components of the blood by reducing lipid levels, increasing or decreasing the coagulation time, or dissolving thrombi.

For some cardiovascular diseases, drug therapy requires the use of drugs that are outside the scope of cardiovascular pharmacology. Antimicrobial and anti-inflammatory agents are routinely used in the treatment of diseases of the cardiovascular system. In addition, autonomic drugs (i.e., sympathomimetics, sympatholytics, antimuscarinics) are major drugs used in the treatment of diseases of the cardiovascular system.

SUMMARY

The cardiovascular system delivers oxygen and nutrients to cells of the body, removes metabolic waste products from cells, and transports other substances from one part of the body to another. Both microscopic and macroscopic cardiovascular structures are involved in the completion of these functions. The degree to which the functions are carried out depends on normal cardiac physiology.

Specialized myocardial cells are responsible for the generation and distribution of electric cardiac impulses throughout the myocardium. A cardiac cycle is the result of these impulses and consists of the relaxation period, ventricular filling period, and ventricular systole. Cardiovascular function is under the control of three regulatory mechanisms: the nervous system, reflexes, and peripheral circulation.

EFFECTS OF DRUGS ON CARDIAC FUNCTION

▶ Help the heart muscle overcome the force that opposes ventricular ejection (**afterload**)

▶ Increase or decrease the volume of blood in the ventricle at the end of diastole (**preload**)

▶ Affect **automaticity**—ability of cardiac cells to initiate electric impulses

▶ Change the rate at which cardiac cells generate electric impulses (**chronotropic effect**)

▶ Alter the conductivity of a nerve fiber (**dromotropic effect**)

▶ Change the force of cardiac muscle fiber contraction (**inotropic effect**)

REFERENCES

1. Gauthier, D.K. (1991). Anatomy and physiology of the heart. In Kinney, M.R., Packa, D.R., Andreoli, K.G., & Zipes, D.P. (Eds.). *Comprehensive cardiac care* (7th ed.) (pp. 1-10). St. Louis: C.V. Mosby.
2. Funkhouser, S.W. (1990). Cardiovascular anatomy and physiology. In Thelan, L.A., Davie, J.K., & Urden, L.D. (Eds.). *Textbook of critical care nursing: Diagnosis and management* (pp. 133-156). St. Louis: C.V. Mosby.
3. Richardson, S. (1990). Physiological anatomy of the cardiovascular system. In Hudak, C.M., Gallo, B.M., & Benz, J.J. (Eds.). *Critical care nursing: A holistic approach* (pp. 79-88). Philadelphia: J.B. Lippincott.
4. Guyton, A.C. (1992). *Human physiology and mechanisms of disease* (5th ed.). Philadelphia: W.B. Saunders.
5. Guyton, A.C. (1991). *Textbook of medical physiology* (8th ed.). Philadelphia: W.B. Saunders.
6. Hole, J. (1993). *Human anatomy and physiology* (6th ed.). Dubuque, IA: Wm. C. Brown.
7. Seeley, T., Stephens, T., & Tate, P. (1992). *Anatomy and physiology* (2nd ed.). St. Louis: Mosby–Year Book.
8. Marieb, E.N. (1991). *Essentials of human anatomy and physiology* (3rd ed.). Redwood City, CA: Benjamin/Cummings.
9. Tortora, G., & Grabowski, S. (1993). *Principles of anatomy and physiology* (7th ed.). New York: Harper Collins.
10. Wilson, J.W. (1990). *Anatomy and physiology in health and illness* (7th ed.). New York: Churchill Livingstone.

11. Garfein, O.B. (Ed.) (1990). *Current concepts in cardiovascular physiology.* San Diego: Academic Press.
12. Opie, L.H. (1991). *The heart: Physiology and metabolism* (2nd ed.). New York: Raven Press.

BIBLIOGRAPHY

Ahrens, T. (1991). *Critical care: Certification preparation and review* (2nd ed.). Norwalk, CT: Appleton & Lange.

Esberger, K.K., & Hughes, S.T. (1989). *Nursing care of the aged.* Norwalk, CT: Appleton & Lange.

Gary, L.C., & Guzetta, C.E. (1992). Cardiac monitoring and dysrhythmias. In Dossey, B.M., Guzetta, C.E., & Kenner, C.V. (Eds.). *Critical care nursing: Body-mind-spirit* (3rd ed.) (pp. 157-187). Philadelphia: J.B. Lippincott.

Guzetta, C.E., & Dossey, B.M. (Eds.) (1991). *Cardiovascular nursing: Assessment and intervention.* St. Louis: C.V. Mosby.

Hurst, W., Logue, R.B., Rackley, C.E., Schlant, R.C., Sonnenblick, E.H., Wallace, A.G., & Wenger, N.K. (Eds.) (1989). *The heart* (7th ed.). New York: McGraw-Hill.

Huszar, R.J. (1988). *Basic dysrhythmias: Interpretation and management.* St. Louis: C.V. Mosby.

Kay, G.N., & Bubien, R.S. (1992). *Clinical management of cardiac arrhythmias.* Gaithersburg, MD: Aspen.

Marino, P.L. (1991). *The ICU book.* Philadelphia: Lea & Febiger.

Ross, J.R. (Ed.) (1991). Cardiovascular system. In West, J.B. (Ed.). *Physiological basis of medical practice* (12th ed.) (pp. 110-289). Baltimore: Williams & Wilkins.

Saksena, S., & Goldschlager, N. (Eds.) (1990). *Electrical therapy for cardiac arrhythmias.* Philadelphia: W.B. Saunders.

Urden, L.D., Davie, J.K., & Thelan, L.A. (1992). *Essentials of critical care nursing.* St. Louis: C.V. Mosby.

Zipes, D.P., & Jalife, J. (Eds.) (1990). *Cardiac electrophysiology: From cell to bedside.* Philadelphia: W.B. Saunders.

 Drugs That Affect Vascular Tone

SONJA HOWARD • NORMA L. PINNELL

✹ Drugs Used to Treat Angina Pectoris

LEARNING OBJECTIVES:

Explain the relationship between angina and the myocardial oxygen supply.

Describe the two main types of angina pectoris.

Develop a plan of care for the client requiring drug therapy for angina pectoris.

Discuss the pharmacokinetic and pharmacodynamic properties of nitroglycerin.

List common undesired clinical responses associated with organic nitrates.

Identify other organic nitrates used to treat angina pectoris.

Discuss the use of β-adrenergic blockers and calcium channel blockers in the treatment of angina.

KEY TERMS:

Nitrate tolerance, typical angina, variant angina

✹ Peripheral and Cerebral Vasodilators

LEARNING OBJECTIVES:

Describe the use of drugs in the treatment of peripheral and cerebral vascular insufficiency.

Discuss the pharmacokinetic and pharmacodynamic properties of papaverine hydrochloride.

Identify common undesired clinical responses associated with papaverine hydrochloride.

CONCEPTS AND TERMS TO REVIEW

Review Chapter 29 for an overview of the cardiovascular system.

Reexamine the meaning of *preload* and *afterload*.

Study the impact of atherosclerosis and coronary artery blood flow.

Review the effects of the autonomic nervous system on the circulatory system.

---

*B*lood flow within systemic circulation is governed by the difference in pressure gradients within the circulatory system. Fluid always flows from an area of higher pressure to an area of lower pressure. The high-pressure gradient of the circulatory system begins in the arterial tree and ends with low-pressure gradient in the venous system.

Control of the rate of blood flow through the circulatory system is regulated by a number of factors. Some mechanisms (e.g., diameter of the vessel, elastic recoil ability of the vessel wall, viscosity of the blood) impede or cause resistance to the flow. In addition, three mechanisms—local, neural, and humoral control—influence blood flow by direct effects on the vessels.

Local control of blood flow in all body tissues is governed by the tissue's need for perfusion and nutrition. The tissues regulate flow independently of the autonomic nervous system through metabolic autoregulation, which is produced by a lack of oxygen or accumulation of tissue metabolites. **Neural control** of blood flow is regulated by the sympathetic branch of the autonomic nervous system. The sympathetic pathway begins in the vasomotor center located in the lower pons and medulla. All blood vessels, with the exception of capillaries, are supplied with sympathetic nerve fibers. The sympathetic nerve fibers secrete norepinephrine, a potent vasoconstrictive neurotransmitter. Vasoconstriction of arterioles produces an increase in arterial blood pressure, and venoconstriction increases venous return to the heart. In addition, various substances (e.g., epinephrine, bradykinin, serotonin) released into or circulating in the blood provide **humoral control** over blood flow. These substances either produce vasoconstriction or vasodilation.[1-3]

Several disease conditions cause inappropriate vasoconstriction or vasodilation of blood vessels. Some of these conditions can be treated with drugs. This chapter focuses on drugs that enhance blood flow, specifically those used to treat angina, peripheral insufficiency, and cerebral insufficiency. Drugs that reduce blood flow, vasodilators, are discussed briefly.

DRUGS USED TO TREAT ANGINA PECTORIS

Since the oxygen requirement of the heart is greater than that of most of the body's other organs, any increase in the cardiac workload results in an increase in the heart's oxygen consumption. Three factors—contractile state of the heart, cardiac rate, and wall tension of the myocardium—determine myocardial oxygen demand. The more forcefully the heart contracts, the more energy it uses, and the more adenosine triphosphate (ATP) it requires. Likewise, the faster the heart beats and the greater the wall tension of the myocardium, the more oxygen the heart consumes. Angina pectoris occurs when the myocardial demand for oxygen exceeds the supply provided by the coronary arteries.[4]

Types of Angina Pectoris

Angina is usually caused by coronary artery disease (CAD). CAD results from atherosclerosis of the coronary arteries. (Fig. 30–1 illustrates some of the factors that precipitate CAD and some of the pathologic processes produced by CAD.) Angina caused by diseases of coronary arteries can be subdivided into two types: typical and variant.

Typical angina, also called *classic* or *exertional angina,* is brought about by conditions that increase myocardial oxygen consumption such as physical exertion, emotional stress, exposure to cold, or eating large meals. Typical angina occurs in clients with significant atherosclerotic lesions of the coronary arteries. Pharmacologic treatment of typical angina is directed at relief of acute pain and prevention of its recurrence. Sublingual nitroglycerin is used for the treatment of acute anginal attacks. Prophylactic treatment of angina includes the use of long-acting organic nitrate preparations, β-adrenergic blockers, or calcium blockers.

Variant angina (spastic or Prinzmetal's angina) develops at rest rather than during physical exertion. It frequently follows a diurnal rhythm, often occurring in the early morning. Variant angina is probably produced by spasm of one or more coronary arteries. This spasm is usually associated with atheromatous CAD. Drug therapy is directed at relaxing the coronary artery spasm, which usually is accomplished with sublingual nitroglycerin. Long-term prophylactic therapy usually includes the use of organic nitrates or calcium channel blockers.[4,5]

NURSING CONSIDERATIONS

Care of the individual with angina takes place in a variety of health care settings (e.g., clinic, emergency department, hospital). Regardless of the setting, you must organize your care within the steps of the nursing process.

Assessing Care of the client who requires antianginal drugs begins with a thorough health history and physical inventory. As you take the **health history,** inquire about chest pain or discomfort. Determine the precipitating causes, frequency, and duration of the pain and relief mechanisms. This information helps differentiate angina from other cardiac problems. For example, a pain that comes on shortly after exercise or a regular meal may be angina, but pain that follows a dinner at a Chinese restaurant could be a reaction to monosodium glutamate (MSG).[6] Determine if the pain is dull, sharp, stabbing, or cramping. Ask the client to show you where it hurts. Ask if the pain radiates to other parts of the body. Question the client about dyspnea. Assess for a history of hypertension, arrhythmias, previous cardiac disease, peripheral edema, or syncope.

Collect and analyze a drug history to help identify factors associated with drug side effects or inappropriate drug usage. Assess the client's lifestyle, occupation, eating and smoking habits, and psychosocial status. Collect a family health history to determine if CAD or other vascular disease exists.

After the health history, proceed to the **physical assessment.** Inspect the client's chest; palpate the point of maximum impulse or intensity. Auscultate the chest; listen to the heart's rhythm and count the number of beats for 1 minute. Assess the client's blood pressure and respiratory character and rate.

Diagnosing Nursing diagnoses are determined after analysis of the assessment data. Possible nursing diagnoses for the client requiring antianginal drugs follow:

• Knowledge deficit regarding vasodilators and their use in the control of angina.

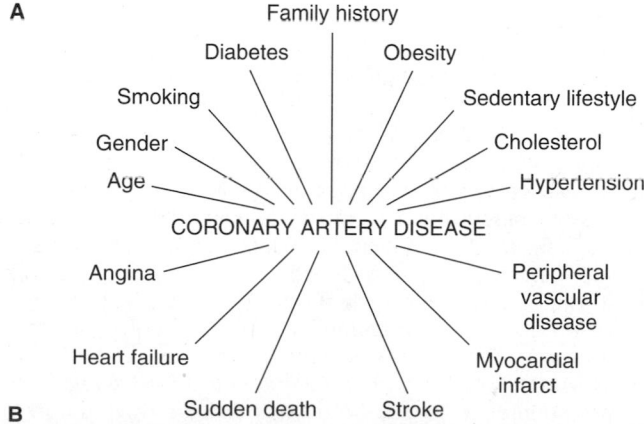

FIGURE 30–1 Risk factors **(A)** and pathologic processes **(B)** associated with coronary artery disease.

- Activity intolerance related to imbalance between oxygen supply and demand.
- Alteration in comfort related to increased cerebral blood flow (headaches) produced by nitrate therapy.
- High risk for injury related to postural or orthostatic hypotension produced by nitrate therapy.
- Anxiety related to required change in lifestyle, altered self-esteem, and changed locus of control.
- Alteration in family process related to change, for example, in family member's ability to function, drug therapy costs.

Planning A plan of care must be developed with goal-related expected outcomes. Client teaching is directed at increasing the knowledge base of the client or significant other to achieve effective drug therapy.

Nitrates come in a variety of dosages and dosage forms. Therefore teaching is highly individualized based on the prescribed drug preparation. Teach the client how the drug will be used. (See Table 30–2 for information on the various dosage forms.) Discuss times and dosages of drugs for both control of an acute attack and prevention of recurrence. Provide information on desired and undesired clinical responses. Stress the importance of taking the drug as prescribed. Make certain that the client knows to contact the primary care provider if he or she is not pain free. Instruct the client not to discontinue nitrates without the advice of the primary care provider.

Instruct the client to carry nitroglycerin prescribed on an "as-needed" basis with him or her at all times. Remind clients receiving sublingual or translingual nitroglycerin for acute attacks to rest after drug administration. Since sublingual nitroglycerin can be taken before stressful situations, help the client identify events that produce stress. If appropriate, instruct the client to take a sublingual tablet 5 to 10 minutes before the event. Review the application procedure for topical drug preparations. To avoid accidental absorption of the drug from skin surfaces of fingers and hands, instruct the client to use an applicator. Tell the client to rotate sites of topical ointments or transdermal patches to decrease the risk of dermatologic problems.

Plan to review the pathophysiology of angina with the client or significant other. Encourage questions and provide educational material from dietary and other hospital personnel when appropriate. Instruct the client to avoid stress, both physical and mental, and provide information on relaxation techniques.

Expected outcomes appropriate for this client include the following:

- Client relates sign and symptoms that indicate need for nitrate therapy.
- Client experiences a lack of chest pain when using a nitrate prophylactically.
- Client verbalizes knowledge of disease process as it relates to prescribed drug.
- Client discusses action of and undesired responses to prescribed drug.
- Client demonstrates how to administer prescribed drug.

- Client remains injury free.
- Client indicates decreased fatigue and increased ability to perform activities of daily living.

Implementing Since these drugs are available in a variety of dosage forms and dosages, you must read the prescription order carefully. Next you must read the drug label and manufacturer's insert, noting the recommended method of administering the drug. For example, when nitroglycerin is administered intravenously, it must be diluted in 5% dextrose or 0.9% sodium chloride.

Evaluating Review the expected outcomes with the client or significant other. Determine if there is a decrease in anginal pain. Evaluate the client's level of understanding of the treatment plan. Determine if changes in lifestyle have occurred.

Organic Nitrates

The therapeutic properties of nitrogen-containing compounds were first observed by Sir Lauder Brunton in 1857. Today there are four organic nitrates used in the treatment of angina: nitroglycerin (glyceryl trinitrate), pentaerythritol tetranitrate, erythrityl tetranitrate, and isosorbide dinitrate.

All four of these compounds are polyol esters of nitric acid and are highly lipid soluble. The prototype and most thoroughly investigated drug in the group is nitroglycerin. However, the other three drugs are thought to act by an identical mechanism and differ only in their pharmacokinetic properties.[4]

Organic Nitrate Prototype
NITROGLYCERIN

As previously indicated, nitroglycerin is effective in treating both typical and variant angina.

Pharmacotherapeutics Nitrates have been used for the last 130 years to treat and control the symptoms of angina pectoris. Within the last 15 years, nitrates also have been shown to limit infarct size and to benefit the treatment of severe intractable heart failure, cardiogenic shock, severe mitral and aortic regurgitation, hypertensive episodes, and portal hypertension.[7]

Pharmacokinetics As with all of the nitrates, the onset and duration of action of nitroglycerin are influenced by the route of administration and dosage form. For example, the onset of action with intravenous (IV) nitroglycerin occurs within 1 to 2 minutes; the duration of action is 3 to 5 minutes. Nitroglycerin administered via a transdermal patch has an onset of action within 30 to 60 minutes, with a duration of action of approximately 12 to 24 hours. Although nitroglycerin is rapidly absorbed from the gastrointestinal (GI) tract, the oral dosage form is not recommended since the drug is extensively metabolized before it reaches the liver. (See Table 30–1 for a summary of pharmacokinetics properties of various nitroglycerin preparations.) Plasma-protein binding of nitroglycerin is approximately 60%. Although therapeutic blood levels have not been established, the biologic half-life ranges from 1 to 4 minutes, resulting in low plasma concentrations. Nitroglycerin is metabolized in the liver, producing nitrate

TABLE 30–1

Pharmacokinetic Properties of Various Nitroglycerin Dosage Forms

Dosage Form	Onset (min)	Duration
IV	1–2	3–5 min
Sublingual tablets	1–3	30–60 min
Translingual spray	2	30–60 min
Transmucosal tablets	3	5 h
Oral sustained-release tablets or caplets	40	4–8 h
Topical ointment	20–60	2–12 h
Transdermal system	40–60	13–24 h

derivatives and inorganic nitrites.[7] Excretion is through the kidney.

Pharmacodynamics Nitroglycerin has no direct effect on cardiac muscle and does not directly elicit changes in either the rate or the inotropic state of the heart. It acts as a venous dilator at low concentrations and as an arterial dilator at high concentrations. Nitroglycerin reduces venous return (preload) and decreases cardiac output (afterload). It lowers systolic pressures and peripheral resistance and enhances oxygen supply by dilation of coronary arteries and inhibition of coronary spasm.[7] Therapeutic dosages of IV nitroglycerin cause a reduction in systolic, diastolic, and mean arterial blood pressure. IV nitroglycerin also produces a reduction in elevated central venous and pulmonary capillary wedge pressures and may improve the cardiac index. Systemic vascular resistance is also lowered.[8–10]

Pharmaceutics Nitroglycerin is available in a variety of dosage forms. **Sublingual nitrate tablets** are used for rapid relief of anginal pain. Doses may be repeated every 5 minutes for 15 minutes in acute attacks. If pain persists after three doses, the primary care provider should be contacted. **Translingual spray** is used much the same way as sublingual tablets. The dosage is usually one or two metered sprays under the tongue.

Transdermal nitroglycerin is continuously absorbed into circulation. Topical nitroglycerin is also available in **ointment** form, which also allows continuous absorption. The greatest decrease in the workload of the heart occurs with these topical preparations. Nitroglycerin is also available for IV infusion. **IV nitroglycerin** dosages must be titrated slowly to avoid hypotension and a decrease in arterial oxygenation.[11,12]

Undesired Clinical Responses Headache is the most common undesired clinical response. It is caused by pulsations in dilated temporal and meningeal arteries. The headaches usually subside within a few days, especially if the dose is decreased.[8,9,13]

Disappearance of headaches may be the first indication of **nitrate tolerance.** Nitrate tolerance apparently is related to the availability of receptor sites within vascular tissue. During long-term administration, systems clearance and vascular metabolism may be decreased as a result of metabolite interaction. This decreases the availability of receptor sites for conversion and results in vascular tolerance. Tolerance may be reversed with short periods (8 to 24 hours) of nitrate withdrawal. In addi-

tion, using the smallest effective dose or alternating nitrates with other vasodilators delays the occurrence of tolerance.[14,15]

Several undesired responses stem from changes in the cardiovascular system. Orthostatic or postural hypotension, which is characterized by weakness, dizziness, and fainting, may occur if the client suddenly changes position. Reflex tachycardia due to the decrease in blood pressure can cause palpitations and exacerbation of angina. Venous pooling may cause ankle edema in some clients.

In addition, contact dermatitis from transdermal patches or topical ointment has been reported. Nitroglycerin ointments may also cause topical allergic reactions. Organic nitrates can affect nonvascular smooth muscles, producing bronchodilation or relaxation of the biliary tract (Fig. 30–2).[11]

Contraindications and Precautions Because IV nitrates can increase the severity of hypovolemia, nitroglycerin is not recommended for use by individuals with hypotension or hypovolemia. In addition, ethanol intoxication has developed in clients who receive high doses of IV nitroglycerin over a long period of time.

Since nitrates can increase intracranial pressure, their use in clients with head trauma or cerebral hemorrhage is not recommended. Neither should nitroglycerin be used in clients with inadequate cerebral circulation. Nitroglycerin may also aggravate angina caused by hypertrophy or cardiomyopathy.

Drug-Drug and Drug-Environment Interactions Alcohol taken concurrently with nitroglycerin can accentuate transient episodes of syncope. Additionally, when oral nitroglycerin is combined with calcium channel blockers, β-adrenergic blockers, and other hypotensive drugs, severe hypotension may occur.

Most nitroglycerin preparations must be stored at controlled room temperatures between 15° and 30° C. Extremes in temperature and humidity can alter drug potency. In addition, nitroglycerin degrades when exposed to light or air. Therefore tablets should be stored in an amber container with the cap tightly closed. Since the drug loses its potency over time, unused sublingual tablets should be discarded every 3 to 6 months.

Nitroglycerin readily migrates into many plastics. To avoid absorption of nitroglycerin into plastic parenteral solution containers, dilute IV nitroglycerin solution in glass parenteral solution containers. Additionally, some filters and IV tubings absorb nitroglycerin. It is estimated that some tubings absorb 40% to 80% of the total amount of nitroglycerin in the diluted solution for infusion. Thus you must read the manufacturer's insert and use the least absorptive tubing available.

Infusion pumps represent an additional problem. The special tubing required by IV nitroglycerin is less pliable than conventional tubing. This may keep the infusion pump from adequately occluding the tubing, resulting in excessive flow at low-infusion-rate settings. You must remove transdermal patches before defibrillation or cardioversion since arcing has been reported. This can result in burns to the client and damage to the paddles.[11]

Life-Span Considerations No long-term animal studies have examined the effects of organic nitrates. Since it is not known whether it causes fetal harm when administered during pregnancy, nitroglycerin should be adminis-

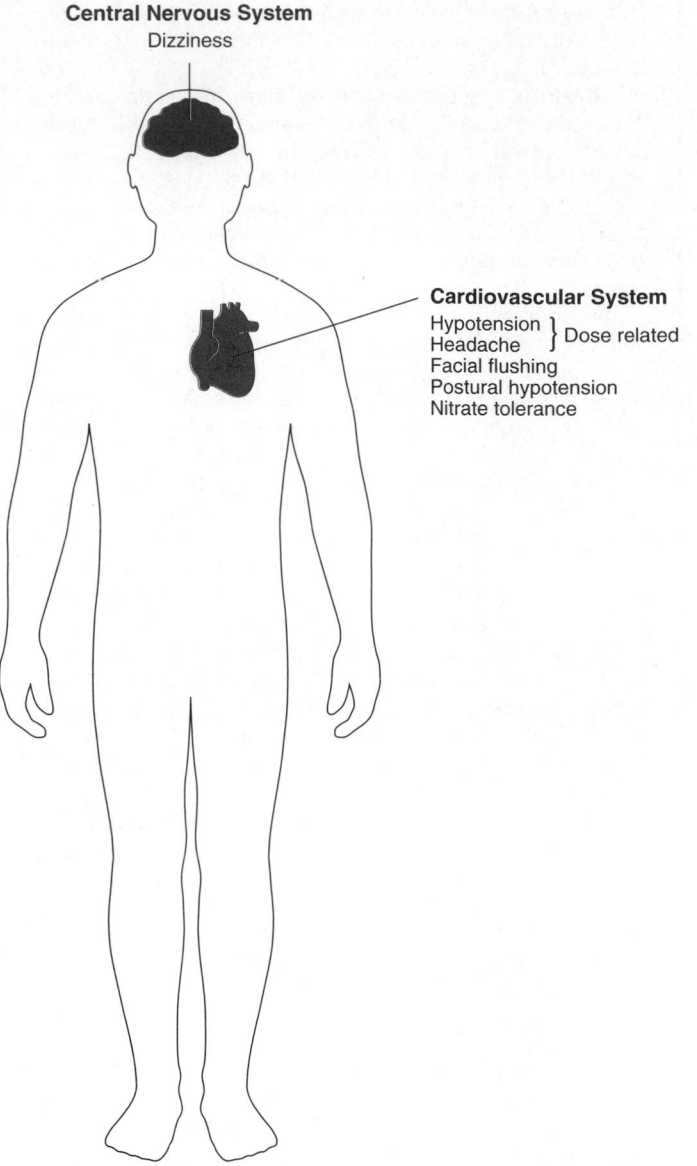

Central Nervous System
Dizziness

Cardiovascular System
Hypotension ⎫ Dose related
Headache ⎭
Facial flushing
Postural hypotension
Nitrate tolerance

FIGURE 30–2   Common undesired responses associated with organic nitrates.

tered to pregnant women only if clearly needed. In addition, caution should be used when prescribing organic nitrates for nursing mothers because many drugs are excreted in breast milk. It has not been established if nitrates are safe or effective in children.[11]

Venous responsiveness to nitrates does not appear to alter with age; therefore the pharmacodynamic properties are not expected to alter. However, decreased baroreflex function causes an increased tendency for posturally related side effects to occur in elderly clients. In addition, therapy in this age group must be titrated since the elderly are prone to chronic diseases that predispose them to other undesired drug reactions.[7]

Specific Drug-Related Nursing Considerations
Clients receiving IV nitroglycerin are monitored carefully, usually in an intensive care unit or on a monitored floor. Inspect the parenteral solution carefully for discoloration

and particulate matter. If either exists, return the solution to the pharmacy. IV nitroglycerin should be administered via an infusion pump that is capable of exact and constant delivery of the drug. The drug dosage is titrated based on client response (e.g., degree of pain relief, blood pressure findings). Monitor the client's blood pressure and pulse rate carefully. Prolonged hypotension may result in poor perfusion to vital organs or thrombus formation. Since IV nitroglycerin is extremely short acting, discontinuation of the drug in the case of severe hypotension is usually the only therapy needed.

Include the following points when teaching the client receiving prophylactic sublingual nitroglycerin:
• Carry sublingual tablets for immediate use if needed.
• Keep tablets in original container, tightly closed.
• Store tablets in a cool, dry place.
• Discard unused tablets after 3 to 6 months.
• Avoid excessive activity in cold weather.
• Avoid overeating.
• Minimize exposure to stressful situations.
• Use stress-reducing activities when possible.
• Continue medical follow-up as instructed.
• Report to primary care provider if angina persists.

❧ NURSING RESEARCH

Rayn, M., Gallagher S., & Wandel, J. (1992). Effect of nitropaste administration times on sleep and nocturnal angina. *Applied Nursing Research, 5*(2), 84–86.

The purpose of this study was to investigate the influence of nitroglycerin paste application on the client's sleep and nocturnal angina. A convenience sample of 33 subjects (18 males and 15 females) with coronary artery disease participated in the study. These subjects received their nitroglycerin paste application every 4 hours on one night and every 6 hours the following night.

Clinical nurses recorded the presence of environmental stimuli and physical discomforts on the two nights. They also noted the occurrence of nocturnal angina. Subjects were asked to rate the quality and quantity of their sleep on the two consecutive nights. Subjects' reports were compared using tests for paired scores. Findings revealed that the subjects slept better and longer without nocturnal angina on the 6-hour schedule.

STUDENT ACTIVITIES

• Determine the scheduling of nitroglycerin paste applications at your assigned agency.
• Review the charts of five clients receiving nitroglycerin paste during the night and record the frequency of nocturnal angina.   ❧

MISCELLANEOUS NITRITES AND ORGANIC NITRATES

Amyl nitrite is the only nitrite used to treat angina. It is provided in an easily crushed vial with a woven cover and is administered by breaking the vial and inhaling the contents.

Table 30–2
Organic Nitrate Prototype Drug: Nitroglycerin

Drug Name	Dosage and Route of Administration	Nursing Considerations
NITROGLYCERIN (Nitro-Bid, Nitrostat, Nitrocap, Nitroglyn, Nitrogard, Nitrodisc, Transderm-Nitro)		**Assess** Determine activities that produce angina. Assess duration, frequency, and quality of pain. Obtain blood pressure in both arms with client lying and standing. Collect complete drug history; nitroglycerin interacts with calcium channel antagonists, channel β-adrenergic blockers, acetylcholine, norepinephrine. Ask client about history of allergic reaction to organic nitrates, history of severe anemia, closed-angle glaucoma, postural hypotensioin, head trauma, and increased intracranial pressure; they are contraindications to use of nitroglycerin. Determine client's use of alcohol; concurrent use of alcohol can cause severe hypotension and cardiovascular collapse. Determine if client is pregnant; nitroglycerin is classified as a Pregnancy Category C drug.
HOW SUPPLIED Sublingual tablet: 0.15 mg (1/400 gr), 0.3 mg (1/200 gr), 0.4 mg (1/150 gr), 0.6 mg (1/100 gr)	**SUBLINGUAL** One tablet dissolved under tongue at first indication of angina; may repeat dosage q5min for a total of three tablets	**Implement** **SUBLINGUAL DOSAGE FORM** Instruct client to place one tablet under tongue at first indication of angina. Teach client that dosage may be repeated q5 min for a total of three tablets. Instruct client to notify physician and go to the nearest emergency department if pain increases or continues. Teach client to expel any unused drug from the mouth when the pain is relieved. Store at room temperature. Teach client to discard unused drug q6 mo and replace with new prescription.
Extended-release capsules: 2.5, 6.5, 9 mg	**EXTENDED-RELEASE CAPSULES** Usual starting dose, 2.5 mg bid to tid; increase dosage by 2.5-mg increments bid or qid over period of days to weeks	**EXTENDED-RELEASE CAPSULES** Monitor client's pulse and blood pressure when drug is initiated or dosage increase is required. Teach client not to chew or crush capsule; capsule must be swallowed whole.
Extended-release transmucosal tablets: 1, 2, 3 mg	**TRANSMUCOSAL TABLET** 1–2 mg q3-5h	**EXTENDED-RELEASE TRANSMUCOSAL TABLET** Instruct client not to chew or swallow tablet. Teach client to place tablet between lip and gum or between cheek and gum. Instruct client to expel from mouth any unused drug once pain has subsided.
Translingual spray: 0.4 mg per metered dose	**TRANSLINGUAL SPRAY** 0.4–0.8 mg as needed to total of three metered doses within 15 min	**TRANSLINGUAL SPRAY** Instruct client to use no more than three metered doses within 15 min. Tell client to use drug as prophylactic 5–10 min before activities. Teach client to seek medical attention promptly if chest pain is not relieved.
Topical ointment: 2% in lanolin-petrolatum base	**TOPICAL OINTMENT** 25–50 mm (1–2 in) q8h; may increase up to 100–125 mm (4–5 in) q4h (25 mm [1 in] of ointment contains 15 mg nitroglycerin)	**TOPICAL OINTMENT** Spread ointment with the applicator in a thin, uniform layer on clean, dry, hairless skin of the upper arm or body. Do not apply with fingers.

Table continued on following page.

TABLE 30–2 *Continued*
Organic Nitrate Prototype Drug: Nitroglycerin

Drug Name	Dosage and Route of Administration	Nursing Considerations
NITROGLYCERIN—CONT'D Transdermal system: release rate available—2.5, 5, 7.5, 10, 15 mg/24 h; this is also commonly written 0.1, 0.2, 0.3, 0.4, 0.6, 0.8 mg/h	**TRANSDERMAL SYSTEM** Initial dose, usually 5 mg/24 h (10 cm² system)	**TRANSDERMAL SYSTEM** Apply to skin site free of hair; avoid area with cuts or irritation. Apply to areas not subject to excessive movement; do not place below knee or elbow. Rotate site to prevent irritation. Reduce dosage and frequency of administration gradually over 4–6 wk when terminating treatment to prevent withdrawal reactions.
IV solution: 5 mg/ml supplied in 1-ml, 5-ml, and 10-ml vials; also available in solutions (5% dextrose) as 25 mg/250 ml, 50 mg/250 and 500 ml, 100 mg/250 ml, 200 mg/500 ml	**IV** Adult: initial dose at 5 µg/min; increase q3-5 min by 5 µg/min; if no response noted at 20 µg/min, increase dosage by increments of 10–20 µg/min, no fixed optimum dosage	**IV INFUSION** Dilute IV solution in 5% dextrose or 0.9% sodium chloride solution. Never mix IV solution with other drugs. Administer diluted preparation via infusion pump. Monitor blood pressure, pulse, and client response continuously. **Monitor** Monitor blood pressure, pulse, and client response. Assess for undesired clinical responses (e.g., headache, lightheadedness). Assist with ambulation if necessary. Discontinue drug if blurred vision or dry mouth occurs. **Evaluate** Evaluate whether client's angina has subsided or disappeared.

Amyl nitrite is effective in 30 seconds and lasts for 3 to 5 minutes; it may be repeated as needed. Because amyl nitrite can cause reflex tachycardia and hypotension, it is rarely used today. In addition, the sexual stimulation experienced when amyl nitrite is inhaled has resulted in abuse of this drug. Amyl nitrite should be stored in a cool place (8° to 15° C) and protected from light. If properly stored, the drug is stable for 2 years.[11]

Another organic nitrate used to control or prevent angina is isosorbide dinitrate (Isordil). **Isosorbide dinitrate** is available in several dosage forms, including sublingual tablets, oral tablets, sustained-action capsules and tablets, and chewable tablets. The sublingual tablets are used to treat acute angina attacks, whereas the other forms prevent angina and improve exercise tolerance. (See Table 30–3).

β-Adrenergic Blockers

Nitrates and β-blockers are often prescribed together because their effects complement each other—nitrates increase coronary blood flow, and β-blockers prevent reflex tachycardia.[17] β-Adrenergic blockers act by inhibiting substances such as norepinephrine and epinephrine.[9] This action slows the heart rate, lowers systolic blood pressure, and decreases cardiac contractility, thus reducing oxygen requirements. β-Adrenergic blockers are also used to treat hypertension and arrhythmias.[18,19] These drugs are discussed in more detail in Chapter 32.

Calcium Channel Blockers

Calcium channel blockers have emerged as an important addition to the pharmacologic therapy of angina.[9] The effects of calcium channel blockers are greatest in cells that depend on intracellular influx of calcium for activation. They are found in cardiac tissue and smooth muscle. The AV and SA nodes are depolarized mainly by the calcium flow. Cardiac contractility depends on the movement of calcium ions through specific channels. Calcium-blocking agents inhibit this movement and thereby decrease cardiac contractibility and impulse formation. When calcium is inhibited, smooth muscles relax, and this helps prevent coronary artery vasospasm.[17] Calcium inhibition also reduces afterload and depresses myocardial contractility. Both actions reduce the heart's oxygen consumption. Thus calcium blockers directly increase coronary blood flow and myocardial perfusion and decrease myocardial oxygen re-

TABLE 30–3
Miscellaneous Organic Nitrates

Drug Name	Dosage and Route of Administration	Nursing Considerations
Isosorbide Dinitrate (Dilatrate, Isordil, Sorbitrate) HOW SUPPLIED Sublingual tablet: 2.5, 5, 10 mg Chewable tablet: 5, 10 mg Oral tablet: 5, 10, 20, 30, 40 mg Sustained-release tablet and capsule: 40 mg	**Acute Angina, Prophylactic Dose When Attack is Likely** Sublingual or chewable tablet: usual initial dose, 2.5–5 mg sublingual or 5 mg chewable; repeat at 5- to 10-min intervals; no more than three doses in 15–30 min **Acute Prophylactic Management of Angina** Initially, 5–20 mg tid or qid Maintenance, 10–40 mg q6h; last dose no later than 7 PM to minimize intolerance	**Assess** Determine activities or emotional states that produce angina. Assess duration, location, frequency, and quality of pain. Obtain blood pressure of client both lying and standing. Take a medical history to include history of hypersensitivity to nitrates, severe anemia, closed angle glaucoma, postural hypotension, head trauma, increased intracranial pressure; they are contraindications to use of isosorbide. Determine client use of alcohol; concurrent use of alcohol can cause severe hypotension and cardiovascular collapse. Determine if client is pregnant; this is Pregnancy Category C drug. **Implement** Do not crush chewable tablets before administering. Teach client not to crush or chew sublingual tablets. Client should dissolve tablets under tongue and not swallow medication. **Monitor** Monitor blood pressure. Assist with ambulation if necessary. Discontinue drug if blurred vision or dry mouth occurs. **Evaluate** Observe client for efficacy of drug. See isosorbide dinitrate.
Isosorbide Mononitrate (Ismo, Monoket, Imdur) HOW SUPPLIED Tablets: 10, 20 mg Extended-release tablets: 60 mg	**Angina Pectoris** TABLETS 20 mg bid given 7 h apart; may initiate with 5 mg, increased to 10 mg by day 2 or 3 EXTENDED-RELEASE TABLETS 30-60 mg/d; may increase to 120 mg/d	

quirements.[20] Calcium channel blockers are also used as antiarrhythmic drugs. They are discussed in more detail in Chapter 32.

CONCEPT REVIEW

Angina pectoris is usually the result of coronary artery disease. Angina occurs when the myocardial oxygen supply does not meet myocardial oxygen demand.

Drug therapy for angina is directed at treating acute angina attacks and preventing their recurrence.

Organic nitrates are commonly prescribed to treat angina. Nitroglycerin is the prototype drug for this group.

Nitroglycerin has no direct effect on cardiac muscle and does not directly elicit changes in either the rate or the inotropic state of the heart. Nitroglycerin lowers systolic pressures and peripheral resistance and enhances oxygen supply by dilation of coronary arteries and inhibition of coronary spasm.

PERIPHERAL AND CEREBRAL VASODILATORS

Vasodilators are sometimes prescribed in the treatment of peripheral vascular disease and cerebral insufficiency. In both situations the drug therapy is not curative but is symptomatic. The prototype peripheral and cerebral vasodilator is papaverine hydrochloride.

PERIPHERAL CEREBRAL VASODILATOR PROTOTYPE
PAPAVERINE HYDROCHLORIDE

Papaverine is an alkaloid prepared synthetically or obtained from opium. However, it is neither chemically nor pharmacologically similar to morphine since it has no addictive properties.

Pharmacotherapeutics The principal use for papaverine is for the relief of cerebral and peripheral ischemia. It has also been prescribed to treat cardiac ischemia.

Pharmacokinetics Papaverine is effective by all routes of administration. However, some studies indicate that the extended-release dosage forms may be poorly and erratically absorbed. Oral tablets and capsules are readily absorbed from the GI tract, and peak levels of the drug occur within 1 to 2 hours. Approximately 90% of the drug is bound to plasma protein. Papaverine is metabolized by the liver and excreted in the urine.

Pharmacodynamics Papaverine relaxes the smooth musculature of large blood vessels, especially coronary, systemic peripheral, and pulmonary arteries. It has direct vasodilating action on cerebral blood vessels. It increases cerebral blood flow and decreases cerebral vascular resistance in normal individuals.[11]

Pharmaceutics Papaverine is available in capsule, tablet, and parenteral solutions.

Undesired Clinical Responses. Although occurring rarely, nausea, abdominal discomfort, anorexia, constipation, malaise, vertigo, headache, and skin rash have been reported with papaverine use.[11]

Contraindications and Precautions Papaverine should be used with caution in individuals with glaucoma, sickle cell anemia, or severe coagulation defects.

Drug-Drug and Drug-Environment Interactions Concurrent administration of papaverine and levodopa in clients with Parkinson's disease can diminish the effects of the levodopa. The parenteral solutions of papaverine are incompatible with lactated Ringer's solution and aminophylline. Oral dosage forms should be stored in a tightly covered, light-resistant container. Parenteral solution vials should not be refrigerated.

Life-Span Considerations Safety in pregnancy and usage in children have not been established. It is not known if the drug is excreted in breast milk.

Specific Drug-Related Nursing Considerations Monitor the client's blood pressure and pulse before and during the course of therapy. When the client is receiving IV drug therapy with papaverine, monitor his or her electrocardiogram for AV blocks. Also monitor hepatic function test results.

Instruct the client to take the drug as prescribed. Explain to both the client and family that the dose should be taken on time. If a dose is omitted, instruct the client *not* to double the next dosage. If dizziness or drowsiness is experienced, advise the client to avoid activities that require alertness.

TABLE 30–4
Peripheral and Cerebral Vasodilators

Drug Name	Dosage and Route of Administration	Nursing Considerations
PAPAVERINE HYDROCHLORIDE (Cerespan, Genabid, Pavabid, Pavacap Unicells, Pavacin) **HOW SUPPLIED** Multiple-dose vials: 30 mg/ml, 10 ml, with 0.5% chlorobutanol Ampules: 60 mg in 2 ml Capsules: 150 mg Tablets: 30, 60, 100, 150, 200 mg	*Oral* Tablets: 100–300 mg three to five times daily Timed-release capsules: 150 mg q12h; if necessary, 150 mg q8h or 300 mg q12h *Parenteral* 30–120 mg q3h; IV route recommended for immediate effect	Oral medications should be taken during or after meals or with milk or antacid to reduce nausea. Teach client not to chew or crush timed-release forms. Inform client that alcohol may intensify dizziness and drowsiness. Client should use caution when performing tasks that require alertness. Give IV form slowly over 1 to 2 min. Monitor pulse and blood pressure of client receiving papaverine parenterally. Notify physician if any adverse signs and symptoms become pronounced.
Cyclandelate (Cyclan, Cyclospasmol) **HOW SUPPLIED** Capsules: 200, 400 mg Tablets: 200, 400 mg	*Oral* Initial dose: 200–400 mg qid Maintenance dose: 400–800 mg/d in two to four divided doses	Use with caution in clients with glaucoma. Have client take with or after meals to reduce GI distress. Store in tightly closed container.

Administer oral tablets and capsules with meals, milk, or antacids to prevent GI discomfort. Oral sustained-action capsules should not be chewed or crushed. Administer IV papaverine solution slowly to avoid tachycardia, dizziness, facial flushing, and hypotension.

MISCELLANEOUS VASODILATORS

Ethaverine hydrochloride and **cyclandelate** are both closely related chemically to papaverine. They are used to treat peripheral and cerebral vascular insufficiency associated with arterial spasm. (See Table 30–4.)

CONCEPT REVIEW

Drugs used to treat peripheral vascular disease and cerebral insufficiency do not cure; they treat the symptoms of the disorder.

Papaverine hydrochloride is the prototype for this group of drugs. It relaxes the smooth musculature of large blood vessels, especially coronary, systemic peripheral, and pulmonary arteries. It also has direct vasodilating action on cerebral blood vessels, increasing cerebral blood flow and decreasing cerebral vascular resistance in normal individuals.

SUMMARY

Angina, peripheral vascular disease, and cerebral insufficiency are the result of diminished arterial blood flow. These conditions are usually caused by atherosclerosis or vasospasm. Drug therapy, although not a cure for these diseases, can reduce symptomatology. Organic nitrates are the primary drugs used to relieve acute angina attacks and to prevent their recurrence. Vasodilators such as papaverine hydrochloride are used in the treatment of peripheral vascular disease and cerebral insufficiency.

REFERENCES

1. Guyton, A.C. (1991). *Textbook of medical physiology* (8th ed.). Philadelphia: W.B. Saunders.
2. Seeley, R., Stephens, T., & Tate, P. (1992). *Anatomy and physiology* (2nd ed.). St. Louis: Mosby–Year Book.
3. Monahon, F., Drake, T., & Neighbors, M. (1994). *Nursing care of adults*. Philadelphia: W.B. Saunders.
4. Higgins (1992). In C.M. Smith and A.M. Reynard (Eds.), *Textbook of pharmacology*. Philadelphia: W.B. Saunders.
5. Abrams, J. (1991). Angina pectoris mechanisms, diagnosis, and therapy. *Nursing Clinics of North America, 9,* 89–97.
6. Morton, L. (1991). Perfecting the art of cardiac assessment. *RN Magazine, 54*(12), 28–35.
7. Kelly, J., & O'Malley, K. (1992). Nitrates in the elderly. Pharmacological considerations. *Drugs—Aging, 2*(1), 14–19.
8. Gold, M.E. (1991). Pharmacology of the nitrovasodilators. *Nurisng Clinics of North America, 26,* 437–449.
9. Fleury, J. (1992). Long-term management of the patient with stable angina. *Nursing Clinics of North America, 27,* 205–227.
10. Kuhn, M. (1992). Nitrates. *AACN–Clinical Issues in Critical Care Nursing, 3,* 409–422.
11. Data Pharmaceutica, Inc. (1993). *1993 physicians' genRx.* Smithtown, NY: Author.
12. U.S. Pharmacopeial Convention. (1990). *The United States pharmacopeia* (22nd rev.). Rockville, MD: Author.
13. Yakabowich, M. (1992, September). Administering nitrates. *Nursing '92,* 52–54.
14. Kalman, J.M. (1990). Nitrate tolerance: A new look at an old problem. *Focus on Critical Care, 17,* 407–409.
15. Elkayam, U. (1991). Tolerance to organic nitrates: Evidence, mechanisms, clinical relevance, and strategies for prevention. *Annals Internal Medicine, 114,* 667–677.
16. Ryan, M., Gallagher, S., & Wandel, J. (1992). Effect of nitropaste administration times on sleep and nocturnal angina. *Applied Nursing Research, 5*(2), 84–86.
17. Gleeson, B. (1991, January). Loosening the grip of anginal pain. *Nursing '91,* 33–39.
18. Parmley, W.W., & Weart, C. (1991). Ca channel blockers: The new, the tried-and-true, *Patient Care, 26*(9), 32–34.
19. Dennis, K.E., Froman, D., Morrison, A.S., Holmes, K.D., & Howes, D.G. (1991). Beta blocker therapy: Identification and management of side effects. *Heart and Lung, 20,* 459–463.
20. Clark, B.K. (1992). Beta-adrenergic blocking agents: Their current status. *Clinical Issues in Critical Care Nursing, 3,* 447–480.

BIBLIOGRAPHY

Beer, M.H., Sliwkowski, J., Brooks, J. (1992). Compliance with medication orders among the elderly after hospital discharge. *Hospital Formulary, 27,* 720–724.

Edwards, L.C., & Louie, E.K. (1992). Stable angina: Review of therapies to prevent, reduce, or interrupt the ischemic process. *Hospital Formulary, 27,* 355–375.

Green, E. (1992). Solving the puzzle of chest pain. *American Journal of Nursing, 92*(1), 32–37.

Kinoshita, M., & Sakai, K. (1990). Pharmacology and therapeutic effects of nicorandil. *Cardiovascular Drugs Therapy, 4,* 1075–1088.

Porterfield, L.M., & Porterfield, J.G. (1990). Understanding cardiovascular drug interactions. *Focus on Critical Care, 17,* 412–416.

Sutton, M., & Jeffrey, B. (1992). Acquired methemoglobinemia from amyl nitrite inhalation. *Journal of Emergency Nursing, 18*(1), 8–9.

Udho, T. (1991). Medical therapy of stable angina pectoris. *Cardiology Clinics, 9*(1), 73–85.

CHAPTER 31

Cardiac Glycosides

NORMA L. PINNELL

⊛ **Pharmacotherapeutics of Cardiac Glycosides**

LEARNING OBJECTIVE: Describe the clinical indications for cardiac glycosides.

KEY TERMS:

Cardiac glycosides, congestive heart failure, digitalis glycosides

⊛ **General Characteristics of Cardiac Glycosides**

LEARNING OBJECTIVE: Summarize the general characteristics of cardiac glycosides.

KEY TERMS:

Aglycone, negative chronotropic effects, negative dromotropic effects, positive inotropic effects

⊛ **Pharmacodynamics of Cardiac Glycosides**

LEARNING OBJECTIVES:

Describe both the mechanical and electric effects of cardiac glycosides.

Differentiate between the direct and indirect effects of cardiac glycosides.

KEY TERM: Sodium-potassium-ATPase pump

⊛ **Physiologic Response to Cardiac Glycosides**

LEARNING OBJECTIVE: Describe the physiologic response of the body to cardiac glycosides.

⊛ **Medical Management of Clients Receiving Cardiac Glycosides**

LEARNING OBJECTIVE: Identify factors the nurse should monitor in clients receiving cardiac glycosides.

⊛ **General Nursing Considerations**

LEARNING OBJECTIVES:

Develop a teaching plan for a client beginning cardiac glycoside drug therapy.

Develop a discharge plan for a client receiving cardiac glycosides.

KEY TERMS:

Digitalizing dose, maintenance dose, pulse deficit

⊛ **Cardiac Glycoside Prototype**

LEARNING OBJECTIVES:

Describe the pharmacokinetic qualities of digoxin.

List signs and symptoms of toxicity and/or adverse effects from cardiac glycosides.

Describe the use of digoxin immune FAB (ovine) in the treatment of digitalis toxicity.

Identify common contraindications associated with the use of cardiac glycosides.

List three drugs that interact with cardiac glycosides.

⊛ **Other Cardiac Glycoside Drug**

LEARNING OBJECTIVE: Differentiate between the pharmacokinetic properties of digoxin and digitoxin.

⊛ **Life-Span Considerations**

LEARNING OBJECTIVE: Describe life-span considerations associated with cardiac glycosides.

*C*ardiac glycosides are naturally occurring compounds obtained from the leaves of *Digitalis purpurea* (purple foxglove) and *Digitalis lanata* (white foxglove). Because of their presence in digitalis plants, these drugs are also known as digitalis glycosides.

Cardiac, or **digitalis, glycosides** are among the oldest prescription drugs. Early accounts of the use of digitalis derivatives are found in the Ebers Papyrus (1500 BC), in early Chinese writings, in early Roman records (AD 1000), and in early chronicles that date back to 1542. As early as 1785 records show foxglove (*Digitalis* spp.) plant leaves were used to treat **congestive heart failure (CHF),** called *dropsy* at the time.[1]

PHARMACOTHERAPEUTICS OF CARDIAC GLYCOSIDES

Cardiac glycosides are prescribed to treat CHF, atrial fibrillation and flutter, and paroxysmal atrial tachycardia. This chapter focuses on their use in the treatment of CHF.

CHF is produced by conditions that increase preload, increase afterload, or reduce myocardial contractility. When these conditions occur, the left ventricular stroke volume is reduced. As ventricular end-diastolic volumes increase, there is a corresponding rise in the left ventricular end-diastolic pressure. This increase in pressure causes an elevation of the left atrial pressure and a corresponding elevation in the pulmonary venous and pulmonary capillary pressures. If the hydrostatic pressure in the pulmonary capillary system exceeds oncotic pressure, fluid transudation into the interstitial tissue occurs. Further elevation of pulmonary pressure may cause fluid seepage into the alveoli and the development of pulmonary edema.[2]

When the heart fails, mean arterial pressure and cardiac output decrease, and circulatory failure ensues. The body's response to heart failure consists of three primary compensatory mechanisms: increased autonomic sympathetic adrenergic activity; activation of the renin-angiotensin-aldosterone system; and ventricular hypertrophy. These compensatory mechanisms are attempts to maintain cardiac output by affecting preload, afterload, and myocardial contractility.

Enhanced sympathetic tone results in elevated peripheral vascular resistance, increased venous tone, redistribution of blood flow, and reduced renal perfusion. An elevation in peripheral vascular resistance and venous tone increases afterload and preload. Decreased glomerular filtration rate as a result of reduced renal blood flow and activation of the renin-angiotensin-aldosterone system cause sodium and water retention. Retention of sodium and water also increases preload. With the increase in preload, ventricular dilation and stretching of the cardiac fibers occur, thus increasing the force of contraction and causing myocardial hypertrophy.[2-5]

Initially these mechanisms are usually sufficient to maintain cardiac output at normal or near-normal levels. However, after sustained increases in preload and afterload or as the degree of heart failure progresses, compensation becomes less effective. Eventually cardiac decompensation occurs, and the heart is unable to eject blood and meet the metabolic and energy demands of the peripheral tissue.

With the beginning of decompensation, respiratory and heart rates increase; urinary output declines; skin and extremities cool; and diaphoresis occurs. As the client's status deteriorates, intestinal peristalsis slows, causing nausea, vomiting, and abdominal pain. Arterial CO_2 tension ($PaCO_2$), arterial oxygen tension (PaO_2), and arterial O_2 saturation (SaO_2) fall, and blood glucose levels rise. The client's level of consciousness and mental processes decrease, and mood changes occur.[6]

Drug therapy is used in an attempt to stabilize the client's hemodynamic status. In the past cardiac (digitalis) glycosides and diuretics were the only drugs available to relieve the clinical manifestation of heart failure. Now newer inotropic drugs such as phosphodiesterase III inhibitors, angiotensin-converting enzyme (ACE) inhibitors, sympathomimetic amines, and vasodilators are used.[4,7-11] (See Chapter 30 for discussion of these drug categories.)

USE OF PHOSPHODIESTERASE III INHIBITORS TO TREAT CONGESTIVE HEART FAILURE

Phosphodiesterase III inhibitors, such as amrinone (Inocor) and milrinone (Primacor), are used for short-term treatment of severe congestive heart failure. Because these drugs inhibit phosphodiesterase III, intracellular cyclic AMP (cAMP) accumulates. (Normally, phosphodiesterase III degrades cAMP). The cAMP increases myocardial contractility and promotes vasodilation.

Amrinone is used for 2 to 3 days in clients who have not responded to diuretics, cardiac glycosides, and vasodilators. The initial intravenous dose is 0.75 mg/kg administered over 2 to 3 minutes. The maintenance dose is 5 to 10 µg/kg/min. Amrinone should be protected from light and should not be mixed with glucose-containing solutions. Constant monitoring of the client is required.

GENERAL CHARACTERISTICS OF CARDIAC GLYCOSIDES

The objectives for treatment of CHF are to improve cardiac performance (contractility and output), to reduce cardiac workload, and to correct related impairments in organ function and fluid balance. When administered in therapeutic doses, cardiac glycosides increase the force of cardiac contraction and improve cardiac output. The delivery of oxygen to body tissues and of blood flow to the kidneys is improved, and renal filtration and urinary output are subsequently increased. The results of these actions include improved coronary perfusion and reduced total circulating blood volume, thus improving cardiac performance and reducing the physiologic changes produced by the failing heart.

Differences in the pharmacokinetic and pharmacodynamic properties among the various digitalis glycosides are due to variations in water and lipid solubility. For example, digitoxin (Crystodigin, Purodigin) is lipid soluble and thus absorbed completely from the gastrointestinal (GI) tract. Digoxin (Lanoxin) is less lipid soluble and not as well absorbed as digitoxin.[12]

Chemically, digitalis glycosides are composed of a sugar and an **aglycone.** Sugar molecules enhance water solubility and cell permeability; the chemical structure of the sugar portion influences glycoside potency and the dose-response relationship. Aglycone is responsible for the cardiac effects associated with glycosides.[12] Minor structural differences among the digitalis drugs create the metabolic differences. All cardiac glycosides are potent in very low doses, and their effects on the heart are dose related. In addition, cardiac glycosides have a low therapeutic index; a dose adequate for therapeutic effect can produce signs of toxicity. All cardiac glycosides produce **positive inotropic effects** and **negative chronotropic** and **dromotropic effects.** The degree of inotropic action increases progressively with an increasing dose until toxic effects are manifested.

PHARMACODYNAMICS OF CARDIAC GLYCOSIDES

Since the pharmacodynamic activities of the various cardiac glycoside drugs are considered identical, each drug is not discussed separately. Instead, a summary of the pharmacodynamic activities of the drug category is presented.

Cardiac glycosides are the oldest and most widely used inotropic agents. They have significant effects on the heart, altering both the mechanical and electric components of cardiac function. These glycosides act on cardiac muscle to stimulate the force of cardiac contraction, a **positive** inotropic effect. This effect is produced by inhibition of the **sodium-potassium-ATPase** (Na⁺K⁺ATPase) **pump,** which normally maintains the sodium and potassium concentration differences across the cell membrane. Pump inhibition increases intracellular sodium, which inhibits further entry of sodium and activates the **sodium-calcium exchange mechanism.** Calcium accumulation occurs within the cardiac cells. This accumulation

---

EFFECTS OF CARDIAC GLYCOSIDES ON CARDIAC FUNCTION

Atrial and Ventricular Muscle Fibers
Minimum direct or indirect effects on the electric activity of cardiac muscle; myocardial contractility increased by inhibition of sodium-potassium-ATPase pump

SA Node
Slows pacemaker activity by increased vagal activity and decreased sympathetic activity

AV Node
Decreases conduction through AV node and increases the refractory period of the node; effects result from direct effect (inhibition of sodium-potassium-ATPase pump) and indirect effects (increased vagal influence and decreased sympathetic activity)

Purkinje Fibers
Direct action on fibers to increase automaticity

---

makes increased intracellular calcium available to the contractile elements of the myocardium, causing the heart to contract with increased force. By increasing contractile force of the heart, cardiac output is normalized or at least improved. Secondary to the increase in cardiac output is a decrease in preload and end-diastolic volume.

In addition to increasing cardiac contractility, cardiac glycosides alter the electric impulse generation and conduction in the heart. The electric effects of cardiac glycosides are complex. The exact effects depend, in part, on the cardiac status, drug dosage, and tissue involved. In addition to therapeutic effects, serious toxicity can be caused by the glycosides' effect on impulse generation and conduction.

Glycosides alter the electric activity of noncontractile tissue (sinoatrial [SA] and atrioventricular [AV] nodes and Purkinje fibers) and the activity of the atrial and ventricular muscle. Direct effects of digitalis on cardiac electric activities include reduction of resting membrane potential, reduction of action potential duration, and decrease in the maximum rate of rise in phase 0. These actions can promote increased automaticity and slower depolarization. Inhibition of the Na⁺K⁺ATPase pump also produces direct effects on the electric properties of cardiac tissues.

Indirect parasympathomimetic actions of cardiac glycosides are largely responsible for the effects on the sinus and AV nodes. The two primary indirect effects by which cardiac glycosides alter cardiac electric activity are increased vagal influence and reflexive reduction in sympathetic tone. By stimulating the parasympathetic division of the autonomic system, vagal tone is increased. This vagal effect slows the heart rate, increases the refractory period, and slows conduction through the AV node and junctional tissue. The decreased conduction through the AV node is considered a **negative** dromotropic effect.

A reduction in sympathetic tone and increased sensitization of the myocardium to acetylcholine also occur. These two changes cause a decrease in the heart rate, a **negative** chronotropic effect. The combined effects on the vagal nerve and sympathetic tone also decrease automaticity of the SA node.[12]

PHYSIOLOGIC RESPONSE TO CARDIAC GLYCOSIDES

Once the client is established on the therapeutic regimen, significant improvement in cardiac function usually occurs. Cardiac glycosides improve exercise tolerance, reduce the signs and symptoms associated with heart failure, and reduce the frequency of clinical decompensation (Fig. 31–1).[3,12]

Cardiovascular System

Multiple sites are involved in the action of glycosides on the cardiovascular system. In the heart, contractility increases be-

cause of the direct positive inotropic action of the drug. Stroke volume increases, heart rate decreases slightly, and ventricular emptying improves. These factors reduce the workload of the heart and leave less blood in the ventricles during diastole. Thus a decrease in the heart size results in clients with cardiomegaly.

Cardiac glycosides alter the client's blood pressure by action on the autonomic nervous system (ANS). Glycosides produce direct α-adrenergic vasoconstriction action on peripheral vessels and a central sympathetic or reflex action. These responses are dose related. Smooth muscles of veins are also affected; glycosides act directly on the smooth muscle to induce constriction.

Renal System

As the stroke volume and cardiac output increase, an increase in renal blood flow occurs. The improved blood flow increases the glomerular filtration rate, resulting in increased urinary output and sodium excretion.

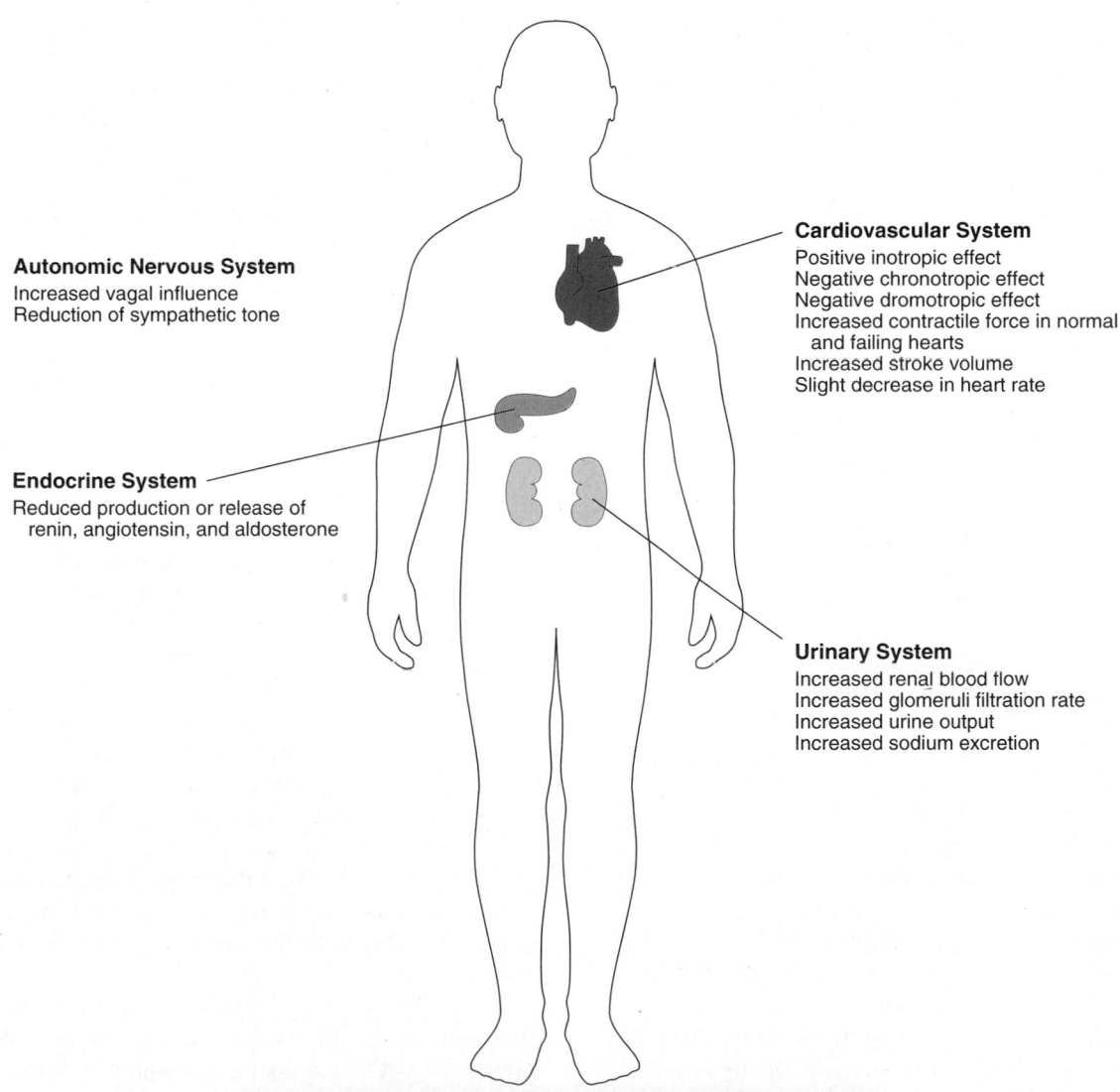

Autonomic Nervous System
Increased vagal influence
Reduction of sympathetic tone

Endocrine System
Reduced production or release of
   renin, angiotensin, and aldosterone

Cardiovascular System
Positive inotropic effect
Negative chronotropic effect
Negative dromotropic effect
Increased contractile force in normal
   and failing hearts
Increased stroke volume
Slight decrease in heart rate

Urinary System
Increased renal blood flow
Increased glomeruli filtration rate
Increased urine output
Increased sodium excretion

FIGURE 31–1   Physiologic responses to cardiac glycosides.

Hormonal Effects

As the blood flow to the kidneys improves, hormonal changes occur. Renin release by the kidneys diminishes. This reduction in renin release decreases the formation of angiotensin II. With the reduction in angiotensin II, decreased release of the hormone aldosterone occurs. Since aldosterone causes the kidneys to retain more sodium and water, the reduction helps to reduce fluid volume excess in the body.

MEDICAL MANAGEMENT OF CLIENTS RECEIVING CARDIAC GLYCOSIDES

Individuals receiving cardiac glycosides require close monitoring. Physicians often order the determination of glycoside plasma levels, electrocardiograms (ECGs), and serum potassium levels to help determine the client's response to a specific drug and/or drug dose.

Knowing glycoside plasma levels aids in determining therapeutic and toxic effects and assessing client compliance. However, the relationship between plasma levels and clinical response is not the same with each client. Several factors can alter plasma levels, including electrolyte imbalance, renal disorders, age, and thyroid conditions. The time that the blood sample is drawn is also important. Because of these factors, plasma levels should be evaluated in conjunction with current symptoms, other laboratory tests, and ECG results.[3,12,13]

The primary effects on the ECG in clients receiving therapeutic levels of cardiac glycosides are PR-interval prolongation, QT shortening, ST depression, and T-wave depression. With digitalis toxicity, premature ventricular contractions, progressive bradycardia, and progressive slowing of AV conduction are seen.[12] You must monitor the client's ECG carefully for these changes.

Potassium depletion increases the sensitivity of cardiac muscles to the effects of cardiac glycosides and reduces the tubular secretion of the glycoside. Therefore monitoring the potassium levels of clients prone to low serum potassium levels is important. Clients receiving loop or thiazide diuretics, glucocorticoids, or mineralocorticoids or those who are chronic users of laxatives are prone to potassium depletion.

CONCEPT REVIEW

Cardiac glycosides are used primarily to treat CHF.
Cardiac glycosides produce a positive inotropic effect, a negative dromotropic effect, and a negative chronotropic effect on the heart.
Direct and indirect cardiac effects are produced by cardiac glycosides.
Therapeutic doses of cardiac glycosides decrease the workload of the heart, improve cardiac contractility, and increase renal blood flow.
Knowing plasma levels and serum potassium levels and ECGs helps determine the client's response to a specific drug and/or drug dose.

PLASMA LEVELS OF CARDIAC GLYCOSIDES

Digoxin
Therapeutic levels: 0.5-2.0 ng/ml
Toxic levels: >2.5 ng/ml

Digitoxin
Therapeutic levels: 15-25 ng/ml
Toxic levels: >35 ng/ml

▨ NURSING CONSIDERATIONS

Managing the care of a client who is receiving cardiac glycosides is a challenge. Nursing care focuses on the initiation of the prescribed drug therapy and evaluation of the client's response to the drug. Although some clients begin their therapy in a community setting (home, nursing home, extended care facility, etc.), most clients require hospitalization until their condition stabilizes. The intensity of the nursing care varies with the client's baseline status, type of drug prescribed, route of administration prescribed, and concomitant use of other drugs.

Assessing A health history and physical assessment should be completed by the nurse to provide baseline data about the client. During the health history interview, determine if the client has experienced any recent weight gain, swelling of hands and feet, difficulty sleeping, or the need to sleep with additional pillows. Ask the client if there has been an increase or decrease in urinary output, shortness of breath, presence of a cough, palpitations, fatigue, dizziness, confusion, or exercise intolerance. Determine if the client has a history of smoking. Assess the client's lifestyle activities; ask if these activities are affected by the current health status.

As a part of the health history, collect a nutritional and drug history. The nutritional history helps determine the client's daily dietary intake of sodium. In addition, since anorexia occurs in clients with CHF, the history will provide general information about the individual's nutritional status. During the drug history, collect information on all prescription and over-the-counter (OTC) drugs used by the client. Identify the use of any drug that may interact with glycosides such as barbiturates, antacids, antineoplastic agents, potassium-wasting diuretics, or quinidine. In addition, assess for concurrent health problems, especially those that might contraindicate cardiac glycoside therapy such as impaired renal or hepatic function, electrolyte imbalances, hypothyroidism, or prior cardiac disease.

During the physical examination, specifically assess aspects that would reflect the cardiac status of the individual. Since performance of the respiratory system is dependent on cardiovascular function, assess for increased respiratory rate, increased respiratory effort, and/or adventitious breath sounds.

During the cardiovascular assessment, assess pulse rate and rhythm, peripheral pulses, neck vein distention, presence of edema, abdominal distention, body weight, skin color and temperature, and level of consciousness. (Review a nursing assessment book for detailed information on physical and cardiovascular assessment.)

🎋 NURSING RESEARCH

Dunbar, S., Marchette, L., & Salerno, E. (1988). Circadian rhythms and timing of digoxin administration. *The Journal of Cardiovascular Nursing, 2*(4), 1-11.

The purpose of this study was to determine the effects of oral digoxin administered at two different times. The following hypotheses were tested: (1) serum digoxin levels are higher when digoxin is administered in the evening rather than in the morning, and (2) the clinical effects of digoxin are greater when it is administered in the evening rather than in the morning.

A total of 26 subjects ranging in age from 79 to 99 years met the criteria for the study. Six men and 14 women (N = 20) completed the study. There was no statistically significant difference between 9:00 AM and 9:00 PM serum levels of digoxin. However, in some subjects, great individual variation in response was seen. There was also no significant differences in clinical effects of digoxin as measured by heart rate, blood pressure, or ECG variations.

STUDENT ACTIVITIES

- Establish when oral digoxin is administered in your assigned agency.
- Determine what time routine serum digoxin levels are drawn.
- Learn the bases for these procedures.
- Monitor three or four clients who are receiving oral digoxin. Check and record blood pressure, pulse, ECG findings, and serum digoxin levels for several days. Analyze data for any patterns of response.
- Share research findings with nurses on your assigned division.

Diagnosing Once the database has been established, the data are analyzed and nursing diagnoses developed. Depending on the data, several nursing diagnoses may be appropriate for an individual receiving cardiac glycosides for CHF. These diagnoses include the following:
- Self-care deficit related to fatigue and shortness of breath.
- Altered sleep and rest pattern related to difficulty breathing.
- Excess fluid volume related to excess sodium intake.
- Altered respiratory function related to increased respiratory secretions.
- Altered tissue perfusion related to decreased blood flow and immobility.
- Altered health maintenance related to knowledge deficit about drug regimen, diet, activity.

- Anxiety related to change in self-concept, change or threat to health status, threat of death.
- High risk for infection related to altered body defense mechanisms associated with drug therapy.
- Altered nutrition: less than body requirement related to digoxin-induced nausea and anorexia.

Planning For the client with CHF, it is important to reduce the oxygen requirements of the body. Plan your care carefully so that you can avoid activities that might compromise the client's myocardial function. Assess the client frequently, monitoring carefully for the presence of symptoms. Adjust the client's plan of care to correspond with his or her response to therapy. As with any plan, consult the client and family before establishing specific goals, objectives, and interventions. Client participation in the planning of care usually increases compliance.

During this phase, you must also develop individualized teaching and discharge plans for the client and establish expected outcomes. Expected outcomes that can be discussed with the client include the following:
- Client will perform activities of daily living (ADL) without undue fatigue.
- Client will demonstrate tolerance to increased activity.
- Client will maintain adequate rest and sleep.
- Client will maintain fluid volume balance.
- Client will plan a diet in accordance to prescribed sodium, caloric, and/or fluid restrictions.
- Client will plan a modified activity schedule.
- Client will demonstrate proper technique for monitoring radial pulse rate.
- Client will discuss components of the drug therapy plan.
- Client will describe plans for follow-up medical care.

Implementing Nursing therapies are directed initially at safe administration of the prescribed drug. If therapy with cardiac glycosides is for a client with long-standing, mild heart failure, gradual digitalization is usually preferred. The simplest method to produce gradual digitalization is to place the client on a **maintenance dose.** Maintenance doses produce maximum effect in approximately 1 week of digoxin therapy and 1 month of digitoxin therapy.

If a more rapid response is desired, an initial **loading** or **digitalizing dose** is administered. Onset of action and peak effects vary with the type of cardiac glycoside and route of administration. For example, onset of action from an intravenous (IV) loading dose of digoxin occurs within 15 to 30 minutes after dosing. Peak effects occur within $1^1/_2$ to 5 hours after dosing. Onset of action from an IV loading dose of digitoxin occurs within 25 minutes to 2 hours, and the peak effects occur within 4 to 12 hours. Rapid digitalization should be avoided when the slow method suffices. After the loading dose, the client is placed on a daily maintenance dose. This dose is gradually adjusted to achieve the desired therapeutic benefit for the client. If plasma levels are ordered, have the samples drawn at least 3 to 4 hours after an IV dose of digoxin and at least 6 to 8 hours after an oral dose.

Cardiac glycosides are potent in very low doses and have a low therapeutic index. Read the orders and drug labels carefully—at least three times. Be careful not to confuse digoxin and digitoxin. Before administering a cardiac glycoside, the apical pulse rate is counted for 1 full minute. In addition to the rate, note the rhythm and regularity of the beat. The physician usually establishes a desired pulse range for the client. (The most frequently used pulse range is 60 to 110 beats/min.) If the pulse rate exceeds the upper limit or drops below the lower limit, do not administer the drug before notifying the physician. A decrease in pulse rate is usually associated with increased plasma glycoside levels. An abrupt increase in pulse rate can be associated with early indications of drug toxicity.

In some clients with atrial flutter or fibrillation the physician may specify checking an apical-radial pulse rate. In these clients, a **pulse deficit** (apical pulse is faster than radial pulse) usually exists. With cardiac glycoside therapy, the goal is to lower the pulse deficit to zero. To obtain an accurate apical-radial pulse, two nurses must take the pulse simultaneously, one counting the apical pulse and the other counting the radial pulse.

Cardiac glycosides should be administered at the same time each day. Before establishing an administration time, consult the client and establish a time that is compatible with that individual's lifestyle. Since the drug can be given either with or between meals, a midday administration time is recommended if it does not conflict with the client's home schedule. Administering the medication around noon allows the client time to be up and active before the pulse rate is assessed. If the drug is administered between meals, provide the client with a snack to lessen gastric irritation.

If a parenteral dose is prescribed, the IV route is the preferred route of administration. Both the subcutaneous (SC) and intramuscular (IM) routes produce tissue irritation. Cardiac glycosides administered in the deltoid muscle cause severe pain at the injection site and increase creatine phosphokinase (CPK) levels, which complicate interpretation of enzyme elevation. Therefore this route is **not** recommended. Instead, inject the drug into a large muscle mass (gluteus maximus or ventrogluteal muscle) to decrease the chance of muscle fasciculations and necrosis. If the client is experiencing current signs of CHF, the absorption rate from parenteral routes is uncertain. In these cases and in emergencies, the IV route is usually prescribed.

Preparing the client and the family for self-care requires a well-organized and comprehensive teaching/discharge plan. The teaching plan should be initiated as early as possible. Many episodes of recurring heart failure and/or drug toxicity possibly could be prevented if clients are prepared to follow the prescribed drug therapy and dietary and activity restrictions and to recognize recurring symptoms of cardiac failure or adverse drug response.

Teach the client the name, dosage, action, frequency of administration, and adverse effects of the prescribed cardiac glycosides. Discuss with the client the expected benefits of the drug therapy. Review all medications the client is taking, and

---

TEACHING/DISCHARGE PLAN

The following information should be taught to the client and family:

1. Monitor for and report signs and symptoms of recurring heart failure:
   - Weight gain over a short period of time: 1-2 pounds (0.45-0.90 kg) in 1 day or 5 pounds (2.25 kg) in 1 week
   - Loss of appetite
   - Shortness of breath
   - Orthopnea
   - Swelling of ankles, feet, or abdomen
   - Persistent cough
   - Frequent nighttime urination
2. Take cardiac glycoside as prescribed:
   - Check pulse rate daily before taking the drug.
   - If the rate is less than 60 beats/min or more than 110 beats/min, notify the physician or clinic before taking the drug.
   - Drug can be taken with or between meals.
   - If drug taken between meals, be sure to eat a snack with the drug to lessen gastric irritation.
   - Try to take the cardiac glycoside at the same time each day.
   - Store the drug in a tightly covered, light-resistant container.
   - Store the drug out of reach of children
   - Do not take cardiac glycoside concurrent with antacids, antidiarrheals, or laxatives.
   - Check with your physician or pharmacist before taking other medications.
   - If you forget to take your cardiac glycoside, check with your physician. You should not take two doses in the same day.
   - Do not discontinue the drug without checking with the physician.
   - Monitor for and report signs of adverse effects and cardiac glycoside toxicity (loss of appetite, nausea, vomiting, weakness, fatigue, visual changes, cardiac changes, headaches, fatigue, malaise, depression, disorientation, confusion, etc.) to the physician or clinic.
3. Eat high-potassium foods (orange juice, bananas, spinach, cantaloupe, watermelon, dates, raisins, apples, prunes, beans, potatoes, squash) unless taking a potassium-sparing diuretic, ACE inhibitor, or potassium supplement.
4. Wear a medical identification tag or bracelet indicating you are taking a cardiac glycoside.

stress the importance of taking the drugs exactly as prescribed. Demonstrate to the client and a family member how to take a radial pulse. Have them practice and do a return demonstration to determine their level of understanding. Instruct the client to consult with the pharmacist before each drug refill to ensure that the prescribed cardiac glycoside is from the same manufacturer. (Drugs from different manufacturing companies can display differences in bioavailability.) Also instruct the client to check the prescription carefully for right drug and dosage.

Discuss with the client the importance of maintaining an adequate potassium level. Review sources of dietary potassium and provide the client with a list of these sources. Some clients with cardiac conditions may also need instruction on sodium restricted diets, weight reduction diets, and low cholesterol diets. Provide these clients with appropriate information and refer them to a dietician if possible.

Refer elderly or debilitated clients or individuals with inadequate home supervision to a home health agency. For these clients, a periodic pill count should be done to evaluate compliance and to detect accidental overdose.

Evaluating Evaluation of the effectiveness of drug therapy in clients with CHF is based in part on the client's clinical response. To help you determine his or her response, you should monitor the following: daily weights, intake and output, pedal edema, abdominal girth, vital signs, breath sounds, activity tolerance, and heart rate and rhythm. Once the client has been established on drug therapy, expect to see an increase in urinary output with an accompanying weight loss. Tachycardia lessens; cardiac rhythm becomes more regular; and adventitious breath sounds disappear. The client should experience increased activity tolerance and decreased fatigue and weakness.

Review the expected outcomes previously developed with the client to determine if the plan of care was effective. Determine which of the outcomes were accomplished and decide with the client what additional interventions are needed.

To evaluate the client's response to the teaching plan, have the individual demonstrate the procedure for taking a radial pulse. Ask the client to describe the signs and symptoms of adverse reactions and drug toxicity and to tell you what to do if these signs and symptoms occur. Describe possible scenarios to the client and ask him or her to describe how he or she should respond in these situations. Remember that knowledge increases compliance and can prevent this client from returning to the health care facility with drug toxicity and/or recurring heart failure.

CONCEPT REVIEW

Nursing care focuses on monitoring the client's response to the drug therapy and teaching the client to manage self-administration of the drug.

An initial loading or digitalizing dose is administered if rapid response is desired.

Cardiac glycosides are potent in very low doses and have a narrow therapeutic index.

Always check the apical pulse before administering the drug.

If the pulse rate is below 60 or above 110, notify the physician before administering the drug.

CARDIAC GLYCOSIDE PROTOTYPE

DIGOXIN

In this section of the chapter the prototype for cardiac glycosides, digoxin, is discussed. Information on the pharmacokinetic qualities, adverse reactions, side effects, toxic effects, contraindications, and drug-drug and drug-nutrient interactions is included.

Pharmacokinetics Understanding the absorption, distribution, biotransformation, and excretion of digoxin is important. Knowledge of the half-life, onset of action, and time of peak action for this drug helps you provide safe, effective care.

ABSORPTION Digoxin comes from the foxglove plant, *D. lanata.* It is less lipid soluble than other cardiac glycosides; therefore it is not as well absorbed from the GI tract. The GI absorption of digoxin is a passive process, and the degree of oral absorption depends on the dosage form (tablet, liquid, or capsule) used. Sixty to 80% of an oral dose of a standard digoxin tablet is absorbed. When digoxin tablets are taken after meals, the rate of absorption is slowed, but the total amount of the drug absorbed is usually unchanged. However, if taken with meals high in bran fiber, the amount absorbed may be reduced.

From 70% to 85% of elixirs are absorbed, and capsules containing digoxin solution are absorbed almost completely (90% to 100% absorption). With parenteral administration, 70% to 85% of the drug is absorbed with the IM route.

DISTRIBUTION After drug administration, a 6- to 8-hour distribution phase occurs. Approximately 20% to 25% of plasma digoxin is bound to plasma proteins, allowing more rapid diffusion of the drug out of the bloodstream and into the tissues. Digoxin concentrates in most body tissues, particularly erythrocytes, heart, skeletal muscle, kidney, liver, intestine, and pancreas. This extracardiac binding accounts for several drug interactions that occur with individuals receiving digoxin. Serum digoxin concentrations are not significantly altered by large changes in fat tissue weight; distribution space correlates best with lean body weight.

Digoxin does cross both the blood-brain barrier and the placenta. At the time of birth, serum concentration in the newborn is similar to the serum level in the mother. Cardiac glycosides are also found in breast milk.

After administration of a digoxin tablet or capsule, onset of action occurs within 30 minutes to 2 hours; peak effects occur in 2 to 6 hours. Maximum effect for tablets and elixirs is 6 to 8 hours. After IV administration, onset of action occurs within 15 to 30 minutes; peak effects occur in 1 to 4 hours. After IM administration, onset of action occurs in 30 minutes to 2 hours; peak effects occur in 2 to 6 hours.

BIOTRANSFORMATION A small percentage of digoxin is metabolized by the liver and GI flora into metabolites that exhibit cardiac activity. The remaining digoxin is excreted unchanged. In individuals with normal renal function, digoxin has a half-life of 1½ to 2 days.

EXCRETION As indicated previously, most digoxin in the bloodstream (75% to 85%) is excreted unchanged by the kidney. The quantity of digoxin eliminated at any time is proportional to the total body content. In addition, renal excretion is proportional to the glomerular filtration rate and is largely independent of urinary flow. Adjustment of dosage is essential if renal function is impaired[14–16] (See Table 31–1 Characteristics of Digoxin and Digitoxin for a comparison of the two major cardiac glycosides.)

Side Effects and Digitalis Toxicity Because of the small difference between therapeutic doses and doses that cause side effects, it is not unusual for clients to experience drug-related difficulties at one time or another. **Side effect symptoms** usually are vague and may be confused with recurring signs and symptoms of heart failure. Allergic reactions such as rashes are rare. However, gynecomastia may result from the estrogen-like activity of these drugs (Table 31–2).

Adverse effects associated with these drugs are usually referred to as **digitalis toxicity.** Toxicity can result from many factors, including accumulation of maintenance doses, rapid loading or digitalization, impaired liver and/or renal function, age extremes, electrolyte imbalance, hypothyroidism (slows biotransformation of drug), and concurrent therapy with other drugs affecting the heart. The signs and symptoms of digitalis toxicity fall into two main categories: noncardiac and cardiac.

NONCARDIAC MANIFESTATIONS GI and neurologic disturbances are the major noncardiac manifestations of digitalis toxicity. Central nervous system (CNS) effects from cardiac glycosides are significant sources of major toxic effects. Anorexia, nausea, and vomiting are the result of stimulation of the chemoreceptor trigger zone in the CNS. Weakness, fatigue, and fainting also originate in the CNS. In addition, visual disturbances such as dimness of vision,

double vision, blind spots, flashing lights, or altered color vision occur. They usually occur later than nausea, vomiting, and anorexia. Psychologic disturbances range from mood alterations to hallucinations or psychoses.

CARDIAC MANIFESTATIONS Alterations in cardiac function are the most common and most serious forms of digitalis toxicity. Bradycardia and arrhythmias, including extrasystoles, sinus arrhythmias, paroxysmal atrial and ventricular tachycardia, atrial flutter, and atrial and ventricular

---

ADMINISTRATION AND DOSAGE OF DIGOXIN IMMUNE FAB

▶ Initially the total amount of digoxin or digitoxin in the client's body is determined in milligrams.

▶ The amount of digoxin or digitoxin in the client's body is divided by 0.6. The resulting figure represents the number of vials of digoxin immune fab (Digibind) to administer. (Each 40-mg vial of digoxin immune fab will bind with approximately 0.6 mg of digoxin or digitoxin.)

▶ Each vial is reconstituted with 4 ml of sterile water.

▶ The solution is mixed gently to avoid foaming the medication. The final concentration is 10 mg/ml. The solutions may be stored at 7.7° C (46° F) for 4 hours after reconstitution.

▶ The medication is infused intravenously over a 30-minute period through a 0.22 μm inline filter.

▶ Single IV bolus can be used if digoxin serum levels are markedly elevated.

TABLE 31–1
Pharmacokinetic Characteristics of Digoxin and Digitoxin

DIGOXIN (LANOXIN)	**DIGITOXIN (CRYSTODIGIN)**
Absorption	**Absorption**
Less lipid soluble GI absorption with tablets: 60%-80%	Lipid soluble GI absorption with tablets: 90%-100%
Distribution	**Distribution**
Plasma protein binding: 20%-25% Onset of action: 30 min-2 h with oral dosage form Peak action: 2-6 h with oral dosage form Concentrates in most body tissues Therapeutic plasma concentration: 0.5-2 ng/ml Crosses blood-brain barrier Crosses placenta	Highly bound to albumin: 86%-97% Onset of action: 1-4 h with oral dosage form Peak action: 6-12 h with oral dosage form Therapeutic plasma concentrations: 10-25 ng/ml
Biotransformation	**Biotransformation**
Small amount metabolized in liver Half-life: 1½-2 days Two major metabolites: digoxigenin mono-digitoxiside; digoxigenin bis-digitoxiside	Metabolized in liver Half-life: 5-9 days Major metabolite: digoxin
Excretion	**Excretion**
Primarily excreted by kidneys Excreted in unchanged state	Unmetabolized drug excreted in bile; reabsorbed and recycled to liver until complete metabolism occurs Excretion independent of renal function

TABLE 31–2
Prototype and Major Drug in Category

Drug Name	Dosage and Route of Administration	Nursing Considerations

DIGOXIN
HOW SUPPLIED
Lanoxin tablets
  125 µg (0.125 mg) scored tablets
  250 µg (0.25 mg) scored tablets
  500 µg (0.5 mg) scored tablets
Lanoxicaps (liquid digoxin in capsules)
  50 µg (0.05 mg)
  100 µg (0.1 mg)
  200 µg (0.2 mg)
Lanoxin elixir pediatric
  50 µg (0.05 mg)/ml
Lanoxin injection
  500 µg (0.5 mg) in 2 ml
Lanoxin injection pediatric
  100 µg (0.1 mg)/ml
	Dosage is highly individualized and based on age, renal function, and lean body weight.
	ADULTS
	Loading
	Oral: 0.75-1.25 mg in divided doses
	IV: 0.5-1.0 mg in divided doses
	Maintenance
	Oral: 0.25-0.5 mg/d
	IV: 0.25 mg/d
	ADULTS >65
	Maintenance: 0.125 mg/d
	PREMATURE INFANTS
	Loading IV: 0.025 mg/kg divided into three doses over 24 h
	Maintenance IV: 0.01 mg/kg/d divided into q12h doses
	NEONATES <1 MO
	Loading
	Oral: 0.035 mg/kg/d in divided doses q8h
	IV: 0.02-0.03 mg/kg/d divided over 24 h
	Maintenance: 0.01 mg/kg/d orally in divided doses q12h
		Assess
		Obtain baseline heart rate and rhythm and blood pressure values.
		Question client about past use of cardiac glycosides before administering loading dose.
		Ask client about existing renal problems.
		Determine if client is pregnant; cardiac glycosides are classified as Pregnancy Category C.
		
		Implement
		Doublecheck prescribed dose.
		Use care not to confuse digoxin and digitoxin.
		Divide loading dose over first 24 h unless prescribed otherwise.
		Take apical-radial pulse for full minute before administering loading dose if pulse deficit exists.
		Direct IV injection is administered undiluted or diluted in D_5W or sodium chloride (0.9%) solution.
		Tablets may be crushed and mixed with food or fluid.
		Measure elixir dosage forms with specially calibrated droppers supplied with drug.
		Take radial pulse for full minute before administering maintenance dose.

CHILDREN 1 MO-2 Y *Loading* Oral: 0.035-0.06 mg/kg/d divided into three doses IV: 0.03-0.05 mg/kg/d in divided doses *Maintenance:* 0.01-0.02 mg/kg/d orally in divided doses q12h	**CHILDREN >2 Y** *Loading* Oral: 0.02-0.04 mg/kg/d in divided doses q8h IV: 0.015-0.035 mg/kg/d in divided doses *Maintenance:* 0.012 mg/kg/d orally in divided doses q12h	**Monitor** Monitor intake and output ratio during digitalization period. Monitor electrolyte levels. Monitor client closely for signs of toxicity (e.g., nausea, vomiting, anorexia, bradycardia, arrhythmias, confusion, headache, depression). **Evaluate** Record and report significant changes in client's status. Therapeutic serum concentration level is 0.5-2.0 ng/ml.
DIGITOXIN (CRYSTODIGIN) **HOW SUPPLIED** 0.05 mg scored tablets 0.1 mg scored tablets	**ADULTS** *Loading* Oral: 0.2 mg bid (slow digitalization) Oral: 0.6 mg initially, followed by 0.4 mg and then 0.2 mg at intervals of 4-6 h *Maintenance:* 0.05-0.3 mg orally daily	**Implement** Take apical pulse for 1 full min before administering. If prescribed by IM route, inject deep into gluteal muscle. Inject no more than 0.4 mg into any single IM site. Protect drug from light. Store at controlled room temperatures (15°-30° C). Store in airtight container. **Evaluate** Therapeutic serum concentration level is 15-25 ng/ml.

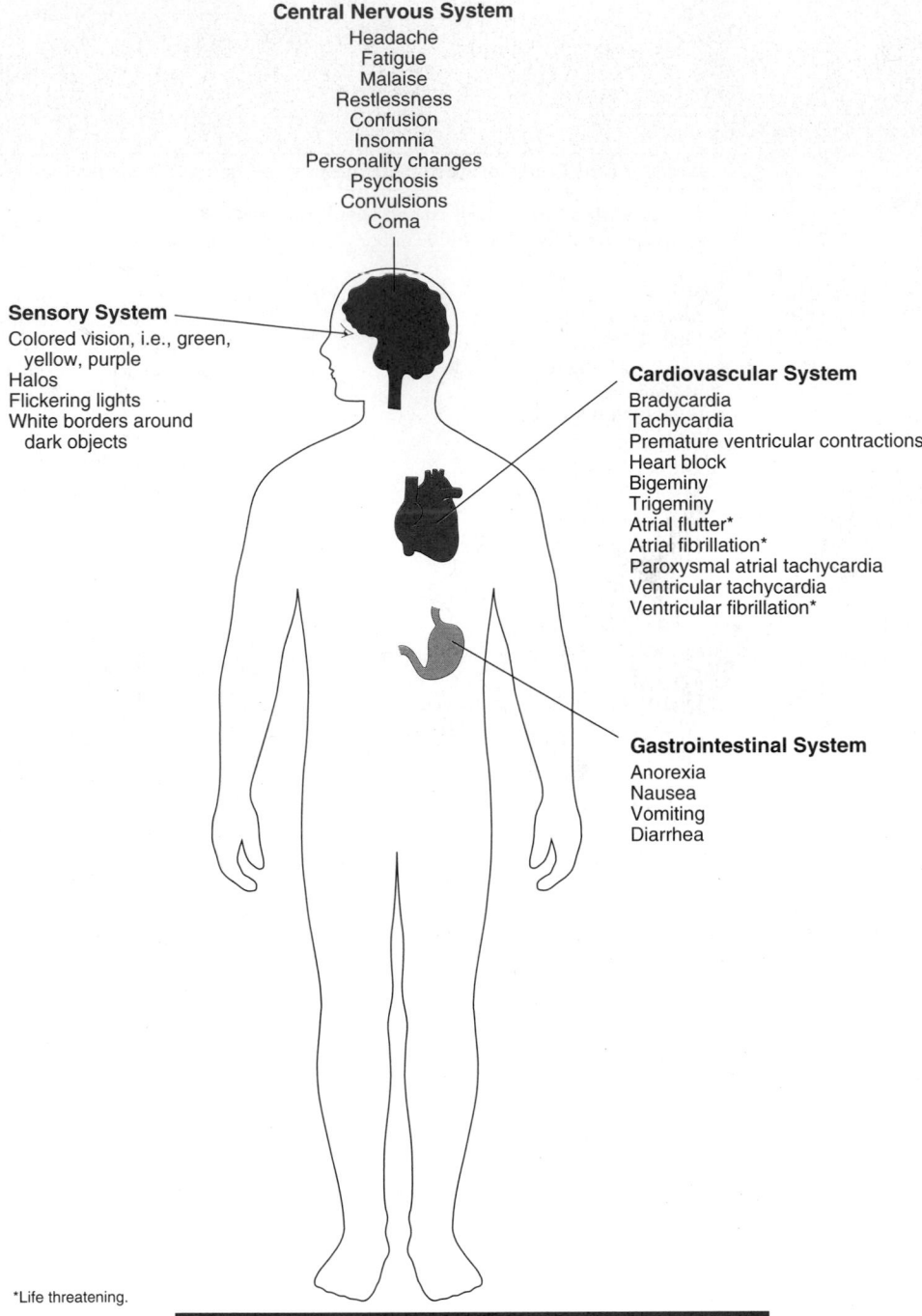

Central Nervous System
Headache
Fatigue
Malaise
Restlessness
Confusion
Insomnia
Personality changes
Psychosis
Convulsions
Coma

Sensory System
Colored vision, i.e., green,
  yellow, purple
Halos
Flickering lights
White borders around
  dark objects

Cardiovascular System
Bradycardia
Tachycardia
Premature ventricular contractions
Heart block
Bigeminy
Trigeminy
Atrial flutter*
Atrial fibrillation*
Paroxysmal atrial tachycardia
Ventricular tachycardia
Ventricular fibrillation*

Gastrointestinal System
Anorexia
Nausea
Vomiting
Diarrhea

*Life threatening.

FIGURE 31–2   Clinical manifestations of digitalis toxicity.

fibrillation, are possible. All cardiac changes are detected best by the ECG.[4,17]

MEDICAL MANAGEMENT OF DRUG TOXICITY Stopping the drug is the first step in managing toxicity. Further treatment depends on the manifestations of the toxicity. If the symptoms of digitalis toxicity become life threatening, digoxin immune fab (ovine) (Digibind) is administered to neutralize the drug (Fig. 31–2).

Digoxin immune fab is composed of digoxin-binding fragments derived from ovine antidigoxin antibodies. The drug attaches itself to unbound digoxin. As active extra-

cellular digoxin levels fall as a result of the binding process, digoxin is released from its receptor sites on cells. The newly released digoxin is also bound to the antibody.

Reversal of the signs and symptoms of digitalis toxicity usually occurs within 30 minutes and complete resolution of symptoms within 3 to 4 hours. Digoxin immune fab is excreted in the urine and has a biologic half-life of 9 to 10 hours. Total elimination of digoxin immune fab from the body may take from 15 hours to 1 week, depending on the renal function of the client. Clients requiring redigitalization must wait 2 to 3 days until any remaining digoxin immune fab is cleared from their body.[18,19]

Contraindications and Precautions Cardiac glycoside use is contraindicated in clients with ventricular fibrillation. In addition, these drugs should be used with caution in clients with renal impairment and/or electrolyte imbalances. These individuals develop digitalis toxicity and/or arrhythmias more frequently.[15]

Interactions Administration of cardiac glycosides must be monitored carefully since drug-drug and drug-nutrient interactions can occur (Table 31–3).

DRUG-DRUG INTERACTIONS The most common drug-drug interactions are reduced absorption and enhanced bioavailability of cardiac glycosides. Any client with an alteration in GI, cardiac, renal, or liver function is at risk of an adverse drug interaction.[20] Drug therapy in these individuals should be monitored carefully and drug dosage modified as needed.

Several drug categories potentially can produce serious drug-drug interactions with cardiac glycosides: diuretics, antacids, antibiotics, and other cardiac drugs. Some cardiac arrhythmias are treated successfully with a combination of digoxin and quinidine sulfate. However, adding quinidine sulfate (Quinidex, Cin-Quin) to the drug regimen of a client already receiving digoxin causes the digoxin levels to rise, often to toxicity levels. The serum

TABLE 31–3

Drugs that Interact with Cardiac Glycosides

Drug Name/ Category	Effects on Cardiac Glycosides	Mechanism Involved	Nursing Considerations
Quinidine sulfate (Quinidex)	Serum digoxin and digitoxin levels rise.	Renal excretion of digoxin inhibited Nonrenal clearance of digoxin reduced Digoxin displaced from tissue-binding sites	Maintenance dose of cardiac glycoside should be reduced. Monitor renal function and cardiac status. Monitor serum digoxin levels. Serum digoxin levels usually return to baseline level 48-72 h after quinidine is discontinued. Monitor for signs and symptoms of digoxin toxicity. Quinidine should not be discontinued suddenly.
Amiodarone (Cordarone)	Serum levels of digoxin rise during loading doses of amiodarone.	Total body clearance of digoxin reduced Volume distribution of glycoside affected Nonrenal clearance of digoxin decreased	Monitor serum digoxin levels. Monitor renal function. Monitor for signs and symptoms of digoxin toxicity for 1-3 wk after amiodarone is started since amiodarone has an unusually long half-life.
Calcium channel blockers (verapamil, diltiazem)	Serum digoxin level increase.	Renal and nonrenal clearance of digoxin reduced Volume of distribution reduced	Assess for bradycardia. Monitor serum digoxin levels. Elevation of serum glycoside levels may take 1 wk to appear with verapamil. Glycoside dose should be reduced by one third to one half. Monitor ECG for AV nodal depression or prolonged PR interval.
Potassium-wasting thiazide and loop diuretics (furosemide, chlorothiazide)	Hypokalemia increases sensitivity of myocardium to glycoside	Low plasma K$^+$ level caused by diuretics leads to increased myocardial uptake of glycoside Tubular secretion of digoxin reduced	Monitor K$^+$ levels. Assess for signs and symptoms of hypokalemia. Consult with physician about use of K$^+$ supplements. Encourage dietary intake of K$^+$.
Antacids	Serum level of glycoside decreases.	Calcium, magnesium, and aluminum antacids bind with digoxin, impairing absorption of drug	Administer digoxin first. Administer antacid 2-4 h later. Teach client proper administration technique.
Antilipidemic agents (cholestyramine colestipol)	Concentration of glycoside decreases.	Absorption of digoxin diminished	Give antilipidemic agent at least 2 h before digoxin. Monitor serum digoxin levels. Digoxin dose may be increased.

digoxin concentration begins to rise early in the treatment with quinidine sulfate, and it returns to a baseline level approximately 48 to 72 hours after quinidine sulfate is discontinued. When the client is receiving both of these drugs, the digoxin maintenance dose should be reduced. Quinidine sulfate should not be discontinued abruptly; the resultant drop in serum digoxin can precipitate cardiac failure. Studies have shown that digitoxin also interacts with quinidine sulfate but less extensively.

Calcium channel blockers such as verapamil (Calan, Isoptin) and diltiazem (Cardizem, Dilacor) interact with digoxin to increase the serum concentration level of digoxin. As with quinidine sulfate, it is recommended that the digoxin dose be decreased while the client is receiving both types of drugs.

Excessive reduction in the heart rate occurs when β-adrenergic blockers interact with cardiac glycosides. This drug-drug interaction is additive in nature; both drugs have similar effects on the heart rate, and the combination produces an increased effect. The β-adrenergic blocker can worsen cardiac failure because of its negative inotropic action.

Toxicity is a significant hazard when a thiazide or loop diuretic and a digitalis glycoside are given concurrently. These diuretics cause a loss of potassium from the body, resulting in a drop in serum potassium levels. A low serum potassium level can increase the myocardial uptake of digitalis and reduce the tubular secretion of digoxin, increasing the half-life of the drug. Any physical condition or drug that lowers serum potassium levels has the same potential of predisposing the client to digitalis toxicity.

The oral absorption of glycosides can be severely reduced by antacids that contain aluminum, magnesium, and calcium. Kaolin-pectin, an antidiarrheal mixture, can also reduce absorption. These drugs should be administered at different times to ensure adequate absorption, or digoxin capsules instead of tablets should be prescribed. Cholestyramine, an antilipidemic agent, also significantly reduces absorption of cardiac glycosides. Cholestyramine and digoxin should be given 2 to 4 hours apart.

Antibiotics such as an aminoglycoside and erythromycin alter the action of digoxin in the body. Oral aminoglycosides decrease the effect of the cardiac glycoside by altering its absorption. Serum levels of digoxin should be monitored carefully since separating the times of administration for these drugs does not avoid interaction. Conversely, erythromycin increases the effects of digoxin.[20–22]

Drug-Nutrient Interactions Even though food in the stomach delays the absorption of digoxin, administering the drug with meals is not contraindicated. However, some foods should be avoided since they significantly alter its absorption and action. For example, bran in the diet decreases the concentration of the drug. Hypokalemia induced by the ingestion of large amounts of natural licorice may enhance the action of cardiac glycosides and cause drug toxicity. If the client's diet is high in vitamin D, a hypercalcemic state may be induced. Hypercalcemia can potentiate the effects of the cardiac glycoside and produce cardiac arrhythmias. Digoxin-induced anorexia does occur with some clients. This is usually an indication of an adverse reaction to the drug, and medical intervention is required.[22,23]

OTHER CARDIAC GLYCOSIDE DRUG

Digitoxin is the other cardiac glycoside. This drug is from the foxglove plant, *D. purpurea*. It is rarely used but does provide an alternative drug for oral therapy of CHF. Although digoxin and digitoxin have identical mechanisms of actions, digitoxin differs from the prototype in several ways.

Digitoxin is completely absorbed and extensively recycled through the liver and bowel. It has a greater plasma protein–binding capacity and a much longer half-life than digoxin; thus digitoxin has a slower onset of action. Most of digitoxin is eliminated by hepatic metabolism and is excreted in the urine as a cardiac-inactive metabolite. Some of the drug is excreted unchanged in the urine.

Hepatic function is an important consideration for clients receiving this drug. Since digitoxin naturally remains in the body longer, dosage adjustment and careful assessment for toxicity are important.

LIFE-SPAN CONSIDERATIONS

Cardiac glycosides are used in children for the same indications as for adults. The response to a given dose varies with age, size, and renal and/or liver function. As in adults, the dosage must be individualized. Digoxin is the cardiac glycoside most frequently used with children. Divided daily doses of digoxin should be given to infants and children younger than 10 years of age; adult dosages adjusted to the child's weight should be given to children older than 10. Neonates vary in tolerance of digoxin, depending on their degree of maturity. Premature and immature infants are especially sensitive to the effects of the drug.

Since very small doses are given to children, each dose should be verified with another nurse before it is administered. As with the adult, a pulse range for the child is established by the physician or institution. Usually the cardiac glycoside is withheld if the pulse is below 90 to 110 in an infant or small child.[24]

Since digoxin crosses the placental barrier, fetal monitoring is essential. In addition, digoxin is excreted in breast milk. Concentrations of digoxin found in breast milk may equal those in maternal blood. Careful monitoring of the infant is required.

Digoxin is widely used in older adults. The pharmacokinetics of digoxin are altered with age. Absorption is slower and peak concentration time delayed. The volume of distribution is reduced in proportion to the diminished lean body mass. In addition, because these individuals may have age-related alterations in hepatic and liver function, the half-life of digoxin is prolonged. Thus the elderly client is predisposed to digitalis toxicity.

Dosages are frequently reduced because of decreased liver and/or kidney function, decreased lean body weight, and advanced cardiac disease. Loading doses are proportionally less for the elderly client, with 0.01 mg/kg a commonly seen dose. Maintenance dosages should be based on renal function.

Serum concentrations drawn at least 6 hours after drug administration can be used as a guide to future treatment.

Generally the older adult can be maintained on as little as 0.065 mg/d.[25] In elderly clients with renal failure and/or receiving concurrent administration of other cardiac drugs such as quinidine sulfate, nifedipine (Procardia), or verapamil (Calan, Isoptin), dosages may be reduced by as much as 50%. See Table 31–3 for drugs that interact with cardiac glycosides.

SUMMARY

Cardiac or digitalis glycosides are naturally occurring compounds obtained from the leaves of *D. purpurea* (purple foxglove) and *D. lanata* (white foxglove). They are among the oldest prescription drugs. Cardiac glycosides are prescribed to treat congestive heart failure, atrial fibrillation and flutter, and paroxysmal atrial tachycardia.

When administered in therapeutic doses, cardiac glycosides increase the force of cardiac contraction and improve cardiac output, improving the delivery of oxygen to body tissues and organs. This improved cardiac performance reduces the physiologic changes produced by the failing heart.

Nursing care focuses on the initiation of the prescribed drug therapy and evaluation of the client's response to the drug. The intensity of the nursing care varies with the client's baseline status, type of drug prescribed, route of administration prescribed, and concomitant uses of other drugs.

REFERENCES

1. Aronson, J.K. (1985). *An account of the foxglove and its medical uses, 1785-1985.* New York: Oxford University Press.
2. Price, S.A., & Wilson, L.M. (1992). *Pathophysiology: Clinical concepts of disease processes* (4th ed.). St. Louis: Mosby–Year Book.
3. Nagelhout, J.J. (1991). Pharmacologic treatment of heart failure. *Nursing Clinics of North America, 26,* 401-415.
4. Schwertz, D.W., & Plano, M.R. (1990). New inotropic drugs for treatment of congestive heart failure. *Cardiovascular Nursing, 26*(2), 7-11.
5. Wright, S.M. (1990). Pathophysiology of congestive heart failure. *Journal of Cardiovascular Nursing, 4*(3), 1-16.
6. Murphy, T.G., & Bennett, E.J. (1992). Low-tech, high-touch perfusion assessment. *American Journal of Nursing, 92,* 36-40, 42, 44, 46.
7. Galvao, M. (1990). Role of angiotensin-converting enzyme inhibitors in congestive heart failure. *Heart and Lung: Journal of Critical Care, 19,* 505-513.
8. Kelleher, R.M. (1989). Cardiac drugs: New inotropes. *Critical Care Nursing Clinics of North America, 1,* 391-397.
9. Kelly, R.A. (1990). Cardiac glycosides and congestive heart failure. *American Journal of Cardiology, 65*(10), 10E-16E.
10. Schron, E.B., & Friedman, L.M. (1990). Cardiovascular options for the 1990s. *Geriatric Nursing: American Journal of Care for the Aging, 11,* 187-190.
11. Stanley, R. (1990). Drug therapy of heart failure. *Journal of Cardiovascular Nursing, 4*(3), 17-34.
12. Smith, C.M., & Reynard, A.M. (1992). *Textbook of pharmacology.* Philadelphia: W.B. Saunders.
13. Pagana, K.D., & Pagana, T.J. (1992). *Mosby's diagnostic and laboratory test reference.* St. Louis: Mosby–Year Book.
14. Excerpta Medica, Inc. (1990). *The internist's compendium of drug therapy.* Lawrenceville, NJ: CORE Publishing Division.
15. U.S. Food and Drug Administration (1993). *1993 Physicians' genr$_x$.* New York: Data Pharmaceutica.
16. Williams, R., Brater, C., & Mordenti, J. (Eds.). (1990). *Rational therapeutics: A clinical pharmacologic guide for the health professional.* New York: Marcel Dekker.
17. Manoguerra, A.S. (1990). Digoxin therapy. *Emergency, 22*(10), 27, 29-31.
18. Riddle, K., & Lee, A.J. (1989). Drug update Digibind: Emergency treatment for digitalis toxicity. *Journal of Emergency Nursing, 15,* 266-268.
19. Schakenbach, L., & Arft, P. (1989). Digoxin toxicity treated with digibind. *Critical Care Nurse, 9*(5), 16-17, 20, 22.
20. Porterfield, L.M., & Porterfield, J.G. (1990). How digoxin interacts with other drugs: A practical guide. *Nursing 90, 20*(1), 50-51.
21. Porterfield, L.M., & Porterfield, J.G. (1990). Understanding cardiovascular drug interactions. *Focus on Critical Care, 17,* 412-416.
22. Mathewson, M.K. (1989). Drug interaction. *Critical Care Nurse, 8*(4), 86-88, 90-93.
23. Litteral, J. (1990). What are the clinically important drug-nutrient interactions? *Pediatric Nursing, 6,* 594-596.
24. Baker, L.K. (1992). Pharmacologic manipulation of preload, afterload, and contractility in the young. *Journal of Cardiovascular Nursing, 6*(3), 12-29.
25. Stolley, J.M., Buckwalter, K.C., & Fjordbak, B. (1990). Iatrogenesis in the elderly: Drug-related problems. *Journal of Gerontological Nursing, 17*(9), 12-17.

BIBLIOGRAPHY

Abrams, W.B. (1990). Cardiovascular drugs in the elderly. *Chest: The Cardiopulmonary Journal, 98,* 980-986.

Dennison, R.D. (1990). Understanding the four determinants of cardiac output—Heart rate, preload, afterload, and contractility. *Nursing 90, 20*(7), 34-42.

Dobbs, J., O'Neill, C., Deshmukh, A., Nicholson, & Dobbs, S. (1991). Serum concentration monitoring of cardiac glycosides. *Clinical Pharmacokinetics, 20,* 175-193.

Feagins, C., & Daniel, D. (1991). Management of congestive heart failure in the home setting: A guide to clinical management and patient education. *Journal of Home Health Care Practice, 4*(1), 31-37.

Jarvis, C. (1992). *Physical examination and health assessment.* Philadelphia: W.B. Saunders.

Jessup, M., Lakatta, E.G., Leier, C.V., & Santinga, J.T. (1990). Managing CHF in the older patient. *Patient Care, 24*(5), 55-58, 61-62, 65.

Kennedy, G. (1990). Captopril in the treatment of chronic CHF. *Critical Care Nurse, 10*(2), 39-42, 44, 46.

Kieber, F., Niemoller, L., Fischer, M., & Doering, W. (1991). Influence of severity of heart failure on the efficacy of angiotensin-converting enzyme inhibition. *American Journal of Cardiology, 68*(14), 121D-126D.

Kruck, F. (1991). Acute and long term effects of loop diuretics in heart failure. *Drugs, 41*(Suppl 3), 60-68.

Northridge, D.B., & Dargie, H.J. (1990). Quinapril in chronic heart failure. *American Journal of Hypertension, 3*(11), 2838-2878.

CHAPTER 32

Antiarrhythmic Drugs

KIM LITWACK • ROBERT J. KIZIOR • NORMA L. PINNELL

⚙ **Classification of Antiarrhythmic Drugs**
LEARNING OBJECTIVE: Summarize general characteristics of the various classes of antiarrhythmic drugs.
KEY TERM: Membrane stabilizer

⚙ **Nursing Considerations**
LEARNING OBJECTIVE: Develop a plan of care for a client requiring antiarrhythmic drug therapy.

⚙ **Class Ia Antiarrhythmic Drugs**
LEARNING OBJECTIVES:
Describe the pharmacodynamic and pharmacokinetic properties of class Ia antiarrhythmic drugs.
Identify common undesired clinical responses associated with class Ia antiarrhythmic drugs.
List class Ia antiarrhythmic drugs.
KEY TERMS:
Cinchonism, torsades de pointes

⚙ **Class Ib Antiarrhythmic Drugs**
LEARNING OBJECTIVES:
Describe the pharmacodynamic and pharmacokinetic properties of class Ib antiarrhythmic drugs.
Identify common undesired clinical responses associated with class Ib antiarrhythmic drugs.
Differentiate between class Ia and class Ib antiarrhythmic drugs.

⚙ **Class Ic Antiarrhythmic Drugs**
LEARNING OBJECTIVES:
Describe the pharmacodynamic and pharmacokinetic properties of class Ic antiarrhythmic drugs.
Identify common undesired clinical responses associated with class Ic antiarrhythmic drugs.

⚙ **Class I Antiarrhythmic Drugs**
LEARNING OBJECTIVES:
Describe the pharmacodynamic and pharmacokinetic properties of class I antiarrhythmic drugs.
Identify common undesired clinical responses associated with class I antiarrhythmic drugs.

⚙ **Class II Antiarrhythmic Drugs**
LEARNING OBJECTIVES:
Describe the pharmacodynamic and pharmacokinetic properties of class II antiarrhythmic drugs.
Identify common undesired clinical responses associated with class II antiarrhythmic drugs.
Discuss other therapeutic uses for propranolol, the prototype drug for class II.

⚙ **Class III Antiarrhythmic Drugs**
LEARNING OBJECTIVES:
Describe the pharmacodynamic and pharmacokinetic properties of class III antiarrhythmic drugs.
Identify common undesired clinical responses associated with class III antiarrhythmic drugs.

⚙ **Class IV Antiarrhythmic Drugs**
LEARNING OBJECTIVES:
Describe the pharmacodynamic and pharmacokinetic properties of class IV antiarrhythmic drugs.
Identify common undesired clinical responses associated with class IV antiarrhythmic drugs.
Discuss other therapeutic uses for verapamil, the prototype drug for class IV.

⚙ **Miscellaneous Antiarrhythmic Drugs**
LEARNING OBJECTIVE: Describe other antiarrhythmic drugs.

*C*ardiac arrhythmias are disorders of rate, rhythm, impulse generation, or impulse conduction within the heart. A normal heartbeat is initiated in the sinoatrial (SA) node and follows a consistent pathway of depolarization through the atria, atrioventricular (AV) node, His-Purkinje system, and ventricular myocardium. Electric depolarization of the heart normally is followed by atrial and then ventricular muscular contraction. Numerous factors can cause disturbances in heartbeat, including hypoxia, electrolyte imbalance, trauma, inflammation, and drugs. One way of categorizing arrhythmias follows: abnormal rates of sinus rhythm, abnormal sites of impulse initiation, or disturbances in conduction pathways.[1] (See box for summary of some of the different types of arrhythmias.)

This chapter presents information on the major classes of antiarrhythmic drugs. Prototypes for each class are described and specific drug-related nursing interventions provided.

CLASSIFICATION OF ANTIARRHYTHMIC DRUGS

Antiarrhythmic drugs are usually grouped into six classes, depending on their action and effect on the cardiac electric properties. Most antiarrhythmic drugs seem to preferentially depress areas exhibiting abnormal pacemaker activity or conduction while having little effect on healthy cardiac tissue.

Class I

Class I antiarrhythmic drugs, also referred to as **membrane stabilizers,** affect sodium channels. Because of their differing effects on sodium channels, drugs in this group are subdivided into three subgroups.

Drugs in **class Ia** include quinidine, procainamide, and disopyramide. These drugs apparently block the rapid inward flux of sodium ions. By allowing fewer sodium ions to pass through the cardiac membrane, membrane responsiveness is reduced and depolarization slowed. **Class Ib** includes lidocaine, tocainide, phenytoin, and mexiletine. These drugs control ventricular arrhythmias and decrease ventricular conduction automaticity by blocking both activated and inactivated sodium channels. The relative selectivity of these drugs for inactivated sodium channels explains their affinity for diseased cardiac tissue. Unlike drugs in Class Ia, these drugs have little

effect on membrane responsiveness. **Class Ic** contains the newest class I antiarrhythmic drugs (e.g., flecainide, lorcainide, and propafenone). These drugs decrease myocardial membrane responsiveness to sodium, slowing conduction velocity.[2,3] A relatively new drug, moricizine hydrochloride, is classified as a class I antiarrhythmic drug.

Class II

Class II antiarrhythmic drugs are the β-adrenergic blockers. This group includes propranolol, acebutolol, and esmolol. These drugs block myocardial β-adrenergic receptors, reducing or antagonizing the actions of endogenous, circulating catecholamines. Class II drugs also have direct membrane effects: at high concentrations they block sodium channels and depress membrane responsiveness. These drugs depress both automaticity and conduction of cardiac impulses. They decrease heart rate and produce vasodilation; this action decreases blood pressure and reduces myocardial oxygen requirements.[3]

Since not all class II drugs are specific to β_1-receptors, their antagonism of β_2-receptors may produce bronchospasm and bronchoconstriction, particularly in asthmatic clients. Newer drugs (i.e., esmolol, metoprolol, acebutolol, and atenolol) are β_1 specific; thus they avoid the risks of pulmonary complications.

Class III

Class III antiarrhythmic drugs include bretylium, amiodarone, and sotalol. These drugs control supraventricular and ventricular arrhythmias by reducing the refractory period and action potential duration without affecting conduction time or depressing cardiac contractility.[4,5]

Class IV

Class IV antiarrhythmic drugs include the calcium channel blockers, specifically verapamil and IV diltiazem. These drugs inhibit the inward passage of calcium ions across cardiac membranes. Class IV drugs help control supraventricular tachyarrhythmias, especially those involving the AV node.[4,5]

CONCEPT REVIEW

Antiarrhythmic drugs are classified into six major classes. Drugs in class I (i.e., Ia, Ib, and Ic) slow the rate of impulse conduction by blocking cardiac sodium channels. Class II drugs block myocardial β-adrenergic receptors. Class III drugs specifically prolong refractoriness; and drugs in class IV inhibit passage of calcium across cardiac cell membranes.

▦ NURSING CONSIDERATIONS

The purpose of antiarrhythmic therapy is to alleviate symptoms, restore hemodynamic stability, and prevent recurring arrhythmias.

Assessing During the **health history** seek information about the client's current cardiovascular status. Ask about sleep and rest patterns, strength and endurance, and ability to perform activities of daily living. Question the client about anorexia, nausea, and vomiting. Complete a risk factor analysis and determine the client's knowledge of the disease process and treatment modalities. Review the client's chart for documentation of a cardiac history and pertinent diagnostic studies (e.g., serum electrolyte levels, serum acid-base level).

During the **physical assessment** check the vital signs and examine the result of the electrocardiogram (ECG). Auscultate the lungs for rales. Check for signs of mental changes (e.g., confusion, disorientation, memory loss, or changes in the level of consciousness). These changes can be associated with decreased cardiac output.

Diagnosing Potential nursing diagnoses for the client receiving or requiring antiarrhythmic therapy incude the following:
- Knowledge deficit regarding treatment plan.
- Anxiety related to disease process or dependence on drug therapy.
- Activity intolerance related to decreased oxygenation.
- High risk for noncompliance related to economic stress of long-term drug therapy.
- High risk for injury related to hypotension associated with drug therapy.
- Alteration in bowel elimination, diarrhea or constipation, related to drug therapy.

Planning In acute care settings much of the plan of care is directed toward achieving hemodynamic and respiratory stability. In an ambulatory setting the client ideally is well controlled, and the focus of the plan is on client education and maintenance of health.

Planning requires the establishment of expected outcomes specific to the individual client. Appropriate outcomes follow:
- Client experiences decreased episodes of dyspnea, angina, and arrhythmias.
- Client demonstrates a measurable increase in activity tolerance.
- Client identifies factors affecting activity intolerance.
- Client participates in treatment plan.
- Client verbalizes an understanding of the disease process.
- Client verbalizes decreased levels of anxiety.

Implementing If the arrhythmia is acute and the client is symptomatic, initial interventions are directed toward prompt recognition of the arrhythmia, elimination of any readily identifiable cause, and administration of the appropriate antiarrhythmic drug. Usually in the acute situation drugs are administered intravenously to allow rapid stabilization and normalization of cardiac functions.

If the arrhythmia is chronic, nursing actions are directed toward client teaching to reinforce the treatment plan. Assess the client's compliance and his or her understanding of the disease process.

Evaluating In the acute care setting ongoing evaluation of cardiopulmonary stability is necessary. Effectiveness of medical therapy is based on symptomatology, ECG results, and therapeutic serum levels of the prescribed drugs. Use the expected client outcomes to guide evaluation of nursing interventions. If the outcomes have been met, the diagnosis is resolved. If, despite interventions, the outcome is not met, reevaluate the nursing interventions or redefine the outcomes. In an ambulatory setting evaluate the client for tolerance of therapy, possible undesired clinical responses from the drugs, and the status of the underlying disease process.

CLASS IA ANTIARRHYTHMIC DRUGS

As indicated previously, class Ia antiarrhythmic drugs act on receptors in the cardiac sodium channels to reduce sodium entry during cardiac membrane depolarization.

CLASS IA ANTIARRHYTHMIC PROTOTYPE

QUINIDINE

Quinidine is a natural alkaloid.

Pharmacotherapeutics Quinidine (e.g., Quinaglute Dura-Tabs, Quinidex Extentabs) is used to control acute and chronic supraventricular arrhythmias. Its use is indicated in the prevention of supraventricular tachyarrhythmias, including atrial fibrillation, paroxysmal atrial tachycardia (PAT), and other atrial arrhythmias. Quinidine is also used to suppress premature ventricular contractions (PVCs).[6]

Pharmacokinetics Quinidine is rapidly absorbed after oral administration. Peak plasma levels after oral administration depend on the dosage form used (i.e., 1 to 3 hours after quinidine sulfate and up to 5 hours after quinidine gluconate). Duration of action is usually 6 to 8 hours or longer. After intramuscular (IM) administration, maximal effects may occur within $\frac{1}{2}$ to $1\frac{1}{2}$ hours. Onset of action occurs more quickly after intravenous (IV) administration. The therapeutic serum level of quinidine is 2 to 6 μg/ml.

Quinidine is primarily metabolized (60% to 80% of a dose) in the liver. The drug is hydroxylated to inactive metabolites and is eliminated in the urine. As a result of this dependence on hepatic metabolism and renal clearance, toxic levels may occur in clients with impaired hepatic or renal function. Elimination half-life ranges from 4 to 10 hours, with a mean of 6 to 7 hours.[2,3]

Pharmacodynamics Quinidine suppresses cardiac arrhythmias by depressing myocardial excitability, conduction velocity, and myocardial contractibility. Quinidine also prolongs the effective refractory period.

Pharmaceutics Quinidine is administered orally, IM, and IV. Quinidine is administered over a range of dosages depending on the arrhythmia being treated. Table 32–1 summarizes information on dosage forms, dosages, and route of administration.

Undesired Clinical Responses Quinidine has a low therapeutic index, and undesired clinical responses are predictable if plasma levels become excessive. As plasma concentrations increase above 2 μg/ml, the PR interval, QRS complex, and QT interval become prolonged. Abnormal lengthening of the QT interval is a sign of quinidine toxicity. It is sometimes followed by a rhythm known as **torsades de pointes,** a dangerous arrhythmia that can lead to ventricular fibrillation and death.[2,3]

Common undesired responses associated with quinidine include nausea, vomiting, diarrhea, vague abdominal pain, and anorexia. **Cinchonism** is a unique complex of side effects associated with quinidine toxicity. Manifestations of cinchonism include headaches, tinnitus, visual disturbances, and vertigo.[3] Administration of quinidine can also produce fever, which disappears when the drug is discontinued. Thrombocytopenia is a rare occur-

rence. Platelet counts usually return to normal within 2 to 7 days after drug discontinuation.

In some clients quinidine produces profound hypotension when administered intravenously, probably because of peripheral vasodilation from α-adrenergic blockade. Occasionally clients develop idiosyncratic reactions to quinidine. These reactions include syncope and sudden death. The syncope may reflect the development of ventricular arrhythmias caused by delayed intraventricular conduction of cardiac impulses.[7] Figure 32–1 illustrates

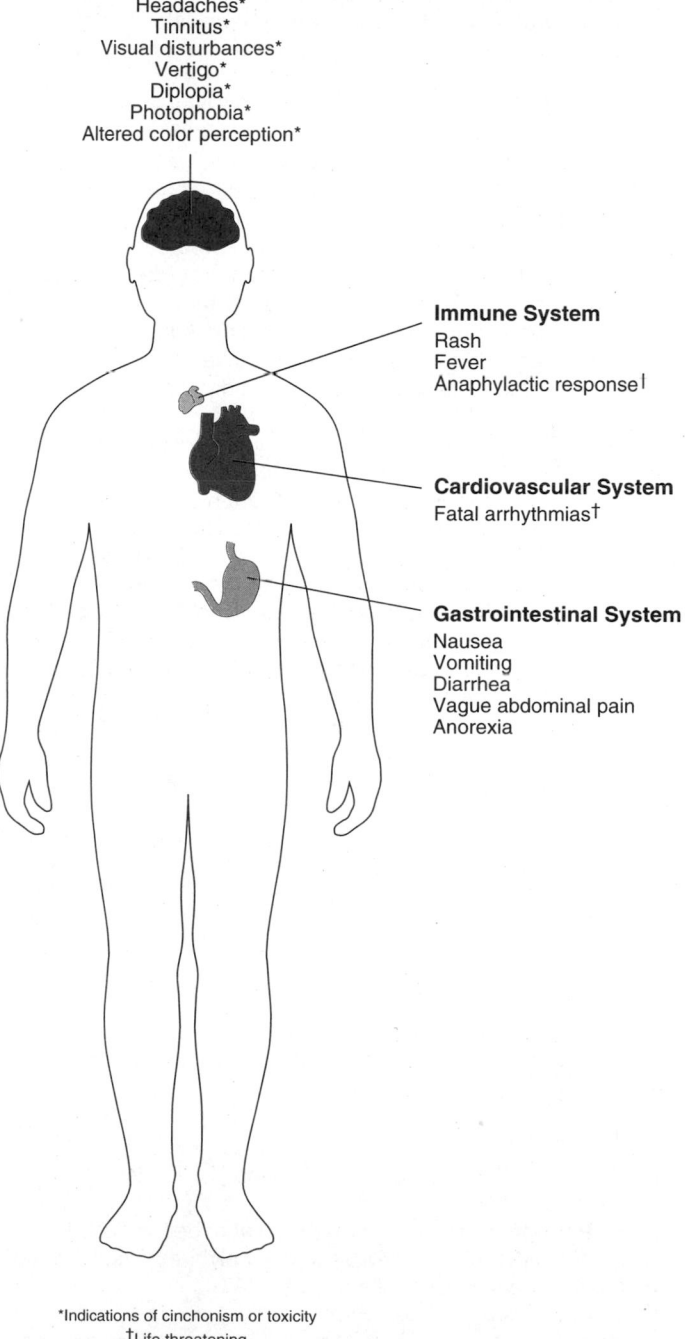

Central Nervous System
Headaches*
Tinnitus*
Visual disturbances*
Vertigo*
Diplopia*
Photophobia*
Altered color perception*

Immune System
Rash
Fever
Anaphylactic response[‖]

Cardiovascular System
Fatal arrhythmias[†]

Gastrointestinal System
Nausea
Vomiting
Diarrhea
Vague abdominal pain
Anorexia

*Indications of cinchonism or toxicity
†Life threatening

FIGURE 32–1   Common undesired clinical responses associated with quinidine.

common undesired clinical responses associated with quinidine.

Contraindications and Precautions Quinidine should not be administered to individuals allergic to it. Its use is not recommended in individuals with a history of prolonged QT intervals and those with evidence of atrioventricular heart block.[7] Quinidine use is also contraindicated in clients with digoxin toxicity. It should be used with caution in clients with myasthenia gravis, a history of thrombocytopenia, or hepatic or renal dysfunction.

Drug-Drug, Drug-Nutrient, Drug-Environment Interactions Quinidine increases the effects of neuromuscular blocking agents, digoxin, and coumadin. On the other hand, drugs such as cimetidine, propranolol, thiazide diuretics, sodium bicarbonate, carbonic anhydrase inhibitors, and antacids increase the effects of quinidine. Barbiturates, phenytoin, rifampin, and nifedipine may decrease the effects of quinidine. In addition, combining quinidine with other drugs with vasodilating properties (e.g., nitroglycerin) can exaggerate orthostatic hypotension.

Quinidine may be administered without regard to meals or food. The presence of food may decrease gastrointestinal (GI) symptoms produced by the drug. Some quinidine preparations (e.g., quinidine sulfate) must be dispensed in tight, light-resistant containers. Most preparations may be stored at controlled room temperature between 15° and 30° C.[7]

Life-Span Considerations Quinidine should be used during pregnancy only when potential benefits outweigh the risk. Caution should be used when administering the drug to nursing women. Safe use in children has not been established. Elderly clients may have age-related renal impairment and thus require dosage reduction.

Specific Drug-Related Nursing Considerations Clients beginning therapy with quinidine require ECG monitoring to assess for correction of the arrhythmia and to monitor for any increase in PR or QRS intervals. If PR or QRS intervals increase, the drug dose usually is reduced. Once long-term therapy is established, serum levels should be followed.

If the drug is administered intravenously, injection must be done slowly and the drug diluted to prevent hypotension and myocardial depression. Be aware that IM injection of the drug is painful. Aspirate before the IM injection to avoid inadvertent IV injection. Table 32–1 provides additional nursing considerations.

CLASS IA ANTIARRHYTHMIC PROTOTYPE

PROCAINAMIDE

Procainamide (Procan SR, Pronestyl) is also a major class Ia antiarrhythmic drug.

Pharmacotherapeutics Procainamide is used primarily in the treatment of ventricular arrhythmias. It is also used to treat atrial fibrillation and PAT.

Pharmacokinetics Procainamide is well absorbed from the entire small intestinal surface and is rapidly absorbed after IM administration. Peak plasma levels after oral administration occur within 90 to 120 minutes and within 15 to 60 minutes after IM administration. Peak levels occur within several minutes after an IV infusion is started. The therapeutic serum level for procainamide is 3 to 10 μg/ml. However, higher levels may be needed in clients with sustained ventricular tachycardia.

Procainamide is metabolized in the liver to an active metabolite, N-acetyl procainamide (NAPA). Approximately 25% of the dose is converted to NAPA. This percentage may increase in clients with impaired renal function. The elimination half-life of procainamide is 2½ to 4½ hours.[7]

Pharmacodynamics Procainamide, like quinidine, depresses myocardial excitability, conduction velocity, and automaticity. Procainamide also prolongs the effective refractory period but usually does not have any effect on myocardial contractility.[6]

Pharmaceutics Procainamide is administered orally as tablets, capsules, and extended-release tablets. It is available in parenteral solution for IM injection or IV infusion. Table 32–1 summarizes information about dosage forms, dosages, and routes of administration.

Undesired Clinical Responses Hypotension, especially in the conscious client, may occur after IV administration. It occurs less frequently with IM administration and rarely after oral administration. Because of transiently high plasma levels, procainamide may also produce central nervous system (CNS) depression or tremor. Blood dyscrasias (agranulocytosis, bone marrow depression, neutropenia, thrombocytopenia) have been reported at a rate of approximately 0.5%. Most have been noticed within the first 12 weeks of therapy.

During long-term therapy or in clients who are slow acetylators, procainamide may cause a systemic lupus erythematosus–like syndrome. This syndrome, which is characterized by fever, chills, joint pain or swelling, pain with breathing, and sometimes arthritis, occurs in approximately 30% of the clients. This condition is usually reversible with discontinuation of the drug. Approximately 80% of the clients receiving procainamide show an increased antinuclear antibody (ANA) titer.

Like quinidine, procainamide can cause progressive widening of the QRS complex, prolonged QT and PR intervals, and increasing AV block. If these situations develop, the drug should be held or discontinued. Other side effects reported with procainamide include diarrhea, loss of appetite, dizziness, or lightheadedness. Rarely confusion, depression, or hallucinations occur.[5,7,8]

Contraindications and Precautions Use of procainamide is contraindicated in clients hypersensitive to the drug. Its use also is contraindicated in clients with complete heart block, lupus erythematosus, and torsades de pointes (a ventricular arrhythmia). Procainamide should be used with caution in clients with bundle branch block, severe digoxin toxicity, congestive heart failure (CHF), myasthenia gravis, or impaired renal impairment.

Drug-Drug and Drug-Environment Interactions When administered concurrently, quinidine may increase the effects and plasma levels of procainamide, thus increasing procainamide toxicity. Lidocaine administered concurrently may cause an additive cardiodepressive action, which may lead to conduction abnormalities. In addition, the effects of neuromuscular blocking agents may be prolonged or enhanced when administered concurrently.

Procainamide should be stored at room temperature. It must be protected from excessive heat and moisture.

Life-Span Considerations Procainamide is classified as a Pregnancy Category C drug. Although it crosses the placenta, it is unknown if it can cause fetal harm. The drug and its metabolite are excreted in breast milk. Safety and efficacy in children have not been established. Elderly clients may be more susceptible to hypotensive effects and may require lower doses or longer dosing intervals.

Specific Drug-Related Nursing Considerations Obtain a baseline ECG and vital signs. In addition, assess the ECG throughout therapy. Monitor the serum drug levels to prevent toxicity, and assess for polyarthralgia, arthritis, pleuritic pain, fever, neuralgia, and skin lesions since these symptoms suggest drug-induced systemic lupus erythematosus. During IV administration the client should be recumbent and the blood pressure monitored continuously. Table 32–1 provides additional nursing considerations associated with procainamide.

MISCELLANEOUS DRUGS IN CATEGORY

Disopyramide (Norpace, Norpace CR) has actions similar to those of quinidine. It is used in the treatment of ventricular arrhythmias (e.g., ventricular tachycardia and supraventricular tachycardia). Most common undesired responses associated with disopyramide are dry mouth, blurred vision, constipation, urinary retention, or hesitancy, which are anticholinergic effects of the drug. Additionally, disopyramide has a negative inotropic effect, which may lead to severe hypotension or exacerbation of CHF. Table 32–1 summarizes information on dosage forms, dosages, routes of administration, and nursing considerations.

TABLE 32–1

Class Ia Antiarrhythmic Drugs: Clinical Considerations

Drug Name	Dosage and Route of Administration	Nursing Considerations
QUINIDINE **Quinidine Sulfate** (Quinora, Quinidex Extentabs) **How Supplied** Tablets: 200, 300 mg Tablets (extended release): 300 mg **Quinidine Gluconate** (Quinaglute Dura-Tabs, Quinalan) **How Supplied** Tablets (sustained release): 324, 330 mg Injection: 80 mg/ml, 10-ml vial **Quinidine Polygalacturonate** (Cardioquin) **How Supplied** Tablets: 275 mg	**Quinidine Sulfate** **ADULTS** *Initial Dose* Premature atrial, ventricular contractions: oral—200–300 tid or qid Paroxysmal supraventricular tachycardia: oral—400–600 mg q2-3h until arrhythmia terminated Atrial flutter: oral—individual titration Conversion of atrial fibrillation: oral—200 mg q2-3h for five to eight doses, increased if needed and tolerated *Maintenance Dose* **ADULTS** Oral: 200–300 tid or qid **CHILDREN** Oral: 30 mg/kg/24 h or 900 mg/m²/24 h in five divided doses **Quinidine Sulfate Extended Release** **ADULTS** Oral: 300–600 mg q8-12h **Quinidine Gluconate** **ADULTS** Oral: 324–648 mg q6-12h IM: initial dose, 600 mg; then 400 mg as often as q2h prn IV: 800 mg in 40 ml 5% dextrose solution given at rate of 1 ml/min with ECG and blood pressure (BP) monitoring **Quinidine Polygalacturonate** **ADULTS** Oral: initial dose, 275–825 mg q3-4h for three or four doses; additional doses increased by 137.5–275 mg every third or fourth dose until restoration of rhythm; usual maintenance dose, 275 mg bid or tid **CHILDREN** Oral: 8.25 mg/kg five times/d	**Assess** Assess for preexisting conditions that may preclude use of drug (e.g., complete AV block; digoxin toxicity, hypotension, congestive heart failure). Determine if client is pregnant; quinidine is classified as Pregnancy Category C drug. Determine if client is breast-feeding; drug is distributed in breast milk. **Implement** Do not crush or chew sustained-release tablets. Administer with food if gastrointestinal (GI) upset occurs. Use parenteral solution only if clear and colorless. Solution is stable for 24 h at room temperature when diluted with 5% dextrose solution. For IV infusion, dilute 800 mg with 40 ml 5% dextrose solution to provide concentration of 16 mg/ml. Administer IV dosage with client in supine position. Monitor BP and ECG continuously during IV infusion. For IV injection, administer at rate of 1 ml (16 mg)/min. Take BP and apical-radial pulse above administering oral dosage form. **Monitor** Monitor for undesired clinical responses (e.g., abdominal pain, nausea, diarrhea, vomiting, hypotension, tinnitus, blurred vision, vertigo, sweating, headache, hearing loss). Monitor input and output (I&O), complete blood count (CBC), serum potassium, hepatic/renal function studies. Monitor blood pressure. **Evaluate** Evaluate for control of arrhythmias being treated.

Table continued on following page.

TABLE 32–1 *Continued*
Class Ia Antiarrhythmic Drugs: Clinical Considerations

Drug Name	Dosage and Route of Administration	Nursing Considerations
PROCAINAMIDE HYDROCHLORIDE Pronestyl **HOW SUPPLIED** Tablets: 250, 375, 500 mg Capsules: 250, 375, 500 mg Injection: 500 mg/ml vials	**ADULTS** *Atrial Arrhythmias* Oral: initial dose, 1.25 g; then 750 mg in 1–2 h; then 500 mg–1 g q2-3h as needed; usual maintenance dose, 500 mg–1 g q4-6h as needed *Ventricular Arrhythmias* Oral: 50 mg/kg/d in eight equally divided doses *Usual Parenteral Dosage* IM: 50 mg/kg/d in divided doses q3-6h IV: example of IV loading dose—1 g in 100 ml 5% dextrose solution infused over 1 h followed by maintenance dose of 2–6 mg/min (2 g in 250 ml 5% dextrose solution equals 8 mg/ml concentration) **CHILDREN** Oral: 15–50 mg/kg/d divided q3-6h IM: 20–30 mg/kg/d divided q4-6h IV: loading dose, 3–6 mg/kg; maintenance dose, 20–80 μg/kg/min continuous infusion	**Assess** See quinidine with following exception: unknown whether or not drug is distributed in milk. **Implement** Do not crush or break sustained-released tablets. Use solution only if clear, colorless, or light yellow. Discard solution if discolored or darkened or if it contains precipitate. For direct IV injection, dilute with 5% dextrose solution; administer at rate not to exceed 25–50 mg/min. For IV infusion, add 1 g to 250–500 ml 5% dextrose solution; provides concentration of 2–4 mg/ml. Infuse at 1–3 ml/min. Check blood pressure q5-10min during infusion. If blood pressure falls in excess of 15 mm Hg, discontinue drug and contact physician. Take BP and apical-radial pulse before administering oral dosage form. Administer drug at regular intervals throughout 24 h. Teach client to contact physician if fever, joint pain, or signs of upper respiratory infection occur. Instruct client not to use nasal decongestants or over-the-counter (OTC) cold preparations without consulting primary care provider.
Procainamide Hydrochloride Extended Release (Procan SR, Pronestyl-SR) **HOW SUPPLIED** Tablets: 250, 500, 750, 1000 mg	**Procainamide Hydrochoride Extended Release** *Ventricular Arrhythmias* Oral: 50 mg/kg/d in four divided doses	**Monitor** Monitor for undesired clinical responses (e.g., abdominal pain, nausea, diarrhea, vomiting, dizziness, weakness, rapid ventricular rate, fever, joint pain, pleuritic chest pain). Monitor I&O. **Evaluate** Monitor for therapeutic serum level (3–10 μg/ml).

CONCEPT REVIEW

Quinidine and procainamide are the prototype drugs for Class Ia.

Quinidine is associated with many undesirable clinical responses, including ECG changes (e.g., prolonged PR interval, QRS complex, and QT interval), nausea, vomiting, and diarrhea.

Procainamide may cause the same ECG changes as quinidine. In addition, procainamide may produce hypotension, especially after IV administration of the drug. Blood dyscrasias and systemic lupus erythematosus–like syndrome may occur with prolonged therapy.

CLASS IB ANTIARRHYTHMIC DRUGS

Class Ib antiarrhythmic drugs control ventricular arrhythmias and decrease ventricular conduction automaticity by blocking both activated and inactivated sodium channels.

CLASS IB ANTIARRHYTHMIC PROTOTYPE

LIDOCAINE HYDROCHLORIDE

Lidocaine hydrochloride is also used for production of local or regional anesthesia.

Pharmacotherapeutics Lidocaine (Xylocaine) use is indicated in the acute management of ventricular arrhythmias such as those resulting from acute myocardial infarction or digoxin toxicity.

TABLE 32–1 *Continued*

Class Ia Antiarrhythmic Drugs: Clinical Considerations

Drug Name	Dosage and Route of Administration	Nursing Considerations
Disopyramide Phosphate (Norpace, Norpace CR) **HOW SUPPLIED** Capsules: 100, 150 mg Extended-release capsules: 100, 150 mg	**ADULTS** Initial dose, 300 mg (200 mg for weight <50 kg) Usual maintenance dose: 150 mg q6h (100 mg q6-8h for weight <50 kgh) Maximum dose: up to 1600 mg/d NOTE: Creatinine clearance value is used to adjust dosage interval in patient with renal impairment. **CHILDREN** <1 y: 10–30 mg/kg/d in four divided doses 1–4 y: 10–20 mg/kg/d in four divided doses 4–12 y: 10–15 mg/kg/d in four divided doses 12–18 y: 6–15 mg/kg/d in four divided doses **Extended Release** 300 mg q12h (200 mg q12h for weight <50 kg) for maintenance use only	**Assess** See quinidine with following exception: assess for preexisting conditions that may preclude use (e.g., urinary retention, second- or third-degree AV block, cardiogenic shock, narrow-angle glaucoma). **Implement** Drug may be administered without regard to food and is absorbed best 1 h before or 2 h after meals. Do not crush or break extended-release capsules. Before administering drug, instruct client to void to reduce risk of urinary retention. Take BP and apical-radial pulse before administering oral dosage form. Teach client to report shortness of breath or cough. Instruct client not to use nasal decongestants or OTC cold preparations without consulting primary care provider. **Monitor** Monitor I&O. Monitor for indications of CHF or evidence of edema. Monitor for undesired clinical responses (e.g., dry mouth, dry nose and eyes, urinary hesitancy, constipation, blurred vision, dizziness, fatigue, muscle weakness). **Evaluate** Monitor for therapeutic serum level (2–8 µg/ml).

Pharmacokinetics Lidocaine is ineffective when administered orally since 60% to 70% of the drug is metabolized by the liver before reaching systemic circulation. After IM administration, lidocaine achieves a therapeutic serum level within 5 to 15 minutes. The duration of action is approximately 2 hours. With an IV injection, lidocaine's onset of action is within minutes (45 to 90 seconds). The duration of action after an IV bolus injection is 10 to 20 minutes. Therefore lidocaine usually is administered by IV infusion to maintain a sustained therapeutic serum level of 1.5 to 6 µg/ml.

Lidocaine is extensively metabolized in the liver to two active metabolites, which also have convulsant properties. Lidocaine is excreted primarily in the urine. Therefore the drug must be used with caution in clients with impaired hepatic or kidney function or conditions such as CHF that can alter liver function. The half-life of lidocaine is 1 to 2 hours; it is increased to 3 hours or longer after prolonged IV infusion.[9]

Pharmacodynamics Lidocaine has a direct action in the ventricles, decreasing depolarization, automaticity, and excitability. The effective refractory period of Purkinje fibers and ventricular muscle is also decreased. Lidocaine has no effect on the autonomic nervous system. In addition, contractility, AV conduction velocity, and absolute refractory period are not altered by lidocaine.[10]

Pharmaceutics Lidocaine is available in parenteral solutions for IV and IM administration. Table 32–2 summarizes information on dosage forms, dosages, and routes of administration.

Undesired Clinical Responses The incidence of side effects associated with lidocaine is largely correlated with the serum concentration of the drug. The therapeutic serum concentration of 1.5 to 6 µg/ml may be associated with mild CNS or cardiovascular effects (e.g., anxiety, nervousness, dizziness, drowsiness, feelings of heat, cold, or numbness). As the serum level increases to 6 to 8 µg/ml, the client may experience blurred vision, nausea or vomiting, tinnitus, tremors, or twitching. When serum concentrations are greater than 8 µg/ml, respiratory depression, severe dizziness, fainting, hypotension, decreased cardiac output, bradycardia, seizures, and coma are manifested.

Contraindications and Precautions Lidocaine use should be avoided in clients with Adams-Stokes syndrome or severe heart block, including AV and SA block. Its use is also contraindicated in clients with hypersensitivity to local anesthetics. Lidocaine should be used with caution in clients with CHF, incomplete heart block, sinus bradycardia, Wolff-Parkinson-White syndrome, or reduced hepatic blood flow.

Drug-Drug and Drug-Environment Interactions
Lidocaine may prolong or potentiate the effects of neuromuscular blocking drugs. β-Blockers increase the serum concentration of lidocaine, thus increasing the risk of toxicity. Cimetidine may decrease renal clearance of lidocaine, increasing serum concentration and the risk of toxicity. Phenytoin may have an added cardiac depressant effect, may increase hepatic metabolism, and may decrease the serum concentration of lidocaine.

Lidocaine solutions must be stored at controlled room temperatures, 15° to 30° C.[7]

Life-Span Considerations Lidocaine is classified as a Pregnancy Category B drug. It readily crosses the placental barrier. Lidocaine is also excreted in breast milk. It should be used during pregnancy only if its use is clearly indicated; caution must be used when it is administered to a nursing mother. Safety and efficacy in children have not been established. Elderly clients are more prone to undesired responses.

Specific Drug-Related Nursing Considerations
Since lidocaine use is indicated for acute suppression of ventricular arrhythmias, continuous ECG monitoring is essential. PR and QRS intervals should be assessed since an increase in the intervals may require reduction of the infusion rate or discontinuation of the drug. Table 32–2 provides additional nursing considerations.

MISCELLANEOUS DRUGS IN CATEGORY

Phenytoin, which was presented as a prototype drug in Chapter 21, is used to treat digoxin-induced arrhythmias. Phenytoin reduces automaticity, especially in the ventricles, and increases AV conduction. The most common undesired responses are sedation, ataxia, and nystagmus. If administered too rapidly by IV infusion, it may cause hypotension, arrhythmias, and cardiac arrest.

Mexiletine hydrochloride depresses the automaticity and refractoriness or ventricular tissue and shortens repolarization, which reduces irritability and prevents ectopic beats. Mexiletine is used to treat symptomatic ventricular arrhythmias (e.g., sustained ventricular tachycardia). The most common undesired clinical responses are nausea, vomiting, diarrhea, constipation, tremor, dizziness, sleep disturbances, psychosis, and convulsions. Several of the undesired clinical responses are dose related and reversible by reducing the dosage or discontinuing the drug. Since mexiletine is metabolized by the liver, clients with liver dysfunction need lower dosages. The toxic serum level is greater than 2 μg/ml. If the client is taking cimetidine, it can slow the clearance of mexiletine and thus elevate serum levels of the cardiac drug.[11]

Tocainide hydrochloride may slow the heart rate. It reduces the rate and rise of phase 0 of the action potential and shortens the duration of the phase. It is used to treat ventricular arrhythmias. The most common undesired clinical responses are nausea, vomiting, anorexia, lightheadedness, tremors, vertigo, and numbness. Coughing, wheezing, shortness of breath, bradycardia, and hypotension may also occur. In addition, tocainide may cause serious blood dyscrasias, pulmonary fibrosis, and pneumonitis. The toxic serum level is greater than 15 μg/ml. Tocainide enhances the effects of digoxin, quinidine, and β-blockers. The drug should be ad-

ministered with food to prevent nausea and abdominal upset. The client should be taught to count the pulse and to notify the primary care provider if the rate is less than 60 beats per minute after two consecutive counts.[11] Table 32–2 contains additional information about Class Ib antiarrhythmic drugs.

CONCEPT REVIEW

Lidocaine has a direct action in the ventricles, decreasing depolarization, automaticity, and excitability. The effective refractory period of Purkinje fibers and ventricular muscle is also decreased.

Lidocaine is associated with undesired clinical responses associated with drug serum concentrations. Low serum concentrations may produce mild CNS or cardiovascular effects, whereas high serum concentrations may produce seizures, respiratory depression, and coma.

CLASS IC ANTIARRHYTHMIC DRUGS

Class Ic antiarrhythmic drugs decrease myocardial membrane responsiveness to sodium, slowing conduction velocity. This is a relatively new group of antiarrhythmic drugs.

CLASS IC ANTIARRHYTHMIC PROTOTYPE
FLECAINIDE ACETATE

Flecainide (Tambocor) is the prototype of class Ic antiarrhythmic drugs.

Pharmacotherapeutics Flecainide is effective for suppressing supraventricular and ventricular tachyarrhythmias.

Pharmacokinetics Flecainide is almost completely absorbed from the GI tract after oral administration. Peak serum concentration levels occur within approximately 3 hours. The therapeutic serum level is 0.2 to 1 μg/ml. Toxic serum levels are greater than 1 μg/ml. Flecainide is metabolized in the liver and is eliminated primarily in the urine. The elimination half-life is approximately 20 hours, with a range of 12 to 27 hours.

Pharmacodynamics Flecainide slows atrial, AV, Purkinje, and intraventricular conduction, decreasing myocardial excitability, conduction velocity, and automaticity. Flecainide also prolongs the refractory period. It has little effect on repolarization.[11]

Pharmaceutics Flecainide is administered orally. It is available in tablets. Table 32–3 contains information about dosage forms, dosages, and routes of administration.

Undesired Clinical Responses Common undesired clinical responses include nausea, constipation, dizziness, lightheadedness, visual disturbances, fatigue, and headaches. The most serious side effect is a proarrhythmic effect, including worsened ventricular tachycardia, increased PVCs, or new supraventricular arrhythmias. Flecainide may also produce ECG changes

TABLE 32–2

367

Class Ib Antiarrhythmic Drugs: Clinical Considerations

Drug Name	Dosage and Route of Administration	Nursing Considerations
LIDOCAINE (Xylocaine) **HOW SUPPLIED** Automatic injection device: 300 mg Ampules: 10, 40 mg/ml Vials: 10, 20, 40, 100, 200 mg/ml Syringes: 10, 20, 40, 100, 200 mg/ml IV infusion: 2, 4, 8 mg/ml	ADULTS IM: 300 mg; may repeat in 60–90 min IV: loading dose, 1 mg/kg (usually 50–100 mg); may repeat in 5 min; maximum, 300 mg in any 1-h period IV infusion: after loading dose, 20–50 μg/kg/min at rate of 1–4 mg/min CHILDREN IV: loading dose, 1 mg/kg; may repeat in 5 min; maximum, 3 mg/kg total dose IV infusion: after loading dose, 20–50 μg/kg/min at rate of 1–4 mg/min	**Assess** Assess for preexisting conditions that may preclude lidocaine's use (e.g., Adams-Stokes syndrome, severe heart block, CHF, reduced hepatic blood flow). Determine if client is pregnant; lidocaine is classified as a Pregnancy Category B drug. Determine if client is nursing; drug is distributed in breast milk. **Implement** For IM injections, use 10% (100 mg/ml) concentration; drug is labeled for IM use. Administer IM injection in deltoid muscle. For IV injection, use 1% (10 mg/ml) or 2% (20 mg/ml) concentration. Administer IV injection at 25–50 mg/min rate. For IV infusion, prepare solution by adding 1 g to 1 L 5% dextrose solution for 1 mg/ml or 0.1% concentration. Administer IV infusion at rate of 1–4 mg/min. Assess for pain at site of IM injection or IV infusion. Monitor ECG constantly during IV infusion. **Monitor** Monitor I&O and electrolyte serum level. Monitor blood pressure for hypotension. Monitor for undesired clinical responses (e.g., anxiety, nervousness, dizziness, drowsiness, numbness, blurred vision, nausea, decreased cardiac output, bradycardia). **Evaluate** Monitor for therapeutic serum level (1.5–6 μg/ml).
Phenytoin (Dilantin) **HOW SUPPLIED** Injection: 50 mg/ml	ADULTS IV injection: 50–100 mg q10-15min as needed but not to exceed 15 mg/kg total dose; administer slowly at rate not to exceed 50 mg/min	See Table 21–1. **Implement** Administer by direct IV injection; do not add to IV infusion. Administer IV injection at rate that does not exceed 50 mg/min in adults. Administer 50 mg over 2–3 min for elderly clients. IV injection is very painful; flush vein with sterile saline solution through same IV needle or catheter after each IV injection.
Mexiletine Hydrochloride (Mexitil) **HOW SUPPLIED** Capsules: 150, 200, 250 mg	ADULTS Oral: initial dose, 200 mg q8h (400 mg, then 200 mg in 8 h for rapid control of ventricular arrhythmia); usual maintenance dose, 200–300 mg q8h; maximum, 400 mg q8h; lower doses may be required in patients with severe liver impairment	**Assess** Assess for preexisting conditions that may preclude mexiletene's use (e.g., cardiogenic shock, second- or third-degree AV block, CHF, sick sinus syndrome). Determine if client is pregnant or breast-feeding; drug is distributed in breast milk and classified in Pregnancy Category B. **Implement** Administer with food or antacid to reduce GI distress. Assess pulse for irregular rate, strength, weakness. **Monitor** Monitor for dizziness, syncope, hand tremor, and GI distress, which are indications of undesired responses. **Evaluate** Check for therapeutic serum level of 0.5–2 μg/ml.
Tocainide Hydrochloride (Tonocard) **HOW SUPPLIED** Tablets: 400, 600 mg	ADULTS Oral: initial dose, 400 mg q8h; usual maintenance dose, 1200–1800 mg/d in three divided doses; clients with renal or hepatic impairment may be adequately treated with <1200 mg/d	**Assess** Determine if client is pregnant; tocainide is classified as a Pregnancy Category C drug. Determine if client has preexisting conditions that preclude use of drug (e.g., hypersensitivity to local anesthetics, second- or third-degree block, CHF). **Implement** Do not crush or break film-coated tablets. Administer drug with food to decrease GI upset. Assess sleeping client for night sweats. Assess hand movement for sign of tremor. **Monitor** Monitor fluid and electrolyte serum levels. Monitor ECG for cardiac changes. **Evaluate** Check for therapeutic serum level (3–10 μg/ml).

(e.g., prolonged PR intervals or widening of the QRS complex).[12]

Contraindications and Precautions Flecainide should not be used in clients with second- or third-degree AV block or right bundle branch block associated with a left hemiblock without a pacemaker. It should be used with caution in clients with impaired liver function or sick sinus syndrome.

Drug-Drug Interactions Taken concurrently with digoxin or β-blockers, flecainide may cause sinus bradycardia. Disopyramide and verapamil use may increase the risk of CHF since all of these drugs have a negative isotropic effect. Flecainide can potentiate the action of amiodarone when administered concurrently. Serum levels of both drugs must be monitored carefully.

Life-Span Considerations Flecainide is classified as a Pregnancy Category C drug. It is distributed in breast milk.

Specific Drug-Related Nursing Considerations Review with the client and family signs and symptoms of CHF such as dyspnea, cough, weight gain, and edema. Teach the client how to take a pulse and to notify the primary care provider if his or her pulse falls below 60 or becomes irregular. Table 32–3 contains additional nursing considerations associated with flecainide.

MISCELLANEOUS DRUGS IN CATEGORY

Propafenone hydrochloride (Rythmol) is also classified as a class Ic antiarrhythmic agent for the treatment of ventricular and supraventricular arrhythmias. This drug is an oral sodium channel blocker that reduces upstroke velocity of the action potential and decreases conduction velocity in the atria, ventricles, and Purkinje fibers.

Propafenone is well absorbed from the GI tract, attaining peak plasma concentration within 1 to 3½ hours. The drug is metabolized in the liver to active metabolites and is eliminated in urine and feces. Propafenone's half-life is 2 to 10 hours in most individuals and is 10 to 32 hours in clients who do not metabolize the drug well.

Propafenone use is contraindicated in clients with uncontrolled CHF or bronchospastic disease. It should be used with caution in clients with impaired renal or hepatic function. The most undesired clinical responses are a proarrhythmic effect (e.g., ventricular tachyarrhythmias), angina, bradycardia, and CHF. Other common responses include dizziness, taste change (bitter or metallic), blurred vision, constipation or diarrhea, nausea or vomiting, and unusual tiredness or weakness.[13]

TABLE 32–3

Class Ic Antiarrhythmic Drugs: Clinical Considerations

Drug Name	Dosage and Route of Administration	Nursing Considerations
FLECAINIDE ACETATE (Tambocor) HOW SUPPLIED Tablets: 50, 100, 150 mg	***Paroxysmal Supraventricular Tachycardia or Paroxysmal Atrial Fibrillation or Flutter*** ADULTS Oral: 50 mg q12h; may increase by 50 mg bid q4d; maximum dose, 300 mg/d ***Sustained Ventricular Tachycardia*** ADULTS Oral: 100 mg q12h; may increase by 50 mg bid q4d; maximum dose, 400 g/d; lower doses may be required in patients with severe renal impairment	**Assess** Determine if client has preexisting conditions that preclude drug use (e.g., cardiogenic shock, right bundle branch block, second- or third-degree block). Assess if client is pregnant or breast-feeding; flecainide is classified as a Pregnancy Category C drug and is distributed in breast milk. **Implement** Scored tablets may be crushed. Assess hand movement for sign of tremor. **Monitor** Question client about visual disturbances, headache, GI upset. Monitor I&O and ECG changes. **Evaluate** Monitor for therapeutic serum level of 0.2–1 μg/ml.
Propafenone (Rythmol) HOW SUPPLIED Tablets: 150, 300 mg	ADULTS Oral: initial dose, 150 mg q8h; may increase at minimum of 3–4 d to 225 mg q8h and up to 300 mg q8h if necessary	**Assess** Determine if client is pregnant; drug is classified in Pregnancy Category C. Assess for preexisting conditions that preclude its use (e.g., CHF, cardiogenic shock, disorders of impulse or condition, electrolyte imbalance). **Implement** Scored tablets may be crushed. Give without regard to meals; food may increase serum concentrations. **Monitor** Monitor for undesired clinical responses (e.g., nausea, vomiting, constipation, blurred vision). Monitor ECG for changes. **Evaluate** Check for therapeutic serum level (0.06–1 μg/ml).

Monitor the client's heart sounds and pulses for rate, rhythm, and quality. Assess for indications of agranulocytosis; specifically observe for indications of an infection. Table 32–3 contains additional information about propafenone.

CLASS I ANTIARRHYTHMIC DRUGS

The class I antiarrhythmic category is limited to one primary drug, moricizine hydrochloride.

CLASS I ANTIARRHYTHMIC PROTOTYPE

MORICIZINE HYDROCHLORIDE

Moricizine hydrochloride (Ethmozine) is classified as a class I antiarrhythmic drug. It is a phenothiazine derivative recently approved by the Food and Drug Administration (FDA) for use in the United States.[14]

Pharmacotherapeutics Moricizine is used to suppress documented life-threatening ventricular arrhythmias (e.g., sustained ventricular tachycardia).

Pharmacokinetics Moricizine is well absorbed after oral administration, with peak serum levels occurring within ½ to 2 hours. Moricizine is extensively metabolized in the liver and is eliminated in urine and feces via bile excretion. The elimination half-life for moricizine is 1½ to 3½ hours.

Pharmacodynamics Moricizine resembles class Ia antiarrhythmic drugs in the intensity of its effect on the sodium channel. However, moricizine also shortens the action potential duration in ventricular tissue.[14] It is possible that moricizine has potent local anesthetic activity and a membrane stabilizing effect. It also decreases excitability, conduction velocity, automaticity, and the effective refractory period.

Pharmaceutics Moricizine is administered orally. The suggested dosage is 600 to 900 mg/d in three divided doses. Within this range the dosage may be adjusted in increments of 150 mg/d at 3-day intervals. It is supplied in 200-, 250-, and 300-mg tablets.

Undesired Clinical Responses The drug is well tolerated, with a low incidence of adverse effects.[12] The more serious undesired responses are similar to those that occur with flecainide (e.g., new or exacerbated arrhythmias, CHF, sinus arrest, coma, and respiratory failure). Other common responses include dizziness, blurred vision, diarrhea, dry mouth, headache, nausea, vomiting, and unusual tiredness or weakness.

Contraindications and Precautions Moricizine should not be used in clients with second- or third-degree AV block or right bundle branch block associated with a left hemiblock without a pacemaker. It should be used with caution in clients with impaired liver function or sick sinus syndrome.

Drug-Drug Interactions When they are administered concurrently, cimetidine may increase plasma concentrations of moricizine. If administered concurrently with theophylline, moricizine may increase theophylline clearance and decrease serum theophylline concentration.

Life-Span Considerations Moricizine is classified as a Pregnancy Category B drug. In addition, it is distributed in breast milk.

Specific Drug-Related Nursing Considerations Monitor the ECG for cardiac changes, particularly an increase in PR and QRS intervals. Assess the pulse for strength, weakness, and irregular rate. Inform the client not to discontinue the drug abruptly.

CLASS II ANTIARRHYTHMIC DRUGS

Class II antiarrhythmic drugs are also called *β-adrenergic blockers*. β-Blockers (e.g., propranolol, esmolol, acebutolol) are used to treat hypertension, angina, and cardiac arrhythmias.[7]

CLASS II ANTIARRHYTHMIC PROTOTYPE

PROPRANOLOL

Propranolol (Inderal) is a synthetic drug approved for a variety of medical conditions, including hypertension, angina pectoris, arrhythmias, migraines, myocardial infarction, and hypertrophic subaortic stenosis.

Pharmacotherapeutics Propranolol is used primarily to slow the ventricular response to atrial fibrillation or paroxysmal supraventricular tachycardia. The primary emergency indication for propranolol is to control recurrent ventricular tachycardia, recurrent ventricular fibrillation, or rapid supraventricular arrhythmias refractory to other therapy. PVCs are also suppressed by propranolol.[2]

Pharmacokinetics Propranolol is well absorbed after oral administration. However, systemic bioavailability is low because of significant first-pass metabolism in the liver. Time to peak action is approximately 1 to 1½ hours. Propranolol is metabolized in the liver and eliminated in the urine. Its elimination half-life is 3 to 5 hours.[6]

Pharmacodynamics β-Adrenergic blockers reduce the effect of circulating catecholamines by blocking their ability to bind to β-receptors. Propranolol is a nonselective drug, affecting both β_1- and β_2-receptors. It has a negative inotropic, negative chronotropic, and negative dromotropic effect.[6,15]

Pharmaceutics Propranolol is administered orally or intravenously. The IV route usually is prescribed when the client is unable to take the oral drug or when a rapid observable effect is desired. Table 32–4 contains additional information about dosage forms, dosages, and routes of administration.

Undesired Clinical Responses Major toxic effects of β-blockers are bradycardia and hypotension. Additional symptoms of overdose include severe dizziness or fainting, an irregular heartbeat, AV block, asystole, seizures, respiratory depression, and bronchospasm (especially in individuals with a history of chronic obstructive pulmonary disease [COPD]). Other responses are decreased sexual ability, drowsiness, trouble sleeping, unusual tiredness, weakness, swelling of ankles and feet, shortness of breath, mental depression, and reduced peripheral circulation.[3,7,15] Figure 32–2 illustrates common undesired clinical responses associated with β-adrenergic blockers.

Contraindications and Precautions Use of β_1-blockers is contraindicated in clients with overt cardiac failure, second- or third-degree AV heart block, sinus bradycardia, cardiogenic shock, or hypersensitivity to β-blockers. Since β-blockers are nonselective, their use is

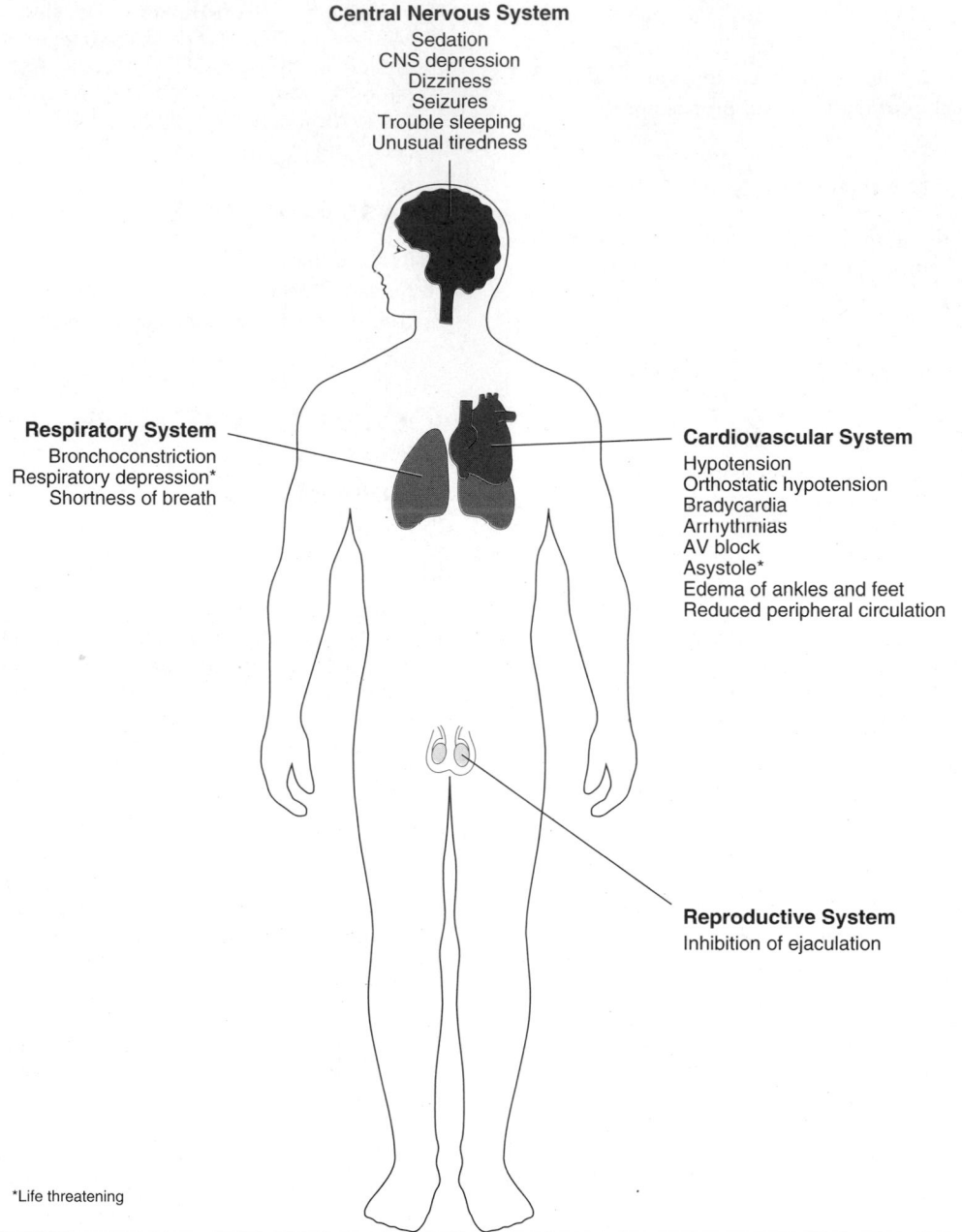

Central Nervous System
Sedation
CNS depression
Dizziness
Seizures
Trouble sleeping
Unusual tiredness

Respiratory System
Bronchoconstriction
Respiratory depression*
Shortness of breath

Cardiovascular System
Hypotension
Orthostatic hypotension
Bradycardia
Arrhythmias
AV block
Asystole*
Edema of ankles and feet
Reduced peripheral circulation

Reproductive System
Inhibition of ejaculation

*Life threatening

FIGURE 32–2   Common undesired clinical responses associated with β-Adrenergic blockers.

contraindicated in clients with bronchial asthma or bronchospasm, including severe COPD. The drug should be used with caution in clients with CHF or a history of mental depression. Because it may mask signs of hypoglycemia, propranolol is used with caution in individuals with diabetes mellitus. It also should be used with caution in clients with hyperthyroidism since it may mask symptoms of tachycardia.[7]

Drug-Drug and Drug-Environment Interactions Concurrent use of propranolol with oral hypoglycemic drugs or insulin may impair glycemic control. Calcium channel blockers (verapamil, diltiazem) may cause symptomatic bradycardia, and nifedipine may produce excessive hypotension. In addition, combining propranolol with other antiarrhythmic drugs such as calcium channel blockers and digitalis may produce profound AV block or increase the pharmacodynamic effects of propranolol. Dopamine, dobutamine, albuterol, and isoetharine administered concurrently may decrease the β-blocking effects of propranolol.

IV solution must be stored at room temperature. The solution should be dispensed in tightly closed, light-resistant containers.[7]

Life-Span Considerations Propranolol is classified as a Pregnancy Category C drug. Since the drug is excreted in breast milk, caution should be exercised when administering it to nursing mothers. Safety and effectiveness in children have not been established. Safety in pregnancy has not been established; therefore use only when benefits clearly outweigh risks.[7]

Specific Drug-Related Nursing Considerations Before the administration of propranolol, assess the client's vital signs and particularly note the heart rate. Instruct the client to take the drug daily, preferably at the same time each day. Remind him or her not to discontinue the drug abruptly; encourage the client to refill prescriptions in a timely manner. Instruct the client to monitor his or her weight weekly and to report any significant weight gain (2 kg). Encourage the client to avoid OTC drugs unless approved by the primary care provider.

MISCELLANEOUS DRUGS IN CATEGORY

Esmolol hydrochloride (Brevibloc) is a beta-1, cardioselective adrenergic blocking drug. It has a rapid onset (within minutes) and short duration of action. The distribution and elimination half-life is 9 minutes. Esmolol is metabolized by esterases located in red blood cells and is excreted in the urine.

Esmolol is especially useful in the management of supraventricular tachycardia. It is also effective in the management of acute myocardial ischemia. Esmolol decreases the heart rate, contractility, and after load, thereby decreasing the oxygen demand of the heart.

Esmolol is administered by bolus injection or continuous IV infusion. Bolus doses of 25 to 35 mg or 500 μg/kg are titrated according to need and general condition of the client. The recommended dilution for continuous IV infusion is two 2.5-g ampules in 500 ml diluent (5% dextrose or 0.9% sodium chloride solution), giving a concentration of 10 mg/ml. Doses greater than 200 μg/kg/min are not recommended.

The most common undesired clinical response is hypotension, characterized by dizziness and sweating. Other side effects include confusion, erythema and swelling at the injection site, cold hands and feet, anxiety, nervousness, headache, or nausea and vomiting.[16]

TABLE 32–4
Class II Antiarrhythmic Drugs: Clinical Considerations

Drug Name	Dosage and Route of Administration	Nursing Considerations
PROPRANOLOL (Inderal) **HOW SUPPLIED** Tablets: 10, 20, 40 mg Solution, oral: 4, 8 mg/ml Injection: 1 mg/ml	**ADULTS** Oral: 10–30 mg tid or qid; dose adjusted as needed IV: 1–3 mg (given at rate not to exceed 1 mg/min); may repeat after 2 min and again in 4 h **CHILDREN** Oral: 0.5–1 mg/kg/d in two to four divided doses IV: 0.01–0.1 mg/kg (up to maximum of 1 mg/dose); repeat q6-8h if necessary	**Assess** Assess for preexisting conditions that preclude use of the drug (e.g., overt cardiac failure, second or third-degree heart block, cardiogenic shock, hypotension). Determine if client is pregnant or breast-feeding; drug is distributed in breast milk and is classified in Pregnancy Category C. **Implement** Scored tablets may be crushed. Administer at same time each day. Administer undiluted for direct injection. Do not exceed 1 mg/min injection rate. For IV infusion, each 1 mg may be diluted in 10 ml 5% dextrose in water. Administer 1 mg over 10–15 min. **Monitor** Monitor for undesired clinical responses (e.g., bradycardia, hypotension, decreased sexual ability, drowsiness, insomnia, tiredness, weakness, edema in ankles and feet, shortness of breath, mental depression, reduces peripheral circulation).
Esmolol (Brevibloc) **HOW SUPPLIED** Injection: 10 mg/ml vials; 250 mg/ml ampules	Dose is established by series of loading and maintenance doses. **ADULTS** IV: loading dose, 0.5 mg/kg/min for 1 min followed by maintenance infusion of 0.05 mg/kg/min for 4 min; sequence repeated with a 0.05-mg increment in maintenance dose if adequate response not observed at end of 5 min; as desired response approached, loading dose may be omitted, increments decreased to 0.025 mg or less, and interval between titration steps increased to 10 min; range of maintenance infusion, 0.05–0.2 mg/kg/min.	**Assess** Determine if client is pregnant; esmolol is classified as Pregnancy Category C drug. **Implement** Use only clear and colorless-to-light yellow solution. After dilution, parenteral solution is stable for 24 h. Discard parenteral solution if it is discolored or if precipitate forms. Administer IV infusion by controlled infusion device. Do not use butterfly needles or small veins. Dilute to concentration of 10 mg/ml or less to prevent vein irritation. Assess BP and apical pulse immediately before drug is administered. If pulse rate is 60/min or below or systolic BP is below 90 mm/Hg, contact primary care provider. **Monitor** See acebutolol.

Table continued on following page.

TABLE 32–4 *Continued*
Class II Antiarrhythmic Drugs: Clinical Considerations

Drug Name	Dosage and Route of Administration	Nursing Considerations
Acebutolol (Sectral) **HOW SUPPLIED** Capsules: 200, 400 mg	ADULTS Oral: initial dose, 200 mg bid; gradually increase dose; usual maintenance dose, 600–1200 mg/d Avoid doses >800 mg/d in the elderly	**Assess** Assess for conditions that may preclude drug's use (e.g., heart failure, cardiogenic shock, heart block greater than first degree, severe bradycadia). Determine if client is pregnant or breast-feeding; acebutolol is distributed in breast milk and is classified as Pregnancy Category B drug. **Implement** Assess BP and pulse before administering drugs. Assess for bradycardia and hypotension during therapy. Assess pulse for strength, weakness, irregular rate. Teach client to rise slowly from lying to sitting position. Teach client to check BP and pulse before taking drug. **Monitor** Monitor for undesired clinical responses (e.g., nausea, dizziness, diaphoresis, headache, fatigue). Monitor ECG for cardiac arrhythmias, particularly shortening of QT interval and prolongation of PR interval.

Acebutolol (Sectral) is a β-adrenergic blocking agent used to control PVCs. It is also used in treatment of supraventricular arrhythmias and ventricular tachycardia. Acebutolol is administered orally, 400 to 1200 mg/d, in divided doses. Table 32–4 provides additional information about β-blockers.

CONCEPT REVIEW

Propranolol is the prototype for class II antiarrhythmic drugs.

Propranolol is associated with many undesired clinical responses, with the major toxic ones bradycardia and hypotension. Bronchospasm may also occur, especially in clients with a history of COPD.

CLASS III ANTIARRHYTHMIC DRUGS

The class III antiarrhythmic drugs are three distinct medications: bretylium, amiodarone, and sotalol.[17,18] Because each drug has multiple actions different from one another, they cannot be used interchangeably.

Bretylium

Bretylium (Bretylol) is used for the prophylaxis and treatment of ventricular fibrillation and life-threatening ventricular arrhythmias refractory to first-line treatment.

Pharmacokinetics After IM injection, the peak serum concentration occurs within 1 hour. After IV administration, antifibrillatory effects occur within minutes, whereas suppression of ventricular arrhythmias occurs 20 minutes to 2 hours after administration. Bretylium is eliminated unchanged in the urine. Its elimination half-life is 5 to 10 hours.

Pharmacodynamics The exact mechanism of action for bretylium is unknown. Its ability to suppress ventricular fibrillation rapidly may be due to a direct effect. Also, the drug causes sympathetic nerve stimulation, which produces an initial release of norepinephrine followed by blockade of norepinephrine release. This blockage may contribute to suppression of ventricular arrhythmias.

Pharmaceutics Bretylium is administered either IM or by IV injection or infusion. When administered IM, no more than 5 ml should be injected at any one site. In addition, injection sites should be rotated to avoid tissue destruction. When administered IV, bretylium is usually diluted in at least 50 ml of 5% dextrose or 0.9% sodium chloride solution. (When used in treating life-threatening ventricular fibrillation, undiluted bretylium is administered as rapidly as possible.) Dosages vary with the type of arrhythmias treated.[2] Table 32–5 contains additional information on dosage forms, dosages, and routes of administration.

Undesired clinical responses Hypotension and orthostatic hypotension occur routinely with the use of bretylium, but rarely is the hypotension symptomatic. Also, an initial increase in the frequency of arrhythmias and transient hypertension may occur because of the initial release of norepinephrine. This response to norepinephrine may last from a few minutes to an hour; it usually is reduced by decreasing the rate of administration. In addition, nausea and vomiting may occur, especially if bretylium is given over less than an 8-minute period.

Contraindications and precautions Bretylium should be used with caution in clients with aortic stenosis or severe pulmonary hypertension and in clients with reduced cardiac output, impaired renal function, or known sensitivity to bretylium.

Drug-drug interactions Digoxin toxicity may be aggravated by the initial release of norepinephrine produced by bretylium. Additionally, procainamide or quinidine may counter the inotropic effect of bretylium and increase hypotension.[2]

Life-span considerations   Studies have not been done in pregnant women, and it is not known if bretylium is excreted in breast milk. Safety and effectiveness in children have not been established.

Specific drug-related nursing considerations   When bretylium is administered intravenously, the recommended dilution is one part bretylium to four parts dextrose or normal saline solution. This is done to prevent the nausea and vomiting associated with rapid IV injection.

Amiodarone Hydrochloride (Cordarone)

The antiarrhythmic drug amiodarone is widely prescribed in the hospital setting.

Pharmacotherapeutics   Amiodarone is used to suppress and prevent recurrent life-threatening ventricular arrhythmias (e.g., ventricular fibrillation, hemodynamically unstable ventricular tachycardia). It is also used for the prophylaxis and treatment of supraventricular arrhythmias refractory to conventional treatment.[19]

Pharmacokinetics   Amiodarone is incompletely absorbed from the GI tract. Peak serum concentration occurs within 3 to 7 hours. However, the onset of action may take from 2 to 3 days to 2 to 3 months, even with loading doses. The therapeutic plasma concentration is 1 to 2.5 μg/ml; however, the therapeutic effect is difficult to predict by plasma concentration, and toxicity may occur even at therapeutic concentrations. The toxic serum level is greater than or equal to 3.5 μg/ml.[11]

Amiodarone is metabolized extensively in the liver to an active metabolite. The main route of elimination is via hepatic excretion into bile. The elimination half-life is biphasic, with an initial half-life of $2\frac{1}{2}$ to 10 days and a terminal half-life of 26 to 107 days.

Pharmacodynamics   Amiodarone prolongs the duration of the action potential of atrial and ventricular muscles and Purkinje fibers. It prolongs the plateau phase of repolarization. The heart rate slows and prolongs the effective refractory period.[11]

Pharmaceutics   Amiodarone is given orally. Usually a loading dose of 600 to 1600 mg is administered for 1 to 3 weeks. This dose is followed by a maintenance dose of 200 to 400 mg/d, depending on the particular arrhythmia being treated. Table 32–5 provides additional information on dosage forms, dosages, and routes of administration.

TABLE 32–5
Class III Antiarrhythmic Drugs: Clinical Considerations

Drug Name	Dosage and Route of Administration
BRETYLIUM (Bretylol) HOW SUPPLIED Injection: 50 mg/ml	ADULTS IM: Initial dose, 5–10 mg/kg undiluted, repeated q1-2h if necessary; usual maintenance dose, 5–10 mg/kg undiluted q6-8h
	Life-threatening Ventricular Fibrillation IV (rapid): 5 mg/kg undiluted, followed by 10 mg/kg q15–30min if necessary, up to a total of 30 mg/kg/d
	Unstable Ventricular Tachycardia IV infusion: initial dose (diluted) 5–10 mg/kg, over 10–30 min; may repeat in 1–2h; usual maintenance dose (diluted), 5–10 mg/kg over 10–30 min q6h or continuous IV infusion of 1–2 mg/min
	Other Ventricular Arrhythmias IV infusion (diluted): initial dose 5–10 mg/kg over 10–30 min repeated q1-2h prn; usual maintenance dose (diluted), 5–10 mg/kg over 10–30 min q6-8h or continuous infusion of 1–2 mg/min
SOTALOL (Betapace) HOW SUPPLIED Tablets: 80, 160, 240 mg	ADULTS Oral: initial dose, 80 mg bid, gradually increased; usual maintenance dose, 160–320 mg/d in two or three divided doses; maximum dose, 480 mg/d (640 mg/d in life-threatening arrhythmias); dosing interval increased in renally impaired clients.
AMIODARONE (Cordarone) HOW SUPPLIED Tablets: 200 mg	ADULTS
	Ventricular arrhythmias Oral: initial dose 800–1600 mg/d in divided doses for 1–3 wk (or longer); reduce dose to 600–800 mg/d for 1 mo, then decrease to usual maintenance dose, 400 mg/d adjusted as necessary
	Supraventricular arrhythmias ADULTS Oral: initial dose 600–800 mg/d for 1 wk, then decrease to 400 mg/d for 3 wk; usual maintenance dose, 200–400 mg/d CHILDREN Oral: initial dose, 10 mg/kg/d for 10 d, then reduce to 5 mg/kg/d for several wk; gradually decrease to lowest maintenance dose, 2.5 mg/kg/d

Undesired clinical responses Common responses associated with amiodarone include neurotoxicity (numbing or tingling in fingers or toes and weakness in arms or legs), ataxia, pulmonary toxicity (pulmonary fibrosis or pneumonitis), new or exacerbated arrhythmia, photosensitivity, constipation, and anorexia. The loss of appetite may lead to weight loss, nausea, and vomiting.

Other side effects include a blue-gray coloring of skin on arms, face, and neck, hypothyroidism or hyperthyroidism, pain and swelling in the scrotal area, and blurred vision. In addition, the client may experience sinus bradycardia, taste disturbances (bitter or metallic taste), dizziness, flushed face, decreased sexual ability, and sexual disinterest.[11]

Contraindications and precautions Amiodarone use is contraindicated in clients without a pacemaker who have pre-existing second- or third-degree AV block, bradycardia with syncope, or sinus node function impairment. It should be used with caution in clients with liver impairment, CHF, hypokalemia, and impaired thyroid function.

Drug-drug and drug-nutrient interactions Amiodarone administration may increase the hypoprothrombinemic effect of warfarin. This effect may persist for several months after amiodarone is discontinued. Concurrent administration with digoxin may increase digoxin serum levels and produce digoxin toxicity. Concurrent administration with phenytoin may increase phenytoin serum levels.

The client should take amiodarone with food.

Interference with laboratory studies Amiodarone alters results of thyroid function studies (thyroid-stimulating hormone) because of the release of inorganic iodine and its interference with thyroxine metabolism.

Life-span considerations Amiodarone is classified as a Pregnancy Category D drug. It is not recommended for use in pregnancy or nursing mothers.

Specific drug-related nursing considerations Instruct the client to have an eye examination every 1 to 2 years. Tell client to avoid prolonged exposure to the sun and to use a sunscreen product with a value greater than skin protection factor (SPF) 15. Monitor liver and thyroid function test results and the ECG while the client is receiving amiodarone; compare the results with baseline findings. Because pneumonitis is possible, advise the client to report cough, fever, painful breathing, or shortness of breath.

Sotalol Hydrochloride (Betapace)

Sotalol was recently released by the FDA for use in the treatment of a variety of ventricular and supraventricular tachyarrhythmias. The drug's dominant action is the result of combined nonselective β-adrenergic antagonism (class II effect) and monophasic prolongation of the action potential duration in all cardiac tissues (class III effect). Sotalol causes less left ventricular depression than propranolol and has a low incidence of toxicity.

Sotalol is absorbed rapidly, with the plasma concentration peaking at 2½ to 4 hours. The drug is excreted unchanged by the kidneys; its average elimination half-life is 12 hours. A ma-

jor undesired clinical response associated with sotalol is torsades de pointes. Sotalol may also cause bradycardia, AV block, CHF, and bronchospasm.[20,21]

CONCEPT REVIEW

Bretylium, amiodarone, and sotalol are three class III antiarrhythmic drugs. The primary action of these drugs is prolongation of the action potential duration in all cardiac tissues.

Bretylium is associated with several undesired clinical responses, including hypotension and postural hypotension; nausea and vomiting may occur with rapid IV infusion.

The most common undesired clinical responses associated with amiodarone are neurotoxicity, ataxia, possible pneumonitis, and new or exacerbated arrhythmias.

Sotalol is a relatively new drug. Its most serious side effect is torsades de pointes.

CLASS IV ANTIARRHYTHMIC DRUGS

Class IV antiarrhythmic drugs are also called *calcium channel blockers* or *calcium channel antagonists*. Of the nine calcium channel blockers available, only verapamil and IV diltiazem are approved for the treatment of arrhythmias. Calcium channel blockers are also indicated for treatment of hypertension and angina pectoris.

CLASS IV ANTIARRHYTHMIC PROTOTYPE

VERAPAMIL

Verapamil is the prototype for class IV antiarrhythmic drugs.[22-24]

Pharmacotherapeutics Verapamil (Calan, Isoptin, Verelan) is used in the treatment and prophylaxis of paroxysmal supraventricular tachycardia. In addition, it is indicated in the treatment of rapid ventricular rates in clients with atrial flutter or fibrillation.

Pharmacokinetics Verapamil is well absorbed from the GI tract but undergoes first-pass metabolism in the liver. Peak serum concentrations occur within 1 to 2 hours when using tablets; this time is prolonged to 5 to 9 hours when using extended-release preparations. The onset of action with oral tablets is 1 to 2 hours; it is usually less than 2 minutes after IV administration. Verapamil is eliminated primarily in the urine. The elimination half-life with oral administration ranges from 4½ to 12 hours and from 2 to 5 hours after IV administration.

Pharmacodynamics Verapamil, like other calcium channel blockers, inhibits calcium ion entry across cell membranes. Thus by causing a reduction of intracellular calcium concentration in cardiac and vascular smooth muscle, the calcium blockers dilate arteries and arterioles. They may decrease heart rate and contractility and slow AV nodal conduction. Verapamil also prolongs the effective refractory period.

Pharmaceutics Verapamil is administered orally or by IV injection. When given orally, its initial dose is 40 to 120 mg three times a day, with a range of 240 to 480 mg/d. Extended-release preparations are approved only for treatment of hypertension.

The usual IV dose is 5 to 10 mg, with a repeat dose of 10 mg in 30 minutes if necessary. IV verampamil must be administered over at least 2 minutes with continuous ECG and blood pressure monitoring. Some clients develop a rapid ventricular rate when experiencing atrial flutter or fibrillation; marked hypotension, bradycardia, or asystole may occur. Table 32–6 provides additional information about dosage forms, dosages, and routes of administration.

Undesired Clinical Responses Undesired clinical responses vary among the various calcium channel blockers. Undesired responses associated with verapamil include skin rash, possible CHF or pulmonary edema, bradycardia, hypotension, edema of feet and ankles, constipation, dizziness or lightheadedness, nausea, and unusual tiredness or weakness. Figure 32–3 illustrates common undesired clinical responses associated with calcium channel blockers.

Contraindications and Precautions Verapamil use is contraindicated in clients with second- or third-degree AV block, SA nodal function impairment (sick sinus syndrome), Wolff-Parkinson-White syndrome accompanied by atrial flutter or fibrillation, or severe hypotension. Caution should be used in clients with extreme bradycardia, heart failure, or hypersensitivity to verapamil.

Drug-Drug Interactions When calcium channel blockers are administered concurrently with β-adrenergic blockers, additive effects may occur. The SA and AV conduction is prolonged, resulting in severe hypotension or bradycardia. Verapamil may increase the serum concentration and toxicity of cyclosporine, quinidine, and digoxin.[25]

Life-Span Considerations Verapamil is classified as a Pregnancy Category C drug. It should be used during pregnancy only when clearly indicated and benefits

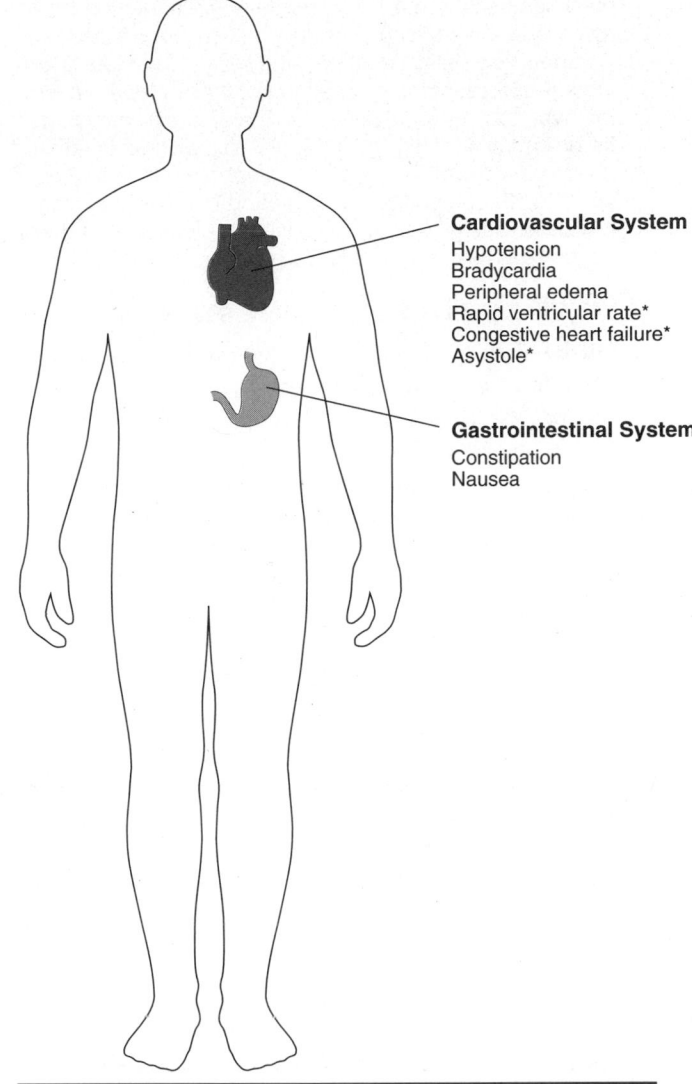

Cardiovascular System
Hypotension
Bradycardia
Peripheral edema
Rapid ventricular rate*
Congestive heart failure*
Asystole*

Gastrointestinal System
Constipation
Nausea

FIGURE 32–3   Common undesired clinical responses associated with calcium channel blockers.

TABLE 32–6
Class IV Antiarrhythmic Drugs: Clinical Considerations

Drug Name	Dosage and Route of Administration
VERPAMIL (Calan, Isoptin, Verelan) **HOW SUPPLIED** Tablets: 40, 80, 120 mg Injection: 5 mg/2 ml	**ADULTS** Oral: initial dose, 40–120 mg tid; usual maintenance dose, 240–480 mg/d; initial dose of 40 mg three tid for patients with hepatic impairment, poor left ventricular function, and the elderly IV: initial dose, 5–10 mg over 2 min; may repeat in 30 min with dose of 10 mg; administer over 3 min in elderly to avoid untoward drug effects **CHILDREN** IV Infants up to 1 y: 0.1–0.2 mg/kg over 2 min; may repeat in 30 min 1–15 y: 0.1–0.3 mg over 2 min, not to exceed 5 mg; may repeat in 30 min, not to exceed 10 mg
Diltiazem (Cardizem) **HOW SUPPLIED** Injection: 25 mg/ml	**ADULTS** IV: initial dose, 0.25 mg/kg over 2 min; may repeat 15 min after completion of initial dose at dose of 0.35 mg/kg; additional doses individualized IV infusion: initially 10 mg/h begins immediately after last IV injection; may increase by 5 mg/h up to maximum of 15 mg/h; may continue for up to 24 h

outweigh risks to the fetus. Since it is excreted in breast milk, its use in nursing women is not recommended.

Specific Drug-Related Nursing Considerations Obtain a baseline blood pressure. Check blood pressure for hypertension and pulse for bradycardia immediately before administering the drug. Assist with ambulation if dizziness occurs. Assess for peripheral edema. Teach client to change positions slowly and to rise slowly from a lying to a sitting or standing position. Monitor for a therapeutic serum level, 0.1 to 0.3 μg/ml.

MISCELLANEOUS DRUGS IN CATEGORY

Diltiazem (Cardizem) is used in prophylaxis and treatment of supraventricular tachyarrhythmias. It also controls the ventricular rate in clients with atrial flutter or fibrillation.

For use in clients with arrhythmias, diltiazem must be administered intravenously. The usual dose is 0.25 mg/kg of body weight over a 2-minute period. If the client's response is inadequate, a second IV bolus of 0.35 mg/kg may be administered. For continued reduction in heart rate in clients with atrial flutter or fibrillation, an IV infusion is administered. Initially the infusion rate is 10 mg/h; it may be increased in 5 mg/h increments up to 15 mg/h. A diltiazem infusion should not be continued longer than 24 hours.

CONCEPT REVIEW

Verapamil represents the class IV antiarrhythmic drugs, also known as *calcium channel blockers*. With the exception of diltiazem for IV use, verapamil is the only agent in this class.

More serious undesired responses associated with verapamil include bradycardia, AV block, and CHF.

MISCELLANEOUS ANTIARRHYTHMIC DRUGS

Digoxin is used to treat arrhythmias, specifically atrial flutter, atrial fibrillation, and supraventricular tachycardia. It suppresses arrhythmias by decreasing AV node conduction; digoxin produces a direct action on the AV node by increasing parasympathetic impulses to the node. Digoxin also decreases automaticity of the SA node. The usual dosage is 1 to 1.5 mg given in three to four divided doses over a 24-hour period. Maintenance dosage is 0.125 to 0.5 mg/d. (See Chapter 31 for a complete discussion of digoxin and its use to treat CHF.)

Adenosine (Adenocard) is a new, potent antiarrhythmic drug capable of slowing AV node conduction. It is used to treat paroxysmal supraventricular tachycardia. In addition, adenosine is used to diagnose wide QRS-complex regular tachycardias. The drug's onset and duration of action are measured in seconds; its half-life is 0.6 to 10 seconds.

Adenosine is administered only by IV bolus through an antecubital or other large proximal vein. The IV injection is followed immediately by a saline solution bolus. The usual dose is 6 mg given by rapid (within 2 seconds) IV injection. If the drug is not effective within 1 to 2 minutes, a repeat dose of 12 mg is administered and repeated if needed.

Adenosine should not be administered to clients with bradycardia or second- and third-degree AV blocks. Its use is not recommended for clients with tachycardia or bradycardia syndromes. Undesired clinical responses include facial flushing, headache, hypotension, dyspnea, chest pain, nausea, and bradycardia, which usually resolve within 1 to 2 minutes because of the drug's brevity of action. Sinus arrest, sometimes lasting several seconds, can also occur.[26–28]

SUMMARY

Antiarrhythmic drugs are usually grouped into six classes, depending on their action and effect on the cardiac electric properties. Most antiarrhythmic drugs seem preferentially to depress areas exhibiting abnormal pacemaker activity or conduction while having little effect on healthy cardiac tissue.

Class I antiarrhythmic drugs, also referred to as *membrane stabilizers,* affect sodium channels. Because of the differing effects on sodium channels, this group is subdivided into three subgroups. Drugs in class Ia appear to block the rapid inward flux of sodium ions. By allowing fewer sodium ions to pass through the cardiac membrane, membrane responsiveness is reduced, and depolarization is slowed. Class Ib drugs control ventricular arrhythmias and decrease ventricular conduction automaticity by blocking both activated and inactivated sodium channels. Class Ic contains the newest class I antiarrhythmic drugs. These drugs decrease myocardial membrane responsiveness to sodium, slowing conduction velocity. A relatively new drug, moricizine hydrochloride, is classified as a class I antiarrhythmic drug.

Class II antiarrhythmic drugs are the β-adrenergic blockers. These drugs block myocardial β-adrenergic receptors, reducing or antagonizing the actions of endogenous, circulating catecholamines. They also have direct membrane effects; at high concentrations they block sodium channels and depress membrane responsiveness.

Class III antiarrhythmic drugs control supraventricular and ventricular arrhythmias by reducing the refractory period and action potential duration without affecting conduction time or depressing cardiac contractility. Class IV antiarrhythmic drugs include the calcium channel blockers. These drugs inhibit the inward passage of calcium ions across cardiac membranes.

REFERENCES

1. Copstead, L.C. (1995). *Perspectives on pathophysiology.* Philadelphia: W.B. Saunders.
2. Adult advanced cardiac life support. (1992). *Journal of American Medical Association, 268,* 2199–2241.
3. Lathers, C.M., & O'Rourke, D.K. (1992). Antiarrhythmic agents. In C.M. Smith & A.M. Reynard (Eds.), *Textbook of Pharmacology* (pp. 505–553). Philadelphia: W.B. Saunders.
4. Melmor, K.L., Morrelli, H., Hoffman, B.B., & Nierenberg, D. (Eds.). (1992). *Clinical pharmacology: Basic principles in therapeutics* (3rd ed.). New York: McGraw-Hill.
5. DiPalma, J., & DiGregorio, C.J. (1990). *Basic pharmacology in medicine.* New York: McGraw-Hill.

6. Weiner, B. (1991). Hemodynamic effects of antidysrhythmic drugs. *Journal of Cardiovascular Nursing, 5*(4), 39–48.

7. Data Pharmaceutica, Inc. (1993). *1993 physicians' genRx.* Smithtown, NY: Author.

8. Lucas, W.J., Maccioli, G., & Mueller, R. (1990). Advances in oral antiarrhythmic therapy: Implications for the anaesthetist. *Canadian Journal of Anaesthesia, 37,* 94–101.

9. U.S. Pharmacopeia Convention. (1990). *The United States pharmacopeia* (22nd rev.). Rockville, MD: Author.

10. Hilleman, D.E., Mohiuddin, S.M., Mooss, A., Hunter, C., Destache, C., & Sketch, M. (1992). Comparative pharmacodynamics of intravenous lidocaine in patients with acute and chronic ventricular arrhythmias. *Annals of Pharmacotherapeutics, 26,* 763–777.

11. Berry, S.L., & Schleicher, C. (1992). Adjusting the beat. *American Journal of Nursing, 92*(6), 28–32.

12. Morganroth, J. (1992). Early and late proarrhythmia from antiarrhythmic drug therapy. *Cardiovascular Drugs and Therapy, 6*(1), 11–14.

13. Bryson, H.M., Palmer, K., Langtry, H., & Fitton, A. (1993). Proprofenone. A reappraisal of its pharmacology, pharmacokinetics, and therapeutic use in cardiac arrhythmias. *Drugs, 45*(1), 85–130.

14. Vanerio, G., & Maloney, J. (1992). Moricizine: Pharmacodynamic, pharmacokinetic, and therapeutic profile of a new antiarrhythmic. *Cleveland Clinic Journal of Medicine, 59*(1), 79–86.

15. Dennis, K.E., Froman, D., Morrison, A.S., Holmes, K.D., & Howes, D.G. (1991). Beta blocker therapy: Identification and management of side effects. *Heart and Lung, 20,* 459–463.

16. Maree, S.M. (1992). Esmolol: A unique beta adrenergic antagonist. *Journal of Neuroscience Nursing, 22*(2), 121–124.

17. Singh, B., & Ahmed, R. (1994). Class III antiarrhythmic drugs. *Current Opinion in Cardiology, 9*(1), 12–22.

18. Wit, A., & Coromilas, J. (1993). Role of alteration in refractoriness and conduction in the genesis of reentrant arrhythmias. Implications for antiarrhythmic effects of class III drugs. *American Journal of Cardiology, 72*(16), 3F–12F.

19. Roden, D. (1993). Pharmacokinetics of amiodarone: Implications for drug therapy. *American Journal of Cardiology, 72*(16), 45F–50F.

20. Dunnington, C. (1993). Sotalol hydrochloride (Betapace): A new antiarrhythmic drug. *American Journal of Critical Care, 2,* 397–406.

21. Dual action against ventricular dysrhythmias. (1993). *American Journal of Nursing, 93*(7), 56–57.

22. Triggle, D. (1992). Drugs affecting calcium—regulation and actions. In C.M. Smith & A.M. Reynard (Eds.), *Textbook of Pharmacology* (pp. 467–476). Philadelphia: W.B. Saunders.

23. Rising, J.B. (1990). Review of calcium-channel blockers. *U.S. Pharmacology, 15,* 37–41, 44, 46.

24. Hopkins, S. (1994). A guide to calcium channel blockers. *Nursing Standard, 8*(20), 30–31.

25. Hedman, A., Angelin, B., Arvidson, A., et al. (1991). Digoxin-verapamil interaction: Reduction of biliary but not renal digoxin clearance in humans. *Clinical Pharmacology and Therapeutics, 49,* 256–262.

26. Murphy, T. (1992). Adenosine: Slow down and take a look. *American Journal of Nursing, 92*(11), 22–24.

27. Nagelhout, J.J. (1992). Adenosine: Novel antiarrhythmic therapy for supraventricular tachycardia. *AANA Journal, 60,* 287–292.

28. Severson, A.L., & Meyer., T. (1992). Treatment of paroxysmal supraventricular tachycardia with adenosine: Implications for nursing. *Heart and Lung: Journal of Critical Care, 21,* 350–356.

BIBLIOGRAPHY

Bennett, B., & Singh, S. (1992). Management of ventricular arrhythmia: Then and now. *American Journal of Critical Care, 1*(3), 107–114.

Calcium antagonists and gingival overgrowth. (1994). *Nurses' Drug Alert, 18*(6), 44.

Campbell, J.K. (1993). Diagnosis and treatment of cluster headache. *Journal of Pain and Symptom Management, 8,* 155–164.

Clark, B.K. (1992). Beta-adrenergic blocking agents: Their current status. *Clinical Issues in Critical Care Nursing, 3,* 447–480.

Donnelly, A.J. (1991). Pharmacodynamics of parenteral antiarrhythmic agents: Part 2. *AORN Journal, 54*(1), 121–125, 128–130.

Hahnel, J., Linder, K., Schurmann, C., Prengel, A., & Ahnefeld, F. (1990). Plasma lidocaine levels and PAO_2 with endobronchial administration: Dilution with normal saline or distilled water? *Annals of Emergency Medicine, 19,* 1314–1317.

Hanisch, D., & Perron, L. (1992). Complex dysrhythmias in infants and children. *AACN—Clinical Issues in Critical Care Nursing, 3,* 255–269.

Lanuza, D.D., & Dunbar, S.B. (1993). Circadian rhythms: Implications for cardiovascular nursing and drug therapy. *Journal of Cardiovascular Nursing, 8*(1), 63–79.

Murphy, T. (1993). Digoxin toxicity: Ventricular dysrhythmias to watch for. *American Journal of Nursing, 93*(12), 37–41.

Singh, B. (1993). Controlling cardiac arrhythmias by lengthening repolarization: Historical overview. *American Journal of Cardiology, 72*(16), 18F–24F.

Taylor, D., Wilkins, G., Herbison, & Flannery, E. (1992). Interaction between corticosteroid and β-agonist drugs: Biochemical and cardiovascular effects in normal subjects. *Chest, 102,* 519–524.

Ujhelyi, M. (1993). Spotlight article: Quinidine enhances digitalis toxicity at therapeutic serum digoxin levels. *Heart and Lung: Journal of Critical Care, 22,* 560–562.

CHAPTER 33

Antihypertensive Drugs

DONNA HENRY • NORMA L. PINNELL

⊛ Hypertension

LEARNING OBJECTIVES:
Define the term *hypertension.*
Describe the two major classifications of hypertension.
KEY TERMS:
Diastolic blood pressure, essential hypertension, hypertension, primary hypertension, secondary hypertension, systolic blood pressure

⊛ Nursing Considerations

LEARNING OBJECTIVE: Develop a plan of care for a client requiring antihypertensive drugs.

⊛ Drugs Used to Treat Hypertension

LEARNING OBJECTIVE: Discuss the rationale behind drug selection for hypertension.
KEY TERM: Monotherapy

⊛ Diuretics

LEARNING OBJECTIVE: Describe the use of diuretics in the treatment of hypertension.

⊛ Drugs With Central Sympatholytic Action

LEARNING OBJECTIVES:
Describe the pharmacokinetic and pharmacodynamic properties of methyldopa.
Discuss the undesired clinical responses associated with methyldopa therapy.
Summarize major nursing considerations associated with methyldopa therapy.
Identify two other central-acting sympatholytic drugs.

⊛ Ganglionic Blockers

LEARNING OBJECTIVES:
Describe the pharmacokinetic and pharmacodynamic properties of mecamylamine hydrochloride.
Discuss the undesired clinical responses associated with mecamylamine hydrochloride.
Discuss the use of trimethaphan in the treatment of hypertension.
Summarize major nursing considerations associated with mecamylamine hydrochloride and trimethaphan therapy.

⊛ Drugs With Peripheral Sympatholytic Action

LEARNING OBJECTIVES:
Describe the use of β-adrenergic blockers in the treatment of hypertension.
Discuss the pharmacodynamic properties of prazosin, the prototype α-adrenergic blocker.
List major undesired clinical responses associated with prazosin.
Differentiate between α-adrenergic blockers and β-adrenergic blockers.
Explain the pharmacodynamics of labetalol hydrochloride, the prototype α-β–adrenergic blocker.
Explain the pharmacodynamics of reserpine, the prototype adrenergic neuron blocker.
Summarize major nursing considerations associated with peripheral sympatholytic drugs.
KEY TERM: Norepinephrine depletor

⊛ Drugs Inhibiting Catecholamine Synthesis

LEARNING OBJECTIVE: Discuss the therapeutic value of metyrosine.

⊛ Direct Vasodilators

LEARNING OBJECTIVES:
Explain the physiologic effect of direct vasodilators.
Differentiate between vasodilators used for moderate hypertension and those used in hypertensive emergencies.

⊛ ACE Inhibitors

LEARNING OBJECTIVES:
Discuss pharmacodynamic properties of angiotensin converting enzyme (ACE) inhibitors.
Identify major ACE inhibitors used to treat hypertension.

⊛ Calcium Channel Blockers

LEARNING OBJECTIVES:
Discuss the therapeutic value of calcium channel blockers in the treatment of hypertension.
Identify major calcium channel blockers used to treat hypertension.

*A*rterial blood pressure is the pressure generated by the heart as it contracts and ejects blood into the systemic arterial vascular system. As blood passes through the vascular system, the pressure decreases. By the time the blood returns to the right atrium, the pressure is almost dissipated. This pressure reduction is due to the resistance to flow offered by the vascular system.

The arterioles create most of the resistance in the circulatory system. Arterioles are innervated by both the sympathetic and parasympathetic divisions of the autonomic nervous system. Baseline vasoconstriction is produced by a tonic level of sympathetic discharge. Altering the rate of sympathetic discharge increases vasoconstriction or causes vasodilation.[1]

This chapter presents information about a variety of drugs used to treat hypertension. It also provides an overview of nursing care required by the individual receiving antihypertensive drug therapy.

HYPERTENSION

Arterial blood pressure is recorded as a systolic and a diastolic value. **Systolic blood pressure** reflects maximum pressure in the aorta and major arteries during ventricular ejection of blood. This pressure averages 120 mm Hg in healthy adults. **Diastolic blood pressure** reflects the minimum pressure in the aorta during the preejection rest period just before ventricular contraction. The average diastolic blood pressure in the healthy adult is 80 mm Hg.[1]

Definition of Hypertension

Hypertension is defined as blood pressure persistently elevated above 140 mm Hg systolic or 90 mm Hg diastolic.[1] Age, race, and obesity affect hypertensive mechanisms and therapy.[2] Blood pressure rises consistently with age, beginning at levels as low as 50/40 mm Hg in newborns and increasing to more than 200 mm Hg in some elderly individuals.[3] However, excessively elevated blood pressures should not be considered a normal consequence of aging. Elevated systolic or diastolic blood pressure in the elderly is a significant problem. This problem is compounded because the pathophysiology of hypertension in the elderly may differ from that of younger individuals.[4]

Hypertension is also influenced by race. It occurs two to three times more frequently in African-Americans than in Caucasians, and elevated blood pressures appear earlier in African-Americans. In addition, their target organ damage is more severe than that of individuals of European, Hispanic, or Native-American descent.[5,6]

Classification of Hypertension

Hypertension is classified as either primary (essential) or secondary hypertension. **Primary,** or **essential, hypertension** represents 90% of all diagnosed cases of hypertension and usually develops between 25 and 55 years of age. Primary hypertension is subdivided into benign, which has a slow onset and is initially asymptomatic, and malignant, which is characterized by a sudden onset of symptoms and accelerated progression of the disease. **Secondary hypertension** is the result of an underlying known cause that impairs peripheral blood flow, alters cardiac output, or increases blood viscosity. When the underlying cause is treated, the hypertension resolves.[7]

NURSING CONSIDERATIONS

Contact with clients with hypertension is common; therefore you must be prepared to provide thorough, comprehensive care to these individuals.

Assessing   During the **health history** assess the following points:
- Family history of hypertension or cardiovascular disease
- History of weight gain
- Dietary history, including sodium intake, fat intake, and alcohol use
- Presence of other cardiovascular risk factors (e.g., smoking, sedentary lifestyle, obesity)
- Psychologic, cultural, and sociologic factors that may influence blood pressure control
- Present support system
- Environmental factors that may influence blood pressure control
- Clinical manifestations of cardiovascular disorders
- Client's level of knowledge

During the **physical assessment** assess his or her blood pressure while the client is lying, sitting, and standing. Take the measurements in both arms to determine baseline data. Note any differences bilaterally and compare the findings with previous data.

Palpate the apical pulse and peripheral pulses to determine rate, rhythm, and amplitude. Palpate extremities for edema. Auscultate heart and pulmonary sounds and examine the neck for distended veins, carotid bruits, or enlarged thyroid. Examine the abdomen for masses and bruits. Perform a funduscopic examination for retinal changes.

Diagnosing   After analysis of the data base, develop suitable nursing diagnoses. Nursing diagnoses appropriate for the client requiring antihypertensive drugs follow:
- Knowledge deficit regarding drug treatment plan.
- Health maintenance, altered, related to inadequate knowledge about the disease process.

- Nutrition, altered, more than body requirements related to high sodium, fat, or caloric intake.
- High risk for noncompliance related to cost of therapy and undesired responses to drugs.
- Self-esteem, disturbance, related to hypertensive disease state and dependency on drug therapy.
- High risk for injury related to orthostatic hypotension associated with drug therapy.

Planning Teaching is an important part of this client's care and must be initiated early. Because of the chronicity of hypertension, clients need clear, practical learning guidelines about the effective management of high blood pressure. The guidelines should include information about the disease and its management. Use written material with illustrations to introduce the subject of hypertension to a newly diagnosed client. Plan on teaching the client to monitor and record his or her own blood pressure. Provide specific material about the drug treatment plan; include information on drug dosage, dosage schedule, expected response to therapy, and undesired clinical responses.

With the client, identify expected outcomes, which might include the following:

- Client verbalizes drug action, dosage schedule, and undesired clinical responses associated with the drug.
- Client participates in the treatment plan.
- Client states accurate information about appropriate diet plan.
- Client denies feelings of dependency and inadequacy.
- Client's vital signs are within his or her normal range.
- Client remains injury free.

Implementing During hospitalization monitor the client's vital signs, intake and output, and daily weight. Observe the client for indications of orthostatic hypotension. If the client complains of dizziness with position changes, teach the client to move slowly (i.e., move from lying position to sitting position before standing).

Teach the client self-care measures; encourage participation in the treatment plan and decision making. Allow time for questions and clarification of concerns. Encourage the family or significant other to participate in the treamtent plan. If appropriate, refer the client to a support group.

Evaluating Evaluate the effectiveness of the plan of care by comparing the client's status with the expected outcomes. Review the outcomes with the client to determine if changes are necessary. Effectiveness of the treatment plan is determined by the status of the client's vital signs, weight, and fluid balance.

DRUGS USED TO TREAT HYPERTENSION

In the past drug therapy was based on a specific plan of treatment, **stepped care,** which involved the initial use of diuretics and the sequential addition of antiadrenergic drugs and vasodilators if pressure failed to respond to therapy. This method did not take into account all of the variables that influence initial therapy.

Currently an attempt is made to individualize the therapeutic plan. One drug known to be effective as a **monotherapy** and compatible with the client's condition is selected. The starting dose of this drug is low. Several weeks or even longer should be allowed before deciding dosage changes are necessary. If the initial drug is ineffective, another drug is substituted instead of adding drugs to the treatment plan.[8] Monotherapy is effective in controlling blood pressure for approximately 40% to 60% of the individuals with mild primary hypertension.[9]

DIURETICS

Thiazide and related sulfonamide diuretics are the most frequently prescribed drugs in the treatment of hypertension. These drugs increase the excretion of sodium and water by decreasing their reabsorption in the kidneys. Diuretics are especially useful for hypertension associated with obesity, chronic renal failure, or congestive heart failure (CHF).

There are both advantages and disadvantages to the use of diuretics in the treatment of hypertension. Advantages include ease of administration, low cost, and proven efficacy. Disadvantages include sexual dysfunction and metabolic side effects (e.g., hyperglycemia, hypokalemia, hyperlipidemia, hypomagnesemia).[10] (See Chapter 36 for a complete discussion of diuretics.)

DRUGS WITH CENTRAL SYMPATHOLYTIC ACTION

Centrally acting α_2-agonist drugs decrease sympathetic outflow and thereby reduce blood pressure. Stimulation of α_2-receptors in the central nervous system (CNS) decreases sympathetic nervous activity and enhances baroreceptor reflexes. In response to the baroreceptor reflex, the CNS causes peripheral vasodilation, which decreases peripheral vascular resistance, reducing the heart rate, force of contraction, and cardiac output.[11-13]

α_2-Agonists also decrease norepinephrine release and stimulate receptors in the kidney to reduce renin release. A reduction in norepinephrine results in a decreased heart rate, decreased force of cardiac contraction, and peripheral vasodilation. Activation of the renin-angiotensin-aldosterone system results in vasoconstriction. (See the section on ACE inhibitors later in this chapter.) Reduction of renin promotes vasodilation and helps reduce blood pressure.[12]

SYMPATHOLYTIC PROTOTYPE
METHYLDOPA

Methyldopa (Aldomet) is one of the oldest central-acting sympatholytic drugs. It is not prescribed as frequently as it once was.

Pharmacotherapeutics Methyldopa is used in the management of moderate to severe hypertension. The drug is equally effective in managing hypertension in African-Americans and Caucasians.[14]

Pharmacokinetics Methyldopa has variable absorption from the gastrointestinal (GI) tract after oral administration. An average of 25% is absorbed unchanged. Biotransformation of the drug occurs in the liver and the intestine. The main metabolite, mono-0-sulfate conjugate, is formed in the liver. Other metabolites are formed in the intestine. Methyldopa and its metabolites are weakly bound to plasma proteins. The drug crosses the placenta in humans and is distributed into milk.

After oral administration peak plasma levels occur in 3 to 6 hours. The elimination half-life is approximately 2 hours; however, antihypertensive effects persist for up to 24 hours. Approximately 70% of the absorbed drug and its major metabolite are excreted in the urine. Unabsorbed drug is excreted in the feces unchanged. Excretion is essentially complete in 36 hours. Delayed excretion and accumulation of mono-0-sulfate occur in clients with renal insufficiency. The drug is removed by dialysis.

Plasma concentration and antihypertensive therapeutic effect generally do not correlate. Maximum decrease in blood pressure occurs in 4 to 6 hours. In most clients optimum blood pressure response occurs 12 to 24 hours after an adequate oral dosage level is attained. After discontinuation of the drug, blood pressure returns to pretreatment levels within 24 to 48 hours. After intravenous (IV) administration, blood pressure decline begins in 4 to 6 hours. The effect lasts 10 to 16 hours (Table 33–1).[11–13]

Pharmacodynamics The mechanism of action of methyldopa is not completely understood but probably is due to an effect on the CNS. Methyldopa is metabolized to α-methyl norepinephrine, which lowers blood pressure by stimulation of central inhibitory α-adrenergic receptors. Methyldopa causes some reduction of plasma renin activity, which may contribute to the hypotensive effect. Methyldopa also causes a net reduction in the tissue concentrations of serotonin, dopamine, norepinephrine, and epinephrine. The overall effect on the body is a decrease in total peripheral vascular resistance. Minimal change in cardiac output and heart rate is produced.

Pharmaceutics Methyldopa is supplied orally in tablets and an oral suspension. Methyldopate hydrochloride, the parenteral form, is available for IV use. Methyldopa is also available in fixed combination preparations with chlorothiazide (Aldoclor) and with hydrochlorothiazide (Aldoril).

Undesired Clinical Responses The most common side effect of methyldopa is drowsiness. This sedative effect, which occurs most commonly early in therapy, subsides as therapy is continued. However, if the dosage is increased, it may recur. Clients may experience a decrease in mental acuity, including forgetfulness, difficulty concentrating, and difficulty performing simple tasks. Other common undesired responses include orthostatic hypotension, sodium and water retention, and nasal congestion. Bradycardia, aggravation of angina, pericarditis, and myocarditis have also occurred.

Clients less frequently experience nightmares, reversible mild psychosis or depression, GI symptoms, and skin eruptions. Failure to ejaculate, decreased libido, and breast enlargement or tenderness have occurred in males. In females lactation and amenorrhea have been reported infrequently. The client's urine may darken when exposed to air because of the breakdown of methyldopa to its metabolites. A positive Coombs' test result, liver dysfunction, and hemolytic anemia have occurred with prolonged therapy.[11,12,14] Figure 33–1 illustrates undesired clinical responses associated with most central-acting sympatholytic drugs.

Contraindications and Precautions Methyldopa use is contraindicated in clients with active hepatic disease or a history of prior methyldopa-liver disorders. The drug should be used with caution in clients with a history of impaired hepatic or renal function. Sulfite sensitivity with allergic-like reactions may occur in susceptible individuals.

Drug-Drug and Drug-Environment Interactions Methyldopa interacts with several drugs. It may potentiate the effects of levodopa, causing increased hypotension. Concomitant administration with lithium may cause lithium toxicity. Concurrent administration with tolbutamide may impair the metabolism of tolbutamide. Methyldopa in combination with haloperidol may produce dementia and increased sedation.

Since methyldopa is decomposed by oxidizing agents, the oral suspension should be stored in a tight, light-resistant container. The parenteral solution is stable at pH 3.5 to 6.0 for 24 hours in most IV fluids.

Life-Span Considerations Methyldopa is classified as a Pregnancy Category B drug. It should be used during pregnancy only when clearly needed. Since the drug is excreted in breast milk, it should be used with caution in nursing mothers. Lower dosages should be prescribed initially to elderly individuals to avoid syncope.

Specific Drug-Related Nursing Considerations Do not administer it intramuscularly (IM) or subcutaneously (SC) because methyldopa has unpredictable absorption from these routes. IV solution must be administered slowly. Watch for paradoxic pressor effect during IV infusion.

Expect variable blood pressure response in the first 12 to 24 hours and then stabilization as maximal antihypertensive effect occurs. Monitor and record blood pressure and pulse. Report to the primary care provider if blood pressure is elevated over the target pressure after 2 days of therapy because dosage adjustment may be needed.

Advise the client to make positional changes slowly and to avoid prolonged standing. Instruct the client to report continuous dizziness or lightheadedness because dosage adjustment may be necessary. Weigh or instruct the client to weigh daily. Inspect lower extremities or other dependent areas for edema. Advise the client to report "swelling" or weight gain.

Teach the client that urine may darken after exposure to air; assure the client that this response is not an indication of a problem. Explain the sedative effect, including mentation changes, to the client. Instruct the client not to drive or operate hazardous machinery during this period of therapy. For nonambulatory clients, teach and provide safety precautions such as use of side rails, call light, and supervised activity. Reassure the client that these effects are reversible.

Advise the client to consult his or her primary care provider if prolonged general tiredness, fever, or jaundice is experienced. A direct Coombs' test may be done before and during therapy at 6- and 12-month intervals. (See Table 33–2 for a summary of information about dosage forms, dosages, routes of administration, and nursing considerations.)

TABLE 33–1
Summary of Pharmacokinetic Properties

Drug	Route	Onset of Action	Peak Action	Duration of Action
CENTRAL-ACTING SYMPATHOLYTIC DRUGS				
Methyldopa (Aldomet)	Oral	2 h	4–6 h	12–24 h
Methyldopate hydrochloride	IV	Immediate	4–6 h	10–16 h
Clonidine hydrochloride (Catapres)	Oral	30–60 min	2–4 h	12–24 h
Guanabenz acetate (Wytensin)	Oral	60 min	2–4 h	6–12 h
Guanfacine hydrochloride (Tenex)	Oral	1–2 h	1–4 h	24 h
GANGLIONIC BLOCKERS				
Mecamylamine hydrochloride (Inversine)	Oral	30 min–2 h	3–5 h	6–12 h
Trimethaphan camsylate (Arfonad)	IV	Immediate	1–2 min	10–30 min
α-ADRENERGIC BLOCKERS				
Prazosin (Minipress)	Oral	2 h	2–4 h	6–12 h
Terazosin (Hytrin)	Oral	15 min	1–2 h	12–24 h
Doxazosin mesylate (Cardura)	Oral	30 min	2–6 h	24 h
β-ADRENERGIC BLOCKERS				
Propranolol (Inderal)	Oral	30 min	2–4 h	8–12 h
Metoprolol (Lopressor, Toprol XL)	IV	Immediate	2 min	15 min
	Oral	>1 h	$1^{1}/_{2}$ h	13–19 h
Atenolol (Tenormin)	IV	Minutes	20 min	5–8 h
	Oral	1 h	2–4 h	24 h
Nadolol (Corgard)	IV	Immediate	5 min	7 h
	Oral	>3 h	3–4 h	20–24 h
Penbutolol (Levatol)	Oral	15 min	$1^{1}/_{2}$–3 h	20–24 h
Timolol maleate (Blocadren)	Oral	30 min	1–3 h	12 h
Pindolol (Visken)	Oral	<1 h	1 h	24 h
Acebutolol (Sectral)	Oral	1 h	$2^{1}/_{2}$–$3^{1}/_{2}$ h	24–30 h
Carteolol hydrochloride (Cartrol)	Oral	<1 h	1–3 h	24 h
MIXED α-β–BLOCKERS				
Labetalol (Normodyne, Trandate)	Oral	20 min–1 h	1–4 h	8–12 h
	IV	2–5 min	5–15 min	2–4 h
NOREPINEPHRINE DEPLETORS				
Reserpine (Serpasil)	Oral	2 h	6–12 h	6–24 h
Guanadrel sulfate (Hylorel)	Oral	2 h	4–6 h	10 h
Guanethidine monosulfate (Ismelin)	Oral	Variable	6–8 h	24–48 h
DIRECT VASODILATORS				
Hydralazine hydrochloride (Apresoline)	Oral	20–30 min	30 min–2 h	6–8 h
	IM	10–20 min	1 h	
	IV	5–20 min	10–30 min	
Minoxidil (Loniten)	Oral	30 min	2–3 h	24–72 h
Sodium nitroprusside (Nipride)	IV	$^{1}/_{2}$–1 min	1 min	3–5 min
Diazoxide (Hyperstat)	Oral	1 h	4 h	8 h
CALCIUM CHANNEL BLOCKERS				
Amlodipine (Norvasc)	Oral	Gradual	6–12 h	>24 h
Diltiazem hydrochloride (Cardizem SR)	Oral	30 min–1 h	6–12 h	24 h
Nicardipine hydrochloride (Cardene SR)	Oral	20 min	30 min–2 h	8 h
Nifedipine (Procardia, Adalat)	Oral	10 min	30 min	4–6 h
Verapamil hydrochloride (Calan, Isoptin, Verelan)	Oral	30 min	1–2 h	4–8 h
	IV	Immediate	3–5 min	2–5 h
Felodipine (Plendil)	Oral	<2 h	$2^{1}/_{2}$–5 h	11–16 h
Isadipine (DynaCirc)	Oral	2 h	1.5 h	8 h
ACE INHIBITORS				
Enalapril (Vasotec)	Oral	1 h	4–8 h	24 h
Captopril (Capoten)	Oral	15 min	30 min–$1^{1}/_{2}$ h	6–12 h
Benazepril (Lotensin)	Oral	1 h	2–6 h	24 h
Fosinopril (Monopril)	Oral	1 h	2–6 h	24 h
Lisonopril (Prinivil, Zestril)	Oral	1 h	6–7 h	24 h
Quinapril (Accupril)	Oral	1 h	2–6 h	24 h
Ramipril (Altace)	Oral	1 h	2–4 h	24 h

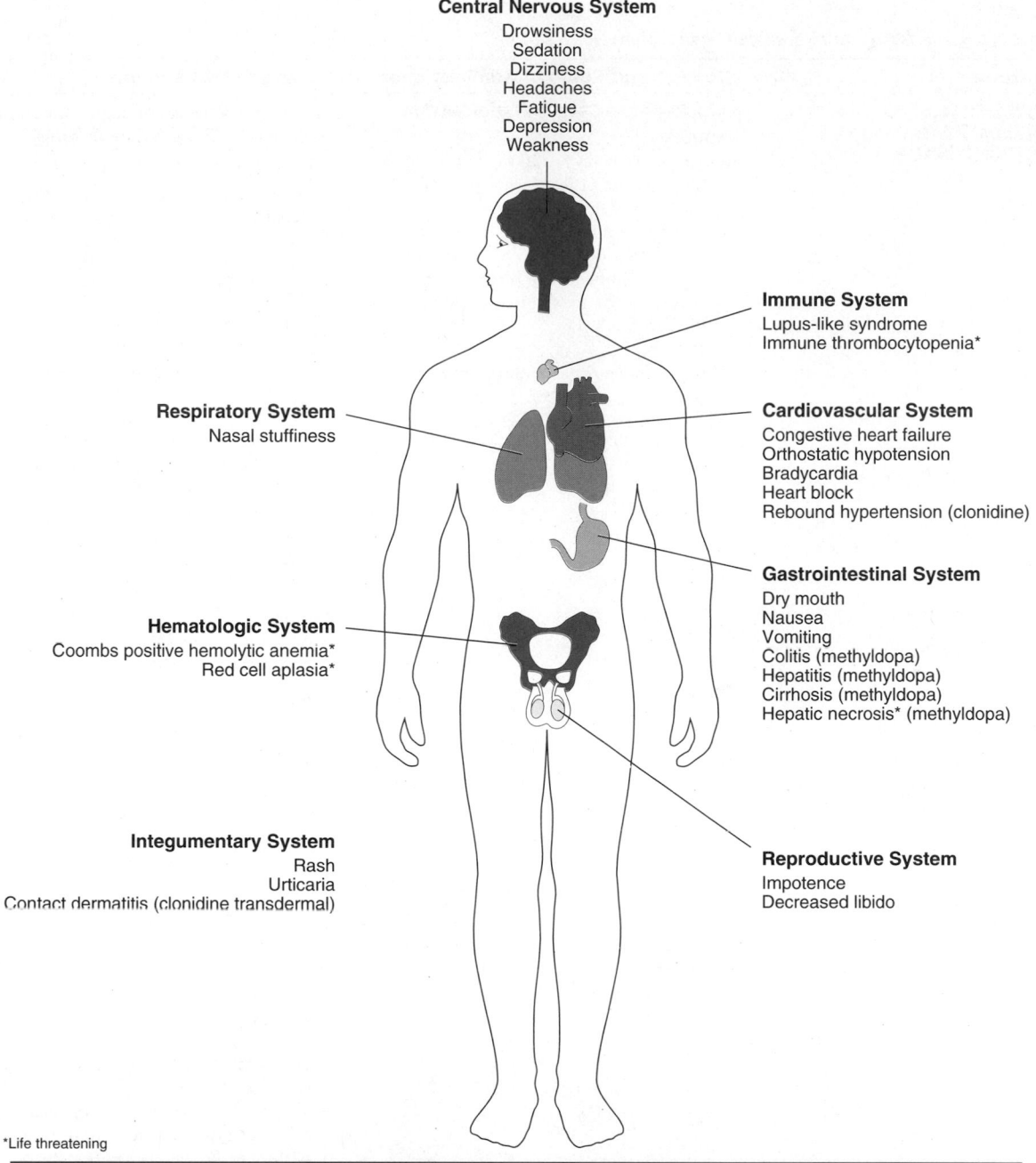

Central Nervous System
Drowsiness
Sedation
Dizziness
Headaches
Fatigue
Depression
Weakness

Immune System
Lupus-like syndrome
Immune thrombocytopenia*

Respiratory System
Nasal stuffiness

Cardiovascular System
Congestive heart failure
Orthostatic hypotension
Bradycardia
Heart block
Rebound hypertension (clonidine)

Gastrointestinal System
Dry mouth
Nausea
Vomiting
Colitis (methyldopa)
Hepatitis (methyldopa)
Cirrhosis (methyldopa)
Hepatic necrosis* (methyldopa)

Hematologic System
Coombs positive hemolytic anemia*
Red cell aplasia*

Integumentary System
Rash
Urticaria
Contact dermatitis (clonidine transdermal)

Reproductive System
Impotence
Decreased libido

*Life threatening

FIGURE 33–1   Common undesired clinical responses associated with central-acting sympatholytic drugs.

MISCELLANEOUS DRUGS IN CATEGORY

Clonidine (Catapres), guanabenz (Wytensin), and guanfacine (Tenex) are also drugs with central sympatholytic action. **Clonidine,** like methyldopa, is not prescribed as frequently as it was in the past. Clonidine stimulates central α_2-adrenergic receptors at the postsynaptic site. This reduces sympathetic tone, resulting in a decline in blood pressure and pulse rate. The most frequent undesired clinical responses are sedation and dryness of the mouth due to reduced salivary flow rate. Abrupt withdrawal of clonidine has produced rebound hypertensive crisis similar to that seen with pheochromocytoma. Clonidine is considered a potent antihypertensive drug.

However, its use is limited by significant undesired clinical responses.[8] Clonidine comes in fixed combination with the thiazide diuretic chlorthalidone, Combipres.

Clonidine is available in a transdermal dosage form. Once every 7 days, apply the transdermal system to a hairless area of intact skin on upper arm or torso. Use a different site with each application and be certain to remove the old system. If the system loosens during the 7 days, apply an adhesive overlay directly over the system. The antihypertensive effect of the transdermal system may not begin for 2 to 3 days after the initial application. During this period oral antihypertensive drugs may be administered concurrently.

TABLE 33–2
Antihypertensive Drugs with Central Sympatholytic Actions

Drug Name	Dosage and Route of Administration	Nursing Considerations
METHYLDOPA, METHYLDOPATE HYDROCHLORIDE (Aldomet) **HOW SUPPLIED** Tablets: 125, 250, 500 mg Parenteral: 250 mg/5 ml	***Moderate to Severe Hypertension*** ADULTS Oral: initial therapy, 250 mg bid or tid for 2 d; increase or decrease at intervals of 2 d until adequate response achieved Maintenance dose: 500 mg–2 g daily in two to four divided doses, maximum of 3 g; if combined with other antihypertensive drugs, maximum of 500 mg in divided doses CHILDREN Oral: 10 mg/kg/d, or 300 mg/m^2 in two to four divided doses Maximum dose: 65 mg/kg/d, 2 g/m^2, or 3 g daily, whichever is less	See text for nursing considerations common to all central sympatholytic drugs. ***Assess*** Drug is contraindicated in clients with active hepatic disease, history of methyldopa-induced liver abnormalities, or direct Coombs'-positive hemolytic anemia. Drug is classified in Pregnancy Category B. ***Implement*** Elderly clients or individuals with impaired renal function may need decreased dosage. Instruct client that urine may darken after exposure to air. Drug is supplied in a suspension dosage form to facilitate pediatric administration. Parenteral solution is added to 100 ml of 5% dextrose solution or in a concentration of 100 mg/10 ml. Infuse slowly over 30–60 min. *Do not* administer IM or SC. ***Monitor*** Monitor hemoglobin and hematocrit levels and direct Coombs' test results.
Clonidine (Catapres, Catapres TTS) **HOW SUPPLIED** Tablet: 0.1, 0.2, 0.3 mg Transdermal patch: 0.1, 0.2, 0.3 mg	***Oral*** ADULTS Initial dose: 0.1 mg bid Maintenance dose: 0.2–1.2 mg/d Maximum dose: 2.4 mg/d CHILDREN 4–25 μg/kg/d in divided doses q6h Increase at intervals of 5–7 d ***Transdermal*** Start with 0.1 mg/24 h applied once q7d; if after 1 wk blood pressure reduction is not achieved, add another 0.1 mg or use larger transdermal system	***Assess*** Assess for contraindications (e.g., severe coronary insufficiency, cerebrovascular disease, Raynaud's disease) before initiating therapy. Determine if client is pregnant or breast-feeding. Clonidine is excreted in breast milk and is classified as a Pregnancy Category C drug. ***Implement*** Elderly clients require lower doses. Instruct client in proper application of transdermal system. Instruct client to check for local skin reactions. Teach safety precautions necessary with sedative side effects. Advise client that constipation, headache, fatigue, and dizziness tend to diminish within 4 to 6 wk of therapy. Instruct client in symptomatic management of undesired responses. Advise client not to miss doses or discontinue drug without consulting the prescriber. ***Monitor*** Monitor blood pressure carefully.

TABLE *33–2 Continued*

Antihypertensive Drugs with Central Sympatholytic Actions

Drug Name	Dosage and Route of Administration	Nursing Considerations
Guanabenz (Wytensin) HOW SUPPLIED Tablets: 4, 8 mg	ADULTS 4 mg bid; increase in increments of 4–8 mg/d q1–2wk Maximum dose: 32 mg bid Usual maintenance dose: 8–16 mg/d CHILDREN >12 Y 4–24 mg/d (0.08–0.2 mg/kg/d) in two divided doses Not recommended for children <12 y	**Assess** Determine if client is pregnant; drug is classified in Pregnancy Category C. Assess for history of severe coronary insufficiency, recent myocardial infarction, cerebrovascular disease, or hepatic or renal failure. **Implement** Advise client not to discontinue drug; rebound hypertension may occur. Administer last dose of day at bedtime to ensure overnight control and to minimize daytime drowsiness.
Guanfacine Hydrochloride (Tenex) HOW SUPPLIED Tablets: 1, 2 mg	**Mild to Moderate Hypertension** Oral: 1 mg at bedtime; may be increased to 2 and then 3 mg/d after 3 or 4 wk Not recommended for children <12 y of age	**Assess** Assess for contraindications; see guanabenz. Determine if client is pregnant; drug is classified in Pregnancy Category B. **Implement** Guanfacine is used in clients already receiving thiazide diuretic. Instruct client not to discontinue drug; rebound hypertension may develop within 2–4 d after drug is stopped. Remind client to take drug at bedtime to minimize somnolence. **Monitor** Monitor blood pressure carefully.

Instruct client to store this drug safely and to discard used transdermal systems where they cannot be retrieved by toddlers or small children. Accidental overdose can occur from chewing on new or used systems because some active drug is still present in the used system.

Guanabenz, a guanadine derivative, has a structure and mode of action similar to that of clonidine. The most frequent undesired clinical responses are drowsiness, sleepiness, dizziness, and headache. Guanabenz is considered a moderately effective antihypertensive drug. However, because of its relatively high incidence of symptomatic side effects, it should not be considered first-line therapy.[8]

Guanfacine is also a guanadine derivative that lowers blood pressure by a mechanism similar to that of clonidine and guanabenz. Its therapeutic uses and effectiveness, undesired clinical responses, and drug interactions are basically the same as those of clonidine and guanabenz.[8]

CONCEPT REVIEW

Central-acting sympatholytic drugs are potent α_2-adrenergic agonists that reduce central vasoconstrictor outflow.

Methyldopa, the prototype, reduces total peripheral resistance but produces minimal changes in cardiac output and heart rate.

Clonidine, guanabenz, and guanfacine reduce total peripheral resistance, cardiac output, and heart rate. Unlike methyldopa, these drugs act peripherally on presynaptic nerve endings to reduce norepinephrine release.

GANGLIONIC BLOCKERS

Ganglionic blockers compete with acetylcholine for cholinergic receptors at the autonomic ganglia. This competition for receptors blocks transmission of both sympathetic and parasympathetic ganglia. Through sympathetic blockade, ganglionic blockers cause vasodilation, increased peripheral blood flow, and decreased blood pressure. This relatively nonspecific blockade of the autonomic nervous system results in many potential undesired responses. Therefore these drugs are used for hypertensive emergencies and when moderately severe or severe hypertension is refractory to other treatment.[8,15]

GANGLIONIC BLOCKER PROTOTYPE

MECAMYLAMINE HYDROCHLORIDE

Mecamylamine hydrochloride (Inversine) is a secondary amine.

Pharmacotherapeutics Mecamylamine is used in the management of moderately severe to severe primary hypertension and in uncomplicated cases of malignant hypertension. The drug should not be used in clients with mild, moderate, or labile hypertension.

Pharmacokinetics Mecamylamine is almost completely absorbed from the GI tract after oral administration. Onset of action is gradual, occurring in 30 minutes to 2 hours. Duration of action is 6 to 12 hours or longer. The drug crosses the placenta and the blood-brain barrier. The rate of renal elimination is markedly influenced by the pH of the urine. Alkaline urine reduces and acidic urine promotes renal excretion. Approximately 50% of the drug is excreted unchanged in the urine within 24 hours if the urine is acidic (see Table 33–1).[15]

Pharmacodynamics Mecamylamine is a potent oral ganglionic blocker that reduces blood pressure through sympathetic blockade. The antihypertensive effect is predominantly orthostatic, but supine blood pressure is also significantly reduced. Heart rate generally increases but may decrease if tachycardia was present before the drug was administered. Because of reduced venous return, resulting from peripheral vasodilation and peripheral pooling of blood, cardiac output is decreased. Splanchnic and cerebral blood flow is decreased; skeletal muscle blood flow is unchanged. Renal blood flow may increase, decrease, or be unchanged. Because parasympathetic blockade also occurs, atony of the bladder and GI tract, cycloplegia, mydriasis, xerostomia, and anhidrosis generally result.[15]

Pharmaceutics Mecamylamine is supplied as scored tablets for oral administration.

Recommended Dosage

- Therapy is usually started with 2.5 mg bid. The dose is increased by 2.5 mg at intervals of not less than 2 days until desired response is obtained.
- Two to 3 days of therapy are needed before the full effect of the drug is achieved.

Undesired Clinical Responses Mecamylamine produces numerous undesired responses because of its nonspecific beta blockade. Adynamic ileus is the most serious adverse effect. Other GI symptoms include anorexia, nausea, vomiting, constipation, dry mouth, and dysphagia. CNS effects include weakness, fatigue, sedation, and headache. Rarely tremor, mental aberrations, choreiform movements, and seizures have occurred. Mecamylamine does cause postural hypotension, especially when the client arises in the morning. In addition, nasal congestion, dilated pupils, blurred vision, decreased libido, impotence, dysuria, and urinary retention occur.[15]

Contraindications and Precautions Mecamylamine use is contraindicated in clients with coronary insufficiency, compromised renal or cerebral blood flow, uremia, glaucoma, or organic pyloric stenosis. It is also contraindicated in clients with known hypersensitivity and those with chronic pyelonephritis who are receiving antibiotics or sulfonamides. Sodium depletion, fever, infection, hemorrhage, or excessive heat may potentiate drug effects.

Life-Span Considerations Mecamylamine is classified as a Pregnancy Category C drug. Mecamylamine crosses the placental barrier. Pregnancy also potentiates the hypotensive effect of the drug. Because the drug passes into breast milk, either the drug or breast-feeding should be discontinued to avoid effects on the infant.

Drug-Drug, Drug-Nutrient, Drug-Environment Interactions The antihypertensive effects of mecamylamine can be increased by diuretics, other hypotensive drugs, and alcohol. Drugs such as sodium bicarbonate and acetazolamide that increase urinary pH may cause mecamylamine toxicity. Generally mecamylamine should not be administered concurrently with antibiotics and sulfonamides.

Sodium intake should not be restricted with mecamylamine therapy. Sodium depletion may result in excessive hypotension. The drug should be administered in a consistent pattern in relation to meals. An additional fall in blood pressure may occur after a meal. This fall may be due to inability of vascular reflexes to compensate for dilation of splanchnic blood vessels.

Vigorous exercise, excessive heat, and excessive perspiration with sodium depletion also potentiate the drug's hypotensive effects. Clients who exercise, especially outdoors in warm weather, are especially at risk for hypotensive episodes.

Specific Drug-Related Nursing Considerations For safe home administration, clients who can use a sphygmomanometer must be given instructions to reduce or omit a dose if blood pressure readings fall below a designated level. Teach clients not monitored by actual blood pressure readings to use faintness or lightheadedness as the criterion. The designated level and orthostatic symptoms and dosage adjustment are directed by the primary care provider. Teach the client not to make other changes without consulting the care provider.

The drug should be administered after meals to produce gradual absorption and smoother control of blood pressure. Instruct the client to take the drug on a consistent pattern in relation to meals. Since blood pressure response to mecamylamine is increased in the morning, the morning dose is usually relatively small. Larger dosages are prescribed at noontime and in the evening.

Teach clients about the possibility of postural dizziness, especially when arising in the morning. Instruct clients to change position slowly and to lie down if dizziness persists. Advise clients that the hypotensive effect of mecamylamine may be increased by excessive heat, fever, infection, vigorous exercise, or sodium depletion. Instruct clients not to restrict sodium during drug therapy. Be aware that surgery, anesthesia, hemorrhage, and pregnancy may also potentiate hypotensive effects of mecamylamine.

The most serious undesired response to mecamylamine is adynamic ileus. Instruct the client to report frequent, loose bowel movements or abdominal distention. Assess bowel sound quality regularly.

MISCELLANEOUS DRUGS IN CATEGORY

Trimethaphan camsylate (Arfonad) is a short-acting, potent ganglionic blocker used during hypertensive emergencies and specific surgical procedures to induce hypotension. It is administered only intravenously via an infusion pump. The onset of action for this drug is immediate, and peak action occurs in 5 minutes, with a duration of action of 10 to 15 minutes. A systolic blood pressure of 100 mm Hg is usually attained within 10 minutes. After discontinuation of the drug, the blood pressure begins to increase in 3 to 5 minutes. The drug probably is metabolized by pseudocholinesterase. It is excreted by the kidneys.[8,15] Trimethaphan camsylate use is contraindicated in clients with anemia, hypovolemia, shock, asphyxia, or respiratory insufficiency. The drug is classified as a Pregnancy Category D drug; it does cause fetal harm, and its use should be avoided during pregnancy.

- Trimethaphan is initiated at a dose of 3 to 4 mg/min then individualized with a range of 0.3 to 6 mg/min.

Always dilute the concentrated drug. Use an infusion pump with a microdrip regulator that allows precise measurement of the flow rate of the IV infusion. Freshly prepare the IV solution and discard any unused portion. Do not use the infusion fluid as a vehicle for simultaneous administration of other drugs. The blood pressure should be measured every 2 minutes during initial therapy and every 5 minutes during maintenance. Monitor respiratory status closely. Assess for indication of adequate oxygenation. Since the drug causes pupillary dilation, this sign is not an adequate indicator of cerebral oxygenation.

CONCEPT REVIEW

Ganglionic blockers compete with acetylcholine for cholinergic receptors at the autonomic ganglia.

Through sympathetic blockade, ganglionic blockers cause vasodilation, increased peripheral blood flow, and decreased blood pressure.

Mecamylamine and trimethaphan are two ganglionic blockers used to treat hypertension.

DRUGS WITH PERIPHERAL SYMPATHOLYTIC ACTION

Adrenergic blockers of the peripheral nervous system reduce blood pressure by reducing tonic neural vasoconstriction.

β-Adrenergic Blockers

β-Adrenergic receptor blocking agents, commonly called *β-blockers,* compete with β-agonists for β_1- or β_2-receptor sites. β_1-Receptors are primarily in the heart. They are also present at sympathetic nerve endings where they are associated with increased norepinephrine release. In the kidney they increase renin release; in fat cells they increase lipolysis. β_2-Receptors are present in bronchial and vascular smooth muscle. They are also present in skeletal muscle where they increase potassium uptake and glycogenolysis. In the liver β_2-receptors increase glycogenolysis, and in the pancreas they are associated with increased insulin release.

β-Blockers that block either β_2 (cardioselective) or β_1 and β_2 (nonselective) receptors are used as antihypertensive drugs. These drugs reduce blood pressure by blocking sympathetic effects on the heart, thus decreasing the heart rate and cardiac output. They also decrease blood pressure by blocking adren-

TABLE 33–3
β-Adrenergic Blockers Used to Treat Hypertension

Drug Name	Usual Daily Dosage
Atenolol (Tenormin)	25–100 mg/d; decrease in presence of renal failure
Betaxolol (Kerlone)	10–20 mg once a day
Bisoprolol (Zebeta)	5–20 mg/d
Carteolol (Cartrol)	2.5–10 mg/d
Metoprolol (Lopressor, Toprol XL)	Initial: 100 mg/d; maintenance: 100–450 mg/d; Toprol XL: 50–100 mg/d
Nadolol (Corgard)	40–320 mg/d; decrease in presence of renal failure
Penbutolol (Levatol)	10–40 mg/d
Pindolol (Visken)	10–60 mg/d
Propranolol (Inderal)	40–160 mg bid or tid; reduce in presence of liver failure
Timolol (Blocadren)	20–60 mg/d

ergic nerve-mediated release of renin, thereby decreasing peripheral vascular resistance.

β-Blockers have been designated as suitable drugs for initial monotherapy since 1984. However, because of the undesired clinical responses (e.g., fatigue, lethargy, depression, diminished mental acuity, and decreased exercise tolerance), β-blockers are being used with more discretion than in the past. They are considered the drugs of choice in obese clients and in younger clients with hyperdynamic circulation. β-Blockers are specifically recommended for clients who have experienced ischemic heart disease, angina, or myocardial infarction because they reduce the risk of subsequent episodes.

β-Blockers are used cautiously to treat hypertension in clients with asthma, insulin-dependent diabetes mellitus, peripheral vascular disease, hypertriglyceridemia, or CHF. Use of β-blockers affecting β_2-adrenergic receptors that mediate bronchodilation is contraindicated for clients with chronic bronchitis, emphysema, or asthma. In addition, the response to β-blockers is generally poor in the elderly and African-Americans.[2,14,16–18] Table 33–3 summarizes information about β-blockers commonly prescribed for hypertension. See Chapter 32 for more information on β-adrenergic blockers.

🌿 NURSING RESEARCH

Potema, K.M., Fogg, L.F., Fish, A.F., & Kravitz, H.M. (1993). Blood pressure reactivity in the evaluation of resting blood pressure and mood responses to pindolol and propranolol in hypertensive patients. *Heart and Lung: Journal of Critical Care, 22,* 383–391.

The purpose of this exploratory study was to evaluate the relationship of blood pressure reactivity during exercise to treatment responsiveness to two commonly used β-adrenergic blockers, propranolol and pindolol. A convenience sample of 19 white male subjects with mild to moderate essential hypertension was studied.

All antihypertensive drugs were gradually discontinued, and the subjects were free of all prescription drugs for 2 weeks. Subjects were randomly assigned to a propranolol-pindolol or a pindolol-propranolol group. Each 4- to 6-week treatment phase was preceded by a 2-week placebo phase. At the end of the initial placebo phase and each active drug treatment phase, subjects were assessed for depression and mood disturbances. Subjects were also given a graded exercise test on a cycle ergometer.

Subjects demonstrating high diastolic blood pressure reactivity to exercise required high doses of β-blockers for resting diastolic blood pressure reduction. These subjects also demonstrated the least change in mood at high doses. Similar patterns were found for the relationship of systolic blood pressure reactivity and blood pressure and mood responsiveness to drug treatment. However, these findings were not statistically significant.

STUDENT ACTIVITIES

- Discuss findings of this study with a clinical nurse specialist. Inquire about depression and mood disturbances assessed in clients receiving β-blockers.
- Review five charts of clients receiving β-blockers for hypertension. Graph systolic and diastolic blood pressure readings, noting time of day, level of physical activity, and relationship to mealtime.

α-Adrenergic Blockers

α_1-Adrenergic blockers act generally by blocking the sympathetic vasoconstrictor impulses at α_1-adrenergic receptors in vascular smooth muscle. This widening of the vessel lumen causes decreased peripheral vascular resistance and a reduction in blood pressure.

Since these drugs do not block the presynaptic α_2-receptors, which inhibit excessive norepinephrine release, accelerated heart rate and increased cardiac output do not occur. Reduction of preload by venous dilation and of afterload by arterial dilation makes these drugs therapeutic in the treatment of CHF, causing regression of left-ventricular hypertrophy. α_1-Adrenergic blockers lower total cholesterol, low-density lipoprotein (LDL) cholesterol, and triglyceride levels, thus influencing the total cholesterol–high-density lipoprotein (HDL) cholesterol ratio.[8,12,20–22]

α-ADRENERGIC PROTOTYPE

PRAZOSIN HYDROCHLORIDE

Prazosin (Minipress), a quinazoline derivative, is considered a selective blocker on postsynaptic α_1-receptors.

Pharmacotherapeutics Prazosin is used alone or in combination with other drugs in the management of hypertension. Some clinicians consider prazosin suitable first-line therapy because of its generally benign side effect profile, minimal adverse metabolic effects, and improved lipid profiles. The drug is being evaluated for use in clients with refractory CHF, vasospasm associated with Raynaud's disease, and prostatic outflow problems.[15]

Pharmacokinetics Prazosin is well absorbed from the GI tract. The presence of food may delay absorption but does not affect the extent of absorption. The absolute bioavailability of prazosin averages 48% to 68%. It is widely distributed in body tissues. Approximately 92% to 97% of the drug in plasma is bound to protein.

After oral administration of prazosin, the plasma concentration reaches a peak in approximately 3 hours. The drug's half-life is 2 to 3 hours. Prazosin is extensively metabolized by the liver to active metabolites. The drug is excreted as unchanged drug (5% to 11%) and metabolites. Approximately 90% of the drug is excreted in feces via bile and the remainder in urine. Elimination is slower in clients with CHF (see Table 33–1).

Pharmacodynamics As previously indicated, prazosin selectively blocks postsynaptic α_1-adrenergic receptors. This causes dilation of both resistance (arterioles) and capacitance (veins) vessels. Both supine and standing blood pressure are decreased. Blood pressure begins to decrease within 2 hours after oral administration. The duration of antihypertensive effect is 10 hours.[8,15]

Pharmaceutics Prazosin is available in capsules for oral administration. It is prepared in a fixed combination with a thiazide diuretic, polythiazide (Minizide). See Table 33–4 for information about dosage and route of administration.

Undesired Clinical Responses Syncope episodes with sudden loss of consciousness have occurred with prazosin therapy, probably because of an excessive postural hypotensive effect. Syncope episodes occur most commonly within 30 to 90 minutes of the initial dose of the drugs and are called *"first-dose" effect*. The incidence of first-dose effect is greatest in individuals receiving an initial dose of 2 mg or more.

In addition to postural symptoms, dizziness, palpitations, headache, drowsiness, weakness, lack of energy, and nausea are frequent undesired clinical responses. Less common reactions include edema, dyspnea, nasal congestion, epistaxis, arthralgia, urinary frequency, impotence, rash pruritus, alopecia, lichen planus, fever, blurred vision, dry mouth, conjunctivitis, tinnitus, vomiting, diarrhea, constipation, and abdominal discomfort. Positive antinuclear antibody (ANA) titer, transient fall in leukocyte count, increased serum uric acid and blood urea nitrogen (BUN) levels, and abnormal liver function test results have also been reported.[8,11,12,15]

Contraindications and Precautions Prazosin should be used with caution in clients with chronic renal failure. In addition, injury could result if syncope occurs when the client is operating machinery or driving motor vehicles.

Drug-Drug, Drug-Nutrient, Drug-Environment Interactions Increased hypotension can be expected if prazosin is administered concomitantly with diuretics or other hypotensive drugs, particularly β-adrenergic blockers. Prazosin can be administered without regard to food intake. It should be stored in tightly closed, light-resistant containers.

Life-Span Considerations Prazosin is classified as a Pregnancy Category C drug. It should be used with caution during pregnancy and lactation. Safety and efficacy in children have not been established.

Specific Drug-Related Nursing Considerations
Check initial dosage carefully. Only 1-mg capsules are used; the 2-mg and 5-mg capsules are not used for initial therapy. Monitor the client closely during this initial period. If syncope occurs, place the client in a recumbent position and monitor vital signs. Explain to the client that the first-dose effect is usually self-limiting and in most cases does not recur.

Teach clients that postural dizziness and palpitations may occur, especially early in therapy. Instruct clients to avoid situations in which injuries may happen and to avoid operating motor vehicles or machinery 12 to 24 hours after the first dose, after a dosage increase, and after interruption of therapy when treatment is resumed. Teach clients to use caution when rising from a sitting or lying position. Explain factors that increase postural hypotension such as over-warm environments, hot baths, and standing for long periods. Advise clients to consult the prescriber if dizziness is persistent or bothersome since dosage adjustment may be necessary.

MISCELLANEOUS DRUGS IN CATEGORY

Terazosin (Hytrin) is a postsynaptic α_1-blocker used to treat mild to moderate hypertension. It is similar chemically to prazosin. Terazosin differs from prazosin in that its water solubility is 25 times greater and its elimination half-life is approximately three times that of prazosin. Terazosin also has a slower onset of action. These features allow for once-daily dosing. Terazosin is also used in the treatment of benign prostatic hypertrophy.[21–23]

Doxazosin (Cardura), like prazosin and terazosin, is a quinazoline acting as a postsynaptic alpha-1 competitive antagonist. Peak levels of doxazosin occur 2 to 3 hours after the first dose. Doxazosin has extensive first-pass hepatic metabolism. The elimination of the drug is slow, with a terminal half-life of approximately 22 hours. Maximal antihypertensive effects are observed 2 to 6 hours after an oral dose.

Two α_1-adrenergic blockers, phentolamine mesylate and phenoxybenzamine hydrochloride are used only for hypertension associated with pheochromocytoma. **Phentolamine mesylate** (Regitine) is supplied only in a parenteral dosage form. It is administered IV or IM for the diagnosis of pheochromocytoma (Regitine blocking test) and for prevention and control of hypertensive episodes associated with stress in perioperative situations. **Phenoxybenzamine** (Dibenzyline) is an oral preparation used to control episodes of hypertension and sweating in clients with pheochromocytoma. Table 33–4 provides a summary of dosage and routes of administration for α_1-adrenergic blockers.

α-β-Adrenergic Blockers

Mixed α_1- and β-adrenergic blockers combine effects described for α_1-adrenergic blockers and β-adrenergic blockers. The prototype for this drug category is labetalol hydrochloride.

🦋 Nursing Research

Malsch, E., Katonah, J., Gratz, I., & Scott, A. (1991). The effectiveness of labetalol in treating postoperative hypertension. *Nurse Anesthesia, 2*(2), 65–71.

Surgical clients often exhibit increased arterial blood pressure during the postanesthetic recovery period. Although these transient increases in blood pressure are usually benign, significant morbidity and mortality can result. The purposes of this study were to determine the frequency of postoperative hypertension in one particular recovery room and to determine the efficacy of labetalol as an antihypertensive drug in this setting.

Data were gathered through a retrospective review of 465 client records. In addition, a prospective study was conducted of the treatment protocols for 30 postoperative hypertensive clients. These clients were treated with graduated IV injections of labetalol.

Nearly 20% of the clients admitted to this particular recovery room had blood pressures in the range of the study's criteria for hypertension. Labetalol was effective in controlling clients' blood pressure within an average of 25 minutes. The blood pressures remained effectively controlled for 24 hours postoperatively.

STUDENT ACTIVITIES

- Review postoperative records of 10 clients not diagnosed with hypertension. Check the baseline blood pressure for each individual. Compare this value with the blood pressure readings in the postanesthetic period. Determine how many individuals had significant increases in arterial blood pressure postoperatively. 🦋

α-β–ADRENERGIC BLOCKER PROTOTYPE

LABETALOL HYDROCHLORIDE

Labetalol hydrochloride (Normodyne, Tranlate) received Food and Drug Administration (FDA) approval in 1984.

Pharmacotherapeutics Parenteral labetalol is used to treat severe hypertensive urgencies and emergencies. This drug is more effective than β-blockers in African-Americans and elderly clients. Labetalol has also been used to lower blood pressure and relieve symptoms in clients with pheochromocytoma.

Pharmacokinetics Labetalol is completely absorbed from the GI tract; peak plasma levels occur 1 to 2 hours after oral administration. Steady-state plasma levels during repetitive dosing are reached by the third day of therapy. Because of extensive first-pass metabolism by the liver, bioavailability of oral dosages is only 25%. However, bioavailability is increased when the drug is administered with food. Labetalol is approximately 50% protein bound. The plasma half-life for oral dosages is 6 to 8 hours.

Labetalol is metabolized mainly through conjugation to glucuronide metabolites. These metabolites are present in plasma and are excreted in the urine and bile.

TABLE 33–4

Drugs with Peripheral Sympatholytic Action

Drug Name	Dosage and Route of Administration	Nursing Considerations
α-ADRENERGIC BLOCKER PRAZOSIN HYDROCHLORIDE (Minipress) HOW SUPPLIED Capsules: 1, 2, 5 mg	ORAL Initial dose: 1 mg bid or tid Maintenance dose: usual range, 6–15 mg/d in divided doses **Acute Management of Severe Hypertension** 1–2 mg; repeat in 1 h if necessary	**Implement** Check dosage carefully in initial therapy. Only 1-mg capsules are used. Prazosin may be administered without regard to food intake. Administer first dose at bedtime to minimize risk of fainting from first-dose syncope. Dry mouth may be relieved by sugarless gum or sips of tepid water. Advise client that use of alcohol may increase postural hypotension.
Terazosin Hydrochloride (Hytrin) HOW SUPPLIED Tablets: 1, 2, 5, 10 mg	ORAL Initial dose: 1 mg at bedtime Maintenance dose: 1–5 mg/d	**Implement** Instruct client that somnolence or drowsiness may occur with drug. Tablets may be crushed. Give first dose at bedtime. If initial dose is given during daytime, client must remain recumbent for 3 to 4 h. Advise client that noncarbonated beverage, unsalted crackers, or dry toast may relieve nausea. Measure blood pressure 2–3 h after dosing and at end of dosing interval (24 h) to see if maximum and minimum responses are similar. Full therapeutic effect may not occur for 3 to 4 wk.
Doxazosin Mesylate (Cardura) HOW SUPPLIED Tablets: 1, 2, 4, 8 mg	ORAL Initial dose: 1 mg daily; dosage may be gradually increased to 2, 4, 8, 16 mg Increases beyond 4 mg increase risk of excessive postural effects	**Implement** Postural effects most likely to occur 2 to 6 h after a dose. Standing blood pressures should be taken at 2, 6, and 24 h after dose to evaluate response to drug.
Phenoxybenzamine Hydrochloride (Dibenzyline) HOW SUPPLIED Capsules: 10 mg	**Treatment in Pheochromocytoma** ORAL Initial dose: 10 mg bid; increase dosage daily to 20–40 mg bid or tid	**Implement** Monitor blood pressure. Assist with ambulation if dizziness occurs. Advise client to avoid drinking alcoholic beverages. Do not use epinephrine. Instruct client to avoid use of over-the-counter cough and cold medications. Advise client that side effects tend to diminish as therapy continues.
Phentolamine Mesylate (Regitine) HOW SUPPLIED Vial: 5 mg phentolamine mesylate and 25 mg lyophilzed mannitol/ vial	**Treatment in Pheochromocytoma** IV Adults: 5 mg 1–2 h before surgery Children: 1 mg 1–2 h before surgery **Diagnosis of Pheochromocytoma** IV Adults: 2.5–5 mg Children: 1 mg	**Implement** Position client supine for pheochromocytoma test. Administer drug IM or rapidly IV when blood pressure is stabilized. If drug is given IV, record blood pressure (BP) immediately and at 30-sec intervals for 3 min; then at 60-sec intervals for 7 min. Expect preinjection pressure to return within 15–30 min. If drug is administered IM, record BP q5min for 30–45 min. Positive pheochromocytoma test result is indicated by decrease in BP >35 mm Hg systolic and >25 mm Hg diastolic pressure. Negative pheochromocytoma test result is indicated by no BP change, elevated BP, or BP elevated 35 mm Hg systolic and 25 mm Hg diastolic.

TABLE 33–4 *Continued*
Drugs with Peripheral Sympatholytic Action

Drug Name	Dosage and Route of Administration	Nursing Considerations
α-β-ADRENERGIC BLOCKERS **LABETALOL HYDROCHLORIDE** (Normodyne, Trandate) **HOW SUPPLIED** Tablets: 100, 200, 300 mg Parenteral: 5 mg/ml	**ADULTS** *Oral* Initial dose: 100 mg bid; titrate by standing BP; increase dosage in increments of 100 mg bid q2–3d Maintenance dose: 200–400 mg bid Severe hypertension may require doses of 1200–2400 mg/d in divided doses bid or tid *Parenteral* IV bolus: 20 mg over 2 min, then 40–80-mg increments q10min until desired BP is attained or total of 300 mg is injected IV infusion: dilute drug in IV fluid, 40 ml (200 mg) in 160 ml or 40 ml in 250 ml, and administer at 2 mg/min (2 ml/min or 3 ml/min, respectively) Usual effective dose: 50–200 mg; total dose of 300 mg may be required	***Implement*** Labetalol is not compatible with 5% sodium bicarbonate solution. Take baseline BP before giving initial oral dose. Tablets may be crushed. Tablets may be administered without regard to food intake. Observe client closely during first 4 h when peak is expected. Take standing BP qh three times with initial dose and dosage increases. For IV injection, give over 2 min at 10-min intervals. Check BP immediately before IV bolus and recheck at 5 and 10 min after injection. Monitor BP continuously during IV infusion. For IV infusion, dilute 200 mg in 160 ml 5% dextrose solution, 0.9% NaCl solution, or other compatible IV fluid to produce concentration of 1 mg/ml. Administer IV infusion at rate of 2 mg/min initially. Rate is adjusted according to blood pressure. After drug is discontinued, check BP at 5-min intervals for 30 min, 30-min intervals for 2 h, and hourly for 6 h. Keep client supine during IV infusion and for 3 h after.
ADRENERGIC NEURON BLOCKERS **RESERPINE** (Serpasil, Serpalan) **HOW SUPPLIED** Tablets: 0.1, 0.25, 1 mg	**ADULTS** Initial dose: 0.5 mg/d for 1–2 wk Maintenance dose: 0.1–0.25 mg/d **CHILDREN** 20 μg/kg/d to maximum of 0.25 mg/d	***Implement*** Monitor BP carefully so lowest effective dose is identified. Caution client about sedative effects. Monitor client for indications of depression. Instruct client to report signs of upper GI distress immediately.
Guanethidine Monosulfate (Ismelin) **HOW SUPPLIED** Tablets: 10, 25 mg	**ADULTS** *Ambulatory Clients* Initial dose, 10 mg/d; increase dose q5–7d based on supine, standing, and post exercise BP measurements Maintenance dose: 25–60 mg/d *Hospitalized Clients* Initial dose: 25–50 mg; increase by 25–50 mg/d or qod to maximum of 300 mg *Severe Hypertension* Loading dose regimen: give drug tid at 6-h intervals over 1–3 d Maintenance dose: ⅟₇ to ⅕ of total loading dose required **CHILDREN** Initial dose: 0.2 mg/kg/24 h (6 mg/m²/24 h) as single dose; increase by 0.2 mg/kg/24 h q7–10d; maximum: 3 mg/kg/24 h	***Implement*** During initial therapy and dosage increases, take BP supine, after standing 10 min and immediately after exercising. Advise client of risk for postural hypotension. Teach specific safety factors (e.g., change position slowly).
Guanadrel Sulfate (Hylorel) **HOW SUPPLIED** Scored tablets: 10, 25 mg	Initial dose: 10 mg/d; adjust dosage weekly or monthly Maintenance dose: 20–75 mg/d in two divided doses; higher dosages may be administered tid or qid	See guanethidine monosulfate.

Approximately 55% to 60% of the unchanged drug or its metabolites is excreted in the urine within 24 hours; 30% is excreted in feces within 4 days. Elimination of the drug is not altered with decreased hepatic or renal function. However, bioavailability is increased in clients with impaired hepatic function because of decreased first-pass metabolism (see Table 33–1).[8,15,17]

Pharmacodynamics Labetalol is a nonselective β-adrenergic blocker and a selective α_1-adrenergic blocker. However, the β-adrenergic blocking activity of labetalol is greater than the α-adrenergic blocking activity. The principal physiologic action of labetalol is to block competitively the adrenergic stimulation of β-receptors within the myocardium and bronchial and vascular smooth muscle and of α_1-receptors within vascular smooth muscle.

Labetalol produces dose-related reduction in blood pressure without reflex tachycardia or significant reduction in heart rate. After oral administration of the drug, the hypotensive effect is usually apparent within 20 minutes to 2 hours. Duration of action is also dose dependent—8 to 12 hours for a 200-mg dose and 12 to 24 hours for a 300-mg dose. With direct IV dosing, the hypotensive effect occurs within 2 to 5 minutes; peak action occurs in 5 to 15 minutes, and duration of action is 2 to 4 hours.[8,15,25]

Pharmaceutics Labetalol is available for oral administration in tablet form. It is also available in multidose vials and single-dose, prefilled syringes for IV use. Labetalol is available in fixed combinations with the thiazide diuretic hydrochlorothiazide (Normozide) for oral administration. See Table 33–4 for information on dosage forms, route of administration, and dosages.

Undesired Clinical Responses Most undesired clinical responses with labetalol are mild and transient and occur early in therapy. The most frequent cardiovascular effect is symptomatic orthostatic hypotension. This occurs most often with initiation of oral therapy or when a client is tilted upward or assumes an upright position within 3 hours of an IV dose. Atrioventricular conduction arrhythmias have occurred.

Edema, bradycardia, dizziness, drowsiness, headache, fatigue, lethargy, nightmares, or vivid dreams have been reported. Paresthesia, usually mild transient tingling of scalp and skin, has occurred early in therapy. Occasionally dyspnea, wheezing, bronchospasm, nasal congestion, and coryza-like symptoms occur. Signs of hepatocellular injury, a rare response, or CHF require withdrawal of the drug.[8,15]

Contraindications and Precautions Labetalol use is contraindicated in clients with bronchial asthma. It should also be used with caution in clients with chronic bronchitis, emphysema, and diabetes mellitus. Its use is contraindicated in clients with overt cardiac failure, severe bradycardia, heart block greater than first degree, and cardiogenic shock. Labetalol is used with caution in clients scheduled for surgery. Notify the anesthetist or anesthesiologist of this drug use because increased hypotension is expected with the anesthesia.

Drug-Drug, Drug-Nutrient, Drug-Environment Interactions Additive effects occur if labetalol is administered concurrently with diuretics and other hypotensive drugs. When administered concurrently with calcium channel blockers, undesired and therapeutic effects may be additive. Labetalol antagonizes the reflex tachycardia produced by nitroglycerin; an additive hypotensive effect may also occur.

Synergistic hypotensive effect occurs with use of IV labetalol and halothane anesthesia. Concomitant administration of cimetidine increases the bioavailability of labetalol, and concomitant administration of glutethimide decreases its bioavailability.

Labetalol parenteral solution, which is stable for 24 hours, should be protected from freezing and light. The parenteral solution should not be mixed with 5% sodium bicarbonate. Tablets should be stored in well-sealed containers and protected from moisture. Labetalol can be administered without regard to food. However, food does increase its bioavailability.[15,17,26]

Life-Span Considerations Labetalol is classified as a Pregnancy Category C drug. It has been used orally in the management of hypertension during pregnancy and intravenously in clients with severe hypertension in pregnancy without undesired effects. Safety of labetalol has not been established in children. In the elderly it is more effective than β-blockers.

Specific Drug-Related Nursing Considerations Take baseline blood pressure before the **initial oral dose.** After the initial dose, measure standing blood pressure every hour for the first 3 hours. Observe client closely during the first 4 hours when peak action is expected. Assess blood pressure 12 hours after the dose to determine duration of effectiveness.

Immediately before an **IV bolus** check the blood pressure. Measure the blood pressure 5 and 10 minutes after the injection. Maximum effect usually occurs within 5 minutes of each injection.

During **IV infusion** the blood pressure and electrocardiogram (ECG) should be monitored continuously and rate of flow titrated according to the client's response. Rapid or excessive falls in systolic or diastolic pressures are not desired. Advise the client that scalp tingling may occur at the beginning of treatment. Explain that this is usually a mild transient effect. Monitor the blood pressure at 5-minute intervals for 30 minutes, then at 30-minute intervals for 2 hours, then hourly for 6 hours, and then as necessary thereafter. Keep the client supine during IV therapy and for 3 hours after the drug is discontinued. Expect a substantial fall in blood pressure when the client moves to an upright position. Supervise initial activity. Oral drug therapy is usually initiated when the supine diastolic pressure begins to increase.

Instruct clients to take the drug as prescribed and not to discontinue the drug without consulting the prescriber. Advise clients to report persistent side effects. Teach clients signs and symptoms of hepatic injury (i.e., pruritus, dark urine, jaundice, anorexia, right upper quadrant tenderness, unexplained "flulike" symptoms, and CHF). Explain the importance of reporting these responses immediately.

CONCEPT REVIEW

Drugs with peripheral sympatholytic action are divided into three subclassifications: β-adrenergic blockers, α-adrenergic blockers, and α-β–adrenergic blockers.

These adrenergic blockers of the peripheral nervous system reduce blood pressure by reducing tonic neural vasoconstriction.

β-Adrenergic blockers compete with β-agonists for β$_1$- and β$_2$-receptor sites.

α$_1$-Adrenergic blockers act generally by blocking the sympathetic vasoconstrictor impulses at α$_1$-adrenergic receptors in vascular smooth muscle.

α-β–Adrenergic blockers have both selective α$_1$- and nonselective β-adrenergic receptor blocking actions.

Adrenergic Neuron Blockers

Adrenergic neuron blockers inhibit sympathetic vasoconstriction by depleting catecholamine (epinephrine and norepinephrine) stores in the adrenergic nerve endings. They also inhibit norepinephrine release from neuronal storage sites in response to nerve stimulation. Depletion or inhibition of norepinephrine causes relaxation of vascular smooth muscle, which decreases total peripheral resistance. Prolonged therapy causes pooling of peripheral blood and reduces venous return. This results in decreased cardiac output, bradycardia, and hypotension.[8]

ADRENERGIC NEURON BLOCKER PROTOTYPE

RESERPINE

Reserpine (Serpasil) is a refined alkaloid of rauwolfia derivatives. Reserpine and rauwolfia alkaloids are sometimes classified as **norepinephrine depletors.**

Pharmacotherapeutics Reserpine is used in the treatment of mild to moderate hypertension. It generally is most effective when used with a diuretic. Reserpine has also been used for symptomatic treatment of agitated psychotic states in clients who require an antihypertensive drug or who cannot take phenothiazine.[15]

Pharmacokinetics After absorption from the GI tract, reserpine is widely distributed. The drug concentrates in tissues with high lipid content. Reserpine crosses the blood-brain barrier and the placenta. It is also distributed into breast milk. Ninety-six percent of the drug is bound to plasma proteins. Bioavailability of reserpine is 50%. Reserpine has a slow onset and a long duration of action. Full effects of fixed oral doses are usually delayed for at least 2 to 3 weeks. Reserpine is metabolized in the liver to inactive metabolites, which are excreted primarily in the urine. Unchanged alkaloid is excreted primarily in the feces (see Table 33–1).[8,15]

Pharmacodynamics Reserpine depletes epinephrine and norepinephrine and 5-hydroxytryptamine stores in many organs, including the brain and adrenal medulla. As a result of this action, sympathetic inhibition occurs, which results in vasodilation.

With usual doses of reserpine, postural hypotension does not occur. However, the decreased cardiac output may decrease renal blood flow. In addition, the increased parasympathomimetic activity produced by this drug results in increased GI motility, increased gastric acid secretion, and miosis. Reserpine produces a tranquilizing effect, probably related to depletion of 5-hydroxytryptamine and catecholamines from the brain.

Pharmaceutics Reserpine is available for oral administration in tablet form. The drug is also available as a fixed combination drug with hydralazine hydrochloride and hydrochlorothiazide (Hydropres), with hydroflumethiazide (Salutensin), and with methyclothiazide (Diutensen-R). See Table 33–4 for information about dosages and route of administration.

Undesired Clinical Responses The most common undesired responses associated with the CNS are drowsiness, lethargy, or fatigue. Mental depression may occur and is considered a serious side effect of this drug. Depressive reactions occur more frequently in clients receiving high doses (>0.25 mg/d) and after 2 to 8 months of therapy at usual doses. Headache, dizziness, nervousness, anxiety, increased dreaming, and nightmares have occurred.

Other undesired clinical responses include dry mouth, abdominal cramps, diarrhea, nausea, vomiting, anorexia, or an increased appetite. Increased gastric acid secretion may activate peptic ulcers. Blurred vision, lacrimation, ptosis, uveitis, glaucoma, optic atrophy, and conjunctival infection have occurred. Pruritus, rash, thrombocytopenia purpura, impotence, gynecomastia, decreased libido, breast engorgement, and muscular aches have also been noted.

Chronic drug therapy may increase serum prolactin levels and decrease urinary excretion of catecholamines, 17-ketosteroids, 17-hydroxycorticosteroid, and vanillylmandelic acid. In addition, sodium and water retention occurs, which may result in both weight gain and tolerance to the hypotensive effect of the drug.[8,15]

Contraindications and Precautions Reserpine use is contraindicated in clients with mental depression or a history of mental depression, especially those with suicidal tendencies. The drug is also contraindicated for clients with active peptic ulcers or ulcerative colitis. It should be used with caution in clients with a history of gallstone; the drug may precipitate biliary colic.

Drug-Drug, Drug-Nutrient, Drug-Environment Interactions Additive hypotensive effects may occur with diuretics, other hypotensive drugs, and general anesthesia. Reserpine may add to the β-adrenergic blocking activity of propranolol. In combination with monoamine oxidase inhibitors or methotrimeprazine, reserpine may cause excitation and hypertension. Concomitant administration of CNS depressants with reserpine may cause additive depressant effect. In addition, tricyclic antidepressants may decrease the antihypertensive effect of reserpine. Concurrent use with digitalis and quinidine has produced cardiac irregularities.[15]

Reserpine should be stored in a light-resistant container. The drug should be administered with food or milk to decrease GI discomforts.

Life-Span Considerations Reserpine is classified as a pregnancy Category C drug. Safe use during pregnancy or lactation has not been established. Although the drug has been used with children, this practice is not recommended.

Specific Drug-Related Nursing Considerations The drug dosage is adjusted according to the client's response. The dose is increased in small increments at intervals of at least 10 days. Maintain a careful record of blood pressure and pulse readings. Teach ambulatory clients to take their own pulse and to report bradycardia.

Advise the client to use caution during early therapy because of the sedative drug effects. Teach clients and family members to report despondency, early morning awakening, anorexia, impotence, or self-deprecation. Be alert to somatic complaints that may mask depression.

Instruct the client not to drink alcohol or take other CNS depressants without consulting the primary care provider. Teach the client to take the drug with food or milk. Instruct the client to note weight changes and corresponding blood pressure changes. Have the client check for edema of hands and feet.

MISCELLANEOUS DRUGS IN CATEGORY

Guanethidine monosulfate (Ismelin) reduces blood pressure by inhibiting postganglionic nerve release of norepinephrine to sympathetic stimulation. Guanethidine reduces cardiac output, venous tone, and venous return, thus producing hypotension. The principal undesired clinical response associated with guanethidine is postural hypotension. Currently, guanethidine is rarely prescribed; however, a few clients still are treated with this drug.[8]

Guanadrel sulfate (Hylorel) reduces blood pressure by the same mechanism as guanethidine. Like guanethidine, it does not enter or act through the CNS. Like guanethidine, guanadrel is rarely prescribed today.[8] Table 33–4 provides additional information about adrenergic neuron blockers.

CONCEPT REVIEW

Unlike the other drugs with peripheral sympatholytic action, adrenergic neuron blockers deplete the norepinephrine supplies or inhibit the norepinephrine release from neuronal storage sites in response to nerve stimulation.

Reserpine is the prototype of this category. Before modern drugs were developed, reserpine and rauwolfia alkaloids were important antihypertensive drugs, particularly for clients with moderate to severe hypertension. Currently, except in unusual circumstances, drugs with fewer undesired clinical responses are prescribed.

DRUGS INHIBITING CATECHOLAMINE SYNTHESIS

These drugs suppress urinary catecholamine and catecholamine-metabolite excretion.

CATECHOLAMINE SYNTHESIS INHIBITOR PROTOTYPE
METYROSINE

Metyrosine (Demser) is a potent antihypertensive drug that produces significant undesired clinical responses.

Pharmacotherapeutics Metyrosine's use has been re-

stricted to clients with pheochromocytoma. It is not recommended for the treatment of essential hypertension.

Pharmacokinetics Metyrosine is well absorbed from the GI tract and is excreted unchanged in the urine. Maximum effect from a given dose of drug occurs after 1 to 3 days. Conversely, effects last for 3 to 5 days after discontinuation of the drug.

Pharmacodynamics Metyrosine inhibits tyrosine hydroxylase, the principal rate-limiting enzyme in catecholamine biosynthesis. This step blocks the conversion of tyrosine to dopa.

Pharmaceutics Metyrosine is available in 250-mg capsules for oral administration.

Recommended Dosage
- Recommended initial dosage for adults and children 12 years of age and older is 250 mg qid.
- Dosage may be increased by 250 to 500 mg every day to a maximum of 4g/d in divided doses.
- Phenoxybenzamine, an α-adrenergic blocker, frequently is administered concurrently.

Undesired Clinical Responses Undesired clinical responses of metyrosine primarily involve the CNS. They include sedation, anxiety, depression, confusion, hallucinations, and disorientation. GI side effects, including diarrhea, nausea, vomiting, anorexia, and abdominal pain, may also occur. Other undesired clinical responses include gynecomastia, galactorrhea, sexual impotence, increased prolactin levels, eosinophilia, liver enzyme elevations, nasal stuffiness, dry mouth, and hypersensitivity reactions.

Contraindications and Precautions Metyrosine should be used with care in clients with renal impairment. Its use is contraindicated in clients with hypersensitivity to the compound.

Drug-Drug and Drug-Nutrient Interactions Caution should be observed in administering metyrosine to clients receiving phenothiazines or haloperiodol because of the risk of extrapyramidal effects. To minimize the risk of crystalluria, clients should maintain water intake sufficient to achieve a daily urinary volume of 2000 ml or more.

Interference With Laboratory Results False increases in urinary catecholamines may be observed because of the presence of drug metabolites.

Life-Span Considerations Use of metyrosine in children less than 12 years of age has been limited. Its use during pregnancy and lactation has not been studied. It is not known if the drug has a teratogenic effect or if it is excreted in human milk.[8,27]

Specific Drug-Related Nursing Considerations Monitor blood pressure carefully. Encourage the client to maintain sufficient water intake.

DIRECT VASODILATORS

Direct vasodilators exert a direct vasodilator effect on vascular smooth muscle. This effect is more pronounced on arteries than on veins. This peripheral vasodilator effect results in decreased arterial blood pressure, which frequently is accompanied by reflex increase in heart rate, cardiac output, and stroke volume. Sodium and water retention may also occur. Because of these effects, concomitant administration of diuretics and β-blockers is recommended.

DIRECT VASODILATOR PROTOTYPE

HYDRALAZINE HYDROCHLORIDE

Hydralazine (Apresoline) is a widely prescribed antihypertensive drug, particularly in conjunction with a β-blocker and diuretic.

Pharmacotherapeutics Hydralazine is used in the management of moderate to severe hypertension. The parenteral preparation may be used for the management of severe hypertension when oral administration is not possible or the need to lower the blood pressure is urgent. The drug is being evaluated for use in reducing afterload in the treatment of CHF and severe aortic insufficiency and after valve replacement.

Pharmacokinetics Hydralazine is rapidly absorbed after oral ingestion. Protein binding is 87%, and bioavailability is 30% to 50%. Peak plasma concentrations occur 30 to 120 minutes after an oral dose. The drug is widely distributed; it crosses the placenta and is excreted in human milk. Duration of action is 6 to 12 hours. Hydralazine is metabolized in the GI mucosa and during the first pass through the liver. The metabolites of hydralazine are inactive. Hydralazine is excreted in the urine as active drug (12% to 14%) and metabolites; approximately 10% of the drug is excreted in feces (Table 33–1).[15,27]

Pharmacodynamics Hydralazine, through direct relaxation of vascular smooth muscle, exerts a peripheral vasodilator effect. Hydralazine also alters cellular calcium metabolism, interfering with calcium movement within the vascular smooth muscle. The preferential dilation of arterioles, as compared to veins, minimizes postural hypotension and promotes an increase in cardiac output. Hydralazine increases plasma renin activity, which results in increased sodium and water retention with the renin-angiotensin-aldosterone mechanism. Coronary, cerebral, and renal blood flow remains the same or increases.[15,17,26]

Pharmaceutics Hydralazine is available in tablets for oral administration. It is available as a parenteral solution for IM or IV administration. The drug is also available in fixed combination with hydrochlorothiazide (Apresazide, Hydralazide) and with hydrochlorothiazide and reserpine (SER-AP-ES). Table 33–5 summarizes information about the dosages and routes of administration of hydralazine.

Undesired Clinical Responses Most undesired clinical responses are reversible with dosage reductions. The most common responses are headache, nausea, anorexia, vomiting, diarrhea, palpitations, tachycardia, and angina pectoris. Less frequent responses include constipation, paralytic ileus, hypotension, paradoxic pressor response, edema, dyspnea, peripheral neuritis, dysuria, nasal congestion, and psychotic reactions. Systemic lupus erythematosus has occurred, especially in clients receiving large dosages and prolonged drug therapy.

Contraindications and Precautions Hydralazine use is contraindicated in clients with coronary artery disease and mitral valvular rheumatic heart disease. Its use is also contraindicated in clients with known hypersensitivity. Hydralazine should be discontinued gradually to avoid rebound hypertension in clients with marked reduction in blood pressure. It should be used with caution in clients with advanced renal damage.

Drug-Drug, Drug-Nutrient, Drug-Environment Interactions Serum levels of β-blockers, metoprolol, propranolol, and hydralazine are increased when they are administered concurrently with hydralazine. In addition, the pharmacologic effects of hydralazine may be decreased by indomethacin.

Administration of hydralazine with food results in higher plasma drug levels. Hydralazine parenteral solution may change color after contact with metal (e.g., when the drug is removed from a vial with a syringe and metal needle). Discolored solutions should not be used.

Life-Span Considerations Hydralazine is classified as a Pregnancy Category C drug. If it is used for hypertensive crisis of pregnancy, monitor fetal parameters and maternal vital signs continuously. The drug is relatively safe for use in pregnancy if carefully titrated.[28] Although the drug has been used with children, safety and efficacy for this age group have not been established.

Specific Drug-Related Nursing Considerations Instruct clients to take the drug with meals. After preparing an hydralazine injection, administer the drug as soon as possible to avoid color changes of the drug solution.

Monitor clients closely during initiation of therapy because reflex tachycardia may occur. Additionally, angina may be precipitated in susceptible clients. Advise the client to report weight increase, edema, or breathing difficulties. Instruct the client that combination drug therapy with hydralazine is common. Emphasize the importance of taking all drugs as prescribed.

Because of the risk of lupuslike syndrome, complete blood count and ANA studies should be done before and periodically during drug therapy. If peripheral neuritis occurs, pyridoxine may be added to the treatment regimen since the neuritis apparently is an antipyridoxine effect.

MISCELLANEOUS DRUGS IN CATEGORY

Several additional drugs with vasodilating actions are important in the treatment of hypertension. Information about the dosage, routes of administration, and nursing considerations for these drugs is summarized in Table 33–4.

Minoxidil (Loniten, Minodyl) is a potent direct vasodilator whose mechanism of action is believed to be the same as hydralazine. However, minoxidil is significantly more potent and has a longer duration of action than hydralazine. As a result, the direct arteriolar vasodilation in the absence of venous dilation leads to a marked increase in reflex sympathetic activity and in sodium and water retention. Because of its potency, minoxidil has been used for severe and malignant forms of hypertension and for treatment-resistant hypertension.[8]

Eighty percent of the clients receiving minoxidil experience enhanced hair growth, presumably because of the regional increase in cutaneous blood flow. Hair growth is most conspicuous on the face, although it occurs over the entire body. The skin may darken and wrinkle as well. These changes are partially reversible over time, even when the drug is continued. Advise the client to report tachycardia, rapid weight gain, shortness of breath, angina, severe indigestion, dizziness, or fainting.[8,15]

Sodium nitroprusside (Nipride, Nitropress) is used in IV solutions for the treatment of hypertensive emergencies.

TABLE 33–5
Direct Vasodilators Used to Treat Hypertension

Drug Name	Dosage and Route of Administration	Nursing Considerations
HYDRALAZINE HYDROCHLORIDE (Apresoline) HOW SUPPLIED Tablets: 10, 25, 50, 100 mg Parenteral solution: 1-ml vials— 20 mg/ml	ORAL *Adults* Initial dose, 10 mg qid for 2–4 d; increase to 25 mg qid for balance of first week; increase to 50 mg qid for subsequent therapy Maintenance dose: lowest effective dose; 300–400 mg/d may be required *Children* Initial dose, 0.75 mg/kg/d in four divided doses; increase over next 3–4 wk to maximum of 7.5 mg/kg or 200 mg/d PARENTERAL *Adults* IM: 10–50 mg; repeat as necessary IV: 10–20 mg; repeat as necessary *Children* 0.4–1.25 mg/kg/d divided in four to six doses Initial parenteral dose should not exceed 20 mg **Pregnancy-induced Hypertension** IV: 5 mg, followed by 5–10 mg q20–30min	**Assess** Assess for contraindications to therapy (e.g., coronary artery disease, mitral valvular rheumatic heart disease). Determine if client is pregnant; drug is classified as Pregnancy Category C drug. **Implement** Monitor blood pressure carefully. Instruct client to report persistent palpitations, edema, weight gain, arthralgia, chest pain, fever. Explain need for periodic blood tests. Assess fetal parameters when used with pregnant client. **Monitor** Monitor hemoglobin and red blood count for reduced levels. Monitor white blood count for leukopenia, eosinophilia, and agranulocytosis.
Minoxidil (Loniten, Minodyl) HOW SUPPLIED Scored tablets: 2.5, 10 mg	ADULTS AND CHILDREN >12 Y Initial dose: 5 mg daily; increase at 3-d intervals to 10, 20, and 40 mg daily in one to two doses Maintenance dose: 10–40 mg/d to maximum of 100 mg/d CHILDREN <12 Y Initial dose: 0.2 mg/kg/d (maximum 5 mg); increase at 3-d intervals Maintenance dose: 0.25–1 mg/kg/d in one or two doses to maximum 50 mg/d	**Assess** Assess for contraindications to therapy (e.g., pheochromocytoma, acute myocardial infarction). Determine if client is pregnant; minoxidil is classified as Pregnancy Category C drug. **Implement** Monitor blood pressure closely. Explain to client that enhanced hair growth and darkening of the skin may occur. Advise client to report tachycardia, rapid weight gain, shortness of breath, angina, dizziness, fainting.
Sodium Nitroprusside (Nipride, Nitropress) HOW SUPPLIED Powder: 50 mg/vial	IV *ONLY* Start infusion at 0.3 µg/kg/min; gradually titrate upward every few minutes until blood pressure control or *maximum infusion rate* of 10 µg/kg/min is achieved; if adequate reduction in blood pressure does not occur within 10 min at maximum infusion, drug should be discontinued	**Assess** Assess for contraindications to therapy. Determine if client is pregnant; sodium nitroprusside is classifed as Pregnancy Category C drug. Determine if client is breast-feeding; do not administer if woman is breast-feeding. **Implement** Dilute 50 mg of powdered drug in 2–3 ml of 5% dextrose solution; further dilute in 100–250 ml of 5% dextrose solution. Read manufacturer's directions carefully to determine alternative reconstituting procedures. Administer IV solution through controlled infusion device, microdrip regular device, or similar device that allows precise measurement of flow rate. Do not administer other drugs in same solution as nitroprusside. Use freshly prepared solution; it will have faint brownish tint.

TABLE 33–5 *Continued*
Direct Vasodilators Used to Treat Hypertension

Drug Name	Dosage and Route of Administration	Nursing Considerations
		Discard solution if highly colored. Wrap solution container in aluminum foil to protect from light. It is not necessary to cover drip chamber and tubing. Expect hypotensive effect within 1–2 min of adequate infusion. Monitor blood pressure continuously. Titrate dose to maintain hypotensive effect. Do not exceed maximum dose. Hypotensive effect ceases rapidly after infusion is stopped.
Diazoxide (Hyperstat) HOW SUPPLIED Ampule: 15 mg/ml (300 mg and 20 ml equal one ampule)	**IV** ONLY All ages: 1–3 mg/kg up to maximum of 150 mg in single injection q5–15min until adequate reduction in pressure is achieved (diastolic <100 mm Hg)	**Assess** Determine if client is pregnant or breast-feeding. Safety for use in pregnancy has not been determined; drug is classified in Pregnancy Category C. Client should not use if breast-feeding. **Implement** Administer "minibolus" dose into peripheral vein. Do not administer IM or SC or into body cavity. Use warm compresses to infusion site if extravasation occurs. Solution is alkaline and irritating to tissue. Monitor blood pressure closely until stable, then hourly. Keep client supine during and for 1 h after drug administration. Assess standing blood pressure in ambulatory clients. **Monitor** Observe client for hyperglycemia; check serum glucose levels. Monitor for fluid retention.

Nitroprusside produces both arteriolar and venous dilation. This action is produced by interference with the intracellular flux of calcium.

Nitroprusside has almost an immediate onset of action that becomes maximal in 1 to 2 minutes. The most frequent undesired clinical response is hypotension. Nausea, vomiting, headache, sweating, restlessness, confusion, and palpitations may occur if the hypertension is reduced rapidly. These responses may be avoided by slow and careful titration of the IV infusion. Rebound hypertension also commonly occurs with nitroprusside.

Diazoxide (Hyperstat) is also used for hypertensive emergencies. This drug is an IV nondiuretic thiazide that, like minoxidil, acts directly on arterioles. Diazoxide has a marked antinatriuretic effect. Undesired clinical responses of diazoxide are similar to those of hydralazine and minoxidil. In addition, diazoxide may produce marked hyperglycemia and hyperosmolarity.

CONCEPT REVIEW

Metyrosine inhibits catecholamine synthesis. Specifically, it inhibits tyrosine hydroxylase, the principal rate-limiting enzyme in catecholamine biosynthesis. This action blocks the conversion of tyrosine to dopa.

Metyrosine is used to treat clients with pheochromocytoma. It is not recommended for the treatment of essential hypertension.

Direct vasodilators exert a direct vasodilator effect on vascular smooth muscle. With most vasodilators, this effect is more pronounced on arteries than on veins. This peripheral vasodilator effect results in decreased arterial blood pressure.

Hydralazine is the prototype for direct vasodilators. It is used to treat moderate to severe hypertension.

Other direct vasodilators (i.e., minoxidil, sodium nitroprusside, and diazoxide) are used to treat malignant hypertension and hypertensive emergencies.

ACE INHIBITORS

Angiotensin-converting enzyme (ACE) inhibitors act principally through suppression of the renin-angiotensin-aldosterone system. Renin, synthesized by the kidney, is released into circulation; it acts on a plasma globulin substrate to produce angiotensin I. Angiotensin I is converted by ACE to angiotensin II. Angiotensin II is a potent vasoconstrictor; it also stimulates release of aldosterone, increasing retention of sodium and water. ACE inhibitors block the conversion of angiotensin I to angiotensin II, preventing vasoconstriction and reducing total peripheral vascular resistance.[1,3]

ACE inhibitors appear to reverse left-ventricular hypertrophy in hypertensive clients. Cardiac output is unchanged or increased; renal blood flow is increased. These drugs do not affect exercise tolerance or sexual function.

ACE inhibitors are recommended in the initial treatment of mild to moderate hypertension when use of diuretics or β-blockers is contraindicated. ACE inhibitors are frequently used to treat hypertension in diabetics since these drugs may reduce proteinuria and help slow progression of nephropathy. They are also used to treat hypertension accompanied by CHF since they reduce afterload and improve myocardial function.[2,25]

Response to ACE inhibitors apparently is greater in Orientals and whites. African-Americans and the elderly, regardless of race, tend to have low-renin hypertension and respond less well to monotherapy with ACE inhibitors.[2,5,25]

ACE INHIBITOR PROTOTYPE
ENALAPRIL MALEATE

Enalapril (Vasotec) received FDA approval in 1985.

Pharmacotherapeutics Enalapril is used to treat mild to moderate hypertension. It is effective alone or in combination with other antihypertensive drugs, especially thiazide diuretics. Enalapril is also indicated as adjunct therapy in the management of heart failure.[29,30]

Pharmacokinetics After oral administration approximately 60% of enalapril is absorbed. Absorption is not affected by food. Peak serum concentration of enalapril occurs within 1 hour. Enalapril is hydrolyzed to enalaprilat, a more potent ACE inhibitor. Peak serum concentration of enalaprilat occurs in 3 to 4 hours. Enalapril crosses the blood-brain barrier poorly, if at all, and does not accumulate in any tissues. The drug crosses the placenta and is distributed into breast milk.

Enalapril is eliminated primarily in the urine (54%) as enalapril and enalaprilat. Ninety-four percent of the drug is eliminated in the urine and feces within 24 hours (see Table 33–1).

Pharmacodynamics Enalapril, after hydrolysis to enalaprilat, inhibits ACE. Inhibition of ACE results in decreased plasma angiotensin II, which leads to decreased vasopressor activity and to decreased aldosterone secretion. Decreased aldosterone secretion results in small increases of serum potassium.

In most clients onset of antihypertensive activity is 1 hour after oral administration, with peak reduction of blood pressure in 4 to 6 hours. Duration of action is approximately 24 hours. Cardiac output, heart rate, renal blood flow, and glomerular filtration rate are unchanged.[8,15]

Pharmaceutics Enalapril is available as tablets for oral administration. A parenteral solution, enalaprilat, is available for IV use. Enalapril is also available in a fixed combination with hydrochlorothiazide (Vaseretic). Table 33–6 summarizes information about dosages and routes of administration.

Undesired Clinical Responses Enalapril may cause a profound reduction in blood pressure after the first dose, especially in severely salt- or volume-depleted clients and clients with CHF. Other cardiovascular side effects include chest pain, orthostatic hypotension, palpitations, and arrhythmias.

A chronic nonproductive cough occurs frequently. It usually resolves within 1 to 4 days after drug discontinuation. The incidence of coughing is higher in women. Bronchitis, dyspnea, and less frequently asthma, bronchospasm, and upper respiratory infection may also occur.

GI symptoms include abdominal pain, diarrhea, vomiting, nausea, dry mouth, impaired sense of taste, glossitis, anorexia, constipation, melena, hepatitis, pancreatitis, and jaundice. Dizziness, fatigue, vertigo, syncope, and infrequently, nervousness, sleep disturbances, paresthesia, and other mental status changes have occurred.[8,15]

Contraindications and Precautions Enalapril use is contraindicated in clients with a history of angioedema related to previous treatment with ACE inhibitors. Enalapril administered to some hypertensive clients with renal impairment has resulted in increased BUN and serum creatinine levels. The drug should be used with caution in these individuals, and their renal function should be monitored carefully.

Drug-Drug, Drug-Nutrient, Drug-Environment Interactions Antacids may decrease the bioavailability of enalapril, and rifampin and indomethacin may decrease its effects. When administered concomitantly with enalapril, serum levels of digoxin and lithium are increased. Coadministration of enalapril with potassium preparations or potassium-sparing diuretics increases the risk for hyperkalemia. The pharmacologic effects of enalapril are increased by phenothiazine drugs.

Food does not interfere with enalapril absorption. The drug should be stored in tightly closed containers to protect it from moisture.

Life-Span Considerations Enalapril is classified as a Pregnancy Category C drug during the first trimester and a Category D drug during the second and third trimesters. Use of enalapril during the second and third trimesters has been associated with fetal and neonatal morbidity and mortality. The drug should be discontinued as soon as possible when pregnancy is known or suspected. Since enalapril is detected in human milk in small amounts, caution should be exercised when it is administered during lactation. Safety and efficacy in children have not been established.

Specific Drug-Related Nursing Considerations Enalapril is usually administered once a day. Symptomatic hypotension does not commonly occur. However, be alert for this effect if the client is already taking a diuretic. Take the blood pressure before administering the dose to help evaluate consistency of control. In some clients the antihypertensive effect may diminish toward the end of the dosing interval. Report blood pressure elevations to the primary care provider; dosage increase or twice-daily dosing may be indicated.

TABLE 33–6
ACE Inhibitors Used to Treat Hypertension

Drug Name	Daily Adult Dosage
Enalapril (Vasotec)	2.5–40 mg in one or two doses
Benazepril (Lotensin)	5–40 mg in one or two doses
Captopril (Capoten)	12.5–450 mg in two or three doses
Fosinopril (Monopril)	10–40 mg in one or two doses
Lisinopril (Prinivil, Zestril)	5–40 mg in one dose
Quinapril (Accupril)	5–80 in one or two doses
Ramipril (Altace)	1.25–20 mg in one or two doses

TABLE 33–7
Calcium Channel Blockers Used to Treat Hypertension

Drug Name	Daily Adult Dosage
Diltiazem	
Cardizem SR	120–360 mg in two doses
Cardizem CD	120–360 mg in one dose
Dilacor XR	120–480 mg in one dose
Verapamil	
Calan	120–480 mg in two or three doses
Calan SR	120–480 mg in one or two doses
Verelan	120–480 mg in one dose
Amlodipine (Norvasc)	2.5–10 mg in one dose
Felodipine (Plendil)	5–20 mg in one dose
Isradipine (DynaCirc)	5–10 in one or two doses
Nicardipine	
Cardene	60–120 mg in three doses
Cardene SR	60–120 mg in two doses
Nifedipine (Procardia XL)	30–90 mg in one dose

> Because the drug increases serum potassium levels, teach clients not to use potassium-containing salt substitutes without consulting the care provider. Teach the client common undesired clinical responses, and advise him or her to report persistent problems.

MISCELLANEOUS DRUGS IN CATEGORY

Several other ACE inhibitors are used to treat hypertension, including benazepril (Lotensin), captopril (Capoten), fosinopril (Monopril), lisinopril (Prinivil, Zestril), quinapril (Accupril), and ramipril (Altace). The pharmacodynamic properties of these drugs are similar. **Captopril** is effective in both mild and severe forms of renin-dependent hypertension. Because of the absence of undesired clinical responses, it often is used as a first-line drug. Captopril is also available in combination with hydrochlorothiazide.

Lisinopril is the lysine analog of enalapril and is similar in characteristics. In contrast to enalapril, lisinopril does not require conversion by the liver to the active form.[8,15,31,32]

CALCIUM CHANNEL BLOCKERS

Increased intracellular calcium activates contraction of smooth muscle and increases vascular reactivity to vasoconstrictor substances. Calcium channel blockers prevent the influx of calcium ions into vascular muscle, decreasing peripheral vascular resistance and blood pressure. Blood flow to vital organs, including the heart, CNS, and kidneys, is not compromised.

Calcium channel blockers are suitable as initial treatment of hypertension when use of β-blockers or diuretics is contraindicated. Since these drugs do not depend on the renin-angiotensin-aldosterone system, they are particularly useful in clients with low-renin hypertension. Calcium channel blockers are also suitable for hypertensive diabetic clients because at low and moderate dosages, they have few metabolic adverse effects. These drugs, especially nifedipine, can treat cyclosporine-related hypertension. Table 33–7 summarizes the usual adult dosages for calcium channel blockers commonly prescribed for hypertension. See Chapter 32 for more information on calcium channel blockers.[15,17,33]

CONCEPT REVIEW

Angiotensin-converting enzyme (ACE) inhibitors act principally through suppression of the renin-angiotensin-aldosterone system.

ACE inhibitors are recommended in the initial treatment of mild to moderate hypertension when use of diuretics or β-blockers is contraindicated.

Increased intracellular calcium activates contraction of smooth muscle and increases vascular reactivity to vasoconstrictor substances. Calcium channel blockers prevent the influx of calcium ions into vascular muscle, thus inhibiting vasoconstriction.

SUMMARY

Many drug groups are used to treat hypertension. In most situations drug selection is based on the drug's ability to be effective without producing undesired clinical responses. Currently prescribers attempt to achieve monotherapy; that is, they try to reduce the client's hypertensive state with one drug instead of a combination of drugs. However, even with this goal, many clients receive more than one antihypertensive drug. For example, diuretics and β-blockers are frequently used as adjunct therapy for the client.

REFERENCES

1. Copstead, L.C. (1995). *Perspectives on pathophysiology.* Philadelphia: W.B. Saunders.
2. Weir, M. (1991). Impact of age, race, and obesity on hypertensive mechanisms and therapy. *American Journal of Medicine, 90*(5A), 3S–14S.
3. Guyton, A.C. (1991). *Textbook of medical physiology* (8th ed.). Philadelphia: W.B. Saunders.
4. Lopez, L. (1991). Hypertension in the elderly: Conventional wisdom revisited. *Pharmacotherapy, 11,* 225–236.
5. American Heart Association. (1993). *1993 heart and stroke facts.* Dallas: Author.

6. Fifth report of the Joint National Committee on Detection, Evaluation, and Treatment of High Blood Pressure. (1993). *Archives of Internal Medicine, 153*(2), 154.

7. Monahan, F.D., Drake, T., & Neighbors, M. (Eds.). (1994). *Nursing Care of Adults.* Philadelphia: W.B. Saunders.

8. Case, D. (1992). Drugs Used in the treatment of hypertension. In C.M. Smith & A.M. Reynard (Eds.), *Textbook of pharmacology* (pp. 589–621). Philadelphia: W.B. Saunders.

9. Hockenberry, B. (1991). Multiple drug therapy in the treatment of essential hypertension. *Nursing Clinics of North America, 26,* 417–435.

10. Rodman, M.J. (1991, February). Hypertension: Step-care management. *RN,* 24–31.

11. Tjoa, H.I., & Kaplan, N.M. (1990). Treatment of hypertension in the elderly. *Journal of American Medical Association, 264,* 1015–1018.

12. Itskovitz, H.D. (1991). Alpha₁ blockers: Safe, effective treatment for hypertension. *Postgraduate Medicine, 89*(8), 89–112.

13. Bledsoe, B.E. (1990). Hypertensive emergencies: Performing under pressure. *Journal of Emergency Medical Services, 9,* 66–74, 76–77.

14. Taylor, R.B. (1990). Patient profiling: Individualization of hypertension therapy. *American Family Physician, 42*(Suppl. 5), 29S–36S.

15. McEvoy, G.K., & Litvak, K. (Eds.). (1992). *AHFS drug information.* Bethesda, MD: American Society of Hospital Pharmacists.

16. Johannsen, J.M. (1993). Update: Guideline for treating hypertension. *American Journal of Nursing, 93*(3), 29–42.

17. Solomon, J. (1994, January). Hypertension: New drug therapies. *RN,* 26–33.

18. Trottier, D.J., & Kochar, M.S. (1992). Hypertension and high cholesterol: A dangerous synergy. *American Journal of Nursing, 92*(11), 40–43.

19. Potema, K.M., Fogg, L.F., Fish, A.F., & Kravitz, H.M. (1993). Blood pressure reactivity in the evaluation of resting blood pressure and mood responses to pindolol and propranolol in hypertensive patients. *Heart and Lung: Journal of Critical Care, 22,* 383–391.

20. Grimm, R.H. (1991). Antihypertensive therapy: Taking lipids into consideration. *American Heart Journal, 122,* 910–918.

21. Black, H.R., Chrysant, S., Curry, C., Frishman, W., et al. (1992). Antihypertensive and metabolic effects of concomitant administration of terazosin and methyclothiazide for the treatment of essential hypertension. *Journal of Clinical Pharmacology, 32,* 351–359.

22. Achari, R., Laddu, A. (1992). Terazosin: A new alpha adrenoreceptor blocking drug. *Journal of Clinical Pharmacology, 32,* 520–523.

23. Lepor, H., Meretyk, S., & Knapp-Maloney, G. (1992). The safety, efficacy and compliance of terazosin therapy for benign prostatic hyperplasia. *Journal of Urology, 147,* 1554–1557.

24. Malsch, E., Katonah, J., Gratz, I., & Scott, A. (1991). The effectiveness of labetalol in treating postoperative hypertension. *Nurse Anesthesia, 2*(2), 65–71.

25. Fleg, J.L., Gavras, I.H., Langford, H.G., & Pecker, M.S. (1990, February 15). Fine points of hypertension therapy. *Patient Care,* 171–197.

26. Schrank, K.S. (1991, April). Avoiding "over shoot" in therapeutic options. *Consultant,* 39–47.

27. Data Pharmaceutica, Inc. (1993). *1993 physicians' genRx.* Smithtown, NY: Author.

28. Rcmuzzi, G., & Ruggenenti, P. (1991). Prevention and treatment of pregnancy-associated hypertension: What have we learned in the last 10 years? *American Journal of Kidney Disease, 18,* 285–305.

29. Deglin, J.H., & Deglin, S. (1992). Hypertension: Current trends and choices in pharmacotherapeutics. *AACN–Clinical Issues in Critical Care Nursing, 3,* 507–526.

30. Townsend, R.R., & Holland, O.B. (1990). Combination of converting enzyme inhibitor with diuretic for the treatment of hypertension. *Archives of Internal Medicine, 150,* 1175–1183.

31. Wiseman, L., & McTavish, D. (1994). Trandolapril: A review of its pharmacodynamic and pharmacokinetic properties, and therapeutic use in essential hypertension. *Drugs, 48,* 71–90.

32. Fernancdz, P., & Snedden, W. (1992). The pharmacodynamic responses of hypertensive patients to quinapril therapy. *Canadian Journal of Cardiology, 8*(2), 189–194.

33. Murphy, M. (1992). Selecting optimum antihypertensive therapy: Indications for choosing a calcium channel blocker. *American Journal of Medicine, 93,* 385–445.

BIBLIOGRAPHY

Anastos, D., Charney, P., Charon, R.A., Cohen, E., Jones, C.Y., Marte, C., Swiderski, D.M., Wheat, M.E., & Williams, S. (1991). Hypertension in women: What is really known? *Annals of Internal Medicine, 115,* 287–293.

Caralis, P.V. (1990). Hypertension in the Hispanic-American population. *American Journal of Medicine, 88*(Suppl. 3B), 9–16S.

Donnelly, R., Elliott, H., Meredith, P., Howie, C., & Reid, J. (1992). Combination of nifedipine and doxazosin in essential hypertension. *Journal of Cardiovascular Pharmacology, 19,* 479–486.

Hildreth, C. (1992). Hypertension in blacks: Disease characteristics and unique needs. *Consultant, 32*(2), 109–111, 115.

Mangino, M.W. (1991). Hypertension in elders: Clinical diagnosis and treatment considerations . . . isolated systolic hypertension. *Journal of Gerontological Nursing, 17*(12), 14–22.

Manos, J. (1991). A long-term study of doxazosin in the treatment of mild or moderate essential hypertension in general medical practice. *American Heart Journal, 121*(1), 346–351.

Trottier, D., & Kochar, M. (1993). Managing isolated systolic hypertension. *American Journal of Nursing, 93*(10), 51–53.

CHAPTER 34

Drugs Affecting Plasma Lipids and Coagulation Factors

ELIZABETH A. BUCK • JACQUELYN M. CLEMENT

⊛ **Composition of Blood**

LEARNING OBJECTIVES:

Describe the major components of blood.
Identify the cellular components of blood.

KEY TERMS:

Albumin, cholesterol, endomitosis, erythrocytes, globulins, leukocytes, lipoproteins, saturated fatty acids, triglycerides, unsaturated fatty acids

⊛ **Hemostatic Process**

LEARNING OBJECTIVES:

List four mechanisms of hemostasis.
Summarize the coagulation process.
Discuss the role of vitamin K in coagulation.
Identify the two countermechanisms to blood clotting.

KEY TERMS:

Aggregation, agglutination, coagulation factors, extrinsic pathway, intrinsic pathway, platelets, platelet degranulation, thrombin

⊛ **Antilipidemic Drugs**

LEARNING OBJECTIVES:

Describe the relationship of lipoproteins and the risk of atherosclerosis.
Summarize data that should be included in the assessment of the client receiving antilipidemic drugs.
Design a plan of care for the client receiving antilipidemic drugs.
List the six major categories of antilipidemic drugs.
Summarize pharmacokinetic and pharmacodynamic properties for each category.
List major undesired clinical responses to each category.

KEY TERM: Enterohepatic circulation

⊛ **Anticoagulant Drugs**

LEARNING OBJECTIVES:

Discuss the action of heparin and warfarin on the coagulation cascade.

Contrast the pharmacodynamic properties of heparin and warfarin.
Describe laboratory tests used to evaluate therapeutic effectiveness of heparin and warfarin.
Develop a plan of care for the client receiving an anticoagulant drug.

KEY TERMS:

Antithrombin III, prothrombin time, partial thromboplastin time, protamine sulfate, white-clot syndrome

⊛ **Antiplatelet Drugs**

LEARNING OBJECTIVES:

Identify the two major antiplatelet drugs.
Describe the major pharmacokinetic and pharmacodynamic properties of each drug.
Summarize common undesired clinical responses for each drug.

KEY TERMS:

Aspirin-tolerance test, bleeding time test

⊛ **Thrombolytic Drugs**

LEARNING OBJECTIVES:

Discuss the importance of early initiation of thrombolytic drugs.
List contraindications to thrombolytic therapy.
Discuss pharmacokinetic and pharmacodynamic properties of major thrombolytic drugs.

KEY TERMS:

Plasmin, plasminogen, plasminogen activators

⊛ **Antihemophilic, Antihemorrhagic, and Hemostatic Drugs**

LEARNING OBJECTIVES:

Describe the goals of therapy with antihemophilic drugs.
List three topical hemostatic drugs.

The incidence of heart disease has increased rapidly during the 1900s. Approximately 80% of all heart disease results from ischemic heart disease, which is produced by coronary atherosclerosis. Coronary atherosclerosis is linked to several risk factors, including hyperlipidemia.

This chapter contains a review of blood components (i.e., plasma and cellular elements) and the processes of hematopoiesis and hemostasis. After reviewing the physiology of these topics, drugs that affect these processes are discussed: antilipidemic drugs, anticoagulant drugs, antiplatelet drugs, thrombolytic drugs, and antihemophilic and hemostatic drugs.

COMPOSITION OF BLOOD

Whole blood is composed of two portions: plasma, a watery liquid that contains dissolved substances, and formed elements, which are cells and cell fragments.

Plasma

Plasma comprises 55% to 60% of the total blood volume and is composed of 91% to 92% water and 7% to 9% solids. Plasma proteins are the primary solid contained in the plasma. These proteins are albumin, globulins, and clotting factors; the most abundant clotting factor is fibrinogen. **Albumin** is the most plentiful plasma protein, comprising 53% of the total plasma proteins. Albumin is synthesized in the liver and provides colloid osmotic pressure in the blood vessels. **Globulins** comprise 43% of the plasma proteins and are synthesized in the lymphoid tissue. Only 4% of the plasma proteins are composed of fibrinogen. Plasma also contains inorganic and organic constituents.[1,2]

In addition, plasma lipids, which are required by most cells for the manufacture and repair of plasma membranes, are contained in the blood and are circulated as complexes combined with plasma proteins, **lipoproteins.** Major forms of lipids include triglycerides, phospholipids, cholesterol, and fatty acids.

Cholesterol is endogenously produced and is ingested through saturated fats from animal sources in the diet. It is used in the production of steroid hormones and is required by most cells for manufacturing and repairing plasma membranes. Most of the cholesterol in the bloodstream is in an esterified form. Cholesterol is excreted into the bile.

Triglycerides are the most abundant lipids and come from both animal and vegetable sources. They are composed of three fatty acids and one glycerol molecule. There are two types of fatty acids: saturated and unsaturated. The carbon atoms of **saturated fatty acids** are bound to as many hydrogen atoms as possible. **Unsaturated fatty acids** can be either monounsaturated, containing one double-bonded carbon atom (oleic acid), or polyunsaturated, containing more than one double-bonded carbon atom (omega 3, omega 6, and linoleic acid).[3,4] In addition, substances called *apoproteins* (lipid-acceptor proteins) bind with triglycerides to form lipoproteins.

Through a series of chemical reactions in the liver, several lipoproteins are produced:

- **Very low-density lipoprotein (VLDL)** contains primarily triglyceride and protein
- **Low-density lipoprotein (LDL)** contains primarily cholesterol and protein
- **High-density lipoprotein (HDL)** contains primarily phospholipids and protein

High levels of VLDL and LDL are directly related to an increased risk of atherosclerosis, whereas HDL is believed to be protective, delaying or even preventing atherogenesis. HDL contains more protein and less lipid than the other lipoproteins. HDL is broken into two subfractions, HDL_2 and HDL_3, both of which are predictors for the risk of myocardial infarction (MI).[5]

Cellular Components

There are three primary cellular components in blood: erythrocytes (red blood cells), leukocytes (white blood cells), and platelets (thrombocytes). **Erythrocytes** are the most abundant cells in the blood, comprising approximately 48% of the blood volume in men and 42% of the blood volume in women. There are approximately $4\frac{1}{2}$ to $5\frac{1}{2}$ million erythrocytes/mm³ in human blood. The main functions of erythrocytes are to transport gases such as oxygen and CO_2 to and from tissues and to help maintain acid-base balance through the buffering action of hemoglobin. Hemoglobin is the major component of erythrocytes and is composed of iron and protein.

Leukocytes are the body's primary defense against infection. In addition, these cells remove cellular debris. There are approximately 5000 to 10,000 leukocytes/mm³ of blood. The five types of leukocytes can be classified in two ways: according to their structure or according to their function. Granulocytes (neutrophils, basophils, and eosinophils) contain granules in their cytoplasm. These granules contain enzymes that kill microorganisms and break down cellular debris; their primary function is phagocytosis. Agranulocytes (monocytes, macrophages, and lymphocytes) do not contain granules. Monocytes and macrophages are phagocytic.[1,2]

Platelets, or thrombocytes, are not true cells but are "cytoplasmic fragments" without a nucleus; therefore they are not capable of mitotic division. Platelets develop from megakaryocytes through a unique process of proliferation called **endomitosis.** These cells do not develop into two daughter cells; instead they break into fragments. A hormone known as *thrombopoietin* or *platelet-stimulating factor* stimulates the pluripotential stem cells in the bone marrow to become committed megakaryocytes and stimulates other cells further along in the maturation process of platelets to differentiate more quickly. Approximately 150,000 to 400,000 platelets/mm³ are in the blood; one third of them is available in a reserve pool. The life span of platelets is only 10 days. Platelets circulate in the blood in an inactive state and are essential for blood coagulation and control of bleeding.[1,2,6]

HEMOSTATIC PROCESS

The four mechanisms of hemostasis are (1) vasoconstriction; (2) formation of a platelet plug; (3) activation of the coagulation cascade; and (4) formation of the blood clot.

Vasoconstriction

Whenever a blood vessel is injured, local vasoconstriction occurs immediately. This vasospasm lasts approximately 20 to 30 minutes so that the response of the platelets and clotting factors can begin.

Formation of Platelet Plug

Whenever a vessel is damaged, collagen becomes exposed. **Platelets** are attracted to the collagen and adhere to it rapidly so that the platelets clump together in a process called **aggregation** or **agglutination.** A platelet plug forms within 3 to 5 minutes of an injury.

The interaction of platelets with collagen causes the platelets to release various biochemical mediators. Two of them, serotonin and histamine, cause temporary vasoconstriction of the injured vessel. Another mediator, adenosine diphosphate (ADP), promotes platelet adherence by making their membranes rough and sticky. In addition, these mediators stimulate more **platelet degranulation.**

Two other mediators work together to ensure platelet aggregation continues at the site of the injury and to prevent platelets' adhering to normal vascular endothelium. One of them, thromboxane A₂, is synthesized and released by the degranulated platelets. This substance causes vasoconstriction and promotes further platelet degranulation and the production of more ADP. The second, prostacyclin₂, is synthesized and released by uninjured endothelial cells in vessel walls. It acts as a thromboxane antagonist, promoting vasodilation and preventing further platelet degradation. One other factor, called *platelet factor 4* or *heparin-neutralizing factor,* is also released by the degranulating platelets. This substance enhances clot formation at the site of the injury.[1,2]

Activation of Coagulation Cascade

Blood **coagulation factors,** with the exception of tissue thromboplastin and calcium, are plasma proteins and circulate in the bloodstream in an inactive state. These factors are listed in Table 34–1 according to the internationally standardized nomenclature. The factors are numbered according to the order of their discovery, not the order in which they participate in the clotting cascade. The liver is responsible for the synthesis of coagulation factors with the exception of part of factor

TABLE 34–1
Blood Coagulation Factors

Factors	Other Designations
I	Fibrinogen
II	Prothrombin
III	Tissue factor; tissue thromboplastin
IV	Calcium
V	Proaccelerin; labile factor
VI	This factor is no longer considered a distinct part of coagulation
VII	Stable factor; serum prothrombin conversion accelerator
VIII	Antihemophilic globulin; antihemophilic factor
IX	Christmas factor
X	Stuart factor: Stuart-Prower factor
XI	Plasma thromboplastin antecedent (PTA)
XII	Hageman factor
XIII	Fibrin stabilizing factor
Prekallikrein	Fletcher factor
High-molecular-weight kininogen	Contact activation cofactor

From Copstead, L.C. (1995). *Perspectives on pathophysiology.* Philadelphia: W.B. Saunders, p. 288.

VIII. Factors II, VII, IX, and X depend on vitamin K for synthesis and normal activity.[2,3,6]

There are two mechanisms in the coagulation pathway. The first, called the **intrinsic pathway,** is activated by the exposure of factor XII to the collagen from damaged blood vessel endothelium. It is measured by the activated partial thromboplastin time (APTT). The second mechanism, the **extrinsic pathway,** is activated when tissue thromboplastin, which is released from damaged endothelial cells, comes into contact with factor VII. It is measured by the prothrombin time (PT). Both of these pathways lead to a common pathway when each has activated factor X (Fig. 34–1).

CONCEPT REVIEW

Whole blood is composed of two portions: plasma, a watery liquid that contains dissolved substances, and formed elements, which are cells and cell fragments.

Major forms of lipids include triglycerides, phospholipids, cholesterol, and fatty acids. Cholesterol is endogenously produced and is ingested through saturated fats from animal sources in the diet.

Triglycerides are the most abundant lipids and come from both animal and vegetable sources. They are composed of three fatty acids and one glycerol molecule. There are two types of fatty acids: saturated and unsaturated.

The four mechanisms of hemostasis are (1) vasoconstriction; (2) formation of a platelet plug; (3) activation of the coagulation cascade; and (4) formation of the blood clot.

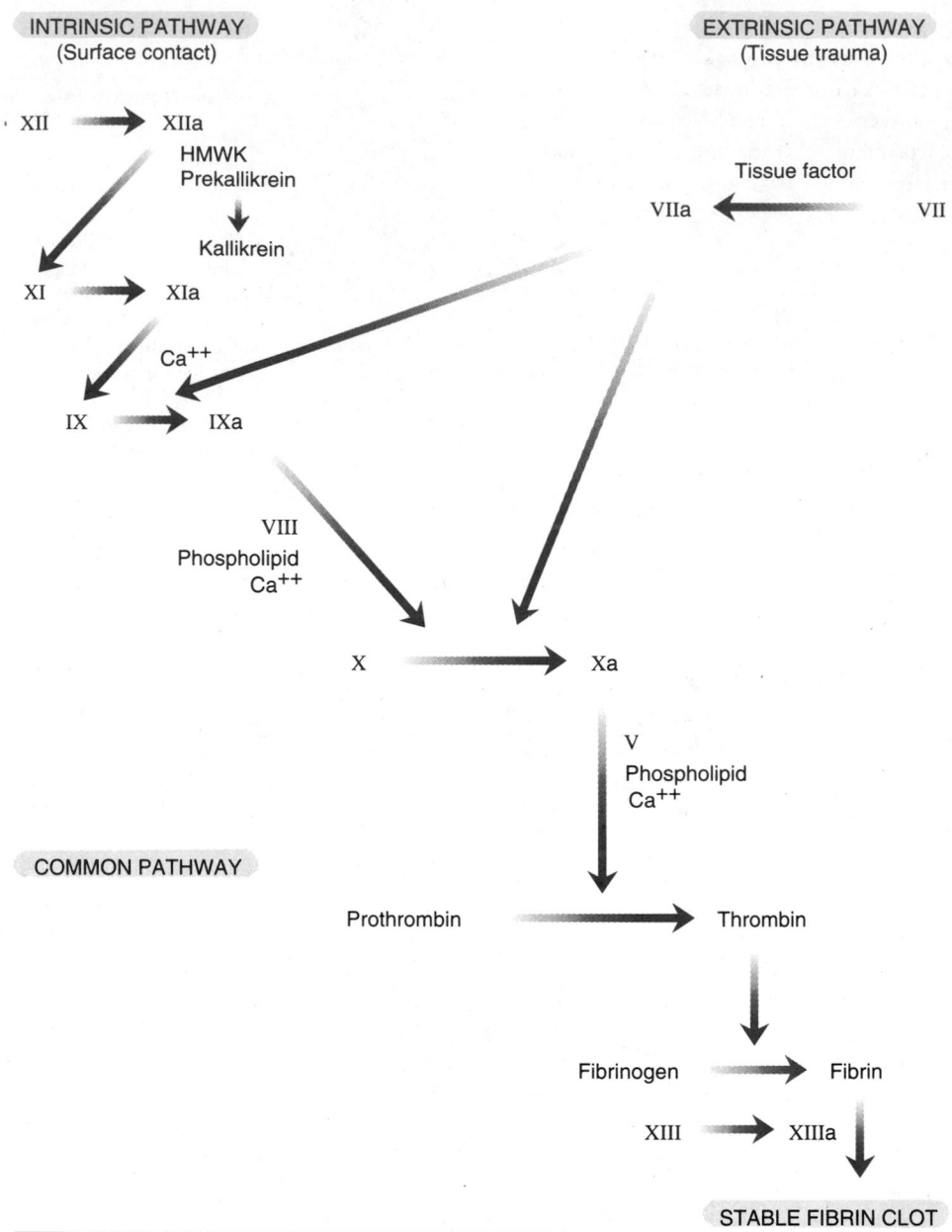

INTRINSIC PATHWAY
(Surface contact)

EXTRINSIC PATHWAY
(Tissue trauma)

COMMON PATHWAY

STABLE FIBRIN CLOT

FIGURE 34–1   Major events in the formation of a fibrin clot. Some factors have both an active and inactive form; the letter *a* after the Roman numeral designates the active form. (HMWK, high-molecular-weight kininogen.) (From Copstead, L.C. [1995]. *Perspectives on Pathophysiology.* Philadelphia: W.B. Saunders, p. 289.)

Formation of the Blood Clot

Within the common pathway, factor Xa, in the presence of Factor V, calcium, and phospholipid, converts prothrombin (factor II) to thrombin. **Thrombin** is the most powerful enzyme in the coagulation process. It converts fibrinogen into fibrin. The strands of fibrin become entwined and turn the blood into a gel. The rest of the nine clotting factors accelerate the clotting process.[3,4]

The body has two built-in countermechanisms to blood clotting: (1) antithrombins such as endogenous heparin, which antagonize the powerful coagulant, thrombin, preventing its formation or inactivating it; and (2) fibrinolysis, which is initiated when plasminogen is activated to plasmin.

ANTILIPIDEMIC DRUGS

A high fat intake through the diet has been associated with the development of hyperlipidemia. Familial dyslipoproteinemias are caused by a genetic defect. In addition, several disease processes can cause hyperlipidemia: pancreatitis, diabetes mel-

TABLE 34–2
Types of Hereditary Hyperlipoproteinemia

Type	Description	Lipoprotein Patterns	Drug Therapy
I	Exogenous hyperlipidemia Hyperchylomicronemia Fat-induced hypertriglyceridemia	Chylomicrons elevated Cholesterol normal Triglycerides increased three times normal	None
IIa	Familial hypercholesterolemia Familial hyperbetalipoproteinemia	LDL elevated; normal levels of VLDL Triglycerides normal	Cholestyramine, colestipol, nicotinic acid, probucol, neomycin
IIb	Combined hyperlipoproteinemia Carbohydrate-induced hyper-triglyceridemia	LDL and VLDL elevated Triglycerides elevated	Clofibrate, nicotinic acid, probucol, colestipol, lovastatin, gemfibrozil, cholestyramine
III	Familial dysbetalipoproteinemia Broad-beta hyperlipidemia	Broad-beta lipoproteins (remnants of chylomicron) elevated Triglycerides elevated	Clofibrate, gemfibrozil, nicotinic acid, estrogens
IV	Endogenous hyperlipemia Hypertriglyceridemia	VLDL elevated Triglycerides elevated	Clofibrate, nicotinic acid, gemfibrozil
V	Mixed hyperlipemia Carbohydrate- and fat-induced hypertriglyceridemia	Chylomicrons elevated VLDL elevated Triglycerides elevated three times normal	Clofibrate, nicotinic acid, gemfibrozil, progesterone

litus, hypothyroidism, nephrosis, and systemic lupus erythematosus. Table 34–2 summarizes the different types of hereditary hyperlipidemia.

Since high concentrations of lipoproteins in the bloodstream contribute to coronary disease, administration of antilipidemic drugs can be critical in the long-range health status of individuals. These drugs use various mechanisms to decrease the levels of lipoproteins.

▣ NURSING CONSIDERATIONS

The nurse plays an important role in the treatment of hyperlipidemia. Client education and support are essential to compliance with drug and diet therapy.

Assessing During the initial **health history** question the client about lifestyle factors such as dietary intake of fats, smoking, exercise regimen, past history of dieting, and changes in body weight over time. In addition, gather information about family history of elevated cholesterol levels and personal history of hypertension, angina, MI, or diagnosis of coronary artery disease.

Collect a detailed nutritional assessment. Have the client record all food intake, with estimated quantities, for a period of at least 1 week. Make certain that the client knows to record snacks also. Analyze the data to determine the client's total intake of dietary fat.

Assess the client's exercise habits. Collect information about routine activities such as walking, participation in exercise classes, and regular sports activities. In addition, gather information about activities related to the client's employment situation such as lifting, walking, sitting, and eating in restaurants. Since stress contributes to hyperlipidemia, include lifestyle analysis in the overall nurse-client discussion. Include information such as the client's perception of stressors, family responsibilities, potential financial pressures, and maintenance of a balance of leisure and work.

Gather detailed information about the client's use of the health care system for health promotion and disease prevention (e.g., regular cholesterol screening and blood pressure evaluations). Laboratory data to obtain include total cholesterol levels and lipoprotein fractionation (HDL, LDL, and triglyceride levels).

Finally, review the systems with the client. Specifically ask the client about shortness of breath, chest pain, and altered circulation or feeling in the lower extremities.

During the **physical assessment** include measurement of body frame size and body weight. In addition, calculate the percentage of body fat.

Diagnosing Based on the data collected, the following may be appropriate nursing diagnoses for the individual receiving antilipidemic drugs:

• Alteration in nutrition: more than body requirements related to poor eating habits and lack of regular exercise program.

• Alteration in nutrition: less than body requirements related to undesired response to drug therapy.

• High risk for altered cardiopulmonary tissue perfusion related to plaque formation.

• High risk for decreased cardiac output related to increased body weight and decreased cardiac efficiency.

• Ineffective management of therapeutic regimen related to decreased access to regular health care, economic barriers, family lifestyle demands, patterns of poor health care, knowledge deficits, and social support deficits.

• Noncompliance related to health beliefs, cultural influences, and economic constraints.

• High risk for activity intolerance related to failure to adhere to exercise program, lifestyle, presence of other disease processes, and economic barriers.

Planning Client teaching should include individualized

nutrition education compatible with the client's physical, economic and lifestyle needs. Remind the client of his or her ability to control this important risk factor for heart disease by limiting the daily fat intake to no more than 25% of the total daily caloric intake.

For overweight clients, address dietary myths such as the efficacy of fast-weight-loss diets and diet pills. Plan a sound weight-reducing diet with the client and individuals in his or her social support system. Consider scheduling a consultation with a dietitian or nutritionist.

Design an exercise program compatible with the client's age, lifestyle and daily routine, overall health status, likes and dislikes, and economic status. Encourage regular exercise. Consider scheduling a consultation with an exercise physiologist.

To aid adherence to the program developed, encourage the client to maintain daily logs of dietary intake and of exercise, including type of exercise and length of time engaged in exercising. Graphs to monitor progress are helpful in encouraging the maintenance of these programs.

Plan to teach the client about the actions, undesired responses, and possible complications of any prescribed antilipidemic drugs. Instruct the client to take the prescribed antilipidemic drug as directed by the primary care provider. Reinforce the need for regular follow-up evaluation of the response to the drug therapy.

Include immediate family members or significant others who may be responsible for cooking, meal planning, and food shopping in any client education programs. Also educate these individuals about the importance of the client's adhering to an exercise regimen.

During the planning phase expected outcomes must be developed. Possible outcomes include the following:

• Client adheres to a regular exercise program.
• Client adheres to recommended dietary restrictions.
• Client demonstrates behavior to improve circulation (e.g., cessation of smoking, relaxation techniques).
• Client demonstrates an increase in activity tolerance.
• Client participates in the therapeutic regimen.

Implementing Document the client's baseline data such as body weight, serum cholesterol level, estimated daily fat intake, daily caloric needs, and exercise pattern. These data provide a benchmark against which to determine the client's progress.

Initiate consultations with a nutritionist, exercise physiologist, and other appropriate support groups. Monitor the client for any side effects or adverse reactions to the antilipidemic drugs.

Evaluating Evaluate adherence to the prescribed health care regimen by monitoring the client's serum cholesterol levels, rate of weight loss as compared to the individual client's goal, the amount of fat intake reported in the client's food diary, and the exercise recorded in the client's exercise log. In addition, review the outcomes with the client to determine if changes in the plan of care are needed.

Bile Acid Sequestrant Resins

Bile, a substance secreted by the liver, contains electrolytes, water, cholesterol, bilirubin, and bile salts, which are conjugated bile acids. The bile salts are responsible for emulsification and absorption of fats in the intestine. Most of the bile salts are reabsorbed in the terminal ileum and are returned to the liver through the portal circulation for reuse. This process is called the **enterohepatic circulation.** This concept is important for understanding the action of the bile acid sequestrant resins used in the treatment of hyperlipidemia.

BILE ACID SEQUESTRANT RESIN PROTOTYPE

CHOLESTYRAMINE

Pharmacotherapeutics Cholestyramine (Questran) has been effective in treating type IIa hypercholesterolemia. Other uses of this drug include the treatment of diarrhea and of pruritis associated with bile acid accumulation in the skin and the binding of toxicologic agents.

Pharmacokinetics Cholestyramine is hydrophilic but insoluble in water. It is not absorbed from the gastrointestinal tract. The level of cholesterol in the serum begins to decrease within 7 to 9 days after the initiation of therapy, with the maximum effect at 21 days. After discontinuation of the drug, the cholesterol level returns to the client's previous baseline level within 1 month. The drug is not metabolized or excreted in the urine; it is excreted in the feces as an insoluble complex with bile acids.

Pharmacodynamics Bile acid sequestrant resins act by binding bile acids and inhibiting their reabsorption and enterohepatic cycling. In addition, these drugs increase fecal absorption of bile acids. Another mechanism of action is the promotion of LDL catabolism, which results in increased bile acid formation. The reduced level of bile acids promotes apoprotein B catabolism and increases conversion of cholesterol to bile acids, which causes an increased rate of LDL removal.[7,8]

Pharmaceutics Cholestyramine is prepared in several oral dosage forms, including a powder and tablets. It can be administered once or twice daily. Table 34–3 contains additional information about dosage forms, dosages, and routes of administration.

Undesired Clinical Responses Common undesired responses to cholestyramine include constipation, heartburn, nausea, vomiting, and stomach discomfort. Infrequently the client experiences a bloated feeling, hiccups, diarrhea, headache, dizziness, rapid weight loss, severe stomach pain, black or tarry stools, tongue soreness, or a skin rash. Vitamin deficiencies such as of folic acid, vitamin A, D, E, or K occur with chronic use, as does a deficiency in calcium.

Life-threatening side effects are those that occur with an allergic reaction. They include hives, wheezing, or difficulty breathing.

Contraindications and Precautions Cholestyramine is not recommended for clients having hyperlipoproteinemia types III, IV, or V, hypersensitivity, or complete biliary obstruction.

Drug-Drug, Drug-Nutrient, and Drug-Environment Interactions Cholestyramine may interfere with the absorption of some antibiotics, thiazide diuretics, and digoxin. If the client is taking anticoagulants concurrently, cholestyramine may decrease their effect.

Normal fat digestion and fat absorption may be altered during cholestyramine therapy, which can decrease or stop the absorption of the fat-soluble vitamins. Because of the potential deficiency of vitamin K, hypoprothrombinemia may occur, producing increased bleeding tendencies. The powder should be stored at room temperature and away from heat and moisture.

Life-Span Considerations There are no well-controlled studies of cholestyramine use in pregnant women. The drug should be used with caution in nursing women since the lack of fat-soluble vitamin absorption may affect the nursing infant. The safety and effectiveness in children are unknown.

Specific Drug-Related Nursing Considerations Teach the client to take cholestyramine just before or with meals. Dissolve the powder in 2 to 6 ounces (60 to 180 ml) of beverage such as water, milk, or juice. Twirl the glass gently at first to avoid clumping the powder, and then stir it gently to obtain a uniform suspension. Rinse the glass with additional liquid to ensure the full dose has been taken. See box for summary of instructions for the client about cholestyramine.

MISCELLANEOUS DRUGS IN CATEGORY

Colestipol hydrochloride (Colestid) is also an exchange resin; it is used as an adjunct to diet and exercise to lower cholesterol levels. Colestipol binds bile acids in the intestines and forms a complex excreted in the feces. Colestipol also is used in the treatment of digitalis overdose and antibiotic-associated pseudomembranous colitis.

Colestipol is not absorbed to any significant extent. It causes a decrease in plasma cholesterol concentrations within 24 to 48 hours. The maximum reduction in serum cholesterol levels usually occurs after the client has taken colestipol for 1 month.

Colestipol, like cholestyramine, is dispensed in powder form and must be dissolved in liquid. Other drugs should be taken at least 1 hour before or 4 hours after colestipol to minimize interference with their absorption.

Undesired clinical responses to colestipol include black, tarry stools and severe abdominal pain with nausea and vomiting. Clients should contact their primary care provider immediately if these side effects develop. Constipation and weight loss are also possible, as are belching, bloating, and diarrhea.

Like cholestyramine, colestipol may interfere with normal fat absorption and therefore the absorption of the fat-soluble vitamins A, D, E, and K. Vitamin K deficiency may produce hypoprothrombinemia, which can be corrected by the use of supplemental vitamin K. In addition, colestipol binds with vitamin B_{12}–intrinsic factor complex, folic acid, and iron citrate.[8] See the box on p. 408 for instructions for the client receiving colestipol.

CLIENT INSTRUCTIONS ABOUT CHOLESTYRAMINE

1. Undesired clinical responses:
   Common responses: Constipation, heartburn, nausea, vomiting, stomach discomfort
   Infrequent responses: Bloated feeling, hiccups, diarrhea, headache, dizziness, rapid weight loss, severe stomach pain, black or tarry stools, tongue soreness, skin rash
   Life-threatening responses: Hives, wheezing, or difficulty breathing
   Responses with chronic use: Folic acid deficiency; deficiency of vitamins A, D, E, and K; calcium deficiency

2. Do not take this drug if you have had an allergic reaction to it in the past.

3. If you have phenylalanine deficiency or phenylketonuria, do not take Questran Light, which contains aspartame.

4. If you are taking other drugs, cholestyramine may affect their absorption. In addition, if you are taking anticoagulants, this drug may decrease their effect. Be sure to check with your primary care provider before taking this drug with others.

5. **Powder:** Take just before or with meals. Do *not* take it in the dry form. Mix in 4 to 6 ounces of any beverage. Make sure it is completely dissolved.

6. Store the powder at room temperature away from heat and moisture.

Nicotinic Acid

Pharmacotherapeutics Nicotinic acid (niacin) is a water-soluble vitamin that has antilipidemic action. It is used as an adjunct to nondrug therapies in the treatment of types II, III, IV, and V hyperlipoproteinemia. Niacin can decrease the levels of VLDL by up to 40%.[9]

Pharmacokinetics The peak serum concentration of niacin occurs in 30 to 70 minutes. It has a half-life of 45 minutes and is metabolized in the liver.

Pharmacodynamics The normal physiologic role of niacin is as a part of coenzymes involved in tissue respiration. The exact mechanism of action by which it decreases serum lipid levels is not known. However, there are several possible explanations: inhibition of hepatic synthesis of lipoproteins containing apolipoprotein B-100, promotion of lipoprotein lipase activity, and reduction of free fatty acid mobilization from adipose tissue with an increase in fecal output of sterols.

Pharmaceutics Niacin is available in oral (tablets, sustained-action capsules) and parenteral dosage forms. The dosage for niacin is gradually increased from 100 mg administered three times per day to an average dose of 1 g three times per day, with a maximum dosage of 6 to 9 g per day.

CLIENT INSTRUCTIONS ABOUT COLESTIPOL

1. Continue to take the drug as ordered to lower your cholesterol level. In addition, your health care professional will assist you with both a weight-reduction diet that is low fat, low carbohydrate and low cholesterol and an exercise program.

2. Let your health care professional know if you have *ever* had an allergic reaction to colestipol.

3. Tell your primary care provider if you have any of the following health problems: angina, bleeding problems, constipation, gallstones, heart or blood vessel disease, hemorrhoids, stomach ulcer, or other stomach problems.

4. Tell your primary care provider if you are taking any of the following types of drugs: anticoagulants, drugs for heart disease, penicillins, tetracyclines, thiazide diuretics, or vitamins. Do not take *any* other drug unless specifically prescribed by your primary care provider.

5. Take this drug exactly as prescribed. Do not skip any doses or take more than is prescribed.

6. Contact your primary care provider immediately if you develop black, tarry stools or severe stomach pain with nausea and vomiting. Also contact your primary care provider as soon as possible if you develop constipation or an unusual loss of weight.

7. Other less serious side effects include belching, bloating, diarrhea, nausea or vomiting, or stomach pain.

8. Store this drug away from moisture and at room temperature.

Undesired clinical responses Intense flushing may occur while plasma niacin levels are increasing. Administering 325 mg of aspirin 30 minutes before each dose of niacin can decrease the flushing.[9] Pruritis and GI upset are also frequent symptoms after taking oral niacin.

Contraindications and precautions Niacin use is contraindicated in clients with known hypersensitivity, hepatic dysfunction, active peptic ulcer, or arterial bleeding.

Drug-drug, Drug-nutrient, drug-environment interactions Antihypertensive drugs may have an additive vasodilating effect to niacin and produce postural hypotension. Niacin may increase the action of ganglionic blockers.

Niacin should be administered with meals if GI symptoms occur. The client should avoid sunlight if skin lesions are present.

Life-span considerations Use of niacin during pregnancy or lactation or in women of childbearing age requires caution.

Specific drug-related nursing considerations Advise clients that flushing occurs after drug administration. Teach clients to remain recumbent if postural hypotension occurs. Counsel them to abstain from alcohol. The drug must be kept out of the reach of children.

HMG-CoA Reductase Inhibitors

3-Hydroxy-3-methylglutaryl coenzyme A (HMG-CoA) reductase inhibitors comprise a relatively new class of drugs used to lower the LDL levels. They inhibit HMG-CoA reductase, an essential enzyme in the synthesis of cholesterol.

HMG-CoA REDUCTASE INHIBITOR PROTOTYPE

LOVASTATIN

Pharmacotherapeutics Lovastatin (Mevacor) is used as an adjunct therapy in the treatment of primary hypercholesterolemia (types IIa and IIb) and mixed hyperlipidemia.

Pharmacokinetics Lovastatin is incompletely absorbed from the GI tract; absorption is increased if the drug is administered on an empty stomach. At least 95% of the drug is bound to protein. Lovastatin is hydrolyzed in the liver to an active metabolite. It has a half-life of 3 hours and is eliminated primarily in feces.[8]

The therapeutic effect of lovastatin occurs within 3 days to 2 weeks. The maximum therapeutic effect occurs within 4 to 6 weeks. Cholesterol levels return to the client's baseline within 4 to 6 weeks after the client stops taking the drug.

Pharmacodynamics As indicated previously, drugs in this category interfere with cholesterol synthesis. Lovastatin effectively reduces both normal and elevated LDL levels and reduces levels of apolipoprotein B, VLDL, and plasma triglycerides. Lovastatin also increases HDL levels. In some clients it may be necessary to use lovastatin in combination with colestipol, a bile acid–binding resin, to decrease cholesterol levels below 240 mg/dl.

Pharmaceutics Lovastatin is available as uncoated tablets for oral administration. Table 34–3 contains additional information about dosage forms, dosage, and route of administration.

Undesired Clinical Responses Common undesired responses to lovastatin include headache, excessive gas, diarrhea, or constipation. Infrequently clients experience nausea, indigestion, stomach pain, dizziness, insomnia, blurring of vision, skin rash, muscle cramps or pain, or unusual tiredness or weakness. Chronic use of lovastatin may, in rare cases, result in liver disorders.[7]

Contraindications and Precautions Individuals with hypersensitivity to lovastatin or with active liver disease should not receive the drug. This drug may significantly increase serum transaminase levels, so clients with a history of liver disease and those who consume substantial quantities of alcohol should be monitored carefully. In addition, the drug is prescribed with caution in clients with hypotension, hormonal abnormalities, a seizure disorder, or an active infection.[8]

Drug-Drug, Drug-Nutrient, Drug-Environment Interactions Gemfibrozil, cyclosporine, erythromycin, and nicotinic acid should not be used in combination with any HMG-CoA reductase inhibitor. These combinations may result in myopathy and rhabdomyolysis, with or without acute renal failure. Lovastatin should be administered with food. The drug should be stored in a tightly closed, light-resistant container. Storage temperature should be between 5° and 30° C.[8]

Life-Span Considerations Clients should not take lovastatin if they are pregnant or breast-feeding. HMG-CoA

CLIENT INSTRUCTIONS ABOUT LOVASTATIN

1. Undesired clinical responses:
   Common responses: Headache, excessive gas, diarrhea, or constipation
   Infrequent responses: Nausea, indigestion, stomach pain, dizziness, insomnia, blurred vision, skin rash, muscle cramps or pain, unusual tiredness or weakness
   Responses with chronic use: Liver disorders without symptoms (rare)

2. Do not take lovastatin if you have had an allergic reaction to it in the past. Do not take this medicine if you are pregnant or breast-feeding or have active liver disease.

3. If you have any of the following health problems, notify your health care professional before taking lovastatin: low blood pressure, hormonal abnormalities, a seizure disorder, an active infection, or a history of liver disease.

4. Do not stop taking this medication without first checking with your primary care provider.

5. Closely follow the diet your health care professional has prescribed for you.

6. Do not take this drug with gemfibrozil, cyclosporine, erythromycin, or nicotinic acid.

7. Be sure to take this drug with food.

8. Store this drug at room temperature away from heat and moisture.

reductase inhibitors decrease the synthesis of cholesterol, which is needed for normal fetal development.

Specific Drug-Related Nursing Considerations Instruct the client not to stop taking this drug without consulting the primary care provider. Advise the client to store the drug at room temperature and away from heat and moisture. Teach the client to take the drug with food. See the box for summary of points to teach the client.

MISCELLANEOUS DRUGS IN CATEGORY

Several new HMG-CoA reductase inhibitors are available, including pravastatin sodium (Pravachol), fluvastatin (Lescol), and simvastatin (Zocor). **Simvastatin** is used as adjunctive therapy in clients with primary hypercholesterolemia. Its pharmacokinetic and pharmacodynamic properties are similar to those of lovastatin. Undesired clinical responses associated with simvastatin include rash, pruritus, alopecia, dyspepsia, flatus, abdominal pain, heartburn, liver dysfunction, and pancreatitis. The client may also experience muscle cramps, myalgia, headache, and vertigo. The usual dose is 5 to 10 mg in the evening; the usual range is 5 to 40 mg/d.

Pravastatin also is used as adjunctive therapy in clients with primary hypercholesterolemia. It is poorly absorbed from the GI tract and is only 50% protein bound. Pravastatin is metabolized in the liver. The drug has a half-life of 2.7 hours and is excreted in feces via the biliary system. Pravastatin is gener-

ally well tolerated. Undesired clinical responses such as nausea, vomiting, diarrhea, constipation, and flatulence are usually mild and transient. Pravastatin is classified as a Pregnancy Category X drug. The initial adult dose is 10 to 20 mg/d at bedtime; the dosage range is 10 to 40 mg/d at bedtime. Pravastatin may be administered without regard to meals.

Fluvastatin is chemically distinct from other HMG-CoA reductase inhibitors. When administered orally, it is almost completely absorbed. However, because of extensive first-pass metabolism and biliary excretion, less than 30% reaches systemic circulation. Circulating fluvastatin is almost completely bound to proteins, primarily albumin. Fluvastatin is bound to bile acid–binding resins. Therefore if the two are used concurrently, the drugs should be administered 2 hours apart if fluvastatin is administered first and at least 4 hours apart if a resin is administered first. Concurrent use of cimetidine, ranitidine, or omeprazole increases serum concentrations of fluvastatin. The recommended initial daily dose is 20 mg administered in the evening. Maximum effect occurs in approximately 4 weeks.[10]

Gemfibrozil

Pharmacotherapeutics Gemfibrozil (Lopid) is an effective antihyperlipidemic agent in the treatment of types II and IV hyperlipoproteinemia.

Pharmacokinetics Gemfibrozil is well absorbed, with peak serum levels at 1 to 2 hours. Approximately 99% of the drug circulates bound to proteins. Two inactive metabolites are produced through metabolism in the liver. The kidney excretes approximately 70% of the drug in an unchanged state. The half-life of gemfibrozil is 1.4 hours.[7–9]

Pharmacodynamics Gemfibrozil decreases LDL and VLDL levels. It is more effective in lowering triglyceride levels than cholesterol levels. Gemfibrozil also increases the HDL levels. The probable mechanism of action is decreased production of triglycerides in the liver through inhibition of peripheral lipolysis and decreased hepatic extraction of plasma free fatty acids. It is similar in structure to clofibrate.[8]

Pharmaceutics Gemfibrozil is available in tablet form for oral administration. The manufacturer recommends a dosage of 1200 mg/d in two divided doses administered 30 minutes before both the morning and evening meals. Table 34–3 contains additional information about antilipidemic drugs.

Undesired clinical responses Common undesired responses to gemfibrozil include stomach discomfort, a bloated feeling, and nausea. Less frequently clients experience diarrhea, vomiting, sores in the mouth, tiredness, skin rash, fever, sore throat, severe stomach pain, and muscle pain or cramps.

Contraindications and precautions Use of gemfibrozil is contraindicated in clients with known hypersensitivity to the drug. In addition, clients with preexisting gallbladder disease or hepatic or severe renal dysfunction should not receive gemfibrozil.

Gemfibrozil should be used with caution in obese clients and only after more conservative therapies such as diet, exercise, and weight loss have been tried. It should be used with caution in clients with diabetes and hypothyroidism and only after control of these conditions has been established.

Drug-drug, drug-nutrient, drug-environment interactions   Caution should be used when anticoagulants are administered concurrently with gemfibrozil. The dosage of the anticoagulant should be reduced to maintain the PT at the desired level. As previously indicated, gemfibrozil should be administered 30 minutes before morning and evening meals. A low-fat diet is recommended. Gemfibrozil should be stored below 30° C.[8]

Interference with diagnostic studies   Gemfibrozil use may increase the levels of aspartate aminotransferase (AST), alanine aminotransferase (ALT), alkaline phosphatase, bilirubin, creatine kinase (CK), and lactate dehydrogenase (LDH). Its use may decrease the hemoglobin, hematocrit, potassium, and leukocyte counts.

Life-span considerations   Gemfibrozil is classified as a Pregnancy Category B drug. It is not known if the drug is excreted in breast milk. Safety and efficacy in children and adolescents have not been established.

Specific drug-related nursing considerations   Teach the client common undesired clinical responses associated with gemfibrozil (e.g., nausea, stomach discomfort, bloating). Instruct the client to notify a primary care provider if she is pregnant or has any kind of liver or kidney disorder. Counsel the client about the necessity of taking the drug as prescribed, 30 minutes before morning and evening meals. Advise the client not to stop taking the drug without the primary care provider's knowledge.

Probucol

Pharmacotherapeutics   Probucol (Lorelco) is used as a cholesterol-lowering drug in combination with dietary restrictions in clients with primary hypercholesterolemia (types IIa and IIb). Probucol is used as an alternative to bile acid sequestrant drugs. It has not, however, been shown to lower the incidence of coronary heart disease.

Pharmacokinetics   Approximately 10% of probucol is absorbed orally. The serum cholesterol level begins to decrease within 5 to 7 days after initiation of the drug, with the maximum effect occurring between 20 and 50 days. After the drug is discontinued, the serum cholesterol level reaches its baseline level within 25 days. The drug collects in adipose tissue and is excreted primarily in the bile and feces.[8,9]

Pharmacodynamics   The chemical structure of probucol is unlike that of any other cholesterol-lowering drug. It lowers the total serum cholesterol level and has relatively little effect on serum triglycerides. Probucol increases the fractional rate of LDL catabolism. Increased excretion of fecal bile acids and inhibition of early stages of cholesterol biosynthesis occur.[8]

Pharmaceutics   Probucol is available as tablets for oral administration. The normal adult dose is 500 mg twice daily with both the morning and evening meals. Its use should be discontinued if there has been no substantial lowering of cholesterol levels within 3 to 4 months of therapy. If the drug is effective, it can be administered for an indefinite period of time. Table 34–3 contains additional information on antilipidemic drugs.

Undesired clinical responses   The side effects of probucol include nausea, vomiting, increased appetite, diarrhea, flatulence, decreased taste and smell, and abdominal pain and cramps. In addition, hyperuricemia, paresthesia, dizziness, insomnia, headache, depression, blurred vision, impotence, sweating, pruritis, rash, and conjunctivitis may occur.[8]

Contraindications and precautions   Probucol use is contraindicated in clients hypersensitive to it. It should not be used in clients with recent myocardial damage, serious ventricular arrhythmias, syncope of unknown or cardiovascular origin, or an abnormally long QT interval.

An electrocardiogram (ECG) should be obtained before starting treatment with probucol to assess the QT interval and heart rate. In addition, potassium and magnesium levels should be assessed; if they are low, they should be treated before starting probucol.

Drug-drug, drug-nutrient, drug-environment interactions   Concurrent administration of clofibrate and probucol is not recommended since the lowering of HDL cholesterol may be pronounced. Following a diet low in cholesterol and saturated fat during therapy is recommended. Probucol should be stored in a dry place; excessive heat should be avoided. A tightly closed, light-resistant container with child-resistant closure should be used.[8]

Interference with diagnostic studies   Probucol may elevate hepatic enzyme levels and increase bilirubin, creatinine, blood urea nitrogen, and blood glucose levels. It may decrease hemoglobin, hematocrit, and eosinophil levels and produce thrombocytopenia.[11]

Life-span considerations   Probucol is classified as a Pregnancy Category B drug. Birth control should be practiced while taking probucol. It is not known if probucol is excreted in breast milk. Safety and effectiveness in children have not been established.[8]

Specific drug-related nursing considerations   Teach the client to take the drug with meals. Assess him or her for numbness or swelling of face, hands, and feet. Teach the client proper storage of the drug.

Clofibrate

Pharmacotherapeutics   Clofibrate (Atromid S) effectively treats several types of hyperlipidemia: types IIb, III, IV, and V.

Pharmacokinetics   Clofibrate is rapidly absorbed. It is metabolized in the liver. Between 95% and 99% of an oral dose is excreted in the urine as free and conjugated clofibric acid. Excretion usually occurs within 48 hours of administration. The onset of hyperlipidemic effects is usually within 2 to 5 days.[8]

Pharmacodynamics   Clofibrate decreases the VLDL lipoprotein fraction, which is rich in triglycerides, and the LDL fraction of cholesterol. The drug may inhibit release of lipoproteins, potentiate action of lipoprotein lipase, and increase the fecal excretion of neutral sterols.[8]

Pharmaceutics   Clofibrate is available in capsules for oral administration. The usual oral dosage of clofibrate is 1 to 2 g/d in two to four divided doses. Table 34–3 contains additional information on antilipidemic drugs.

Because the drug is excreted in the kidneys, the dosage is decreased for clients with renal failure. The interval between administration of the drug should be increased proportionally to the amount of renal failure present (i.e., mild renal failure, every 5 to 12 hours; moderate renal failure, every 12 to 18 hours; and severe renal failure, every 24 to 48 hours).

Undesired clinical responses The side effects of clofibrate include a number of GI effects: nausea, vomiting, dyspepsia, diarrhea, flatulence, and epigastric pain. In addition, clients may experience thrombophlebitis, angina, pulmonary embolism, fatigue, weakness, headache, dizziness, cholelithiasis, arthralgias, myopathy, nephrotoxicity, and impotence.

Contraindications and precautions The only contraindication to the use of clofibrate is primary biliary cirrhosis. The drug should be given cautiously to clients with peptic ulcers, cardiovascular disease, and hepatic and renal function impairment.

Two additional precautions deserve further attention. There is an increased risk, approximately 67%, for the development of cholesterol gallstones in clients receiving clofibrate

TABLE 34–3
Antilipidemic Drugs

Drug Name	Dosage and Route of Administration	Nursing Considerations
BILE ACID SEQUESTRANT RESINS CHOLESTYRAMINE (Questran, Questran Light) **HOW SUPPLIED** Powder: 9-g packet, 378-g can (each packet or level scoopful contains 4 g anhydrous cholestyramine resin) "Light" for oral suspension: 5-g packet, 210-g can (each packet or scoopful contains 4 g anhydrous cholestyramine resin)	**ADULTS** Initial dose: 1 packet or 1 level scoopful (4 g anhydrous cholestyramine resin) once or twice/d **MAINTENANCE DOSE:** 2–4 packets or scoopfuls (8–16 g cholestyramine)/d divided into two doses; increase dose gradually to a maximum of six packets or scoopfuls/d (24 g anhydrous cholestyramine resin)	***Assess*** Inquire about diseases contributing to increased blood cholesterol level and about possible history of biliary obstruction. Ask client if she is pregnant or breast-feeding. Cholestyramine may interfere with absorption of necessary vitamins. Ask about other drugs client may be taking, especially digitalis; cholestyramine may interfere with other drugs' absorption, and discontinuation of cholestyramine in client using digitalis may trigger toxicity. Ask about history of sensitivity to cholestyramine. Obtain baseline levels of serum cholesterol, serum triglyceride, and electrolytes. ***Implement*** Always mix powder with water or other fluid (60–180 ml fluid per packet or scoopful). Twirl glass gently at first and then stir gently. Rinse glass with additional liquid to ensure full dose is administered. Administer at mealtime if possible. Give other drugs 1 h before or 4–6 h after cholestyramine. Teach client to complete full drug course and not to omit or change doses. ***Monitor*** Obtain periodic serum cholesterol level readings. Observe for undesired clinical responses (e.g., constipation, GI distress, headache). Assess skin and mucous membranes for rash or irritation. Encourage client to drink several glasses of water between meals. ***Evaluate*** Assess laboratory values for effect.
Colestipol (Colestid) **HOW SUPPLIED** 5-g packets; 300-, 500-g cans (one scoopful equals 5 g colestipol)	**ADULTS** Initial dose: 5 g once or twice daily; increase by 5 g at 1- or 2-mo intervals to a maximum of 30 g/d 5–30 g/d given once or in divided doses	Same as for cholestyramine.

Table continued on following page.

TABLE 34–3 *Continued*
Antilipidemic Drugs

Drug Name	Dosage and Route of Administration	Nursing Considerations
HMG-COA REDUCTASE LOVASTATIN (Mevacor) HOW SUPPLIED Tablets: 10, 20, 40 mg	ADULTS Initial dose: 20 mg with the evening meal; may increase dose gradually at 4-wk intervals Maintenance dose: 20–80 mg/d in single or divided doses; maximum recommended dose, 80 mg/d; adjust dosage to response **Clients Taking Immunosuppressive Drugs** Initial dose: 10 mg/d Maintenance dose: not to exceed 20 mg/d **Clients with Renal Insufficiency** Dosage >20 mg/d may be considered *cautiously*	**Assess** Assess for contraindications to the drug (e.g., active liver disease, chronic alcoholism). Determine if client is pregnant or breast-feeding. Lovastatin is classified as Pregnancy Category X drug and should not be administered to pregnant or nursing women. Inquire whether client is receiving anticoagulant therapy. Obtain baseline serum transaminase levels. **Implement** Administer drug with foods. Instruct client to store drug at room temperature; away from heat and moisture. Teach client to consult with primary care provider before starting or stopping other medication. Teach client to report unexplained muscle tenderness, pain, or weakness, especially if accompanied by malaise or fever. **Monitor** Monitor for undesired clinical responses (e.g., headache, excessive gas, diarrhea, constipation, blurred vision). Obtain results of liver function tests (ALT, AST) q6wk for 3 mo, q8wk for 9 mo, then periodically. Assess for rash or pruritis. Monitor temperatures at least twice a day.
Pravastatin Sodium (Pravachol) HOW SUPPLIED Tablets: 10, 20, 40 mg	ADULTS Initial dose: 10 or 20 mg/d at bedtime Maintenance dose: 10–40 mg/d at bedtime **Elderly Client or Client with Liver or Renal Dysfunction** 10 mg/d at bedtime; may increase to 20 mg/d if needed	Same as lovastatin.

as compared to those who do not receive this drug. In addition, the drug should be administered with caution in clients who have had an MI. Significant cardiovascular toxicity, including arrhythmias, claudication, thromboembolism, and angina, has been observed in these individuals.[12]

Drug-drug and drug-environment interactions Clofibrate should not be administered concurrently with warfarin because it increases the PT. This drug also increases the effects of sulfonylureas and insulin. When administered concurrently with probenecid, the toxicity of clofibrate is increased. Concurrent administration of rifampin and clofibrate decreases the effects of clofibrate.

Clofibrate should be stored at room temperature at approximately 25° C. Excessive heat should be avoided.[8]

Life-span considerations Clofibrate is classified as a Pregnancy Category C drug. Its use is contraindicated in lac-

tating women since an active metabolite of the drug has been measured in breast milk. Safety and efficacy in children have not been established.[8]

Specific drug-related nursing considerations Instruct the client to take clofibrate with meals to avoid gastric irritation. In addition, advise the client to continue to follow prescribed diets and to consult the primary care provider before discontinuing the drug. Instruct the client to report any genitourinary symptoms such as decreased libido, impotence, dysuria, proteinuria, oliguria, and hematuria.

Dextrothyroxine

Dextrothyroxine (Choloxin) is an isomer of the thyroid hormone, thyroxine.

Pharmacotherapeutics Dextrothyroxine is effective in treating the type II hyperlipidemias. However, it has deleterious cardiovascular effects and is used only in clients who are euthyroid with no known heart disease.

Pharmacokinetics Dextrothyroxine is poorly absorbed from the GI tract and is distributed to most body tissues. It is excreted in the feces and the urine. Its half-life is approximately 18 hours.

Pharmacodynamics The exact mechanism of action of dextrothyroxine is not known. It may intensify the conversion of cholesterol to bile salts in the liver so that they are lost in the feces. This drug decreases hyperlipoproteinemia 2 to 3 weeks after it is initiated. After it has been discontinued, the serum lipids return to their baseline levels in 6 weeks to 3 months.

Pharmaceutics Dextrothyroxine is available in tablets for oral administration. The usual initial oral dose for clients with normal thyroid function is 1 to 2 mg/d. Depending on its therapeutic effect, dextrothyroxine is increased in increments of 1 to 2 mg/d at intervals of at least 1 month. The usual recommended maintenance dose is 4 to 8 mg/d.[8,12]

Undesired clinical responses Possible side effects associated with dextrothyroxine include symptoms of chronic poisoning by iodine or iodides and an allergic reaction to Food, Drug, and Cosmetic Act (FD&C) yellow dye No. 5, which is in tablets of dextrothyroxine. In addition, GI complaints of dyspepsia, nausea, vomiting, diarrhea, constipation, and anorexia have been reported.

Contraindications and precautions Contraindications for dextrothyroxine use include known or suspected heart disease (e.g., angina, MI, arrhythmias, rheumatic heart disease, and heart failure), advanced hepatic or renal disease, history of iodism, and hypertension.

Keep the following precautions in mind when a client is receiving dextrothyroxine. This drug may increase the mortality rate in clients with either known cardiac disease or those with high risk because of family history or other factors such as age, sex, obesity, smoking, and hypertension. In addition, clients undergoing surgery should discontinue the drug at least 2 weeks before the procedure is undertaken.[12]

Drug-drug interactions Dextrothyroxine should not be given with thyroid replacement drugs. The drug may potentiate the effects of anticoagulants on PT. Antidiabetic drug dosage may need an increase during dextrothyroxine therapy.[8]

Life-span considerations Dextrothyroxine is classified as a Pregnancy Category B drug. It should not be administered to pregnant or breast-feeding clients. Birth control should be practiced during the period of administration. Safety and effectiveness with children have not been established.[8,13]

Specific drug-related nursing considerations Instruct the client to notify the primary care provider if chest pain, diarrhea, excessive sweating, rash, acne, insomnia, headache, or visual disturbance occurs.

CONCEPT REVIEW

Lifestyle factors and family and personal history are important areas to assess in clients receiving antilipidemic drugs. Individualized nutritional and exercise programs should be developed for each client.

There are several different types of antilipidemic drugs. The pharmacotherapeutic use of these drugs is to lower cholesterol or triglyceride levels. Many of these drugs produce GI distress; antilipidemic drugs are used with caution in clients with hepatic or renal disease.

ANTICOAGULANTS

Anticoagulants interfere with the normal clotting processes to prevent clot formation or the extension of existing clots. The two primary drugs in this category are heparin and warfarin. Each of these drugs acts on a different mechanism in the coagulation cascade, although each produces the same general anticoagulant effect. Because the drugs vary in their specific pharmacodynamic properties, different laboratory tests are used to determine each drug's effectiveness. In addition, the drugs have varying durations of action and are administered by various routes. These characteristics are among the factors considered when determining specific anticoagulant therapy.

▦ NURSING CONSIDERATIONS

As with other drugs, the nurse's role in client education about anticoagulant therapy is important. In addition, assessing baseline data and monitoring the client during therapy are essential.

Assessing During the **health history** question the client about past medical problems; especially ask about venous thrombosis, pulmonary embolism, episodes of systemic embolism, unstable angina, MI, thrombolysis, atrial fibrillation, cerebrovascular accident, valvular heart disease, or prosthetic heart valves. In addition, ask about the occurrence of unusual bleeding, heavy menstrual cycles, hypertension, gastric or other GI bleeding, hematuria, nosebleeds, bleeding gums, or hemoptysis.

During therapy with anticoagulants the **physical assessment** parameters focus on symptoms specific to the skin, GI tract, and genitourinary tract. Be alert for petechiae, bruises, and prolonged bleeding after an injection or a venipuncture. Report the presence of any fresh or increased bleeding at wound sites. When assessing bleeding of the GI tract, observe for any oropharyngeal bleeding, bleeding gums after oral hygiene, hematemesis, abdominal swelling, tarry stools, or bright red blood in the stools. If GI bleeding of any type is suspected, test the stool for occult blood. The most obvious symptom of genitourinary tract bleeding is pink-tinged, bright red, or tea-colored urine. A urinalysis will detect the presence of microscopic erythrocytes.

In addition, monitor orthostatic blood pressure changes, pulse rates, and hemoglobin and hematocrit levels. A significant decrease in the systolic blood pressure between lying in bed and sitting or standing (more than 20 mm Hg difference) may signify a volume loss caused by bleeding.[14] Along with these changes in blood pressure, assess the client for dizziness, changes in vision, and increased heart rate. A drop in both the hemoglobin and hematocrit levels occurs if bleeding is present.

The client who is receiving anticoagulants may have any of the following laboratory tests performed:

1. **Activated partial thromboplastin time (APTT)** This blood test measures the intrinsic and common coagulation pathways. The APTT evaluates fibrinogen, prothrombin, and factors V, VIII, IX, X, XI, and XII. The APTT is prolonged if any of these factors is decreased. The APTT results are reported in seconds, along with a control value, which is dependent on specific chemicals used in the laboratory.[15]

2. **Prothrombin time (PT)** This blood test measures the extrinsic and common coagulation pathways. The PT evaluates fibrinogen, prothrombin, and factors V, VII, and X. The PT is prolonged if any of these factors is decreased. The PT results are reported in seconds, along with a control value, which is dependent on specific chemicals used in the laboratory. The normal PT is equal to the control value.[15]

Diagnosing Clients receiving anticoagulant drugs may have the following nursing diagnoses:

• High risk for injury related to decreased clotting ability.
• Altered protection related to abnormal blood coagulation from anticoagulant therapy.
• Anxiety related to change in health status or dependency on drug therapy.
• Individual ineffective coping related to inadequate support systems.
• Fear related to unfamiliarity with drug regimen.
• Altered health maintenance related to lack of economic resources for prescribed drugs.

Planning Client education is crucial. Teach the client about actions, undesired clinical responses, and complications of anticoagulant drugs. Alert the client to safety measures associated with therapy. For example, encourage the client to use electric shavers, rather than razor blades, to decrease the risk of cuts and prolonged bleeding. Recommend that the client use a soft-bristled toothbrush for oral hygiene. Assess the client's environment for items that could cause injury (e.g., throw rugs or electric cords). Counsel the client to use extreme caution if knives are used in the kitchen for cooking and to wear foot coverings at all times to avoid injury. Instruct the client to wear a Medic-Alert bracelet or carry an identification card indicating that he or she is receiving anticoagulant therapy.

Establish expected outcomes. Possible outcomes follow:

• Client remains free of injury.
• Client demonstrates problem-solving skills.
• Client identifies options and possible resources.
• Client describes drug action, undesired clinical responses, drug schedule, and precautions associated with anticoagulant therapy.
• Client participates in treatment plan.

Implementing Document any signs or symptoms of bleeding and notify the primary care provider if they occur. Monitor vital signs and report any changes that could signify bleeding. Be aware of laboratory data such as the PT and the APTT results that indicate the effects of the anticoagulant therapy. Review laboratory results daily and transmit this information during change-of-shift reports. Anticipate that anticoagulant orders will be prescribed on a daily basis according to the daily PT or APTT levels. Be alert to changes in dosages.

Evaluating Daily PT and APTT results reveal the level of anticoagulation achieved with the therapy. Review the expected outcomes with the client. Were the outcomes achieved? If not, what changes in the care plan are required?

Parenteral Anticoagulant Drug: Heparin Sodium

Heparin is a naturally occurring substance present in the mast cells.

Pharmacotherapeutics Heparin is used to treat already existing conditions and to prevent the development of further pathophysiologic complications. Existing conditions include unstable angina, acute myocardial infarction (AMI), selected cases of disseminated intravascular coagulation (DIC), and fetal growth retardation in pregnant women. Heparin is also used in the prevention of venous thrombosis, pulmonary embolism, mural thrombosis after MI, coronary artery rethrombosis after thrombolysis, exercise-induced asthma, and thrombosis in intravenous (IV), extracorporeal devices or hemodialysis.

Pharmacokinetics Heparin is poorly absorbed through the GI tract; hence it is given parenterally, either IV or subcutaneously (SC). It has irregular absorption when administered intramuscularly (IM). Heparin is extensively bound to plasma proteins such as LDLs, globulins, and fibrinogen. It binds to sites on endothelial cells and displaces platelet factor IV, a protein that neutralizes heparin.

Heparin's half-life is dose dependent; its anticoagulant effect occurs within 20 to 30 minutes after an SC injection and is immediate when administered IV. Duration of action is approximately $1\frac{1}{2}$ hours but is prolonged in clients with hepatic dysfunction. Heparin is metabolized in the liver and is excreted by the kidney. It does not cross the placenta and produces no deleterious effects in the fetus or newborn. Its anticoagulant effects are reversed within hours of stopping an IV infusion of heparin.[8,16]

Pharmacodynamics Heparin acts primarily through the inactivation of thrombin, which is necessary for the activation of clotting factors V and VIII. It potentiates the activity of **antithrombin III,** a plasma cofactor. Only approximately one third of the heparin binds to antithrombin III, and it is this portion that is responsible for most of the anticoagulant effect. The remaining two thirds has minimal anticoagulant activity.[16,17]

Pharmaceutics Heparin is available in parenteral solutions for IV and SC injections. Heparin is available in a variety of concentrations (e.g., 1000 U/ml, 40,000 U/ml). Heparin is also used in an aerosolized form to treat asthma.[18] Anticoagulant therapy usually is continued for 7 to 10 days; it should be overlapped with oral anticoagulant therapy for 3 to 5 days. Heparin dosages are altered to maintain the APTT in

he range of 1.5 to 2.5 times the normal value (e.g., 70 seconds).[12] Table 34–5 provides additional information about
dosage forms, dosages, and routes of administration.

 ## Nursing Research

Kleiber, C., Hanrahan, K., Fagan, C.L., & Zittergruen, M.
(1993). Heparin vs. saline for peripheral IV locks in children.
Pediatric Nursing, 19, 405–409.

The purpose of this study was to determine the efficacy
of saline solution versus heparin flush solution in maintaining peripheral IV locks in a pediatric population. A
prospective, randomized, double-blind design was used.
Subjects were infants more than 28 days of age and children. A sample of 124 peripheral IVs were flushed with
either saline solution or heparin in saline solution.

The heparin and saline groups were comparable for
total hours' duration of the IV and for incidence of complications. The study's conclusion is that saline solution
is efficacious in maintaining the patency of peripheral
IV locks in children more than 28 days of age.

STUDENT ACTIVITIES

- Review the procedure manual in your assigned agency.
  Determine the procedure for "flushing" peripheral intermittent IV devices.
- Determine the basis for the procedure and if other
  techniques have been tried.

Undesired clinical responses   Of the several side effects
to heparin therapy, the most common is hemorrhage. Four
variables influence bleeding during treatment with heparin: (1)
dose of heparin; (2) client's anticoagulant response; (3)
method of administration; and (4) other client-related factors
(e.g., serious concurrent illness, chronic heavy consumption of
alcohol, concomitant use of aspirin, renal failure, IM injections, elderly age group, and gender). The primary sites where
bleeding occurs are the GI tract, the skin, and the genitourinary tract.[16,20]

The treatment for minor bleeding is to discontinue use of
the drug. For major hemorrhages a transfusion with fresh
whole blood or fresh frozen plasma is indicated. In severe cases
protamine sulfate can be given (see box).

Another common side effect of heparin therapy is thrombocytopenia, which occurs in approximately 5% to 10% of clients receiving heparin. The platelet count can decrease to
100,000 to 150,000 (normal value: 195,000 to 450,000).
Clients are usually asymptomatic with this condition, and it
generally resolves without treatment in 1 to 5 days, even with
continued heparin therapy. Despite the benign nature of this
condition, the client's platelet count should be monitored
every other day.

In a client with thrombocytopenia that has a delayed onset,
occurring 6 to 8 days after the initiation of heparin therapy,
the platelet count can decrease below 100,000. In this case the
heparin causes the formation of antiplatelet antibodies, which

---

PROTAMINE SULFATE

Protamine sulfate injection should be administered by
very slow IV injection over a 10-min period in doses
not to exceed 50 mg. The dosage of protamine sulfate should be guided by blood coagulation studies.

Protamine sulfate is intended for injection without further dilution; if further dilution is desired, D₅W or
normal saline solution may be used.

Data from Data Pharmaceutica, Inc. (1993). *1993 physicians' genRx.*
Smithtown, NY: Author.

---

cause the platelets to aggregate. This in turn causes clotting
and embolization. Heparin-induced arterial thrombosis can
occur, which is called the **white-clot syndrome** in which a clot
made of platelets, fibrin, and leukocytes forms.[8]

Other side effects of heparin therapy include osteoporosis,
skin necrosis, alopecia, hypersensitivity reactions, hypoaldos-
teronism, vasospasm, and hyperkalemia.

Contraindications and precautions   Heparin should
never be administered to clients with known hypersensitivity
to the drug, those who are actively bleeding, those with blood
dyscrasias, or those who have hemophilia or other blood disorders. Heparin should be used cautiously in clients who have
allergies, renal and hepatic diseases, hypertension during menstruation, diabetes mellitus, or renal insufficiency. This latter
category of client is more susceptible to heparin-induced hy-
poaldosteronism and hyperkalemia; the clients' potassium levels should be monitored frequently.[8,12]

Drug-drug and drug-environment interactions   One of
the primary drugs that interacts with heparin with potentially
dangerous consequences is aspirin. The use of aspirin has resulted in increased operative and postoperative bleeding in clients who receive the very high doses of heparin required during open heart surgery. However, the risk of adding a short
course of aspirin to a regular therapeutic dose of heparin is
much lower and is acceptable in clients with ischemic heart
disease.[16]

Other drugs that interact with heparin include anisindione,
chlordiazepoxide, diazepam, digitoxin, dihydroergotamine, lorazepam, oxazepam, propranolol, and tobramycin. Many
drugs, including antibiotics, inactivate heparin; therefore other
drugs should never be infused in the same line with a heparin
drip. In addition, heparin should never be mixed with any
other drugs in a single syringe for IV injection. Table 34–4
provides a summary of other drugs that interact with heparin.

Heparin sodium should be stored at room temperature.

Life-span considerations   Heparin is classified as a
Pregnancy Category C drug. It is not excreted in human milk.
Elderly women over the age of 60 years are at greater risk for
bleeding complications.

Specific drug-related nursing considerations   If the client is receiving heparin therapy through continuous infusion,

TABLE 34–4
Drugs That Interact With Heparin

Drug Name	Response to Interaction With Heparin	Nursing Considerations
Anistreplase	May cause prolonged APTT	Be alert to increased bleeding; monitor APTT.
Antithrombin III	May increase anticoagulant effect in clients with hereditary antithrombin III deficiency	Be alert to increased bleeding and report it immediately to the physician.
Aspirin	Increases anticoagulant effects	Generally instruct clients to avoid aspirin use while receiving heparin; acetaminophen may be a suitable substitute for aspirin. Be alert for abnormal bleeding in clients who must receive aspirin and heparin together.
Gentamicin	Prolonged APTT without any significant loss of anticoagulant activity. Decreased activity of gentamicin with concurrent administration of heparin	Do not mix gentamicin and heparin in the same syringe or give them together in the same IV line.
Nitroglycerin (NTG)	Decreased effect of heparin. Marked increase in sensitivity to heparin with withdrawal of NTG	Monitor APTT closely in clients receiving both drugs, with higher doses of heparin being used to prevent inadequate anticoagulation. Heparin dose should be reduced when NTG dose is discontinued to avoid hemorrhage.
Warfarin	Concurrent use of both drugs may result in a prolonged PT	PT may not provide an accurate gauge for warfarin doses while the client is receiving heparin.

use an infusion pump and carefully monitor the drip rate to ensure that the proper dose is administered. If the client is receiving SC injections of heparin, inspect injections sites for excessive bruising, intradermal bleeding, discomfort, or prolonged bleeding after the injection has been administered.

Although the abdomen is usually the preferred site for SC injections of heparin, using the thigh and arm as sites does not alter the drug's effectiveness. In addition, no increased bruising is associated with the alternate sites.[21]

🦎 NURSING RESEARCH

Fahs, P.S., & Kinney, M. (1991). The abdomen, thigh, and arm sites for subcutaneous sodium heparin injections. *Nursing Research, 40,* 204–207.

The purpose of this study was to evaluate the effectiveness of three SC heparin injection sites. One-hundred one subjects, ranging in age from 20 to 94 years, were randomly placed in one of three groups. Group A received injections in the abdomen, group B in the thigh, and group C in the arm. Each subject received three injections at one site. APTT was measured before initiation of heparin and 4 hours after the first injection. Bruising was measured at 48, 60, and 72 hours after the injection.

There were no statistically significant differences among the groups for either changes in APTT or bruising at 60 and 72 hours after the injection. Therefore the clinical practice of using the abdomen as the primary site for SC heparin injections was not supported.

STUDENT ACTIVITIES

- Determine the procedure for using SC injections of heparin in your assigned clinical agency.
- Based on your knowledge of heparin, identify parameters to consider in future studies. 🦎

MISCELLANEOUS DRUGS IN CATEGORY

Recently clinical trials of **low-molecular-weight heparin solutions** have been conducted. The mean molecular weight of regular heparin is approximately 12,000 to 16,000 daltons as compared to 4000 to 5000 daltons in the low-molecular-weight heparin. The anticoagulant effect of low-molecular-weight heparin is equal to or greater than that of continuous IV heparin. In addition, it can be administered SC once daily and has fewer incidents of hemorrhagic side effects. Because of these factors, it may be used to treat uncomplicated venous thrombosis without hospitalization, thereby saving considerable health care costs.[17,22]

Oral Anticoagulant Drug: Warfarin Sodium

Pharmacotherapeutics Clinical use of warfarin (Coumadin, Panwarfin, Sofarin) include primary and secondary prevention of venous thromboembolism, treatment and prophylaxis of pulmonary embolism, and prevention of systemic embolism in clients with prosthetic heart valves or atrial fibrillation. In addition, warfarin is used in the prevention of stroke and recurrent infarction and death in clients with AMI.

Pharmacokinetics Orally administered warfarin is absorbed rapidly and extensively from the GI tract. Ninety-seven

TABLE 34–5
Parenteral Anticoagulant Drugs

Drug Name	Dosage and Route of Administration	Nursing Considerations
Heparin Sodium (Liquaemin Sodium) **HOW SUPPLIED** Injection: 1000, 2500, 5000, 7500, 10,000, 20,000 U/ml; 5000 U/0.5 ml; single-dose syringe in varying concentrations; single- or multiple-dose vials	**Intermittent Intravenous Therapy via Heparin Lock** Initial dose: 10,000 U; subsequent doses, 4000–10,000 U q4–6h **Continuous IV Infusion** Bolus: 5000–10,000 U; then infuse at 100 U/h **Prophylaxis of Postsurgical Thromboembolism** IV 5000 U 2 h before surgery and 500 U q8-12h after surgery for 7 d or until ambulation (whichever is longer) **Surgery of Heart and Blood Vessels** IV initial dose: no less than 150 U/kg of body weight; 150–400 U/kg, depending on estimated length of surgery **Blood Transfusion** 400–600 USP U/dl whole blood **Subcutaneous Dosage** **ADULTS** Initial dose: 5000 U IV injection and 10,000–20,000 U SC Maintenance dose: 8000–10,000 U q8h or 15,000–20,000 U q12h **CHILDREN** Initial dose: 100 U/kg (IV drip) q4h *or* 20,000 U/m^2/24 h continuously	**Assess** Assess for contraindications to drug (e.g., renal or hepatic disease, diabetes mellitus, known hypersensitivity). Inquire whether the client is pregnant. Heparin is classifed as a Pregnancy Category C drug. Cross-check dose with coworker. Obtain activated partial thromboplastin time (APTT) before administering and 24 h after initiating therapy, then q24-48h for first week, and one to two times/wk for first month. **Implement** For IV administration, use of continuous IV drip is preferred. Dilute infusion in isotonic sterile saline, 5% dextrose in water, or lactated Ringer's solution. Invert container at least six times to ensure mixing. For SC administration, inject above iliac crest or in abdominal fat layer (but not within 2 in of umbilicus), withdraw needle rapidly, and apply pressure for 1–2 min. Rotate injection sites. Teach client to use electric razor, soft toothbrush. Teach client not to use any over-the-counter drug without consulting primary care provider and to wear or carry identification bracelet. **Monitor** Monitor APTT and blood pressure carefully. Assess for occult blood, AST, ALT. Monitor for undesired clinical responses (e.g., GI or genitourinary bleeding, thrombocytopenia, alopecia, skin necrosis). With continuous IV infusion, monitor coagulation time q4h in early stages. With intermittent IV infusion, test coagulation time before each injection in early stages. **Evaluate** Assess for APTT in therapeutic range. Assess for platelet count in range of 195,000–450,000.

percent of warfarin circulates bound to plasma proteins. It reaches its maximum plasma concentration in 90 minutes and has a plasma half-life of 36 to 42 hours. Warfarin accumulates rapidly in the liver and is excreted in the urine and bile. The anticoagulant effect of warfarin is delayed until all of the circulating clotting factors are cleared. The anticoagulant effect occurs within 24 hours, but its peak anticoagulant effect is delayed for 72 to 96 hours because of the longer plasma half-lives of factors II, IX, and X.[23] This is why it is essential to overlap treatment with heparin with warfarin for 3 to 5 days when a client will be receiving warfarin therapy on a continuing basis.

Once use of the medication has been discontinued, the duration of its anticoagulant effects depends on the resynthesis of the vitamin K–dependent clotting factors (II, VII, IX, and X). This usually occurs within 4 to 5 days.

Pharmacodynamics Warfarin acts as a vitamin K antagonist. It interferes with hepatic vitamin K–dependent carboxylation and limits the activation of the vitamin K–dependent coagulation proteins: prothrombin and factors VII, IX, and X in the liver. Mechanisms that may produce some variability in the anticoagulant effect of warfarin include differences in the affinity of the receptor, availability of vitamin K, and levels of vitamin K–dependent coagulation factors. Hereditary resistance to warfarin has been described.[9,23,24]

Pharmaceutics Warfarin sodium is available as tablets for oral administration. The usual oral dose is 2 to 10 mg/d. Dosage is adjusted to maintain a PT of 1.3 to 2 times the control value. Take the weight and age of the client into consideration when deciding the initial therapy; heavier weight tends to increase the dosage needed, and age tends to decrease the dosage needed. The timing of the dose is not crucial; the client may take this drug on either a full or empty stomach. Table 34–7 provides additional information on dosage forms, dosages, and routes of administration.

Undesired clinical responses Bleeding is one of the most common side effects of treatment with warfarin. Additional side effects include hematoma formation, hemopericardium, renal tubular necrosis, jaundice, tissue necrosis, vasculitis, alopecia, urticaria, dermatitis, fever, nausea, diarrhea, abdominal cramping, systemic cholesterol microembolism, and hypersensitivity reaction. Figure 34–2 illustrates common undesired clinical responses associated with warfarin. See the box for information about the antidote to excessive warfarin.

Contraindications and precautions The risk of bleeding is influenced by the dose of warfarin administered, the client's underlying disease, and the concomitant use of aspirin. Clients with a history of stroke, GI bleeding, atrial fibrillation, or other serious coexisting conditions are also at an increased risk of bleeding.

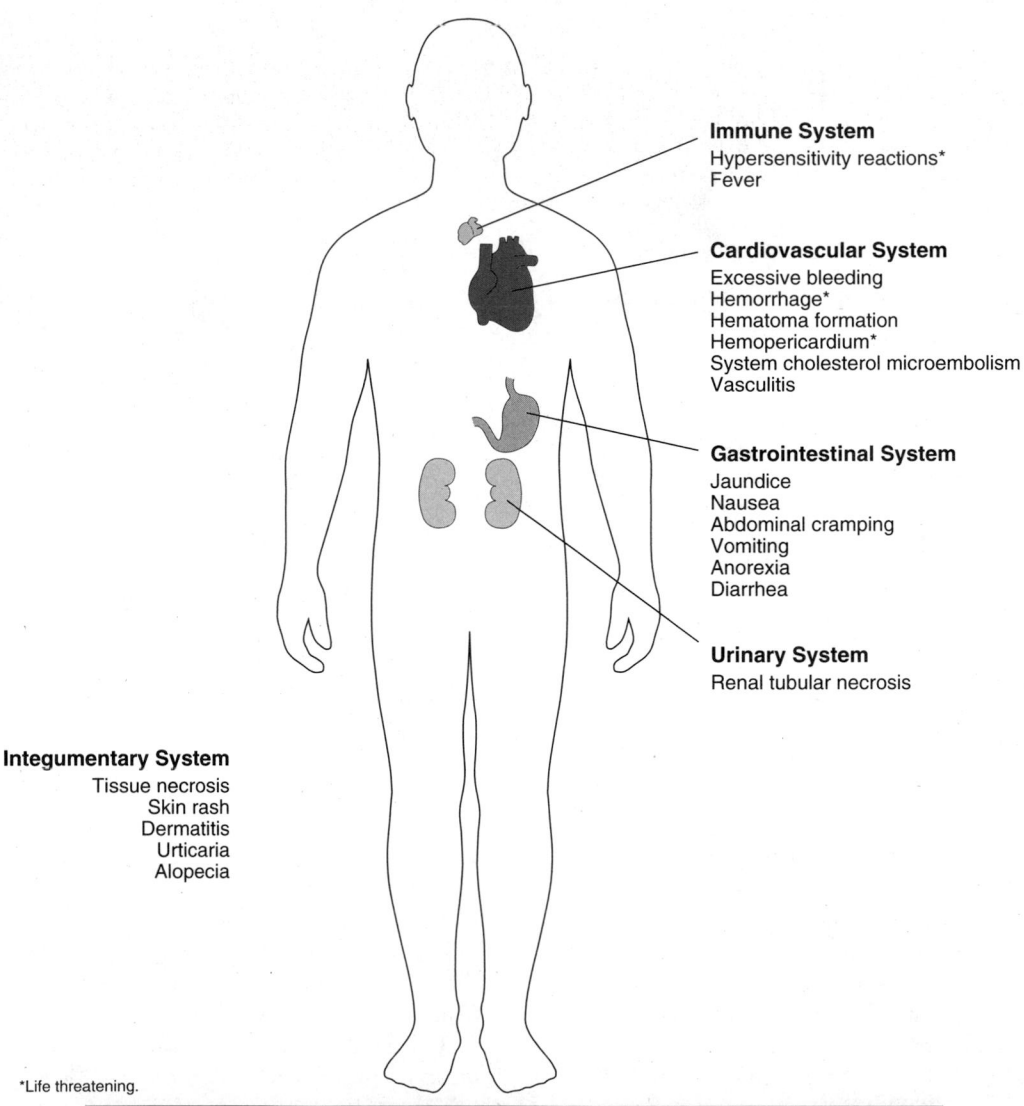

Immune System
Hypersensitivity reactions*
Fever

Cardiovascular System
Excessive bleeding
Hemorrhage*
Hematoma formation
Hemopericardium*
System cholesterol microembolism
Vasculitis

Gastrointestinal System
Jaundice
Nausea
Abdominal cramping
Vomiting
Anorexia
Diarrhea

Urinary System
Renal tubular necrosis

Integumentary System
Tissue necrosis
Skin rash
Dermatitis
Urticaria
Alopecia

*Life threatening.

FIGURE 34–2 Common undesired clinical responses associated with warfarin.

ANTIDOTE TO EXCESS WARFARIN

▶ If bleeding complications occur, warfarin therapy should be discontinued and vitamin K (phytonadione) administered.

▶ Mild hemorrhage: 2.5–10 mg PO, IM, or IV of vitamin K.

▶ Severe hemorrhage: 10–15 mg IV of vitamin K; repeat q4h as needed.

There are numerous contraindications to warfarin therapy. Clients with lesions of the genitourinary or GI tract, hepatic disease, cerebrovascular accident, malignant hypertension, and retinopathy should not receive warfarin. Other contraindications include pregnancy, esophageal varices, threatened abortion, eclampsia, preeclampsia, recent surgical trauma to the brain, eye, or spinal cord, recent lumbar block anesthesia, arterial aneurysm, infective endocarditis or acute pericarditis, and pericardial effusions. Clients with congenital clotting factor defects (hemophilia) or acquired clotting factor defects (liver disease, obstructive jaundice), thrombocytopenia, or blood dyscrasias are not candidates for warfarin therapy. In addition, other factors that make warfarin therapy inappropriate include the presence of inadequate laboratory facilities for monitoring the drug's effectiveness, unsupervised senility, alcoholism, psychosis, or lack of client cooperation.

Drug-drug, drug-nutrient, and drug-environment interactions Any condition that causes changing levels of vitamin K can affect the action of warfarin. For example, dietary in-

gestion of vitamin K in green, leafy vegetables decreases the effectivness of the drug. Fat malabsorption, when absorption of vitamin K is decreased, potentiates the action of warfarin.[23] In addition, hypermetabolic states such as those produced by fever or hyperthyroidism increase the responsiveness to warfarin because of increased catabolism of the vitamin K–dependent coagulation factors.[23,24]

Warfarin sodium should be protected from light. It should be stored at controlled room temperature (15° to 30° C) and dispensed in a tight, light-resistant container. Drug interactions that potentiate or interfere with the actions of warfarin are summarized in Table 34–6.

Life-span considerations Warfarin is classified as a Pregnancy Category X drug. It does cross the placenta and is distributed in breast milk. Conflicting data about the increased risk of bleeding in the elderly client receiving warfarin therapy exist. The recommended dosage for elderly clients does decrease with advancing age.

Specific drug-related nursing considerations The PT should be determined for a client receiving warfarin. This is the only laboratory test that measures the effectiveness of warfarin. The therapeutic goal is approximately 1.2 to 1.5 times control. Changes in PT do not occur for approximately 24 hours; PT usually takes several days to reach the therapeutic range.

Provide the client specific information about the risks of taking warfarin, and emphasize the dangers of excessive bleeding. Instruct the client on the importance of making regular visits to the primary care provider so that proper, safe doses of warfarin can be determined. Remind the client to carry identification cards or Medic-Alert bracelets, to avoid excessive

TABLE 34–6
Drugs That Interact With Warfarin

Drugs Altering Warfarin Absorption	Drugs Interacting With Warfarin Distribution	Drugs Affecting Hepatic Metabolism and Excretion of Warfarin	Drugs Affecting Pharmacodynamic Mechanisms of Warfarin
Cholestyramine	Chloral hydrate	Allopurinol	Androgens
Colestipol	NSAIDs	Amiodarone	Broad-spectrum antibiotics
	Phenytoin	Barbiturates	Clofibrate
	Sulfonamides	Carbamazepine	Corticosteroids
	Sulfonylureas	Cimetidine	Gemfibrozil
		Ciprofloxacin	NSAIDs
		Disulfiram	Oral contraceptives
		Erythromycin	Parenteral cephalosporins
		Ethanol	Quinine
		Griseofulvin	Quinidine
		Metronidazole	Thyroid drugs
		Omeprazole	Vitamin E
		Phenylbutazone	Vitamin K
		Phenytoin	
		Primidone	
		Ranitidine	
		Rifampin	
		Sulfamethoxazole	
		Sulfinpyrazone	

Data from references 23–26.

TABLE 34–7
Oral Anticoagulant Drugs

Drug Name	Dosage and Route of Administration	Nursing Considerations
WARFARIN (Coumadin, Panwarfin) **HOW SUPPLIED** Tablets: 1, 2, 2.5, 5, 7.5, 10 mg	Dosage individualized according to results of one-stage PT Recommended initial dose: 2–5 mg/d Usual maintenance dose: 2–10 mg/d	***Assess*** Assess for contraindications to drug (see text). Inquire whether client is pregnant or breast-feeding; warfarin is classified as Pregnancy Category X drug, and its use is contraindicated. ***Implement*** Cross-check dose with coworker. Determine PT before drug is administered and daily after initiating therapy. After stabilization, obtain PT results q4-6wk. Instruct client about importance of regular visits to primary care provider. Advise client to carry identification card or Medic-Alert bracelet. (See box, "Client Instructions About Warfarin," for additional teaching needs.) ***Monitor*** Monitor client for undesired clinical responses (e.g., bleeding, hematoma, jaundice, alopecia, urticaria, fever, nausea, diarrhea, vasculitis). ***Evaluate*** Assess for PT of 1.3 to 2 times control value.

CLIENT INSTRUCTIONS ABOUT WARFARIN

1. Undesired clinical responses:
   Mild responses: Reduced appetite, scalp hair loss, nausea, vomiting, mild stomach cramps, diarrhea, skin rash
   Severe responses: Bleeding from gums or nose, unusually heavy menstrual bleeding, excessive bleeding from cuts or wounds, easy bruising, purplish areas on skin, internal bleeding,* bluish color of toes, skin rash or hives, severe or persistent stomach pain, fever, sore throat, yellowing of eyes or skin, pain during urination, decreased amount of urine, mouth sores or ulcers

2. **Contraindications**
   a. Do not take warfarin if you have had an allergic reaction to it in the past.
   b. Do not take warfarin if you are or think you may be pregnant.

3. **Precautions**
   a. Regular visits to your primary care provider for blood tests that will determine the proper, safe dose are mandatory while taking warfarin.
   b. Take the prescribed dose; do not take less or more than what is prescribed.

4. Carry an identification card or wear a Medic-Alert bracelet stating you are taking warfarin.

5. Do not take any other medications while taking warfarin without checking with your primary care provider.

6. Avoid ingesting excessive amounts of alcohol.

7. Do not make any changes in your normal diet while taking warfarin. If your primary care provider provides you with a specific diet, adhere to it closely.

*Symptoms of internal bleeding: blood in urine or stools, vomiting blood, coughing up blood, constipation, severe headache, joint swelling or pain, abdominal swelling.

amounts of alcohol, and to follow any specifically recommended diet. Detailed client teaching information is found in the box on the opposite page.

CONCEPT REVIEW

The two primary anticoagulant drugs are heparin and warfarin sodium. Heparin sodium is usually administered SC or IV. Warfarin is administered orally.

Both drugs potentially can produce excessive bleeding. Usual sites of bleeding include the GI and genitourinary tracts and the skin.

Dosages for heparin are based on APTT findings, whereas doses for warfarin are based on PT results. Protamine sulfate is used to counteract bleeding in clients receiving heparin, and vitamin K is used in those receiving warfarin.

ANTIPLATELET DRUGS

Antiplatelet drugs generally inhibit the aggregation of platelets in the clotting process, thereby prolonging the bleeding time. They may be used in conjunction with anticoagulants. The effects of antiplatelet drugs are ideal in the prophylaxis of long-term complications after MIs, coronary revascularization, and cerebrovascular accidents.

▣ NURSING CONSIDERATIONS

Assessing   During the **health history** of a client receiving antiplatelet drugs inquire about the recurrence of symptoms of coronary artery disease, transient ischemic attacks (TIAs), or vascular problems. Specifically focus on the presence of any symptoms that the client had previous to the drug therapy. For example, if a client was prescribed an antiplatelet drug as a result of episodes of TIAs, ask about the presence of symptoms such as dizziness, loss of consciousness, weakness, fainting, slurred speech, and visual changes.

During a **physical assessment** observe for symptoms of antiplatelet toxicity such as GI bleeding, bruising, or hematuria. In addition, physical signs of the recurrence of the disease process for which the antiplatelet drugs were prescribed should be investigated. For example, clients who had a history of deep vein thrombosis should be assessed for the possible presence of recurring thrombosis.

The primary laboratory test performed on clients receiving antiplatelet drugs is the bleeding time. Platelet aggregation, which normally results in clotting, is inhibited by the use of antiplatelet drugs; however, the number of platelets in the blood is not decreased by these drugs. The **bleeding time test** measures platelet and vascular function. It is conducted by making a small superficial incision on the forearm and noting the time it takes for the bleeding to stop. Antiplatelet therapy prolongs the bleeding time.

Diagnosing   The following nursing diagnoses are appropriate for a client receiving antiplatelet drugs:
- High risk for injury related to decreased clotting ability.
- Anxiety related to lack of knowledge about drug therapy.
- Noncompliance related to inability to adhere to drug regimen.
- Self-esteem disturbance related to dependency on drug therapy.

Planning   Information in the teaching plan for clients receiving antiplatelet drugs includes the goal of drug therapy relative to the underlying disease process and the need to report any incidents of abnormal bleeding such as bleeding gums, vomiting of blood, tarry stools, or hematuria. In addition, instruct the client on the side effects, complications, and precautions specific to the prescribed drug.

Expected appropriate outcomes include the following:
- Client remains free of injury.
- Client verbalizes decreased anxiety levels.
- Client describes drug action, undesired clinical responses, and precautions associated with prescribed drug.
- Client participates in treatment plan.
- Client demonstrates adaptation to changes that have occurred.

Implementing   Document the presence of any undesired responses, complications, or recurrence of symptoms of the underlying disease process. Be alert to any possible interactions with other drugs that might be prescribed for the client.

Evaluating   Monitor the client for resolution or recurrence of the symptoms of the underlying disease process. Monitor the bleeding time test results on a frequency appropriate to the client's condition. Review expected outcomes with the client to determine effectiveness of the plan of care. Revise the plan as needed, based on findings.

ANTIPLATELET DRUG PROTOTYPE

ASPIRIN

As a nonsteroidal antiinflammatory drug (NSAID), aspirin (salicylic acid; ASA, Ecotrin, Empirin) is discussed in depth in Chapter 51. This section presents only information associated with its use as an antiplatelet drug.

Pharmacotherapeutics Aspirin is widely used as a prophylactic antithrombotic agent, primarily in the prevention of recurring TIAs in men and MIs in both sexes.

Pharmacokinetics   The average bleeding time in normal subjects increases after the ingestion of 650 mg of aspirin. Its effects persist for as long as 4 days.[27] See Chapter 51 for additional information on the pharmacokinetics of aspirin.

Pharmacodynamics Aspirin prevents the production of thromboxane A_2, which is necessary for maximum platelet aggregation.[27]

Pharmaceutics Aspirin is manufactured by a variety of drug companies. It is available in several dosage forms, including tablets and enteric-coated, timed-release, and buffered preparations. Although most clients receive 5 grains of aspirin daily or every other day for antiplatelet effect, recent research suggests that even 1 grain daily may be sufficient.

Undesired Clinical Responses Common side effects of aspirin therapy are easy bruising, hematemesis, melena, and epistaxis. Other responses include thrombocytopenia, agranulocytosis, leukopenia, neutropenia, hemolytic anemia, and increased APTT, PT, and bleeding time. (See Chapter 51 for information on salicylism or salicylate poisoning.)

Contraindications and Precautions See Chapter 51.

Drug-Drug and Drug-Nutrient Interactions Aspirin use increases the risk of bleeding in clients treated with warfarin or tissue plasminogen activator. Effects of aspirin are diminished when administered concurrently with antacids, steroids, and urinary alkalizers. Clients consuming alcohol or receiving heparin therapy may experience increased blood loss. Anticoagulants, insulin, and methotrexate manifest increased effects when given with aspirin. In addition, administration of aspirin with probenecid, spironolactone, sulfinpyrazone, and sulfanilamides leads to reduced effects of these drugs. One of the most common drug interactions, that of aspirin in combination with steroids or other antiinflammatory drugs, results in the development of gastric ulcer.

Life-Span Considerations See section in Chapter 51.

Specific Drug-Related Nursing Considerations As previously indicated, the bleeding time is a test that measures platelet and vascular function. When bleeding time is used to assess the effect of aspirin, it is called an **aspirin tolerance test.** Advise the client receiving long-term, large doses of aspirin that an aspirin tolerance test may be regularly ordered.

For best results, instruct the client to take aspirin 30 minutes before or 2 hours after meals. However, if gastric symptoms occur, it may be taken with food or milk.

Dipyridamole

Pharmacotherapeutics The primary indication for dipyridamole (Persantine) therapy is in combination with aspirin or warfarin in the prevention of postoperative thromboembolic complications after cardiac valve replacement. Other uses include prevention of recurrent TIAs, MIs, and coronary bypass graft occlusion.

Pharmacokinetics An oral dose of dipyridamole reaches its average peak concentration in approximately 75 minutes. Its alpha half-life is 40 minutes; this is the initial decrease in the serum level immediately after achievement of peak concentration. The beta half-life, which is the final drop in total plasma concentration, is approximately 10 hours long. Dipyridamole is metabolized in the liver and excreted with the bile.[8,12]

Pharmacodynamics Dipyridamole is a platelet adhesion inhibitor. Its mechanism of action is not completely understood but may relate to inhibition of erythrocyte uptake of adenosine. In addition, dipyridamole decreases vascular resistance, especially in the coronary vessels.

Pharmaceutics Dipyridamole is available in 25-, 50-, and 75-mg tablets for oral administration. See Table 34–8 for additional information on dosage forms, dosages, and routes of administration.

Undesired clinical responses Side effects and adverse reactions to dipyridamole are usually minor and transient. The

TABLE 34–8
Antiplatelet Drugs

Drug Name	Dosage and Route of Administration
ASPIRIN (ASA, Ecotrin, Empirin)	**ADULTS:** 1300 mg/d in divided doses of 650 mg bid or 325 mg qid, not to exceed 12 tablets or caplets in 24 h
HOW SUPPLIED Tablets: 325 mg Caplets: 325 mg	**CHILDREN 6–12 Y:** 325 mg q4h, not to exceed five tablets or caplets in 24 h <6 y: consult primary care provider
Dipyridamole (Persantine) HOW SUPPLIED Tablets: 25, 50, 75 mg	75–100 mg qid as adjunct to warfarin therapy
Pentoxifylline (Trental) HOW SUPPLIED Tablets: 400 mg	Usual dosage: 400 mg tid with meals; 400 mg bid may be used if digestive and central nervous system effects occur
Ticlopidine (Ticlid) HOW SUPPLIED Tablets: 250 mg	Recommended dose: 250 mg bid

most common response is hypotension. Rare reactions include diarrhea, vomiting, flushing of skin, pruritis, headache, dizziness, weakness, fainting, syncope, nausea, and anorexia. Even more rare are angina pectoris and liver dysfunction. All of these side effects cease with withdrawal of the drug.

Contraindications and precautions The only identified contraindications for dipyridamole are hypersensitivity and hypotension.

Drug-drug and drug-environment interactions Additive anti-platelet effects occur when dipyridamole is administered in combination with aspirin and NSAIDs. Increased bleeding may occur when it is given with warfarin. The drug should be stored at room temperature.

Life-span considerations Dipyridamole is classified as a Pregnancy Category C drug. It should be administered during pregnancy only if clearly needed and only after the safety of the fetus has been determined. Since it is excreted in human milk, dipyridamole should be administered to nursing women only with extreme caution. Adequate studies have not been conducted to demonstrate safety and effectiveness in children below the age of 12 years.[8]

Specific drug-related nursing considerations Monitor the client for the most common side effect, which is a reduction in blood pressure. Instruct the client to take the drug on an empty stomach, preferably 1 hour before or 2 hours after meals. Advise the client that dizziness may occur until he or she is stabilized; therefore caution should be used during hazardous activities.

MISCELLANEOUS DRUGS IN CATEGORY

Pentoxifylline (Trental) increases blood flow to the microcirculation by decreasing the viscosity of the blood. This mechanism results in enhanced tissue oxygenation. The exact chemical action of the drug is unclear; however, it does cause dose-related hemorrhagic effects, a decrease in blood viscosity, and an increase in erythrocyte flexibility. In clients with peripheral artery disease, particularly intermittent claudication, the use of this drug has resulted in significantly improved tissue oxygen levels.

Pentoxifylline is available in 400-mg controlled-release tablets. This drug is usually prescribed three times a day with meals. Undesired clinical responses that occur occasionally include heartburn, indigestion, epigastric pain, nausea, and dizziness. Headache, hand tremor, and vomiting have also been reported. Adverse reactions include angina, palpitations, tachycardia, and arrhythmias.[8]

Special nursing considerations for clients receiving pentoxifylline include monitoring the clients' blood pressure and respirations, especially in clients who are also taking antihypertensives.

CONCEPT REVIEW

Antiplatelet drugs generally inhibit the aggregation of platelets in the clotting process, thereby prolonging the bleeding time. These drugs have been prescribed in the prophylaxis of long-term complications after MIs, coronary revascularization, and cerebrovascular accidents.

Aspirin and dipyridamole are the main antiplatelet drugs currently prescribed. Therapy with these drugs is long term. Thus thorough client education is essential to ensure compliance with the treatment.

THROMBOLYTIC DRUGS

Thrombolytic drugs were introduced for use in the clinical setting in the early 1980s and have since revolutionized the early treatment of AMIs. With the advent of thrombolytics, it became possible to arrest the MI as it was occurring, thus preventing the damage that was inevitable before the introduction of these drugs. Use of thrombolytic drugs is now considered a standard treatment for AMI by both the American College of Cardiology and the American Heart Association.[28,29]

General Characteristics

Thrombolytic drugs are **plasminogen activators. Plasminogen** is an inactive proenzyme present in human serum that is incorporated in the fibrin mesh of a blood clot (thrombus). Plasminogen activators convert plasminogen to **plasmin,** which is an active enzyme that degrades fibrin, fibrinogen, and factors V and VIII. This breakdown results in the by-products, fibrinogen degradation products (FDPs), and in dissolution of the clot. In addition, high levels of FDPs interfere with platelet aggregation, which increases the likelihood of a hypocoagulable state. Depletion of α_2-antiplasmin also occurs.[29] α_2-Antiplasmin inactivates plasmin and decreases its circulating level.

Each of the thrombolytic drugs has unique biochemical structure and effects. They are usually classified as first-, second-, and third-generation drugs. Streptokinase and urokinase are first-generation drugs; tissue-type plasminogen activator (t-PA), anisoylated plasminogen streptokinase activator complex (APSAC), and prourokinase or single-chain urokinase plasminogen activator (SCU-PA) are second-generation drugs; and third-generation thrombolytic agents are synergic combinations, hybrids, chimerics, and fibrin-tagged antibody preparations. Third-generation agents are those currently under investigation.[29]

General Contraindications

There are several absolute contraindications for the use of all thrombolytic agents. With thrombolytic drugs, there is a high risk for cranial bleeding. Therefore use of these drugs is contraindicated in clients with the following conditions:

- **History of cerebrovascular accident:** the clot may be present in a weakened or damaged cerebral vessel.
- **Uncontrolled hypertension:** small clots may form in tears produced by high intravascular pressure.
- **Recent intracranial or intraspinal surgery:** clots are part of the normal healing process.
- **Arteriovenous malformation and aneurysm:** vessel walls may be weakened because of high intravascular pressure within these abnormal vessels, and small tears may develop where clots adhere.
- **Intracranial tumors:** tumors may be highly vascular, and some actually may produce plasminogen activator.

Since there is a high risk for internal hemorrhaging with use of thrombolytic drugs, the following conditions prevent the use of these drugs: GI or retroperitoneal bleeding and history of blood dyscrasias such as thrombocytopenia or hemophilia.[30]

▨ NURSING CONSIDERATIONS

Assessing   When obtaining a **health history** from the client, review all the signs and symptoms of MI, including the onset of chest pain and its nature, intensity, location, and duration. Did it occur during exercise or at rest? What, if any, medications were administered and did they relieve the symptoms? Is there a prior history of chest pain or MI or a family history of heart disease?

Clients suspected of having an AMI after undergoing examination using a 12-lead ECG and after **physical assessment** are evaluated for thrombolytic therapy to assess the benefits of thrombolytic therapy versus its risks. In addition to the contraindications previously discussed, clients are at high risk if any of the following have occurred during the 10 days before treatment: major surgery, GI or genitourinary bleeding, cardiopulmonary resuscitation (CPR) for more than 10 minutes' duration, moderately high blood pressure, mitral stenosis with atrial fibrillation, acute pericarditis, subacute bacterial endocarditis, severe renal or hepatic disease, pregnancy, diabetic hemorrhagic retinopathy, or current anticoagulant therapy.

Cardiac enzyme testing should be done whenever potential heart muscle damage is suspected. Baseline coagulation studies are also a routine part of the laboratory work, as is obtaining type and crossmatch information. Type and crossmatch results are obtained in the event that severe bleeding occurs as a result of the thrombolytic therapy.

Diagnosing The following nursing diagnoses are appropriate for clients who receive thrombolytic therapy:
- Altered tissue perfusion related to occlusion of coronary artery(ies).
- Pain related to ischemia or death of myocardial tissue.
- Anxiety related to uncertainty of outcome of acute episode.
- Decreased cardiac output related to possible arrhythmias and decreased contractility.
- Ineffective breathing pattern related to anxiety, pain, and hypoxia.
- Fear related to knowledge deficit and unfamiliar surroundings.
- High risk for impaired gas exchange related to decreased cardiac output and impaired respiratory status.
- High risk for injury (hemorrhage) related to side effects of thrombolytic therapy.

Planning Thrombolytic therapy is effective if initiated within 6 hours of the onset of chest pain that cannot be relieved. Since thrombolytic therapy is given in an acute setting such as the emergency room or in a critical care unit, client teaching opportunities are limited. If he or she is conscious, inform the client of all procedures in as much detail as possible given the nature of the acute episode and the time factors involved in treatment. Keep the client's family aware of the treatment as soon as possible so they may participate in decision making as appropriate.

Expected outcomes for the client receiving thrombolytic therapy follow:
- Client reports decreased levels of pain.
- Client appears relaxed and reports anxiety is reduced.
- Client displays improved hemodynamic stability (e.g., stabilized blood pressure, cardiac output, urinary output).
- Client establishes effective respiratory pattern.
- Client demonstrates lessened fear.
- Client remains free of injury.

Implementing A number of general guidelines can be followed by the health care provider in implementing thrombolytic therapy. All of them should be followed in light of each client's individual history of anticoagulant use and aspirin ingestion at home.

The client should have at least two large-bore IV lines and a heparin lock in place in preparation for thrombolytic therapy. Ideally any required laboratory testing should be done on blood drawn from the heparin lock, not from the site of thrombolytic infusion. Because of the high risk for bleeding with thrombolytic therapy, avoid any injections, arterial sticks, or venipunctures. If they are necessary, select only compressible sites. After the needle stick, place pressure over the site for at least 5 minutes and monitor the site frequently thereafter.

Be alert to any signs of bleeding, particularly from the GI tract, gingiva, and IV sites. Intracranial bleeding is also possible, and the client's level of consciousness should be monitored closely.

Evaluating Note the clinical signs of reperfusion. The most characteristic signs of reperfusion include relief of chest pain, reduction in the ST segment elevation, which may not occur for 24 hours after therapy, and peak cardiac creatine kinase (CK-MB) levels in less than 12 hours.[28]

First-Generation Thrombolytic Drugs

STREPTOKINASE

Pharmacotherapeutics The clinical uses of streptokinase (Kabikinase, Streptase) include treatment of pulmonary embolism, deep vein thrombosis, arterial thrombosis, arterial venous cannula occlusion, and coronary artery thrombosis. In addition, this is one of the drugs of choice to reperfuse coronary arteries after an AMI. Other uses include the lysis of pulmonary microemboli and extensive iliofemoral thrombi.

Pharmacokinetics Streptokinase is not absorbed orally or rectally. The duration of its fibrinolytic effect disappears within a few hours, but its effect on coagulation can persist for 12 to 24 hours because of a decrease in plasma levels of fibrinogen and an increase in circulating fibrin degradation products. The pharmacologic half-life of streptokinase is 18 minutes, and its elimination half-life is approximately 83 minutes.[8,12,28] During this time the enzyme is biochemically active, although it is not detected in the serum.

Pharmacodynamics Streptokinase is a potent fibrinolytic agent that dissolves intravascular fibrin clots. It is a bacterial protein produced by β-hemolytic group B streptococci. Streptokinase acts with plasminogen to produce an "activator" complex that converts plasminogen into the proteolytic enzyme plasmin. Plasmin then hydrolyzes fibrin into polypeptides and hydrolyzes fibrinogen, factor V, factor VIII, and other plasma proteins. As a result of therapy, the client experiences systemic hypocoagulation for 24 to 36 hours or until clotting protein levels return to their baseline.[32]

Pharmaceutics Streptokinase is available in 250,000, 600,000 and 750,000 IU for IV administration. These solutions must be reconstituted with normal saline or D_5W solution before administration. The dosage of streptokinase varies according to its use. Lower doses are used for arterial thrombosis or embolism, deep vein thrombosis, and pulmonary embolism. An initial bolus of 250,000 IU is given over 30 minutes. The normal dose for maintenance is 100,000 IU/h. To treat AMIs, a continuous infusion of 1,500,000 IU is given over 60 minutes. Table 34–9 summarizes information on dosage forms, dosages, and routes of administration.

Undesired clinical responses Adverse effects of streptokinase may occur in any of the body systems. However, the most dangerous adverse effect is intracranial bleeding, which may manifest in the early stages as agitation, confusion, and depression. Another adverse reaction directly related to hemorrhage is hemopericardium. In addition, clients may experience hypotension, not as a result of hemorrhage, but as a result of the action of bradykinin, causing vasodilation.[32] (Bradykinin

TABLE 34–9
Thrombolytic Agents

Drug Name	Dosage and Route of Administration
Streptokinase	**Acute Evolving Transmural Myocardial Infarction**
(Kabikinase, Streptase)	IV infusion: 1,500,000 IU within 60 min of onset of symptoms
HOW SUPPLIED	Intracoronary infusion: 20,000 IU bolus followed by 2000 IU/min for 60 min (total dose, 140,000 IU)
Lyophilized powder: 50 ml in infusion bottles (1,500,000 IU) or 6.5-ml vials of 250,000, 750,000, or 1,500,000 IU	**Pulmonary Embolism, Deep Vein Thrombosis, Arterial Thrombosis or Embolism**
	250,000 IU in peripheral vein over 30 min; then 100,000 IU/h for 24–72 h
	Arteriovenous Cannula Occlusion
	250,000 IU streptokinase in 2 ml of solution instilled slowly into each occluded limb of the cannula; clamp off for 2 h; aspirate contents of cannula's limbs, flush with saline solution, reconnect cannula
Urokinase	**Pulmonary Embolism**
(Abbokinase)	Initial dose: 4400 IU/kg at a rate of 90 ml/h over a period of 10 min; follow with continuous infusion of 4400 IU/kg/h at a rate of 15 ml/h for 12 h; flush with 0.9% sodium chloride or 5% dextrose solution; follow with anticoagulant therapy
HOW SUPPLIED	
Sterile lyophilized preparation: 250,000 IU urokinase/25 mg mannitol/250 mg albumin (human)/50 mg sodium chloride per vial; 5000 IU/ml after reconstitution	**Lysis of Coronary Artery Thrombi**
	Administer bolus dose of heparin ranging from 2500–10,000 U; then infuse combination of three reconstituted urokinase vials and 500 ml of 5% dextrose solution injection at a rate of 4 ml/min (6000 IU/min) for periods up to 2 h; average total dose, 500,000 IU
	IV Catheter Clearance
	Add 1 ml of reconstituted drug to 9 ml sterile water for injection (final dilution 5000 IU/ml); use 1 ml of the preparation for each catheter-clearing procedure; may also use 5000-IU vial
Alteplase (Tissue Plasminogen Activator (t-PA))	**Acute Myocardial Infarction**
(Activase)	Recommended dose: 100 mg (6–10 mg as bolus, balance; infused over 90 min)
HOW SUPPLIED	Clients < 65 kg: 1.25 mg/kg administered over 1.5 h as described above
Sterile, lyophilized powder: 20-mg and 50-mg vials with vacuum and 100-mg vials without vacuum	**Pulmonary Embolism**
	Recommended dose: 100 mg by IV infusion over 2 h, followed by heparin therapy
Anistreplase	**Acute Myocardial Infarction**
(Eminase)	Recommended dose: 30 U administered only by IV injection over 2–5 min into IV line or vein
HOW SUPPLIED	
Sterile lyophilized powder: 30-U vials	

production results from the high plasmin levels initiated during therapy.)

Because streptokinase is manufactured from foreign protein, allergic reactions present a concern. Allergic reactions include fever, chills, shivering, urticaria, itching, rash, hives, bronchospasm, and anaphylaxis. Because of the possibility of an allergic reaction, the client frequently is premedicated with a corticosteroid; this drug may be repeated during the treatment. Other adverse reactions include headache, musculoskeletal pain, flushing, nausea, pyrexia, phlebitis, and spontaneous bleeding in any system.

Contraindications and precautions Contraindications to streptokinase therapy were discussed previously. Streptokinase is classified as nonselective because it has a low specificity for fibrin. In addition, it activates both circulating and fibrin-bound plasminogen. Because of both of these factors, streptokinase produces a systemic lytic state, which makes treatment of any bleeding complications more difficult.[29] Therefore any arterial invasive procedures should be avoided before and after treatment. If an arterial procedure is necessary,

only the radial or brachial, not the femoral, arteries should be used, with pressure applied for at least 30 minutes, followed by use of a pressure dressing. The puncture site should be assessed frequently for evidence of bleeding. Invasive venous procedures should be avoided as much as possible.

Drug-drug interactions Other drugs that alter the blood's coagulation should be given with caution when an individual receives streptokinase. If a client has been treated with heparin, an APTT of less than twice the control should be achieved before he or she receives streptokinase. Concurrent use of IV heparin is contraindicated during IV infusion of streptokinase. However, it may be administered during intracoronary administration of streptokinase. In addition, drugs that interfere with platelet function (e.g., dextran, aspirin, indomethacin, phenylbutazone) should be used cautiously. Aminocaproic acid reverses the action of streptokinase.[12]

Vials should be stored at room temperature. Reconstitute vials immediately before use. The solution for direct IV administration must be used within 8 hours of reconstitution.

Life-span considerations Streptokinase is classified as a

Pregnancy Category C drug. It is not known if the drug crosses the placenta or is distributed in breast milk.

Specific drug-related nursing considerations When reconstituting streptokinase with sodium chloride or dextrose solution, roll or tilt the bottle. Avoid shaking the solution since to do so promotes foaming and flocculation.

Observe carefully for infiltrates and phlebitis at the infusion site. In the event that phlebitis does occur, it is usually treated by diluting the infusing solution. Monitor the client's blood pressure closely since hypotension increases the oxygen demand of the myocardium, nullifying the effects of the streptokinase and possibly extending the infarction.

MISCELLANEOUS DRUGS IN CATEGORY

Urokinase (Abbokinase) is used in the treatment of pulmonary embolism, coronary artery thrombi, and AMIs. It also is used in clearing IV catheters.

The fibrinolytic activity of urokinase begins immediately after IV administration and can last for up to 24 hours. The serum half-life is 10 to 20 minutes.[12,29] The drug is metabolized in the liver; a small amount of it is found in bile and urine.

Urokinase is a naturally occurring protein manufactured by the epithelial cells of the urinary tract. It directly activates plasminogen and is nonselective for fibrin or fibrin-bound plasminogen. It therefore causes plasminogen to convert extensively to plasmin, causing a systemic lytic state. Plasminogen and fibrinogen levels decrease, and there is an increase in the amount of circulating fibrinogen and fibrin split products that may persist for 12 to 24 hours.

The dosage of urokinase varies with the disorder treated. It can be given as an IV bolus to treat pulmonary emboli and AMIs or through an occluded central venous catheter.

Because it is a human enzyme, urokinase does not cause allergic reactions or antibody formation. In addition, it does not cause hypotension when given as an IV bolus.

Second-Generation Thrombolytic Drugs

TISSUE PLASMINOGEN ACTIVATOR

Pharmacotherapeutics Tissue plasminogen activator (t-PA), or alteplase, is very effective in the treatment of AMIs. It has been used to treat both basilar artery occlusions and pulmonary emboli.[12]

Pharmacokinetics Distribution of t-PA in the body is rapid. The pharmacologic half-life of t-PA is between 5 and 8 minutes; its beta half-life is 15 minutes. It is quickly cleared from the circulation by the liver; therefore when an infusion of t-PA is discontinued, the lytic state lasts for approximately 30 minutes. Recanalization of an occluded artery occurs fairly rapidly, usually between 15 and 60 minutes. Thrombolytic activity is correlated with the blood concentration.[12,29]

Pharmacodynamics Tissue plasminogen activator is an endogenously produced enzyme that is cloned through recombinant techniques. It produces fibrin-enhanced conversion of plasminogen to plasmin. It does not convert plasminogen in the absence of fibrin. The drug binds to fibrin in a thrombus and converts the entrapped plasminogen to plasmin; it does not catabolize circulating fibrinogen. The drug is classified as selective and does not produce systemic lytic states.[12,29]

Pharmaceutics The available forms of t-PA include a powder for injection (20 and 50 mg per vial). The dose of t-PA is adjusted according to the client's body weight. It is administered only intravenously. It is administered as a bolus, followed by an infusion that lasts 1.5 hours. As with all thrombolytic agents, treatment should begin as soon as possible after the onset of AMI symptoms.[12,33]

Undesired clinical responses Because t-PA is a human enzyme, it does not produce allergic reactions or antibody formation. The client may receive repeated doses of t-PA.

Some side effects and adverse reactions include GI, genitourinary, intracranial, retroperitoneal, and surface bleeding, sinus bradycardia, ventricular tachycardia, accelerated idioventricular rhythm, urticaria, and rash.

Contraindications and precautions Clients with hypersensitivity to t-PA, active internal bleeding, recent cerebrovascular accidents, aneurysms, uncontrolled hypertension, or surgery or trauma to the intracranial or intraspinal areas should not receive t-PA.

Drug-drug interactions Clients receiving heparin, acetylsalicylic acid, or dipyridamole may experience increased bleeding with t-PA. No other drugs should be added to an IV solution of t-PA.

Life-span considerations Caution should be used when administering t-PA to pregnant or lactating women and children.

Specific drug-related nursing considerations During the infusion of t-PA, monitor the client for signs of cardiac reperfusion such as resolution of chest pain. In addition, assess for signs of bleeding such as hematuria, GI bleeding, or gingival bleeding. Also monitor laboratory values such as fibrinogen levels and levels of fibrinogen degradation products.

ANISOYLATED PLASMINOGEN STREPTOKINASE ACTIVATOR COMPLEX

Pharmacotherapeutics The primary therapeutic value of anisoylated plasminogen streptokinase activator complex (APSAC), or anistreplase (Eminase), is in the treatment of AMIs.

Pharmacokinetics The half-life of APSAC is 90 to 105 minutes. Its fibrinolytic effect lasts 4 to 6 hours after administration.[12]

Pharmacodynamics APSAC is a synthetic compound consisting of equal amounts of streptokinase bound to human lysine plasminogen, which has a greater affinity for fibrin than the endogenous plasminogen with which streptokinase usually binds.[29] Through chemical reactions, the drug activates the conversion of plasminogen to plasmin. It is semiselective for fibrin, although it does produce a systemic lytic state similar to that of streptokinase.

Pharmaceutics APSAC is available in a freeze-dried powder form of 30 U/vial. As with other thrombolytic agents used in the treatment of AMIs, APSAC should be administered as quickly as possible after the onset of symptoms. It is administered intravenously in a 30-unit bolus over 2 to 5 minutes. Reperfusion occurs within 45 minutes.

Undesired clinical responses Side effects and adverse reactions associated with APSAC include decreased hematocrit level and GI, genitourinary, intracranial, retroperitoneal, and surface bleeding.

APSAC has the same type of immunologic effects as streptokinase—allergic reactions and hypotension—although they are milder than with streptokinase. There is also the rare possibility of viral transmission because the drug is prepared using heated human plasma.[29]

Contraindications and precautions APSAC should not be administered to clients hypersensitive to the drug. Other contraindications include active internal bleeding, intraspinal or intracranial surgery, neoplasms of the central nervous system, severe hypertension, and cerebral embolism, thrombosis, or hemorrhage.

APSAC should be given with caution to clients with arterial emboli from the left side of the heart, ulcerative colitis or enteritis, renal disease, hepatic disease, hypocoagulation, chronic obstructive pulmonary disease, subacute bacterial endocarditis, or rheumatic valvular disease.

Drug-drug and drug-environment interactions When APSAC is administered with aspirin, indomethacin, phenylbutazone, or anticoagulants, the potential for bleeding increases.

APSAC in its powder form should be stored in the refrigerator. After reconstitution, it should be used within 30 minutes.

Life-span considerations With use of APSAC, the risk of intracranial hemorrhage increases in elderly clients, especially those over 70 years of age. There is an increased rate of mortality in clients over 65 years of age who have received APSAC. It should be used cautiously in these clients and only when the therapeutic benefits outweigh the risks.[12]

Specific drug-related nursing considerations Reconstitute APSAC only with sterile water for injection, rather than bacteriostatic water. Slowly add 5 ml of diluent to powder; direct the stream of diluent against the side of the vial; then gently roll the vial to mix the powder and diluent.

During an infusion of APSAC, monitor the client carefully for the occurrence of reperfusion arrhythmias. Assess for bleeding, signs and symptoms of allergic reactions, hypotension, or an anaphylactoid reaction. Avoid the use of invasive procedures such as injections and rectal temperatures.

ANTIHEMOPHILIC, ANTIHEMORRHAGIC, AND HEMOSTATIC DRUGS

Many antihemophilic, antihemorrhagic, and hemostatic drugs are used to treat hemophilia. Hemophilia is an X-linked recessive disease caused by a deficiency in clotting factors. It is present only in males; women are the carriers of the disease. There are three major types of hemophilia: (1) hemophilia A, or classic hemophilia, in which factor VIII is deficient or absent; (2) Christmas disease, or hemophilia B, in which factor IX is defi-

cient or absent; and (3) von Willebrand's disease, in which factor VIII is deficient and platelets are dysfunctional.[3,4] Hemophilia C, occurring primarily in the Jewish population, is a deficiency of factor XI.

Abnormal bleeding is the hallmark sign of this disease. Spontaneous bleeding usually occurs when the factor activity level is below 1%. Bleeding into the joints (hemarthrosis) and deep tissue bleeding are two types of spontaneous bleeding that occur in clients with severe hemophilia.

The goals of hemophilia therapy are to prevent and treat bleeding. Replacement of the deficient factors is the primary mode of treatment. Each product used to treat hemophilia is discussed below.

▨ NURSING CONSIDERATIONS

Assessing Many of the clients treated for hemophilia are children or adolescents. When obtaining a **health history** from these individuals, gather information about their growth and development, especially posture, movement, gait, abnormalities in joints, and spinal or neurologic changes.

Include in the **physical assessment** the vital signs, especially the heart rate and temperature. An elevated temperature may indicate infection, whereas an increased heart rate may reflect the body's compensation for anemia, which can result from bleeding in the hemophiliac client. Tachypnea and hypotension may signal the body's need for more oxygen and hypovolemia, respectively. In addition, signs of inflammation such as redness, swelling, or tenderness in a joint indicate previous or current bleeding. Since blood disorders affect almost all body systems, assess all systems in the body. In conducting the assessment, focus on particular effects produced by hemophilia: blood loss, bleeding, and hypoxia.

Pertinent laboratory data to obtain include factor VIII and factor IX coagulant assay results. These factors decrease in clients with hemophilia and von Willebrand's disease. Factor XI decreases in clients with hemophilia C. Another laboratory test to perform on these clients is the thrombin time. This test provides a rapid but imprecise estimation of plasma fibrinogen levels and measures the time it takes for plasma to clot when thrombin is added to it.[15]

Diagnosing Pertinent nursing diagnoses for a hemophiliac client follow:

- High risk for fluid volume deficit related to abnormal bleeding.
- High risk for injury related to activity inappropriate for the disease process.
- Impaired physical mobility related to repeated bleeding into joints.
- High risk for peripheral neurovascular dysfunction related to decreased blood flow to the extremity.
- Altered protection related to abnormal clotting factors.
- Altered self-esteem related to dependence on medication and changes in appearance.
- Pain related to bleeding into joints.

Planning Teach clients and their families about the disease process. Efforts, including the avoidance of any contact sports, should be made to protect the client from injury. Families should be aware that hemophilia is a lifelong problem; family activities should be planned with safety factors and appropriate limitations in mind. Should bleeding in a joint occur, the client should go immediately to the emergency room for treatment.

Implementing Document all bleeding episodes from bruises and hematomas to frank hemorrhage and the client's response to treatment. If joint damage does occur, especially in children, schedule the appropriate orthopedic and sports medicine consultations to minimize degenerative joint changes.

Evaluating Evaluate the efficacy of treatment by determining the cessation of bleeding. In addition, regularly evaluate laboratory data, including the thrombin time and clotting factors assay results. Other useful laboratory test results are the hemoglobin and hematocrit. The hematocrit determination, along with the direct Coombs' test, can detect intravascular hemolysis in clients with blood types A, B, or AB. In addition, observe clients for fever, chills, tachycardia, rapid breathing, backache, hematuria, increased serum bilirubin level, and reticulocyte level.

Antihemophilic Drug: Factor VIII

Pharmacotherapeutics Antihemophilic factor (AHF), or factor VIII (H.T. Factorate, H.T. Factorate Generation II, Hemofil T, Humate-P, Koate-HS, Koate-HT, Monoclate, Profilate), is used for treating clients with hemophilia A. It treats or prevents episodes of bleeding by replacing the missing clotting factor, thus reducing or eliminating the need for administration of large volumes of plasma. This reduces the client's risk for hypovolemia or hypoproteinemia. In its cryoprecipitate form, AHF also treats von Willebrand's disease.

Pharmacokinetics Factor VIII is cleared rapidly from the blood. It has a half-life of 4 hours.

Pharmacodynamics Factor VIII is an essential component for the conversion of prothrombin to thrombin along the intrinsic pathway. It is critical in the maintenance of effective hemostasis.

Pharmaceutics The dosage of factor VIII is adjusted to the client's weight, severity of the deficiency, and amount of bleeding that has occurred. Multiple donors are used when preparing factor VIII concentrates. It is refrigerated and reconstituted just before use and should be used within 3 hours of reconstitution. Plastic syringes should be used for administration of factor VIII because the drug clings to glass surfaces.

Undesired clinical responses The primary side effects of factor VIII administration are related to allergic reactions and the rate at which the substance is infused. Although most allergic reactions are mild, clients may experience anaphylaxis, febrile reactions, and hemolysis as hypersensitivity reactions to factor VIII. Other possible adverse effects include headache, paresthesias, somnolence, lethargy, hypotension, tachycardia, dizziness, nausea, vomiting, transient chest discomfort and cough, bronchospasm, disturbed vision, thrombosis, viral hepatitis, and acquired immunodeficiency syndrome (AIDS).

Transfusion-transmitted infectious diseases have occurred in clients receiving factor VIII because of the need for multiple donors for each dose. These instances have decreased, however, because the drug is heat treated and because new techniques have been developed to yield a purer drug. Clients can develop inhibitors to factor VIII.

Contraindications and precautions Caution should be used when factor VIII is administered to clients with hepatic disease or when large or frequently repeated doses are administered to clients whose blood types are A, B, and AB. Since factor VIII may contain small amounts of A and B isohemagglutinins, a life-threatening hemolytic reaction may result.

Drug-drug and drug-environment interactions Clients should avoid taking aspirin concurrently because of the potential for increased bleeding. As previously indicated, factor VIII is refrigerated and reconstituted just before use.

Life-span considerations Safe use of factor VIII during pregnancy has not been established. It should be used cautiously in neonates and infants.

Specific drug-related nursing considerations Clients with hemophilia should be vaccinated against hepatitis B.

Monitor vital signs during the infusion of factor VIII. If flushing, headache, or blood pressure or pulse changes occur, slow the infusion or stop it altogether.

If cryoprecipitate factor VIII is used, keep it frozen until ready for use. Thaw the preparation to room temperature by placing it in a warm water bath at temperatures no greater than 37° C. Higher temperatures can be destructive to factor VIII activity.

MISCELLANEOUS DRUGS IN CATEGORY

Factor IX complex preparations also contain factors II, VII, and X and are used to treat hemophilia B in which there is a deficiency of factor IX.

Factor IX has a half-life of approximately 24 hours. The dosage of factor IX complex is individualized according to the client's laboratory work. It is given IV at a rate not more than 3 ml/min. It should be administered within 3 hours after reconstitution.

The most serious undesired clinical responses to factor IX complex are the possible development of thrombosis or DIC. In addition, less serious side effects (e.g., fever and chills) can occur.

Antiinhibitor coagulant complex consists of clotting factors and is used to treat clients with factor VIII deficiency or those with inhibitors to factor VIII. This drug is administered IV as an infusion. The usual adult dose is 25 to 100 U/kg and is based on the site and degree of hemorrhage.

Allergic reactions are the primary side effects of this drug. In addition, flushing, headaches, and blood pressure and heart rate changes can occur if the infusion is administered too quickly. These symptoms dissipate once the infusion has been slowed or discontinued for a period of time.

Hemostatic Drugs

Several drugs and agents are used to increase clotting during an acute hemorrhage. They can be either systemic or topical.

SYSTEMIC HEMOSTATIC AGENT: AMINOCAPROIC ACID

Pharmacotherapeutics Aminocaproic acid (Amicar) is used in the treatment of hyperfibrinolytic states such as bleeding after surgical procedures. It is also used as an adjunctive therapy in the treatment of hemophilia.

Pharmacokinetics Aminocaproic acid is rapidly absorbed from the GI tract and readily penetrates erythrocytes and other body cells. It reaches its peak serum level in 2 hours. The majority of the drug is excreted by the kidneys in an unmetabolized form within 12 hours.

Pharmacodynamics Aminocaproic acid is classified as a plasminogen inhibitor. It inhibits the activation of plasminogen and thereby decreases its conversion to plasmin. This action decreases fibrinolysis.

Pharmaceutics Aminocaproic acid is available in an injection form of 250 mg/ml, in a tablet form of 500 mg, and in a syrup form of 250 mg/ml. In adults therapy is initiated with either an oral or IV loading dose of 5 g; after the initial dose, 1 to 1.25 g/h is administered if needed. Dosage should not exceed 30 g/d.

Undesired clinical responses The primary side effects of aminocaproic acid are the formation of thromboses, arrhythmias, convulsions, and renal failure. Additional side effects are numerous and include dysuria, frequency, oliguria, ejaculatory failure, menstrual irregularities, nausea, vomiting, abdominal cramps, diarrhea, rash, headache, dizziness, malaise, fatigue, hallucinations, delirium, psychosis, orthostatic hypotension, muscle weakness, bradycardia, tinnitus, nasal congestion, and conjunctival suffusion.

Contraindications and precautions The use of aminocaproic acid is contraindicated if there is any evidence of intravascular clotting, hypersensitivity, abnormal bleeding, postpartum bleeding, and upper urinary tract bleeding. Caution should be used in clients with moderate renal disease, hepatic disease, thrombosis, and cardiac disease.

Drug-drug interactions Aminocaproic acid should not be mixed with any other drugs in solution. When it is administered concurrently with estrogens and oral contraceptives, increased coagulation is a possible result.

Interference with diagnostic studies Serum potassium and CK levels may increase in clients receiving aminocaproic acid.

Life-span considerations Caution should be used in treating neonates and infants and in clients who are pregnant.

Specific drug-related nursing considerations Assess the client's vital signs during drug administration and monitor clotting studies. Monitor the client frequently for the occurrence of any type of thrombotic complication such as leg tenderness, chest pain, or dyspnea.

Teach the client to observe and report any symptoms of bleeding such as bleeding gums, bruising, hematuria, blood in the stools, or blood in emesis. In addition, advise the client to report signs of myopathy. Counsel the client to change positions slowly to decrease the possibility of orthostatic hypotension.

TOPICAL HEMOSTATIC AGENTS

Topical hemostatic agents are used to control capillary bleeding. They have three actions: (1) to stimulate hemostasis; (2) to form artificial clots; and (3) to provide a matrix that facilitates clot formation.

Absorbable gelatin sponge is a sterile gelatin that absorbs blood. It is used in the control of surgical bleeding when suturing is not possible. It is placed in strips within the wound and is completely absorbed within 6 weeks. It should be moistened with saline or thrombin solution before its application. Since this agent enlarges as it absorbs blood, it should not be overused in a wound. It does not affect the healing process of the scar.

Nursing considerations for the use of absorbable gelatin sponges include assessing the wound for redness, tenderness, or discharge and for recurrence of bleeding.

Oxidized cellulose is surgical gauze that has been treated with cellulosic acid, which reacts with hemoglobin to form a clot. It is fully absorbed within 2 to 7 days; it may take longer to absorb larger amounts. It is used to control bleeding in organs and is contraindicated for surface bleeding because it inhibits epithelial tissue growth. In addition, it inhibits bone regeneration and should not be used in the treatment of fractures.

Thrombin, thromboplastin, and **human fibrin foam** agents are naturally occurring clotting factors that are used topically to control bleeding, usually after dental surgery.

SUMMARY

Seven major drug categories affecting plasma lipids and coagulation factors are discussed in this chapter. Each drug is used to treat or prevent specific clinical problems. The nurse must become familiar with primary drugs in each group.

Depending on the type of hyperlipidemia, cholesterol in the blood can be reduced by bile acid sequestrant resins or nicotinic acid, both of which physically remove cholesterol from the gut; HMG-CoA reductase inhibitors that interfere with cholesterol synthesis; gemfibrozil, which decreases LDL and VLDL levels and increases HDL levels; probucol, which lowers total serum cholesterol; clofibrate, which decreases the VLDL lipoprotein fraction and the LDL fraction; or dextrothyroxine, which intensifies the conversion of cholesterol to bile salts that are excreted in feces.

Anticoagulants (mainly heparin and warfarin) operate on different parts of the coagulation cascade to prevent clotting. Heparin acts through inactivation of thrombin and potentiation of activity of antithrombin III. Its dosage is based on PTT test results. Warfarin interferes with vitamin K–dependent carboxylation and limits the activation of vitamin K–dependent coagulation proteins. Dosage is based on PT results. With both drugs, hemorrhage is the most common undesired clinical response, occurring mainly in the GI tract, the genitourinary tract, or the skin.

Antiplatelets inhibit the aggregation of platelets, prolonging bleeding time. They may be used with anticoagulants. Thrombolytics convert plasminogen to plasmin, an enzyme that degrades fibrin, fibrinogens, and factors V and VIII and dissolves clots. It is the drug of choice in treatment of AMI but carries a high risk for internal hemorrhage. The antihemophilics, antihemorrhagics, and hemostatic drugs are used primarily in treatment of hemophilia. Their purpose is to enhance the clotting ability of the blood.

REFERENCES

1. Seeley, T., Stephens, T., & Tate, P. (1992). *Anatomy and physiology* (2nd ed.). St. Louis: Mosby–Year Book.
2. Tortora, G., & Grabowski, S. (1993). *Principles of anatomy and physiology* (7th ed.). New York: Harper Collins.
3. Copstead, L.C. (1995). *Perspectives on pathophysiology.* Philadelphia: W.B. Saunders.
4. McCance, K.L., & Huether, S.E. (1990). *Pathophysiology: The biologic basis for disease in adults and children.* St. Louis: CV Mosby.
5. Stampfer, M.J., Sacks, F.M., Salvini, S., Willett, W.C., & Hennekens, C.H. (1991). A prospective study of cholesterol, apolipoproteins, and the risk of myocardial infarction. *New England Journal of Medicine, 325,* 373–381.
6. Furie, B., & Furie, B.C. (1992). Molecular and cellular biology of blood coagulation. *New England Journal of Medicine, 326,* 800–806.
7. Milander, M.M., & Kuhn, M. (1992). Lipid-lowering drugs. *AACN–Clinical Issues in Critical Care Nursing, 3,* 494–506.
8. Data Pharmaceutica, Inc. (1993). *1993 physicians' genRx.* Smithtown, NY: Author.
9. Woodley M., & Whelan, A. (Eds.). *Manual of medical therapeutics* (27th ed.). Boston: Little, Brown.
10. Abramowicz, M. (Ed). (1994). Fluvastatin for lowering cholesterol. *The Medical Letter on Drugs and Therapeutics, 36*(923), 45–46.
11. Huang, S.H., Kessler, C., McCulloch, C., & Dasher, L.A. (1989). *Coronary care nursing* (2nd ed.). Philadelphia: W.B. Saunders.
12. Micromedex. (1993). *Drug Evaluation Monographs* (Vol 78). Author.
13. U.S. Pharmacopeia Convention. (1990). *The United States pharmacopeia* (22nd rev.). Rockville, MD: Author.
14. Morton, P.G. (1993). *Health assessment in nursing* (2nd ed.). Springhouse, PA: Springhouse.
15. Chernecky, C., Krech, R., & Berger, B. (1993). *Laboratory tests and diagnostic procedures.* Philadelphia: W.B. Saunders.
16. Weitz, J. (1994). New anticoagulant strategies: Current status and future potential. *Drugs, 48,* 485–497.
17. Hirsch, J. (1991). Heparin. *New England Journal of Medicine, 324,* 1565–1574.
18. Ahmed, T., Garrigo, J., & Danta, I. (1993). Preventing bronchoconstriction in exercise-induced asthma with inhaled heparin. *New England Journal of Medicine, 329,* 90–95.
19. Kleiber, C., Hanrahan, K., Fagan, C.L., & Zittergruen, M. (1993). Heparin vs. saline for peripheral IV locks in children. *Pediatric Nursing, 19,* 405–409.
20. Heparin therapy: Monitoring is mandatory. (1990). *Emergency Medicine,* May, 36, 43.
21. Fahs, P.S., & Kinney, M.R. (1991). The abdomen, thigh, and arm as sites for subcutaneous sodium heparin injections. *Nursing Research, 40,* 204–207.
22. Hull, R., Raskob, G., Pineo, G., Green, D., et al. (1992). Subcutaneous low-molecular-weight heparin compared with continuous intravenous heparin in the treatment of proximal-vein thrombosis. *New England Journal of Medicine, 326,* 975–982.
23. Hirsch, J. (1991). Oral anticoagulants. *New England Journal of Medicine, 324,* 1865–1875.
24. Loken, S., & Shioshita, G. (1992). Factors that influence therapeutic anticoagulation control. *Nurse Practitioner Forum, 3*(2), 95–104.
25. Tatro, D. (Ed.). (1991). *Drug interaction facts.* St. Louis: J.B. Lippincott.
26. Stults, B.M., Dere, W.H., & Caine, T.H. (1989). Long-term anticoagulation indications and managements. *Western Journal of Medicine, 151,* 414–429.
27. George, J.N., & Shattel, S.J. (1991). The clinical importance of acquired abnormalities of platelet function. *New England Journal of Medicine, 324,* 27–39.
28. Aragon, D., & Martin, M. (1993). What you should know about thrombolytic therapy for acute MI. *American Journal of Nursing, 93*(9), 24–31.
29. Kline, E.M. (1990). Pharmacologic review of thrombolytic agents. *Critical Care Nursing Clinics of North America, 2,* 613–626.
30. Niemyski, P., & Hellstedt, L.F. (1989). Patient selection and management in thrombolytic therapy: Nursing implications. *Critical Care Nursing Quarterly, 12*(2), 8–24.
31. Burns, D. (1993). Review of thrombolytic use in acute myocardial infarction, pulmonary embolism, and cerebral thrombosis. *Critical Care Nursing Quarterly, 15*(4), 1–12.
32. Majoros, K.A. (1993). Comparisons and controversies in clot buster drugs. *Critical Care Nursing Quarterly, 16*(2), 46–49.
33. Cole, P.L. (1991). Thrombolytic therapy: Then and now. *Heart and Lung, 20,* 542–551.

BIBLIOGRAPHY

Bell, L., et al. (1992). Cholesterol-lowering effects of calcium carbonate in patients with mild to moderate hypercholesterolemia. *Archives of Internal Medicine, 152,* 2441–2444.

Crussell-Porter, et al. (1993). Low-dose fluconazole therapy potentiates the hypoprothrombinemic response of warfarin sodium. *Archives of Internal Medicine, 153,* 102–104.

Fihn, S., et al. (1993). Risk factors for complications of chronic anticoagulation: A multicenter study. *Annals of Internal Medicine, 118,* 511–520.

Marsalla, J. (1992). Nursing alert: Simultaneous use of heparin and nitroglycerin infusion. *Critical Care Nurse, 12*(5), 134, 136.

Ostrow, C.L. (1992). Thrombolytics. *AACN–Clinical Issues in Critical Care Nursing, 3,* 423–436.

Porterfield, L.M., & Porterfield, J.G., (1990). Understanding cardiovascular drug interactions. *Focus on Critical Care, 17,* 412 416.

Rapaport, E. (1991). Overview: Rationale of thrombolysis in treating acute myocardial infarction. *Heart and Lung: Journal of Critical Care, 20,* 538–541, 590–593.

Templin, K., Shively, M., & Riley, J. (1993). Accuracy of drawing coagulation samples from heparinized arterial lines. *American Journal of Critical Care, 2*(1), 88–95.

Trottier, D.J., & Kochar, M.S. (1992). Hypertension and high cholesterol: A dangerous synergy. *American Journal of Nursing, 92*(11), 40–43.

Tuten, S.H., & Gueldner, S.H. (1991). Efficacy of sodium chloride verus dilute heparin for maintenance of peripheral intermittent intravenous devices. *Applied Nursing Research, 4*(2), 63–71.

Drugs Affecting the Renal System

CHAPTER 35

OVERVIEW OF
The Renal System

ELIZABETH A. BUCK

⊛ Gross Anatomy of the Kidneys

LEARNING OBJECTIVE: Identify gross anatomic structures of the kidneys.

KEY TERMS:

Major calyx, minor calyx, papillae, renal cortex, renal medulla, renal pelvis, renal pyramids, ureter, urethra

⊛ Renal Circulation

LEARNING OBJECTIVE: Describe the circulation of the renal system.

⊛ Functional Unit of the Kidney: The Nephron

LEARNING OBJECTIVES:

Identify the anatomic structures of the nephron.

Discuss the vascular system and tubular system of the nephron.

KEY TERMS:

Bowman's capsule, collecting ducts, convoluted tubules, fenestrae, glomerular membrane, glomerulus, loop of Henle, peritubular capillaries, vasa recta capillaries

⊛ Functions of the Renal System

LEARNING OBJECTIVES:

Define specific terms associated with the formation of urine.

Explain the mechanisms involved in urine formation.

Summarize the three mechanisms involved in regulation of glomerular filtration rate (GFR).

Describe how the kidneys regulate hydrogen ion balance.

Discuss how the kidneys regulate calcium and phosphate balance.

Explain the influence of the kidneys on the activation of vitamin D_3.

Explain the impact of the kidneys on regulation of systemic blood pressure.

Summarize the functions of erythropoietin.

KEY TERMS:

Angiotensin II, diffusion, filtrate, filtration, hydrostatic pressure, osmosis, osmotic pressure, tubular reabsorption, tubular secretion

⊛ Drugs Affecting the Renal System

LEARNING OBJECTIVE: Describe the effects of drugs on the renal system.

CONCEPTS AND TERMS TO REVIEW

Review an anatomy and physiology textbook for additional information about the renal system.

Review the definition of *filtration, secretion, osmosis, osmolality,* and *reabsorption.*

When the body metabolizes nutrients, body cells produce wastes, including CO_2, excess water, heat, and nitrogen. In addition, essential ions such as sodium, potassium, chloride, sulfate, phosphate, and hydrogen build up in excess amounts. These excesses and metabolic waste products must be eliminated from the body.

The urinary or renal system assists with the maintenance of homeostasis within the human body. It helps to maintain the normal concentrations of water and electrolytes within body fluids and to regulate the pH and volume of body fluids. The renal system also helps to control red blood cell production and blood pressure.

Gross anatomy of the kidney, renal circulation, anatomy and physiology of the nephron, and major functions of the renal system are presented in this chapter. Knowledge of this information will help you to understand the relationship between drug therapy and renal function. In addition, most drugs are excreted or eliminated from the body through the renal system. An understanding of this system will enhance your ability to assess possible renal complications.

GROSS ANATOMY OF THE KIDNEYS

The kidneys, two bean-shaped organs, are located in the posterior aspect of the abdomen. They are positioned on either side of the vertebral column at the level of T-12 to L-3 vertebrae. Since the right kidney lies below the liver, the left kidney is usually positioned higher than the right. Fat, muscle, and a fibrous outer covering protect the kidneys from injury[1-3] (Fig. 35–1).

The outer portion of the kidney, the **renal cortex,** lies just beneath the fibrous outer covering. Glomeruli, proximal and distal tubules, collecting ducts, and parts of the loop of Henle are contained in the cortex. Beneath the cortex is the **renal medulla;** the medulla contains the remaining portions of the loop of Henle, collecting ducts, and vasa recta.[4] **Renal pyramids,** 12 to 18 coneshaped masses of collecting ducts, divide the medulla. The bases of the pyramids lie on the boundary between the cortex and the medulla. Apices of the pyramids spread toward the renal pelvis, forming **papillae.** These papillae have multiple openings on their surfaces through which urine empties into the renal pelvis. Groups of papillae empty into a **minor calyx;** several minor calyces merge to form a **major calyx** (Fig. 35–2).

Eventually the major calyces merge to form the **renal pelvis,** an extension of the upper end of the ureter. A **ureter** leads from each kidney to the **urinary bladder.** From the floor of the urinary bladder, a connecting tube, the **urethra,** extends to the exterior of the body. In females the urethra is approximately 4 cm long. In males it is approximately 20 cm long. Immediately below the urinary bladder, the male urethra passes through the prostate gland and penis. The male urethra also carries semen during ejaculation.[5]

RENAL CIRCULATION

Renal blood flow is approximately 1200 ml/min. This amount represents 20% to 25% of the total cardiac output. **Renal arteries** deliver the blood supply to the kidneys. These arteries branch off the abdominal aorta and enter the kidney through the **hilum.** Each renal artery further divides into segmental arteries *(interlobar, arcuate, and interlobular arteries).* Segmental arteries branch into progressively smaller vessels *(afferent arterioles, efferent arterioles, and peritubular capillaries)* that supply all areas of the renal parenchyma. The renal venous system parallels the arterial system. Blood leaves the kidneys through the interlobular veins. These veins connect with the interlobar veins. The interlobar veins eventually become the right and left renal veins and empty into the inferior vena cava.[5,6]

FUNCTIONAL UNIT OF THE KIDNEY: NEPHRON

More than 1 million nephrons are in each kidney. Each nephron is composed of a vascular system and a tubular system (Fig. 35–3).

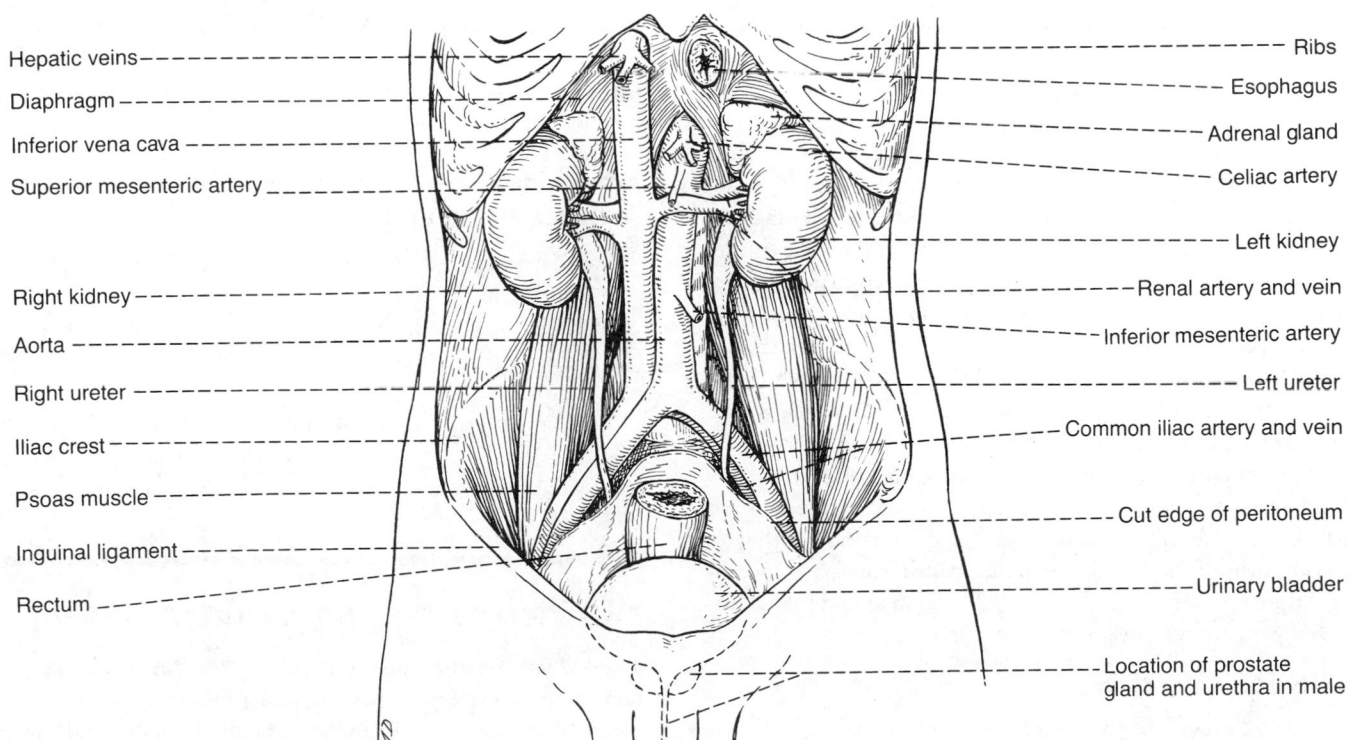

Hepatic veins — Diaphragm — Inferior vena cava — Superior mesenteric artery —

Right kidney — Aorta — Right ureter — Iliac crest — Psoas muscle — Inguinal ligament — Rectum —

— Ribs — Esophagus — Adrenal gland — Celiac artery — Left kidney — Renal artery and vein — Inferior mesenteric artery — Left ureter — Common iliac artery and vein — Cut edge of peritoneum — Urinary bladder — Location of prostate gland and urethra in male

FIGURE 35–1   Anatomic locations of the organs of the urinary system. (From Black, J., & Matassarin-Jacobs, E. [1993]. *Luckmann and Sorensen's medical-surgical nursing: A psychophysiologic approach* [4th ed.]. Philadelphia: W.B. Saunders.)

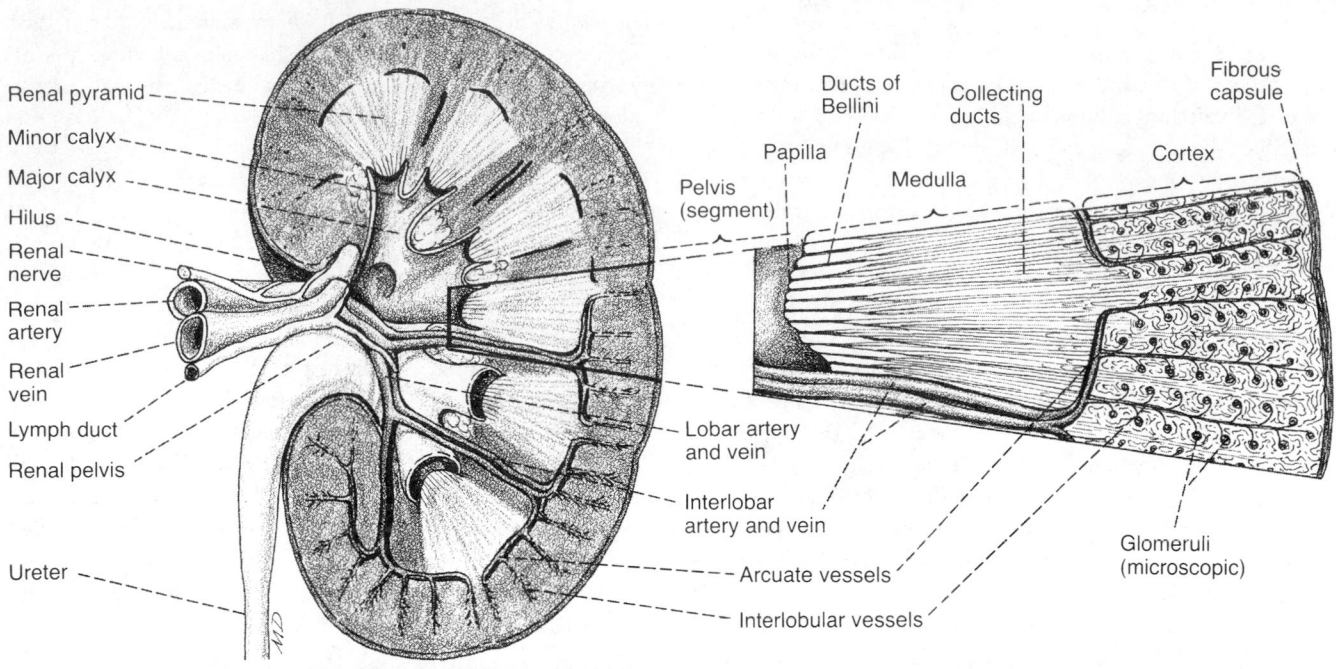

FIGURE 35–2 Anatomy of the kidney. *Inset,* Enlargement of a segment of the kidney. (From Black, J., & Matassarin-Jacobs, E. [1993]. *Luckmann and Sorensen's medical-surgical nursing: A psychophysiologic approach* [4th ed.]. Philadelphia: W.B. Saunders.)

Vascular System

The vascular system contains glomeruli, peritubular capillaries, and vasa recta capillaries. **Glomeruli** are networks of parallel capillaries. Fluid filters from the glomerulus through the **glomerular membrane.** Endothelial cells comprise the first of three cellular layers in the glomerular membrane. These cells are perforated by tiny "windows," **fenestrae,** which allow easy filtration of water and solutes from the blood. The **basement membrane,** the middle layer, is selectively permeable, allowing passage of only certain substances. The outer epithelial layer is the inner layer of the Bowman's capsule. This layer has specialized cells called **podocytes** (foot cells), which form clefts called **slit pores.** These pores allow water and crystalloids (solutes with small molecular weight) to pass through them. Larger molecules such as white blood cells, red blood cells, and albumin are too large to pass through these pores.[3,4]

A second capillary bed, the **peritubular capillaries,** surrounds the tubular system. These capillaries play an important role in the reabsorption and excretion of fluid and electrolytes during urine formation. **Vasa recta capillaries** are a specialized portion of the peritubular capillary system and play an integral part in the concentration of urine.

Tubular System

The tubular component of the nephron consists of the Bowman's or glomerular capsule, proximal convoluted tubules, descending and ascending limbs of the loop of Henle, distal convoluted tubules, and collecting ducts. A saclike structure, the **Bowman's capsule,** surrounds the glomerulus. After the filtrate leaves the Bowman's capsule, it enters the **proximal convoluted tubules** and then the **descending** and **ascending limbs of the loop of Henle.** From the loop of Henle, the filtrate enters the **distal convoluted tubules** and, finally, the **collecting ducts.** The collecting ducts pass through the papillae and empty into the minor calyx and major calyx.[1,5,6]

CONCEPT REVIEW

Renal blood flow represents 20% to 25% of the total cardiac output each minute.

Filtration occurs in the renal corpuscle, which consists of the glomerulus and the glomerular or Bowman's capsule.

From the capsular space, the filtrate passes into the renal tubule. The renal tubule consists of a proximal convoluted tubule, loop of Henle, and distal convoluted tubule.

FUNCTIONS OF THE RENAL SYSTEM

The kidneys are the most important organs in the renal system. They excrete most of the end products of the body's metabolic processes, regulate the amount of body fluids, and control the concentrations of most body fluid elements. In addition, the kidneys assist with the regulation of arterial blood pressure, production of red blood cells, and activation of vitamin D_3.

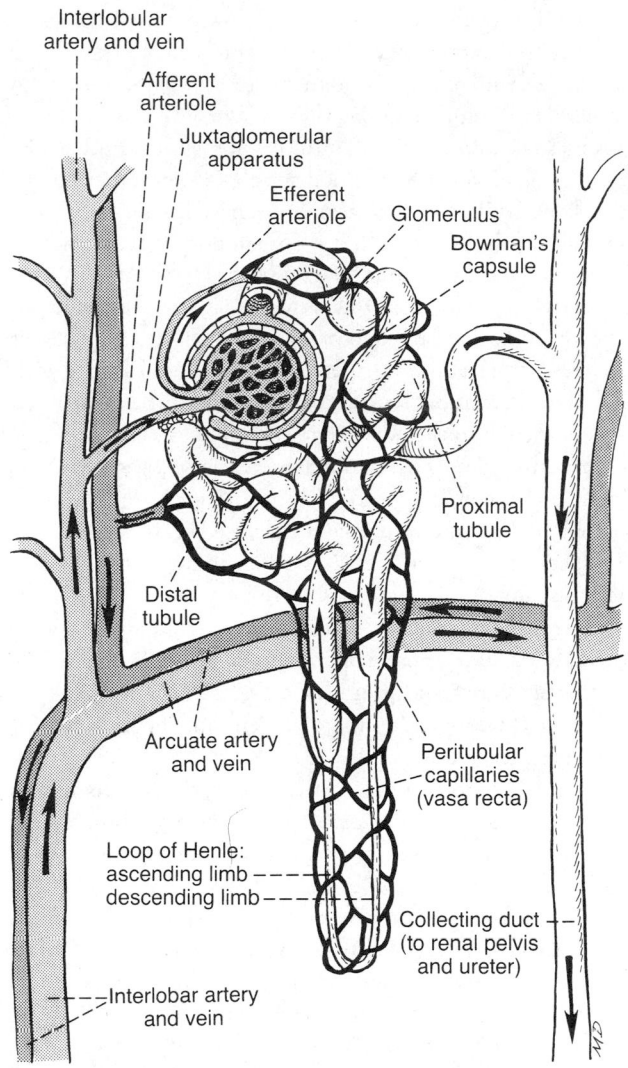

FIGURE 35–3   Anatomy of the nephron. (From Black, J., & Matassarin-Jacobs, E. [1993]. *Luckmann and Sorensen's medical-surgical nursing: A psychophysiologic approach* [4th ed.]. Philadelphia: W.B. Saunders.)

Interlobular artery and vein
Afferent arteriole
Juxtaglomerular apparatus
Efferent arteriole
Glomerulus
Bowman's capsule
Proximal tubule
Distal tubule
Arcuate artery and vein
Peritubular capillaries (vasa recta)
Loop of Henle: ascending limb descending limb
Collecting duct (to renal pelvis and ureter)
Interlobar artery and vein

MAJOR FUNCTIONS OF THE KIDNEYS
▶ Regulation of fluid and electrolyte balance
▶ Excretion of metabolic waste products
▶ Regulation of arterial blood pressure
▶ Regulation of hydrogen ion balance
▶ Regulation of calcium and phosphate balance
▶ Secretion of erythropoietin

Formation of Urine

As indicated previously, the functional unit of the renal system is the nephron. Nephrons remove selected amounts of water and solutes, regulate blood pH, and remove toxic wastes from the blood. One product of this process is urine. Urine is composed primarily of water. However, it also contains varying amounts of electrolytes and breakdown products of proteins. Urine formation involves three principal processes: filtration, reabsorption, and secretion.

GLOMERULAR FILTRATION

Filtration is the movement of water and solutes from an area of higher pressure to an area of lower pressure. Blood pressure forces water and dissolved blood components through the vascular system of the nephron. The semipermeable mem-

brane of the glomerulus allows only certain electrolytes (sodium, potassium, and chloride), organic molecules (creatinine, urea, and glucose), and water to pass through it. Albumin, other plasma proteins, and white and red blood cells are not filtered because of their large size. The fluid that is filtered through the glomerular membrane is called the **glomerular filtrate.** It has the same composition as the plasma except there are no plasma proteins.

The **glomerular filtration rate (GFR)** is the amount of glomerular filtration that occurs within a given period of time. It is usually 125 ml/min or 180 L/d. In the glomerulus blood filtering depends on three main pressures. Glomerular-blood hydrostatic pressure is the most important. (**Hydrostatic pressure** is the force that a fluid under pressure exerts against the walls of its container.) Glomerular-blood hydrostatic pressure is the blood pressure in the glomerular capillaries—approximately 60 mmHg.

Capsular hydrostatic pressure and blood-colloid osmotic pressure oppose the glomerular-blood hydrostatic pressure. *Capsular hydrostatic pressure,* approximately 15 mmHg, develops as the filtrate is forced into the capsular space between the walls of the glomerular capsule. As a result of this pressure, some filtrate is forced back into the capillary. *Blood-colloid osmotic pressure,* approximately 27 mmHg, is caused by the presence of proteins in the blood plasma. The greater the plasma protein concentration, the greater is the osmotic pressure. (**Osmotic pressure** is the amount of hydrostatic pressure necessary to counterbalance the osmotic movement of water across a semipermeable membrane.[2,7,8]) The sum of capsular hydrostatic pressure and blood-colloid osmotic pressure normally is less than the hydrostatic pressure in the glomerular capillaries. Therefore the net pressure favors filtration.

Determination of the GFR is possible with a creatinine clearance test. **Creatinine,** an end product of muscle metabolism, is released into the bloodstream at a relatively constant rate. Under normal circumstances, creatinine is completely filtered into the glomerular filtrate and is not reabsorbed. The creatinine clearance test measures blood and urine samples to determine the rate at which creatinine is cleared from the blood by the kidneys. **Clearance** specifically means the amount of blood cleared of creatinine in 1 minute; clearance is independent of urinary flow rate. Normal creatinine clearance is 100 to 120 ml/min in the adult.[9]

TUBULAR REABSORPTION

As the filtrate passes through the renal tubules, approximately 99% of it is reabsorbed. This movement of water and solutes back into the blood of the peritubular or vasa recta capillaries is called **tubular reabsorption.** Although the rate of reabsorption differs in various parts of the tubular system, most reabsorption occurs in the proximal convoluted tubule of the nephron. Processes used in reabsorption include both passive and active transport. Passive transport processes include osmosis and diffusion. (**Osmosis** is the movement of water across a semipermeable membrane from an area of higher water concentration to an area of lower water concentration. **Diffusion** is the movement of solutes from an area of greater concentration to an area of lesser concentration.) Active transport of solutes requires the expenditure of energy.[2,6]

Glucose, amino acids, urea, sodium, potassium, calcium, chloride, and bicarbonate are reabsorbed by both active and passive processes. Water reabsorption occurs by the passive process of osmosis. Small proteins and peptides are usually reabsorbed by **pinocytosis,** a process in which substances are engulfed by the cell membrane.[8]

TUBULAR SECRETION

The third process involved in urine formation is tubular secretion. **Tubular secretion** removes materials from the blood and adds them to the filtrate. Initially substances diffuse into the interstitial tissue. The substances then move into the tubular lumen by either active or passive transport. Secreted substances include hydrogen ions, potassium ions, ammonium ions, and creatinine. Tubular secretion helps to rid the body of certain materials and to control the blood pH.[5,8]

CONCEPT REVIEW

Nephrons form urine by glomerular filtration, tubular reabsorption, and tubular secretion.

The primary force behind glomerular filtration is glomerular-blood hydrostatic pressure.

Most substances in blood are filtered by the glomerular capsule. Blood cells and plasma proteins are not normally filtered.

GFR represents the amount of filtrate formed in both kidneys per minute.

Regulation of GFR

GFR is increased by increased blood flow into the glomerular capillaries. Glomerular blood flow depends on the systemic blood pressure and the diameter of the afferent and efferent arterioles. Three major mechanisms regulate these two factors: renal autoregulation of GFR, neural regulation, and hormonal regulation.

Renal autoregulation of GFR　Renal autoregulation is intrinsic. It operates completely within the kidneys to maintain a relatively constant renal blood flow despite fluctuations in the systolic blood pressure. Renal autoregulation causes dilation of the afferent arteriole that increases blood flow to the glomerulus. Simultaneously, the efferent arteriole constricts, causing a back flow of blood into the glomerulus. Both actions result in a maintenance of blood supply to the glomerulus and a constant GFR. Autoregulation does have limitations. It cannot continue indefinitely, and it does not occur at all when the mean arterial pressure falls below 70 mmHg.[2]

Neural regulation　Diminished fluid volume results in a decrease in the arterial blood pressure. The decrease in pressure activates baroreceptors in the carotid sinus and in the aortic arch. These receptors send impulses through the sympathetic nervous system to the adrenergic receptors in the afferent and efferent arterioles. The sympathetic activity causes vasoconstriction of the afferent and efferent arterioles, decreasing the renal blood flow and resulting in decreased GFR. As a result of these actions, total peripheral resistance in the rest of the body increases, and arterial blood pressure increases.[6,8]

Hormonal regulation　Within the nephron exists an area (**juxtaglomerular apparatus**) of specialized cells. These cells, the **macula densa** and **granular cells,** assist in the control of renin secretion. Renin, a proteolytic enzyme, helps to regulate blood pressure and maintain GFR.[3]

Intrarenal baroreceptors in the macula densa recognize diminished renal blood flow or decreased concentration levels of sodium. When this occurs, granular cells are stimulated to release renin. Through a series of chemical reactions that occur outside the kidney, renin stimulates the production of **angiotensin II,** a potent vasoconstrictor. Angiotensin II causes an increase in arterial blood pressure and stimulates the release of **aldosterone,** a mineralocorticoid from the adrenal cortex. Aldosterone conserves sodium by increasing its reabsorption in the renal tubules. Increased plasma sodium levels cause additional reabsorption of water. As a result, the circulating blood volume increases, thus elevating the blood pressure.[1,6,8]

Regulation of Hydrogen Ion Balance

The body maintains normal blood pH (7.35 to 7.45) despite continual production of more acids than bases by metabolic reactions. Nephrons of the kidneys help regulate acid-base balance by secreting hydrogen ions. The kidneys' response to an imbalance is much slower than the response by the respiratory system or the chemical buffers in the bloodstream.[5,8] (Additional information on acid-base balance and disorders of acid-base balance is located in Chapter 74.)

Regulation of Calcium and Phosphate Balance

Calcium is found in plasma in three forms: ionized, bound to plasma proteins, and attached to anions. Forty-five percent of the body's calcium is in an ionized, biologically active form. Forty percent is bound to plasma proteins, and 15% is attached to such anions as citrate and phosphate. Calcium bound to plasma proteins cannot be filtered because of the large size of the plasma proteins. The remaining calcium is filtered and reabsorbed through the kidney.

Activation of Vitamin D₃

Vitamin D_3 forms through the action of ultraviolet radiation on the skin. However, it is inactive until it undergoes chemical transformation in the kidney. The active form of vitamin D_3 is called *1,25 dihydroxycholecalciferol (1,25-$(OH)_2D_3$)*. Its major action is to stimulate active absorption of calcium and phosphate from the intestine.

Secretion of Erythropoietin

Ninety percent of the body's erythropoietin is synthesized by the kidneys; the remaining 10% is synthesized in the liver. Hypoxia within the kidneys is the stimulus for erythropoietin secretion. Once renal cells detect a decrease in the oxygen-carrying capacity of the blood, the kidneys secrete erythropoietin. Erythropoietin stimulates the bone marrow to produce red blood cells. A negative-feedback system regulates erythropoietin secretion. If excessive erythropoietin is present, its release by renal cells diminishes.[10]

CONCEPT REVIEW

Filtration rate varies with the filtration pressure.

Glomerular blood flow depends on renal autoregulation, hormonal regulation, and neural regulation.

Stimulation of the macula densa causes the afferent arterioles to dilate and the juxtaglomerular cells to release renin.

Reabsorption of solutes such as sodium and glucose causes reabsorption of water.

Chemicals not needed by the body are discharged into the urine by tubular secretion.

DRUGS AFFECTING THE RENAL SYSTEM

Drugs or their metabolites are excreted from the body by glomerular filtration, tubular reabsorption, and tubular secretion. Several factors affect the excretion process. For example, drugs bound to proteins cannot filter through the glomeruli. Water-soluble drugs easily filter into the glomerular filtrate.

Some drugs specifically act on the kidney. These drugs include diuretics, hyperuricemic agents, vasopressin (antidiuretic hormone [ADH]), and synthetic erythropoietin. All diuretics produce the same response in the body, excretion of water. However, the pharmacodynamics of these drugs are not all the same. (Diuretics are discussed in depth in Chapter 36.) Hyperuricemic drugs act to decrease the level of uric acid within the bloodstream. These drugs inhibit renal tubular reabsorption of uric acid or the synthesis of uric acid. (Chapter 37 contains information on hyperuricemic drugs.)

Vasopressin, a hormone, is released from the posterior pituitary gland. It acts directly on the collecting ducts of the nephron to increase water reabsorption. This hormone is either prepared synthetically or acquired from animal sources. (Vasopressin is discussed in more depth in Chapter 40.) Recently a synthetic erythropoietin has been developed. This drug is administered to clients who have disorders affecting the production of red blood cells.

Drugs given for their effects on other organs and body systems also may affect the functioning of the renal system. Some drugs may temporarily alter renal function; other drugs are **nephrotoxic.** Nephrotoxic drugs cause damage to various structures within the kidney. Kidney damage caused by these drugs can be permanent and eventually result in renal failure. When potentially nephrotoxic drugs are administered, the nurse should monitor laboratory values that measure renal function such as blood urea nitrogen and serum creatinine.

SUMMARY

The urinary tract or system is composed of the kidneys, ureters, bladder, and urethra. Within the body, the kidneys perform several essential functions that maintain homeostasis. Kidneys help maintain the normal concentrations of water and electrolytes within body fluids and regulate the pH and volume of body fluids. The kidneys also help control red blood cell production, vitamin D_3 activation, and blood pressure.

Drugs such as diuretics, hyperuricemic agents, and vasopressin are prescribed because of their action on the kidneys. However, drugs administered for other purposes may have side effects that involve the kidneys. In addition, most drugs are excreted through the urine and therefore must pass through the kidneys. Any drug that passes through the kidneys has the potential of damaging them. Nurses must be aware of the actions of all drugs and carefully monitor laboratory values to assess renal function.

REFERENCES

1. Chmielewski, C. (1992). Renal anatomy and overview of nephron function. *ANNA Journal, 19,* 34-38.
2. McCance, K.L., & Huether, S.E. (1990). *Pathophysiology: The biologic basis for disease in adults and children.* St. Louis: C.V. Mosby.
3. Vander, A.J. (1991). *Renal physiology* (4th ed.). New York: McGraw-Hill.
4. Ulrich, B.T. (1989). *Nephrology nursing: Concepts and strategies.* Norwalk, CT: Appleton & Lange.
5. Hole, J.W. (1993). *Human anatomy and physiology* (6th ed.). Dubuque, IA: Wm. C. Brown.
6. Guyton, A.C. (1991). *Textbook of medical physiology* (8th ed.). Philadelphia: W.B. Saunders.
7. Metheny, N.M. (1992). *Fluid and electrolyte balance: Nursing consideration* (2nd ed.). Philadelphia: J.B. Lippincott.
8. Tortora, G., & Grabowski, S. (1993). *Principles of anatomy and physiology* (7th ed.). New York: Harper Collins.
9. Chernecky, C.C., Krech, R., & Berger, B. (1993). *Laboratory tests and diagnostic procedures.* Philadelphia: W.B. Saunders.
10. Schwartz, A.B., Prior, J., Terzian, L., & Kahn, B. (1988). Erythropoietin for the anemia of chronic renal failure. *AFP, 37,* 211-215.

BIBLIOGRAPHY

Black, J.M., & Matassarin-Jacobs, E. (1993). *Luckmann and Sorensen's medical-surgical nursing: A psychophysiologic approach* (4th ed.). Philadelphia: W.B. Saunders.

Guyton, A.C. (1992). *Human physiology and mechanisms of disease* (5th ed.). Philadelphia: W.B. Saunders.

Ignatavicius, S., & Bayne, M.V. (1991). *Medical-surgical nursing: A nursing process approach.* Philadelphia: W.B. Saunders.

Lehne, R. (1994). *Pharmacology for nursing care* (2nd ed.). Philadelphia: W.B. Saunders.

Monahan, F., Drake, T., & Neighbors, M. (1994). *Nursing care of adults.* Philadelphia: W.B. Saunders.

Price, S.A., & Wilson, L.M. (1992). *Pathophysiology: Clinical concepts of disease processes.* St. Louis: C.V. Mosby.

Seeley, R., Stephens, T., & Tate, P. (1992). *Anatomy and physiology* (2nd ed.). St. Louis: Mosby–Year Book.

CHAPTER 36

Diuretics

JEANNE E. CATANZARO

⊛ **Diuretics**

LEARNING OBJECTIVES:

Discuss classification of diuretics.

Identify four pharmacotherapeutic uses for diuretics.

Summarize major undesired clinical responses
associated with diuretic therapy.

Plan care for a client receiving diuretic therapy.

KEY TERMS:

Aquaretics, diuretic, edema, kaliuretic, natriuretic,
solute diuretic, water diuretic

⊛ **Diuretics Acting on Distal Convoluted
Tubular Site: Thiazides**

LEARNING OBJECTIVES:

Identify site of action for thiazide diuretics.

Summarize essential information about the thiazide
diuretics.

⊛ **Diuretics Acting on the Loop of Henle Site:
Loop Diuretics**

LEARNING OBJECTIVES:

Identify site of action for loop diuretics.

Summarize essential information about loop diuretics.

Describe the mechanism that produces hypochloremic
alkalosis.

KEY TERM: Hypochloremic alkalosis

⊛ **Diuretics Acting on Terminal Distal
Convoluted Tubule and Cortical Collecting
Duct: Potassium-Sparing Diuretics**

LEARNING OBJECTIVES:

Identify site of action for potassium-sparing diuretics.

Summarize essential information about potassium-
sparing diuretics.

Differentiate between aldosterone antagonists and
nonaldosterone antagonists.

KEY TERMS:

Aldosterone antagonist, nonaldosterone antagonist

⊛ **Diuretics Acting at Proximal Convoluted
Tubule Site**

LEARNING OBJECTIVES:

Identify the action site for osmotic diuretics.

Summarize essential information about osmotic
diuretics.

Describe the mechanism of osmosis.

CONCEPTS AND TERMS TO REVIEW

Review anatomy and physiology of the renal system.

Review renal transport systems responsible for maintaining sodium and water balance and acid-base
homeostasis.

Review the function of the Na^+-K^+-ATPase pump.

Reexamine the function of carbonic anhydrase.

Review mechanisms involved with osmosis, capillary
fluid pressure, capillary oncotic pressure, and interstitial oncotic pressure.

---

*D*iuretics are among the first synthetic drugs used clinically. Their discovery is one of the most significant advances in twentieth century medicine. Additionally, they are
among the safest and most sophisticated therapeutic agents.

This chapter discusses four major groups of diuretics. Their
pharmacologic properties, therapeutic uses, undesired clinical
responses, and possible drug interactions are considered. Special consideration is given to the application of the nursing
process.

DIURETICS

A **diuretic** is any factor capable of producing an increase in
urinary volume. Even ingestion of large quantities of fluids is

a diuretic since doing so increases urinary output. As these fluids are ingested, the volume in the vascular compartment increases, which increases renal plasma flow and glomerular filtration rate.

Pharmacologic agents that function as diuretics usually do not increase glomerular filtration rate. Instead, they interfere with the reabsorption of sodium, which decreases the amount of tubular fluid reabsorbed. As a result, natriuresis and diuresis occur.

Classification of Diuretics

Diuretics are classified according to mechanism of action or site of action. The mechanism of action classification is further divided into solute and water diuretics.

Solute diuretics   Solute diuretics produce diuresis by altering the concentration of solutes in the body. These diuretics primarily act on sodium or potassium or both. **Natriuretic** agents promote excretion of large amounts of sodium in the urine, thus reducing fluid volume. **Kaliuretic** agents produce the excretion of potassium in the urine.

Water diuretics   Agents that inhibit the action of vasopressin on the renal tubule are water diuretics or **aquaretics.** A series of vasopressin analogs is being developed; however, their effectiveness on humans has not been proved.[1,2]

Site of action   Classification according to site of action, which is the classification system used for this chapter, describes the effects of the drug on the nephron. In other words, where along the nephron does the drug interfere with sodium reabsorption? Knowledge of the physiology of the nephron is essential as a basis for understanding the effects of diuretics. See box for a summary of nephron physiology relevant to diuretic pharmacology. Figure 36–1 illustrates the site of action of the various diuretic groups.

Pharmacotherapeutics

Diuretics are clinically indicated for two main purposes: to decrease peripheral and pulmonary edema and to lower blood pressure. However, because diuretics are ion-transport inhibitors, they affect nonrenal tissue also. Some of these actions contribute to undesired clinical responses, but others are clinically useful and are discussed later in the chapter.

Edema is defined as swelling of the interstitial space and indicates an expanded volume in the interstitial fluid. Edema is caused by increased capillary fluid pressure, decreased capillary oncotic pressure, or increased interstitial oncotic pressure.[3] In edematous states diuretics mobilize tissue fluids by decreasing plasma volume.

Hypertension, or the elevation of systolic or diastolic blood pressure or both was discussed in Chapter 33. Hypotensive effects are produced by a reduction in sodium and body fluid. Initially this decreases blood volume and cardiac output and produces a negative state of sodium balance. However, with consistent use, sodium balance, cardiac output, and plasma volume return to normal. However, there is a persistent decrease in peripheral vascular resistance.[4]

SUMMARY OF NEPHRON PHYSIOLOGY

Proximal Tubule
Secretion of organic acids
Bicarbonate and carbonic anhydrase–dependent sodium reabsorption
Isotonic reabsorption of sodium chloride and water

Thick-ascending Limb of Loop of Henle
Reabsorption of sodium, chloride, potassium, calcium
Impermeable to water
Transport important for concentrating and diluting urine

Cortical Distal Tubule
Reabsorption of sodium and chloride
Impermeable to water in absence of vasopressin
Transport critical to urine dilution, not urine concentration

Collecting Tubule
Secretion of potassium and hydrogen ion
Stimulation by aldosterone of sodium reabsorption; hydrogen and potassium secretion
Potassium secretion increased by elevated bicarbonate levels in the tubular fluid

Data from Levine S. (1989). Diuretics. *Medical Clinics of North America, 73,* 271-282.

Undesired Clinical Responses

Major undesired clinical responses associated with all groups of diuretics are concentration changes of major electrolytes, fluid volume changes, and changes in uric acid levels. (Unit 18 contains additional information about fluid, electrolyte, and nutritional balance.)

Concentration changes of major electrolytes   The major electrolytes affected by diuretics are sodium, potassium, calcium, and magnesium. Sodium deficit (**hyponatremia**) produced by diuretics is usually mild. However, in some clients with impaired renal function or receiving concurrent drug therapy that also affects sodium levels, the condition may be severe. Drugs that stimulate antidiuretic hormone (ADH) such as morphine, barbiturates, and nicotine or drugs that stimulate thirst such as antihistamines and tricyclic antidepressants should be avoided.[3] Figure 36–2 illustrates some of the common indications of electrolyte imbalances associated with orally administered diuretics.

The body does not have an efficient mechanism for conserving potassium. Even when potassium is needed for normal body function, the kidneys continue to eliminate 40 to 50 mEq of potassium daily in the urine. This may eventually cause **hypokalemia.** Early indications of hypokalemia are nonspecific. Later, skeletal muscles become weak; reflexes are decreased or absent. Cardiac disturbances also accompany hy-

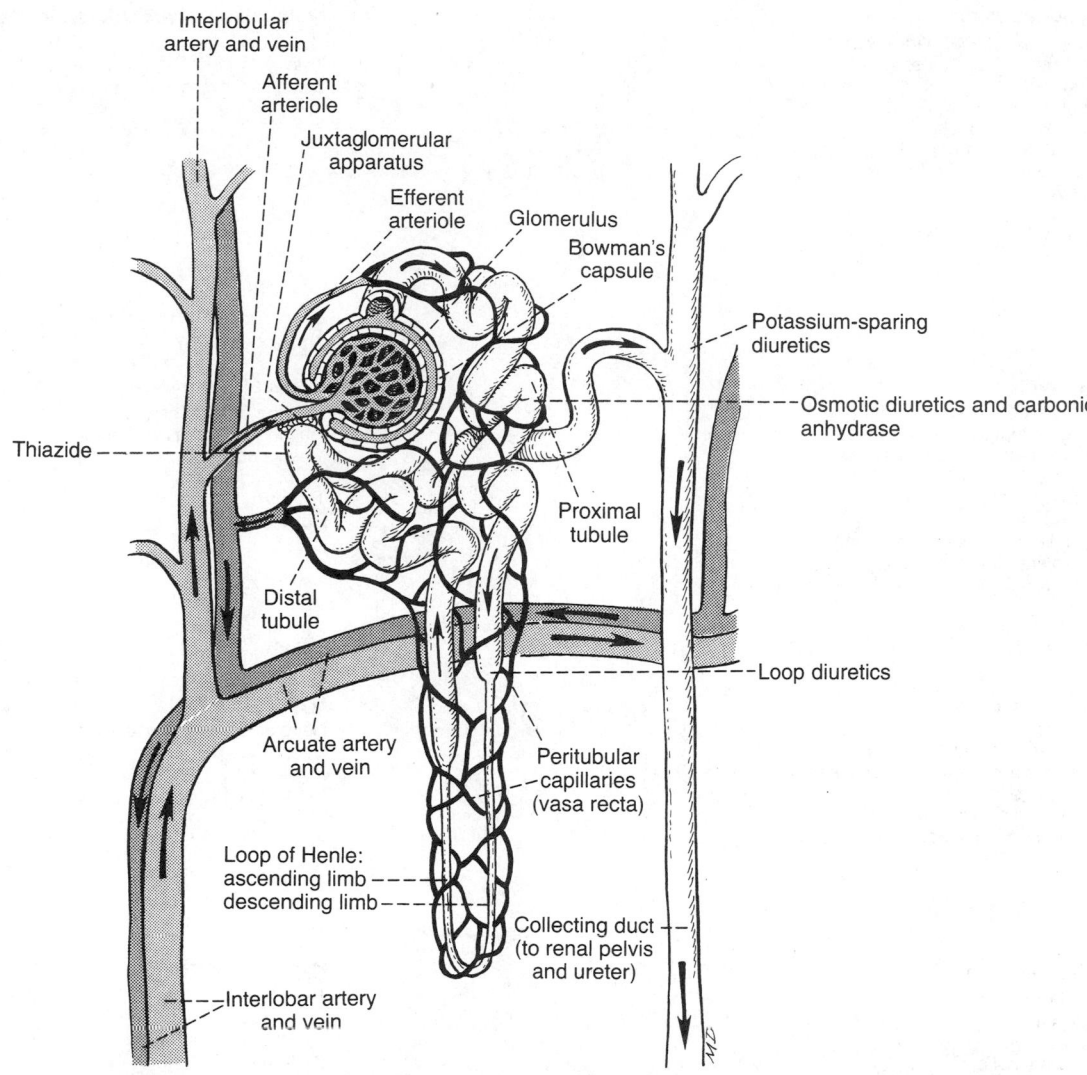

Interlobular
artery and vein

Afferent
arteriole

Juxtaglomerular
apparatus

Efferent
arteriole

Glomerulus

Bowman's
capsule

Potassium-sparing
diuretics

Osmotic diuretics and carbonic
anhydrase

Thiazide

Proximal
tubule

Distal
tubule

Loop diuretics

Arcuate artery
and vein

Peritubular
capillaries
(vasa recta)

Loop of Henle:
ascending limb
descending limb

Collecting duct
(to renal pelvis
and ureter)

Interlobar artery
and vein

FIGURE 36–1   Site of action of diuretics. Diuretics selectively interfere with ion transport along the nephron. Osmotic diuretics and carbonic anhydrase act mainly at the proximal convoluted tubule. Loop diuretics inhibit sodium reabsorption in cells in the thick ascending limb of the loop of Henle. Thiazide diuretics act primarily in the first part of the distal convoluted tubule. Action of potassium-sparing diuretics occurs in the terminal distal convoluted tubule and cortical collecting duct. (From Black, J., & Matassarin-Jacobs, E. (1993). Luckmann and Sorensen's Medical-Surgical Nursing: A Psychophysiologic Approach. Philadelphia: W.B. Saunders.)

pokalemia (e.g., weak pulse, atrial and ventricular arrhythmia, heart block).[3] Potassium loss occurs with loop and thiazide diuretics; it does not occur with potassium-sparing diuretics.

Diuretics also have important effects on calcium levels. Loop diuretics increase calcium excretion, producing **hypocalcemia;** thiazide diuretics decrease calcium excretion and can produce **hypercalcemia.** Some potassium-sparing diuretics also increase urinary calcium.[5]

Thiazide and loop diuretics also enhance the excretion of magnesium, which can produce magnesium deficit (**hypomagnesemia**). The clinical picture of hypomagnesemia varies from client to client. Most frequently seen symptoms include tremor, athetoid or choreiform movements, tetany, a positive Chvostek or Trousseau sign, excessive neuromuscular irritability, and convulsions. Potassium-sparing diuretics conserve magnesium.[3,5]

Fluid volume changes   With the use of any diuretic, fluid volume deficit (**hypovolemia**) can occur. The degree of deficit and rapidity of occurrence influence the severity of the situation.

Changes in uric acid levels   Approximately 65% to 70% of the clients treated with diuretics develop elevated uric acid levels (**hyperuricemia**). Hyperuricemia is due to plasma volume depletion and inhibition of uric acid excretion.[5]

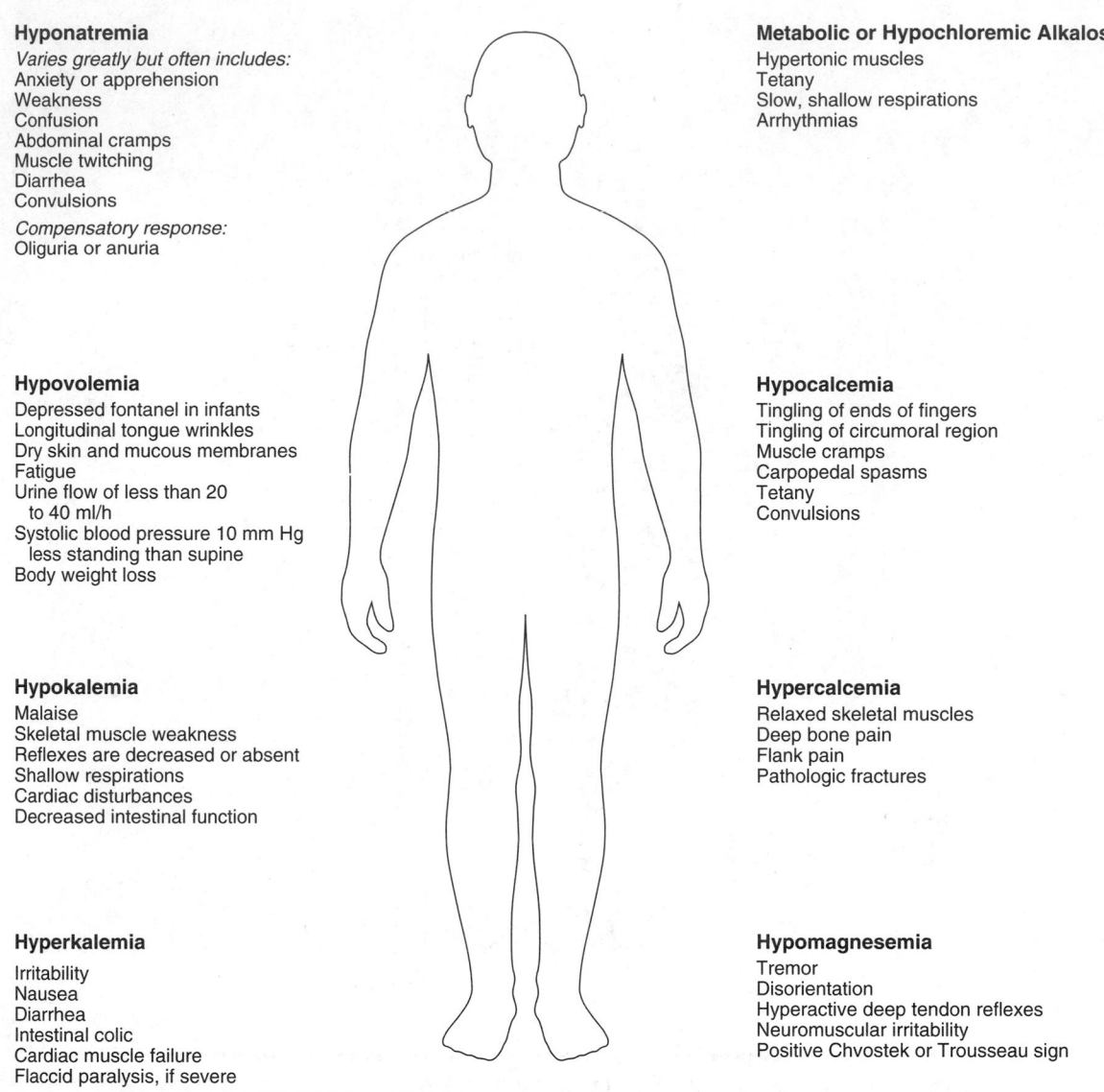

Hyponatremia

Varies greatly but often includes:
Anxiety or apprehension
Weakness
Confusion
Abdominal cramps
Muscle twitching
Diarrhea
Convulsions

Compensatory response:
Oliguria or anuria

Metabolic or Hypochloremic Alkalosis
Hypertonic muscles
Tetany
Slow, shallow respirations
Arrhythmias

Hypovolemia
Depressed fontanel in infants
Longitudinal tongue wrinkles
Dry skin and mucous membranes
Fatigue
Urine flow of less than 20
   to 40 ml/h
Systolic blood pressure 10 mm Hg
   less standing than supine
Body weight loss

Hypocalcemia
Tingling of ends of fingers
Tingling of circumoral region
Muscle cramps
Carpopedal spasms
Tetany
Convulsions

Hypokalemia
Malaise
Skeletal muscle weakness
Reflexes are decreased or absent
Shallow respirations
Cardiac disturbances
Decreased intestinal function

Hypercalcemia
Relaxed skeletal muscles
Deep bone pain
Flank pain
Pathologic fractures

Hyperkalemia
Irritability
Nausea
Diarrhea
Intestinal colic
Cardiac muscle failure
Flaccid paralysis, if severe

Hypomagnesemia
Tremor
Disorientation
Hyperactive deep tendon reflexes
Neuromuscular irritability
Positive Chvostek or Trousseau sign

FIGURE 36–2   Major undesired clinical responses associated with diuretic therapy. Effects may be organ specific or systemic.

▨ NURSING CONSIDERATIONS

Care of the client receiving diuretic drug therapy is based on the phases of the nursing process.

Assessing   Collect a complete **health history.** Question the client about weight gain, abnormal swelling of hands, feet, or around eyes, frequency of voiding, color and odor of urine, and preexisting conditions that may contraindicate diuretic therapy (e.g., pregnancy, renal or liver failure, gout).

Review the client's drug history to determine potential drug-drug interactions. Drugs such as lithium, nonsteroidal anti-inflammatory agents (NSAIDs), angiotensin converting enzyme (ACE) inhibitors, and digoxin can potentiate interactions. Also obtain a dietary history and review it for possible excess intake of sodium.

Collect baseline vital signs and body weight, and review serum electrolyte, serum glucose, blood urea nitrogen (BUN), serum osmolality, and creatinine clearance levels, urinary specific gravity, and electrocardiogram findings. Hematocrit reflects the proportion of blood plasma to red blood cells; fluid loss causes hemoconcentration and fluid gain causes hemodilution. Serum osmolality reflects the actual number of osmotically active particles in the blood. Fluid loss increases serum osmolality because particles become more concentrated; fluid excess decreases serum osmolality because particles become diluted. A rise in BUN frequently indicates a fluid deficit. A fluid deficit also causes more concentrated urine and specific gravity greater than 1.030. Fluid excess dilutes urine, leading to a specific gravity of less than 1.010.[3]

Objective data for the **physical assessment** are gathered via inspection, palpation, percussion, and auscultation. Inspect the color of the client's skin and mucous membranes. An individual's skin color depends on race, ethnic background, and lifestyle. It is an indication of cardiac output and circulation.

Inspect for evidence of edema. Edema is most evident in dependent parts of the body (i.e., feet, ankles, sacral area). Palpate for edema by pressing your thumb firmly against the surface of the skin over the tibia or ankle malleolus. If the pressure leaves a dent in the skin, pitting edema is present. Usually a 4-point scale is used to grade the severity of edema, 1+ for mild edema and 4+ for deep, pitting edema. Edema masks both normal skin color and changes associated with pathologic conditions because the fluid lies between the surface and the pigmented and vascular layers.[6]

Edema that disappears with elevation of the extremity may be caused by gravity flow or interruption of the venous return to the heart as a result of constricting clothing. Pitting edema does not disappear with elevation of the extremity, and it may indicate fluid overload or a pathologic condition such as congestive heart failure.

Also assess for mobility and turgor of the skin. Pinch up a large fold of skin on the anterior chest under the clavicle. *Mobility* describes the skin's ease of rising; it is decreased when edema is present. *Turgor* is the skin's ability to return to place promptly when released; this reflects elasticity of the skin. Skin turgor decreases with dehydration; the pinched skin recedes slowly or "tents" and stands by itself.[6]

If pulmonary edema is suspected, a thorough respiratory assessment is needed. Note shape and configuration of the chest wall. Palpate the chest to determine symmetry of expansion and tactile fremitus. Percuss and auscultate the lung fields; note any abnormal findings.

Diagnosing After completion of the data base, the data are analyzed and nursing diagnoses developed. Nursing diagnoses related to clients receiving diuretic therapy may include the following:

- Fluid volume excess related to excess sodium intake or retention of sodium and water.
- Fluid volume deficit related to increased urinary output after initiation of diuretic therapy.
- High risk for injury related to dizziness and orthostatic hypotension.
- High risk for impaired skin integrity related to presence of edema.
- Noncompliance related to insufficient information about drug regimen.
- Urge incontinence related to irritation of bladder stretch receptors from increased urinary volume.
- Altered nutrition: less than body requirements related to excessive potassium loss.

Planning Client teaching is a major component of the planning phase. Include in the teaching plan information about drug administration, prevention of complications, and evaluation of therapeutic results. Take the client's lifestyle into consideration when planning the drug schedule for the home. The client should be instructed to take once-daily doses of diuretics early in the day, shortly after awakening. This mini-

mizes interruption of evening activities and eliminates the potential for nocturia. If drugs are taken more than once daily, recommend that the last dose of the day be administered as early in the day as possible.

Include in the plan information about self-medication with over-the-counter (OTC) drugs. Teach the client to check with the primary care provider or pharmacist before taking other pharmacologic agents. OTC drugs such as laxatives, cathartics, and antacids may enhance symptoms of dehydration and electrolyte imbalance.

Discuss with the client the importance of reducing dietary intake of sodium. Limiting sodium in the diet allows greater effectiveness of the prescribed diuretic and may permit the use of smaller dosages. Clients requiring only a mild sodium restriction have a great deal of freedom in food selection and may lightly salt most foods during preparation. However, salt should not be used at the table. Clients with more restrictive sodium diets must limit their intake of commercially processed foods that contain sodium benzoate, monosodium glutamate, and baking powder. Salt substitutes are sometimes used to make low-sodium diets more palatable. Many commercial salt substitutes contain potassium and must be used cautiously in clients with a tendency toward hypokalemia. Inform the client that a variety of commercial seasoning mixtures that do not contain sodium or potassium is available.

Client's receiving potassium-wasting diuretics must also be taught methods of maintaining serum potassium levels. Teach clients **not** receiving potassium supplement to include potassium-rich foods such as citrus fruits, tomatoes, bananas, dates, and apricots in their daily diet.

Since diuretics deplete fluid volume, there is a potential for orthostatic hypotension. Teach the client or caregiver the importance of regular monitoring of the client's blood pressure. Advise the client to rise slowly from a lying or sitting position to prevent orthostatic hypotension. Advise the client to limit or avoid alcohol intake and to avoid strenuous exercise in hot weather. In addition, teach the client to monitor the apical pulse rate and report any episodes of palpitations or irregularities.

To prevent complications associated with drug therapy, teach the client the major signs and symptoms of hypokalemia. Advise the client to report symptoms such as drowsiness, confusion, lethargy, anorexia, and muscle weakness immediately. Hyponatremia is another potential problem for clients taking diuretics. Inform the client that clammy skin, decreased skin turgor, thirst, salt craving, and a generalized feeling of weakness are signs of excessive sodium loss.

Hypoglycemia is a concern for diabetic or prediabetic clients. Advise the diabetic client that changes in diet and drug requirements might be needed. Encourage the client to monitor serum glucose levels carefully and to report symptoms of hypoglycemia or hyperglycemia.

Follow-up appointments with the primary care provider are of extreme importance. Inform the client that evaluation of blood pressure, serum electrolytes, electrocardiogram, and edema determines if dosage adjustment is needed.

Teach the client methods of evaluating the drug's effectiveness. Tell the client to weigh daily, preferably upon rising, after voiding, and before eating. For purposes of consistency in weight evaluation, instruct the client that the same amount of clothing should be worn and the same scale used. Teach the client to maintain a record of daily weight. Identify what weight changes should be reported to the primary care provider (Table 36–1).

Expected outcomes must also be developed during the planning phase. Possible expected outcomes for the client receiving diuretic therapy include the following:

- Client verbalizes understanding of dietary restrictions.
- Client demonstrates behaviors to monitor deficit.
- Client demonstrates behaviors to reduce risk factors and protect self from injury.
- Client demonstrates behavior to prevent skin breakdown.
- Client participates in the treatment plan.
- Client verbalizes understanding of causative factors for hypokalemia.

Implementing   Carefully monitor the client's fluid intake and urinary output. Urinary output less than 30 ml per hour may indicate renal failure. Weigh the client daily and monitor the client's blood pressure regularly. Since the client is at risk for developing orthostatic hypotension, assess the client's pressure in both sitting and lying positions. The blood pressure should be taken in the same arm and with the same cuff to ensure accuracy.

Monitor the client's serum electrolyte, glucose, and renal function tests frequently. Assess for signs and symptoms of hypokalemia such as drowsiness, muscle cramps, hyporeflexia, and paresthesias. Monitor glucose and uric acid levels of clients with a history of diabetes or gout.

Inspect the client's abdomen, sacrum, and extremities daily for the presence of or change in the amount of edema. (This is also an accurate method for evaluating drug effectiveness.) Since clients with edema are often immobile, assess the lower extremities for signs of a thrombophlebitis (i.e., pain, redness, and swelling in the calf).

TABLE 36–1

Teaching Plan for Diuretic Therapy

Objectives	Content	Teaching Activities	Evaluation
1. Demonstrate an understanding of diuretic therapy.	Diuretics used to prevent or control fluid retention when heart is decompensated	Include significant other in all teaching. Determine level of previous knowledge. Identify and reinforce previous knowledge. Explain diuretic's action. Explain the reason for using diuretic when the heart is decompensated.	Client can explain that diuretics will increase urinary output and thus reduce fluid in the lungs and edema in general.
2. Demonstrate safe self-medication procedure.	Dosage and administration schedule	Explain the importance for using correct dosage. Give specific instructions on how to measure correct drug dosage. Give written schedule for administration.	Client can measure correct dosage and outline dosage schedule, action expected, and reportable side effects.
3. Demonstrate an understanding of the need for accurate daily weight.	Procedure for weighing client on same scale, same amount of clothes, same time each day; significance of weight gain	Explain the importance of keeping daily weight. Have client demonstrate weighing procedure. Explain keeping a record of weight.	Client can demonstrate weighing procedures, record weight. Client can explain why weighing each day is important.
4. Demonstrate an understanding of the type of diuretic.	Specific diuretic	Explain basic action of drug.	Client can verbalize type and action of diuretic.
5. Demonstrate an understanding of common diuretic undesired clinical responses and need to report them.	Side effects: hyponatremia, hypokalemia, nausea, vomiting, diarrhea, skin rash, weakness, headache; Specific side effects of each drug; foods high in potassium and potassium supplements Responses or reactions to report	Include only those untoward effects that come from the particular diuretic the client is taking. Explain importance of reporting them. Discuss diuretic in terms of loss or conservation of potassium. Give client a list of foods high in potassium. Explain use of potassium supplements.	Client can explain the common side effects of diuretic. Client can verbalize the need to report side effects. Client can outline dosage and schedule for potassium supplement. Client can list specific foods high in potassium.

Evaluating With diuretic therapy, a decrease in the client's blood pressure, weight, and edema is expected. In addition, initial changes in electrolyte levels occur. You must evaluate laboratory findings on a regular basis (see box). These findings reflect the effectiveness of the therapy (i.e., reduced sodium levels) and are early indications of possible undesired clinical responses (e.g., reduced potassium levels).

CONCEPT REVIEW

Most diuretics act by blocking sodium reabsorption in the nephron. This causes an increase in sodium excretion and an obligatory increase in urine.

Diuretics are primarily used to treat peripheral and pulmonary edema and to reduce systolic or diastolic blood pressure or both.

The most common undesired clinical responses associated with diuretic therapy are altered concentrations of major electrolytes, changes in fluid volume, and elevation in uric acid levels.

DIURETICS ACTING ON DISTAL CONVOLUTED TUBULAR SITE: THIAZIDES

Thiazide diuretics have been in use for 30 years; these synthetic drugs are chemically related to the sulfonamides. They are further classified as short-acting, medium-acting, and long-acting. All thiazides act within the distal convoluted tubule, and all are highly protein bound.

THIAZIDE PROTOTYPE

HYDROCHLOROTHIAZIDE

Hydrochlorothiazide (HydroDIURIL, Esidrix, Oretic), the prototype of this group of drugs, is one of the most commonly used thiazides.

Pharmacotherapeutics Thiazide diuretics are commonly used for initial management of all degrees of hypertension. Used alone, they can reduce blood pressure up to 10 to 15 mm Hg. However, in clients with moderate-to-severe hypertension combination therapy with an antihypertensive agent is usually necessary.[7] These drugs are also used to treat edema associated with failure of the right side of the heart, mild-to-moderate failure of the left side of the heart, and drug-induced edema related to the use of estrogens and corticosteroids.[8]

Diabetes insipidus is an endocrine disorder in which the client produces unusually large amounts of dilute urine each day. This leads to other symptoms such as excessive thirst, dehydration, and electrolyte imbalance. Thiazide diuretics reduce urinary volume in these individuals by approximately 40%. In addition, urinary osmolarity increases. This is believed related to sodium depletion and decreased plasma volume.[1]

Thiazides are also used to treat hypercalciuria. In this condition calcium excretion in the urine is so elevated that stones can form and block the tubules, leading to potentially serious kidney damage. Thiazides may reduce urinary excretion of calcium by as much as 50%.[9]

Pharmacokinetics Hydrochlorothiazide is a short-acting thiazide. It is rapidly absorbed from the gastrointestinal (GI) tract after oral administration and produces a diuretic effect within 2 hours. Peak effect usually occurs in approximately 4 hours and lasts approximately 6 to 12 hours. The plasma half-life for hydrochlorothiazide is 5 to 14 hours. It is not metabolized but is eliminated rapidly by the kidneys. At least 61% of an oral dose is eliminated unchanged within 24 hours.[10]

Pharmacodynamics Hydrochlorothiazide acts on the distal convoluted tubule to inhibit slightly the ion pumps that participate in sodium and chloride reabsorption. This indirectly inhibits water reabsorption and increases urinary volume. Therapeutic doses of thiazides increase urinary potassium and magnesium excretion and decrease urinary calcium excretion. Therefore serum levels of potassium and magnesium diminish, and serum calcium levels increase.

Hydrochlorothiazide can significantly decrease renal tubular secretion of uric acid, causing serum uric acid levels to rise and increasing the client's potential for gout. In diabetic clients dosage adjustments of insulin or oral hypoglycemic drugs may be required since thiazides inhibit pancreatic insulin release, causing elevated blood glucose levels.

Thiazides have been associated with increased serum levels of cholesterol and triglycerides. The mechanism for this effect on lipid levels is not fully known; however, proper diet reduces its occurrence.[11]

Pharmaceutics Hydrochlorothiazide is available as an oral solution, oral concentrate, and tablet. Doses depend on therapeutic use (Table 36-2).

Undesired Clinical Responses The most common undesired clinical responses associated with hydrochlorothiazide are fluid or electrolyte imbalance or both (i.e., hyponatremia, hypochloremic alkalosis, and hypokalemia). Clients may experience generalized weakness, hypotension, vertigo, and dizziness. In addition, some clients develop signs and symptoms of gout.

Less common undesired clinical responses include palpitations, ventricular arrhythmias, and GI symptoms such as severe pain accompanied by nausea and vomiting. GI symptoms may indicate thiazide-induced pancreatitis. In some clients this reaction affects the liver, causing jaundice and hepatitis.

Some clients experience hypersensitivity reactions to hydrochlorothiazide. Responses such as photosensitivity, purpura, urticaria, rash, vasculitis, and anaphylactic reactions have been noted. In addition, blood dyscrasias such as leukopenia, thrombocytopenia, aplastic anemia, hemolytic anemia, and neutropenia may occur.[10]

Contraindications and Precautions Thiazide diuretic use is contraindicated in clients with sulfonamide hypersensitivity. These drugs must also be used with caution in clients with severe renal disease. In the presence of a creatinine clearance of 25 to 30 ml/minute, thiazide diuretics lose their potency. Therefore their use is contraindicated in azotemic clients.

Drug-Drug and Drug-Environment Interactions When administered concurrently, the following drugs may interact with thiazide diuretics:

- Alcohol, barbiturates, or narcotics (potentiate orthostatic hypotension)
- Antidiabetic drugs (inhibit insulin release)
- Other antihypertensive drugs (potentiate hypotensive action)
- CNS depressants, phenothiazines, and tricyclic antidepressants (potentiate orthostatic hypotension)
- Corticosteroids (intensify electrolyte imbalance)
- Calcium-containing products (produce hypercalcemia)
- NSAIDs (reduce diuretic, natriuretic, and antihypertensive effects)[10]

Clients receiving hydrochlorothiazide must limit their alcohol intake and avoid natural licorice. They also require a high-potassium and low-sodium diet.

Interference With Laboratory Tests Thiazide diuretics should be discontinued before conducting tests for parathyroid function.

Life-Span Considerations Hydrochlorothiazide should not be administered to pregnant women or women who are breast-feeding. The drug is classified as a Pregnancy Category B drug. Hydrochlorothiazide is administered to children. Pediatric dosages are approximately 1 mg per pound of body weight per day in two doses.

Thiazides are routinely used to treat hypertension in the elderly. However, fluid volume depletion side effects may aggravate renal or hepatic insufficiency in this age group.[12] In addition, hydrochlorothiazide has an increased effect in elderly clients as a result of reduction in baroreceptor response and venous tone in this age group.[13]

Specific Drug-Related Nursing Considerations The drug should be administered with food to decrease GI discomfort. Watch closely for signs and symptoms of fluid volume depletion and hyponatremia. Monitor serum potassium levels, and observe for the indications of hypokalemia. Administer potassium supplements as ordered to maintain acceptable serum levels and encourage the client to eat potassium-rich foods.

Clients receiving digoxin and thiazide therapy have an increased risk for developing digitalis toxicity. Therefore frequent assessment of serum digoxin levels and the client's apical pulse is necessary. If the apical pulse is below 60 beats per minute, assess for other symptoms of digoxin or digitalis toxicity.

Teach the client to monitor for symptoms of hypomagnesemia such as agitation, confusion, tachycardia, hypotension, muscle cramps, and muscle twitching. Instruct clients to report at once severe abdominal pain, yellowish color to the skin, and urinary discoloration; these may be signs of hepatic or pancreatic damage.

MISCELLANEOUS DRUGS IN CATEGORY

Approximately 10 other diuretics have pharmacologic properties similar to those of hydrochlorothiazide. They differ mainly in terms of their potency and duration of action. In addition, hydrochlorothiazide is one of the active ingredients in many drug combinations (e.g., lisinopril, hydrochlorothiazide; methyldopa, hydrochlorothiazide; metoprolol).

Three variants of the thiazides are in clinical use: chlorthalidone (Hygroton), metolazone (Diulo, Zaroxolyn), and indapamide (Lozol). **Chlorthalidone** is similar to thiazide diuretics except for its prolonged half-life (several days). Peak plasma concentrations occur in 2 to 4 hours. It is more potent than hydrochlorothiazide in inhibiting carbonic anhydrase. It is excreted unchanged by the kidneys. **Metolazone,** like the loop diuretics, is more potent than thiazides and retains its natriuretic effect in clients with advanced renal failure. Its onset of action is 1 hour and duration of action 18 to 24 hours. **Indapamide** belongs to the indolone class and is not chemically a thiazide. However, its pharmacologic properties are similar to those of hydrochlorothiazide, and it is frequently used as an alternative to thiazide therapy. Indapamide is very lipid soluble and undergoes extensive metabolism; urinary elimination of unchanged drug is minimal. In addition, indapamide has a long duration of action.[5,14] Table 36–2 summarizes clinical uses, dosage, and route of administration of various thiazide and thiazide-like drugs.

CONCEPT REVIEW

Thiazide diuretics inhibit sodium reabsorption in the distal convoluted tubular site. Diuresis occurring with these drugs is associated with increased water, sodium, potassium, chloride, bicarbonate, and phosphate excretion.

Common undesired clinical responses associated with thiazides involve changes in electrolyte concentration and fluid volume depletion.

DIURETICS ACTING ON THE LOOP OF HENLE SITE: LOOP DIURETICS

Loop, or high-ceiling, diuretics are the most potent diuretics available. They produce the greatest volume of diuresis and

TABLE 36–2
Thiazide and Thiazide-Like Diuretics: Clinical Uses, Dosage, and Route of Administration

Drug Name	Clinical Use, Dosage, Route of Administration
HYDROCHLOROTHIAZIDE (HydroDIURIL, Esidrex, Oretic) HOW SUPPLIED Tablets: 25, 50, and 100 mg Solution: 50 mg/5 ml Intensol solution: 100 mg/ml	*Edema* ADULTS 25-200 mg/d; in divided doses if total dose exceeds 100 mg/d INFANTS <2 y 12.5-37.5 mg/d CHILDREN 2-12 y 37.5-100 mg/d *Hypertension* Initially 12.5–25 mg/d; maintenance 12.5–50 mg/d
Chlorothiazide (Diuril) HOW SUPPLIED Tablets: 250 and 500 mg Suspension: 250 mg/5 ml IV: 500 mg/2 ml Available with reserpine (Diupres) and methyldopa (Aldoclor)	*Edema* Oral: 0.5–1 g once or twice daily *Hypertension* Oral: 0.5-2 g/d *Edema or Hypertension* IV: 0.5-1 g/d once or twice daily for emergency use or for clients unable to take oral drug
Bendroflumethiazide (Naturetin) HOW SUPPLIED Tablets: 5 and 10 mg	*Edema* 2.5-20 mg/d *Hypertension* Initially 5-20 mg/d; maintenance 2.5-15 mg/d
Chlorthalidone (Hygroton) HOW SUPPLIED Tablets: 25, 50, and 100 mg	*Edema* Initially 50-100 mg/d; maintenance usually 100 mg/d *Hypertension* Initially 25 mg/d; maintenance up to 100 mg/d
Trichlormethiazide (Metahydrin, Naqua, Niazide) HOW SUPPLIED Tablets: 2 and 4 mg Available with reserpine (Metatensin)	*Edema* 1-4 mg/d *Hypertension* 2-4 mg/d
Metolazone (Diulo, Mykrox, Zaroxolyn) HOW SUPPLIED Tablets: 2.5, 5, and 10 mg; Mykrox, 0.5 mg	*Edema* 5-20 mg/d *Hypertension* 2.5-5 mg/d; Mykrox: 0.5–1 mg/d
Methyclothiazide (Enduron, Aquatensen, Ethon) HOW SUPPLIED Tablets: 2.5 and 5 mg	*Edema* 2.5-10 mg/d *Hypertension* 2.5-5 mg/d
Indapamide (Lozol, Indolone) HOW SUPPLIED Tablets: 1.25, 2.5 mg	*Edema* Initially 2.5 mg/d; if necessary increase to 5 mg/d maximum after 1 wk *Hypertension* Initially 1.25 mg/d; if necessary, increase to 2.5 mg; then 5 mg/d at 4-wk intervals

have the highest potential for causing undesired clinical responses. This group includes the prototype furosemide (Lasix) and three related drugs, ethacrynic acid (Edecrin), torsemide (Demadex), and bumetanide (Bumex). These drugs act principally along the thick ascending limb of the loop of Henle and have similar pharmacokinetics. Like the thiazides, they are classified as potassium-wasting diuretics.[15] Additionally, all three drugs are weak acids, extensively bound to plasma protein, and reach their tubular site of action via the same mechanism.

LOOP DIURETIC PROTOTYPE
FUROSEMIDE

Furosemide (Lasix) and bumetanide are the most commonly prescribed loop diuretics. Both drugs have similar efficacy rates and undesired clinical responses. Since furosemide has a significantly lower cost, it is usually prescribed as the first-line drug.[15]

Pharmacotherapeutics Loop diuretics are superior to other diuretics when the objective is to eliminate large quantities of fluid rapidly. These drugs are used in the treatment of edema associated with congestive heart failure, particularly severe failure of the left side of the heart. They are also useful in the treatment of edema associated with renal failure or hepatic cirrhosis and ascites. These drugs remain effective when creatinine clearance falls below 25 ml per minute.

Since fluid volume depletion is more common with loop diuretics, they are not routinely used to treat primary hypertension. Loop diuretics may be selected for treatment of hypertensive crisis caused by acute fluid overload. However, in most hypertensive emergencies the blood pressure is high because of vasoconstriction; therefore the objective is to dilate blood vessels rather than reduce fluid volume.[16]

Pharmacokinetics Furosemide is well absorbed from the GI tract. Its protein binding is greater than 95%. Onset of action occurs within 30 minutes to 1 hour; time to peak action occurs in 1 to 2 hours, and it has a 4- to 6-hour duration of action. The drug's bioavailability is 40% to 60%. It is metabolized by the liver. Fifty to 60% of the drug is excreted unchanged in the urine.[15]

When administered intravenously, furosemide's onset of action is approximately 5 minutes. The duration of action for IV doses is decreased to 2 to 3 hours. Sixty to 80% of the drug is excreted unchanged in the urine.[15]

Pharmacodynamics Loop diuretics act directly on the thick ascending limb of the loop of Henle to inhibit sodium and chloride reabsorption. The net result is a 20% to 35% increase in the fractional excretion of sodium. This leads to a depletion of plasma volume and total body potassium. The fluid volume depletion causes an increase in the plasma concentration of renin, angiotensin, and aldosterone. Aldosterone stimulates the medullary

collecting tubule to secrete both potassium and hydrogen ion, worsening the potassium deficit and causing metabolic alkalosis. Potassium depletion stimulates proximal tubular synthesis of ammonium and increases the concentration of that urinary buffer. Loop diuretics also diminish tubular calcium reabsorption.[1,15]

Pharmaceutics Loop diuretics are available in tablets, suspension, and injectable form. Doses depend on the therapeutic use. Table 36–3 summarizes clinical uses, dosage, and routes of administration.

Undesired Clinical Responses Many undesired clinical responses related to use of loop diuretics are identical to those for thiazides. However, risks and severity of responses differ because of drug potency. When used aggressively, loop diuretics can cause a syndrome called **hypochloremic alkalosis** or *contraction alkalosis.* (The term *contraction* implies that extracellular fluid volume has shrunk excessively because of fluid shifts from the bloodstream into the urine.) Along with the excess sodium and water loss, large amounts of chloride ions are excreted, leading to hypochloremia. Bicarbonate remains in the bloodstream, causing metabolic alkalosis. When hypochloremic alkalosis occurs, hypotension develops. Water depletion elevates the concentration of cells and protein in the blood, resulting in an elevated hematocrit and elevated BUN and creatine levels.

Loop diuretics can damage the auditory nerve, leaving the client with mild to severe, temporary or permanent hearing impairments. The risk is less with furosemide or bumetanide than with ethacrynic acid. In addition, the client may complain of vertigo, tinnitus, headache, and blurred vision.

TABLE 36–3
Loop Diuretics: Clinical Use, Adult Dosage, and Route of Administration

Drug Name	Clinical Use, Adult Dosage, Route of Administration
FUROSEMIDE (Lasix) HOW SUPPLIED Tablets: 20, 40, and 80 mg Solution: 10 mg/ml, 40 mg/5 ml IM, IV: 10 mg/ml	**Edema** Oral: 20-80 mg initially in single dose; titrate in 20- to 40-mg increments for maintenance; maximum 600 mg/d in divided doses IV or IM: 20-40 mg; repeat 20 mg at 2-h intervals prn **Hypertension** Oral: initially 40 mg bid; adjust dose as needed
Bumetanide (Bumex) HOW SUPPLIED Tablets: 0.5, 1, and 2 mg IM, IV: 0.25 mg/ml	**Edema** Oral: initially 0.5-2 mg/d as single dose; increase up to 10 mg if needed; manufacturer recommends alternating 3-4 days on drug and 1- or 2-day rest period; maximum of 10 mg/d IM or IV: initially 0.5-1 mg; repeat q2-3h as needed; do not exceed 10 mg/d
Ethacrynic Acid, Ethacrynate Sodium (Edecrin, Edecrin Sodium) HOW SUPPLIED Tablets: 25 and 50 mg IV: 50 mg/vial	**Edema** Oral: initially 50-100 mg/d of ethacrynic acid, usually in divided doses IV: 50 mg or 0.5–1 mg/kg; maximum single dose 100 mg
Torsemide (Demadex) HOW SUPPLIED Tablets: 5, 10, 20, and 100 mg IV: 10 mg/ml	**Hypertension** Oral: initially 5 mg; may increase to 10mg/d in 4–6 wk **Edema** Oral or IV: 5–20 mg up to 200 mg/d

Chronic use of furosemide diuretics may lead to hypokalemia, hyponatremia, hyperuricemia, hyperglycemia, and hypomagnesemia. Additionally, furosemide can induce acute interstitial nephritis and cause gout and diabetes.[10]

Contraindications and Precautions Loop diuretic use is contraindicated in clients allergic to sulfonamide antibiotics. Both classes have similar chemical structure, and exposure may cause hepatic and pancreatic symptomatology.[17]

Drug-Drug, Drug-Nutrient, Drug-Environment Interactions Numerous **drug-drug interactions** are possible with loop diuretics. For example, like the thiazides, loop diuretics increase the risk of digitalis toxicity. Pharmacodynamic interactions between loop diuretics and aminoglycosides increase the risk of ototoxicity and nephrotoxicity. Furosemide administered concurrently with lithium increases tubular resorption of lithium; therefore serum levels of lithium must be monitored closely.[18] There is also the risk of potentiating the action of antihypertensive agents, which leads to hypotension. In addition, concurrent use of furosemide and metolazone (Zaroxolyn), a thiazide-like drug, may result in profound diuresis and excessive electrolyte loss.[17,19]

Other types of interactions include increased potassium loss associated with concurrent use of corticosteroids, reduced effectiveness of uricosuric agents caused by elevation of serum uric acid levels, and impaired loop diuretic action with the use of NSAIDs, caused by decreased prostaglandin synthesis. Diabetics taking loop diuretics may require increased dosages of oral hypoglycemics or insulin. Since furosemide IV infusion solution is not compatible with atropine, diazepam, gentamicin, dobutamine, and several other drugs, it should be prepared in a separate syringe and infused through a separate line.[10]

Drug-nutrient interactions are also possible. Drug absorption is delayed when furosemide is administered with food. Since the drug increases urinary excretion of sodium, potassium, magnesium, and calcium, various nutritional deficiencies are possible. The client should be advised to consume foods rich in potassium and magnesium and low in sodium.

A few **drug-environment interactions** occur with furosemide. The drug should be stored at a controlled room temperature. Prepackaged syringes should be protected from light, and the injection solution discarded if it is discolored.[10]

Life-Span Considerations Loop diuretics should not be given to pregnant women or women who are breastfeeding. Furosemide is classified as a Pregnancy Category C drug, and it does appear in human milk. Loop diuretics, including furosemide, are used with children. However, daily doses greater than 6 mg per kilogram are not recommended.[10]

Use of loop diuretics in the elderly has a greater risk of causing excessive diuresis with circulatory collapse and possibly thrombosis or embolism. These clients are also less tolerant of rapid changes in blood pressure, and rapid or excessive diuresis often causes urinary incontinence.[17]

Specific Drug-Related Nursing Considerations Monitor clients who are also receiving digitalis for digitalis toxicity, which may result from the potassium-depleting effect of the loop diuretic. Instruct the client to report

symptoms such as tinnitus, dizziness, or hearing loss. Vestibular damage associated with the use of furosemide may be partially or completely reversed if the drug is discontinued.[8]

Administer IV furosemide slowly—over 1 to 2 minutes. Since the oral form contains sorbitol, it may cause diarrhea, especially in children.[10]

MISCELLANEOUS DRUGS IN CATEGORY

The other frequently prescribed loop diuretic is **bumetanide.** This drug's onset of action is 5 to 10 minutes. Diuresis is completed within 4 hours, and urinary volumes are greater than those achieved with furosemide. Bumetanide is more potent than furosemide. For example, 1 mg of bumetanide promotes a sodium loss of 82 mEq; 40 mg of furosemide produces a sodium loss of 65 mEq. In addition, the side effects' profile is more favorable, and oral dosage forms of the drug are absorbed better than furosemide.[2] Administer IV doses of bumetanide over 1 to 2 minutes, and monitor the blood pressure every 15 minutes after infusion.

Ethacrynic acid is not as frequently prescribed as in the past. Of the three loop diuretics described in this section, ethacrynic acid is thought to pose the greatest risk of ototoxicity.[17] Ethacrynic acid displaces anticoagulants from binding sites, increasing the anticoagulant effect.[18] Administer an IV dose at a rate of 10 mg or less over 1 minute, or infuse the total dose over 30 minutes. Monitor blood pressure every 15 minutes after infusion. Also check the infusion site frequently since thrombophlebitis is common.

Torasemide is a new loop diuretic. It differs from furosemide and related loop diuretics because of its longer elimination half-life and longer duration of action. A once-daily oral dose of torasemide reduces body weight, edema, and symptoms of heart failure. Torasemide is well tolerated, and only mild and transient undesired clinical responses have been reported.[20]

CONCEPT REVIEW

Loop diuretics are potent therapeutic drugs with a rapid onset of action.

Furosemide and bumetanide are the most commonly prescribed loop diuretics. They have similar efficacy rates, despite bumetanide's being 40 times more potent than furosemide. Both of these drugs have similar undesired clinical responses and are easily dosed and administered.

DIURETICS ACTING AT TERMINAL DISTAL CONVOLUTED TUBULE AND CORTICAL COLLECTING DUCT: POTASSIUM-SPARING DIURETICS

Unlike most other major classes of diuretic drugs, potassium-sparing diuretics do not cause a loss of potassium by way of the kidneys. These drugs act to conserve potassium by reducing its distal tubular secretion in conjunction with sodium reabsorption.

There are two subcategories of potassium-sparing diuretics: **aldosterone antagonists** and **nonaldosterone antagonists.** Spironolactone, a steroid, is the only aldosterone antagonist. Triamterene (an organic acid) and amiloride (an organic base) are nonaldosterone antagonists.[5]

NONALDOSTERONE ANTAGONIST PROTOTYPE

TRIAMTERENE

Triamterene (Dyrenium) is a pteridine that originally was synthesized as a folic acid antagonist.

Pharmacotherapeutics Triamterene is indicated in the treatment of edema associated with congestive heart failure, cirrhosis of the liver, and the nephrotic syndrome. It is also used to treat steroid-induced edema, idiopathic edema, and edema caused by secondary hyperaldosteronism.

Triamterene may be used alone or in combination with a potassium-wasting diuretic. This combination increases the natriuretic effect of the other drugs but blocks kaliuresis and hydrogen excretion, thus reducing the risk of hypokalemia and metabolic alkalosis.[10]

Pharmacokinetics Triamterene is rapidly absorbed, with less than 50% of the oral dose reaching the urine. The drug's onset of action is 2 to 4 hours after ingestion. Peak serum levels occur in 3 hours. Triamterene is metabolized in the liver, and 21% of the drug dose is recovered in the urine.[10]

Pharmacodynamics Triamterene inhibits the reabsorption of sodium ions in exchange for potassium and hydrogen ions. It acts in the section of the distal tubule that is under the control of adrenal mineralocorticoids. This produces mild diuretic and antihypertensive effects.[10]

Pharmaceutics Triamterene is available in gelatin capsules for oral administration. Table 36–4 summarizes clinical uses, dosage, and routes of administration.

Undesired Clinical Responses Some of the undesired clinical responses associated with triamterene are hypersensitivity, hyperkalemia, hypokalemia, and azotemia. Clients may complain of headache, anorexia, nausea and diarrhea.

Contraindications and Precautions Potassium-sparing diuretic use is contraindicated in the client with hyperkalemia or impaired renal function or with concomitant use of other potassium-sparing diuretics or potassium supplements.

Drug-Drug Interactions The most common drug-drug interactions involve concurrent administration of a potassium-sparing diuretic and either lithium, digitalis, NSAIDs, or ACE inhibitors. Response to these interactions may be life threatening.[17]

Interference With Laboratory Tests Triamterene and quinidine have similar fluorescence spectra. Therefore triamterene interferes with fluorescent measurement of quinidine.

Life-Span Considerations Triamterene should not be administered to pregnant women or women who are breast-feeding. It is classified as a Pregnancy Category B drug. Safety and effectiveness in children have not been

TABLE 36–4

Potassium-Sparing Diuretics: Clinical Use, Dosage and Route of Administration

Drug Name	Clinical Use, Dosage, Route of Administration
TRIAMTERENE (Dyrenium)	*Edema, Hypertension, Hypokalemia*
HOW SUPPLIED Capsules: 50 and 100 mg	Initially 100 mg bid; maximum 300 mg/d
Amiloride (Midamor)	*Edema, Hypertension, Hypokalemia*
HOW SUPPLIED Tablets: 5 mg	5 mg/d; adjunct therapy with potassium-wasting diuretic or other antihypertensive drug; increase to 20 mg/d for poorly controlled hypokalemia
SPIRONOLACTONE (Aldactone)	*Edema*
HOW SUPPLIED Tablets: 25, 50, and 100 mg	100 mg/d in single or divided doses
	Hypertension
	50-100 mg/d in single or divided doses; use with potassium-wasting diuretic
	Hypokalemia
	25-100 mg/d

established. Hyperkalemia is more likely to occur in elderly clients if urinary output is reduced.[17]

Specific Drug-Related Nursing Considerations Remind the client to avoid foods high in potassium since the drug conserves potassium.

MISCELLANEOUS DRUGS IN CATEGORY

Amiloride (Midamor) has the same pharmacologic actions as triamterene. It is a basic compound that has approximately 50% bioavailability after oral administration. Its absorption is significantly decreased by food. The drug is essentially unmetabolized and is excreted in the urine. Amiloride is the weakest of the potassium-sparing diuretics with respect to effect on urinary sodium excretion. It is frequently used in combination with other diuretics.

ALDOSTERONE ANTAGONIST PROTOTYPE

SPIRONOLACTONE

Spironolactone (Aldactone) is a steroidal analog of the natural hormone aldosterone. It is this structure that is responsible for its mechanism of action via competition for binding to aldosterone receptors.

Pharmacotherapeutics Spironolactone is effective in the treatment of primary aldosteronism. It may be used to treat congestive heart failure since hyperaldosteronism commonly occurs with this disease. Hypokalemia and alkalosis are counteracted by the administration of spironolactone (Table 36–4).

Pharmacokinetics Spironolactone begins to act in 8 hours. It is almost completely metabolized to active metabolites. The metabolites have a half-life of 17 to 22 hours, thus extending the effects of spironolactone for several days. The effect of any change in dosage peaks in 3 to 4 days.[5] Metabolites of spironolactone are excreted primarily in urine, but small amounts are excreted in bile.[10]

Pharmacodynamics Spironolactone is a competitive antagonist for the aldosterone receptor in the cortical collecting tubules. It binds to the receptor, preventing normal receptor site activity. Antagonism of aldosterone causes sodium excretion and potassium conservation. Spironolactone has little effect in the absence of aldosterone. It also increases calcium excretion through a direct action on tubular transport.[5]

Pharmaceutics Spironolactone is available in tablet form for oral administration.

Undesired Clinical Responses Spironolactone produces gynecomastia in addition to hyperkalemia and hyperchloremic acidosis. GI symptoms such as cramping and diarrhea have been reported, as have drowsiness, lethargy, headache, and skin eruptions.[10]

Contraindications and Precautions Spironolactone is contraindicated for clients with anuria, acute renal insufficiency, impaired renal function, or hyperkalemia.

Drug-Drug and Drug-Environment Interactions Spironolactone should not be administered with other potassium-sparing diuretics because of the risk of severe hyperkalemia. When used in combination with antihypertensive drugs, the dose of the antihypertensive is usually reduced to prevent excessive hypotensive action. If spironolactone is administered concurrently with digoxin, there is a possibility of digoxin toxicity since tubular secretion of digoxin is decreased. Taking spironolactone with salicylates reduces the effectiveness of the diuretic.

Spironolactone tablets must be stored at temperatures between 15° and 30° C. They should be dispensed in tight, light-resistant, and child-resistant containers.

Life-Span Considerations Spironolactone or its metabolites may cross the placental barrier. Therefore the benefit of its use must be weighed against the risk to the fetus. One of the active metabolites for this drug appears in milk. Spironolactone is used to treat edema in children.

DIURETICS ACTING AT PROXIMAL CONVOLUTED TUBULE SITE

Both osmotic diuretics and carbonic anhydrase inhibitors act mainly at the proximal convoluted tubule. Osmotic diuretics act as a nonabsorbable solute; carbonic anhydrase inhibitors prevent reabsorption of filtered sodium bicarbonate.

Osmotic Diuretics

Substances in this group include mannitol, urea, organic acids, and glucose. Osmotic diuretics act by increasing the osmolality of the plasma, glomerular filtrate, and tubular fluid to decrease the reabsorption of fluid and electrolytes, increase the excretion of water, chloride, and sodium, and slightly increase the excretion of potassium.[17]

OSMOTIC DIURETIC PROTOTYPE
MANNITOL

Mannitol (Osmitrol, Mannitol) is the most widely used osmotic diuretic.

Pharmacotherapeutics Since mannitol does not promote sodium excretion to any extent, it is not useful in clients in edematous states. It is most often used as a diuretic in clients with acute oliguria in an attempt to prevent acute renal failure. When used for other conditions such as increased intracranial pressure or to reverse cerebral edema, the resultant diuresis is considered a predictable side effect.[17]

Pharmacokinetics Osmotic diuretics are rapidly distributed to the extracellular fluid after IV administration. Only approximately 7% to 10% of the mannitol dose is metabolized and reabsorbed by the renal tubules. The remaining mannitol is filtered by the glomeruli and excreted unchanged in the urine. Diuresis occurs 1 to 3 hours after administration, with peak effect in 30 minutes to 2 hours and a duration of action of 3 to 10 hours. In clients with normal renal function mannitol is eliminated quickly (half-life is 1.2 hours).[17]

Pharmacodynamics Mannitol is a nonabsorbable solute that acts along the entire nephron. Its primary site of action is the proximal tubule. Mannitol induces diuresis by elevating the osmolarity of the glomerular filtrate, hindering the tubular reabsorption of water and increasing the excretion of sodium and chloride. Mannitol is also a vasodilator; it increases both glomerular filtration and renal plasma flow.[2]

Pharmaceutics Mannitol is available in sterile solution for intravenous (IV) infusion. Table 36–5 summarizes information about drug preparations, dosage, and route of administration.

Undesired Clinical Responses Common adverse reactions to the osmotic diuretics include transient expansion of plasma volume during infusion, electrolyte imbalances, volume depletion, cellular dehydration, headache, and nausea and vomiting. Osmotic diuretics may also cause angina-like chest pain, blurred vision, rhinitis, and urinary retention.[10]

Contraindications and Precautions Because osmotic diuretics temporarily increase blood volume, they cannot be used in clients with impaired cardiac function or congestive heart failure. Their use is also contraindicated in clients with acute renal failure, active intracranial hemorrhage, and severe dehydration.[2]

Drug-Drug Interactions No significant drug interactions occur with the use of osmotic diuretics. However, they can accelerate the excretion of virtually any drug that is eliminated by the kidneys, interfering with the drug's duration of action.[17]

Life-Span Considerations Osmotic diuretics should not be given to pregnant women or women who are breast-feeding. Mannitol is classified as a Pregnancy Category C drug. Use in children less than the age of 12 years old has not been established. Elderly clients must be carefully evaluated for dizziness, disorientation, and confusion while receiving osmotic diuretics.[17]

Specific Drug-Related Nursing Considerations Monitor fluid intake and output accurately since drug therapy is based on the hourly urinary flow rate. In addition, monitor the client for fluid volume overload if urinary output is less than 30 to 50 ml per hour. Assist the client to maintain an adequate fluid intake to promote renal function. Offer frequent mouth care, ice chips, or hard candy to relieve thirst if client is receiving nothing by mouth.

Administer mannitol through an in-line filter. Observe

TABLE 36–5

Osmotic Diuretics and Carbonic Anhydrase Inhibitors: Clinical Uses, Dosage, and Route of Administration

Drug	Clinical Use, Adult Dosage, Route of Administration
OSMOTIC DIURETICS **MANNITOL** (Mannitol, Osmitrol) HOW SUPPLIED IV: 5%, 10%, 15%, 20%, 25%	***Prevention, Treatment of Acute Renal Failure*** IV: 50-100 g as a 5%-25% solution; infuse slowly; rate adjusted to maintain urinary output of >30 ml ***Reduction of Intracranial Pressure*** IV: 1.5-2 g/kg as a 15%-25% solution infused over 30-60 min ***Reduction of Intraocular Pressure*** IV: 1.5-2 g/kg as a 20% solution; infuse over 30 min
CARBONIC ANHYDRASE INHIBITORS **ACETAZOLAMIDE** (Diamox, Diamox Sequels) HOW SUPPLIED Tablets: 125 and 250 mg Sustained-release capsule: 500 mg Injection solution: 500 mg/vial (sodium salt)	***Edema*** Oral: usually 250-375 mg in AM; intermittent dosing (2 days on drug, 1 day off drug) reduces refractoriness when long-term therapy is anticipated ***Chronic Open-Angle Glaucoma*** Oral: usually 250-1000 mg/d in divided doses if daily dose >250 mg; sustained-release capsule, 500 mg, may be given bid ***Acute Angle-Closure Glaucoma*** Oral: usually 500 mg initially, then 125-250 mg q4h IV: 500 mg for prompt reduction of intraocular pressure (dilute 500 mg with 5 ml sterile water and administer slowly; may be diluted further and administered over 4-8 h)
Dichlorphenamide (Daranide) HOW SUPPLIED Tablets: 50 mg	***Glaucoma*** Oral: 100-200 mg initially, then 100 mg q12h until ocular pressure reduced adequately; maintenance 25-50 mg one to three times daily
Methazolamide (Neptazane) HOW SUPPLIED Tablets: 25 and 50 mg	***Glaucoma*** Oral: 50-100 mg bid or tid

infusion site for local irritation, extravasation, or signs of potential thrombophlebitis. Never administer blood products through IV lines used for osmotic diuretics since this causes pseudoagglutination. Product should not be exposed to excessive heat and must be protected from freezing.[8]

MISCELLANEOUS DRUGS IN CATEGORY

Another drug in this class is **urea.** It is used less frequently than mannitol since high doses are necessary to increase urinary output. Urea can be administered orally, although it has a very unpleasant taste. Ureaphil, a sterile 30% solution, can be given intravenously to reduce intracranial pressure. It is very irritating to the tissues and can cause local pain, tissue necrosis, and possible thrombophlebitis if it extravasates.[17]

Carbonic Anhydrase Inhibitors

Carbonic anhydrase inhibitors are considered weak diuretics. They are used for clinical conditions in which induction of negative sodium balance is unimportant. Although carbonic anhydrase inhibitors are among the weakest natriuretic agents, they are potent kaliuretic agents.[14]

CARBONIC ANHYDRASE INHIBITOR PROTOTYPE

ACETAZOLAMIDE

Acetazolamide (Diamox) was the first widely used oral diuretic and is considered the prototype for this class of di-

uretics. It acts principally in the proximal tubule, directly distal to the glomerulus. Acetazolamide is a nonbacteriostatic sulfonamide possessing a chemical structure and pharmacologic activity distinctly different from the bacteriostatic sulfonamides.[10]

Pharmacotherapeutics The major clinical uses for acetazolamide are to treat chronic simple (open-angle) glaucoma and to lower intraocular pressure preoperatively in clients with acute angle-closure glaucoma. Aqueous humor contains a large concentration of bicarbonate ion, and inhibition of carbonic anhydrase significantly reduces the rate of its formation.[14]

Acetazolamide occasionally is used as a diuretic to manage mild edema, especially if the edema probably will be short lived. It is not the preferred treatment for clients with chronic or severe edema or hypertension since its effects are self-limiting and are generally accompanied by systemic acidosis.[1]

Acetazolamide is used as adjunctive therapy for some forms of epilepsy, primarily petit mal seizures in children. The metabolic acidosis that develops after acetazolamide administration is thought to suppress the abnormal brain activity that elicits seizure activity[21] (Table 36–5).

Pharmacokinetics Acetazolamide is well absorbed from the GI tract. After absorption, it is widely distributed throughout tissues and the central nervous system. Peak plasma levels occur approximately 2 hours after administration or 6 to 8 hours after administration with sustained-release oral dosage forms. Because it is an organic acid diuretic, it is tightly bound to plasma proteins, undergoes negligible filtration, and is secreted by the proximal tubule organic acid transport system.[5] Acetazolamide has a long half-life (13 hours) and usually can be administered on a once- or twice-daily basis with chronic therapy. It is excreted unchanged in the urine.[17]

Pharmacodynamics Normally both the production of hydrogen ion within the cell and its removal from the tubular fluid are catalyzed by the enzyme carbonic anhydrase. Inhibition of this enzyme leads to inhibition of hydrogen ion secretion, diminished bicarbonate reabsorption, and diminished sodium reabsorption.[1]

Continued diuresis of sodium, potassium, bicarbonate, and water diminishes the plasma volume and plasma potassium and bicarbonate. As a result, hypokalemia and metabolic acidosis develop.[1] Inhibition of carbonic anhydrase is not limited to renal tissues but also occurs in other tissues such as the eyes where it decreases the formation of vitreous humor.[2]

Pharmaceutics Carbonic anhydrase inhibitors are available in tablets, sustained-release capsules, and an injectable form. Generally clients should not be administered more than 1 g per day.[14] Table 36–5 summarizes drug preparations, usual adult dosages, and routes of administration.

Undesired Clinical Responses Only a few toxic effects have been observed with carbonic anhydrase inhibitors; the most notable is the loss of potassium, leading to hypokalemia. In addition, chronic use may lead to hyponatremia and volume depletion. Generally these responses do not occur unless the client is taking other diuretics concurrently or there is a preexisting fluid and electrolyte imbalance. In large doses acetazolamide may produce drowsiness and paresthesias. The most common major clinical toxicity associated with carbonicanhydrase inhibitors is hyperchloremic metabolic acidosis.[5,14]

Contraindications and Precautions Contraindications for this class of diuretics include severe liver or kidney disease, chronic pulmonary disease, adrenocortical insufficiency, hyperchloremic acidosis, and chronic noncongestive angle-closure glaucoma. Caution is recommended when using in clients with diabetes and gout.[17]

Carbonic anhydrase inhibitors have a sulfa composition and should not be administered to clients with a history of allergic reactions to sulfonamides. Symptoms of an allergic reaction include fever, rashes, crystalluria, and blood dyscrasias.

Drug-Drug Interactions Carbonic anhydrase inhibitors make the urine alkaline and may enhance the action of drugs such as amphetamines, catecholamines, procainamide, quinidine, and tricyclic antidepressants. In addition, this class of diuretics can decrease the effects of lithium, barbiturates, salicylates, oral hypoglycemics, and insulin.

Severe hypokalemia can result with the combination of carbonic anhydrase inhibitors and other diuretics, corticosteroids, and amphotericin B. In addition, carbonic anhydrase–induced hypokalemia may augment digitalis toxicity.[17] Coadministration of phenytoin has been reported to result in drug-induced osteomalacia.[5]

Life-Span Considerations Studies with animals have shown that acetazolamide causes fetal malformations or death. Although no studies have demonstrated evidence this occurs with humans, the potential risks outweigh the possible benefits, particularly in the first trimester of pregnancy. Acetazolamide is classified as a Pregnancy Category D drug. Its safety has not been proved for use in women who are breast-feeding. Its safety and effectiveness in children have not been established.[10]

Use of acetazolamide in the elderly may reduce visual acuity whether used for glaucoma or other purposes. Assistance with ambulation may be required by these clients.[17]

Specific Drug-Related Nursing Considerations Assessment of allergies related to sulfonamides and client history or familiar history of diabetes is of utmost importance. To monitor for hematologic reactions common to all sulfonamides, a baseline CBC and platelet count should be obtained before initiating drug therapy. Similar studies should be completed at intervals throughout drug therapy. In addition, monitor levels of serum electrolytes, BUN, uric acid, creatinine, and blood and urinary glucose.

Monitor client for signs of orthostatic hypotension, signs of numbness, tingling, or excessive malaise. Advise client to report the sensation of "not feeling well" to the physician who then can monitor for acidosis, blood dyscrasias, or hypokalemia. Advise client to watch for signs of kidney stone formation (i.e., renal colic, hematuria, and oliguria). Encourage the client with a history of gout to increase intake of fluids to prevent the risk of renal calculi.[8]

MISCELLANEOUS DRUGS IN CATEGORY

Related drugs in this class are **dichlorphenamide** (Daranide) and **methazolamide** (Neptazane). Methazolamide is a derivative of acetazolamide; both methazolamide and dichlorphenamide are used as adjunctive treatment of chronic simple glaucoma. Although diuretic effects can occur, these drugs are not used as diuretics. These related drugs have the same undesired clinical responses and contraindications as acetazolamide[17] (Table 36–5).

CONCEPT REVIEW

Both osmotic diuretics and carbonic anhydrase inhibitors act mainly at the proximal convoluted tubule.

The major use of osmotic diuretics is to increase urinary flow rate. These diuretics act by increasing osmotic force in tubular fluid.

Carbonic anhydrase inhibitors act by noncompetitive inhibition of renal carbonic anhydrase. When this enzyme is inhibited, there is a decrease in hydrogen ion to exchange for sodium, and less sodium enters the tubule. These drugs are weak diuretics.

SUMMARY

The kidneys are the primary organs that excrete water-soluble substances from the body, including products of metabolism, electrolytes, and foreign substances. They play an important part in maintaining the osmotic pressure of the blood and optimum concentrations of individual constituents of plasma and other body fluids.

Diuretics act in various sites to (1) increase glomerular filtration, (2) inhibit reabsorption of sodium and chloride by direct action on the tubules, and (3) inhibit reabsorption of sodium by an indirect mechanism. Nursing implications for clients receiving diuretic therapy include monitoring intake and output, daily weight, and status of edema. In addition, the nurse must assess carefully for indications of electrolyte and fluid volume imbalances and for drug interactions.

REFERENCES

1. Levine, S. (1989). Diuretics. *Medical Clinics of North America, 73,* 271-282.
2. Mende, C. (1990). Current issues in diuretic therapy. *Hospital Practice, 25*(Suppl. 1), 15-21.
3. Metheny, N. (1992). *Fluid and electrolyte balance: Nursing considerations* (2nd ed.). Philadelphia: J.B. Lippincott.
4. Mujais, S.K., Nora, N.A., & Levin, M.L. (1992). Principles and clinical uses of diuretic therapy. *Progress in Cardiovascular Diseases, 35,* 221-245.
5. Smith, C.M., & Reynard, A.M. (1992). *Textbook of pharmacology.* Philadelphia: W.B. Saunders.
6. Jarvis, C. (1992). *Physical examination and health assessment.* Philadelphia: W.B. Saunders.
7. Moser, M. (1992). Diuretics and cardiovascular risk factors. *European Heart Journal, 13*(Suppl. G), 72-80.
8. Kellick, K. (1992). Diuretics. *AACN—Clinical Issues in Critical Care Nursing, 3*(2), 472-482.
9. Mendyka, B. (1992). Fluid and electrolyte disorders caused by diuretic therapy. *AACN—Clinical Issues in Critical Care Nursing, 3*(3), 672-680.
10. U.S. Pharmacopeial Convention. (1990). *The United States pharmacopeia* (22nd rev.). Rockville, MD: Author.
11. Andersson, O.K., et al. (1991). Metabolic adverse effects of thiazide diuretics: The importance of normokalemia. *Journal of Internal Medicine, 91*(229) (Suppl. 2), 89-96.
12. MacLennan, W. (1989). Update: Diuretic therapy in the elderly. *Comprehensive Therapy, 15*(6), 19-24.
13. Tideiksaar, R. (1990). Principles of drug therapy in the elderly. *Physician Assistant, 14*(2), 29-30, 33-34, 45-46, 52.
14. Jacobson, H. (1987). Diuretics: Mechanisms of action and uses. *Hospital Practice,* (December), 129-156.
15. Ujhelyi, M. (1991). Loop diuretics: A practical guide to their use and selection. *Connecticut Medicine, 55*(3), 162-165.
16. Achhammer, I. (1991). Low dose loop diuretics in essential hypertension. Experience with torasemide. *Drugs, 41*(Suppl. 3), 80-91.
17. Kastrup, E.K. (Ed). (1993). *Facts and Comparisons.* St. Louis: J.B. Lippincott.
18. Mathewson, M. (1989). Drug interactions. *Critical Care Nurse, 9*(4), 84, 86-88, 90-93.
19. Brater, D. (1991). Clinical pharmacology of loop diuretics. *Drugs, 41*(Suppl. 3), 14-22.
20. Kruck, F. (1991). Acute and long term effects of loop diuretics in heart failure. *Drugs, 41*(Suppl. 3), 60-68.
21. Goodman, A., Gilman, G., Rall, T., Niles, A., & Taylor, P., (Eds.). (1990). *Goodman and Gilman's: The pharmacological basis of therapeutics* (8th ed.). New York: Pergamon Press.

BIBLIOGRAPHY

Aranda, P. (1990). Diuretics and the treatment of systemic hypertension. *American Journal of Cardiology, 65*(17), 72-76.
Cauley, J., et al. (1993). Effects of thiazide diuretic therapy on bone mass, fractures, and falls. *Annals of Internal Medicine, 118,* 666-673.
Clarke, R. (1991). Indapamide: A diuretic of choice for the treatment of hypertension. *American Journal of the Medical Sciences, 301,* 215-220.
Di Somma, S., Liquori, V., Petitto, M., et al. (1990). Hemodynamic interactions between diuretics and calcium antagonists in the treatment of hypertensive patients. *Cardiovascular Drug Therapy, 4,* 1151-1156.
Ellison, D. (1991). The physiologic basis of diuretic synergism: Its role in treating diuretic resistance. *Annals of Internal Medicine, 114,* 886-894.
Evans, J. (1990). Diuretics for elderly patients. *Journal of Hypertension—Supplement, 8*(2), S33-S37.
Freis, E. (1990). The cardiotoxicity of thiazide diuretics: Review of the evidence. *Journal of Hypertension—Supplement, 8*(2), S23-S32.
Moser, M. (1990). Controversies in the management of hypertension: Diuretic use in the 1990s. *Physician Assistant, 14*(5), 85-88.
Nicholls, M.G. (1990). Interaction of diuretics and electrolytes in congestive heart failure. *American Journal of Cardiology, 65*(10), 17E-21E.
Wittner, M., Di Stefano, A., Wangemann, P., & Greger, R. (1991). How do loop diuretics act? *Drugs, 41*(Suppl. 3), 1-13.

Hyperuricemic Drugs

KAREN C. JOHNSON-BRENNAN

⊛ **Uric Acid Synthesis**
LEARNING OBJECTIVE: Describe the synthesis of uric acid.
KEY TERM: Purine

⊛ **Renal Excretion of Uric Acid**
LEARNING OBJECTIVE: Identify the renal processes involved in the excretion of uric acid.
KEY TERM: Urate

⊛ **Hyperuricemia**
LEARNING OBJECTIVE: Differentiate between primary and secondary hyperuricemia and gout.
KEY TERMS:
Gout, hyperuricemia

⊛ **Progression of Hyperuricemia**
LEARNING OBJECTIVE: Summarize the progression of hyperuricemia through the three clinical stages.
KEY TERMS:
Acute gout, asymptomatic hyperuricemia, tophaceous gout, tophi

⊛ **Hyperuricemic Drugs**
LEARNING OBJECTIVE: Identify the three categories of drugs used to treat hyperuricemia.

⊛ **General Nursing Considerations**
LEARNING OBJECTIVE: Plan care for the client receiving hyperuricemic drugs.

⊛ **Uricosuric Drugs**
LEARNING OBJECTIVES:
Summarize essential information about the prototype drug probenecid.
Explain the rationale for increasing fluid intake for the client receiving a uricosuric drug.

⊛ **Uric Acid Synthesis Inhibitor**
LEARNING OBJECTIVE: Summarize essential information about the prototype drug allopurinol.

⊛ **Drugs that Terminate the Inflammatory Response**
LEARNING OBJECTIVES:
Provide the rationale for terminating the inflammatory response in an individual in an acute gout episode.
Summarize essential information about the prototype drug colchicine.

CONCEPTS AND TERMS TO REVIEW

Review the physiology of the renal system.
Reexamine the physiologic processes of filtration, reabsorption, and secretion.
Review renal handling of uric acid.

The condition hyperuricemia, elevation of serum uric acid, is usually chronic, with periods of acute episodes. Treatment involves drug and nondrug measures. This chapter discusses the three groups of drugs used to lower serum uric acid levels. This information provides a basis for providing nursing care for the client receiving treatment with hyperuricemic drugs.

URIC ACID SYNTHESIS

Breakdown of DNA, RNA, and adenosine triphosphate (ATP) provides a constant source of the metabolite **purine.** At a cellular level, purines are synthesized to purine nucleotides. These nucleotides are used in the synthesis of nucleic acids, ATP, cyclic adenosine monophosphate (cAMP), and cyclic guanosine monophosphate. Uric acid is a breakdown product of purine nucleotides. Synthesis of uric acid, which occurs in the liver, is triggered by the action of xanthine oxidase. The average individual produces approximately 600 to 700 mg of uric acid per day.[1-3]

RENAL EXCRETION OF URIC ACID

Uric acid circulates in the bloodstream in the form of a uric acid salt, **urate.** The major organs for the excretion of urate are the kidneys. Two thirds of uric acid salt cleared from the blood appears in urine; the remaining third appears in intestinal secretions. Plasma protein binding of uric acid is less than 10%. The remainder is filtered freely at the glomerulus.[3] With a glomerular filtration rate of 125 ml per minute, 3.8 mEq per minute of uric acid is filtered.[1] Uric acid undergoes both absorption by an organic anion transport mechanism and excretion within the renal tubules.

HYPERURICEMIA

Hyperuricemia is an excess of uric acid in the blood. **Gout** is the disease process that results from hyperuricemia. Hyperuricemia and gout are classified as either primary or secondary. **Primary hyperuricemia** or **gout** is the result of an endogenous metabolic disorder that causes overproduction of uric acid. Some studies suggest that it is caused by a genetic error. For example, the genetic disorder **Lesch-Nyhan syndrome** involves purine metabolism and is transmitted as an X-linked recessive trait. As a consequence of improper purine metabolism, extreme hyperuricemia occurs, resulting in physical and mental retardation, compulsive self-mutilation, choreoathetosis, and impaired renal function. Studies also suggest that primary gout may be a multifactorial inherited disease.[4]

Several factors produce **secondary hyperuricemia** or **gout,** which is more common than the primary condition. Diseases such as leukemias and other malignancies in which nucleic acid breakdown is increased lead to hyperuricemia. In addition, diseases such as renal failure or dysfunction may cause impaired renal excretion of uric acid. Hyperuricemia may also develop during starvation diets or as an undesired clinical response to some drugs such as thiazide and loop diuretics and cytotoxic agents.[4–7]

PROGRESSION OF HYPERURICEMIA

There are three clinical stages in hyperuricemia: asymptomatic hyperuricemia, acute gout or acute gouty arthritis, and tophaceous gout or chronic tophaceous gouty arthritis.

Asymptomatic Hyperuricemia

During **asymptomatic hyperuricemia** the serum uric acid level is elevated but an inflammatory response, arthritic symptoms, tophi, and renal stones are not present. The client may remain asymptomatic throughout life.

Acute Gout

Although the serum uric acid range is only slightly higher in men than in women, men have an increased incidence of **acute gout.** Obesity is also implicated in the incidence of gout. The typical client with gout is an obese, middle-aged male who may have cardiovascular risk factors such as hypertension, hyperlipidemia, or atherosclerosis.

A sudden increase of hyperuricemia usually triggers an acute episode. However, in susceptible individuals trauma, drugs, and alcohol can also initiate an attack. As uric acid reaches a certain concentration, it crystallizes, forming insoluble precipitates that are deposited in connective tissues throughout the body. The body treats these crystal deposits as foreign material and activates the inflammatory response. Leukocytes travel to the area, engulf the crystals, and release a variety of inflammatory substances, some of which are acidic. The resulting regional drop in pH enhances formation of additional uric acid crystals.

Pain is the primary symptom of this response. A few hours after the onset of pain, the affected joint becomes hot, red, and extremely tender. Slight swelling may also occur. Common sites are the base of the great toe, heel, ankle, instep of the foot, knee, wrist, or elbow.

Because the pain is so intense during an acute attack, most clients seek medical attention. However, even without treatment the inflammatory response may subside. During the acute episode the serum uric acid level may be normal or only slightly elevated because uric acid has precipitated into the joint as crystals. Consequently, a positive diagnosis of gout is based on finding uric acid crystals in a sample of joint fluid, not on the serum uric acid level.[2,4,8]

Tophaceous Gout

Tophaceous gout is the third clinical stage. This stage of the disease can begin as early as 2 years or as late as 35 years after an initial acute attack. Progressive and prolonged elevated uric acid serum levels eventually cause urate crystal deposits **(tophi)** in cartilage, synovial membranes, tendons, and soft tissue. Each tophus consists of a deposit of urate crystals and a mass of mononuclear phagocytes.

Large crystal deposits form under the skin, producing visible nodules. Crystals can form in the blood vessels, impairing blood flow. Depending on the extent of damage, the impaired blood flow can lead to coronary artery disease, renal ischemia, and renal failure. Crystals may also form in the urine, especially if urinary output is low. Although these crystals are not especially painful, they can accumulate and produce renal stones (calculi), causing obstruction, dilation, and atrophy of the proximal tubules. Crystals that form in joints produce a corrosive action that eventually destroys the surface of the joint. As a result, chronic gouty arthritis develops, with inflammation, joint deformity, and decreased joint mobility.[2–4]

HYPERURICEMIC DRUGS

Major drug categories used in the treatment and prevention of hyperuricemia and gout are uricosurics, uric acid synthesis inhibitors, and drugs that terminate the inflammatory response. There is one major drug used to inhibit the production of uric acid: allopurinol. Uricosuric drugs (e.g., probenecid) promote urinary excretion of uric acid by blocking its reabsorption from the proximal tubule. Colchicine is the drug of choice to treat the inflammatory process that accompanies acute gout. Because it reduces inflammation, colchicine also alleviates pain and enhances joint mobility.[8,9]

CONCEPT REVIEW

Hyperuricemia develops if uric acid excretion is diminished or uric acid synthesis is increased. Clinical stages of this disorder are asymptomatic hyperuricemia, acute gout, and tophaceous gout.

With asymptomatic hyperuricemia, the serum uric acid level is elevated, but signs and symptoms are not apparent. Acute gout is the result of uric acid crystal deposits in joints. In a client with chronic tophaceous gout urate deposits are in a variety of tissues, producing deformities and limiting mobility.

Three main categories of drugs are used to treat hyperuricemia and gout: uricosuric drugs, uric acid synthesis inhibitors, and drugs that terminate the inflammatory response.

⌨ NURSING CONSIDERATIONS

Usually the nurse is not in contact with the client diagnosed with hyperuricemia. However, the client with acute gout may be hospitalized during attacks. In addition, the client with tophaceous gout may require hospitalization and home care for treatment of complications associated with the disease.

Assessing Obtain a complete **health history** that includes previous and currently existing health problems. Since diets high in purines can elevate serum uric acid levels, question the client about dietary patterns. Collect a drug history to determine if the client is receiving prescription drugs such as thiazide diuretics or cytotoxic agents. Ask about over-the-counter (OTC) drug use since some OTC drugs (e.g., salicylate and salicylate-containing drugs) can precipitate or aggravate an attack of gout. Ask the client to describe recent stressors since an acute attack can be precipitated by illness, trauma, or strenuous exercise. Question the client about previous episodes. Determine if there is a history of gouty arthritis in the family. Query the client about any recent weight gain.

Before the **physical assessment** collect a thorough pain assessment. The client's pain may be so excruciating that palpation of the affected extremity or assessment of joint mobility is not possible. Asking the client to describe the level of pain on a scale of 1 to 10 is helpful. Look for nonverbal clues of pain such as rigid body posturing or facial grimacing to provide additional assessment data.

Weigh the client since overweight and obesity are common in clients with gout. Do not estimate the client's weight or ask the client for an estimation. Assess the general fluid status of the client by inspecting mucous membranes, checking skin turgor, and observing and palpating for the presence or absence of edema.

Inspect the affected extremity for appearance of the involved joint(s) and for evidence of soft-tissue deposits. Nodular swelling may be visible in the subcutaneous tissues overlying the joints. The joint may be red. In addition, a low-grade fever is usually present. Review the results of diagnostic tests such as serum uric acid level, sedimentation rate, and 24-hour urinary uric acid level.

Diagnosing Analyze the data base and formulate appropriate nursing diagnoses. Diagnoses appropriate for the client receiving hyperuricemic drugs include the following:

- Pain related to joint inflammation and swelling.
- Impaired physical mobility related to painful joint(s).
- Activity intolerance related to pain.
- Diarrhea related to effects of antigout drugs.
- High risk for fluid volume deficit related to diarrheal effects of antigout drugs.
- Noncompliance of drug therapy related to drug side effects.
- Knowledge deficit regarding drug and dietary restrictions.
- Ineffective individual coping related to acute or chronic illness.

Planning Treatment is directed at relieving the pain and symptoms of the acute attack and lowering the serum uric acid level so that future attacks are prevented or modified. Long-term treatment goals include prevention of joint deformity, immobility, and systemic damage caused by tophaceous gout.

Client teaching is always an important nursing intervention. Develop a teaching plan that provides information about the disease, treatment measures, and health promotion methods. Instruct the client about the nature of the disease. Describe prescribed treatment measures. Include such information on drug therapy as action of drugs, anticipated response to therapy, and possible undesired clinical responses associated with drug therapy.

Dietary restrictions of purines are not prescribed for all clients. Before providing instructions to the client, discuss this topic with the primary care provider. If dietary restriction of purines is prescribed, provide the client with a list of high-purine foods such as organ meats (e.g., brains, liver, and sweetbreads). (See the box for a list of high-purine foods.)

Health promotion measures include avoidance of alcohol and salicylates and maintenance of adequate fluid intake. Alcohol causes direct cellular toxic effects that increase serum uric acid levels. Alcohol can also predispose the client to dehydration because of its inhibitory effect on antidiuretic hormone (ADH). In general, salicylates antagonize the effects of uricosuric drugs and therefore should be avoided. Provide the client or caregiver with a list of prescription and OTC drugs that contain salicylates. Dehydration is also a problem. It aggravates the client's condition and may precipitate formation

---

HIGH-PURINE FOODS

Anchovies	Liver
Bouillon	Mussels
Broth	Sardines
Gravies	Scallops
Heart	Sweetbreads
Kidney	Yeast

of renal calculi. Advise the client to ingest at least 2 to 3 L of fluid per day and to pay special attention to fluid intake during periods of exercise or hot weather and when receiving uricosuric drugs. Since an acid urinary pH may also promote formation of renal calculi, advise the client to avoid drinking vitamin C preparations or juices such as cranberry juice that may acidify the urine.

Since obesity is a factor in the incidence of hyperuricemia, a weight loss program is advisable. Arrange for a dietary consultation if necessary. Stress the need for lifelong monitoring and drug therapy.

Expected outcomes are based on the nursing diagnoses and the plan of care. Appropriate outcomes include the following:
- Client reports that pain is relieved or controlled.
- Client demonstrates behaviors that enable resumption of activities.
- Client reports an increase in activity tolerance.
- Client reestablishes normal pattern of bowel functioning.
- Client verbalizes understanding of factors causing fluid volume deficit.
- Client participates in the development of the treatment plan.
- Client identifies ineffective coping behaviors.

Implementing Nursing actions that assist in pain relief are very important in caring for clients with gout. Administer analgesics (other than those containing salicylates) in a timely fashion. Administer antigout drugs with meals or with milk to reduce possible side effects of gastric distress.

Usually the affected extremity is elevated, and cold compresses are applied to reduce pain and swelling of the affected joint(s). As the client's level of pain permits, instruct and assist the client with passive and active range of motion exercises. Monitor the client's fluid status by checking blood pressure, intake and output, and daily weight. Assess the client for symptoms of flank pain or darkened or bloody urine that could indicate renal stone formation.

Evaluating Evaluation is based on the expected client outcomes. Relief of pain is evidenced by client report and by a relaxed body posture and increased joint mobility. The affected area should appear less swollen and inflamed. A stable fluid status is evidenced by consistent body weight, adequate skin turgor, and moist mucous membranes. Expect a reduction in serum uric acid levels (see box). Additionally, the client should describe the rationale for drug therapy and identify drugs and foods to avoid.

CONCEPT REVIEW

The nurse's role in the care of the client with acute or tophaceous gout focuses on relief of pain, prevention of complications, and client education.

Teach the client the importance of avoiding alcohol and drugs containing salicylates. In addition, stress the importance of adequate (2 to 3 L per day) fluid intake.

URICOSURIC DRUGS

Uricosuric drugs act to enhance renal excretion of uric acid by blocking tubular reabsorption of urate. The prototype is probenecid (Benemid) and a related drug is sulfinpyrazone (Anturane). The primary use of these drugs is management of chronic hyperuricemia. Uricosuric drugs do not have anti-inflammatory or analgesic properties and thus are of no use in the treatment of acute gouty attacks.[11]

URICOSURIC PROTOTYPE
PROBENECID

Probenecid (Benemid) was initially developed as an agent to inhibit renal tubular secretion of penicillin, thereby increasing serum plasma level of penicillin two to four times. It still is used to augment penicillin and cephalosporin therapy.

Pharmacotherapeutics As mentioned previously, uricosurics are of no value in the symptomatic treatment of acute gout. In fact, it may take several months of uricosuric therapy before serum uric acid levels decrease to a level sufficient to reduce symptoms of chronic gouty arthritis or frequent gout attacks. Therefore therapy with probenecid begins once the acute phase has been suppressed with an anti-inflammatory drug.

In some instances serum uric acid levels increase during initiation of probenecid therapy. Initial low blood levels or subtherapeutic levels may favor displacement of tissue stores of uric acid into the blood. There may even be mobilization of uric acid deposits from existing tophi. If an acute attack occurs while the client is taking probenecid, the drug should be continued and an anti-inflammatory drug added. Abrupt discontinuance of probenecid would cause a drastic increase in serum uric acid levels and aggravation of symptoms. For some clients a fixed-dose combination drug of probenecid and colchicine (ColBenemid) is available and can be started once the acute attack has been suppressed.[12]

Pharmacokinetics Probenecid is rapidly absorbed after oral administration and reaches peak plasma levels in 2 to 4 hours. Probenecid is transported in the blood mainly bound to plasma proteins. The free fraction of the drug is filtered at the glomerulus and is reabsorbed in the proximal tubule by an organic anion transport mecha-

---

URIC ACID SERUM AND URINE LEVELS
Uric Acid Serum Levels
Adult female: 2.4-6.0 mg/dl
Adult male: 3.4-7.0 mg/dl
Children: 2.5-5.5 mg/dl
Uric Acid Urinary Levels
Adult female: 250-750 mg/24 h
Adult male: 250-800 mg/24 h

Data from Chernecky, C., Krech, R., Berger, B. (1993).[10]

nism. Probenecid has a relatively short half-life of 6 to 12 hours.[12,13]

Pharmacodynamics Probenecid is a uricosuric and renal tubular blocking agent. It inhibits tubular reabsorption of urate, thus increasing the urinary excretion of uric acid and decreasing serum urate levels. Uric acid is both secreted and reabsorbed in the proximal tubule by the same organic anion transport mechanism that reabsorbs probenecid. Probenecid competes with uric acid for reabsorption, thus enhancing renal excretion of uric acid. Normal therapeutic doses of probenecid can nearly double urate excretion in clients with gout. Even higher levels of urate excretion can be achieved with high-dose probenecid therapy.[12]

Pharmaceutics Probenecid is administered orally and is available as 500-mg tablets. It is also available in fixed combination with colchicine (500 mg and 0.5 mg, respectively) as ColBenemid, Colabid, or Proben-C for treatment of chronic gouty arthritis or frequently recurring acute attacks.

Undesired Clinical Responses Probenecid is usually well tolerated with few undesired clinical responses. Some clients have reported gastrointestinal (GI) problems such as nausea, vomiting, diarrhea, constipation, and abdominal distress. Presence of a fever or rash may indicate a hypersensitivity reaction and the possibility of future anaphylactic reactions. (See Fig. 37–1 for a summary of undesired clinical responses associated with probenecid.)

Contraindications and Precautions Probenecid should not be administered to someone with a known hypersensitivity to the drug. Because probenecid can increase the risk of uric acid stone formation, it should be administered cautiously in clients with poor renal function or with a history of renal stones. It should also be used with caution in clients with known peptic ulcer disease.

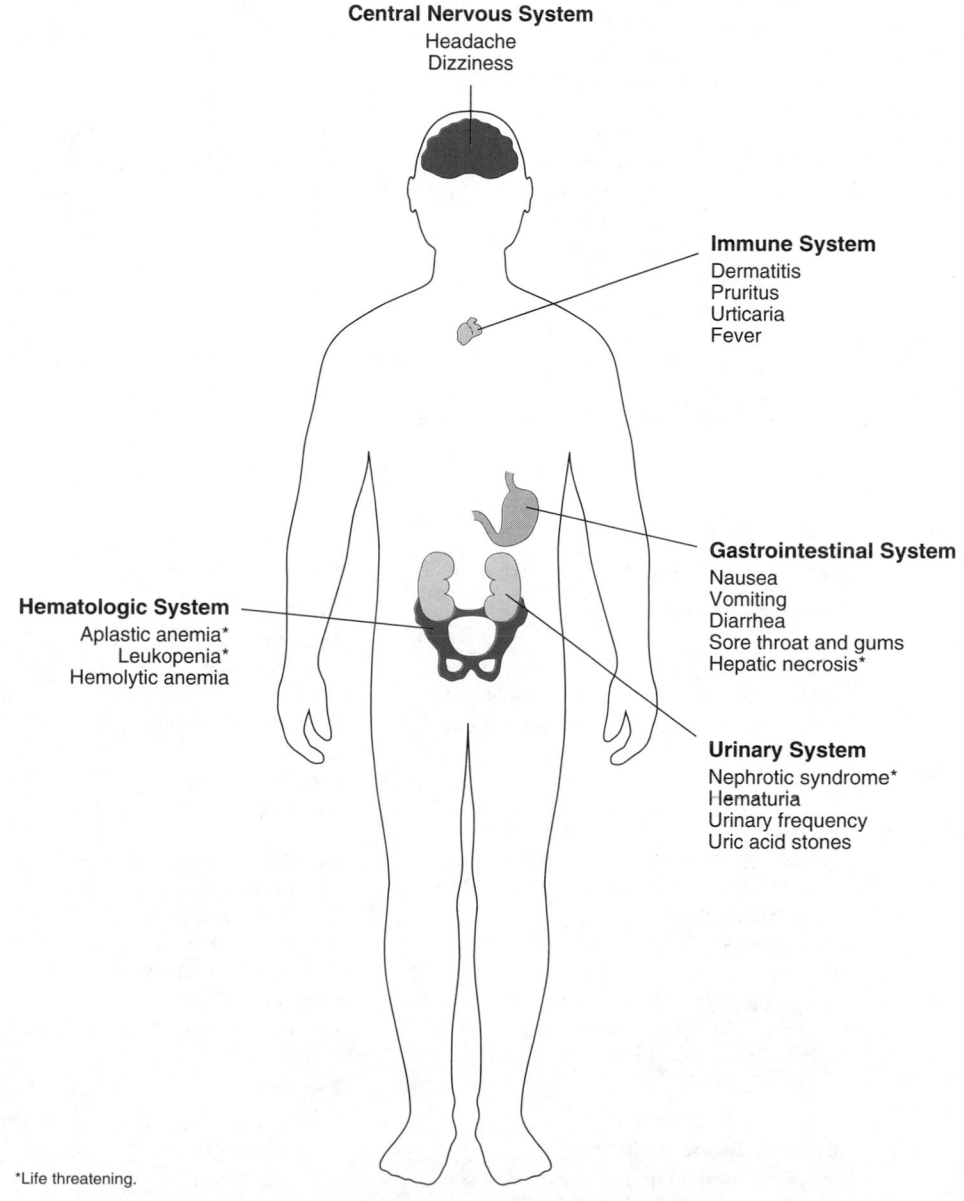

Central Nervous System
Headache
Dizziness

Immune System
Dermatitis
Pruritus
Urticaria
Fever

Gastrointestinal System
Nausea
Vomiting
Diarrhea
Sore throat and gums
Hepatic necrosis*

Hematologic System
Aplastic anemia*
Leukopenia*
Hemolytic anemia

Urinary System
Nephrotic syndrome*
Hematuria
Urinary frequency
Uric acid stones

*Life threatening.

FIGURE 37–1   Undesired clinical responses associated with probenecid.

Drug-Drug, Drug-Nutrient, Drug-Environment Interactions Salicylates and thiazide diuretics antagonize the action of uricosurics. Probenecid potentiates the action of penicillin and cephalosporin antibiotics and is sometimes used as adjunctive therapy in severe cases of infection. Additionally, probenecid potentiates the action of sulfonylurea-type oral hypoglycemic agents. Diabetics who require uricosuric therapy may require dosage adjustment in one or both drugs. Probenecid inhibits elimination of methotrexate and can cause methotrexate toxicity.

High-purine foods, alcohol, and caffeine should be avoided. These substances can increase uric acid levels in the blood. Foods such as vitamin C and cranberry juice should also be avoided. These liquids acidify the urine and increase the risk of renal calculi formation. The client should increase fluid intake during hot weather to prevent dehydration.[12,13]

Life-Span Considerations Probenecid is not recommended for children less than 2 years of age. When administered to older children, it is used as an adjunct to antibiotic therapy. Probenecid crosses the placental barrier; therefore both maternal and fetal risks must be considered. Its use is discouraged in nursing mothers. As with most drugs, probenecid therapy should be monitored carefully in the older population. Those with renal impairment are at increased risk for the development of uric acid stones.

Specific Drug-Related Nursing Considerations Encourage the client to drink sufficient fluids to maintain a urinary output of at least 2 L per day. Anticipate that drugs such as sodium bicarbonate or potassium citrate may be prescribed to alkalinize the urine. This increases the excretion of probenecid and decreases the risk of urinary stone formation. Urinary alkalinizers also act to increase the solubility of uric acid in the urine. However, these drugs must be used with caution. Sodium bicarbonate may aggravate symptoms of hypertension or congestive heart failure in the client with cardiac dysfunction. Potassium citrate increases the risk of hyperkalemia.

Monitor the diabetic client carefully for symptoms of hypoglycemia. Finger-stick serum glucose testing is preferred over urinary glucose monitoring since probenecid may cause false-positive readings with some tests (e.g., Clinitest) but not others (e.g., Clinistix, Diastix, Testape).

MISCELLANEOUS DRUGS IN CATEGORY

Sulfinpyrazone (Anturane) is an active metabolite of the anti-inflammatory drug phenylbutazone. It has the same mechanism of action and characteristics as probenecid, but it is longer acting and more potent. Sulfinpyrazone has mild anti-inflammatory action and is not intended for relief of acute attacks. It is indicated for chronic gouty arthritis or intermittent gouty arthritis. Sulfinpyrazone has become available as an inhibitor of platelet aggregation in the prophylactic treatment of myocardial infarct.[13]

The drug is rapidly absorbed after oral administration, and effects may be noted within 30 to 60 minutes. Duration of action is 4 to 8 hours. Sulfinpyrazone is highly protein bound and is excreted in the urine almost totally unchanged.

Sulfinpyrazone shares similar nursing considerations with probenecid. However, it is more likely to cause gastric distress. Therefore instruct clients to take the drug with milk or meals. Since sulfinpyrazone does inhibit platelet aggregation, monitor for evidence of bleeding such as hematuria, bleeding gums, or easy bruising. Serious bleeding may occur if the client is also receiving an anticoagulant drug such as warfarin sulfate.

TABLE 37–1
Uricosuric Drugs: Prototype and Related Drug

Drug	Dosage and Route of Administration	Nursing Considerations
PROBENECID (Benemid) HOW SUPPLIED Coated tablet: 500 mg Uncoated tablet: 0.5 g	***Chronic Hyperuricemia*** ADULTS Initially 0.25 g bid for 1 wk; then 0.5 g bid; maximum dose 2 g/d in four divided doses ***Adjunctive Therapy with Penicillin or Cephalosporin*** ADULTS 1 g bid or 500 mg qid CHILDREN Initially 25 mg/kg/d; then 40 mg/kg/d in four divided doses; children over 50 kg may receive adult dose ***Gonorrhea*** ADULTS 3.5 g ampicillin PO with 1 g probenecid *or* 1 g probenecid PO 30 min before IM injection of 4.8 million U aqueous penicillin G procaine	***Assess*** Assess for indications of acute symptoms; drug is not recommended until acute attack has subsided. Determine if client has preexisting renal dysfunction. ***Implement*** Administer with food or milk to decrease GI distress. Encourage compliance and provide ongoing support since therapy is usually lifelong. Encourage fluid intake of 2 to 3 L/d. Instruct client to avoid vitamin C and cranberry juice, which can acidify urine. ***Monitor*** Monitor urinary pH with nitrazine paper. Monitor intake and output. ***Evaluate*** Evaluate serum and urinary uric acid levels.
Sulfinpyrazone (Anturane) HOW SUPPLIED Capsules: 200 mg Uncoated tablets: 100 mg	***Chronic Gouty Arthritis*** Initially 200-400 mg/d in two divided doses; maintenance 400 mg daily in two divided doses	Same as probenecid

Salicylates are contraindicated because they interfere with the uricosuric effect of sulfinpyrazone and inhibit platelet aggregation.

Sulfinpyrazone is available as 100- or 200-mg capsules. The initial dose is 200 to 400 mg daily in two divided doses. This dosage may be gradually increased to a full maintenance dose (400 mg in two divided doses) in 1 week. If an acute attack of gout occurs during initiation of therapy, colchicine or another anti-inflammatory drug should be added.[13] Table 37–1 summarizes information about uricosuric drugs.

Benzbromarone is a relatively new uricosuric drug. It has greater potency than sulfinpyrazone and is particularly effective in clients with renal dysfunction.

CONCEPT REVIEW

Uricosuric drugs inhibit uric acid reabsorption.
Probenecid is the most widely used uricosuric. However, sulfinpyrazone is longer acting, and benzbromarone has greater potency.
Clients receiving uricosuric drugs must maintain a high fluid intake.

URIC ACID SYNTHESIS INHIBITOR

A uric acid synthesis inhibitor is used for long-term treatment of hyperuricemia. By reducing the circulating pool of uric acid, the frequency of gouty attacks is reduced.

URIC ACID SYNTHESIS INHIBITOR PROTOTYPE

ALLOPURINOL

Allopurinol (Zyloprim) is the only major drug used to inhibit the production of uric acid.

Pharmacotherapeutics As with uricosuric drugs, allopurinol is not used to treat acute gout attacks. Allopurinol is used to prevent attacks in individuals with hyperuricemia. It is the drug of choice for hyperuricemic clients with renal insufficiency or calculi. Allopurinol is also used prophylactically in clients with leukemia and other forms of cancer. As indicated previously, these clients are at risk of hyperuricemia caused by the increased production and turnover of white blood cells. In addition, allopurinol prevents tophi formation or uric acid nephropathy associated with radiation or chemotherapy.

Allopurinol is effective in clients refractory to uricosurics or with an intolerance to uricosuric therapy. When administered in conjunction with uricosuric drugs, smaller doses of each drug may be used. Allopurinol is also effective in lowering uric acid levels in clients receiving thiazide diuretics.

Allopurinol may increase acute gouty attacks during initiation of therapy because of mobilization of uric acid from existing tophi. Therefore concurrent therapy with an anti-inflammatory drug is warranted. Urinary alkalinization and optimal fluid intake during this time help maximize drug effectiveness and decrease the risk of urinary tract stone formation.[4,14,15]

Pharmacokinetics Allopurinol is well absorbed but not strongly bound to plasma proteins. Its half-life (2 to 3 hours) is shorter than the half-life of its active metabolite, oxypurinol (18 to 20 hours). Allopurinol is distributed extensively in the body except for the central nervous system; it is eliminated mainly by metabolism. A small amount of unchanged drug may be excreted in the feces and in the urine.[3]

Pharmacodynamics Allopurinol is a competitive inhibitor of xanthine oxidase. It decreases the serum level of uric acid and increases the serum level of the xanthine oxidase precursors, hypoxanthine and xanthine. Allopurinol is metabolized by xanthine oxidase to oxypurinol, an active metabolite. Treatment with allopurinol results in a decrease in the plasma level of uric acid and its urinary excretion. Because of the xanthine oxidase inhibition, serum levels of hypoxanthine and xanthine increase, as does the urinary excretion of these substances.[3,14]

Pharmaceutics Allopurinol is administered orally. It is available in 100- and 300-mg tablets.

Undesired Clinical Responses Undesired clinical responses to allopurinol are somewhat more severe than to uricosuric drugs. The most common undesired response is a skin rash. Skin reactions can be severe and at times fatal; therefore allopurinol should be discontinued at the first sign of a rash. Concurrent use of certain antibiotics such as ampicillin increases the risk of skin eruptions. Other common undesired responses include diarrhea, nausea, increased serum alkaline phosphatase, and increased aspartate aminotransferase (AST; SGOT) and alanine aminotransferase (ALT; SGPT). In addition, cataract formation, bone marrow suppression, and drowsiness have been reported.

As noted previously, the incidence of acute gout attacks may increase during initiation of allopurinol therapy. Initiating therapy in low doses and gradually increasing the dosage are helpful steps in modifying this untoward response. In addition, maintenance doses of an anti-inflammatory drug reduce the incidence of acute gout.[12,13]

Contraindications and Precautions Clients who have developed a severe hypersensitivity reaction to allopurinol should not be restarted on the drug. The drug is used with caution in clients with preexisting hepatic or renal dysfunction.

Drug-Drug, Drug-Nutrient, Drug-Environment Interactions The most important drug-drug interactions with allopurinol therapy occurs with the concurrent administration of mercaptopurine and azathioprine. The oxidation of these drugs is inhibited by allopurinol, and it may be necessary to reduce their doses by as much as 75%. Allopurinol may also potentiate the effects of drugs such as oral anticoagulants, oral hypoglycemics, phenytoin, and theophylline by inhibiting their hepatic metabolism. In addition, urinary acidifying drugs such as sodium phosphate, potassium phosphate, vitamin C, and ammonium chloride may increase the potential for renal calculi formation.[3,12]

Drug-nutrient and drug-environment interactions are also possible. Allopurinol may increase iron absorption and hepatic iron stores. Additionally, ultraviolet rays may increase the risk of cataracts.

Life-Span Considerations Allopurinol is used with caution in pregnant or nursing mothers. It is classified as a Pregnancy Category C drug. Allopurinol is rarely indi-

TABLE 37–2
Uric Acid Synthesis Inhibitor

Drug	Dosage and Route of Administration	Nursing Considerations
ALLOPURINOL (Lopurin, Zyloprim) HOW SUPPLIED Uncoated tablet: 100 and 300 mg	***Chronic Management of Gout*** 100-300 mg/d for mild cases; 300-600 mg/d in divided doses for more severe cases ***Prevention of Drug-induced Hyperuricemia*** Usually 300 mg/d ***Adjunct Therapy with Chemotherapeutic Drugs*** ADULTS 600-800 mg/d in two divided doses; after 2 to 3 d dosage may be reduced to 100-300 mg/d CHILDREN 6-10 years of age: 150-300 mg/d; <6 y of age: 150 mg/d	***Assess*** Assess for indications of acute symptoms. Determine if client has preexisting renal dysfunction. ***Implement*** Administer after meals. Caution client to discontinue drug and to consult care provider if skin rash occurs. Encourage fluid intake of 2 to 3 L/d. Instruct client not to double dose if one dose is missed. Advise client to have periodic eye examinations. Caution against driving or using heavy machinery if drowsiness occurs. Advise client to avoid ultraviolet exposure, which may increase risk of cataracts. ***Monitor*** Monitor BUN and creatinine levels. Monitor intake and output. ***Evaluate*** Evaluate serum and urinary uric acid levels.

cated for use in children except those with secondary hyperuricemia from malignancy. As with most drugs, it may be necessary to modify the dosage in the elderly because of renal, hepatic, or other disease states.[12,13]

Specific Drug-Related Nursing Considerations Review with the client possible undesired clinical responses and actions to take. Instruct the client to observe for evidence of skin eruptions such as a maculopapular rash. If any skin reaction or pruritus is noted, tell the client to discontinue the drug immediately and contact the primary care provider. Since cataract formation can occur as a result of ultraviolet rays, advise the client to have periodic eye examinations and to avoid ultraviolet exposure. Caution the client against driving or using heavy machinery if drowsiness occurs.

Optimizing fluid intake in these clients places them at increased risk for the development of fluid overload. Carefully monitor fluid status. Report any change in urinary output or change in color or odor of urine. Monitor serum blood urea nitrogen (BUN) levels and creatinine results. Table 37–2 summarizes information about allopurinol.

CONCEPT REVIEW

Allopurinol is the major uric acid synthesis inhibitor. It inhibits xanthine oxidase, thus decreasing plasma uric acid and increasing plasma hypoxanthine and xanthine.

Treatment with allopurinol should not be started until the acute gout attack has subsided.

DRUGS THAT TERMINATE THE INFLAMMATORY RESPONSE

Drugs used to treat the inflammation associated with acute gout are administered during the attack and are used prophylactically to prevent or modify future attacks. Colchicine and indomethacin are the major anti-inflammatory drugs used in the treatment of gout.

ANTI-INFLAMMATORY PROTOTYPE
COLCHICINE

Colchicine is the prototype anti-inflammatory drug for gout. It was first introduced in the therapy of gout in 1763 by Von Stoorck. Benjamin Franklin, who suffered from gout, is credited with its introduction into the United States.

Pharmacotherapeutics Colchicine is extremely effective in the treatment of acute gouty arthritis, relieving symptoms in approximately 95% of cases. In fact, since it is not effective as an anti-inflammatory agent in the absence of gout, it has been used to confirm the diagnosis of gout.[16,17]

Pharmacokinetics Colchicine is rapidly absorbed, and peak plasma concentrations occur within $\frac{1}{2}$ to 2 hours after oral administration. The drug is partially metabolized in the liver. Both its metabolites and the unchanged drug enter the GI tract via bile and intestinal secretions. Colchicine is excreted mainly in the feces, with 10% to 20% excreted in the urine. It has an extended presence in the body, giving rise to potential cumulative toxicity. The activity of colchicine is enhanced by alkalinizing agents and is inhibited by acidifying agents.[13,16,17]

Pharmacodynamics Colchicine is an alkaloid obtained from *Colchicum autumnale* (autumn crocus). Although its exact anti-inflammatory mechanism is not known, it is believed that colchicine exerts its pain-relieving effects by inhibiting leukocyte migration into the involved area. This impairs phagocytic breakdown of white blood cell membranes and subsequent release of tissue-damaging enzymes that cause inflammation. Additionally, the synthesis and release of acid metabolites by leukocytes is prevented, retarding further uric acid deposition in the affected joint.[2,4,15] Pain, swelling, and redness are relieved within 12 hours, and most clients are symptom free within 48 to 72 hours after oral administration.

Pharmaceutics Colchicine may be administered orally or intravenously; however, the oral route is preferred. It is not administered intramuscularly or subcutaneously because it causes severe tissue irritation. Additionally, IV solutions are administered cautiously because extravasation can cause severe pain and tissue necrosis.

To avoid possible cumulative effects, a course of therapy is usually not repeated within 3 days. With IV administration the chance of toxicity is even greater. Any IV order lasting more than 24 hours or exceeding the recommended daily limit of 4 mg per day should be questioned.

Undesired Clinical Responses Some drugs affect cells that are rapidly proliferating. With colchicine, the GI tract is particularly affected. In fact, 80% of the clients receiving colchicine experience GI reactions (e.g., nausea, vomiting, diarrhea, abdominal pain). Some clients learn to titrate doses of colchicine based on GI response. Because of its similarity to drugs used in chemotherapy, colchicine may also cause alopecia, agranulocytosis, and bone marrow suppression with aplastic anemia.

Contraindications and Precautions Because colchicine is a known GI irritant, it is contraindicated in clients with peptic ulcer or inflammatory bowel disease. It is also contraindicated in clients with serious renal or cardiac disorders.

Drug-Drug, Drug-Nutrient, Drug-Environment Interactions Colchicine may potentiate the effect of narcotics, sedatives, antidepressants, or antihistamines, producing oversedation. In addition, colchicine can cause vitamin B_{12} malabsorption. The drug should be stored in a tightly closed, light-resistant container.

Life-Span Considerations Colchicine crosses the placental barrier and may cause fetal malformations or death. It is not known whether it is excreted in breast milk. The safety and efficacy of colchicine in children have not been established. It should be used with caution in the elderly, especially those with known cardiac or renal disorders. Doses are generally decreased in the elderly.

Specific Drug-Related Nursing Considerations Colchicine is most effective when given at the first sign of an acute attack of gout. Encourage the client to carry a supply of the drug at all times and instruct him or her to begin the prescribed dose at the first indication of an acute attack. The initial dose is one or two 0.6-mg tablets, followed by one tablet every hour or two tablets every 2 hours until pain is relieved or until nausea, vomiting, or diarrhea occur. If colchicine is administered for chronic gout, it is administered 0.5 to 0.6 mg once to three times daily.

Instruct the client to maintain a fluid intake of at least 2 to 3 L per day. Prevention of fluid deficit helps prevent renal damage and uric acid stone formation. Instruct the client to report hematuria or oliguria. Administer colchicine with meals to minimize GI effects, and instruct the client to report profuse or bloody diarrhea immediately. Monitor the client closely for indications of drug overdose. Indications include profuse bloody diarrhea and intense abdominal pain. These signs and symptoms may be followed by generalized hemorrhage, shock, renal failure, and neuromuscular paralysis.

If the IV dosage form is prescribed, dilute the colchicine preparation with normal saline solution as directed. Do not dilute with dextrose solution or a bacteriostatic agent. Administer the solution slowly over 2 to 5 minutes; monitor the site for pain, warmth, redness, or signs of extravasation.

MISCELLANEOUS DRUGS IN CATEGORY

Indomethacin (Indocin) and **phenylbutazone** (Butazolidin) are also anti-inflammatory drugs used to reduce the inflammation and pain associated with acute gouty arthritis. These drugs are discussed in Chapter 51.

CONCEPT REVIEW

Anti-inflammatory drugs are used to relieve pain and inflammation associated with acute gout. These drugs also decrease the formation of uric acid crystals by a regional or local increase in pH.

Colchicine is the prototype for drugs in this group. It is considered a disease-specific drug. Major undesired clinical responses associated with colchicine include nausea, vomiting, diarrhea, and abdominal pain.

SUMMARY

Drug therapy for hyperuricemia and gout include the use of uricosuric drugs, uric acid synthesis inhibitors, and anti-inflammatory drugs. These drugs reduce the amount of serum or local uric acid or both, relieving signs and symptoms of the current attack and preventing or modifying future attacks. The nurse's role requires providing adequate client education about the prescribed drugs and about measures to prevent possible complications.

REFERENCES

1. Guyton, A.C. (1991). *Textbook of medical physiology* (8th ed.). Philadelphia: W.B. Saunders.
2. McCance, K.L., & Huether, S. (1994). *Pathophysiology: The biologic basis for disease in adults and children.* St. Louis: Mosby–Year Book.
3. Smith, C.M., & Reynard, A.M. (Eds.). (1992). *Textbook of pharmacology.* Philadelphia: W.B. Saunders.
4. Kelley, W.N., Fox, I., & Palella, T.D. (1989). Crystal-associated synovitis. In W.N. Kelley, E.D. Harris, S. Ruddy, & C. Sledge (Eds.). *Textbook of rheumatology* (3rd ed.). Philadelphia: W.B. Saunders.

5. Agudelo, C.A., & Wise, C.M. (1991). Gout and hyperuricemia. *Current Opinion in Rheumatology, 3,* 684-691.

6. Conger, J.D. (1990). Acute uric acid nephropathy. *Medical Clinics of North America, 74,* 859-871.

7. Wolfe, F. (1991). The misdiagnosis of gout and hyperuricemia. *Journal of Rheumatology, 18,* 1232-1234.

8. Vawter, R.L. (1992). Rational treatment of gout. Stopping an attack and preventing recurrence. *Postgraduate Medicine, 91*(2), 115-118.

9. Star, V.L., & Hochberg, M.C. (1993). Prevention and management of gout. *Drugs, 45,* 212-222.

10. Chernecky, C., Krech, R., & Berger, B. (1993). *Laboratory tests and diagnostic procedures.* Philadelphia: W.B. Saunders.

11. Gray, M.A. (1993). Antigout medications. *Orthopaedic Nursing, 12*(4), 53-55.

12. U.S. Pharmacopeial Convention. (1990). *The United States pharmacopeia* (22nd rev.). Rockville, MD: Author.

13. Data Pharmaceutica, Inc. (1993). *1993 physicians' genRx.* Smithtown, New York: Author.

14. Urivetzky, M., Braverman, S., Motola, J.A., & Smith, A.D. (1990). Absence of effect of allopurinol on oxalate excretion by stone patients on random and controlled diets. *Journal of Urology, 144*(1), 97-98.

15. Edwards, N.L. (1991). Drugs to lower uric acid levels: How to avoid misuse in gouty arthritis. *Postgraduate Medicine, 89*(2), 111-116.

16. Groff, G.D., Franck, W.A., & Raddatz, D.A. (1990). Systemic steroid therapy for acute gout: A clinical trial and review of literature. *Seminars in Arthritis & Rheumatism, 19,* 329-336.

17. Moreland, L.W., & Ball, G.V. (1991). Colchicine and gout. *Arthritis & Rheumatism, 34,* 782-786.

BIBLIOGRAPHY

Famaey, J.P. (1988). Colchicine in therapy. State of the art and new perspectives for an old drug. *Clinical and Experimental Rheumatology, 6,* 305-317.

Milillo, K.D. (1993). Interpretation of laboratory values in older adults. *Nurse Practitioner: American Journal of Primary Health Care, 18*(7), 59-67.

Moser, M. (1992). Diuretics and cardiovascular risk factors. *European Heart Journal, 13*(Suppl. G), 72-80.

Puig, J.G., Michan, A.D., Jimenez, M.L., et al. (1991). Female gout. Clinical spectrum and uric acid metabolism. *Archives of Internal Medicine, 151,* 726-732.

Shulkin, D., & DeTore, A.W. (1990). When laboratory tests are abnormal and the patient feels fine. *Hospital Practice, 25*(7), 85-86, 89-90, 92.

Yeomans, A.C. (1991). Assessment and management of gouty arthritis. *Nurse Practitioner: American Journal of Primary Health Care, 16*(4), 25-26.

Zell, S.C. (1989). Evaluation of allopurinol use in patients with gout. *American Journal of Hospital Pharmacy, 46,* 1813-1816.

Drugs Affecting the Endocrine System

OVERVIEW OF
The Endocrine System

JOAN M. KULPA

⊛ Hormones

LEARNING OBJECTIVES:

Differentiate between circulating and local hormones.

Describe the major classifications of hormones.

Distinguish between the two mechanisms of hormonal action.

Explain the negative feedback mechanism involved in the control of hormonal secretions.

KEY TERMS:

Endocrine, exocrine, fixed-membrane-receptor mechanism, homeostasis, hormone, mobile-receptor mechanism, negative feedback

⊛ Hypothalamus and Pituitary Gland

LEARNING OBJECTIVES:

Describe the functions of the hypothalamus.

Explain the relationship between the hypothalamus and pituitary gland.

Summarize the functions of the anterior and posterior pituitary gland hormones.

KEY TERMS:

Adenohypophysis, factor, hypophysis, neurohypophysis

⊛ Thyroid Gland

LEARNING OBJECTIVES:

Describe the formation, storage, and release of the thyroid gland hormones.

Summarize the functions of the thyroid gland hormones.

KEY TERMS:

Calcitonin, follicular, parafollicular, thyroxine, triiodothyronine

⊛ Parathyroid Glands

LEARNING OBJECTIVES:

Explain the relationship between the thyroid gland hormones and the parathyroid gland.

Summarize the functions of the parathryoid glands hormones.

KEY TERM: Parathormone

⊛ Adrenal Glands

LEARNING OBJECTIVES:

Describe the three types of hormones secreted by the adrenal glands.

Summarize the functions of mineralocorticoids and glucocorticoids.

Explain the functions of gonadocorticoids.

KEY TERMS:

Adrenal cortex, adrenal medulla, cortisol, epinephrine, glucocorticoids, gonadocorticoids, mineralocorticoids, norepinephrine, renin-angiotensin system

⊛ Pancreas

LEARNING OBJECTIVE: Describe the functions of insulin and glucagon in the body.

KEY TERMS:

Glucagon, insulin, islets of Langerhans, somatostatin

⊛ Pharmacologic Use of Hormones

LEARNING OBJECTIVE: Discuss the pharmacologic use of hormones.

CONCEPTS AND TERMS TO REVIEW

Review section on endocrine system in an anatomy and physiology book.

Review section in Chapter 25 on action of epinephrine and norepinephrine as neurotransmitters or neurohormones.

$\mathcal{T}$he endocrine system, along with the nervous system, is responsible for maintaining a constant environment, or **homeostasis,** in the body. In general, the endocrine system is concerned with the control of different metabolic functions in the body such as the rate of chemical reactions in the cells or the transport of substances through cell membranes. Some effects produced by the endocrine system occur in seconds, whereas other effects are not apparent for several days.

The endocrine system contains the pituitary gland, thyroid gland, parathyroid glands, adrenal glands, and pineal gland. Several organs of the body, including the hypothalamus, thymus, pancreas, ovaries, testes, and placenta, contain endocrine tissue but are not endocrine glands exclusively. This chapter provides an overview of the hypothalamus, pituitary gland, thyroid gland, parathyroid glands, adrenal glands, and the islets of Langerhans in the pancreas. The reproductive glands, or gonads, and their hormones are discussed in Chapter 61.

Knowledge of normal anatomy and physiology of these glands and organs is necessary for safe drug administration and helps correlate drug therapy and endocrine function (Fig. 38–1). In addition, an understanding of this information helps you assess for the manifestations of hormonal disturbances.

HORMONES

Within the body are two kinds of glands: exocrine and endocrine. **Exocrine glands** excrete their products externally into ducts. **Endocrine glands** secrete their products (hormones) internally, directly into body fluids. **Hormones,** chemical transmitting substances, are released in minute amounts from cells in endocrine glands directly into body fluids. These substances are distributed by the blood and produce physiologic changes in other cells in the body.[1]

Hormones help maintain a constant internal environment, or homeostasis, in the body. Hormones can modify the rate of chemical reactions occurring in the cell, and they can selectively alter plasma membrane permeability. This latter action influences the transport of essential nutrients, electrolytes, and water across the plasma membrane.

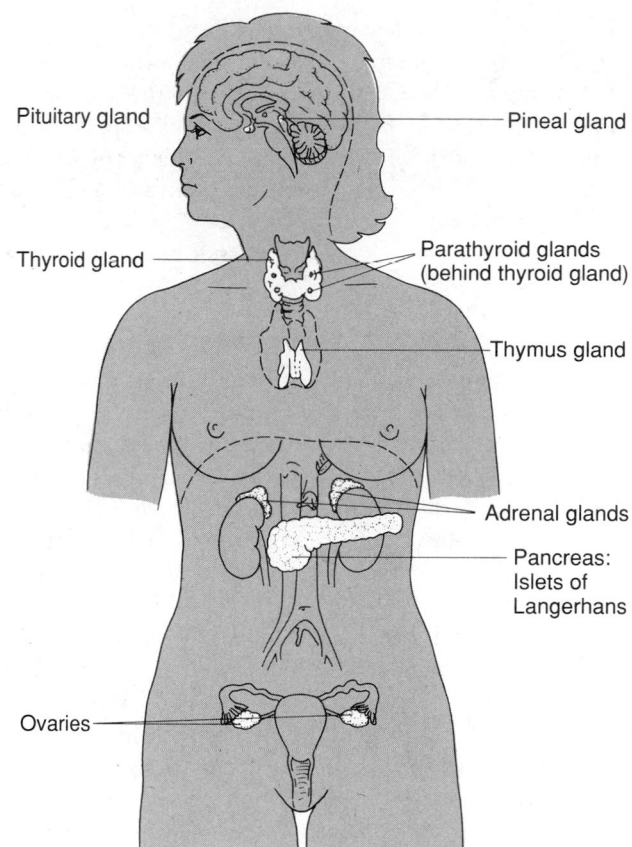

FIGURE 38–1   Anatomic loci of principal endocrine glands of the body. (From Guyton, A.C. [1993]. *Textbook of medical physiology* [8th ed.]. Philadelphia: W.B. Saunders.)

Circulating and Local Hormones

Circulating hormones, or endocrines, pass into the blood and act on distant target cells. **Local hormones** act on target cells close to the site of release. Local hormones are usually inactivated quickly. Circulating hormones remain in the blood for a few minutes or a few hours until inactivated by the liver and excreted by the kidneys.[2]

Classification of Hormones

The chemical composition of hormones can serve as a basis for their classification. Chemically, there are four classes of hormones: steroids, biogenic amines, proteins and peptides, and eicosanoids. **Steroid hormones** (e.g., cortisol, aldosterone) are derived from cholesterol. **Biogenic amines** are the simplest hormone molecules. Several hormones in this classification are synthesized by modification of the amino acid tyrosine. Thyroxine and triiodothyronine, thyroid hormones, are examples of biogenic amines. **Peptides** and **proteins** consist of chains of amino acids. Peptides are smaller (<20 amino acids) than proteins (>20 amino acids). Angiotensin and thyrotropin-releasing hormones are examples of peptides. Insulin and adrenocorticotropin represent the proteins. The most recently discovered class of hormones is the **eicosanoids.**

Eicosanoids are important local hormones. Prostaglandins and leukotrienes are the two major types of eicosanoids.[1,2]

Mechanisms of Hormonal Action

Two general mechanisms by which hormones bring about homeostatic control have been identified: **cyclic adenosine monophosphate (cAMP)–mediated** and **intracellular protein synthesis.** With cAMP the plasma membrane of the target cell contains a receptor specific for a hormone. The hormone, or first messenger, interacts with the cell at the specific receptor site. This hormone-receptor interaction activates adenylate cyclase, an enzyme present in the cell membrane. Once activated, adenylate cyclase catalyzes the conversion of intracellular adenosine triphosphate (ATP) to cAMP. As a result, a variety of physiologic effects may occur, depending on which biochemical changes are associated with the hormone involved. For example, liver enzymes may be activated, or the permeability of cell membranes may be altered. The cAMP mechanism is associated with the water-soluble (amine) hormones. It is also known as the **fixed-membrane-receptor mechanism.**

Hormones that increase intracellular protein synthesis must combine with protein receptors inside the cell. After entering a target cell, the hormone binds to and activates an **intracellular receptor.** Within the cell nucleus, the hormone-receptor complex binds to DNA. Interaction between the hormone-receptor complex and DNA causes transcription of specific genes on the DNA and production of new messenger RNA. The newly transcribed RNA passes into the cytoplasm and begins synthesizing protein. Enzymes that catalyze the initiating hormone's responses are produced as a result of the **mobile-receptor mechanism.**[1-4]

Control of Hormonal Secretions

Most hormone secretion is regulated by a closed-loop negative-feedback system. **Negative feedback** produces an effect opposite to that of the initiating stimulus. For example, if the blood glucose level is too high (initiating stimulus), the islets of Langerhans in the pancreas are stimulated to produce insulin. Insulin inhibits glucose production by the liver and lowers the blood glucose level, an effect directly opposite to the initiating stimulus.

Positive-feedback systems (the initiating stimulus is reinforced) are relatively rare in the human body. An example of positive feedback involves edema of the brain. With cerebral edema, cerebral blood vessels compress, causing decreased blood flow and ischemia of the tissues. A vicious cycle is then set in motion. Arteriolar dilation with increased capillary pressure results from the ischemia. Increased capillary pressure leads to more edema and magnifies the initial problem.[4]

Some hormones also show evidence of response to internal biorhythms. Most internal biorhythms occur every 24 hours and are called **circadian rhythms.** Circadian rhythms of the adrenocorticotropic hormone (ACTH) and cortisol are well documented. Levels of these hormones in individuals who work days are highest in the morning and lowest in the evening. The pattern is reversed for those who work nights.[3]

CONCEPT REVIEW

Each kind of hormone has a special molecular structure.
Hormones only affect specific target cells that have receptor sites for a given hormone.
Chemically, hormones are classified as *steroids, biogenic amines, peptides* or *proteins,* and *eicosanoids.*
Most hormonal secretion is regulated by negative-feedback systems.

HYPOTHALAMUS AND PITUITARY GLAND

The hypothalamus is a major anatomic structure with a myriad of centers that influence autonomic responses, somatic activity, and endocrine activity. Located between the two lobes of the thalamus, the hypothalamus provides the connecting link between the nervous system and the endocrine system. It receives input from several regions of the brain, including the limbic system, cerebral cortex, and thalamus. It also receives

sensory signals from internal organs. Cells in the hypothalamus synthesize at least nine different hormones and the pituitary gland secretes seven more. Together they play important roles in regulation of growth, development, metabolism, and homeostasis.[2,5]

The hypothalamus secretes its releasing or inhibiting hormones or factors in response to internal and external environmental stimuli. (The term *hormone* applies to identified chemical compounds. If the chemical nature of the substance is not known, the term **factor** is used.) Subsequent production of hormones by the pituitary gland is dependent on these hypothalamic releasing and inhibitory hormones (or factors).[4]

Major releasing or inhibitory hormones and factors are thyrotropin releasing hormone (TRH), corticotropin releasing factor (CRF), growth hormone releasing factor (GH-RF), and growth hormone inhibiting factor (GH-IF). Releasing or inhibiting hormones or factors are transported in the blood from the hypothalamus to the pituitary gland through the hypothalamic-hypophyseal portal system. Direct neural control regulates the release of the antidiuretic hormone (ADH), which is produced by the hypothalamus and stored in the posterior pituitary lobe.[4,6]

The pituitary gland **(hypophysis)** is located in the sella turcica, a depression in the sphenoid bone. It is connected to the hypothalamus by the hypophyseal stalk (infundibulum). The pituitary gland is divided into two lobes: the anterior lobe **(adenohypophysis)** and the posterior lobe **(neurohypophysis).**

Anterior Pituitary Gland (Adenohypophysis)

The anterior lobe comprises approximately 75% of the entire gland. This lobe is the source of a variety of hormones including thyroid-stimulating hormone (TSH), ACTH, melanocyte-stimulating hormone (MSH), and growth hormone (GH). Follicle-stimulating hormone (FSH), luteinizing hormone (LH), and prolactin are also produced by the anterior pituitary lobe (Table 38–1).

Posterior Pituitary Gland (Neurohypophysis)

The posterior lobe of the pituitary gland does not produce hormones. It contains axon terminals of secretory neurons of the hypothalamus. Neurosecretory cells in the hypothalamus produce ADH and oxytocin. These hormones are transported to axon terminals in the neurohypophysis and are stored (Table 38–2).

THYROID GLAND

The thyroid gland, located just below the larynx, is composed of two lobes that are positioned on either side of the trachea. Connecting the lobes is a mass of tissue, the **isthmus,** which spans the trachea anteriorly just inferior to the cricoid cartilage.

TABLE 38–1

Anterior Pituitary Gland Hormones: Principal Actions and Associated Hypothalamic Regulating Hormones

Hormone	Principal Actions	Associated Hypothalamic Hormones
Human growth hormone (hGH)	Growth of body cells; protein anabolism; elevation of blood glucose concentration	Growth hormone releasing hormone (GH-RH); growth hormone inhibiting hormone (GH-IH); secretion also stimulated by thyrotropin releasing hormone (TRH)
Thyroid-stimulating hormone (TSH)	Controls secretion of thyroid hormones by thyroid gland	Thyrotropin releasing hormone (TRH)
Adrenocorticotropic hormone (ACTH)	Controls secretion of some hormones (mainly cortisol) by adrenal cortex	Corticotropin releasing hormone (CRH)
Follicle-stimulating hormone (FSH)	In females initiates development of ova and induces ovarian secretion of estrogens; in males stimulates testes to produce sperm	Gonadotropin releasing hormone (Gn-RH)
Luteinizing hormone (LH)	In females, together with FSH, stimulates ovulation and formation of corpus luteum, which secretes estrogens and progesterone; in males stimulates interstitial cells in testes to develop and produce testosterone	Gondadotropin releasing hormone (Gn-RH)
Prolactin	In females, together with other hormones, initiates and maintains effect of luteinizing hormone in promoting milk secretion by mammary glands	Prolactin inhibiting hormone; prolactin releasing hormone
Melanocyte-stimulating hormone (MSH)	Stimulates dispersion of melanin granules in melanocytes	Melanocyte-stimulating hormone releasing hormone; melanocyte-stimulating hormone inhibiting hormone

TABLE 38–2

Posterior Pituitary Gland Hormones: Principal Actions and Control of Secretion

Hormone	Principal Actions	Control of Secretion
Oxytocin	Stimulates contraction of smooth muscle cells of pregnant uterus during labor; stimulates contraction of contractile cells of mammary glands for milk ejection	Neurosecretory cells of hypothalamus secrete oxytocin in response to uterine distention and stimulation of nipples.
Antidiuretic hormone (ADH)	Principal effect: decreases urinary volume; also raises blood pressure by constricting arterioles during severe hemorrhage	Neurosecretory cells of hypothalamus secrete ADH in response to low water concentration of the blood, pain, stress, trauma, anxiety, acetylcholine (ACh), nicotine, morphine, some anesthetics, and tranquilizers; alcohol inhibits secretion

Formation, Storage, and Release of Hormones

Two types of cells, **follicular** and **parafollicular,** make up thyroid tissue. Thyroid follicular cells actively remove iodide from the blood and store it in an iodinated colloidal protein called **thyroglobulin. Tyrosine,** a thyroid hormone precursor, is also stored in the thyroglobulin. These cells then synthesize **thyroxine (T_4)** and **triiodothyronine (T_3)** by attaching iodines to the amino acid tyrosine. Parafollicular cells, or C (clear) cells, produce **calcitonin (CT),** a hormone involved in calcium homeostasis.[2,3]

Release of thyroid hormones is regulated primarily by negative feedback. When circulating T_3 and T_4 levels become too low, the hypothalamus releases TRH. The anterior pituitary lobe responds by secreting TSH, which stimulates follicular cells to secrete more of their hormones into the blood. Most of the circulating T_3 and T_4 is bound to a serum protein, thyroxine-binding globulin. Only minute amounts of T_3 and T_4 are free to enter tissue cells and exert their efforts.

Actions of Thyroid Hormones

T_3 and T_4 increase the rate of activity in all body tissues, thus increasing the basal metabolic rate (BMR). As a result, protein, carbohydrate, lipid, and vitamin metabolism increases; the growth rate in growing children increases; and mental processes accelerate. On a cellular level, the number and activity of mitochondria increase. In addition, some cell membranes become more permeable to the transport of both sodium and potassium.

Parafollicular cells produce calcitonin only when excess calcium is in the blood. Calcitonin inhibits bone resorption of calcium. It also acts on the loop of Henle to allow filtering of calcium and its excretion in the urine. Calcitonin's effects are not dependent on a functioning parathyroid gland, nor does calcitonin influence the release or action of the parathyroid hormone.[3]

PARATHYROID GLANDS

Four small parathyroid glands are embedded in the dorsal surface of the thyroid lobes, one gland in the upper and lower pole of each lobe. Two types of cells, the **chief cell** and the **oxyphil cell,** make up the parathyroid glands. Chief cells are responsible for the production of parathormone; the function of the oxyphil cells is not clear.

Parathormone regulates both calcium and phosphate metabolism. It increases calcium and phosphate absorption from the bone and decreases renal excretion of calcium. Parathormone stimulates the activity of osteoclasts that break down bone tissue, releasing calcium and phosphate into the blood. It increases the rate at which kidneys remove calcium and magnesium during urine formation and return the substances to the blood. Parathormone inhibits the transport of phosphates from urine into the blood. Therefore more phosphates are lost through urine formation than are gained from bone destruction. Parathormone also promotes the formation of the hormone **calcitriol,** an active form of vitamin D (1,25-dihydroxy cholecalciferol; vitamin D_3). Calcitriol increases the rate of calcium, phosphate, and magnesium absorption from the gastrointestinal tract into the blood. This results in an increase in serum calcium and magnesium concentrations and maintenance of normal phosphate levels.[1-3]

CONCEPT REVIEW

The pituitary gland, which is attached to the base of the brain, has an anterior lobe and a posterior lobe. Most pituitary secretions are controlled by the hypothalamus.

The adenohypophysis secretes GH, prolactin, TSH, ACTH, FSH, and LH.

The two hormones of the neurohypophysis, ADH and oxytocin, are produced in the hypothalamus.

Thyroxine, triiodothyronine, and calcitonin are produced by the cells of the thyroid gland.

Parathyroid glands produce parathormone.

ADRENAL (SUPRARENAL) GLANDS

The adrenal (suprarenal) glands rest on the superior poles of the kidneys. Each gland is composed of two distinct types of tissue, medulla and cortex. Each type of tissue secretes different hormones.

Adrenal Medulla

The inner portion of tissue, the **medulla,** represents approximately 10% of the total gland. This layer of tissue consists of hormone-producing cells, the chromaffin cells. Chromaffin cells receive direct innervation from preganglionic neurons of the sympathetic branch of the autonomic nervous system (ANS). Principal hormones synthesized by the adrenal medulla are **epinephrine** and **norepinephrine.** Secretion of epinephrine constitutes approximately 80% of the total hormones synthesized by the gland. Both epinephrine and norepinephrine are sympathomimetic; they mimic the sympathetic division of the ANS.

Adrenal Cortex

Ninety percent of the adrenal gland is the **cortex,** the outer layer of tissue. This layer is further divided into three histologically distinct zones: the outer *(zona glomerulosa),* the middle *(zona fasciculata),* and the inner *(zona reticularis)* zones. Mineralocorticoids are secreted by the outer zone, glucocorticoids by the middle zone, and gonadocorticoids by the inner zone. All hormones synthesized and secreted by the adrenal cortex are steroids. Homeostasis requires the presence of both mineralocorticoids and glucocorticoids.[1,2,4]

Mineralocorticoids. Mineralocorticoids are essential for fluid and electrolyte balance. Production of aldosterone represents approximately 95% of mineralocorticoid activity. Aldosterone acts on certain tubule cells in the kidneys to increase the reabsorption of sodium and the excretion of potassium. Since aldosterone helps to maintain sodium and water balance, it also promotes normal cardiac output and blood pressure.[2,7]

Secretion of aldosterone is under the control of several different mechanisms operating simultaneously. One such mechanism is the **renin-angiotensin system.** Renin is released in response to a decrease in blood volume or a sodium deficiency that precipitates a drop in blood pressure. Once secreted, renin converts a plasma protein, angiotensinogen, to angiotensin I. As blood flows through lung capillaries, angiotensin-converting enzyme changes angiotensin I into angiotensin II. Angiotensin II stimulates the release of aldosterone.

Other mechanisms involved in the control of aldosterone secretion include serum potassium concentration, extracellular fluid sodium ion concentration, and the pituitary hormone ACTH. Aldosterone is released from the adrenal cortex in response to elevated serum potassium levels. This action causes the kidneys to excrete excess potassium. Extracellular sodium ion concentration and ACTH play a minor role in the control of aldosterone secretion.

Glucocorticoids Glucocorticoids, principally **cortisol** (hydrocortisone), are secreted in response to the pituitary output of ACTH. In humans there is a daily pattern of ACTH and cortisol plasma levels. During periods of stress, the hypothalamus is stimulated to secrete CRF. This factor causes the pituitary to release more ACTH that further stimulates the secretion of cortisol by the adrenal cortex.

Physiologic effects from the glucocorticoids are diverse, affecting virtually all body tissues. Some of the main effects are those produced by cortisol on carbohydrate, protein, and fat metabolism. Cortisol affects carbohydrate metabolism by mobilizing amino acids for gluconeogenesis and decreasing cellular glucose use in the body. It also increases the activity of enzymes required for glucose production and inhibits glycolytic enzymes. These actions provide glucose to meet the body's immediate needs; they also promote glycogen storage in the liver.[1,8]

Cortisol also affects protein and fat metabolism. It decreases protein synthesis and increases protein catabolism. The action of cortisol mobilizes amino acids that are used by the liver during the period of increased gluconeogenesis and plasma protein production. Cortisol also increases the concentration of plasma fatty acids.

All phases of the inflammatory response are blocked by cortisol. This leads to decreased edema, warmth, redness, and pain in the affected area. Individuals requiring long-term therapeutic use of glucocorticoids have an increased risk of infection and delayed healing.

Gonadocorticoids   Adrenal sex hormones (**gonadocorticoids**) are produced by cells in the inner zone (zona reticularis) of the cortex. Although the hormones of this group are androgens, some of them are converted into female hormones (estrogens) by the skin, liver, and adipose tissue. Adrenal androgens supplement the sex hormones from the gonads.[2,5] Androgens and estrogens are discussed in more detail in Chapters 61 through 63.

Adrenocortical suppression   Therapeutic administration of glucocorticoids suppresses the adrenal cortex and the production of ACTH by the anterior lobe of the pituitary gland. Prolonged high-dose corticosteroid therapy can lead to acute adrenal insufficiency. If the steroid therapy is abruptly discontinued, the adrenal insufficiency may be life threatening.

The smallest dose of glucocorticoids that achieves the desired effect is prescribed in an attempt to minimize the risk of adrenal insufficiency. In addition, the drug is gradually discontinued. This process gives the adrenal cortex and pituitary gland time to regain function.[9]

PANCREAS: THE ISLETS OF LANGERHANS

The endocrine portion of the pancreas consists of the **islets of Langerhans.** Islets include three types of hormone-secreting cells: beta, alpha, and delta. Beta cells secrete **insulin;** alpha cells secrete **glucagon;** and delta cells secrete **somatostatin.** Insulin and glucagon are peptide hormones. Insulin lowers the blood glucose level, and glucagon raises the blood glucose level. Insulin also makes cell membranes more permeable to amino acids and electrolytes such as potassium, magnesium, and phosphate. Somatostatin helps regulate carbohydrate by inhibiting the secretion of glucagon.

Glucagon

Both the pancreas and liver are involved in the negative-feedback mechanism that regulates glucagon and insulin. When the blood glucose level drops below normal, alpha cells

secrete glucagon. Glucagon accelerates the conversion of glycogen into glucose (glycogenolysis) in the liver. It also promotes the conversion of other nutrients into glucose in the liver (gluconeogenesis).

Glucagon acts by increasing cAMP levels that cause production of an enzyme, phosphorylase. This enzyme breaks glycogen molecules down to glucose for release into the bloodstream. Glucagon is also involved in breaking down adipose tissue into fatty acids and glycerol.[1,4]

Insulin

The main effect of insulin is exactly opposite that of glucagon. Insulin acts on the liver to stimulate the formation of glycogen from glucose and to inhibit the conversion of noncarbohydrates into glucose. Insulin also accelerates the transport of glucose into cells that possess insulin receptors.

In addition, insulin promotes the transport of amino acids into cells and increases the synthesis of proteins. The exact mechanism involved in the transport of amino acids is unknown. However, without insulin, protein synthesis and storage cease, and protein catabolism increases. Insulin also affects the metabolism of fats by stimulating the adipose cells to synthesize and store fat. Insulin is required for conversion of glucose to triglycerides. The triglycerides are then stored in the adipose tissue.

CONCEPT REVIEW

Epinephrine and norepinephrine are secreted by the adrenal medulla. These hormones are synthesized from tyrosine and are closely related to each other chemically.

Epinephrine and norepinephrine produce effects similar to those of the sympathetic branch of the ANS.

The adrenal cortex produces a variety of steroids, including aldosterone, cortisol, and adrenal sex hormones.

PHARMACOLOGIC USES OF HORMONES

Hormones are comonly used to replace hormones lacking in an individual; to achieve effects beyond normal replacement; and to test the response of a target organ. Examples of replacement therapy include the use of insulin to treat diabetes mellitus, thyroxine to treat hypothyroidism, and cortisol to treat adrenal insufficiency. The most common example of using a hormone to achieve effects beyond normal replacement is the use of adrenal corticosteroids for their anti-inflammatory effects.

Several tests use hormones to evaluate the function of their respective target organs. For example, ACTH is administered to an individual suspected of having adrenal insufficiency. The

TABLE 38–3

Summary of Endocrine Glands, Hormones, and Effects on Target Tissues

Gland	Hormone	Effects on Target Tissues
Hypothalamus	Release or inhibiting hormones	Regulates anterior pituitary hormones
Pituitary		
Anterior lobe	Thyrotropic hormone (TSH)	Secretion of T_3 and T_4 by thyroid gland
	Adrenocorticotropic hormone (ACTH)	Production of steroids by adrenal cortex
Posterior lobe	Antidiuretic hormone (ADH, vasopressin)	Promotes renal reabsorption of water, decreasing urinary output
Thyroid	Thyroxine (T_4)	Increases metabolic activity of almost all body cells; stimulates metabolism of carbohydrates, fats, and proteins
	Triiodothyronine (T_3)	
	Thyrocalcitonin	Decreases calcium levels; increases phosphate levels
Parathyroid	Parathormone (PTH)	Increases calcium levels; decreases phosphate levels
Adrenal cortex	Glucocorticoids (e.g., cortisol)	Stimulates carbohydrate, fat, and protein metabolism
	Mineralocorticoids (e.g., aldosterone)	Increases sodium retention and potassium excretion
Pancreas		
Islets of Langerhans	Insulin	Maintains blood glucose by promoting carbohydrate, fat, and protein metabolism
	Glucagon	Promotes glycogenolysis
	Somatostatin	Decreases insulin and glucagon secretion

NOTE: This table contains only those glands and hormones discussed in Chapter 38. Please refer to other sources for a full discussion of all glands and hormones in the human endocrine system.

normal response is an increase in serum cortisol levels. If the serum cortisol levels remain low, it means that the adrenal cortex has not responded to the ACTH and adrenal insufficiency exists. [10]

SUMMARY

The endocrine system, in concert with the nervous system, is responsible for regulating and maintaining homeostasis. Glands that secrete hormones into the blood constitute the endocrine system. These hormones regulate the body's metabolic activities.

Secretion of most hormones is controlled by a negative-feedback mechanism. Negative feedback is a self-regulating mechanism that sustains hormonal activities within prescribed ranges. Once hormones reach their target tissue, they act on the cells by either the fixed-membrane-receptor (cAMP) mechanism or intracellular protein synthesis. Normally the response of the target tissue corrects whatever imbalance exists, and homeostasis is achieved (Table 38–3).

Pharmacologic uses of hormones include replacement therapy and diagnosis of endocrine dysfunction. Regardless of the reason for administering hormones, clients must be carefully monitored and assessed.

REFERENCES

1. Goodman, H.M. (1988). *Basic medical endocrinology*. New York: Raven Press.
2. Tortora, G., & Grabowski, S. (1993). *Principles of anatomy and physiology* (7th ed.). New York: Harper Collins.
3. Bullock, J., Boyle, J., & Wang, M.B. (1991). *Physiology* (2nd ed.). Baltimore: Williams & Wilkins.
4. Guyton, A.C. (1991). *Textbook of medical physiology* (8th ed.). Philadelphia: W.B. Saunders.
5. Hole, J.W. (1993). *Human anatomy and physiology* (6th ed.). Dubuque, IA: Wm. C. Brown.
6. Rhoades, R., & Pflanzer, R. (1989). *Human physiology*. Philadelphia: W.B. Saunders.
7. Guyton, A.C. (1992). *Human physiology and mechanisms of disease* (5th ed.). Philadelphia: W.B. Saunders.
8. Carola, R., Harley, J.P., & Noback, C.R. (1992). *Human anatomy and physiology* (2nd ed.). New York: McGraw-Hill.
9. Haynes, R.C. (1990). Adrenocorticotropic hormones: Adrenocortical steroids and their synthetic analogs; Inhibitors of the synthesis and action of adrenocortical hormones. In Gilman, A.G., Rall, T.W., Nies, A.S., & Taylor, P. (Eds.). *The pharmacological basis of therapeutics* (pp. 1431-1462). New York: Pergamon Press.
10. Chernecky, C.C., Krech, R., & Berger, B. (1993). *Laboratory tests and diagnostic procedures*. Philadelphia: W.B. Saunders.

BIBLIOGRAPHY

Black, J.M., & Matassarin-Jacobs, E. (1993). *Luckmann and Sorensen's medical-surgical nursing: A psychophysiologic approach* (4th ed.). Philadelphia: W.B. Saunders.
Ignatavicius, S., & Bayne, M.V. (1991). *Medical-surgical nursing: A nursing process approach*. Philadelphia: W.B. Saunders.
Reasner, C.A. (1990). Adrenal disorders. *Critical Care Nursing Quarterly, 13*(3), 67-73.
Seeley, R., Stephens, T., & Tate, P. (1992). *Anatomy and physiology* (2nd ed.). St. Louis: Mosby–Year Book.
Sikes, P.J. (1992). Endocrine responses to the stress of critical illness. *AACN: Clinical Issues in Critical Care Nursing, 3*, 379-391.

CHAPTER 39

Drugs Used to Regulate Blood Glucose Levels

JULIA ANN RAITHEL

● **Pancreatic Functions**

LEARNING OBJECTIVE: Describe the exocrine and endocrine functions of the pancreas.

KEY TERMS:

Glucagon, insulin, somatostatin

● **Hyperglycemia and Hypoglycemia**

LEARNING OBJECTIVE: Identify causes of hyperglycemia and hypoglycemia.

KEY TERMS:

Hyperglycemia, hypoglycemia

● **Diabetes Mellitus**

LEARNING OBJECTIVES:

Summarize the pathophysiology involved in diabetes mellitus.

Compare the two major types of diabetes mellitus: insulin-dependent diabetes mellitus (IDDM) and non-insulin-dependent diabetes mellitus (NIDDM).

Discuss the management of diabetes mellitus.

Explain four methods of monitoring serum glucose levels.

KEY TERMS:

Gestational diabetes mellitus, insulin-dependent diabetes mellitus, ketone bodies, ketoacidosis, ketosis, non-insulin-dependent diabetes mellitus, renal threshold

● **Drug Therapy for Insulin-Dependent Diabetes Mellitus**

LEARNING OBJECTIVES:

Differentiate among the different sources of insulin.

Contrast the different insulin preparations.

Describe the primary methods of insulin delivery.

KEY TERM: United States Pharmacopeia (USP)

● **Nursing Considerations in the Care of Insulin-Dependent Diabetics**

LEARNING OBJECTIVE: Develop a plan of care for the client requiring insulin therapy.

● **Insulin**

LEARNING OBJECTIVES:

Discuss the pharmacodynamic properties of insulin.

Contrast and compare the pharmacokinetic properties of the various forms of insulin.

KEY TERMS:

Dawn phenomenon, flocculation, insulin allergy, insulin resistance, lipotrophy, lipohypertrophy, sliding scale, Somogyi effect

● **Drug Therapy for Non-Insulin-Dependent Diabetes Mellitus**

LEARNING OBJECTIVES:

Develop a plan of care for a client requiring therapy with oral hypoglycemic drugs.

Describe the pharmacokinetic and pharmacodynamic properties of sulfonylureas.

KEY TERMS:

Biguanide, hyperosmolar hyperglycemic nonketotic coma, sulfonylurea

● **Drugs Used to Increase Blood Glucose Levels**

LEARNING OBJECTIVES:

Discuss causes of hypoglycemia.

Describe appropriate nursing care for a client requiring drug therapy to increase blood glucose levels.

Describe the pharmacokinetic and pharmacodynamic properties of glucagon.

KEY TERMS:

Chronic reactive hypoglycemia, hyperinsulinism, insulin reaction, postprandial hypoglycemia

Maintenance of blood glucose levels within certain limits is vital for the survival of humans. All animal cells can metabolize glucose in some way. However, brain, blood cells, and muscles are the major consumers of glucose. For example, approximately 60% to 70% of endogenous glucose production is used exclusively for the energy requirements of the brain. Blood glucose is regulated by the actions of insulin, which is secreted by the pancreas, and hormones such as glucagon, epinephrine, norepinephrine, cortisol, and growth hormone.

Drugs that help regulate blood glucose are designed to support the natural functions of the body, including raising or lowering the serum glucose level. Raising the serum glucose level is mainly accomplished by glucagon. Lowering serum glucose level can be accomplished by the administration of insulin or oral hypoglycemic drugs. These drugs are the focus of this chapter.

PANCREATIC FUNCTIONS

The pancreas, located behind the stomach and between the spleen and duodenum, is composed of tissue for exocrine and endocrine functions. Exocrine function includes the production of enzymes used in the digestion of proteins, carbohydrates, and fats. This production is the responsibility of the acinar cells. Endocrine function is produced by a cluster of cells called the *islets of Langerhans.*

There are 1 to 2 million islets in the adult human pancreas; each islet is about 0.3 mm in diameter.[1] These islets consist of three major cell types: alpha, beta, and delta. The delta cells secrete **somatostatin,** which inhibits the release of glucagon and insulin and prolongs the absorption time of nutrients into the blood. Alpha cells are responsible for the production of glucagon. **Glucagon** elevates serum glucose level by the process of gluconeogenesis.[1]

Beta cells, the most prominent islet cell type, secrete insulin. **Insulin,** a metabolic hormone, has a profound effect on the use of glucose by body cells. Additionally, insulin promotes protein and fat metabolism and is the primary hormone responsible for controlling the storage and use of cellular nutrients. Important target tissues for the actions of insulin include the liver, muscle, and fat.

HYPERGLYCEMIA AND HYPOGLYCEMIA

The term **hyperglycemia** is used to describe an excess of glucose in the blood. Hyperglycemia can result from pancreatic diseases, hormonal abnormalities, drug- or chemical-induced reactions, insulin receptor abnormalities, certain genetic syndromes, and certain malnutrition-related problems. The most common pathology that causes hyperglycemia is diabetes mellitus.

Hypoglycemia occurs when the serum glucose level is lower than 80 mg/dl. Hypoglycemia in nondiabetic clients is usually caused by metabolic diseases that interfere with glucose metabolism. Among these diseases are genetic disorders; liver, pituitary, thyroid, or adrenal disorders; and pancreatic tumors.

DIABETES MELLITUS

More than 11 million individuals in the United States have diabetes mellitus, a disorder of chronic abnormal fuel metabolism, and the incidence of the disorder continues to increase yearly. It is not a single disease but a syndrome with several causes, all characterized by elevated blood glucose. A deficiency in the secretion of insulin or failure of the body's cells to respond to the insulin being produced (insulin resistance) results in diabetes mellitus. Although the metabolism of protein and fat is affected, carbohydrate use is the most profound and apparent alteration.[2]

Pathophysiology

Normally as food is consumed, it is converted into glucose and other energy precursors by the digestive system and is absorbed into the circulatory system. As the glucose is absorbed into the blood, the serum glucose level rises. This elevated blood glucose level stimulates insulin secretion. The increased level of insulin facilitates the transport of glucose into target cells and promotes the storage of glucose as glycogen in liver and muscle. The rate of insulin secretion is designed to produce a stable serum concentration of glucose, usually 80 to 120 mg/dl.[3] An increased level of insulin also enhances fat deposition in adipose tissue, inhibits protein degradation, and accelerates the processes of amino acid transport into cells and protein synthesis. When plasma glucose levels begin to fall, the process is reversed.

Without sufficient insulin, normal carbohydrate metabolism is impaired. Although the blood glucose rises to excessive levels, hyperglycemia, the lack of insulin prevents cells from receiving the needed glucose for intracellular metabolic functions and prevents storage of excess glucose and glycogen. Elevated serum glucose pulls water from the cells into the blood, causing cellular dehydration. With the expanded blood volume, renal perfusion is increased, and polyuria occurs. Without treatment, cells starve from the lack of glucose in spite of the hyperglycemia in the blood.

With the continued absence of insulin, fat stores are metabolized into free fatty acids and glycerol. These free fatty acids and glycerol are referred to as **ketone bodies;** the presence of excessive ketone bodies in the blood is called **ketosis.** If this accumulation continues, **diabetic ketoacidosis (DKA)** occurs, which can result in coma and death.

The lack of insulin also causes an increase in the amount of stored triglycerides in the liver. An excess of triglycerides causes a fatty liver and results in the conversion of some fatty acids into phospholipids and cholesterol. As a result, serum levels of triglycerides, phospholipids, and cholesterol are elevated, which can result in atherosclerosis.

Without insulin, protein synthesis and storage stop. Catabolism of protein increases, and amino acids are released into the blood where they are converted into glucose, resulting in additional hyperglycemia. As the serum glucose level continues to rise, some glucose filters out of the blood and is excreted in the urine (**glycosuria**). The protein catabolism results in protein wasting, weight loss, and weakness.[2,4] See box below for a summary of some of the physiologic changes that occur with insufficient insulin.

Classifications of Diabetes Mellitus

Criteria for diagnosis of diabetes mellitus in the nonpregnant adult include (1) a random plasma glucose level of 200 mg/dl or above plus classic clinical manifestations of diabetes; (2) a fasting plasma glucose level of 140 mg/dl or greater on at least two occasions; and (3) a fasting plasma glucose level of less than 140 mg/dl plus a sustained elevated plasma glucose level during at least two oral glucose tolerance tests. The criteria for diagnosing children differ from adults. In children a fasting glucose level greater than 100 mg/dl, a 1-hour glucose level greater than 160 mg/dl, and a 2-hour level greater than 140 mg/dl are diagnostic of diabetes mellitus.[5]

Two major types of diabetes mellitus are recognized: insulin-dependent diabetes mellitus and non-insulin-dependent diabetes mellitus. These terms are used to describe the pathogenesis of the disorder, not the treatment. **Insulin-dependent diabetes mellitus** (type I; IDDM) comprises approximately 10% of the diabetic population. It is believed that IDDM results from autoimmune destruction of pancreatic beta cells in genetically predisposed individuals. Although IDDM can develop at any age, it most commonly occurs before the age of 30

years. IDDM frequency is characterized by a rather abrupt onset of clinical manifestations, which include polydipsia, polyuria, dehydration, weight loss, polyphagia, fatigue, weakness, and blurred vision.

Non-insulin-dependent diabetes mellitus (type II; NIDDM) is more common after the age of 30 years. Although individuals with NIDDM may have low, normal, or even excessive levels of insulin in the bloodstream, the insulin is ineffective in controlling blood glucose. Hyperglycemia results from insulin resistance. Usually the onset of NIDDM is gradual. Frequently the client is overweight and has a family history of diabetes. Clinical manifestations of NIDDM are less severe than those of IDDM. The client may eventually seek medical intervention for symptoms such as dry mouth and skin, increased lethargy, slowly healing cuts, irritability, blurred vision, vaginal and bladder infections, and excessive sweating. For clients with NIDDM, drugs that increase insulin secretion from the pancreas or increase cellular membrane sensitivity to glucose or do both are prescribed. Table 39–1 contains a summary of common characteristics of IDDM and NIDDM.

An additional type of diabetes mellitus is referred to as **gestational diabetes mellitus.** This condition develops during pregnancy in a woman not previously diagnosed with the disease. Since plasma glucose levels tend to fall during pregnancy, criteria are different for this group of clients. The diagnosis of gestational diabetes is made if two plasma glucose values during a glucose tolerance test equal or exceed the following: fasting serum glucose level, 105 mg/dl; 1-hour serum glucose level, 190 mg/dl; 2-hour serum glucose level, 165 mg/dl; and 3-hour serum glucose level, 145 mg/dl.[5] Gestational diabetes mellitus often requires both dietary changes and exogenous insulin. After delivery, many women do not require continuation of insulin injections.

Management of Diabetes Mellitus

There is no cure for diabetes mellitus, but it can be controlled using a treatment plan of drugs, diet, and exercise.

Exercise   Exercise increases the permeability of the cell membrane to glucose. It also decreases the need for insulin for glucose transportation into cells.[1] This reduces the amount of insulin required by the individual. In addition, consistent exercise increases the lean body mass (muscle) and decreases adipose tissue.[6] Exercise should be performed at approximately the same time each day and should consist of the same amount of exercise. Consistency is important to prevent excessive lowering of the glucose level.[7]

Nutrition   Since clients with NIDDM tend to be overweight, weight reduction is beneficial. In fact, adherence to a dietary program allows some NIDDM clients to avoid drug therapy. For IDDM clients, dietary control is equally important, but these clients generally need to prevent weight loss.[6]

Many of the complications associated with diabetes mellitus such as cardiovascular changes, neuropathy, and nephropathy are secondary to inadequate metabolic control of diabetes. Dietary focus generally has been on limiting hyperglycemia, but serum lipid levels are also important.[8] Therefore dietary in-

---

PHYSIOLOGIC ALTERATIONS RELATED TO INSUFFICIENT INSULIN

▶ Impaired carbohydrate metabolism

▶ Decreased transfer of glucose into cells for intracellular metabolic functions

▶ Reduced storage of excess glucose and glycogen

▶ Expanded blood volume, producing an increase in renal perfusion and polyuria

▶ Increased metabolism of fat into fatty acids and glycerol

▶ Increased storage of triglycerides in liver

▶ Reduced protein synthesis and storage

▶ Increased protein catabolism, producing an increase in released amino acids

▶ Increased gluconeogenesis, resulting in increased levels of glucose

▶ Increased level of glucose filtered out of blood by kidneys, producing glycosuria

TABLE 39–1
Comparison of IDDM and NIDDM

Insulin-dependent Diabetes Mellitus: Type I	Non-insulin-dependent Diabetes Mellitus: Type II
DEFINITION	
Absolute deficiency of insulin from the pancreatic beta cells	Relative lack of insulin or resistance to its effects
ONSET	
Can occur at any age	Commonly occurs after age 30 y
Commonly occurs before age 30 y	Gradual onset
Abrupt onset	
CLINICAL MANIFESTATIONS	
Elevated serum glucose level	Frequently asymptomatic
Glycosuria	Elevated serum glucose level
Polyuria	Dry mouth and skin
Ketonuria	Increased lethargy
Polydipsia	Irritability
Polyphagia	Susceptibility to infection
Susceptibility to infection	Slow wound healing
Poor wound healing	Blurred vision
Frequently underweight	Excessive sweating
	Obese
CLINICAL MANAGEMENT	
Insulin dependent	Not insulin dependent, although insulin may be required, especially with stressful events
Diet	
Exercise	Oral hypoglycemic drugs
Routine monitoring of serum glucose level	Diet
	Exercise
	Weight loss

ADA NUTRITIONAL RECOMMENDATIONS

The client should:

Achieve and maintain ideal body weight

Derive 55% to 60% of total caloric intake from carbohydrates

Consume foods containing unrefined carbohydrates with fiber

Consume modest amounts of sucrose if this does not alter control of body weight

Limit daily protein intake for adults to 0.8 g/kg of body weight

Limit total daily fat intake to <30% of total calories

Limit cholesterol to <300 mg/d

Limit daily sodium intake to 3000 mg/d or less

take of fat and cholesterol must be monitored. See box for a summary of nutritional recommendations from the American Diabetes Association (ADA).

Drug therapy Drugs used to treat diabetes mellitus consist of two categories: insulin and oral hypoglycemic drugs. Insulin must be used for IDDM clients and for clients with NIDDM whose serum glucose level is high in spite of diet therapy and oral hypoglycemia drugs.

Pancreatic transplantation This form of treatment ranges from transplantation of the entire pancreas to transplantation of islet cells. Unfortunately, there are major obstacles to transplantation therapy, including the lack of transplantable tissue and posttransplantation rejection of the pancreatic tissue.

Monitoring Serum Glucose Levels

Several methods are available for monitoring the serum glucose level of an individual. Results from these various methods are used to confirm the diagnosis of diabetes mellitus or to evaluate the effectiveness of the treatment plan.

Urine testing for glucose Testing the urine for glucose is no longer considered an accurate measurement of diabetic control. Usually kidneys do not filter out excess glucose until the serum glucose level is higher than 175 mg/dl, the minimum **renal threshold.** This means that a client's blood glucose level must be greater than 175 mg/dl before the result of the urine test for glucose is positive. Another problem is the differences observed in individual renal thresholds. For example, the elderly frequently have higher renal thresholds, but the threshold is lowered during pregnancy.[6–8] Furthermore, false-positive and false-negative results can occur if the client is receiving certain drugs.

Despite these problems, some clients are unable or unwilling to use other methods. For these clients, several agents are available. Each product contains instructions and a color chart for reading the results. The client should be instructed to use a fresh, double-voided urine specimen.

Urine testing for ketones   Since individuals with IDDM are prone to developing ketosis, their urine frequently is tested for ketones. In addition, any client testing urine for glucose should test for ketones if the urinary glucose level is 1% or higher. Several products are available for testing urine for ketones or for acetone, one form of ketone.

Fasting serum glucose level   A fasting blood sugar, or fasting serum glucose, level indicates the amount of glucose in the blood. To improve the accuracy of the test, the client must fast, except for water, for at least 8 hours before the test.

Postprandial glucose level   In this test a serum glucose level is measured 2 hours after the client eats a meal. Results that are 140 mg/dl or higher require additional diagnostic tests to determine if diabetes mellitus is present.[6,8]

Oral glucose tolerance   The oral glucose tolerance test is used to diagnose diabetes mellitus. After the client fasts for 10 hours, an initial fasting blood sugar level is determined. The client then drinks a solution containing 75 g of glucose. (In children the quantity of glucose administered is 1.75 g/kg, up to a maximum of 100 g.) Serum glucose levels are then determined at specific time intervals up to 3 hours. If the 2-hour value is greater than 200 mg/dl, diabetes is diagnosed.[5,7]

Glycosylated hemoglobin   Glycosylated hemoglobin provides an accurate index of the client's average serum glucose level for a 100- to 120-day period before the test. Glycohemoglobin is formed when serum glucose combines with the hemoglobin. This reaction is not reversible. Therefore the amount of glycohemoglobin reflects the amount of exposure to serum glucose during the life span of the red blood cell. Elevated serum glucose results in higher levels of glycohemoglobin. Although this test can be used as an indicator of overall control of the glucose level, false high values can be obtained in clients with uremia and hyperlipidemia.[6,8]

Self–blood glucose monitoring   In self–blood glucose monitoring a drop of the client's capillary blood is placed on a reagent strip, which is inserted into a meter device that reads the intensity of the color on the strip. The greater the intensity of color, the higher the serum glucose level.

This test is used by care providers to determine changes in the client's serum glucose when clinical manifestations of hypoglycemia or hyperglycemia occur. It is also used to facilitate attaining control in clients with IDDM and gestational diabetes. The frequency of testing varies with the client's condition and the treatment regimen used. However, unnecessary testing increases the financial cost to the client. Since this procedure requires contact with blood specimens, universal precautions are needed. Suggestions for improving the accuracy of testing include the following[10]:

- Be certain that blood drop completely covers the test area on the reagent strip.
- Avoid adding additional blood once the initial drop of blood has been placed on the reagent strip.
- Follow manufacturer guidelines to determine the length of time to leave the blood in contact with reagent strip.

- Check calibration of meter using test strips or test solutions.
- Clean the meter, especially at the infrared light source.
- Protect the meter and reagent strips from temperatures higher than 35.4° C (95.8° F).

With the advent of the reagent strip test, self-monitoring of serum glucose levels by the client became possible. Use of this procedure is recommended for clients with IDDM; its value for clients with NIDDM has not been shown. In some situations the client is taught to manipulate insulin, diet, and exercise based on the test results.

CONCEPT REVIEW

Diabetes mellitus is a disorder of chronic abnormal fuel metabolism. It is considered a syndrome and is characterized by elevated blood glucose levels.

A deficiency in the secretion of insulin or a failure of the body's cells to respond to the insulin produced (insulin resistance) produces diabetes mellitus.

Diabetes mellitus is classified as IDDM and NIDDM, based on the pathogenesis of the disorder.

DRUG THERAPY FOR INSULIN-DEPENDENT DIABETES MELLITUS

Insulin was isolated in 1921 by Frederick Banting and Charles Best. Through a series of experiments, they were able to obtain pancreatic extracts that were successful in decreasing the concentration of blood glucose in diabetic dogs. This pancreatic extract was first administered to a human in 1922.

In the years that followed, chemical procedures were developed to isolate insulin and to produce it commercially from bovine (beef) or porcine (pork) pancreatic glands. These early insulin preparations were relatively impure and frequently caused allergic reactions because of the presence of protein contaminants such as proinsulin and to species' differences. Early products also only lowered blood glucose levels for a few hours. Continued modification has resulted in insulin products that are more pure, have varying lengths of action, and are chemically similar to human insulin.

Sources of Insulin

Commercial insulins still are derived from beef or pork pancreas. Although these insulins are similar to human insulin, they have a slightly different amino acid structure. Insulin produced from pork pancreas is more similar to human insulin than is beef. Additionally, allergic reactions are less common with purified pork insulin.

Semisynthetic human insulin derived from pork pancreas and synthetic **human insulin** derived from recombinant deoxyribonucleic acid (DNA) are also available. Semisynthetic insulin is manufactured by chemically modifying the amino acids of pork insulin. Synthetic human insulin is manufactured by using recombinant DNA from strains of *Escherichia coli*. This type of insulin has the same number and sequence of amino acids as the insulin produced by the human pancreas.

Most newly diagnosed diabetic clients and all clients receiving premixed insulins use human insulin. Although some clients have allergic reactions to synthetic human insulin, it is less immunogenic than animal insulins.[11-13]

Insulin Preparations

Insulin is available in many forms. The different forms are made by the addition of zinc, protamine, or both in the presence of a suitable buffer. These modifications delay absorption of insulin from a subcutanous site, resulting in extended duration of action. Based on duration of action, insulin preparations are divided into three categories: short, intermediate, and long acting. In addition, each insulin preparation is classified as *purified* (less than 10 parts per million of proinsulin) or *unpurified*.[5,10]

Potency of insulin is expressed as **United States Pharmacopeia (USP)** units. All types of insulin are prepared in solutions of two different strengths, U-40 and U-100. The numbers after the U indicate the number of units per milliliter (i.e., U-100 contains 100 units of insulin per milliliter). Most insulin currently in clinical use is U-100. If the client requires large dosages of insulin, a preparation of U-500 (500 U/ml) is available.[5]

Methods of Insulin Delivery

The usual route of insulin administration is by subcutaneous injection. Continuous subcutaneous insulin infusion (CSII), with bolus dosages of insulin administered before each meal, most closely resembles the insulin pattern in nondiabetic humans. Regular insulin can be delivered intravenously. Intravenous administration of insulin is recommended in clients with acute conditions such as diabetic ketoacidosis or hyperosmolar nonketotic coma. Intramuscular injections have been used in the treatment of diabetic ketoacidosis if intravenous infusion capabilities are not available.[5]

Intranasal delivery of insulin has been tried. However, studies indicate that nasal irritation occurs in most clients using intranasal aerosolized insulin. An additional disadvantage to this dosage form is that five to ten times the usual dose is required. Insulin enclosed in a chemical complex that resists digestion, thereby allowing oral administration, and a transdermal delivery system are also being investigated.[13]

Insulin Regimen

The specific regimen prescribed for each client is based on several factors, including the age and weight of the client, presence of other medical problems or disabilities, and the philosophy of the health care team. The conventional insulin regimen involves the daily injection of insulin in the morning. With some clients, a second injection is needed in the evening.

Currently greater emphasis is placed on achieving near-normalization of blood glucose levels (normoglycemia) with fewer periods of hypoglycemia. To achieve this condition, multiple injections of insulin may be required. A regimen of self–blood glucose monitoring and administration of split and mixed insulin dosages or multiple daily injections of regular insulin combined with an intermediate- or long-acting insulin is frequently prescribed. The multiple dosage regimen or intensified insulin therapy allows greater flexibility in meal patterns and reduces the incidence of hypoglycemia. In addition, research has suggested that normoglycemia prevents, delays, or reverses some of the chronic complications associated with diabetes.[8,14] (See Fig. 39–1 for examples of intensified insulin therapy.)

CONCEPT REVIEW

Commercial insulins are derived from beef or pork pancreas. Semisynthetic insulin, manufactured by chemically modifying the amino acids of pork insulin, and synthetic human insulin, manufactured by using recombinant DNA from strains of *E. coli,* are also available.

Based on duration of action, insulin preparations are divided into three categories: short, intermediate, and long acting. Potency of insulin is expressed as USP units. All types of insulin are prepared in solutions of two different strengths: U-40 and U-100.

Most insulin is administered subcutaneously. However, regular insulin is also administered intravenously.

■ NURSING CONSIDERATIONS

Managing the care of a client receiving insulin is a challenge. Nursing care focuses on the initiation of the prescribed insulin regimen and evaluation of the client's response to the drug. Many clients newly diagnosed with diabetes mellitus require hospitalization until their condition stabilizes. Diabetic clients are also admitted to the hospital for regulation of their treatment plan. Many clients require follow-up nursing care in their home.

Assessing As with any client, you must complete a health history and physical assessment to obtain baseline data about the client. During the **health history** interview, determine when the initial diagnosis of diabetes mellitus was made. Assess the client's current lifestyle activities and determine the effect of the client's health status on these activities. Collect a current drug history, including information on all prescription and over-the-counter drugs. Review this information carefully and identify drugs that can alter the action of insulin. Assess for complications related to diabetes mellitus such as neuropathy, nephropathy, or retinopathy or to the prescribed medical regimen. Assess the client's ability to perform psychomotor skills such as self-monitoring of glucose levels or self-injection.

Determine the client's knowledge level regarding diabetes mellitus and the treatment plan. Assess psychosocial aspects such as role changes, use of support systems, and presence of financial concerns. Evaluate the client's ability to cope with a chronic illness that involves changes in lifestyle. During the interview attempt to establish a trust relationship. Without this,

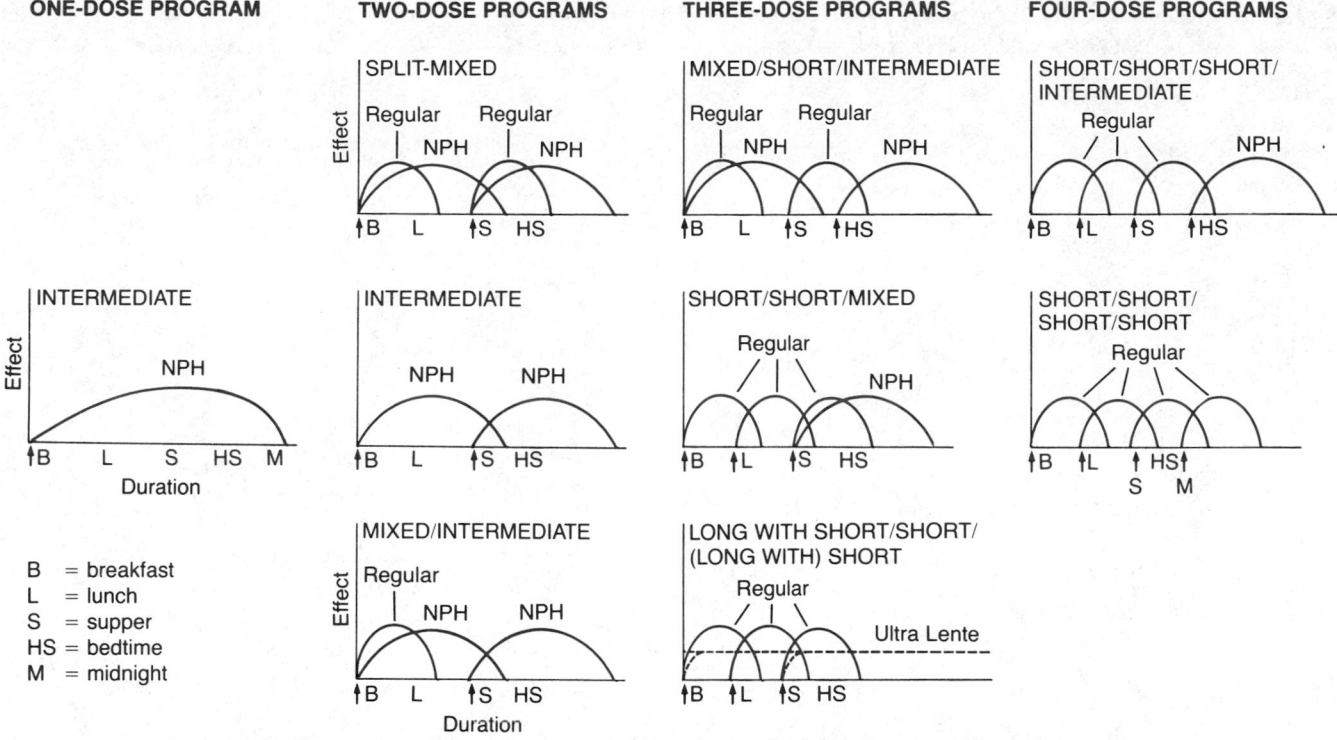

ONE-DOSE PROGRAM   **TWO-DOSE PROGRAMS**   **THREE-DOSE PROGRAMS**   **FOUR-DOSE PROGRAMS**

B = breakfast
L = lunch
S = supper
HS = bedtime
M = midnight

FIGURE 39–1   Insulin regimens. One injection per day of short-acting or intermediate-acting insulin may be enough to control blood glucose levels. However, split doses (two, three, or four injections of the daily dose) or mixed doses (a mixture of short- and longer-acting insulins) may give better control. (From Ignatavicius, D.D., & Bayne, M. [1991]. *Medical-surgical nursing.* Philadelphia: W.B. Saunders.)

the client may be unwilling to express fears and concerns that affect self-care.

Although a complete **physical assessment** is usually indicated in all clients, specifically assess aspects that reflect the status of the client with diabetes mellitus. High-risk areas include the integumentary, sensory, cardiovascular, genitourinary, and reproductive systems.

Diagnosing   Once the database has been established, analyze the data and develop appropriate nursing diagnoses. Based on the outcome of the data analysis, several nursing diagnoses are appropriate for the client receiving insulin. These diagnoses include the following:

• Altered health maintenance related to knowledge deficit regarding treatment plan.
• High risk for infection related to alterations in circulation and elevated serum glucose levels.
• Altered nutrition: less than body requirements related to insulin deficiency.
• Powerlessness related to perceived lack of control over illness.
• Anxiety related to change in self-concept and change or threat to health status.
• Knowledge deficit regarding treatment plan.
• High risk for injury related to changes in neuromuscular and sensory systems.

• High risk for altered skin integrity related to decreased tissue perfusion.

Planning   Focus the plan of care on the client's response to the disease process and treatment plan. The plan must also prepare the client or the client's significant other or both for self-care. Teaching plans are developed based on the needs of the client. If the client is newly diagnosed, a complete teaching/discharge plan is needed. Previously diagnosed clients usually benefit from a review of insulin administration technique, foot and skin care, and self-monitoring of blood glucose levels. As with any plan, consult the client and family before establishing specific goals, expected outcomes, and interventions.

Expected outcomes appropriate for the client receiving insulin include the following:

• Client plans a diet in accordance with prescribed fat, protein, and carbohydrate restrictions.
• Client demonstrates proper administration of insulin.
• Client demonstrates proper technique for monitoring blood glucose levels.
• Client describes plans for follow-up medical care.
• Client explains clinical manifestations of and treatment for hypoglycemia.
• Client demonstrates foot care procedures.
• Client identifies the resources available to promote positive adaptation to chronic illness.

ASSESSMENT OF CLIENTS WITH *IDDM*

Health History

SUPPORT SYSTEMS—ASSESS:

Presence of and support offered by significant others

Client's knowledge of support groups such as American Diabetes Association and Juvenile Diabetes Foundation

Type of health insurance coverage

Client's coping and problem-solving skills

KNOWLEDGE OF DISEASE—DETERMINE IF

CLIENT KNOWS:

When disease was diagnosed

Type of diabetes mellitus

Complications related to disease or drug therapy

Signs and symptoms of hypoglycemia and hyperglycemia

Need for follow-up care

KNOWLEDGE OF TREATMENT PLAN

Insulin therapy—determine if client knows:

Type of insulin used

Dosage regimen

Administration technique

Undesired clinical responses associated with prescribed insulin preparation

Proper storage of insulin

Measures to take when traveling

Risk for interactions with other drugs

Diet therapy—assess client's knowledge of:

Number of calories prescribed

Food exchanges

Menu planning

Scheduling of meals

Activity and exercise—determine client's:

Usual activity level

Type of work

Amount and type of recreational activities

Daily exercise pattern

SELF-CARE ACTIVITIES: ASSESS CLIENT'S KNOWLEDGE ABOUT:

Technique for blood glucose monitoring

Response to indications for hypoglycemia or hyperglycemia

Skin care measures

Foot care measures

Need for regular eye examinations

Actions to take when ill

Physical Assessment

INTEGUMENTARY SYSTEM—ASSESS FOR:

Signs of infection

Atrophy or hypertrophy at injection sites

Color and temperature of lower extremities

Presence of calluses or ulcers on feet

Healing ability of wounds

SENSORY SYSTEM—DETERMINE:

Visual acuity

Sensations of pain and touch in extremities, especially legs and feet

Presence of numbness or tingling in extremities

CARDIOVASCULAR SYSTEM—ASSESS:

Blood pressure and pulse

Pattern of blood pressure readings

Presence of chest or leg pain with exercise or rest

Indications of decreased circulation; check peripheral pulses and skin temperature

GENITOURINARY SYSTEM—ASSESS FOR:

Indications of urinary tract infection (e.g., burning during urination, frequency, hematuria)

Presence of polyuria, glycosuria, or ketonuria

Volume of urinary output

REPRODUCTIVE SYSTEM—DETERMINE:

Presence of impotence

Presence of frequent vaginal infections

• Client explains prescribed medical regimen.
• Client explains selected exercise pattern.

Implementing Nursing therapies initially are directed toward safe administration of the prescribed drug. Since insulin is destroyed by gastrointestinal (GI) enzymes, the parenteral route is the standard method of administration.

PREPARATION OF INSULIN INJECTION. Before preparing the insulin injection, check the written order for the insulin dosage. Read the label on the insulin vial carefully; determine the drug's expiration date and source (i.e., pork, beef, and the type of insulin preparation). Do not change the type and preparation of insulin without guidance from the primary care provider since this action may require an alteration in the dosage. Do not use insulin that has changed color or is clumped or granular in appearance. When modified insulin preparations are used, gently invert the bottle several times or rotate the insulin vial between both hands until the sediment in the bottom is suspended in the solution. Avoid shaking the vial since this action creates bubbles or foam. If refrigerated insulin is used, warm the insulin to room temperature before administering. Using cold insulin can lead to lipodystrophy, reduced rates of absorption, and local reactions.

Always use a syringe that coordinates with the potency of insulin that will be administered. Disposable plastic syringes are available with calibrations for U-100 or U-40 insulin. Each syringe holds 1 ml of solution. Usually a 26-gauge, ½-inch needle is directly attached to the disposable syringe. In some agencies two nurses are required to check the prepared insulin dose before administration.

ROTATION OF INJECTION SITES. Rotation of injection sites is required to prevent tissue damage. Common anatomic locations for injections include arms, thighs, back, and ab-

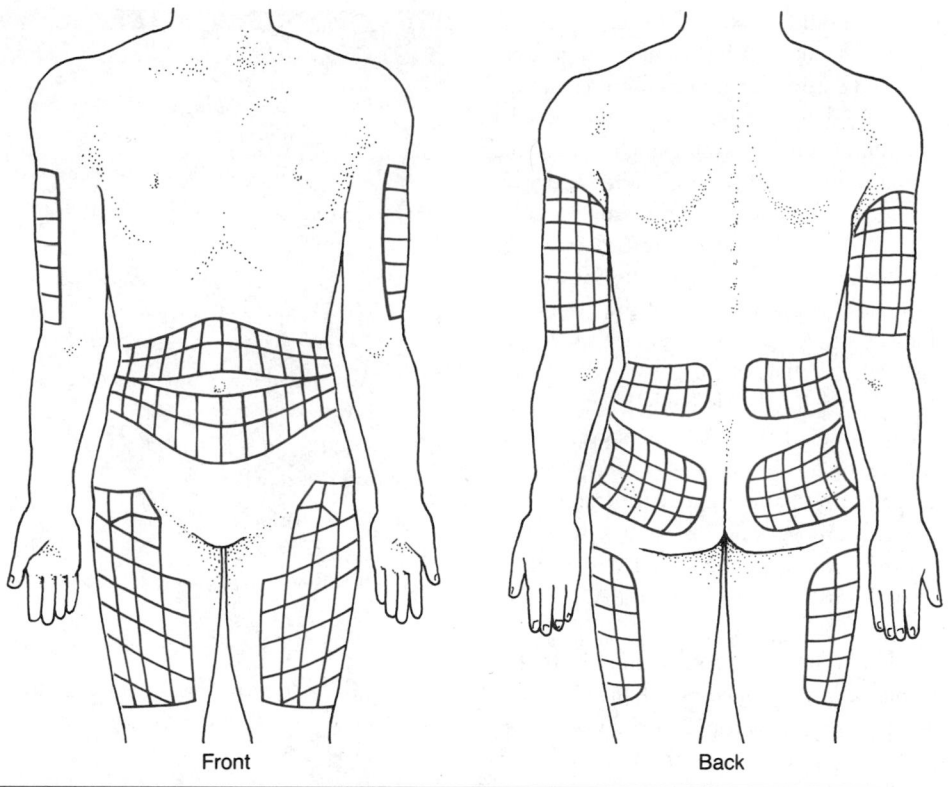

FIGURE 39–2   Common insulin injection sites. (From Ignatavicius, D.D., & Bayne, M. [1991]. *Medical-surgical nursing.* Philadelphia: W.B. Saunders.)

domen (Fig. 39–2). At one time it was recommended that the anatomic location be changed for each injection. However, since insulin absorption varies according to the location used, the preferred practice is to stay at one location for 1 week or more. Within that location (e.g., the right arm), the actual injection site is changed each time. Each injection site should be at least ½ to 1 inch away from a previous site. With this rotation, every anatomic location has a 4- to 6-week period of nonuse. Some practitioners recommend that only the abdomen be used for insulin injections since research has shown that insulin absorption is more complete in this area.

METHODS OF INSULIN DELIVERY. **Subcutaneous injections** are administered between the subcutaneous fat and muscle. Cleanse the injection site carefully and allow the skin surface to dry completely before the injection since alcohol precipitates insulin. Base the angle of injection on the client's body weight; usually, a 45- to 90-degree angle is used. (With a ½-inch needle, a 90-degree angle is preferred.) After injecting the insulin, withdraw the needle and apply pressure to the injection site; do not rub the area.[15]

Regular insulin may also be administered by intravenous push or by continuous intravenous infusion. When administered by **intravenous push,** administer the insulin slowly with an infusion rate of less than 50 units per minute. Do not mix regular insulin with other drugs; known incompatibilities exist between insulin and aminophylline, barbiturates, dobutamine, methylprednisolone, and phenytoin.

With **continuous intravenous infusion,** the dosage is calculated by units per hour. Since insulin adheres to intravenous tubing, flush the intravenous tubing with 50 ml of insulin and intravenous saline solution before beginning the insulin infusion. Use a drop counter or infusion pump to ensure careful rate regulation. Since equipment malfunction can occur, count the intravenous drip rate every hour. Monitor the serum glucose levels closely. Usually the continuous infusion is discontinued as the serum glucose level approaches normal to avoid hypoglycemia.

Continuous subcutaneous insulin infusion is prescribed for some clients. Two types of subcutaneous infusion pumps are available: a closed-loop pump and an open-loop pump. A closed-loop insulin pump samples the client's blood, determines the blood glucose level, and, based on the results, injects a predetermined amount of insulin. However, since the closed-loop insulin pump is large, the open-loop pump usually is prescribed. The open-loop insulin pump does not determine the serum glucose level. Instead, this is done with a portable, self-monitoring meter. Usually the open-loop insulin infuser consists of a syringe containing regular insulin, a small electronic pump, an infusion rate selector, a small rechargeable battery, and a small plastic catheter with a needle.[5] The open-loop pump either can administer a prescribed dosage of insulin automatically at a set time or can be manually activated to give the prescribed dosage.

The syringe on the pump is refilled every 1 to 3 days.

Needle sites for injections should be rotated at least every 3 days since longer usage at one site has been linked to greater occurrence of infections. To ensure continuous, uninterrupted service, a daily check of the battery supply is recommended. An added safety factor on most pumps is a locking mechanism that prevents inadvertent alteration of settings. With a highly motivated client, the open-loop insulin pump can provide consistent control of the serum glucose level, thus decreasing the complications associated with diabetes mellitus. However, the cost and the risk of possible dislodgment of the needle or kinking of the infusion tubing without the client's knowledge prevent the use of this device with all clients.

STORAGE OF INSULIN. Insulin that is being used can remain unrefrigerated since it maintains its potency at room temperature (15° to 30° C or 59° to 86° F) for long periods. However, sudden temperature changes and temperature extremes should be avoided. All surplus insulin preparations should be stored in a refrigerator. Opened vials of insulin should be replaced every 4 to 6 weeks and the unused portion of insulin discarded.

MIXING INSULIN PREPARATIONS. Insulins should not be mixed unless doing so has been prescribed by the primary care provider. Mixing insulin preparations usually produces better control of serum glucose levels and decreases the number of daily injections. However, since various buffers are added to the insulins, mixing can produce problems. The most obvious problem is the formation of a precipitate. In addition, buffers in one insulin preparation can neutralize the effectiveness of other insulin preparations.

PREPARATION FOR SELF-CARE. Preparing the client and family for self-care requires a well-organized and comprehensive teaching/discharge plan. Teaching should be initiated as early as possible. When clients are prepared to follow the prescribed drug and dietary therapy and to recognize signs and symptoms of adverse drug response, the number of hyperglycemia and hypoglycemia episodes is diminished.

Include in the teaching plan information about the pathology of IDDM and the role of insulin. Provide the client the name, dosage, action, frequency of administration, storage, and undesired clinical responses of the prescribed insulin preparation. Discuss with the client the expected benefits of the drug therapy. Review all drugs the client is taking and stress the importance of taking the drugs exactly as prescribed. Emphasize the need to contact the primary care provider before drugs are discontinued or new drugs are added to the drug regimen. Recommend to the client that he or she wear a medical identification tag or bracelet at all times. Caution the client to avoid the use of alcohol.

Demonstrate proper foot and skin care to the client and family member or significant other. Provide these individuals with written instructions about the care of specific skin problems (e.g., lesions, dryness). Demonstrate how to monitor blood glucose levels and administer insulin. Have the client (or individual administering insulin in the home) practice and perform a return demonstration to determine the level of understanding. When teaching the injection technique, include the following important points:

MIXING INSULIN PREPARATIONS

▶ Do not mix insulins from different species (e.g., pork insulin with beef insulin).

▶ Do not mix insulins if purity level is different.

▶ Do not mix insulins produced by different manufacturers.

▶ Avoid combining any buffered insulin (all brands of NPH, protamine zinc insulin, Humulin BR, and all Nordisk insulins) with any Lente preparation.

▶ Avoid combining protamine zinc insulin and regular insulin.

▶ Semilente, Lente, and Ultralente insulins may be mixed together in any ratio.

▶ Combination of NPH and regular insulin produces a stable mixture. This is the mixture of choice for short-acting and intermediate-acting insulin combinations.

▶ Mixture of NPH and regular insulin should be administered within 5 minutes of preparation.

▶ Mixture of Lente insulin and regular insulin should be administered immediately after preparation to avoid binding of the regular insulin.

▶ Regular insulin should always be drawn into the syringe first when insulins are mixed.

▶ Order in which insulins are drawn into solution should not be altered.[5,16]

- Use as many available anatomic locations as possible.
- Do not return to the same anatomic location more frequently than every 4 to 6 weeks.
- Avoid the use of the inner thigh, inner arm, and midline area of the abdomen.
- Depending on the amount of subcutaneous tissue at the injection site, use either a 45- or 90-degree injection angle.
- Allow ½ to 1 inch between injection sites in an anatomic location.

To reduce equipment expense, some clients reuse disposable syringes. This practice is not recommended since maintenance of sterile techniques becomes difficult. In addition, since the needle cannot be changed, the needle becomes dull, resulting in tissue damage at the injection sites.

Discuss with the client the importance of establishing and maintaining a daily exercise pattern. Review the dietary plan with the client and arrange for a dietitian to assist the client with menu planning. Exercise should not be performed at the peak time of insulin action, and the client should exercise no sooner than 20 minutes to 1 hour after mealtime. In addition, insulin should not be injected into the extremity that is exercised since drug absorption is enhanced.[7]

Be certain to discuss complications associated with diabetes mellitus (e.g., increased susceptibility to infection, vascular occlusion, and neuropathy). Provide the client with health pro-

---

TEACHING/DISCHARGE PLAN

The following information should be taught to the client and family or significant other:

1. In the home setting monitor the supply of insulin and syringes carefully to avoid running out. Do not change brands, preparations, or potency of insulin when getting prescription refills. Any change in insulin may result in a need to adjust dosage.
2. Carry supplies (insulin, syringes, alcohol, and cotton balls) directly with you when traveling. In addition, carry a prescription for your insulin in case supplies are lost. Since travel may result in sudden temperature changes, pay close attention to the environmental temperature of the insulin.
3. Follow-up care in the home may be needed. If so, arrangements can be made for a home health or visiting nurse. Make contact with available community resources such as the American Diabetes Association or local support groups as advised by primary care provider or nurse.

---

motion measures associated with these complications. Explain to the client the signs and symptoms of hyperglycemia and hypoglycemia. Provide written instructions regarding actions to take if these signs and symptoms are detected. Review with the client what actions to take if he or she becomes ill or unable to eat. Instruct the client to notify his or her primary care provider if the illness is severe or persistent.

NURSING RESEARCH

Weinbacher, F.M., Littlejohn, C.E., & Conley, P.F. (1990). Growth of bacteria in prefilled syringes stored in home refrigerators. *Applied Nursing Research, 3*(2), 63–67.

It has been the practice of home health nurses to prefill insulin syringes for visually impaired diabetic clients. After preparing the syringes, the nurses would leave a 1- to 2-week supply of prefilled syringes in the client's refrigerator.

The safety of this practice has come under question. To address this concern, syringes prefilled with U-100 Humulin insulin were stored in three different home refrigerators. To simulate actual client conditions, the temperature of the home refrigerators was not controlled but was determined to be 77° F. The controlled temperature of the laboratory refrigerator was −2° to +11° C (28° to 51.8° F).

Cultures from 96 prefilled syringes were taken at weekly intervals for a total of 4 weeks from both the home and laboratory refrigerators. A very low incidence of bacterial contamination was found; however, it was not statistically significant at $P <.05$. The bacterial growth that was found in the syringes consisted of normal skin flora.

The amount of bacterial contamination, although not statistically significant, was greater in syringes stored in home refrigerators at 77° F. No growth was found in syringes stored in the laboratory at 41° F. When the amount of bacterial growth from the uncontrolled home refrigerator was compared to the amount in an earlier study by the same researcher, it was found that the level of contamination of prefilled syringes was highest at room temperature of 98.6° F.

Although the results were not statistically significant, the authors noted a concern that any amount of bacterial contamination could be potentially harmful. Additional research is needed to determine the optional temperature to store prefilled syringes in the home and the influence of possible bacterial toxins and resistant organisms in prefilled syringes. Also, research is needed into the possibility of having the insulin vial contain an additive that would retard bacterial growth. It is possible that use of prefilled syringes is safe, but refrigeration is important for storage because it inhibits bacterial growth.

STUDENT ACTIVITIES

• Check the procedure for insulin storage in your assigned agency. Talk with an individual responsible for quality control within the agency and ask about the measures used to ensure proper insulin storage.
• Contact four local home health agencies and determine if they prefill syringes. If they do leave prefilled syringes, ask to review their policy for this procedure.

Evaluating Evaluating the effectiveness of drug therapy in clients with diabetes mellitus is based on the client's clinical response. To help determine the response, you or the client should monitor daily weights, serum glucose levels, and glycosylated hemoglobin levels.

To evaluate the effectiveness of the client's plan of care, review the expected outcomes previously developed with the client. To evaluate the effectiveness of your teaching, ask the client to demonstrate the procedures for testing serum glucose and administration of insulin injections and to describe the signs and symptoms of hypoglycemia and hyperglycemia. Describe possible scenarios to the client and ask him or her to describe how he or she should respond in these situations.

INSULIN

As previously indicated, insulin is the primary drug used to treat IDDM.

Pharmaceutics, Pharmacokinetics, and Specific Nursing Considerations

Individual preparations of insulin differ in their pharmaceutic and pharmacokinetic characteristics. The absorption rate of insulin administered subcutaneously varies according to the type of insulin preparation and the condition and location of the injection site. Usually absorption is most rapid from the abdominal areas, less rapid from the arm, and least rapid from the leg. However, if the client exercises the arms and legs after injecting insulin into them, absorption is faster.[12] Other factors that delay or decrease insulin absorption include the presence of circulatory problems (e.g., edema or hypotension), lipodystrophy, smoking, and injection of refrigerated insulin. Even though insulin is distributed widely throughout the body, some insulin is bound and inactivated by peripheral tissues. The majority of insulin is metabolized in the liver and kidneys. Although some insulin undergoes tubular reabsorption, most insulin is filtered by the renal glomeruli and excreted by the kidneys.[3,17–19]

SHORT-ACTING INSULINS

Solutions of regular and modified short-acting insulin are available. **Regular insulin** in purified beef, purified pork, unpurified pork, unpurified beef-pork combination, and recombinant DNA human form is accessible in the United States. It is usually administered subcutaneously and has an onset of action within 30 to 60 minutes of the injection.[12] Regular insulin is the only type of insulin that is administered intravenously. Intravenous administration is especially helpful in unstable diabetic clients or in clients whose requirements for insulin change rapidly. Regular insulin may be mixed with other insulin preparations when administered subcutaneously or intramuscularly. Mixing slightly prolongs the effects of the short-acting insulin.

A special formula of buffered regular insulin (**Humulin BR**) has been developed for use in the subcutaneous infusion pump. This insulin preparation has less potential for crystal formation in the tubing. Humulin BR insulin should not be directly injected by syringe. In addition, mixing Humulin BR with other insulin products should be avoided since the interaction between buffers creates a significant change in insulin action.[3]

Semilente (insulin zinc suspension, prompt) is a modified short-acting insulin. It is available in unpurified beef-pork combination, unpurified pork, and purified pork preparations; no human preparations are presently available. Semilente insulin is used infrequently. When prescribed, the preparation is usually in solutions that combine 30% short-acting insulin (Semilente) and 70% long-acting insulin (Ultralente). This mixture forms an intermediate-acting insulin (Lente). Since Semilente has a longer duration of action than regular insulin, it is not recommended for emergency or intravenous usage.[12,13]

Nursing considerations specific for clients receiving short-acting insulins include the following:

- Administer regular insulin 30 to 45 minutes before a meal. This allows the drug to reach a therapeutic level before the client eats.
- Do not administer short-acting insulin if the blood glucose level is below 70 mg/dl or if signs of hypoglycemia are present.
- Monitor the client carefully for signs and symptoms of hypoglycemia, especially near the peak action time of the insulin.

Regular insulin is frequently administered as part of a sliding scale. With a **sliding scale,** the dosage of insulin is based on the serum glucose level at the time of administration. At specific time intervals (e.g., every 4 hours), the client's serum glucose level is determined by laboratory analysis, bedside-monitoring devices, or self-monitoring meters. Once the serum glucose level is obtained, the sliding scale order is checked and the insulin dosage determined. For example, the order may read, "If the client's serum glucose level is 250 to 275 mg/dl, administer 8 U of regular insulin. If the serum glucose level is 276 to 300 mg/dl, administer 12 U of regular insulin."

During periods of clinical instability, a client with NIDDM might require injections of short-acting insulin. The anxiety level of these individuals is lessened if a clear explanation regarding the injections is provided. For information concerning onset, peak, and duration of action of short-acting insulin preparations, refer to Table 39–2.

INTERMEDIATE-ACTING INSULINS

Intermediate-acting insulins are produced by combining insulin with protamine, a protein from fish, or zinc. These additives prolong the action time of the insulin. Intermediate-acting insulins are administered only subcutaneously; their onset of action is 1 to 2 hours after the injection.

NPH (isophane insulin suspension) insulin is the most widely used intermediate-acting insulin. NPH insulin contains protamine and a small amount of zinc. It is available in unpurified beef, unpurified beef-pork combination, purified beef, purified pork, semisynthetic, and recombinant DNA human preparations.

The human NPH insulin preparation has a slightly shorter duration of action and faster onset of action than NPH pork insulin. In a few cases the human NPH insulin has produced a white precipitate, referred to as **flocculation** or frosting, that adheres to the vial. Although the exact cause of flocculation is unknown, excessive environmental heat, prolonged use of the vial, and vigorous mixing of the solution have been identified as contributing factors. Since flocculation decreases the potency of the insulin, if present, the insulin should not be used.[13,18]

Because NPH insulin has a longer onset of action, it is not used for initial treatment of diabetic ketoacidosis or emergencies.[19] NPH insulin may be mixed with regular insulin, which slows the absorption and the onset of action of the regular insulin.[3]

NPH and regular premixed insulin products are now available. This mixture is available in purified pork, semisynthetic, and recombinant DNA human preparations. Each preparation contains a fixed ratio of 30% regular insulin and 70% NPH insulin. This mixture retains the properties of both insulins. A premixed preparation of 50% regular and 50% NPH should be available in the United States shortly.[18] Additional premixed preparations are available in Europe.

Use of premixed insulin can reduce the number of errors made when using the standard mixing technique. This is especially true for clients who are visually impaired or have difficulty with hand coordination. However, since the ratio of NPH to regular insulin is fixed, the client's insulin needs must match the ratio of the premixed preparation.

Lente (insulin zinc suspension) insulin is another intermediate-acting preparation. As indicated earlier, Lente insulin is a mixture of 30% short-acting insulin zinc suspension (Semilente) and 70% long-acting insulin zinc suspension (Ultralente). As with NPH insulin, this insulin should not be used for emergencies. Additionally, Lente insulin should be mixed only with other Lente products. Mixtures of Lente insulin and regular insulin are subject to binding because of the zinc used to form Lente preparations.[17] Binding of the two insulins (regular and Lente) yields an uncertain concentration of the regular insulin.

Nursing considerations specific for clients receiving intermediate-acting insulins include the following:

- Monitor for hypoglycemia during mid- or late afternoon. With these preparations, the onset of hypoglycemia is less obvious, but the hypoglycemic episodes are more prolonged.[13]
- Observe clients receiving Lente insulin for adequate nutritional intake. The lengthy action time (12 to 18 hours) of the insulin produces additional risks for hypoglycemia.
- Incorporate evening snacks into the meal plan if the client receives an intermediate-acting insulin before supper. In these individuals the blood glucose level may drop to dangerously low levels during sleep, around midnight.

Intermediate-acting insulins normally have a cloudy appearance. To ensure correct suspension of the preparation, gently mix the solution by rotating the insulin vial between both hands. In addition, observe the vial for the white precipitate, flocculation, previously mentioned. For information concerning onset, peak, and duration of action of intermediate-acting insulin preparations, refer to Table 39–2.

LONG-ACTING INSULINS

Long-acting insulins are modified insulin preparations. These products have a very slow onset of action (4 to 8 hours) and a prolonged duration of action (18 to 72 hours). Long-acting insulins are seldom used alone. They most frequently are combined with short-acting insulins to provide blood glucose control throughout the entire day and night.[3] Because of their prolonged action time, it can be difficult to determine the optimal dosage. In addition, the client's blood glucose level may decrease during sleep and go undetected. Irritability, nightmares, and diaphoresis during the night may signal the occurrence of hypoglycemia.

Protamine zinc insulin (PZI) suspension contains more modifying protamine and zinc than intermediate-acting insulin. Because of the presence of these substances, clients receiving PZI are more prone to hypersensitivity reactions. PZI is available in unpurified beef-pork combination and purified beef preparations. Protamine zinc insulin is not suitable for use during emergencies or intravenous administration. Additionally, hypoglycemic reactions from PZI are unpredictable.

Ultralente (extended zinc suspension) insulin does not contain modifying protein, thus reducing the incidence of sensitivity reactions. Currently, Ultralente is the most widely used long-acting insulin. It is available in unpurified beef-pork combination, unpurified beef, purified beef, and biosynthetic human preparations. Because of its prolonged action time, it is rarely used alone. Ultralente may be combined with human regular, Lente, or Semilente insulins.

Nursing considerations for clients receiving long-acting insulins include the need to know each product's onset and duration of action. In addition, consistency in activity and nutritional intake for the client is very important. Human regular insulin and Ultralente insulin should be prepared in separate syringes. If there is a written order to mix the two insulins, administer the mixture immediately to preserve the effects of the short-acting insulin.[17] For information about onset, peak, and duration of action of long-acting insulin preparations, refer to Table 39–2.

Pharmacodynamics

Injected insulin mimics the effect of endogenous insulin. Insulin regulates the serum glucose level by controlling the metabolism of proteins, carbohydrates, and fats. At the cellular level, insulin increases the permeability of the cell's membrane to allow the required glucose, fatty acids, and amino acids to enter. Insulin acts as a catalyst to stimulate enzymes and chemicals required for cellular function and energy production. It also converts excess glucose into glycogen or fat for storage and maintains a constant glucose level by changing glycogen into glucose. In addition, insulin promotes the storage of fat by combining α-glycerophosphate (a product of glucose metabolism) with fatty acids to form triglycerides. It also increases the amount of body protein by facilitating the transportation of amino acids into the cell for protein synthesis.

Undesired Clinical Responses[13,19-21]

Clients can manifest undesired clinical responses to the insulin product itself or to the effect of the insulin on metabolism. Some of the side effects of insulin itself include lipotrophy, lipohypertrophy, insulin allergy, and insulin resistance. **Lipotrophy** is wasting of subcutaneous fat at the site of repeated insulin injections. On manual palpation, lipotrophic areas feel depressed or hollow. Lipotrophy probably is caused by an immune response. The condition is less prevalent when purified insulins are used.[3] With lipotrophy, irregular absorption of insulin occurs. To correct the condition, insulin is injected directly into the atrophied area. Repeated injections are administered around the atrophied area causing hypertrophy

TABLE 39–2
Insulin Preparations

Drug	Onset of Action (h)	Peak Action (h)	Duration of Action (h)	Description
SHORT ACTING				
Regular Insulin				
Iletin II R	½	2–4	4–6	Pork (purified)
Iletin II R	½	2–4	4–6	Beef (purified)
Iletin I R	½	2–4	4–6	Beef-pork mixture
Humulin R	½	2–3	3–6	DNA biosynthetic
Humulin BR*	½	2–3	3–6	DNA biosynthetic
Velosulin	½	2–3	4–6	Pork (purified)
Velosulin human	½	1–3	3–6	Semisynthetic
Regular	½–1	2½–5	4–6	Pork (purified)
Novolin R	½–1	2–4	3–6	Human
Semilente (Prompt Insulin Zinc Suspension)				
Iletin I/S	1–2	3–8	8–10	Beef-pork mixture
Iletin S/H	1–2	3–8	8–10	Human
Semilente	½–1	5–10	8–10	Beef
INTERMEDIATE ACTING				
NPH (Isophane Insulin Suspension)				
Iletin II N	1–2	6–12	12–14	Pork (purified)
Iletin I N	1–2	6–12	12–14	Beef-pork mixture
Humulin	1–2	6–12	10–12	DNA biosynthetic
Insulatard NPH	1–2	6–12	12–14	Pork
Insulatard NPH/H	1–2	4–10	10–12	Semisynthetic
NPH	1–1½	6–12	12–14	Beef
Novolin N	1–2	4–10	10–12	Human
Lente (Insulin Zinc Suspension)				
Iletin II L	1–3	6–12	14–16	Pork (purified)
Iletin IL	1–3	6–12	14–16	Beef-pork mixture
Iletin II L/H	1–3	4–12	12–18	Human
Lente	1–2	8–12	14–16	Beef
Novolin L	2½	8–12	12–18	Human
NPH and Regular Premixed Insulin Mixtard†				
Mixtard (30%R/70%N)	½+	2–4/8±	6–8/12–14	Pork (purified)-human mixture
Novolin mix (30%R/70%N)	½+	2–4/8±	6–8/12–14	
LONG ACTING				
Ultralente (Extended Insulin Zinc Suspension)				
Iletin I U	4–6	Minimal	24–36	Beef-pork mixture
Iletin II U/H	4–6	Minimal	18–20	Human
Ultralente	4–6	Minimal	24–36	Beef
Humulin Ultralente	4	Minimal	18–20	Human
Protamine Zinc Insulin (PZI) Suspension				
Protamine Zinc and Iletin	4–6	Minimal	36–72	Pork (purified)
Protamine Zinc and Iletin	4–6	Minimal	36–72	Beef (purified)
Protamine Zinc and Iletin I	4–6	Minimal	36–72	Pork-beef mixture

*Used for subcutaneous insulin pumps only.
†Initard 50%R/50%N is being investigated by the Food and Drug Administration.

of the underlying fat tissue, which eventually fills in the hollow depression.[11]

In contrast, **lipohypertrophy** is a nonimmune phenomenon involving localized hypertrophy of subcutaneous fat. As with lipotrophy, this condition occurs at the site of repeated injections. Although purified insulin and human products may contribute to lipohypertrophy, it is more common when unpurified insulin preparations are used. With lipohypertrophy, the involved area becomes raised; the skin becomes thicker, and the absorption of insulin at that particular site decreases. Lipohypertrophy lessens if a different site for injection is used.

Insulin allergy, a hypersensitivity reaction to insulin, is common and usually transient. Local reactions at the injection site may develop 1 to 2 weeks after therapy begins or 1 to 12 hours after an insulin injection. An allergic local response includes itching, swelling, redness, stinging, and warmth at the injection site. If local irritation is severe or persistent, a change in the insulin source may be needed. Anaphylactic responses are rare, although systemic urticaria has occurred. Because hypersensitivity is often due to noninsulin protein contaminants, use of the purified insulins has greatly reduced the incidence of insulin allergy. Additionally, clients highly sensitive to insulin can be densensitized with subcutaneous administration of small and frequent doses of insulin.

Insulin resistance is a rare complication of insulin therapy. A client with insulin resistance is unable to achieve blood glucose control with usual dosages. Instead, extremely high insulin requirements, sometimes more than 200 units per day, are required. This is frequently a self-limited condition and may clear spontaneously after several months.[22]

Undesired clinical responses related to the metabolic effects of insulin are common. **Hypoglycemia,** a blood glucose level at or below 60 mg/dl, is the most frequently occurring undesired response to insulin therapy.[21] Common causes of hypoglycemia include missed meals or erratic meal timing, excessive insulin dosage, and unplanned exercise. Occasional hypoglycemic episodes may occur with no demonstrable cause.

There are three clinical classifications of hypoglycemia: mild, moderate, and severe. With **mild hypoglycemia,** the individual feels symptoms but is not sufficiently impaired to interfere with normal activities or self-treatment. During a mild episode the blood glucose level usually decreases to approximately 50 mg/dl, and the client experiences clinical manifestations, which include shakiness, tremulousness, diaphoresis, lightheadedness, nervousness, circumoral pallor, visual disturbances, tachycardia, palpitations, hunger, and weakness. With **moderate hypoglycemia,** the individual exhibits symptoms of obvious impairment of mental or motor functioning but is still alert enough to seek self-treatment. During a moderate episode the blood glucose decreases to approximately 40 mg/dl. Clinical manifestations include inability to concentrate, increased lethargy, mood and behavioral changes, confusion, tingling or numbness of extremities, slurred speech, lack of motor coordination, and headache. When the blood glucose level reaches 30 mg/dl, the individual still can be aroused but is unable to perform simple tasks. Below this level, the individual is unable to initiate self-treatment and needs the assistance of another individual. With **severe hypoglycemia,** the individual is unable to move and displays jerky movements and disoriented behavior. Unconsciousness, seizures, coma, irreversible brain damage, and death may occur.

Initial treatment of hypoglycemia includes determining the actual blood glucose level. This can be done by the client or nurse using a self-monitoring device. If the blood glucose level is 60 mg/dl, 15 g of carbohydrate are administered. Fifteen grams of carbohydrate is equivalent to one of the following: 4 ounces of unsweetened orange or grapefruit juice; 8 ounces of skim, 2%, or whole milk; or 4 ounces of grape juice. (Grape juice is recommended for clients with renal failure instead of orange juice.) If a hospitalized client sustains a severe hypoglycemia episode, dextrose 50% in water ($D_{50}W$) may be administered by intravenous bolus.

If the hypoglycemic episode occurs at or near bedtime, treatment should be followed with a snack. Beneficial snacks include one peanut butter and crackers packet, one cheese and crackers packet, or 4 ounces of milk and two graham crackers. These complex carbohydrates raise the serum glucose slowly, and their effect lasts a long time.

Hyperglycemic rebound (**Somogyi effect**) may develop when a client chronically receives overdoses of insulin. Somogyi effect is characterized by wide differences in the early morning and postprandial glucose levels. Typically early morning hypoglycemia is followed by postprandial hyperglycemia.[23] The blood glucose level drops below normal in response to excess insulin. This results in lipolysis, gluconeogenesis, and glycogenolysis, which produces a rebound hyperglycemia and ketosis. The danger of the Somogyi effect is that the client or health care professional may assess the situation as hyperglycemia and increase the insulin dosage. Clients experiencing the Somogyi effect may report headaches when awakening and recall night sweats or nightmares. The treatment involves lowering the insulin dosage and closely monitoring the blood glucose level.[5,23]

More common in adolescents and adult diabetics is the **dawn phenomenon**—an increase in hepatic glucose output on awakening. The dawn phenomenon is believed mediated by nocturnal surges of growth hormone that cause a rise in the blood glucose level. The awakening client manifests hyperglycemia and ketonuria. Treatment for the dawn phenomenon is an adjustment in the timing of insulin administration or an increase in the insulin dosage or both.[23]

Hyperglycemia is the result of missed insulin injections or may develop with the progression of diabetes. It occurs most frequently in the newly diagnosed client but can occur in clients who have had diabetes mellitus for a long time. If hyperglycemia is left untreated, it can progress to diabetic ketoacidosis (DKA).

DKA requires prompt recognition and treatment. Although there is no uniformly accepted definition of **DKA,** commonly accepted elements of the condition include the following:

· Presence of metabolic acidosis resulting in an arterial pH of less than 7.3
· Elevated plasma ketone level
· Blood glucose concentration greater than 300 mg/dl

Clinical manifestations of DKA include persistent nausea, rapid respirations (early), Kussmaul respirations (deep breathing) associated with a fruity, acetone odor as the acidosis increases, flushed face, parched lips and tongue, dry skin, drowsy to stuporous mental state, and diminished reflexes.[20]

Treatment includes fluid replacement, insulin therapy, electrolyte replacement, and monitoring the client's condition[5,7,13]:

· **Fluid replacement:** Initially 0.9% normal saline solution (NS) is infused rapidly at 1 L/h for 1 to 4 hours. Subsequent fluid replacement is with 0.5 NS. When blood glucose level falls to 250 mg/dl, replacement is with 5% dextrose in 0.5 NS.
· **Insulin:** Initial administration is an intravenous bolus of 0.1 U/kg regular insulin followed by 5 to 10 U/h regular insulin by intravenous infusion. The intravenous infusion rate is titrated to lower the blood glucose level by 75 to 100 mg/dl/h.

- **Electrolyte replacement:** Potassium chloride is added to the intravenous fluids unless the client is hyperkalemic. Sodium bicarbonate may be needed if the pH of the blood is less than 7.1
- **Monitoring:** It is recommended that the blood glucose level be monitored every 1 to 2 hours until DKA is resolved. The arterial blood gas (ABG) levels are checked hourly until the pH is greater than 7.2. Thereafter, the ABG levels are checked only if the client is not improving clinically. Usually urinary output is monitored hourly.

Contraindications and Precautions

The major contraindication to insulin therapy involves hypersensitivity to the source of the drug. It must be determined whether the client is allergic to pork or beef before insulin preparations from these sources are administered.

Drug-Drug, Drug-Nutrient, Drug-Environment Interactions[3,9,11]

A variety of drugs interfere with insulin therapy. Drug-induced hypoglycemia is caused by numerous drugs, including ethanol, β-adrenergic blockers, and salicylates. The primary action of ethanol is to inhibit gluconeogenesis; this action is observed in all individuals, even if diabetes mellitus is not present. Diabetic clients receiving β-adrenergic blockers may develop hypoglycemia because these drugs inhibit the effects of catecholamine on gluconeogenesis and glycogenolysis. β-Adrenergic blockers may also mask the tachycardia associated with a fall in the blood glucose level. Salicylates exert their hypoglycemic effect by enhancing the sensitivity of pancreatic beta cells to glucose, which increases insulin secretion.[24,25] For additional drugs that may produce hypoglycemia, see box.

An equally large number of drugs can cause hyperglycemia in nondiabetic individuals or impair metabolic control in diabetic clients. Some of these drugs (e.g., epinephrine, glucocorticoids, barbiturates, and oral contraceptives) have direct effects on the peripheral tissues opposite to the actions of insulin.[3,24] Other drugs produce hyperglycemia directly by inhibiting insulin secretion (e.g., phenytoin, clonidine, calcium channel blockers) or indirectly by depleting intracellular potassium (e.g., diuretics). Nicotinic acid decreases the absorption of insulin administered subcutaneously, thus increasing the blood glucose level. Clients should not smoke for 30 minutes after the injection of insulin. See box for additional drugs that cause hyperglycemia.

Drug-nutrient interactions are also important.[9,13] Most individuals receiving insulin are given a meal plan that includes three meals and an evening snack. Consumption of the evening snack is important in preventing possible hypoglycemia during the night. In addition, the intake of fiber and fat must be monitored carefully.

In the United States the average diet contains 10 to 20 g of dietary fiber. High-fiber diets of 40 to 50 g of fiber per day, especially of the water-soluble variety, improve carbohydrate metabolism. The client should include beans, peas, nuts, green leafy vegetables, whole-grain cereals, and fruits in the daily meal plans. Fruits and vegetables should be eaten raw to maximize the fiber effect.

DRUGS THAT MAY INTERFERE WITH INSULIN THERAPY	
Drug-Induced Hypoglycemia	**Drug-Induced Hyperglycemia**
Naproxen	Somatotropin
Clofibrate	Thyroid hormone
Bromocriptine mesylate	Glycogen
Mebendazole	Epinephrine
Captopril	Diazoxide
Disopyramide	Phenytoin
Acetaminophen	Clonidine
Dicumarol	Morphine sulfate
Monoamine oxidase inhibitors	Heparin sulfate
Chloramphenicol	Levodopa
Isoniazid	Lithium carbonate
Oxyphenbutazone	Furosemide
Probenecid	
Indomethacin	
Theophylline	

A fat-modified diet lessens the risk for atherosclerosis that is so common in diabetic clients. The total fat intake should be restricted to less than 30% of the total calories, and the cholesterol content should be less than 300 mg per day.

Aspartame is probably the safest sweetener for diabetics. However, since it is broken down by heat, it should not be used in baking or cooking. Long-term ingestion of saccharin has a potential for bladder carcinogenicity. It use in children and pregnant women should be restricted.

Drug-environment interactions also occur with insulin. Insulin can lose its potency if exposed to extreme temperatures (i.e., above 32° C [89.6° F] or below 3.5° C [38° F]).[11] At room temperature the potency of insulin is stable up to 1 year. However, most manufacturers recommend replacing open vials every 3 months and storing surplus insulin in the refrigerator.

Life-Span Considerations

Since IDDM can occur in any age group, nursing care must be adjusted to meet the client's developmental and chronologic age.

Infancy through childhood Infants and toddlers require very small dosages of insulin. Sometimes a dose of 2 U of U-100 insulin or less may be prescribed. If greater flexibility and accuracy of dosage are needed, an insulin concentration of U-25 or U-50 may be used. In addition, low-dosage syringes are available. As indicated earlier, most insulin syringes are calibrated to hold 1 ml of solution. Low-dosage syringes are calibrated to hold 0.5 ml or less.

Infants and toddlers cannot tell their parents when they are experiencing symptoms of hypoglycemia. Therefore more frequent testing of the blood glucose level is needed. Even the collection of capillary blood samples can be difficult in this age group because of the size of the fingers and movement of the hands and body. If necessary, the caregiver can collect blood samples from heels or earlobes. Since small children usually eat a higher proportion of their total daily calories at breakfast, the amount of regular insulin administered before breakfast is higher than other dosages during the day. Uncertain or finicky eating styles of the child may contribute to a low or difficult-to-control blood glucose level.[26]

When hypoglycemia does occur in young children, an early clinical manifestation may be a seizure. Therefore caregivers must be alerted to this possibility. In addition, some children experience transient hemiparesis after the seizure episode. Usually there is marked improvement in the hemiparesis within 6 hours and complete resolution within 24 hours.[26] To treat the hypoglycemia, an oral form of glycogen usually is used.

With preschool-age children, the unpredictable food intake and activity level combine to increase the possibility of hypoglycemia. Usually a multiple-injection regimen of mixed short- and intermediate-acting insulins is used to maintain a serum glucose level of 100 to 200 mg/dl.[26] Approximately 60% to 65% of the total daily insulin dosage is administered before breakfast; the remainder is administered before supper. As children in this age group begin to express interest, they should be taught to self-administer their insulin (with supervision).[11]

Adolescence   The goal for this age group is that the individual assumes responsibility for self-care. However, socialization needs and peer group pressure present many temptations to the adolescent. Providing education and assistance in coping with the disorder is important. Emphasis should be on how the individual is similar to, not different from, other adolescents.

During periods of growth spurt, insulin requirements generally increase substantially. Therefore insulin requirements should be reviewed regularly. Determining periodic glycosylated hemoglobin findings is useful since the test reflects the overall consistency of diabetic control. In addition, frequent monitoring by the finger-stick glucose meter helps maintain a consistent blood glucose level. Once again, a multiple-injection regimen is preferred.

Elderly   Changes in the diet and activity level combine to make control of blood glucose levels difficult in this age group. In addition, decreased visual acuity and motor coordination may impair the client's ability to perform self-injection or self-monitoring of blood glucose levels.

With the elderly, hyperosmolar nonketotic coma is more common than DKA. (See the section "Drug Therapy for Non-insulin-dependent Diabetes Mellitus" for additional information about hyperosmolar nonketotic coma.) The client often has an impaired sense of thirst or a physical disability that limits the intake of water. With a lack of fluid intake, osmotic diuresis results, causing a hyperosmolar imbalance of the blood. However, there is sufficient insulin to prevent ketosis.[27] In addition, many clients in this age group begin experiencing the chronic complications such as renal failure, neuropathy, and macrovascular and microvascular changes in the circulatory system related to long-standing diabetes.

Pregnancy   As previously indicated, gestational diabetes appears during pregnancy and generally disappears as soon as the pregnancy ends.[28] Gestational diabetes occurs in 2% to 3% of pregnancies and often is diagnosed in the third trimester. The cause is related to the physiologic changes that occur during pregnancy. Hormones produced during pregnancy (e.g., estrogen, progesterone) increase insulin requirements, whereas the placenta simultaneously promotes insulin catabolism. Insulin is required if the hyperglycemia is not lowered by diet. Use of oral hypoglycemia drugs is not recommended since these drugs cross the placenta and could harm the fetus. Usually insulin requirements begin to decrease 24 to 72 hours after delivery and return to prepregnancy levels in approximately 6 weeks.[13]

In pregnant clients with preexisting diabetes mellitus, the risk of fetal and neonatal complications (e.g., congenital malformations, fetal death) is increased. These complications are generally related to the severity of the client's diabetes. During the first trimester of pregnancy insulin requirements are usually unchanged or even slightly decreased. However, insulin requirements increase during the second and third trimesters.

To ensure the health of the mother and fetus, self-monitoring of blood glucose levels by the client is essential. Stringent control of blood glucose levels is very important and may require more frequent insulin injections. The usual schedule for the pregnant woman includes two injections, one before breakfast and the other before the evening meal. These injections consist of a short- and intermediate-acting insulin mixture. In some clients additional injections may be required for ideal control.[13]

Surgery and the Client Requiring Insulin

More than 50% of the clients with diabetes mellitus require surgical intervention during their lifetime. The perioperative care for these clients varies with the level of metabolic control that exists preoperatively. Generally it is recommended that a blood glucose level between 120 and 200 mg/dl be maintained.

If the client is receiving nothing by mouth before surgery, the preferred technique is to administer regular insulin intravenously with a glucose solution. In this case usually no subcutaneous insulin is administered. In the initial postoperative period the client's serum glucose level usually is evaluated every 4 hours, and insulin is administered according to a sliding scale. The client's usual diet and insulin regimen should resume as soon as possible.[5,13]

CONCEPT REVIEW

Nursing care focuses on the initiation of the prescribed insulin regimen and evaluation of the client's response to the drug.

The plan of care must involve teaching that prepares the client for self-care. If the client is newly diagnosed, a complete teaching/discharge plan is needed. Previously diagnosed clients usually benefit from a review of insulin administration technique, foot and skin care, and self-monitoring of blood glucose levels. Insulin is administered parenterally. Extreme care must be taken during the preparation and administration of insulin.

DRUG THERAPY FOR NON-INSULIN-DEPENDENT DIABETES MELLITUS

In clients with NIDDM the pancreas can produce limited amounts of endogenous insulin. However, the amount produced is not sufficient to maintain blood glucose levels within normal values. This may be due to insufficient production of insulin, excessive intake of carbohydrates, or increased hepatic glucose production. In addition, in some clients, NIDDM is caused by the production of antibodies to either the insulin or the insulin receptor in the cell membrane. In this situation the insulin is destroyed or inactivated before it can be bound to the glucose for transportation into the cell.[5,29–31]

Oral Hypoglycemic Drugs

Oral hypoglycemic drugs generally are more effective in diabetic clients who are 30 years old or older at the time of onset, who are obese or of normal weight, and who are not using insulin or have been controlled with less than 40 units per day. Additionally, oral hypoglycemic drugs are more effective in individuals who have been diabetic for 5 years or less.[19]

However, even in these individuals, the blood glucose level is not well controlled in 15% to 30% of clients.[13] Many are eventually switched from oral hypoglycemic drugs to insulins. These treatment failures may occur at the beginning of therapy or develop gradually as the client's system becomes less sensitive to the drugs. The exact reason for treatment failure is not clear. It may be associated with pancreatic beta cell death or failure. In addition, nonobese clients are more prone to therapeutic failure than obese clients.[32]

Currently in the United States the **sulfonylureas** are the major oral drugs available for treating NIDDM. Systematic studies were done to isolate insulin, but the hypoglycemic effect of sulfonylureas was accidentally discovered. In 1942 it was observed that some sulfonamides caused hypoglycemia in experimental animals. After further study, carbutamide was marketed as the first clinically useful sulfonylurea for the treatment of NIDDM. However, because the drug produced adverse effects on the bone marrow, carbutamide was later withdrawn from the market. Presently, there are more than 20 different drugs in the sulfonamide class.[3]

A second group of drugs, **biguanides,** are also capable of lowering blood glucose levels. However, the first drug in this category, phenformin, was withdrawn from usage in the United States because of the increased occurrence of lactic acidosis.[3] Newer drugs of this type are currently being investigated. For example, metformin was recently approved in the United States and is being used in Canada and Europe. Metformin does not stimulate the release of insulin, but it may increase the sensitivity of insulin receptors in the peripheral cells. Therefore the result is an increase in transferred glucose from the blood into the cells for metabolic function.[19]

NURSING CONSIDERATIONS

Clients with NIDDM are first treated with exercise and diet. If this regimen fails to maintain control over the client's serum glucose level, one of the oral hypoglycemic drugs is started. However, exercise and diet control remain important components of the treatment plan.

Assessing   As with IDDM, assessment is required to determine baseline data about the client. This assessment includes the basic parameters noted in the box. In addition, it is important to assess the client's knowledge of how NIDDM differs from IDDM, why a oral hypoglycemic agent is being used, if and when insulin may be required, and possible drug interactions with the oral hypoglycemic agent.

Since many individuals are older and obese at the time of initial diagnosis, assessment for early clinical manifestations of complications becomes significant. High-risk systems include the integumentary, sensory, cardiovascular, genitourinary, and reproductive. In addition, the individual may already have a disease process before developing NIDDM. Therefore you must determine the potential impact of NIDDM on previous medical conditions. Elderly clients may need assistance with the treatment plan (e.g., dietary changes, foot care, drug administration). Therefore the presence or absence of an adequate support system is important. You also should determine if the client is aware of available community agencies.

Diagnosing   After you have collected the database, the client's needs are formulated into nursing diagnoses. Although all nursing diagnoses are individualized to the client, the diagnoses listed for the client with NIDDM are appropriate for this client also.

Planning   Planning care for the client with NIDDM must involve the client since many of the interventions are self-care in nature. Once again the support system must be included. Plan teaching activities so that the client is not overwhelmed. Teach or review information about nutrition, drug therapy, foot and skin care, and self-monitoring of blood glucose levels. Time must be allowed for practice of blood glucose testing. Adapt self-care measures to the client's ability. For example, the use of a mirror to check the feet prevents the client's having to bend over to evaluate the condition of skin.

Expected outcomes appropriate for the client receiving oral hypoglycemic drugs include the following:
- Client plans a diet in accordance with prescribed carbohydrate, protein, and fat restriction.
- Client demonstrates correct technique for monitoring blood glucose level.
- Client expresses plans for continued follow-up care.
- Client explains administration and side effects of oral hypoglycemic drugs.
- Client explains clinical manifestations and treatment for hypoglycemia.

Teaching/Discharge Plan for Client with IDDM

The following information should be taught to the client and family or significant other:

1. Insulin
   - Type of insulin(s), dosage, and administration schedule
   - Onset, peak, and duration of action for prescribed insulin(s)
   - Danger of omitting meals or snacks
   - Care and storage of insulin and syringes
   - Technique for preparing and administering insulin
   - Injection sites and intrasite rotation pattern
   - Use of other prescription or over-the-counter drugs
2. Exercise
   - Benefits of an exercise program and the need to maintain a consistent exercise pattern
   - Tell client to:
     Exercise after a meal
     Carry a source of rapid-acting carbohydrate
     Avoid injecting insulin into muscle mass that will be exercised
     Monitor serum glucose level before and after exercise
     Wear or carry diabetic identification
     Avoid exercising alone
3. Nutrition
   - Benefits of eating according to prescribed dietary pattern
   - Teach client:
     To schedule meals and snacks to prevent hypoglycemia and hyperglycemia
     How to plan meals
     How to measure portion size
     How to select foods when eating out
4. Self-monitoring blood glucose testing
   - Schedule for testing blood glucose levels
   - Testing during periods of illness: check blood glucose level every 4 hours or more often if needed; check urine for ketones every 4 hours if blood glucose level is 250 mg/dl
   - Testing procedure
   - Storage of reagent strips
   - Technique for cleaning the monitor or meter
   - Method for recording the results
5. Hypoglycemia
   - Common causes: too much medication or medication administered at wrong time; delayed, missed, or inadequate food intake; increased activity or exercise; and alcohol ingestion
   - Signs and symptoms: restlessness, tachycardia, shakiness, sweating, pallor, hunger, irritability, headache, confusion, memory difficulties, and nervousness
   - Treatment of mild or moderate hypoglycemia: 15 g of simple glucose (4 to 6 crackers; ½ cup sugar-free pudding, 1 slice of bread, ½ cup cooked cereal, 1 small piece of fruit, ½ cup canned fruit, ½ tube of glucose gel, 3 glucose tablets)
6. Hyperglycemia and diabetic ketoacidosis
   - Common causes: missed insulin injections, illness
   - Signs and symptoms of ketoacidosis: flushed, dry skin; rapid, deep breathing; acetone breath; lethargy; nausea; vomiting; decreased level of consciousness; and hyperglycemia, usually 300 mg/dl
   - Treatment of both conditions
7. Sick day rules
   - When to call the primary care provider: vomiting or diarrhea continues more than 4 hours; poor food or fluid intake continues for more than 24 hours; illness lasts for more than 24 to 48 hours; elevated blood glucose levels with increased thirst and urination develop; urinary ketones are present in moderate to large amounts, and progressive drowsiness occurs
   - Drugs: continue usual insulin dosage
   - Diet: continue with regular meal plan if possible; if unable to eat from a normal meal plan, eat 50 to 100 g of easily digested carbohydrates (e.g., orange juice, regular soda, applesauce, pudding); drink small amounts of fluids every 10 to 15 minutes, and record all food and liquids
   - Monitoring: check blood glucose level a minimum of every 4 hours; check urine for ketones if blood glucose is >250 mg/dl
8. Chronic complications
   - Common complications: neuropathy, retinopathy, infections, atherosclerosis, cardiovascular disease
   - Common risk factors: smoking, hypertension, elevated serum cholesterol, lack of exercise.

• Client identifies resources available to promote positive adaptation to a chronic illness.

Implementing NIDDM clients must understand that drug therapy does not cure diabetes mellitus. Provide the client with a clear explanation of the actions of the prescribed drug and a description of the desired response. Include information about dosage, timing of administration, and drugs to avoid while receiving hypoglycemic drugs.

Since insulin injections are not required, some clients may believe that the disease is not "serious." Explain to the client that chronic complications related to diabetes mellitus, such as cardiovascular diseases, do occur with NIDDM. Although hypoglycemia does not commonly occur with oral hypoglycemic drugs, clients still must be aware of its symptoms and treatment.

Oral hypoglycemic drugs are more effective when administered before meals. If a client requires multiple dosages, the drug is usually administered before breakfast and the evening meal. Remind the client that only the prescribed amount should be taken.

Evaluating The effectiveness of the treatment regimen is based on the clinical response of the client. Of great importance are the client's serum glucose level, glycosylated hemoglobin level, and weight. In addition, the presence or absence of long-complications reflects the effectiveness of the treatment regimen.

To evaluate the client's plan of care, review the expected outcomes with the client. Determine if the client can explain the role of oral agents in a client with NIDDM. Have the client state drugs to avoid taking with an oral hypoglycemic agent. Ask the client about the signs of hypoglycemia and the treatment for it. Have the client demonstrate knowledge of dietary requirements by planning 24 hours of meals. Also ask the client to demonstrate self-monitoring of the blood glucose level.

ORAL HYPOGLYCEMIC PROTOTYPE

SULFONYLUREAS

As previously indicated, the prototype for oral hypoglycemic drugs is the sulfonylurea group. Although these drugs are sulfonamide derivatives, they do not have antibacterial actions.

Pharmacotherapeutics First-generation sulfonylureas include acetohexamide (Dymelor), chlorpropamide (Diabinese), tolazamide (Tolinase), and tolbutamide (Orinase). These drugs were among the first sulfonylureas available to treat NIDDM. Second-generation compounds are glyburide (DiaBeta, Micronase) and glipizide (Glucotrol). These drugs have been used in the United States since 1983.[32] Second-generation sulfonylureas are more potent that the first-generation drugs; therefore smaller dosages are required. Generally, use of second-generation sulfonylureas is recommended if the client is a newly diagnosed diabetic.

Pharmacokinetics The pharmacokinetics of all sulfonylureas is similar. Most are effectively absorbed from the GI tract, metabolized by the liver, and excreted in the urine. The primary therapeutic differences among these drugs are the duration of action and their relative potencies.[13] All first-generation sulfonylureas except tolbutamide have active metabolites. This makes tolbutamide especially helpful in clients with impaired renal function.

The duration of action and half-lives of second-generation sulfonylureas are more predictable. In addition, the first-generation sulfonylureas are carried in the plasma as ions bound to albumin as is common with many other drugs. This means the first-generation drugs compete for binding sites, which creates the potential for many drug-drug interactions.[32] Second-generation drugs are transported in the plasma nonionically bound to albumin and do not compete for binding sites with other drugs. Thus they are safer to use in clients who take multiple medications.[32]

Pharmacodynamics Sulfonylureas are *not* a form of oral insulin. These drugs indirectly lower the individual's serum glucose level by enhancing production of insulin and by stimulating the release of insulin from still-active pancreatic beta cells. Sulfonylureas may help slow or decrease the conversion of glycogen into glucose by the liver, thus inhibiting glycogenolysis and gluconeogenesis. In addition, the sulfonylureas increase the number of insulin receptors on peripheral cells and increase the sensitivity of the receptors to insulin. This means that less insulin is required to maintain cellular metabolism.[3,19,32] First-generation sulfonylureas exert their greatest effect by stimulating insulin release. Second-generation drugs have their maximal effect on cellular receptors.[32]

Undesired Clinical Responses Undesired clinical responses are uncommon with sulfonylureas. The most frequent reactions to sulfonylureas are associated with the GI tract. The client may experience nausea, vomiting, anorexia, diarrhea, or constipation. GI symptoms may be lessened by reducing the dosage (if possible) or by splitting the dosage. In some instances the symptoms spontaneously disappear. Other reactions to sulfonylureas include dizziness, headache, transient rash, pancytopenia, and hemolytic anemia. Figure 39–3 illustrates common undesired clinical responses associated with sulfonylureas.

Concerns common to all first-generation sulfonylureas include skin reactions, allergic reactions, and intolerance to alcohol. Skin reactions, although rare, include sensitivity to sunlight. Some clients experience a rash or a sunburn on skin directly exposed to the sun. Intolerance to alcohol, although it may occur with any of the sulfonylureas, is more common if the client is taking chlorpropamide. The reaction is disulfiram-like. Skin flushing is the most common manifestation, but nausea and vomiting may also occur.

Hypoglycemia may occur with any of the sulfonylureas. Usually the low serum glucose level is due to insufficient dietary intake, weight loss, increased activity, lessening of previous stress, or impaired renal or hepatic function.[32] These reactions usually are more common in the elderly.

Hyperosmolar hyperglycemic nonketotic coma results from an extreme elevation of the blood glucose level with only slight, if at all, elevation of ketone bodies. This condition is due to the presence of sufficient insulin to suppress ketogenesis but insufficient insulin to prevent hyperglycemia.[20] Hyperosmolar hyperglycemic nonketotic coma usually occurs in individuals who are more than 60

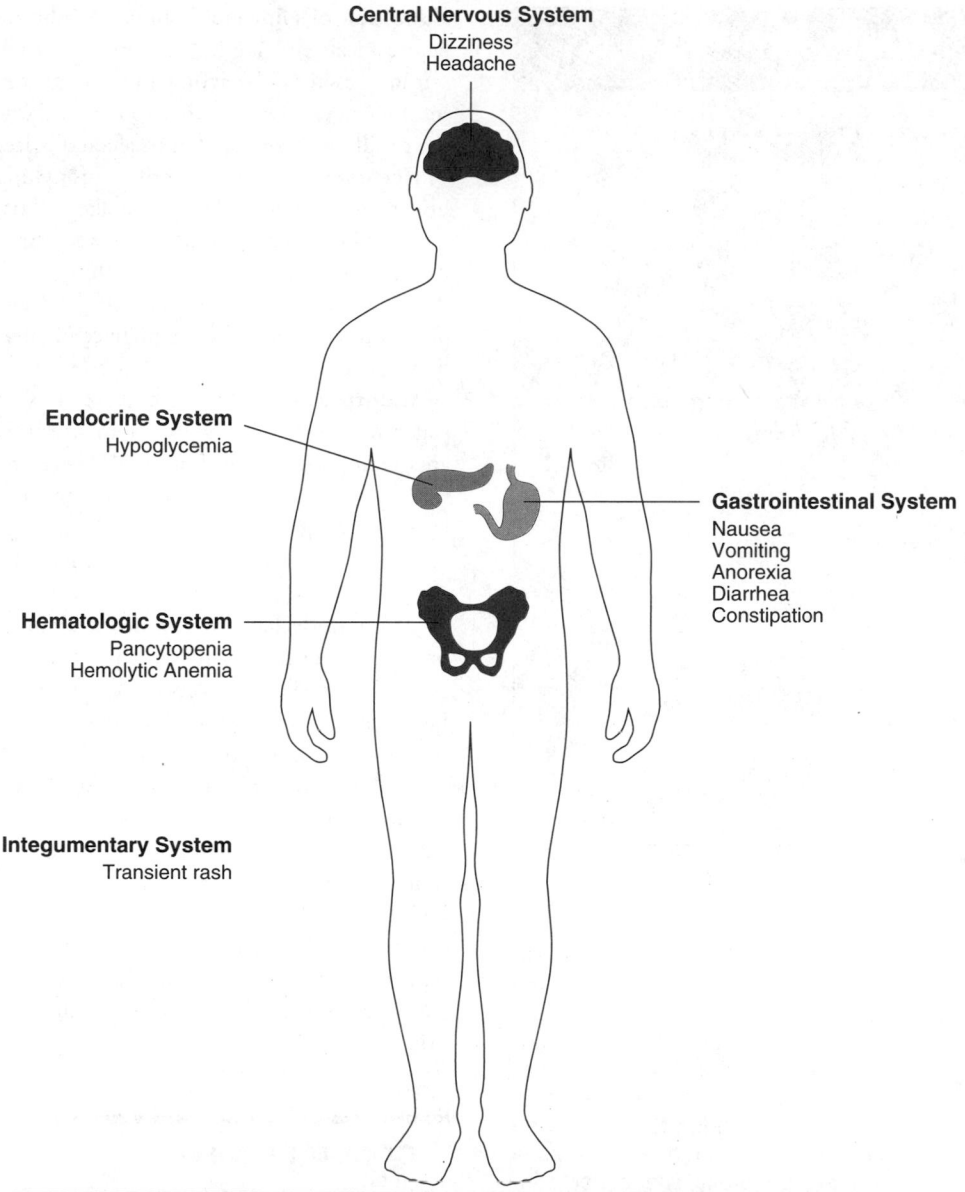

Central Nervous System
Dizziness
Headache

Endocrine System
Hypoglycemia

Gastrointestinal System
Nausea
Vomiting
Anorexia
Diarrhea
Constipation

Hematologic System
Pancytopenia
Hemolytic Anemia

Integumentary System
Transient rash

FIGURE 39–3   Common undesired clinical responses associated with sulfonylureas.

years of age with diagnosed NIDDM. (Although it occurs more commonly in diabetic clients, it also can occur in nondiabetic clients.) Polydipsia and polyuria are present for several days to several weeks and can result in severe dehydration, especially if the client is unable to obtain replacement fluids. Treatment involves administration of large amounts of intravenous fluids, insulin, and potassium replacement. The mortality rate is high (10% to 20%). However, the cause of death is usually the complicating illness (e.g., infection) rather than the metabolic abnormality.[13]

Contraindications and Precautions Sulfonylurea drugs usually are not prescribed for clients with severe hepatic or renal disease, and these drugs have been associated with an increased incidence of death from cardiovascular disease. In addition, caution is advised for clients who are allergic to sulfa drugs since a cross-sensitivity may occur.[33]

Drug-Drug and Drug-Nutrient Interactions Because of the type of albumin binding, drug-drug interactions are more common with first-generation sulfonylureas. Some of these interactions potentiate the action of the sulfonylurea, resulting in hypoglycemia. Common drugs that lower the blood glucose level when administered concurrently with a sulfonylurea drug include antibacterial sulfonamides, salicylates, warfarin, and monoamine oxidase inhibitors. Conversely, drugs (e.g., diazoxide) may interact with sulfonylureas to raise the blood glucose level, resulting in hyperglycemia. (See box on p. 494 for additional drugs that interact with sulfonylurea drugs to produce hypoglycemia or hyperglycemia.) Glipizide is the only oral hypoglycemic agent whose absorption is altered by food.[34]

Life-Span Considerations Even though the sulfonylureas have few undesired clinical responses, they are not recommended for certain population groups. For exam-

---

DRUGS THAT INTERACT WITH SULFONYLUREA DRUGS[24,25]

Drugs That Interact to Produce Hypoglycemia

Anabolic steroids	Allopurinol
Chloramphenicol	Probenecid
Histamine antagonists	Clofibrate
Tricyclic antidepressives	Sulfinpyrazone
Guanethidine	Sulfonamides
Monoamine oxidase inhibitors	Salicylates
Phenylbutazone	

Drugs That Interact to Prolong Hypoglycemia or Mask Indications of Hypoglycemia

β-Blockers
Clonidine

Drugs That Interact to Produce Hyperglycemia

Corticosteroids
Glucagon
Rifampin
Thiazide diuretics
Diazoxide
Barbiturates
Estrogens
Dextrothyroxine

---

ple, sulfonylureas are not recommended for use with pregnant diabetic clients since they do not provide the strict control needed to prevent fetal abnormalities and mortality. Additionally, some sulfonylureas are transferred to breast milk. A nursing infant could develop hypoglycemia, resulting in central nervous system damage. Sulfonylureas are also not recommended for clients who are coping with severe trauma, infection, or very stressful situations. These individuals generally are better controlled with insulin.

Surgery and the Client Requiring Sulfonylureas Although specific orders must be obtained from the primary care provider, oral hypoglycemic drugs are generally discontinued 24 to 72 hours before surgery. Doing so helps prevent the possibility of intraoperative hypoglycemia.[34] Once the oral drugs have been discontinued, the client is placed on a low dosage of intermediate-acting insulin or on a sliding scale with regular insulin. Close monitoring of the client's blood glucose level is required regardless of the insulin regimen used.

MISCELLANEOUS DRUGS IN CATEGORY

Glyburide has a low incidence of serious side effects. GI symptoms, specifically nausea, are most common. Glyburide should not be prescribed for clients with hepatic or renal insufficiency because of the presence of some active metabolites.

Glipizide is considered 100 times more potent than tolazamide. It is less toxic than most first-generation drugs and produces a mild diuretic effect. Since the presence of food delays absorption of glipizide, it must be administered 30 minutes before meals. It may be used in elderly clients with caution, but its use should be avoided if any client has hepatic or renal insufficiency. There is no hyponatremia with this drug, and the disulfiram-like reaction to alcohol is less.

Acetohexamide is the only sulfonylurea compound with uricosuric properties, which makes it useful for NIDDM clients who also have gout. However, this drug is excreted in the form of an active metabolite; thus its use should be avoided if a client has renal insufficiency. If the drug accumulates in the plasma to elevated levels, hypoglycemia may occur. It is rarely prescribed anymore.

Chlorpropamide's length of action is 1 to 3 days. It causes water retention with hyponatremia, especially in elderly clients taking a thiazide diuretic.[13] Therefore it is seldom used with elderly clients or clients with renal insufficiency. Since facial flushing after ingestion of alcohol occurs, the drug usually is not prescribed for clients who routinely ingest alcohol.

Tolazamide has fewer water-retaining effects than chlorpropamide, so it is useful in NIDDM clients who have congestive heart failure, hepatic cirrhosis, or fluid retention. However, it is more slowly absorbed, so effects on blood glucose levels do not appear for several hours.

Tolbutamide is rapidly oxidized by the liver into an inactive form. This property necessitates using doses of the drug before each meal.[22] Because of the drug's short duration of action, it is particularly safe for elderly clients and clients with impaired renal or hepatic function.[34] Studies have shown that certain generic products have unequal dissolution rates that may result in variation of the therapeutic blood levels.[13] Table 39–3 summarizes information about common sulfonylurea drugs.

CONCEPT REVIEW

First-generation sulfonylurea drugs include acetohexamide, chlorpropamide, tolazamide, and tolbutamide. These drugs must be used carefully in elderly clients and clients with liver or renal disease.

Second-generation sulfonylurea drugs include glipizide and glyburide. These drugs are more potent than the first-generation sulfonylureas and are generally the preferred drugs for treating type II diabetes mellitus.

DRUGS USED TO INCREASE BLOOD GLUCOSE LEVELS

Drugs sometimes are used to increase the blood glucose level of clients experiencing hypoglycemia.

Hypoglycemia

Hypoglycemia, an abnormally low level of blood glucose, may result from an excessive rate of removal of glucose from the blood or from decreased secretion of glucose into the

TABLE 39–3
Oral Hypoglycemic Drugs

Drug	Dosage and Pharmacokinetic Properties	Nursing Considerations
Acetohexamide (Dymelor) HOW SUPPLIED Coated tablet: 250, 500 mg Uncoated tablet: 250, 500 mg	Initial dose: 0.25–1.5 g/d in one or two doses Maximum dose: 1.5 g/d in one or two doses Onset of action: 1 h Peak action: 6–8 h Duration of action: 12–24 h	Acetohexamide belongs to sulfonylurea class. Administer before meal. Reduce dosage in clients with renal disorder. Drug is in Pregnancy Category C. Observe for undesired clinical responses: mild headaches, nausea, vomiting, anorexia, malaise, hemolytic anemia. Store at controlled room temperature (15° to 30° C).
Tolazamide (Tolinase) HOW SUPPLIED Uncoated tablet: 100, 250, 500 mg	Usual initial dose: 100–250 mg daily with first meal, determined by fasting blood glucose Maximum dose: 1000 mg/d Maintenance dose: 100–1000 mg/d, with average of 250–500 mg/d When more than 500 mg needed, divide dosage between breakfast and evening meal Onset of action: 4–6 h Peak action: 7 h Duration of action: 12–24 h	Tolazamide belongs to sulfonylurea class. Administer before meal. Drug is in Pregnancy Category C. Observe for undesired clinical responses: nausea, epigastric fullness, heartburn, allergic skin reactions, hematologic reactions. Store at controlled room temperature (15° to 30° C).
Tolbutamide (Orinase) HOW SUPPLIED Uncoated tablet: 250, 500 mg	Usual initial dose: 1–2 g/d Maximum dose: 3 g/d Usual maintenance dose: 0.25–3 g/d Onset of action: 1 h Peak action: 4½–6½ h Duration of action: 6–12 h	Tolbutamide belongs to sulfonylurea class. Administer before meal. Short duration of action makes drug safer for elderly clients. Drug is in Pregnancy Category C. Observe for undesired clinical response: nausea, epigastric fullness, heartburn, allergic skin reactions, hematologic reactions. Store at controlled room temperature (15° to 30° C).
Chlorpropamide (Diabinase) HOW SUPPLIED Uncoated tablet: 100, 250 mg	Initial dose: 250 mg/d (older patients, 100–125 mg/d) Maintenance dose: 250 mg/d usually, with range of 100–500 mg/d Onset of action: 1 h Peak action: 3–6 h Duration of action: up to 60 h	Chlorpropamide belongs to sulfonylurea class. Administer before meal. Drug is in Pregnancy Category C. Drug is not recommended for nursing mothers. Observe for undesired clinical responses: pruritis, nausea, diarrhea, vomiting, anorexia, hunger, hematologic reactions. Store below 30° C.
Glipizide (Glucotrol) HOW SUPPLIED Uncoated tablet: 5, 10 mg	Initial dose: 5 mg given 30 min before breakfast (2.5 mg for elderly or those with liver disease); adjust by increments of 2.5–5 mg as determined by blood and urinary glucose levels; dose may be divided Maximum dose: 40 mg/d Maintenance dose: determined by blood and urinary glucose level; doses between 15 and 30 mg/d should be divided Onset of action: 1–1½ h Peak action: 2–4 h Duration of action: 10–16 h	Glipizide belongs to sulfonylurea class. Administer before meal. Reduce dosage if elderly client has renal or hepatic disease. Drug is in Pregnancy Category C. Observe for undesired clinical responses: nausea, diarrhea, constipation, allergic skin reactions, hematologic reactions. Store below 30° C.
Glyburide (Micronase) HOW SUPPLIED Uncoated tablet: 1.25, 1.5, 2.5, 3, 5 mg	Initial dose: 2.5–5 mg (1.25 mg in the elderly or those with renal or hepatic insufficiency) determined by blood and urinary glucose levels Maintenance dose: 1.25–20 mg/d in one or two doses Maximum dose: 20 mg/d Divide dosage if daily amount exceeds 10 mg Onset of action: 2–4 h Peak action: 10 h Duration of action: 24 h	Glyburide belongs to sulfonylurea class. Administer before meal. Reduce dosage if client is elderly or has renal or hepatic disease. Drug is in Pregnancy Category C. Observe for undesired clinical responses: liver function abnormalities, nausea, epigastric fullness, heartburn, allergic skin reactions, hematologic reactions, blurred vision, changes in visual accommodation, metabolic reactions. Store at controlled room temperature (15° to 30° C).

blood. Hypoglycemia may be tolerated for a brief time without symptoms. However, if the blood glucose level remains very low for a prolonged period, signs and symptoms of cerebral dysfunction develop, including mental confusion, hallucinations, convulsions, and coma. Early indications of hypoglycemia include tachycardia, weakness, malaise, sweating, tremulousness, lightheadedness, and anxiety. These signs and symptoms result from increased secretion of epinephrine, a normal response to hypoglycemia.[35]

Specific treatment of hypoglycemia depends on the primary cause. If **hyperinsulinism** is due to a tumor or hyperplasia of the islets of Langerhans, surgical intervention is necessary. **Chronic reactive,** or **postprandial, hypoglycemia,** believed a precursor of diabetes mellitus, develops suddenly after ingestion of a high-carbohydrate meal. It is characterized by a blood glucose level of 50 mg/dl or less. Treatment for this form of hypoglycemia includes a diet high in protein and fat and low in carbohydrate. An acute episode of hypoglycemia, or **insulin reaction,** demands emergency treatment with intravenous injections of glucose. An alternative treatment method includes the use of glucagon.

Nursing Considerations

Nursing care centers first on providing support to clients as possible causes of hypoglycemia are ruled out. Once the diagnosis is made and the immediate situation is under control, education of the client becomes the priority intervention. Client education focuses on prevention and treatment of future hypoglycemic responses.

HYPOGLYCEMIA ANTAGONIST PROTOTYPE

GLUCAGON

The prototype for this drug category is glucagon.

Pharmacotherapeutics Glucagon can be used to treat insulin reactions or hypoglycemia in diabetic clients. It is effective only if liver glycogen is available. This makes the drug ineffective in clients with chronic states of hypoglycemia, starvation, and adrenal insufficiency.

Pharmacokinetics When produced synthetically, glucagon must be administered parenterally because it is inactivated by gastric enzymes. Glucagon is degraded by the liver and kidneys and has a plasma half-life of 3 to 6 minutes.[3] The hyperglycemic effect is relatively brief and occurs more gradually than that of dextrose.[13]

Pharmacodynamics Glucagon, a polypeptide hormone produced by the pancreas, accelerates the synthesis of cyclic adenosine monophosphate (AMP) and increases phosphorylase activity in the liver. It promotes the breakdown of glycogen from cell stores (glycogenolysis) and the release of newly formed glucose from the liver. Glucagon also increases the uptake of amino acids by the liver and inhibits glycogen synthetase, resulting in greater gluconeogenesis. In addition, hepatic and adipose tissue lipolysis is enhanced by activation of adenyl cyclase, producing free fatty acids and glycerol, which further stimulate glyconeogenesis and ketogenesis.

Pharmaceutics Glucagon is supplied by the manufacturer as a dry powder that must be reconstituted with the accompanying diluent. The mixed solution is administered only if it is clear. The mixture remains stable for 24 hours at room temperature and 48 hours if refrigerated. Emergency kits containing a vial of glucagon (1 U equals 1 mg) and a syringe prefilled with suitable diluent are available by prescription.

Although glucagon usually is administered subcutaneously, it may be administered intravenously or intramuscularly. Intravenous glucagon is administered with only 5% dextrose solutions instead of normal saline solution since glucagon forms a precipitate in saline solutions. Glucagon is also incompatible with potassium chloride and calcium chloride, which are often found in intravenous fluids.

Dosage Information The usual adult dosage is 0.5 to 1 mg (1 mg glucagon equals 1 U glucagon). For children, the dosage is 0.025 mg/kg. If no response occurs in the client, the appropriate dose may be repeated every 5 to 20 minutes for a total of three doses.

Intravenous solutions are administered at a rate of 1 mg or less per minute.

Undesired Clinical Responses Undesired clinical responses, which include rash, dizziness, nausea, or vomiting, are usually not severe. Hypokalemia also may occur.

Life-Span Considerations Safe use during pregnancy and in nursing women has not been established.

MISCELLANEOUS DRUGS IN THIS CATEGORY

Clients with diabetes mellitus are encouraged to carry a simple carbohydrate at all times because of the possibility of hypoglycemia. The following glucose products are convenient to carry. **Glucose** (Glutose, Insta-Glucose), a monosaccharide, is rapidly absorbed from the GI tract and quickly distributed to the tissues. This product provides 4 calories per gram. It must be swallowed since it is not absorbed from the buccal cavity. For adults, a dosage of approximately 10 to 20 g is prescribed. An additional dosage of this drug can be administered in 10 minutes if necessary. Use in children should be only under the direction of a primary care provider. The only noted side effect is nausea; no drug interactions have been reported.[13]

Diazoxide (Proglycem) is a nondiuretic thiazide. For treatment of hypoglycemia, it is administered orally. Diazoxide produces a prompt rise in blood glucose by directly inhibiting insulin secretion. It is used to counteract hyperinsulinism in clients with conditions such as an insulin tumor (insulinoma). In addition, diazoxide may be used to treat severe hypertension.

Absorption of diazoxide occurs with both the oral and intravenous routes of administration. It is protein bound, metabolized in the liver, and excreted by the kidneys. Onset of action is within 1 hour and duration of action is 8 to 12 hours. Undesired clinical responses associated with diazoxide include sodium retention and a decrease in urinary output, which can result in edema of hands or feet, weight gain, and congestive heart failure in susceptible individuals. Oral diazoxide may potentiate the effects of antihypertensives, although the effect on blood pressure is not marked when this drug is used alone. Hyperglycemia or ketoacidosis can occur with overdose. Undesired clinical responses associated with diazoxide include

GI irritation, thrombocytopenia, neutropenia, and tachycardia. Excessive growth of hair occurs most frequently in children with chronic use and is reversible when the drug is discontinued.[3]

SUMMARY

Two major types of diabetes mellitus have been identified, IDDM and NIDDM. With type I diabetes mellitus (IDDM), there is an absolute lack of endogenous insulin. In clients with type II (NIDDM) the insulin is defective or the cellular receptors fail to respond to the insulin. In either situation medical therapy centers on exercise, diet, and drugs.

Exogenous insulin, which is available from a variety of sources, is required for all type I diabetics. In addition, many type II clients require insulin therapy. Insulin products are classified according to their length of action as short-, intermediate-, and long-acting insulins. All insulin products are administered parenterally to prevent inactivation by gastric enzymes.

Clients with type II diabetes mellitus, or NIDDM, are treated with diet, exercise, and oral hypoglycemic drugs. These drugs lower the blood glucose level by stimulating the release of insulin from the pancreas or increasing the sensitivity of peripheral cells to insulin or by doing both. Presently in the United States, sulfonylureas are the major oral hypoglycemic drugs used.

REFERENCES

1. Guyton, A.C. (1991). *Textbook of medical physiology* (8th ed.). Philadelphia: W.B. Saunders.
2. Eisenbarth, G.S., & Kahn, C.R. (1990). Etiology and pathogenesis of diabetes mellitus. In K. Becker (Ed.), *Principles and practice of endocrinology and metabolism* (pp. 1074–1084). Philadelphia: J.B. Lippincott.
3. Kahn, C.R., & Schechter, Y. (1990). Insulin, oral hypoglycemic agents, and the pharmacology of the endocrine pancreas. In A. Gilman et al. (Eds.) *The pharmacological basis of therapeutics* (8th ed.) (pp. 1463–1495). New York: Pergamon Press.
4. McCance
5. Nair, K., & Karki, S. (1992). Carbohydrate metabolism. In C. Smith & A. Reynard (Eds.), *Textbook of pharmacology* (pp. 741–771). Philadelphia: W.B. Saunders.
6. Campbell, R.G., & Brillon, D.J. (1991). Diabetes mellitus. In J. Kassirer (Ed.), *Current therapy in internal medicine* (3rd ed.) (pp. 1270–1275). Philadelphia: B.C. Decker.
7. Ignatavicius, D., & Bayne, M. (1991). *Medical-surgical nursing: A nursing process approach* (pp. 1585–1623). Philadelphia: W.B. Saunders.
8. Weir, G.C., & O'Hare, J.A. (1990). Evaluation of metabolic control in diabetes. In K.. Becker (Ed.), *Principles and practice of endocrinology and metabolism* (pp. 1094–1098). Philadelphia: J.B. Lippincott.
9. American Diabetes Association. (1992). Nutritional recommendations and principles for individuals with diabetes mellitus. *Diabetes Care, 15* (Suppl. 2), 21–28.
10. Monahan, F., Drake, T., & Neighbors, M. (1994). *Nursing care of adults* (pp. 1222–1258). Philadelphia: W.B. Saunders.
11. Burke, E. (1991). Insulin. In D. Guthrie & R. Guthrie (Eds.), *Nursing management of diabetes mellitus* (pp. 102–121). Philadelphia: J.B. Lippincott.
12. Skyler, J.S. (1988). Insulin pharmacology. In R.A. Rizza & D.A. Greene (Eds.), *The medical clinics of North America* (pp. 1337–1351).
13. American Medical Association. (1990). *Drug evaluations annual 1991.* Milwaukee: Author.
14. Hirsch, I., & Farkas-Hirsch, R. (1993). Type I diabetes and insulin therapy. *Nursing Clinics of North America, 28,* 9–23.
15. Burden, M. (1994). A practice guide to insulin injections. *Nursing Standards, 8*(29), 25–29.
16. Weinbacher, F.M., Littlejohn, C.E., & Conley, P.F. (1990). Growth of bacteria in prefilled syringes stored in home refrigerators. *Applied Nursing Research, 3*(2), 63–67.
17. Anderson, J.H., & Campbell, R.K. (1990). Mixing insulins in 1990. *The Diabetes Educator, 16,* 380–385.
18. Hollander, P. (1991). Premixed insulins: How do they compare with other insulin preparations? *Postgraduate Medicine, 89*(4), 52–54, 57–58, 61.
19. Steil, C.F., & Deakins, D.A. (1990). Today's insulins. *Nursing '90, 20*(8), 34–39.
20. George, K., & Alberti, M.M. (1990). Diabetic acidosis, hyperosmolar coma, and lactic acidosis. In K. Becker (Ed.), *Principles and practice of endocrinology and metabolism* (pp. 1175-1187). Philadelphia: J.B. Lippincott.
21. Haeften, T., & Gerich, J. (1990). Complications of insulin therapy. In K. Becker (Ed.), *Principles and practice of endocrinology and metabolism* (pp. 1112–1118). Philadelphia: J.B. Lippincott.
22. Karam, J.H., Salber, P.R., & Forsham, P.H. (1991). Pancreatic hormones and diabetes mellitus. In F. Greenspan (Ed.), *Basic and clinical endocrinology* (3rd ed.) (pp. 613–633). Norwalk, CT: Appleton & Lange.
23. O'Hare, J., & Weir, G. (1990). Insulin therapy. In K. Becker (Ed.), *Principles and practice of endocrinology and metabolism* (pp. 1102–1109). Philadelphia: J.B. Lippincott.
24. Hansten, P., & Horn, J. (1990). *Drug interactions and updates.* Malvern, PA: Lea & Febiger.
25. Tatro, D.S. (Ed.). (1990). *Drug interaction facts.* St. Louis: J.B. Lippincott.
26. Kushion, W., Salisbury, P., Seitz, K., & Wilson, B. (1991). Issues in the care of infants and toddlers with insulin-dependent diabetes mellitus. *The Diabetes Educator, 17*(2), 107–110.
27. Griffiths, R., Trujillo, A., & Tuck, M. (1989). Diabetes mellitus: How it differs in geriatric patients. *Consultant, 29*(8), 23–29.
28. Jovanovic-Peterson, L., & Peterson, C. (1990). Diabetes mellitus and pregnancy. In K. Becker (Ed.), *Principles and practice of endocrinology and metabolism* (pp. 1187–1194). Philadelphia: J.B. Lippincott.
29. Melkus, G. (1993). Type II non-insulin-dependent diabetes mellitus. *Nursing Clinics of North America, 28,* 25–33.
30. Raymond, N., & D'Eramo-Melkus, G. (1993). Non-insulin-dependent diabetes and obesity in the Black and Hispanic population: Culturally sensitive management. *Diabetes Educator, 19,* 313–317.
31. Wilson, B. (1994). What nurses don't know about managing NIDDM. *MEDSURG-Nursing, 3*(2):152–154.
32. Guthrie, B., & Guthrie, R. (1991). *Nursing management of diabetes mellitus* (3rd ed.). New York: Springer.
33. Ganda, O.P., & Weir, G.C. (1990). Oral hypoglycemic agents. In K. Becker (Ed.), *Principles and practice of endocrinology and metabolism* (pp. 1099–1102). Philadelphia: J.B. Lippincott.
34. Steil, C., & Deakins, D. (1992). What you and your patient need to know about oral hypoglycemics. *Nursing '92, 22*(11), 34–39.
35. Comi, R.J., & Gorden, P. (1990). Hypoglycemic disorders in the adult. In K. Becker (Ed.), *Principles and practice of endocrinology and metabolism* (pp. 1198–1205). Philadelphia: J.B. Lippincott.

BIBLIOGRAPHY

Albisser, A., & Sperlich, M. (1992). Adjusting insulin. *Diabetes Educator, 18,* 211–222.

American Diabetes Association. (1992). Gestational diabetes mellitus. *Diabetes Care, 15*(Suppl. 2), 5–6.

Avery, M.D., & Rossi, M.A. (1994). Gestational diabetes. *Journal of Nurse Midwifery, 39*(2; Supplement), 9S–19S, 3S–8S.

Bressler, R., & Johnson, D. (1992). New pharmacological approaches to therapy of NIDDM. *Diabetes Care, 15,* 792–801.

Drass, J. (1992). What you need to know about insulin injections. *Nursing '92, 22*(11), 40–43.

Elshaw, E.B., Young, E., Saunders, M., McGurn, W., & Lopez, L. (1994). Utilizing a 24-hour dietary recall can culturally specific diabetes education in Mexican Americans with diabetes. *Diabetes Educator, 20,* 228–235.

Hamera, E. (1992). Diabetes mellitus. *Annual Review of Nursing Research, 10,* 55–75.

Macheca, M.K. (1993). Diabetic hypoglycemia: How to keep the threat at bay. *American Journal of Nursing, 93*(4), 26–30.

McAvoy, K.H. (1991). Oral hypoglycemic agents in the management of non-insulin-dependent diabetes mellitus among the elderly. *Diabetes Educator, 17,* 411–413.

Mulcahy, K. (1992). Hypoglycemic emergencies. *Clinical Issues in Critical Care Nursing, 3,* 361–369.

Petzinger, R. (1992). Diabetes aids and products for people with visual or physical impairment. *Diabetes Educator, 18,* 121–138.

Saltiel-Berzin, R. (1992). Managing a surgical patient who has diabetes. *Nursing '92, 22*(4), 34–42.

Sauve, D., & Kessler, C. (1992). Hyperglycemic emergencies. *Clinical Issues in Critical Care Nursing, 3,* 350–360.

Schwab, T., Meyer, J., & Merrell, R. (1994). Measuring attitudes and health beliefs among Mexican American with diabetes. *Diabetes Educator, 20,* 221–227.

Yeager, T. (1992). Diabetes in children. *Journal of Home Health Care Practice, 4*(3), 46–51.

CHAPTER 40

DRUGS AFFECTING
Hypothalamic and Pituitary Functions

PAMELA E. HUGIE • NORMA L. PINNELL

⊛ **Functions of the Hypothalamus and Pituitary Gland**

LEARNING OBJECTIVE: Describe functions of the hypothalamus and pituitary gland.

⊛ **Drugs Used to Treat Anterior Pituitary Disorders**

LEARNING OBJECTIVES:

Discuss pharmacodynamic and pharmacokinetic properties of corticotropin.

Discuss pharmacodynamic and pharmacokinetic properties of growth hormone.

Develop a plan of care for the client receiving drugs for an anterior pituitary disorder.

KEY TERMS:

Adrenocorticotropin, growth hormone, primary adrenocortical deficiency, secondary adrenocortical deficiency

⊛ **Drugs Used to Treat Posterior Pituitary Disorders**

LEARNING OBJECTIVES:

Discuss the pharmacokinetic and pharmacodynamic properties of vasopressin.

Identify aspects that must be taught to the client receiving vasopressin.

KEY TERM: Diabetes insipidus

CONCEPTS AND TERMS TO REVIEW

Read Chapter 38 for an overview of the endocrine system.

Read the section in Chapter 62 that contains information about oxytocin, a posterior pituitary hormone or drug.

Reexamine the functions of adrenocorticotropin, growth hormone, and vasopressin.

Review the pathologies produced by a deficit of these hormones.

---

*T*herapeutic interventions that use hypothalamic and pituitary hormones are limited and include diagnostic testing, replacement therapy, and control of excessive secretions. With the exception of dopamine, all hypothalamic and pituitary hormones are proteins. This makes the hormones expensive and difficult to obtain in amounts large enough to use therapeutically. In addition, protein increases the risk of aller-

gic reactions. These problems make replacement with peripheral target organ hormones (e.g., glucocorticoids and thyroid hormones) and hormones from biologic sources (e.g., gonadotrophins) safer and more economical.[1]

In general, drugs produced to replace hormones are either obtained from natural sources or synthesized. Their effects and undesired effects are the same as those produced by the body's natural hormone. This chapter provides information on two anterior pituitary hormones or drugs, corticotropin and growth hormone, and one posterior pituitary hormone or drug, vasopressin. The other posterior hormone, oxytocin, is presented in Chapter 62 as the prototype drug for uterine stimulants.

FUNCTIONS OF THE HYPOTHALAMUS AND PITUITARY GLAND

As indicated in Chapter 38, the hypothalamus is a major anatomic structure with a myriad of centers that influence autonomic responses, somatic activity, and endocrine activity.

The hypothalamus is located between the two lobes of the thalamus and provides the connecting link between the nervous system and the endocrine system. Cells in the hypothalamus synthesize at least nine different hormones; the pituitary gland secretes seven more. Together, the glands play important roles in regulation of growth, development, metabolism, and homeostasis.[2,3]

The hypothalamus secretes its releasing or inhibiting hormones or factors in response to internal and external environmental stimuli. All hormones or factors released by the hypothalamus have the pituitary gland as the target organ and do not seem to affect other organs in a direct manner. Subsequent production of hormones by the pituitary gland depends on these hypothalamic releasing and inhibitory hormones (factors). Major releasing or inhibitory hormones and factors are summarized in the box. These hormones or factors are transported in the blood from the hypothalamus to the pituitary gland via the hypothalamic-hypophyseal portal system. Direct neural control regulates the release of the antidiuretic hormone (ADH), which is produced by the hypothalamus and stored in the posterior pituitary lobe.[4] The pituitary gland (hypophysis) is divided into two lobes: the anterior lobe (adenohypophysis) and the posterior lobe (neurohypophysis).

FUNCTIONS OF HYPOTHALAMIC HORMONES

▶ *Corticotropin releasing hormone (CRH):* produces release of corticotropin during periods of stress

▶ *Gonadotropin releasing hormone (Gn-RH):* causes release of gonadotropins

▶ *Growth hormone releasing factor (GH-RF):* produces release of growth hormone when body level of growth hormone falls to low levels

▶ *Growth hormone release inhibiting hormone (GH-RIH):* releases as a response to increased levels of growth hormone in the body and causes pituitary to stop releasing growth hormone

▶ *Melanocyte stimulating hormone releasing factor (MSH-RF):* stimulates the pituitary to release melanocyte stimulating hormone

▶ *Melanocyte-stimulating hormone inhibiting factor:* inhibits pituitary release of melanocyte-stimulating hormone

▶ *Prolactin releasing factor (PRF):* stimulates pituitary to release prolactin

▶ *Prolactin inhibitory factor (PIF):* inhibits release of prolactin from the pituitary

▶ *Thyrotropin releasing hormone (TRH):* stimulates pituitary to release thyroid-stimulating hormone; active during times of stress or when increased metabolism is needed

---

DRUGS USED TO TREAT ANTERIOR PITUITARY DISORDERS

The anterior pituitary lobe is the source of a variety of hormones, including thyroid-stimulating hormone, growth hormone (GH), adrenocorticotropin, and melanocyte-stimulating hormone. In addition, follicle-stimulating hormone, luteinizing hormone, and prolactin are produced by the anterior pituitary lobe. (See Table 38–1 for a summary of the principal actions of these hormones.)

▣ NURSING CONSIDERATIONS

Because functions of hormones released by the anterior pituitary gland vary significantly, it is difficult to identify general nursing considerations. However, some commonalities exist among all clients receiving anterior pituitary hormones or drugs.

Assessing Assessment of the client before administration of any drug is essential. A thorough **health history** with particular emphasis on the client's history of allergies must be obtained. Ask the client what signs and symptoms made him or her seek medical care. Collect a complete drug history; ask about over-the-counter (OTC) and street drugs. In addition, ask the client and family about any family health history that may be significant. Assess the client for preexisting disease conditions that may contraindicate usage of the prescribed drug.

Perform a complete **physical assessment.** Pay special attention to the status of the cardiovascular, respiratory, and renal systems. Check the blood pressure in standing and lying positions. Assess the client's skin color and turgor and degree of jugular vein distention. Carefully assess lung sounds and determine the intake and output ratio.

Diagnosing After careful assessment of the client, analyze the data and generate nursing diagnoses. Some nursing diagnoses that may apply to the client follow:
- Knowledge deficit regarding drug therapy.
- Anxiety related to, for example, uncertainty of treatment plan, disease process.

Planning Proper planning is important with the client receiving hormone therapy. Teaching or the discharge plan must include information such as consequences of discontinuing drug therapy abruptly, physical changes to expect, and physical changes that must be brought to the primary care provider's attention. Suggest that the client wear a Medic-Alert bracelet. Teach the client to avoid use of OTC drugs and to consult with the primary care provider before adding any drug to the drug regimen.

Expected outcomes include the following:
- Client verbalizes information regarding drug therapy schedule.
- Client demonstrates appropriate drug administration techniques.
- Client verbalizes undesired clinical responses associated with prescribed drug.
- Client describes decreased levels of anxiety.

Implementing Administer the drug according to specification and monitor the client for allergic reactions and undesired clinical responses. Observe the client for expected response to drug therapy and record your observations.

Evaluating Evaluation of the effectiveness of the drug regimen is important. Review the expected outcomes with the client to determine if they were met. Drug therapy is effective if the client's clinical status improves and the client is compliant with the drug regimen.

Adrenocorticotropin

Inadequate secretion of **adrenocorticotropin (ACTH)** from the pituitary gland results in adrenal insufficiency and decreased production of adrenocortical hormones.[5]

ADRENOCORTICOTROPIN PROTOTYPE

CORTICOTROPIN

Corticotropin (e.g., ACTH, Corticotropin), a large polypeptide, is a sterile lyophilized ACTH preparation. It is extracted from the pituitaries of mammals (usually pigs) used as food sources by humans. The ACTH preparation stimulates the adrenal cortex to release cortisol, corticosterone, several weakly androgenic steroids, and a small amount of aldosterone.[6]

Pharmacotherapeutics Preparations of corticotropin are used to diagnose adrenocorticoid function and to treat conditions responsive to glucocorticoid therapy. Plasma ACTH levels are elevated in pathologies of the adrenal gland, **primary adrenocortical deficiency.** In clients with **secondary adrenocortical deficiency,** which is caused by hyposecretion of ACTH from the pituitary, serum ACTH levels are low. A corticotropin stimulation test is used to differentiate primary from secondary adrenocortical deficiency. After an injection of corticotropin, plasma cortisol values rise in clients with secondary insufficiency.[1,5]

Therapeutic use of corticotropin is hampered by the drug's short duration of action and required route of administration. In addition, its effects are less predictable than those of exogenous glucocorticoids, and it is effective only in those clients with adequate adrenal function.[1,6] Medical indications for corticotropin therapy include acute exacerbations of multiple sclerosis, rheumatic disorders, collagen diseases, allergic reactions, leukemias, lymphomas, and ulcerative colitis.

Pharmacokinetics Since corticotropin is destroyed by proteolytic enzymes in the digestive tract, it must be administered by injection. Corticotropin is rapidly removed from the plasma by many tissues. Although the precise distribution is unknown, it is believed that the hormone does not cross the placenta.

Corticotropin has an onset action of 5 minutes, a duration of action 2 to 4 hours, and a half-life of less than 20 minutes. The cortisol concentration in the plasma is increased after a period of several hours, but the maximum stimulation of the adrenal cortex may not be achieved until after a few days of therapy. The exact mechanism of metabolism is unknown but probably occurs at receptor sites in the liver and kidneys. The hormone is excreted by the kidneys in the urine.[7]

Pharmacodynamics Corticotropin functions in an enzymatic manner to stimulate the adrenal cortex to synthesize and secrete adrenocortical hormones. The physiologic effects are exhibited in the relief of symptoms of insufficient cortisol, including increased energy levels and stabilized fluid and electrolyte balance. Corticotropin also has antiinflammatory and immunosuppressant effects.

Pharmaceutics Dosages of corticotropin are highly individualized and adjusted frequently according to physiologic response of the client and client compliance. Corticotropin is administered intramuscularly (IM) or subcutaneously (SC). If prescribed for an adrenal crisis, the drug is administered intravenously over an 8-hour period (see Table 40–1).

Undesired Clinical Responses Unless the client is hypersensitive to the drug, short-term administration of corticotropin, even in massive dosages, is unlikely to produce harmful effects. However, undesired clinical responses are associated with chronic use of more than 40 U/day. Effects on the central nervous system include seizures, vertigo, headache, personality changes, and mental disturbances with euphoria, mood swings, and psychosis. Impaired wound healing, thinning of the skin, petechiae, ecchymoses, facial erythema, increased perspiration, and hyperpigmentation may occur. The client may develop hypertension, congestive heart failure, necrotizing angiitis, sodium retention, fluid volume overload, calcium and potassium loss, hypokalemic alkalosis, and negative nitrogen balance. The major gastrointestinal (GI) tract involvement includes perforation and hemorrhage of peptic ulcers.[7,8]

Long-term therapy with corticotropin may suppress pituitary release of corticotropin, which may produce adrenocortical hyperplasia, decreased glucose tolerance, suppression of growth in children, steroid myopathy, and muscle weakness. Figure 40–1 illustrates common undesired clinical responses associated with corticotropin therapy.

Contraindications and Precautions Use of corticotropin is contraindicated in clients with Cushing's syndrome. Since it exacerbates symptoms, its use is contraindicated in clients with diabetes mellitus and psychotic or psychopathic disorders. Its use also is contraindicated in clients with active tuberculosis (TB) and acquired immune deficiency syndrome because it decreases immunity and in clients with active peptic ulcers because it increases the risk of perforation and hemorrhage. In addition, because of the decreased immunity, the client should not have any immunizations with live vaccines during the course of the drug therapy. Individuals sensitive to porcine products may experience an allergic response from corticotropin.

Corticotropin should be used with caution in clients with hypertension or congestive heart failure because of the risk for sodium and water retention. It also is used with caution in clients with myasthenia gravis because it may cause muscle weakness.[7,8]

Drug-Drug Interactions Drugs that induce hepatic enzymes (e.g., barbiturates, phenytoin, and rifampin) may increase glucocorticoid metabolism and reduce corticosteroid effects. When given concomitantly with cyclophosphamide, corticotropin may inhibit hepatic enzymes that activate cyclophosphamide into its alkylating metabolites. In addition, larger dosages of salicylates, insulin, oral antidiabetic drugs, and oral anticoagulants may be

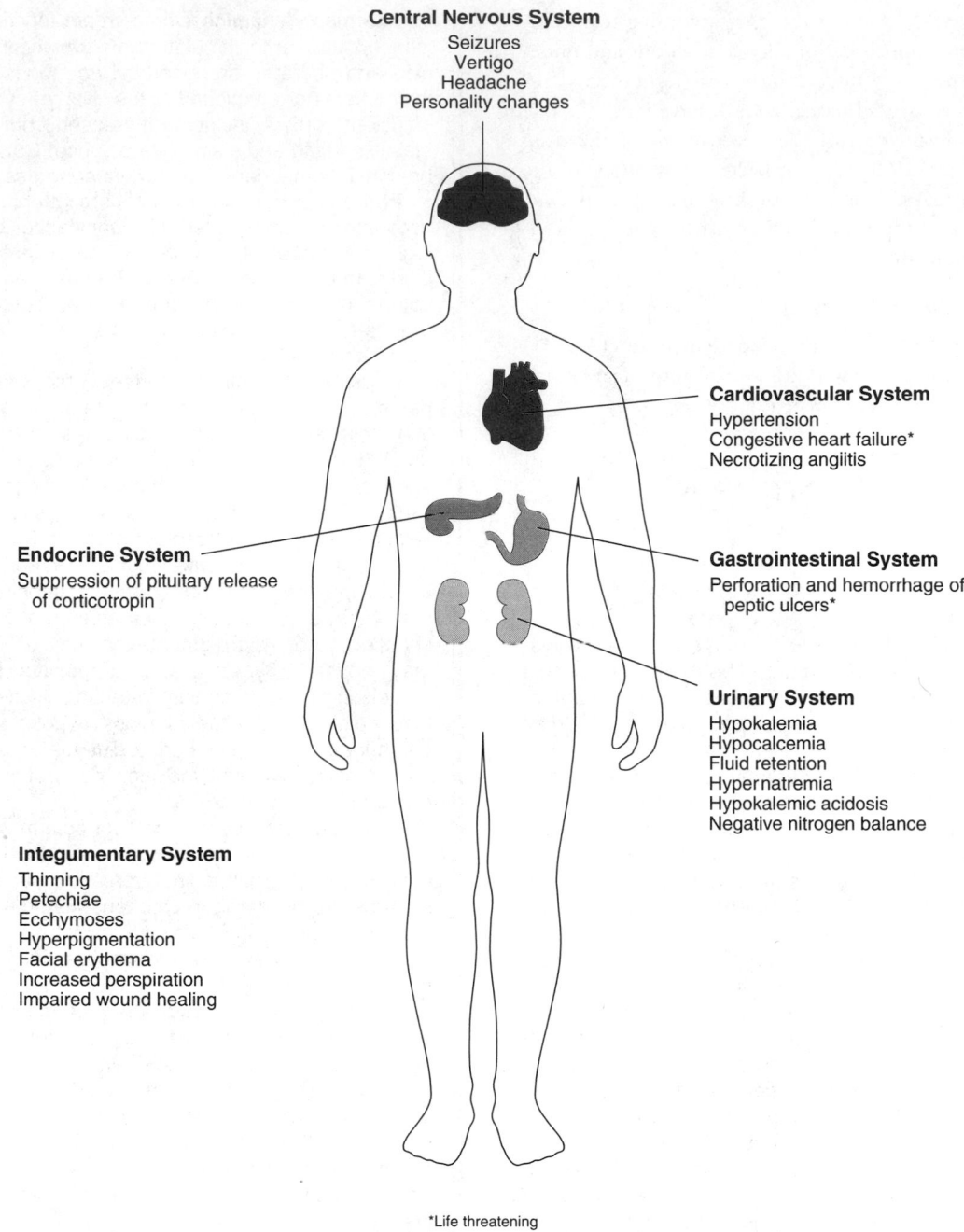

Central Nervous System
Seizures
Vertigo
Headache
Personality changes

Cardiovascular System
Hypertension
Congestive heart failure*
Necrotizing angiitis

Endocrine System
Suppression of pituitary release
   of corticotropin

Gastrointestinal System
Perforation and hemorrhage of
   peptic ulcers*

Urinary System
Hypokalemia
Hypocalcemia
Fluid retention
Hypernatremia
Hypokalemic acidosis
Negative nitrogen balance

Integumentary System
Thinning
Petechiae
Ecchymoses
Hyperpigmentation
Facial erythema
Increased perspiration
Impaired wound healing

*Life threatening

FIGURE 40–1   Common undesired clinical responses associated with corticotropin.

required because of the effect of corticotropin. Corticotropin use results in a decreased response to skin testing.

Concomitant use of corticotropin with potassium-depleting diuretics may enhance potassium wasting. Corticotropin also decreases radioactive iodine uptake. It should be gradually discontinued before therapy with radioactive iodine.[6–8]

Life-Span Considerations Corticotropin is classified as a Pregnancy Category C drug; it is not known if this drug is excreted in human milk. Prolonged use of corticotropin in children inhibits skeletal growth.[8] Corticotropin is used with caution in geriatric clients because of increased problems of chronic illness.

Specific Drug-Related Nursing Considerations Question the client about hypersensitivity to any corticosteroids or porcine proteins. Obtain baseline weight and blood pressure. Review results of cholesterol and electrolyte tests and TB skin testing.

Monitor the client's intake and output and daily weight. Assess for edema. Evaluate food tolerance and bowel activity. Report hyperacidity promptly. Watch for hypocalcemia (muscle twitching, cramps, positive Chvostek's

TABLE 40–1
ATCH Preparations

Drug Name	Dosage and Route of Administration	Nursing Considerations
CORTICOTROPIN (ACTH, Acthar) HOW SUPPLIED Powder for injection: 25, 40 U *Corticotropin Repository* (Acthar Gel) HOW SUPPLIED Repository injection: 40, 80 U/ml *Corticotropin Zinc* (Cortrophin Zinc) HOW SUPPLIED IM: 40-U vial	Dosages are highly individualized for corticotropin **Treatment Purposes** IM or SC: 20 U qid **Corticotropin Gel** IM or SC: 40–80 U q24-72 h **Diagnostic Purposes** IV Adults: 10–25 U in 500 ml D5W solution infused over 8 h IM OR SC Adults: 20 U qid *Acute Exacerbation of Multiple Sclerosis* IM Adults: 80–120 U/d for 2 or 3 weeks *Infantile Spasms* IM Infants: 20–40 U/d or 80 U qod for 3 mo (or 1 mo after cessation of seizures)	**Assess** Assess carefully for contraindications (e.g., osteoporosis, systemic fungal infections, history or presence of peptic ulcer, hypertension). Determine if client is pregnant; corticotropin is classified as a Pregnancy Category C drug. Obtain baseline values for blood pressure, height, weight, and electrolyte studies. **Implement** Reconstitute at the time of use with sterile water or NaCl solution. Refrigerate reconstituted solution and use within 24 h. Warm gel dosage form to room temperature; use a large-gauge needle and administer slowly deep IM. Be alert to signs and symptoms of infection. Teach client to carry card with identification of drug and dose, primary care provider's name and phone number. Advise client not to take aspirin or other drug without consulting primary care provider. **Monitor** Monitor for undesired clinical responses (e.g., fluid and electrolyte disturbance, muscle weakness, impaired wound healing, hypertension, convulsions). Monitor for allergic reactions. Monitor intake and output and daily weight and assess for edema. **Evaluate** Monitor urinary and plasma corticosteroid values. A rise in these values provides evidence of stimulatory effect of the drug.
Cosyntropin (Cortrosyn) HOW SUPPLIED Powder for injection: 0.25 mg	**Diagnostic Purposes** IM Adults: 0.25–0.75 mg one time Children less than 2 y: 0.125 mg one time IV INFUSION Adults: 0.25 mg in 5% dextrose or 0.9% NaCl solution; infuse at rate of 0.04 mg/h	See corticotropin

sign) and hypokalemia (muscle weakness, tingling—especially of lower extremities). Protect the client from unnecessary exposure to pathogens. Good handwashing technique is important. Monitor the client for indications of an infection.

Teach client to carry identification with information about the drug and primary care provider. Instruct client to notify prescriber of fever, sore throat, muscle weakness, sudden weight gain, or edema. Ask dietitian to provide dietary instructions; usually a sodium-restricted diet high in vitamin D, protein, and potassium is prescribed. Teach client to inform dentist or other care provider of drug therapy.[9] Table 40–1 provides a summary of nursing considerations associated with corticotropin therapy.

CONCEPT REVIEW

ACTH stimulates the adrenal cortex to release cortisol, corticosterone, aldosterone, and weak androgenic steroids.

Preparations of ACTH are used for the diagnosis of adrenocorticoid function and for the treatment of conditions responsive to glucocorticoid therapy.

Growth Hormone

Commercially available preparations of human growth hormone (hGH) include natural hormones (i.e., Humatrope, Nutropin) and methionyl–human growth hormone (i.e., Protropin, Somatonorm, and Norditropin). Preparations produced in bacteria through recombinant DNA technology—Protropin, Nutropin, and Humatrope—are approved for human use in the United States.[10]

GROWTH HORMONE PROTOTYPE
SOMATREM

Somatrem (Protropin) has 192 amino acid residues and contains the identical sequence of amino acids constituting pituitary-derived hGH plus an additional amino acid.

Pharmacotherapeutics Exogenous **growth hormone (GH)** is used to increase the growth rate in clients with growth failure or delayed physiologic development due to insufficient endogenous GH secretion. Exogenous GH is ineffective when impaired growth results from other causes or after puberty when the epiphyses of the long bones have closed. When GH is administered to adults with adult-onset pituitary insufficiency caused by pituitary tumors, a marked increase in serum lipoprotein concentrations occurs. Specifically, studies have shown that the high-density lipoprotein cholesterol increases, and low-density lipoprotein cholesterol remains unchanged.[11]

Pharmacokinetics Somatrem is administered by IM or SC injections. Serum GH levels are greater after an SC abdominal injection than after an SC thigh injection.[12] Individual absorption rates vary considerably. In circulation, GH is extensively bound to a high-affinity growth hormone–binding protein. Binding to this protein extends the half-life of GH in circulation. The elimination half-life of GH is between 2 and 3 hours. Ninety percent of the drug is metabolized in the liver and excreted by the kidneys. Little intact GH is excreted in the urine. Metabolism and excretion are more rapid in adults than in children.[10]

Pharmacodynamics Somatrem stimulates growth of linear bone, skeletal muscle, and organs. It increases red blood cell mass by stimulating erythropoietin. Most of somatrem's actions are mediated at the target site by somatomedins, which are liver-synthesized hormones.

Pharmaceutics All GH preparations are delivered by injection. IM and SC routes are equally effective. However, SC injections are preferred because they are less painful.

Dosage Dosage of somatrem must be individualized for each individual. A dosage and schedule of up to 0.1 mg/kg of body weight administered three times per week are recommended.

Undesired Clinical Responses On a local level there may be pain and swelling at the injection site. Approximately 30% of all somatrem-treated clients develop persistent antibodies to GH. In addition, somatrem may depress thyroid function and insulin production.[7]

Contraindications and Precautions Somatrem use is contraindicated in clients with hypersensitivity to the drug. It is also contraindicated in clients with closed epiphyses or actively growing intracranial lesions.

Somatrem must be used with care in clients with a family history of diabetes mellitus since it may precipitate a hyperglycemic episode in susceptible individuals. It should be used in hypothyroid clients only when the client is stabilized in an euthyroid state. Untreated hypothyroidism may interfere with the growth response to somatrem.

Drug-Drug and Drug-Environment Interactions GH reduces the activity of type I and type II mixed-function oxidase enzymes in the liver. This reduction potentially can alter drug metabolism. Use of somatrem concomitantly with adrenocorticoids, glucocorticoids, or corticotropin may inhibit growth response. Use of somatrem with anabolic steroids, androgens, estrogens, or thyroid hormones may accelerate epiphyseal maturation.

Before and after reconstitution with bacteriostatic water for injection, somatrem must be refrigerated. An expiration date is stated on the label of the vial. Reconstituted vials should be used within 14 days of reconstitution.

Interference with Laboratory Tests Somatrem reduces glucose tolerance and total protein and thyroid function test results (thyroxine-binding capacity and radioactive iodine uptake).

Life-Span Considerations Somatrem is classified as a Pregnancy Category C drug. Animal reproduction studies have not been conducted with this drug. It is not known if the drug is excreted in human milk.

Specific Drug-Related Nursing Considerations Assess the client and family for preexisting diabetes mellitus or hypothyroidism. Document the client's growth rate for the past 6 to 12 months. Assess the client's emotional status and coping abilities.

Give consideration to additional nursing diagnoses for this client such as anxiety related to need for multiple injections; body image disturbance related to effects of drug; and self-esteem disturbance related to growth deficit. Help the client understand the physical changes that drug therapy produces. Encourage the client to verbalize concerns and ask questions.[13]

Somatrem is available as a lyophilized powder. To prepare the solution, inject the bacteriostatic water for injection that is supplied with the powder into the vial containing the powder. Swirl the vial to mix the solution. Use a gentle rotary motion. Do not shake the solution. Shaking pushes air bubbles into the solution and results in inaccurate dosing. After reconstitution the solution should be clear. Do not use cloudy solutions.

Once therapy has started, record the client's height and weight at regular intervals. Monitor thyroid function tests and observe the client for glucose intolerance.

MISCELLANEOUS DRUGS IN CATEGORY

The pharmacotherapeutic uses and pharmacodynamic properties of **somatropin, biosynthetic** (Humatrope and Nutropin) are the same as for somatrem. The dosage for Humatrope is individualized; it should not exceed 0.06 mg/kg of body weight three times per week. Dosage for Nutropin is 0.3 ml/kg/d administered subcutaneously for seven days.

CONCEPT REVIEW

Growth hormone (GH) has two main actions: increased growth and metabolic alterations. The increased growth factor affects almost all tissues of the body. The metabolic effects are caused by direct action of GH on the liver, muscle, and adipocytes.

The primary use of GH is as replacement therapy in children who lack GH.

DRUGS USED TO TREAT POSTERIOR PITUITARY DEFICIENCIES

Hormones secreted by the posterior portion of the pituitary gland are actually produced by nerve cells in the hypothalamus. They are stored in the posterior pituitary and released for use in the body. These hormones include vasopressin, or ADH, and oxytocin (see Table 38–2).

Diabetes Insipidus

Diabetes insipidus results from insufficient ADH. With insufficient ADH, the collecting ducts and tubules of the kidney are almost impermeable to water. This condition prevents reabsorption of water and allows loss of water into the urine. In a client with diabetes insipidus the urinary specific gravity remains almost constant between 1.002 and 1.006. The urinary output is usually 4 to 6 L per day but can be as great as 12 to 15 L per day, depending on the client's intake. The increased output results in fluid and electrolyte imbalance. Treatment includes replacing ADH, assuring adequate fluid replacement, and diagnosing and treating the underlying pathology.[14]

⊞ NURSING CONSIDERATIONS

The basis of care in any situation is an individualized plan of care. The plan begins with a thorough assessment.

Assessing   Begin care of the client by collecting a complete **health history.** Assess for contraindications to drug therapy (e.g., epilepsy, asthma, history of heart failure). Determine the client's intake and output ratio. Obtain information about preexisting health problems and a family health history. During the **physical assessment** measure the client's blood pressure. Record the client's weight and collect a urine specimen. Determine the urinary specific gravity and review the laboratory reports of serum electrolyte levels. Conduct a complete neurologic examination.

Diagnosing   Nursing diagnoses appropriate for the client receiving vasopressin include the following:

- High risk for fluid volume excess related to administration of vasopressin.
- Knowledge deficit regarding drug administration and effects.

- Altered nutrition, less than body requirement, related to nausea, vomiting, and abdominal cramps produced by vasopressin.
- High risk for decreased cardiac output related to arrhythmias produced by vasopressin.

Planning   Teaching is an important part of this client's care. Teach him or her the name, dose, and frequency of the drug administration. Since the vasopressin is administered parenterally or intranasally, the client must learn the proper technique for administering the drug. The client must also learn to monitor his or her own intake and output.

Appropriate expected outcomes follow:

- Client maintains an appropriate fluid balance.
- Client describes drug action and undesired clinical responses.
- Client demonstrates proper drug administration technique.
- Client maintains desired body weight.

Implementing   Since several dosage forms for the drug are available, you must read the package insert that accompanies the drug. Be careful to prepare the drug as recommended by the manufacturer.

Observe the client for fluid volume excess and electrolyte imbalance. Monitor the client for undesired clinical responses (e.g., nausea, vomiting, headaches). Assess the client's cardiovascular function frequently.

Evaluating   Review the expected outcomes and determine if they were met. Observe for relief of symptoms. The therapeutic regimen is considered effective if the intake and output ratio is stabilized, the fluid volume is balanced, and electrolyte levels and serum osmolality are stabilized.

Antidiuretic Hormone

ADH increases the permeability of the collecting ducts and tubules to water and allows reabsorption of most of the water as the tubular fluid passes through the ducts, thereby conserving water. Vasopressin is also a potent vasoconstrictor.

ANTIDIURETIC HORMONE PROTOTYPE

VASOPRESSIN

Vasopressin is a polypeptide containing nine amino acids. It is obtained from bovine and porcine posterior pituitaries.

Pharmacotherapeutics   Vasopressin is used primarily in the treatment of diabetes insipidus caused by nonproduction of natural ADH. Nonproduction of ADH may be due to hypothalamic or pituitary trauma, malignancy, or other factors.

Large doses of ADH cause contraction of most smooth muscle tissues in the body, including most of the intestinal musculature, the bile ducts, and the uterus. Based on this action, it sometimes is used to relieve postoperative intestinal gas distention. Vasopressin has also been administered IV or intraarterially as an adjunct in the treatment of acute, massive hemorrhage caused by ruptured esophageal varices, peptic ulcer disease, esophageal laceration, or intestinal perforation. Use of vasopressin in suction situations is a temporary measure intended to decrease portal venous pressure.[6]

Pharmacokinetics Vasopressin is destroyed by trypsin in the GI tract and therefore must be given parenterally. Distribution is throughout the extracellular fluid. Vasopressin's onset of action is 1 minute after IV administration. The effects last 2 to 8 hours with SC administration and 6 to 12 hours with IM administration. Metabolism of vasopressin occurs in the liver and kidneys. Excretion is via the urine.

Pharmacodynamics Vasopressin binds to receptors on the surface of the collecting duct cells and regulates the threshold for water reabsorption by the distal tubules, collecting tubules, and collecting ducts. This action results in urine concentration due to increased water reabsorption.

Pharmaceutics Vasopressin is available in parenteral solutions and an intranasal preparation (Table 40–2).

Undesired Clinical Responses Adverse effects associated with low doses of vasopressin are infrequent. However, undesired responses increase in frequency and severity with high doses. The most important adverse reaction with vasopressin is water intoxication. Excessive fluid volume may affect the cardiovascular system, the genitourinary system, and the GI system. It may produce increased blood pressure, bradycardia, arrhythmias, peripheral vascular constriction or collapse, decreased cardiac output, and myocardial ischemia or infarction.

Hypersensitivity reactions have been reported occasionally in clients receiving vasopressin therapy. Symptoms of these reactions include hives, bronchoconstriction, fever, rash, wheezing, cardiac arrest, and anaphylaxis. When vasopressin is administered IV, there are reported problems with thrombosis formation, which leads to infarction and necrosis of the organ or tissue supplied by that vessel (e.g., coronary thrombosis, venous thrombosis, infarction of the small bowel, and cutaneous gangrene).[6]

TABLE 40–2
Vasopressin Preparations

Drug Name	Dosage and Route of Administration	Nursing Considerations
VASOPRESSIN (Diapid, Pitressin) **HOW SUPPLIED** IM, SC solution: 10 U/0.5 ml, 20 U/ml IV solution: 20 U/ml Nasal spray: lypressin 0.185 mg/ml	**Abdominal Distention** **IM** Adults: 5 U (0.25 ml) initially; increase to 10 U (0.5 ml) at subsequent injections if necessary; give at 3- to 4-h intervals Children: reduce dosage proportionately **Abdominal Roentgenography** Usual dose, two injections of 10 U each given 2 h and ½ h before films are exposed **Diabetes Insipidus** **IM** 5–10 U (0.25–0.5 ml) repeated two or three times daily as needed **INTRANASALLY** Dosage and interval between treatments must be determined for each patient	**Assess** Assess for contraindications (e.g., epilepsy, migraine, asthma, heart failure). Determine if client is pregnant; vasopressin is classified as a Pregnancy Category C drug. Establish baseline values for weight, blood pressure, electrolytes, and specific gravity. **Implement** For IV infusion, dilute with 5% dextrose or 0.9% NaCl solution to concentration of 0.1–1 U/ml. Give client one to two glasses of water at time of administration to reduce side effects. Teach client to report headache, chest pain, shortness of breath. Teach client to monitor intake and output. Be alert for early indications of water intoxication (drowsiness, headache, listlessness). Evaluate injection site for erythema and pain. **Monitor** Monitor intake and output. Monitor for undesired clinical responses (e.g., abdominal cramps, nausea, vomiting, tremor, sweating, headaches). **Evaluate** Evaluate success of therapy by reduction in polyuria.
Desmopressin (DDAVP, Stimate) **HOW SUPPLIED** Nasal solution: 0.1, 0.5 mg/ml Injection: 4 μg/ml	**Diabetes Insipidus** **INTRANASAL** Adults: 0.1–0.4 ml/d Children 3 mo–12y: 0.05–0.3 ml/d **SC, IV** Adults: 0.5–1 ml/d	See vasopressin with following exception: Administer by direct IV injection.

Contraindications and Precautions Vasopressin use is contraindicated in clients with precarious fluid and electrolyte balance, including preoperative and postoperative polyuria clients, renal disease clients, and comatose clients. The drug should be used with caution in clients who would be adversely affected by the smooth muscle constriction, including pregnant women and clients with bowel obstruction or heart disease.

Drug-Drug Interactions Lithium, epinephrine, demeclocycline, heparin, and alcohol block the antidiuretic action of vasopressin in varying degrees. Chlorpropamide, carbamazepine, clofibrate, tricyclic antidepressants, phenformin, urea, and fludrocortisone potentiate the antidiuretic action of vasopressin and require decreased dosage of vasopressin. Barbiturate sedation and cyclopropane anesthesia have a synergistic effect with vasopressin.

Life-Span Considerations Vasopressin is not likely to produce tonic uterine contractions that could be deleterious to the fetus or threaten a pregnancy. However, it is classified as a Pregnancy Category C drug and should be used only when clearly indicated during pregnancy. Vasopressin is used with caution in pediatric and geriatric clients since they are more susceptible to fluid volume disturbance and more sensitive to the effects of vasopressin.

Specific Drug-Related Nursing Considerations You must monitor the client's response to vasopressin because the dosage is highly individualized. Document carefully the client's intake and output, weight, blood pressure, and pulse. Be alert for early indications of water intoxication (e.g., drowsiness, listlessness, headache). If they occur, withhold the drug and report the findings to the primary care provider.

MISCELLANEOUS DRUGS IN CATEGORY

Desmopressin acetate (DDAVP, Stimate) is a synthetic analog of ADH. Its therapeutic uses are the same as those of vasopressin. In addition, because of its dose-dependent increase in plasma factor VIII (antihemophilic factor), desmopressin is used to treat hemophilia A and B and von Willebrand's disease.

Desmopressin is available in a liquid dosage form for intranasal administration. It is administered via a nasal rhinyle, a flexible catheter used to measure the liquid. Once the drug is drawn into the catheter, one end is placed in the client's nose and the other end in the client's mouth. The client then blows into the catheter to deposit the drug in the nasal passageways. Clients receiving the drug in this manner must be observed for chronic rhinopharyngitis. Desmopressin is also available as a parenteral solution for IV administration.

Lypressin (Diapid) is a synthetic nasal spray. Since it is synthetic, it is free of oxytocin impurities and foreign proteins. Therefore it is less likely to produce allergic reactions and other undesired clinical responses than vasopressin. The usual dosage of lypressin is one to two sprays in each nostril four times a day. Dosage is usually based on urinary output and degree of thirst.

CONCEPT REVIEW

Vasopressin has two main actions. In the kidneys it reduces urine formation, thus conserving water. It is also a potent vasoconstrictor.

The primary therapeutic use of vasopressin is as hormone replacement therapy in clients with central diabetes insipidus and for the control of polyuria caused by head trauma.

SUMMARY

The secretion of pituitary cells is influenced by hormones released by the hypothalamus. Hormones of the anterior pituitary can be divided into three major groups based on structural similarities; those related to growth hormone, those related to thyroid-stimulating hormone, and those that produce adrenocorticotropin. Both endogenous and exogenous growth hormones increase growth and metabolic processes. Both endogenous and exogenous ACTH stimulate the adrenal cortex to release its hormones.

Hormones of the posterior pituitary gland are vasopressin and oxytocin. Vasopressin reduces urine formation and contracts smooth muscles through the body. Oxytocin plays an integral role in lactation. (Oxytocin is discussed in Chapter 62.)

REFERENCES

1. Simasko, S. (1992). Pituitary hormones. In C. Smith and A. Reynard (Eds.), *Textbook of Pharmacology* (pp. 664–682). Philadelphia: W.B. Saunders.
2. Tortora, G., & Grabowski, S. (1993). *Principles of anatomy and physiology* (7th ed.). New York: Harper Collins College Publishers.
3. Hole, J.W. (1993). *Human anatomy and physiology* (6th ed.). Dubuque, IA: Wm. C. Brown.
4. Guyton, A.C. (1991). *Textbook of medical physiology* (8th ed.). Philadelphia: W.B. Saunders.
5. Lee, L.M., & Gumowski, J. (1992). Adrenocortical insufficiency: A medical emergency. *AACN—Clinical Issues in Critical Care Nursing, 3*, 319–330.
6. McEvoy, G. (Ed.). *American Hospital Formulary Service.* Bethesda, MD: American Society of Hospital Pharmacists.
7. U.S. Pharmacopeial Convention. (1990). *The United States pharmacopeia* (22nd rev.). Rockville, MD: Author.
8. Data Pharmaceutica, Inc. (1993). *1993 physicians' genRx.* Smithtown, NY: Author.
9. Hodgson, B., Kizior, R., & Kingdom, R. (1995). *Nurse's drug handbook–1995.* Philadelphia: W.B. Saunders.
10. Strobl, J., & Thomas, M. (1994). Human growth hormone, *Pharmacological Reviews, 46*(1), 1–18.
11. Eden, S., Wiklund, O., Oscarsson, J., Rosen, T., & Bengtsson, B. (1993). Growth hormone treatment of growth hormone deficient adults results in a marked increase in Lp (a) and HDL cholesterol concentrations. *Arteriosclerosis-Thrombosis, 13*, 296–301.
12. Laursen, T., Jorgensen, J., & Christiansen, J. (1994). Pharmacokinetics and metabolic effects of growth hormone injected

subcutaneously in growth hormone deficient patients: Thigh versus abdomen. *Clinical Endocrinology Oxford, 40,* 373–378.

13. Wardhaugh, B. (1992). Evaluating growth hormone treatment. *Nursing Standards, 6*(48), 33–36.
14. Black, J.M., & Matassarin-Jacobs, E. (1993). Luckmann and Sorensen's medical-surgical nursing: A psychophysiologic approach (4th ed.). Philadelphia: W.B. Saunders.

BIBLIOGRAPHY

Barbieri, R. (1991). Critical drug appraisal: Nafarelin. *Drug Therapy, 21*(6), 23–24, 30–31.

Gaedeke, M.K. (1993). Evaluating T.S.H. thyroid-stimulating hormone. *Nursing, 23*(10), 72.

Growth hormone and nutritional support: Adverse metabolic effects. *Nutrition in Clinical Practice, 7*(1), 27–30.

Gupta, K., Shetty, K., Agra, J., Cuisinier, M., Rudman, I., & Rudman, D. (1994). Human growth hormone effect on serum IGF-I and muscle function in poliomyelitis survivors. *Archives of Physical Medicine and Rehabilitation, 75,* 889–894.

Rao, M., Gross, G., Strebel, B., Halaris, A., Huber, G., Braunig, P., & Marler, M. (1994). Circadian rhythm of tryptophan, serotonin, melatonin, and pituitary hormones in schizophrenia. *Biological Psychiatry, 35*(3), 151–163.

Reasner, C. (1990). Anterior pituitary disease. *Critical Care Nursing Quarterly, 13*(3), 62–66.

Sikes, P.J. (1992). Endocrine responses to the stress of critical illness. *AACN—Clinical Issues in Critical Care Nursing, 3,* 379–391.

Winkel, C. (1994). Gonadotropin-releasing hormone agonists. Current uses for these increasingly important drugs. *Postgraduate Medicine, 95*(6), 111–118.

Wise, B., & Case, B. (1994). Recombinant human growth hormone. *ANNA-Journal, 21*(1), 87–89.

CHAPTER 41

DRUGS AFFECTING
Thyroid and Parathyroid Functions

PAMELA E. HUGIE • NORMA L. PINNELL

⊛ **Functions of the Thyroid Gland**

LEARNING OBJECTIVES:

Describe the functions of the thyroid hormone, thyroxine.

Explain the physiologic mechanism that stimulates thyroxine release.

Discuss the production of thyroxine by the thyroid gland.

KEY TERMS:

Calcitonin, triiodothyronine, thyroxine

⊛ **Disorders of the Thyroid Gland**

LEARNING OBJECTIVE: Describe major disorders of the thyroid gland.

KEY TERMS:

Hyperthyroidism, hypothyroidism, thyroiditis

⊛ **Drug Therapy for Thyroid Hormone Deficiency or Excess**

LEARNING OBJECTIVES:

List general characteristics of drugs used to treat thyroid disorders.

Develop a plan of care for the client being treated for a thyroid hormone excess or deficiency.

Discuss the pharmacokinetics and pharmacodynamics of levothyroxine sodium, the prototype for treating thyroid hormone deficiencies.

Explain the physiologic bases for undesired responses associated with levothyroxine sodium.

Discuss the pharmacokinetics and pharmacodynamics of propylthiouracil.

Explain the physiologic bases for undesired responses associated with propylthiouracil.

Provide the rationale for prescribing radioactive iodines in the treatment of thyroid excess.

⊛ **Functions of the Parathyroid Glands**

LEARNING OBJECTIVE: Describe the function of the parathyroid hormone, parathormone.

KEY TERM: Parathormone

⊛ **Disorders of the Parathyroid Glands**

LEARNING OBJECTIVE: Describe major disorders of the parathyroid glands.

KEY TERMS:

Hyperparathyroidism, hypoparathyroidism

⊛ **Drugs Used to Treat Parathyroid Disorders**

LEARNING OBJECTIVES:

Develop a plan of care for the client requiring drug therapy for hyperparathyroidism.

Explain the pharmacokinetic and pharmacodynamic properties of calcitonin.

Provide the physiologic rationale for undesired responses to calcitonin.

CONCEPTS AND TERMS TO REVIEW

Review Chapter 39 for information on the functions of thyroxine.

Reexamine the physiologic mechanism that stimulates thyroxine release.

Investigate the production of thyroxine by the thyroid gland.

Review the function of the parathyroid hormone, parathormone.

Reexamine the physiologic mechanism that stimulates parathormone release.

---

*D*isturbances of thyroid function are among the most commonly diagnosed endocrine disorders. Many are autoimmune disorders. Disturbances of parathyroid functions are uncommon but potentially life threatening. Normal thyroid and parathyroid functions and common disorders of these glands are described briefly in this chapter. The main focus of the chapter is the drug therapy and related nursing responsibilities associated with the treatment of these disorders.

FUNCTIONS OF THE THYROID GLAND

Microscopic spherical sacs, follicles, fill most of the thyroid gland. Within the follicles, follicular cells manufacture **thyroxine (T_4),** and **triiodothyronine (T_3).** These hormones are referred to as *thyroid hormones.* Their primary function is to control the metabolic activity of cells in the body. Figure 41–1 illustrates the physiologic effects of thyroxine and triiodothyronine. Parafollicular cells in the gland produce **calcitonin,** which influence calcium homeostasis.

The thyroid gland is the only endocrine gland that stores its secretory product in large quantity, normally approximately a 100-day supply. Stored thyroid hormones are secreted in response to stimulation from the hypothalamus and pituitary glands. The hypothalamus releases thyrotropin-releasing hormones, which stimulates the anterior pituitary to release thyroid-stimulating hormone (TSH). TSH, in turn, stimulates the thyroid to secrete its own hormones, T_3 and T_4.[1]

DISORDERS OF THE THYROID GLAND

Several disorders of the thyroid gland require drug therapy, including thyroiditis, hypothyroidism, and hyperthyroidism. Drug therapy is also used to treat certain types of goiters and neoplasms. **Thyroiditis** is an inflammation of the thyroid gland characterized by enlargement of the gland. With some forms of thyroiditis (i.e., chronic or Hashimoto's thyroiditis), hypothyroidism may develop. Individuals with this form of thyroiditis may require thyroid hormone therapy.

Hypothyroidism is a metabolic disorder usually characterized by a deficiency in circulating thyroid hormones. The condition is further classified as primary, secondary, and tertiary hypothyroidism. **Primary hypothyroidism** results from a functional deficiency produced by atrophy of the thyroid gland or by partial or complete absence of the gland as the result of surgery, radiation, or drug therapy. **Secondary hypothyroidism** is the result of pituitary insufficiency, and **tertiary hypothyroidism** is caused by hypothalamic insufficiency. Clinical manifestations of hypothyroidism include fatigue, hoarseness, cold intolerance, decreased sweating, cool and dry skin, facial puffiness, and dull, sparse, brittle hair. Slowing of mental processes and motor activity, constipation, decreased appetite, and weight gain also occur.

Hyperthyroidism is a disorder of hypermetabolism resulting from exposure of body tissues to excess amounts of circulating thyroid hormones. Its clinical manifestations include exaggerated alertness, nervousness, irritability, insomnia, a feeling of apprehension, emotional liability, and euphoria. There are also weight loss, fine muscle and tongue tremors, impaired coordination, and heat intolerance.[2,3]

DRUG THERAPY FOR THYROID HORMONE DEFICIENCY AND EXCESS

A deficiency of thyroid hormone requires replacement therapy. Therefore drugs that contain T_4, T_3, or both are administered. These preparations are naturally occurring hormones or synthetic derivatives. Thyroid hormone excess is treated with two primary groups of drugs: antithyroid drugs and radioactive iodines.

▨ NURSING CONSIDERATIONS

The client with a thyroid disorder may not require hospitalization but instead be treated on an outpatient basis. Therefore it is essential that nursing care be well planned and organized.

Assessing   As with any client, obtaining a complete **health history** is critical. Ask specifically about the onset of early symptoms. Did fatigue, lethargy, or somnolence occur, or did the client note insomnia, increased alertness and activity, agitation, and inability to concentrate? Ask the client about changes in appearance, behavior, or mental processes.

Question the client about preexisting health problems (e.g., cardiovascular disease, uncorrected adrenal insufficiency). Include in the health history a complete drug history. Many drugs (e.g., estrogens, salicylates, lithium, diazepam, furosemide, cimetidine, glucocorticoids) alter the results of test used to diagnose thyroid disorders. Also determine if the client smokes. Recent studies have demonstrated that smoking may produce antithyroid effects (i.e., inhibition of iodide transport, inhibition of the movement of iodine into the thyroid, and increased iodide efflux).[4]

During the **physical assessment** obtain baseline height and weight. Compare current weight with presymptomatic weight. Note vital signs and apical heart rate to determine the cardiovascular status of the client. Auscultate for hypo- or hyperactive bowel sounds. Assess for clinical manifestations specific to hypothyroidism (e.g., subnormal basal temperature, easy bruising, impaired wound healing, decreased respiratory rate,

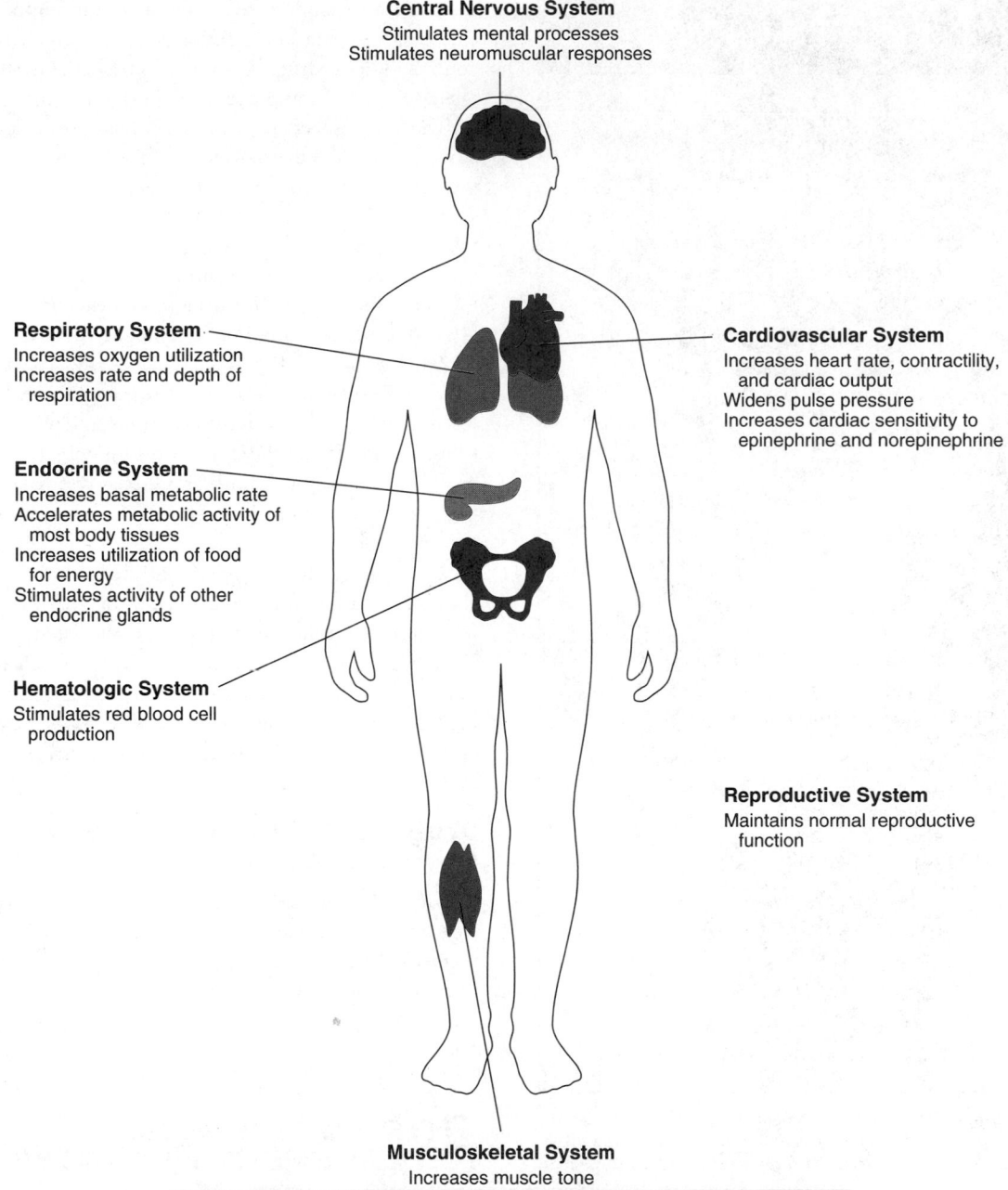

Central Nervous System
Stimulates mental processes
Stimulates neuromuscular responses

Respiratory System
Increases oxygen utilization
Increases rate and depth of
respiration

Cardiovascular System
Increases heart rate, contractility,
and cardiac output
Widens pulse pressure
Increases cardiac sensitivity to
epinephrine and norepinephrine

Endocrine System
Increases basal metabolic rate
Accelerates metabolic activity of
most body tissues
Increases utilization of food
for energy
Stimulates activity of other
endocrine glands

Hematologic System
Stimulates red blood cell
production

Reproductive System
Maintains normal reproductive
function

Musculoskeletal System
Increases muscle tone

FIGURE 41-1   Physiologic effects of thyroxine and triiodothyronine.

bradycardia, and dry, coarse, inelastic skin). Assess for possible indications of hyperthyroidism (e.g., warm, moist skin, bounding pulse, tachycardia, systolic hypertension, tachypnea, and exophthalmos). Test deep tendon reflexes for hyperreflexia. Assess for fine muscle and eyelid tremors. If possible, compare current handwriting with an earlier sample; changes in handwriting can help detect hand tremors associated with hyperthyroidism.

Physical assessment of the individual must include inspection, palpation, and auscultation of the thyroid gland. Inspect the trachea for deviation from midline; inspect the contour and symmetry of the lower anterior portion of the neck. Ask

the client to extend the neck slightly; observe the thyroid while the patient is swallowing. Palpate the thyroid for size, shape, consistency, symmetry, tenderness, and the presence of any nodules. The lobes of the thyroid gland should be symmetric, feel rubbery, and be free of nodules or tenderness.[2,3] Review diagnostic findings. See box on p. 512 for summary of significant diagnostic studies.

Diagnosing   Analysis of data and development of nursing diagnoses are next. Appropriate nursing diagnoses include the following:

• Activity intolerance related to fatigue and lethargy of hypothyroid state.

TESTS USED TO DIAGNOSE THYROID DISORDERS

▶ Serum T_4: Total thyroxine as determined by radioimmunoassay or competitive binding techniques; evaluates thyroid function; normal range—4.5–13 µg/dl

▶ Serum T_3: Free and bound or total serum content of T_3; more accurate indicator of hyperthyroidism than T_4; normal range—70–220 ng/dl

▶ Thyroxine-binding globulin (TBG): Serum levels of TBG provide an assessment of thyroxine-binding capacity; normal value—12–18 µg/dl

▶ T_3 resin uptake test: Amount of hormone bound to TBG; normal range—25%–35%; this percentage indicates one third of available sites on TBG are occupied by thyroid hormone; if percentage is higher than 35%, the number of free sites are low, indicating hyperthyroidism

▶ TSH radioimmunoassay: Level of circulating TSH secreted by anterior pituitary gland; used to differentiate between pituitary dysfunction and primary thyroid dysfunction; normal values—10 µIU/ml

▶ Thyrotropin-releasing hormone stimulation: Direct means of testing response of TSH to TRH; normally TRH stimulates increased TSH production

▶ Radioactive iodine uptake: Rate of iodine uptake by thyroid gland

▶ Thyroid scan: Visual representation of localization of radioactivity; helps determine location, size, and shape of thyroid gland

▶ Protein-bound iodine: Serum proteins are precipitated, washed, and measured for iodine content

Data from Monahan, F.D., Drake, T., & Neighbors, M. (1994). *Nursing care of adults*. Philadelphia: W.B. Saunders; and Price, S., and Wison, L.M. (1992). *Pathophysiology: Clinical concepts of disease processes* (4th ed.). St. Louis: Mosby–Year Book.

- Fatigue related to insomnia and hyperactivity of hyperthyroid state.
- Disturbance in body image related to inability to cope with physical changes associated with thyroid disorder.
- Altered nutrition related to change in body metabolism associated with drug therapy.
- Knowledge deficit regarding drug actions and undesired clinical responses.

Planning   Teaching and discharge plans are important for the client receiving drugs that affect the thyroid gland. Prepare a plan for teaching the client the dosage, drug schedule, expected action, and undesired clinical responses of prescribed drug. Include in the plan signs or symptoms that must be reported to the primary care provider (e.g., shortness of breath, insomnia, and nervousness). Since thyroid hormone prepara-

tions are not standardized, emphasize the importance of not changing preparations. Instruct the client that over-the-counter (OTC) drugs or mineral supplements should not be taken without the approval of the primary care provider.

The final aspect of planning is establishing expected outcomes. Possible outcomes include the following:
- Client reports energy level sufficient to meet activities of daily living.
- Client verbalizes decreased anxiety level.
- Client experiences temperature regulation.
- Client controls weight through diet, exercise, or both.
- Client describes importance of maintaining drug therapy.

Implementing   Reinforce and clarify the primary care provider's explanations of the expected outcomes of treatment. Encourage the client to ask questions and verbalize expectations. During initial therapy, monitor vital signs, weight, heat or cold tolerance, and fluid and electrolyte balance. In addition, monitor thyroid function tests concurrently with drug administration.

Evaluating   Review the expected outcomes with the client. Evaluation of the effectiveness of thyroid agent therapy relies heavily on the client's report of alleviated symptoms that brought him or her to seek help initially. The client should report an increase in activity tolerance, a change in appetite, an increased pulse, temperature, and blood pressure. If no changes occur or if excessive changes occur, question the effectiveness of the dosage.

Drugs Used to Treat Thyroid Hormone Deficiency

Thyroid hormone replacement therapy is used to treat thyroid hormone deficiency. The primary objective of this treatment is to establish a normal metabolic state. The dosage for hormone replacement is based on the client's serum TSH concentration.

THYROID HORMONE REPLACEMENT PROTOTYPE
LEVOTHYROXINE SODIUM

The desired action of levothyroxine sodium is stabilization of the client's metabolic rate without complications of hyperthyroidism.

Pharmacotherapeutics   Levothyroxine sodium is used for replacement of deficient hormone in clients with primary, secondary, tertiary, or congenital hypothyroidism. It is used as replacement therapy in clients with simple (nontoxic) goiter or chronic lymphocytic (Hashimoto's) thyroiditis. It is used also for treatment or myxedema coma or stupor. Evidence of increased responsiveness may occur in 6 to 8 hours. Levothyroxine sodium is administered in suppression tests to differentiate suspected hyperthyroidism from euthyroid and is used in the diagnosis of hyperthyroidism or Graves' disease.

Pharmacokinetics   After oral administration, levothyroxine sodium (Eltroxin, Levoxyl, Levothroid, Levoxine, Synthroid, T_4) has variable absorption, 50% to 80%, from the gastrointestinal (GI) tract. After intramuscular (IM) administration, absorption is variable and poor. Levothyroxine is distributed into most body tissues and fluids; highest concentrations occur in the liver and kidneys. Metabolism occurs in the liver where the drug is conjugated with glucuronic and sulfuric acids. Elimination is through the bile, with 20% to 40% of the drug excreted unchanged in the feces. Levothyroxine has a slow onset and long duration of action. The plasma half-life is 6 to 7 days. Full effects of the drug may not occur for 2 to 3 weeks.[5,6]

Pharmacodynamics Levothyroxine sodium binds to receptors throughout the body and has a principal effect of increasing the metabolic rate of body tissues. It promotes gluconeogenesis and increases the use and mobilization of glycogen stores. The drug stimulates protein synthesis and promotes cell growth and differentiation.

Pharmaceutics Levothyroxine sodium is available as uncoated tablets for oral administration. It is also available in parenteral solution for IM or intravenous (IV) administration. Table 41–1 summarizes information about dosage forms and dosages.

Undesired Clinical Responses Undesired responses to levothyroxine sodium are due to overdose and are manifested mainly as signs and symptoms of hyperthyroidism. (Fig. 41–2).

Contraindications and Precautions Clients receiving levothyroxine sodium must be closely monitored, and their thyroid function status must be routinely assessed. Since thyroid drugs increase oxygen demand, they must be used with extreme caution in clients with angina pectoris or other cardiovascular disease. Frequently these in-

TABLE 41–1

Drugs Used to Treat Thyroid Hormone Deficiencies

Drug Name	Dosage and Route of Administration	Nursing Considerations
LEVOTHYROXINE SODIUM (Eltroxin, Levoxyl, Levothroid, Levoxine, Synthroid) **HOW SUPPLIED** Synthetic preparation of T_4 Uncoated tablets: 25, 50, 75, 88, 100, 112, 125, 137, 150, 175, 200, 300 μg IV solution: 200, 500 μg/vial	**_Hypothyroidism_** ADULTS, ELDERLY Oral: initial dose, 0.05 mg/d; increase by 0.025 mg q2-3wk Maintenance: 0.075–0.125 mg/d IV or IM: initial dose, 0.05–0.1 mg/d **_Myxedema Coma or Stupor_** ADULTS, ELDERLY IV: Initial dose, 0.4 mg; follow with 0.1–0.2 mg daily supplement **_Thyroid Suppression Therapy_** ADULTS, ELDERLY Oral: 2.6 μg/kg/d for 7–10 d Usual parenteral dosage for adults (except in myxedemic coma): one half previously established oral dosage **_Congenital Hypothyroidism_** ORAL Children >12 y: 0.15 mg/d Children 6–12 y: 0.1–0.15 mg/d Children 1–5 y: 0.075–0.1 mg/d Children 6–12 mo: 0.05–0.075 mg/d Infants 0–6 mo: 0.025–0.05 mg/d	**_Assess_** Check results of thyroid function studies. Determine presence of preexisting diseases (e.g., hypertension, angina pectoris). Determine if client is pregnant; levothyroxine is classified as Pregnancy Category A drug. Collect complete drug history; drug interacts with cholesteramine, oral anticoagulants, phenytoin, for example. Question client for hypersensitivity to aspirin, lactose, and tartrazine. **_Implement_** Administer at same time each day to maintain hormone levels. Administer before breakfast. Reconstitute 200 or 500 μg vial with 5 ml 0.09% NaCl to provide concentration of 40 or 100 μg/ml, respectively. Shake solution until clear. Do not mix parenteral drug with other IV solutions. Use mixed solution immediately and discard unused portion. Observe sleep pattern. Teach client not to discontinue drug abruptly; replacement therapy for hypothyroidism is lifelong. Instruct client not to change brands. Teach client how to monitor own pulse rate. Tell parents that children may have reversible hair loss or increased aggressiveness during first few months of therapy. **_Monitor_** Monitor pulse for rate and rhythm; report pulse rate >100. Observe for indications of excessive dosage (e.g., weight loss, palpitations, tremors, nervousness, headache, insomnia, menstrual irregularities). **_Evaluate_** Effectiveness is noted by diminished clinical manifestations of hypothyroidism.

Table continued on following page.

TABLE 41–1 *Continued*
Drugs Used to Treat Thyroid Hormone Deficiencies

Drug Name	Dosage and Route of Administration	Nursing Considerations
Liothyronine (Cytomel, Triostat) **HOW SUPPLIED** Synthetic preparation of T_3 Tablets: 5, 25, 50 µg Parenteral solution: 10 µg/ml packaged in 1-ml vials	**Hypothyroidism** **ADULTS** Oral: initial dose, 25 µg/d; increase by 12.5–25 µg q1-2wk **ELDERLY** Oral: initial dose, 5 µg/d; may increase by 5 µg/d q1-2wk Maintenance: 25–75 µg/d **Myxedema** **ADULTS, ELDERLY** Oral: initial dose 5 µg/d; increase by 5–10 µg q1-2wk Maintenance: 50–100 µg/d **Nontoxic Goiter** **ADULTS, ELDERLY** Oral: initial dose, 5 µg/d; increase by 5–10 µg/d q1-2wk Maintenance: 75 µg/d **T_3 Suppression Test** **ADULTS, ELDERLY** Oral: 75–100 µg/d for 7 d, then repeat ^{131}I thyroid uptake test **Congenital Hypothyroidism** **CHILDREN** Oral: initial dose, 5 µg/d; increase by 5 µg/d q3-4d **MAINTENANCE** Infant: 20 µg/d Children of 1 y: 50 µg/d Children >3 y: full adult dose **Myxedema Coma, Precoma** Dosages based on client's clinical status; administer IV dose at least 4 h, but no longer than 12 h, apart **ADULTS, ELDERLY** IV initial dose, 25–50 µg (10–20 µg in client with cardiovascular disease); total dose, at least 65 µg/d	See levothyroxine sodium with following additions: Refrigerate parenteral dosage forms. Store oral tablets at room temperature. Do not administer IM or subcutaneously (SC). Change to oral dose as soon as a client is stabilized. When changing *from* another thyroid preparation, discontinue other thyroid drug first and begin liothyronine at low dose. When changing *to* another thyroid preparation, continue liothyronine for several days.
Liotrix (Thyrolar) **HOW SUPPLIED** Synthetic T_4 plus synthetic T_3 in a 4:1 fixed ratio Tablets: various dosages Thyrolar <table><tr><td>Strength (grains [gr])</td><td colspan="2">Content (µg)</td></tr><tr><td></td><td>T_4</td><td>T_3</td></tr><tr><td>¼</td><td>12.5</td><td>3.1</td></tr><tr><td>½</td><td>25</td><td>6.25</td></tr><tr><td>1</td><td>50</td><td>12.5</td></tr><tr><td>2</td><td>100</td><td>25</td></tr><tr><td>3</td><td>150</td><td>37.5</td></tr></table>	**Hypothyroidism without Myxedema** **ADULTS** Oral: initial dose, ¼ gr/d before breakfast; increase by ¼ gr bi-weekly or monthly as needed **Myxedema or Hypothyroidism with Cardiovascular Disease** ¼ gr/d Maintenance: 1–2 gr/d **ELDERLY** Initial dose, 25% to 50% usual adult dose; may double dose at 6- to 8-wk intervals if necessary **CHILDREN** See package insert or United States Pharmacopeia Drug Information (USPDI)	

TABLE 41–1 *Continued*

Drugs Used to Treat Thyroid Hormone Deficiencies

Drug Name	Dosage and Route of Administration	Nursing Considerations
Thyroid (Armour Thyroid, S-P-T, Thyrar) **HOW SUPPLIED** Desiccated animal thyroid glands Capsules: 1, 2, 3, 5 gr Tablets: various dosages	**Hypothyroidism** **ADULTS, ELDERLY** Oral: initial dose, 30 mg/d; increase 15 mg q2-3wk Maintenance: 60–120 mg/d **Thyroid Cancer** **ADULTS, ELDERLY** Oral: larger doses required than used for replacement therapy **Congenital Hypothyroidism** **ORAL** Children >12 y: >90 mg/d Children 6–12 y: 60–90 mg/d Children 1–5 y: 45–60 mg/d Infants 6–12 mo: 30–45 mg/d Infants 0–6 mo: 15–30 mg/d	See levothyroxine sodium.

dividuals require reduced dosages. In clients with adrenal insufficiency and hypothyroidism, the adrenal insufficiency must be corrected first since thyroid hormones increase the tissue demand for adrenocortical hormone.

Drug-Drug and Drug-Nutrient Interactions Numerous drugs interact with levothyroxine sodium, including nonsteroidal antiinflammatory drugs (NSAIDs), oral anticoagulants, antihyperglycemic drugs, sympathomimetic drugs, cholestyramine resins, estrogens, and ferrous sulfate. Several NSAIDs can lower serum thyroid hormone concentrations, principally by interfering with the binding of T_4 and T_3 to serum carrier proteins. Clients taking these drugs remain euthyroid.[7] Hypothyroidism reduces the severity of diabetes mellitus; therefore a smaller dosage of the prescribed antihyperglycemic drug is necessary. With administration of levothyroxine sodium, increasing the dosage of insulin or oral antidiabetic agents may be necessary. Additionally, cholestyramine binds both T_3 and T_4 in the intestine, impairing absorption of these thyroid hormones. Four to 5 hours should elapse between administration of cholestyramine and thyroid hormones.[5]

Since levothyroxine sodium increases catabolism of vitamin K–dependent clotting factors, it potentiates the hypoprothrombinemic effect of oral anticoagulants. Clients receiving levothyroxine sodium and oral anticoagulants should be monitored closely for excessive bleeding. In addition, prothrombin time evaluation should be performed frequently.

Several antiepileptic drugs change the serum levels of thyroid hormones. In one study it was reported that a decrease in T_4 serum levels, free T_4 index, and T_3 was observed in clients receiving therapeutic doses of pheno-

barbital, carbamazepine, sodium valproate, and diphenylhydantoin. Another study concluded that diphenylhydantoin causes a decrease in peripheral thyroid hormone levels.[8,9]

Simultaneous ingestion of ferrous sulfate and thyroxine causes a variable reduction in thyroxine efficiency that is clinically significant in some clients. The interaction probably is caused by the binding of iron to thyroxine.[10]

Thyroid preparations should be taken on an empty stomach. In addition, the client should avoid ingesting cabbage, kale, and brussel sprouts.[11]

Life-Span Considerations The incidence of congenital hypothyroidism in infants from hypothyroid mothers is 1:4000. Signs and symptoms of congenital hypothyroidism include large anterior and posterior fontanel, dry skin, feeding problems, hypothermia, failure to gain weight, skin mottling, respiratory problems, persistence of mild jaundice, thick tongue, hoarse cry, and umbilical hernia. Without administration of a thyroid drug, the infant develops cretinism. When a thyroid drug is administered, close control of the dosage is essential to guarantee optimum growth and development.[12]

Studies have shown that only minimal amounts of thyroid hormones are distributed into the milk. Even so, thyroid hormone replacement drugs should be used with caution in nursing women. Levothyroxine sodium is classified as a Pregnancy Category A drug, indicating these hormones do not readily cross the placental barrier. However, recent studies have shown that prenatal thyrotropin-releasing hormones administered to women in preterm labor increase thyroid hormones and prolactin in preterm fetuses to levels similar to those normally occur-

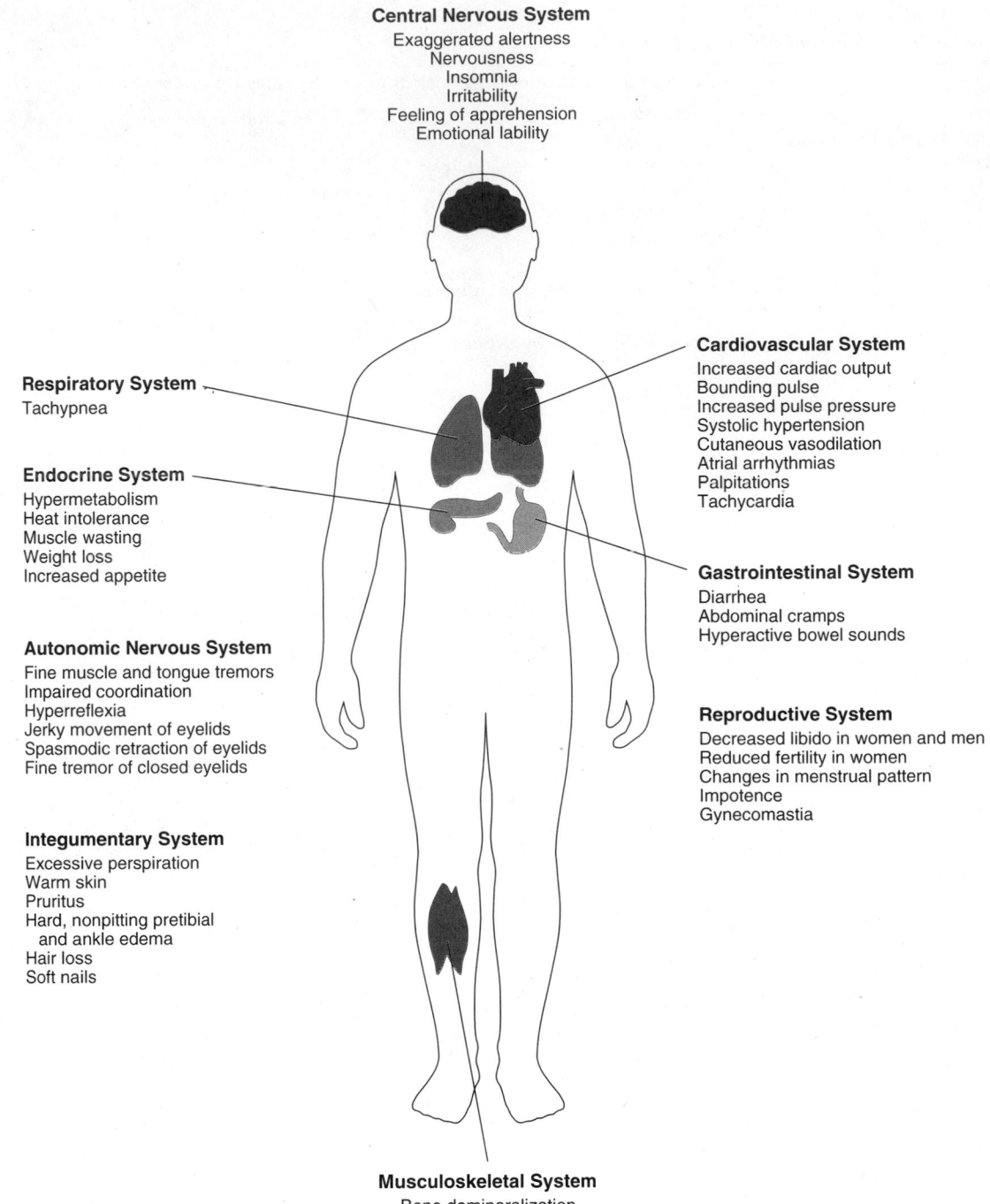

Central Nervous System
Exaggerated alertness
Nervousness
Insomnia
Irritability
Feeling of apprehension
Emotional lability

Cardiovascular System
Increased cardiac output
Bounding pulse
Increased pulse pressure
Systolic hypertension
Cutaneous vasodilation
Atrial arrhythmias
Palpitations
Tachycardia

Respiratory System
Tachypnea

Endocrine System
Hypermetabolism
Heat intolerance
Muscle wasting
Weight loss
Increased appetite

Gastrointestinal System
Diarrhea
Abdominal cramps
Hyperactive bowel sounds

Autonomic Nervous System
Fine muscle and tongue tremors
Impaired coordination
Hyperreflexia
Jerky movement of eyelids
Spasmodic retraction of eyelids
Fine tremor of closed eyelids

Reproductive System
Decreased libido in women and men
Reduced fertility in women
Changes in menstrual pattern
Impotence
Gynecomastia

Integumentary System
Excessive perspiration
Warm skin
Pruritus
Hard, nonpitting pretibial
   and ankle edema
Hair loss
Soft nails

Musculoskeletal System
Bone demineralization

FIGURE 41–2   Undesired responses to drugs used to treat thyroid deficiency.

ring at term. These findings have particular significance for prevention of newborn lung disease.[13]

Thyroid drugs must be administered with care to geriatric clients who are more susceptible to thyroid hormones and have more contraindicating disorders.[14]

Specific Drug-Related Nursing Considerations Levothyroxine should be administered as a single morning dose before the client eats. Monitor his or her changes in pulse and blood pressure. Withhold the dose and instruct the client to withhold the dose and notify primary care

provider if the pulse rate is higher than 100 beats per minute or its rhythm is irregular.

Since hypothyroid clients are particularly sensitive to thyroid drugs, hormone replacement therapy is started at low doses and gradually increased. Monitoring dosages, documenting effects, and communicating with the client are critical.

The myocardial health of the client also is a critical factor. Clients who are hypothyroid for a long period of time usually have elevated serum cholesterol levels, atherosclerosis, and coronary artery disease. While the client remains in a hypothyroid state and his or her metabolism is subnormal, the myocardial oxygen demands are easily met in spite of coronary artery disease. However, with administration of the drug, an increase in metabolism and in myocardial oxygen demand occurs, which may result in myocardial ischemia or infarction. Any complaints of chest pain or angina must be reported. In such instances the thyroid hormone usually is discontinued immediately and after investigation of the angina, restarted at lower levels.

If drug therapy is effective, a rise in serum T_4 and T_3 should occur. The resin T_3 uptake test should show an increased percentage of occupied sites on thyroxine-binding globulin (TBG). Monitoring TSH assay findings also is important. TSH findings are independent of TBG changes that result from pregnancy and from use of birth control pills or estrogen. In addition, these findings are not artificially elevated by the levothyroxine treatment itself.[15]

MISCELLANEOUS DRUGS IN CATEGORY

Other drug preparations used to treat thyroid deficiency include liotrix, liothyronine, and thyroid. **Liothyronine** (Cytomel, Triostat) is a synthetic preparation of T_3. The pharmacologic effects of liothyronine are similar to those of levothyroxine; however, it has a shorter half-life and duration of action and is more expensive. Since liothyronine's effects develop quickly, it is useful in the treatment of conditions requiring rapid results (e.g., myxedema coma or stupor). **Liotrix** (Thyrolar) is a mixture of synthetic T_4 and T_3 in a 4:1 ratio. This preparation produces plasma levels of T_4 and T_3 similar to those occurring naturally.[16]

Thyroid (Armour Thyroid, S-P-T) is a natural thyroid product that consists of desiccated animal thyroid glands. Standardization of this preparation is based on the presence of iodine, levothyroxine, and liothyronine. The ratio of levothyroxine to liothyronine is not less than 5:1. Although currently this preparation is not routinely prescribed for clients starting therapy, it still is used for clients who have been taking the drug for years.

Drugs Used to Treat Thyroid Hormone Excess: Antithyroid Drugs

The most common form of primary hyperthyroidism is Graves' disease. Toxic nodular goiter, secreting adenoma of the thyroid gland, subacute thyroiditis, pituitary adenoma that secretes excess TSH, overtreatment of hypothyroidism, and thyroid-stimulating drugs can also cause symptoms of hyperthyroidism. To date, no treatment for the basic cause of hyperthyroidism has been discovered. Treatment follows three directions: (1) pharmacologic therapy, using antithyroid drugs and other agents that control the manifestations of hyperthyroidism; (2) radiation to destroy thyroid tissue; and (3) surgery with removal of most of the thyroid gland.

ANTITHYROID DRUG PROTOTYPE
PROPYLTHIOURACIL

Propylthiouracil belongs to the antithyroid drug category and serves as prototype of the group. Only one other antithyroid drug, methimazole, currently is prescribed.

Pharmacotherapeutics Propylthiouracil can be used alone to treat Graves's disease, and it can be prescribed concomitantly with radioactive iodine until the effects of the radioactive iodine occur. Propylthiouracil is also administered before thyroid gland surgery to suppress thyroid hormone synthesis.

Pharmacokinetics Propylthiouracil is rapidly absorbed after oral administration. Therapeutic effects begin within 30 minutes. Plasma half-life of the drug is approximately 2 hours. As a result, propylthiouracil must be administered several times each day. Approximately 35% of the drug is excreted in the urine within 24 hours.[5,6]

Pharmacodynamics Propylthiouracil inhibits the synthesis of thyroid hormones during the second stage of formation (i.e., the mono- and diiodination of tyrosyl residues). Thus iodine in a reduced form does not react with tyrosine to form iodotyrosine.[16] Propylthiouracil does not inhibit the action of thyroid hormones already formed and present in the thyroid gland or circulation. It also does not interfere with exogenously administered thyroid hormones.

Pharmaceutics Propylthiouracil is available as coated and uncoated tablets. The usual schedule of administration is three to four times per day. See Table 41–2 for information about dosage and route of administration.

Undesired Clinical Responses Undesired clinical responses include agranulocytosis, granulocytopenia, and thrombocytopenia. Aplastic anemia, drug fever, and a lupuslike syndrome may occur. In addition, rash, nausea, arthralgia, headache, dizziness, and paresthesias are common.

Contraindications and Precautions Use of propylthiouracil is contraindicated in the presence of hypersensitivity to the drug. Clients receiving the drug must be under close supervision and must be monitored for indications of blood dyscrasias. Particular care must be taken with clients receiving other drugs capable of producing agranulocytosis.

Drug-Drug, Drug-Nutrient, Drug-Environment Interactions When they are administered concurrently, the activity of anticoagulants may be potentiated by the anti-vitamin K activity of propylthiouracil. Propylthiouracil must be stored at controlled room temperatures (15° to 30° C). While receiving the drug, the client may need to restrict seafood and iodine products.

Life-Span Considerations Propylthiouracil is classified as a Pregnancy Category D drug. It readily crosses the placenta and has caused neonatal hypothyroidism and goiter. If this drug is used during pregnancy or if the client becomes pregnant while receiving the drug, the client should be warned of the potential hazard to the fetus. Propylthiouracil also enters breast milk and is contraindicated for nursing mothers.

Specific Drug-Related Nursing Considerations The health history should focus on signs and symptoms related to accelerated or exaggerated metabolism. Changes in appearance, appetite, weight, and emotional state are common. Note any preexisting condition that may contraindicate the use of an antithyroid drug (e.g., lactation or hypersensitivity). Note conditions that warrant cautious use of antithyroid drugs (e.g., tuberculosis or use of a granulocytopenic drug). Determine vital signs, weight, fluid and electrolyte status, and energy level. Assess the status of the thyroid gland as previously discussed.

Administer the prescribed dosage at evenly spaced time intervals around the clock. Monitor the client's pulse and weight daily, and teach the client to take a resting pulse daily. Monitor the client for a hypersensitivity reaction that may develop during the first 3 weeks of treatment or for potentially fatal agranulocytosis that may develop 4 to 8 weeks into the treatment. Monitor hematologic studies for evidence of bone marrow suppression. Also teach the client to assess for skin eruptions, itching, enlarged lymph glands, and unusual bleeding.

Warn the client against using OTC drugs that contain iodine (e.g., cough medicine) without checking with the primary care provider. Teach the client to consult with the primary care provider about using iodized salt and eating shellfish. See Table 41–2 for additional information about nursing care of the client receiving propylthiouracil.

MISCELLANEOUS DRUGS IN CATEGORY

The other antithyroid drug, **methimazole** (Tapazole), is similar to propylthiouracil. It is readily absorbed from the GI tract. Approximately 95% of the drug is bioavailable and insignificantly bound to protein. Methimazole is concentrated in the thyroid gland. Clinical effects last up to 3 hours, and the half-life is 6 to 9 hours. Excretion occurs in the urine, with 10% unchanged drug. Like propylthiouracil, use of methima-

TABLE 41–2
Drugs Used to Treat Thyroid Hormone Excess

Drug Name	Dosage and Route of Administration	Nursing Considerations
THIOUREYLENE DRUGS PROPYLTHIOURACIL (Prophylthiouracil) **HOW SUPPLIED** Coated tablet: 50 mg Uncoated tablet: 50 mg	ADULTS Initial dose, 300–400 mg/d Maintenance: 100–150 mg/d CHILDREN 6–10 y: initial dose, 50–150 mg/d >10 y: initial dose, 150–300 mg/d Maintenance dose: determine by response	*Assess* Determine if client is pregnant; drug classified in Pregnancy Catergory D group. Determine if woman is nursing; drug is excreted in milk. Obtain baseline weight and pulse. Review results of serum T_3 and T_4 studies. *Implement* Assess pulse and weight daily. Administer at 8-h intervals. Check with prescriber to determine if seafood or iodine products must be restricted. Teach client to check resting pulse daily to monitor therapeutic response. Teach client to report weight gain, cold intolerance, or depression, which may indicate hypothyroidism. Teach client to report excessive bruising or bleeding, which may indicate hypothrombinemia. Teach client to report fever, headaches, skin eruptions, or sore throat, which could indicate agranulocytosis. *Monitor* Monitor for undesired clinical responses (e.g., skin rash, agranulocytosis, urticaria, nausea, vomiting, loss of hair, pruritus). Monitor complete blood count and differential findings. Monitor prothrombin time. *Evaluate* Observe for decreased indications of hyperthyroidism: decreased pulse rate, decreased intolerance to heat, diminished restlessness. Anticipate decreased serum T_3 and T_4 levels with effective therapy (normal serum T_3, 70–220 ng/dl; normal serum T_4, 4.5–11.5 μm/dl). Anticipate a decrease in serum resin T3 uptake findings (normal, 25% to 35%).

TABLE 41–2 *Continued*

Drugs Used to Treat Thyroid Hormone Excess

Drug Name	Dosage and Route of Administration	Nursing Considerations
Methimazole (Tapazole) **HOW SUPPLIED** Uncoated tablet: 5, 10 mg	Dosage is divided into three equal doses at 8-h intervals. **ADULTS** Mild hyperthyroidism: initial dose, 15 mg Moderately severe hyperthyroidism: initial dose, 30–40 mg Severe hyperthyroidism: initial dose, 60 mg Mainenance dose: 5–15 mg/d **CHILDREN** Initial daily dose: 0.4 mg/kg of body weight Maintenance dose: approximately one half of initial dose	Same as propylthiouracil
RADIOACTIVE ISOTOPES OF IODINE RADIOACTIVE IODINE,[131]I (Iodotope, generic sodium iodide ^{131}I) **HOW SUPPLIED** Capsules: 0.8–100 mCi Oral solution: 3.5–150 mCi	**Hyperthyroidism** Oral: 4–20 mCi (148–740 mBq) **Thyroid Carcinoma** Oral: 50–200 mCi (7.4 GBq)	**Implement** Observe radiation precautions for 24 h after treatment for hyperthyroidism and for 3 d after treatment for thyroid cancer. Explain to client that hypothyroidism may develop. Assess client for signs and symptoms of thyroid crisis. Observe client for undesired clinical responses (e.g., thyroiditis, temporary exacerbation of hyperthyroidism). **Monitor** Monitor white blood count for changes indicative of radiation leukemia. Monitor prothrombin time.

zole is contraindicated for nursing mothers. Methimazole crosses the placenta more readily than propylthiouracil; therefore if treatment for thyroid excess is needed during pregnancy, propylthiouracil is preferred.

Drugs Used to Treat Thyroid Hormone Excess: Radioactive Iodines

The most frequently used radioactive iodine is an isotope of stable iodine, [131]I.

RADIOACTIVE IODINE PROTOTYPE
RADIOACTIVE IODINE 131

Pharmacotherapeutics Radioactive iodine is used for the treatment of hyperthyroidism and thyroid cancer. With treatment of Graves' disease, use of radioactive iodine has resulted in a need for retreatment of 25% to 34% of the clients, and hypothyroidism occurs in 70% to 100% of treated clients.[17,18]

Pharmacokinetics Radioactive iodine is absorbed readily from the GI tract and is distributed into the extracellular fluid. It is selectively concentrated in the thyroid gland where it is bound to tyrosyl residues of thyroglobulin. It also concentrates in the stomach, salivary glands,

and lactating breast. Radioactive iodine is metabolized by the thyroid into protein-bound iodine. It has a potential half-life of 8 days and is excreted by the kidneys.[16] Onset of action occurs in approximately 2 to 4 weeks; peak effect is noted within 2 to 4 months.

Pharmacodynamics Thyroid tissue has an affinity for iodine and picks up the radioactive iodine. The ^{131}I destroys the thyroid tissue. The end result is that there is less thyroid tissue to produce thyroid hormone and therefore less circulating hormone. A decrease in circulating hormone results in a decrease of peripheral symptoms of hyperthyroidism. Relief of symptoms does not occur until 6 to 8 weeks after treatment.

Pharmaceutics ^{131}I is available in capsules and solution for oral administration. Both preparations are odorless and tasteless. The dosage for radioactive iodine is determined by thyroid mass and rate of thyroidal iodine uptake. Dosages are adjusted to as low a level as possible. High doses of radioactive iodine result in greater likelihood of cure but earlier and more frequent onset of hypothyroidism. Lower doses result in less hypothyroidism but a greater incidence of treatment failure that necessitates re-treatment with radioiodine or drug therapy or both.

Undesired Clinical Responses Radioactive iodine causes destruction of thyroid tissue and a decrease in hormone levels. It also produces a change in the pituitary-thyroid axis. These changes continue for a long time after termination of radioactive iodine treatment. Radiation-induced malignancy, usually of the bone marrow and urinary bladder, after radioactive iodine therapy is also possible. This phenomenon, which does not occur frequently, may take several weeks to develop.[16]

Contraindications and Precautions Concurrent administration or recent use (1 to 2 weeks) of iodide products is contraindicated for clients who receive [131]I. Iodine raises the plasma inorganic iodide concentration and lowers the fraction of the dose of ^{131}I taken up by the thyroid.

Drug-Drug, Drug-Nutrient, Drug-Environment Interactions As previously indicated, iodine interferes with the thyroid gland's uptake of radioactive iodine. Therefore ingestion of iodide products, shellfish, and iodized salt should be avoided. In addition, the client should fast the night before receiving ^{131}I since food delays absorption of the drug.

Environmental considerations are important for the client receiving radioactive iodine. After receiving radioactive iodine for hyperthyroidism, the client's urine and saliva are slightly radioactive for 6 to 8 hours. Full radiation precautions, according to the protocol of the facility, must be instituted during this time. After receiving radioactive iodine for thyroid cancer, the client's urine, saliva, and perspiration remain radioactive for 3 days. During this time the client is isolated, and disposable eating utensils and linens are used.

Life-Span Considerations Radioactive iodine is not recommended for persons under age 30 years unless circumstances rule out other forms of therapy. In children there is a higher risk of delayed hypothyroidism. Its use is contraindicated during pregnancy since exposure of the fetus to the radioactive iodine after the first trimester may damage the immature thyroid gland. In addition, radioactive iodine is not recommended for use in lactating women because it enters the breast milk. Radioactive iodine therapy is also more stressful on geriatric clients.

Specific Drug-Related Nursing Considerations Emotional support of the client receiving ^{131}I is important. Assure the client that his or her dosage is carefully regulated. Tell the client what to expect after therapy and the warning signs and symptoms of hypothyroidism. Emphasize to the client and family that the client requires lifelong follow-up after treatment with radioactive iodine. Explain the radiation precautions and encourage the client and family to ask questions. Determine the family's preparation for isolation procedures in the home.

Although you may not administer the radioactive iodine, knowledge of proper procedures is essential. Instruct the client receiving the drug for hyperthyroidism to use appropriate disposal methods when coughing and expectorating. The client receiving radioactive iodine for thyroid cancer must be instructed to save his or her urine in lead containers for 24 to 48 hours. The urine is then analyzed to determine the amount of radioactive material excreted. Encourage the client to drink fluids to facilitate excretion of the radioactive isotope. Warn the client who is discharged less than 7 days after a radioactive iodine dose for thyroid cancer to avoid close, prolonged contact with small children. Instruct the client not to sleep in the same room with another individual for 7 days after treatment because of an increased risk of thyroid cancer in the other individual.

MISCELLANEOUS DRUGS USED TO TREAT HYPERTHYROIDISM

In addition to antithyroid drugs and radioactive iodine, nonreactive iodide products are available for thyroid therapy. These iodide products include **potassium iodide solution, sodium iodide,** and **strong iodine solution.** Nonreactive iodine is not recommended as a sole treatment for hyperthyroidism since effects from the drug are usually transient and incomplete. Undesired clinical responses to iodine include skin reactions, angioedema, vasculitis, and drug fever. In some individuals iodine produces a syndrome, iodism, with irritation of the eyes, nose, and throat and symptoms resembling those of a bad cold.[16]

Another group of drugs used in the treatment of hyperthyroidism is **β-adrenergic blockers.** β-Blockers have been used to modify the severity of the hyperadrenergic symptoms produced by hyperthyroidism. Although their exact mechanism of action in clients with hyperthyroidism is unknown, it is known that they antagonize β-receptor–mediated effects of catecholamines. β-Blockers are effective in treating hypermetabolic symptoms in clients with a variety of hyperthyroid states. They are also administered concurrently with antithyroid drugs and radioactive iodide and in conjunction with surgery to treat Graves' disease and toxic nodular goiters.[19]

CONCEPT REVIEW

Thyroid hormones (T_3 and T_4) are produced in follicular cells of the thyroid gland. The synthesis and secretion of thyroid hormones are stimulated by TSH from the pituitary.

Manifestations of hypothyroidism are due to generalized decreases in metabolism. Treatment centers on hormone replacement therapy.

Hyperthyroidism may be primary or secondary to pituitary hypersecretion of TSH. High levels of T_3 and T_4 confirm the diagnosis of hyperthyroidism. Treatment includes β-blockers to control adrenergic symptoms, antithyroid drugs to reduce thyroid production, and radioactive iodine to destroy thyroid cells.

FUNCTIONS OF THE PARATHYROID GLANDS

The parathyroid glands, which are located on the posterior surface of the thyroid gland, secrete the parathyroid hormone, **parathormone.** The primary function of this hormone is regulation of the body's calcium and phosphate levels. Parathyroid hormone has a half-life of only a few minutes. Therefore it must be secreted constantly to maintain serum calcium levels within a margin of homeostasis. Serum calcium levels are raised by action of the parathyroid hormone on three target sites: the bones, the kidneys, and the GI tract.

In the bones the hormone stimulates osteoclast activity, causing breakdown of the bone and increased resorption of calcium from the bones. In the kidneys parathyroid hormone acts directly on the renal tubules to increase reabsorption of calcium and to promote excretion of phosphate. In the intestines parathyroid hormone activates vitamin D, which acts directly on the intestinal mucosa to increase absorption of dietary calcium. Vitamin D is essential for intestinal absorption of dietary calcium and its use by the body.[1,2]

DISORDERS OF THE PARATHYROID GLANDS

Hypoparathyroidism is an acute or chronic disorder of calcium metabolism. It is produced by inadequate secretion of parathormone or failure of target cells to respond to parathormone. The most common cause of hypoparathyroidism is damage to or accidental removal of the parathyroid glands during thyroid gland surgery or irradiation or surgical removal of the parathyroid glands. Decreased parathyroid hormone causes decreased calcium resorption from the bones, decreased intestinal absorption, and decreased reabsorption of calcium in the renal tubules with increased phosphate retention. Although treatment depends on the severity of the condition, both acute and chronic hypoparathyroidism require calcium replacement therapy.[2]

Hyperparathyroidism causes increased tubular resorption of calcium and increased phosphate excretion, which contribute to hypercalcemia and hypophosphatemia. As a result of the hypercalcemia, renal calculi frequently develop. Excess parathormone also increases bone resorption, resulting in decalcification of the bone. Increased concentrations of serum ionized calcium decrease neuromuscular excitability. Transmission of neuromuscular impulses is slowed. Calcium is deposited in tissues throughout the body.[2]

DRUGS USED TO TREAT PARATHYROID DISORDERS

The major drug groups used to treat parathyroid disorders are calcium regulators, which decrease the serum calcium concentration, and vitamin D, which increases the serum calcium levels. **Calcitriol,** a synthetic vitamin D analog, is active in the regulation of calcium absorption from the GI tract and in the use of calcium in the body. Calcitriol is used in the treatment of hypoparathyroidism. (See Chapters 73 and 74 for a discussion of calcium and vitamin D.)

Calcium Regulators

The major drugs used as calcium regulators are calcitonin and etidronate sodium.

CALCIUM REGULATOR PROTOTYPE

CALCITONIN

Calcitonin is a polypeptide hormone secreted by the perifollicular cells of the thyroid glands in mammals and by the ultimobranchial gland in birds and fish. It has a molecular weight of approximately 3600. Calcitonin is commercially available as calcitonin, human, and calcitonin, salmon. Calcitonin, salmon, is approximately 50 times more potent than calcitonin, human, on a weight-to-weight basis. Both derivatives are prepared synthetically.[5,6]

Pharmacotherapeutics Calcitonin, human, is indicated for the treatment of symptomatic Paget's disease of the bone. Relief of bone pain associated with Paget's disease usually begins 2 to 8 weeks after the start of therapy. (Paget's disease is a chronic, progressive metabolic bone disease of unknown cause.) Other therapeutic uses of calcitonin, human, include treatment of hypercalcemia in cancer clients, vitamin D intoxication, and hyperphosphatemia. Calcitonin, salmon, is indicated for the treatment of symptomatic Paget's disease of the bone, hypercalcemia, and postmenopausal osteoporosis. In addition, one study reported the use of calcitonin, salmon, in clients with metastatic cancer and pain refractory to traditional treatments. Eight of nine subjects reported pain relief after subarachnoid injection. The duration of the pain relief varied from 1 hour to 5 days.[20–24]

Pharmacokinetics Calcitonin is destroyed in the GI tract and therefore must be administered parenterally. The exact distribution is unknown. It is metabolized in the kidneys, blood, and peripheral tissues. Onset of action after IV administration is immediate; onset of action after IM or SC administration is 15 minutes. Peak action occurs in 4 hours, and duration of action is 24 hours.

Pharmacodynamics When calcitonin is administered, the serum calcium level is lowered, and urinary excretion of calcium, phosphorus, and sodium increases.

Pharmaceutics Calcitonin, human, and calcitonin, salmon, are supplied in dosage forms for parenteral administration. Table 41–3 summarizes dosage information about both forms of calcitonin.

Undesired Clinical Responses Undesired clinical responses associated with the clinical use of calcitonin are infrequent and mild. These responses usually involve the GI tract and include transient nausea, with or without vomiting, anorexia, diarrhea, epigastric discomfort, and abdominal pain. Flushing of the face, ears, hands, and feet commonly occurs within minutes of a calcitonin injection. This reaction is diminished if the drug is administered at bedtime. Tenderness or tingling of the palms and soles has also been reported.

Contraindications and Precautions The most important contraindication for calcitonin administration is allergies. Since calcitonin, salmon, is a protein, allergies to it occur more frequently. Skin testing should be considered before therapy in clients with multiple allergies.

Drug-Drug Interactions Calcitonin may be antagonized by calcium and vitamin D. Concurrent administration of theophylline and isoproterenol results in increased bone resorption.

Life-Span Considerations The safe use of calcitonin in pediatric clients is not established. Calcitonin is not recommended for breast-feeding mothers since it does inhibit lactation. It should not be prescribed for women who are or may become pregnant since it may decrease fetal birth weight. Dosages must be monitored more closely with geriatric clients.

Specific Drug-Related Nursing Considerations Ask the client about his or her family medical history. Primary hyperparathyroidism occurs in a number of familial syndromes. Specifically ask about relatives with symptoms such as ulcer disease, bone disease, kidney stones, or any form of endocrine disorder. Collect a drug history, including information about prescription and OTC drugs. Thiazide diuretics and excessive vitamin D intake can produce hypercalcemia. Determine what symptoms caused the client to seek medical attention. Usual manifestations include headache, drowsiness, flank pain, and muscle weakness. Ask about bone pain or fractures or arthritis and unexplained recent weight loss.

The drug should be administered at bedtime to minimize nausea and vomiting. Parenteral calcium must be readily available during the first doses. Monitor serum calcium levels and assess for signs of hypocalcemic tetany (e.g., muscle twitching, tetanic spasms, convulsions). Watch for signs of hypercalcemic relapse (e.g., bone pain, renal stones, polyuria, anorexia, nausea, vomiting, thirst, constipation, lethargy, bradycardia).

Teach the client the proper way to self-administer the drug. Encourage regular visits to the doctor. Remind the client to administer a missed dose as soon as possible. Remind the client being treated for postmenopausal osteoporosis to take calcium and vitamin D supplements. Teach the client the signs of hypercalcemia and hypocalcemia. See Table 41–3 for additional nursing considerations.

TABLE 41–3

Drugs Used to Treat Hyperparathyroidism

Drug Name	Dosage and Route of Administration	Nursing Considerations
CALCITONIN, HUMAN (Cibacalcin) **HOW SUPPLIED** SC solution: 0.5 mg/syringe	Recommended starting dosage: 0.5 mg daily, SC Dosage adjustments are based on client response	*Assess* Determine if client is pregnant; calcitonin is classified as Pregnancy Catergory C drug. Asses for hypersensitivity to fish before administering calcitonin, salmon. *Implement* Inspect parenteral solutions for particulate matter and discoloration. Use reconstituted solutions within 6 h. Teach client and family proper injection technique. Develop plan for rotation of injection sites. Store calcitonin, salmon, in refrigerator at 2° to 8° C. Do not store calcitonin, human, at temperatures >25° C; no refrigeration is required. Protect parenteral solution from light. Explain to client that nausea and flushing are transient. Teach client and family signs and symptoms of allergic reaction and actions to take. *Monitor* Monitor serum calcium levels. Monitor for indications of hypocalcemia. *Evaluate* Base effectiveness of drug therapy on reduction of clinical signs and symptoms.
CALCITONIN, SALMON (Calcimar, Miacalcin) **HOW SUPPLIED** Parenteral solution: 100 and 200 U/ml	*Paget's Disease* Initial dose: 100 IU (0.5 ml)/d IM or SC *Hypercalcemia* Initial dose: 4 IU/kg body weight q12h IM or SC Maximum dose: 8 IU/kg body weight q6h *Postmenopausal Osteoporosis* 100 IU/d SC or IM Supplemental calcium carbonate, 1.5 g daily, and vitamin D, 400 U daily, recommended	

MISCELLANEOUS DRUGS IN CATEGORY

Etidronate disodium (Didronel, EHDP) is a synthetic, oral calcium-level modifier. The advantages it has over calcitonin are in its oral administration and in the lack of allergic reactions. It is prescribed primarily to decrease bone resorption. Etidronate blocks the growth of calcium hydroxyapatite crystals by binding to calcium phosphate.

CONCEPT REVIEW

Parathyroid hormone regulates serum calcium levels. Low serum levels of ionized calcium stimulate parathyroid hormone release.

Hyperparathyroidism results in high serum calcium levels and bone demineralization. Calcitonin is used to lower serum calcium levels.

Hypoparathyroidism results in low serum levels, which increase neuromuscular excitability. Treatment includes calcium and vitamin D supplementation.

SUMMARY

Thyroid hormones affect metabolism, cardiac function, growth, and development. During infancy and childhood, thyroid hormones promote maturation. An absence of these hormones can produce dwarfism and permanent mental impairment. In adults deficiency of thyroid hormone can produce hypothryoidism, myxedema, or cretinism. Excess thyroid hormone secretion produces hyperthyroidism. Most thyroid disorders are treated by drug therapy or surgery or both.

Parathyroid hormone (parathormone) is released in response to low levels of plasma calcium. A reduction in parathyroid hormone produces hypoparathyroidism. An excess in parathyroid hormone results in hyperparathyroidism. Both conditions result in an imbalance in serum calcium levels. Hyperparathyroidism is treated by surgical removal of the parathyroid glands or administration of calcitonin or both.

REFERENCES

1. Tortora, G., & Grabowski, S.R. (1993). *Principles of anatomy and physiology* (7th ed.). New York: Harper Collins College Publisher.
2. Monahan, F.D., Drake, T., & Neighbors, M. (1994). *Nursing care of adults*. Philadelphia: W.B. Saunders.
3. Price, S., & Wison, L.M. (1992). *Pathophysiology: Clinical concepts of disease processes* (4th ed.). St. Louis: Mosby–Year Book.
4. Fukayama, H., Nasu, M., Murakami, S., & Sugawara, M. (1992). Examination of antithyroid effects of smoking products in cultured thyroid follicles: Only thiocyanate is a potent antithyroid agent. *ACTA-Endocrinology of Copenhagen, 127,* 520–525.
5. Data Pharmaceutica, Inc. (1993). *1993 physicians' genRx*. Smithtown, NY: Author.
6. U.S. Pharmacopeial Convention. (1990). *The United States pharmacopeia* (22nd rev.). Rockville, MD: Author.
7. Bishnoi, A., Carlson, H., Gruber, B., Kaufman, L., Bock, J., & Lidonnici, K. (1994). Effects of commonly prescribed nonsteroidal anti-inflammatory drugs on thyroid hormone measurements. *American Journal of Medicine, 96,* 235–238.
8. Gomez, J., Cardesin, R., Virgili, N., Moreno, I., Navarro, M., & Montana, E. (1989). Thyroid function parameters and TSH in patients treated with anticonvulsant drugs. *Annals of Medicine International, 6,* 235–238.
9. Curran, P., & DeGroot, L. (1991). The effect of hepatic enzyme-inducing drugs on thyroid hormones and the thyroid gland. *Endocrinology Reviews, 12*(2), 135–150.
10. Campbell, N., Hasinoff, B., Stalts, H., Rao, B., & Wong, N. (1992). Ferrous sulfate reduces thyroxine efficacy in patients with hypothyroidism. *Annals of Internal Medicine, 117,* 1010–1013.
11. Trovato, A., Nuhlicek, D., & Midtling, J. (1991). Drug-nutrient interactions. *American Family Physician, 44,* 1651–1657.
12. Becks, G.P., & Burrow, G.N. (1991). Thyroid disease and pregnancy. *Medical Clinics of North America, 75*(1), 121–150.
13. Ballard, P., Ballard, R., Creasy, R., Padbury, J., Polk, D., Bracken, M., Moya, F., & Gross, I. (1992). Plasma thyroid hormones and prolactin in premature infants and their mothers after prenatal treatment with thyrotropin-releasing hormone. *Pediatric resident, 32,* 673–678.
14. Levy, E.G. (1991). Thyroid disease in the elderly. *Medical Clinics of North America, 75*(1), 152–167.
15. Nordyke, R., & Gilbert, F. (1990). Management of primary hypothyroidism. *Comprehensive Therapy, 16*(7), 28–32.
16. Carr, E., & Spaulding, S. (1992). Thyroid hormones and drugs that affect the thyroid. In C.M. Smith & A.M. Reynard (Eds.), *Textbook of pharmacology* (pp. 645–663). Philadelphia: W.B. Saunders.
17. Feliciano, D. (1992). Everything you wanted to know about Graves' disease. *American Journal of Surgery, 164,* 404–411.
18. Solomon, B., Glinoer, D., Lagasse, R., & Wartofsku, L. (1990). Current trends in the management of Graves' disease. *Journal of Clinical Endocrinology and Metabolism, 70,* 1518–1524.
19. Geffner, D.L., & Hershman, J.M. (1992). Beta-adrenergic blockade for the treatment of hyperthyroidism. *American Journal of Medicine, 93,* 61–68.
20. Kim, T. (1991). Primary hyperparathyroidism. *Orthopaedic Nursing, 13*(3), 17–28.
21. Blanchard, J., Menk, E., Ramamurphy, S., & Hoffman, J. (1990). Subarachnoid and epidural calcitonin in patients with pain due to metastatic cancer. *Journal of Pain and Symptom Management, 5*(1), 42–45.
22. Freeman, D. (1992). Drug treatment for Paget's disease of the bone. *Physician Assistant, 16,* 125–126, 135–137.
23. Orr, P.M. (1993). Salmon calcitonin. *Orthopaedic Nursing, 12*(5), 15–17, 70.
24. Meythaler, J.M., Tuel, S.M., & Cross, L. (1993). Successful treatment of immobilization hypercalcemia using calcitonin and etidronate. *Archives of Physical Medicine and Rehabilitation, 74,* 316–319.

BIBLIOGRAPHY

Carusso, D., & Mazzaferri, E. (1992). Intervention in Graves' disease. Choosing among imperfect but effective treatment options. *Postgraduate Medicine, 92*(8), 117–124, 128–129, 133–134.

Feliciano, D. (1992). Everything you wanted to know about Graves' disease. *American Journal of Surgery, 164,* 404–411.

Figge, J., Leinung, M., Goodman, A., Izquierdo, R., et al. (1994). The clinical evaluation of patients with subclinical hyperthyroidism and free triiodothyronine (free T$_3$) toxicosis. *American Journal of Medicine, 96,* 229–234.

Gupta, A., Eggo, M.C., Uetrecht, J.P., Cribb, A.E., Daneman, D., et al. (1992). Drug-induced hypothyroidism: The thyroid as a target organ in hypersensitivity reactions to anticonvulsants and sulfonamides. *Clinical Pharmacology and Therapeutics, 51*(1), 56–67.

Ibis, E., Wilson, C., Collier, B., Akansel, G., Isitman, A., & Yoss, R. (1992). Iodine[131] contamination from thyroid cancer patients. *Journal of Nuclear Medicine, 33,* 2110–2115.

Laing, R., & Saunders, M. (1992). A case of lung carcinoma induced by radioactive iodine given for disseminated thyroid carcinoma. *Clinical Oncology and Radiology, 4,* 394–395.

McMorrow, M. (1992). The elderly and thyrotoxicosis. *AACN Clinical Issues in Critical Care Nursing, 3*(1), 114–119.

Papo, T., Oksenhendler, E., Izembart, M., Legar, A., & Lauvel, J. (1992). Antithyroid hormone antibodies induced by interferon-alpha. *Journal of Clinical Endocrinology and Metabolism, 75,* 1484–1486.

Stanley, J., & Nayjar, S. (1992). Painful thyroid gland: An atypical presentation of Graves' disease. *Clinical Endocrinology of Oxford, 37,* 468–469.

Surks, M.I., Chopra, I.J., Mariash, C., Nicoloff, J., & Solomon, D. (1990). American Thyroid Association guidelines for use of laboratory tests in thyroid disorders. *Journal of American Medical Association, 263,* 1529–1532.

CHAPTER 42

Adrenal Corticoids

KAREN MUENCH

⊛ **Adrenocortical Hormones**

LEARNING OBJECTIVE: Describe the functions of the adrenal corticoid hormones.

⊛ **Glucocorticoid Drugs**

LEARNING OBJECTIVES:

Describe therapeutic uses of glucocorticoids.

Explain the pharmacokinetic and pharmacodynamic properties of prednisone, the prototype of glucocorticoids.

List clinical manifestations of physiologic and psychologic changes associated with long-term glucocorticoid drug therapy.

Develop a plan of care for the client receiving long-term therapy with glucocorticoids.

KEY TERMS:

Adrenal insufficiency, adrenal suppression

⊛ **Mineralocorticoid Drugs**

LEARNING OBJECTIVES:

Discuss the pharmacokinetics and pharmacodynamic properties of fludrocortisone acetate, the prototype of mineralocorticoids.

List common undesired clinical responses associated with fludrocortisone acetate.

CONCEPTS AND TERMS TO REVIEW

Review anatomy and physiology of the endocrine system.

Review the functions of the adrenal cortex.

Read about adrenocortical insufficiency and Cushing's disease and syndrome in a medical-surgical textbook.

Review functions of endogenous glucocorticoids and mineralocorticoids.

---

*I*n 1934 Edward Kendall and Tadeus Reichstein independently isolated the hormone cortin, and within 2 years, nine more steroids were isolated from the adrenal cortex.[1] It was not, however, until 1948 that scientists were able to produce enough of one of these compounds for use in clinical practice.[2]

This chapter focuses on these compounds, the adrenal corticosteroids. An overview of glucocorticoid and mineralocorticoid drugs is provided. In addition, prednisone, a frequently prescribed glucocorticoid, and fludrocortisone acetate, a mineralocorticoid, are examined in detail. General nursing considerations for clients receiving these drugs and for clients who have recently received corticosteroid therapy are included.

ADRENOCORTICAL HORMONES

The adrenal cortex synthesizes and secretes more than 30 different steroids. These steroids are divided into the glucocorticoids, mineralocorticoids, and androgens. Secretion of these hormones is governed by the negative feedback mechanism of the hypothalamus-pituitary-adrenal (HPA) axis.

Androgens

The small amount of androgens secreted by the adrenal cortex produces the same masculinizing effect as testosterone. These hormones are produced by the adrenal glands of both sexes; thus women normally have a small percentage of male hormones.

Glucocorticoids

Glucocorticoids influence carbohydrate, lipid, and protein metabolism and possess antiinflammatory and immunosuppressive properties. Ordinarily they are produced by the body in increased amounts during stressful times and exercise. Glucocorticoids also prevent defense mechanisms of the body from becoming dangerously overactive by inhibiting the production or action of many of the mediators of inflammation and immunity such as lymphokines, prostaglandins, and histamine. Glucocorticoids also lower serum calcium levels by inhibiting calcium uptake by the renal tubule and gastrointestinal (GI) tract and by redistributing intracellular calcium. This instigates release of increased amounts of parathyroid hormone, which pulls calcium from the bones.[3]

Mineralocorticoids

The naturally secreted mineralocorticoids maintain fluid and electrolyte balance by promoting sodium and water retention and potassium excretion by the distal tubules of the kidney.

GLUCOCORTICOID DRUGS

Glucocorticoids are classified as short, intermediate, and long acting. Table 42–1 summarizes equivalencies and potencies of the three groups of glucocorticoid drugs. Glucocorticoid drugs, which are available in many dosage forms, including oral and parenteral preparations, topical ointments, ophthalmic solutions, respiratory inhalants, and rectal and intranasal preparations, are used to treat a variety of conditions.

Pharmacotherapeutics

Glucocorticoid drugs have three primary uses: (1) as **replacement therapy** for primary adrenal insufficiency (Addison's disease) or secondary adrenal insufficiency due to inadequate HPA axis functioning; (2) as **immunosuppressive therapy,** and (3) as **antiinflammatory therapy** for a wide variety of conditions such as allergic dermatitis, asthma, rheumatoid arthritis, and inflammatory bowel disease. In addition, glucocorticoids are effective in reducing the mortality rate from respiratory distress syndrome in preterm infants when a combination of prenatal maternal corticosteroids and postnatal surfactant therapy to the infant is used.[4]

Common Undesired Clinical Responses

Exogenous glucocorticoids cause the same effects on cellular activities as the naturally produced glucocorticoids; however, prolonged or excessive exposure to exogenous glucocorticoids may produce undesired clinical outcomes. The glucocorticoids stimulate the appetite and thereby increase caloric intake. They also increase the availability of glucose for energy by mobilizing muscle protein for gluconeogenesis and decreasing tissue use of glucose. These combined effects cause the blood sugar level to rise, making clients prone to hyperglycemia. Clients receiving long-term therapy may experience muscle mass loss and muscle weakness as a result of increased protein catabolism.

Additionally, glucocorticoids affect the metabolism of fats. They mobilize fats to free fatty acids for use as energy. They also increase deposits of fat in the thoracic and upper abdominal regions of the body, the face ("moon face"), and the posterior base of the neck ("buffalo hump"). Fat deposits in the upper portion of the body produce a **cushingoid appearance.**

Electrolyte disturbances may occur as a result of increased sodium retention and increased excretion of potassium. Sodium retention is associated with water retention and an increase in fluid volume and blood pressure. Interference with calcium balance and osteoblast formation can cause osteoporotic bone loss and place the client at risk of pathologic fractures.

Another major concern is adrenal insufficiency. During prolonged therapy, there is sufficient circulation of glucocorticoids from exogenous sources that the HPA axis does not stimulate the adrenal gland to produce glucocorticoids, resulting in **adrenal suppression.** If the exogenous source is abruptly discontinued, the adrenal gland is unable to resume its usual activity immediately, thus producing symptoms of **adrenal insufficiency.** The degree of suppression of the adrenal gland varies with the dosage, duration, and type of glucocorticoid preparation administered. Topical preparations pose the least amount of danger. Symptoms of adrenal insufficiency include fever, anorexia, nausea, fatigue, muscle aches, malaise, arthralgia, hypotension, hypoglycemia, dizziness, and fainting.

Adrenal insufficiency may also occur when clients receiving glucocorticoid therapy experience a high level of stress. Ordinarily, adrenal glands respond to stressful situations by increasing the amount of circulating adrenal hormones. However, a suppressed gland cannot respond sufficiently to meet the body's increased needs. Under highly stressful conditions, the client may experience adrenal crisis, **acute adrenal insufficiency.** In this condition both glucocorticoid production and mineralocorticoid production are severely impaired. As a result, critical fluid and electrolyte imbalance can rapidly develop.

Other adverse effects of the glucocorticoids include peptic ulcer formation, cataract development, exaggerated sense of well-being, and steroid-induced psychosis. There is also a 1% incidence of cleft palate when the drugs are administered during the first trimester of pregnancy.[5,6] (Fig. 42–1 illustrates common undesired clinical responses associated with glucocorticoid drugs.)

▨ NURSING CONSIDERATIONS

Nursing care of a client receiving glucocorticoid drugs can be complex, especially if the client is receiving long-term drug therapy.

Assessing Considerable information from the client's health history and physical assessment is needed to plan effective nursing care for the client receiving glucocorticoid drug therapy. To facilitate the presentation of this information, this section is divided into two parts: (1) information needed when a client is started on glucocorticoid drug therapy and (2) information needed when a client is undergoing long-term glucocorticoid therapy.

• **Assessment before initiation of therapy.** Before a client receives glucocorticoid therapy, a history of any of the following must be determined: (1) hypersensitivity to the drug; (2) hepatitis or chronic hepatic disorder; (3) renal impairment (edema is more likely to occur in clients with fixed or de-

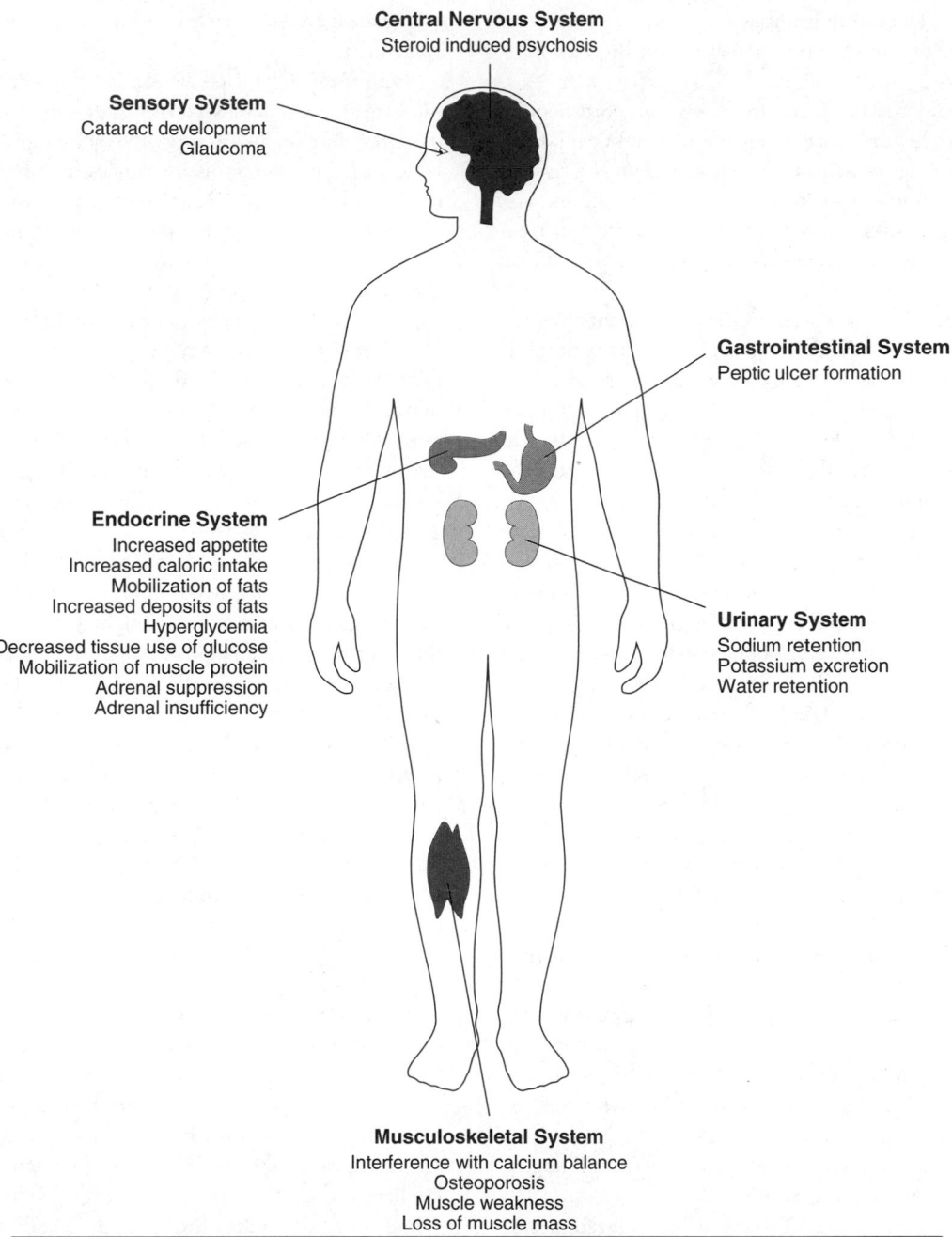

Central Nervous System
Steroid induced psychosis

Sensory System
Cataract development
Glaucoma

Gastrointestinal System
Peptic ulcer formation

Endocrine System
Increased appetite
Increased caloric intake
Mobilization of fats
Increased deposits of fats
Hyperglycemia
Decreased tissue use of glucose
Mobilization of muscle protein
Adrenal suppression
Adrenal insufficiency

Urinary System
Sodium retention
Potassium excretion
Water retention

Musculoskeletal System
Interference with calcium balance
Osteoporosis
Muscle weakness
Loss of muscle mass

FIGURE 42–1   Common undesired clinical responses associated with glucocorticoid drugs.

creased glomerular filtration); (4) unexplained diarrhea or history of having spent time in the tropics (use of glucocorticoids may activate latent amebiasis); and (5) use of drugs that are known gastric irritants (e.g., the nonsteroidal antiinflammatory drugs). Since glucocorticoids decrease the inflammatory response and interfere with the body's usual defense mechanisms, screen the client carefully for signs and symptoms of any preexisting infectious conditions. Glucocorticoids are specifically contraindicated in clients with systemic fungal infections.[6] Additionally, screen for conditions that predispose a client to undesired clinical responses: diabetes mellitus, osteo-

porosis, peptic ulcer disease, gastritis, tuberculosis, hypertension, and psychologic problems.[7]

• **Assessment during long-term therapy.** When clients are receiving long-term glucocorticoid drug therapy, assess for indications of adrenal gland suppression and exaggeration of the usual effects of endogenous glucocorticoid hormones on the body. Note comments from the client about weakness, fatigue, nausea, anorexia, weight loss, vomiting, and diarrhea. Assess for indications of fluid volume depletion: lowered blood pressure, elevated temperature, increased pulse rate, increased respiratory rate, dry skin, and dry mucous membranes. Note laboratory findings such as decreased serum sodium and glucose levels and increased serum potassium levels.[8]

Assess for undesired effects from the glucocorticoids. During the health history, note symptoms of weight gain, nausea, vomiting, edema, muscle weakness, and change in mood or affect (e.g., euphoria, depression, agitation, and insomnia). Assess the client carefully for complaints of gastric distress since long-term glucocorticoid therapy increases the risk of peptic ulcers in some individuals.

During the physical assessment, check the client's weight and blood pressure and assess for peripheral and periorbital edema. Assess infants and children for growth retardation. Observe for redistribution of fat deposits (i.e., increased upper body weight, moon face, buffalo hump) and for structural changes in the face, neck, abdomen, and limbs.[9] Since prolonged use may result in cataracts, glaucoma, or secondary eye infections, check the eyes and visual acuity carefully. Assess for muscle weakness, loss of muscle mass, and muscular aches, which may be associated with protein catabolism. Examine the client for indications of hypokalemia (e.g., muscle cramps or paresthesia). Assess for indications of osteoporosis (e.g., persistent back, hip, or neck pain).[9] Since clients receiving glucocorticoids are more susceptible to hyperlipidemia, assess the vascular system for thrombus formation. Screen the client for impaired wound healing, thin, fragile skin, and ecchymoses and petechiae. Examine the client's skin for acne eruptions; check female clients for facial hair.

Diagnosing Nursing diagnoses appropriate for the client receiving long-term glucocorticoid therapy follow:
• Fluid volume excess related to sodium and water retention.
• High risk for infection related to immunosuppressive action of the drug therapy.
• Alteration in nutrition: more than body requirements related to increased glucose metabolism, increased appetite, and sodium and water retention.
• Alteration in nutrition: less than body requirements related to protein catabolism and potassium loss.
• High risk for impaired skin integrity related to thinning of the dermis and potential for bruising.
• High risk for injury related to bone demineralization and gastric irritation.
• Altered growth and development (children) related to protein catabolism.
• Alteration in body image related to redistribution of body fat, edema, acne, or hirsutism.
• Knowledge deficit regarding long-term corticosteroid management.

Nursing diagnoses appropriate for the client with adrenal insufficiency as a result of long-term glucocorticoid therapy include the following:
• Activity intolerance related to weakness and fatigue.
• Fluid volume deficit related to failure of regulatory mechanisms.
• Alteration in nutrition: less than body requirements related to decreased glucose metabolism.

• Knowledge deficit regarding long-term corticosteroid management.

Planning Client education is an essential component of the care of the client receiving glucocorticoid drug therapy; therefore develop an appropriate teaching plan for each client. Unless the underlying disease process is cured, alert clients receiving short-term glucocorticoid therapy to the possibility of disease recurrence. For clients with conditions such as rheumatoid arthritis and inflammatory bowel disease, provide psychosocial support and comfort measures that assist them in coping with recurrence of pain and disability.

Provide a written time schedule for taking the drug. Frequently glucocorticoid drugs are given on alternate days to minimize suppression of adrenal gland functioning.[6,9] In addition, the drugs are usually discontinued by gradually decreasing the dose; this allows the adrenal gland to regain functioning capacity gradually. The client *must* comply with these dosage schedules.

The client should be knowledgeable about undesired responses. Provide a list of common undesired responses such as edema of hands and ankles, weight gain, polyuria, increased thirst and appetite, change in mood, muscle cramps, heart palpitations, weakness, paresthesia, and bruising. Tell the client that these changes should be reported to the health care provider. Teach the client receiving high doses or prolonged therapy to carry or wear identification containing the drug's name, dosage form, and dosage. Instruct the client to notify all health care providers of his or her corticosteroid use. Additional corticosteroids may be required during stressful situations (e.g., surgery, trauma, tooth extraction, colds, influenza, and infections).[10]

Inform the client that supplemental daily intake of 1500 mg of oral calcium and 400 IU of vitamin D is usually recommended to minimize loss of bone density. In addition, serum calcium levels are monitored for the client receiving vitamin D. Suggest that use of a firm mattress or bedboard may provide comfort if the client experiences osteoporotic pain.[3,9,11]

During the planning phase identify expected outcomes that are appropriate for the client. Possible outcomes follow:
• Client verbalizes understanding of individual dietary restrictions (limited intake of foods high in sodium).
• Client identifies interventions to prevent or reduce the risk of infection.
• Client maintains weight at a satisfactory level for height and body build.
• Client displays timely healing of skin lesions without complications.
• Client verbalizes understanding of body changes.
• Client verbalizes understanding of the drug therapy schedule and describes undesired clinical responses.
• Client reports an increase in activity tolerance.

Implementing Except in emergency situations, glucocorticoids usually are administered in the early morning to coincide with the natural secretion pattern of the adrenal glands.[6,9] In some situations the drug is administered twice a day or more frequently. This dosage may be reduced gradually to once a day and eventually to every other day. At other times, the drug is administered in higher doses as an alternate-day therapy to allow the HPA axis to recover on the day when the drug is not administered.[6]

Be alert to the possibility of frequent changes in dosage and time scheduling. Administering oral glucocorticoid drugs with food may decrease the incidence of gastric irritation. Steroids administered in respiratory inhalants can cause dry mouth, throat irritation, coughing, hoarseness, and fungal infections. Instruct the client to rinse his or her mouth with water or other fluids after using the inhalant to reduce the risk of oral, laryngeal, or pharyngeal fungal infections.[12]

Be alert to rare but serious effects that can occur with high-dose intravenous (IV) drug therapy. These responses include cardiac arrhythmias, fatal cardiac arrest, and circulatory collapse.[6] There have also been reports of temporary paralysis caused by severe muscle fiber degeneration when high-dose IV glucocorticoids and neuromuscular blocking agents are administered concurrently.[13,14]

Evaluating Assess for relief of signs and symptoms that precipitated the use of glucocorticoid drugs. If the drugs are administered as replacement therapy for adrenal insufficiency, the client should experience an increased feeling of well-being and alleviation of problems such as hypovolemia and hypoglycemia. When the client receives the drugs to alleviate inflammatory conditions such as rheumatoid arthritis and asthma, the symptoms caused by the inflammatory process should be relieved. That is, the arthritic client can expect to have less pain and more joint mobility, and the asthmatic client can expect to have less dyspnea. When the drug is given for its immunosuppressive effects, a decrease in lymphocyte production (primarily T4 lymphocytes) should occur. If no undesired clinical responses occur, the client's serum glucose, sodium, potassium, and lipoproteins levels, blood pressure, and body weight should remain within normal limits.

CONCEPT REVIEW

- Hormones synthesized and secreted by the adrenal cortex are divided into the glucocorticoids, mineralocorticoids, and androgens. Secretion of these hormones is governed by the negative feedback mechanism of the hypothalamus-pituitary-adrenal (HPA) axis.
- Glucocorticoids influence carbohydrate, lipid, and protein metabolism and possess antiinflammatory and immunosuppressive properties.
- Glucocorticoid drugs are available in numerous dosage forms and are used to treat a wide variety of conditions.
- Clients receiving long-term glucocorticoid drug therapy are at risk of developing many drug-related physiologic changes.

GLUCOCORTICOID PROTOTYPE

PREDNISONE

Prednisone is classified as an intermediate-acting glucocorticoid drug. It has four times the potency of naturally occurring cortisol.[15]

Pharmacotherapeutics Prednisone has both glucocorticoid and mineralocorticoid activity. However, it is usually prescribed only for its glucocorticoid effects. For this purpose, prednisone is used for adrenal deficiency states as replacement therapy and for its antiinflammatory and immunosuppressive effects.

Prednisone is prescribed for clients with rheumatoid arthritis. It may be used short term at the beginning of treatment to provide symptom management until other drugs become effective, during periods of acute exacerbation, or as long-term low-dose therapy.[16] For clients with rheumatoid arthritis, the antiinflammatory action of prednisone is not curative. The underlying disease process continues its course, and withdrawal of the drug is usually followed by recurrence of the symptoms and for some individuals a significant exacerbation.[9,16]

Prednisone is used in treating respiratory disorders such as severe allergic rhinitis, adult and childhood asthma, and chronic obstructive pulmonary disease (COPD). In addition, nasal sprays containing steroids are the treatment of choice for clients with allergic rhinitis symptoms not relieved by decongestants.[17]

Although the metered-dose inhaler containing steroid aerosols is considered the first line of drug therapy for treating child and adult asthma, some clients need parenteral or oral steroid therapy. Prednisone is the preferred oral preparation since it has approximately a 24-hour duration of effect and causes the fewest side effects. Relatively high doses (30 to 60 mg per day) of prednisone are needed to manage exacerbations of severe asthma. If the drug is used for a short period of time, tapering the dose before discontinuance is not needed.[17–19]

Prednisone generally is not used for the routine treatment of clients with COPD, but IV corticosteroids have been useful in treating actue exacerbations of COPD. As soon as the client's condition stabilizes, the therapy is changed to 40 to 60 mg of prednisone daily, with the goal of withdrawing the drug 7 to 10 days later. Clients who require prolonged therapy are given the lowest possible effective dose. However, even when receiving low doses, these individuals are more susceptible to developing pulmonary infection because of deficiencies in immunoglobulin G.[20,21]

Prednisone, administered early in the course of moderate to severe *Pneumocystis carinii* pneumonia (PCP), can prevent early deterioration of lung function and improve tolerance for antiinfective drug therapy.[22] The use of prednisone for inflammatory bowel disease (ulcerative colitis and Crohn's disease) follows the same approach as its use in rheumatoid arthritis and asthma. That is, prednisone is usually prescribed during acute exacerbations and during the initial attack. When symptoms are relieved, the drug is discontinued as soon as possible.[23] Prednisone is also used to relieve cluster headaches, a condition more rare than migraine headaches. Steroid treatment of acute migraine headaches involves parenteral administration of dexamethasone.[24,25]

Pharmacokinetics   Prednisone administered orally is readily absorbed from the GI tract. It is metabolized in the liver where it is converted to its active form, prednisolone. In general, oral glucocorticoid drugs have high bioavailability, although occasionally asthmatic clients absorb prednisone poorly. In addition, prednisone may not be efficiently converted to prednisolone in clients with severe liver disease. Prednisone has a plasma half-life of 60 minutes and a biologic half-life of 18 to 36 hours. It is excreted by the kidneys.[3,6]

Pharmacodynamics   Prednisone's metabolite, prednisolone, binds to glucocorticoid receptor sites in target cells of the body. Bound receptor sites change form and bind to specific DNA sequences and to proteins in the cell nucleus. Complex interactions then stimulate or inhibit the transcription of specific genes into messenger RNA. The resulting changes in the level of proteins are responsible for the physiologic effects on the client. In some cells production of inhibitory-type proteins (e.g., those proteins needed to build up and stabilize the lysosomal membrane) is stimulated. In other cells such as lymphoid cells, transcription is inhibited entirely, thereby limiting immune and inflammatory responses. Because steroids affect protein synthesis, days may pass before therapeutic effects of oral drug therapy are apparent. Ultimately, the immune response is altered by decreasing the T-helper lymphocyte populations, antibody synthesis, and formation of immune complexes. The inflammatory response is altered by decreasing vascular permeability, inhibiting leukocyte aggregation and arachidonic acid metabolism, and limiting the release of lysosomal enzymes. Prednisone also diminishes the inflammatory response by interfering with some of the essential events of the inflammatory process. Prednisone blocks plasma exudation, inhibits migration of the neutrophils, and inhibits phagocytosis and antibody formation.[3,6,23,26] The exact mechanisms by which the corticosteroids accomplish these activities are not known.

Pharmaceutics   Prednisone is available in tablet, oral solution, and syrup for oral administration. This particular glucocorticoid preparation is not available in a topical or injectable form. Table 42–2 summarizes information about dosage forms and dosages of prednisone.

Undesired Clinical Responses   Usually there is no risk of serious side effects when clients receive glucocorticoid therapy for less than 2 weeks. However, some undesired clinical responses may occur within 2 to 3 days of beginning therapy. These effects include appetite stimulation, slight water retention with weight gain and facial puffiness, and mood changes (i.e., euphoria or depression). With short-term use, these responses disappear 2 to 3 days after the drug is discontinued.[17]

🌾 NURSING RESEARCH

Gift, A.G., Wood, R.M., & Cahill, C.A. (1989). Depression, somatization and steroid use in chronic obstructive pulmonary disease. *International Journal of Nursing Studies, 26*, 281–286.

Steroid therapy has become part of the adjunctive treatment for COPD clients in some settings. Emotional changes have been reported in some individuals while receiving these drugs. However, it is not known if these changes are associated with the pathophysiologic condition or an undesired clinical response to the steroids.

In this study self-reports of depression and somatic complaints were compared between two groups of COPD subjects—20 subjects not receiving steroids and 20 receiving steroids. Both groups demonstrated comparable levels of disease and somatic complaints. Depression was significantly higher in the group receiving steroids when compared to the group not receiving steroids using a Student's t-test. The higher degree of depression among steroid-treated COPD individuals has implications for clinical practice. The emotional status of this group of clients must be monitored and interventions initiated when necessary.

STUDENT ACTIVITIES

- Interview eight clients with COPD, four receiving steroid therapy and four not receiving steroids. Ask them specifically about feelings of depression; determine onset of depression and correlation with drug therapy. Ask each client to rate his or her feelings of depression subjectively on a scale of 1 to 10, with 10 the most severe. Compare the findings to determine which group's members rated themselves as the most depressed.
- Interview a respiratory specialist to determine his or her experience with depression in clients with COPD. 🌾

In clients receiving long-term therapy, prednisone at dosages of 7.5 mg per day or more enhances calcium loss. Loss of calcium increases parathyroid hormone levels, leading to increased bone resorption and decreased bone mineral density. This osteoporotic condition places the client at high risk for fractures of the hips, pelvis, ribs, and vertebrae.[28] Muscle weakness can appear within 1 month of low-dose therapy because corticosteroids cause deterioration of muscle fibers, resulting in loss of muscle strength.[16]

Prednisone interferes with glucose tolerance in 4% to 15% of clients. The risk of corticosteroid-induced diabetes mellitus increases with age and obesity and is higher for individuals with a family history of diabetes or with previous glucose intolerance. Even low-dose therapy can impair glucose tolerance in insulin-dependent diabetics. Because of the mineralocorticoid activity of prednisone, there may also be salt and water retention, resulting in edema and hypertension.

Women and elderly clients are more likely to experience dermatologic undesired responses, which may occur at doses as low as 5 mg per day. Responses include acne, hirsutism, striae, purpura, skin atrophy, spontaneous skin tearing, and delayed wound healing. The most common ophthalmologic response to prednisone is cataract development. Bilateral cataracts have been reported with long-term therapy at doses of less than 10 mg per day. At high doses, prednisone can cause increased intraocular pressure, glaucoma, exacerbation of eye infections, and delayed healing of eye tissue.

High doses of prednisone may cause intestinal perforation and pancreatitis. If clients receiving prednisone therapy experience stressful situations, their risk of developing peptic ulcer disease increases. However, it is unclear if the ulcer formation is from the prednisone or the stress. High doses of prednisone administered for prolonged periods also diminish resistance to microorganisms, increasing the risk of developing infections.

Steroid psychosis, although not frequent, is more likely to occur at doses greater than 40 mg per day. It usually occurs within 15 to 30 days of beginning therapy and is more common in women. The condition is reversed by discontinuing the drug or giving psychotropic medications.

Clients who have taken prednisone in excess of 10 mg per day for longer than 1 year may experience steroid withdrawal syndrome while they are still taking the drug. The primary symptom is aching in muscles and joints. Fever, anorexia, lethargy, and weight loss may also occur. Suppression of the HPA axis may occur in clients taking 20 mg of prednisone per day for 1 week or longer. The degree of HPA axis suppression varies with the dosage and duration of treatment. Children receiving prolonged therapy must be monitored for growth and development.[6,13,16]

Contraindications and Precautions There are no contraindications to replacement glucocorticoid use in clients with adrenocortical insufficiency. However, use of high-dose glucocorticoids as an antiinflammatory is contraindicated in individuals with systemic fungal or bacterial infections or poorly controlled diabetes mellitus. Because of poor antibody response, immunization procedures should not be started while the client is receiving prednisone therapy. Vaccinations with live virus such as smallpox should be avoided.[13,29] In addition, the immune response is diminished, and reactions to skin tests may be suppressed.

Drug-Drug and Drug-Nutrient Interactions Prednisone has the potential of interacting with several drugs (e.g., nonsteroidal antiinflammatory drugs, isoniazid, salicylates, somatrem, cyclosporine, amphotericin B). Concurrent administration of glucocorticoids and nonsteroidal antiinflammatory drugs increases the incidence of peptic ulcer disease. Prednisone decreases the availability of isoniazid, salicylates, and somatrem and increases the availability of cyclosporine. When administered with potassium-depleting diuretics and amphotericin B, the risk of hypokalemia is increased. Concurrent administration may also increase the possibility of digitalis toxicity associated with hypokalemia.[3,6,29]

Prednisone usually is administered without regard to meals. However, it may be administered with food if GI upset occurs.

Altered Laboratory Levels Prednisone may decrease serum calcium, potassium, and thyroxine levels.

It may increase serum cholesterol, lipid, glucose, sodium, and amylase levels.

Life-Span Considerations Administration of glucocorticoids during pregnancy may result in increased fetal deaths and congenital malformation. These drugs are especially contraindicated during the first trimester of pregnancy. Infants born to mothers who have received substantial doses of corticosteroids during pregnancy should be carefully observed for signs of hypoadrenalism.[13,29] In addition, adrenal suppression may occur in breast-feeding infants of mothers receiving steroids.

Specific Drug-Related Nursing Considerations Because the client receiving prednisone may experience impaired wound healing, extra care is needed to prevent infection of surgical wounds and injuries. In addition, because of increased protein catabolism, the client receiving prolonged therapy needs a diet high in protein.

Prednisone's mineralocorticoid activity is more apparent when the drug is administered in large doses. Assess clients receiving high-dose therapy for elevation of blood pressure, salt and water retention, and increased excretion of potassium. Some clients require restricted sodium intake and potassium supplements. Observe clients taking digitalis for indications of digitalis toxicity.

MISCELLANEOUS DRUGS IN CATEGORY

Cortisone and **hydrocortisone** are short-acting glucocorticoid drugs; they have a half-life of 8 to 12 hours. Both drugs are available in oral dosage forms. In addition, hydrocortisone is available in injectable forms for intra-articular, intramuscular (IM), and IV administration. Hydrocortisone retention en-

TABLE 42–1
Equivalencies and Potencies of Glucocorticoid Drugs

Drug	Type	Glucocorticoid Equivalent Dose (mg)	Relative Mineralocorticoid Potency[a]	Plasma Half-Life (h)
SHORT ACTING (8–12h)				
Hydrocortisone	Naturally occurring	20	High	$\frac{1}{2}$
Cortisone		25	High	$1\frac{1}{2}$–2
INTERMEDIATE ACTING (18–36h)				
Prednisone	Synthetic	5	Moderate	1
Prednisolone		5	Moderate	2
Triamcinolone		4	Low	3
Methylprednisolone		4	Low	$1\frac{1}{2}$
LONG ACTING (36–54h)				
Dexamethasone	Synthetic	0.75	Low	$1\frac{1}{2}$
Betamethasone		0.6–0.75	Low	5

[a]Sodium and water retaining; potassium depleting.

TABLE 42–2
Glucocorticoid Drugs

Drug Name	Dosage and Route of Administration	Nursing Considerations
Cortisone (Cortisone Acetate, Cortone Acetate) **HOW SUPPLIED** Scored tablets: 5, 10, 25 mg	*Oral* Adult: initially 25–300 mg/d Maintenance: lowest dosage that maintains clinical response Elderly: lowest effective dose	**Assess** Obtain health history regarding liver and kidney disorders. Determine if client is pregnant; most glucocorticoids are classified as Pregnancy Category C drugs. Ask client about history of eye disorders such as glaucoma or exophthalmos. Ask client about allergic reactions to any of the glucocorticoids. Obtain baseline blood pressure, weight, and respiratory status. Measure and record any preexisting edema. Assess carefully for signs and symptoms of preexisting infections, especially fungal infections. **Implement** Double-check preparation, dosage, and route. Do not confuse prednisone and prednisolone. If client will receive alternate-day oral therapy, explain how it minimizes undesired clinical responses. Administer single daily or alternate-day oral doses in the early morning unless otherwise indicated. Administer oral dosages with meals or snacks to minimize GI upset. Be sure clients receiving long-term therapy wear or carry drug identification information. With high-dose or long-term therapy, avoid discontinuing the drug abruptly. Reconstitute parenteral powder forms according to package insert. Use the correct preparation for IV administration. Many of the injectable preparations are used for IM, soft-tissue, or intra-articular injections but are not for IV use (e.g., hydrocortisone acetate, methylprednisolone acetate, triamcinolone diacetate). Assess patency of IV line before drug infusion. Observe for signs of allergic reactions. **Monitor** Observe for edema and fluid retention. Monitor daily weight and input and output. Monitor blood pressure and pulse. Monitor electrolyte status, especially sodium, potassium, and calcium levels, and serum glucose level. Assess for muscle weakness. Observe for change in mood or affect. Assess surgical or traumatic wounds carefully because healing may be impaired. Observe for signs of GI bleeding and check stools for occult blood. **Evaluate** Report and record improvement in client's initial symptoms. Report and record undesired responses, especially electrolyte imbalance, hypertension, hyperglycemia, and psychosis.

TABLE 42–2 *Continued*
Glucocorticoid Drugs

Drug Name	Dosage and Route of Administration	Nursing Considerations
Hydrocortisone (Cortef, Hydrocortone) HOW SUPPLIED Scored tablets: 5, 10, 20 mg Tablets: 10, 20 mg Oral suspension: 10 mg/5 ml **Hydrocortisone Sodium Succinate** (A-HydroCort, Solu-Cortef) **Hydrocortisone Sodium Phosphate** (Hydrocortone phosphate injection) HOW SUPPLIED Parenteral: 50 mg/ml; 100, 250, 500, 1000 mg/vial	Usual initial dose: 24–240 mg/d	
PREDNISONE (Deltasone, Meticorten, Prednisone Intensol Oral Solution, Liquid Pred Syrup) HOW SUPPLIED Tablets: 1, 2.5, 5, 10, 20, 50 mg Oral solution: 5 mg/ml, 5 mg/5 ml	Usual dose: 5–60 mg/d	Same as above.
Prednisolone (Delta-Cortef, Prelone Syrup, Pediapred) HOW SUPPLIED Tablets: 5 mg Syrup: 15 mg/5 ml **Prednisolone Sodium Phosphate** (Hydeltrasol) HOW SUPPLIED Oral solution: 5 mg/5 ml Parenteral: 20 mg/ml	*Oral* Usual dose: 5–60 mg/d *IV or IM* Usual initial dose: 4–60 mg/d, divided, administered q4–8h *Intra-articular, Intralesional, and Soft Tissue* 2–30 mg; frequency ranges from q3-5d to q2-3 wk	Same as above.
Triamcinolone (Aristocort, Atolone, Kenacort, Kenacort Syrup) HOW SUPPLIED Scored tablets: 1, 2, 4, 8 mg Tablets: 4, 8 mg Syrup: 4 mg/5 ml	*Oral* Initial dose: 3–48 mg/d *IM* 40 mg/wk *Intra-articular or Intrasynovial* Usual dose: 5–40 mg	Same as above.
Methylprednisolone (Medrol) HOW SUPPLIED Tablets: 2, 4, 8, 16, 24, 32 mg **Methylprenisolone Sodium Succinate** (A-Methapred, Solu-Medrol) HOW SUPPLIED Parenteral: 40, 125, 500, 1000, 2000 mg/vial	*Oral* 4–48 mg/d *IM, IV* 10–40 mg IV; subsequent doses IV or IM; 30 mg/kg IV for high-dose therapy	Same as above.
Dexamethasone (Decadron, Dexameth, Dexone, Hexadrol, Dexamethasone Intensol Oral Solution, Decadron Elixir, Hexadrol Elixir) HOW SUPPLIED Tablets: 0.25, 0.5, 0.75, 1, 1.5, 2, 4, 6 mg Elixir: 0.5 mg/5 ml Oral solution: 0.5 mg/5 ml, 0.5 mg/0.5 ml	Usual dose: 0.75–9 mg/d	Same as above.

Table continued on following page.

TABLE 42–2 *Continued*
Glucocorticoid Drugs

Drug Name	Dosage and Route of Administration	Nursing Considerations
Dexamethasone Sodium Phosphate (Decadron Phosphate, Hexadrol Phosphate) **HOW SUPPLIED** Injection: 4, 10, 20, 24 mg/ml	*IM/IV* Adult, elderly: initially 0.5–9 mg/d *Intra-articular, Intralesional, or Soft Tissue* 0.4–6 mg	
Dexamethasone Acetate (Dalalone D.P. Injectable, Decadron-LA suspension) **HOW SUPPLIED** Oral liquid: 0.5 mg/5 ml Parenteral: 8, 16 mg/ml	*IM* Adults, elderly: 8–16 mg; may repeat in 1–3 wk *Intralesional* 0.8–1.6 mg *Intra-articular and Soft Tissues* 4–16 mg; may repeat q1–3 wk	
Betamethasone (Celestone, Celestone Syrup) **HOW SUPPLIED** Scored tablet: 0.6 mg Syrup: 0.6 mg/5 ml	Initial dose: 0.6–7.2 mg/d	Same as above.
Betamethasone Sodium Phosphate (Celestone Phosphate, Cel-U-Jec, Selestoject) **HOW SUPPLIED** Parenteral: 4 mg/vial	Up to 9 mg/d	

ema and intrarectal foam are used to treat inflammatory bowel disease.

In addition to prednisone, the intermediate-acting group of glucocorticoid drugs includes prednisolone, triamcinolone, and methylprednisolone. **Prednisolone** as an oral preparation is used in clients unable to metabolize prednisone. It is frequently prescribed for the treatment of multiple sclerosis. Prednisolone is also available in a variety of injectable forms for intra-articular, IM, and IV use. **Triamcinolone** preparations are used for a wide variety of conditions, including acute leukemia. **Methylprednisolone** is available in oral and injectable dosage forms. High-dose IV infusion of methylprednisolone (30 mg/kg of body weight) is frequently administered to decrease the degree of neurologic impairment in clients with spinal cord injuries.[30]

The long-acting corticosteroids **dexamethasone** and **betamethasone** have a half-life of 36 to 54 hours. Dexamethasone is used to diagnose adrenal insufficiency and to treat cerebral edema. In addition, both of these drugs have been used in women at risk of preterm birth to decrease the incidence of infant respiratory distress syndrome.

Glucocorticoid drugs are available in ophthalmic preparations containing prednisolone or dexamethasone. In addition, more than 90 different topical preparations of glucocorticoids are presently available. Glucocorticoids available as respiratory inhalants include beclomethasone (Beclovent, Vanceril), dexamethasone (Decadron Respihaler), triamcinolone (Azmacort), and flunisolide (AeroBid).[6] Table 42–2 summarizes information regarding dosage forms and dosages of various glucocorticoid drugs.

CONCEPT REVIEW

Prednisone is a frequently prescribed oral glucocorticoid drug. It is used for replacement therapy and for its antiinflammatory and immunosuppressive effects.

Prednisone remains inactive in the body until it is converted to prednisolone.

Prednisone produces a variety of undesired clinical responses. Most of these responses represent exaggerations of the naturally occurring glucocorticoids. In excess this results in Cushing's syndrome.

MINERALOCORTICOIDS

Mineralocorticoids are adrenocortical hormones essential to the maintenance of adequate fluid volume in the extracellular and intravascular fluid compartments, normal cardiac output, and adequate blood pressure levels.

General Characteristics

The primary effects of mineralocorticoids are increasing the reabsorption of sodium and the secretion of potassium in the renal tubules. Secondary effects are related to the reabsorption of water, serum levels of sodium and potassium, anion reabsorption, and secretion of hydrogen ions.

MINERALOCORTICOID PROTOTYPE

FLUDROCORTISONE ACETATE

Fludrocortisone acetate (Florinef) is the only mineralocorticoid available. Although it has potent mineralocorticoid activities, it also has glucocorticoid actions.

Pharmacotherapeutics Fludrocortisone is used in the treatment of primary and secondary adrenocortical insufficiency in clients with Addison's disease and for the treatment of salt-losing adrenogenital syndrome. It has also been used for the management of severe orthostatic hypotension, although this is an unlabeled use.[6]

Pharmacokinetics Fludrocortisone is readily absorbed from the GI tract. It combines with receptor sites in target cells in competition with the glucocorticoids. (It is thought that glucocorticoids and mineralocorticoids use the same receptor sites except in the kidney where there are more mineralocorticoid receptors.[3]) After oral administration, peak concentration occurs in $1\frac{3}{4}$ hours, with plasma half-life lasting $3\frac{1}{2}$ hours and biologic half-life lasting 18 to 36 hours. Mineralocorticoids are excreted by the kidneys.[6,13]

Pharmacodynamics Mineralocorticoids act on the renal distal tubules to enhance the reabsorption of sodium and chloride ions and the excretion of potassium and hydrogen ions. In small doses fludrocortisone causes sodium retention and subsequent hypertension along with increased urinary potassium excretion.

Pharmaceutics Fludrocortisone is available in tablet form for oral administration. Dosage depends on the severity of the disease and the client's response to therapy.

Undesired Clinical Responses Undesired responses to fludrocortisone include hypersensitivity reactions, salt and water retention, potassium loss, drug-induced adrenal insufficiency, and growth and development retardation in children. Dermatologic reactions, including bruising, increased sweating, and allergic rash, have been reported. Cardiovascular effects are edema, hypertension, congestive heart failure, and enlarged heart.

Hypokalemic alkalosis can also occur. Other undesired responses are similar to those of the glucocorticoids.[6,13]

Contraindications and Precautions Clients are at increased risk of infection, and fludrocortisone use is contraindicated if the client has a systemic fungal infection.

Drug-Drug and Drug-Nutrient Interactions Sodium retention and potassium loss may occur more readily if the client has a high dietary salt intake. If edema or hypertension develops, it may be necessary to restrict sodium intake. Since fludrocortisone has glucocorticoid effects, it interacts with the same drugs previously described for prednisone (i.e., digitalis glycosides, amphotericin B, vaccines).[13]

Life-Span Considerations Fludrocortisone is classified as a Pregnancy Category C drug. It should be prescribed to pregnant women only if clearly needed. Infants born to women who have received substantial doses of fludrocortisone during pregnancy should be assessed closely for hypoadrenalism. Corticosteroids are found in the breast milk of lactating women receiving systemic therapy with these drugs; therefore caution should be used when prescribing fludrocortisone to a nursing woman. Safety and effectiveness in children have not been established.[13]

Specific Drug-Related Nursing Considerations Assess the client for a history of renal or cardiovascular dysfunction. Collect and analyze a comprehensive drug history for potential drug-drug interactions. Monitor the client's fluid and electrolyte status carefully. Important assessment parameters during therapy are periodic blood pressure and serum electrolytes findings. Stress to the client the importance of regular follow-up visits. Instruct the client to notify the physician promptly of dizziness, severe or continuing headaches, swelling of feet or lower legs, or unusual weight gain.

As with clients receiving glucocorticoid therapy, individuals receiving fludrocortisone are at risk of acute adrenal insufficiency when they experience stressful situations during or after drug therapy. In addition, the client can rapidly develop hypotension and fluid and electrolyte imbalance if the drug is discontinued abruptly.[8]

RECOMMENDED DOSAGES

Addison's Disease

Usual dose: 0.1 mg daily (dosages ranging from 0.1 mg three times a week to 0.2 mg daily have been used)

If transient hypertension occurs, dose reduced to 0.05 mg daily

Usually administered in combination with a glucocorticoid

Salt-losing Adrenogenital Syndrome

Recommended dose: 0.1–0.2 mg daily

CONCEPT REVIEW

Mineralocorticoids are essential for fluid, sodium, and potassium homeostasis.

Fludrocortisone acetate is the only mineralocorticoid currently available. It is used in combination with glucocorticoids to treat Addison's disease. Fludrocortisone is also used to treat salt-losing adrenogenital syndrome.

SUMMARY

Glucocorticoids are prescribed for replacement therapy and for their antiinflammatory and immunosuppressive properties. Mineralocorticoids are used to restore fluid and electrolyte balance in clients with adrenal insufficiency. Both groups of drugs can cause HPA axis suppression if given for more than 2 weeks, placing the client at risk of adrenal crisis if the drug is withdrawn abruptly or the client experiences a stressful event.

Although short-term glucocorticoid therapy is relatively safe, long-term treatment frequently results in osteoporosis, hypertension, hyperglycemia, and drug-induced cushingoid syndrome. Clients must be carefully monitored for undesired clinical responses. In general, mineralocorticoids cause the body to retain salt and water and excrete potassium, and the glucocorticoids interfere with the inflammatory and immune responses and alter metabolic activities.

REFERENCES

1. Singer, C., & Underwood, E. (1962). *A Short History of Medicine.* New York: Oxford University Press.
2. Weiss, M. (1989). Corticosteroids in rheumatoid arthritis. *Seminars in Arthritis and Rheumatism, 19*(1), 9–21.
3. Baxter, J. (1992). The effects of glucocorticoid therapy. *Hospital Practice, 27*(9), 111–115, 117–118, 123.
4. Jobe, A., Mitchell, B., & Gunkel, H. (1993). Beneficial effects of the combined use of prenatal corticosteroids and postnatal surfactant on preterm infants. *American Journal of Obstetrics and Gynecology, 168,* 508–513.
5. McCance
6. Olin, B., Hebel, S., Dombek, C., Kastrup, E., Cada, D., Covington, T., et al. (1993). *Drug Facts and Comparisons.* St. Louis: Facts and Comparisons.
7. Moeser, P. (1991). Corticosteroid therapy for rheumatoid arthritis. *Postgraduate Medicine, 90*(8), 175–176, 178–179, 182.
8. Epstein, C. (1991). Fluid volume deficit for the adrenal crisis patient. *Dimensions of Critical Care Nursing, 10*(4), 210–217.
9. Hardy, E. (1992). Steroid management in orthopaedic patients. *Orthopaedic Nursing, 11*(6), 27–30.
10. Gotch, P. (1991). The endocrine system. In J. Alspach (Ed.), *Core Curriculum for Critical Care Nursing* (pp. 609–655). Philadelphia: W.B. Saunders.
11. Shaefer, M., & Williams, L. (1991). Nursing implications of immunosuppression in transplantation. *Nursing Clinics of North America, 26,* 291–309.
12. Levin, R. (1991). Advances in pediatric drug therapy of asthma. *Nursing Clinics of North America, 26,* 265–271.
13. Data Pharmaceutica, Inc. (1993). *1993 physicians' genRx.* Smithtown, NY: Author.
14. Hirano, M., Ott, B., Raps, E., Minetti, C., Lennihan, L., Libbey, N., & Bonilla, E. (1992). Acute quadriplegic myopathy: A complication of treatment with steroids, nondepolarizing blocking agents, or both. *Neurology, 42,* 2082–2087.
15. Guyton, A.C. (1991). *Textbook of medical physiology* (8th ed.). Philadelphia: W.B. Saunders.
16. Caldwell, J., & Furst, D. (1991). The efficacy and safety of low-dose corticosteroids for rheumatoid arthritis. *Seminars in Arthritis and Rheumatism, 21*(1), 1–11.
17. Milavetz, G., & Smith, J. (1990). Pharmacotherapy of asthma and allergic rhinitis. *Primary Care, 17,* 685–701.
18. Grossman, J., Sorkness, C., & Joseph, J. (1992). The use of inhaled corticosteroids in patients with asthma. *Physician Assistant, 16*(3), 119–122, 124, 162–164.
19. Schaffer, S. (1991). Current approaches in adult asthma: Assessment, education and emergency management. *Nurse Practitioner, 16*(12), 18, 20, 23–31.
20. Stratton, M., & McCabe, M. (1990) Chronic obstructive pulmonary disease. *Primary Care, 17,* 667–683.
21. Klaustermeyer, W., Gianos, M, Kurohara, M., Dao, H., &
Geiner, D. (1992). IgG subclass deficiency associated with corticosteroids in obstructive lung disease. *Chest, 102,* 1137–1142.
22. Anastasi, J. (1992). Why give corticosteroids for *Pneumocystis carinii* pneumonia? *American Journal of Nursing, 92*(2), 30, 32.
23. Cooke, D. (1991). Inflammatory bowel disease: Primary health care management of ulcerative colitis and Crohn's disease. *Nurse Practitioner, 16*(8), 27–29, 35–39.
24. Campbell, J. (1993). Diagnosis and treatment of cluster headache. *Journal of Pain and Symptom Management, 8*(3), 155–164.
25. Klapper, J. (1993). The pharmacologic treatment of acute migraine headaches. *Journal of Pain and Symptom Management, 8*(3) 140–145.
26. Kirby, B. (1989). A review of the rational use of corticosteroids. *Journal of International Medical Research, 17,* 493–505.
27. Gift, A.G., Wood, R.M., & Cahill, C.A. (1989). Depression, somatization and steroid use in chronic obstructive pulmonary disease. *International Journal of Nursing Studies, 26,* 281–286.
28. Garton, M., Reid, D. (1993). Bone mineral density of the hip and of the anteroposterior and lateral dimension of the spine in men with rheumatoid arthritis. *Arthritis and Rheumatism, 36,* 222–228.
29. Davis, P.J., Tornatore, K., & Brownie, A. (1992). Adrenal Cortex. In C.M. Smith & A.M. Reynard, *Textbook of Pharmacology* (pp. 717–739). Philadelphia: W.B. Saunders.
30. Aminoff, M. (1993). Nervous System. In L. Tierncy, S. McPhee, M. Papadakis, & S. Schroeder (Eds.), *Current Medical Diagnosis and Treatment.* Norwalk, CT: Appleton & Lange.

BIBLIOGRAPHY

Helfer, E., & Rose, L. (1989). Corticosteroids and adrenal suppression: Characterizing and avoiding the problem. *Drugs, 38,* 838–845.

Hilton, G., and Frei, J. (1991). High-dose methylprednisolone in the treatment of spinal cord injuries. *Heart and Lung, 20,* 670–675.

Hodgson, S. (1990). Corticosteroid-induced osteoporosis. *Endocrinology and Metabolism Clinics of North America, 19*(1), 95–110.

Hood, L.J. (1990). Myasthenia gravis: Regimens and regimen-associated problems in adults. *Journal of Neuroscience Nursing, 22,* 358–364.

LaRocco, A., Amundson, D., Wallace, M., Malone, J., & Oldfield, E. (1992). Corticosteroids for *Pneumocystis carinii* pneumonia with acute respiratory failure. *Chest, 102,* 892–895.

Lee, L., & Gumowski, J. (1992). Adrenocortical insufficiency: A medical emergency. *AACN–Clinical Issues in Critical Care Nursing, 3,* 319–330.

Piper, J., Ray, W., Daugherty, J., & Griffin, M. (1991). Corticosteroid use and peptic ulcer disease: Role of nonsteroidal anti-inflammatory drugs. *Annals of Internal Medicine, 114,* 735–740.

Solheim, K. (1993). Managing prednisone in clients with chronic obstructive pulmonary disease. *Nurse Practitioner Forum, 4*(1), 43–48.

Taylor, R., Wilkins, G., Herbison, M., & Flannery, E. (1992). Interaction between corticosteroid and β-agonist drugs: Biochemical and cardiovascular effects in normal subjects. *Chest, 102,* 519–524.

Van Essen-Zandvliet, E., Hughes, M., Waalkens, H., Duiverman, E., Pocock, S., & Kerrebijn, K. (1992). Effects of 22 months of treatment with inhaled corticosteroids and/or beta-2-agonists on lung function, airway responsiveness, and symptoms in children with asthma. *American Review of Respiratory Disease, 146,* 547–554.

Woods, S. (1990). Cataract development after prolonged use of systemic corticosteroids. *Ophthalmic Nursing Forum, 6*(2), 1–4, 6–8.

Drugs Affecting the Respiratory System

CHAPTER 43

OVERVIEW OF
The Respiratory System

JULIA ANN RAITHEL

⊛ Structures of the Respiratory System

LEARNING OBJECTIVES:

Describe the functions of the structures that comprise the upper airway.

Summarize the functions of the structures that comprise the lower airway.

KEY TERMS:

Alveolar ducts, alveolar sacs, alveolus, bronchus, cilia, parietal pleura, respiratory bronchioles, respiratory membrane, surfactant, terminal bronchioles, visceral pleura

⊛ Mechanics of Pulmonary Ventilation

LEARNING OBJECTIVES:

Explain the physiology involved in the process of inspiration.

Describe the physiology involved in the process of expiration.

Summarize the mechanics of airway resistance.

KEY TERMS:

Airway resistance, compliance, expiration, inspiration, pulmonary ventilation

⊛ Pulmonary Volumes and Capacities

LEARNING OBJECTIVE: Differentiate between pulmonary volumes and pulmonary capacities.

KEY TERMS:

Expiratory reserve volume, inspiratory reserve volume, residual volume, tidal volume, total lung capacity, vital capacity

⊛ Alveolar Ventilation

LEARNING OBJECTIVES:

Describe the physiology involved in external and internal respiration.

List arterial blood gas values.

KEY TERMS:

Alveolar ventilation, arterial blood gases, diffusion, oxyhemoglobin, partial pressure of a gas

⊛ Regulation of Respiration

LEARNING OBJECTIVES:

Summarize the functions of the respiratory center in regulation of respiration.

Describe the role of central and peripheral chemoreceptors in the regulation of respiration.

Explain the effect of the inflation reflex on the regulation of respiration.

KEY TERMS:

Apneustic center, chemoreceptors, respiratory center, pneumotaxic center, stretch receptors

⊛ Effects of Drugs on the Respiratory System

LEARNING OBJECTIVE: Summarize the use of pharmacologic agents on disorders of the respiratory system.

CONCEPTS AND TERMS TO REVIEW

Review the section on the respiratory system in an anatomy and physiology book.

Review the definition of and mechanisms involved in diffusion.

With the first breath at the time of birth, respiration becomes the only body function with both automatic and voluntary control. Usually an individual breathes without conscious awareness until a stressor such as vigorous physical activity or disease occurs. In these circumstances additional respiratory effort is needed to provide the required oxygen.

The main function of the respiratory system is to conduct

air into the lungs, deliver oxygen via capillary membranes to the blood, and remove carbon dioxide (CO_2). This role, which helps to determine the quality of life for an individual, is performed on the average of 15 times per minute for as long as the individual is alive. Additional functions of the respiratory system include regulation of the acid-base balance in the blood, filtration of particles from the air, and production of surfactant. The lungs also transform biochemical substances found in the blood (i.e., the conversion of angiotensin to renin) and produce prostaglandin in response to tissue hypoxia and anaphylaxis.[1]

The respiratory system is directly affected by environmental conditions. The pathology that results from poor air quality is one of the major causes of respiratory diseases. Not only is the structure of the lungs affected, but the ability to exchange CO_2 and oxygen is impaired by exposure to air pollution. Additionally, functions of the respiratory system affect other body systems (e.g., cardiovascular), and other body systems (e.g., renal) affect respirations. The interdependency of the respiratory system with other systems of the body cannot be overlooked since the effects of pharmacologic agents are not limited to one system.

STRUCTURES OF THE RESPIRATORY SYSTEM

The respiratory system is divided into two anatomic areas: the upper and lower airways or tracts. Those organs outside the thorax constitute the upper airway, and those within the thorax comprise the lower airway.

Upper Airway

The upper airway consists of the nose, nasal cavity, sinuses, pharynx, and larynx (Fig. 43–1). The **nose** is covered with skin

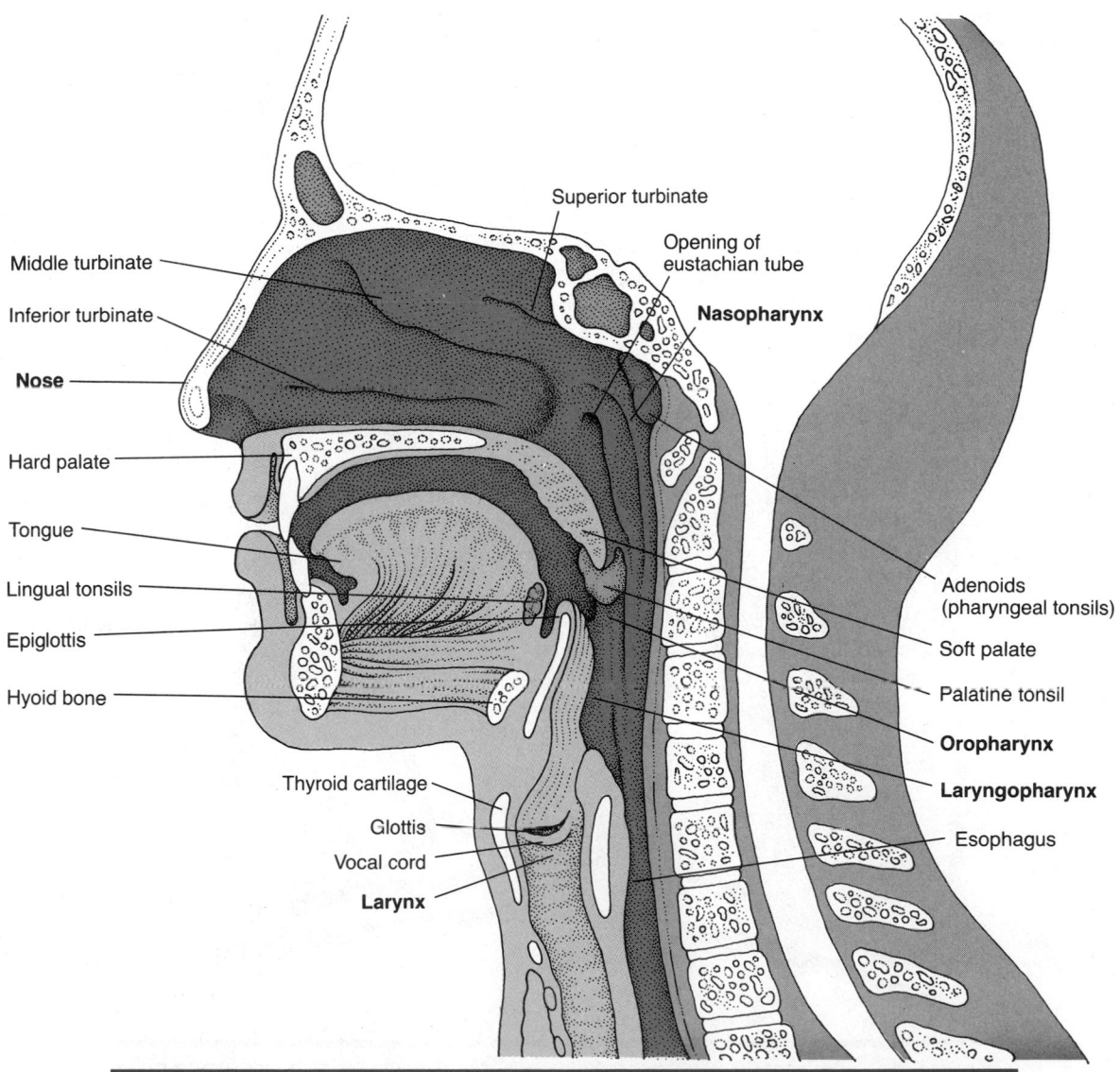

Superior turbinate
Opening of eustachian tube
Nasopharynx
Middle turbinate
Inferior turbinate
Nose
Hard palate
Tongue
Lingual tonsils
Epiglottis
Hyoid bone
Adenoids (pharyngeal tonsils)
Soft palate
Palatine tonsil
Oropharynx
Laryngopharynx
Esophagus
Thyroid cartilage
Glottis
Vocal cord
Larynx

FIGURE 43–1   Structures of the upper respiratory system. (From Ignatavicius, D.D., & Bayne, M. [1991]. *Medical-surgical nursing*. Philadelphia: W.B. Saunders.)

and is supported internally by bone and cartilage. Air enters and leaves the nose through two external nares or nostrils. The **nasal cavity,** a hollow space behind the nose, is divided medially by the nasal septum.

Opening into the nasal cavity are four sets of paranasal **sinuses.** The nose and nasal sinuses warm, moisten, and filter inhaled air, house olfactory receptors, and promote vocal resonance. Mucous membrane lining the nasal cavity contains cilia, or nasal hair, and a sticky mucus. As air passes through the cavity, large particles such as dust and bacteria are filtered out. The sinuses, which are also lined with mucous membranes, drain into the nasal cavities. Infection of the sinuses can occur as a result of microorganisms in the nasal cavity.

The tongue, pharynx, and tonsils are housed in the upper throat. Although the tongue is not considered a part of the upper airway, it can interfere with respiration. If the tongue becomes displaced backward against the posterior wall of the throat, it can block the airway. The **pharynx** (throat) is located behind the oral cavity and between the nasal cavity and the larynx. It provides passage for air during breathing and for food and fluids during swallowing. It also aids in producing the

sounds of speech. Functionally, the pharynx is divided into the nasopharynx, oropharynx, and laryngopharynx.

The **larynx** is an enlargement in the airway at the top of the trachea and below the pharynx. This structure is primarily composed of muscles and cartilages. Attached to the upper border of cartilage is the **epiglottis.** When the epiglottis is open or in an upright position, it allows air to enter the larynx. During swallowing, the epiglottis is pressed downward, partially covering the opening into the larynx. This action prevents food and fluids from entering the airways and obstructing air flow. Two **vocal cords** are attached to the inner walls of the larynx. Vibration of the vocal cords produces phonation.[2–4]

Lower Airway

The lower airway consists of the trachea, bronchi, bronchioles, and lungs (Fig. 43–2). Functionally, this section of the airway is divided into two portions: conducting airways and respiratory units. Conducting airways include the trachea, right and left mainstem bronchi, bronchioles, and terminal

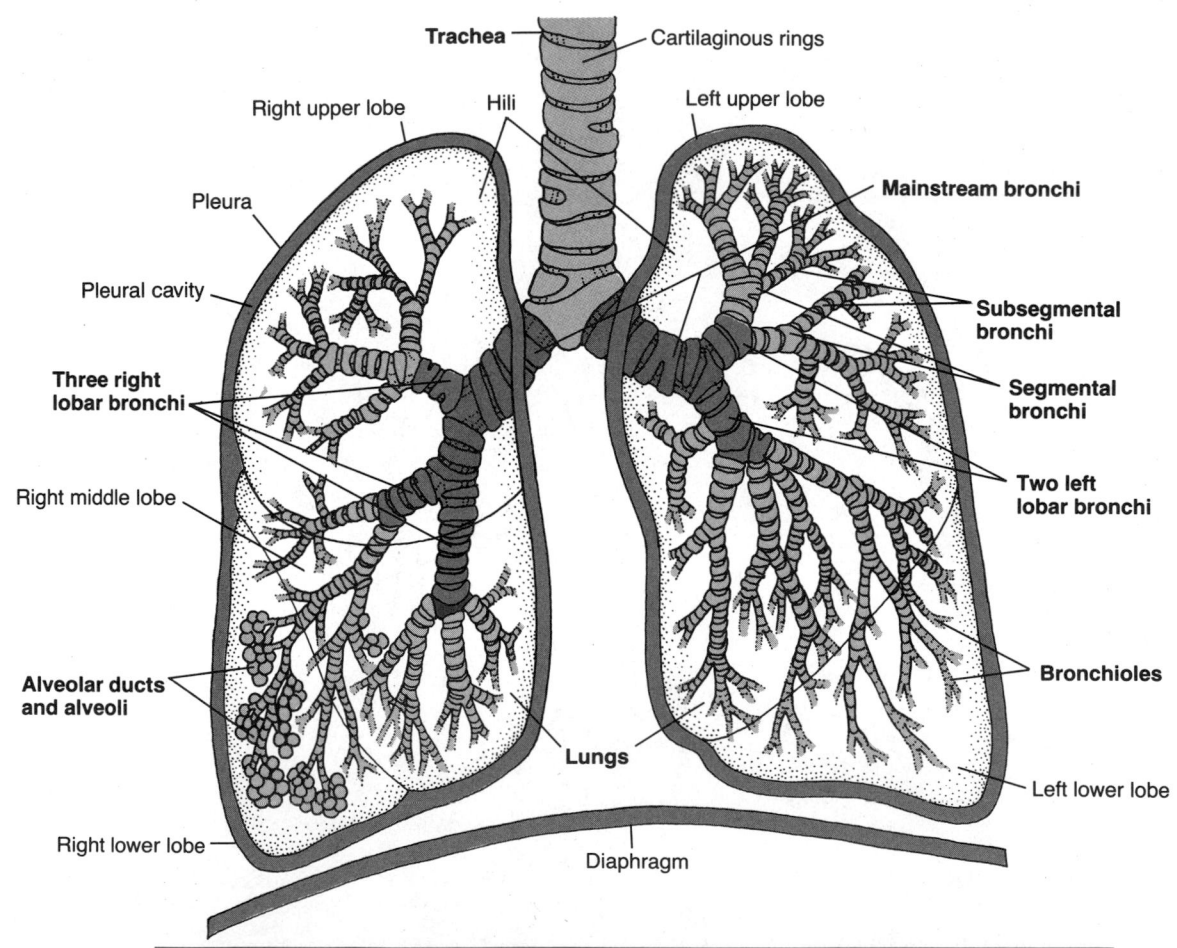

FIGURE 43–2 Structures of the lower respiratory system. (From Ignatavicius, D.D., & Bayne, M. [1991]. *Medical-surgical nursing.* Philadelphia: W.B. Saunders.)

bronchioles. Respiratory bronchioles, alveolar ducts, alveolar sacs, and alveoli make up the respiratory units.

CONDUCTING AIRWAYS

The **trachea,** the largest air passageway, is 2 to 3 cm in diameter and 12 to 13 cm long.[5] It is composed of C-shaped pieces of cartilage. The open ends of these incomplete rings are directed posteriorly; the gaps between their ends are closed by smooth muscle. This smooth muscle allows the nearby esophagus to expand slightly during the swallowing of food. At the same time, the C-shaped cartilage rings prevent closure or collapse of the airway. During coughing, the trachea narrows slightly, increasing the velocity of the expired air to dislodge foreign particles.[1] The trachea eventually divides into the right and left mainstem bronchi.

Both the **right** and **left maintstem bronchi** arise from the trachea at the level of the fifth vertebra. They are composed of cartilage similar to that found in the trachea. The right mainstem bronchus is short and separates from the trachea at a vertical angle. Food or other material aspirated into the lower airways lodges more frequently on the right side.

Approximately 100 ml of **mucus** is produced daily by bronchial glands located in the mainstem bronchi. The composition of this mucus is 95% water.[1] Epithelial cells lining the bronchi are ciliated. The **cilia** move in a rapid, upward wavelike motion to propel the mucus that is produced by the bronchial glands toward the oropharynx. Dust and other particles not previously trapped are removed from the lungs by this process. Once the particles reach the large airways, the cough and sneeze reflexes expel them from the respiratory tract. Chemicals such as sulfur dioxide, anesthetics, and cigarette smoke decrease mucociliary action.[6] Once the mucociliary action is impaired, the lungs and lower airways are exposed to agents that directly damage the cells and diminish respiratory functions.

A short distance from its origin, each mainstem bronchi divides into secondary or **lobar bronchi.** They divide into **segmental bronchi;** each of these branches supplies a segment of the lung. The segmental bronchi divide into smaller **bronchioles** that enter the lobules of the lung. Gradually, the bronchioles branch into the **terminal bronchioles.** As the respiratory tract progressively divides, several changes occur. The original cartilage gradually changes to smooth muscle, and the diameter of the airways becomes smaller. As the diameter of individual airways lessens, the total surface area of the airways progressively increases. In the large airways normal air flow is fairly rapid, but it becomes progressively slower as the diameter of the bronchi decreases.[4,7]

RESPIRATORY UNITS

Respiratory units include the respiratory bronchioles, alveolar ducts, alveolar sacs, and individual alveoli. These structures are located at the end of the terminal nonrespiratory bronchioles (Fig. 43–3). The respiratory units are the principle sites of gas exchange.

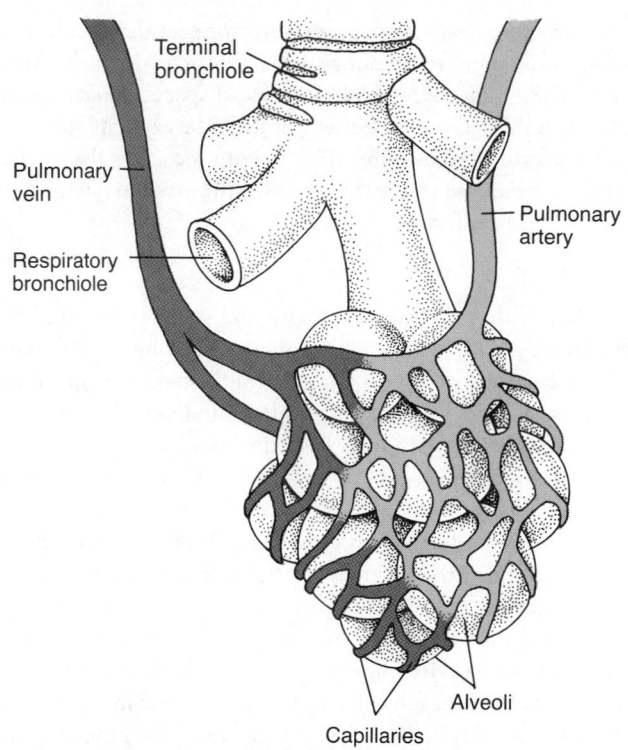

FIGURE 43–3 Terminal and respiratory bronchioles. (From Ignatavicius, D.D., & Bayne, M. [1991]. *Medical-surgical nursing.* Philadelphia: W.B. Saunders.)

Two or more **respiratory bronchioles** branch from each terminal bronchiole. These tubes are short and have diameters of approximately 0.5 mm. A few alveoli project from their sides, enabling the respiratory bronchioles to engage in gas exchange. From each respiratory bronchiole extend two to 10 long, branched **alveolar ducts.** Around the circumference of the alveolar ducts are numerous alveoli and alveolar sacs. An **alveolus** is a cup-shaped outpouching of the alveolar ducts. **Alveolar sacs** are two or more alveoli that share a common opening.[4,7]

Alveolar sacs resemble clusters of grapes. Approximately 300 million alveoli are present in the adult lungs. These alveoli have a collective volume of approximately 2500 ml.[8] Each alveolar sac is surrounded by elastic connective tissue and is supplied by pulmonary capillaries along with lymphatic vessels.

The cellular composition of alveoli includes two types of epithelial cells: type I and type II. Type I cells are flat squamous cells that form the alveolar membrane that is the site of oxygen and CO_2 diffusion. These cells are very susceptible to injury and cannot be replaced.[9] Type II cells produce surfactant. **Surfactant** is a phospholipid film that reduces the surface tension inside the alveoli, prevents total collapse of the alveoli during expiration, and allows easier inflation of the lungs. A continuous supply of surfactant is necessary for the lung to maintain normal function. Absence of this fluid may be the cause of several respiratory diseases.[1]

Tiny openings (Kohn's pores) interconnect the alveoli. The presence of these pores allows even air distribution between the alveoli.[10] The alveoli wall, interstitial space, capillary basement membrane, and endothelial wall of the capillary make up the **respiratory membrane.** This membrane is less than 1 μm thick; any increase in the thickness diminishes the rate of oxygen and CO_2 diffusion.

LUNGS

Lying within the thoracic cavity and separated by the mediastinum are the **lungs.** These organs are cone shaped, with the wider base near the diaphragm and the narrower apices toward the clavicle. Each lung is divided into lobes. The left lung has two lobes; the right lung has three lobes. Each lobe is partitioned into lobules, which further divide into progressively smaller segments that eventually terminate at the alveolar sacs.

Covering the lungs is the **pleural membrane.** This membrane is composed of two layers: the **visceral pleura** and the **parietal pleura.** The visceral pleura covers the lungs; the parietal pleural lines the inside of the thoracic cavity. A potential space (**pleural cavity**) lies between the visceral and parietal pleura. A very thin film of serous fluid present in the pleural cavity lessens the friction that occurs when the lungs expand during inspiration.

Within the lungs are two separate circulatory systems: the pulmonary and bronchial. The chief function of the **pulmonary circulation** is to receive venous (unoxygenated) blood from the right ventricle. This blood flows past the alveolus through the pulmonary capillaries to receive oxygen and remove CO_2. After it is oxygenated, the blood returns to the left atrium and then enters the left ventricle. The left ventricle pumps the oxygenated blood throughout the body by systemic arteries.

The **bronchial circulatory system** originates from the thoracic aorta. This system is relatively small and is located deep within the lung tissue. Its primary purpose is to provide a continuous supply of oxygenated blood and nutrients to the tissues of the lungs. Lung tissues require nutrients and oxygen to maintain cellular function the same as other body cells. Bronchial circulation has no role in the oxygenation of the blood and removal of CO_2.

The **lymphatic system** also plays an important function within the lungs. This system drains excess fluid and protein from the interstitial spaces and removes inhaled particles and/or microorganisms from the lungs. Lymphatic vessels are located both superficially and deeply within the lung tissue. Although lymph flow is generally slow, the rate of flow is facilitated by respiratory movements and the presence of valves inside the vessel. The flow rate increases if there is excessive fluid in the lungs such as occurs with pulmonary edema.

MECHANICS OF PULMONARY VENTILATION

Although the respiratory system has many important functions, one of the most vital is pulmonary ventilation. The term **pulmonary ventilation** refers to the process of inspiration and expiration. This movement of air into and out of the lungs is aided by the muscles of ventilation.

Inspiration

Inspiration, which is an active process, involves the downward contraction of the diaphragm while the external intercostal muscles move upward and outward to expand the thoracic cavity. This expansion of the thoracic cavity creates a negative pressure gradient; pressure inside the lungs is less than atmospheric pressure outside the lungs. This negative pressure gradient encourages the flow of inspired air toward the alveoli. At the end of inspiration but before the start of expiration, the pressure outside and inside the lungs are equal. With expiration, the pressure inside the lungs becomes greater than the atmospheric pressure, and airflow out of the lungs is accomplished.

Inspiration is facilitated by compliance of the lung tissue. **Compliance** refers to the stretchability or elasticity of the lungs. Elastin and collagen fibers present within the parenchyma of the lung stretch with inspiration. Certain conditions such as obesity, kyphosis, or muscle paralysis reduce the expansibility or compliance of the lungs. When this reduction occurs, additional work by the ventilatory muscles is needed to open the airway. Increased lung compliance is also a concern. With increased compliance, the lung tissues, especially the alveoli, lose elasticity and remain distended. This occurs with chronic obstructive pulmonary diseases and in older individuals as part of the aging process.

The muscles of inspiration can become fatigued if their energy supply is exceeded. When this occurs, the individual usually complains of dyspnea. With vigorous exercise or cardiopulmonary diseases that alter the energy needs, accessory muscles (scalene and sternomastoid) are used to assist in the expansion of the thoracic cavity.[7,11]

Expiration

Expiration is a passive event resulting from elastic recoil of the lungs. As the respiratory muscles relax from the work of inspiration, air is released from the lungs. As the lungs deflate, the pressure inside the lungs becomes greater than atmospheric air. This pressure gradient encourages air to flow out of the lungs. In clients with some respiratory diseases, expiration becomes an active process often involving exhaling air through pursed lips, which prolongs the period for exhalation.

CONCEPT REVIEW

Structures in the respiratory system include the nose, pharynx, larynx, trachea, bronchi, and lungs.

These structures act with the cardiovascular system to supply oxygen to and remove CO_2 from the blood.

Gas exchange by diffusion occurs across the alveolar-capillary or respiratory membrane.

Airway Resistance

As indicated previously, the size of the airways affects the flow of air into and out of the lungs. **Airway resistance** is inversely proportional to the diameter of the airway itself. A large airway offers little resistance, whereas a small airway results in greater resistance. Any factor that increases the amount of airway resistance increases the amount of energy needed by the ventilatory muscles to force air into and out of the airways.

Several other factors affect airway resistance, including the actions of the autonomic nervous system, epinephrine, histamine, and mechanical blockage. Sympathetic nervous system stimulation relaxes the smooth muscle of the airways and allows the diameter of the airway to increase. On the other hand, parasympathetic nervous system stimulation causes smooth muscle contraction, resulting in a narrower airway and increased resistance. Epinephrine and histamine also have opposite effects on the respiratory system. Epinephrine relaxes the smooth muscles of the airways and decreases airway resistance; histamine causes bronchospasm or contraction and increases airway resistance. Overproduction of mucus, tumors, or large foreign materials also decrease the diameter of the airways because of blockage.[3,4]

PULMONARY VOLUMES AND CAPACITIES

Lung volumes and capacities reflect the effectiveness of ventilation. **Pulmonary volumes** are measurements of air movement by the lungs. When several measurements of lung volumes are combined together, the combinations are called **lung capacities.** All pulmonary volumes and capacities are smaller in women than in men. Lung volumes and capacities are also affected by lung compliance, muscular effort, aging, and pulmonary disease. Pulmonary function tests are used to measure lung volumes and capacities.[2]

Pulmonary Volumes

Some of the major pulmonary volumes are tidal volume, inspiratory reserve volume, expiratory reserve volume, and residual volume. **Tidal volume** refers to the volume of gas inspired or expired with each normal breath. The tidal volume of an adult is approximately 500 ml. **Inspiratory reserve volume** is the extra volume of air that can be inspired over and beyond the normal tidal volume. The extra volume of air that can be forcefully expired at the end of a normal expiration is the **expiratory reserve volume. Residual volume** is the amount of air remaining in the lungs after a forced expiration.[2,11]

Pulmonary Capacities

The major pulmonary capacities are vital capacity and total lung capacity. The **vital capacity** is the combination of the inspiratory reserve volume, the tidal volume, and the expiratory reserve volume. This is the maximum amount of air that an individual can expel from the lungs after maximum inspiration. **Total lung capacity** is the vital capacity plus the residual volume.[2,3]

ALVEOLAR VENTILATION

The importance of the respiratory system is its ability to renew the air in the gas exchange areas of the lungs continually. These areas include the alveoli, alveolar sacs, alveolar ducts, and respiratory bronchioles. The rate at which new air reaches these areas is called **alveolar ventilation.**

Gas Exchange

When inspired air reaches the alveoli, gas exchange begins. **Gas exchange** involves the diffusion of oxygen and CO_2 across the alveoli and capillary membranes. This exchange of gases is accomplished by diffusion. (**Diffusion** is a passive process in which gas molecules move from an area of higher concentration to an area of lower concentration.)

Within the respiratory system, there is a mixture of gases. Therefore the **total pressure** acting on the surfaces of the respiratory passages is directly proportional to the molecular concentration of all these gases together. The rate of diffusion of each separate gas within the mixture is directly proportional to the pressure caused by the gas alone, which is called the **partial pressure of the gas.** Partial pressures of alveolar gases are difficult to determine because of the numerous variables affecting alveolar ventilation. However, the value for partial pressure of oxygen (PO_2) is usually 100 mmHg, and the value for partial pressure of CO_2 (PCO_2) is 40 mmHg.[3,9]

PO_2 is greater in the alveoli than in the mixed venous blood in the pulmonary capillary. As a result, oxygen readily diffuses across the small distance between the alveolus and the capillary. Once inside the capillary, most of the oxygen combines with the hemoglobin. (Hemoglobin is the major constituent of red blood cells and is the means by which oxygen is transported in the blood to the tissues.) When the oxygen combines with the hemoglobin, the resulting complex is called **oxyhemoglobin.** When the PO_2 in the arterial blood reaches 80 mmHg or above, the hemoglobin of the red blood cells is almost fully saturated.

As blood flows through the body, oxygen dissociates itself from the hemoglobin and diffuses from the arterial capillary into the cells. This action occurs because cells have a lower concentration of oxygen than the arterial capillary blood. As the PO_2 begins to fall, the level of hemoglobin saturation decreases, and the amount of oxygen available to the cells decreases. An arterial PO_2 of 40 mmHg results in a hemoglobin saturation of 75%, which is approximately the same as that of venous blood.[2]

As oxygen is used during cellular metabolic processes, CO_2 is released. Since CO_2 concentration is higher within the cell, diffusion into the venous blood occurs. Once diffused into the blood, CO_2 is transported in three forms: dissolved in the plasma, coupled with hemoglobin and carbaminohemoglobin, and changed to bicarbonate. When it reaches the alveoli, the bicarbonate combines with carbonic acid, which dissociates and diffuses into the alveoli. It is then removed from the lungs by exhalation.[2,7]

Arterial Blood Gases

Arterial blood gases (ABGs) are measured to determine the effectiveness of gas exchange, alveolar ventilation, and level of arterial blood oxygenation. For this test, an arterial blood sample is obtained from a radial, brachial, or femoral artery. The blood sample is analyzed for hydrogen ion concentration, partial pressures of dissolved oxygen and CO_2, and percentage of oxygen bound to the hemoglobin.[11]

REGULATION OF RESPIRATION

The basic ventilatory rate is 14 to 18 respirations per minute. However, acute and chronic increases in oxygen demand may occur. Acute increases are caused by conditions such as fever or physical exercise; chronic increases occur with diseases such as hyperthyroidism. To respond to these changes in oxygen demands, the body must be able to control pulmonary ventilation. This task is accomplished by the respiratory center, chemical regulation, and the inflation reflex.

Respiratory Center

Breathing is controlled by a poorly defined group of neurons in the brain stem called the **respiratory center.** Components of the respiratory center are widely scattered throughout the pons and medulla oblongata. One of the functions of this center is to control the basic rhythm of respiration. Neurons in the dorsal respiratory group emit impulses that initiate the onset of inspiration. These neurons remain inactive during expiration. Neurons in the ventral group generate impulses that increase inspiratory movement. Two other areas, the apneustic

Arterial Blood Gases	
pH	7.35–7.45
$PaCO_2$, PCO_2	35–45 mm Hg
PaO_2, PO_2	80–100 mm Hg
Oxygen saturation	95%–100%

$PaCO_2$ = partial pressure of CO_2 in arterial blood; PCO_2 = partial pressure of CO_2; PaO_2 = partial pressure of oxygen in arterial blood; PO_2 = partial pressure of oxygen.

and pneumotaxic centers, help limit inspiration. The **pneumotaxic center** continuously transmits inhibitory impulses to the inspiratory area. Neurons in the **apneustic center** coordinate the transition between inspiration and expiration.[2,4,7]

Chemical Regulation

Central and peripheral chemoreceptors determine the concentration of CO_2 and oxygen in the blood. **Central chemoreceptors** in the medulla are sensitive to changes in serum CO_2 levels. When CO_2 levels increase, the medullary center stimulates ventilation. A rapid change in the CO_2 concentration has a significant effect on the respiratory rate, but chronic elevation of CO_2 concentration has very little effect.[2]

Peripheral chemoreceptors, located in the carotid body and aortic arch, are sensitive to the amount of oxygen in the blood. Ventilatory rate approximately doubles when the arterial PO_2 decreases to 60 mmHg. This hypoxic drive is critical in diseases accompanied by chronic elevation in the arterial PCO_2 level.

Inflation Reflex

Located in the walls of the bronchi and bronchioles are **stretch receptors.** When these receptors become stretched during overinflation of the lungs, nerve impulses are sent through the vagus nerves to the inspiratory and apneustic areas. This innervation has an inhibiting influence on both of these areas. The result is that expiration occurs. As air leaves the lungs, the lungs deflate, and the stretch receptors are no longer stimulated. As a result, the inspiratory and apneustic areas are not inhibited and a new inspiration begins. This reflex is called the *inflation reflex* or **Hering-Breuer reflex.**

CONCEPT REVIEW

The partial pressure of a gas is the pressure exerted by that gas in a mixture of gases. It is symbolized by p.

Each gas in a mixture of gases exerts its own pressure as if the other gases were not present.

External respiration is the exchange of gases between alveoli and pulmonary blood capillaries.

Internal respiration is the exchange of gases between tissue blood capillaries and tissue cells.

The respiratory center regulates respirations.

Several factors, including oxygen and CO_2 levels, autonomic nervous system stimulation, and cortical influences, modify the respiratory center activity.

EFFECTS OF DRUGS ON THE RESPIRATORY SYSTEM

A variety of drugs is used to treat respiratory disorders. As with any clinical situation, the type of medication, dosage form, and route of administration vary with the client's clinical situation. Drug categories used in the treatment of respiratory disorders include mucokinetics, bronchodilators, antitussives, nasal decongestants, and antihistamines. Some drugs in these categories are available as over-the-counter medications.

Mucokinetic drugs promote the removal of abnormal or excessive secretions from the respiratory airways. This is accomplished by thinning the secretions, which facilitates their removal by ciliary action and/or the cough reflex.

Bronchodilators are used when ineffective airway clearance exists. Ineffective airway clearance occurs most commonly with pulmonary diseases that cause a decrease in the diameter of the bronchioles. The diminished diameter of the bronchioles usually results from contraction or spasm of bronchial smooth muscle, mucous hypersecretion, and/or mucosal inflammation.

Antitussive drugs are used to suppress coughing. Some antitussive drugs act on the cough center in the medulla oblongata; others act peripherally by lessening the irritation of the respiratory tract.

Nasal decongestants are used to shrink engorgement of nasal mucous membranes that commonly occurs secondary to upper respiratory infections. Most nasal decongestants produce drowsiness as a side effect. In addition, rebound engorgement of the nasal membranes can occur.

Antihistamines decrease inflammation of the mucous membranes within the respiratory tract. These drugs are administered to relieve the symptoms associated with immune responses.

SUMMARY

Cells continually use oxygen and release CO_2. Exchange of these gases is the primary function of the respiratory system. The respiratory system removes oxygen from the atmosphere, transports oxygen to the lungs, exchanges oxygen for CO_2 in the alveoli, and returns the CO_2 to the atmospheric air. The cardiovascular system transports the gases via the blood between the lungs and the cells. In addition to respiration, the respiratory system provides one form of acid-base balance.

Acute and chronic respiratory disorders are widespread and affect every age group. Although there are many causes of respiratory disorders, the most significant factors involve air pollution. Drug therapy for treatment of many respiratory disorders is available over-the-counter.

REFERENCES

1. Kersten, L.D. (1989). *Comprehensive respiratory nursing.* Philadelphia: W.B. Saunders.
2. Guyton, A. (1991). *Textbook of medical physiology* (8th ed.). Philadelphia: W.B. Saunders.
3. Guyton, A. (1992). *Human physiology and mechanisms of disease* (5th ed.). Philadelphia: W.B. Saunders.
4. Hole, J. (1993). *Human anatomy and physiology* (6th ed.). Dubuque, IA: Wm. C. Brown.
5. Creager, J. (1992). *Human anatomy and physiology.* Dubuque, IA: Wm. C. Brown.
6. Sexton, D.L. (1990). Anatomy and physiology. In Sexton, D. (Ed.). *Nursing care of the respiratory patient* (pp. 1-39). Norwalk, CA: Appleton & Lange.
7. Tortora, G., & Grabowski, S. (1993). *Principles of anatomy and physiology* (7th ed.). New York: Harper Collins.
8. Bullock, L., & Rosendahl, P.P. (1988). *Pathophysiology: Adaptations and alterations in function* (2nd ed.). Glenview, IL: Scott, Foresman.
9. George, R.B. (1990). Alveolar ventilation, gas transfer, and oxygen delivery. In George, R., Light, R., Matthay, M., & Matthay, R. (Eds.). *Chest medicine: Essentials of pulmonary and critical care medicine* (pp. 57-70). Baltimore, MD: Williams & Wilkins.
10. Wilson, S.F., & Thompson, J.M. (1990). *Respiratory disorders.* St. Louis: C.V. Mosby.
11. Seeley, R., Stephens, T., & Tate, P. (1992). *Anatomy and physiology* (2nd ed.). St. Louis: Mosby–Year Book.

BIBLIOGRAPHY

Clausen, J. (1989). Clinical interpretation of pulmonary function tests. *Respiratory Care, 34,* 638-645.

Crapo, R. (1989). Reference values for lung function tests. *Respiratory Care, 34,* 626-633.

Ignatavicius, D., & Bayne, M. (1991). *Medical-surgical nursing.* Philadelphia: W.B. Saunders.

Lindell, K., & Wesmiller, S. (1989). Using arterial blood gases to interpret acid-base balance. *Orthopaedic Nursing, 8*(3), 31-34.

Preusser, B., Lash, J., Stone, K., Winningham, M., Gonyon, D., & Nickel, J. (1989), Quantifying the minimum discard sample required for accurate arterial blood gases. *Nursing Research, 38,* 276-279.

Ries, A. (1989). Measurement of lung volumes. *Clinical Chest Medicine, 10*(2), 177-186.

Rosen, R., & Bone, R. (1990). Treatment of acute exacerbations in chronic obstructive pulmonary disease. *Medical Clinics of North America, 74,* 691-700.

Spyr, J., & Preach, M.A. (1990). Pulse oximetry: Understanding the concept, knowing the limits. *RN Magazine, 53*(5), 38-45.

West, J. (1990). *Respiratory physiology* (4th ed.). Baltimore: Williams & Wilkins.

CHAPTER 44

Nasal Decongestants, Antitussives, and Mucolytics

BARBARA B. HODGSON • NORMA L. PINNELL

⊛ **Pathologic Conditions Requiring Drug Therapy**
LEARNING OBJECTIVES:
Describe the causes of inflammation and swelling of the nasal mucous membranes.
Discuss the process that leads to nasal congestion.
Explain the physiologic basis for a productive cough.
Identify common signs and symptoms associated with a cold, rhinitis, allergic rhinitis, and sinusitis.
KEY TERMS:
Allergic rhinitis, nasal congestion, dry and nonproductive cough, congested and nonproductive cough, rhinitis, congested and productive cough, sinusitis, common cold

⊛ **Nursing Considerations**
LEARNING OBJECTIVE: Develop a plan of care for a client with severe allergic rhinitis.

⊛ **Nasal Decongestants**
LEARNING OBJECTIVES:
Describe the pharamcodynamics of nasal decongestants.
Name the contraindications and precautions for use of these drugs.
KEY TERM: Rebound phenomenon

⊛ **Antihistamines**
LEARNING OBJECTIVES:
Describe the histamine response.
Name the five groups of antihistamines.

⊛ **Antitussives**
LEARNING OBJECTIVES:
Describe the difference between the narcotic and nonnarcotic cough suppressants.
Name the site of action of antitussive drugs.
KEY TERM: Paradoxical reaction

⊛ **Expectorants**
LEARNING OBJECTIVES:
Describe the effects of expectorants on the respiratory tract.
List the contraindications to use of expectorants.

⊛ **Mucolytics**
LEARNING OBJECTIVES:
Name the common compound useful in thinning pulmonary secretions and correcting dehydration when given by inhalation or orally.
List special materials to use and to avoid when administering mucolytics by nebulization.
KEY TERM: Stomatitis

⊛ **Combination Cold Remedy Preparations**
LEARNING OBJECTIVES:
Explain the benefits and disadvantages of using combination cold remedies.
Name the usual combination of ingredients in such drug preparations.

CONCEPTS AND TERMS TO REVIEW

Read Chapter 43 for an overview of the respiratory system.
Read Chapter 49 for information on immune response.
Read sections on allergic rhinitis, common colds, and sinusitis in a medical-surgical textook.

---

*D*rugs discussed in this chapter are among the most frequently self-prescribed drugs. In addition, they are widely prescribed by primary care providers for a variety of medical problems (e.g., allergic rhinitis, sinusitis, colds, rhinitis, nasal congestion). Nasal decongestants, antitussives, and mucolytic drugs relieve symptoms; they are not curative. Although they are considered relatively safe by the general public, care must be taken to avoid excessive use or administration to individuals with certain conditions, including hypertension, diabetes mellitus, and cardiac disease.

PATHOLOGIC CONDITIONS REQUIRING DRUG THERAPY

The common cold, rhinitis, allergic rhinitis, nasal congestion, sinusitis, and coughing may all require drug therapy. Major symptoms of **rhinitis** are sneezing, runny nose (rhinorrhea), nasal itching, and nasal congestion. **Allergic rhinitis** is a type I hypersensitivity reaction that occurs in response to inhaled antigens, with symptoms localized to the nasal mucosa and conjunctiva. Typical symptoms of allergic rhinitis are a profuse watery nasal discharge, sneezing, swelling of the nasal mucosa, and itching of the nose and palate. The **common cold,** or coryza syndrome, is an infectious process of the upper respiratory tract, which can be caused by 80 to 100 different viruses. Colds can produce a wide variety of symptoms that include nasal discharge with nasal congestion, sneezing, watery eyes, coughing, fever, chills, and a sore throat. **Nasal congestion,** which is associated with rhinitis, allergic rhinitis, and the common cold, results from dilation of the blood vessels in the nasal mucosa. The dilation causes mucous membrane engorgement, stimulating an increase in mucous secretion. Acute **sinusitis,** inflammation of a sinus cavity, produces fever, chills, nasal obstruction, and pain and tenderness over the involved sinus.[1]

The act of **coughing** is a protective reflex action that provides a means of dislodging and ejecting foreign particles or excess mucus from the respiratory passageways. A cough can be categorized as dry and nonproductive, congested and nonproductive, or congested and productive. A **dry and nonproductive cough** does not produce sputum; this cough is not associated with chest congestion. A **congested and nonproductive cough** is associated with chest congestion and a scant amount of mucus. The **congested and productive cough** is associated with chest congestion and expectoration of mucus. This type of cough generally should not be suppressed.

▨ NURSING CONSIDERATIONS

The nursing process helps establish a data base regarding the client's level of health, health practices, past illnesses and related experiences, and health care goals. The nursing process is the framework for providing client care.

Assessing The first step in establishing a data base is to obtain a **health history** with attention to environmental aspects and client comfort. The client's history may include nasal congestion, postnasal drip, nasal discharge, sneezing, sore throat, headache, itchy eyes, lacrimation, earache with decreased hearing, upper respiratory tract infection, or allergies. If a nasal discharge is present, note the amount, color, and thickness. Question the client about the duration and extent of nasal congestion and about factors that precipitate or relieve the symptoms. Symptoms of rhinitis may be present, or the client may have a cough related to a cold or an allergy. There may be a history of nonproductive cough or an overactive cough, which may interrupt the client's sleep or produce muscular pain. Assess the type, severity, and frequency of the cough. If the cough is productive, note the color, odor, viscosity, and amount of sputum. Determine factors that trigger or relieve the cough.

Obtain information about smoking. Determine how long the client has smoked and how many packs per day. If the client does not currently smoke, ask if he or she has ever smoked. Because many respiratory problems are associated with pollutants such as asbestos, fumes, organic dust particles, and chemicals, obtain information about the client's occupational and geographic environment.

Obtain information about any family history of allergy and prior testing for or treatment of allergy. Determine if symptoms occur year-round or only in a particular season. Ask if there are times when symptoms are more pronounced such as certain times of the year or month or if symptoms occur more often under certain weather conditions.

During the **physical assessment** assess breath sounds. Take the client's temperature and check for tenderness over the sinuses. Palpate for enlarged cervical lymph nodes. Inspect the throat; observe for redness, swelling, and drainage.

Diagnosing The nursing diagnosis deals with the client's response to the illness or condition. Appropriate nursing diagnoses follow:

- Ineffective airway clearance related to allergic reaction.
- Altered oral mucous membrane related to decreased fluid intake, irritation, allergic reaction.
- Fatigue related to disturbed sleep pattern from coughing.
- Fluid volume deficit related to decreased consumption of oral fluids or to fever.

Planning After formulating the nursing diagnoses, develop strategies to prevent, minimize, or correct the problems identified. Develop teaching plans that include information on drug dosage, schedule, and administration technique. With input from the client, identify appropriate expected outcomes.

Based on the nursing diagnoses, expected outcomes for the client may include the following:

- Client identifies the need to drink eight or more glasses of fluid per day.
- Client does not drive or engage in activities that may be affected by the sedative effect of the drug.
- Client relates factors that contribute to allergic reaction.
- Client reports decreased levels of fatigue.
- Client describes factors that may result in the rebound phenomenon associated with use of nasal decongestants.

Implementing Advise the client that adequate fluid intake is essential; recommend he or she drink at least eight or more glasses of fluids per day. Talk with the client about the benefits of proper nutrition, especially the impact of ingesting fruits and vegetables. Counsel the client about the need for additional rest and sleep during periods of illness.

Since many individuals self-medicate coughs, colds, and rhinitis, discuss with the client the hazards of using over-the-counter (OTC) drugs. If the client is receiving prescription drugs, advise him or her to consult with the primary care provider or pharmacist before taking OTC drugs. Review with the client the proper method for administering nasal sprays or drops (see box on p. 548).

🌿 NURSING RESEARCH

Conn, V. (1991). Self-care actions taken by older adults for influenza and colds. *Nursing Research, 40*(3), 176–180.

The purpose of this study was to examine self-care behaviors that older adults use to manage colds and flu symptoms. Interviews were conducted with 160 subjects aged 65 to 94 years. A large number and variety of cold- and influenza-related self-care actions were reported. Drug administration was common; 79% of subjects took drugs for colds, and 95% took drugs to treat flu symptoms.

STUDENT ACTIVITIES

- Interview 10 adults over the age of 65. Ask about actions taken during their last cold or flu episode. Note the number and variety of OTC drugs used.
- Interview pharmacists in local pharmacies. Determine the most frequently used OTC remedies (e.g., cold medicine, decongestants, antacids).

Evaluating Assess the therapeutic effects of antihistamines by monitoring for the reversal of allergic symptoms: itchy, watery eyes, runny nose, urticaria, or rash.

Antitussives should produce therapeutic reversal of cough. Assess for resolution of cough, a decrease in frequency and duration of coughing spells, and the client's ability to sleep better at night.

The effectiveness of nasal decongestants allows the client to breathe more readily by reversing nasal congestion, postnasal drip, nasal discharge, and sneezing. Monitor the client for rebound congestion.

CONCEPT REVIEW

Nasal congestion is a common complaint from allergic, viral, bacterial, or fungal causes. It results from dilation of blood vessels in the nasal mucosa and resulting engorgement of the mucous membranes, with an increase in mucus secretion.

Nasal congestion accompanies rhinitis, allergic rhinitis, and sinusitis.

The cough reflex is a protective mechanism for clearing excess secretions from the tracheobronchial tree.

NASAL DECONGESTANTS

Nasal decongestants act by stimulating α-adrenergic receptors on the smooth muscle of nasal blood vessels. Stimulation of these receptors causes vasoconstriction that results in shrinkage of swollen membranes. Response from topical application of decongestant is rapid and intense. After use of oral decongestants, vasoconstriction is delayed and less intense. Nasal decongestants can relieve symptoms associated with rhinitis, allergic rhinitis, sinusitis, and colds.[2-4]

NASAL DECONGESTANT PROTOTYPE

PHENYLEPHRINE HYDROCHLORIDE

Phenylephrine hydrochloride (Alconefrin, Neo-Synephrine) is also present in fixed-combination forms with zinc sulfate, an astringent (Zincfrin); with pyrilamine maleate, an antihistamine (Prefrin-A); with sulfacetamide, an antiinfective (Vasosulf); with pheniramine maleate, an antihistamine (Dristan); and with naphazoline, a vasoconstrictor, and pyrilamine, an antihistamine (4-Way Nasal Spray).

Pharmacotherapeutics Although phenylephrine is used to relieve nasal congestion associated with the common cold, hay fever, sinusitis, or other upper respiratory allergies, it also is used as adjunctive therapy for middle ear infections by decreasing congestion around the eustachian tubes. Ear blockage and pressure pain during air travel also respond to use of nasal decongestants.

Pharmacokinetics Absorption after intranasal administration is minimal. Nasal decongestion may occur within 15 or 20 minutes and may persist for 2 to 4 hours. Phenylephrine has a half-life of $2\frac{1}{2}$ hours. The pharmacologic effects of phenylephrine are partially terminated by uptake of the drug into tissues. Phenylephrine is metabolized in the liver and intestine by the enzyme monoamine oxidase (MAO) and is excreted primarily in the urine.

Pharmacodynamics Phenylephrine acts predominantly by a direct effect on α-adrenergic receptors of vascular smooth muscle, producing constriction of blood vessels. This vasopressor action reduces blood flow, fluid exudation, and mucosal edema.

Pharmaceutics Phenylephrine solutions are available in spray or drop form with strengths of 0.125%, 0.16%, 0.2%, 0.25%, 0.5%, and 1%; it is available in a strength of 0.5% in jelly form (Table 44–1).

Undesired Clinical Responses Stinging, burning, and drying of nasal mucosa may occur with the use of nasal drops or sprays. Prolonged nasal use (longer than 3 to 5 days) may produce chronic nasal congestion or rhinitis. Occasionally mild central nervous system (CNS) stimulation occurs in the form of restlessness, nervousness, tremors, headache, and insomnia, particularly in those clients hypersensitive to sympathomimetics. Large

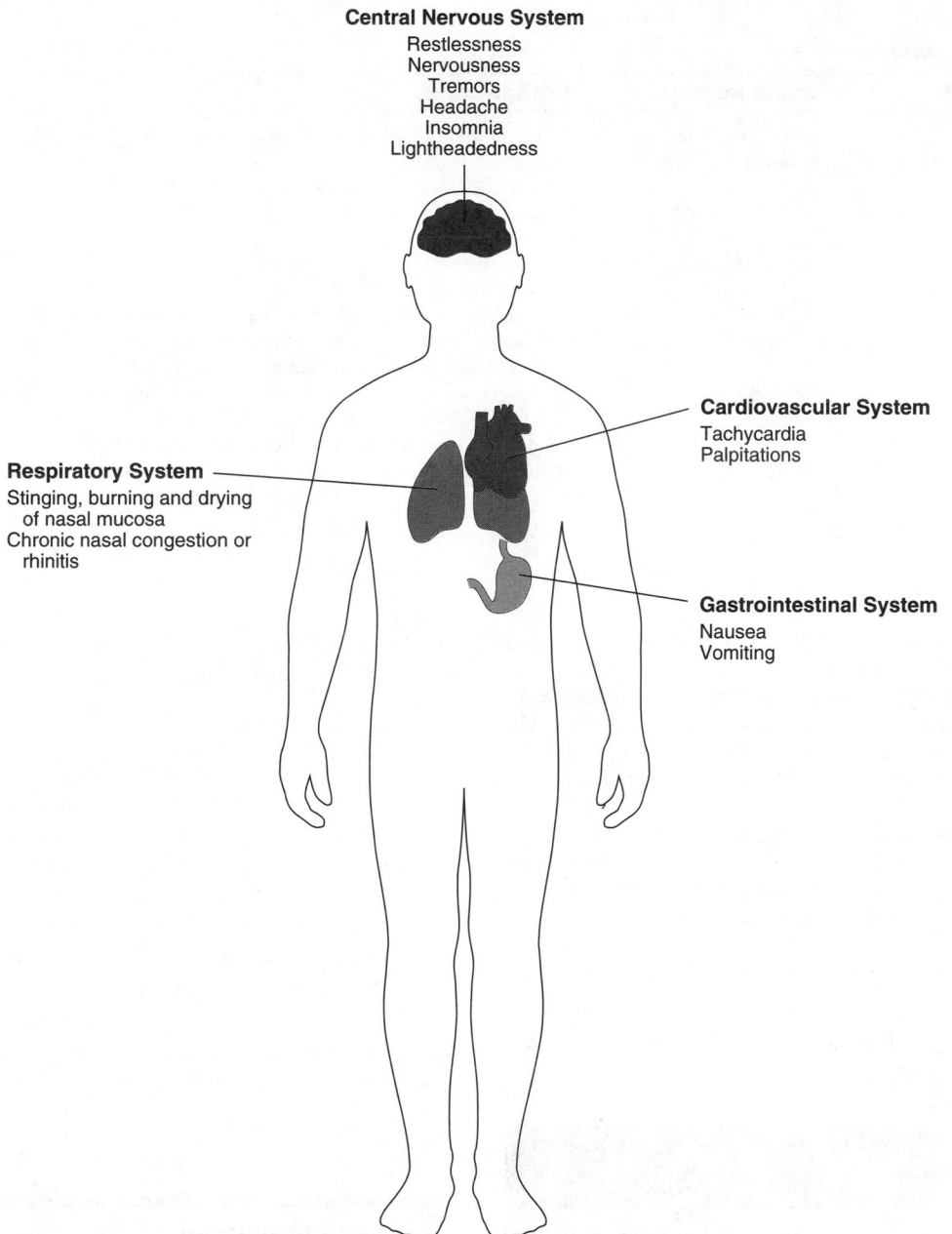

Central Nervous System
Restlessness
Nervousness
Tremors
Headache
Insomnia
Lightheadedness

Cardiovascular System
Tachycardia
Palpitations

Respiratory System
Stinging, burning and drying
of nasal mucosa
Chronic nasal congestion or
rhinitis

Gastrointestinal System
Nausea
Vomiting

FIGURE 44–1   Undesired clinical responses associated with use of nasal decongestants.

doses may produce tachycardia, palpitations (particularly in those with cardiac disease), lightheadedness, nausea, and vomiting. Undesired clinical responses to nasal sprays are illustrated in Figure 44–1.

Contraindications and Precautions Use of phenylephrine is contraindicated in individuals with previous hypersensitivity to sympathomimetics manifested by insomnia, dizziness, weakness, tremor, or arrhythmias. It should not be used concurrently with monoamine oxidase inhibitor (MAOI) therapy and should be used with caution in clients with marked hypertension, cardiac disorders, advanced arteriosclerotic disease, type I (insulin-dependent) diabetes mellitus, or hyperthyroidism.

Drug-Drug Interactions Tricyclic antidepressants (e.g., amitriptyline) may increase the cardiovascular effects of phenylephrine. Phenylephrine may decrease the effect of methyldopa. It may have mutually inhibitory effects with concurrent use of β-blockers. Concurrent use of digoxin may increase the risk of arrhythmias. Ergonovine or oxytocin may increase the vasoconstrictive effect of phenylephrine, whereas MAOIs may increase its vasopressor effects.[5,6]

Life-Span Considerations Phenylephrine is classified as a Pregnancy Category C drug. It is not known if the drug is excreted in human milk. Overdosage in clients greater than 60 years of age may result in hallucinations,

TABLE 44–1
Nasal Decongestants

Generic Name	Brand Name(s)	Dosage Range
Phenylephrine	Neo-Synephrine	Adult, children >12 y: two or three sprays or drops in each nostril q3-4h
Phenylpropanolamine	Propagest	Adults: 25 mg q4h
		Children 6–12 y: 12.5 mg q4h
		Children 2–6 y: 6.25 mg q4h
Sustained release		Adults: 75 mg q12h
Pseudoephedrine	Afrin, Drixoral	Adults, children >12 y: 60 mg q4-6h
Sustained release		Adults: 120 mg q12h
Naphazoline	Privine	Adults, children >12 y: one or two drops in each nostril q3h
Oxymetazoline	Afrin, Allerest	Adults, children >6 y: two or three sprays or drops (0.05% solution) bid
		Children 2–5 y: two or three drops (0.025% solution) bid
Propylhexedrine	Benzedrex	Adults, children >6 y: one or two inhalations in each nostril no more than q2h
Tetrahydrozoline	Tyzine	Adults, children >6 y: two drops (0.1% solution) q3-4h
		Children 2–6 y: two or three drops (0.05% solution) q4-6h
Xylometazoline	Otrivin	Adults, children >12 y: two or three drops or sprays (0.1% solution) q8-10h
		Children 2–12 y: two or three drops (0.05%) q8-10h

CNS depression, and seizures. This drug should be used with caution in children.

Specific Drug-Related Nursing Considerations Nasal decongestants can be administered directly via drops, sprays, and oral inhalation or systemically by the oral route. Topically the onset of action is rapid because of the direct stimulation of the nasal mucosa, but topical forms of the drug should not be used for more than 3 to 5 days because of the high risk of **rebound phenomenon,** through which the nasal passages become extremely congested when the drug's duration of action ends.

MISCELLANEOUS DRUGS IN CATEGORY

Numerous nasal decongestants are available. Table 44–1 contains information about some of these drugs. Corticoste-

INTRANASAL CORTICOSTEROIDS FOR ALLERGIC RHINITIS

Several corticosteroid nasal sprays are available for the treatment of allergic rhinitis. These sprays decrease allergen-induced and nonimmune nasal hyperreactivity. Many of the corticosteroid sprays are marketed in an aerosol metered-dose inhaler.

Examples of corticosteroid nasal sprays follow:

- Beclomethasone: 42 μg or one inhalation in each nostril bid to qid
- Budesonide: 32 μg or two inhalations in each nostril bid
- Flunisolide: 25 μg or two inhalations in each nostril bid
- Triamcinolone acetonide: 55 μg or two inhalations in each nostril once daily or bid

Data from Abramowicz, M. (Ed.). (1994). Intranasal budesonide for allergic rhinitis. *The Medical Letter, 36,* 63–64; Mabry, R.L. (1992). Topical pharmacotherapy for allergic rhinitis: New agents. *Southern Medical Journal, 85*(2), 149–154; Ratner, P.H., Paull, B.R., Findlay, S.R., et al. (1992). Fluticasone propionate given once daily is as effective for seasonal allergic rhinitis as beclomethasone dipropionate given twice daily. *Journal of Allergy and Clinical Immunology, 90*(3, Part I), 285–291.

roid nasal sprays are also available; some of them and their usual dosages are listed in the box.

OTC PREPARATIONS

Because of their popular use and their lack of serious side effects when used topically, many preparations have been released for direct sale to the public. Some of the products approved by the Food and Drug Administration (FDA) as safe and effective topical nasal decongestants are oxymetazoline hydrochloride (0.05%, 0.025%; Afrin, Dristan Nasal Spray); phenylephrine hydrochloride (0.125%, 0.25%, 1%; Neo-Synephrine); and xylometazoline hydrochloride (0.1%, 0.05%; Otrivin). OTC oral decongestant products include phenylephrine (in Dristan), phenylpropanolamine (e.g., in Sine-Off, Sinutab, Comtrex), and pseudoephedrine (e.g., in Fedahist).

CONCEPT REVIEW

Nasal decongestants are adrenergic drugs that shrink the mucous membranes, improving drainage and reducing stuffiness. They may be used as adjunctive therapy in treating middle ear infections or to lessen ear blockage during air travel.

Actions of nasal decongestants are restricted largely to the nasal mucosa.

Nasal decongestants must be used with caution in clients receiving MAOI therapy and those with hypertension or cardiac disease.

ANTIHISTAMINES

Histamine is produced by the body and is responsible for the inflammatory response. Mast cells and basophils contain large amounts of histamine. When histamine is released because of a hypersensitivity reaction or tissue injury, the smooth muscles and vascular system increase blood flow by dilating the capillaries. Fluid escapes from the capillaries into the tissues, producing swelling.

Antihistamines block the histamine effects at various receptor sites in the body. Antihistamines are divided chemically into five groups: ethanolamines, ethylenediamines, alkylamines, piperazines, and phenothiazines. All groups differ somewhat in their sedative, gastrointestinal (GI), anticholinergic, and antiemetic effects, but all have the same basic mechanism of action and same major undesired clinical responses. Antihistamines are discussed at length in Chapter 50.

ANTITUSSIVES

Antitussive drugs are used to alleviate coughing; they act either on the central or peripheral nervous system or on the mucosa locally.

Centrally Acting Antitussives

Centrally acting antitussive drugs apparently act by depressing the cough center in the medulla of the brain. Antitussives of this type are subdivided into two classes: narcotic and non-narcotic.

Narcotic antitussives Codeine is one of the most commonly used antitussive drugs. For cough suppression, it is used in lower doses than for pain relief. At low doses, undesired responses are reduced, as is the risk for addiction. The average dose is between 10 and 20 mg for adults. Opioids such as morphine and hydromorphone also suppress the cough reflex, but their usefulness is limited by side effects. In addition, they can cause drug dependence. (See Chapter 19 for information on

narcotic drugs.) Synthetic narcotic alkaloids (i.e., hydrocodone bitartrate) are marketed in tablet and syrup forms.

Non-narcotic antitussives These drugs are probably as effective as the narcotic agents. **Dextromethorphan hydrobromide** is the most frequently used non-narcotic antitussive. It is a chemical analog of codeine but does not have its analgesic or addictive properties. Dextromethorphan is used as a component of antitussive drug combinations and frequently is used in OTC preparations.

When used as a cough suppressant, 15 to 30 mg of dextromethorphan is considered equivalent in effect to 8 to 15 mg of codeine. It is well absorbed orally from the GI tract, with an onset of action between 15 to 30 minutes and a duration of action between 3 to 6 hours.[5,7,8]

Diphenhydramine is also a non-narcotic antitussive.

Peripherally Acting Antitussives

Peripherally acting antitussives act in numerous ways. Most drugs in this category have no specific local effects. However, one drug, benzonatate, is a potent local anesthetic.

PERIPHERALLY ACTING ANTITUSSIVE PROTOTYPE
BENZONATATE

Pharmacotherapeutics Benzonatate (Tessalon Perles) is used for the symptomatic relief of cough, including that with acute respiratory conditions (e.g., pneumonia) and with chronic diseases (e.g., bronchial asthma).

Pharmacokinetics The onset of action of benzonatate occurs in 15 to 20 minutes, and its effect lasts 3 to 8 hours. It has no inhibitory effect on the respiratory center.

Pharmacodynamics Benzonatate anesthetizes the stretch receptors in the respiratory passages, the lungs, and the pleura, thereby reducing cough production.

TABLE 44–2
Antitussives

Generic Name	Brand Name(s)	Dosage Range
NARCOTIC ANTITUSSIVE		
Codeine		Adults: 10–20 mg q4-6h
		Children 6–12 y: 5–10 mg q4-6h
		Children 2–6 y: 2.5–5 mg q4-6h
NON-NARCOTIC ANTITUSSIVES		
Dextromethorphan	Robitussin	Adults, children >12 y: 10–30 mq q4-6h
		Children 6–12 y: 5–10 mg q4h or 15 mg q6-8h
		Children 2–6 y (syrup): 2.5–7.5 mg q4-8h
Sustained-action liquid		Adults: 60 mg q12h
		Children 6–12 y: 30 mg q12h
		Children 2–5 y: 15 mg q12h
Diphenhydramine	Benylin	Adults: 25 mg q4h
		Children 6–12 y: 12.5 mg q4h
		Children 2–6 y: 6.25 mg q4h
Benzonatate	Tessalon Perles	Adults, children >10 y: 100 mg tid
Dextromethorphan and benzocaine (fixed-combination)	Vicks Formula 44	Adults, children >12 y: two lozenges q4h
		Children 3–12 y: one lozenge q4h

Pharmaceutics Benzonatate is available in capsule form. Capsules should not be chewed or broken but must be swallowed whole. If the capsules are chewed or broken in the mouth, oropharyngeal anesthesia occurs quickly (Table 44–2).

Undesired Clinical Responses Occasional undesired clinical responses to benzonatate include drowsiness, sense of chilliness, headache, GI upset, constipation, and a sensation of burning in the eyes. Rarely noted is a mild hypersensitivity reaction (pruritus or skin eruption). **Paradoxical reaction** (restlessness, insomnia, euphoria, nervousness, tremors) has been noted, which may proceed to clonic convulsions followed by profound CNS depression.

Contraindications and Precautions There are no significant contraindications or precautions to the use of benzonatate.

Drug-Drug Interactions. Potentiated CNS effects occur when benzonatate is used with CNS depressants, including alcohol.

Life-Span Considerations. The elderly are more likely than those in other age groups to have a sensation of burning in the eyes with use of benzonatate. The safe use of this drug in pregnant women or during lactation has not been established.[5,6]

Specific Drug-Related Nursing Considerations Assess the client's history for known hypersensitivity to the drug. If possible, determine the cause of the coughing. Caution the client about operating a car or other machinery since the drug may cause drowsiness or dizziness.

MISCELLANEOUS DRUGS IN CATEGORY

Table 44–2 contains additional information about antitussives.

OTC PREPARATIONS

Codeine, dextromethorphan, and diphenhydramine hydrochloride have been recommended by the FDA as safe and effective drugs. Stringent controls have been placed on codeine-containing nonprescription products.[9]

CONCEPT REVIEW

The two types of centrally acting cough suppressants are narcotic (codeine and hydrocodone) and non-narcotic. They work within the CNS to reduce the frequency and the intensity of the cough. Paradoxical reaction may occur with this drug group.

Peripherally acting antitussives work primarily through receptors within the respiratory tract. Many of them such as benzonate produce mild analgesic or anesthetic action on respiratory tract mucosa.

EXPECTORANTS

Expectorants render the cough more productive by stimulating the flow and reducing the viscosity of respiratory tract secretions. The loosened respiratory tract fluid is moved toward the pharynx by ciliary motion and by coughing.

EXPECTORANT PROTOTYPE
GUAIFENESIN, OR GLYCERYL GUAIACOLATE

Pharmacotherapeutics Guaifenesin (Anti-tuss, Genatuss, Robitussin) is used for the symptomatic relief of respiratory conditions characterized by dry, nonproductive cough. It is also used in the presence of mucus in the respiratory tract. Expectorants should not be used for persistent coughs such as those occurring with smoking, asthma, or emphysema or if a cough is accompanied by excessive secretions.

Pharmacokinetics After ingestion guaifenesin is well absorbed from the GI tract. It is metabolized in the liver and is excreted in the urine.

Pharmacodynamics Guaifenesin enhances the output of respiratory tract fluid by reducing adhesiveness and surface tension, allowing the removal of viscous mucus. The nonproductive cough becomes more productive and less frequent.

Pharmaceutics Guaifenesin is available in syrup, liquid, tablet, capsule, and sustained-release capsule form. The tablets are scored and may be crushed; the capsule form must be swallowed whole.

Undesired Clinical Responses Nausea and vomiting may occur with overdosage. Dizziness, headache, and rash may occur.

Contraindication and Precautions Guaifenesin should not be prescribed for individuals with known hypersensitivity to guaifenesin.

Drug-Drug Interactions Guaifenesin may increase renal clearance for urate and thereby lower serum uric acid levels. It may increase urinary 5-hydroxyindoleacetic acid and interfere with the interpretation of its testing for the diagnosis of carcinoid syndrome.[6]

Life-Span Considerations. Guaifenesin is classified as a Pregnancy Category C drug. It is not known whether the drug is excreted in human milk.

Specific Drug-Related Nursing Considerations The client taking guaifenesin should contact a primary care provider if the cough persists for longer than 1 week. Some coughs such as those associated with bronchitis may take weeks to abate. The client should also contact a primary care provider if the cough is accompanied by a high fever, rash, or persistent headache.

MISCELLANEOUS DRUGS IN CATEGORY

Other expectorants are available, including ammonium chloride and terpin hydrate. **Ammonium chloride** is thought to increase the amount of respiratory tract fluid through reflex stimulation of bronchial mucous glands resulting from irritation of the gastric mucosa. This drug can produce toxicity in clients with severe renal or hepatic failure.

Terpin hydrate is a volatile oil derivative. It probably acts by direct stimulation of the lower respiratory tract secretory glands. Terpin hydrate elixir contains a significant amount of alcohol and must be used with caution. Undesired clinical responses include nausea and vomiting.

Table 44–3 contains additional information about expectorants.

TABLE 44–3
Expectorants

Generic Name	Name Brand(s)	Dosage Range
Guaifenesin	Anti-tuss	Adults: children >12 y: 100–400 mg q4h Children 6–12 y: 100–200 mg q4h Children 2–6 y: 50–100 mg q4h
Terpin hydrate		Adults: 85–170 mg tid or qid Children 10–12 y: 85 mg tid or qid Children 5–9 y: 40 mg tid or qid Children 1–4 y: 20 mg tid or qid
Potassium iodide		Adults: 300–1000 mg after meals bid or tid

CONCEPT REVIEW

Expectorants stimulate the flow and reduce the viscosity of respiratory tract secretions. Their use is limited, and they should not be used for more than 7 days without consultation with the primary care provider. They are not intended for treatment of cough associated with smoking, asthma, or emphysema or for treatment of cough accompanied by excessive secretions.

MUCOLYTICS

When secretions are tenacious, the liquefying action of a mucolytic agent may make the secretions easier to eliminate and may produce enhanced ciliary action. Water given by inhalation or orally is useful, particularly when secretions are thickened by dehydration, and it appears to soothe and cleanse mucous membranes. Various chemical agents are sometimes added to the water used for inhalation to reduce the viscosity of mucus.

MUCOLYTIC PROTOTYPE
ACETYLCYSTEINE

Pharmacotherapeutics Acetylcysteine (Mucomyst, Mucosil) is used as adjunctive treatment for abnormally viscid mucous secretions present in clients with acute and chronic bronchopulmonary disease or pulmonary complications of cystic fibrosis. It is also used as part of tracheostomy care and in the treatment of acetaminophen overdose.

Pharmacokinetics After oral inhalation or intratracheal instillation, most of acetylcysteine is involved in a sulfhydryl-disulfide reaction. The remainder of the drug is absorbed from pulmonary epithelium. After oral administration, it is readily absorbed from the GI tract. It is metabolized in the liver.

Pharmacodynamics The sulfhydryl group in acetylcysteine directly splits disulfide linkage of mucoproteins. It reduces the viscosity of pulmonary secretions and facilitates their removal by coughing, postural drainage, and mechanical means. Acetylcysteine also maintains and restores the hepatic concentration of glutathione, which is necessary for inactivation of hepatotoxic acetaminophen metabolite.

Pharmaceutics Acetylcysteine is provided for nebulization or as an oral solution. During nebulization the 20% solution may be diluted with 0.9% NaCl or sterile water for injection. The 10% solution may be administered undiluted. Orally, give a 5% solution diluted in a 1:3 ratio with cola, soft drink, or juice. The oral solution may be given through a duodenal tube.

Undesired Clinical Responses Bronchospasm occurs rarely with the administration of acetylcysteine and is relieved quickly with the use of a bronchodilator. **Stomatitis** (erythema of mucous membranes, dry mouth, burning of oral mucosa) and rhinorrhea also occur rarely. A large dosage may produce severe nausea and vomiting.

Contraindications and Precautions Use acetylcysteine with caution in clients with bronchial asthma, in the elderly, and in debilitated clients with severe respiratory insufficiency.

Drug-Drug and Drug-Environment Interactions A light-purple color may result in an opened bottle, but it does not impair the safety or effectiveness of the medication. After exposure to air, the solution should be refrigerated and used within 96 hours. A slight, disagreeable odor from the solution may be noticed during the initial administration, but the odor disappears quickly. Avoid contact with iron, copper, or rubber (reacts with acetylcysteine). Instead, use parts made of glass, plastic, aluminum, chromed metal, sterling silver, or stainless steel.

Life-Span Considerations It is not known whether acetylcysteine crosses the placenta or is excreted in breast milk.

Specific Drug-Related Nursing Considerations Assess the client's pretreatment respirations for rate, depth, and rhythm. Have suction equipment available in case the client cannot clear the airway. If bronchospasm occurs, discontinue the treatment and notify the prescriber. Monitor rate, depth, rhythm, and type of respiration (abdominal, thoracic). Check sputum for color, consistency, and amount. Assess lung sounds for rhonchi, wheezing, or rales.

CONCEPT REVIEW

Water given by inhalation or orally is perhaps the most useful agent in eliminating mucous secretions.

Chemical agents for inhalation to reduce mucous viscosity are called *mucolytics*.

During nebulization care must be taken to use equipment that will not react with the drug.

TABLE 44-4

*Examples of OTC Cold Remedy Preparations**

Product	Dose Form	Decongestant	Antihistamine	Cough Suppressant	Expectorant
Actifed Plus	Capsule Tablet	Pseudoephedrine hydrochloride, 30 mg	Triprolidine hydrochloride, 1.25 mg	—	—
Alka-Seltzer Plus	Tablet	Phenylpropanolamine bitartrate, 24 mg	Chlorpheniramine maleate, 2 mg	—	—
Cheracol Plus	Liquid	Phenylpropanolamine hydrochloride, 25 mg/15 ml	Chlorpheniramine maleate, 4 mg/15 ml	Dextromethorphan hydrobromide, 20 mg/15 ml	—
Comtrex	Caplet Tablet Liquid Liquid-gel	Pseudoephedrine hydrochloride *or* Phenylpropanolamine hydrochloride (dosages vary according to dosage form)	Chlorpheniramine maleate 0.65 mg/5 ml–2 mg	Dextromethorphan hydrobromide, 3.35 mg/5 ml– 10 mg	—
Contac Nightime Cold	Liquid	Pseudoephedrine hydrochloride, 10 mg/5 ml	Doxylamine succinate, 1.25 mg/5 ml	Dextromethorphan hydrobromide, 5 mg/5 ml	—
4-Way Cold	Tablet	Phenylpropanolamine hydrochloride, 12.5 mg	Chlorpheniramine maleate, 2 mg	—	—
Kophane Cough and Cold Formula	Syrup	Phenylpropanolamine hydrochloride, 5 mg/5 ml	Chlorpheniramine maleate, 0.5 mg/5 ml	Dextromethorphan hydrobromide, 10 mg/5 ml	Ammonium chloride, 90 mg/5 ml
Novahistine DMX	Syrup	Pseudoephedrine hydrochloride, 30 mg/5 ml	—	Dextramethorphan hydrobromide 10 mg/5 ml	Guaifenesin, 100 mg/5 ml
Tylenol Cold Medication	Liquid	Pseudoephedrine hydrochloride, 10 mg/5 ml	Chlorpheniramine maleate, 0.67 mg/5 ml	Dextromethorphan hydrobromide, 5 mg/5 ml	—

*All ingredients in preparations are not listed.

COMBINATION COLD REMEDY PREPARATIONS

Cold remedies are designed to provide decongestion and dry the nasal mucous membranes. Various mixtures are combined, but when a therapeutic amount of one agent is given, the other drugs in the mixture generally are added at a higher- or lower-than-optimal therapeutic level. A combination of two fractional doses, as opposed to a full dose of a single ingredient from a given classification of drug, apparently is therapeutically inadequate. However, if the client suffers from multiple symptoms, particularly during the early stages of a cold, use of a mixture provides a more convenient and less expensive means of providing relief than does the use of several agents. In most cases such cold remedy preparations contain a decongestant, an antihistamine, and an analgesic.[9–11]

Table 44–4 provides a sampling of the great variety of available mixtures of OTC cold preparations

SUMMARY

Effects of the common cold and of allergies (particularly environmentally produced allergies) cause not only symptoms for the sufferer but also a loss of productive days at work or school. With the assistance of antihistamines to reduce allergic symptoms, nasal decongestants to ease breathing, and antitussives to reduce the cough, the effects of the common cold and allergies are lessened, enabling individuals to function.

REFERENCES

1. Monahan, F.D., Drake, T., & Neighbors, M. (1994). *Nursing care of adults*. Philadelphia: W.B. Saunders.
2. Engle, J.P. (1992). Topical nasal decongestants. *American Pharmacy 32*(5), 33–37.
3. Jackson, R.T. (1991). Mechanism of action of some commonly used nasal drugs. *Otolaryngology—Head and Neck Surgery 104*(4), 433–440.
4. Ziering, R.W., & Klein, G.L. (1992). Allergic rhinitis. Measures to control the misery. *Postgrad-Medicine 91*(1), 225–227, 231–232.
5. United States Pharmacopeia Dispensing Information (USPDI). (1992). *Drug information for the health care professional*. Rockville, MD: US Pharmacopeial Convention.
6. United States Food and Drug Administration. (1993). *Physician's GenRx*. Smithtown, NY: Author.
7. Gilman, A.G., et al. (Eds.). (1990). *Goodman and Gilman's: The*

pharmacological basis of therapeutics (6th ed). New York: Macmillan.

8. Lehne, R.A. (1994). *Pharmacology for nursing care* (2nd ed.). Philadelphia: W.B. Saunders.

9. American Pharmaceutical Association. (1990). *Handbook of non-prescription drugs* (9th ed). Washington, D.C.: Author.

10. Hutton, N., et al. (1991). Effectiveness of an antihistamine-decongestant combination for young children with the common cold: A randomized, controlled clinical trial. *Journal of Pediatrics, 118*, 125–130.

11. Gadomski, A., & Horton, L. (1992). The need for rational therapeutics in the use of cough and cold medicine in infants. *Pediatrics 89*(4, Part 2), 774–776.

BIBLIOGRAPHY

Anastasio, G., & Harston, P. (1992). Fetal tachycardia associated with maternal use of pseudoephedrine, an over-the-counter oral decongestant. *Journal of American Board of Family Practice, 5,* 527–528.

Beck, R.A., Mercado, D.L., Seguin, S.M., Andrade, W.P., & Cushner, H. (1992). Cardiovascular effects of pseudoephedrine in medically controlled hypertensive patients. *Archives of Internal Medicine, 152,* 1242–1245.

Macknin, J.L. (1992). Respiratory infections in children. What helps and what doesn't? *Postgrad-Medicine, 92*(2), 235–238, 243, 247–250.

New antihistamine/decongestant combination. (1994). *Drug Therapy: Prescribing Strategies in Primary Care, 24*(7), 15.

Norman, P.S. (1991). Allergic rhinitis: Combined therapy improves control. *Consultant, 31*(8), 25–29.

Sperber, S.J., Hendley, J.O., Hayden, F.G., Riker, D.K., et al. (1992). Effects of naproxen on experimental rhinovirus colds. A randomized, double-blind, controlled trial. *Annals of Internal Medicine, 117*(1), 37–41.

Wawrose, S., Tami, T., & Amoils, P. (1992). The role of guaifenesin in the treatment of sinonasal disease in patients infected with the human immunodeficiency virus (HIV). *Laryngoscope, 102,* 1225–1228.

Woolbert, L.F. (1990). Do antihistamines and decongestants prevent otitis media? *Pediatric Nursing, 16*(3), 265–267.

Zenk, K.E., & Ma, H. (1990). Pharmacologic treatment of otitis media and sinusitis in pediatrics. *Journal of Pediatric Health Care, 4*(6), 297–303.

CHAPTER 45

Bronchodilating Drugs and Related Agents

NORMA L. PINNELL • BARBARA J. WIRICK

⊛ **Nursing Considerations**

LEARNING OBJECTIVES:

Identify nursing diagnoses appropriate for a client requiring the use of bronchodilating drugs.
Describe appropriate techniques for administering nasal drops or inhalant therapy to children.

⊛ **Bronchodilators**

LEARNING OBJECTIVES:

Describe the pharmacodynamic properties of sympathomimetic bronchodilators.
List major undesired clinical responses associated with the use of sympathomimetic bronchodilators.
Explain the pharmacodynamic and pharmacotherapeutic properties of methylxanthine bronchodilators.

Describe common undesired clinical responses associated with methylxanthine bronchodilators.
Describe pharmacokinetic and pharmacodynamic properties of ipratropium bromide.
Discuss therapeutic uses of ipratropium bromide.

⊛ **Corticosteroids**

LEARNING OBJECTIVE: Describe pharmacotherapeutic and pharmacodynamic properties of corticosteroids.

⊛ **Mast Cell Stabilizers**

LEARNING OBJECTIVES:

Describe pharmacokinetic and pharmacodynamic properties of cromolyn sodium.
Discuss therapeutic uses of cromolyn sodium.

CONCEPTS AND TERMS TO REVIEW

Read Chapter 43 for an overview of the anatomy and physiology of the respiratory system.

Review Chapter 25 for an overview of the autonomic nervous system.

Read the appropriate sections in Chapters 26 and 27 on drugs affecting the parasympathetic and sympathetic nervous system.

Read appropriate sections in Chapter 42 on corticosteroid drugs.

---

*T*housands of individuals each year are treated for respiratory diseases and abnormalities. Routinely treated diseases include restrictive pulmonary diseases, obstructive pulmonary diseases, and chronic obstructive pulmonary disease. A number of drugs are available for the treatment of these diseases.

This chapter addresses general characteristics of these drugs, major prototypes, and nursing considerations. Consideration is also given to life-span aspects of drug therapy and to drug, diet, and environmental interactions.

▦ NURSING CONSIDERATIONS

Since many respiratory diseases require long-term care and follow-up, the client must be prepared for self-care.

Assessing Obtain a complete **health history** from clients being treated with respiratory drugs. Include in the history information on the present complaint, including signs and symptoms, length of the present illness, precipitating events, and treatment measures. Determine if the client has a history of respiratory illnesses; include questions about asthma, allergies, chronic airway diseases, and pneumonia. Determine if the client has a cough; have the client describe the cough. Is it a congested and nonproductive cough? Is it a congested and productive cough? If it is productive, assess color, odor, consistency, and amount of expectorate. Obtain a smoking history; include how long the client has smoked and the number of packs per day.

Collect a drug history; include all prescription and over-the-counter (OTC) drugs that the client is currently taking or has taken in the past. If the client is receiving drugs that affect the respiratory system, determine the dosages, frequency of use, and effectiveness of the drug. Also assess the client's compliance with the drug regimen.

After taking a careful history, perform a **physical assessment.** Pay particular attention to the respiratory system. Examine the ears, nose, and throat for redness, swelling, pain, and drainage. Auscultate the lungs bilaterally in all lobes and anteriorly and posteriorly. Note breath sounds. Are wheezes, rales, crackles, or rhonchi (gurgles) present? Are there decreased breath sounds in any of the areas assessed? Assess the client's respiratory effort. Is the client's breathing labored? Are there retractions when breathing? If so, what type of retractions are seen? Supraclavicular retractions in an adult and intercostal retractions with nasal flaring in infants and children may be evident. Observe the client's skin color. Look for pallor and cyanosis. Check for central cyanosis by inspecting the mucous membranes of the mouth. Labored breathing accompanied by retractions or cyanosis is a medical emergency, and treatment with oxygen and appropriate medical therapy should be begun immediately.

Diagnosing   After obtaining a thorough history and physical assessment, formulate nursing diagnoses based on analysis of the assessed data. Appropriate diagnoses include the following:

* Ineffective airway clearance related to excessive thick mucous secretions.
* Activity intolerance related to inadequate oxygenation.
* Anxiety related to dyspnea or lack of knowledge of treatment plan.
* High risk for altered health maintenance related to lack of knowledge of pharmacologic therapy.
* Knowledge deficit regarding drug therapy.
* Self-esteem disturbance related to reliance on drug therapy.

Planning   Focus the plan of care on the individual client and the nursing diagnoses formulated. Develop discharge and teaching plans that help the client adjust to the drug regimen. Provide a thorough explanation of the drug regimen in terms that the client can understand. Teach the client the name and dosage schedule of the drug. Explain to the client the drug's actions, undesired clinical responses, and signs and symptoms to report to the primary care provider.

Many drugs used to treat respiratory diseases are administered topically via inhalation. Therefore you must teach the client how to administer the prescribed drugs properly. The box summarizes a teaching plan on the use of the metered dose inhaler (MDI).

Develop expected outcomes with the client. Appropriate outcomes follow:

* Client's airway is clear, and lung sounds are clear to auscultation.

INSTRUCTIONS ON USE OF METERED DOSE INHALER

1. Shake the inhaler well. Make sure the canister and mouthpiece are firmly connected.

2. Hold the mouthpiece securely between index finger and thumb.

3. Tilt head back slightly and exhale fully.

4. Close the lips around the mouthpiece or a spacer, or hold the canister 1 or 2 inches away from your mouth.

5. Breathe in deeply and slowly and at the same time depress the top of the canister fully.

6. Hold your breath as long as is comfortably possible (10 seconds) to disperse the medicine in the lungs. Remove the inhaler before exhaling slowly.

7. Wait 1 minute between puffs, shake the inhaler again, and repeat.

8. If using a steroid inhaler, use a spacer or rinse your mouth after each use to prevent fungal infection (thrush) in the mouth.

9. Cleanse the mouthpiece in warm water daily and dry it thoroughly to prevent the growth of bacteria.

10. Use the inhaler as prescribed and do not exceed the dose. If difficult breathing persists or if symptoms of dryness of mouth and throat, headache, nervousness, tremor, or dizziness occur, contact your primary care provider.

---

* Client's respiratory rate is within normal range.
* Client has increased tolerance to exercise.
* Client complies with the pharmacologic regimen.
* Client demonstrates an understanding of the drugs, dosages, schedule, and side effects.

Implementing   Care measures may involve instilling nose drops or administering drugs via inhalation or aerosol. For infants, toddlers, and young children, changes in the administration technique are needed (see box on p. 558). Basically all drugs presented in this chapter may be used in the elderly population. However, care must be taken to assess elderly clients' cardiovascular, neurologic, renal, and hepatic function. Significant alterations in any of these systems dictates whether drugs should be used. In addition, monitor the elderly closely for adverse reactions.

Evaluating   Evaluate the effectiveness of the plan of care and the treatment plan. Determine if expected outcomes were met. If expected outcomes were not met, determine what changes are needed in the plan.

🦅 NURSING RESEARCH

Tetersell, M.J. (1993). Asthma patients knowledge in relation to compliance with drug therapy. *Journal of Advanced Nursing,* *18*(1), 103–113.

NOSE DROP ADMINISTRATION AND INHALATION TECHNIQUES FOR INFANTS, TODDLERS, AND YOUNG CHILDREN

Nose Drops

Nose drops are instilled in the same manner for children as for adults. The individual lies in a supine position, and the head is hyperextended. The drops should be given at room temperature to avoid discomfort of the nasal membranes. Gentle pressure can be applied to the tip of the nose to open the nostrils further. The drops should be instilled into the nares without coming into contact with either nostril or any other part of the face. The client should remain in the same position for approximately 2 minutes after the instillation to allow gravity to assist penetration of the drops into the swollen mucous membranes of the nasal passages. Discourage clients' vigorous sniffing, for doing so could result in sucking the medication into the sinuses.

YOUNG INFANTS

Placing the infant in a football hold may facilitate the procedure. This position allows primary support of the infant's weight by the nurse's hip while one hand supports the head and the other hand is free to administer the drops. The infant could also lie supine on the parent's or nurse's lap with the head tilted down. When nose drops are given to relieve congestion, administer them before feedings so that the infant who is an obligatory nose breather may do so during feedings.

OLDER INFANTS AND TODDLERS

Administration of nose drops to this age child requires the help of two individuals unless the child is wrapped in a mummy restraint. Elevating the shoulders on a pillow allows the head to fall back comfortably and facilitates administration of the nose drops. The second individual stabilizes the child's head.

PRESCHOOLERS

These children are often willing to lie supine across the parent's lap with the head extended downward to one side.

SCHOOLAGERS AND ADOLESCENTS

Clients in this age group often lie across their bed with their heads extended over the edge. This position is easy for them to maintain independently, and the hyperextension of the head should prevent the strangling sensations caused by medication trickling down the throat.

Nasal Inhalation

Nasal inhalation most commonly is used in children with respiratory airway disease, particularly those with asthma and cystic fibrosis. The prescribed drug is mixed with a designated amount of normal saline solution and is placed into a nebulizer, which is connected to either oxygen or compressed air. The nebulized drug is administered over a 10- to 15-minute period, depending on the gas flow.

YOUNG INFANTS

The nebulizer is attached to a mask that can be held over the mouth and nose of the infant. Infants who are held, rocked, and talked to usually accept this aerosol treatment without fussing.

OLDER INFANTS AND TODDLERS

These children often resist having the mask against their face and struggle vigorously and cry. They usually are less frightened if held by the parent and the mask is used as a toy between treatments. The parents can desensitize the struggling child to the mask by taking turns holding the mask over their own faces in a game. Some children respond better to delivery of the mist through a nebulizer tube held near the nose or mouth.

OLDER TODDLERS AND PRESCHOOLERS

These children should have ample opportunity to become acquainted with the equipment before it is used on them. They respond positively to having the treatment demonstrated on a parent. If they can hold the mask themselves or at least help do so, they are less likely to struggle against it.

SCHOOLAGERS AND ADOLESCENTS

Children in these age groups usually respond positively to having the responsibility for choosing the delivery method and doing self-administration after the drug has been added to the nebulizer. The older child can inhale the mist through a mouthpiece on the tube.

This study was undertaken to determine the relationship of client knowledge to compliance in treatment of moderate-to-severe asthma. Thirty-nine of 100 subjects were noncompliant with the therapeutic regimen. The level of knowledge did not correlate with the level of compliance. On the contrary, the highest compliers reported never having received an explanation about their asthma. Explanations about asthma were generally not well understood, especially when the explanations were given by nurses. Only 34.4% were deemed objectively to know how to manage an attack, and this knowledge did correlate with the ability to forestall an asthma attack.

Factors involved in noncompliance were feelings that taking the drugs was not necessary, client forgetfulness, reluctance to use inhalers in public, and a preference for tablets rather than inhalers. The study concludes there is a great need for improved client education about asthma.

STUDENT ACTIVITIES

- Prepare a client education chart to explain asthma and its treatment.
- Use this chart with three individuals with no prior knowledge about asthma. After presenting the information, ask questions to determine the extent of their understanding of the subject.

BRONCHODILATORS

Bronchodilating drugs work by dilating the airways of the respiratory tree, thereby making air exchange and respiration easier for the client. They do this by a number of mechanisms, depending on the classification of the particular bronchodilator. For example, methylxanthines act by blocking the destruction of cyclic adenosine monophosphate (AMP). Common methylxanthine derivatives are caffeine and theophylline. Sympathomimetic drugs such as albuterol act as selective β_2-agonists to relax pulmonary smooth muscle and cause bronchodilation. Anticholinergic drugs reverse the effects of the autonomic nervous system on the pulmonary tree and smooth musculature, producing a dilating effect on the respiratory airways.

Sympathomimetic Bronchodilators

Sympathomimetic bronchodilators are also called β_2-*agonists*. The drug category was presented in detail in Chapter 27.

Sympathomimetic Bronchodilator Prototype

ALBUTEROL

Albuterol (Proventil, Ventolin) is an effective and widely used bronchodilator.

Pharmacotherapeutics Albuterol frequently is prescribed for treatment of asthma. It is also prescribed to prevent exercise-induced bronchospasm.

Pharmacokinetics Albuterol's onset of action begins within 1 to 2 minutes of aerosol administration. Maximal bronchodilation occurs within $\frac{1}{2}$ to 2 hours after two breaths of albuterol. The duration of action is 3 to 6 hours, which is also its half-life. Excretion is via the kidneys, with approximately one fourth excreted unchanged.[2]

When administered orally, albuterol is well absorbed from the gastrointestinal (GI) tract. Onset of action is less than 30 minutes. Peak action occurs in 2 to 3 hours; duration of action is 4 to 8 hours. The half-life is 5 to 6 hours, although it may vary and is dose dependent. Albuterol is metabolized in the liver and excreted in the urine.[3]

Pharmacodynamics As a selective β_2-agonist, albuterol, particularly in the inhaled form, stimulates the β_2-receptors located on bronchial smooth muscle, causing bronchodilation. Although it is selective for β_2-receptors, it is not exclusive. Therefore occasionally β_1-receptors are inadvertently stimulated, which results in albuterol's most common side effect, tachycardia. Albuterol is not an effective prophylactic agent.[4,5]

Pharmaceutics Albuterol is available in a variety of dosage forms, including syrup, uncoated tablets, and sustained-release tablets for oral administration. It is available for use in an MDI.[6]

Albuterol is administered at dosages of 90 μg per puff or via handheld nebulizers. The nebulizer dose is 2.5 to 10 mg of drug diluted in 3 ml of normal saline solution. Both inhaled routes are usually administered every 4 to 6 hours.

When administered orally, the usual adult dose is 2 to 4 mg three or four times per day. The drug is also being administered experimentally via endotracheal tube to relieve bronchospasm induced by inhalation anesthetics.

Undesired Clinical Responses The most serious undesired clinical responses to albuterol are due to β_1-receptor stimulation. β_1-Receptor sites are found mainly in the heart. As a result of β_1-receptor stimulation in the heart, albuterol produces side effects such as tachycardia, palpitations, arrhythmias, angina, and hypertension. Additional side effects are mostly related to central nervous system (CNS) stimulation: nervousness, anxiety, headache, dizziness, and insomnia. Hyperglycemia may also occur.[5]

Contraindications and Precautions Oral administration of albuterol has a greater risk of producing hypokalemia, particularly with large doses. Albuterol should be used with caution in clients with hyperthyroidism, coronary artery disease, and diabetes mellitus. In addition, albuterol may inhibit uterine contractions and complicate labor and delivery.

Drug-Drug, Drug-Nutrient, Drug-Environment Interactions Concomitant use of albuterol with other adrenergic aerosols should be avoided whenever possible because of the risk of paradoxical bronchospasm. Albuterol should not be used in combination with β-blockers since β-blockers oppose the action of albuterol. Concomitant use of albuterol with other sympathomimetic drugs should be avoided because of the additive effect and increased risk for side effects.

The efficacy of oral albuterol with respect to meals has not been established. Administration times should be adjusted based on client responsiveness to therapy.

Albuterol tablets and syrup should be stored between 2° and 30° C. Albuterol sustained-release tablets must be protected from excessive moisture. Inhalation albuterol must be stored between 15° and 30° C. Failure to use the drug within this temperature range may result in improper dosing.[6]

Life-Span Considerations Albuterol is classified as a Pregnancy Category C drug. It is not known if the drug is excreted in human breast milk. Safety and effectiveness of albuterol tablets have not been established for children below the age of 6 years. In addition, safety and effectiveness of sustained-release tablets in children below the age of 12 years has not been established.[6,7]

Specific Drug-Related Nursing Considerations Frequent pulmonary assessment is needed to analyze the effectiveness of albuterol therapy. Teach the client how to use and clean the MDI. Encourage the client to comply with the recommended dosage at scheduled intervals. Advise him or her not to add other drugs to the regimen without consulting the primary health care provider. Caution the client to avoid use of OTC drugs such as Primatene Mist and Bronkaid Mist. These preparations do not selectively stimulate β_2-receptors and therefore produce more side effects. Duration of action of these OTC products is extremely short.[2] If symptoms do not improve, instruct the client to consult the primary care provider.

Instruct the client to avoid excessive use of caffeine derivatives (e.g., chocolate, coffee, tea, cola, cocoa). Counsel him or her to avoid smoking and smoke-filled areas. See Table 45–1.

MISCELLANEOUS DRUGS IN CATEGORY

Other sympathomimetic bronchodilators include epinephrine, terbutaline sulfate, isoetharine, bitolterol mesylate, pirbuterol, and isoproterenol. Epinephrine and isoproterenol are used less frequently since the advent of safer and more effective β_2-selective adrenergic agonists. **Salmeterol xinafoate** (Serevent), a long-acting β_2-selective adrenergic agonist, has also been approved for maintenance treatment of asthma.[8,9] This drug is stronger, acts faster, and lasts twice as long as albuterol. Some studies suggest that salmeterol also produces fewer undesired clinical responses.[10]

TABLE 45–1
Sympathomimetic Bronchodilators

Drug Name	Dosage and Route of Administration	Nursing Considerations
ALBUTEROL (Proventil, Ventolin) HOW SUPPLIED Solution for inhalation: 0.5% in bottles of 20 ml; fill each Solution for inhalation: 0.083% in unit-dose bottles of 3 ml; fill each 17-g canisters: containing 200 metered inhalations, each delivering 90 μg albuterol Syrup: 2 mg albuterol/5 ml Tablets: 2 and 4 mg Tablets, extended release: 4 mg	**Nebulizer** ADULTS AND CHILDREN >12 Y Usual dose: 2.5 mg (3 ml reconstituted) tid or qid; deliver over 5–15 min **Inhalation** **Acute Episodes of Bronchospasm or Prevention of Asthmatic Symptoms** ADULTS AND CHILDREN >4 Y Usual dose: two inhalations repeated q4-6h; one inhalation may be sufficient **Prevention of Exercise-Induced Bronchospasm** ADULTS AND CHILDREN >12 Y Usual dose: inhalations 15 min before exercise **Oral Syrup** ADULTS AND CHILDREN >14 Y 2 or 4 mg qid; if no response, may adjust cautiously up to 8 mg qid CHILDREN 6–14 Y 2 mg tid or qid; if no response, adjust upward, not to exceed 24 mg/d CHILDREN 2–6 Y 0.1 mg/kg tid, not to exceed 2 mg tid; if no response, adjust upward, not to exceed 0.2 mg/kg or 4 mg tid ELDERLY Initial dose: 2 mg tid or qid **Tablets** ADULTS AND CHILDREN >12 Y 2 or 4 mg tid or qid; maximum, 8 mg qid CHILDREN 6–12 Y 2 mg tid or qid; maximum, 24 mg/d in divided doses ELDERLY 2 mg tid or qid **Extended Release Tablets** ADULTS AND CHILDREN >12 Y 4–8 mg q12h; do not exceed 32 mg/d	**Assess** Assess lung sounds for wheezing and rales. Monitor rate, depth, rhythm, type of respiration. Assess the quality and rate of the pulse. **Implement** Provide emotional support (clients are often anxious about symptoms). Instruct the client in proper use of the inhaler, including not taking more than two inhalations at one time and rinsing the mouth after inhalations. Tell the client to increase fluid intake to decrease the viscosity of lung secretions. Teach client not to alter dose or frequency without knowledge and consent of primary care provider. Teach client about potentially fatal paradoxical bronchospasm caused by overuse of drug. **Monitor** Obtain results of periodic serum drug levels. Instruct the client to report any adverse effects such as nausea and vomiting, headache, chest pain, or palpitations as soon as possible. **Evaluate** Assess resolution and control of asthmatic symptoms. See albuterol.
Terbutaline Sulfate (Brethine, Bricanyl) HOW SUPPLIED Micronized powder in an inert propellant: 75 mg (equals approximately 300 actuations); each actuation delivers approximately 0.20 mg terbutaline sulfate Tablets: 2.5 and 5 mg Ampules: 1 mg/ml for SC injection	**Inhalation** ADULTS AND CHILDREN >12 Y One inhalation q60sec to a total of two inhalations q4-6h **Oral Dose** ADULTS 5 mg at 6-h intervals tid, not to exceed 15 mg in 24 h; dosage may be reduced to 2.5-mg doses if side effects are severe CHILDREN 12–15 Y 2.5 mg at 6-h intervals tid, not to exceed 7.5 mg in 24 h Not recommended for children <12 y old **SC Dose** Initial dose: 0.25 mg in lateral deltoid area; after 15–30 min another 0.25 mg may be administered; total dose in 4 h not to exceed 0.5 mg	

TABLE 45-1 *Continued*
Sympathomimetic Bronchodilators

Drug Name	Dosage and Route of Administration	Nursing Considerations
Bitolterol Mesylate (Tornalate) **HOW SUPPLIED** Metered dose inhaler: 16.4-g (15 ml) self-contained aerosol units	ADULTS AND CHILDREN >12 Y **Relief of Bronchospasm** Two inhalations at an interval of 1–3 min followed by a third inhalation if needed **Prevention of Bronchospasm** Two inhalations q8h, not to exceed three inhalations q6h or two inhalations q4h	See albuterol.
Pirbuterol (Maxair) **HOW SUPPLIED** Pressured canister of 80, 300, or 400 inhalations, 0.2 mg pirbuterol per actuation	ADULTS AND CHILDREN >12 Y Usual dose: two inhalations q4-6h, not to exceed a total daily dose of 12 inhalations; some clients may need only one inhalation q4-6h	See albuterol.
Salmeterol Xinafoate (Serevent) **HOW SUPPLIED** Aerosol adaptor: 6.5 g; 60 metered actuations	*Not for use in treating acute bronchospasm* **Maintenance of Bronchodilation** ADULTS AND CHILDREN >12 Y, ELDERLY Two inhalations (42 µg) morning and evening approximately 12 h apart **Prevention of Exercise-Induced Bronchospasm** Two inhalations at least 30 min before exercise	Same as albuterol. Use with extreme caution in clients taking MAO inhibitors or tricyclic antidepressants.
Isoetharine (Bronkosol, Dey-Dose) **HOW SUPPLIED** Vial: 10 or 15 ml with oral nebulizer bottle of 10 or 30 ml	**Hand-bulb Nebulizer** ADULTS AND ELDERLY Three to seven inhalations undiluted; may repeat up to five times/d **Metered-dose Inhalation** ADULTS AND ELDERLY One or two inhalations q4h; wait 1 min before administering second inhalation **Intermittent Positive-Pressure Breathing, Oxygen Aerolization** ADULTS AND ELDERLY 0.5–1 ml of 0.5% solution (or 0.5 ml of a 1% solution) diluted 1:3	See albuterol.

Methylxanthine Bronchodilators

Caffeine is the most widely known methylxanthine agent; however, the prototype drug is theophylline.

METHYLXANTHINE BRONCHODILATOR PROTOTYPE

THEOPHYLLINE

Theophylline has been the cornerstone drug for treating asthma for years.

Pharmacotherapuetics Theophylline (Aerolate, Bronkodyl, Elixophyllin, SR, Theo-Dur) is indicated in the treatment of bronchoconstriction associated with asthma, chronic bronchitis, and emphysema. It has limited usefulness for treatment of acute asthma, but theophylline can decrease the frequency and severity of symptoms in clients with chronic asthma.

Pharmacokinetics Theophylline's onset of action is 30 to 60 minutes. In adults theophylline's half-life is approximately 8 hours. Several variables (e.g., smoking, age, and overall health of the client) can affect the half-life. The half-life of theophylline in children is approximately 4 hours. Duration of action is up to 24 hours. Theophylline is metabolized in the liver and excreted in the urine.[2,11]

Pharmacodynamics Theophylline is a bronchodilator and a vasodilator. It increases cardiac output and heart rate, improves contractility of the diaphragm, and accelerates mucous transport by the cilia. The exact mechanism responsible for these actions is unknown.[2] Theophylline also inhibits phosphodiesterase, which breaks down the cyclic AMP that constricts the bronchi. This action dilates the bronchi and enables greater air exchange.

Pharmaceutics Theophylline is available in elixir, syrup, uncoated sustained-action tablet, capsule, sustained-action capsule, coated and uncoated tablets, and oral solution for oral administration. It is available in parenteral solution for intravenous (IV) administration.[6]

Undesired Clinical Responses One of the earliest signs of toxicity with theophylline administration is CNS stimulation. The symptoms include headaches, irritability, insomnia, tremors, and agitation. Serious toxicity can lead to grand mal seizures. Stimulation of the cardiovascular system produces palpitations, flushing, tachycardia, and

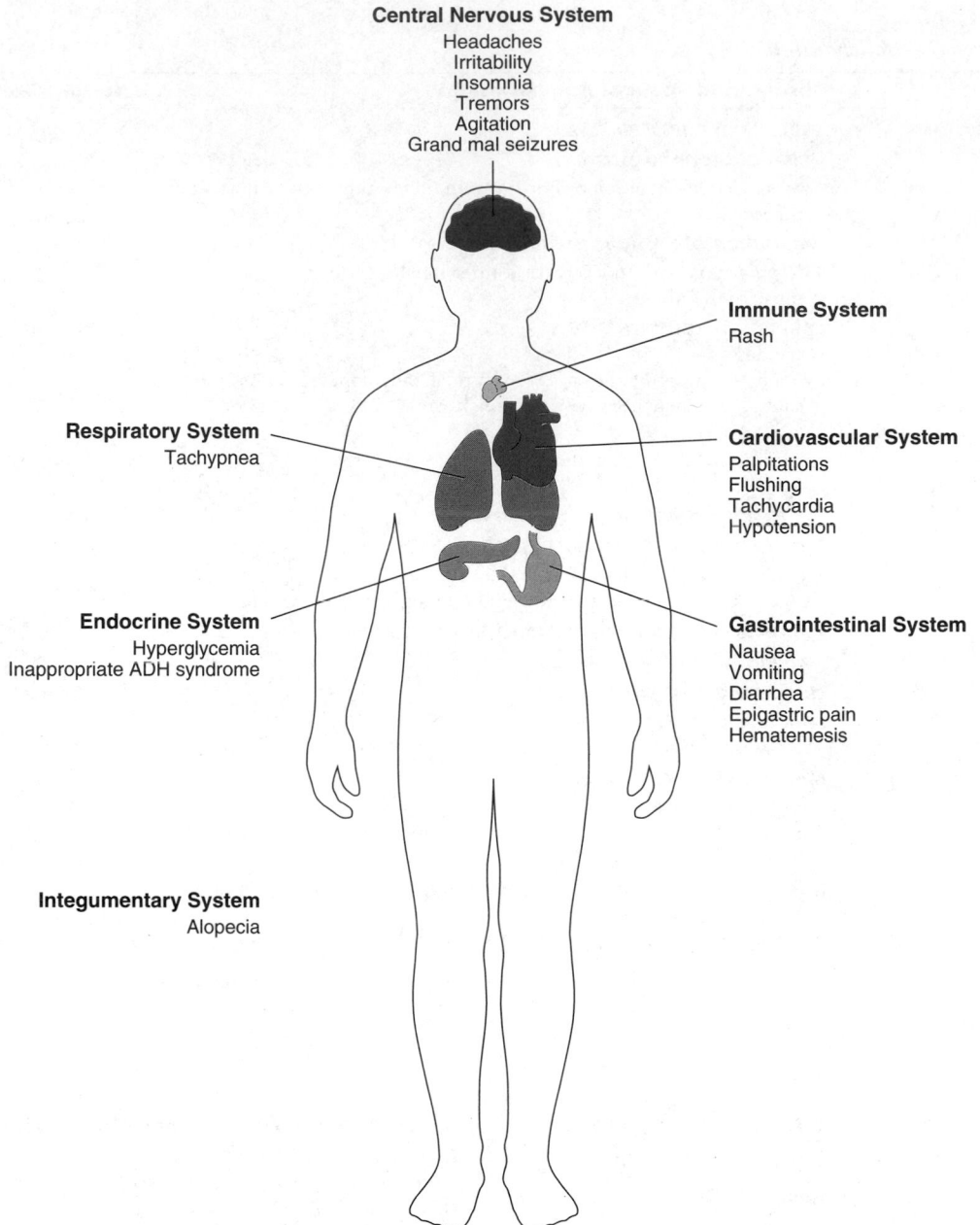

Central Nervous System
Headaches
Irritability
Insomnia
Tremors
Agitation
Grand mal seizures

Immune System
Rash

Respiratory System
Tachypnea

Cardiovascular System
Palpitations
Flushing
Tachycardia
Hypotension

Endocrine System
Hyperglycemia
Inappropriate ADH syndrome

Gastrointestinal System
Nausea
Vomiting
Diarrhea
Epigastric pain
Hematemesis

Integumentary System
Alopecia

FIGURE 45–1   Common undesired clinical responses associated with methylxanthine drugs.

hypotension. Nausea, vomiting, diarrhea, epigastric pain, and hematemesis may be problems for some clients. Figure 45–1 illustrates common undesired responses associated with methylxanthine drugs.[5,6]

Contraindications and Precautions Upper respiratory tract infections in children receiving theophylline slow the clearance rate of the drug. Thus these clients experience more toxic side effects.[11,12] Theophylline use is contraindicated in individuals hypersensitive to it or its components. Its use also is contraindicated in clients with peptic ulcer disease and in individuals with seizure disorders.[6]

Drug-Drug, Drug-Nutrient, and Drug-Environment Interactions If theophylline is administered after a high-

carbohydrate, low-protein or a low-carbohydrate, high-protein meal, theophylline clearance is altered. Clearance of the drug usually is increased by cigarette or marijuana smoking.[2]

The action of theophylline may be altered by many drugs, including cimetidine, ciprofloxacin, allopurinol, erythromycin, oral contraceptives, and rifampin.[13] See the box for factors that affect theophylline serum levels.

Life-Span Considerations Theophylline is classified as a Pregnancy Category C drug. It is distributed into breast milk and may cause irritability or other signs of toxicity in nursing infants. Use in infants has not been sufficiently studied to support its use in this group. If used,

FACTORS AFFECTING THEOPHYLLINE SERUM LEVELS

Factors Increasing Serum Levels

High-carbohydrate, low-protein diet
Obesity
Congestive heart failure
Liver disease
Chronic obstructive pulmonary disease
Acute viral infections
Older age (>55 y)
Influenza A vaccine
Drugs
    Allopurinol
    Cimetidine
    Ciprofloxacin
    Erythromycin preparations
    Propranolol hydrochloride

Factors Decreasing Serum Levels

Cigarette smoking
Eating charcoal-broiled meat
Low-carbohydrate, high-protein diet
Young age (1–16 y)
Drugs
    Ketoconazole
    Phenobarbital
    Phenytoins

Data from references 2 and 4.

dosages must be tritrated carefully.[6] Clearance of theophylline varies with the individual. Generally clearance is lower in clients greater than 55 years of age.

Specific Drug-Related Nursing Considerations
Serum levels provide the only reliable method for determining the appropriate theophylline dose. Serum levels should be monitored every 6 to 12 months, more frequently if undesired responses occur. Therapeutic blood levels of theophylline are 5 to 15 μg/ml. If the serum level approaches 20 μg/ml, serious side effects may occur.

Observe for potential toxicities, especially if the client is very ill. Assess respiratory status and breath sounds to gauge the effectiveness of theophylline treatment. When giving IV theophylline, monitor the cardiac status, including the blood pressure, since toxicity may be more rapid with IV administration.

Teach the client to take the drug with food or an antacid if GI symptoms occur. (However, food must be low in fat.) Encourage client compliance. Advise the client to take only the prescribed dose at the prescribed intervals to prevent serious side effects and toxicities.

MISCELLANEOUS DRUGS IN CATEGORY

Aminophylline is also a xanthine bronchodilator. It is a mixture of theophylline and a base; it has the pharmacodynamic properties of theophylline. Aminophylline is available in parenteral solution for IV injection. It is available as a rectal suppository and in a variety of oral dosage forms. See Table 45–2.

TABLE **45–2**
Methylxanthine Bronchodilators

Drug Name	Dosage and Route of Administration	Nursing Considerations
THEOPHYLLINE (Theo-Dur, Aerolate, Slo-bid, Theolair) **HOW SUPPLIED** Tablets: 100, 125, 200, 250, and 300 mg Sustained-action tablets: 100, 200, 300, and 450 mg Capsules: 100 and 200 mg Sustained-action capsules: 50, 65, 75, 125, 130, 200, 260 and 300 mg Syrup: 80 mg/15 ml and 150 mg/15 ml Elixir: 80 mg/15 ml Solution: 80 mg/15 ml and 150 mg/15 ml	**Loading Dose** ADULTS AND CHILDREN >1 Y 5 mg/kg; then begin maintenance dose **Maintenance Dose** ADULTS AND CHILDREN >25 KG Initial dose: 200 mg q12h; increase dose approximately 25% at 3-d intervals to minimum effective dose, not to exceed 450 mg q12h in adults >70 kg, 300 mg q12h in adults and children 35–70 kg, and 250 mg q12h in children 25–35 kg Doses vary among brand names; see package insert	**Assess** Assess anxiety level of client and offer emotional support. Take baseline rate, depth, rhythm, type of respiration, quality and rate of pulse. Assess lung sounds for rhonchi, wheezing, or rales. Observe color of lips, fingernails for cyanosis. **Implement** Teach client to increase fluid intake to decrease lung secretion viscosity. Encourage client to avoid caffeine, smoking, and smoky areas. Advise client that charcoal-broiled food and a high-protein, low-carbohydrate diet may decrease theophylline level. Teach client not to alter dosage and frequency without consent of prescriber. **Monitor** Have client report promptly any adverse affects such as nausea and vomiting, headache, chest pain, or palpitations. Obtain periodic serum drug levels to ensure they remain therapeutic (5–15 μg/ml). **Evaluate** Observe for resolution and control of asthmatic symptoms.

Anticholinergic Drugs

Advanced understanding of the autonomic control of airways and development of synthetic analogs of atropine have increased the use of anticholinergic drugs to achieve bronchodilation.[14]

ANTICHOLINERGIC DRUG PROTOTYPE

IPRATROPIUM BROMIDE

Ipratropium bromide (Atrovent) is an atropine derivative. It is a relatively weak bronchodilator.

Pharmacotherapuetics Ipratropium use is indicated in the maintenance therapy of clients with chronic bronchitis and emphysema. It is not indicated for the treatment of acute episodes of bronchoconstriction in which a rapid response is desirable.

Pharmacokinetics Ipratropium is for inhalation; it is not absorbed well systemically. Onset of action is within 15 minutes; peak action occurs in 1 to 2 hours, and duration of action is 3 to 6 hours. The half-life of ipratropium is 2 hours after administration.[6]

Pharmacodynamics Normally, efferent fibers pass down the vagus nerve to ganglia in the airway wall. Stimulation of these fibers results in contraction of airway smooth muscle and mucous glands and mast-cell mediator release. Ipratropium inhibits these changes by antagonizing the action of acetylcholine, the neurotransmitter released from the vagus nerve.[2] Bronchodilation after inhalation of ipratropium is primarily a local, site-specific effect.[6]

Pharmaceutics Ipratropium is available for administration as an aerosol or inhalant. The usual dose of ipratropium is two inhalations (36 μg) four times a day. Clients may take additional inhalations as required. Total number of inhalations should not exceed 12 in 24 hours.[6]

Undesired Clinical Responses Ipratropium is not readily absorbed into the systemic circulation either from the surface of the lung or from the GI tract. Thus adverse reactions are rare. The most common ones are nervousness, dizziness, headache, dry mouth, and cough.[2]

Contraindications and Precautions Use of ipratropium is contraindicated in clients with hypersensitivity to atropine, and it should be used with caution in clients with glaucoma or bladder neck obstruction.

Drug-Drug and Drug-Environment Interactions Ipratropium should not be stored at temperatures greater than 30° C. Excessive humidity also should be avoided. Ipratropium has been administered concomitantly with other drugs, including sympathomimetic bronchodilators, methylxanthine bronchodilators, steroids, and cromolyn sodium without adverse drug reactions.[6]

Life-Span Considerations Ipratropium is classified as a Pregnancy Category B drug. It is not known if it is excreted in human milk. Safety and effectiveness in children below the age of 12 years have not been established.[6]

Specific Drug-Related Nursing Considerations Ongoing pulmonary assessment is essential for clients receiving ipratropium therapy to aid in determining the effectiveness of the therapeutic regimen. Advise the client that ipratropium is not for occasional use; encourage the client to follow dosing recommendations carefully. Counsel the client not to spray ipratropium in the eyes; to do so causes temporary blurred vision due to the anticholinergic activity on the pupils.

CONCEPT REVIEW

Bronchodilating drugs work by dilating the airways of the respiratory tree, thereby making air exchange and respiration easier for the client.

Methylxanthines act by blocking the destruction of cyclic AMP. Common methylxanthine derivatives are caffeine and theophylline.

Sympathomimetic drugs such as albuterol act as selective β_2-agonists to relax pulmonary smooth muscle and cause bronchodilation.

Anticholinergic drugs reverse the effects of the autonomic nervous system on the pulmonary tree and smooth musculature, producing a dilating effect on the respiratory airways.

CORTICOSTEROIDS

As a primary drug category, corticosteroids are discussed in Chapter 42. In the present chapter, content focuses on the use of corticosteroids to treat respiratory diseases.

Pharmacotherapeutics Most experts consider asthma an inflammatory disorder of the airway, with inflammation caused by allergy or other stimuli. The inflammation leads to bronchial hyperresponsiveness and airflow obstruction.[10,15] Inhaled corticosteroids apparently provide more effective therapy than regular use of β_2-selective adrenergic drugs. In fact, low doses of inhaled corticosteroids can decrease the dosage of systemic steroids needed for clients with severe asthma.[16] Oral or injected corticosteroids are the most effective drugs available for acute exacerbations of asthma. Corticosteroids are also used to treat allergic rhinitis and bronchopulmonary dysplasia and to control acute episodes of bronchitis.[17,18]

Pharmacodynamics Regular, continuous use of inhaled corticosteroids suppresses inflammation, decreases bronchial hyperresponsiveness, and decreases symptoms of chronic asthma. Many mechanisms have been proposed to explain these actions. For example, it has been suggested that corticosteroids interfere with arachidonic acid metabolism and synthesis of leukotrienes and prostaglandins.[2,15]

Pharmaceutics For the treatment of asthma, corticosteroids are administered orally, parenterally, or topically via inhalation dosage forms. Table 45–3 provides additional information on dosage forms, dosages, and routes of administration.

Undesired clinical responses With high doses of inhaled corticosteroids, suppression of the hypothalamic-pituitary-adrenal axis can occur. In addition, dysphonia and oral or esophageal candidiasis can occur as a result of local deposition of the drug. In children continuous daily use of inhaled corticosteroids can slow growth. Prolonged daily use of oral corticosteroids can produce glucose intolerance, weight gain, increased blood pressure, bone demineralization, cataracts, immunosuppression, and decreased growth in children.[16,19]

Specific drug-related nursing considerations Teach client being treated with inhaled corticosteroids to rinse their mouth after inhalation; this can decrease both local and systemic adverse effects of inhaled steroids. Teach individuals receiving steroids to wear a Medic-Alert bracelet or warning card to alert emergency health care providers that they are using steroids.[2]

If both an inhaled bronchodilator and an inhaled steroid are used, teach the client to administer the bronchodilator and then the steroid. Dilation of the airways allows the inhaled steroid to permeate more deeply into the lungs.[2]

CONCEPT REVIEW

Corticosteroids are used to treat a variety of respiratory problems, including acute episodes of bronchitis and asthma, allergic rhinitis, and bronchopulmonary dysplasia.

Corticosteroids decrease inflammation and bronchial hyperresponsiveness. It has been suggested that corticosteroids interfere with arachidonic acid metabolism and synthesis of leukotrienes and prostaglandins.

TABLE 45–3
Corticosteroids

Drug Name	Dosage and Route of Administration	Nursing Considerations
Beclomethasone Dipropionate (Beclovent, Beconase, Vanceril, Vancenase) **HOW SUPPLIED** Inhalation aerosol for oral use only: 16.8-g canister with 200 metered inhalations Inhalation aerosol for nasal use only: 16.8-g canister with 200 metered inhalations Nasal spary: 0.042%, bottle with 25 g of suspension	**Beclovent** ADULTS AND CHILDREN >12 Y Usual dose: 84 μg tid or qid or 168 μg bid Maximum daily intake: 840 μg in adults CHILDREN 6–12 Y Usual dose: 42–84 μg tid or qid or 168 bid Maximum daily intake: 420 μg **Beconase or Vancenase Nasal Spray** ADULTS AND CHILDREN >6 Y One to two inhalations each nostril bid Total daily dose: 168–336 μg	**Assess** Inquire about hypersensitivity to corticoids or components of corticoids. Assess lung sounds and status of sinus passages. Ask whether the client is pregnant; drug is classified in Pregnancy Category C. **Implement** Have the client clear nasal passages before use. Shake the container well before use. If client is using bronchodilators, have him or her use this spray before the corticosteroid to enhance its effect. Teach client to rinse the mouth after use. Instruct client not to change the dosage schedule and to taper use under supervision. **Monitor** Expect improvement in symptoms within several days. Tell client to contact prescriber if sore throat or mouth develops or if there is no improvement. Severe bronchospasm is a rare consequence. **Evaluate** Assess for lessening of symptoms. See beclomethasone.
Flunisolide (Aerobid, Nasalide) **HOW SUPPLIED** Canister of 100 metered inhalations (250 μg flunisolide/inhalation) Solution 0.025%: 25-ml bottle containing 6.25 mg (0.25 mg/ml) flunisolide	INHALATION ADULTS, ELDERLY: two inhalations bid (morning and evening) to a maximum of four inhalations bid CHILDREN 6–15 Y Two inhalations bid INTRANASAL ADULTS, ELDERLY Initially two sprays each nostril bid; may increase to two sprays tid to maximum of eight sprays each nostril/d CHILDREN 6–14 Y Initially one spray tid or two sprays bid to maximum of four sprays each nostril/d Maintenance dose: smallest dose possible to control symptoms	

Table continued on following page.

TABLE 45–3 *Continued*
Corticosteroids

Drug Name	Dosage and Route of Administration	Nursing Considerations
Triamcinolone Acetonide (Aristocort, Azmacort, Kenalog) **HOW SUPPLIED** Sterile suspension: 25 mg/ml micronized triamcinolone diacetate for IM use Canister of 240 metered doses (100 μg triamcinolone per inhalation)	**For Control of Severe or Incapacitating Allergic Conditions Intractable to Conventional Treatment** Initial dose: 3–60 mg/d, depending on specific disease entity treated Usual parenteral dosage range: one third to one half the oral dose, given q12h **Control of Bronchial Asthma** **INHALATION** **ADULTS AND ELDERLY:** two inhalations tid to qid **CHILDREN 6–12 Y:** one to two inhalations tid to qid **MAXIMUM DOSE:** 12 inhalations/d	See beclomethasone. Use is contraindicated in client with fungal infection, history of tuberculosis. Do not give IV; give deep IM in gluteus maximus.
Prednisone or Prednisolone (Pediapred, Hydeltra-T.B.A.) **HOW SUPPLIED** Oral liquid: 6.7 mg prednisolone sodium phosphate/5 ml; 120-ml bottle Sterile suspension: 20 mg/ml in 1- or 5-ml vial Tablets: 2.5, 5, 10, 20, and 50 mg	4–60 mg/d determined by client condition and response	See beclomethasone and triamcinolone.

AEROSOLIZED DEOXYRIBONUCLEASE FOR CYSTIC FIBROSIS

The sputum of individuals with cystic fibrosis is more viscous than normal, partly because it contains large quantities of DNA that has been released from disintegrated neutrophils. Deoxyribonuclease, which normally is produced in small amounts by the pancreas and salivary glands, breaks extracellular DNA into smaller fragments, making the sputum less viscous. Recombinant human deoxyribonuclease (rhDNase) I is available as a purified solution and is used to treat cystic fibrosis.

Inhalation of rhDNase once or twice a day apparently is well tolerated. Undesired responses include hoarseness, pharyngitis, laryngitis, rash, chest pain, and conjunctivitis. The major disadvantage of the therapy is cost.

Data from reference 20.

MAST CELL STABILIZERS

This group of drugs acts by inhibiting the release of mediators from sensitized mast cells, thus explaining the name *mast cell stabilizers.*

MAST CELL STABILIZER PROTOTYPE
CROMOLYN SODIUM

Cromolyn sodium can have a major impact on clients with mild-to-moderate asthma.

Pharmacotheraputics Cromolyn is effective in preventing seasonal allergic asthma, perennial allergic asthma, animal-induced asthma, exercise-induced asthma, occupational asthma, and irritant-induced asthma.[21] The key to successful therapy with cromolyn is to treat the client prophylactically. For example, the client should receive the drug 7 to 10 days before the anticipated allergen season.

Pharmacokinetics Only about 8% of the inhaled cromolyn dose is absorbed. Onset of action occurs within 15 minutes; duration of action is 4 to 6 hours. Cromolyn is poorly absorbed from the GI tract. It is rapidly excreted in equal proportions in the urine and the bile.[6]

Pharmacodynamics Cromolyn acts by inhibiting release of mediators from mast cells after exposure to an antigen. It can also interrupt the migration of eosinophils into the inflammatory site and decrease the number of eosinophils or eosinophil products. These actions decrease airway hyperresponsiveness in some clients with asthma. Cromolyn has no bronchodilating action and is useful only for prophylaxis.[16]

Pharmaceutics Cromolyn is primarily administered by inhalation method. However, it is available in aerosol spray, nasal solution, and opthalmic solution. It is also available in capsule form for oral administration. Table 45–4 provides additional information on dosage forms, dosages, and routes of administration.

Undesired Clinical Responses The most common undesired clinical responses associated with inhalation therapy are bronchospasm, cough, nasal congestion, throat irritation, and wheezing. Clients receiving cromolyn sodium orally may experience pruritus, nausea, diarrhea, and myalgia.

TABLE 45–4
Mast Cell Stabilizers

Drug Name	Dosage and Route of Administration	Nursing Considerations
CROMOLYN SODIUM (Gastrocrom, Intal, Nasalcrom) HOW SUPPLIED Capsules: 20 mg for use with Spinhaler Capsules (oral): 100 mg Inhaler: 8.1-g or 14.2-g canister (800 μg/inhalation) Nebulizer solution: double-ended glass ampule containing 20 mg cromolyn sodium in water Nasal solution: 13-ml and 26-ml bottles; 40 mg/ml	**Inhaler** **Treatment of Severe Asthmatic Symptoms or Antigen-Induced Bronchospasm** ADULTS AND CHILDREN >5 Y Two metered sprays qid at regular intervals **Prevention of Antigen Reaction** Two metered sprays 10–15 min (not >60 min) before exposure **Nasal Spray** ADULTS AND CHILDREN >6 Y One spray each nostril tid or qid at equal intervals; may be increased to six times/d **Nebulizer** **Management of Bronchial Asthma** ADULTS AND CHILDREN >2 Y Usual dose, 20 mg by nebulization qid at regular intervals **Prevention of Exercise- or Antigen-Induced Asthma** 20 mg shortly before exposure **Oral** ADULTS 2 capsules qid	**Assess** Assess lung sounds for wheezing, rhonchi, or rales. Assess quality and rate of pulse. Give emotional support if client is anxious. Drug is in Pregnancy Category B. **Implement** Advise client to take drug at regular intervals and not to take more than prescribed drug amount. (Excessive use may produce paradoxical bronchoconstriction.) Instruct client in the use and care of inhaler and Spinhaler. Teach client to increase fluid intake to decrease viscosity of lung secretions. **Monitor** Periodically assess pulmonary status and arterial blood gas levels. Observe lips and fingernails for cyanosis. Observe for clavicular retractions, hand tremor. **Evaluate** Assess for resolution of symptoms.
Nedocromil (Tilade) HOW SUPPLIED 16.2-g canister containing 112 inhalations	ADULTS AND CHILDREN >12 Y Initial dose: two inhalations qid (14 mg/d) Maintenance dose: may be able to reduce to two inhalations tid or bid	See cromolyn sodium.

Contraindications and Precautions Oral cromolyn is used with caution in clients with impaired hepatic or renal function. It should not be administered to individuals with known hypersensitivity to the drug.

Drug-Environment Interactions Cromolyn capsules, inhalation aerosol, and nasal solutions should be stored between 15° and 30° C. The nebulizer dosage form should be stored between 15° and 25° C. It must also be protected from light.[6]

Life-Span Considerations Cromolyn is classified as a Pregnancy Category B drug. It is not known if the drug is excreted in human milk. In term infants up to 6 months of age, the dosage should not exceed 20 mg/kg/d. Its use in children less than 2 years old should be reserved for clients with severe disease.[6]

Specific Drug-Related Nursing Considerations Providing proper education on the use and care of the inhaler is important. Package inserts with instructions for use of the inhaler are usually included. Review the instructions with the client and allow for questions. Emphasize that cromolyn capsules supplied with the inhaler are *not* to be taken orally. If the client is aware of what triggers the bronchospasm, teach him or her to use the inhaler before the anticipated exposure to the substance.

MISCELLANEOUS DRUGS IN CATEGORY

Nedocromil sodium (Tilade) is chemically unrelated to cromolyn but has similar pharmacodynamic and pharmacokinetic properties. Nedocromil is ineffective in relieving acute asthma attacks but is effective in lessening the severity of chronic asthma. This drug is also used to treat exercised-induced asthma and allergic rhinitis.[22]

Systemic bioavailability of inhaled nedocromil is low; the plasma concentration peaks in 20 to 40 minutes. Plasma half-life is approximately 2 hours. Adverse effects of the drug include bad taste, headache, and nausea. If the client experiences a cough or bronchospasm in response to the drug, therapy should be stopped.[23]

CONCEPT REVIEW

Cromolyn sodium has been used successfully to treat several types of asthma.

The mechanism of action of mast cell stabilizers is not completely understood. These drugs probably stabilize mast cell membranes, preventing mast cell degranulation and mediator release.

SUMMARY

Drugs discussed in this chapter are used primarily to prevent bronchoconstriction or bronchospasm. In clients with occasional episodes of bronchospasm or those with exercise-induced asthma, aerosolized β_2-adrenergic agonists are probably the drugs of choice. However, in clients who experience daily symptoms, preventive therapy with inhaled cromolyn sodium or inhaled topical corticosteroid is best.

REFERENCES

1. Tetersell, M.J. (1993). Asthma patients knowledge in relation to compliance with drug therapy. *Journal of Advanced Nursing, 18*(1), 103–113.
2. Reinke, L.F., & Hoffman, L. (1992). How to teach asthma co-management. *American Journal of Nursing, 92*(10), 40–48.
3. Hodgson, B., Kizior, R., & Kingdon, R. (1995). *1995 nurse's drug handbook.* Philadelphia: W.B. Saunders.
4. Smith, C.M., & Reynard, A.M. (Eds.). (1992). *Textbook of pharmacology.* Philadelphia: W.B. Saunders.
5. U.S. Pharmacopeial Convention. (1990). *The United States pharmacopeia* (22nd rev.). Rockville, MD: Author.
6. Data Pharmaceutica, Inc. (1993). *1993 physician's genRx.* Smithtown, NY: Author.
7. Tinkelman, D.G., & Naspitz, C.K. (1993). *Childhood asthma: Pathophysiology and treatment.* New York: Marcel Dekker.
8. Pearlman, D.S., et al. (1992). A comparison of salmeterol with albuterol in the treatment of mild-to-moderate asthma. *New England Journal of Medicine, 327*, 1420–1425.
9. Abramowicz, M. (Ed). (1994). Salmeterol. *The Medical Letter on Drugs and Therapeutics, 36*(921), 37-39.
10. Weiss, E.B., & Stein, M. (Eds.). (1993). *Bronchial asthma: Mechanisms and therapeutics* (3rd ed.). Boston: Little, Brown.
11. Olin, B.R., Hebel, S.K., Dombek, C.E., & Kastrup, E.K. (Eds.). (1992). *Facts and Comparisons* (46th ed.). St. Louis: J.B. Lippincott.
12. Shilalukey, K., Robieux, I., Spino, M., et al. (1993). Are current pediatric dose recommendations for intravenous theophylline appropriate? *Journal of Asthma, 30*(2), 109–121.
13. Fraser, I.M., Buttoo, K.M., Walker, S.E., Stewart, J.H., & Gabul, N. (1993). Effects of cimetidine and ranitidine on the pharmacokinetics of a chronotherapeutically formulated once daily theophylline preparation (Uniphyl). *Clinical Therapeutics, 15*, 383–393.
14. Zamary, R.K., & Gross, N.J. (1989). Anticholinergic drugs for obstructive pulmonary disease. *Choices in Respiratory Management, 19*(6), 141–146.
15. Lipworth, B. (1993). Clinical pharmacology of corticosteroids in bronchial asthma. *Pharmacology and Therapeutics, 58*, 173–209.
16. Abramowicz, M. (Ed.). (1993). Drugs for ambulatory asthma. *The Medical Letter on Drugs and Therapeutics, 35*(889), 11–14.
17. Avent, M.L., Cal, P., & Ransom, J. (1994). The role of inhaled steroids in the treatment of bronchopulmonary dysplasia. *Neonatal Network Journal of Neonatal Nursing, 13*(3), 83–89.
18. Knopper, D.C., & Mackanjee, M. (1994). Current strategies in the management of bronchopulmonary dysplasia: The role of corticosteroids. *Neonatal Network Journal of Neonatal Nursing, 13*(3), 53–60.
19. Greenberger, P.A. (1992). Corticosteroids in asthma: Rationale, use, and problems, *Chest: The Cardiopulmonary Journal, 101,* 4185–4215.
20. Abramowicz, M. (Ed.). (1994). Aerosolized deoxyribonuclease for cystic fibrosis. *The Medical Letter on Drugs and Therapeutics, 36*(920), 34–35.
21. Creticos, P.S. (1993). Drug therapy of asthma. In C.M. Smith & A.M. Reynard (Eds.), *Textbook of pharmacology* (pp. 1056–1058). Philadelphia: W.B. Saunders.
22. Parish, R.C., & Miller, L.J. (1993). Nedocromil sodium. *Annals of Pharmacotherapeutics, 27*, 599–606.
23. Puff of prevention for asthma. (1993). *American Journal of Nursing, 93*(12), 53.

BIBLIOGRAPHY

Bella, L.A.D. (1992). Steroidphobia. *American Journal of Nursing, 92*(2), 26–29.
Harman, C.M. (1992). Status asthmaticus: The need for early intervention, aggressive management. *Consultant, 32*(1), 54–58.
Irwin, R.S., Curley, F.J., & French, C.L. (1993). Difficult-to-control asthma: Contributing factors and outcome of a systematic management protocol. *Chest: The Cardiopulmonary Journal, 103,* 1662–1669.
Marin, M.G. (1994). Update: Pharmacology of airway secretion. *Pharmacological Review, 46*(1), 35–59.
McDonald, A.J. (1991). New approaches to emergency management of asthma. *Choices of Respiratory Management, 21*(3), 52–54, 56–58.
Rachelefsky, G., Fitzgerald, S., Page, D., & Santamaria, B. (1993). An update on the diagnosis and management of pediatric asthma. Based on the National Heart, Lung, and Blood Institute expert panel report. *Nurse Practitioner, 18*(2), 51–52, 55, 59–62.
Rau, J.L. (1991). Delivery of aerosolized drugs to neonatal and pediatric patients. *Respiratory Care, 30,* 514–545.
Rumbak, M.J. (1991). New concepts in the treatment of chronic persistent asthma. *Postgraduate Medicine, 90*(3), 81.
Skorodin, M. (1993). Pharmacotherapy for asthma and chronic obstructive pulmonary disease: Current thinking, practices, and controversies. *Archives of Internal Medicine, 153,* 814–828.
Svedmyr, N. (1991). Clinical advantages of the aerosol route of drug administration. *Respiratory Care, 36,* 922–930.

Drugs Affecting the Gastrointestinal System

CHAPTER 46

OVERVIEW OF
The Digestive System

JUDITH K. HEDRICK-THOMPSON

⚛ **Divisions of the Digestive System**

LEARNING OBJECTIVE: Identify the two divisions of the digestive system.

KEY TERMS:

Accessory organs, alimentary canal, gastrointestinal (GI) tract

⚛ **General Characteristics of the GI Tract**

LEARNING OBJECTIVES:

Describe the wall of the alimentary canal.

Name the two types of movements within the GI tract.

Summarize the affect of parasympathetic and sympathetic nerve impulses on digestive actions.

KEY TERMS:

Adventitia, propulsion, serosa tunics

⚛ **Structures of the GI Tract**

LEARNING OBJECTIVES:

List the structures of the GI tract.

Summarize the functions of the mouth, teeth, and tongue.

Describe the regions of the pharynx.

List the parts of the stomach.

List the substances secreted by the glands in the stomach.

List the parts of the small intestine.

Explain two mechanisms that protect the walls of the small intestine from the acidic chyme from the stomach.

List the parts of the large intestine.

Explain how peristalsis in the large intestine differs from peristalsis in the small intestine.

Describe the process of defecation.

KEY TERMS:

Amylase, brush border, chyme, microvilli, rugae, secretin, villus

⚛ **Impact of Drug Therapy on the GI Tract**

LEARNING OBJECTIVE: Discuss the impact of drug therapy on the GI tract.

⚛ **Accessory Organs**

LEARNING OBJECTIVES:

Describe the functions of the liver.

Summarize the functions of the gallbladder.

Explain the role of the pancreas in digestion.

CONCEPTS AND TERMS TO REVIEW

Review the anatomy and physiology of the alimentary canal in an anatomy and physiology textbook.

Determine the pH of gastric secretions and intestinal secretions.

Reexamine the influence of the autonomic nervous system on functions of the GI tract.

Study the process of food and fluid ingestion and the digestion process.

The human body requires a continual source of energy to sustain life. Water, electrolytes, and nutrients needed to produce this energy normally enter the body via the gastrointestinal (GI) tract. As these substances move through the GI tract, digestion occurs. By-products of the digestive process, water, and electrolytes are absorbed and distributed to other organs in the body. These activities are controlled by the nervous and hormonal systems.

This chapter provides an overview of the digestive system with emphasis on the GI tract. A clear understanding of the normal anatomy and physiology of the digestive system provides a basis for understanding pathologic states and the relationship of pharmacologic treatment.

DIVISIONS OF THE DIGESTIVE SYSTEM

The two generally accepted divisions of the digestive system are the GI tract (commonly referred to as the **alimentary**

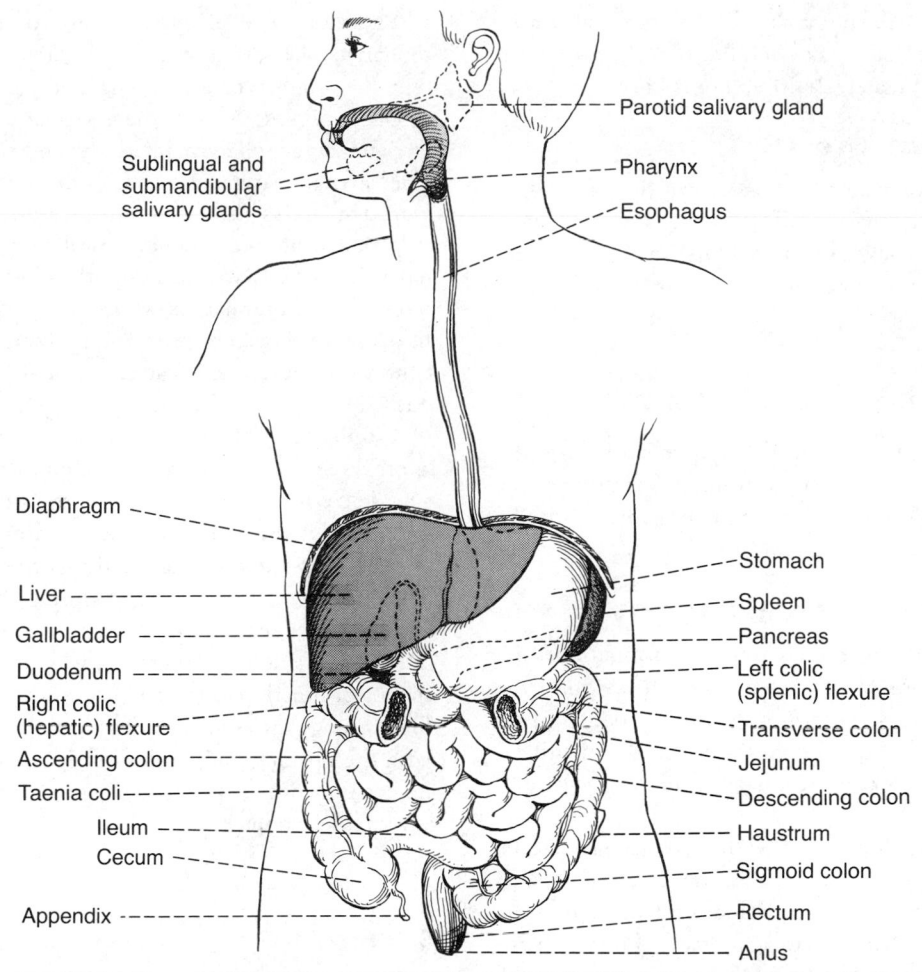

Figure 46–1   The digestive system. (From Black, J.M., Matassarin-Jacobs. E. [1993]. *Luckmann and Sorensen's medical-surgical nursing: A psychophysiologic approach* [4th ed.]. Philadelphia: W.B. Saunders.)

canal) and the accessory organs. The **GI tract** begins at the mouth and ends at the anus (Fig. 46–1). In an adult it is more than 8.5 m long. Propulsion of food, mechanical and chemical digestion, absorption of food, and storage and expulsion of wastes are some of the functions of the GI tract. Teeth, tongue, salivary glands, liver, gallbladder, and pancreas are some of the **accessory organs** of the digestive system.

GENERAL CHARACTERISTICS OF GI TRACT

From the esophagus to anus, the wall of the GI tract has the same basic structure, innervation, and types of muscle movement. These similarities help simplify the study of this portion of the human body.

Structure of the GI Wall

Four distinct layers, or **tunics,** form the wall of the GI tract. These four tunics are present in all areas of the tract from the esophagus to the anus. The innermost layer, the **mucous membrane,** consists of surface epithelium, underlying connec-

tive tissue, and a small amount of smooth muscle. A thick connective tissue layer, the **submucosa,** which contains nerves, blood vessels, and small glands, lies beneath the mucosa. Vessels within this layer nourish the surrounding tissues and carry away absorbed materials. The next tunic is the **muscularis.** It consists of an inner layer of circular smooth muscle and an outer layer of longitudinal smooth muscle. Within the upper esophagus, the muscles are striated, and in the stomach are three layers of smooth muscles. The fourth layer of the GI tract is a connective tissue layer called either the **serosa** or the **adventitia.** Cells of this layer protect underlying tissue and secrete serous fluid, which keeps the outer surface of the GI tract moist.[1,2]

Movement Within the GI Tract

Movement within the tract is of two types: segmental contraction and propulsion. Segmental contractions are ringlike contractions that produce back-and-forth motion. These rhythmic contractions mix the food with digestive juices and break the food into smaller pieces. **Propulsion** in the tract is the movement of food from one end of the tract to the other.

Propelling movements include a wavelike motion called *peristalsis*. The total time that it takes food to travel the length of the GI tract is approximately 24 to 36 hours.[1,2]

Innervation of the GI Tract

The GI tract is innervated by branches of the parasympathetic and sympathetic divisions of the nervous system. These nerve fibers are responsible for maintaining muscle tone and regulating the strength, rate, and velocity of muscular contractions.[1]

STRUCTURES OF THE GI TRACT

The parts of the digestive system through which food passes are the mouth, pharynx, esophagus, stomach, small intestine, and large intestine. Each of these structures has a specific function.

Mouth and Accessory Organs

At the proximal end of the GI tract is the mouth or oral cavity. Major functions carried out by structures within the oral cavity include speech, nutrient ingestion, initiation of digestion, and swallowing. Key structures within the mouth include the hard and soft palates, salivary glands, tongue, and teeth.[1,2]

Mouth The mouth is lined with mucous membrane; muscle, fat, areolar tissue, nerves, vessels, and salivary glands lie beneath the membrane. The hard and soft palates form the roof of the mouth; the hard palate, comprised of bone, is situated anteriorly. Attached to the posterior portion of the hard palate is the soft palate. This structure serves as a partition between the mouth and nasopharynx and forms the palatine arches and uvula. During swallowing, the soft palate moves upward and closes the opening to the nasopharynx; this prevents food and fluid from entering the cavity.

Accessory organs Salivary glands, the tongue, and teeth are accessory organs of the oral cavity. The parotid, submaxillary, and sublingual glands produce most of the saliva in the mouth. Saliva, a mixture of mucus, thin serous secretions, and amylase, lubricates food particles and serves as a protective shield for the mouth. The enzyme **amylase** begins the process of carbohydrate digestion.

An adult normally has 32 teeth that play a role in digestion and speech. Teeth assist digestion by cutting, tearing, grinding, and chewing food. This action provides more surface area for enzymatic action. The tongue manipulates food, assists swallowing, determines sensation and taste, cleanses teeth and gums, and aids in the production of sound and speech. Intrinsic and extrinsic muscles control the tongue's shape, position, and movements.

Pharynx and Esophagus

The pharynx, or throat, serves as the entrance to both the respiratory and digestive systems. Connected to the distal end of the pharynx is the esophagus. Functions of the esophagus are associated only with the digestive system.

Pharynx The pharynx consists of three parts: the nasopharynx, the oropharynx, and the laryngopharynx. Normally only the oropharynx and laryngopharynx transmit food. The oropharynx connects with the nasopharynx superiorly, the larynx and laryngopharynx inferiorly, and the mouth anteriorly. The laryngopharynx extends from the oropharynx to the esophagus and is posterior to the pharynx.[2]

Swallowing mechanism Swallowing occurs after food has been chewed and mixed with saliva. The tongue forces food into the oropharynx while a small cartilage, the epiglottis, closes the larynx to prevent aspiration. Pharyngeal muscles contract while the esophageal sphincter relaxes and food is pushed into the esophagus.

Esophagus The esophagus, a hollow, muscular tube, is approximately 25 cm long in the adult. Proximally, the esophagus is connected to the pharynx by the *pharyngoesophageal sphincter*. The esophagus then passes through the mediastinum and connects to the stomach at the gastroesophageal sphincter. These sphincters are open only during the act of swallowing and remain closed at other times to prevent reflux.

Transportation of food from the mouth into the stomach is the major function of the esophagus. Peristaltic activity moves food through the esophagus. This activity must be coordinated with the opening and closing of the sphincters. Vagus nerve innervation, which stimulates contraction of smooth muscle within the esophagus, is responsible for most of this coordination.[3]

Stomach

The stomach, a J-shaped, pouchlike organ, hangs under the diaphragm in the upper left portion of the abdominal cavity. It is approximately 25 to 30 cm long and 10 cm wide. At full capacity, the stomach is capable of holding approximately 1 L.

Structure of the stomach The stomach is divided into the cardiac, fundic, body, and pyloric regions (Fig. 46–2). Located between the stomach and esophagus is the gastroesophageal sphincter. The **cardiac region** is a small area near the esophageal opening. The **fundic region** acts as a temporary storage area. Adjacent to the fundic region is the main region of the stomach, the **body region.** The **pyloric region** (antrum) of the stomach narrows as it approaches the small intestine. Located between the stomach and the small intestine is the pyloric sphincter.[1,3,4]

Gastric secretions The mucous coat (tunica mucosa) or innermost lining of the stomach is arranged in longitudinal folds **(rugae),** which expand for stomach distention. Five types of cells are located within this lining. These cells (surface mucous cells, parietal cells, chief cells, and endocrine cells) secrete substances that protect the lining of the stomach or aid in digestion. Total daily secretion by these cells is 2 to 3 L.[2,3]

- **Surface mucous cells** or **mucous neck cells** secrete a viscous, alkaline mucus that coats the lining of the stomach for protection.
- **Parietal cells** produce hydrochloric acid and an intrinsic factor. Hydrochloric acid activates pepsin, which initiates

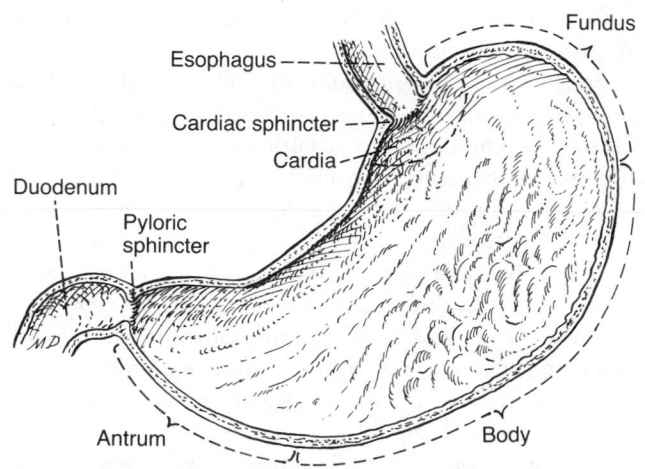

FIGURE 46–2   Anatomy of the stomach. (From Black, J.M., Matassarin-Jacobs, E. [1993]. *Luckmann and Sorensen's medical-surgical nursing: A psychophysiologic approach* [4th ed.]. Philadelphia: W.B. Saunders.)

protein digestion. The intrinsic factor facilitates absorption of vitamin B_{12} in the small bowel.

- **Chief cells** secrete pepsinogen, which mixes with hydrochloric acid to form pepsin.
- **Endocrine cells** secrete regulatory hormones (i.e., gastrin and secretin) that stimulate or inhibit gastric secretion.

Gastric absorption   The stomach wall is impermeable to the passage of most materials into the blood. However, the stomach does absorb water, glucose, electrolytes, certain drugs, and alcohol.

Gastric emptying   Ingested food and fluid are retained in the stomach until thoroughly mixed with gastric secretions and converted to a semifluid material known as **chyme.** Mixing is accomplished by the muscular peristaltic activity of the stomach. Rate of stomach emptying is determined by pH, amount of fat, osmolarity, consistency, and temperature of the stomach content. For instance, meals high in solids, fat, and protein are slow to empty, whereas a tepid, isotonic liquid moves at a faster pace.

Small Intestine

The small intestine is the major organ for digestion and absorption of nutrients. It extends from the pyloric sphincter to the beginning of the large intestine. With its many loops and coils, it fills much of the abdominal cavity.

Structure of the small intestine   The small intestine is divided into three anatomic portions: duodenum, jejunum, and ileum. In the adult the duodenum is approximately 25 cm long and 5 cm in diameter. It lies behind the parietal peritoneum and is the shortest portion of the small intestine. Of the remaining portion of the small intestine, the proximal two fifths form the jejunum, and the remainder is the ileum.[1,6,7] The ileocecal valve is located at the junction of the ileum and the large intestine. This one-way valve regulates emptying into the large intestine and prevents reflux into the small intestine.

Throughout its length, the inner wall (mucosal layer) of small intestine is covered by innumerable tiny, fingerlike projections of mucous membrane called **intestinal villi** (Fig. 46–3). Villi average 0.5 to 1.5 cm in length and give the surface of the small intestine a velvety appearance. Each villus consists of a layer of columnar epithelium and a core of connective tissue that contains blood capillaries, a lymphatic capillary, and nerve fibers. At their free surfaces, the epithelial cells possess many cytoplasmic extensions known as **microvilli.** Microvilli comprise the **brush border** that contains enzymes and carrier substances. Together, the submucosal and mucosal coats of the small intestine form numerous circular folds called *valvulae conniventes* or *folds of Kerckring.* These folds, along with villi, create a large absorptive surface.[3,4]

Movement within the small intestine   Both types of muscle contractions, segmental contractions and peristaltic waves, occur regularly in the small bowel. Segmental contractions mix and churn the intestinal contents, redistributing the chyme against the villi. Peristaltic waves propel the chyme

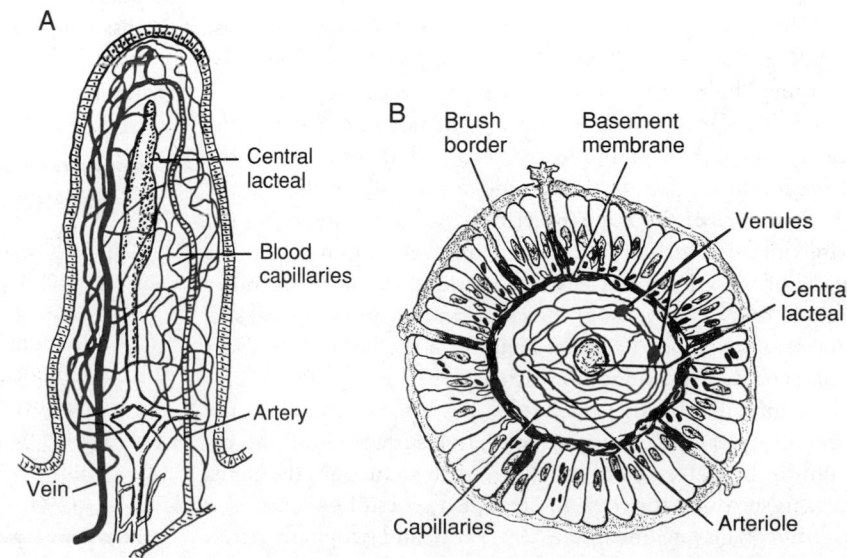

FIGURE 46–3   Functional organization of the villus. **A,** Longitudinal section. **B,** Cross section showing the epithelial cells and basement membrane. (From Guyton, A.C. [1991]. *Textbook of medical physiology* [8th ed.]. Philadelphia: W.B. Saunders.)

through the bowel. Normal peristaltic waves occur almost continuously, propelling the intestinal contents at a rate of 2 to 25 cm per minute.[2-4,6]

Secretions within the small intestine The small intestine receives secretions from the pancreas and liver. In addition, cells in the small intestine secrete intestinal enzymes and mucus. These secretions protect the lining of the small intestine and assist with the digestive process.

Several secretions protect the small intestine from the acidic content from the stomach. **Brunner's glands,** located in the submucosa within the proximal portion of the duodenum, secrete large quantities of viscid, alkaline mucus. Intestinal glands at the bases of the villi also secrete large amounts of a watery fluid that has a pH of 6.5 to 7.5. In addition, when the acidic chyme enters the duodenum, the pancreas is stimulated to secrete a large quantity of fluid containing a high concentration of bicarbonate ions. The stimulus for the pancreas is **secretin,** a peptide hormone. Secretin is released into the blood from the duodenal mucous in response to the acid in chyme. The gallbladder also delivers alkaline bile in the presence of fatty and amino acids.

Digestive enzymes are embedded in the surfaces of microvilli in the intestinal mucosa. These enzymes—peptidases, sucrase, maltase, lactase, and intestinal lipase—break down food molecules before absorption occurs. **Peptidases** split peptides into amino acids; **sucrase, maltase,** and **lactase** split the disaccharides—sucrose, maltose, and lactose—into the simple sugars (monosaccharides) of glucose, fructose, and galactose. **Intestinal lipase** splits fats into fatty acids and glycerol.[1,8,9].

Absorption within the small intestine Absorption of monosaccharides, amino acids, fatty acids, glycerol, electrolytes, and water occurs throughout the small intestine. The jejunum is the major organ of nutrient absorption. Most fats, proteins, and vitamins are absorbed in this area, as are carbohydrates not absorbed in the stomach and duodenum. The ileum absorbs any nutrients not absorbed in the duodenum or jejunum. It is also the only area of absorption for vitamin B_{12} complex and bile salts.[7,8]

Large Intestine

The large intestine (colon) comprises the cecum, the ascending, transverse, descending, and sigmoid colon, and the rectum. This portion of the alimentary tract is approximately 1.5 m long. It begins in the lower right side of the abdominal cavity where the ileum joins the cecum. The distal end of the large intestine opens to the outside of the body as the anus.

Structure of the large intestine Although the wall of the large intestine includes the same four layers common to other parts of the GI tract, it has some unique features. The outer serosal coat covers most of the colon and forms peritoneal sacs enclosing fat appendices that hang from the bowel. The muscular coat has two smooth muscle layers that are gathered into three muscular bands *(teniae coli)*. These bands run along the anterior, posterior, and posteroinferior surfaces from the cecum to the rectosigmoid junction. At this junction, the bands fuse to surround the rectum, creating a series of pouches. The submucosal layer contains arteries, veins, and lymphatic vessels

and attaches the muscular coat to the mucosal layer. The inner mucosal layer has no villi.[1,3,6,8]

Functions of the large intestine The colon has two major functions: to absorb water and electrolytes from the chyme remaining in the alimentary canal and to form and store feces until defecation occurs. The large intestine has little or no digestive functions. Absorption in this area is usually limited to water and electrolytes.

Secretions of the large intestine Water, mucus, potassium, and bicarbonate are secreted by cells in the large intestine. These secretions lubricate and protect the mucosa and help bind the fecal matter together. The rate of mucous secretion is controlled by mechanical stimulation from chyme and by parasympathetic impulses.

Movements of the large intestine Mixing action of the bowel content continues as in the small intestine but at a slower rate. The mixing movements break the fecal matter into segments and turn the matter so that all portions are exposed to the intestinal mucosa. This promotes water and electyrolyte absorption. Peristaltic waves in this area are different from those in the small intestine. Waves occur only two or three times each day. **Mass movement** (large segment of intestinal wall constricts vigorously) forces the intestinal contents toward the rectum.[1]

When the feces is pushed into the rectum, the **defecation reflex** occurs. As a result, peristaltic waves in the descending colon are stimulated, and the internal anal sphincter relaxes. As internal abdominal pressure increases, the external anal sphincter relaxes, and the feces is forced to the outside. The internal sphincter is not under voluntary control. However, the external sphincter that surrounds the anal canal is striated muscle and can be voluntarily constricted or relaxed.

Feces Fecal content consists of bile pigments, mucus, unabsorbed minerals, cellulose, undigested fats, toxins, epithelial cells, potassium, chloride, sodium, bicarbonate, and water. Normal intestinal flora include *Escherichia coli, Enterobacter aerogenes, Clostridium perfringens,* and *Lactobacillus bifidus.* These bacteria putrefy remaining proteins and indigestible residue, synthesize certain vitamins, and convert urea salts for reabsorption. Bacterial concentration is much higher in the distal portion of the colon. This increased concentration of bacteria contributes to the formation of flatus and the odor of the feces.[3,6]

CONCEPT REVIEW

The digestive system consists of the mouth, pharynx, esophagus, stomach, small intestine, large intestine, and anus.

Functions of the digestive system include ingestion, mastication, propulsion, mixing, secretion, digestion, absorption, and excretion.

Most functions are regulated by the parasympathetic and sympathetic nervous systems and hormonal mechanisms.

ACCESSORY ORGANS

Accessory organs discussed in this chapter are the liver, gallbladder, and pancreas. These organs play major roles in the functions of the digestive system.

Liver

The liver, the largest organ in the body, is located in the right upper abdominal quadrant, just below the diaphragm. It is enclosed in a fibrous capsule and is divided into a large right lobe and a smaller left lobe. Each lobe is divided into thousands of microscopic **lobules,** the functional units of the liver.[10]

The liver has many important metabolic activities. For example, it plays a major role in carbohydrate, lipid, and protein metabolism. Its converts glucose to glycogen, glycogen to glucose, and noncarbohydrates to glucose. The liver's effects on lipid metabolism include oxidation of fatty acids and synthesis of lipoproteins, phospholipids, and cholesterol. In protein metabolism, the liver forms urea, synthesizes blood proteins, and converts various amino acids to other amino acids. The liver also plays a role in the storage of vitamins and minerals and in detoxification of substances harmful to the body.

The secretion of bile is the liver function most important to digestion. **Bile,** a yellowish green liquid, is continuously secreted by the hepatic cells. It contains water, bile salts, bile pigments, and various electrolytes. Bile reduces the acidity of chyme, stimulates intestinal motility, and aids in utilization of protein and carbohydrates. In addition, bile emulsifies fat, increases lipase activity, and increases absorption of the fat soluble vitamins A, D, and K.[1,10]

Gallbladder

The gallbladder, a pear-shaped organ, is located on the inferior surface of the liver. It is connected to the cystic duct that joins the hepatic duct to form the common bile duct, which leads to the duodenum. The gallbladder stores and concentrates bile between meals; it has a capacity of 30 to 50 ml. Bile is released into the duodenum when the gallbladder is stimulated by the hormone **cholecystokinin,** which is secreted by the intestinal mucosa when fat is present.[1,8,10]

Pancreas

The endocrine functions of the pancreas are described in Chapter 38. However, this organ also has an exocrine function—the secretion of a digestive juice. Structurally, the pancreas is 10 to 22 cm long and extends horizontally across the posterior abdominal wall. Pancreatic acinar cells that comprise the bulk of the pancreas produce pancreatic juice. These cells release their secretions into a pancreatic duct. The pancreatic duct connects with the duodenum and delivers pancreatic juice by way of the ampulla of Vater (the same lumen that drains the common bile duct).[1,3]

Pancreatic juice contains enzymes (trypsin, chymotrypsin, carboxypeptidase, amylase, lipase, and cholesterol esterase) that split carbohydrates, proteins, fats, and nucleic acids. In addition, pancreatic juice has a high bicarbonate ion concentration. The presence of the bicarbonate ions helps neutralize chyme. Secretin from the duodenum and cholecystokinin from the intestinal wall stimulate the release of pancreatic juice.[1,8,10]

IMPACT OF DRUG THERAPY ON THE GI TRACT

The GI tract is used as a route of drug administration and as a target for pharmacologic treatment of GI disorders. Drugs used to treat disorders of the upper GI tract include antisecretory agents, acid neutralizers, antiflatulents, antiemetics, and digestants. Antisecretory agents and acid neutralizers are used to prevent problems associated with increased secretion of hydrochloric acid. Gaseous distention of the upper GI tract is treated with antiflatulent drugs, and antiemetics are used to control nausea and vomiting. Digestants are used to treat conditions in which altered absorption and metabolism of nutrients exist. Drugs used to treat lower GI disorders are directed at treatment of constipation, diarrhea, and flatulence.

Many drugs produce side effects and adverse reactions associated with the GI tract. Drugs can cause irritability of and damage to the mucosal lining of the tract, decreased production and release of secretions, change in intestinal flora, and decreased motility. Common symptoms related to these effects are nausea, vomiting, diarrhea, abdominal discomfort, and constipation. In addition, drugs can alter or delay absorption of nutrients.

SUMMARY

The principal function of the GI tract is to provide the body with fluid, nutrients, and electrolytes. Normally the GI tract is the source of intake for the body. Electrolytes, hormones, and enzymes secreted by the GI tract break down materials ingested through the mouth. These ingested products move through the digestive system as additional digestion of food and fluids occurs. In addition, end products of digestion are absorbed into the bloodstream. The GI tract also disposes of the wastes from the digestive process.

REFERENCES

1. Hole, J. (1993). *Human anatomy and physiology* (6th ed.). Dubuque, IA: Wm. C. Brown.
2. Tortora, G., & Grabowski, S. (1993). *Principles of anatomy and physiology* (7th ed.). New York: Harper Collins.
3. Guyton, A. (1991). *Textbook of medical physiology* (8th ed.). Philadelphia: W.B. Saunders.
4. Guyton, A. (1992). *Human physiology and mechanisms of disease* (5th ed.). Philadelphia: W.B. Saunders.
5. Broadwell, D. (1989). Gastrointestinal system. In Thompson, J.M. (Ed.). *Mosby's manual of clinical nursing* (2nd ed.). St. Louis: Mosby–Year Book.
6. Seeley, R., Stephens, T., & Tate, P. (1992). *Anatomy and physiology* (2nd ed.). St. Louis: Mosby–Year Book.
7. West, J.B. (1991). *Best and Taylor's physiological basis of medical practice* (12th ed.). Baltimore: Williams & Wilkins.
8. Creager, J. (1992). *Human anatomy and physiology.* Dubuque, IA: Wm. C. Brown.
9. Whitney, E., Cataldo, C., & Rolfes, S. (1991). Digestion, ab-

sorption, and transport. *Understanding Normal and Clinical Nutrition, 3,* 43-65.

10. Soloman, E., & Phillips, G. (1987). *Understanding human anatomy and physiology.* Philadelphia: W.B. Saunders.

BIBLIOGRAPHY

Ahern, H.L., & Rice, K.T. (1991). How do you measure gastric pH? *American Journal of Nursing, 91,* 70.

Garcia, G. (1992). Gastrointestinal disorders. In Melman, K.L., Morrelli, H.F., Hoffman, B.B., & Nierenberg, D.W. (Eds.). *Melman and Morrelli's clinical pharmacology: Basic principles in therapeutics* (3rd ed.) (pp. 219-232). New York: McGraw-Hill.

Ignativicius, D.D., & Bayne, M.V. (1991). *Medical-surgical nursing: A nursing process approach.* Philadelphia: W.B. Saunders.

Massoni, M. (1990). Nurses' GI handbook. *Nursing '90, 20*(11), 65-80.

O'Toole, M.T. (1990). Advanced assessment of the abdomen and gastrointestinal problems. *Nursing Clinics of North America, 25,* 771-776.

CHAPTER 47

DRUGS AFFECTING THE
Upper Gastrointestinal Tract

DONNA HENRY

⊛ **Gastric Physiology**
LEARNING OBJECTIVES:
List the four types of cells found in the tunica mucosal lining.
Name the three types of receptors on the surface of parietal cells.
KEY TERMS:
Cephalic phase, gastric phase

⊛ **Common Upper Gastrointestinal Tract Disorders**
LEARNING OBJECTIVE: Describe common upper gastrointestinal (UGI) tract disorders.
KEY TERMS:
Hypersecretion, hyposecretion, peptic ulceration, pyrosis

⊛ **Nursing Process**
LEARNING OBJECTIVE: Plan care appropriate for a client receiving drugs that affect the UGI tract.
KEY TERMS:
Dysphagia, eructation, flatulence

⊛ **Upper Gastrointestinal Protective Agents**
LEARNING OBJECTIVES:
Describe the physiologic response of the body to each subclassification of UGI protective agents.
Summarize essential information about the prototype drug for each subclassification.
Outline a plan of care for a client receiving a UGI protective agent.
KEY TERMS:
Acid neutralizing capacity, antacid, milk-alkali syndrome, proton pump

⊛ **Antibacterial Drugs**
LEARNING OBJECTIVE: Describe the use of antibacterial drugs in the treatment of peptic ulcer disease.

⊛ **Antiflatulents**
LEARNING OBJECTIVE: Describe the use of antiflatulents in the treatment of upper and lower GI disorders.

⊛ **Digestants**
LEARNING OBJECTIVE: Summarize the action of each subclassification of digestants.

⊛ **Antiemetics**
LEARNING OBJECTIVES:
Describe the physiologic mechanism involved in the emetic process.
Explain the mechanism of action for each group of antiemetics.

⊛ **Emetics and Adsorbents**
LEARNING OBJECTIVE: List major therapeutic uses for emetics and adsorbents.

*H*ealth concerns related to the upper gastrointestinal (GI) tract are among the most common problems seen by the nurse. Dyspepsia, gas, heartburn, acid indigestion, and sour stomach are common complaints of a large portion of the population. These symptoms are distressing in themselves, but they may also herald more significant health problems such as gastritis, peptic ulcer disease (PUD), gastroesophageal reflux disease (GERD), cholecystitis, cholelithiasis, or pancreatitis. Clients may also experience upper GI tract symptoms such as anorexia, nausea, vomiting, and flatulence secondary to systemic illness, surgery, and drug therapy.

This chapter focuses on drugs that affect the upper GI tract. These drugs are administered to relieve symptoms and/or prevent symptoms from occurring.

GASTRIC PHYSIOLOGY

The stomach is divided into the cardiac, fundic, body, and pyloric regions. The tunica mucosa gastris, or mucous lining of the stomach, contains four types of cells: surface mucous cells, parietal cells, chief cells, and endocrine cells. These cells secrete substances that protect the lining of the stomach or aid in digestion.

The surface of the parietal cell contains three types of receptors: H_2 receptors for histamine, receptors for acetylcholine (ACh), and receptors for gastrin. Receptor-site stimulation by histamine sets in motion a chain of events that results in secretion of hydrogen ion. When the other two receptor types are activated, the cellular membrane becomes more permeable to calcium, and secretion of hydrochloric acid increases.

What sets this chain of events into motion? Acid secretion is initiated by the anticipation of eating (**cephalic phase**). During the cephalic phase, excitation of the vagus nerve liberates ACh and gastrin, which activate the parietal cells. Once the food reaches the stomach and mucosal exposure to protein occurs, gastrin is released (**gastric phase**), and additional hydrochloric acid is secreted. As the digestive process continues, the decrease in antral pH inhibits the further release of gastrin.[1,2]

COMMON UPPER GASTROINTESTINAL TRACT DISORDERS

Common conditions of the upper GI tract are hypersecretion and hyposecretion, inflammatory disorders, ulcers, and disorders of digestion. **Hypersecretion** of the parietal and chief cells exposes the mucosal lining of the GI tract to excessive hydrochloric acid and pepsinogen. When hydrochloric acid comes into contact with the mucosa, injury to small vessels occurs, with edema, hemorrhage, and possible ulcer formation. Thickening and erythema of the mucosal lining also occur.

If this condition persists, the mucosal lining becomes atrophic and thin. Continued deterioration and atrophy lead to loss of function of the parietal cells (**hyposecretion**). Because the mucosal lining has thinned, **peptic ulceration**—a break in continuity of esophageal, gastric, or duodenal mucosa—may occur.[3]

Heartburn (**pyrosis**) is among the most common symptoms encountered in clinical practice. It may be due to the occasional reflux that occurs with swallowing and after meals or may indicate reflux esophagitis.[4]

◼ NURSING CONSIDERATIONS

The nurse has an important role in the diagnosis and treatment of upper GI disorders. This role is challenged by the client's use of over-the-counter (OTC) treatments, home remedies, and other drug therapies. Providing client education about the disorder, drug therapy, and self-care is paramount. Evaluation of compliance and expected outcomes is ongoing.

Assessing Begin your assessment by gathering a **health history.** This information provides direction for the physical assessment. Include in your assessment interview a review of physical symptoms.

Ask the client about the presence of **dysphagia** or **odynophagia** (painful swallowing). If this condition exists, the client may report a feeling of food's "sticking" in the throat or chest. Ask if the client is experiencing **eructation** (belching) or **flatulence** (gastric or intestinal gas). Question the client about feelings of fullness in the thorax or abdomen and how positional changes affect these symptoms. Ask if the client experiences heartburn. If he or she does, ask about its frequency and duration and radiation of the discomfort.

Pain, anorexia, nausea, vomiting, and weight loss are also common symptoms associated with upper GI conditions. If pain is present, question the client about the relationship of the pain to food and fluid ingestion. Note the time of the day or night that the pain occurs. Assess the pain characteristics and note the terms (e.g., burning, gnawing, or stabbing) used by the individual. Ask the client if the nausea is precipitated by any particular event. Inquire about weight pattern changes. Be specific; ask for number of pounds lost or gained in a specific time frame. Question the client about the characteristics of any emesis; determine the color, odor, and presence of formed material in the emesis. Also ask the client about frequency and timing of emesis.

When symptoms are related to food or fluid intake, determine what was ingested. For example, right upper quadrant pain may be reported after ingestion of a high-fat meal, indicating a gallbladder disorder. Food patterns should also be assessed. Irregular meal patterns and eating rapidly are frequently associated with increased GI complaints. A diet history, including ethnic or religious influences, is important.

Because problems with ingestion and digestion in the upper GI tract affect elimination, ask about changes in bowel elimination patterns and characteristics of stools. Ask the client about drug reactions and allergies. Since many drugs are capable of causing upper GI problems, carefully assess the use of prescription and nonprescription drugs. Also inquire about home remedies. Baking soda for indigestion and mineral oil and lemon juice for "gallbladder trouble" are common home remedies.

Family history and lifestyle patterns are relevant to this assessment. Note use of alcohol and nicotine specifically. Chronic alcoholism is the principal cause of acute and chronic pancreatitis and cirrhosis. There is an increased incidence of gastritis, gastric and duodenal ulcers, and reflux esophagitis in heavy smokers and alcoholics.

Begin the **physical assessment** with the oral cavity and throat. An edentulous state, caries, or periodontal disease may alter mastication of food and increase GI symptoms. Look for signs of infection or dehydration. Inspect the mouth for a coated tongue, decreased or absent salivation, and/or halitosis.

Place the client in a supine position. Observe the abdomen for distention, ascites, and prominence of abdominal veins. Since percussion and palpation may alter peristalsis, auscultate the abdomen for bowel sounds first. Palpate the abdomen for tenderness and enlargement of the liver. Examine sequentially, moving from the right upper quadrant to the left upper quadrant, then to the left lower quadrant and right lower quadrant. Palpate painful areas last. If ascites is suspected, assess for a fluid wave by palpating one flank while gently tapping the other side of the abdomen. If ascites is present, a wave is felt by the palpating hand as fluid washes against the abdominal wall. Also measure abdominal girth if distention or ascites is present.[5]

Weigh the client and measure his or her height; compare these findings with standard weight and height charts. Clients who weigh 20% or more under ideal body weight are considered underweight. Compare infant and child weights to appropriate growth tables.

Diagnosing   Analysis of the data is the basis for determining nursing diagnoses. Some common diagnoses for clients receiving drugs for GI disorders are as follows:

- Knowledge deficit related to lack of exposure to information about drug therapy.
- Sleep pattern disturbance related to pain.
- Pain related to increased gastric acidity in GI tract.
- Altered nutrition, less than body requirements, related to nausea, vomiting, and anorexia.
- Constipation related to decreased motility of GI tract associated with drug therapy.
- Anxiety related to possibility of long-term drug therapy.
- Altered health maintenance related to lack of material resources.
- Noncompliance related to lack of understanding of medical diagnosis and/or drug regimen.

Planning   Clients with upper GI tract disorders usually require a variety of diagnostic tests. Include in your plan an explanation of the purpose and procedure for each test. Be prepared to supply written explanations and directions to supplement verbal information. Advise clients that these same tests may be used to monitor response to drug therapy.

The plan of care should include material that explains or reinforces explanations about the medical diagnosis, its cause, and its treatment. Stress areas in which the client can have a positive impact in controlling symptoms or enhancing cure. Provide written information about the condition to clients when appropriate.

In client populations in which UGI problems can be anticipated, check records for prescribed prophylactic therapy. If no drug therapy is ordered, consult with the primary care provider about appropriate treatment. For example, anticipate receiving orders for preoperative and postoperative clients that include administering prophylactic antisecretory and antiemetic drugs. Critically ill clients may need antisecretory drugs, acid buffers, cytoprotective agents, or combination therapy. These individuals may also need antiemetics. Plan to share with the client information about the availability of and expected effects of prophylactic drugs.

Clients with upper GI tract problems usually need dietary instructions. The diet history, which contains information on religious and cultural preferences, will direct your teaching in this area. Instruct the client to eliminate known GI irritants from the diet until symptoms are controlled. Teach the client to reintroduce these foods cautiously into the diet one at a time. In general, advise clients to avoid ingesting caffeine, alcohol, high-fat foods, and large meals.

Teaching plans should include strategies that help the client decrease stress and initiate appropriate lifestyle changes. Teach the client the value of planned programs of exercise and provide instructions on relaxation techniques. On the basis of the client's lifestyle history you can refer him or her to appropriate resources. For example, support groups for alcohol abstinence, eating disorders, and smoking cessation are available.

All clients need information about their drug therapy. Include in your teaching information on drug administration, expected response to therapy, and common undesired responses. Because drug interactions may occur, the client taking these drugs on an ambulatory basis needs particular attention. Assist the client to make a list of all drugs being used. Assign specific times for administration of each drug. When developing this plan, take into consideration the client's schedule. Review precautions related to expected side effects (e.g., drowsiness associated with some antiemetics). List symptoms that the client should report immediately to the primary care provider. Remind the client not to take OTC drugs without consulting the primary care provider. Instruct the client not to substitute OTC drugs for prescription drugs or specific nonprescription drugs recommended by the prescriber.

Include expected outcomes in the plan of care. When possible, develop these goals with the client. Outcomes for clients requiring drugs that affect the upper GI tract might include the following:

- Client verbalizes heartburn relief within 30 minutes of antacid ingestion.
- Client demonstrates progressive weight gain toward goal weight.
- Client maintains desired weight.

- Client reports relief of nocturnal pain and improvement in sleep pattern.
- Client returns to normal patterns of bowel functioning.
- Client verbalizes dosing schedule, expected response to drug therapy, and undesired responses to report.
- Client complies with prescribed drug therapy.

Implementing Follow the specific recommendations for drug administration. For example, many of these drugs must be administered 30 min to 1 hour before meals. Some must be administered at bedtime to be effective.

Initiate intake and output (I and O) records, food intake records, and daily weights on all clients. To improve accuracy, clients should be weighed at the same time each day, on the same scale, and in comparable clothing. Since infants and older adults are at the greatest risk for developing fluid and electrolyte imbalances, I and O records for these clients should be reviewed at least every 4 hours. Instruct the client treated at home to keep self-records. If possible, provide a sample format for data collection.

Many of these drugs alter production and/or composition of gastric secretions. Therefore you may be asked to test gastric secretions for occult blood or to measure the pH level of the secretions. This information helps monitor the client's status and response to drug therapy. Also observe the client for signs of infection, especially oral, nasopharyngeal, and respiratory infections. Drugs that increase gastric pH (antisecretory agents and acid neutralizers) can produce a significant increase in intragastric concentration of viable bacteria.

Evaluating Observe, report, and record therapeutic responses and undesired clinical responses to the drug therapy. Determine the status of the client's initial symptoms. Is the gastric pain and/or discomfort lessened? Is the gastric pH maintained at proper level? Have eructation and flatulence diminished? Review the expected outcomes with the client and determine the status of each. Alter the plan of care based on your evaluation findings.

UPPER GASTROINTESTINAL PROTECTIVE AGENTS

As previously mentioned, many conditions of the UGI tract result from an imbalance of the mucosal protective properties and the secretion of hydrochloric acid. For example, because the esophagus has no protective barrier to gastric acids, reflux of acid from the stomach can result in GERD or erosive esophagitis. Although the stomach has a mucosal protective barrier, the mucosal lining can be damaged by ingestion of drugs such as salicylates or nonsteroidal anti-inflammatory drugs (NSAIDs), toxins, infections, or ischemia. Without this protection, back diffusion of gastric acid (hydrogen ions [H^+]) into the gastric mucosa occurs, and the ulceration process begins.[3]

Pharmacotherapeutics

Drug therapy is directed at the control of gastric acidity to alleviate symptoms, promote healing, and reduce ulcer recurrences. A variety of drugs may be used, either alone or in combination. **Antisecretory drugs** reduce the secretion of hydrochloric acid, and **acid neutralizers** buffer the hydrochloric acid, raising pH and decreasing injury to the mucosal lining. **Cytoprotective drugs** protect the mucosa from the effects of acid. In addition, **antibacterial drugs** are used to diminish the effects of *Helicobacter pylori* in the GI tract.

General Characteristics

Reduction of inflammation of the mucosal lining (esophagitis or gastritis) is usually accomplished within 2 weeks after initiation of drug therapy. Healing of peptic ulcers and reversal of symptoms or conditions caused by GERD is expected within 4 to 8 weeks with acid neutralizers, antisecretory drugs, or cytoprotective drugs. Pain relief is expected within 2 weeks. The clinical efficacies of these drugs, with minor exceptions, are comparable. H_2-receptor antagonists (antisecretory drugs), sucralfate (a cytoprotective drug), and antacids (acid neutralizers) heal more than 90% of duodenal ulcers in 6 to 8 weeks. H_2-receptor antagonists heal 80% of gastric ulcers in 8 weeks and more than 90% by 12 weeks.[6]

Antisecretory Drugs: H_2-Receptor Antagonists

Histamine H_2-receptor antagonists are competitive blockers of histamine at the H_2-receptor sites. Histamine H_2 stimulates receptors in parietal cells in the mucosal lining of the stomach to release hydrochloric acid. H_2 antagonists occupy the H_2-receptor sites of the parietal cells, blocking stimulation by histamine H_2.

H_2-receptor antagonists also indirectly diminish the effects of gastrin and ACh through the blockade of histamine H_2. These drugs inhibit both daytime and nocturnal basal gastric acid secretion. They also inhibit gastric acid secretion stimulated by food, pentagastrin, caffeine, and insulin[7] (Fig. 47–1).

H_2-RECEPTOR ANTAGONIST PROTOTYPE

CIMETIDINE

Cimetidine (Tagamet), the first H_2-receptor antagonist available in the United States, was introduced in 1977. It is considered a first-generation H_2-receptor antagonist.

Pharmacotherapeutics Cimetidine is used to treat PUD, GERD, and hypersecretory gastric conditions. It is also used for maintenance therapy to prevent recurrence of ulcers and prophylactically in critically ill and preoperative and postoperative clients to prevent stress ulcers.

Pharmacokinetics Cimetidine is rapidly absorbed after oral administration. Peak plasma concentration occurs within 1 hour after oral administration and immediately after intravenous (IV) administration. Onset of action is 30 minutes by the oral route and 10 minutes by IV route. The half-life is approximately 2 hours in clients with normal renal function. Comparable periods of therapeutically effective blood levels are provided by both oral and parenteral (IV and intramuscular [IM]) administration. Steady-state blood concentrations resulting from continuous infusion of cimetidine are determined by the infusion rate (milligrams

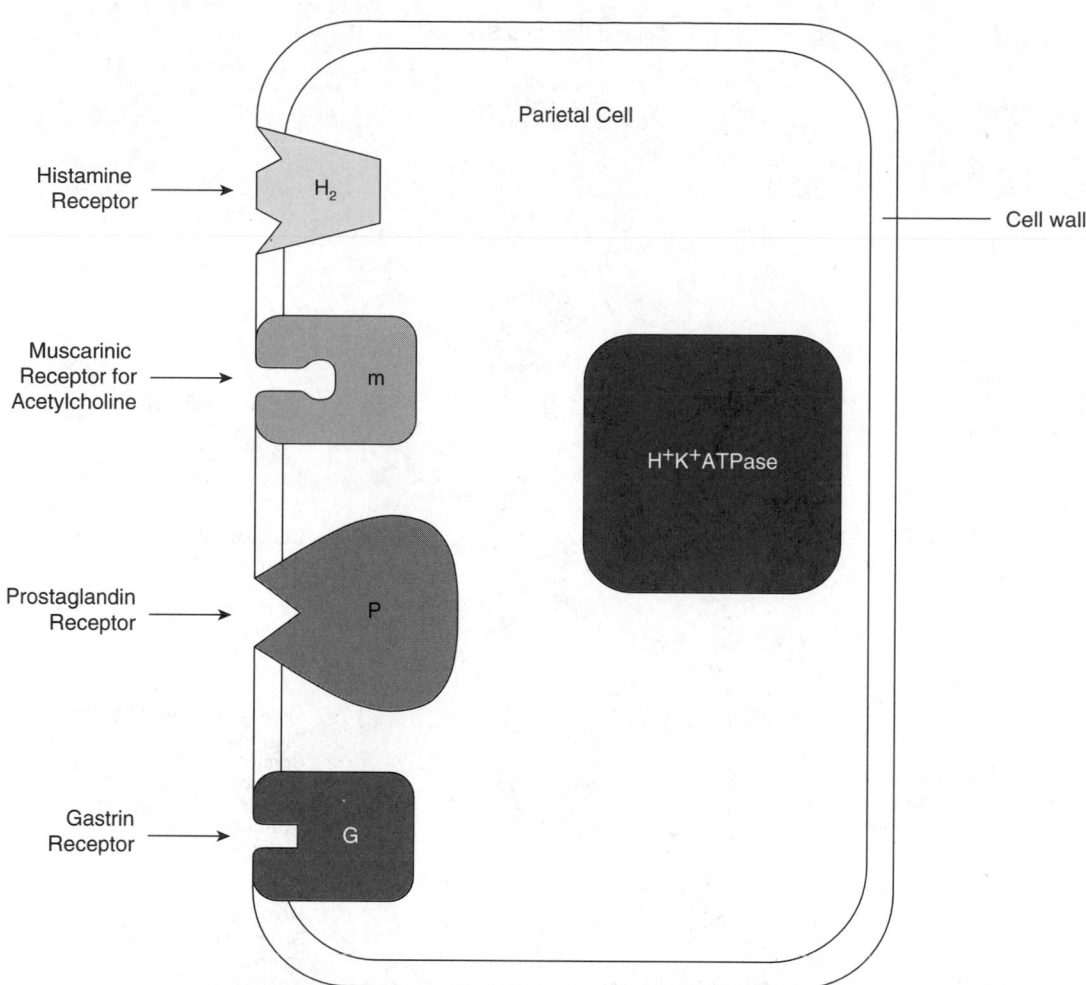

FIGURE 47–1   Action sites of gastric antisecretory drugs. Histamine H_2-receptor antagonists occupy H_2-receptor sites, blocking stimulation of histamine. Antimuscarinic drugs form a competitive blockade of muscarinic receptors, diminishing gastric acid secretion. Synthetic prostaglandin E_1 forms a reversible bond with prostaglandin-receptor sites, increasing bicarbonate and mucus production. Pump inhibitors block the final step of acid production by nonreversible inhibition of $H^+K^+ATPase$.

per hour) and the clearance of the drug in the individual client.

Cimetidine is distributed to all body systems. Plasma protein binding is minimal (15% to 20%). The drug undergoes hepatic first-pass metabolism. Approximately 30% to 40% of the drug is metabolized in the liver, resulting in 60% to 70% bioavailability. After oral administration 48% of the drug is excreted unchanged in the urine within 24 hours. After parenteral administration, 75% of the unchanged drug is excreted in the urine within 24 hours. Drug dosage usually is decreased in clients with decreased renal function. Approximately 10% of the drug is excreted in the feces.[8,9]

Pharmacodynamics Cimetidine produces its pharmacologic effects in the same manner as other H_2-receptor antagonists. A 300-mg dose of cimetidine reduces basal gastric acid secretion by 90% and reduces meal-stimulated acid secretion by 66%. Effective inhibition of basal gastric acid secretion lasts for 4 to 5 hours. Cimetidine also reduces total gastric secretory volume and raises the mean gastric pH. Pepsin is reduced pro-

portionately to the reduction in total gastric volume. Cimetidine does not affect gastric emptying, lower esophageal sphincter (LES) tone, or biliary or pancreatic secretion.[7,9]

Pharmaceutics Cimetidine is available in oral and parenteral dosage forms. Oral preparations include tablets and liquid forms of the drug.

Undesired Clinical Responses Headaches, dizziness, and somnolence are the undesired clinical responses reported most frequently. However, transient central nervous system (CNS) effects may occur in clients who are elderly or severely ill or who have decreased hepatic or renal function. The CNS effects include reversible mental changes such as confusion, anxiety, disorientation, agitation, psychosis, depression, and hallucinations. These responses are usually noted 2 to 3 days after initiation of cimetidine and disappear within 3 to 4 days after discontinuation of the drug. In some situations the effects are mild, and drug discontinuation is not necessary. Other adverse effects of cimetidine include diarrhea, nausea, rash, and muscular aches[8,9] (Fig. 47–2).

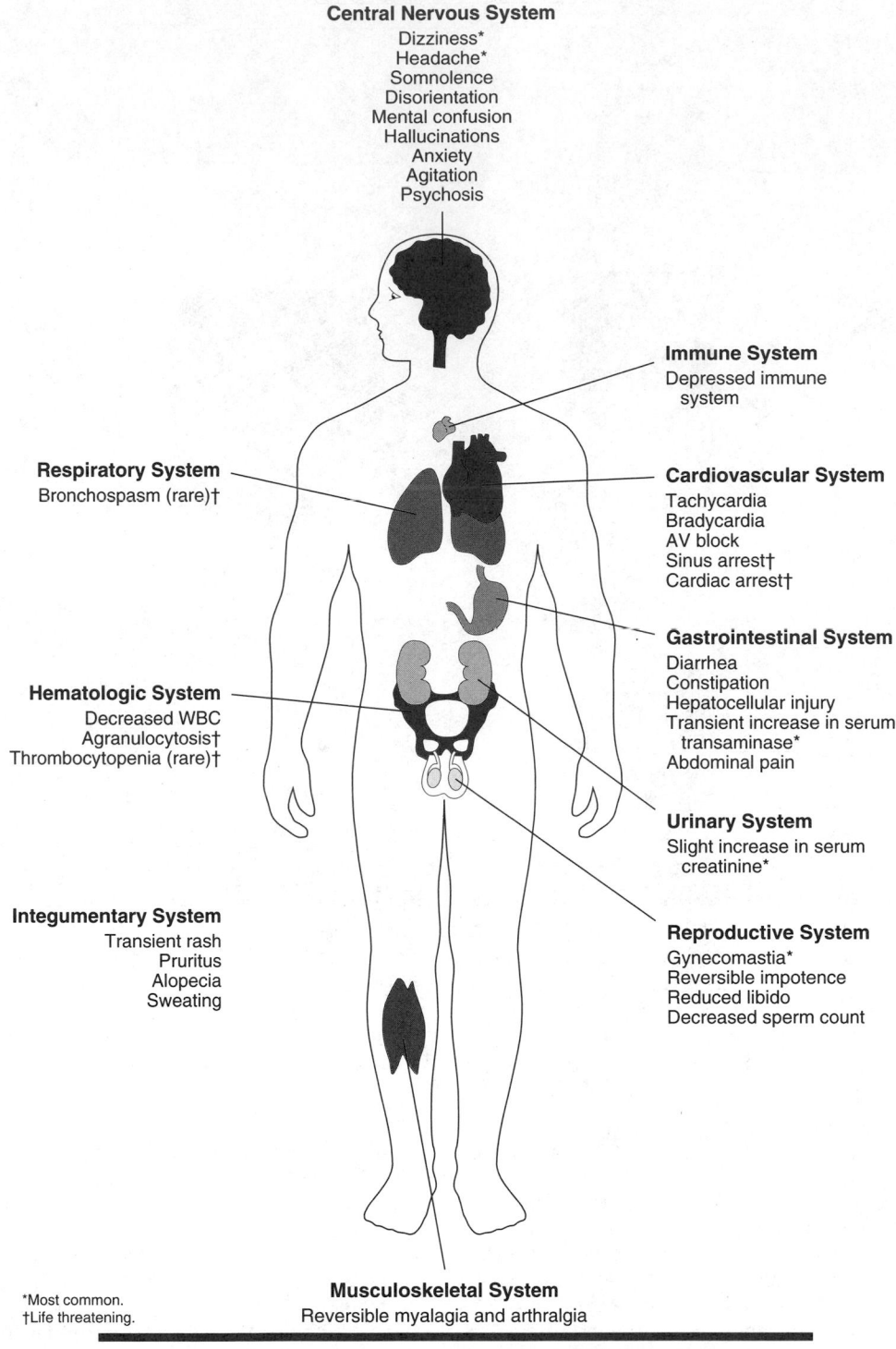

Central Nervous System
Dizziness*
Headache*
Somnolence
Disorientation
Mental confusion
Hallucinations
Anxiety
Agitation
Psychosis

Immune System
Depressed immune
system

Respiratory System
Bronchospasm (rare)†

Cardiovascular System
Tachycardia
Bradycardia
AV block
Sinus arrest†
Cardiac arrest†

Gastrointestinal System
Diarrhea
Constipation
Hepatocellular injury
Transient increase in serum
transaminase*
Abdominal pain

Hematologic System
Decreased WBC
Agranulocytosis†
Thrombocytopenia (rare)†

Urinary System
Slight increase in serum
creatinine*

Integumentary System
Transient rash
Pruritus
Alopecia
Sweating

Reproductive System
Gynecomastia*
Reversible impotence
Reduced libido
Decreased sperm count

*Most common.
†Life threatening.

Musculoskeletal System
Reversible myalagia and arthralgia

FIGURE 47–2   Undesired clinical responses associated with cimetidine.

Cimetidine has been reported to affect other H$_2$-receptor sites, notably the androgen receptor sites. The drug displaces testosterone from its receptor site and exerts a weak antiandrogenic effect. Alopecia has been noted, and mild bilateral gynecomastia and breast soreness have occurred in men. Decreased libido, reversible impotence, and decreased sperm count have also been reported.[9]

Drug-Drug, Drug-Nutrient, Drug-Environment Interactions   In the liver cimetidine reversibly inhibits the

microsomal enzyme oxidase system of cytochrome P-450 (microsomal P-450 system). This system produces drug-metabolizing enzymes. By inhibition of the system, cimetidine reduces the hepatic metabolism of some drugs and delays their elimination, thus increasing their pharmacologic effects.[8,9]

Cimetidine decreases the clearance of such drugs as meperidine (Demerol), phenytoin (Dilantin), diazepam (Valium), theophylline, warfarin (Coumadin), and ethanol. Theophylline, warfarin, and phenytoin are of particular clinical significance because of their narrow therapeutic range and low therapeutic-to-toxic ratio. Cimetidine also decreases serum levels of digoxin and decreases oral absorption of the antimicrobial drug ketoconazole (Nizoral). Concomitant administration of antacids decreases cimetidine absorption.

Life-Span Considerations Use of cimetidine in children less than 16 years is not recommended unless the potential benefits outweigh the risks. Cimetidine has been used with good outcomes to treat peptic esophagitis secondary to GERD and chronic duodenal ulcer in children. However, additional data are needed in this population.

Use of the drug is not recommended during pregnancy and lactation. Cimetidine is excreted in human milk. Teratogenic effects are not known because controlled studies in pregnant women are not available. In animal studies cimetidine crossed the placental barrier.[8,9]

Specific Drug-Related Nursing Considerations Generally maintenance drug therapy is given at bedtime. Administering the drug at bedtime reduces nocturnal hypersecretion, a significant factor in ulcer formation. Since late evening meals or snacks increase nocturnal gastric secretions, they should be avoided. The bedtime dose of cimetidine is not accompanied by food intake. However, daytime doses are usually taken with meals. If the client is also receiving antacid therapy, separate cimetidine and antacid administration by 1 hour.

Administer IV cimetidine slowly, since rapid IV infusion can produce cardiovascular side effects. If hypotension and bradycardia occur, they usually resolve within 24 hours of drug discontinuance. In rare instances, atrioventricular block and cardiac arrest have occurred.

MISCELLANEOUS DRUGS IN CATEGORY

Ranitidine hydrochloride (Zantac), famotidine (Pepcid), and nizatidine (Axid) are second-generation drugs. Unlike cimetidine, **ranitidine** exerts its action more specifically on the H_2 receptors of the GI tract. It is also more potent than cimetidine. Because ranitidine does not easily penetrate the blood-brain barrier, CNS effects are rare. In fact, significant side effects are uncommon. In addition, the administration of ranitidine concomitantly with other drugs produces few drug-drug interactions. Since ranitidine is a weak inhibitor of hepatic drug-metabolizing enzymes, it has minimal effects on the metabolism of other drugs.[8]

Ranitidine is administered orally, intramuscularly, and intravenously. After an oral dose of 150 mg of ranitidine, 50% of the drug is absorbed. The elimination half-life is 2 to 3 hours. The principal route of excretion is the urine.[8,9]

Famotidine and **nizatidine** are similar to ranitidine. Antiandrogenic effects are noted infrequently with these drugs. Famotidine and nizatidine do not affect the cytochrome P-450 microsomal enzyme system and therefore do not affect hepatic metabolism of other drugs. See Tables 47–1 and 47–2 for additional information on antisecretory drugs.

Antisecretory Drugs: Antimuscarinic Drugs

Antimuscarinic drugs produce a variety of responses in the body. (A general discussion of antimuscarinic drugs appears in Chapter 26.) In the treatment of upper GI disorders, the desired responses are diminished gastric acid secretion and decreased motility of the GI tract. They are achieved through competitive blockade of muscarinic receptors.

Most antimuscarinic drugs used to treat GI disorders are synthetic. Synthetic drugs have a more selective effect on the GI tract than naturally occurring antimuscarinic agents have, however, even with increased selectivity, high drug doses are required to inhibit gastric acid secretion. Doses are so high that muscarinic blockade is produced throughout the body. For this reason, antimuscarinic drugs such as **propantheline bromide** (Pro-Banthine), **clidinium bromide** (Quarzan), and **hyoscyamine sulfate** (Donnamar, Levsin, Pasmex, etc.) are used as part of an adjunctive therapy plan. Information about these drugs is summarized in Table 47–2.

Antisecretory Drugs: Pump Inhibitor and Substituted Benzimidazole

The newest class of antisecretory agents is substituted benzimidazole, called **pump blockers** or **proton pump inhibitors.** The final step in the formation of gastric acid is energized by the enzyme hydrogen/potassium adenosine triphosphatase (H^+/K^+ATPase). This enzyme causes exchange of hydrogen ions (H^+) (protons) for potassium ions (K^+) across the parietal cell membrane. This exchange system, the **proton pump,** maintains gastric acidity. Pump inhibitors block this final step of acid production by nonreversible inhibition of H^+/K^+ATPase.[3,6,10,11]

PUMP INHIBITOR PROTOTYPE
OMEPRAZOLE

Omeprazole (Prilosec) is the prototype for pump inhibitors.

Pharmacotherapeutics Omeprazole is used to treat duodenal ulcers, erosive esophagitis associated with GERD, and hypersecretory conditions.

Pharmacokinetics Since omeprazole is acid labile, the drug is supplied in enteric-coated granules that are not absorbed until the granules leave the stomach. Absorption of the granules in the intestine is rapid, with peak plasma levels occurring within $\frac{1}{2}$ to $3\frac{1}{2}$ hours. Hepatic first-pass metabolism reduces the drug's bioavailability to 30% to 40%. With repeated dosages, there is a slight increase in bioavailability. Protein binding is approximately 95%.

Omeprazole is almost completely metabolized in the liver through the microsomal P-450 system. The plasma half-life is 30 to 60 minutes, with appropriately 77% of the drug excreted as metabolites in the urine. The remainder of the drug is excreted through the biliary system into the feces. Drug clearance is slowed in clients with renal or hepatic disease.[8,9,12]

Pharmacodynamics As indicated previously, substituted benzimidazole suppresses gastric acid secretion by specific inhibition of the H^+/K^+ATPase system. These enzymes are present at the secretory surface of the gastric parietal cell. The antisecretory effect of the drug is dose

TABLE 47–1

Interactions Associated With Upper Gastrointestinal Protective Agents

Drug Name and Category	Drug-Drug, Drug-Nutrient, Drug-Environment Interactions	Nursing Considerations
H₂-RECEPTOR ANTAGONISTS		
Cimetidine (Tagamet)	Simultaneous administration with antacids decreases absorption of cimetidine.	Separate administration of antacids and cimetidine by 1 h.
	Cimetidine decreases clearance of meperidine (Demerol), diazepam (Valium), ethanol, phenytoin (Dilantin), quinidine, theophylline, warfarin, propranolol (Inderal), lidocaine, tricyclic antidepressants, and salicylates.	Instruct client to decrease or eliminate intake of alcohol. Monitor therapeutic effects on concomitantly administered drugs. Monitor prothrombin time if client is receiving concomitant warfarin.
	It decreases serum levels of digoxin. It reduces effectiveness of sucralfate.	Monitor serum levels of digoxin, theophylline, and phenytoin. Instruct client not to take OTC drugs without consulting primary care provider.
	It decreases clearance of caffeine.	Instruct client to decrease or eliminate caffeine intake.
	Food delays absorption and prolongs drug effects.	Administer drug with meals. Administer drug at bedtime to help control nocturnal secretion of gastric acid.
Ranitidine hydrochloride (Zantac)	Ranitidine inhibits acetaminophen metabolism.	Assess for acetaminophen toxicity.
Nizatidine (Axid)	Antacids containing aluminum hydroxides, magnesium hydroxides, and simethicone may decrease absorption.	Note contents of concomitantly administered antacids.
Famotidine (Pepcid)	See nizatidine	See nizatidine
PROTON PUMP INHIBITORS		
Omeprazole (Prilosec)	Omeprazole prolongs elimination of diazepam, warfarin, and phenytoin.	Monitor serum levels of drugs.
	It interferes with absorption if drugs need a specific gastric pH for absorption.	Monitor prothrombin time of clients receiving warfarin. Observe client closely for desired therapeutic effects of concomitantly administered drugs.
	Food decreases passage from stomach and delays onset of drug action.	Administer before meals and teach client the reason for before-meal dosing.
Lansoprazole (Prevacid)	Sucralfate delays absorption and reduces bioavailability	Administer lansoprazole at least 30 min before sucralfate
	Food decreases absorption	Administer before meals.
PROSTAGLANDIN		
Misoprostol (Cytotec)	Antacids may decrease total availability of misoprostol.	Separate concomitant antacid drug therapy by 1 h.
	Meals decrease plasma level of drug but do not decrease drug effectiveness. Food decreases undesired GI effects.	Administer drug with meals and at bedtime.
CYTOPROTECTIVE AGENT		
Sucralfate (Carafate)	Sucralfate decreases absorption of cimetidine, ranitidine, phenytoin, tetracycline, digoxin, and theophylline.	Instruct client to take other drugs 2 h before sucralfate. Do not administer antacids within ½ h of sucralfate.
	It contains small amounts of aluminum. If it is administered with other drugs containing aluminum, accumulation of aluminum may occur.	Use caution with aluminum-containing antacids; observe for signs of aluminum accumulation.
	Antacids interfere with sucralfate action. Food interferes with drug action.	Instruct client to take drug on an empty stomach.

related and inhibits both basal and stimulated acid secretion.

Onset of action per oral dose is 1 hour, with maximum effect occurring within 2 hours. Inhibition of gastric acid secretion is approximately 50% in 24 hours and lasts up to 72 hours. The relatively long duration of action is thought to be due to prolonged binding to the parietal $H^+/K^+ATPase$. When the drug is discontinued, secretory activity gradually returns to normal over 3 to 5 days.[6,9,12]

Pharmaceutics Omeprazole is supplied only in 20-mg delayed-release capsules.

Undesired Clinical Responses Omeprazole is used for short-term therapy (4 to 8 weeks). It is not recommended for maintenance therapy after treatment of ulcer or GERD. In clinical trials, symptoms reported in 1% or more of clients were diarrhea, abdominal pain, nausea, vomiting, constipation, headache, dizziness, upper respiratory infection, cough, rash, and back pain.[8,9]

Contraindications and Precautions Omeprazole is contraindicated in clients with known hypersensitivity to any component of the formulation.

Drug-Drug, Drug-Nutrient, Drug-Environment Interactions To prevent drug-nutrient interaction, omeprazole should be taken before eating. The delayed-release capsule is swallowed whole; it must not be opened, chewed, or crushed.

Because omeprazole produces extreme and prolonged inhibition of gastric acid secretion, it may interfere with absorption of drugs dependent on gastric pH (e.g., iron salts, ampicillin). Omeprazole also increases the plasma concentration of diazepam, phenytoin, and warfarin by inhibiting oxidative metabolism of them.[8,9]

Life-Span Considerations Omeprazole is classified as a Pregnancy Category C drug. Therefore the drug should be used by pregnant women only if the potential benefits justify the potential risk to the fetus. It is not known if the drug is excreted in human milk. Safety and effectiveness in children have not been established. Elimination is decreased and bioavailability increased in the elderly.[9]

Specific Drug-Related Nursing Considerations Since the drug must be swallowed whole, consult with the primary care provider if the client has swallowing difficulty. Since this drug is used for short-term therapy, note the date that therapy is started so the expected drug discontinuance date is known. Carefully note GI symptoms present when drug therapy is initiated. These baseline data make identification of desired and undesired clinical responses easier. Since drug clearance or elimination is diminished in elderly clients or clients with renal or hepatic dysfunction, observe these individuals closely for adverse effects. A second proton pump inhibitor, **lansoprazole** (Prevacid), has been introduced. Tables 47–1 and 47–2 contain additional information about omeprazole and lansoprazole.

Antisecretory Drugs: Prostaglandins

A deficiency of prostaglandin in the gastric mucosa diminishes bicarbonate and mucus secretion and may lead to mucosal damage. Synthetic prostaglandin E_1 (PGE_1) reversibly binds to prostaglandin-receptor sites in gastric parietal cells, mimicking the effects of naturally occurring prostaglandin E.

As a result, bicarbonate and mucus production is increased. This increase in bicarbonate and mucus production protects the gastric mucosal lining. Synthetic PGE_1 also inhibits gastric acid secretion.[6,13]

PROSTAGLANDIN PROTOTYPE

MISOPROSTOL

In late 1988 the drug misoprostol (Cytotec) was introduced. At present, it is the only approved synthetic PGE_1.

Pharmacotherapeutics Misoprostol is indicated for the prevention of NSAID-induced and aspirin-induced gastric ulcers in clients at high risk. These clients include the elderly, those with concomitant debilitating disease or a history of ulcer, women with rheumatoid arthritis, smokers, and abusers of alcohol.[6,10,11,13]

Pharmacokinetics Misoprostol is rapidly absorbed after oral administration. Protein binding of misoprostol acid is less than 90%. Peak plasma concentration is reached in approximately 12 minutes, and plasma steady state is achieved within 2 days. Half-life of the drug is 20 to 40 minutes. Misoprostol does not affect the microsomal P-450 system, but the drug does undergo deesterification to misoprostol acid, which is responsible for its clinical activity. Eighty percent of the drug is excreted in the urine.[8,9]

Pharmacodynamics Misoprostol has the same mucosal protective properties previously described. It also inhibits basal and nocturnal gastric acid secretion and acid secretion in response to food, histamine, pentagastrin, and coffee. Onset of action is 30 minutes, and the duration is at least 3 hours.

Pharmaceutics Misoprostol is supplied in uncoated 100- and 200-μg tablets.

Undesired Clinical Responses Frequent side effects are diarrhea, abdominal pain, nausea, vomiting, dyspepsia, and flatulence. Headache and constipation may also occur. The toxic dose of misoprostol has not been determined. Clinical signs that may indicate an overdose include sedation, tremor, convulsions, dyspnea, abdominal pain, diarrhea, fever, palpitations, hypotension, or bradycardia.

Contraindications and Precautions Use of the drug is contraindicated in women who are pregnant, and it must be used cautiously in women of childbearing potential. Use of misoprostol is also contraindicated in clients with a history of allergy to prostaglandins.

Drug-Drug, Drug-Nutrient, Drug-Environment Interactions Antacids produce several problems when administered to clients receiving misoprostol. Total availability of the drug is reduced with concomitant use of antacids. Although this effect does not appear clinically significant, it is recommended that antacids not be given at the same time as misoprostol. In addition, when antacids containing magnesium are administered concurrently with misoprostol, the incidence of diarrhea may increase. Misoprostol does not interfere with the therapeutic effects of NSAIDs or aspirin. There is also no effect on the intrinsic factor output. (Intrinsic factor is secreted from the parietal cells of the gastric glands and is necessary for absorption of cyanocobalamin, vitamin B_{12}.) Food causes lower serum levels of the drug but does not interfere with the action at the gastric receptor cells.[9,11,13]

Life-Span Considerations Misoprostol is classified as a Pregnancy Category X drug. Women have reported

TABLE 47–2

Upper Gastrointestinal Protective Agents: Prototypes and Major Drugs in Category

Drug Name	Dosage and Route of Administration	Nursing Considerations
H₂-RECEPTOR ANTAGONIST: CIMETIDINE (Tagamet) **HOW SUPPLIED** Coated tablet: 200, 300, 400, and 800 mg Liquid: 300 mg/5 ml IV: 300 mg/50 ml; 150 mg/50 ml IM, IV: 300 mg/2 ml; 300 mg/8 ml	**Peptic Ulcer** Oral: 800 mg hs or 300 mg qid with meals and hs or 400 mg AM and hs *Maintenance:* 400 mg hs **Hypersecretory Condition** Oral: 300 mg qid with meals and hs; may increase to maximum of 2400 mg/24 h **Gastroesophagogeal Reflux Disease** IM: 300 mg q6-8h Intermittent IV infusion: 300 mg q6-8h Continuous IV infusion: 37.5 mg/h or 900 mg/24 h diluted in 100-1000 ml	**Assess** Assess client for risk of drug-drug interactions. Assess client for preexisting renal or hepatic dysfunction. Determine if client is pregnant; drug classified as Pregnancy Category B drug. **Implement** Administer oral drug with meals or at hs. Store oral dosage form at controlled room temperature (15° to 30° C) in a tight, light-resistant container. Dilute 300 mg of cimetidine injection solution in 0.9% NaCl injection solution or other compatible IV solution to total volume of 20 ml. Inject over a period of not less than 5 min. If premixed, no additional solution is needed. Use mixtures within 48 h; store at room temperature. With volume <250 ml, use of a volumetric pump is recommended. If in plastic container, solution may appear opaque when first opened. This opaqueness will disappear gradually and does not affect drug. Do not add other drugs to premixed cimetidine in plastic containers. Advise client there may be transient pain at injection site. Instruct client to report signs of thrombocytopenia (sore throat, fever, unusual bleeding, bruising, unusual tiredness or weakness). **Monitor** Observe for oropharyngeal, respiratory, or gastric infection since concentration of intragastric bacteria increases with increased intragastric pH. Assess client for undesired clinical responses such as tinnitus, taste disorder, diarrhea, constipation, headache, dizziness, disorientation, gynecomastia, reversible impotence, and thrombocytopenia. Monitor serum creatinine level. Monitor complete blood count (CBC). Monitor alanine transaminase (ALT) and aspartate transaminase (AST). **Evaluate** Evaluate for diminished gastric symptoms.
Rantidine Hydrochloride (Zantac) **HOW SUPPLIED** Syrup: 15 mg/ml Uncoated tablets: 150 mg, 300 mg IM, IV: 25 mg/ml, 5 mg/10 ml	**Peptic Ulcer** Oral: 150 mg bid or 300 mg hs *Maintenance:* 150 mg hs **Gastroesophageal Reflux Disease** Oral: 150 mg bid	**Assess** See cimetidine. **Implement** Dilute for IV bolus with 0.9% NaCl injection or compatible solution to a concentration no greater than 2.5 mg/ml. Infuse at a rate no greater than 4 ml/min. Rapid infusion might cause bradycardia. For intermittent IV infusion, dilute drug with 100 ml of compatible solution. Administer over 20 min.

TABLE 47–2 *Continued*

Upper Gastrointestinal Protective Agents: Prototypes and Major Drugs in Category

Drug Name	Dosage and Route of Administration	Nursing Considerations
Rantidine Hydrochloride—Continued	**Hypersecretory Conditions** Oral: 150 mg bid or more frequently, based on need; up to 6 g/24 h IM or IV bolus: 50 mg q6-8h Intermittent IV Infusion: 50 mg q6-8h, not to exceed 400 mg/24 h Continuous IV infusion: 6.25 mg/h NOTE: For clients with severely impaired renal function (creatinine clearance <50 ml/min), recommended dose is 150 mg/24 h.	**Implement—Continued** Premixed solution requires no dilution. Administer over 15-20 min. If administered via primary IV fluid system, discontinue primary solution during premixed infusion. Store injection solution at 4°-30° C. Protect from light. Store premixed solution at 2°-25° C. Be aware that false-positive test results for urinary protein with Multistix may occur. **Monitor** Monitor urinary output. Monitor creatinine clearance reports. Monitor ALT values daily from day 5 to end of therapy. **Evaluate** Evaluate for diminished gastric symptoms.
Famotidine (Pepcid) HOW SUPPLIED Granule (reconstituted): 40 mg/5 ml Coated tablet: 20 mg, 40 mg Uncoated tablet: 20 mg, 40 mg IV: 10 mg/ml	**Peptic Ulcer** Oral: 40 mg hs or 20 mg bid for 4-8 wk **Maintenance and Prophylaxis for Duodenal Ulcer** Oral: 20 mg hs **Hypersecretory Conditions** Oral: 20 mg q6h; increase dose on individualized basis IV bolus: 20 mg q12h Intermittent IV infusion: 20 mg q12h NOTE: Dose may be reduced in clients with severe renal insufficiency (creatinine clearance <10 ml/min)	**Assess** See cimetidine. **Implement** Antacids may be administered concomitantly with famotidine. Shake oral suspension 5-10 s before use. Discard unused oral suspension after 30 d. For IV bolus, dilute 2 ml (10 mg/ml) with compatible IV solution to total volume of 5-10 ml. Infuse over more than 2 min. For intermittent infusion, dilute 20 mg with 100 ml of D_5W or other compatible IV solution. Infuse over 15-30 min. Use solution within 48 h. Observe for irritation at injection site. Safety and effectiveness in children have not been established. **Monitor** Monitor for adverse reactions to drug: headache, dizziness, diarrhea, constipation. See cimetidine. **Evaluate** See cimetidine.
Nizatidine (Axid) HOW SUPPLIED Gelatin capsule: 150 mg, 300 mg	**Duodenal Ulcer** Oral: 300 mg hs or 150 mg bid *Maintenance:* 150 mg hs NOTE: Dose may be reduced to maximum of 150 mg/24 h or administered qod or q3d in clients with moderate (creatinine clearance, 20-50 ml/min) to severe (creatinine clearance >20 ml/min) renal insufficiency.	**Assess** See cimetidine with following exception: nizatidine is classified as a Pregnancy Category C drug. **Implement** False-positive test results for urobilinogen with Multistix may occur during therapy with nizatidine. **Monitor** Monitor creatinine clearance, AST, and ALT results. **Evaluate** See cimetidine.
ANTIMUSCARINIC DRUGS: CLIDINIUM BROMIDE (Quarzan) HOW SUPPLIED Gelatin capsule: 2.5 mg, 5 mg	Dosage individualized according to severity of symptoms	**Assess** Determine hypersensitivity to antimuscarinic drugs.

Table continued on following page.

TABLE 47–2 *Continued*
Upper Gastrointestinal Protective Agents: Prototypes and Major Drugs in Category

Drug Name	Dosage and Route of Administration	Nursing Considerations
ANTIMUSCARINIC DRUGS: CLIDINIUM BROMIDE—CONT'D	***Adjunctive Therapy in Peptic Ulcer Disease*** Usual dose: 2.5-5 mg tid or qid before meals and hs Aged or debilitated client: 2.5 mg tid before meals	**Assess—Continued** Assess for preexisting glaucoma, obstructive uropathy, obstructive GI disease, unstable cardiovascular status, myasthenia gravis. Determine if client is pregnant; safety in pregnancy has not been established. **Implement** Inform client that drug may produce drowsiness or blurred vision. Caution client about activities that require mental alertness. Encourage client to maintain adequate fluid intake to diminish risk of constipation. Suggest client suck on hard candy to decrease dryness of mouth. **Monitor** Monitor for undesired clinical responses: dryness of mouth, blurring vision, urinary hesitancy, constipation, tachycardia, palpitations. **Evaluate** Evaluate client for diminished gastric discomfort.
Hyoscyamine sulfate (Anaspaz, Levsin, etc.) **HOW SUPPLIED** *Oral* Gelatin sustained-action capsule: 0.375 mg Elixir: 0.125 mg/5 ml Solution: 0.125 mg/ml Uncoated tablet: 0.125 and 0.15 mg *Sublingual:* Uncoated tablet: 0.125 mg *Injection Solution:* IM, IV, SC: 0.5 mg/ml	Dosage individualized according to severity of symptoms ***Adjunctive Therapy in Peptic Ulcer Disease*** CHILDREN >12 Y AND ADULTS Oral: One to two tablets q4h or as needed; not to exceed 12 tablets in 24 h; 1-2 teaspoonsful q4h or as needed; not to exceed 12 teaspoonsful in 24 h *IV, IM, SC:* 0.5-1.0 ml (0.25-0.5 mg); may be repeated CHILDREN 2-12 Y Oral: ¼ to 1 teaspoonful q4h or as needed; not to exceed 6 teaspoonsful in 24 h NOTE: Drug dosage for children <2 y of age is based on body weight. Check specific directions that accompany drug.	**Assess** See clidinium bromide with this exception: hyoscyamine sulfate is classified as a Pregnancy Category C drug. **Implement** Some oral tablets may be chewed. Check specific directions that accompany drug. Caution client about danger of high environmental temperature; heat prostration can occur. See clidinium bromide. **Monitor** See clidinium bromide. **Evaluate** See clidinium bromide.
Propantheline bromide (Pro-Banthine, Probamide) **HOW SUPPLIED** Sugar-coated tablet: 7.5 mg, 15 mg	Dosage individualized according to client. ***Adjunctive therapy in Peptic Ulcer Disease*** ADULTS Oral: Usual initial dosage is 15 mg administered 30 min before each meal and 30 mg hs Geriatric clients and clients with mild manifestations: 7.5 mg tid	**Assess** See clidinium bromide with this exception: propantheline bromide is classified as a Pregnancy Category C drug. **Implement** Caution client about danger of high environmental temperature; heat prostration can occur. Store drug below 30° C. See clidinium bromide. **Monitor** See clidinium bromide. **Evaluate** See clidinium bromide.

TABLE 47–2 *Continued*

Upper Gastrointestinal Protective Agents: Prototypes and Major Drugs in Category

Drug Name	Dosage and Route of Administration	Nursing Considerations
PROTON PUMP INHIBITORS: OMEPRAZOLE (Prilosec) HOW SUPPLIED Gelatin sustained-action capsule: 20 mg	***Active Duodenal Ulcer/ Gastroesophageal Reflux Disease*** Oral: 20 mg before meals for 4-8 wk ***Hypersecretory Condition*** Oral: 60 mg before meals; may increase to 120 mg tid based on individual response	**Assess** Assess client for risk of drug-drug interactions. Determine baseline data about GI symptoms. Determine if client is pregnant; omeproazole is classified as a Pregnancy Category C drug. **Implement** Instruct client that capsule must be swallowed whole. The capsule must not be opened or crushed. Closely observe client with renal or hepatic dysfunction for undesired clinical responses. **Monitor** Monitor client for undesired clinical response: diarrhea, abdominal pain, nausea, vomiting, constipation, headache, dizziness, upper respiratory infection, rash, and back pain. **Evaluate** Evaluate for decreased gastroesophageal symptoms.
Lansoprazole (Prevacid) HOW SUPPLIED Capsules, delayed release: 15 and 30 mg	***Duodenal Ulcer*** Oral: 15 mg/d before eating for 4 wk ***Erosive Esophagitis*** Oral: 30 mg/d before eating for 8 wk ***Hypersecretory Condition*** Oral: 60-80 mg/d	See omeprazole *except:* Pregnancy Category B. No dosage adjustment with renal disease.
PROSTAGLADIN: MISOPROSTOL (Cytotec) HOW SUPPLIED Uncoated tablet: 100 and 200 μg	***Prevention of NSAID- and Aspirin-induced Gastric Ulcers*** Oral: 100-200 μg qid with meals and hs	**Assess** Assess if client is allergic to prostaglandins. Determine if client is pregnant; misoprostol can produce uterine contractions and is classified as a Pregnancy Category X drug. **Implement** Check result of serum pregnancy test before administering drug. Avoid administering concomitantly with antacids. Instruct client not to share drug with others. **Monitor** Monitor client for undesired clinical responses: diarrhea, abdominal pain, nausea, vomiting, dyspepsia, flatulence. **Evaluate** Evaluate client for absence of gastric ulcer symptoms.

spotting, cramps, hypermenorrhea, menstrual disorder, and dysmenorrhea. The drug produces uterine contractions, which can result in partial or complete miscarriage. Because of the threat of miscarriage, a woman must have a negative serum pregnancy test result before initiation of the drug therapy. After the negative report has been received, drug therapy is initiated on the second or third day of the next normal menstrual period. No teratogenic effects are known. In addition, safety in children younger than 18 years of age has not been established.[6,8,9]

Specific Drug-Related Nursing Considerations
Female clients must receive both verbal and written warnings of the abortifacient properties of misoprostol. Assess females of childbearing age for adequacy of contraceptive information and practices. Instruct the female client to discontinue the drug immediately if pregnancy is suspected

or confirmed and to contact the primary care provider. Also, instruct the client not to share this drug with any other individual; emphasize the risk to females who are capable of conceiving. Tables 47–1 and 47–2 contain additional information about misoprostol.

CONCEPT REVIEW

Antisecretory drugs reduce the secretion of hydrochloric acid.

The four groups of antisecretory drugs are H$_2$-receptor antagonists, antimuscarinic drugs, pump inhibitors, and prostaglandins.

Histamine H$_2$-receptor antagonists are competitive blockers of histamine at the H$_2$-receptor sites.

Antimuscarinic drugs inhibit gastric acid secretion and excessive motility of the GI tract through competitive blockade of muscarinic receptors.

Synthetic PGE$_1$ reversibly binds to prostaglandin-receptor sites in gastric parietal cells, causing increased production of bicarbonate and mucus.

Pump inhibitors suppress gastric acid secretion by specific inhibition of the H$^+$/K$^+$ATPase enzyme system.

Cytoprotective Drugs

Cytoprotective drugs act locally to cover and protect a peptic ulcer site to allow healing.

CYTOPROTECTIVE PROTOTYPE
SUCRALFATE

Sucralfate (Carafate) is the only drug classified as cytoprotective.

Pharmacotherapeutics Sucralfate is used for short-term treatment of gastric and duodenal ulcers. Drug therapy usually heals an ulcer in 4 to 8 weeks. At that time a lower dose of sucralfate may be used to prevent recurrence of the ulcer. The drug is also used to treat peptic esophagitis and chronic duodenal ulcers in children.

Studies show that sucralfate is also effective in preventing stress bleeding in critically ill clients. In addition, fewer incidents of nosocomial pneumonia were reported in long-term ventilated clients who received sucralfate instead of antacids or H$_2$-receptor antagonists. Sucralfate does not cause the gastric alkalization that can lead to an overgrowth of gastric and oropharyngeal gram-negative bacilli.[14-18]

Pharmacokinetics Sucralfate is only minimally absorbed from the GI tract. Therefore it exerts a local effect rather than a systemic one. The small amounts of sucralfate that are absorbed are excreted primarily in the urine.[8]

Pharmacodynamics In an acid environment, sucralfate forms a pastelike material that binds to the proteinaceous exudate at the ulcer site. This ulcer-adherent complex is highly viscous and adhesive; it covers the ulcer site and protects it against further attack by acid, pepsin, and bile salts. Administered in recommended doses, sucralfate inhibits pepsin activity in gastric juice by

32%. It also adsorbs bile salts. The onset of the local effect is rapid, and the duration is up to 6 hours after administration.[9,10]

Pharmaceutics Sucralfate is supplied in 1-g tablets and suspension for oral administration.

Undesired Clinical Responses Because only small amounts of sucralfate are absorbed systemically, adverse effects are not common. The most commonly reported undesired clinical response is constipation. Other GI effects include indigestion, flatulence, gastric discomfort, nausea, vomiting, and dry mouth.[10,12]

Contraindications and Precautions Since small amounts of aluminum contained within sucralfate are absorbed from the GI tract, sucralfate must be used with caution in some clients. For example, clients with chronic renal failure or those receiving dialysis have impaired excretion of absorbed aluminum. In addition, aluminum does not cross dialysis membranes because it is bound to albumin. Therefore aluminum accumulates in the body, and toxicity may occur.[8]

Drug-Drug, Drug-Nutrient, Drug-Environment Interactions Sucralfate interferes with the action of several oral drugs, including digoxin, phenytoin, theophylline, ciprofloxacin (Cipro), cimetidine, ranitidine, and tetracycline. This interference results from sucralfate's binding to the other drug in the GI tract.[9,10]

Life-Span Considerations Sucralfate is classified as a Pregnancy Category B drug. Because of the local rather than systemic action of sucralfate, the drug has been used safely in pregnant women and the elderly. Safety and effectiveness in children and nursing mothers have not been established.[9]

Specific Drug-Related Nursing Considerations For treatment of duodenal ulcers, the recommended adult oral dosage of sucralfate is 1 g four times a day. The drug is administered on an empty stomach. It is considered safe to prescribe antacids as needed with sucralfate therapy. However, the antacid should not be taken less than 30 min before or after sucralfate. Teach the client receiving other drugs the importance of taking these drugs at least 2 hours before the sucralfate. Assist the client to establish a realistic schedule of drug dosing. Assess the client carefully for therapeutic effects of any drug used concomitantly with sucralfate. If problems are noted, consult with the primary care provider immediately.

If GI side effects occur, assess the client's food and fluid intake to determine if dosage alterations or a change in dosing schedules might alleviate symptoms. If there are no contraindications, increasing fluids and dietary fiber may help with constipation and flatulence. Effectiveness of drug therapy is based on x-ray or endoscopic examinations.

Gastric Acid Neutralizers

As previously mentioned, gastric acid neutralizers (antacids) buffer the hydrochloric acid, raising pH and decreasing injury to the mucosal lining. These drugs have been used in the treatment of GI disorders for hundreds of years.

Pharmacotherapeutics Antacids are used in the treatment of acute and chronic upper GI disorders. They are also used in the prophylactic treatment of GI bleeding and stress ulcers.

Antacid preparations Antacids are inorganic salts formed by a combination of a cation with an anion. Common cations are magnesium, aluminum, sodium, and calcium. Anions include hydroxide, bicarbonate, citrate, carbonate, oxide, and phosphate. After dissolution in gastric acid, antacids release the anion, which partially neutralizes the hydrochloric acid.[3,6,9]

Sodium is an ingredient in many antacids. However, **sodium bicarbonate** is the only sodium antacid. It is a short-acting, potent antacid and is sometimes used for temporary relief of symptoms of overeating and indigestion.

Sodium bicarbonate reacts rapidly with hydrochloric acid to form sodium chloride, carbon dioxide, and water. Acid neutralization occurs immediately. Each level $\frac{1}{2}$-teaspoon dose neutralizes 20.9 mEq of acid.[12]

Each gram of sodium bicarbonate contains 12 mEq of sodium. Excess sodium and bicarbonate are readily absorbed. Therefore sodium bicarbonate use is contraindicated for chronic or prolonged therapy because of the risk of sodium overload or systemic alkalosis. In addition, chronic administration of sodium bicarbonate with milk or calcium leads to an increase in calcium absorption and may precipitate the **milk-alkali syndrome,** which is characterized by hypercalcemia, renal insufficiency, and metabolic alkalosis. Symptoms include nausea, vomiting, headache, mental confusion, and anorexia. Since the undesired clinical responses associated with sodium bicarbonate outweigh its usefulness, its use is not encouraged.[8,9,12]

Calcium antacids have limited usefulness for long-term treatment because they cause gastric hypersecretion and acid rebound. **Calcium carbonate** is the most common calcium antacid.

Calcium carbonate exerts rapid, prolonged, and potent neutralization of gastric acid. It has the highest acid-neutralizing capacity of all antacids. Calcium carbonate reacts with gastric acid to form carbon dioxide, water, and calcium chloride. Acid neutralization is reversible, and systemic alkalosis is not a major risk.[12,19]

As previously indicated, calcium carbonate reacts with hydrochloric acid to form calcium chloride, which is highly soluble and available for absorption while in the stomach. After several days of antacid ingestion, enough calcium may be absorbed to produce hypercalcemia, with resultant neurologic symptoms, renal calculi, and decreased renal function. In addition, the milk-alkali syndrome can occur with calcium carbonate therapy. The risk of developing this syndrome is increased by prolonged administration of calcium carbonate or concomitant administration of sodium bicarbonate or homogenized milk containing vitamin D. Therefore long-term therapy with calcium carbonate is not recommended.[9,12,19]

Aluminum can be administered in the hydroxide, carbonate, phosphate, or aminoacetate form. It is most often administered in the hydroxide form, which has the greatest neutralizing capacity. The reaction of gastric acid and aluminum hydroxide produces aluminum chloride and water. In the small intestine the aluminum chloride is coverted to a poorly absorbable aluminum salt. Aluminum also combines with dietary phosphate in the intestine forming insoluble, nonabsorbable aluminum phosphate, which eventually is excreted in the feces.[3,9,20]

The main undesired clinical response associated with aluminum hydroxide is constipation. However, aluminum is absorbed from the GI tract. In individuals with impaired renal function, systemic toxicity can occur.

Magnesium salts with antacid properties are the oxide, carbonate, hydroxide, and trisilicate forms. Of them, the hydroxide, carbonate, and oxide forms are the most potent.

Magnesium antacids react with gastric acid to form magnesium chloride and water. Magnesium chloride is partially absorbed and rapidly eliminated by the kidneys. In the presence of renal disease, magnesium may accumulate, causing **hypermagnesemia.** Hypermagnesemia is manifested by hypotension, nausea, vomiting, depressed reflexes, muscle paralysis, respiratory depression, and coma. Magnesium that does not combine to form magnesium chloride is changed in the small intestine to soluble but poorly absorbed salts that are responsible for osmotic diarrhea. This diarrhea may affect fluid and electrolyte balance systemically.[3,6,21]

Magnesium-aluminum combinations are frequently used as antacids. The usual combination is magnesium hydroxide and aluminum hydroxide. The total neutralizing capacity of this combination appears to be equivalent to the sum of the capacities of the active ingredients. Five milliliters of magnesium and aluminum hydroxide suspension neutralizes 27.2 mEq of acid. The normal gastric pH of approximately 1.0 is raised to between 4.0 and 5.0. Since the activity of pepsin is decreased at pH levels greater than 1.5 to 2.5, magnesium and aluminum hydroxide combinations also suppress pepsin.[10,12]

The combination of aluminum hydroxide and magnesium hydroxide decreases the alterations associated with bowel elimination. Aluminum hydroxide is constipating, and magnesium hydroxide has a laxative effect. In combination, a balance is achieved. However, constipation and mild diarrhea may occur in some susceptible clients.

Because both salts are present, magnesium-aluminum combinations have the potential for the undesired clinical responses of either drug. If excretion of aluminum and magnesium is impaired by renal insufficiency or failure, elevated aluminum levels and hypermagnesemia may occur. The administration of aluminum and magnesium hydroxide does not induce acid-base disturbance in clients with normal renal functions. In clients with impaired renal function, moderate to severe metabolic alkalosis may occur.

Pharmaceutics Antacids are available as chewing gums, tablets, lozenges, powders, and liquids. Solid-dosage forms must be chewed before they can disintegrate and react with gastric acid. Liquid antacids are suspensions composed of fine particles in a vehicle.

Dosage recommendations Antacids should be administered on a regular schedule and not just in response to GI discomfort. Dosage is individualized, based on the product, the disorder being treated, and the client. However, the usual dosing schedule is seven times a day—1 and 3 hours after meals and at bedtime.

Antacids neither neutralize all of the stomach acid nor bring the pH to 7.0. At a pH of 2.3, 90% of the acid has been neutralized, and at a pH of 3.3, 99% has been neutralized. The **acid-neutralizing capacity (ANC)** of an antacid is expressed as milliequivalents per milliliter. (ANC is determined by the milliequivalents of hydrochloric acid needed to keep an antacid suspension at a pH of 3.0 for 2 hours in vitro.[3,6,9]) The ANC of a single dose usually ranges from 20 to 80 mEq. To provide maximum benefits, treatment should elevate gastric pH above 5. At this pH, pepsin activity is also inhibited.[22] Table 47–3 summarizes some of the major antacids and antacid combinations and indicates each drug's ANC.

Drug-drug interactions Antacids affect many concomitantly administered drugs. Antacids can form insoluble complexes with some drugs or alter drug absorption or elimination. Raising the gastric pH with antacids alters disintegration, dissolution, solubility, and ionization of enteric-coated or weakly acidic or basic drugs. These factors result in either increased or decreased absorption of the other drug involved in the interaction. In addition, antacid-induced changes in the urinary pH increase the excretion of weakly acidic and weakly basic drugs. Antacids interact with tetracyclines and other antibiotics, digoxin, digitoxin, quinidine, indomethacin (Indocin), levodopa, anticoagulants, estrogen, progestogen, and sucralfate.

Drug selection The selection of an antacid is based on the client and the GI disorder being treated. However, when making the selection, the following should also be considered: Is the antacid **efficient?** The drug should have a high ANC. Only a small amount of the drug should be required to neutralize large amounts of gastric acid. Is the antacid **effective?** The drug should exert a prolonged effect without a rebound increase in gastric secretion. Is the antacid **safe?** The drug should not interfere with acid-base or electrolyte balance. It should not prevent the absorption or excretion of nutrients or other drugs that the client is receiving. Is the antacid **inexpensive?** Because most antacid therapy lasts several weeks, it is important that the drug be low in cost. Is the antacid **palatable?** Compliance is enhanced if the taste of the antacid is appealing.

General nursing considerations Antacid therapy is

TABLE 47–3
Major Antacids and Antacid Combinations*

Product	Al(OH)₃	Mg(OH)₂	CaCO₃	Na/mg	ANC (mEq)	Other Content
Alka-Seltzer Tablets				311	10.6	958 mg sodium bicarbonate, 832 mg citric acid, 312 mg potassium bicarbonate
Amphojel Suspension	320			2.3	10	Saccharin, simethicone, sorbitol
Camalox Suspension	225	200	250	1.15	18.5	
Di-Gel Liquid	200	200		<5	10.5	20 mg simethicone, sorbitol, saccharin
Di-Gel Chewable Tablets		128	280	<5	9	20 mg simethicone
Gaviscon Chewable Tablets	80			19	0.5	70 mg sodium bicarbonate, 200 mg alginic acid
Gaviscon-2 Chewable Tablets	160			36.8	1	40 mg magnesium trisilicate, 400 mg alginic acid, 140 mg sodium bicarbonate
Gelusil Liquid	200	200		0.7	12	25 mg simethicone, sodium saccharin, sorbitol
Gelusil-II Liquid	400	400		1.3	24	30 mg simethicone, sodium saccharin, sorbitol
Maalox Chewable Tablets	200	200		0.7	9.7	
Maalox Plus Extra Strength Suspension	500	450		1.65	29.05	40 mg simethicone, sodium saccharin, sorbitol
Marblen Tablets			520	3		400 magnesium carbonate
Mylanta Suspension	200	200		0.68	11.5	20 mg simethicone
Mylanta Double Strength Suspension	400	400		1.14	25.4	40 mg simethicone, potassium citrate, sodium saccharin, sorbitol
Riopan Suspension				0.3	15	540 mg magaldrate (aluminum magnesium hydroxide)
Rolaids Chewable Tablets				50	7.5-8	350 mg dihydroxyaluminum sodium carbonate, magnesium stearate
Rolaids Calcium Rich Chewable Tablets			550	0.4	11	Magnesium stearate
Titralac Plus Liquid			500	0.0005	11	20 mg simethicone
Tums Chewable Tablets			500	≤2	10	
Tums E-X Extra Strength Chewable Tablets			750	≤2	15	

ANC = acid neutralizing capacity.
*Content in mg/5 ml, tablet, or capsule.

sometimes viewed as a time-consuming task—a task that requires the nurse to prepare and administer a small quantity of liquid, usually 5 ml, seven or more times a day. In reality, antacid therapy is an essential component in the treatment of upper GI disorders, and proper administration of these drugs determines the effectiveness of the therapy.

Before administering the antacid, read the label carefully to determine the proper method of administration. Shake all liquid preparations thoroughly before dispensing. Instruct the client to chew antacid tablets completely and to follow administration of the drug with a glass of water.

In some situations the dosage is titrated according to gastric pH measurements. For these clients, a nasogastric (NG) tube is inserted, and stomach content is aspirated for a baseline pH reading. After the reading, the antacid is instilled and the NG tube clamped for 1 hour. At that time another pH determination is done. If the pH is less than 4.0 to 5.0, further antacid is administered; the tube is clamped, and the pH is checked again in 1 hour. Increasing amounts of antacid are given until the target pH is achieved.[3]

Because of the high risk for drug-drug interactions, antacids should not be administered concomitantly with other drugs. Instead, administer other drugs 1 hour before or 2 hours after administration of an antacid. In addition, in preparation for discharge, provide the client verbal and written instructions about the dosing schedule of all prescribed drugs.

The most common undesired clinical response associated with antacid therapy is alteration in bowel elimination. Instruct the client to report diarrhea or constipation. If diarrhea occurs, assess the dosing schedule and consult with the primary care provider. If constipation occurs, increase the client's fluid and fiber intake unless there are contraindications to this approach.

Assess carefully for other possible undesired clinical responses. Be alert for signs of hypophosphatemia—decreased stroke volume; diminished cardiac output; slow, weak peripheral pulses; skeletal muscle weakness; and increased tendency to bleed. Look for electrocardiogram (ECG) changes, bradycardia, hypotension, widening pulse pressure, lethargy, decreased deep tendon reflexes, and respiratory depression as signs of hypermagnesemia. Elevated tissue levels of aluminum can lead to encephalopathy and osteomalacia.[3,6,9]

Be alert for symptoms of hypercalcemia, including nausea, vomiting, anorexia, weakness, headache, dizziness, and change in mental status. The milk-alkali syndrome can occur within 2 to 90 days of calcium alkali ingestion. During the acute phase, if the calcium and alkali are discontinued, the condition is reversible. In clients with chronic milk-alkali syndrome, reduced renal function may persist.[12,19]

Client compliance is of primary concern with antacid therapy. Many preparations are available OTC, and the client may be tempted to substitute an OTC drug for a prescribed drug. Because OTC antacid drugs are readily available and relatively inexpensive, the client may overuse them. Some clients may discontinue the antacid use, questioning the value of a drug that is available to the general public. Client education about expected therapeutic effects and the efficacy of antacids may

---

TEACHING THE CLIENT ABOUT SELF-TREATMENT WITH ANTACIDS

The following information should be taught to the client and family:

- Check with primary care provider or pharmacist before starting self-prescribed antacid therapy if you are currently taking other drugs.
- Do not use self-prescribed antacids longer than 2 weeks. If relief is not obtained in that length of time, a primary care provider should be contacted.
- Do not exceed dosage recommendations on the label or package.
- Store the drug out of the reach of children.
- Be aware that antacids may cause diarrhea and constipation.
- Use products with low-sodium content if on sodium restriction. Antacid products must be labeled with their sodium content if they contain more than 0.2 mEq (4.6 mg) of sodium per dose.
- Be aware that antacid tablets have less neutralizing capacity.
- Chew tablets thoroughly and follow them with a full glass of water.
- Dissolve effervescent tablets in water and allow most of the bubbles to subside before drinking the liquid.

---

prevent some compliance problems. If dosing schedule or taste is a problem, consult with the primary care provider to determine if another preparation or drug form can be used.

Because of availability of antacids, many clients self-medicate without an evaluation by an appropriate health care provider. Clients should be assessed for nonprescribed antacid use and advised of the need for evaluation of persistent symptoms. Teaching guidelines for these clients are included in the box.

ANTIBACTERIAL DRUGS

Clinical studies have established a link between *Helicobacter pylori* infection and gastric acid secretion. However, even after clinical trials involving various antisecretory drugs and antibiotics, an optimal, well-tolerated treatment plan against *H. pylori* infection has not been established.[23,24]

At present, a combination drug plan appears most effective. Treatment plans are combining antibiotics, acid pump inhibitors or prostaglandins, and bismuth subsalicylate (Pepto-Bismol). Studies do not indicate that H_2-receptor antagonists have any effect against *H. pylori* infection; but omeprazole (an acid pump inhibitor) appears to have some bacteriostatic action. In one study a combination therapy of omeprazole and amoxicillin eradicated *H. pylori* in 50% to 80% of the clients with duodenal ulcer. In another, bismuth salts, amoxicillin, and tinidazole eradicated the infection in 69% of the cases. Studies have also shown that when *H. pylori* infection is eradicated, long-term ulcer recurrence rates are reduced.[25,26]

CONCEPT REVIEW

The cytoprotective drug sucralfate has high efficacy and few undesired clinical responses or drug interactions and does not alter gastric pH.

Antacids are inorganic salts formed by a combination of a cation with an anion. Common cations are magnesium, aluminum, sodium, and calcium. Anions include hydroxide, bicarbonate, citrate, carbonate, oxide, and phosphate.

H. pylori infection in the GI tract increases gastric acid secretion. Certain antibacterial drugs are used to eradicate the infection.

ANTIFLATULENTS

Antiflatulents are used to relieve symptoms of gaseous discomfort or flatulence in the upper and lower GI tract. Flatulence is associated with eating too fast, air swallowing, postoperative gaseous distention, functional dyspepsia, peptic ulcer disease, and colic.

Currently **simethicone** is the only approved antiflatulent. It is marketed as Mylicon in a chewable tablet or drop form. Simethicone is also combined with antacids, antispasmodics, and digestants in various drug preparations. Simethicone exerts its action in the stomach and the intestine. It alters the surface tension of gas bubbles, enabling them to break or coalesce into a form that can be eliminated more easily by belching or flatus. Simethicone also has a defoaming action that disperses and prevents the formation of mucous-surrounded gas pockets in the GI tract. The drug is not absorbed from the intestinal tract and is eliminated in the feces.

Simethicone is usually administered after each meal and at bedtime. Advise the client to seek consultation if symptoms persist or relief is inadequate. Instruct the client to eat slowly, chew food thoroughly, and eat smaller, more frequent meals to help decrease gas distress. Instruct the client to avoid smoking and gum chewing, which are associated with increased air swallowing. Parents should be advised to consult their infant's primary health care provider before administering simethicone to him or her. With approval, the drug may be mixed with 1 ounce of cool water, infant formula, or other liquid to facilitate administration to the infant.

DIGESTANTS

Gastric acids and digestive enzymes are necessary to aid digestion of fats, proteins, and carbohydrates. Drug therapy is initiated when there is a relative or absolute deficiency of these normally occurring substances. Digestant drugs include hydrochloric acid, pepsin, pancreatic enzymes, cellulase, and bile extracts. Many drug preparations are combinations of these agents. Combination digestant drugs may also include anticholinergics, barbiturates, antihistamines, or antiflatulents in small doses.

Gastric Digestants or Acidifiers

Gastric digestants or acidifiers restore the normal acidic environment to the stomach. This action increases the precipitation of casein and enhances the conversion of pepsinogen into pepsin. Gastric digestants also inhibit the multiplication of bacteria in the stomach.

Once gastric acidifiers such as **hydrochloric acid** and **glutamic acid hydrochloride** enter the stomach, they act in the same manner as endogenous hydrochloric acid. When the food mass containing these acids reaches the duodenum, pancreatic juice neutralizes the acid.

Pancreatic Enzymes

Pancreatic enzymes (i.e., lipase, amylase, chymotrypsin, and trypsin) aid in the digestion of fats, carbohydrates, and proteins. When availability of pancreatic enzymes is decreased, replacement therapy is required. Pancreatic enzyme deficiency is caused by pancreatectomy, cystic fibrosis, pancreatitis, and obstruction of the pancreatic duct.

PANCREATIC ENZYME PROTOTYPE

PANCRELIPASE

Pancrelipase (Cotazym, Protilase, Zymase, etc.) catalyzes the hydrolysis of fats into glycerol and fatty acids, protein into proteoses and derived substances, and starch into dextrins and sugars. The active ingredients of the drug—lipase, amylase, and protease—are obtained from the pancreas of hogs. Pancrelipase is supplied for oral use in capsule, tablet, or powder form. Dosage is adjusted according to the severity of the pancreatic enzyme deficiency. The drug is administered with meals or snacks. Since pancrelipase is inactivated by the presence of acids in more than trace amounts, most dosage forms are specially treated to protect the drug from the effects of gastric acid.[8]

Undesired Clinical Responses The most frequently reported undesired clinical responses are nausea, abdominal cramps, and diarrhea. With extremely high doses, hyperuricemia and hyperuricosuria have been reported. Use of the drug is contraindicated in clients allergic to pork protein.

Life-Span Considerations Pancrelipase is classified as a Pregnancy Category C drug. Safety in pregnancy and lactation has not been established. As individuals with cystic fibrosis have longer life expectancies, the need for this drug in pregnancy may become more common.

Drug-Drug, Drug-Nutrient, Drug-Environment Interactions Pancrelipase is not administered concomitantly with antacids and H_2-receptor antagonists. The inhibition of gastric acid secretion by these drugs prevents gastric-acid inactivation of conventional enzyme preparations (i.e., those without enteric coating) and thus increases the effects of pancrelipase. The drug should be stored at room temperatures (15° to 30° C) in a tightly closed, dry container.

Nursing Considerations Do not crush the capsules or enteric-coated tablets and instruct the client not to chew them. If dysphagia is a problem, open capsules and sprinkle the contents on a small amount of soft food that can be swallowed without chewing. (The pH of the food must be > 6.0. A lower pH dissolves the protective shell that coats the drug particles and begins inactivation of the drug.) Instruct the client to swallow the food immediately and to follow it with juice or water. Teach the client that the drug may irritate the oral mucous membranes with prolonged contact. Powders are mixed in liquids or in food. Teach clients how to handle powders safely to avoid inhalation and skin contact.

ANTIEMETICS

Nausea and vomiting are protective mechanisms controlled by the CNS. The emetic process has three components: nausea, retching, and vomiting. **Nausea** is a subjective phenomenon experienced as an unpleasant wavelike sensation in the back of the throat, the upper gastric region, or the abdomen. It is accompanied by gastric stasis. Nausea often precedes retching and vomiting.

Retching is the labored movement of the diaphragm and abdominal muscles. These rhythmic, spasmodic movements alter intrathoracic pressure and facilitate vomiting. **Vomiting** is the forceful expulsion of the contents of the stomach, duodenum, or jejunum. GI retroperistalsis is responsible for the forceful oral expulsion of gastric contents. Increased intrathoracic pressure created by the diaphragm and abdominal muscles facilitates the process.

The emetic process results from the stimulation of a complex reflex coordinated by the emetic center. This emetic center, also called the *vomiting center,* is located in the medulla oblongata. When the vomiting center is excited, it induces emesis by sending impulses to the salivation and respiratory centers and the pharyngeal, GI, and abdominal muscles.

The vomiting center can be stimulated from several neurologic pathways. Impulses are received from (1) the chemoreceptor trigger zone (CTZ), located in the fourth ventricle of the brain; (2) the vagal viscera; (3) other sympathetic afferents from the viscera; (4) the labyrinth in the inner ear (vestibular apparatus); and (5) the cerebral cortex and limbic system. These neurologic pathways that converge on the emetic center contain distinct types of neurotransmitter receptors. These receptors respond to specific chemicals, including dopamine, histamine, ACh, serotonin, norepinephrine, and glutamine. The receptor sites and chemical stimulators are summarized in Table 47–4.[27-29]

Antiemetics antagonize or block the emetogenic receptors to prevent or treat nausea and vomiting from various causes. Frequently antiemetic combinations are more beneficial than single-drug treatment. Antiemetics are usually more effective when administered prophylactically to prevent emesis instead of to suppress emesis that has begun.

TABLE 47–4
Emetic Center Neurotransmitter Receptors and Stimulators

Receptor Sites	Chemical Stimulators
Chemoreceptor trigger zone	Dopamine
Vomiting center	Acetylcholine
	Norepinephrine
	Histamine
Vestibular apparatus	Acetylcholine
	Norepinephrine
	Histamine
Vagal afferent nerves	Serotonin
Efferent vagal motor nuclei	Acetylcholine
	Norepinephrine

Many different antiemetics are available. Some of these drugs were originally developed to treat other diseases. Classifications, trade names, and dosages are summarized in Table 47–5. Nursing considerations and major drug groups are discussed below.

Antidopaminergic Drugs

Antidopaminergic agents control vomiting by blocking dopamine receptors in the CTZ. This prevents stimulation of the vomiting center.

Phenothiazines Phenothiazines, major antianxiety and antipsychotic agents, are widely used as antiemetics. These drugs directly affect the CTZ by blocking dopamine receptors. Some of the commonly used phenothiazine antiemetics are prochlorperazine (Compazine), chlorpromazine (Thorazine), promazine (Sparine), and thiethylperazine (Torecan). As a drug category, phenothiazines are discussed in Chapter 20.

Metoclopramide hydrochloride Metoclopramide (Reglan, etc.) stimulates motility of the upper GI tract and blocks dopamine receptors in the CTZ. Metoclopramide is used in the prevention of postoperative nausea and vomiting and nausea and vomiting associated with emetogenic cancer. Metoclopramide is available in tablets, syrup, and injection solution.

The incidence of undesired clinical responses correlates with the dose and duration of therapy. CNS symptoms such as sedation, restlessness, drowsiness, and fatigue are common. In addition, extrapyramidal reactions have been reported.[8,9]

🦥 NURSING RESEARCH

Simms, S., Rhodes, V., & Madsen, R. (1993). Comparison of prochlorperazine and lorazepam antiemetic regimens in the control of postchemotherapy symptoms. *Nursing Research, 42,* 234-239.

The purpose of this study was to compare the antiemetic effectiveness of intravenous prochlorperazine (Compazine) and lorazepam (Ativan) in postchemotherapy management. A convenience sample (N = 24) of

TABLE 47–5

Antiemetics: Classification, Trade Names, Route, Adult Dosage

Class and Generic Name	Example of Trade Name	Route and Adult Dosage
ANTIDOPAMINERGICS		
Phenothiazines		
Chlorpromazine	Thorazine	PO, IM: 10-25 mg q4-6h prn
Prochlorperazine	Compazine	PO, IM: 5-10 mg three or four times per day prn
Thiethylperazine	Torecan	PO, IM: 2-10 mg one to three times per day prn
Others		
Metoclopramide	Reglan	IV: 10-20 mg q2h × 2; then q3h × 3
ANTIHISTAMINES		
Dimenhydrinate	Dramamine	PO, IM: 50-100 mg q4-6h prn
Diphenhydramine	Benadryl	PO, IM, IV: 10-50 mg q4-6h prn
Hydroxyzine	Vistaril, Atarax	IM: 25-100 mg q6h prn
Meclizine	Bonine, Antivert	PO: 25-50 mg q24h prn
Promethazine	Phenergan	PO, IM, IV: 12.5-25 mg q4-6h prn
CANNABINOIDS		
Dronabinol	Marinol	PO: 5-15 mg/m² four to six times per day prn
ANTISEROTONERGIC		
Ondansetron	Zofran	IV: 0.15 mg/kg before chemotherapy, then repeat in 4 and 8 h Oral: 8 mg before chemotherapy, then repeat in 4 and 8 h IV: 4 mg for postoperative nausea and vomiting
Granisetron	Kytril	IV: 10 μg/kg over 5 min only on day of chemotherapy Oral: 1 mg bid only on day of chemotherapy

adult oncology clients was recruited. All subjects were 21 years of age or older.

Two separate antiemetic regimens were established. One regimen included lorazepam, dexamethasone (Decadron), diphenhydramine (Benadryl), and thiethylperazine (Torecan). The other regimen replaced lorazepam with prochlorperazine. The randomized, double-blind crossover study indicated no statistically significant difference between regimens in the control of posttherapy nausea and vomiting. However, findings did support the value of lorazepam in antiemetic regimens since the drug decreases the client's experience of fatigue and pain.

STUDENT ACTIVITIES

- Review the physiologic action of lorazepam and prochlorperazine.
- Identify variables that might influence the client's response to an antiemetic regimen.
- Interview an oncology nurse to determine the antiemetic regimen used in your agency. 🖐

Cannabinoids

The exact antiemetic action of cannabinoids is not clear, but the effect is probably at the vomiting center. High abuse potential and psychoactive side effects have resulted in decreased use of these drugs.

CANNABINOID PROTOTYPE
DRONABINOL

Dronabinol (Marinol) is one of two cannabinoids available. Efficacy of this agent to control vomiting associated with cancer therapy has been examined since the mid-1970s.[29]

Pharmacotherapeutics Dronabinol is not chosen as a first-line antiemetic. The drug is used for control of nausea and vomiting associated with cancer chemotherapy when other methods of treatment have not been successful.

Pharmacokinetics Dronabinol is the principal psychoactive substance present in *Cannabis sativa L* (marijuana). After oral administration, the drug has a systemic bioavailability of 10% to 20% as a result of extensive first-pass metabolism. Numerous metabolites have been identified, including 11-hydroxy-tetrahydrocannabinol (11-hydroxy-THC). This metabolite is psychoactive and appears in plasma in about the same quantities as the parent drug. After oral dosing, the maximum plasma concentrations of dronabinol and 11-hydroxy-THC occur in approximately 2 to 3 hours. The major route of excretion is in the bile. Within 72 hours after oral administration, approximately 50% of the dose is recovered in feces; another 10% to 15% appears in the urine either unchanged or as a metabolite. Renal clearance in clients with normal renal functioning is approximately 10% of the glomerular filtration rate.[9,10,29]

Pharmacodynamics The antiemetic mechanism of action of dronabinol may be related to its effects on opiate receptors, the cortex, and vomiting centers of the brain. The nontherapeutic effects of dronabinol are identical to those of marijuana and other centrally active cannabinoids.

Pharmaceutics The drug is supplied in soft gelatin capsules for oral administration. The capsules are color coded by strength.

Undesired Clinical Responses Most undesired clinical responses stem from the drug's effects on the CNS. Some clients experience a subjective "high," which is characterized by easy laughing, elation, and heightened awareness. Mood changes (i.e., euphoria, detachment, depression, anxiety, panic, and paranoia), changes in cognitive performance and memory, decreased ability to control drives and impulses, distortions in perception of objects and time, and hallucinations may occur. These latter phenomena are more common with larger doses of dronabinol; however, full-blown psychosis may occur in clients receiving doses within the lower portion of the therapeutic range. Dronabinol can also cause tachycardia and hypotension.

While an individual is receiving dronabinol, rapid eye movement (REM) sleep is decreased. After discontinuation, marked rebound of REM sleep occurs. Sleep disturbances may occur for several weeks after discontinuation of high doses of dronabinol.[29]

Contraindications and Precautions Use of the drug is contraindicated in clients whose nausea and vomiting arise from causes other than cancer chemotherapy. Because of the CNS effects, its use is contraindicated in clients with psychiatric disorders. In addition, because of the risk of tachycardia and hypotension, dronabinol must be used with caution in clients with cardiovascular disease. Its use is also contraindicated in clients hypersensitive to sesame oil.

Life-Span Considerations Dronabinol's safe use in pregnancy has not been determined; thus the drug should be used in pregnancy only when clearly needed. Since dronabinol and its metabolites are concentrated and excreted in breast milk, the drug is not administered to women who are breast-feeding.[9,10,29]

Drug-Drug, Drug-Nutrient, Drug-Environment Interactions When the drug is administered concomitantly with alcohol or barbiturates, additive CNS depression occurs.

Specific Drug-Related Nursing Considerations Observe the client closely when therapy is initiated. Because of the high risk for dronabinol to alter the mental state and the variation in individual response, monitoring is essential. Initially the drug should be tried in an inpatient setting, especially if the client has never used dronabinol. If the client has a psychotic experience, provide close supervision in a quiet environment and withhold further doses of the drug until the client is evaluated. If the situation warrants it, dronabinol may be continued at a lower dose. In this event, discuss the experience with the client; the client should share in the decision about further use of dronabinol.

Therapy with dronabinol may continue or recur on an ambulatory basis. Advise the client that the prescription for dronabinol is written for the amount needed for one cycle of chemotherapy. Advise the client of the necessity of having a responsible adult available. Remind the client of the possible mood and adverse behavioral effects that may occur and instruct him or her not to drive or perform hazardous tasks while taking the drug. In addition, remind the client not to take other drugs, including alcohol and barbiturates, without consulting the primary care provider.

Since dronabinol is highly abusable, it is listed as Δ^9-tetrahydrocannabinol under Schedule II of the Controlled Substances Act. The proportion of clients exposed chronically to dronabinol who will develop physical or psychologic dependence is not known. Long-term use of cannabinoids has been associated with disorders of motivation, judgment, and cognition. It is not clear if these symptoms reflect the underlying personalities of the chronic users of this class of drug or if cannabinoids are directly responsible.

A withdrawal syndrome has been observed in some clients within 12 hours after abrupt withdrawal of the drug. The syndrome reaches a peak intensity at 24 hours with symptoms of hot flashes, sweating, rhinorrhea, loose stools, hiccoughs, psychic distress, and insomnia. The syndrome is essentially complete within 96 hours.[29]

Serotonin Antagonists

The majority of the total-body serotonin is located in the GI tract, mainly within the enterochromaffin cells of the mucosal layer. Serotonin (5-hydroxytryptamine) type 3 (5-HT3) receptors are present both peripherally and centrally. Peripherally, the receptors are on vagal nerve afferents and neurons within the GI tract; centrally, the receptors are in the CTZ.

Cytotoxic chemotherapy—drug treatment destructive to cells—appears to be associated with release of serotonin from the enterochromaffin cells in the GI tract. The released serotonin stimulates the vagal afferents and splanchnic nerve receptors through the 5-HT3 receptors that project to the vomiting center. This activation initiates the vomiting reflex. Serotonin antagonists block the afferent stimulus from the gut; they may also act centrally by disrupting afferent transmission through the CTZ.[31]

SEROTONIN ANTAGONIST PROTOTYPE
ONDANSETRON

Ondansetron (Zofran) is a new drug used to suppress nausea and vomiting. It has been extensively evaluated in clinical trials.

Pharmacotherapeutics Ondansetron is indicated for the prevention of nausea and vomiting associated with initial and repeat courses of emetogenic cancer chemotherapy, including high-dose cisplatin (see Chapter 69 for information about cisplatin and other antineoplastic drugs). Studies have shown ondansetron to be more effective than metoclopramide in the prevention of emesis with chemotherapy.

Pharmacokinetics Ondansetron is extensively metabolized, with approximately 5% of the parent compound recovered from the urine. The drug is metabolized by hepatic cytochrome P-450 drug-metabolizing enzymes. In healthy adults the mean elimination half-life is 3 hours and 30 minutes for age group 19 to 40 years, 4 hours and 42 minutes for age group 61 to 74 years, and 5 hours and 30 minutes for age group 75 years and older. In clients more than 75 years of age, a reduction in clearance and an increase in elimination half-life are seen.[8,9,31,32]

Pharmacodynamics Ondansetron is a highly selective 5-HT3-receptor antagonist. It is not certain if the antiemetic action of ondansetron is mediated centrally, peripherally, or in both sites. Ondansetron has not been shown to affect esophageal motility, gastric motility, LES pressure, or small intestine transit time. It has no effect on plasma prolactin concentrations.

Pharmaceutics Ondansetron is available in oral tablets and vials containing 2 mg/ml for IV use.

Undesired Clinical Responses The drug is generally well tolerated. Diarrhea, constipation, headaches, and skin rashes have been reported. Transient elevations in aspartate transaminase (AST) and alanine transaminase (ALT) have occurred, but symptomatic hepatic disease has not. Rare cases of bronchospasm, tachycardia, chest pain, hypokalemia, electrocardiographic alterations, and grand mal seizures have been noted.[32]

Contraindications and Precautions Since drug clearance is reduced and volume distribution is increased in clients with impaired renal or hepatic functioning, drug dose should be decreased to prevent an increase in plasma half-life.

Drug-Drug, Drug-Nutrient, Drug-Environment Interactions Drugs that induce or inhibit the cytochrome P-450 drug metabolizing enzyme system of the liver may change the clearance and thus the half-life of ondansetron.

Life-Span Considerations Administer the drug cautiously in pregnant and lactating women since there have been no well-controlled studies in these groups. No dosage adjustment is required in the elderly; the dosage for children 4 to 18 years of age is the same as for adults. Little information is available about dosage in children 3 years of age or younger.

Specific Drug-Related Nursing Considerations Be alert to alterations in bowel functioning because diarrhea may occur. Before and during therapy, monitor liver enzyme results.

The prescribed IV dose is diluted in 50 ml of 5% dextrose injection or 0.9% sodium chloride injection solution. Administer the first doses over 15 minutes, beginning 30 minutes before the start of the emetogenic chemotherapy. Other doses are given 4 and 8 hours after the first dose. For postoperative nausea and vomiting, ondansetron is administered undiluted over 2 to 5 minutes. Ondansetron is stable at room temperature and under normal lighting conditions for 48 hours.

Since ondansetron is not a dopamine antagonist, it may be particularly beneficial in younger adults, children, and clients who are likely to receive chemotherapy over consecutive days. These clients are all prone to dystonic reactions with antiemetics that are dopamine antagonists.

Antihistamines

Antihistamines block the action of histamine on the vestibular apparatus and the vomiting center. These drugs are useful particularly with motion sickness. **Promethazine** (Phenergan) is the most effective antihistamine for prophylaxis of motion sickness. Other antihistamine drugs used for this purpose include **cyclizine** (Marezine), **diphenhydramine** (Benadryl), **hydroxyzine** (Vistaril), and **dimenhydrinate** (Dramamine). Antihistamine drugs are discussed in Unit 10.

Antimuscarinic Drugs

Scopolamine, a muscarinic antagonist, is the most effective drug for prophylaxis and treatment of motion sickness. The mechanism by which it suppresses motion sickness is unclear. It appears to suppress nerve activity within the labyrinth of the inner ear. This drug is discussed in Chapter 26.

CONCEPT REVIEW

Antiemetics are used for prophylaxis and control of nausea and vomiting. These drugs act by blocking chemically stimulated central and peripheral receptors.

Antiemetics provide symptomatic treatment and are chosen according to the cause of the nausea and vomiting.

Antidopaminergic phenothiazine antiemetics are recommended only for severe nausea and vomiting or intractable hiccoughs.

Cannabinoids and serotonin antagonists (5-HT3) are used to control nausea and vomiting associated with cancer chemotherapy.

Histamine and antimuscarinic antiemetics are effective for treating nausea and vomiting associated with motion. Many of these drugs are available OTC.

EMETICS AND ADSORBENTS

Emetics are generally used in emergency situations when rapid gut emptying is desired. Drugs act by direct stimulation of the CTZ, local irritation of the GI tract, or a combination of the two actions. Induced emesis is used in clients who are awake and who have ingested a toxic substance or a drug overdose. The adsorbent activated charcoal may be used in conjunction with emetics. Both of these drug groups are presented in Chapter 75.

SUMMARY

Upper GI problems that require pharmacologic intervention are common in clients of all ages. Clients may self-medicate with OTC agents or take prescription preparations. The nurse uses the nursing process to assist clients to maximize the safety and effectiveness of drug therapy.

REFERENCES

1. Guyton, A.C. (1991). *Textbook of medical physiology* (8th ed.). Philadelphia: W.B. Saunders.
2. Smith, C.M., & Reynard, A.M. (Eds.). (1992). *Textbook of pharmacology.* Philadelphia: W.B. Saunders.
3. Peterson, W.L. (1990). Pathogenesis and therapy of peptic ulcer disease. *Journal of Clinical Gastroenterology, 12*(Suppl 2P), S1-6.
4. Richter, J.E. (1992). Gastroesophageal reflux: Diagnosis and management. *Hospital Practice, 27*(1), 59-66.

5. O'Toole, M.T. (1990). Advanced assessment of the abdomen and gastrointestinal problems. *Nursing Clinics of North America, 25,* 771-776.

6. Rubin, W. (1991). Medical treatment of peptic ulcer disease. *Medical Clinics of North America, 75,* 981-998.

7. Keithley, J.K. (1991). Histamine H$_2$-receptor antagonists. *Nursing Clinics of North America, 26,* 361-373.

8. Data Pharmaceutica, Inc. (1993). *1993 physicians' genRx.* Smithtown, NY: Author.

9. U.S. Pharmacopeial Convention. (1990). *The United States pharmacopeia* (22nd rev.). Rockville, MD: Author.

10. Olin, B.R., Hebel, S.K., Dombek, C.E., & Kastrup, E.K. (Eds.) (1992). *Facts and comparisons* (46th ed.). St. Louis: J.B. Lippincott.

11. Feldman, M., Maton, P.N., McCallum, R.W., & McCarthy, D.M. (1992). Treating ulcers and reflux: What's new? *Patient Care, 27*(1), 59-66.

12. McEvoy, G.K., & Litvak, K. (Eds.) (1992). *AHFS drug information.* Bethesda, MD: American Society of Hospital Pharmacists.

13. Rogers, A.I. (1990). Medical treatment and prevention of peptic ulcer disease. *Postgraduate Medicine Journal, 88*(5), 57-60.

14. Arguelles-Martin, F., Gonzalez-Fernandez, R., & Gentles, M.G. (1989). Sucralfate versus cimetidine in the treatment of reflux esophagitis in children. *American Journal of Medicine, 86*(6A), 73-76.

15. Chiang, B.L., Chang, M.H., Lin, M.I., Hsu, J.Y., Wang, C.Y., & Wang, T.H. (1989). Chronic duodenal ulcer in children: Clinical observation and response to treatment. *Journal of Pediatric Gastroenterology and Nutrition, 8*(2), 161-165.

16. Rey, J.F., Legras, B., Verdier, A., Vicari, F., & Gorget, C. (1989). Comparative study of sucralfate versus cimetidine in the treatment of acute gastroduodenal ulcer. *American Journal of Medicine, 86*(6A), 116-121.

17. Tryba, M. (1991). Sucralfate versus antacids or H$_2$-antagonists for stress ulcer prophylaxis: A meta-analysis on efficacy and pneumonia rate. *Critical Care Medicine, 19,* 942-949.

18. Weinstein, R.A. (1991). Failure of infection control in intensive care units: Can sucralfate improve the situation? *American Journal of Medicine, 91*(2A), 132S-134S.

19. Texter, E.C. (1989). A critical look at the clinical use of antacids in acid-peptic disease and gastric acid rebound. *American Journal of Gastroenterology, 84*(2), 97-108.

20. Salusky, I.B., Foley, J., Nelson, P., & Goodman, W.G. (1991). Aluminum accumulation during treatment with aluminum hydroxide and dialysis in children and young adults with chronic renal disease. *New England Journal of Medicine, 324,* 527-531.

21. Bauerfeind, P., Cilluffo, T., Armstrong, D., Emde, C., Muller-Duysing, W., Duroux, R., & Blum, A.L. (1990). Fate of antacid gel in the stomach. Site of action and interaction with food. *Digestive Diseases and Sciences, 33,* 553-558.

22. Lehne, R.A. (1994). *Pharmacology for nursing care* (2nd ed.). Philadelphia: W.B. Saunders.

23. Rune, S. (1992). *Helicobacter pylori,* peptic ulcer disease and inhibition of gastric acid secretion. *Digestion, 51*(Suppl 1), 11-16.

24. Di-Napoli, A., Petrino, R., Goero, M., Bellis, D., & Chiandussi, L. (1992). Quantitative assessment of histological changes in chronic gastritis after eradication of *Helicobacteri pylori. Journal of Clinical Pathology, 45,* 796-798.

25. Graham, D., et al. (1992). Effect of treatment of *Helicobacter pylori* infection on the long-term recurrence of gastric or duodenal ulcer: A randomized, controlled study. *Annals of Internal Medicine, 115,* 705-709.

26. Westblom, T., Madan, E., Subik, M.A., et al. (1992). Double-blind randomized trial of bismuth subsalicylate and clindamycin for treatment of *Helicobacter pylori* infection. *Scandinavian Journal of Gastroenterology, 27,* 249-252.

27. Peters, C.A. (1989). Myths of antiemetic administration. *Cancer Nursing, 12,* 102-106.

28. Rhodes, V.A. (1990). Nausea, vomiting, and retching. *Nursing Clinics of North America, 25,* 885-900.

29. Tortorice, P.V. (1990). Management of chemotherapy induced nausea and vomiting. *Pharmacotherapy, 10*(2), 129-145.

30. Simms, S., Rhodes, V., & Madsen, R. (1993). Comparison of prochlorperazaine and lorazepam antemetic regimens in the control of postchemotherapy symptoms. *Nursing Research, 42,* 234-239.

31. Hesketh, P., & Gandara, D. (1991). Serotonin antagonists: A new class of antiemetic agents. *Journal of the National Cancer Institute, 83,* 613-620.

32. Chaffee, B.J., & Tankanow, R.M. (1991). Ondansetron—The first of a new class of antiemetic agents. *Clinical Pharmacology, 10,* 430-446.

BIBLIOGRAPHY

Ahern, H.L., & Rice, K.T. (1991). How do you measure gastric pH? *American Journal of Nursing, 91,* 70.

Bianchi Porro, G., Parente, R., & Sangaletti, O. (1990). Inhibition of nocturnal acidity is important but not essential for duodenal ulcer healing. *Gut, 31,* 397-400.

Hennessy, K. (1989). Nutritional support and gastrointestinal disease. *Nursing Clinics of North America, 24,* 373-382.

McConnell, E.A. (1990). Determining the cause of nausea and vomiting. *Nursing, 20*(12), 74, 77.

Sullivan, P.B., & Thomas, J.E. (1991). *Helicobacter pylori* in children. *Postgraduate Medicine Journal, 67,* 330-333.

Welling, L.R., & Watson, W.A. (1990). The emergency department treatment of dyspepsia with antacids and oral lidocaine. *Annuals of Emergency Medicine, 19,* 785-788.

CHAPTER 48

DRUGS AFFECTING THE
Lower Gastrointestinal Tract

JEAN NELSON

⦿ Drugs Used to Treat Constipation
LEARNING OBJECTIVES:
- Describe six factors that can contribute to constipation.
- Discuss general characteristics of cathartics and laxatives.
- Summarize essential information about the prototype drug for each subclassification.
- Outline a plan of care for a client receiving drug therapy for constipation.

KEY TERMS:
- Cathartic, constipation, encopresis, hyperosmotic, lavage, laxative, osmotic, surfactant

⦿ Drugs Used to Treat Diarrhea
LEARNING OBJECTIVES:
- Explain three factors that can contribute to diarrhea.
- Discuss general characteristics of drugs used to treat diarrhea.
- Summarize essential information about the prototype drug for each subclassification.
- Outline a plan of care for a client receiving drug therapy for diarrhea.

KEY TERMS:
- Diarrhea, opioid

⦿ Drugs Used to Treat Inflammatory Bowel Disease
LEARNING OBJECTIVE: Describe the use of drugs in the treatment of inflammatory bowel disease.

⦿ Drugs Used to Treat Flatulence
LEARNING OBJECTIVE: Describe the use of drugs in the treatment of flatulence.
KEY TERM: Flatulence

CONCEPTS AND TERMS TO REVIEW

Read Chapter 46 for a review of the anatomy and physiology of the lower gastrointestinal tract.

Review the definitions for *osmosis* and *hyperosmotic solution.*

Study the mechanisms involved in normal peristaltic activity.

Review the mechanisms involved in the inflammatory process.

---

*T*he normal physiologic functions of the lower gastrointestinal (GI) tract include motility, absorption, and secretion. Alterations in bowel elimination (constipation or diarrhea) represent changes in one or more of these functions. Although various drugs may be administered for symptomatic relief, drug therapy does not address the underlying cause and in some cases may contribute to or intensify the problem. When an underlying medical condition exists, accurate diagnosis and specific treatment are essential. When lifestyle factors cause altered bowel function, nurses can teach clients how to achieve normal elimination without habitual medication use.

This chapter discusses drugs used to prevent and/or eliminate constipation, diarrhea, and flatulence. In addition, the use of drugs in the treatment of inflammatory bowel disease (IBD) is examined.

DRUGS USED TO TREAT CONSTIPATION

Constipation has been defined as infrequent defecation, hardening of stool consistency, reduced caliber of stool, sense of incomplete evacuation, and necessity for straining with bowel movement. Defecation less than three times weekly is a commonly accepted criterion for the diagnosis of constipation.

Contributing Factors

The most common causes of constipation are lifestyle factors such as inadequate intake of fluids and fiber, insufficient exercise, and hectic schedules with no established time for regular elimination. Other causes include pregnancy, metabolic and endocrine disorders, colonic and rectal disorders, neurologic disorders, and drug side effects. Drugs that may cause constipation are listed in the box.

▣ NURSING CONSIDERATIONS

It is important to follow the steps in the nursing process when organizing care for individuals with constipation.

Assessing During the **health history,** gather a careful description of the client's usual and current bowel elimination pattern. Include information about the frequency, consistency, size, and color of stools. Also ask the client about any related symptoms such as pain, flatulence, difficulty passing stool, or sensation of incomplete evacuation. Question the client about the onset and duration of the elimination problem and any apparent precipitating, aggravating, or mitigating factors.

Pertinent lifestyle factors include usual activities, occupation, type and frequency of exercise, and dietary habits. A 3-day recall of food and fluid consumption provides more specific nutritional information. Ascertain information about past surgeries, past and present illness, and current drug therapy. When questioning the client about drug use, it is vital to include nonprescription drugs, especially laxatives and/or enemas, that the client may be using for self-treatment of the bowel problem. If the client reports constipation, question his or her perception of normal defecation patterns; many describe themselves as constipated when evacuation does not occur every day.

Inspection, auscultation, percussion, and palpation are used during the **physical assessment** of the abdomen. Inspection may reveal distention, surgical scars, hernias, ostomy stomas, and other pertinent findings. Auscultation of bowel sounds may indicate increased or decreased peristalsis. Percussion is helpful in validating the impression of distention. Palpation is used to determine generalized or localized areas of tenderness and the presence of abdominal masses.

Examine the rectal area for local skin irritation, presence of hemorrhoids, and condition of the rectal sphincter. Fecal impaction may be felt during digital rectal examination. A test for occult blood (guaiac test) should be performed on any stool that adheres to the gloved examining finger.

Diagnosing To establish a nursing diagnosis of constipation, the essential factors to consider in data analysis are stool consistency and frequency of defecation. According to the North American Nursing Diagnosis Association (NANDA), the diagnosis of constipation is appropriate when the client is passing hard stools and/or having bowel movements less than three times weekly. Lifestyle patterns revealed in the health history will suggest causative or contributing factors. NANDA suggests a diagnosis of "perceived constipation" when self-prescribed medications and/or enemas are used to produce daily defecation. Other appropriate diagnoses might include the following:

- Constipation related to limited activity.
- Constipation related to inadequate fluid and/or fiber.
- Constipation related to chronic use of laxatives and enemas.
- Constipation related to change in daily routine.
- Constipation related to stress and/or emotional disturbance.
- Altered health maintenance related to chronic use of laxatives.
- Fluid volume deficit related to excessive use of laxatives.

Planning If factors contributing to constipation are identified during assessment and analysis, develop a plan of care that addresses those factors amenable to nursing interventions. The emphasis of the plan is usually on client and family teaching. The long-term expected outcome is the establishment of a regular bowel elimination pattern that is appropriate for the individual client. Short-term expected outcomes include the following:

- Client describes the processes of normal bowel elimination.
- Client relates factors contributing to the problem of constipation (possibly including misuse of laxatives).
- Client describes the rationale for planned corrective measures.

Drugs That May Cause Constipation

Analgesics (opioids and nonsteroidal anti-inflammatory agents)

Antacids that contain aluminum or calcium

Anticholinergic drugs

Antidepressants (tricyclic, monoamine oxidase inhibitors)

Antidiarrheal agents

Antihistamines

Antihypertensives (calcium channel blockers, clonidine, ganglionic blocking agents)

Antiparkinsonian drugs

Barium sulfate

Diuretics

Iron supplements

Laxatives (stimulants and osmotic agents used habitually)

Muscle relaxants

Polystyrene resins

Psychotherapeutic agents (phenothiazines)[1,3]

- Client demonstrates changes in lifestyle as necessitated by contributing factors.
- Client returns to normal patterns of bowel functioning.
- Client demonstrates behaviors to monitor and correct fluid volume deficit.
- Clients adopts lifestyle changes that support individual health-care goals.

Include in the teaching plan information about the causes of constipation. Teach the client measures that promote normal elimination such as ingesting adequate fiber (see box) and fluids and exercising regularly. Teach the client the importance of establishing a regular time for defecation. Emphasize that laxative and cathartic use is contraindicated in the presence of acute abdominal pain.

Provide the client with information about the prescribed drug. Include in the teaching plan the actions of the drug and specific directions for administration. Emphasize the need for eventual weaning.

Implementing Severe constipation may require initial treatment with oral cathartics, rectal suppositories, and/or cleansing enemas. When the acute problem has been resolved, direct nursing interventions toward correcting the causative factors. Assist clients with limited mobility to assume a comfortable position for defecation and to increase their levels of activity. Include in the client's diet adequate fluids and high-fiber foods.

Evaluating On a short-term basis, the success of initial teaching about normal bowel elimination, causes of constipation, and rationale for corrective measures is evaluated by questioning the client to determine his or her level of knowledge. Further evaluation of the plan is based on assessment of objective and subjective data. Important objective findings include the frequency of defecation, fecal consistency, and other observed characteristics of the stool. Significant subjective findings include the presence or absence of complaints of pain, flatulence, and other discomforts associated with constipation. In addition, evaluation includes observation of specific client behaviors such as using drugs correctly, drinking additional fluids, planning menus for home or selecting appropriate foods from the hospital menu, and increasing levels of activity within individual limits.

On a long-term basis, the client hopefully will be able to achieve an individualized normal pattern of bowel elimination without habitual use of drugs. A possible exception is the use of bulk-forming laxatives, which are similar to dietary fiber. In institutional settings evaluation of this outcome is accomplished by observing and documenting the client's bowel eliminations. When the client is at home, outcome achievement is ascertained by self-report of the client and/or family members. Positive reinforcement should be provided for any partial attainment of the desired long-range outcome. The evaluation process includes ongoing assessment, analysis, and revision in the plan of care.

General Characteristics of Category

Drugs used for symptomatic relief of constipation are laxatives or cathartics. These terms denote intensity and duration of action. A **laxative** produces soft stools over a period of time (gentle action), whereas a **cathartic** promotes prompt fluid evacuation (purgative action). The same drug may have either a laxative or cathartic effect in a client, depending on the dosage and sensitivity of the individual. **Stool softeners** help keep stools soft for easy, natural passage. Seven subcatories of laxatives, cathartics, and stool softeners are discussed in this section: bulk-producing drugs, surfactants, lubricants, osmotic laxatives, hyperosmotic laxatives, stimulants, and bowel lavage solutions. All exert their pharmacologic actions locally within the colon itself (Fig. 48–1).

Bulk-producing drugs increase the water content and mass of feces. **Surfactants** have a detergent-like action that facilitates penetration of water and lipids into the stool; **lubricants** are oils that lubricate the outside of the fecal mass and the inside of the bowel wall. **Osmotic** and **hyperosmotic laxatives** produce their effects by drawing water into the gut. **Stimulants** or contact laxatives act on the intestinal wall to increase the amount of fluid and electrolytes within the intestinal lumen. **Bowel lavage solutions** accomplish irrigation of the entire colon with a minimal gain or loss of body fluid.

Bulk-Producing Drugs

Bulk-producing drugs have the same mechanism of action as dietary fiber. They may be used safely in the long-term management of chronic constipation. These laxatives are natural and semisynthetic polysaccharides and cellulose derivatives that swell or dissolve in the intestinal fluid, forming emollient gels that facilitate the passage of the intestinal content.[1,2]

GUIDELINES FOR HIGH-FIBER DIET

▶ Whole grain breads and cereals: at least four servings daily.

▶ Fruits and vegetables, preferably raw: at least 4 servings daily.

▶ 1-2 tablespoons of additional bran may be added daily.

BULK-PRODUCING PROTOTYPE
PSYLLIUM HYDROPHILIC COLLOID[2-5]

Psyllium hydrophilic colloid (Metamucil, Effer-Syllium, Perdiem Fiber) contains no chemical stimulants and is nonaddictive. Although it was once only a prescription drug, psyllium is now available over-the-counter (OTC).

Pharmacotherapeutics Psyllium hydrophilic colloid is used to treat a variety of conditions, including functional constipation, constipation in pregnancy, hemorrhoids, rectal surgery, colostomies, diverticulosis, irritable bowel syndrome (IBS), and chronic diarrhea.

Pharmacokinetics This drug is an indigestible polysaccharide that is not absorbed from the GI tract.

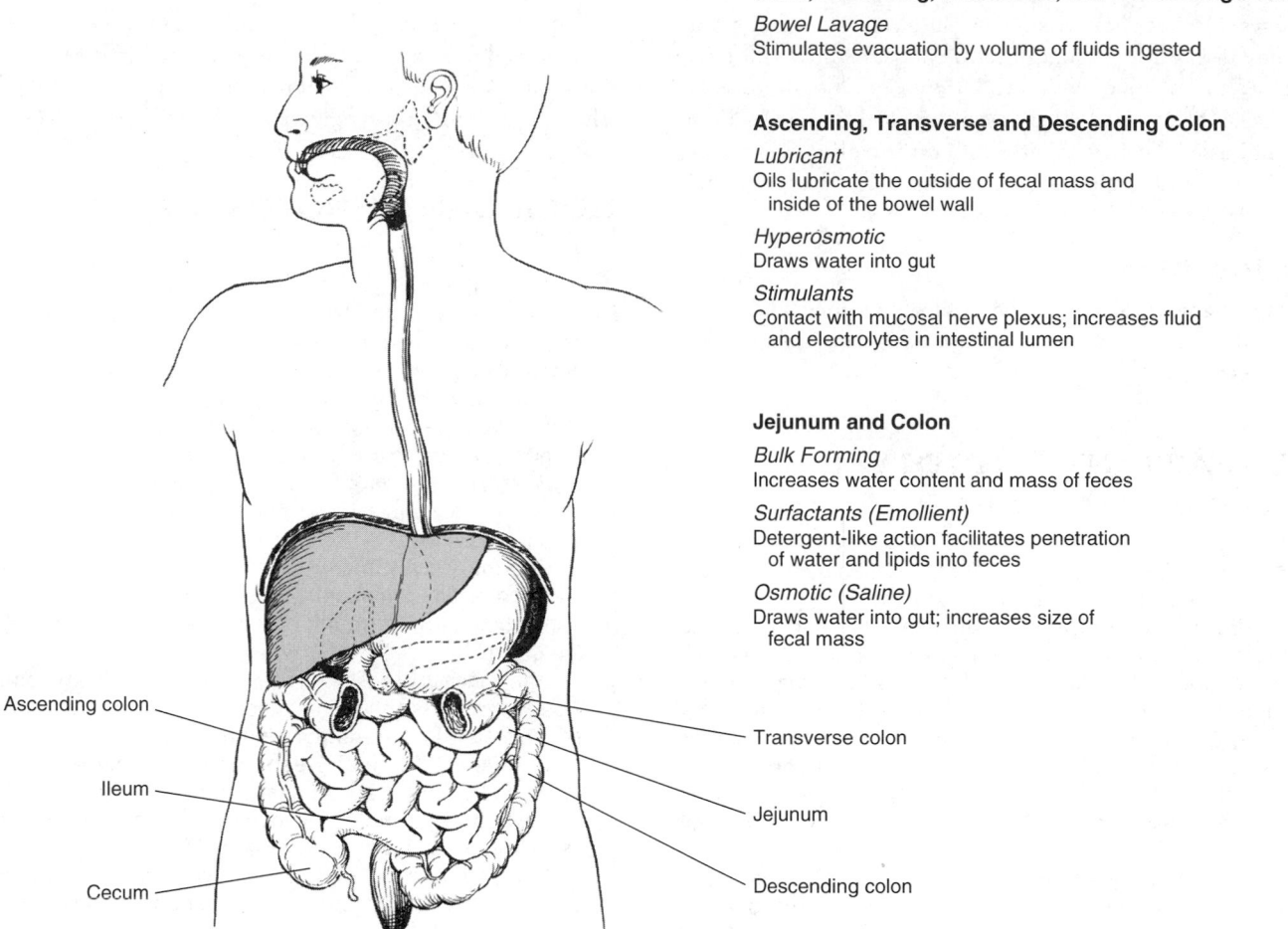

Ileum, Ascending, Transverse, and Descending Colon

Bowel Lavage
Stimulates evacuation by volume of fluids ingested

Ascending, Transverse and Descending Colon

Lubricant
Oils lubricate the outside of fecal mass and
   inside of the bowel wall

Hyperosmotic
Draws water into gut

Stimulants
Contact with mucosal nerve plexus; increases fluid
   and electrolytes in intestinal lumen

Jejunum and Colon

Bulk Forming
Increases water content and mass of feces

Surfactants (Emollient)
Detergent-like action facilitates penetration
   of water and lipids into feces

Osmotic (Saline)
Draws water into gut; increases size of
   fecal mass

Ascending colon

Ileum

Cecum

Transverse colon

Jejunum

Descending colon

FIGURE 48–1   Sites and mechanisms of action of laxatives, cathartics, and stool softeners. (Adapted from Black, J.M., & Matassarin-Jacobs, E. (1993). *Luckmann and Sorensen's Medical-Surgical Nursing: A Psychophysiologic Approach* (4th ed.). Philadelphia: W.B. Saunders.)

Pharmacodynamics Psyllium hydrophilic colloid has a local hydrophilic (water-holding) action. The drug produces soft, bulky stools within 1 to 3 days.

Pharmaceutics Psyllium hydrophilic colloid is supplied as powders, granules, and wafers for oral administration. The powders are available in flavored, effervescent, sugar-free, and low-sodium forms; flavored wafers are also available.

Undesired Clinical Responses Bloating and flatulence are common undesired clinical responses, and bowel obstruction may occur if fluid intake is inadequate. In addition, allergic reactions (urticaria, dermatitis, rhinitis, asthma) may result from inhaling the powder. Esophageal obstruction has occurred in clients who have difficulty swallowing.

Contraindications and Precautions This drug is not recommended for clients with conditions that narrow the bowel lumen. Clients with diabetes should avoid the products that contain sugar, and clients with cardiac or renal disease should avoid products with sodium.

Drug-Drug, Drug-Nutrient Interactions Psyllium may decrease the bioavailability of warfarin sodium (Coumadin). High-fiber foods have the same effect as the drug; therefore if there is an increase in dietary fiber intake, the need for the drug decreases.

Specific Drug-Related Nursing Considerations Stir powders and granules into a glass of liquid and have the client drink the mixture promptly before thickening and hardening occur. Instruct the client to drink an additional glass of fluid after each dose. Explain to the client that an optimum fluid intake of 2 to 3 L per 24 hours is essential to prevent bowel obstruction. Teach the client about the varied dosage forms available.

MISCELLANEOUS DRUGS IN CATEGORY

Other drugs in this group include **calcium polycarbophil** (FiberCon, Fiberall Chewable) and **methylcellulose** (Citrucel). These drugs are similar to psyllium in regard to pharmacokinetics and pharmacodynamics. Calcium polycarbophil is supplied in tablet, powder, and wafer forms. It is indicated for the treatment of constipation associated with IBS and diverticular disease. The calcium content is approximately 150 mg or 7.6 mEq per tablet. Ingestion of this drug in therapeutic dosages increases the risk of hypercalcemia in susceptible clients. If this drug is administered concomitantly with tetracycline, it can bind with the tetracycline and decrease its bioavailability.[6,7] Methylcellulose is supplied in powder form. If administered concomitantly with cardiac glycosides, salicylates, and nitrofurantoin (Macrodantin), it decreases their bioavailability.

Surfactants

Surfactant laxatives are also called **emollient laxatives.** These drugs soften stools for easier passage and are used on a short-term basis.

SURFACTANT PROTOTYPE
DOCUSATE SODIUM[1,2,4,5]

Docusate sodium (Colace, D-S-S, Doxinate) is not officially classified as a laxative. It is classified as a stool softener and is not considered habit forming.

Pharmacotherapeutics Docusate is used in clients with conditions such as cardiovascular disease, hernias, or general debilitation, with colon or rectal surgery, and in other situations in which straining must be avoided.

Pharmacokinetics Docusate is absorbed to a limited extent in the duodenum and proximal jejunum. The remainder of the dose passes through the lower intestinal tract. Metabolic rate and amount of the dosage absorbed are unknown.[3]

Pharmacodynamics Docusate is a surface-acting drug; it lowers the surface tension of the fecal mass. It has a local emollient action and produces soft stools in 1 to 3 days.

Pharmaceutics Docusate is supplied as soft capsules, syrup, and liquid. The liquid dosage form is packaged with a calibrated dropper for oral administration. The liquid dosage form can also be administered as an enema.

Undesired Clinical Responses Oral liquid and syrup dosage forms of the drug may cause throat irritation and nausea. A rash has been reported with some clients. The detergent properties of docusate possibly facilitate the transport of other substances across cell membranes. In addition, chronic active liver disease has occurred with prolonged use (8 months or longer) of the drug.

Drug-Drug and Drug-Environment Interactions Docusate increases the absorption of digoxin, quinidine, mineral oil, and salicylates. Docusate capsules should be stored at controlled room temperatures of 15° to 30° C.

Specific Drug-Related Nursing Considerations Encourage the client to increase fluid and fiber intake. To decrease the bitter taste associated with docusate liquid, administer the liquid in half a glass of milk or fruit juice.

MISCELLANEOUS DRUGS IN CATEGORY

Other drugs in this group include **docusate potassium** (Dialose) and **docusate calcium** (Surfak). These drugs are similar to docusate sodium in regard to pharmacodynamics. One advantage these two drugs offer is that they do not contain sodium.

Lubricants

Liquid petrolatum and other digestible plant oils coat fecal contents and prevent absorption of fecal water in the GI tract. Lubricants are used on a short-term basis in situations in which clients must avoid straining.[1,2]

LUBRICANT PROTOTYPE
MINERAL OIL[3,8-10]

Minimal difference exists among the various lubricant laxatives. However, emulsions of mineral oil penetrate and soften fecal matter more effectively than nonemulsified preparations.

Pharmacotherapeutics Mineral oil can be used in clients with cardiovascular disease, rectal or abdominal surgery, hemorrhoids, hypertension, and fecal impaction.

Pharmacokinetics As indicated previously, mineral oil is an indigestible liquid hydrocarbon with limited absorption.

Pharmacodynamics Mineral oil has a coating and lubricating action on fecal matter and bowel wall. Fecal transit time is more rapid, and less water is absorbed in the colon.

Pharmaceutics The oil is available in liquid and emulsion forms for oral administration. The liquid form is also administered in oil-retention enemas.

Undesired Clinical Responses Oral administration of mineral oil may cause nausea in some clients. In addition, when large doses of mineral oil are administered, seepage of oil through the anal sphincter may result in rectal irritation. Another danger is lipid pneumonia, which occurs after oral ingestion and subsequent aspiration of oil droplets.

Undesired clinical responses are usually associated with repeated and prolonged use. In these situations significant absorption of mineral oil may occur, especialy if emulsified products are used. If oil droplets reach the mesenteric lymph nodes, oil deposits occur in the intestinal mucosa, liver, and spleen where they produce a typical foreign body reaction.[3]

Contraindications and Precautions Mineral oil should not be administered at bedtime or to very young, elderly, or debilitated clients. Development of lipid pneumonia is more common under these circumstances.

Drug-Drug and Drug-Nutrient Interactions The actions of the oral anticoagulant warfarin sodium is increased when used with mineral oil. Mineral oil also impairs the absorption of the fat-soluble vitamins A, D, E, and K. Mineral oil should not be administered to pregnant clients because the availability of vitamin K to the fetus is decreased. In addition, mineral oil should not be taken with meals because it may delay gastric emptying.

Specific Drug-Related Nursing Considerations Chill oral preparations of mineral oil and administer the oil with juice or other beverage. Caution the client to swallow the liquid carefully and not to recline for 2 hours to prevent aspiration. A cleansing enema is frequently administered 30 to 60 minutes after an oil-retention enema.

Osmotic Laxatives

Osmotic laxatives are also called **saline laxatives.** The active ingredients in these laxatives are relatively nonabsorbable salts. The salts include magnesium salts (magnesium hydroxide, magnesium citrate, and magnesium sulfate), sodium salts (sodium phosphate and sodium potassium), and potassium salts (potassium bitartrate and potassium phosphate).[2,11]

OSMOTIC LAXATIVE PROTOTYPE

MAGNESIUM HYDROXIDE

Magnesium hydroxide (e.g., Milk of Magnesia) laxatives are used in acute situations. They should not be used for the long-term management of constipation.

Pharmacotherapeutics Magnesium hydroxide is used for acute constipation, removal of harmful substances such as poisons and parasitic worms, and stool specimen collection.

Pharmacokinetics The magnesium salt in magnesium hydroxide is poorly absorbed from the GI tract.

Pharmacodynamics Osmotic action of the magnesium salts draws water into the intestine, increasing the size of the fecal mass. As the fecal mass increases in size, stretch receptors in the intestinal wall are stimulated; this stimulation increases propulsive movements. Magnesium hydroxide may also increase GI motility and secretion by stimulating the release of cholecystokinin. Administered in low doses, magnesium hydroxide produces a soft to semisoft stool in 6 to 12 hours, a laxative effect. In high doses bowel evacuation occurs in 2 to 6 hours, a cathartic effect.

Pharmaceutics Magnesium hydroxide is available in plain and flavored oral suspensions and chewable tablets.

Undesired Clinical Responses Abdominal cramping and diarrhea may occur with magnesium hydroxide. In addition, these laxatives can cause substantial fluid loss, which may result in dehydration and electrolyte imbalance.

Contraindication and Precautions Although the absorption of magnesium hydroxide is limited, some magnesium is absorbed. Therefore magnesium can accumulate to toxic levels in clients with renal dysfunction.

Drug-Drug Interactions Magnesium hydroxide decreases the bioavailability of tetracycline and digoxin.

Specific Drug-Related Nursing Considerations To prevent dehydration, increase the client's fluid intake. Also discourage habitual use of magnesium hydroxide; habitual use can lead to dependence. In addition, since magnesium exerts a depressant effect on the central nervous system (CNS) and neuromuscular activity, assess the client for muscle weakness and electrocardiogram changes.

MISCELLANEOUS DRUGS IN CATEGORY

Other laxatives in this group include sodium phosphate, magnesium citrate, and magnesium sulfate. **Sodium phosphate** (Fleet Phospho-soda) is available in oral and rectal dosage forms. The usual oral adult dose (20 to 30 ml) contains 96.5 mEq of sodium and should be administered with caution to clients ingesting sodium-restricted diets. When administered rectally (e.g., Fleet enema), up to 10% of the sodium content may be absorbed. The use of phosphate salts in children less than 2 years of age can result in hypercalcemia.

Citrate of magnesium contains magnesium salts. The usual adult dose of 200 ml produces bowel evacuation within ½ to 3 hours. Magnesium citrate is more palatable if administered chilled.

Hyperosmotic Laxatives

Hyperosmotic laxatives have limited therapeutic use. The major laxative in this group is glycerin in suppository form. **Glycerin suppositories** are used for infants and adults and usually produce bowel evacuation within 30 minutes. The laxative effect of these suppositories is caused by the osmotic action of the glycerin. In addition, the suppositories contain sodium stearate, which acts as a local irritant on the colon.

Stimulants or Contact Laxatives

Stimulant or contact laxatives are divided into two groups: anthraquinone and diphenylmethane laxatives. **Anthraquinone compounds** are the active ingredients in cascara sagrada and senna. The most common **diphenylmethane laxatives** agents are bisacodyl and phenolphthalein.

DIPHENYLMETHANE GROUP PROTOTYPE

BISACODYL

Bisacodyl (e.g., Dulcolax) was introduced as a cathartic as a result of structure-activity studies of phenolphthalein-related compounds.

Pharmacotherapeutics Bisacodyl is used in the treatment of acute constipation. It is recommended for cleaning the colon before and after surgery and before radiologic examinations.

Pharmacokinetics Enteric-coated tablets of bisacodyl pass through the stomach intact and are converted to an active metabolite by intestinal and bacterial enzymes. Approximately 5% of the drug is absorbed and excreted in the urine; a small amount may be excreted in the bile.[1,2]

Pharmacodynamics Practically insoluble in water or a saline medium, bisacodyl exerts its action in the colon on contact with the mucosal nerve plexus. Bisacodyl produces an increase in the amount of fluid and electrolytes in the intestinal lumen. Bowel evacuation occurs in 6 to 10 hours. Rectal suppositories act directly on the intestinal wall with results in 15 to 60 minutes.[8–10]

Pharmaceutics Bisacodyl is available in enteric-coated tablets and rectal suppositories.

Undesired Clinical Responses Bisacodyl may produce abdominal cramping and diarrhea. In addition, fluid loss may lead to dehydration and electrolyte imbalance. Long-term use of the drug results in atrophy of colonic mucosa. Bisacodyl suppositories may cause a burning sensation, and with continued use, proctitis may develop.[11]

Drug-Drug and Drug-Nutrient Interactions If administered concurrently with antacids or milk, the enteric coating can dissolve, causing gastric irritation. If concurrent use of milk and antacids is necessary, bisacodyl should be administered no sooner than 1 hour after these substances.

Specific Drug-Related Nursing Considerations
Enteric-coated tablets prevent gastric irritation; therefore the tablets should not be broken or chewed. Encourage the client to consume additional fluids to prevent dehydration. Habitual use should be discouraged since dependence may develop.

MISCELLANEOUS DRUGS IN DIPHENYLMETHANE GROUP

Phenolphthalein (e.g., Ex-Lax, Phenolax) is similar in structure and actions to bisacodyl. The drug exerts its stimulating effect mainly on the colon, but the activity of the small intestine may also be increased. Phenolphthalein is effective in small doses and usually is active in 6 to 8 hours. The drug passes through the stomach unchanged and is dissolved by bile salts and alkaline intestinal secretions. Approximately 15% of the dose is absorbed; the rest is excreted unchanged in the feces. Some of the absorbed drug appears in the urine. If the urine is sufficiently alkaline, it turns a pink to red color. Similarly, the drug excreted in the feces causes a red discoloration of the feces.[5,11]

ANTHRAQUINONE GROUP PROTOTYPE

CASCARA SAGRADA

The actions of this laxative are similar to those of bisacodyl and phenolphthalein. Systemic absorption of the active ingredient produces a harmless yellowish-brown or pink color to the urine. Feces are colored light red. Prolonged use of cascara sagrada can cause reversible discoloration of colonic mucosa (melanosis coli).

Cascara sagrada is available as a fluid extract. The extract is very bitter but is more reliable than solid dosage forms. The aromatic cascara fluid extract is less active and less bitter.

MISCELLANEOUS DRUGS IN STIMULANT OR CONTACT CATEGORY

Castor oil is the only stimulant or contact laxative that acts on the small intestine. It acts quickly, producing a stool of watery consistence. Castor oil is not used for routine treatment of constipation but is used for bowel preparation before radiologic procedures. To reduce the bitter, unpleasant taste of castor oil, it can be chilled or mixed with fruit juice.

Bowel Lavage Solution

Bowel lavage solutions are not available without a prescription.

BOWEL LAVAGE PROTOTYPE

POLYETHYLENE GLYCOL SOLUTION

Polyethylene glycol solution (GoLYTELY, CoLyte) contains a mixture of polyethylene glycol, potassium chloride, sodium chloride, sodium sulfate, and sodium bicarbonate.

Pharmacotherapeutics Polyethylene glycol solutions are used to treat severe constipation. They are also used for bowel preparation before diagnostic procedures and in clients with drug overdose. These solutions can be used safely in clients who are dehydrated or sensitive to electrolyte imbalances.[11]

Pharmacokinetics Polyethylene glycol is an isosmotic solution that is not absorbed. Bowel evacuation begins approximately 1 hour after initial ingestion of the solution.

Pharmacodynamics Since this is an isosmotic solution, water and electrolytes are neither absorbed from nor secreted into the intestinal tract. Evacuation is stimulated by the large volume of solution ingested.[1,3]

Pharmaceutics The solution is prepared by mixing a powder containing the ingredients previously mentioned with 4 L of water.

Undesired Clinical Responses Nausea, cramps, and a feeling of fullness are common.

Contraindications and Precautions Use of polyethylene glycol solution is contraindicated in the presence of acute abdominal pain, obstruction, perforation, or toxic megacolon.

Drug-Drug Interaction Any oral medication given within 1 hour of the solution will be irrigated out and not absorbed.

Specific Drug-Related Nursing Considerations The solution is more palatable if chilled or served over ice. Instruct the client that rapid drinking, 250 to 300 ml every 10 minutes for 2 to 3 hours, is preferred to sipping. Inform the client that no solid food should be taken while bowel cleansing is in progress.

Miscellaneous Laxatives

Lactulose (Chronulac). Lactulose is a semisynthetic disaccharide. It is poorly absorbed and cannot be digested by intestinal enzymes. In the colon resident bacteria metabolize the drug to lactic, formic, and acetic acids. These acids exert a mild osmotic action and produce a soft-formed stool in 1 to 3 days. The adult dose is 15 to 60 ml per day. Lactulose should be used with caution in clients with diabetes mellitus. In addition to the laxative effects, lactulose traps and facilitates excretion of ammonia, thus reducing serum ammonia levels in individuals with chronic liver disease.[11,12] See Table 48–1 for information on commonly used laxatives.

Life-Span Considerations

USE OF LAXATIVES DURING PREGNANCY AND LACTATION

Constipation during pregnancy is caused by intestinal smooth muscle relaxation associated with progesterone secretion, mechanical compression of the bowel by the enlarging uterus, and the effects of iron supplements. Pregnant clients should attempt to maintain regular bowel elimination through ingestion of fluids and fiber and by regular exercise. If these measures are not effective, the health care provider should be consulted. Usually bulk-forming laxatives and surfactants are considered the drugs of choice. Castor oil is not recommended during pregnancy since it may cause uterine contractions. Mineral oil is also contraindicated since it may interfere with fat-soluble vitamin absorption.

TABLE 48–1
Laxatives

Group Generic Name	Trade Names	Routes/Dosages
Bulk-Forming Laxatives		
Psyllium hydrophilic colloid	Metamucil, Fiberall, Effer-Syllium	ADULTS Oral—2.5-4 g one to three times daily CHILDREN Oral—one half of adult dose
Methylcellulose	Citrucel	ADULTS Oral: 2 g one to three times daily CHILDREN 6-12 Y Oral: 1 g tid or qid
Calcium polycarbophil	Fibercon, Fiberall Chewable, Mitrolan	ADULTS Oral: 1 g one to four times daily CHILDREN 6-12 Y Oral: 0.5 g one to four times daily CHILDREN 2-6 Y Oral: 0.5 g one to two times daily
Surfactants		
Docusate sodium	Colace, D-S-S, Doxinate	ADULTS AND CHILDREN >12 Y Oral: 50-360 mg/d Enema: 50-100 mg (5-10 ml) of drug in retention or flushing enema CHILDREN 2-12 Y Oral: 50-150 mg/d CHILDREN <2 Y Oral: 25 mg/d
Docusate potassium	Dialose	ADULTS Oral: 100-300 mg/d CHILDREN ≤6 Y Oral: 100 mg/d
Docusate calcium	Surfak	ADULTS AND CHILDREN >12 Y Oral: 240 mg/d CHILDREN 2-12 Y Oral: 50-150 mg/d CHILDREN <2 Y Oral: 25 mg/d
Lubricants Mineral oil		ADULTS Oral: 15-45 ml Oil retention enema: 120 ml CHILDREN >6 Y Oral: 10-15 ml of emulsion Oil retention enema: 60 ml
Osmotic Laxatives		
Magnesium hydroxide suspension	Milk of Magnesia	ADULTS Oral: 30-60 ml CHILDREN ≥2 Y Oral: 5-30 ml
Sodium phosphate solution	Fleet Phospho-Soda, Fleet enema	ADULTS Oral: 20-30 ml CHILDREN Oral: 5-15 ml
Magnesium citrate		ADULTS Oral: 240 ml; repeat as needed CHILDREN Oral: 120 ml; repeat as needed
Hyperosmotic Laxatives Glycerin		ADULTS AND CHILDREN >6 Y Rectal suppository: 3 g Enema: 5-15 ml INFANTS AND CHILDREN <6 Y Rectal suppository: 1-1.5 g Enema: 2-5 ml

Table continued on following page.

TABLE 48–1 *Continued*
Laxatives

Group Generic Name	Trade Names	Routes/Dosages
Bowel Lavage		**Bowel Evacuation**
Polyethylene glycol solution	CoLyte, GoLYTELY	**ADULTS** Oral: 4 L over 3-4 h: 240-300 ml (8-10 oz) q10min **Severe Constipation** **ADULTS** Oral: 500 ml/d for 5 d
Stimulants		
DIPHENYLMETHANES		
Bisacodyl	Dulcolax	**ADULTS** Oral: up to 30 mg Rectal: one suppository **CHILDREN >6 Y** Oral: 5 mg Rectal: one half suppository
Phenolphthalein	Correctol, Ex-Lax, Feen-a-Mint	**ADULTS** oral: 30-270 mg **CHILDREN ≥6 Y** Oral: 30-60 mg **CHILDREN 2-5 Y** Oral: 15-20 mg
ANTHRAQUINONES		**Granules**
Senna	Senokot, Perdiem	**ADULTS** Oral: up to 4 tsp/d **CHILDREN >27 KG** Oral: one half adult dose **PREGNANT OR ELDERLY CLIENT** Oral: one half adult dose **Syrup** **ADULTS** Oral: 2-3 tsp hs (up to 30 ml/d) **PREGNANT OR ELDERLY CLIENT** Oral: one half adult dose **CHILDREN 5-15 Y** Oral: 1-2 tsp hs (up to 20 ml/d) **CHILDREN 1-5 Y** Oral: ½-1 tsp hs (up to 10 ml/d) **INFANTS 1-12 MO** Oral: ¼-½ tsp hs (up to 5 ml/d) **Tablets** **ADULTS** Oral: 2 tablets (up to 8/d) **CHILDREN >27 KG** Oral: one half adult dose **PREGNANT OR ELDERLY CLIENT** Oral: one half adult dose **Rectal** **ADULTS** One suppository; may repeat in 2 h
Cascara sagrada		**ADULTS** Oral: 5 ml **CHILDREN ≥2 Y** Oral: 2.5 ml **CHILDREN 2 Y** Oral: 1-2 ml
Castor oil		**ADULTS** Oral: 15-60 ml **CHILDREN ≥2 Y** Oral: 5-15 ml **CHILDREN <2 Y** Oral: 1-5 ml

Nursing mothers should also try to regulate their bowel elimination without the use of laxatives. Bulk-forming agents and surfactants are considered safe. Use of the anthraquinones (senna, cascara, and casanthranol) should be avoided because they are excreted in breast milk.[2,13,14]

USE OF LAXATIVES WITH PEDIATRIC CLIENTS

Stool patterns vary widely in children. Normally neonates pass more than four stools a day during the first week of life. This rate declines to one or two stools per day by 4 years of age. Such factors as increased emotional distress, family conflict, changes in diet, febrile illness, or recent travel can alter bowel habits in children. Since constipation in children can be a complex problem difficult to detect and manage, parents should be taught to note any deviation from the child's normal pattern of defecation.[2,15]

A significant number of children have chronic functional constipation. This condition, which sometimes begins in infancy, tends to be self-perpetuating. Large, hard stools are retained because defecation is painful. Chronic distention of the rectum and colon gradually decreases the child's awareness of the need to defecate. This results in more retention, water absorption, and hardening of the stool. As the rectum becomes dilated, liquid stool oozes around the hard mass as involuntary **encopresis** (soiling).[16–18]

In general, when constipation has been diagnosed, treatment takes place in three phases: (1) evacuation of the hard stool by using enemas and/or laxatives; (2) establishment of regular elimination of soft stools using laxatives and dietary counseling; and (3) establishment of regular bowel habits with the use of little or no medication. For all of these measures, the child's age should be considered and the primary health care provider consulted.

USE OF LAXATIVES WITH ADULT CLIENTS

Although bowel function is usually good in young adults, hectic lifestyles may result in habits that eventually contribute to constipation. These habits include failure to establish a regular time and place for defecation, inadequate dietary fiber intake, and insufficient exercise. Self-medication with laxatives often begins in middle age as many adults assume increasingly sedentary lifestyles. Teaching about diet, exercise, and stress management assists many adults to maintain normal bowel elimination without dependence on drugs.

USE OF LAXATIVES WITH ELDERLY CLIENTS

Since intestinal motility decreases with aging, constipation is common in the older age group. Poor appetite, difficulty chewing, and reduced activity also contribute to the problem. Many elderly individuals use laxatives habitually to evacuate themselves. These individuals should be encouraged to regulate bowel elimination by dietary modification and exercise regimens.

For clients requiring laxatives, bulk-forming agents are taken to supplement dietary fiber, and surfactants are often used on a short-term basis. Since osmotic agents and stimulant or contact laxatives may cause significant fluid and electrolyte loss, they should be used sparingly. Use of lubricant laxatives in this age group is also discouraged. The danger of aspiration and lipid pneumonia exists with mineral oil use, and castor oil is too harsh for use in the elderly.[10,19]

CONCEPT REVIEW

Constipation is frequently caused by lifestyle factors such as inadequate intake of fluids and fiber, insufficient exercise, hectic schedules with no established pattern for defecation, and excessive use of laxatives and enemas.

When constipation is treatable without the use of drugs, the primary role of the nurse is client education.

Most laxatives, cathartics, and stool softeners discussed in this section are available without a prescription. Selection of an appropriate OTC drug should be based on the client's age and clinical status.

DRUGS USED TO TREAT DIARRHEA

Since the frequency of bowel movements varies with the individual, diarrhea cannot be defined by number of stools per day. Usually, **diarrhea** is characterized by an increase in the frequency of profuse, watery, loose stools during a limited period. An abnormal increase in passage of formed stools can also be considered diarrhea.[2,8]

Contributing Factors

Acute diarrhea usually results from a bacterial or viral infection. Acute diarrhea can also be caused by an overgrowth of pathogens secondary to antibiotic suppression of normal flora (superinfection) or as an undesired clinical response to drug therapy (see box). If severe, acute diarrhea can cause substantial fluid and electrolyte loss and be fatal, especially in infants and young children. Diarrhea that accompanies **food poisoning** results from eating food or fluids contaminated by microbes during preparation, serving, and/or storage. **Traveler's diarrhea** occurs in individuals who travel to countries where

---

DRUGS THAT MAY CAUSE DIARRHEA

- Antacids containing magnesium
- Antihypertensives such as guanethidine, methyldopa, and reserpine
- Antimicrobials
- Antineoplastic drugs
- Bile acids
- Cardiac glycoside
- Cholinergic agonists and cholinesterase inhibitors
- Osmotic laxatives
- Quinidine
- Stimulant laxatives[2,13]

enteric pathogens are prevalent. Common causes of **chronic diarrhea** include malabsorption, IBD, and surgical procedures that shorten the intestinal tract (short-gut syndrome) or cause rapid stomach emptying (dumping syndrome).[4,13]

⁂ NURSING CONSIDERATIONS

Nursing care for an individual receiving antidiarrheal drugs is based on assessing, diagnosing, planning, implementing, and evaluating.

Assessing A thorough health history and physical assessment should be performed. (See also Nursing Considerations in previous section on Constipation.) Question the client with acute diarrhea about exposure to infected individuals and/or possible carriers of enteric infection, consumption of potentially contaminated food or water, and/or travel to foreign counties. A sexual history is also pertinent since diarrhea may be a manifestation of gay bowel syndrome in male homosexuals. Include in the physical assessment a careful examination of the skin and mucous membranes; this provides important information about hydration status.

Diagnosing Data analysis focuses initially on the client's pattern of defecation and state of hydration. If the defecation pattern includes loose or watery stools and/or increased frequency of defecation to more than three times daily, a nursing diagnosis of diarrhea is appropriate. Possible nursing diagnoses associated with clients receiving drug therapy for diarrhea include the following:

• Fluid volume deficit related to diarrhea.
• Impaired skin integrity related to excess fluid loss.
• Diarrhea related to drug therapy (state specific cause).
• Constipation related to excessive or improper use of antidiarrheal drugs.

Planning For the client with diarrhea, essential elements of the care plan should include maintenance of adequate hydration, gradual progression to a regular diet, maintenance of skin integrity, and limited use of prescribed drugs. Expected outcomes are based on the appropriate client-oriented nursing diagnoses and include the following:

• Client maintains fluid volume at a functional level as evidenced by adequate urinary output, moist mucous membranes, and prompt capillary refill.
• Client demonstrates behaviors to prevent impaired skin integrity.
• Client reestablishes normal pattern of bowel functioning.
• Client verbalizes understanding of factors contributing to constipation.

Implementing Initially, parenteral fluid use may be indicated to help the client achieve adequate hydration. When solid food is permitted, a bland or low-residue diet may be prescribed (see box).

Antidiarrheal drugs are intended for use on a short-term basis only. Instruct the client and/or family caregiver in the action of any prescribed drugs and the specific directions for administration.

Evaluating Evaluation of the plan is based on assessment of objective and subjective data. Important objective findings

---

> ### GUIDELINES FOR BLAND OR LOW-RESIDUE DIET
>
> Teach the client to select a balanced diet from the following items:
>
> ▶ Dairy products: milk, buttermilk, yogurt, cottage cheese, cheddar cheese*
>
> ▶ Eggs: cooked, poached, or scrambled
>
> ▶ Meats: fish or fowl; ground beef or lamb
>
> ▶ Soups: strained soups or broths
>
> ▶ Vegetables: well-cooked without skins; potatoes—boiled, mashed, or baked
>
> ▶ Fruits: cooked or canned without skins; strained juices
>
> ▶ Breads and cereals: refined breads and cereals; rice; pastas
>
> ▶ Margarine or butter
>
> ▶ Desserts: ice cream, custard, frozen yogurt, pudding, gelatin, plain cake, or cookies*
>
> *Dairy products should be restricted if they precipitate diarrhea in the individual.

---

include the frequency of defecation, fecal consistency, and other observed characteristics of the stool. Significant subjective findings include the presence or absence of complaints of abdominal cramping, flatulence, and other discomforts associated with diarrhea. In addition, evaluate the client's ability to use prescribed drugs correctly and plan menus for home use. Also evaluate the status of the expected outcomes.

General Characteristics of Category

Most antidiarrheal drugs are **opioids** or **anti-inflammatory agents** (Table 48–2). Both of these groups act by decreasing intestinal motility, lengthening transit time, and increasing absorption of fluids and electrolytes. Some nonprescription drugs act as adsorbents, but the therapeutic value of these agents is questionable. An antisecretory hormonal agent is under extensive study for its potential benefit in the treatment of severe, refractory diarrhea.

Opioid Antidiarrheal Drugs

Opioid drugs are the most effective antidiarrheal drugs. Several opioid preparations—diphenoxylate, difenoxin, loperamide, paregoric, and opium tincture—are approved for treatment of diarrhea.[11] Diphenoxylate (Lomotil) and loperamide (Imodium) are used the most frequently.

OPIOID ANTIDIARRHEAL PROTOTYPE

DIPHENOXYLATE HYDROCHLORIDE

Diphenoxylate hydrochloride (Logen, Lonox, Lomotil) is chemically related to the narcotic meperidine (Demerol). For antidiarrheal use, diphenoxylate is combined with a subtherapeutic amount of atropine sulfate, an anticholinergic agent. Atropine sulfate is added to discourage deliberate overdosing. This combination is classified as a Schedule V controlled substance by federal law.[5]

Pharmacotherapeutics Diphenoxylate is used only in the treatment of acute, self-limiting diarrhea.

Pharmacokinetics Diphenoxylate is insoluble in water. However, in humans diphenoxylate is rapidly and extensively metabolized by ester hydrolysis to diphenoxylic acid, which is biologically active. Diphenoxylate is excreted in the urine and has a half-life of approximately 12 hours.[5]

Pharmacodynamics Depressant action on receptors in the GI tract produces decreased intestinal motility and lengthens transit time. CNS depression may also occur, but it is minimal when the recommended dosage schedule is followed.

Pharmaceutics Diphenoxylate with atropine is available in tablet or liquid form for oral administration.

Undesired Clinical Responses Nervous system effects such as depression, euphoria, confusion, sedation, restlessness, and headache have been reported. In addition, allergic responses such as anaphylaxis, urticaria, and pruritus can occur. Since the drug contains atropine, hyperthermia, tachycardia, urinary retention, flushing, and dryness of the skin and mucous membranes are possible.

Contraindications and Precautions Diphenoyxlate with atropine should be used with caution in clients with acute bowel infection or inflammation, glaucoma, or prostatic hypertrophy. This drug is classified as a Pregnancy Category C drug.

Drug-Drug Interactions Diphenoxylate with atropine potentiates the action of other CNS depressants such as alcohol, barbiturates, and tranquilizers. Concurrent use with monoamine oxidase inhibitors (MAOIs) may precipitate hypertensive crisis.

Specific Drug-Related Nursing Considerations Assess the client for dehydration and provide appropriate fluid replacement if needed. Since the liquid dosage form of diphenoxylate has an unpleasant taste, administer the drug in a beverage of the client's choice. Monitor the client's response to the drug; clinical improvement is usually observed within 48 hours. Anticipate that the dosage will be reduced once initial control of the diarrhea has been achieved.

MISCELLANEOUS DRUGS IN CATEGORY

Loperamide hydrochloride (Imodium A-D) is indicated for the control and symptomatic relief of acute, nonspecific diarrhea. It acts by slowing intestinal motility and by affecting water and electrolyte movement through the bowel. The drug is poorly absorbed and does not readily cross the blood-brain barrier. Loperamide has minimal potential for abuse and is not classified as a controlled substance. It is available without prescription in capsule and liquid forms for oral administration.[2,20]

Paregoric, **camphorated opium tincture,** is a dilute solution of powdered opium and morphine sulfate. It acts by decreasing hydrochloric acid secretion and stomach motility and increasing antral tone. Paregoric also decreases propulsive contractions in the small intestine. Since the drug contains both opium and morphine, it is classified as a Schedule III Controlled Substance.[4,5,11]

Sometimes, paregoric is administered in combination with **kaolin** and **pectin.** The kaolin adsorbs irritants and forms a protective coating on the intestinal mucosa. Pectin acts to consolidate the stool. The mixture of the three drugs effectively controls diarrhea and colicky cramps.

Anti-Inflammatory Antidiarrheal Drugs

Bismuth subsalts are used in antidiarrheal preparations as adsorbents, astringents, protectives, and anti-inflammatory agents.

ANTI-INFLAMMATORY ANTIDIARRHEAL PROTOTYPE
BISMUTH SUBSALICYLATE

Bismuth subsalicylate (Pepto-Bismol) is a nonprescription drug. It is the only available bismuth subsalicylate.

Pharmacotherapeutics Bismuth subsalicylate is used in the treatment of nonspecific acute diarrhea and enterotoxic bacterial diarrhea. It is also used in the prevention and treatment of traveler's diarrhea.

Pharmacokinetics Bismuth subsalicylate is a salt that partially dissociates in the stomach. The salicylate is absorbed in the small intestine and reaches peak serum levels in 1 to 2 hours. It is excreted in the urine. Even when repeated doses of bismuth subsalicylate are given, steady-state blood levels generally remain lower and safer than those that occur with acetylsalicylic acid (aspirin) ingestion. The bismuth forms other salts that pass into the colon and react with the hydrogen sulfide produced by anaerobic bacteria. This action produces bismuth sulfide, an insoluble black salt that imparts a dark color to the feces.[21,22]

Pharmacodynamics The anti-inflammatory action of the salicylate inhibits motility and secretion in the lower intestinal tract. Bismuth subsalicylate also binds the toxins of certain bacteria (*Escherichia coli* and *Vibrio cholerae*) and may have some antimicrobial activity.[22]

Pharmaceutics Bismuth subsalicylate is available in chewable tablets and flavored liquid for oral administration.

Undesired Clinical Responses This drug may cause fecal impaction in infants and elderly individuals. If ingested in large doses, the salicylate may cause ringing in the ears, a sign of salicylism. In addition, bismuth is potentially neurotoxic.

Contraindications and Precautions Bismuth subsalicylate use is contraindicated in clients allergic to acetylsalicylic acid. Because of the danger of Reye's syndrome, its use is also contraindicated in children and teenagers with viral infections.

Drug-Drug Interactions Bismuth subsalicylate decreases the bioavailability of tetracycline. The drug also has an additive effect with other salicylates, thus increasing the likelihood of salicylism.

Specific Drug-Related Nursing Considerations Instruct the client to chew the tablets or allow them to dissolve in the mouth. Suggest to the client that the liquid dosage form be mixed with a beverage. Advise the client that the drug imparts a gray or black color to the tongue and feces. For individuals traveling abroad, suggest they carry a kit containing bismuth subsalicylate and an antimicrobial agent for prophylactic use.[23,24]

Adsorbent Antidiarrheal Drugs

The main GI adsorbents used are activated charcoal, aluminum hydroxide, attapulgite, bismuth subsalts, kaolin, magnesium trisilicate, and pectin. Adsorbents are the most frequently used type of drugs in nonprescription antidiarrheal preparations.

ADSORBENT ANTIDIARRHEAL DRUG PROTOTYPE

ACTIVATED ATTAPULGITE

Activated attapulgite (Kaopectate) is a nonspecific antidiarrheal drug; it does not treat the underlying cause of the diarrhea.

Pharmacotherapeutics Despite the common use of attapulgite for treatment of nonspecific diarrhea, there is insufficient evidence to support its effectiveness.

Pharmacokinetics Attapulgite is similar to kaolin, a hydrated nonabsorbable aluminum clay.

Pharmacodynamics Although the adsorbent clay produces stools with a more normal appearance, body fluid loss may remain unchanged, and electrolyte loss may actually increase. The claim that adsorbents facilitate removal of bacterial toxins has not been substantiated.

Pharmaceutics Attapulgite is available in liquid form and chewable tablets for oral administration.

Undesired Clinical Responses Attapulgite may increase fecal excretion of sodium and potassium.

Drug-Drug and Drug-Nutrient Interactions Activated attapulgite decreases the bioavailability of any oral drug administered within a 2- to 3-hour period. This drug can also interfere with nutrient absorption.

Specific Drug-Related Nursing Considerations Clients intending to purchase nonprescription antidiarrheal remedies should be advised that adsorbents have no established therapeutic value. Loperamide and bismuth subsalicylate, also available without prescription, have demonstrated effectiveness.

Hormonal Antisecretory Antidiarrheal Drugs

Use of hormonal antisecretory drugs for treatment of diarrhea is still in the investigational phase.

HORMONAL ANTISECRETORY ANTIDIARRHEAL PROTOTYPE

OCTREOTIDE ACETATE

Octreotide (Sandostatin) is classified primarily as an antineoplastic drug. Octreotide exerts pharmacologic actions similar to those of the natural hormone somatostatin.[4,5]

Pharmacotherapeutics Octreotide is used as an investigational drug to treat severe, refractory diarrhea. Some of the conditions that cause this problem are acquired immunodeficiency syndrome (AIDS), graft-versus-host disease, hormone-secreting tumors, severe enterotoxic infections, short-gut syndrome, and dumping syndrome.[25–28]

Pharmacokinetics After subcutaneous (SC) injection, octreotide is absorbed rapidly and completely from the injection site. Peak plasma concentration is achieved within 30 minutes. Intravenous (IV) administration produces peak plasma concentration within 4 minutes. Distribution of the drug is rapid. Approximately 32% of a dose is excreted unchanged into the urine; the remainder is eliminated in the bile and by proteolysis.

Pharmacodyamics Octreotide is described as the "universal inhibitor of secretory cells."[28] It decreases the secretion of various gastroenteropancreatic hormones. It also decreases motility and increases fluid and electrolyte absorption.

Pharmaceutics Octreotide is available in sterile parenteral solution for IV and SC use.

Undesired Clinical Responses Common side effects include transient nausea and cramping. Localized discomfort at the injection site may also occur. Since octreotide decreases emptying of the gallbladder, gallstones may form. Octreotide also alters pancreatic secretion of insulin and glucagon.

Contraindications and Precautions Octreotide use is contraindicated in children because it suppresses the growth hormone. It is classified as a Pregnancy Category B drug.

Drug-Drug, Drug-Nutrient, and Drug-Environment Interactions Insulin dosage in diabetic clients usually needs adjustment. There is also evidence that octreotide acetate alters absorption of dietary fats in some clients. In addition, ampules and vials should be stored in the refrigerator; they can be stored at room temperature only for the day of their administration.

Specific Drug-Related Nursing Considerations Blood glucose levels should be monitored carefully, especially in diabetic clients. Caregivers in the home setting need instruction in the technique of deep SC injection.

MISCELLANEOUS DRUGS USED TO TREAT DIARRHEA

Diarrhea is a significant complication for the client being fed through a tube. In an attempt to alleviate this problem, bulk-forming laxatives are added to enteral feedings. The primary drug used is psyllium hydrophilic mucilloid, which was discussed previously in the chapter.[29,30]

🌿 NURSING RESEARCH

Heather, D.J., Howell, L., Montana, M., Howell, M., & Hill, R. (1991). Effect of bulk-forming cathartic on diarrhea in tube-fed patients. *Heart & Lung, 20*, 409-413.

The purpose of this study was to determine if bulk-forming cathartics administered to tube-fed patients would result in firmer stools. A convenience sample of 49 patients receiving tube feedings was used; 25 subjects were assigned to an experimental group and 24 to a control group. Subjects in the experimental group received 5 ml of a psyllium preparation in their tube feedings three times daily for 6 days. Stool consistency was measured on a seven-point scale. When the two groups were compared, the hypothesis that administration of the psyllium preparation would lead to firmer stool consistency was supported. No apparent difference in stool frequency was noted.

STUDENT ACTIVITIES

• Determine the procedure for enteral feedings in your assigned agency.
• Request permission to monitor the elimination pattern of six clients receiving enteral nutrition through a nasogastric or nasoduodenal tube. Note frequency and consistency of stools.

Life-Span Considerations

Life-span considerations must be addressed whenever antidiarrheal drugs are prescribed.

USE OF ANTIDIARRHEAL DRUGS DURING PREGNANCY AND LACTATION

If diarrhea develops during pregnancy or lactation, it should be managed without drugs whenever possible. Use of opioids, which cause CNS depression, is especially undesirable. In addition, bismuth subsalicylate use should be avoided because of the salicylate component.

USE OF ANTIDIARRHEAL DRUGS WITH PEDIATRIC CLIENTS

Fluid replacement is crucial when diarrhea develops in infants and toddlers since it can lead to life-threatening dehydration. However, antidiarrheal drugs have limited value in this age group, and there is concern about possible toxicity. Although there are suggested pediatric dosages for diphenoxylate with atropine and for loperamide, the World Health Organization does not recommend giving either of these drugs to children.[31]

USE OF ANTIDIARRHEAL DRUGS WITH ADULT CLIENTS

Young and middle-aged adults who are in good general health may use antidiarrheal drugs safely on a short-term basis within the guidelines described in this section. Dehydration is less likely to occur in this age group than in young children and the elderly.

USE OF ANTIDIARRHEAL DRUGS WITH ELDERLY CLIENTS

Diarrhea in older adults can easily lead to serious fluid volume deficit. Fluid replacement must be undertaken with caution so that volume overload does not occur. Since glaucoma and prostatic hypertrophy are both common in geriatric clients, combination drugs such as Lomotil that contain atropine must be used with discretion.

CONCEPT REVIEW

Since many OTC antidiarrheal drugs are available, diarrhea is frequently self-treated by clients.
Clients should be cautioned that diarrhea can result in loss of fluid and electrolytes.
Causative factor, age, and physical condition of the client must be considered before recommending an antidiarrheal drug.
Antidiarrheal drugs are classified as *specific* and *nonspecific*. Specific antidiarrheal drugs treat the causative factor.

DRUGS USED TO TREAT INFLAMMATORY BOWEL DISEASE

There are two forms of IBD: Crohn's disease and ulcerative colitis. Treatment of these diseases depends on the severity of the symptoms. Severe IBD requires surgery. When the condition is mild, it usually can be managed with dietary measures and drugs. The most commonly prescribed drugs are sulfasalazine and glucocorticoids. These drugs may be used alone or in combination.

INFLAMMATORY BOWEL DISEASE DRUG PROTOTYPE

SULFASALAZINE

Sulfasalazine (Azulfidine) belongs to the same chemical family as the sulfonamide antibiotics. However, sulfasalazine is classified as an *anti-inflammatory agent.*

Pharmacodynamics After oral administration approximately one third of the dose of sulfasalazine is absorbed in the small intestine. The remaining drug enters the colon where the compound is split into 5-aminosalicylic acid (5-ASA) and sulfapyridine. It is the 5-ASA that is responsible for the drug's anti-inflammatory actions.[5]

Undesired Clinical Responses The most common responses associated with sulfasalazine are anorexia, headache, nausea, vomiting, and gastric distress. Less frequent undesired clinical responses include skin rash, pruritus, fever, urticaria, and hemolytic anemia.[4,5]

Pharmaceutics Sulfasalazine is available as plain-coated, uncoated, and enteric-coated tablets. The drug dosage is adjusted to each individual's response and tolerance. **Initial therapy** for adults usually consists of 3 to 4 g daily. For children 2 years of age and older, 40 to 60 mg per kilogram of body weight is recommended. **Maintenance dose** for the adult is usually 2 g per day, and for children 2 years of age and older, 30 mg per kilogram of body weight is recommended. **The drug must be given in evenly divided doses over a 24-hour period. The interval between doses should not exceed 8 hours.[3,4]**

Glucocorticoids

Glucocorticoids decrease the body's inflammatory response. When present in large amounts, glucocorticoids inhibit the release of histamine and counteract potentially de-

TABLE 48–2
Antidiarrheal and Antiflatulent Drugs

Group and Generic Name	Trade Names	Routes/Dosages
Opiate Antidiarrheal Drugs		
Diphenoxylate with atropine	Lomotil	**ADULTS** Oral: 5-10 mg three to four times daily **CHILDREN 2-12 Y** Oral: 0.3-0.4 mg/kg/d in divided doses; liquid dosage form only
Paregoric (camphorated opium tincture)		**ADULTS** Oral: 5-10 ml, maximum of qid **CHILDREN** Oral: 0.25-0.5 ml/kg; maximum of qid
Loperamide	Imodium A-D	**ADULTS** Oral: initial dose, 4 mg; then 2 mg after each loose stool; then 2-4 mg one to two times daily; maximum 16 mg/d **CHILDREN 2-5 Y (13-20 KG)** Oral: first day, 1 mg tid **CHILDREN 5-8 Y (20-30 KG)** Oral: first day, 2 mg bid **CHILDREN 8-12 Y (>30 KG)** Oral: First day, 2 mg tid **CHILDREN 2-12 Y** Follow first day's dose with 1 kg/10 kg after each loose stool; do not exceed first day doses
Anti-Inflammatory Antidiarrheal Drugs		
Bismuth subsalicylate	Pepto-Bismol	**ADULTS** Oral: 30 ml or two tablets initially; repeat q30-60 min up to 8 doses per 24 h **CHILDREN 3-6 Y** Oral: 5 ml/initially **CHILDREN 6-9 Y** Oral: 10 ml initially **CHILDREN 9-12 Y** Oral: 15 ml or one tablet initially
Adsorbent Antidiarrheal Drugs		
Activated attapulgite or kaolin and pectin	Kaopectate	**ADULTS** Oral: 2 tbsp or two caplets initially followed by 1 tbsp or two caplets after each loose stool (maximum of 12 caplets or 14 tbsp in 24 h) **CHILDREN 6-12 Y** Oral: 1 tbsp or one caplet initially, followed by ½ tbsp or one caplet after each loose stool (maximum of six caplets or 7 tbsp in 24 h) **CHILDREN 3-6 Y** Oral: ½ tbsp after each loose stool (maximum of seven doses in 24 h)
Hormonal Antisecretory Antidiarrheal Drugs		
Octreotide acetate	Sandostatin	**ADULTS** SC: initial dose, 50 μg; increase according to client's response IV: dose individually determined
Antiflatulent Drug		
Simethicone	Mylicon, Phazyme, Gas-X; also an ingredient in many antacids	**ADULTS** Oral: 40-125 mg qid

structive reactions. Glucocorticoids are discussed further in Chapter 42.

DRUGS USED TO TREAT FLATULENCE

Flatulence refers to the presence of excessive gas in the intestinal tract. It is an exaggeration of the normal process of gas production by bacterial fermentation in the colon. Complaints of flatulence are related to excessive gas production, decreased motility causing distention, increased motility causing rapid expulsion, and/or increased sensitivity on the part of the client. It is a common complaint in postoperative clients and in individuals with IBS. Gas-forming foods that contain certain indigestible carbohydrates have also been implicated.

Antiflatulents alter the surface tension of gas bubbles, causing them to coalesce. The coalesced bubbles are dispersed and expelled more readily, producing symptomatic relief of discomfort. The prototype for this drug group is simethicone (Table 48–2).

ANTIFLATULENT PROTOTYPE
SIMETHICONE

Simethicone (Mylicon, Gas-X, Phazyme) is an inert silicone substance that is not absorbed from the GI tract. It is excreted unchanged in the feces. Simethicone is available in oral liquids and as both tablets and chewable tablets. Undesired clinical responses are rare, but nausea has been reported.

SUMMARY

The problems of constipation and diarrhea have many causes but are often related to lifestyle factors, in which case the focus of the nursing care is on client education. In many instances clients self-treat these conditions with OTC drugs. Again, the role of the nurse is to educate the client about safe use of these products.

REFERENCES
1. Robinson, B.L., & Hecht, G. (1992). Constipation. In R.E. Rakel (Ed.), *1992 Conn's current therapy* (pp. 17-19). Philadelphia: W.B. Saunders.
2. American Pharmaceutical Association (1990). *Handbook of nonprescription drugs* (9th ed.). Washington, DC: Author.
3. American Medical Association (1992). *Drug evaluations.* Chicago: Author.
4. U.S. Pharmacopeial Convention (1990). *The United States pharmacopeia* (22nd rev.). Rockville, MD: Author.
5. Data Pharmaceutica, Inc. (1993). *1993 physicians' genRx.* Smithtown, NY: Author.
6. Snape, W.J. (1989). The effect of methylcellulose on symptoms of constipation. *Clinical Therapeutics, 11,* 572-579.
7. Swartz, M.L. (1989). Citrucel (methylcellulose/bulk-forming laxative). *Gastroenterology Nursing, 12*(1), 50-52.
8. Garcia, G. (1992). Gastrointestinal disorders. In K.L. Melman, et al. (Eds.), *Melman and Morrelli's clinical pharmacology: Basic principles in therapeutics* (3rd ed.). (pp. 219-232). New York: McGraw-Hill.
9. Karig, A.W., & Hartshorn, E.A. (1991). *Counseling patients on their medications.* Hamilton, IL: Intelligence Publications.
10. Yakabowich, M. (1990). Prescribe with care: The role of laxatives in the treatment of constipation. *Journal of Gerontological Nursing, 16*(7), 4-11.
11. Lehne, R.A. (1994). *Pharmacology for nursing care* (2nd ed.). Philadelphia: W.B. Saunders.
12. Lederle, F.A., Busch, D.L., Mattox, K.M., West, M.J., & Aske, D.M. (1990). Cost-effective treatment of constipation: A randomized double-blind comparison of sorbitol and lactulose. *American Journal of Medicine, 89,* 597-601.
13. Brunton, L.L. (1990). Agents affecting gastrointestinal water flux and mobility, digestants, and bile acids. In R. Goodman, E.W. Gilman, T. Rall, A. Nies, & P. Taylor (Eds.), *Goodman and Gilman's the pharmacological basis of therapeutics* (8th ed.) (pp. 914-932). New York: Pergamon Press.
14. Rayburn, W.F., & Zuspan, F.P. (Eds.) (1991). *Drug therapy in obstetrics and gynecology* (3rd ed.). St. Louis: C.V. Mosby.
15. Evans, K. (1990). Pediatric management problems: Chronic constipation. *Pediatric Nursing, 16,* 590-591.
16. Ellett, M.L. (1990). Constipation/encopresis: A nursing perspective. *Journal of Pediatric Health Care, 4*(3), 141-146.
17. Sprague-McRae, J.M. (1990). Encopresis: Developmental, behavioral and physiological considerations for treatment. *Nurse Practitioner, 15*(6), 8-24.
18. Gleghorn, E.E. (1991). No-enema therapy for idiopathic constipation and encopresis. *Clinical Pediatrics, 30,* 669-672.
19. Cheskin, L.J., & Schuster, M.M. (1990). Constipation. In W.R. Hazzard, R. Andres, E.L. Bierman, & J.P. Blass (Eds.), *Principles of geriatric medicine and gerontology* (2nd ed.) (pp. 1161-1167). New York: McGraw-Hill.
20. Ericsson, C.D., & Johnson, P.C. (1990). Safety and efficacy of loperamide. *American Journal of Medicine, 88*(Suppl. 6A), 10S-14S.
21. Bierer, D.W. (1990). Bismuth subsalicylate: History, chemistry, and safety. *Reviews of Infectious Diseases, 12*(Suppl. 1), S3-S8.
22. Gorbach, S.L. (1990). Bismuth therapy in gastrointestinal disease. *Gastroenterology, 99,* 863-875.
23. Gryboski, J.D., & Kocoshis, S. (1990). Effect of bismuth subsalicylate on chronic diarrhea in childhood: A preliminary report. *Reviews of Infectious Diseases, 12*(Suppl. 1), S36-S40.
24. Steffen, R. (1990). Worldwide efficacy of bismuth subsalicylate in the treatment of traveler's diarrhea. *Reviews of Infectious Diseases, 12*(Suppl. 1), S80-S86.
25. Ely, P., Dunitz, J., Rogosheske, J., & Weisdorf, D. (1991). Use of somatostatin analogue, octreotide acetate, in the management of acute gastrointestinal graft-versus-host disease. *American Journal of Medicine, 90,* 707-710.
26. Flanning, M., et al. (1991). Pilot study of sandostatin (octreotide) therapy of refractory HIV-associated diarrhea. *Digestive Diseases and Sciences, 36,* 476-480.
27. Greenberg, R.N. (1991). Effects of somatostatin analog SMS 201-995 on enterotoxigenic diarrhea. *Digestive Diseases and Sciences, 36,* 1768-1773.
28. Pon, D., & Dong, B.J. (1990). Octreotide use in AIDS. *DICP, The Annals of Pharmacotherapy, 24,* 951-952.
29. Heather, D.J., Howell, L., Montana, M., & Howell, M. (1991). Effect of a bulk-forming cathartic on diarrhea in tube-fed patients. *Heart & Lung, 20,* 409-413.
30. World Health Organization (1990). The rational use of drugs in the management of acute diarrhoea in children. Geneva: Author.

BIBLIOGRAPHY

Balistreri, W.F. (1990). Oral rehydration of acute infantile diarrhea. *American Journal of Medicine, 88*(Suppl. 6A), 30S-33S.
Camp-Sorrell, D. (1991). Controlling adverse effects of chemotherapy. *Nursing, 21*(4), 34-42.
Castle S.C., Cantrell, M., Israel, D.S., & Samuelson, M.J. (1991). Constipation prevention: Empiric use of stool softeners questioned. *Geriatrics, 46*(11), 84-86.

Davidson, L.J., Belknap, D.C., & Flournoy, D.J. (1991). Flow characteristics of enteral feeding with psyllium hydrophilic mucilloid added. *Heart & Lung, 20,* 404-408.

Fifield, M.Y. (1991). Relieving constipation and pain in the terminally ill. *American Journal of Nursing, 91*(7), 18-19.

Hanham, S. (1990). Management of constipation. *Nursing: The Journal of Clinical Practice, Education, and Management, 4*(17), 28-31.

Oral rehydration therapy: The best response to diarrheal dehydration. (1991). *Journal of Emergency Nursing, 17*(2), 99-101.

Ross, D. (1990). Constipation among hospitalized elders. *Orthopaedic Nursing, 9*(3), 73-77.

Schmelzer, M. (1990). Effectiveness of wheat bran in preventing constipation of hospitalized orthopaedic surgery patients. *Orthopaedic Nursing, 9*(6), 55-59.

Wadle, K.R. (1990). Diarrhea. *Nursing Clinics of North America, 25,* 901-908.

Williams, S.G., & DiPalma, J.A. (1990). Constipation in the long-term care facility. *Gastroenterology Nursing, 12*(3), 179-182.

Drugs Affecting the Body's Defense System

CHAPTER 49

OVERVIEW OF
Biologic Defense Mechanisms

MARGUERITE NEWTON • ROBYN RICE

⊛ **Nonspecific Defense Mechanisms**

LEARNING OBJECTIVES:

Distinguish between specific and nonspecific defenses against infection.

Name three external nonspecific defense mechanisms.

Identify the major phagocytic cells in the blood and other tissues.

Describe the process of phagocytosis.

Summarize the steps in the inflammatory response.

KEY TERMS:

Chemotaxis, complement system, inflammation, interferon, lymphocyte, lymphokines, macrophage, margination, opsonization, phagocytosis, reticuloendothelial system

⊛ **Internal Specific Defense Mechanisms**

LEARNING OBJECTIVES:

Describe the functions of antibodies and immunoglobulins.

Explain what is meant by humoral-mediated immunity.

Summarize the cell-mediated immune response.

Distinguish between active and passive immunity.

KEY TERMS:

Active acquired immunity, allergen, antibody, antigen, immunogen, immunoglobulin, passive acquired immunity

⊛ **Biologic Defense Mechanisms in Fetus and Newborn**

LEARNING OBJECTIVE: Discuss the biologic defense mechanisms of the fetus and newborn.

⊛ **Effects of Aging on Biologic Defense Mechanisms**

LEARNING OBJECTIVE: Summarize the effects aging has on biologic defense mechanisms.

⊛ **Autoimmune Diseases**

LEARNING OBJECTIVE: Identify three autoimmune diseases.

⊛ **Effects of Drugs on Body's Defense System**

LEARNING OBJECTIVE: Describe the impact of drugs on the body's defense system.

CONCEPTS AND TERMS TO REVIEW

Review the lymphatic system and immunity in an anatomy and physiology textbook.

Review origin of T cells and B cells.

Review process for T-cell and B-cell activation.

Review humoral-mediated and cell-mediated immunity.

Review definitions of the following terms: *allergen, antigen, antibody, phagocytosis,* and *vaccine.*

---

*T*here are numerous biologic defense mechanisms within the human body. These mechanisms are considered either nonspecific or specific. Nonspecific mechanisms are nonselectively directed against any foreign substance; specific mechanisms respond to specific foreign substances. Nonspecific and specific mechanisms are further divided on the basis of where the lines of defense are formed in relation to the human body—externally or internally.

The function of these biologic defense mechanisms is to protect the body (self) from invasion by nonself materials.

Thus the body's ability to distinguish self from nonself is critical. This recognition of self from nonself is accomplished by specific protein molecules embedded in the cell membrane of all human body cells.

This chapter provides an overview of external and internal nonspecific defense mechanisms and internal specific defense mechanisms. Life span changes within the body's defense mechanisms and autoimmune diseases are also discussed. An understanding of this information is essential for safe and effective drug administration.

NONSPECIFIC DEFENSE MECHANISMS

The body has general physical responses and structures that deter invading organisms. These responses and structures are further classified as external and internal nonspecific defense mechanisms.

External Nonspecific Defense Mechanisms

Most external nonspecific defense mechanisms are classified as anatomic, chemical, and mechanical barriers. **Anatomic barriers** include the skin, nasal hairs, eyelids, and eyelashes, which provide structural protection for the body. Mucous membranes that line the respiratory, gastrointestinal (GI), and genitourinary (GU) tracts are also anatomic barriers. These membranes secrete mucus that protects by lubricating the surface of the membranes, trapping foreign material, and neutralizing the effects of bacteria and other agents. **Mechanical barriers** include fever, coughing, sneezing, vomiting, and excretory processes. Perspiration, tears, gastric juice, vaginal secretions, and saliva are considered **chemical barriers.** Perspiration contains antibacterial and antifungal substances and lactic acid, which discourage growth of gram-positive bacteria. The acidity of gastric juices and vaginal secretions also deters bacterial infections. An additional external defense mechanism is the body's normal **microbic flora,** which retards the colonization of other potentially harmful organisms.[1]

Internal Nonspecific Defense Mechanisms

Once a foreign agent penetrates the external lines of defense, it is met by a complex array of internal nonspecific defense mechanisms, including phagocytosis and inflammation. Both of these processes involve cellular components of the blood (white blood cells [WBCs]) and cells and molecules of the reticuloendothelial system (RES). Interferons, the complement system, and opsonization are also important in the internal nonspecific defense process.

CELLULAR COMPONENTS OF BLOOD

Six different types of WBCs (leukocytes) normally appear in the blood: polymorphonuclear neutrophils, polymorphonuclear eosinophils, polymorphonuclear basophils, monocytes, lymphocytes, and an occasional plasma cell. Although most of their work is outside the circulatory system, leukocytes use the

---

NONSPECIFIC DEFENSE MECHANISMS

External Defense Mechanisms	Internal Defense Mechanisms
Anatomic barriers	Leukocytes
Skin	Neutrophils
Nasal hairs	Eosinophils
Eyelids and eyelashes	Basophils
Mucous membranes	Monocytes
	Lymphocytes
Mechanical Barriers	
Fever	Plasma cells
Coughing	Phagocytosis
Sneezing	
Vomiting	Reticuloendothelial system
	Inflammatory response
Chemical Barriers	
Perspiration	Interferons
Tears	Complement system
Gastric juices	
Vaginal secretions	Opsonization
Saliva	

---

blood for transportation to sites of infection. These cells are distinguished by their size, shape of their nucleus, nature of their cytoplasm, and staining characteristics.[2,3]

The three types of polymorphonuclear cells (neutrophils, eosinophils, and basophils) have a granular appearance and are called **granulocytes.** These cells develop in the red bone marrow; they have a short life span, averaging approximately 12 hours. Out of the total circulating leukocytes, **neutrophils** account for 54% to 62% and **eosinophils** for 1% to 3%. The **basophils** usually account for less than 1% of the total number of leukocytes.[2]

Monocytes and lymphocytes are called *agranulocytes.* **Monocytes** are the largest cells found in the blood. These cells usually arise from the red bone marrow and live for several weeks or even months. Monocytes comprise 3% to 9% of the circulating leukocytes. Granulocytes and monocytes are the two major types of leukocytes that fight infection.

Monocytes give rise to **macrophages,** which are large phagocytic cells. Macrophages attach themselves to various tissues and to the inner walls of blood and lymphatic vessels. These cells can divide and produce new macrophages. This group of phagocytic cells constitutes the reticuloendothelial tissue or the RES, which is discussed later in the chapter.[2-4]

Lymphocytes are formed in the organs of the lymphatic system and in the red bone marrow. These cells account for 25% to 33% of the circulating leukocytes. Lymphocytes have a long life span that may extend for years.

PHAGOCYTOSIS

The most important function of the neutrophils and macrophages is phagocytosis. **Phagocytosis,** the engulfment and destruction of invading organisms, begins as soon as neutrophils enter the inflamed area. Neutrophils are mature cells; they can usually phagocytize five to 20 bacteria before becoming inactivated and dying.

Mobile macrophages must be activated by the immune system before they begin to phagocytize invading organisms and neutralize toxins. It may take several days to several weeks before the macrophages dominate the phagocytic cells in the inflamed tissue. Macrophages are more powerful phagocytes than neutrophils; they are often capable of phagocytizing as many as 100 bacteria. In addition, macrophages are able to engulf larger particles than neutrophils.[3–5]

Lymphokines, a series of protein mediators, are formed by T lymphocytes of the lymphoid tissue (Table 49–1). Lymphokines such as interleukin-2 and interleukin-3 activate macrophages throughout the body. They slow or stop the migration of macrophages from the inflamed tissue, causing macrophages to accumulate at the site. Lymphokines also enhance the actions of the macrophages, causing more efficient phagocytosis.[3–6] Once a foreign particle has been phagocytized by the neutrophils or macrophages, **lysosomal enzymes** immediately begin to digest the particle.

RETICULOENDOTHELIAL SYSTEM

The **RES,** also known as the *mononuclear phagocyte system,* consists of phagocytic macrophage cells that are scattered throughout various body tissues. The macrophage cells of the RES ingest foreign particles and damaged host tissues. They are classified as either mobile or stationary. Mobile (wandering) macrophages travel in connective tissues (histiocytes) or the bloodstream (monocytes) to phagocytize foreign material or debris. Stationary (fixed) macrophages reside in specific tissues such as lymphoid tissue, spleen, liver, bone marrow, lungs, and blood vessels. These fixed cells engulf and destroy foreign material in the fluids and tissues of their environment.[2,3]

INFLAMMATORY RESPONSE

When the body sustains an injury, all the nonspecific defense mechanisms are directed toward isolating the effects of the injury, protecting against microbial invasion at the site, and preparing the site for healing. This process is called **inflammation.** The inflammatory response can be initiated by any type of injury and begins within seconds of injury.

Local clinical manifestions of the inflammatory response include redness, heat, swelling, and pain. These manifestations coincide with the amount or degree of tissue destruction. The inflammatory response begins with transitory vasoconstriction followed immediately by vasodilation. This increased blood flow **(hyperemia)** causes redness and heat. Serous fluids and proteins leak into the interstitial spaces, causing swelling of the tissue, **edema.** Soon fibrinogen clots form and "wall off" tissue spaces and lymphatics in the inflamed area. This response delays the spread of foreign organisms to other areas of the body.

During the early stages of the inflammatory response, large numbers of neutrophils quickly invade the inflamed tissues. Monocytes also enter the affected area. Since the number of circulating monocytes is low, the buildup of monocytes at the

TABLE 49–1
Mediators of Immune System

Mediator	Effect
Skin reactive factor	Facilitates cell recruitment from circulation for the inflammatory response
Macrophage-activating factor (MAF)	Attracts macrophages to the site and increases ability to adhere to cell surfaces
Macrophage aggregation factor	Results in clumping of macrophages
Proliferation inhibitory factor	Prevents growth of particular antigenic cells
Cytophilic antibody	Facilitates binding of macrophages to antigens
Interleukin-1	Stimulates differentiation of T-cell growth and differentiation of B cells
Interleukin-2	Stimulates proliferation and growth of cytotoxic (killer) T cells, helper T cells, and suppressor T cells
Interleukin-3	Promotes growth of mast cells and other blood cells
Interleukin-4	Stimulates growth and proliferation of cytotoxic T cells, suppressor T cells, mast cells, and macrophages
Interleukin-5 Interleukin-6	Stimulates growth of B cells and differentiaton to plasma cells and antibodies
Neutrophil, eosinophil, and basophil chemotactic factors	Attract macrophages
Migration inhibitory factor (MIF)	Maintains macrophages at antigen site
Lymphocyte inhibitory factor	Maintains lymphocytes at antigen site
Lymphotoxin	Causes lysis of the antigen
Leukocyte inhibitory factor (LIF)	Maintains leukocytes at antigen site
Lymphocyte blastogenic factor	Stimulates lymphocytes and attracts lymphocytes to the site
Histamine releasing factor	Stimulates histamine release from basophils
Transfer factor	Promotes nonsensitized lymphocytes' response to antigens
Interferon	Produces response to viral antigens
Prostaglandins (PGs)	PGE_1 increases vascular permeability; PGE_2 attracts leukocytes to the site

inflamed area occurs more slowly than that of neutrophils. Two processes, chemotaxis and margination, cause both neutrophils and macrophages to move toward the inflamed tissues. With **chemotaxis,** a chemical that attracts neutrophils and macrophages is released from the injured tissue. The chemotactic substance increases the permeability of the walls of the blood vessels, allowing the leukocytes to leave the blood vessels and migrate into the inflamed area. In **margination,** the inflamed tissues produce a substance that causes neutrophils to adhere to capillary walls.[7]

As the inflammatory process continues, pus formation occurs. **Pus** is a by-product of inflammation. It is a protein-rich liquid composed of destroyed tissue, neutrophils, and invading organisms. As the infection is suppressed, pus either undergoes autolysis and is absorbed by surrounding tissue or is drained out of the inflamed cavity.

Inflammatory responses also produce systemic manifestations, including fever, malaise, nausea, vomiting, diarrhea, and hematologic changes. When injured, the body releases substances known as *endogenous pyrogens* at the inflammatory site. These substances circulate to the temperature-regulating center in the hypothalamus and reset the body's temperature set point. The adjustment in the set point causes the body to increase heat production and decrease heat loss. The fever response is a part of the defense mechanisms of the body and helps increase the production of antimicrobial agents. Hematologic changes include elevations in leukocytes (**leukocytosis**) and blood fibrinogen levels.[1,5,8,9]

INTERFERONS

Various tissue cells and sensitized lymphocytes produce proteins known as **interferons** during viral infections. Infected cells release interferon into their surrounding environment where the interferon acts to protect uninfected cells by inhibiting viral replication. Although interferon production is usually associated with viruses, production is not limited to viral infections.

COMPLEMENT SYSTEM

Approximately 20 interacting plasma proteins, many of which are enzyme precursors, make up the **complement system.** Of these 20 plasma proteins, 11 are designated *C1* through *C9, B,* and *D.* These plasma proteins are always present in circulating blood, but the enzyme precursors are inactive. Activation of the complement system occurs through two independent pathways, the classic and alternative pathways.

In the *classic pathway* complement components of C1 through C9 react. Specific antigen-antibody reactions involving immunoglobulin M (IgM) and immunoglobulin G (IgG) can activate this pathway and components of the nonspecific defense system. The *alternate pathway* is triggered by immunoglobulin A (IgA) or tissue injury and follows a different path through C3.

The antigen-antibody interaction or tissue injury that triggers the complement cascade reaction results in products that possess biologic and enzymatic capabilities. Some complement products immobilize immune cells so that they remain on site to battle the antigen. Other products increase vascular permeability, allowing more immune cells into the site. In addition, they help fight invading organisms through chemotaxis, agglutination or clumping of the antigen, opsonization, phagocytosis, and anaphylactic (histamine-mediated reactions) and cytolytic actions of the immune response.[4,6,9,10]

OPSONIZATION

The process of phagocytosis is enhanced by opsonization. **Opsonization** is action by a substance (Opsonin) that coats and binds antigens to the phagocyte. Opsonization is elicited by antibody-antigen and complement interactions. Thus a specific immune response mechanism contributes to the nonspecific mechanism and makes it significantly more efficient.

CONCEPT REVIEW

The body is equipped with external and internal nonspecific defense mechanisms. Inflammation and phagocytosis are examples of internal nonspecific mechanisms.

Inflammation is a tissue response to damage, injury, or infection. The inflammatory response includes localized redness, swelling, heat, and pain.

The most active phagocytes in blood are neutrophils and monocytes. Monocytes give rise to macrophages.

Phagocytic cells associated with linings of blood vessels in the bone marrow, liver, spleen, and lymph nodes constitute the reticuloendothelial tissue.

INTERNAL SPECIFIC DEFENSE MECHANISMS

An internal specific defense mechanism provides protection against a particular microorganism or molecular entity. This type of protection is called **specific immunity.** Together, specific and nonspecific defense mechanisms work to monitor and neutralize invading organisms or potential sources of infection.

Structures and components involved in specific immunity are part of the immune system. The physical reaction to an invading organism, an **antigen** or **immunogen,** is called an *immune response.* Once the antigen or immunogen is detected as a foreign substance, the immune response is activated. Antigens, or immunogens, include viruses, bacteria, fungi, parasites, food, pollen, drugs, vaccines, transplanted tissues, neoplastic cells, and transfused blood products.[4,11,12]

Specific immunity works best when there has been prior exposure to the antigen. Exposure may be acquired in an active or passive manner. **Passive acquired immunity** occurs when immune cells are passed from one individual to another. This immunity is transitory in nature. One example is the passage of maternal immune cells across the placenta to the fetus. Passive acquired immunity also results when gamma globulin is given to an individual exposed to a disease such as hepatitis. The gamma globulin provides temporary protection for the individual. **Active acquired immunity** results when the individual has direct contact with an antigen and the immune response is stimulated. When the individual has a disease, he or she acquires active acquired immunity. In addition, vaccines are examples of active acquired immunity.[1]

Specific immunity is the body's last line of defense. It occurs much more slowly than the inflammatory process and

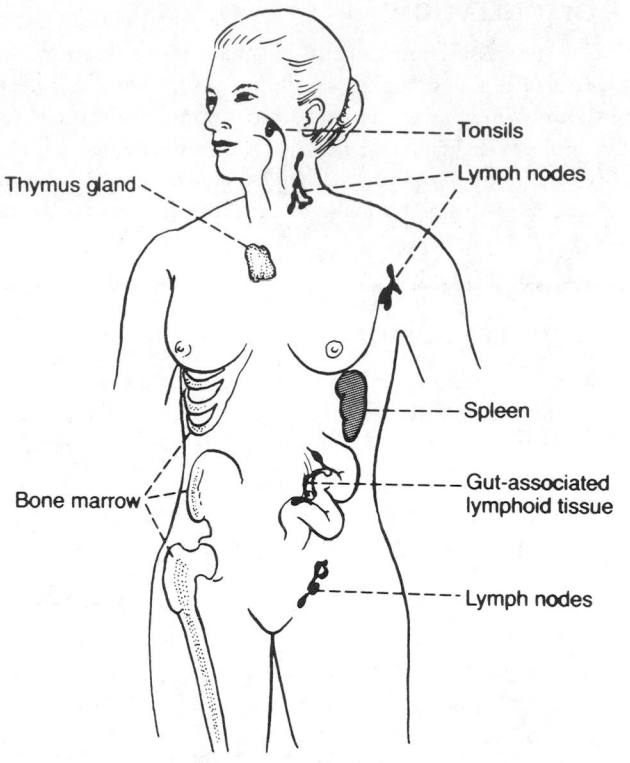

FIGURE 49–1   Organs of the immune system. (From Black, J., & Matassarin-Jacobs, E. [1993]. *Luckmann and Sorensen's medical-surgical nursing: A psychophysiologic approach [4th ed.]. Philadelphia: W.B. Saunders.*)

TABLE 49–2
Immunoglobulins

Classification	Characteristics
IgG	Comprises 75% of immunoglobulins Major component of commercial immunoglobulin Activates complement system Mediates agglutination and opsonization of antigens Transferred across the placenta Enhances phagocytosis Major immunoglobulin produced with reexposure to an antigen Present in interstitial fluid
IgA	Comprises 15% of immunoglobulins Present in secretions: saliva, tears, GI and respiratory secretions Passed to neonate through breast milk
IgM	Comprises 10% of immunoglobulins Present in intravascular fluid Produced first in response to an antigen Fixes complement Not transferred across the placenta
IgD	Comprises 0.2% of total immunoglobulins Small amounts found in serum Function not yet defined
IgE	Comprises 0.004% of total immunoglobulins Found in serum Mediates immediate-type hypersensitivity reactions Elevated in certain parasitic diseases

provides the body long-term protection against invading organisms. The immune system includes stem cells, primary lymphoid organs, and secondary lymphoid organs that produce humoral and cellular immunity.

All blood cells circulating in the body are derived from pluripotential stem cells in the bone marrow. Stem cells are precursors to differentiated blood cells. Through a process of cell division and exposure to growth inducers and differentiation inducers, stem cells mature into erythrocytes, leukocytes, and/or megakaryocytes.[3,6] The primary lymphoid organs are the bone marrow and thymus gland. These structures are the organs that produce immune system cells[5] (Fig. 49–1).

Humoral-Mediated Immunity

Hematopoietic tissue produces stem cells that mature in the bone marrow and become **B cells.** Each B cell is capable of responding to only a specific antigen. B cells that encounter an antigen in the presence of T cells are transformed to plasma cells. Plasma cells possess memory of the antigen and can initiate a strong response with reexposure.[6]

Antibody   When a B cell encounters its specific antigen, antibodies or immunoglobulins are produced. **Antibodies** are serum glycoproteins that fight infection by directly attacking the antigen and by activating the complement system that subsequently destroys the antigen. Antibodies and antigens may also combine to form complexes that cannot bind with host cell receptors.[4]

Immunoglobulin Immunoglobulins are heavy and light chains of polypeptides. There are five types of immunoglobulins: IgM, IgA, IgG, IgE, and IgD (Table 49–2). IgM comprises 5% of the total immunoglobulin. As indicated previously, IgM, IgG, and IgA aid in the activation of the classic and alternate pathways of the complement system.

IgM activates the classic complement pathway and fixes it by binding it to other cells. IgM is the first to respond to an antigen and is active in fighting blood-borne infections. **IgA** is found in secretions such as saliva, tears, and mucus. These secretions provide protection for the mucosal surfaces of the respiratory, digestive, and genital tracts. IgA can activate the alternative complement pathway, and it comprises 17% to 20% of all serum immunoglobulin. **IgG** comprises approximately 75% of the immunoglobulin pool. This immunoglobulin can cross the placenta and is found in the blood and tissues. IgG works by agglutination and/or opsonization and activates the classic pathway of the complement system. IgG levels rise dramatically in response to the second exposure to an antigen.[6,11]

IgE is present in trace amounts and is involved in the response to helminthic parasites. IgE is the major immunoglobulin involved in an allergic response. With second exposure to an **allergen,** IgE binds to mast cells and basophils. These cells burst and release histamine, which causes the urticaria and rhinitis associated with an allergic response. The last immunoglobulin, **IgD,** is less than 1% of the serum immunoglobulin pool. Little is known about its function, but it may aid in assisting B-cell maturation.[11]

Cell-Mediated Immunity

T lymphocytes or T cells provide cell-mediated immunity. Differentiation occurs when stem cells migrate to the thymus where, under hormonal influence, they are transformed to T cells. After migration to the secondary lymphoid organs, they are released to circulate in the blood where they perform a surveillance function. Three types of T cells exist: helper, effector or cytotoxic, and suppressor cells (Fig. 49–2). **Helper cells** serve as the major regulator of virtually all immune functions. They do this by forming a series of protein mediators, called *lymphokines,* that act on other cells of the immune system and on bone marrow cells. In the absence of lymphokines

from the helper T cells, the remainder of the immune system is not functional. Helper cells stimulate the growth and proliferation of effector and suppressor cells. They also stimulate B-cell growth, proliferation, and formation of plasma cells and secretion of antibodies. **Effector cells** attack the antigen and destroy it through lysis. The third type, the **suppressor cell,** decreases the immune response to the antigen and assists the body in differentiation of foreign substances from self. When the body views self-tissue as foreign, the suppressor cells prohibit anti-self antibody production.[4,5,9]

Sensitized T cells are also capable of transferring their antigen sensitivity to other nonsensitized T cells through release of a transfer factor. T cells provide protection from viruses, bacteria, protozoa, fungi, and tumor cells. They are involved in graft-versus-host reactions and delayed hypersensitivity reactions.[9]

Table 49–3 compares humoral-mediated and cell-mediated immunity.

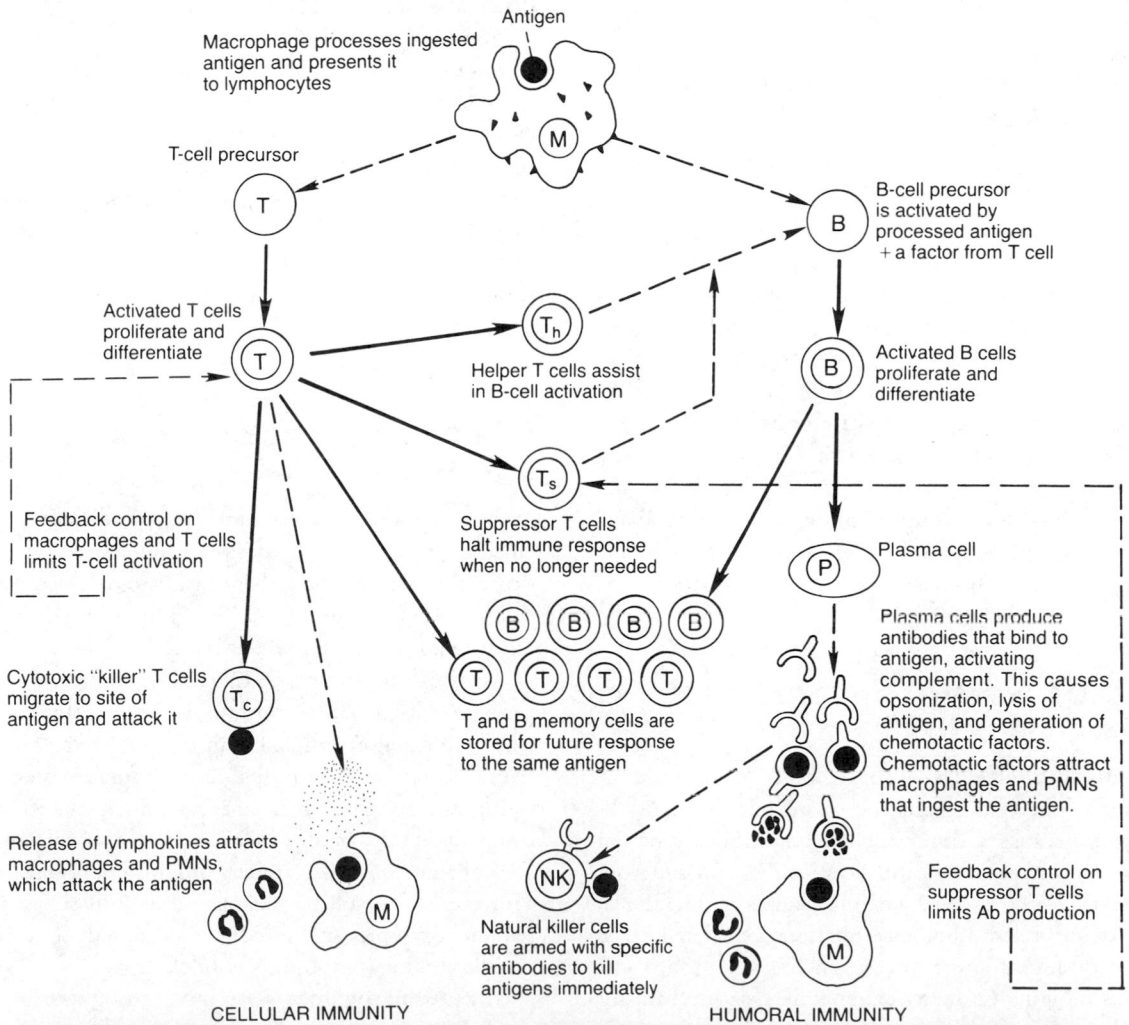

FIGURE 49–2   Overview of cell cooperation in immune response. (From Luckmann, J., & Sorensen, K. [1987]. Medical-surgical nursing [3rd ed.]. Philadelphia: W.B. Saunders.)

TABLE 49–3
Comparison of Humoral-mediated and Cell-mediated Immunity

Humoral-Mediated Immunity	Cell-Mediated Immunity
Short life span	Long life span
Present primarily in blood	Present primarily in lymph tissue
Possesses memory of antigens; reacts immediately with reexposure.	Involved in delayed sensitivity reactions
Synthesizes antibodies in response to antigen	Stimulates macrophages, activates complement, destroys intracellular pathogens Stimulates B-cell antibody production
Transferred via plasma	Transfer unusual
Involved in pyogenic infections, toxic reactions, immune complex disease, anaphylactic shock, transfusion reaction	Involved in graft rejection, tumor surveillance or destruction, viral, fungal, or parasitic infections

BIOLOGIC DEFENSE MECHANISMS IN FETUS AND NEWBORN

In the fetus and newborn, biologic defense mechanisms are immature. During the third trimester of pregnancy, the fetus is capable of producing IgM in response to infection. IgA and IgG production ability at this time is minimal.

Maternal active transport of immunoglobulins provides passive protection for the newborn during the first few months of life. Most of the antibodies from the mother are IgG; these antibodies reach their lowest level in the neonate at 6 months of age when production increases in him or her. The newborn possesses a full number of T cells, but the T cells are not fully functional until the fourteenth week. The complement cascade components, phagocytosis ability of monocytes, and mechanical barriers such as the gag and cough reflex are also diminished in the newborn. This leaves the newborn at risk for infections from invading organisms.[10]

EFFECTS OF AGING ON BIOLOGIC DEFENSE MECHANISMS

Aging diminishes the effectiveness of the body's defense mechanisms. Some of the changes that occur include decreased T-cell population because of diminished cell division; atrophy of the thymus; and increased cytotoxic cell activity. In addition, suppressor T cells are less effective. This causes an increase in the number of anti-self antibodies, which may be related to the development of autoimmune diseases in this age group. The overall effects of aging on many external defense mechanisms such as thinning skin and decreased GI motility also increase the risk of infection.

AUTOIMMUNE DISEASES

Autoimmune disease occurs when there is an abnormal response of the immune system against the body. Normally self-antigens exist in the body. However, when the body begins to see these self-antigens as foreign, the immune system reacts as it would to an invader. Autoimmune diseases can be systemic disorders such as rheumatoid arthritis or organ specific as in ulcerative colitis.

Several factors are thought to contribute to the development of autoimmune disease. A family history of autoimmune disease may be related to inherited human leukocyte antigen (HLA) factors. HLA is an antigen type that recognizes self from nonself. Since more women than men suffer from autoimmune disease, it is thought that female hormones foster the development of the autoimmune response. In research studies with women experiencing a lupuslike disease, removal of the ovaries and treatment with male hormones delayed the onset of symptoms. Tissue injury or surgery may cause transportation of cells through the bloodstream from one area of the body to another where they are seen as foreign. This can produce an autoantibody response. For example, ovarian cells that do not normally circulate in the blood could be introduced after removal of an ovarian cyst.

Some foreign antigens closely resemble self-antigens. When introduced, they stimulate the immune system, which then reacts to the similar self-antigen. The streptococcal antigen closely resembles the heart tissue self-antigen. Any antibodies produced to fight the streptococcal infection can react to the heart self-antigen, producing rheumatic fever. Viral infections may damage cells and allow circulation of antigens, causing an immune response. T cells can also be damaged by viruses, and suppressor T-cell activity can be impaired, resulting in the autoimmune response.[6,13]

EFFECTS OF DRUGS ON BODY'S DEFENSE SYSTEM

Many drugs affect the immune response directly or indirectly. In some cases this is the desired drug action, but with many drugs, this is a side effect that must be monitored. Examples of drugs that affect the immune response are alcohol, steroids, antineoplastic agents, and antibiotics.

Habitual consumption of large amounts of **alcohol** depresses cell-mediated immunity and granulocyte levels. Impaired defenses coupled with the poor nutritional status of many alcoholics result in high infection rates. **Steroids** are often prescribed for their anti-inflammatory actions. These drugs cause a transitory increase in neutrophils and suppression of function and numbers of eosinophils and monocytes. However, the resulting leukopenia may mask signs of an infection. Examples of steroids are dexamethasone (Decadron) and flunisolide (Aerobid, Nasalide).[14]

Antineoplastic agents are immunosuppressive because of their cytotoxic effects. These agents destroy stem cells, thus decreasing WBC levels. Radiation therapy often accompanies the use of chemotherapy to combat malignancies. The resulting leukopenia from the radiation increases the client's susceptibility to infection.[11] Examples of antineoplastic agents are methotrexate (Mexate, Folex) and fluorouracil (Adrucil, 5-FU, 5-Fluorouracil).[14]

SUMMARY

The body's defense system is dynamic and is held in a delicate balance by chemical and cellular factors, with the whole greater than the parts. The nonspecific and specific components work together in a complex fashion to protect the body from foreign antigens. Many factors influence biologic defense mechanisms, including age, trauma, disease, and pharmacologic agents. These factors can profoundly alter the effectiveness of the body's defense system.

REFERENCES

1. Black, J., & Matassarin-Jacobs, E. (1993). *Luckmann and Sorensen's medical-surgical nursing: A psychophysiologic approach* (4th ed.). Philadelphia: W.B. Saunders.
2. Hole, J. (1993). *Human anatomy and physiology* (6th ed.). Dubuque, IA: Wm. C. Brown.
3. Guyton, A.C. (1991). *Textbook of medical physiology* (8th ed.). Philadelphia: W.B. Saunders.
4. McCance, K., & Huether, S. (1990). *Pathophysiology: The biologic basis for disease in adults and children.* St. Louis: C.V. Mosby.
5. Gurka, A. (1989). The immune system: Implications for critical care. *Critical Care Nurse, 9*(7), 24-35.
6. Guyton, A.C. (1992). *Human physiology and mechanisms of disease* (5th ed.). Philadelphia: W.B. Saunders.
7. Seeley, R., Stephens, T., & Tate, P. (1992). *Anatomy and physiology* (2nd ed.). St. Louis: Mosby–Year Book.
8. Gogia, P. (1992). The biology of wound healing. *Ostomy/Wound Management, 38*(9), 12-20.
9. Lockey, R., & Burkantz, S. (1987). *Fundamentals of immunology and allergy.* Philadelphia: W.B. Saunders.
10. Petrucci, K., Booth-Blaemire, E., & Watson, K. (1989). Aging, immunity and critical care nursing. *Critical Care Nursing Clinics of North America, 1,* 787-795.
11. Frey, A. (1991). The immune system and intravenous administration of immune globulins. *Journal of Intravenous Nursing, 14,* 315-329.
12. Washington Univeristy Medical Center (1989). *The immune system—The body in balance.* St. Louis: Author.
13. Porth, C. (1991). *Pathophysiology: Concepts of altered health states* (3rd ed.). Philadelphia: J.B. Lippincott.
14. Lehne, R. (1990). *Pharmacology for nursing care.* Philadelphia: W.B. Saunders.

BIBLIOGRAPHY

Applebaym, J. (1992). The role of the immune system in the pathogenesis of cancer. *Seminars in Oncology Nursing, 8*(1), 51-62.
Cerrato, P.L. (1990). Does diet affect the immune system? *RN Magazine, 53*(6), 67-68.
Gawlikowski, J. (1992). White cells at war. *American Journal of Nursing, 93*(3), 45-51.
Geld, D. (1991). The stem cell. *Scientific American, 265*(6), 86-93.
Jackson, S.A. (1991). The immune system: Basic concepts for understanding transplantation. *Critical Care Nursing Quarterly, 13*(4), 83-88.
Jordan, K. (1990). Interferon: Clinical uses and nursing implications. *Journal of Intravenous Nursing, 13*(6), 388-391.
Noerr, B. (1990). Intravenous immune human serumglobulin. *Journal of Neonatal Nursing, 8*(5), 81-83.
Sheehan, C. (1990). *Clinical immunology: Principles and laboratory diagnosis.* Philadelphia: J.B. Lippincott.
Stroud, M., Swindell, B., & Bernard, G.R. (1990). Cellular and humoral mediators of sepsis syndrome. *Critical Care Clinics of North America, 2*(2), 151-160.
VanBoehmer, H. & Kisielow, P. (1991). How the immune system learns about self. *Scientific American, 265*(4), 74-81.
Van Buren, D.H. (1991). Transplant immunology. *Journal of Urological Nursing, 10*(1), 1076-1085.

CHAPTER 50

Histamine-Receptor Agonists and Antagonists

JANET L. MELNIK STEWART

⊛ **Histamine**

LEARNING OBJECTIVES:

Describe how histamine produces symptoms of allergic or anaphylactic reactions.

Describe the wheal-and-flare response.

Discuss clinical uses of histamine.

KEY TERMS:

Antigen, histamine

⊛ **General Characteristics of Histamine-Receptor Antagonists**

LEARNING OBJECTIVES:

Describe the actions of antihistamines.

Identify subclasses of H_1-receptor antagonists.

Distinguish between first- and second-generation H_1-receptor antagonists.

KEY TERMS:

Antihistamine, histamine-receptor blockers, histamine-receptor antagonists, histamine antagonists, first-generation H_1-receptor antagonists, second-generation H_1-receptor antagonists

⊛ **Pharmacotherapeutics of H_1-Receptor Antagonists**

LEARNING OBJECTIVE: Describe the effects that H_1-receptor antagonists exert on specific body systems.

⊛ **Nursing Considerations**

LEARNING OBJECTIVES:

Describe assessment of clients being considered for antihistamine therapy.

Develop teaching plan for client receiving H_1-receptor antagonists.

Discuss nursing interventions for clients taking antihistamines.

⊛ **First-Generation Antagonists**

LEARNING OBJECTIVES:

Discuss pharmacodynamic and pharmacokinetic properties of the first-generation antagonist prototypes.

Identify major undesired clinical responses and contraindications associated with these drugs.

Describe major nursing considerations related to first-generation antihistamines.

⊛ **Second-Generation Antagonists**

LEARNING OBJECTIVES:

Discuss pharmacodynamic and pharmacokinetic properties of the second-generation antagonist prototypes.

Identify major undesired clinical responses and contraindications associated with these drugs.

Describe major nursing considerations related to second-generation antihistamines.

⊛ **Life-Span Considerations**

LEARNING OBJECTIVE: Discuss the life-span considerations of antihistamines.

Effects of Histamine

Histamine has direct and indirect actions on multiple body systems (Fig. 50–1). Histamine causes constriction of large arteries, veins, and venules and dilation of the minute blood vessels, including the capillaries and the small arterioles. The vasodilation is mediated by both H_1 and H_2 receptors. H_1 receptors have a greater affinity for histamine and mediate a dilator response that has a rapid onset but a brief duration. Stimulation of H_2 receptors produces vasodilation that develops more slowly but is then sustained.

Vasodilation produces flushing of the skin, increased skin temperature, headache, and reduction of systemic blood pressure, which are characteristic symptoms of allergic or anaphylactic reactions. Another effect of histamine on smaller blood vessels is increased capillary permeability, which results in exudation of fluid and plasma proteins into the extravascular spaces and the formation of edema.[5]

Clinical Uses of Histamine

Histamine (as histamine phosphate) has very limited use as a diagnostic agent. Injected intradermally, it causes itching and a wheal-and-flare response; thus it can be used to assess the effectiveness of H_1-receptor antagonist therapy [6] (see Box). It can also be used to diagnose achlorhydria (absence of free hydrochloric acid in the stomach). However, because of its serious and potentially lethal adverse effects, use of histamine phosphate has generally been replaced by the use of pentagastrin in testing gastric acid secretion[6].

GENERAL CHARACTERISTICS OF HISTAMINE-RECEPTOR ANTAGONISTS

Drugs have been developed that can block the effects of histamine on the histamine receptors. These drugs are referred to synonymously as **histamine-receptor antagonists, histamine antagonists,** or **histamine-receptor blockers.**

The H_2-receptor antagonists block the effects of histamine on the H_2 receptors. Although they sometimes have other uses, their main use is in the treatment of peptic ulcers. Research is

---

Although histamine was discovered in 1909, its role still is not fully understood. Conditions produced by excessive histamine release are numerous and include hay fever, urticaria, headaches, rashes, bronchial smooth muscle constriction, rhinorrhea, and rhinitis.

This chapter reviews the process by which histamine is released from its storage sites and the resultant effects that it produces in the body after its release. The limited clinical uses of histamine phosphate as a diagnostic agent are briefly presented. Most of this chapter is devoted to discussion of a group of drugs, the H_1-receptor antagonists. These drugs antagonize the effects of histamine on H_1 receptors.

HISTAMINE

Histamine is an endogenous autocoid that exerts a major role as a mediator in immediate (type I) hypersensitivity and allergic reactions.

Distribution and Release of Histamine

The primary target cells of immediate hypersensitivity reactions are the mast cells (in tissues) and the basophils (in blood) in which histamine is synthesized and stored. Histamine is stored within the secretory granules of the mast cells and basophils along with a heparin-protein complex, eosinophil chemotactic factor of anaphylaxis (ECF-A), neutrophil chemotactic factor, and various enzymes.[1] Mast cells are in the loose connective tissue of all organs, especially around blood vessels, lymphatic vessels, and nerves. The concentration of histamine is especially high in the tissues containing the largest numbers of mast cells: the skin, upper and lower respiratory tracts, and the gastrointestinal (GI) mucosa.[2,3]

When a foreign substance, called an **antigen,** interacts with IgE antibodies bound to the surface of the mast cells and basophils, the cells are damaged. The result is degranulation of the cells and release of the stored histamine and other chemical mediators that form the secretory granules of the cells. Once released, histamine rapidly diffuses into surrounding tissues along with the other released chemical mediators. The released histamine exerts powerful effects on target organs through one of three types of histamine receptors (H_1, H_2, H_3 receptors), and elicits the symptoms characteristically seen in individuals with allergic and anaphylactic reactions.[3,4]

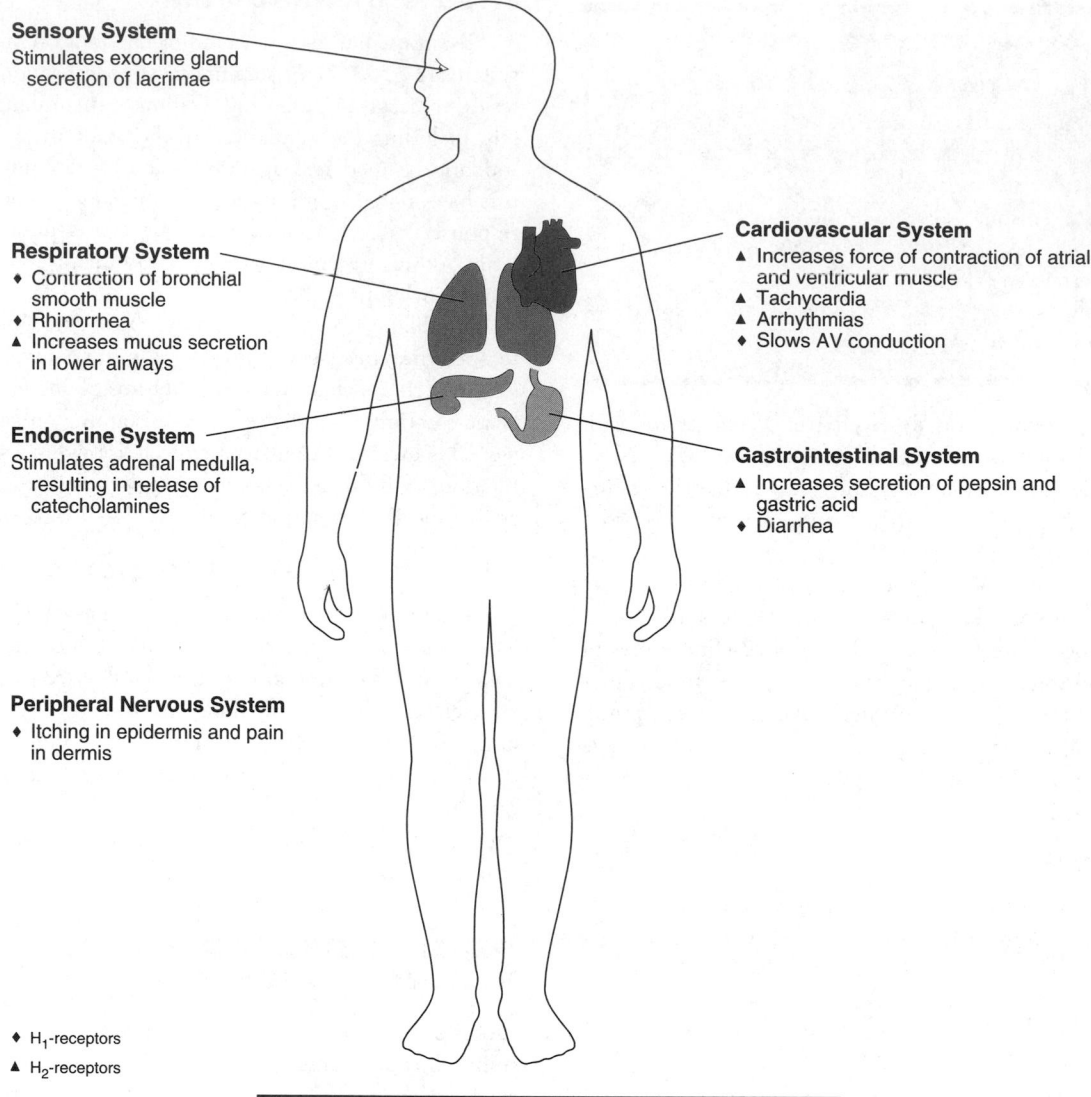

Sensory System
Stimulates exocrine gland
secretion of lacrimae

Respiratory System
♦ Contraction of bronchial
  smooth muscle
♦ Rhinorrhea
▲ Increases mucus secretion
  in lower airways

Cardiovascular System
▲ Increases force of contraction of atrial
  and ventricular muscle
▲ Tachycardia
▲ Arrhythmias
♦ Slows AV conduction

Endocrine System
Stimulates adrenal medulla,
resulting in release of
catecholamines

Gastrointestinal System
▲ Increases secretion of pepsin and
  gastric acid
♦ Diarrhea

Peripheral Nervous System
♦ Itching in epidermis and pain
  in dermis

♦ H₁-receptors
▲ H₂-receptors

FIGURE 50–1   Effects of histamine on body systems.

continuing on drugs that block histamine's effects on H_3 receptors. Most of the effects of histamine on allergic conditions are mediated through the H_1 receptors.[5] Some of histamine's effects such as hypotension, flushing, and headache require the combined use of H_1- and H_2-receptor antagonists to eliminate the response completely.[8] This chapter focuses on the H_1-receptor antagonists.

The term **antihistamine** frequently is used when referring to a drug that acts as an H_1-receptor antagonist. As discussed previously, H_1-receptor antagonists work by blocking H_1-receptor sites, thus preventing the interaction of histamine with the H_1 receptors. The H_1 antagonists do not chemically inactivate or physiologically exert any type of effect on histamine itself, nor do most antihistamines prevent the release of histamine from the cells.

The six subclasses of **first-generation H_1-receptor antagonists** include ethanolamines, alkylamines, phenothiazines, piperidines, ethylenediamines, and piperazines. A subclass of newer, **second-generation H_1-receptor antagonists** has been

developed. These drugs, which are actually piperidine derivatives, are large lipophobic molecules that are extensively protein bound.

In general, all subclasses of the H_1-receptor antagonists have similar actions and can be discussed together. However, some differences exist, not just between the subclasses, but between specific drugs within each subclass. The nurse is responsible for studying the individual drugs before administering them.

CONCEPT REVIEW

When a foreign substance (antigen) interacts with IgE antibodies, cells are damaged, and the histamines stored in the cells are released.

These histamines elicit symptoms seen during allergic and anaphylactic reactions.

PHARMACOTHERAPEUTICS OF H₁-RECEPTOR ANTAGONISTS

The H₁-receptor antagonists are used to treat the symptoms of various immediate (type I) hypersensitivity reactions. The majority of the H₁ antagonists are effective in treating perennial allergic rhinitis and seasonal allergic rhinitis (hay fever). They relieve the rhinorrhea, sneezing, and lacrimation and itching of eyes, nose, and throat that are characteristic symptoms of these conditions. Antihistamines are more effective when pollen counts are low. They are less effective when pollen counts are high, exposure to the allergens is prolonged, or nasal congestion has become pronounced. Use of the nonsedating (second-generation) antihistamines is especially beneficial to clients with perennial allergic rhinitis whose nasal mucosa is constantly inflamed.[9] A number of antihistamines are effective in reducing the rhinorrhea of vasomotor rhinitis, and some are effective in treating allergic conjunctivitis caused by foods or inhaled allergens.

H₁-receptor antagonists can be used to treat the mild, uncomplicated allergic skin manifestations of urticaria and an-

gioedema. Angioedema is usually limited to diffuse, nonpitting edema of the deeper layers of the skin; it sometimes gives a reddish hue to the skin. However, in individuals with severe angioedema that involves edema of mucous membranes, laryngeal edema can become life threatening. These cases require initial treatment with epinephrine followed by adjuvant use of antihistamines.

Similarly, when used in the treatment of anaphylactic reactions, H₁-receptor antagonists act as an adjunct to epinephrine and other standard measures after the acute symptoms of anaphylaxis (sudden loss of blood pressure, urticaria, dyspnea) are under control. Antihistamines are useful in the amelioration of allergic reactions to blood or plasma not caused by ABO incompatibilities or pyrogens; they should not be added to blood that is being transfused.

These drugs are very effective in the treatment of acute urticaria. They are less effective when used to treat chronic urticaria, but some relief is obtained. Certain allergic dermatoses, allergic dermatitis conditions, and dermatographism also respond to treatment with H₁ antagonists. Antihistamines relieve itching, burning, erythema, edema, and skin lesions. Some antihistamines relieve the itching that accompanies pityriasis rosea, poison ivy dermatitis, eczematous dermatitis, pruritus ani and vulvae, and drug rash. Because they do inhibit allergic dermatoses and may suppress the wheal-and-flare response, antihistamine use is usually stopped approximately 4 days before skin testing for allergies is performed.

Dimenhydrinate, promethazine, and the piperazines are very useful as antiemetics and for prophylaxis and treatment of motion sickness, although they produce simultaneous sedation. Dimenhydrinate and meclizine reduce the vertigo associated with Ménière's disease and other vestibular disturbances. The sedative effect of the antihistamines is the basis for their use as preoperative sedatives or as mild nighttime sleep aids. Diphenhydramine is a common ingredient in many of the over-the-counter (OTC) sleep aids. Diphenhydramine reverses the extrapyramidal side effects caused by phenothiazines. Diphenhydramine is also used to treat Parkinson's disease.

Some antihistamines are effective in relieving rhinorrhea and sneezing associated with the common cold. However, use of an H₁-receptor antagonist by itself may not be sufficient to relieve all symptoms adequately, so drug combinations may be prescribed. Additives such as pseudoephedrine, phenylephrine, and phenylpropanolamine have a sympathomimetic effect that produces vasoconstriction and results in nasal decongestion. When codeine is used as an additive, it produces an antitussive (cough suppressant) effect by depressing the medullary cough center in the brain. Although the use of these combination products enhances their effectiveness and expands the range of symptoms that can be relieved, the list of possible side effects increases. The nurse must be aware of the actions and side effects of the additive ingredients so that proper observations are made and appropriate client teaching implemented. The effects of the H₁-receptor antagonists on specific body systems are illustrated in Figure 50–2.

TERMS ASSOCIATED WITH ANTIHISTAMINE THERAPY

Angioedema condition characterized by development of urticaria and edematous areas of skin, mucous membranes, or viscera

Atopic disease allergy for which there is a genetic predisposition

Cold urticaria cold-induced urticarial eruption that may progress to angioedema

Dermatitis inflammation of the skin evidenced by itching, redness, and various skin lesions

Dermatographism abnormal skin condition characterized by wheals that form from tracing on the skin with the fingernail or a blunted instrument; makes skin especially susceptible to irritation and may be associated with urticaria

Dermatosis disease of skin in which inflammation is not necessarily a feature

Flare flush or spreading area of redness that surrounds an area of injured skin; the second reaction in the triple response

Perennial rhinitis nonseasonal inflammation of the nasal mucous membranes; continues indefinitely with variations in severity

Urticaria vascular reaction of the skin characterized by the eruption of pale, short-lived wheals, which are associated with severe itching (synonym: hives)

Vasomotor rhinitis rhinorrhea due to increased secretion of mucus from the nasal mucosa; may be caused by allergy or neurovascular imbalance

Wheal more-or-less round and short-lived elevation of the skin, white in center, with pale red periphery, accompanied by itching; seen in individuals with urticaria, insect bites, anaphylaxis, angioneurotic edema

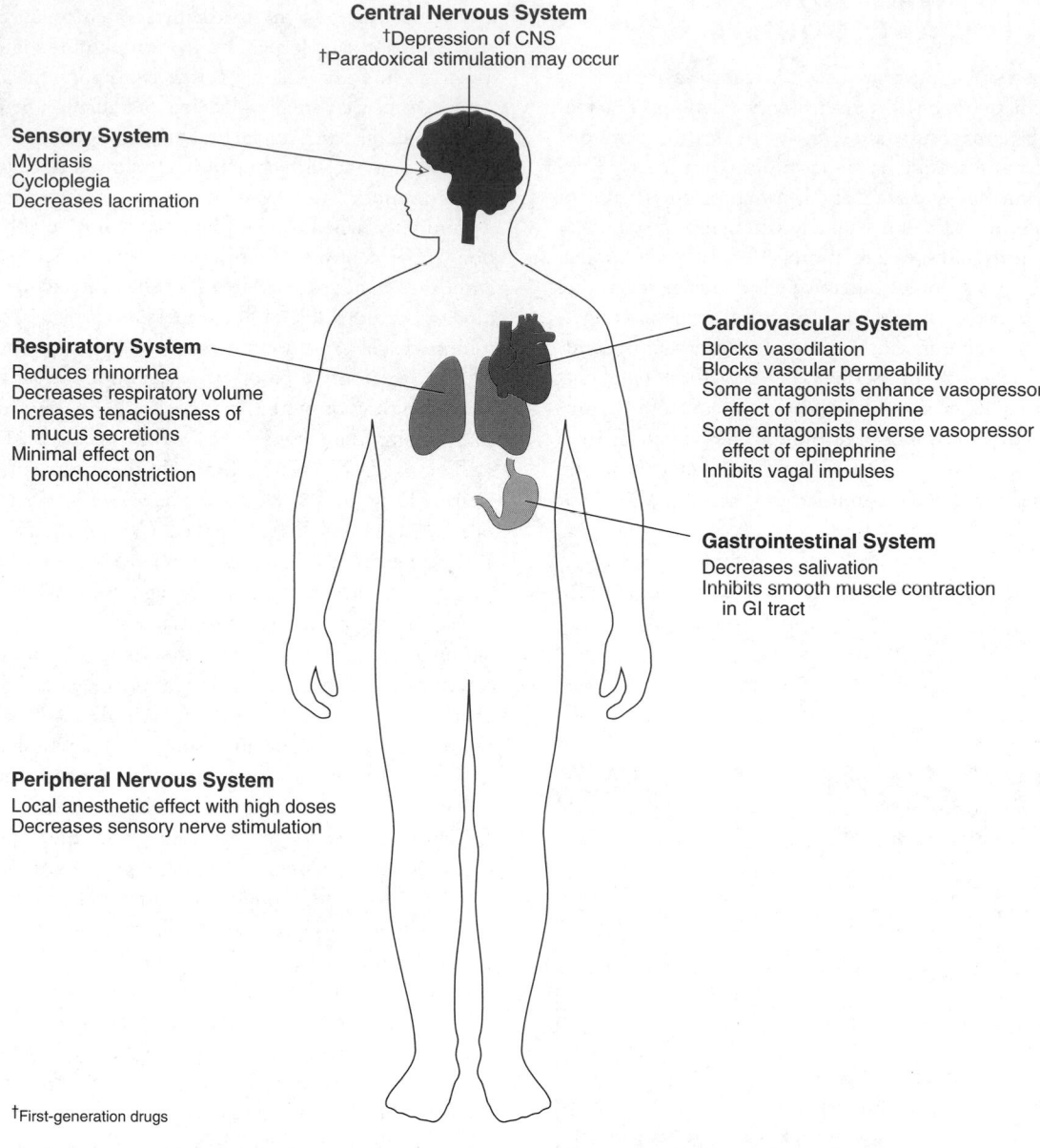

Central Nervous System
†Depression of CNS
†Paradoxical stimulation may occur

Sensory System
Mydriasis
Cycloplegia
Decreases lacrimation

Respiratory System
Reduces rhinorrhea
Decreases respiratory volume
Increases tenaciousness of
 mucus secretions
Minimal effect on
 bronchoconstriction

Cardiovascular System
Blocks vasodilation
Blocks vascular permeability
Some antagonists enhance vasopressor
 effect of norepinephrine
Some antagonists reverse vasopressor
 effect of epinephrine
Inhibits vagal impulses

Gastrointestinal System
Decreases salivation
Inhibits smooth muscle contraction
 in GI tract

Peripheral Nervous System
Local anesthetic effect with high doses
Decreases sensory nerve stimulation

†First-generation drugs

FIGURE 50–2   Effects of H_1-receptor antagonists on body systems.

CONCEPT REVIEW

H_1-receptor antagonists are used to treat the characteristic symptoms of hay fever (rhinorrhea, sneezing, watery and itchy eyes), skin symptoms, and anaphylactic shock.

Additional uses are to prevent motion sickness and to produce mild sedation.

▨ NURSING CONSIDERATIONS

The major responsibility of health care providers caring for clients receiving H_1-receptor antagonists is client education. This is accomplished through assessment of the client's needs and development of interventions that minimize the occurrence of undesired clinical responses.

Assessing   Before therapy with antihistamines is initiated, a thorough nursing **health history** should be obtained. Assess for pregnancy, lactation, history of seizures, and prior adverse reactions from use of antihistamines. For clients prescribed a second-generation antihistamine, assess for a history of arrhythmias or significant hepatic dysfunction. Assess clients for preexisting physical conditions that would either contraindicate or require caution in the use of H_1 antagonists with anticholinergic effects (e.g., narrow-angle glaucoma, stenosing peptic ulcer, symptomatic prostatic hypertrophy, bladder-neck obstruction, urinary retention, pyloroduodenal obstruction, history of bronchial asthma, chronic pulmonary disease, severe cardiovascular disease, hypertension, hyperthyroidism, diminished cough reflex, or central nervous system [CNS] depression from use of alcohol, narcotic analgesics, or barbiturates).

After obtaining the health history, have the client identify all drugs currently in use. Determine possible interactions with H_1 antagonists. Assess the client's knowledge of the condition for which the H_1 antagonists have been prescribed, and ask the client to describe any symptoms. Assess baseline vital signs and results of laboratory and diagnostic studies.

Diagnosing Analyze the data obtained from the nursing health history and develop appropriate nursing diagnoses. Possible nursing diagnoses related to drug therapy follow:

- Health seeking behaviors related to required lifestyle modifications.
- Knowledge deficit regarding correct administration, actions, and side effects of H_1 antagonists.
- Altered oral mucous membranes related to decreased oral secretions associated with use of antihistamines with anticholinergic effects.
- Ineffective airway clearance related to tenacious secretions associated with use of antihistamines with anticholinergic effects.
- High risk for altered health maintenance related to failure to discontinue drugs 2 to 4 days before allergy skin testing.
- High risk for noncompliance with medication regimen related to negative side effects of prescribed medications.
- High risk for injury related to drowsiness, dizziness, or hypotension.
- High risk for injury related to exceeding recommended dosages of antihistamines.
- High risk for altered urinary elimination patterns related to use of antihistamines with anticholinergic effects.
- High risk for altered sexuality patterns related to sexual dysfunction secondary to side effects of selected antihistamines.

Planning When formulating a plan of care for the client, set specific client outcomes. Possible expected outcomes include the following:

- Client experiences relief of symptoms.
- Client achieves and maintains effective airway clearance.
- Client is free from injury, severe side effects, or adverse reactions.
- Client experiences a reduction in discomfort.
- Client maintains adequate nutrition.
- Client adapts to necessary lifestyle alterations.
- Client demonstrates knowledge of safe self-administration of drugs and the need for follow-up care.

A teaching plan should be developed. Information to include in the plan can be organized under four basic points: (1) safety factors, (2) drug side effects, (3) drug administration, and (4) follow-up care.

In the plan, stress the measures to promote safety. Advise the client to store H_1 antagonists in tightly closed, light-resistant containers in a cool, dry location out of the reach of children. Advise the client not to combine the drug with other CNS depressants such as alcohol, analgesics, barbiturates, or tranquilizers. Counsel the client that symptoms of CNS depression (marked drowsiness, dizziness, weakness, slowed reaction times) are common with usual dosages. Teach the client to avoid performing potentially hazardous activities (e.g., driving motor vehicles, operating machinery) that require mental alertness or physical coordination if they experience these symptoms. Advise parents to supervise children who are taking antihistamines while they are engaged in potentially hazardous activities.

Advise the client to make position changes slowly if orthostatic hypotension or dizziness develops. Suggest that the client minimize exposure to individuals with upper respiratory infections. Advise clients with allergies to avoid exposure to known allergens and to practice allergy precautions. Recommend that the client wear an identification bracelet or necklace that indicates substances to which he or she is allergic.

Advise the client with pruritus to keep his or her fingernails trimmed short and smooth. Instruct the client who wears contact lenses that the lenses must be moistened more frequently to prevent corneal abrasions. In addition, lens-cleaning procedures may need modification if characteristics of lacrimal secretions change as a result of using H_1 antagonists.

Teach the client to recognize and prevent drug side effects and how to cope with the unavoidable side effects of antihistamine therapy. Advise the client to avoid the use of caffeine or other stimulants to counteract the CNS depressant effects of antihistamines. Teach the client who experiences palpitations to rest until the symptom subsides and to report this side effect to the primary care provider.

Teach the client about coughing and deep breathing, increasing activity, and increasing fluid intake to 1500 to 2000 ml/d, unless contraindicated, to promote expectoration of secretions. Increasing activity and fluid intake also helps prevent constipation. Advise the client that the use of artificial tears reduces dryness and corneal irritation. Teach the client to practice good oral hygiene and to use sugarless gum or candy to minimize the effects of dry mouth. Advise the client to maintain a schedule of voiding at least every 4 hours to prevent urinary complications. Instruct the client to wear sunscreen, sunglasses, and protective clothing to prevent photosensitivity reactions.

Advise the client about the correct administration of H_1 antagonists: dosage, route, times, desired actions, and side effects. Teach him or her to take the drugs only as directed and not to exceed the recommended dosage. This is especially important with the second-generation drugs, whose duration of action is 12 to 24 hours. Excessive dosages of these drugs can result in severe cardiac events. Instruct the client not to self-regulate dosages of H_1 antagonists and to contact the primary care provider before combining H_1 antagonists with OTC drugs. Instruct the client in the proper administration technique for the prescribed dosage from.

To achieve appropriate follow-up care for the client, advise him or her to report pertinent side effects of H_1 antagonists to the primary care provider. Instruct the client to seek immediate medical attention should an upper respiratory infection develop. In addition, tell him or her to report any voiding difficulties such as painful urination, the sensation of incomplete relief with voiding, or changes in frequency to the health care provider and also to report the development of involuntary muscle movements or insomnia that persists for longer than 2 weeks.

Implementing Nursing interventions must be individualized; they vary according to the client's specific condition and the prescribed medication. Interventions for specific drugs are discussed in Table 50–1.

To promote effective airway clearance, encourage coughing and deep breathing exercises and expectoration of secretions. Assess lung sounds and characteristics of sputum or cough. Unless contraindicated, increase fluid intake to 1500 to 2000 ml/d to decrease the viscosity of secretions. Encourage frequent position changes and increased activity to decrease pooling of secretions.

To promote client safety, monitor blood pressure for hypotension or hypertension and report development of any blood pressure difficulties. Monitor lying and standing blood pressures to detect postural hypotension. Assist with ambulation if the client experiences episodes of dizziness. Monitor pulse for tachycardia, bradycardia, or arrhythmias. Serious cardiac events (death, cardiac arrest, torsade de pointes and other ventricular arrhythmias) have been reported with use of the second-generation antihistamines terfenadine and astemizole. Observe for electrocardiogram (ECG) changes, including prolongation of QT interval, flattened T waves, and ventricular tachycardia, on monitored clients.

Continually assess the client for petechiae, ecchymoses, epistaxis, bleeding gums, excessive or irregular vaginal bleeding, hematuria, or symptoms of GI bleeding. Perform tests for occult blood in urine and stool. Assess for bladder distention and note characteristics of urine—color, amount, frequency. To promote comfort, plan nursing interventions that minimize sleep interruptions. Assess sleep patterns and note complaints of daytime sleepiness or frequent napping.

Do not crush or let the client chew orally administered sustained-release preparations; however, have the client thoroughly chew chewable tablets before swallowing. Avoid administering sustained-release preparations to children less than 12 years of age. Children less than 6 years of age should not be given repeat-action tablets. Syrup preparations are intended for children but may be used by adults who have difficulty swallowing tablets or capsules.

Administer parenteral H_1 antagonists carefully; avoid the use of subcutaneous (SC) injections. Administer these drugs by intramuscular (IM) injection deep into well-developed muscle; rotate IM injection sites. Check syringe and intravenous (IV) solution compatibilities before combining them.

Antihistamines can affect the client's nutritional status or GI function. Administer these drugs with food or milk to decrease GI irritation. Assess clients for complaints of nausea, vomiting, epigastric distress, loss of appetite, or increased appetite. Auscultate bowel sounds and observe for changes in frequency or consistency of bowel movements. Listen for complaints of abdominal pain. If the client is experiencing diarrhea, assess for signs and symptoms of dehydration.

Evaluating   Evaluate to determine if the drug therapy is effective and observe for side effects or adverse reactions. The client should experience relief of the symptoms for which the antihistamines are prescribed. Normal breathing patterns and effective airway clearance should be maintained. Excessive sedation and injury or adverse drug reactions should be avoided. Vital signs should be within normal range. Laboratory and di-

agnostic tests to monitor the client's progress may be ordered. They may include complete blood count (CBC), urine and stool tests, and ECG.

CONCEPT REVIEW

Obtain a thorough health history to identify allergies or other preexisting problems that would contraindicate the use of antihistamines.

Since many of these drugs are available over the counter, teach the client about safety factors, drug side effects, drug administration techniques, and follow-up care. Carefully observe clients receiving antihistamines for side effects or adverse reactions.

FIRST-GENERATION ANTAGONISTS

First-generation H_1-receptor antagonists comprise the older group of histamine blockers. As previously mentioned, this group is divided into several subclasses: ethanolamines, alkylamines, phenothiazines, piperidines, ethylenediamines, and piperazines.

Ethanolamines

ETHANOLAMINE PROTOTYPE
DIPHENHYDRAMINE HYDROCHLORIDE

Pharmacotherapeutics Diphenhydramine (Benadryl) is used to treat all of the conditions presented in the general discussion section.

Pharmacokinetics Diphenhydramine hydrochloride is well absorbed after oral administration. It undergoes first-pass metabolism in the liver; approximately 40% to 60% of an oral dose reaches the systemic circulation unchanged. It can be absorbed percutaneously after topical administration but rarely produces systemic effects or toxicity when administered topically. After oral administration of a single dose, diphenhydramine appears in plasma within 15 minutes. Peak plasma concentrations are reached within 1 to 4 hours. The antihistamine effect (as measured by suppression of the wheal-and-flare response after intradermal injection of histamine) is maximal within 1 to 3 hours and may last for up to 7 hours after administration of a single dose. Sedative effects are maximal within 1 to 3 hours.

Distribution of diphenhydramine has not been fully determined. The drug is 80% to 85% bound to plasma proteins. Half-life ranges from 2.4 to 9.3 hours in healthy adults and is prolonged in clients with cirrhosis of the liver. Diphenhydramine crosses the placenta and has been detected in breast milk. The drug is rapidly and almost completely metabolized. Diphenhydramine and its metabolites are excreted primarily in the urine.[10,11]

Pharmacodynamics Diphenhydramine binds competitively with histamine at the H_1 receptors. This binding is reversible and depends on free-drug plasma concentrations. While it is bound to the receptor, diphenhydramine antagonizes the effects of histamine at the receptor sites. Diphenhydramine is lipophilic and easily crosses the blood-brain barrier, which accounts for its CNS effects. As the drug is metabolized and excreted, the histamine receptors become desaturated, allowing histamine to bind to the receptors. Because of this action, frequent doses of diphenhydramine are required to sustain maximal desired effects.[10]

Pharmaceutics Diphenhydramine usually is administered orally. It can be administered by deep IM injection or IV infusion. It should not be given subcutaneously because of its irritating effects. Diphenhydramine is available in tablet, capsule, elixir, syrup, and injectable formulations. It is also available as topical creams, lotions, and solutions. Table 50–1 provides additional information about dosage forms, dosages, and routes of administration.

Undesired Clinical Responses Diphenhydramine can cause CNS depression; drowsiness occurs in approximately 50% of clients. Figure 50–3 illustrates common undesired clinical responses associated with most first-generation H_1-receptor antagonists.

Contraindications and Precautions Because it exerts a high degree of anticholinergic action, diphenhydramine should be used with caution and its use avoided if possible in clients with narrow-angle glaucoma, prostatic hypertrophy, stenosing peptic ulcer, pyloroduodenal obstruction, or bladder-neck obstruction. It should be used with caution and only under the direction of a primary care provider in clients with asthma or chronic obstructive pulmonary disease (COPD) if clearance of bronchial secretions is a problem. Diphenhydramine should also be used with caution in clients with seizure disorders, hyperthyroidism, cardiovascular disease, hypertension, or liver disease and by pregnant or lactating women. Commercially available formulations may contain sodium bisulfite, which could cause potentially severe allergic reactions in susceptible individuals.[11,12]

Drug-Drug, Drug-Nutrient, Drug-Environment Interactions Diphenhydramine can cause interactions with the following drugs: other antihistamines, anticholinesterases, CNS depressants, corticosteroids, monoamine oxidases inhibitors (MAOIs), hyoscine, or epinephrine (see Table 50–2). Caffeine counteracts the sedative effects of diphenhydramine. In addition, clients receiving diphenhydramine may experience photosensitivity reactions from sunlight exposure. Store the drug at room temperature.

Life-Span Considerations Diphenhydramine is classified as a Pregnancy Category B drug. It should not be administered to newborns or premature infants. Diphenhydramine use is also contraindicated in nursing mothers. In the elderly it is more likely to cause dizziness, sedation, and hypotension.

Specific Drug-Related Nursing Implications Diphenhydramine should be administered orally whenever possible. IM injections must be administered deep IM, and injection sites should be carefully rotated. Diphenhydramine is incompatible with most IV solutions and is syringe-incompatible with some drugs.

MISCELLANEOUS DRUG IN CATEGORY

Dimenhydrinate (Dramamine) remains a treatment choice for symptoms associated with vestibular stimulation. It is used to prevent and treat the nausea, vomiting, and vertigo of motion sickness. It is more effective for motion sickness when administered prophylactically.

Dimenhydrinate is well absorbed after oral administration. The exact distribution and metabolism of the drug are not known. Like other antihistamines, it is probably widely distributed in body tissues. Dimenhydrinate is metabolized in the liver; metabolites and small amounts of unchanged drug are eliminated in the urine. Small amounts of dimenhydrinate may be excreted in breast milk; it does cross the placental barrier.

Dimenhydrinate is available in tablets, chewable tablets, and syrup for oral administration. It is also available in patch form for topical application and in parenteral solutions. After oral administration, the onset of antiemetic action is 15 to 30 minutes. The peak effect is within 1 to 2 hours; duration of action is unknown. Antiemetic effects are almost immediate after IV administration and occur within 20 to 30 minutes after IM administration. Patch dosage forms are used primarily in the prevention of motion sickness.

Drowsiness occurs commonly with administration of dimenhydrinate, especially early in therapy. Excitation may be an early sign of toxicity in children. Other indications of toxicity in adults and children include dilated pupils, flushed face, ataxia, hallucinations, and convulsions.

Advise clients that tolerance to drowsiness usually develops in a few days. During initial therapy safety precautions (e.g., supervised ambulation, side rails) must be available. Instruct clients to avoid hazardous activities that require mental alertness or physical coordination. Caution the client not to drink alcohol or take sedatives or tranquilizers while receiving dimenhydrinate therapy without consulting the prescriber.

Alkylamines

ALKYLAMINE PROTOTYPE
CHLORPHENIRAMINE MALEATE

Pharmacotherapeutics Chlorpheniramine (Teldrin, Chlor-Trimeton) is used in the treatment of seasonal and perennial allergic rhinitis, vasomotor rhinitis, and the common cold.

Pharmacokinetics Chlorpheniramine is well absorbed after oral administration. It appears in the plasma within 30 to 60 minutes after oral administration, and peak plasma concentrations occur within 2 to 6 hours. Antihistamine effect (as measured by suppression of the wheal-and-flare response after intradermal injection of histamine) occurs within 6 hours after a single oral dose and lasts up to at least 24 hours.

Distribution of chlorpheniramine into body tissues and fluids has not been fully determined, but it is known that the drug undergoes rapid and extensive distribution. Approximately 69% to 72% is bound to plasma proteins. Half-life of chlorpheniramine in adults with normal renal and hepatic function ranges from 12 to 43 hours.

The drug is rapidly and extensively metabolized and undergoes significant metabolism in the GI tract and on first-pass metabolism through the liver after oral administration. The drug and its metabolites are almost completely excreted by the urine.[11,12]

Pharmacodynamics See diphenhydramine hydrochloride.

Pharmaceutics Chlorpheniramine may be administered orally or by SC and IM injections or IV infusion. It is available in tablet, chewable tablet, capsule, timed-release tablet, timed-release capsule, syrup, and injectable formulations (see Table 50–1).

Undesired Clinical Responses Chlorpheniramine can cause sedation, drowsiness, dry mouth, hypertension, and blurred vision (see Fig. 50–3).

Contraindications and Precautions Chlorpheniramine possesses a moderate degree of anticholinergic action and should be used with caution in clients with narrow-angle glaucoma, prostatic hypertrophy, stenosing peptic ulcer, pyloroduodenal obstruction, or bladder-neck obstruction. It should be used with caution and only under the direction of a primary care provider in clients with liver disease and during pregnancy and lactation. Individuals with phenylketonuria and others who must restrict their intake of phenylalanine should be warned that some preparations contain aspartame, which is metabolized in the GI tract to phenylalanine after oral ingestion.[11]

Drug-Drug, Drug-Nutrient, Drug-Environment Interactions Chlorpheniramine can cause interactions with the following drugs: anticholinesterases, hyoscine, CNS depressants, corticosteroids, MAOIs, and promethazine (see Table 50–2).

Caffeine counteracts the sedative effects of chlorpheniramine. Clients taking chlorpheniramine may experience photosensitivity reactions from sunlight exposure.

Life-Span Considerations Chlorpheniramine is classified as a Pregnancy Category B drug. Its use is not recommended during pregnancy, especially in the third trimester, or during breast-feeding. Chlorpheniramine

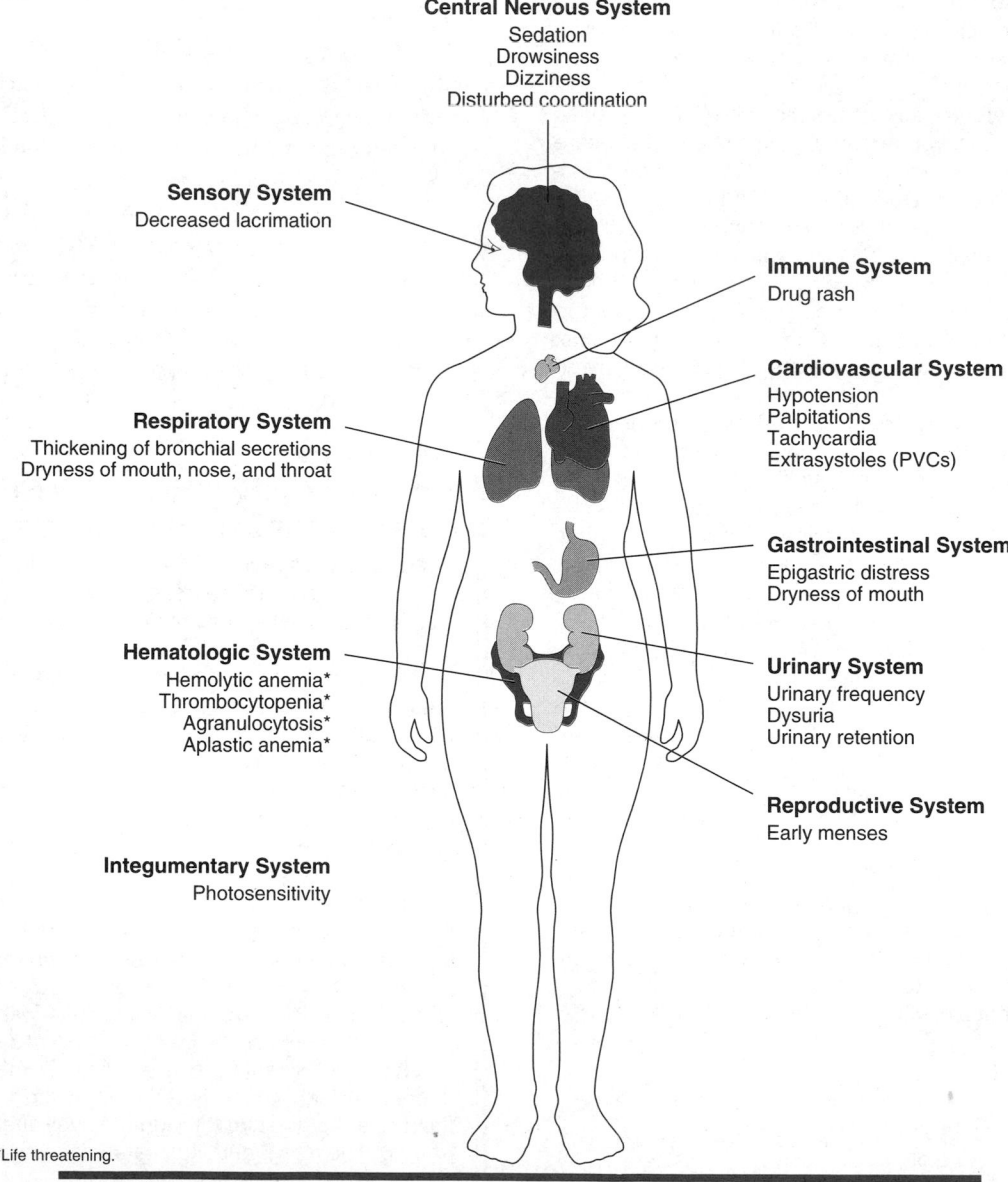

Central Nervous System
Sedation
Drowsiness
Dizziness
Disturbed coordination

Sensory System
Decreased lacrimation

Immune System
Drug rash

Cardiovascular System
Hypotension
Palpitations
Tachycardia
Extrasystoles (PVCs)

Respiratory System
Thickening of bronchial secretions
Dryness of mouth, nose, and throat

Gastrointestinal System
Epigastric distress
Dryness of mouth

Hematologic System
Hemolytic anemia*
Thrombocytopenia*
Agranulocytosis*
Aplastic anemia*

Urinary System
Urinary frequency
Dysuria
Urinary retention

Reproductive System
Early menses

Integumentary System
Photosensitivity

*Life threatening.

FIGURE 50–3 Common undesired clinical responses associated with first-generation H₁-receptor antagonists.

should not be used in children less than 12 years of age unless under direct supervision of a primary care provider.

Specific Drug-Related Nursing Considerations Sustained-release formulations of chlorpheniramine should not be crushed or chewed, and their use is contraindicated in children less than 12 years of age. Monitor the client's blood pressure, especially that of the elderly. Monitor children closely for paradoxical reaction.

Phenothiazines
PHENOTHIAZINE PROTOTYPE
PROMETHAZINE HYDROCHLORIDE

Pharmacotherapeutics Promethazine hydrochloride (Phenergan) is used to treat motion sickness, nausea, and allergic rhinitis. It is also administered for its sedative effect. Promethazine sometimes is used as a component of preoperative or postoperative sedation or as an adjunct to analgesics.

Pharmacokinetics Promethazine is well absorbed from the GI tract. Onset of antihistamine effects (as measured by suppression of the wheal-and-flare response after intradermal injection of histamine) occurs within 20 minutes after oral, IM, or rectal administration and within 3 to 5 minutes after IV administration. Duration of action is variable but may last for 12 hours or longer.

Promethazine is widely distributed in body tissues. It is 76% to 93% protein bound. The drug readily crosses the placenta; distribution into breast milk has not been established. Promethazine is metabolized by the liver and excreted in both urine and feces. Half-life is unknown.[11–13]

Pharmacodynamics See diphenhydramine hydrochloride.

Pharmaceutics Promethazine can be administered by oral, rectal, IM, or IV routes. It is available in tablet, syrup, suppository, and injectable formulations. See Table 50–1 for additional information about dosage forms and dosages.

Undesired Clinical Responses The major and most common adverse reactions to promethazine are pronounced sedation, confusion, and disorientation (see Fig. 50–3).

Contraindications and Precautions Promethazine exerts a high degree of anticholinergic activity. It should be used with caution and its use avoided if possible in clients with narrow-angle glaucoma, prostatic hypertrophy, stenosing peptic ulcer, pyloroduodenal obstruction, or bladder-neck obstruction.

It should also be used with caution in clients with cardiovascular disease, impaired liver function, acute or chronic respiratory function, sleep apnea, and seizure disorders. Commercially available formulations may contain sulfites, which could cause potentially severe allergic reactions in susceptible individuals.

Drug-Drug, Drug-Nutrient Interactions Promethazine can cause interactions with the following: anticholinesterases, hyoscine, CNS depressants, corticosteroids, MAOIs, antacids, anticholinergics, anticonvulsants, antihypertensives, epinephrine, oral antidiabetic drugs, thiazide diuretics, and ototoxic drugs (see Table 50–2). Caffeine counteracts the sedative effects of promethazine.

Life-Span Considerations Although it has been used safely during labor, chronic use of promethazine during pregnancy should be avoided. Safety during lactation has not been established. Elderly clients may require a reduced dosage.

Specific Drug-Related Nursing Considerations Nursing implications related to use of promethazine are varied and extensive. Avoid SC administration because tissue necrosis may result. Anticipate reduction in dosages of analgesics by 25% to 50% when promethazine is used as an adjunct. Observe clients carefully for either CNS depression or paradoxical stimulation; observe for involuntary muscle movements.

Piperidines
PIPERIDINE PROTOTYPE
CYPROHEPTADINE HYDROCHLORIDE

Pharmacotherapeutics Cyproheptadine hydrochloride (Periactin) is used primarily to treat allergy symptoms and pruritus. It has also been used to treat headaches produced by excess histamine in the body.[12,14]

Pharmacokinetics Cyproheptadine is well absorbed after oral administration. Peak plasma concentrations occur 6 to 9 hours after oral administration. Distribution into body tissues and fluids has not been fully determined. The amount of distribution into breast milk is unknown. The drug is almost completely metabolized and is excreted in urine and feces. Half-life of cyproheptadine is unknown.[11,12]

Pharmacodynamics See diphenhydramine hydrochloride.

Pharmaceutics Cyproheptadine is administered orally as tablets and syrup. See Table 50–1 for additional information about dosage forms and dosages.

Undesired Clinical Responses Major adverse reactions to cyproheptadine are drowsiness, sedation, dry mouth, and blurred vision (see Fig. 50–3).

Contraindications and Precautions Cyproheptadine exerts moderate anticholinergic effects and should be used with caution in clients with narrow-angle glaucoma, prostatic hypertrophy, stenosing peptic ulcer, pyloroduodenal obstruction, or bladder-neck obstruction. It should also be used with caution in clients with liver disease or acute asthma and during pregnancy and lactation.

Drug-Drug, Drug-Nutrient, Drug-Environment Interactions Cyproheptadine can cause interactions with the following drugs: anticholinesterases, hyoscine, CNS depressants, corticosteroids, MAOIs, and promethazine. Caffeine counteracts the sedative effects of cyproheptadine. Clients taking cyproheptadine may experience photosensitivity reactions from sunlight exposure.

Life-Span Considerations Cyproheptadine is classified as a Pregnancy Category B drug. Its use is not recommended during pregnancy, especially in the third trimester, or during breast-feeding. Cyproheptadine should not be administered to children less than 14 years of age without direct supervision of primary care provider. Elderly clients may require a reduced dosage.

Specific Drug-Related Nursing Considerations Oral dosage forms of cyproheptadine may be administered with food to decrease GI distress. Monitor the client carefully for CNS effects (e.g., drowsiness, sedation). If severe drowsiness occurs, institute safety measures. Tell client that sugarless gum, sour hard candy, or ice chips may relieve dry mouth.

Ethylenediamines
ETHYLENEDIAMINE PROTOTYPE
TRIPELENNAMINE HYDROCHLORIDE

Pharmacotherapeutics Tripelennamine hydrochloride (PBZ) is primarily used to treat allergic rhinitis. [12,15]

Pharmacokinetics Tripelennamine is well absorbed after oral administration. Peak plasma concentrations are achieved within 2 to 3 hours after oral administration. Distribution of the drug has not been fully determined, but it does cross the placenta. It is almost completely metabolized and is excreted primarily in the urine.

Pharmacodynamics See diphenhydramine hydrochloride.

Pharmaceutics Tripelennamine is administered orally and is available as tablets, elixir, and sustained-release tablets. See Table 50–1 for additional information about dosage forms and dosages.

Undesired Clinical Response Tripelennamine shares the common side effects of other antihistamines. It produces a low degree of anticholinergic effect, so side effects related to anticholinergic activity are limited (see Fig. 50–3).

Contraindications and Precautions Tripelennamine use is contraindicated in clients with hypersensitivity to the drug or antihistamines with similar chemical structure such as pyrilamine. It is also not recommended for use during asthma attacks or for clients who have taken MAO inhibitors within the preceding 2 weeks. Because it has a significant anticholinergic effect, tripelennamine should be used with caution in clients with narrow-angle glaucoma, urinary bladder obstruction, or cardiovascular disease.

Drug-Drug, Drug-Nutrient, Drug-Environment Interactions Tripelennamine should not be administered with the following drugs: anticholinesterases, MAOIs, CNS depressants, corticosteroids, hyoscine, promethazine, or epinephrine (see Table 50–2). Caffeine counteracts the sedative effects of tripelennamine. Clients taking tripelennamine may experience photosensitivity reactions from sunlight exposure.

Life-Span Considerations Tripelennamine should be used with caution in infants and young children. Extended-release tablets should not be used in children. Tripelennamine should be used cautiously or not at all in pregnant or lactating women. Elderly clients may require a reduced dosage.

Specific Drug-Related Nursing Considerations Sustained-release tablets should not be crushed, chewed, or administered to children. See Table 50–2 for additional nursing considerations.

Piperazines
PIPERAZINE PROTOTYPE
HYDROXYZINE HYDROCHLORIDE

Pharmacotherapeutics Hydroxyzine hydrochloride (Atarax, Vistaril) is used in the treatment of anxiety, tension, and hyperkinesia. It sometimes is administered as a part of preoperative and postoperative adjunctive therapy. Hydroxyzine is also prescribed to relieve rashes and pruritus. [12,15]

Pharmacokinetics Hydroxyzine is rapidly absorbed from the GI tract after oral administration. Onset of sedative action occurs 15 to 30 minutes after oral administration. The action peaks in 2 to 4 hours, and sedative effects last for 4 to 6 hours. Hydroxyzine suppresses pruritus and the inflammatory response (wheal-and-flare reaction) for up to 4 days. Distribution of hydroxyzine has not been fully identified. It is unknown whether the drug crosses the placenta or is distributed into breast milk. It is completely metabolized by the liver and excreted by the feces via biliary elimination. Half-life for hydroxyzine is 3 hours.

Pharmacodynamics See diphenhydramine hydrochloride.

Pharmaceutics Hydroxyzine is administered orally and is available in tablet, capsule, syrup, and suspension formulations. See Table 50–1 for additional information about dosage forms and dosages.

Undesired Clinical Responses The primary side effects of hydroxyzine are drowsiness and dry mouth (see Fig. 50–3).

Contraindications and Precautions Hydroxyzine use is contraindicated in clients with hypersensitivity to the drug. It should be used with caution in clients with open-angle glaucoma, urinary retention, or any condition in which anticholinergic effects would be detrimental.

Drug-Drug, Drug-Nutrient Interactions Hydroxyzine can cause interactions with the following drugs: anticholinesterases, hyoscine, CNS depressants, corticosteroids, MAOIs, promethazine, epinephrine, and ototoxic drugs (see Table 50–2). Caffeine counteracts the sedative effects of hydroxyzine.

Life-Span Considerations Hydroxyzine use is contraindicated during early pregnancy, and it is inadvisable during lactation because hydroxyzine's degree of distribution into breast milk is not known. The drug should be used with caution in clients with severe liver disease and in elderly clients.

Specific Drug-Related Nursing Considerations Observe for excessive sedation if hydroxyzine is used with other CNS depressants. See Table 50–3 for additional nursing considerations.

CONCEPT REVIEW

First-generation H_1-receptor antagonists comprise the older group of drugs used to block the effects of histamine. These drugs are divided into six subclasses: ethanolamines, alkylamines, phenothiazines, piperidines, ethylenediamines, and piperazines.

Undesired clinical responses produced by these drugs are numerous and affect many body systems.

Most first-generation drugs are classified as Pregnancy Category B or C drugs; therefore their use during pregnancy is limited.

Administration to children less than 12 years old usually requires supervision and direction from the primary care provider.

TABLE 50–1

First-Generation H$_1$-Receptor Antagonists

Drug Name	Dosage and Route of Administration	Nursing Considerations

ETHANOLAMINES:
 	
DIPHENHYDRAMINE HYDROCHLORIDE
(Benadryl, Benylin)
HOW SUPPLIED
Capsules: 25, 50 mg
Tablets: 25, 50 mg
Elixir: 12.5 mg/ml
Injection: 10 mg/ml, 50 mg/ml
	ORAL DOSES
	Allergic Conditions
	Adults, children >12 y:
	25–50 mg q4-6h, not to exceed 300 mg/24 h
	Children 6–12 y:
	   12.5 mg q4-6h, not to exceed 150 mg/24 h
	   2–6 y: under supervision of primary care provider only—6.25 mg q4-6 h, not to exceed 37.5 mg/24 h
	
	Motion Sickness
	Adults, children >12 y:
	25–50 mg q4-6h, not to exceed 300 mg/24 h; give first dose 30 min before exposure to motion and other doses ac and hs
	Children 6–12 y:
	12.5–25 mg q4-6h, not to exceed 150 mg/24 h (or 5 mg/kg 24 h)
	
	Insomnia
	Adults, children >12 y:
	50 mg hs
	Children 2–12 y with sleep disorders:
	   1 mg/kg 30 min before bedtime
	Safety and efficacy in children <12 y not established
	
	Parkinson's Disease
	Initial dose: 25 mg tid; if needed, increase dosage gradually up to 50 mg qid
	
	PARENTERAL DOSES (IV or deep IM)
	Adults
	10–50 mg; 100 mg as required, not to exceed 400 mg/24 h
	Children
	5 mg/kg/24 h, not to exceed 300 mg/24 h divided into four doses
	
	TOPICAL APPLICATIONS
	Adults, children >2 y
	1% to 2% diphenhydramine cream, lotion, or solution to affected areas tid or qid or as directed by primary care provider
		Assess
		Determine if client has history of general adverse reactions to antihistamines.
		Assess pulse and blood pressure.
		Determine if client has preexisting conditions that contraindicate use of drug (e.g., bronchial asthma, hypotension, severe hypertension, or severe cardiac, pulmonary, or renal disease).
		
		Implement
		Administer orally whenever possible.
		Administer IM injections deep IM.
		Rotate IM injection sites.
		Do not administer SC because tissue necrosis may result.
		Check syringe or IV solution compatibilities because diphenhydramine is incompatible with most IV solutions and is syringe incompatible with some drugs.
		Store injection and elixir preparations in light-resistant containers.
		Do not apply topical preparations to broken or abraded skin.
		Do not use topical preparations on children <2 y of age unless specifically prescribed.
		Syrup formulations may contain ammonium chloride and sodium citrate as expectorants, although their actual therapeutic value is uncertain.
		
		Monitor
		Monitor client for undesired clinical responses (e.g., drowsiness, dizziness, disturbed coordination).
		Monitor blood pressure, especially in elderly since they have an increased risk of hypotension.
		
		Evaluate
		Assess client for reduction in signs and symptoms (e.g., decreased sneezing, increased sleep, decreased conjunctivitis).

Carbinoxamine maleate
(Rondec, Rondec-TR)
Usually combined with other drugs (e.g., dextromethorphan hydrochloride, pseudoephedrine hydrochloride)
HOW SUPPLIED
Oral solutions, tablets, and syrups
	Seasonal and Perennial Allergic Rhinitis; Vasomotor Rhinitis
	Adults
	4–8 mg tid or qid, not to exceed 24 mg/24 h; TR tablets for adults only
	Children
	   >6 y: 4–6 mg tid or qid
	   3–6 y: 2–4 mg tid or qid
	   1–3 y: 2 mg tid or qid or 0.2–0.4 mg/kg/24 h
	Infants: Oral Drops
	   9–19 mo: 1 dropper (1 ml = 2 mg) qid
	   6–9 mo: ¾ dropper (¾ ml = 1.5 mg) qid
	   3–6 mo: ½ dropper (½ ml = 1 mg) qid
		See diphenhydramine.

Table continued on following page.

TABLE 50–1 *Continued*
First-Generation H₁-Receptor Antagonists

Drug Name	Dosage and Route of Administration	Nursing Considerations
Carbinoxamine maleate **Continued**	***Seasonal and Perennial Allergic Rhinitis; vasomotor rhinitis Continued*** *Infants: Oral Drops Continued* 1–3 mo: ¼ dropper (¼ ml = 0.5 mg) qid	
Clemastine fumerate (Tavist, Tavist-1) HOW SUPPLIED Uncoated tablet: 1.34, 2.68 mg Syrup: 0.67 mg/5 ml	***Allergic Rhinitis*** *Adults, children >12 y:* 1.34 mg bid (Tavist tablet); increase as required, not to exceed 8.04 mg/24 h; or 2 tsp syrup bid, not to exceed 12 tsp/24 h *Children 6–12 y:* 1 tsp syrup (0.5 mg) bid; increase as required, not to exceed 6 tsp (3 mg)/24 h ***Urticaria or Angioedema*** *Adults, children >12 y:* 2.68 mg one to three times/d (tablet), not to exceed 8.04 mg/24 h or 4 tsp (2 mg) syrup bid; increase as needed, not to exceed 12 tsp (6 mg)/24 h *Children 6–12 y:* 2 tsp (1 mg) bid; increase as needed, not to exceed 6 tsp (3 mg)/24 h	See diphenhydramine. Safety and efficacy for use in children <12 y have been established for syrup preparation but not for tablets.
Dimenhydrinate (Dramamine) HOW SUPPLIED Tablets and chewable tablets: 50 mg each Liquid: 12.5 mg/5 ml	***Motion Sickness*** ORAL DOSES *Adults, children >12 y:* One or two tablets q4-6h, not to exceed eight tablets/24 h *Children* 6–12 y: one half to one tablet q6-8h, not to exceed three tablets/24 h 2–6 y: one half tablet q6-8h, not to exceed one and one half tablets/24 h *Adults, children >12 y:* 4–8 tsp q4-6h, not to exceed 32 tsp/24 h *Children* 6–12 y: 2–4 tsp q6-8h, not to exceed 12 tsp/24 h 2–6 y: 1–2 tsp q6-8h, not to exceed 6 tsp/24 h Not for use in children <2 y	See diphenhydramine.
ALKYLAMINES: **CHLORPHENIRAMINE MALEATE** (Teldrin, Chlor-Trimeton) HOW SUPPLIED Tablets: 4, 8, 12 mg Tablets, chewable: 2 mg Syrup: 2 mg/5 ml SR Capsules: 8 mg	***Seasonal and Perennial Allergic Rhinitis; Vasomotor Rhinitis; Common Cold (Rhinorrhea, Sneezing)*** TABLETS *Adults, children >12 y:* One 4 mg tablet tid or qid; one SR capsule q12h Not recommended for children <12 y SYRUP *Adults/children >12 y:* 1–2 tsp tid or qid SYRUP *Children* 6–12 y: ½–1 tsp tid or qid, not to exceed 4 tsp/24 h 2–6 y: ½ tsp tid or qid, not to exceed 2 tsp/24 h	**Assess** Inquire about general adverse reactions to antihistamines. **Implement** Administration of tablets and syrup with food delays absorption but does not effect bioavailability. Advise clients with phenylketonuria that certain over-the-counter (OTC) preparations of chlorpheniramine contain aspartame, which is metabolized to phenylalanine in the GI tract after oral ingestion. Sustained-release preparations should not be crushed or chewed, and their use is contraindicated in children <12 y.

TABLE 50–1 *Continued*
First-Generation H₁-Receptor Antagonists

Drug Name	Dosage and Route of Administration	Nursing Considerations
PHENOTHIAZINES: PROMETHAZINE HYDROCHLORIDE (Phenergan) HOW SUPPLIED Tablets: 12.5, 25, 50 mg Syrup: 6.25 mg/5 ml Suppositories: 12.5, 25, 50 mg Injection: 25 mg/ml, 50 mg/ml	**ORAL DOSES** **Allergic Conditions** *Adults* 25 mg hs or 12 .5 mg ac and hs *Children* 25 mg hs, or 6.25–12.5 mg tid (or 0.5 mg/kg hs and 0.125 mg/kg prn) **Motion Sickness** *Adults* 25 mg 30–60 min before travel, second 25-mg dose 8–12 h later; additional doses upon arising in morning and before evening meal for duration of travel *Children* 12.5–25 mg bid **Nausea, Vomiting:** *Adults* 25 mg; repeat doses of 12.5–25 mg q4-6h prn *Children* 0.5 mg/lb or 1 mg/kg **Sedation Adjunct to Analgesics** *Adults* 25–50 mg *Children* 12.5–25 mg **PARENTERAL DOSES** Deep IM injection preferred; IV administration with caution **Allergic Conditions** *Adults* 25 mg *Children <12 y:* Not more than 12.5 mg or 0.5 mg/lb (1 mg/kg) **Nausea, Vomiting** *Adults* 12.5–25 mg q4h *Children* Not more than 6.25–12.5 mg or 0.5 mg/lb (1 mg/kg) **Sedation, Adjunct to Analgesics** *Adults* 25–50 mg *Children* Not more than 12.5–25 mg or 0.5 mg/lb (1 mg/kg)	**Assess** Inquire about general adverse reactions to antihistamines. Assess client for symptoms of either central nervous system (CNS) depression or paradoxical stimulation. Assess clients for allergy to sulfites; some preparations contain sulfites that may produce an allergic reaction, including anaphylaxis and less severe asthmatic attacks in susceptible clients. Assess for history of sleep apnea, family history of sudden infant death syndrome (SIDS), or possibility of Reye's syndrome, any of which contraindicates use. **Implement** Administer orally, rectally, deep IM, or IV. Do not administer SC because tissue necrosis may result. Reduce dosage of analgesics by 25% to 50% when promethazine is used as an adjunct. Tablets and suppositories are not recommended for use in children <2 y. Alert laboratory personnel if client requires blood transfusions because promethazine may interfere with blood typing. **Monitor** Monitor for tachycardia or bradycardia during parenteral administration. Monitor blood pressure (BP) during IV administration. Monitor IV infusion rate carefully; rate should not exceed 25 mg/min. Rapid IV administration may produce transient drop in BP. If hypotension occurs, do not use epinephrine because phenothiazines may reverse its usual pressor effect and cause further lowering of BP. IV administration at the prescribed infusion rate may result in a slight rise in BP. Watch for respiratory depression and diminished cough reflex. **Evaluate** Assess client for reduction in signs and symptoms.

Table continued on following page.

TABLE 50–1 *Continued*
First-Generation H₁-Receptor Antagonists

Drug Name	Dosage and Route of Administration	Nursing Considerations
PROMETHAZINE HYDROCHLORIDE—CONT'D	**PARENTERAL DOSES** *Obstetric Sedation* 50 mg in early stages of labor; 25–75 mg with reduced dose of analgesic repeated once or twice q4h	
Trimeprazine tartrate (Temaril) HOW SUPPLIED Tablets: 2.5 mg Spansules: 5 mg Syrup: 2.5 mg/5 ml	*Allergic Condition* TABLETS AND SYRUP: *Adults* 2.5 mg qid *Children* >3 y: 25 mg hs or tid if needed 6 mo–3 y: 1.25 mg hs or tid if needed SUSTAINED-RELEASE CAPSULE *Adults* 5 mg (one capsule) q12h *Children* >6 y 5 mg (one capsule)/24 h Not for use in children <6 y	**Assess** Inquire about general adverse reactions to antihistamines. See promethazine. **Implement** Teach client to avoid tasks that require alertness or motor skills. Instruct client to avoid drinking alcoholic beverages. **Monitor** Monitor the elderly for hypotension. Assess children for paradoxical reaction. **Evaluate** Assess client for reduction in allergic signs and symptoms.
PIPERIDINES: CYPROHEPTADINE HYDROCHLORIDE (Periactin) HOW SUPPLIED Tablets: 4 mg Syrup: 2 mg/5 ml	*Miscellaneous Allergic Reactions* *Adults* 4 mg tid initially; dosage may be increased as required and tolerated, not to exceed 0.5 mg/kg/24 h in divided doses; most clients require 12–16 mg/24 h and occasionally as much as 32 mg/24 h *Children* 7–14 y: 4 mg bid or tid (or 0.25 mg/kg/24 h in divided doses), not to exceed 16 mg/24 h 2–6 y: 2 mg bid or tid or 0.25 mg/kg/24 h, not to exceed 12 mg/24 h	**Assess** Assess for general allergic reactions to antihistamines. **Implement** Syrup preparations are intended for use in children but may be used by adults who have difficulty swallowing tablets. **Monitor** Monitor blood pressure, especially in elderly; increased risk of hypotension is present. **Evaluate** Assess client for decreased signs and symptoms of allergic reaction.
ETHYLENEDIAMINES: TRIPELENNAMINE HYDROCHLORIDE (PBZ) HOW SUPPLIED Tablets: 25, 50 mg Elixir: 25 mg/5 ml Sustained-release tablets: 100 mg	*Miscellaneous Allergic Reactions* TABLETS AND ELIXIRS *Adults* 25–50 mg q4-6h; increase dosage as required, not to exceed 600 mg/24 h *Children* 5 mg/kg/24 h in divided doses, not to exceed 300 mg/24 h SUSTAINED-RELEASE TABLETS *Adults* 100 mg morning and evening Not for use in children	**Assess** Inquire about general adverse reactions to antihistamines. **Implement** Elixirs are intended for use in children but may be used by adults who have difficulty swallowing tablets. Sustained-release tablets should be swallowed whole and should not be crushed or chewed. Do not administer sustained-release tablets to children.
PIPERAZINES: HYDROXYZINE HYDROCHLORIDE (Atarax, Vistaril) HOW SUPPLIED Capsules: 25, 50, 100 mg Tablets: 10, 25, 50, 100 mg Syrup: 10 mg/5 ml	*Allergic Conditions, Including Pruritis* *Adults* 25 mg tid or qid *Children* >6 y: 50–100 mg/24 h in divided doses <6 y: 50 mg/24 h in divided doses *Sedation* *Adults* 50–100 mg *Children* 0.6 mg/kg	**Assess** Inquire about general adverse reactions to antihistamines. **Implement** Syrup preparations are intended for use in children but may be used by adults who have difficulty swallowing tablets. Shake oral suspension well. Scored tablets may be crushed. **Monitor** Monitor liver and renal function test results for those receiving long-term therapy.

TABLE 50–1 *Continued*
First-Generation H₁-Receptor Antagonists

Drug Name	Dosage and Route of Administration	Nursing Considerations
Meclizine Hydrochloride (Antivert, Bonine) HOW SUPPLIED Tablets: 12.5, 25, 50 mg Chewable tablets: 25 mg	**Motion Sickness** *Adults* 25–50 mg 1 h before travel; subsequent doses of 25–50 mg q24h for duration of travel Not for use in children <12 y **Vertigo** *Adults, children >12 y* 25–100 mg/d in divided doses	**Assess** Inquire about general adverse reactions to antihistamines. **Implement** Chewable tablets should be thoroughly chewed before swallowing.

SECOND-GENERATION H₁-RECEPTOR ANTAGONISTS

Second-generation H₁-receptor antagonists are newer drugs. These drugs usually produce fewer undesired clinical responses than the first-generation drugs. Drugs belonging to this subclass include terfenadine, astemizole, and loratadine.[16]

SECOND-GENERATION H₁-RECEPTOR ANTAGONIST PROTOTYPE

TERFENADINE

Pharmacotherapeutics Terfenadine (Seldane) is used to treat seasonal allergic rhinitis. It provides symptomatic relief of rhinorrhea, sneezing, oronasopharyngeal irritation, itching, lacrimation, and red, irritated, and itching eyes.[12,17]

Pharmacokinetics Approximately 70% of an oral dose of terfenadine is rapidly absorbed from the GI tract after oral administration. Peak plasma concentrations occur in approximately 1 to 2 hours. The onset of antihistaminic effect (as measured by suppression of the wheal-and-flare response induced by intradermal injection of histamine) occurs in 1 to 2 hours. Terfenadine peaks in 3 to 6 hours and lasts for 12 hours or longer. Distribution into human body tissues and fluids has not been fully determined, and it is not known if terfenadine and its metabolites cross the placenta or distribute into breast milk. The drug is 97% protein bound. Terfenadine undergoes extensive first-pass metabolism in the liver and GI tract. Less than 1% of an oral dose of terfenadine reaches the systemic circulation unchanged in healthy adults without liver impairment. Most of terfenadine (60%) and its metabolites are excreted in feces through biliary elimination. It is also excreted in urine.[12,17]

Pharmacodynamics Terfenadine does not compete with histamine at the H₁-receptor sites in the same manner as the first-generation antihistamines. Terfenadine binds slowly to H₁ receptors and also dissociates from the receptors slowly. Terfenadine is lipophobic, and it does not easily cross the blood-brain barrier to produce CNS effects. Instead, in binds selectively to peripheral nervous system receptors.[12,17]

Pharmaceutics Terfenadine is administered orally. It is available in tablet dosage form. Table 50–3 provides additional information about dosage forms and dosages.

Undesired Clinical Responses The most frequent adverse effects with terfenadine are drowsiness, sedation, headache, nausea, vomiting, abdominal pain, and dry mouth. Terfenadine is less likely to cause CNS effects than the first-generation antihistamines. Severe cardiac events (arrhythmias, ventricular tachycardia, torsade de pointes) have been reported, usually associated with excessive dosages. Mild-to-moderate increases in serum alanine aminotransferase (ALT) and aspartate aminotransferase (AST) concentrations have developed in some clients.

Contraindications and Precautions Terfenadine use is contraindicated in clients with significant liver dysfunction and in clients with underlying conditions that might prolong the QT interval (hypokalemia, congenital QT syndrome). Terfenadine use is also contraindicated in clients who are taking erythromycin, ketoconazole, or itraconazole.

Drug-Drug, Drug-Environment Interactions As stated previously, terfenadine should not be used concomitantly with erythromycin, ketaconazole, or itraconazole. This combination could prolongate QT intervals or produce ventricular tachycardia. Exposure to sunlight while taking terfenadine can result in a photosensitivity reaction.

Life-Span Considerations Terfenadine is classified as a Pregnancy Category C drug. The risk of seizures in neonates and premature infants is increased if the drug is used during the third trimester of pregnancy. Terfenadine use may prohibit lactation. Children may experience a dominant paradoxical reaction (e.g., restlessness, insomnia, euphoria, nervousness, tremors).

Specific Drug-Related Considerations Terfenadine should be administered with food or milk to minimize GI irritation. See Table 50–3 for additional nursing considerations.

MISCELLANEOUS DRUGS IN CATEGORY

Astemizole (Hismanal) and loratadine (Claritin) are also second-generation H₁-receptor antagonists. **Astemizole** is well absorbed after oral administration. However, its absorption is reduced by 60% when administered with meals. It is widely distributed throughout the body but does not cross the blood-

TABLE 50–2
Drug-Drug Interactions Associated With H₁-Receptor Antagonists

H₁-Receptor Antagonists	Other Drugs	Results
FIRST-GENERATION DRUGS		
Diphenhydramine, carbinoxamine, clemastine, dimenhydrinate, chlorpheniramine, dexchlorpheniramine, brompheniramine, triprolidine, promethazine, trimeprazine, methdilazine, cyproheptadine, azatadine, phenindamine, tripelennamine, pyrilamine, hydroxyzine, meclizine	Anticholinergics	Antihistamines potentiate CNS depressant and atropine-like effects of anticholinergics.
	Anticholinesterases	Antihistamines antagonize antiglaucoma (miotic) and CNS effects of anticholinesterases.
		Anticholinesterases potentiate the tranquilizing and behavioral changes caused by antihistamines.
	Central nervous system (CNS) depressants (alcohol, barbiturates, general anesthetics, narcotic analgesics, tranquilizers)	Combination results in additive CNS depression.
	Corticosteroids	Corticosteroids increase ocular pressure in long-term therapy.
	Hyoscine (scopolamine)	Enhanced sedative effect of this combination is used in over-the-counter sleep aids.
	Monoamine oxidase inhibitors (MAOs)	MAOs prolong and intensify the anticholinergic effects of antihistamines.
		MAO addition increases the risk of orthostatic hypotension.
	Promethazine	Combination results in additive CNS depression.
Hydroxyzine	Epinephrine	Hydroxyzine inhibits and reverses the vasopressor effects of epinephrine.
Phenothiazines	Antacids	Antacids inhibit gastrointestinal absorption of phenothiazines.
	Anticonvulsants	Some phenothiazines may lower convulsive threshold in susceptible individuals; increased dosages of anticonvulsants may be required.
	Antihypertensives	Phenothiazines may potentiate effect of antihypertensives, resulting in profound hypotension.
	Epinephrine	Phenothiazines block and possibly reverse the vasopressor effect of epinephrine.
	Oral antidiabetics	Phenothiazines may potentiate the hypoglycemic effect of oral antidiabetic agents.
	Thiazide diuretics	Combination may result in severe hypotension and shock.
Dexchlorpheniramine, diphenhydramine, tripelennamine	Epinephrine	These drugs enhance effects of epinephrine.
Dimenhydrinate, hydroxyzine, meclizine, promethazine	Ototoxic drugs (e.g., aminoglycoside antibiotics, aspirin, furosemide, quinine)	Antiemetic action may mask symptoms (nausea and vomiting) of ototoxicity.
SECOND-GENERATION DRUGS		
Terfenadine and loratadine	Erythromycin, ketoconazole, itraconazole	Combination may result in prolongation of QT interval or ventricular tachycardia.

brain barrier. Astemizole is extensively metabolized by the liver. It is primarily (60%) excreted in the feces and to a lesser extent in the urine.

Like other second-generation drugs, astemizole has a delayed onset, peak, and duration of action. Its onset of action is 4 hours or more. Because it is extensively metabolized, peak clinical effects may not occur until several hours after the peak plasma concentration level is reached. The drug requires a prolonged period of time to reach a steady state; thus use of a special dosing schedule is recommended. The dosage is 10 mg/d taken on an empty stomach at least 2 h after meals. Astemizole's duration of action is approximately 24 hours.[12,18]

TABLE 50–3
Second-Generation H₁-Receptor Antagonists

Drug Name	Dosage and Route of Administration	Nursing Considerations
TERFENADINE (Seldane) HOW SUPPLIED Tablets: 60 mg	***Seasonal and Perennial Allergic Rhinitis*** *Adults, children >12 y:* 60 mg bid Safety and efficacy in children <12 y not established	**Assess** Inquire about general adverse reactions to antihistamines. Because terfenadine does not readily cross the blood-brain barrier, anticholinergic side effects are less likely to occur, but the potential still exists. **Implement** Administer with food if gastrointestinal distress occurs. Instruct client not to crush or chew tablets.
Astemizole (Hismanal) HOW SUPPLIED Tablets: 10 mg	***Seasonal and Perennial Allergic Rhinitis; Chronic Idiopathic Urticaria*** *Adults, children >12 y:* Recommended maintenance dosage: 10 mg once daily Safety and efficacy in children <12 y not established	**Assess** Inquire for general adverse reactions to antihistamines. Because astemizole does not readily cross the blood-brain barrier, anticholinergic side effects are less likely to occur, but the potential still exists. **Implement** Administer drug on an empty stomach at least 2 h after a meal, with no additional food intake for at least 1 h after dosing.
Loratadine (Claritin) HOW SUPPLIED Tablets: 10 mg	***Seasonal Allergic Rhinitis*** *Adults, children <12 y* 10 mg once daily on an empty stomach Not for use in children <12 y *Adults With Hepatic Function Impairment* 10 mg qod	**Assess** Inquire about general adverse reactions to antihistamines. **Implement** Teach client to take drug on an empty stomach. Advise client to report blurred vision or eye pain.

Loratadine is approved for treatment of seasonal rhinitis. This drug offers the convenience of once-a-day dosing. In addition, it is less likely to cause drowsiness. Loratadine is rapidly absorbed and converted to an active metabolite. The elimination half-life averages 8 hours for the drug and 28 hours for the metabolite. In clients with chronic alcoholic liver disease, bioavailability of the drug is increased, and elimination of both the drug and metabolite is prolonged. The antihistamine effect of loratadine begins 1 to 2 hours after dosing and lasts more than 24 hours. Food increases loratadine's bioavailability but delays the peak plasma concentration.[19,20] (See Table 50–3 for additional information on second-generation drugs.)

LIFE-SPAN CONSIDERATIONS

Most of the H₁-receptor antagonists are classified in either Pregnancy Category B or C. For some, safety for use during pregnancy has not been established. Benefits for use during pregnancy should clearly outweigh unknown potential hazards to the fetus.

Use of all the H₁-receptor antagonists is contraindicated in newborns and premature infants. Safe use in children of specific antihistamines or specific formulations varies considerably. Supervision and direction are strongly recommended or, in some cases, required with antihistamine administration. Antihistamine use in children may cause diminished mental alertness and physical coordination or paradoxical excitation. Overdosage may cause hallucinations, convulsions, or death. Phenothiazines should be used with caution in children with a history of sleep apnea. Safety and efficacy for use in children less than 12 years of age have not been established for the second-generation antihistamines.

Antihistamines are more likely to produce dizziness, hypotension, sedation, syncope, or toxic confusional states in the elderly. Dosage reduction may be required. Phenothiazines may produce extrapyramidal side effects.

SUMMARY

Histamine is synthesized and stored in mast cells and basophils. It is released when these cells are damaged. Once released, histamine has both direct and indirect actions on multiple body systems. Drugs are used to block the effects of histamine on histamine receptors. These drugs are termed *histamine-receptor antagonists, histamine antagonists,* or *histamine-receptor blockers.*

First-generation H₁-receptor antagonists comprise the older group of drugs used to block the effects of histamine. These drugs are divided into six subclasses: ethanolamines, alkylamines, phenothiazines, piperidines, ethylenediamines, and piperazines. Second-generation drugs (e.g., terfenadine, astemizole, loratadine) have prolonged durations of action and fewer undesired clinical responses.

REFERENCES

1. Hole, J. (1993). *Human anatomy & physiology* (6th ed.). Dubuque, IA: Wm. C. Brown.
2. Seeley, R., Stephens, T., & Tate, P. (1992). *Anatomy & physiology* (2nd ed.). St. Louis: Mosby–Year Book.
3. Guyton, A.C. (1991). *Textbook of medical physiology* (8th ed.). Philadelphia: W.B. Saunders.
4. White, M.V. (1990). The role of histamine in allergic diseases. *Journal of Allergy and Clinical Immunology, 86,* 599–605.
5. Porth, C.M. (1994). *Pathophysiology: Concepts of altered health states* (4th ed.). Philadelphia: J.B. Lippincott.
6. Gilman, A.G., Rall, T.W., Nies, A.S., & Taylor, P. (Eds.). (1990). *Goodman and Gilman's: The pharmacological basis of therapeutics* (8th ed.). New York: Pergamon Press, Inc.
7. Black, J.M., & Matassarin-Jacobs, E. (1993). *Luckmann and Sorensen's medical-surgical nursing: A psychophysiologic approach* (4th ed.). Philadelphia: W.B. Saunders.
8. Simons, F.E. (1989). H_1-receptor antagonists: Clinical pharmacology and therapeutics. *Journal of Allergy and Clinical Immunology, 84,* 845–861.
9. Berman, B.A. (1990). Perennial allergic rhinitis: Clinical efficacy of a new antihistamine. *Journal of Allergy and Clinical Immunology, 86,* 1004–1008.
10. Patterson, R., Grammer, L.C., Greenberger, P.A., & Zeiss, C.R. (Eds.). (1993). *Allergic diseases: Diagnosis and management* (4th ed.). Philadelphia: J.B. Lippincott.
11. Data Pharmaceutica, Inc. (1993). *1993 physicians' genrx.* Smithtown, NY: Author.
12. U.S. Pharmacopeial Convention. (1990). *The United States pharmacopeia* (22nd revision). Rockville, MD: Author.
13. Smith, C., & Reynard, A. (1992). *Textbook of pharmacology.* Philadelphia: W.B. Saunders.
14. Frazier, C.A. (1991). Periactin for headache. *Southern Medical Journal, 84,* 1510.
15. Kaiser, H.B. (1990). H_1-receptor antagonist treatment of seasonal allergic rhinitis. *Journal of Allergy and Clinical Immunology, 86*(Pt. 2), 1000–1003.
16. Ryhal, B.T., & Fletcher, M.P. (1991). The second-generation antihistamines. What makes them different? *Postgraduate Medicine, 89*(6), 87–88, 91–94, 99.
17. Naclerio, R.M., et al. (1990). Terfenadine, an H_1 antihistamine, inhibits histamine release in vivo in man. *American Review of Respiratory Disease, 142,* 167–171.
18. Hodgson, B., Kizior, R., Kingdon, R. (1995). 1995 Nurse's drug handbook. Philadelphia: W.B. Saunders.
19. New Drugs. (1994). Long-lasting relief of hay fever. *American Journal of Nursing, 94*(3), 62–63.
20. Haria, M., Fitton, A., & Peters, D. (1994). Loratadine: A reappraisal of its pharmacological properties and therapeutic use in allergic disorders. *Drugs, 48,* 617–637.

BIBLIOGRAPHY

Conn, V. (1991). Self-care actions taken by older adults for influenza and colds. *Nursing Research, 40,* 176–181.

Culver, S., & Parks, B.R. (1989). Antihistamines in allergic rhinitis. *Pediatric Nursing, 15,* 615–616.

Massey, W.A., & Lichtenstein, L.M. (1990). The effects of antihistamines beyond H_1 antagonism in allergic inflammation. *Journal of Allergy and Clinical Immunology, 86*(Part 2), 1019–1024.

Rafferty, P., & Holgate, S.T. (1989). Histamine and its antagonists in asthma. *Journal of Allergy and Clinical Immunology, 84,* 144–151.

Ruckenstein, M.J., & Harrison, R. (1991). Motion sickness. Helping patients tolerate the ups and downs. *Postgraduate Medicine, 89*(6), 139–144.

Saunders, E.J., & Saunders, J.A. (1990). Drug therapy in pregnancy: the lessons of deithylstilbestrol, thalidomide, and bendectin. *Health Care for Women International, 11,* 423–432.

Simons, F.E. (1990). Recent advances in H_1-receptor antagonist treatment. *Journal of Allergy and Clinical Immunology, 86*(Part 2), 995–999.

Simons, K.J., Martin, T.J., Watson, W.T., & Simons, F.E. (1990). Pharmacokinetics and pharmacodynamics of terfenadine and chlorpheniramine in the elderly. *Journal of Allergy and Clinical Immunology, 85,* 540–547.

Woodward, J.K. (1990). Pharmacology of antihistamines. *Journal of Allergy and Clinical Immunology, 86*(Part 2), 606–612.

Woolbert, L.F. (1990). Do antihistamines and decongestants prevent otitis media? *Pediatric Nursing, 16,* 265–267.

CHAPTER 51

Nonsteroidal, Anti-inflammatory Drugs

MARY MIRCH

⊛ Nonsteroidal, Anti-inflammatory Drugs

LEARNING OBJECTIVES:

Describe three major therapeutic uses for NSAIDs.

Discuss general characteristics of NSAIDs category.

KEY TERMS:

Antipyretics, nonprostaglandin synthetase inhibitor, nonsteroidal anti-inflammatory drug, prostaglandin synthetase inhibitor

⊛ Prostaglandin Synthetase Inhibitors

LEARNING OBJECTIVES:

Explain the pharmacodynamics of PSIs.

Provide the rationale for four major undesired clinical responses associated with PSIs.

Summarize major drug-drug and drug-nutrient interactions associated with PSIs.

Describe essential life-span considerations associated with PSIs.

Develop a plan of care for a client receiving long-term PSI therapy.

Summarize essential information about the pharmacokinetic and pharmacodynamic properties of salicylates.

Summarize essential information about the pharmacokinetic and pharmacodynamic properties of propionic acid derivatives.

Summarize essential information about the pharmacokinetic and pharmacodynamic properties of acetic acid anti-inflammatory drugs.

Describe four miscellaneous PSIs.

KEY TERMS:

Acetic acid derivative, acetylsalicylic acid, anthranilic acid derivative, oxicam, arylacetic acid derivative, phenylalkanoic acid derivative, propionic acid derivative, prostaglandin, pyrrolacetic acid, pyrazolone, Reye's syndrome, salicylate, salicylism

⊛ Nonprostaglandin Synthetase Inhibitors

LEARNING OBJECTIVES:

Identify three major categories of non-PSIs.

Describe the pharmacodynamics of antirheumatic remitting drugs.

Summarize major undesired clinical responses associated with gold salts.

KEY TERMS:

Gold salts, para-aminophenol derivatives

CONCEPTS AND TERMS TO REVIEW

Review the section on nonspecific defense mechanisms of the body in Chapter 49.

Reexamine the physiologic changes that occur during the inflammatory response.

Review the section on pain response in Chapter 19.

Read the section on acetylsalicylic acid in Chapter 19.

Review definitions of the following terms: *chemotaxis, inflammation, leukocytosis, margination*.

The two most important drug categories that inhibit acute or chronic inflammatory response are adrenal glucocorticosteroid hormones (steroidal anti-inflammatory drugs) and nonsteroidal anti-inflammatory drugs (NSAIDs). Since steroidal anti-inflammatory drugs are discussed in Chapter 42, only NSAIDs are included in this chapter.

NONSTEROIDAL ANTI-INFLAMMATORY DRUGS

NSAIDs are subdivided into **prostaglandin synthetase inhibitors (PSIs)** and **nonprostaglandin synthetase inhibitors**

(non-PSIs). Some of the major categories of NSAIDs are listed in the box.

Pharmacotherapeutics

NSAIDs are used to interfere with the inflammatory process and to reduce associated symptoms. In addition, NSAIDs sometimes are prescribed strictly for relief of pain and fever.

Inflammation Numerous chemical mediators are involved in the acute inflammatory response. It is believed that histamine and serotonin initiate the first phase (1 to 1½ hours) of inflammation, and kinin controls the second phase (1½ to 2 hours). Prostaglandins (PGs) probably exert their proinflammatory effects in the late phases of inflammation (2½ to 6 hours). In addition, some PGs (e.g., PGE_2) may contribute to pathologic processes associated with chronic inflammatory disease.[1] (See Chapter 49 for a description of the inflammatory response.)

Pain Pain is usually viewed as a warning of actual or impending tissue injury. The pain sensation is produced when pain receptors (nociceptors) are directly stimulated by prostaglandins and other inflammatory compounds (e.g., histamine, bradykinin, leukotrienes, interleukin).[2] (See Chapter 19 for additional information about pain.)

Fever Fever develops when there is a disturbance in the body's homeostatic mechanisms. When this occurs, the hypothalamus is unable to maintain a balance between heat production and peripheral heat loss. Although dehydration, heat stroke, and certain drugs can elevate body temperature, fever occurs as a result of inflammation or infection. During the infectious and inflammatory processes, endogenous pyrogens are produced within the body. Endogenous pyrogens act directly on the hypothalamus, affecting its thermostatic functions. Drugs designed to reduce fever are referred to as **antipyretics.**

PROSTAGLANDIN SYNTHETASE INHIBITORS

There are several groups of PSIs, including the **carboxylic acids** (**salicylic, acetic, propionic,** and **anthranilic acids**) and the **enolic acids** (**oxicams** and **pyrazolones**).

Pharmacodynamics

PSIs act primarily to prevent the biosynthesis and release of PGs. PGs do not normally exist in the cells but are synthesized from phospholipids and are released when there is trauma to the cell membrane.[3]

Synthesis of PG occurs in two stages: release of arachidonic acid from the phospholipid of the cell membrane and conversion of arachidonic acid to PGs with the assistance of the enzyme cyclooxygenase. PSIs probably block the action of cyclooxygenase.[4] (Figure 51–1 illustrates the conversion of phospholipids to PGs.)

MAJOR CATEGORIES OF NSAIDs

Prostaglandin Synthetase Inhibitors	Nonprostaglandin Synthetase Inhibitors
Salicylates	Para-aminophenols (discussed in Chapter 19)
Propionic acid derivatives	Hyperuricemic drugs (discussed in Chapter 37)
Acetic acids	Antirheumatic remitting drugs
Anthranilic acids	Immunosuppressant drugs (discussed in Chapter 52)
Pyrrolacetic acids	
Oxicams	Antimalarial drugs (discussed in Chapter 60)
Pyrazolones	

Undesired Clinical Responses Common to PSIs

In the individual client the therapeutic response is unpredictable. In addition, numerous undesired clinical responses are common to all PSIs. The most common are gastrointestinal (GI) symptoms, renal impairment, hypersensitivity reactions, and hematologic changes.

Gastrointestinal effects GI effects are among the most common undesired clinical responses associated with long-term PSI therapy. Symptoms involving the GI tract include dyspepsia, epigastric pain, nausea, vomiting, flatulence, and abdominal cramps. In addition, peptic ulceration and GI hemorrhage may occur.[1]

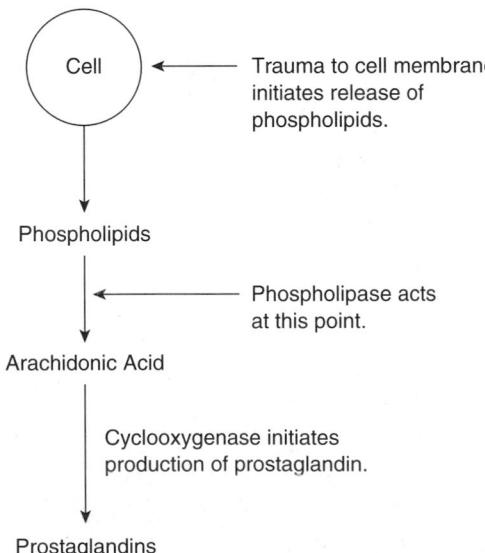

PGE₂ is responsible for fever, edema, redness, and pain. PGE₂ₐ is responsible for vasodilation and uterine contraction.

FIGURE 51–1 Phospholipid conversion to prostaglandins.

Gastic ulceration largely occurs in individuals receiving long-term, high-dose PSI therapy, and is caused by PG synthesis inhibition. Normally PGE_2 increases intestinal motility, inhibits gastric hydrochloric acid secretion, and promotes cytoprotection of the lining of the GI tract. With the inhibition of PGs, these functions are altered.[1,5]

Renal impairment Normally renal PGs participate in many important renal processes such as autoregulation of renal blood flow and glomerular filtration, regulation of renin release, and renal handling of sodium and water. Administration of PSIs can produce sodium and water retention, hyperkalemia, and hypertension. These drugs can cause nephritis, nephrotic syndrome, and papillary necrosis. If the client is hypovolemic, renal pathology is usually more severe.[1,6]

Hypersensitivity reactions Manifestations of hypersensitivity include vasomotor rhinitis, urticaria, bronchial wheezing, and angioneurotic edema. The immune mechanism that produces these reactions is unclear. However, clients who are sensitive to one PSI frequently experience hypersensitivity to other PSIs.[1]

Hematologic changes Prolonged bleeding and prothrombin times may be induced by PSIs. A tendency toward antiplatelet aggregation also occurs.

Additional undesired clinical responses associated with PSIs include headache, dizziness, drowsiness, mental confusion, tinnitus, vertigo, and visual and hearing disturbances. Common undesired responses are summarized in Figure 51–2.

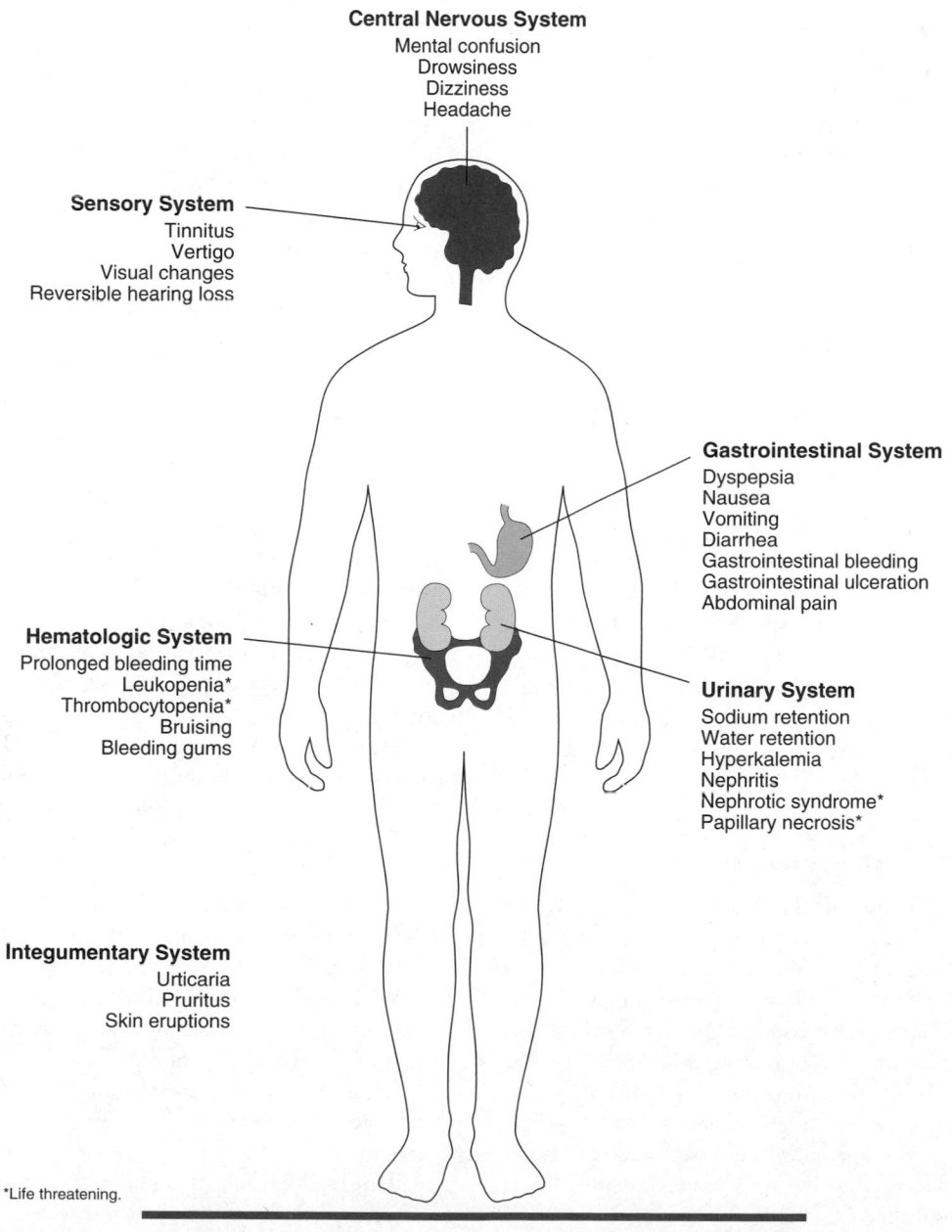

Central Nervous System
Mental confusion
Drowsiness
Dizziness
Headache

Sensory System
Tinnitus
Vertigo
Visual changes
Reversible hearing loss

Gastrointestinal System
Dyspepsia
Nausea
Vomiting
Diarrhea
Gastrointestinal bleeding
Gastrointestinal ulceration
Abdominal pain

Hematologic System
Prolonged bleeding time
Leukopenia*
Thrombocytopenia*
Bruising
Bleeding gums

Urinary System
Sodium retention
Water retention
Hyperkalemia
Nephritis
Nephrotic syndrome*
Papillary necrosis*

Integumentary System
Urticaria
Pruritus
Skin eruptions

*Life threatening.

FIGURE 51–2   Undesired clinical responses common to PSIs.

Drug-Drug and Drug-Nutrient Interactions Common to PSIs

Numerous drug-drug interactions occur with PSIs. Major drugs or drug categories included in these interactions are diuretics, antihypertensive drugs, methotrexate, lithium, other PSIs, anticoagulants, and hyperuricemic drugs. When administered concurrently with PSIs, the natriuretic and hypotensive effects of diuretics are inhibited. This effect possibly is related to the ability of PSIs to inhibit renal PG synthesis. The action of some antihypertensive drugs may be inhibited by the same mechanism. Hyperkalemia and renal failure are possible when PSIs are administered with potassium-sparing diuretics.[1]

If PSIs are administered within a 10-day period before the administration of methotrexate, a decreased excretion rate of methotrexate occurs, possibly causing methotrexate toxicity.[6] In addition, many PSIs influence bleeding time by inhibiting platelet aggregation. Therefore combining PSIs with anticoagulant drugs may potentiate their anticoagulant effect and result in bleeding. In addition, PSIs displace warfarin from plasma protein–binding sites, producing more free drug.[1]

Administration of two or more PSIs at the same time is not recommended. Such a combination increases the incidence of undesired clinical response. In addition, aspirin can displace other PSIs from plasma-binding sites. Caution should be used when PSIs are administered concurrently with lithium or probenecid. When administered with lithium, the risk for lithium toxicity is increased. If probenecid is administered with PSIs, the effects of PSIs are enhanced. Thus the dosage of PSIs must be reduced.[1]

Two undesired clinical responses associated with some PSIs (i.e., irritation or ulceration of the GI tract and tendency toward elevated liver enzymes) make concomitant use with alcohol potentially dangerous. The Food and Drug Administration (FDA) currently is conducting hearings to determine if label warnings against the use of alcohol while taking PSIs are warranted.

Although many individuals taking PSIs experience some GI distress, taking these drugs with food actually delays their absorption. Therefore it is preferred that PSIs be taken approximately 15 to 30 minutes before meals. If GI distress does occur, the drugs may be taken with milk or small amounts of food.

Life-Span Considerations

PSIs are useful in individuals of all ages with acute or chronic inflammatory conditions. However, caution must be taken with the different age groups. For example, some PSIs are fetal teratogenic. Other PSIs have not been studied for use during pregnancy; therefore their effects on the fetus are unknown. Most PSIs are excreted in human milk and should be used with caution by lactating women.

PSIs are frequently used by elderly clients. These drugs can produce reactions in this age group not associated with other clients. For example, many of the PSIs produce depression in the elderly. In addition, the elderly are more prone to GI bleeding and ulceration, renal damage, and central nervous system (CNS) changes. These individuals also develop sodium and fluid retention more easily, which can exacerbate other medical problems such as congestive heart failure. Most PSIs are highly bound to proteins in the blood. When serum protein levels are low, as commonly occurs in the elderly, drugs normally highly bound to protein circulate freely and can produce toxicity.

General Nursing Considerations

The use of PSIs is rising dramatically. Careful assessment and client education are essential for clients receiving these drugs.

Assessing When assessing the client for treatment with a PSI, a detailed description of the presenting symptom(s) must be elicited. Also determine the length of time the condition has been present and what the client has done to eliminate or minimize the problem. Since the inflammatory response produces pain, evaluate the client's pain level and tolerance. (Refer to Chapter 19 for a discussion of pain assessment.)

Specifically ask the client about past and present drug use, including prescription and over-the-counter (OTC) drugs and alcohol or street drugs. If the client has previously taken PSIs, determine his or her reaction to the drug. Did the drug produce therapeutic effects? Did the client have undesired clinical responses? Ask the client specifically about aspirin since an individual allergic to aspirin is at risk of developing cross sensitivities to other NSAIDs. Question the client about preexisting renal, hepatic, or GI problems. Ascertain if the client has any condition that affects the hematologic system. If the client is female, determine if she is pregnant or nursing.

During the physical examination observe for outward signs of inflammation (i.e., erythema, swelling, and warmth). If the inflammatory process is isolated to specific joints, examine each joint carefully. Observe for crepitation, deformity, subluxation, and muscle contractions. Look at affected limbs; note muscle atrophy or decreased subcutaneous tissue. Check the client's vital signs; pay particular attention to the client's body temperature.

Diagnosing After you have analyzed all of the assessment data, develop nursing diagnoses. The following are examples of diagnoses appropriate for a client receiving PSIs:
- Knowledge deficit regarding the use of NSAIDs.
- Health-seeking behaviors related to desire for improved health and decreased pain, discomfort, and swelling.
- Altered nutrition: less than body requirement related to nausea and gastric distress associated with drug therapy.
- Noncompliance related to inappropriate self-treatment.
- High risk for injury related to effects of drug therapy (i.e., inhibited platelet aggregation).
- Pain (chronic) related to inflammation of joints.
- Powerlessness related to perceived lack of control over treatment.

Planning During this phase, develop appropriate teaching plans. Include in the plans information about the disease being treated, the planned treatment, and self-care interventions. Also incorporate information about the prescribed drug therapy. Plans should include the following:

- Correct drug dose
- Schedule for taking the drug
- Desired therapeutic effects of drug
- Undesired clinical responses associated with drug
- Signs and symptoms to report to the primary care provider
- Specific drugs to avoid during therapy
- Proper drug storage, including the need to keep the drug out of the reach of children and confused individuals

If the drug is prescribed on an "as-needed" basis, teach the client to take the drug in the early stages of the inflammatory or pain response.

Include information about nutrition. Encourage the client to consume a diet high in protein, vitamins, and minerals. Teach him or her to avoid alcohol or caffeine since these agents might increase the gastric irritation common with PSIs.

Expected outcomes are also developed during the planning. These outcomes are based on the individual client and the nursing diagnoses used in the plan of care. Possible outcomes for clients receiving PSIs follow:

- Client verbalizes information about drug treatment plan.
- Client maintains desired body weight.
- Client participates in prescribed treatment plan.
- Client remains free of injury.
- Client verbalizes relief from pain.
- Client regularly contacts primary care provider for evaluation of treatment plan.

Implementing   During teaching encourage the client to ask questions and to express fears and concerns. Since many of these drugs are prescribed for long-term treatment, client compliance is essential. Answer questions honestly and reinforce instructions. If needed, initiate social service referrals and inform the client of local and national support groups.

Since NSAIDs are absorbed better in an empty stomach, administer oral drugs 15 to 30 minutes before meals. Ask the client to drink at least 8 ounces of water with the drug to diminish the risk of renal problems. If the client experiences gastric distress, determine if the drug can be administered with small amounts of food or milk.

Baseline hematologic, hepatic, or renal tests should be conducted before drug therapy is initiated. These same measurements should be repeated every 3 to 6 months during long-term therapy. Monitor the client for indications of undesired clinical responses. Clients who complain of stomach pain or burning must be evaluated for gastric irritation or ulceration. Those who experience excessive bruising should be evaluated for a decreased platelet count or decreased ability of the platelets to aggregate.

Evaluating   To evaluate the effectiveness of the plan of care, review the original plan and expected outcomes. If the expected outcomes are unmet, reevaluation of nursing diagnoses, expected outcome, and overall plan is essential. In addition, evaluate the effectiveness of the drug regimen by monitoring the client for decreasing symptoms and increased comfort.

CONCEPT REVIEW

NSAIDS are subdivided into prostaglandin synthetase inhibitors (PSIs) and nonprostaglandin synthetase inhibitors (non-PSIs).

PSIs probably block the action of cyclooxygenase, which is essential for the conversion of arachidonic acid to PGs.

Common undesired clinical responses associated with PSIs are gastric symptoms, renal impairment, hypersensitivity reactions, and hematologic changes.

Salicylates

Salicylic acid is believed to be the active component of salicylates. It has been used for years for its anti-inflammatory, analgesic, and antipyretic properties.

SALICYLATE PROTOTYPE
ACETYLSALICYLIC ACID

In addition to being the prototype for the salicylate group, acetylsalicylic acid (aspirin) is the prototype with which all other NSAIDs are compared. Although aspirin has specific medical indications, its availability as an OTC drug often leads to indiscriminate and hazardous usage.

Pharmacotherapeutics   Aspirin has been beneficial in the treatment of a wide variety of inflammatory disorders, including rheumatic fever, rheumatoid arthritis, osteoarthritis, ankylosing spondylitis, fever, headache, myalgias, and dysmenorrhea. In addition, since the 1980s low aspirin administration has been used to prevent cardiovascular disorders (i.e., coronary thrombosis and cerebrovascular accidents).[7,8] New studies suggest that aspirin reduces the risk of colon cancer and prevents pregnancy-induced hypertension.[9–11]

Pharmacokinetics   Oral dosages of aspirin are rapidly and completely absorbed in the stomach and upper small intestines. After oral dosages peak salicylate levels are reached in 1 to 3 hours. When administered as a suppository, absorption is slower, resulting in lower blood levels of the drug.

After absorption salicylates are highly bound (90%) to albumin. They are distributed to all body tissues and fluids by pH-dependent passive diffusion. Biotransformation of salicylates occurs primarily in the liver where the majority of the drug is converted to water-soluble metabolites. The metabolites are excreted in the urine. The half-life of aspirin varies according to dosage. Low-dose aspirin has a half-life of 3 to 4 hours, whereas larger doses have a half-life of 9 to 16 hours. Aspirin has an increased half-life in the elderly because of altered distribution of the drug.[12] Renal excretion of salicylates is enhanced by urinary alkalization.[1]

Pharmacodynamics   As indicated previously, aspirin is classified as a PSI. As such, it works by inhibiting PG synthesis. Aspirin also inhibits thromboxane A_2 (TXA_2) and prolongs bleeding time. The effects of aspirin are systemic and not generally targeted to specific body organs.

Pharmaceutics Aspirin is manufactured by a variety of drug companies. The desired route of administration is oral in the form of tablets. Timed-release, enteric-coated, and buffered preparations are also available. Topical dosage forms include suppositories for stomal and rectal use and creams and ointments for skin applications (e.g., Aspercream). Aspirin is also available as a gum (e.g., Aspergum).

Undesired Clinical Responses Common undesired clinical responses shared by all PSIs were previously discussed. However, toxic effects associated with aspirin overdose or sensitivity must be considered.

Salicylism, or salicylate poisoning, results from aspirin overdose. In general, mild-to-moderate toxicity occurs with doses between 150 and 250 mg/kg of body weight. Severe-to-lethal toxicity is observed with doses above 250 mg/kg of body weight. Serum salicylate levels vary according to the severity of the toxicity[1] (see box).

Early indications of salicylate intoxication include tinnitus, decreased auditory acuity, headache, sweating, nausea, and vomiting. Respiratory centers in the CNS are directly stimulated by elevated plasma salicylate levels. This stimulation usually causes hyperventilation, which produces respiratory alkalosis. In most individuals the body compensates by increasing renal sodium and potassium bicarbonate excretion.[1]

Salicylism in children produces severe CNS effects, including respiratory depression, marked hyperthermia, vomiting, diarrhea, and sweating. These effects usually cause respiratory and metabolic acidosis, which can lead to convulsions, coma, and death.

Although allergy or hypersensitivity to aspirin does exist, it usually occurs only in susceptible individuals (i.e., those individuals with preexisting asthma or nasal polyps). Manifestations of hypersensitivity include vasomotor rhinitis, urticaria, bronchial wheezing, and angioneurotic edema.[13]

Contraindications and Precautions Aspirin is not recommended for a client with a history of adverse reactions to salicylates. It is also contraindicated in the following situations:

- Clients with hemophilia, bleeding ulcers, or hemorrhagic states
- Clients with a history of nasal polyps, asthma, or rhinitis
- Pregnant clients in the third trimester
- Clients concurrently receiving anticoagulant therapy
- Postoperative client or clients anticipating surgery

Drug-Drug and Drug-Nutrient Interactions Drug-drug interactions for salicylates are numerous. (See previous section, "Drug-Drug and Drug-Nutrient Common to PSIs.") Special concerns involve lithium, antacids, activated charcoal, urinary alkalizers, carbonic anhydrase inhibitors, corticosteroids, exogenous insulin, and β-adrenergic blockers. If salicylates are administered concurrently with lithium, an increase in lithium effect can occur. This is probably due to decreased renal excretion of the lithium.[14] If administered concurrently with aluminium–magnesium hydroxide, the absorption of aspirin is accelerated. However, an antacid containing magnesium and aluminium hydroxide can also increase urinary pH, increasing salicylate clearance and lowering serum salicylate concentrations by 30% to 70%.

Chronic high-dose aspirin therapy, 4 to 5 g/d, can lead to increased ascorbic acid excretion and potassium depletion.[15] In addition, a combination of food and enteric-coated aspirin may delay the absorption of the drug and predispose the client to overdose or poisoning.[16]

Life-Span Considerations It is especially important not to use aspirin during the last 3 months of pregnancy. In general, salicylates cross the placenta barrier and appear in the system of the newborn. These drugs are poorly detoxified and excreted by the neonate, predisposing the newborn to bleeding and salicylate intoxication.

Reye's syndrome was first recognized in 1963. Eventually an association was made between the syndrome and the use of aspirin in children with viral infections. Originally it was thought that Reye's syndrome occurred only with young children. However, it has been determined that adolescents are also at risk. The syndrome, which has a high mortality rate, is characterized by encephalopathy, acute renal failure, and fatty infiltration of the liver.

Specific Drug-Related Nursing Considerations Ask the client to take the drug with 8 ounces of water and to swallow the tablet whole. Encourage the client to remain in a semi-Fowler's or Fowler's position for 15 to 30 minutes after taking the drug. If the client is receiving enteric-coated aspirin, antacids should not be administered 1 to 2 hours before or after the aspirin dose.[17] Encourage the client to consume foods high in potassium and vitamin C to compensate for excess ascorbic acid and potassium excretion.

Monitor serum levels of aspirin and recommend an increase in dosage if symptoms continue. Also monitor carefully for undesired clinical responses, including nausea, vomiting, abdominal pain, tinnitus, dizziness, bruising, bleeding gums, hematuria, hematemesis, melena, and orthostatic changes in vital signs.

MISCELLANEOUS DRUGS IN CATEGORY

Diflunisal and **choline magnesium trisalicylate** are both salicylates. Table 51–1 contains dosage information for these drugs.

PLASMA SALICYLATE LEVELS ASSOCIATED WITH SALICYLISM

Mild salicylate toxicity: 40-70 mg/dl
Moderate salicylate toxicity: 70-150 mg/dl
Severe-to-lethal salicylate toxicity: >150 mg/dl

CONCEPT REVIEW

Acetylsalicylic acid (aspirin) is the prototype for PG cyclooxygenase inhibitors and for salicylates.

Salicylates are absorbed in the stomach and distributed throughout the body bound to albumin. They are metabolized in the liver and excreted by the kidneys.

TABLE 51–1

Prostaglandin Synthetase Inhibitors—Salicylates: Prototype and Major Drugs in Category

Drug and How Supplied	Dosage and Route of Administration	Nursing Considerations
ACETYLSALICYLIC ACID (aspirin—many trade names) **HOW SUPPLIED** Sustained-action coated tablet: 325, 500, 650 mg Sustained-action uncoated tablet: 325, 650 mg Enteric-coated sustained-action tablet: 650 mg Enteric-coated tablet: 81, 165, 650 mg Tablet: 800 mg Rectal suppositories: 120, 200, 325, 650 mg	**Analgesic and Antipyretic** ADULTS 325-650 mg q4h up to 4000 mg/d in divided doses CHILDREN Dose determined by age, from 160 mg q4h to 650 mg q4h **Anti-inflammatory** ADULTS 3.6-5.4 g/d in divided doses CHILDREN 90-130 mg/kg/d in divided doses at intervals of 4-6 h SUPPOSITORIES 1 suppository not more often than q4h	**Assess** Assess for indications of inflammation. Assess for pain level. Assess for concurrent use of drugs that interact with salicylates (e.g., antacids, anticoagulants, insulin). Determine if client is pregnant; drug is not recommended during last 3 mo of pregnancy and is classified as Pregnancy Category D drug. **Implement** Advise client to take drug before pain is out of control. Instruct client to take enteric-coated drug on an empty stomach. Instruct client to take uncoated drug with small amount of food. Teach client to keep drug out of reach of children and confused individuals. Teach client not to crush or chew sustained-action preparations. Advise client to discontinue drug and notify primary care provider if undesired clinical responses occur. Instruct client to notify primary care provider if other prescription or OTC drugs are being used. Store in cool, dry place. Discard drug supply if tablets have a strong vinegar-like odor. **Monitor** Monitor for indications of undesired clinical responses (e.g., abdominal pain, nausea, tinnitus, vomiting, dizziness, bleeding). Monitor urinary output to detect decreased renal clearance. Monitor for indications of salicylism. **Evaluate** Evaluate serum levels. Therapeutic analgesic serum level for acetylsalicylic acid is <100 µg/ml. Therapeutic anti-inflammatory serum level is 100-200 µg/ml for acetylsalicylic acid. Panic level for acetylsalicylic acid is >50 mg/dl. Evaluate client for reduction in signs and symptoms (e.g., decreased body temperature, reduced pain level, decreased indications of inflammation).
Choline Magnesium Trisalicylate (Trilisate) **HOW SUPPLIED** Oral liquid: 500 mg/5 ml Coated tablet: 500, 750, 1000 mg Uncoated tablet: 293 mg/362 mg, 440 mg/544 mg, 500, 750, 1000 mg	**Analgesic or Antipyretic** ADULTS 2000-3000 mg/d in two or three divided doses CHILDREN Usual daily dose, 50 mg/kg/d (for those 37 kg or less), 2250 mg/d for heavier children; give in two divided doses **Anti-inflammatory** ADULTS Initial dose, 1500 mg bid or tid; elderly, 2250 mg divided into three doses CHILDREN Usual daily dose, 50 mg/kg/d (for those 37 kg or less), 2250 mg/d for heavier children; give in two divided doses	Same as for prototype. Drug is equianalgesic to 650 mg of aspirin but has longer duration of action. Evaluate plasma levels. Therapeutic level is 15-30 mg/dl. Plasma half-life is 9-17 h.
Diflunisal (Dolobid) **HOW SUPPLIED** Coated tablet: 250, 500 mg	**Analgesic** Initial dose, 1000 mg, followed by 500 mg q8-12h **Anti-inflammatory** 500-1000 mg daily in two divided doses; maintenance dose should not exceed 1500 mg/d	Same as for prototype. 500 mg of diflunisal is comparable to 650 mg of aspirin. Evaluate for peak effect in 2-3 h.

Drug-drug interactions are common with aspirin since it displaces many drugs bound to plasma protein.

Aspirin is associated with many undesired clinical responses and toxic reactions, including tinnitus, gastric distress, bleeding tendencies, salicylism, and Reye's syndrome.

Acetic Acid Derivatives

Major acetic acid derivatives are indomethacin, sulindac, tolmetin sodium, and diclofenac sodium. The prototype is indomethacin.

ACETIC ACID DERIVATIVE PROTOTYPE
INDOMETHACIN

Indomethacin (e.g., Indocin) has been in use since 1965.

Pharmacotherapeutics Clinically the drug is used to treat osteoarthritis, ankylosing spondylitis, and rheumatoid arthritis. It is also effective in the treatment of acute gouty arthritis, acute bursitis, and acute tendinitis. In addition, intravenous (IV) indomethacin is used to close patent ductus arteriosus in premature infants.

Pharmacokinetics Indomethacin is rapidly absorbed from the GI tract, including the rectal mucosa when administered by suppository. Once absorbed, it is almost entirely bound to plasma proteins. Peak plasma concentration of 1 μg/ml occurs approximately 2 hours after administration of a 25-mg capsule. Indomethacin is distributed to all body fluids and tissues. Generally it has a plasma half-life of 4 to 5 hours. However, half-lives of 12 to 13 hours have been reported. The drug is metabolized in the liver and excreted in the urine (60%) and bile (30% in feces) as unchanged compound and metabolites.[1]

Pharmacodynamics Indomethacin has all of the actions of aspirin but is 20 to 30 times more potent. In addition, indomethacin decreases production of renin by the juxtaglomerular cells of the kidney cortex. It may affect cyclic adenosine monophosphate functions by its inhibitory effect on phosphodiesterase.[1]

Pharmaceutics Indomethacin is available for oral administration in capsule, sustained-action capsule, and suspension dosage forms. It is also available in rectal suppository form and IV solution.

Undesired Clinical Responses Drowsiness and headache are common undesired clinical responses associated with this drug. These discomforts are readily reversed by omitting or lowering the dose of indomethacin. Other responses include GI effects and renal involvement, which were discussed previously in the section, "Undesired Clinical Responses Common to PSIs."

Contraindications and Precautions The use of indomethacin is contraindicated during pregnancy, especially during the last trimester when indomethacin-induced premature closure of the ductus may occur. Its use is contraindicated in clients with hypersensitivity to indomethacin or other PSIs or with bleeding abnormalities. Since indomethacin can cause fluid retention and peripheral edema, it should be used with caution in clients with cardiac dysfunction or hypertension. In addition, use of in-

domethacin suppositories is contraindicated in clients with a history of proctitis or recent rectal bleeding.[1,17]

Drug-Drug Interactions Drug-drug interactions similar to those associated with other PSIs occur with indomethacin. In addition, when indomethacin and diflunisal are administered concurrently, the renal clearance of indomethacin decreases and the plasma level increases. Indomethacin administered concurrently with digoxin can increase the serum concentration and prolong the half-life of digoxin.[17]

Life-Span Considerations Effectiveness of indomethacin in children 14 years of age and younger has not been established. As indicated previously, indomethacin use is contraindicated during pregnancy. The drug crosses the human placenta easily throughout gestation, and small amounts of unchanged drug are found in the amniotic fluid.[18] Since indomethacin is excreted in the milk of lactating mothers, it is not recommended for use in these clients. Caution must be taken when administering the drug to elderly individuals since indomethacin can cause signs of depression in this age group. It is recommended that the maintenance dose for elderly clients be reduced by 25%.[19]

Specific Drug-Related Nursing Considerations Because indomethacin can mask the usual signs and symptoms of infection, assess the client carefully. Indomethacin should be administered immediately after meals, with food, or with antacids.

MISCELLANEOUS DRUGS IN CATEGORY

Other drugs in this category include sulindac, tolmetin sodium, and diclofenac (Table 51–2). **Sulindac** (Clinoril) was developed in an attempt to find an anti-inflammatory drug with fewer side effects than indomethacin. Sulindac itself is biologically inactive. However, during the biotransformation process a sulfide metabolite is formed. This metabolite probably is the pharmacologically active form of the drug. Sulindac possesses all the undesired clinical responses of other PSIs.[1]

Tolmetin sodium (Tolectin) is more potent than aspirin but less potent than indomethacin. Peak plasma levels occur quickly, within 30 to 60 minutes after administration of the drug. It is recommended that the drug be administered immediately after waking and at bedtime with milk or meals.[1,17]

Diclofenac sodium (Voltaren) is absorbed completely but has a high rate of first-pass hepatic metabolism; only 50% to 60% of a dose reaches systemic circulation. Peak plasma concentration levels range from 1 to 2 μg/ml after administration of 25 to 50 mg of the drug. Low circulating plasma diclofenac levels are associated with a lower incidence and severity of classic undesired clinical responses of other PSIs. Diclofenac is distributed throughout all body tissues. It penetrates synovial membranes, reaching joint fluid within 4 hours. This produces synovial fluid concentrations that are higher and last longer than plasma concentrations.[1]

Propionic Acid Derivatives

Propionic acid derivatives share all the properties of the acetic acid PSIs, including rapid absorption and peak plasma concentrations within 1 to 2 hours.[1]

TABLE 51-2

Prostaglandin Synthetase Inhibitors—Acetic Acid Derivatives: Prototype and Major Drugs in Category

Drug Name	Dosage and Route of Administration
INDOMETHACIN (Indocin) **HOW SUPPLIED** Capsule: 25, 50 mg Sustained-action capsule: 75 mg Rectal suppository: 50 mg Suspension: 25 mg/5 ml	**Rheumatoid Arthritis** ADULTS Initial dose, 25 mg bid or tid, increased at weekly intervals to a maximum of 150-200 mg/d in divided doses; use with care in elderly **Bursitis, Tendinitis, Acute Gout** ADULTS Initial dose, 75-150 mg/d in three or four divided doses until symptoms have been controlled for several days CHILDREN Not recommended in children <14 y
Sulindac (Clinoril) **HOW SUPPLIED** Uncoated tablet: 150, 200 mg	**Arthritis, Spondylitis** Initial dose, 150 mg bid; adjust to a maximum dose of 400 mg/d **Bursitis, Tendinitis, Acute Gout** 200 mg bid until response, then reduce; usual therapy, 7-14 d
Tolmetin Sodium (Tolmetin) **HOW SUPPLIED** Capsule: 400 mg Uncoated tablet: 200, 600 mg	ADULTS Initial dose, 400 mg tid, then adjust to a maximum of 600-1800 mg/d divided in three doses CHILDREN 2 Y OR OLDER Initial dose, 20 mg/kg/d; usual maintenance dose, 15-30 mg/kg/d
Diclofenac Sodium (Voltaren) **HOW SUPPLIED** Enteric-coated tablet: 25, 50, 75 mg	**Osteoarthritis or Rheumatoid Arthritis** 100-150 mg/d in divided doses, 50 mg bid or tid or 75 mg bid **Ankylosing Spondylitis** 100-125 mg/d administered as 25 mg qid with an extra 25-mg dose at bedtime if necessary

PROPIONIC ACID DERIVATIVE PROTOTYPE

IBUPROFEN

Ibuprofen (e.g., Motrin, Advil, Nuprin) has been available in Europe since 1967. It was approved for use in the United States in 1974. In 1984 the FDA approved low-dose ibuprofen—200-mg tablets—for OTC use.

Pharmacotherapeutics Ibuprofen is classified as a nonsteroidal anti-inflammatory, mild antispasmodic, and antipyretic drug effective for the symptomatic treatment of rheumatoid arthritis and osteoarthritis and as an analgesic for relief of musculoskeletal pain. Ibuprofen is also effective in the treatment of primary dysmenorrhea.

Pharmacokinetics Ibuprofen is well absorbed in the GI tract. Peak effect of the drug occurs in 1 to 2 hours. It is metabolized in the liver and excreted by the kidneys. The plasma half-life of ibuprofen is approximately 2 to 2½ hours. Excretion of the drug is practically complete within 24 hours of the last dose.

Pharmacodynamics Like other PSIs, ibuprofen inhibits the synthesis of PGs. This action accounts for its anti-inflammatory and antipyretic effects. Ibuprofen also reduces PG levels in menstrual fluid and inhibits uterine contractions.[1]

Pharmaceutics Ibuprofen is administered orally in the form of tablets or in a suspension. Ibuprofen is administered in a wide range of dosages depending on the therapeutic effect desired. When compared to aspirin, 200 mg of ibuprofen is superior to 650 mg of aspirin.

Undesired Clinical Responses Like those of aspirin, the effects of ibuprofen are more general and systemic than local. However, undesired clinical responses do target specific organs (i.e., GI tract or kidneys). GI effects of ibuprofen range from nausea, vomiting, and abdominal pain to ulceration and bleeding. The severity of the symptoms appear to be related to dose.[20] Large dosages of ibuprofen given over an extended time frame may produce renal damage in the form of nephritis with hematuria, proteinuria, or renal failure.[21] Other reported undesired clinical responses include headache, dizziness, drowsiness, blurred vision, diminished visual acuity, and diplopia.

Contraindications and Precautions Individuals allergic to aspirin are cautioned to avoid ibuprofen use because there is evidence of cross sensitivity.

Drug-Drug, Drug-Nutrient, and Drug-Environment Interactions Like other PSIs, ibuprofen interacts with coumarin-type anticoagulants, aspirin, methotrexate, furosemide, and lithium. Most of these interactions are associated with ibuprofen's high level of binding with plasma protein. Drug-nutrient and drug-environment interactions are also possible with ibuprofen. For example, concurrent food ingestion, especially foods high in fiber (e.g., bran, pectin) or carbohydrates, delays ibuprofen's bioavailability.[22] Photosensitivity has been reported in some clients.

Life-Span Considerations Ibuprofen is not recommended during pregnancy or for use in nursing mothers. The FDA has approved its use as an antipyretic in children (6 months to 12 years old) if the following formula is used: 5 mg/kg if the baseline temperature is 102.5° F or below or 10 mg/kg if the baseline temperature is greater than 102.5° F.

Specific Drug-Related Nursing Considerations If the client is experiencing gastric irritation, consult with the primary care provider to determine if the drug can be taken with food or antacids. Because photosensitivity occurs with ibuprofen and other propionic acid derivatives, advise the client to avoid the use of sunlamps and to use sunscreen and protective clothing (e.g., long sleeves, hat with a brim) when in the sun.

Advise the client that ibuprofen may interfere with performance or tasks requiring mental alertness. (Some clients experience dizziness and drowsiness during therapy.) In addition, since visual problems (i.e., diminished acuity, diplopia, disturbance in color vision) are possible, recommend that the client receiving long-term therapy have periodic ophthalmic examinations. Because the client may experience altered bleeding times, advise the client to inform other care providers (i.e., dentists, surgeons) that they are taking the drug.

MISCELLANEOUS DRUG IN CATEGORY

The drug discussed in this section is a PSI. Since only drug-specific information is included, review of the previous general section on PSIs and the information about ibuprofen, the prototype for propionic acid derivatives, would be beneficial (Table 51–3).

Ketoprofen (Orudis) is one of the newer propionic acid derivatives. This drug has an inhibitory effect on PG and leukotriene synthesis, an antibradykinin activity, and a lysosomal membrane-stabilizing action. Ketoprofen is used for chronic treatment of rheumatoid arthritis and osteoarthritis. It

TABLE 51–3

Prostaglandin Synthetase Inhibitors—Propionic Acid Derivatives: Prototype and Major Drug in Category

Drug Name	Dosage and Route of Administration
IBUPROFEN	*Analgesic*
(Motrin, Rufen, Advil, Nuprin)	ADULTS
	200-400 mg q4-6h as needed
HOW SUPPLIED	*Antipyretic*
Coated tablet: 200	400 mg q4-6h
300, 400, 600, 800 mg	*Anti-inflammatory*
Suspension: 100 mg/5 ml	1200-3200 mg/d divided into three or four doses; adjust as low as possible for maintenance dose
	Antipyretic
	CHILDREN
	With fever up to 39° C, 5 mg/kg q6-8h; with fever >39° C, 10 mg/kg q6-8h; maximum daily dose not to exceed 40 mg/kg
Ketoprofen	*Analgesic*
(Orudis)	25-50 mg q6-8h as needed to a total daily dose of 300 mg
HOW SUPPLIED	*Anti-inflammatory*
Capsule: 25, 50, 75 mg	Initial dose, 75 mg tid or 50 mg qid, increase to 150-300 mg/d divided into three or four doses; reduce dose by one half to one third in elderly and those with renal impairment
Capsule, sustained release: 200 mg	

is also prescribed for mild-to-moderate pain and primary dysmenorrhea. The most common undesired clinical responses are dyspepsia, nausea, vomiting, abdominal pain, flatulence, anorexia, and headache. Ketoprofen is classified as a Pregnancy Category B drug. Its use in children is not recommended.

CONCEPT REVIEW

Indomethacin is the prototype for acetic acid derivatives. Other drugs in this category are sulindac, tolmetin sodium, and diclofenac sodium.

Indomethacin is considered a classic example of PG cyclooxygenase inhibitors. It has all of the actions of aspirin but is 20 to 30 times more potent.

Drowsiness and headache are common undesired clinical responses associated with indomethacin use. Other undesired responses include GI effects and renal involvement.

Propionic acid derivatives share all the properties of the acetic acid PSIs, including rapid absorption and peak plasma concentrations within 1 to 2 hours. The prototype for this group is ibuprofen.

Like other PSIs, ibuprofen inhibits the synthesis of PGs. It also reduces PG levels in menstrual fluid and inhibits uterine contractions.

Drug-drug interactions are common with ibuprofen because it displaces other drugs bound to plasma protein.

Ibuprofen is associated with many undesired clinical responses, including tinnitus, gastric distress, renal dysfunction, photosensitivity, and CNS changes.

Miscellaneous Prostaglandin Synthetase Inhibitors

Since all of the drugs in this section are PSIs, properties common to PSIs are not repeated. Only drug-specific information is included in the discussion (Table 51–4). Reviewing the previous general section on PSIs is beneficial.

ARYLACETIC ACID DERIVATIVES

Naproxen, naproxen sodium, and fenoprofen calcium are chemically arylacetic acid derivatives.

Naproxen (Naprosyn) inhibits PG synthesis and has a prominent inhibitory effect on the migration of leukocytes. It is indicated for the treatment of rheumatoid arthritis, osteoarthritis, juvenile arthritis, ankylosing spondylitis, tendinitis, bursitis, and acute gout. It is also used to relieve mild-to-moderate pain and to treat primary dysmenorrhea.

Naproxen must not be used concomitantly with the related drug naproxen sodium since they both circulate in plasma as the naproxen anion. Naproxen is classified as a Pregnancy Category B drug. The safety and effectiveness of naproxen in children below the age of 2 years have not been established.

Naproxen is most effective when taken on an empty stomach (e.g., 1 hour before or 2 hours after meals) (Table 51–5).

Naproxen sodium (Anaprox) is a combination of naproxen and sodium. Sodium accelerates the absorption rate of the drug. Naproxen sodium is indicated in the relief of mild-to-moderate pain and for the treatment of primary dysmenorrhea. It has also been used to treat rheumatoid arthritis, osteoarthritis, ankylosing spondylitis, tendinitis, bursitis, and acute gout. This drug should not be used concomitantly with naproxen. It should be used with caution for clients receiving a sodium-restricted diet.

INTERFERENCE WITH LABORATORY TESTS. Naproxen and naproxen sodium may increase urinary values for 17-ketogenic steroids, and both drugs may interfere with some urinary assays of 5-hydroxyindoleacetic acid (5-HIAA).

Fenoprofen calcium (Fenoprofen, Nalfon) chemically is an arylacetic acid derivative used to treat rheumatoid arthritis and osteoarthritis and to relieve mild-to-moderate pain. It is most effective if administered 30 minutes before or 2 hours after meals. Tinnitus, blurred vision, and decreased hearing have been reported with long-term use of the drug.

PHENYLALKANOIC ACID DERIVATIVE

Flurbiprofen (Ansaid) is a potent PSI. It also increases migration of leukocytes into inflamed tissues and depresses monocyte function. Flurbiprofen is indicated for the acute or long-term treatment of rheumatoid arthritis and osteoarthritis.

Flurbiprofen is well absorbed after oral administration, reaching peak plasma levels in approximately 1½ hours. Administration of flurbiprofen with food alters the rate of drug absorption but does not affect its bioavailability. Amost all of the drug is bound to albumin. Flurbiprofen is extensively metabolized and is excreted primarily in the urine. Excretion is almost complete within 24 hours of the last dose.

Flurbiprofen is considered a Pregnancy Category B drug. Since the drug appears in breast milk, it is not recommended for use in nursing mothers. Common undesired clinical responses include dyspepsia, diarrhea, abdominal pain, nausea, and headache. Major drugs involved in drug-drug interactions with flurbiprofen are antacids, anticoagulants, β-adrenergic blocking agents, cimetidine, digoxin, and diuretics.[17]

ANTHRANILIC ACID DERIVATIVES

Of the anthranilic acid derivatives, only mefenamic acid and meclofenamate sodium are available in the United States. These drugs are also classified as *fenamates* or *fenamic acid derivatives.* Both mefenamic acid and meclofenamate sodium are potent PSIs. Since they are also used as analgesics, they are discussed in Chapter 19. Information about their use as an analgesic is provided in Table 19–1.

Mefenamic acid (Ponstel) is used primarily in the treatment of dysmenorrhea and moderate pain. In the United States it is approved for 7 days of treatment; the usual duration of treatment is 2 to 3 days. It is classified as a Pregnancy Category C drug. Its safety and efficacy in children below the age of 14 years has not been established. Mefenamic acid should be administered with food or milk to decrease GI distress. Un-

desired clinical responses include nausea, vomiting, severe diarrhea, peptic ulceration, facial edema, leukopenia, eosinophilia, agranulocytosis, and pancytopenia.

Meclofenamate sodium (Meclomen) is rapidly absorbed from the GI tract; peak action is within 2 hours. The drug is used to relieve symptoms of acute or chronic rheumatoid arthritis or osteoarthritis. However, since use of meclofenamate sodium is associated with a high incidence of diarrhea and bowel inflammation, it is not recommended as initial treatment for these conditions. Other common undesired clinical responses include dry mouth, sores in the mouth, headache, and sedation. Although administering meclofenamate with meals or milk usually decreases or prevents GI symptoms, doing so can delay absorption of the drug. However, concomitant administration of aluminum or magnesium hydroxide antacids does not appear to interfere with meclofenamate absorption.[1,17] Long-term therapy should be monitored with complete blood count (CBC) and renal and hepatic function studies.

OXICAMS

The primary oxicam is **piroxicam** (Feldene). This drug has potent anti-inflammatory, analgesic, and antipyretic actions derived primarily from its PG synthetase inhibitory properties. Piroxicam appears equivalent to aspirin, indomethacin, and naproxen for long-term treatment of rheumatoid arthritis or osteoarthritis. It is also used in the treatment of acute gouty arthritis, ankylosing spondylitis, and acute musculoskeletal disorders.

Piroxicam is well absorbed after oral administration. Because of its prolonged half-life, single daily dosing is possible. The long plasma half-life also allows plasma concentrations to increase gradually for 7 to 12 days before reaching a therapeutic level. At the level (3 to 8 μg per milliliter), the synovial fluid concentration is approximately equal to the plasma concentration. Piroxicam is 99% bound to plasma protein. It is metabolized by the liver and excreted in urine (65%) and feces (35%).

The most frequent undesired clinical responses are those associated with most PSIs, including GI disturbances, headache, dizziness, and drowsiness. In addition, malaise, somnolence, and reduced hemoglobin and hematocrit levels have been reported. Piroxicam may increase the effects of oral anticoagulant drugs. It also may increase toxic symptoms of diazepam, propranolol, phenylbutazone, and lithium.

PYRROLACETIC ACID DERIVATIVES

Ketorolac tromethamine (Toradol) has analgesic, anti-inflammatory, and antipyretic effects. It inhibits PG synthesis and acts peripherally to relieve pain. Currently ketorolac is the only injectable NSAID available in the United States for pain relief. Because of risks associated with prolonged use, the drug is approved for short-term therapy only.[23]

Administered orally and intramuscularly, ketorolac is quickly absorbed into the blood. Ketorolac may also be administered intravenously. Since ketorolac is 99% bound to plasma protein, it is rapidly distributed throughout the body.

TABLE 51–4
Prostaglandin Synthetase Inhibitors—Miscellaneous Agents

Drug Name	Dosage and Route of Administration
ARYLACETIC ACID DERIVATIVES	
Naproxen	***Analgesic***
(Naprosyn)	Initial dose, 500 mg, followed by 250 mg q8h as required, not to exceed a total daily dose of 1250 mg
HOW SUPPLIED	
Suspension: 125 mg/ml	***Anti-inflammatory***
Coated tablet: 375 mg	ADULTS
Uncoated tablet: 250, 500 mg	250, 375, or 500 mg bid; dose may be increased to 1500 mg/d for limited periods
	CHILDREN
	10 mg/kg total daily dose divided into two doses
Naproxen Sodium	***Analgesic***
(Anaprox)	Initial dose, 550 mg, then 275 mg q6-8h as required, not to exceed 1375 mg/d
HOW SUPPLIED	
Coated tablet: 275, 550 mg	***Anti-inflammatory***
	ADULTS
	275 or 550 mg bid; may increase for limited periods to 1650 mg/d
	CHILDREN
	Recommended total daily dose, 10 mg/kg in two divided doses
Fenoprofen Calcium	***Analgesic***
(Nalfon)	200 mg q4-6h as needed
HOW SUPPLIED	
Capsule: 200, 300 mg	***Anti-inflammatory***
Coated tablet: 600 mg	300-600 mg three or four times daily up to a total daily dose of 3200 mg
Uncoated tablet: 600 mg	
PHENYLALKANOIC ACID DERIVATIVE	
Flurbiprofen	***Anti-inflammatory***
(Ansaid)	200-300 mg total daily dose divided into two, three, or four doses
HOW SUPPLIED	
Uncoated tablet: 50, 100 mg	
ANTHRANILIC ACID DERIVATIVES	
Mefenamic Acid	ADULTS AND CHILDREN >14 Y
(Ponstel)	Initial dose, 500 mg; then 250 mg q6h as needed, usually not to exceed 1 wk
HOW SUPPLIED	
Capsule: 250 mg	
Meclofenamate Sodium	***Anti-inflammatory***
(Meclomen)	Initial dose, 200 mg daily divided into three or four equal doses; increase if necessary to maximum of 400 mg/d in divided doses
HOW SUPPLIED	
Capsule: 50, 100 mg	***Analgesic***
	50 mg q4-6h, not to exceed 400 mg total daily dose
OXICAMS	***Anti-inflammatory for Osteoarthritis and Rheumatoid Arthritis***
Piroxicam	ADULTS
(Feldene)	20 mg in single daily dose or divided; assess effectiveness in 2 wk
HOW SUPPLIED	CHILDREN
Capsule: 10, 20 mg	Dose not established
	Analgesic or Antipyretic
	Not recommended
PYRROLACETIC ACIDS	
Ketorolac Tromethamine	***Analgesic***
(Toradol)	Oral: 10 mg as needed q4-6h for limited duration
HOW SUPPLIED	ADULTS <65 Y
Injection solution: 15 or 30 mg/ml, 60 mg	IV, IM: 30 mg q6h; maximum: 120 mg/24 h
Uncoated tablet: 10 mg	ADULTS >65 Y, RENAL IMPAIRMENT, <50 KG
	IV, IM: 15 mg q6h; maximum: 60 mg/24 h
	Anti-inflammatory
	Not recommended for long-term use

TABLE 51–5
Prostaglandin Synthetase Inhibitors: Pharmacokinetic and Equianalgesic Properties

Drug	Peak Effect	Plasma Half-life (h)	Equianalgesic Properties
Aspirin	1-3 h	Low dose, 3-4 High dose, 9-16	—
Diflunisal	2-3 h	8-12	500 mg superior to 650 mg aspirin
Indomethacin	2 h after oral capsule	Average, 4-5	20-30 times more potent than aspirin
Sulindac	2 h	16	
Tolmetin sodium	30-60 min	1-2	More potent than aspirin
Diclofenac	2-3 h	Mean terminal half-life, 2	Potency approximately equal to that of indomethacin
Ibuprofen	1-2 h	2-2½	200 mg equal to 650 mg aspirin
Fenoprofen calcium	2 h	2-3	200 mg equal to 650 mg aspirin
Ketoprofen	½-2 h	2-4	25 mg superior to 650 mg aspirin and comparable to 400 mg ibuprofen
Naproxen	2-4 h	10-20	250 mg probably comparable to 650 mg aspirin
Naproxen sodium	1-2 h	13-15	275 mg equal to 650 mg aspirin
Mefenamic acid	2-4 h	2	250 mg equal to 650 mg aspirin
Meclofenamate sodium	½-1 h	1-2	—
Piroxicam	3-5 h	Mean, 50 Range, 30-86	—
Ketorolac tromethamine	IM: 50 min Oral: 44 min	IM: 3½-9 for young adults; 5-9 for elderly Oral: 2-9 for young adults; 4-8 for elderly	30 mg equal to 12 mg morphine
Flurbiprofen	1½ h	6	—

The drug is eliminated by hepatic metabolism and urinary excretion.

The most common undesired clinical responses are GI disturbances: nausea, dyspepsia, diarrhea, abdominal pain, and cramping. With long-term oral therapy, gastric ulceration has occurred. In addition, long-term oral therapy can precipitate reversible suppression of platelet aggregation, asthma, and nephrotoxicity.[24,25] Other undesired responses include drowsiness, dizziness, edema, headache, urinary frequency, abnormal taste in the mouth, and blurred vision.

Ketorolac use is contraindicated in clients who developed nasal polyps, angioedema, or bronchospasm from other NSAIDs. The drug should be administered with caution to clients receiving lithium or methotrexate. Ketorolac is classified as a Pregnancy Category C drug. It is not recommended for use during labor and delivery or for lactating women. It also is not recommended in clients with impaired hepatic function or for children. In addition, a lower dose range is usually administered to clients who weigh less than 50 kg, who are over 65 years old, or who have decreased renal function.[24]

Do not use the injectable solution if it is not clear. Discard it if it is slightly yellow. Protect the drug from light and store it at room temperature between 15° and 30° C. Do not mix parenteral ketorolac in a syringe with other drugs without checking a compatibility chart.

Tell the client that ketorolac can cause drowsiness and dizziness and that driving or using heavy equipment while receiving the drug is not recommended. If necessary, instruct the client or significant other about the correct method of administering an intramuscular (IM) injection.

CONCEPT REVIEW

Numerous PSIs are available for use as anti-inflammatory, analgesic, and antipyretic drugs.

These drugs can be subclassified according to their chemical composition: arylacetic acid derivatives (naproxen, naproxen sodium), phenylalkanoic acid derivatives (flurbiprofen), anthranilic acid derivatives (mefenamic acid, meclofenamate sodium), oxicams (piroxicam), and pyrrolacetic acid derivatives (ketorolac trometh-amine).

Undesired clinical responses associated with these drugs include GI disturbances, renal and hepatic dysfunction, CNS changes, bleeding abnormalities, and allergic reactions.

NONPROSTAGLANDIN SYNTHETASE INHIBITORS

Non-PSIs are either weak PSIs or produce their effects by other mechanisms.

Para-Aminophenol Derivatives

The prototype for para-aminophenol derivatives is acetaminophen. This drug was discussed in Chapter 19. Acetaminophen is a weak PG inhibitor. As such, it is used primarily for relief of headaches, dysmenorrhea, myalgias, neuralgias, and fever. It is not an effective anti-inflammatory drug.

❧ NURSING RESEARCH

Morgan, S. (1990). A comparison of three methods of managing fever in the neurologic patient. *Journal of Neuroscience Nursing, 22*(1), 19-24.

The purpose of this quasi-experimental study was to compare the effectiveness of three methods of fever reduction and the effect of each on patient shivering. Twenty-one febrile neurologic patients were randomly placed in one of three temperature reduction groups: acetaminophen only, acetaminophen with tepid water sponging, and acetaminophen with hypothermia blanket.

A temperature reduction protocol was initiated when a subject first became febrile. Rectal temperatures were taken every 15 minutes until the subject's temperature returned to 100° F. Subjects were observed for shivering throughout the procedures.

The analysis revealed no statistically significant difference among the three methods of fever reduction. A chi-square analysis indicated a significant relationship between shivering and the use of a hypothermia blanket.

STUDENT ACTIVITIES

- Read the procedure for fever reduction in neurologic clients in your assigned agency. Determine how the procedure was established.
- Monitor the temperature of two febrile clients. Record the fever reduction strategies used for each client. Determine the length of time required to reduce each client's temperature to 100° F. Determine if the clients experienced shivering.

Antigout or Hyperuricemic Drugs

Gout is caused by hyperuricemia and the deposition of sodium urate crystals in joints. With local urate deposits in joints, local infiltration of granulocytes that phagocytize the urate crystals occurs. Gout is treated by drugs that reduce the inflammatory response or decrease the level of uric acid in the plasma or both, thus decreasing the inflammatory response. Drugs used to treat gout and hyperuricemia were discussed in Chapter 37.

Antirheumatic Drugs

Although several types of arthritis exist, rheumatoid arthritis is unique in that it is a systemic disease of the connective tissue. In clients with rheumatoid arthritis the repeated swelling and inflammation of a joint's synovial membrane progress to the point of tissue destruction.

Treatment includes the use of second-line or disease-modifying antirheumatic drugs. These drugs include gold salts, methotrexate, azathioprine, the antimalarials chloroquine and hydroxychloroquine, sulfasalazine, penicillamine, and cyclophosphamide. Second-line antirheumatic drugs are relatively slow acting, with benefits not appearing for 1 to 6 months. Only injectable gold and cyclophosphamide have

demonstrated the ability to slow or reverse the progression of rheumatoid arthritis.[27] (Cyclophosphamide is discussed in Chapter 69.)

GOLD SALTS

Gold salts have been used to treat rheumatoid arthritis since the 1920s. These agents are valuable because, unlike other NSAIDs, gold retards the progression of bone and articular destruction. The three most commonly used preparations are gold sodium thiomalate, aurothioglucose, and auranofin.

GOLD SALT PROTOTYPE
GOLD SODIUM THIOMALATE

Some primary care providers strongly believe in the use of gold (Myochrysine) as a treatment for rheumatoid arthritis, whereas others believe it is a dangerous toxin. Because of these varying opinions, treatment regimens also vary. Some clients are treated initially with gold salts before bone and articular destruction occurs. With other clients, NSAIDs, steroids, and other drugs are tried before gold salts are prescribed.

Pharmacotherapeutics Gold therapy (chrysotherapy) is indicated in the treatment of **active** rheumatoid arthritis. Gold therapy decreases the pain, swelling, and inflammation of rheumatoid arthritis and slows the progression of the disease. However, it is does not repair damaged tissue.[27,28]

Pharmacokinetics After an IM injection of gold sodium thiomalate, peak plasma concentrations occur in 2 to 6 hours. With initial therapy, the plasma half-life of the drug is approximately 1 week. However, with continued therapy, the plasma half-life is extended for weeks. Gold is 95% bound to plasma protein during the first 7 days but may be transported by erythrocytes after this time. Gold accumulates in many tissues (i.e., synovial membrane, macrophages, skin, and hepatic and renal tubular cells) where it remains for years. Gold is eliminated by the kidneys and in the feces.[1,17,29]

Pharmacodynamics The exact mechanism of action of gold therapy is unknown. However, it appears that gold suppresses the immune response at the local level by decreasing phagocytosis and fibroblast proliferation. It also decreases the activity of monocytes and lymphocytes.[27]

Pharmaceutics Gold sodium thiomalate is administered only intramuscularly. The first dose, a test dose, is generally 10 mg. The second dose is usually 25 mg, and following dosages are between 25 and 50 mg.

Undesired Clinical Responses Undesired clinical responses include a variety of systemic reactions. The most common are dermatitis, skin pigmentation with pruritis, and stomatitis. Other serious responses include renal dysfunction and hematologic reactions (i.e., anemia, leukopenia, and thrombocytopenia). Hypersensitivity and anaphylactic reactions have also been reported (Fig. 51–3).

Contraindications and Precautions Use of gold salts is contraindicated in clients with diabetes mellitus, renal disease, enterocolitis, hepatic dysfunction, congestive heart failure, hypertension, and blood dyscrasias.

Drug-Drug Interactions Since gold therapy can cause bone marrow toxicity, drugs or substances that predis-

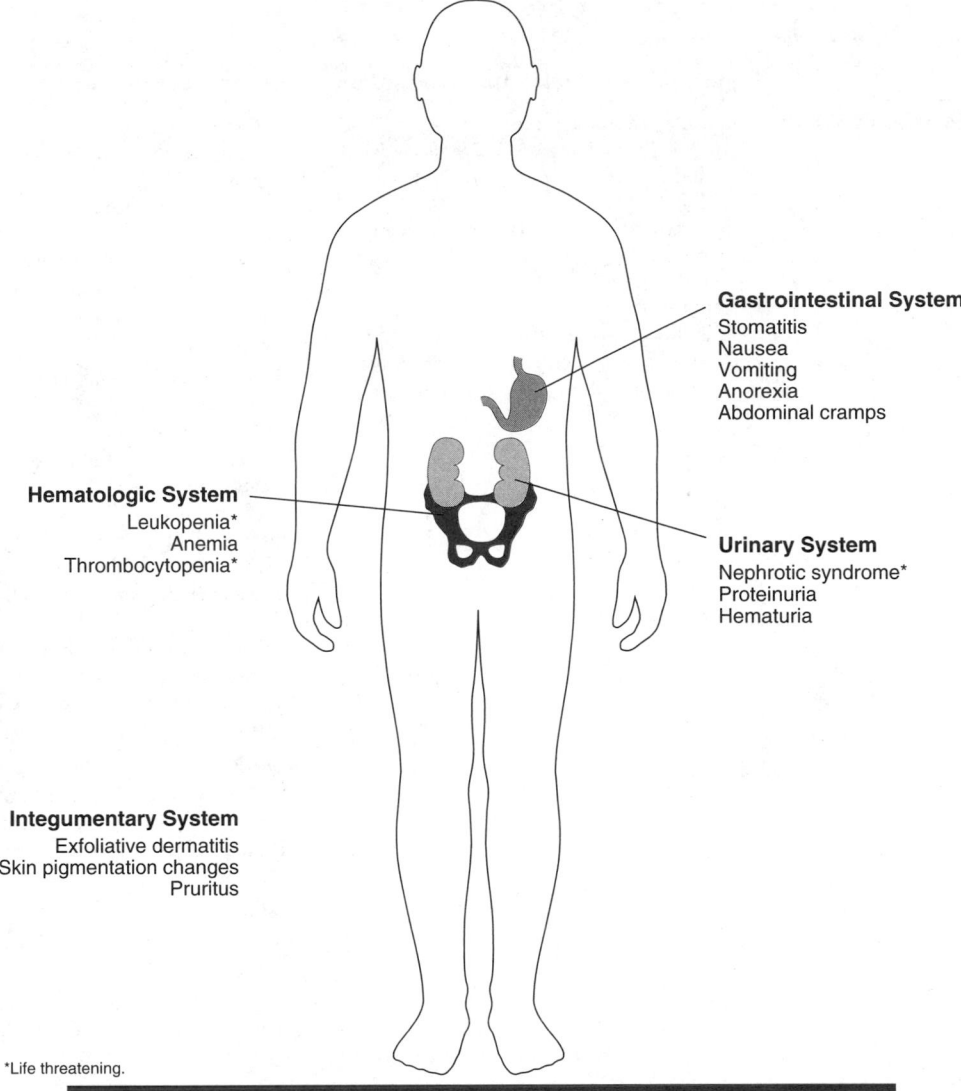

Gastrointestinal System
Stomatitis
Nausea
Vomiting
Anorexia
Abdominal cramps

Hematologic System
Leukopenia*
Anemia
Thrombocytopenia*

Urinary System
Nephrotic syndrome*
Proteinuria
Hematuria

Integumentary System
Exfoliative dermatitis
Skin pigmentation changes
Pruritus

*Life threatening.

Figure 51–3   Undesired clinical responses associated with injectable gold.

pose the client to bone marrow suppression should be avoided. Gold salts should not be used concomitantly with penicillamine because of the risk of toxicities. The safety of coadministration with cytotoxic drugs has not been established.

Life-Span Considerations Gold sodium thiomalate is classified as a Pregnancy Category C drug. The presence of gold has been found in the milk of nursing mothers and in the serum and red blood cells of nursing infants.

Specific Drug-Related Nursing Considerations Injectable gold is administered intramuscularly on a weekly basis until a particular dose of the drug has been given. Continuation of therapy is based on the client's response to the drug. During the injection the client must be in a recumbent position. Ask the client to remain in the recumbent position for at least 10 minutes after the injection. During this time observe the client carefully for indications of an allergic reaction. You should have a chelating agent (e.g., dimercaprol [BAL]) available in case of a toxic or anaphylactic reaction. (A chelating agent is a chemical compound that sequesters and binds metallic ions.)

MISCELLANEOUS DRUGS IN CATEGORY

Aurothioglucose (Solganal) is available in a suspension for IM administration. It has pharmacologic properties similar to those of gold sodium thiomalate. **Auranofin** (Ridaura), an oral gold preparation, has been available since the early 1980s. Although the drug is less toxic than injectable gold, it is also less effective. Auranofin produces most of the same adverse reactions and side effects as injectable gold, with diarrhea its most common side effect.

Additional information about gold salts is summarized in Table 51–6.

CONCEPT REVIEW

Gold salts are used to treat rheumatoid arthritis. They are not used to treat other forms of arthritis.

Gold salts produce their effects by suppressing the immune response on a local level.

TABLE 51–6
Antirheumatic Remitting Drugs—Gold Salts

Drug Name	Dosage and Route of Administration	Nursing Considerations
GOLD SODIUM THIOMALATE (Myochrysine) HOW SUPPLIED Injection solution: 25, 50 mg/ml	ADULTS (AVERAGE SIZE) 10 mg wk 1; 25 mg wk 2; 25-50 mg wk 3 and following, up to cumulative dose of 1 g Maintenance, 25-50 mg every other week for 20 wk; then every third and subsequently every four week indefinitely CHILDREN Initial dose, 10 mg, then 1 mg/kg body weight, not to exceed 50 mg for a single injection; follow adult guidelines	**Assess** Determine if client has preexisting kidney disease. Assess for allergies to gold. Assess for previous exposure to heavy metals. Review findings from diagnostic studies (e.g., RBC, CBC, urea nitrogen, creatinine, specific gravity). **Implement** Discard injectable solution if darkened. (Solution should be pale yellow.) Protect solution from light. Place client in a recumbent position for the injection. Inject drug deep IM. Observe client for at least 10 min after injection. Watch carefully for signs of anaphylaxis. Have a chelating agent (e.g., dimercaprol) available. Explain to client that gold storage in skin may lead to chrysiasis (a bronze or grey-blue color). Teach client to report sore throat, fever, or bruising to primary care provider. **Monitor** Monitor client for indications of blood dyscrasia (e.g., leukopenia, thrombocytopenia). Monitor CBC and platelet count before each injection. **Evaluate** Anticipate improvement will begin after 6-8 wk of treatment.
Aurothioglucose (Solganal) HOW SUPPLIED Suspension: 50 mg/ml	ADULTS 10 mg wk 1; 25 mg wk 2 and 3; 50 mg wk 4 and thereafter until 0.8-1 g given; then 25 or 50 mg 3-4 wk CHILDREN 6-12 Y One fourth of adult dose, governed chiefly by body weight; not to exceed 25-mg dose	Same as for gold sodium thiomalate. Shake suspension well before use.
Auranofin (Ridaura) HOW SUPPLIED Capsules: 3 mg	ADULTS 6 mg/d in either one or two doses; after 6 mo dose may be raised to 9 mg/d (3 mg tid) CHILDREN Not recommended for use in children	**Assess** Same as for gold sodium thiomalate. **Implement** Teach client that diarrhea is a fairly common adverse reaction. **Monitor** Monitor laboratory blood values on a monthly basis. **Evaluate** Anticipate improvement within 3 mo; otherwise drug should be discontinued.

Injectable gold is one of the most toxic second-line antirheumatic drugs, with up to 50% of the clients stopping therapy because of undesired clinical responses.

Primary undesired clinical responses involve the skin, mucous membranes, and hematologic system.

SUMMARY

Inflammation is the body's reaction to tissue damage or injury. The most common symptoms that occur as a result of the inflammatory process are pain, swelling, redness, warmth, tenderness, decreased movement, and impaired, limited, or distorted function. NSAIDs limit the symptoms associated with inflammation. NSAIDs are divided into prostaglandin synthetase inhibitors (PSIs) and nonprostaglandin synthetase inhibitors (non-PSIs).

Aspirin and indomethacin are classic PSIs. These drugs suppress the production of prostaglandins (PGs), which are active components of the inflammatory process. Two popular PSIs available over the counter are aspirin and ibuprofen. Both drugs are capable of producing serious undesired clinical responses.

Non-PSIs include para-aminophenol drugs, antigout or hyperuricemic drugs, and antirheumatic drugs. These drugs are weak PG inhibitors and produce their anti-inflammatory effects by other mechanisms.

REFERENCES

1. Lee, J., & Katayama, S. (1992). Inflammation and nonsteroidal anti-inflammatory drugs. In C.M. Smith & A.M. Reynard (Eds.), *Textbook of pharmacology* (pp. 401-435). Philadelphia: W.B. Saunders.
2. Cross, S. (1994). Pathophysiology of pain. *Mayo Clinic Proceedings, 69,* 375-383.
3. Di Gregorio, G.J., et al. (Eds.) (1990). *Handbook of pain management* (3rd ed.). West Chester, PA: Medical Surveillance.
4. Porth, C.M. (1994). *Pathophysiology: Concepts of altered health state* (4th ed.). Philadelphia: J.B. Lippincott.
5. Garcia Rodriquez, L. (1994). Risk of upper gastrointestinal bleeding and perforation associated with individual nonsteroidal anti-inflammatory drugs. *Lancet, 343,* 769-772.
6. Spilman, P., & Whelton, A. (1992). Nonsteroidal anti-inflammatory drugs: Effects on kidney function and implications for nursing care. *American Nephrology Nurses' Association Journal, 19*(1), 19-25.
7. Hirsh, J., et al. (1992). Aspirin and other platelet-active drugs. The relationship between dose, effectiveness, and side effects. *Chest, 102*(Suppl. 4), 327S-336S.
8. Lekstrom, J.A., and Bell, W.R. (1991). Aspirin in the prevention of thrombosis. *Medicine, 70*(3), 161-178.
9. Imperiale, T., & Petrulis, A. (1991). A meta-analysis of low dose aspirin for the prevention of pregnancy induced hypertension. *Journal of the American Medical Association, 266,* 260-264.
10. Peleg, I., Maibach, H., Brown, S., & Wilcox, C. (1994). Aspirin and nonsteroidal anti-inflammatory drug use and the risk of subsequent colorectal cancer. *Archives of Internal Medicine, 154,* 394-399.
11. Thum, M., et al. (1991). Aspirin and the risk of fatal colon cancer. *New England Journal of Medicine, 325,* 1593-1596.
12. Tideiksaar, R. (1990). Principles of drug therapy in the elderly. *Physician Assistant, 14*(2), 29-42.
13. Lee, T.H. (1992). Mechanism of aspirin sensitivity. *American Review of Respiratory Disease, 145,* S34-S36.
14. Mathewson, M.K. (1989). Drug interactions. *Critical Care Nurse, 9*(4), 86-88, 90-93.
15. Trovato, A., Nuhlicek D., & Midtling, J. (1991). Drug-nutrient interactions. *American Family Physician, 44,* 1651-1657.
16. Pierce, R.P., et al. (1991). Salicylate poisoning from enteric-coated aspirin: Delayed absorption to complicate management. *Postgraduate Medicine, 89*(5), 61-62, 64.
17. U.S. Pharmacopeial Convention. (1990). *United States pharmacopeia* (22nd rev.). Rockville, MD.: Author.
18. Moise, K., Ou, C., Kirshon, B., Cano, L., Rognerud, C., & Carpenter, R. (1990). Placental transfer of indomethacin in the human pregnancy. *American Journal of Obstetrics and Gynecology, 162,* 549-554.
19. Oberbauer, R., Krivanek, P., & Turnheim, K. (1993). Pharmacokinetics of indomethacin in the elderly. *Clinical Pharmacokinetics, 24,* 428-434.
20. Furey, S.A. (1990). Ibuprofen and renal disease. *Annals of Internal Medicine, 113,* 481-482.
21. Griffin, M.R., et al. (1991). Nonsteroidal anti-inflammatory drug use and increased risk for peptic ulcer disease in elderly persons. *Annals of Internal Medicine, 114,* 257-263.
22. McPherson, M. (1989). Drugs and dietary interactions: Guidelines for counseling the home health care patient. *Journal of Home Health Care Practice, 1*(4), 27-29.
23. Cummings, D., & Amadio, P. (1994). A review of selected newer nonsteroidal anti-inflammatory drugs. *American Family Physician, 49,* 1197-1202.
24. Hebert, W., & Scopelitis, E. (1994). Ketorolac-precipitated asthma. *Southern Medical Journal, 87,* 282-283.
25. Perazella, M., & Buller, G. (1993). NSAID nephrotoxicity revisited: Acute renal failure due to parenteral ketorolac. *Southern Medical Journal, 86,* 1421-1424.
26. Morgan, S. (1990). A comparison of three methods of managing fever in the neurologic patient. *Journal of Neuroscience Nursing, 22*(1), 19-24.
27. Boyce, E. (1992). Pharmacology of antiarthritic drugs. *Clinics in Podiatric Medicine and Surgery, 9,* 327-348.
28. Epstein, W.V., et al. (1991). Effect of parenterally administered gold therapy on the course of adult rheumatoid arthritis. *Annals of Internal Medicine, 114,* 437-444.
29. McMahon, J.M. (1992). Gold therapy for rheumatoid arthritis. *Annals of Internal Medicine, 117,* 169-170.

BIBLIOGRAPHY

Bianco, S., Pieroni, M., Refini, R., Robuschi, M., Vaghi, A., & Sestini, P. (1994). Could NSAIDs have a role as antiasthmatic agents? *Drugs, 48,* 9-15.

Brown, R., Wilson, J., Kearns, G., Elihier, V., Johnson, V., & Bertrand, R. (1992). Single-dose pharmacokinetics of ibuprofen and acetaminophen in febrile children. *Journal of Clinical Pharmacology, 32,* 231-241.

Davis, G.C., Cortez, C., & Rubin, B.R. (1990). Pain management in the older adult with rheumatoid arthritis or osteoarthritis. *Arthritis Care and Research, 3*(3), 127-131.

Hollander, D. (1994). Gastrointestinal complications of nonsteroidal anti-inflammatory drugs: Prophylactic and therapeutic strategies. *American Journal of Medicine, 96,* 274-281.

Hough, M., & Waugaman, W. (1993). Ketorolac and propofol administration for prevention of nausea and vomiting in patients undergoing minor gynecologic surgery. *Nurse Anesthesia, 4*(1), 9-17.

Hussar, D.A. (1990). Use of nonprescription medications in the treatment of pain. *American Journal of Pharmacy, 162,* 17-24.

Kauffman, R.E., & Nelson, M.V. (1992). Effect of age on ibuprofen pharmacokinetics and antipyretic response. *Journal of Pediatrics, 121,* 969-973.

Medical Letter, Inc. (1993). Drugs for pain. *Medical Letter: On Drugs and Therapeutics, 35*(887), 1-6.

Murphy, K. (1992). Acetaminophen and ibuprofen: Fever control and overdose. *Pediatric Nursing, 18,* 428-431.

Wilcox, C., Shalek, K., & Cotsonis, G. (1994). Striking prevalence of over-the-counter nonsteroidal anti-inflammatory drug use in patient with upper gastrointestinal hemorrhage. *Archives of Internal Medicine, 154,* 42-46.

CHAPTER 52

Immunosuppressant and Immunostimulant Drugs

JAN HOOT MARTIN • JUDY MALKIEWICZ

⊛ Immunosuppressants

LEARNING OBJECTIVES:

Provide a general description of the drug category *immunosuppressants*.

Develop a plan of care for a client receiving immunosuppressant drugs.

Describe pathologies of the immune system treated with immunosuppressant drugs.

Summarize pharmacokinetic and pharmacodynamic properties of azathioprine, the prototype for cytotoxic immunosuppressants.

Describe causative factors for major undesired clinical responses associated with cytotoxic immunosuppressants.

List two additional cytotoxic immunosuppressant drugs.

Summarize pharmacokinetic and pharmacodynamic properties of cyclosporine, the prototype drug for T-helper cell suppressors.

Describe three major undesired clinical responses associated with cyclosporine.

Identify two clinical uses of antilymphocyte-antithymocyte antibodies.

Discuss the pharmacodynamics of antilymphocyte-antithymocyte antibodies.

Describe two miscellaneous immunosuppressant drugs.

KEY TERMS:

Autoimmune diseases, cycle-specific drugs, immunostimulants, immunosuppressants, isoimmune reaction, phase-specific drugs

⊛ Immunostimulant Drugs

LEARNING OBJECTIVES:

Describe clinical situations that require the use of immunostimulant drugs.

Identify six drugs that produce active immunity.

Identify three drugs that produce passive immunity.

KEY TERMS:

Active immunity, passive immunity, toxoid, vaccine

CONCEPTS AND TERMS TO REVIEW

Read the section on nonspecific defense mechanisms of the body in Chapter 49.

Reexamine the physiologic changes that occur during the inflammatory response.

Review origin of T cells and B cells.

Review process for T-cell and B-cell activation.

Reexamine the functions of the different types of T cells.

Review humoral-mediated and cell-mediated immunity.

Study the concepts of active and passive immunity.

Read section in Chapter 68 that discusses the mitotic cycle of cells.

---

*D*rugs that modify the immune system are generally classified as either immunosuppressants or immunostimulants. **Immunosuppressant drugs** suppress or inhibit the action of the immune system. Historically, until the advent of immunosuppressive drug therapy, tissue transplantation without rejection of the living donor tissue (except tissue from an identical twin) was impossible. Today, with the growing number of specialized immunosuppressive drugs, successful transplantations from relative and nonrelative donors are common. Additionally, therapeutic immunosuppression is developing as a treatment modality for autoimmune disorders resistant to current conventional therapies.

In the treatment or prevention of some disorders, the immune system may need stimulation instead of suppression. In these situations immunostimulant drugs are administered. Some **immunostimulant drugs** (vaccines, toxoids) are used to stimulate the response of the immune system to specific antigens, thus producing active and passive immunity. Other immunostimulant drugs are used to stimulate the immune response in individuals with immune deficiencies. (Immunostimulant drugs used to treat immuno-deficiencies are discussed in Chapter 53.)

IMMUNOSUPPRESSANTS

As previously indicated, immunosupresssant drugs inhibit immune responses. The major compounds used to suppress immune responses are subdivided into several categories, including cytotoxins, T-helper cell suppressors, lymphocyte antibodies, and corticosteroids. Corticosteroids, which are derived from adrenal cortex hormones, are the most widely used immunosuppressant drugs. They are discussed in Unit 9.

General Characteristics of Immunosuppressant Drugs

Ideally an immunosuppressant drug would specifically inhibit one immune response without impairing any other reaction. However, most immunosuppressant drugs do not selectively inhibit a single response. Even though the different drugs affect different components of the immune system, the overall response is generalized immune suppression. In addition, all available immunosuppressant drugs are highly toxic.[1]

Pharmacotherapeutics

As noted in Chapter 49, the biologic defense systems protect against unwanted intrusion from foreign substances. Pathologies occur when the body's defense systems, specifically the components of the immune system, respond inappropriately to a given stimulus.

AUTOIMMUNE DISEASES

Autoimmune diseases occur when components of the immune system are unable to differentiate self from foreign materials. Disorders associated with autoimmunity include rheumatoid arthritis, systemic lupus erythematosus, polymyositis, multiple sclerosis, pernicious anemia, autoimmune hemolytic anemia, and ulcerative colitis. In clients with these disorders, self-antigens cause the production of antibodies. For example, with rheumatoid arthritis the probable self-antigen is IgG, whereas with pernicious anemia the self-antigen is probably on the surface of parietal cells. Clinical manifestations of autoimmune diseases depend on the body systems most affected.[2]

ISOIMMUNE DISORDERS

When the immune system of one individual produces an immunologic reaction against tissues of another individual, an **isoimmune reaction** results. This type of reaction can occur during transfusions, against grafted tissue, or against the fetus during pregnancy. Isoimmune reactions to transfusions cause the client to develop antibodies in response to antigens in the transfused blood. The most severe transfusion reaction involves hemolysis (destruction) of the donor's red blood cells (RBCs) by the recipient's antibodies.[2]

When there is an incompatibility between the blood of an Rh-positive fetus and an Rh-negative mother, a hemolytic isoimmune reaction may occur. In Rh incompatibility, the mother builds immune bodies against the cells of the fetus. These antibodies cross the placenta and enter the fetal circulation. Once in fetal circulation, the antibodies rapidly destroy the erythrocytes of the fetus. In an attempt to compensate for this destruction, the fetus releases immature RBCs, erythroblasts. This isoimmune disorder, erythroblastosis fetalis, can result in the death of the fetus or newborn.[2]

Graft rejection is the body's normal immune response to the invasion of foreign tissue, the transplanted tissue or organ. Although the response is normal, it is not the desired response. During rejection, all components of the immune response work together to destroy the transplanted tissue. The most significant response is caused by the T-lymphocyte or cell-mediated response.

There are three basic types of rejection: hyperacute, acute, and chronic. **Hyperacute rejection** occurs very quickly (from time of the transplant up to 48 hours) and is not treatable with drugs. Removal of the rejected tissue or organ is the only way to stop the reaction. **Acute rejection** occurs usually within 3 months but may occur as late as 2 years after the transplant. With acute rejection the response is primarily a cell-mediated response. Acute rejection is treatable with corticosteroids, azathioprine, cyclophosphamide, antithymocyte globulin, cyclosporine, and OKT_3. Once initiated, immunosuppression therapy is required throughout the remainder of the client's life.

Chronic rejection occurs months or even years after the transplant. Symptoms of chronic rejection are related to gradual deterioration of the transplanted tissue or organ. Antibodies and the complement system are active in this type of rejection. Although immunosuppressant drugs are administered, the treatment usually is not successful.[2]

A different type of rejection occurs when the transplanted material is an allogeneic (individuals of the same species but of different genetic constitution) bone marrow transplant. Most individuals requiring bone marrow transplantation have already received immunosuppressant drugs. Graft-versus-host disease (GVHD) occurs when immunocompetent donor cells are infused into these immunosuppressed recipients. The immunocompetent T lymphocytes from the donated marrow produce the disease.[2,3]

NURSING CONSIDERATIONS

The major responsibility of health care providers caring for clients receiving immunosuppressant drugs involves support of immunocompetence. This is accomplished through assessment of the factors that affect the immune system and development of interventions that minimize further deterioration of the body's defense systems.

Assessing   As with all clients requiring drug therapy, you must obtain a thorough **health history.** Include in the history a review of present and past illness. Your concern is the integrity of the client's immune system. Ask the client about allergies, including food, drugs, insect, or pollen sensitivities. Determine how these allergies affect the client and what measures are used to terminate or diminish the allergic response. Ask the client specifically about rashes, urticaria, scaling, or skin dryness. Question the client about the following: sneezing, rhinitis, nasal stuffiness, itching of the throat, wheezing, frequent cough, or sniffling.

For an infant or young child, direct your questions to the parent or guardian. If the client is an infant, ask if the infant is breast-fed or bottle-fed. (Breast-feeding introduces immunoglobulins into the infant's gastrointestinal [GI] tract, conferring some immunity.) For all children, regardless of age, determine what immunizations they have received. In addition, to prevent unwanted complications to the fetus or newborn, you must determine if the female client is pregnant or nursing.

Since the client will receive immunosuppressant drugs, determine potential sources of infections in the home environment. Ascertain the age of all household members. Is there anyone living in the house with a chronic, low-grade infection (e.g., chronic bronchititis)? If young children live in the house, what is the status of their immunizations against childhood diseases (e.g., measles, mumps, pertussis)? Is the home environment free of major allergens? Ask the client to describe his or her work environment. Is the client exposed to substances that affect the immune system?

Assess the client's social network and support system. Since immunosuppressant therapy is associated with chronic disorders, lifestyle changes are usually required. A support system of family and friends can help the client adapt to these changes. In addition, the support system is available to provide special care associated with either the primary disease or the drug therapy.

Conduct a thorough **physical assessment** before beginning immunosuppressive drug therapy. This information provides a basis for comparing future physical changes. Include an examination of all body systems, with emphasis on those systems expected to benefit from immunosuppressive therapy (e.g., cardiovascular, renal). Inspect all nodal regions. Proceed from head to toe to avoid missing any region. Look for visible lymph node enlargement or color abnormalities. Palpate superficial lymph nodes of the head and neck and of the axillary, inguinal, and popliteal areas.

Review results from diagnostic tests. Common laboratory studies include complete blood count (CBC), RBC indices, leukocyte count, differential white blood cell (WBC) count, platelet count, activated partial thromboplastin time (APTT), and immunoelectrophoresis. In addition, a bone marrow aspiration is usually conducted.

Diagnosing   Data gathered from the nursing history and physical assessment are used to determine nursing diagnoses.

Common diagnoses for clients who require immunosuppressant drug therapy include the following:

- Activity intolerance related to fatigue, weakness, fever, and anorexia associated with drug therapy.
- Body image disturbance related to physical changes (e.g., hirsutism, alopecia) caused by immunosuppressant drugs.
- Coping, ineffective individual, related to inadequate support systems.
- Fluid volume deficit related to diarrhea or vomiting from drug therapy.
- High risk for infection related to suppressed immune response.
- High risk for injury related to suppressed immune response.
- Knowledge deficit.
- Noncompliance related to adverse reactions of drug therapy and high cost of therapy.
- Nutrition, altered, less than body requirements related to inability to ingest adequate nutrients.
- Oral mucous membrane, altered, related to drug therapy.

Planning   Once the nursing diagnoses are established, expected outcomes are developed. Appropriate expected outcomes for the client receiving immunosuppressant drugs follow:

- Client demonstrates a decrease in physiologic signs of activity intolerance.
- Client verbalizes an understanding of body changes.
- Client identifies ineffective coping behaviors.
- Client's fluid volume is maintained at a functional level as evidenced by adequate urinary output, stable vital signs, moist mucous membranes, and adequate skin turgor.
- Client demonstrates techniques and lifestyle changes that promote a self environment.
- Client modifies environment as indicated to enhance safety.
- Client verbalizes understanding of disease process and treatment.
- Client actively participates in treatment plan.
- Client remains free of signs of malnutrition.
- Client reports improved integrity of oral mucosa.

During this phase you should develop a teaching and discharge plan for the client. Because this client usually requires lifelong immunosuppressive drug therapy, you should include in the teaching plan all aspects of care you are now providing for the client (e.g., oral hygiene, protection from infection).

Infections are a significant problem for clients using immunosuppressant drugs. Thus one goal is the prevention and early detection and treatment of infections. Achievement of this goal begins with educating the client about early indications of an infection (e.g., malaise, fatigue, or low-grade fever). The client must know that suppression of the immune system blunts common signs and symptoms of infection. These findings, even a temperature elevation of 37.8° C, are considered significant and must be reported to the primary care provider.

Instruct the client to avoid contact with individuals who have active bacterial or viral infections. Additionally, tell the client to avoid day care settings, hospitals (except when essential), and crowded rooms where ventilation is poor. Swimming and swimming pools, though not specifically contraindicated, should be used with caution, especially if the client is troubled by frequent upper respiratory disorders or external ear infections.

Teach the client to check his or her skin daily. If small cuts, scratches, or scrapes are present, even without erythema, edema, or exudate, instruct the client to clean the areas thoroughly and apply a topical antiseptic or antibiotic ointment. Tell the client to monitor the areas closely.

Include in the teaching plan the importance of routine tartar and plaque removal. Inform the client that the provider of these services must be aware of the client's immunosuppressed state. In addition, the provider must take special care to prevent traumatic injury to the oral mucosa and gums. In some situations prophylactic antibiotic therapy is used to prevent infections from these procedures.

Since the client is also at risk for injury because of the suppressed immune response, provide information about factors that increase his or her risk. Provide a list of interventions that promote a safe physical environment. Discuss with the client the importance of self-monitoring of conditions that can contribute to the occurrence of injury (e.g., diminished vision, fatigue, weakness, dizziness).

The client must thoroughly understand the plan of treatment, including information about the drug therapy. As with all clients, assess the client's current level of knowledge and determine his or her ability to learn. Include in the plan information about the rationale for immunosuppressant therapy; anticipated length of therapy; dosage, frequency, and method of administering the drugs; potential toxic effects of drugs; and therapies that may interfere with drugs. Provide the client with information about follow-up care, which includes routine laboratory studies, and the possibility of changes in the treatment plan. Additionally, develop guidelines to help the client decide when to contact health care providers. In the plan include the phone number of the individual who is available to answer questions or validate information after discharge.

Implementing   Since the client receiving immunosuppressant drugs may experience fatigue, plan your care with rest periods between activities. Suggest to the client that he or she should do the same after discharge. Provide a positive atmosphere and emphasize accomplishments made by the client.

Immunosuppressant drugs can produce significant physical changes in the client. By establishing a therapeutic nurse-client relationship, you convey an attitude of caring. Provide opportunities for listening to the client's concerns and questions, and encourage the client to verbalize his or her feelings. Help the client care for his or her appearance. For example, encourage female clients to use makeup or, if necessary, to wear a wig.

Fluid volume deficit is another problem associated with immunosuppressant therapy. Note the client's liking for fluids and for foods high in fluid content. Recommend that the client restrict his or her intake of caffeine, alcohol, and fluids with high sugar content. These substances can promote diuresis, increasing the fluid volume deficit. Always keep fluids within reach, and encourage regular intake. Monitor urinary specific gravity and intake and output, and weigh the client on a daily basis. Since the client may need to record intake and output at home, assist client or significant other(s) to measure intake and output during the hospitalization.

If the client experiences anorexia or difficulty ingesting adequate nutrients, interventions are needed. Note the client's total daily caloric intake. To assess this information, ask the client or caregiver to maintain a diary of food intake. Provide diet modification as indicated (e.g., mechanical soft diet, small feedings with snacks). If carbohydrates are tolerated, encourage the client to use sugar or honey in beverages. Limit the client's intake of fiber or bulk since these nutrients may lead to early satiety. As much as possible, prevent unpleasant odors or sights that may have a negative effect on the client's appetite. It is also important to provide oral care before and after meals.

Sometimes the client does not eat properly because he or she has developed stomatitis or mucositis. Routinely inspect the oral cavity for sores, lesions, or bleeding. (Remember that you must constantly assess for early indications of infection.) Encourage the client to avoid irritating foods and fluids and temperature extremes (e.g., hot coffee, iced tea). The client should be encouraged to avoid alcohol, smoking, and chewing tobacco. If the client complains of a dry mouth, have the individual chew gum, which stimulates saliva production. You must promote the client's adequate fluid intake to prevent dehydration of the oral mucous membranes. Providing frequent oral care with mouthwash also promotes moist mucous membranes. Use hydrogen peroxide or 2% sodium perborate, sodium chloride, sodium bicarbonate, or alkaline solutions, depending on cause of condition.[4] When cleaning the client's teeth, use a soft bristle brush or sponge- or cotton-tip applicators.

Lifelong compliance by the client is necessary with most immunosuppressant drug therapy regimens, especially when used with transplantation. Unfortunately, immunosuppressant drugs often cause undesired clinical responses that lead the client to discontinue use or reduce drug doses. Assess carefully for undesired responses. Early detection may permit alterations in the type or amount of drug prescribed. With some clients, other drugs (e.g., corticosteroids, antihistamines) are administered concurrently with immunosuppressant drugs to alleviate some of the undesired signs and symptoms. In addition, the high cost of immunosuppressive therapy makes compliance an issue for many individuals. If this is a problem, request an assessment by the agency's social worker.

Evaluating   During this phase determine the efficacy of the drug therapy and the effectiveness of the plan of care. Graft or transplant survival or reduction of pathologies associated with autoimmune disorders is evidence of an effective treatment plan. Although laboratory values that measure cells involved in an immune response (e.g., WBC, T lymphocytes, sedimentation rates, rheumatoid factor) help determine the effectiveness of the drug regimen, subjective and objective assessment data are used more frequently. Also review the expected outcomes of the plan of care with the client and determine if they were achieved. Revise the plan of care based on your findings.

Cytotoxic Immunosuppressant Drugs

Cytotoxic drugs are a group of pharmacologic agents that kill cells capable of self-replication. During an immune response immunologically competent lymphocytes are transferred from a resting state to actively proliferating cells. They are the cells that are the targets for cytotoxic drugs.

Three cytotoxic drugs commonly used for their clinical immunosuppressive activities are azathioprine, methotrexate, and cyclophosphamide. These cytotoxic drugs inhibit all immunologic competent cells to some extent. Thus therapy produces a state of generalized immunosuppression. Additionally, the drugs not only kill lymphocytes but also nonlymphoid proliferating cells.

The lymphocytotoxic activities of the cytotoxic drugs can be related to their action on cells in specific phases of the mitotic cycle. Azathioprine and methotrexate are considered **phase-specific drugs.** These drugs are cytotoxic to cells during a specific phase of the mitotic cycle, specifically the S or DNA-synthetic phase. Cyclophosphamide is classified as **cycle specific;** it is toxic for cells at all stages of the mitotic cycle.[1]

CYTOTOXIC IMMUNOSUPPRESSANT PROTOTYPE

AZATHIOPRINE

As previously indicated, azathioprine (Imuran) is a phase-specific drug. It was first used in 1961 to help prevent tissue and organ transplant rejection. Although its use has waned with the advent of newer immunosuppressants, the historical importance of azathioprine cannot be denied.

Pharmacotherapeutics Azathioprine currently is used as an immunosuppressant in the prevention of transplant rejection, primarily renal homotransplantation. Additionally, lower doses of azathioprine are approved for the treatment of severe rheumatoid arthritis resistant to conventional therapy such as nonsteroidal anti-inflammatory drugs (NSAIDs) and aspirin.[5,6]

Pharmacokinetics Azathioprine, an inactive antimetabolite, is well absorbed after oral administration. Peak levels of the drug occur 1 to 2 hours after oral doses. However, bioavailability of oral doses is estimated as 41% to 44% of that of the intravenous (IV) administration. The half-life of unchanged azathioprine varies from $\frac{1}{2}$ to 1 hour. Azathioprine is rapidly converted to 6-mercaptopurine and other active metabolites. Both azathioprine and 6-mercaptopurine are moderately bound (30%) to serum proteins.[5,7]

Azathioprine and 6-mercaptopurine are rapidly eliminated from the blood and are oxidized or methylated in erythrocytes and the liver. Metabolites are excreted by the kidneys. Neither azathioprine nor 6-mercaptopurine is detectable in urine after 8 hours. However, the estimated elimination half-life of one of the active metabolites, 6-thioguanine nucleotides, is 13 days.[5,6,8]

Pharmacodynamics Azathioprine acts primarily by suppressing both DNA and RNA synthesis during the initial stages of lymphoid cell differentiation. Thus azathioprine decreases the initial proliferation and maturation of both T and B lymphocytes in response to a foreign antigen. Immunosuppressive effects are greater for cellular-mediated immunity than antibody-mediated immunity.[9] Once T and B lymphocytes are produced, the drug has little affect on suppression of the immune response. Therefore azathioprine is most effective in prevention of acute transplant rejection and is of little value in its treatment.[7]

The exact mechanism of action of azathioprine in treatment of rheumatoid arthritis is not fully understood. However, both azathioprine and 6-mercaptopurine inhibit prostaglandin production. In addition, 6-mercaptopurine inhibits local inflammatory reactions.[5]

Pharmaceutics Azathioprine is available in uncoated tablets for oral administration and as Lyphl-Soln for IV infusion. When used to prevent homotransplantation rejection, treatment is initiated at the time of the transplant. However, if deemed necessary, treatment may be initiated 1 to 3 days before transplantation. After transplantation, doses are tapered for maintenance therapy. Usually IV therapy is used initially and then changed to oral administration for long-term therapy.[6]

Dosages of azathioprine are altered based on factors such as renal clearance and degree of bone marrow suppression. Laboratory indicators are WBC and serum creatinine clearance determinations. Dosage usually is decreased when the WBC falls between 5000 and 3000/mm³. The drug is usually discontinued when the WBC drops below 3000/mm³.[3,7,10]

Undesired Clinical Responses When used in the treatment of rheumatoid arthritis, azathioprine has a relatively safe adverse-effect profile. However, because doses required to prevent transplantation rejection are larger than those used for rheumatoid arthritis, 3 to 5 mg/kg daily compared to 1 mg/kg daily, the client's risk of developing toxic undesired responses increases.[5,6] The most frequent toxic effects involve the hematologic and GI systems.

Azathioprine causes myelosuppression characterized by leukopenia and thrombocytopenia and less often by macrocytic anemia, pure red cell aplasias, and reticulocytopenia. These toxic reactions are dose related and reversible when the dosage is decreased or the drug is discontinued.[7,8,10]

Toxic effects on the GI tract include nausea and vomiting. With some clients, diarrhea, fever, malaise, and abdominal pain accompany the nausea and vomiting. In addition, mucositis and hepatotoxicty can occur.[5] Other undesired clinical responses include a predisposition to infection, renal insufficiency, alopecia, and malignancies. Figure 52–1 provides a summary of undesired clinical responses associated with most cytotoxic immunosuppressant drugs.

Contraindications and Precautions Azathioprine should not be administered to clients who have shown hypersensitivity to the drug. Since the risk of neoplasia is increased, azathioprine should not be administered to clients with rheumatoid arthritis previously treated with alkylating agents. Diagnoses of chickenpox, herpes zoster, hepatic dysfunction, infection, or renal insufficiency may contraindicate the use of azathioprine since im-

munosuppressive therapy often accelerates or potentiates the consequences of these disorders. Additionally, live vaccine immunizations, particularly oral poliovirus vaccine, are not given to the client or individuals living in the same household as the client.

The immunosuppressive activity of azathioprine is severely compromised in the client with significantly diminished hepatic function. In these clients the formation of 6-mercaptopurine and other active metabolites by the liver is decreased. Therefore the individual who has undergone liver transplantation requires special consideration, especially when the transplant is being acutely or chronically rejected.[11]

Drug-Drug Interactions Significant drug-drug interactions are possible during the use of azathioprine. For example, xanthine oxidase is necessary for biotransformation of 6-mercaptopurine. As a xanthine oxidase inhibitor, allopurinol prevents this biotransformation and produces toxic levels of azathioprine and its active

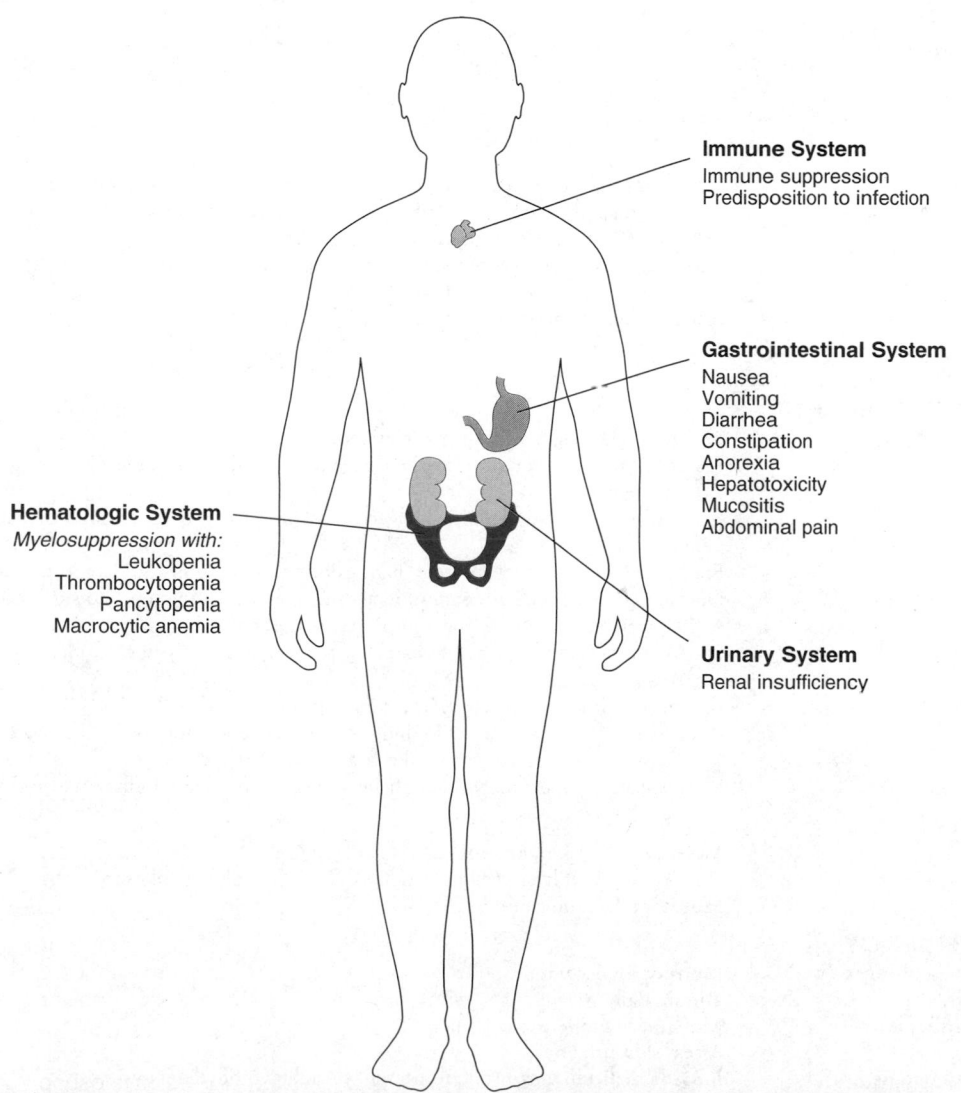

Immune System
Immune suppression
Predisposition to infection

Gastrointestinal System
Nausea
Vomiting
Diarrhea
Constipation
Anorexia
Hepatotoxicity
Mucositis
Abdominal pain

Hematologic System
Myelosuppression with:
    Leukopenia
    Thrombocytopenia
    Pancytopenia
    Macrocytic anemia

Urinary System
Renal insufficiency

FIGURE 52–1 Undesired clinical responses associated with cytotoxic immunosuppressant drugs.

TABLE 52–1

Cytotoxic Immunosuppressant Drugs: Common Undesired Clinical Responses and Associated Nursing Considerations

Undesired Clinical Responses and Their Manifestations	Nursing Considerations
MYELOSUPPRESSION	
Leukopenia (WBC <5000/mm³)	Teach client to maintain adequate nutrition and fluid intake.
Neutropenia (absolute neutrophil count <1000/mm³)	Instruct client to avoid crowds, individuals with infections, or clients recently vaccinated with live or attenuated vaccines.
	Tell client to report immediately any indications of infections: fever >38° C, cough, sore throat, chills, frequent or painful urination.
	Teach client to get adequate rest.
	Instruct client in proper personal hygiene.
	Use strict handwashing technique.
	Monitor WBC and differential.
	Hold dose if WBC <5000/mm³ and notify primary care provider.
	Assess mucous membranes for signs of breakdown.
	Assess wound sites carefully for signs of infections.
	Use strict sterile technique for dressing changes.
Thrombocytopenia	Teach client to report indications of thrombocytopenia (see manifestations of thrombocytopenia this table).
High risk for hemorrhage with platelet count <20,000/mm³	Monitor platelet count.
Risk of fatal central nervous system (CNS) hemorrhage or massive GI hemorrhage with platelet count <10,000/mm³	Avoid needle sticks.
	Teach client to use toothbrush with soft bristles.
Bleeding gums	
Hypermenorrhea	
Tarry-colored stools	
Blood in urine	
Coffee-ground emesis	
Epistaxis	
Hemoptysis	
Anemia	Assess for indications of anemia; monitor hematocrit and hemoglobin values.
Fatigue	Teach client indications of anemia (see manifestations of anemia this table).
Dizziness	Encourage diet high in iron, protein, and vitamins.
Pallor	Encourage ingestion of foods such as liver, lean meats, kidney beans, spinach, whole wheat bread, carrots, apricots, and raisins.
Dyspnea	
Palpitations	Instruct client in good oral hygiene.
Tachycardia	
Sensitivity to cold	
GASTROINTESTINAL EFFECTS	
Nausea	Administer antiemetic drugs as prescribed.
Vomiting	Assess client's current and normal weight, daily caloric intake, diet history, anthropometric measurements.
Anorexia	
Weight loss	Encourage client to use guided imagery, relaxation techniques, or biofeedback to diminish nausea and vomiting.
Oral mucositis	
Altered taste	Encourage intake of high-protein, high-caloric diet when medically appropriate.
Diarrhea	Develop an oral hygiene program, including dental examination, moisturization of mouth, thorough brushing with soft toothbrush, use of topical anesthetics or analgesics.
Constipation	
	During periods of stomatitis, teach client to avoid extremely hot or cold foods, spices, and citrus juices.
	Instruct client to avoid alcohol and smoking.
	If diarrhea occurs, provide scrupulous perineal hygiene, monitor intake and output and electrolytes, and encourage intake of a low-residue diet.
	If constipation occurs, encourage client to increase fluid and bulk intake and increase activity.
HEPATOXICITY	
Jaundice	Monitor urine, skin, and sclera for color changes.
Elevated liver enzymes and bilirubin	Monitor levels of liver enzymes: AST, ALT, GGT, alkaline phosphatase.
	Monitor serum bilirubin level.
RENAL INSUFFICIENCY	
Elevated blood urea nitrogen (BUN), serum creatinine levels	Monitor intake and output.
	Obtain daily weight.
Decreased creatinine clearance	Measure circumference of ankles.
Edema	Assess skin turgor.
Decreased urinary output	Provide meticulous skin care to prevent breakdown of edematous areas.
	Monitor vital signs, including postural blood pressure and apical pulse.
	Auscultate lung sounds.

metabolites. If the client must receive allopurinol, the dosage of azathioprine is usually decreased by as much as 75% to 80%.[7]

Other drugs that interact with azathioprine include captopril, sulfamethoxazole-trimethoprim, and glucocorticoids. Sulfamethoxazole-trimethoprim, which is prescribed to prevent *Pneumocystis carinii* pneumonia in transplant clients, increases the incidence of thrombocytopenia. Captopril, when administered concurrently with azathioprine, worsens leukopenia. Since azathioprine is a steroid-sparing drug, dosage of prescribed glucocorticoid drugs is decreased when the two drugs are administered concurrently.[7,11]

Life-Span Considerations Azathioprine can cause fetal harm when administered to a pregnant woman. It is classified as a Pregnancy Category D drug. The use of the drug in nursing mothers is not recommended. Use of azathioprine is effective in preventing transplant rejection for children. Dosages in these clients are altered based on body weight. Although azathioprine has not been specifically studied with older people, no evidence exists to suggest its effects will be different. However, decreased dosage of azathioprine may be necessary if age-related changes cause decreased renal function.

Specific Drug-Related Nursing Considerations Monitor the client carefully for undesired clinical responses. Common undesired clinical responses and nursing considerations associated with most cytotoxic drugs are summarized in Table 52–1. Table 52–2 provides additional information about doses, routes of administration, and nursing considerations for azathioprine.

MISCELLANEOUS DRUGS IN CATEGORY

Cyclophosphamide (Cytoxan), a cycle-specific drug, is an extremely potent immunosuppressant drug. The drug has more sustained suppressive action on humoral antibody responses than on cellular antibody responses. Cyclophosphamide is used to treat numerous disorders, including rheumatoid arthritis, systemic lupus erythematosus, autoimmune blood dyscrasias, immune-mediated glomerulonephritis, and Wegener's granulomatosis.[1] More information about this drug is presented in Chapter 69 where its use as an alkylating agent in the treatment of neoplastic disorders is discussed.

Methotrexate sodium (Rheumatrex), a phase-specific drug, inhibits dihydrofolate reductase, an enzyme required for conversion of folic acid to its active form. This action inhibits DNA synthesis. Methotrexate is used to treat neoplasms, rheumatoid arthritis, psoriasis, polymyositis, and Reiter's syndrome and to prevent GVHD in bone marrow transplant clients. GI disturbances, hepatic fibrosis, pneumonitis, decreased fertility, and megaloblastic anemia are toxic responses to the drug.[1] Table 52–2 provides additional information about doses, routes of administration, and nursing considerations for methotrexate.

T-Helper Cell Suppressors

Currently only one drug exists in this category: cyclosporine. However, FK 506, a macrolipid antibiotic, functions similarly to cyclosporine.

T-HELPER CELL SUPPRESSOR PROTOTYPE

CYCLOSPORINE

Cyclosporine (Sandimmune) is produced naturally by a fungal species. It is a potent drug and is used for its highly specific immunosuppressive properties. Cyclosporine was approved by the Food and Drug Administration for general use in 1983.[7,8]

Pharmacotherapeutics Cyclosporine is effective in preventing rejection of various types of solid organ transplants, including kidney, liver, pancreas, heart, and liver. It is also effective in preventing problems associated with bone marrow graft rejection and GVHD seen concurrently with bone marrow grafts. Additionally, use of cyclosporine in the treatment of some autoimmune disorders, particularly aplastic anemia, is expanding.[7,12]

Pharmacokinetics Since the oral dosage form of cyclosporine is prepared in a lipid vehicle, this form of the drug is not water soluble. Oral cyclosporine is absorbed primarily in the small intestine. Absorption, which depends on the presence of bile, is slow, variable, and incomplete in both adult and pediatric clients. After oral administration, cyclosporine's bioavailability is approximately 30%.

Cyclosporine is highly bound to erythyrocytes and plasma proteins. Blood distribution depends on drug concentration, hematocrit level, and lipoprotein concentration. Because cyclosporine is highly lipid soluble, it readily crosses most biologic membranes and is extensively distributed throughout the body, especially to fat and liver cells. In children the increased ratio of fat to total body weight results in greater drug distribution.[7,8]

Peak blood levels after oral administration are achieved in 1 to 8 hours. Cyclosporine undergoes extensive metabolism by liver enzymes. Therefore drugs that induce or inhibit liver enzyme activity also affect cyclosporine levels. The half-life of cyclosporine is approximately 7 hours for children and 19 hours for adults. Decreased half-life in pediatric clients is attributed to increased metabolism by the liver and faster rates of elimination. The major elimination route in both adults and children is through feces, with only about 1% of the drug excreted unchanged through the kidneys.[7,8]

Pharmacodynamics Unlike other immunosuppressant drugs, cyclosporine does not cause generalized suppression of bone marrow cell production. It selectively suppresses activation of T-helper cells by blocking the synthesis and secretion of interleukin-2. (Interleukin-2, a protein, is required for the proliferation and growth of antigen-stimulated cells.)[7-11] Cyclosporine also impairs cell-mediated responses without destroying the effector lymphocyte. However, it has minimal or no effect on T-suppressor cells, B lymphocytes, granulocytes, or macrophages.[1] Additionally, it does not prevent immune cells already activated by an antigen from maturing and differentiating. Therefore the drug is of little use in the treatment of chronic transplant rejection.[7]

The effectiveness of cyclosporine is usually increased by the simultaneous administration of moderate doses of corticosteroids. The two drugs appear to act synergistically. Whereas cyclosporine directly inhibits interleukin-2 production, corticosteroids indirectly suppress the synthesis of interleukin-2 by blocking release of interleukin-1.[1]

TABLE 52–2

Cytotoxic Immunosuppressants and T-Helper Cell Suppressors: Prototypes and Major Drugs in Category

Drug Name	Dosage and Route of Administration	Nursing Considerations
CYTOTOXIC IMMUNOSUPPRESSANTS: AZATHIOPRINE (Imuran) **HOW SUPPLIED:** Injection solution: 5 mg/ml Scored tablets: 50 mg	***Transplant: Prophylaxis of Organ Rejection*** Oral: initial dose, 3-5 mg/kg on day of transplant Maintenance: 1-2 mg/kg/d IV: initial dose, 100 mg infused usually within 30-60 min; continue until oral dosage form is tolerated ***Rheumatoid Arthritis*** Oral: initial dose, 1 mg/kg (50-100 mg) in one dose or two divided doses for 6-8 wk, increasing at 4-wk intervals by 0.5 mg/kg/d up to maximum dose of 2.5 mg/kg/d Maintenance dose: lowest possible dose; dose may be decreased in increments of 0.5 mg/kg (approximately 25 mg/d) q4wk	***Assess*** Determine if client is pregnant; azathioprine is classified as a Pregnancy Category D drug. Determine if client is breast-feeding; drug and its metabolites are transferred to breast milk. Collect a complete drug history. ***Implement*** Store drug in cool, dry area; heat and moisture cause drug to break down. Reconstitute IV solution with 0.9% NaCl or D_5W 0.9% normal saline (NS) solution. Administer IV solution by infusion or push: IV push over 5 min or infusion over 30-60 min. Withhold dose if WBC <5000/mm³ and notify primary care provider. Mixed IV solution is stable for 24 h. Avoid direct contact with IV solution; solution may be mutagenic, teratogenic, or carcinogenic to health care provider. Treat drug as a biohazard and dispose of properly. Administer oral dosage form with meals. Advise client to avoid storage of tablets in bathroom or kitchen. ***Monitor*** Monitor for undesired clinical responses. Monitor WBC and differential, platelet count, hematocrit, and hemoglobin. Monitor intake and output. ***Evaluate*** Evaluate for absence of signs and symptoms or organ rejection or reduced signs and symptoms of the immunoinflammatory response.
Methotrexate Sodium (Astra, Folex, Rheumatrex) **HOW SUPPLIED** Injection solution: 250, 50, 25, and 20 mg/vial; 2.5 mg/ml Tablet: 2.5 mg	***Psoriasis*** Recommended starting dose schedules: 1. Weekly single oral, IM, or IV dose of 10-25 mg 2. Divided oral dosages of 2.5 mg at 12-h intervals for three doses once per week Adjust each schedule gradually not to exceed 30 mg/wk; reduce dose to lowest possible amount over greatest length of time ***Rheumatoid Arthritis*** Recommended starting dose schedules: 1. Single oral doses of 7.5 mg/wk 2. Divided oral dosages of 2.5 mg at 12-h intervals for three doses once a week Adjust each schedule gradually not to exceed 20 mg/wk; reduce to lowest possible effective dose	***Assess*** Determine if client is pregnant; methotrexate sodium is classified as a Pregnancy Category X drug. Determine if client is nursing; drug is contraindicated in nursing mothers. Assess hematologic, hepatic, renal, and pulmonary function. ***Implement*** Follow package guidelines for proper handling and disposal. Reconstitute immediately before use. Reconstitute with sterile 5% dextrose or NaCl solution. Store reconstituted solution for up to 24 h at 21° to 25° C. Protect solution from light. Teach client early signs of toxicity. ***Monitor*** Monitor WBC and differential, platelet count, hematocrit, and hemoglobin. ***Evaluate*** Evaluate for reduced signs and symptoms of the immunoinflammatory response.

TABLE 52–2 *Continued*

Cytotoxic Immunosuppressants and T-Helper Cell Suppressors: Prototypes and Major Drugs in Category

Drug Name	Dosage and Route of Administration	Nursing Considerations
T-HELPER CELL SUPPRESSORS: CYCLOSPORINE (Sandimmune) HOW SUPPLIED: Capsule: 25, 100 mg Oral solution: 100 mg/ml IV solution: 250 mg/5 ml	**Transplant: Prophylaxis of Organ Rejection** ADULTS Oral: initial dose, 12-15 mg/kg beginning 4-12 h before transplant; continue dose 1-2 wk after transplant, then reduce by 5% per week, until reach maintenance dose Maintenance: 5-10 mg/kg/d IV: initial dose, 2-6 mg/kg/d beginning 4-12 h before transplant; continue until oral dosage form is tolerated CHILDREN Oral and IV: same dose and dosing regimen as in adults, although children may require and tolerate higher doses than those used in adults	**Assess** Determine if client is pregnant; cyclosporine is classified as a Pregnancy Category C drug. Assess for preexisting hepatic or renal impairment. Collect a complete drug history; cyclosporine interacts with numerous drugs. **Implement** Dilute IV solution with 0.9% NaCl or 5% dextrose solution. Discard diluted IV solution after 24 h. Store drug in original container at temperatures below 30° C. Administer IV solution slowly over 2-6 h. Administer IV solution in glass bottle or syringe to prevent adherence of drug to sides of container. Administer liquid solution in juice or milk, using a glass container. Keep client receiving IV cyclosporine under continuous observation for at least 30 min after start of infusion. Assess client frequently throughout treatment. Keep epinephrine 1:1000 available at the bedside while client is receiving infusion. Administer oral dosage on a consistent schedule with regard to time of day and relation to meal. Advise client to check blood pressure at least weekly. **Monitor** Monitor renal and hepatic function tests: BUN, serum creatinine, serum bilirubin, and liver enzymes. Monitor intake, output, and daily weight. Monitor for undesired clinical responses (e.g., hypertension, nephrotoxicity, gingival hyperplasia, hirsutism). **Evaluate** Evaluate for absence of signs and symptoms of organ rejection.

Pharmaceutics Cyclosporine is available in oral and IV dosage forms. Dosage and route of administration depend on type of transplant, age of client, clinical response to the drug, drug levels, and renal function. Cyclosporine is administered just before transplantation. However, it may be administered for 5 days before living-related-donor transplants when transplant timing is predictable.[7] (See Table 52–2 for dosing information.)

Undesired Clinical Responses Unlike cytotoxic drugs, cyclosporine does not cause myelosuppression. However, acute or chronic renal failure is almost universal in clients receiving this drug. The manifestations of renal failure are dose dependent and generally reversible.[1,10] Other undesired responses include hypertension, hyperglycemia, extremity tremor, anxiety, insomnia, gingi-

val hyperplasia, sensory paresthesia, hirsutism, salt retention, hyperkalemia, hyperuricemia, hypomagnesemia, and fluid retention. Reversible hepatotoxicity, with elevation of the serum bilirubin and transaminase levels, is also common.[1,7]

Contraindications and Precautions Cyclosporine use is contraindicated in clients with herpes zoster, chickenpox, or recent exposure to chickenpox. The drug should be used with care in clients with existing hepatic or renal insufficiency or hyperkalemia. Additionally, clients with malabsorption may not achieve therapeutic levels with oral administration of the drug.

Drug-Drug Interactions Cyclosporine levels are influenced by many other drugs. Drugs that increase the metabolism of cyclosporine (e.g., nafcillin, phenytoin, pheno-

DRUGS THAT AFFECT CYCLOSPORINE SERUM LEVELS

Drugs That Increase the Concentration of Cyclosporine	Drugs That Decrease the Concentration of Cyclosporine
INCREASE ABSORPTION	DECREASE ABSORPTION
Erythromycin	Octreotide acetate
Metoclopramide	Phenytoin
DECREASE METABOLISM	INCREASE METABOLISM
Diltiazem	Nafcillin
Nifedipine HCL	Phenytoin
Verapamil	Phenobarbital
Ketoconazole, fluconazole	Carbamazepine
Erythromycin	Rifampin
FK 506	Prednisone
Oral contraceptives	

barbital) decrease cyclosporine concentration levels. On the other hand, drugs that decrease the metabolism of cyclosporine (e.g., diltiazem, verapamil, ketoconazole) increase the concentration of cyclosporine. Some drugs (e.g., erythromycin, metoclopramide) increase the absorption of cyclosporine, whereas other drugs (e.g., octreotide acetate, phenytoin) decrease the absorption of cyclosporine. Additionally, drugs affecting renal clearance can affect therapeutic blood levels of cyclosporine.[7]

Life-Span Considerations Cyclosporine is classified as a Pregnancy Category C drug. Since it is excreted in breast milk, nursing should be avoided. As indicated in an earlier section, children exhibit different pharmacokinetic properties than adults and are more prone to subtherapeutic drug levels. Pediatric clients generally require more frequent dosing or larger doses per body weight.[7]

Specific studies with the elderly population have not been conducted. At present, no specific age-related changes in therapy are recommended. However, since the elderly are at risk of age-related renal and hepatic dysfunction, they are also at risk for altered metabolism and elimination of cyclosporine.

Specific Drug-Related Nursing Considerations Cyclosporine is potentially toxic at therapeutic concentrations. Monitoring drug concentrations is an important part of your care. At present, several methods of evaluating drug levels are used (e.g., radioimmunoassay, fluorescent polarization immunoassay, and high-pressure liquid chromatography). The therapeutic range differs according to the technique and sample source (e.g., plasma or whole blood). Therefore consistency of measurement techniques and sample source is essential.[7]

Assess the client carefully for indications of drug toxicity or undesired clinical responses. Both nephrotoxicity and hepatotoxicity can indicate transplant rejection as well as drug toxicity. Monitor results of hepatic studies (e.g., serum bilirubin, AST, ALT, GGT, and alkaline phosphatase). In addition, assess the color of the client's urine, skin, and sclera. Monitor renal function. Indications of renal insufficiency include decreased urinary output, increased serum creatinine level, decreased creatinine clearance, edema, hypertension, and increased cyclosporine blood level. Assess the client's daily weight, intake and output, and blood pressure.

If administering the drug parenterally, use *glass* bottles and syringes to prevent drug adherence to the container. Further dilute the oral cyclosporine solution with milk, chocolate milk, or orange juice to make it more palatable. Since the drug will adhere to the sides of the container, have the client pour additional fluid into the glass to ensure assimilation of the full dose. When administering the oral solution to children, dilute the solution in as small an amount of liquid as possible. This decreases the amount of liquid that the child must drink to receive the entire dose. Avoid mixing the drug with formula since this may make the infant refuse the formula. Use of gelatin capsules makes administration of the correct dose simpler and does not require specialized drug administration instruction.

Since cyclosporine can cause gum hyperplasia, instruct the client in proper oral hygiene. In some situations a topical antifungal drug for use in the mouth is prescribed. Body hair changes also occur. The scalp hair becomes thicker, darker, and wavier, and body hair is increased. If necessary, a gentle depilatory may be used. This is especially important in older children and adults. You also must support the client's efforts to cope with a changing self-image.

CONCEPT REVIEW

Cytotoxic drugs kill cells capable of self-replication.

Azathioprine and methotrexate are cytotoxic to cells during the S or DNA-synthesis phase of the mitotic cycle.

Azathioprine blocks synthesis of inosinic acid. The major effect of this action is to impair DNA synthesis. It also suppresses RNA synthesis.

Cyclosporine selectively alters the immunologic actions of T-helper cells.

Cyclosporine does not inhibit bone marrow function. Renal failure is its major toxicity.

Antibodies

Antibodies directed against components of the immune system are administered to suppress immune responses.

POLYCLONAL ANTIBODIES

Polyclonal antibodies are prepared by immunizing animals with human lymphocyte suspensions. If cells from the thymus are used, the preparation is termed *antithymocyte serum (ATS)*. Other antibody solutions are prepared from thoracic duct lymphocytes, splenic cells, or peripheral blood lymphocytes and are referred to as either *antilymphocyte serum (ALS)* or *antilymphocyte globulin (ALG)*.

POLYCLONAL ANTIBODY PROTOTYPE

LYMPHOCYTE IMMUNE GLOBULIN

Lymphocyte immune globulin (Atgam), a lymphocyte-selective immunosuppressant drug, is prepared by immunizing horses with human T lymphocytes. Its primary effect is to impair cell-mediated responses; more specifically, it alters the function of T lymphocytes. Lymphocyte immune globulin is used primarily to treat allograft rejection associated with renal transplantation. It has also been used to treat aplastic anemia. Lymphocyte immune globulin is usually administered concurrently with other immunosuppressant drugs.

Undesired clinical responses associated with the drug include anaphylaxis, chills, fever, itching, erythema, and hemolysis. To decrease the risk of allergic responses, skin testing before the first infusion is recommended. Additionally, epinephrine and other emergency equipment should be available during the infusion. Another concern associated with this drug is chemical phlebitis, which can occur if the drug is infused through peripheral veins. This can be avoided by administering the infusion solution into a high-flow vein.[6,7,12] Table 52–3 describes the administration of this preparation along with recommended dosages and nursing considerations.

MONOCLONAL ANTIBODIES

Monoclonal antibodies are highly selective in their reactions; these preparations are specific to lymphocytic membrane antigens.

MONOCLONAL ANTIBODY PROTOTYPE

MUROMONAB-CD3

Muromonab-CD3 (Orthoclone OKT3) binds to CD3 receptors found only on mature circulating T cells and medullary thymocytes. This action blocks the ability of cells to recognize foreign antigens, inhibiting the generation and function of cytotoxic T cells responsible for graft rejection. The plasma half-life of muromonab is approximately 18 hours, and distribution of the drug is similar to that of albumin.

The majority of clients experience a mild-to-severe "flulike" syndrome with the first doses of muromonab. Typical reactions include fever, chills, headache, nausea, vomiting, diarrhea, and malaise. Reactions often decrease with subsequent injections. Less frequent undesired responses include pulmonary edema in fluid-overloaded clients, marked hypotension, aseptic meningitis, and an acute decline in glomerular filtration rate.[1,6] Table 52–3 describes the administration of muromonab along with recommended dosages and nursing considerations.

Rh₀(D) IMMUNE GLOBULIN

Rh$_o$(D) immune globulin (RhoGAM) is a human antibody directed at the D antigen of the Rh system. The preparation is used to suppress the immune response of nonsensitized Rh$_o$ (D)–negative individuals who are exposed to Rh$_o$ (D)–positive blood. Its most important use is in pregnancy. It is effective for up to 72 hours after delivery in preventing maternal sensitization to Rh antigens. This action inhibits the development of Rh antibody–related diseases such as erythroblastosis fetalis during the next pregnancy. Rh$_o$ immune globulin does not suppress antibody production if the mother has already been sensitized to Rh antigens. This drug should be administered to all nonsensitized Rh-negative women after spontaneous or induced abortions, after ruptured tubal pregnancies, amniocentesis, or any occurrence of transplacental hemorrhage unless the blood type of the fetus has been determined as Rh$_o$ (D) negative. Rh$_o$ immune globulin is also used to prevent sensitization in individuals who received mismatched blood transfusions.[1,6] Table 52–3 provides information about routes of administration, dosages, and nursing considerations.

Miscellaneous Immunosuppressive Drugs

FK 506 was first discovered in 1984 in a fungus growing in northern Japan. FK 506 belongs to the macrolide group, chemicals that originally became known for antibacterial properties. This drug has been used as a primary immunosuppressant most often after liver transplants. However, it has also been administered after kidney, heart, heart-lung, pancreas, lung, small bowel, and islet-cell transplants.

Pharmacokinetic and pharmacodynamic properties of FK 506 are similar to those of cyclosporine. FK 506 inhibits the cell-mediated immune response by blocking the production of interleukin-2 and other lymphokines. Unlike cyclosporine, FK 506 absorption does not require bile. FK 506 is more potent than cyclosporine and appears to have less severe undesired clinical responses. It also has a stronger hepatotrophic effect—it promotes regeneration and repair of the liver.[7,13]

Many other agents with immunosuppressive characteristics are being investigated; however, most are currently in clinical trial studies only. Although not widely used, the newer drugs are responsible for the increased success rate with multiorgan transplantation. The goal of investigators for the newer immunosuppressive drugs is to find substances with very selective suppression effects on the immune system.

Other investigational agents include **cyclosporine G, rapamycin,** a macrolide similar to FK 506, and **RS61443,** a

TABLE 52–3
Antibodies

Drug Name	Dosage and Route of Administration	Nursing Considerations
MONOCLONAL ANTIBODY: **MUROMONAB-CD3** (Orthoclone OKT3) **HOW SUPPLIED** IV solution: 5 mg/5 ml	*Acute Transplant Rejection* IV: 5 mg/d for 10-14 d	**Assess** Assess fluid volume status of client before drug administration: auscultate breath sounds; weigh client to ensure client is within 3% of baseline weight; determine intake and output for past 24 h. **Implement** Anticipate premedicating the client with antihistamine, acetaminophen, and glucocorticoids to alleviate undesired clinical responses. Inspect solution for particulate matter or discoloration. Administer IV bolus over 1 min or less. Administer drug via peripheral or central IV line. Do not infuse with other drugs. Keep equipment and supplies for cardiopulmonary resuscitation on hand during initial therapy. **Monitor** Monitor for undesired clinical responses: pulmonary edema, fever, chills, diarrhea, nausea, vomiting. Monitor intake and output. **Evaluate** Evaluate for diminished indications of rejection.
POLYCLONAL ANTIBODY: **LYMPHOCYTE IMMUNE GLOBULIN** (Atgam) **HOW SUPPLIED** IV solution: 50 mg/ml	*Transplant Rejection* IV: 10-15 mg/kg/d for up to 14 d after transplant *Aplastic Anemia* IV: 10-20 mg/kg/d for 8-14 d	**Assess** Determine if client is pregnant; drug is classified in Pregnancy Category C. **Implement** Do skin testing before first dose. Skin test with 0.1 ml of a 1:1000 dilution in normal saline (NS) solution; inject intradermally. Monitor client and skin test for 30 min-1 h. Positive reaction is erythema or induration >10 mm diameter. Dilute drug with NS solution; use of dextrose or highly acidic infusion solutions is contraindicated. Allow diluted drug to reach room temperature before infusion. Administer drug through a central line, vascular shunt, or arterial venous fistula, using an in-line filter. Infuse IV solution slowly over 4-12 h. Store in refrigerator before and after dilution; discard unused diluted drug after 24 h. Monitor for allergic reactions throughout infusion. Keep appropriate emergency equipment and drugs available. **Monitor** Monitor for undesired clinical responses (e.g., fever, chills, anaphylactic reaction, serum sickness, hematologic disorders). Monitor differential blood count for thrombocytopenia or leukopenia. **Evaluate** Evaluate for diminished indications of organ rejection or improved findings on differential blood count and bone marrow examination.

TABLE 52–3 *Continued*
Antibodies

Drug Name	Dosage and Route of Administration	Nursing Considerations
Rhₒ (D) Immune Globulin (Human) (Gamulin Rh, HypRho-D, MICRhoGAM, Mini-Gamulin Rh, RhoGAM) **HOW SUPPLIED** Single-dose vial Single-dose syringe IM use only Each vial or syringe effectively inhibits the immunizing potential of up to 15 ml of Rh-positive packed red blood cells; to determine the number of vials or syringes to use, divide the volume (ml) of packed red blood cells by 15	**Postpartum Prophylaxis, Miscarriage, Abortion, or Ectopic Pregnancy** *Single Dose* One vial or syringe if fetal packed blood cell volume, which entered the mother's blood because of fetomaternal hemorrhage, is <15 ml (30 ml of whole blood); inject entire contents IM *Multiple Dose* When fetomaternal hemorrhage exceeds 15 ml of packed cells (30 ml whole blood), more than one vial or syringe should be administered; contents of the total number of vials or syringes may be injected as a divided dose at different injection sites at the same time, or the total dosage may be divided and injected at intervals, provided the total dosage is injected within 72 h postpartum **Antepartum Prophylaxis** Usual dose: one vial or syringe IM at 28 wk gestation; one vial or syringe within 72 h after an Rh-incompatible delivery; multiple doses may be necessary as determined by packed red blood cells **Transfusion Accident Procedure** 1. Multiply the volume in milliliters of Rh-positive whole blood administered by the hematocrit of the donor unit; this value equals the volume of packed red blood cells transfused 2. Divide the volume in milliliters of packed red blood cells by 15 to obtain the number of vials or syringes to administer *Single Vial or Syringe Dose* Inject the entire contents IM *Multiple Dose* Contents of the total number of vials or syringes may be injected IM as a divided dose at different injection sites at the same time; or the total dosage may be divided and injected at intervals, provided the total dosage is injected within 72 h after the transfusion accident	**Assess** Immediately postpartum, determine the infant's blood group (ABO, Rhₒ [D]) and perform a direct antiglobulin test. (Use of drug postpartum may interfere with laboratory results.) Confirm that the mother is Rhₒ (D) negative. Use during pregnancy only if clearly needed (drug is Pregnancy Category C). **Implement** Inspect drug visually for particulate matter and discoloration. Administer drug intramuscularly only. Do not give intravenously. Include in the individual's records: 1. Individual's complete identification. 2. ABO and Rh group and date determined. 3. Result of test for prior Rh sensitization. 4. Infant's ABO and Rh group, when known, and result of direct antiglobulin tests; in case of transfusion accident, the ABO and Rh groups of the donor tested and the volume transfused. 5. Notification of individual concerning nature of medication, date, and reason for giving it. 6. Lot number of Rh₀(D) immune globulin (human) and date and location(s) of injection(s) and the number of vials or syringes injected. 7. Adequate documentation if medication is refused by the individual. Store at 2° to 8° C. Do not freeze. **Monitor** Monitor for adverse reactions. Allergic reactions are rare and include low-grade fever and soreness at injection site. Monitor laboratory blood values. **Evaluate** Evaluate for effectiveness of medication.

purine antagonist. RS61443 is compared with azathioprine in effectiveness; however, bone marrow suppression is not as problematic. **Deoxyspergualin** (15-DSG), a guanidine derivative, has shown potent immunosuppressive effect in animal trials. However, since this drug must be administered parenterally, its clinical use will be limited to management of rejection. Finally, widespread use of and success with OKT3 therapy has sparked interest in development of new monoclonal antibodies with fewer side effects. Examples of drugs under investigation include **T10B9, 1A-3A, 33B.1,** and **OKT4A.**[7,14,15]

CONCEPT REVIEW

Antibodies are administered to suppress components of the immune system.

Rhₒ (D) immune globulin, a human antibody, is the most specific immunosuppressant drug available. It is directed at the D antigen of the Rh system.

Polyclonal antibodies impair cell-mediated responses, specifically T-lymphocyte action.

Monoclonal antibodies are highly specific. Their action is specific to lymphocyte membrane antigens.

IMMUNOSTIMULANTS

The influence exerted by immunostimulant drugs varies, depending on the type of immunity modulated and the results expected from the drug therapy. In general, as the name suggests, the body's normal immune response is stimulated in response to foreign protein. Through the use of immunostimulants, clients artificially acquire either active or passive immunity to specific foreign proteins or antigens.

▩ NURSING CONSIDERATIONS

General nursing considerations for the client receiving immunostimulant drugs are similar to those discussed for the client requiring immunosuppressant drugs. Only significant differences are presented in the following section.

Assessing While obtaining the health history, review the client's current health status, including any present illness requiring immunosuppression or chemotherapy. Specifically ask about allergies to chickens, eggs, feathers, sorbitol, antibiotics (especially neomycin and polymyxin), and thimerosal, a mercury derivative, since many vaccines contain these substances. In addition, elicit the client's history of asthma, hay fever, urticaria, or other allergic reactions before or after previous vaccinations. Obtain a complete list of currently prescribed drugs. Drugs that produce immunosuppression usually preclude the concurrent use of vaccines. Furthermore, determining if the female client is pregnant or lactating is always important. Assess the client's temperature before and after immunization. Most vaccinations are delayed in febrile clients, especially those experiencing respiratory tract or other acute infections.

Diagnosing Nursing diagnoses appropriate for clients receiving immunostimulant drugs include the following:
- Knowledge deficit.
- High risk for altered body temperature related to enhanced immune response.
- Sleep disturbance related to discomfort associated with vaccination. (Fretfulness and restlessness frequently occur with infants.)

Planning Proper scheduling of immunizations is necessary to achieve therapeutic effects. Therefore client education is important. When caring for *any* client, assess his or her immunization status and provide information about the immunizations recommended for his or her age group (Table 52–4 and Fig. 52–2).

Implementing Before giving any immunization, read the package insert carefully. Inspect the vaccine and diluent for particulate matter or discoloration. If these changes exist, dis-

TABLE 52–4
Immunization Schedules for Children Not Immunized in Early Infancy (Canada)

Timing	Immunization Against				
FOR CHILDREN 1-6 Y OF AGE					
First visit[3,5]	Diphtheria	Pertussis	Tetanus	Poliomyelitis	Haemophilus influenzae b (HIB)[3]
Interval after first visit					
1 mo	Measles	Mumps	Rubella[2]		
2 mo	Diphtheria	Pertussis	Tetanus	Poliomyelitis	
4 mo	Diphtheria	Pertussis	Tetanus	Poliomyelitis[1]	
16 mo	Diphtheria	Pertussis	Tetanus	Poliomyelitis	
Preschool[6]	Diphtheria	Pertussis	Tetanus	Poliomyelitis	
At age 14-16 y	Diphtheria[4]	Tetanus[4]	Poliomyelitis[1]		
FOR CHILDREN 7 Y OF AGE AND OVER					
First visit[5]	Diphtheria[4]		Tetanus[4]	Poliomyelitis	
Interval after first visit					
1 mo	Measles	Mumps	Rubella[2]		
2 mo	Diphtheria		Tetanus	Poliomyelitis	
14 mo	Diphtheria		Tetanus	Poliomyelitis	
10 y	Diphtheria		Tetanus	Poliomyelitis[1]	

[1]This dose may be omitted if live (oral) polio vaccine is being used exclusively.
[2]Rubella vaccine is also indicated for all girls and women of childbearing age who lack proof of immunity. At all medical visits, the opportunity should be taken to check whether girls and women need rubella vaccine.
[3]Children beginning their series at age 12-14 mo require one dose followed by a booster at age 18 mo. Unimmunized children aged 15-59 mo require only a single dose.
[4]Diphtheria and tetanus toxoid (Td), a combined adsorbed "adult type" preparation for use in persons 7 y of age or more, contains less diphtheria toxoid than preparations given to younger children and is less likely to cause reactions in older persons.
[5]Measles, mumps, and rubella vaccines may also be given at the first visit if it is considered likely that a child will not return for further immunization.
[6]If the last dose of the primary series for diphtheria, tetanus, pertussis, and polio is given after the fourth birthday, this dose may be omitted.
NOTE: The *Canadian immunization guide* (4th ed.) was not available at time of publication. This schedule is based on current practice in Ontario and the most recent publication: National Advisory Committee on Immunization. (1989). *Canadian immunization guide.* (3rd ed.). (Cat. No. H49-8/1989E). Ottawa: Ministry of National Health and Welfare.
From Betz, C., Hunsberger, M., & Wright, S. (1994). *Family-centered nursing care of children* (2nd ed.). Philadelphia: W.B. Saunders.

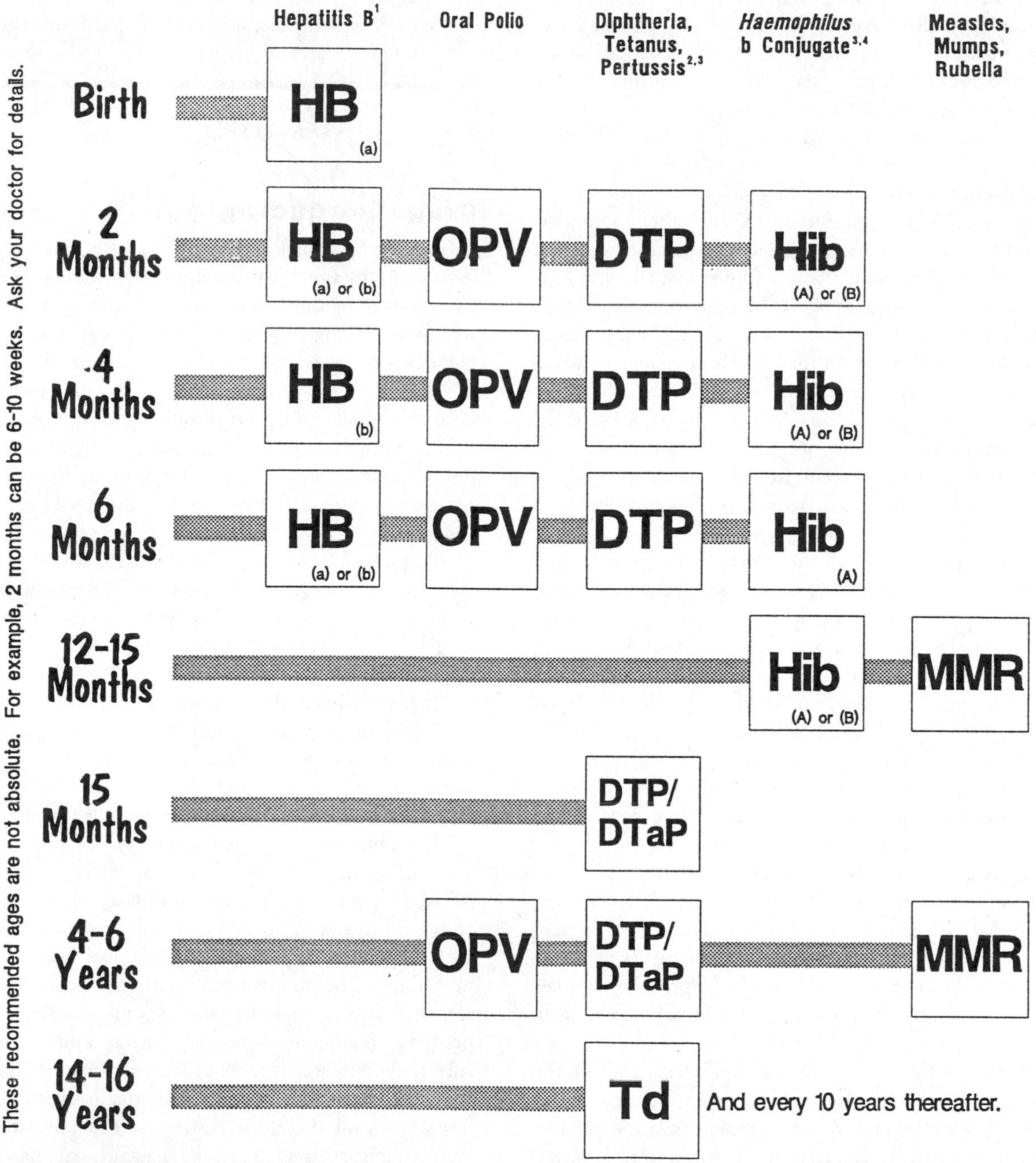

	Hepatitis B[1]	Oral Polio	Diphtheria, Tetanus, Pertussis[2,3]	*Haemophilus* b Conjugate[3,4]	Measles, Mumps, Rubella
Birth	**HB** (a)				
2 Months	**HB** (a) or (b)	**OPV**	**DTP**	**Hib** (A) or (B)	
4 Months	**HB** (b)	**OPV**	**DTP**	**Hib** (A) or (B)	
6 Months	**HB** (a) or (b)	**OPV**	**DTP**	**Hib** (A)	
12-15 Months				**Hib** (A) or (B)	**MMR**
15 Months			**DTP/ DTaP**		
4-6 Years		**OPV**	**DTP/ DTaP**		**MMR**
14-16 Years			**Td**		

Ask your doctor for details. For example, 2 months can be 6-10 weeks. These recommended ages are not absolute.

And every 10 years thereafter.

[1] Hepatitis B vaccine may be given in either of 2 schedules:
  (a) Birth, 1-2 Months, 6-18 Months
  (b) 1-2 Months, 4 Months, 6-18 Months

[2] DTP preparation containing acellular pertussis vaccine (DTaP) is recommended for the 4th and 5th doses, but whole-cell DTP may still be used if DTaP is not available.

[3] Combination DTP/Hib conjugate vaccine may be used when both shots are scheduled simultaneously.

[4] There are 2 schedules for Hib conjugate vaccines:
  (A) HbOC (HibTITER™), PRP-T (ActHIB™), or DTP/HbOC (TETRAMUNE™): 2, 4, 6, & 12-15 Months
  (B) PRP-OMP (PedvaxHIB®): 2, 4, & 12-15 Months

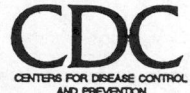

CDC
CENTERS FOR DISEASE CONTROL AND PREVENTION

FIGURE 52–2   Advisory Committee on Immunization Practices (ACIP) recommended immunization schedule (11/93). All recommended vaccines may be given simultaneously.

card the solution. Select the appropriate syringe and needle for the injection. Most immunizations are administered intramuscularly; however, some are administered intradermally and subcutaneously. If the immunizations will be administered intramuscularly, select a sterile needle of sufficient length to reach the muscle mass. The preferred IM sites include the deltoid muscle in older children and adults and the anterolateral aspect of the vastus lateralis in infants less than 2 years of age. Aspirate before injecting to avoid giving the vaccine into a blood vessel.[16]

Since allergic reactions, including anaphylaxis, may occur from vaccines, have epinephrine 1:1000 and other appropriate agents available to treat systemic allergic reactions. According to the National Childhood Vaccine Injury Act, all allergic reactions must be reported to the U.S. Department of Health and Human Services (1-800-822-7967). After the immunization, record the following on the client's permanent medical record: the date of administration; the client's name and address; the title of the individual administering the vaccine; the vaccine manufacturer; and the lot number of the vaccine.[16,17]

Some vaccines can be administered concurrently. Again, read and adhere to the manufacturer's recommendations. If vaccines are administered on the same day, select a different site for each injection. Teach the client or caregiver that live vaccines are shed in the stool and pharyngeal secretions of the client for 6 to 8 weeks after immunization. Also teach the client or caregiver the importance of good handwashing with diaper changes or when handling pharyngeal secretions.

Common minor vaccination reactions include local erythema, warmth, and edema at the injection site. In addition, the client may experience low-grade fever, irritability, and lethargy. Instruct the client or caregiver in the use of antipyretic and analgesic drugs to treat these discomforts.

Killed vaccines usually are not administered to the immunosuppressed client because the expected immunity does not develop. Live vaccines are *never* administered to immunocompromised clients. Additionally, immunosuppressed individuals should be isolated from clients receiving live vaccines for 6 to 8 weeks. The safety of vaccines in pregnant and lactating women has not been established, and vaccinations generally should be avoided in this population.

Evaluating   Keep a written record of the client's immunization with the health care provider and with the client or caregiver. Review the record for completeness. Compliance with recommended immunizations is an important determination of the client's knowledge about immunizations. In addition, evaluation requires a review of any vaccination reaction, the treatment regimen, and the report to the proper authorities.

CONCEPT REVIEW

Immunostimulant drugs are capable of producing active and passive immunity.

The Centers for Disease Control and Prevention has a recommended immunization schedule. This sched-

ule was developed under the guidance of the Advisory Committee for Immunization Practices.

Nursing care for the client receiving immunostimulant drugs includes informing the client of the recommended schedule, administering the prescribed immunizations, and monitoring for allergic reactions.

Drugs Producing Active Immunity

Immunity is a state in which the host is resistant to specific diseases. **Active immunity** develops when immune bodies are actively formed by the host against specific antigens. This type of immunity develops when the host is exposed to modified pathogens or toxins (acquired) or contracts the disease (natural).

Pharmacotherapeutics   Immunizations can protect children and adults against numerous infectious diseases, including poliomyelitis, smallpox, tetanus, diphtheria, measles, mumps, rubella, and influenza. These immunizations not only protect the individuals but also slow the spread of the disease throughout the community.

Pharmacokinetics   Active acquired immunity lasts for years. In some situations a booster dose is required to maintain this long-lasting immunity. For some immunizations serology studies and titers are determined after vaccination to evaluate the effectiveness of the immunization.

Pharmacodynamics   As previously indicated, drugs producing active acquired immunity do so by stimulating the body's natural immune system to produce antibodies to antigens.

Pharmaceutics   Vaccines and toxoids are dosage forms used to confer active acquired immunity. A **vaccine** is a suspension of live attenuated (weakened) or killed microorganisms. Measles, mumps, rubella, and varicella are examples of live attenuated vaccines. Polio (Salk) and influenza vaccines are examples of killed virus vaccines. Once injected or ingested by the host, the vaccine stimulates an immune response that provides resistance against a specific infectious disease. The vaccine also produces immunologic memory—when future exposure occurs, the immune cells recall prior exposure to the antigen and respond. A **toxoid** is a bacterial toxin that has been treated with heat or a chemical agent to destroy its toxic properties without destroying its antigenic qualities. Tetanus toxoid and diphtheria toxoid are examples of treated toxins.[18] Table 52–5 contains information about drug dosage, route of administration, and recommended frequency of administration.

Life-span considerations   Immunizations are administered throughout the life span. For example, hepatitis B, oral polio, diphtheria, tetanus, pertussis, and *Haemophilus* type b conjugate vaccines are administered to infants. Between 12 and 15 months of age, the child receives measles, mumps, and rubella vaccine and another *Haemophilus* type b conjugate vaccine. At the other end of the life span, individuals over the age of 65 are encouraged to receive tetanus boosters, influenza vaccine, and pneumococcal vaccine.[19–22]

Text continued on p. 683.

TABLE 52–5
Drugs Producing Active Immunity

Drug, How Supplied, Dosage, and Route of Administration	Undesired Clinical Responses and Contraindications	Nursing Considerations
Diphtheria, Tetanus Toxoids, and Pertussis Vaccine Adsorbed (DPT) (Acel-Imune, Tri-Immunol) HOW SUPPLIED Injection suspension: 4 U/0.5 ml DOSAGE 0.5 ml IM Dose 1 at 2 mo of age Dose 2 at 4 mo of age Dose 3 at 6 mo of age Dose 4 6-12 mo after third dose	**Undesired Clinical Responses** Local reactions (erythema, induration, tenderness, nodule palpable at injection site for a few weeks) Fever, fretfulness, anorexia, drowsiness, vomiting **Contraindications** Hypersensitivity or allergic reaction to any component of vaccine Child with neurologic symptoms Fever 40.5° C or greater within 48 h of previous immunization Collapse or shocklike state (hypotonic-hyporesponsive episode) within 48 h of previous immunization Persistent, inconsolable crying lasting 3 h or more within 48 h of previous immunization Convulsions with or without fever within 3 d of previous immunization Encephalopathy within 7 days of previous immunization Individual with impaired immune response Individual with coagulation disorder or thrombocytopenia Allergy to mercury; drug contains thimerosal, a mercury derivative	Administer antipyretic at time of injection to reduce febrile response after immunization. Repeat acetaminophen q4-6h for 48-72 h after immunization in children at risk of seizures. Report adverse reactions to U.S. Department of Health and Human Services. Diphtheria toxoid provides protection for 10 y. Tetanus toxoid provides protection for 10 y. Routine immunization for pertussis not recommended in individuals 7 y of age or older. Do not administer partial doses. Delay administration if febrile illness or acute infection exists. Mix suspension before aspirating solution. Aspirate to help avoid inadvertent injection into a blood vessel. Expel antigen slowly; terminate the dose with a small bubble of air (0.1-0.2 ml).
Diphtheria Tetanus Toxoids HOW SUPPLIED Injection suspension: 0.5 ml diphtheria, 0.5 ml tetanus, 6.6 U/5 U, 2 U/ml DOSAGE 0.5 ml IM Dose 1 at 2 mo of age Dose 2 4-8 wk after dose 1 Dose 3 4-8 wk after dose 2 Dose 4 6-12 mo after dose 3	See Diphtheria; Pertussis; Tetanus	See DPT.
Diphtheria, Tetanus Toxoids, and Pertussis Vaccine Adsorbed Combined with Haemophilus b Conjugate Vaccine (Tetramune) HOW SUPPLIED Injection suspension: 5 Lf* units tetanus toxoid, 12.5 Lf units diphtheria toxoid, 4 U pertussis, and 10 μg *H. infuenzae* type b oligosaccharide per 0.5 ml DOSAGE 0.5 ml IM Dose 1 at 2 mo of age Dose 2 at 4 mo of age Dose 3 at 6 mo of age Dose 4 at 15-18 mo of age Dose 5, a DPT booster at 4-6 y of age	**Undesired Clinical Responses** See DPT and *Haemophilus* b. **Contraindications** See DPT and *Haemophilus* b.	See DPT and *Haemophilus* b.

*Lf = limit flocculation unit. The limit flocculation unit is that amount of diphtheria toxin or toxoid that gives the most rapid flocculation with 1 standard unit of diphtheria antitoxin when mixed and incubated in vitro.

Table continued on following page.

TABLE 52–5 *Continued*
Drugs Producing Active Immunity

Drug, How Supplied, Dosage, and Route of Administration	Undesired Clinical Responses and Contraindications	Nursing Considerations
Measles, Mumps, and Rubella Virus Vaccine, Live (M-M-R) HOW SUPPLIED Powder for injection: ≥ 1000 measles TCID$_{50}$,* ≥ 20,000 mumps TCID$_{50}$, and ≥ 1000 rubella TCID$_{50}$ per 0.5 ml dose DOSAGE 0.5 ml SC for all ages	**Undesired Clinical Responses** Burning, stinging at injection site Erythema, induration, tenderness, and regional lymphadenopathy at injection site Malaise, sore throat, cough, rhinitis, headache, dizziness, moderate fever, rash, parotitis, orchitis, nerve deafness, nausea, vomiting, diarrhea, thrombocytopenia, purpura, otitis media, and conjunctivitis Rarely, febrile convulsions, erythema multiforme, optic neuritis, encephalitis, ocular palsies, Guillain-Barré syndrome **Contraindications** Child <15 mo of age Allergy to neomycin Pregnancy Lactating women; transmission of rubella vaccine virus to infants via breast milk has been documented Allergy to eggs; may administer if client is allergic only to chickens or feathers Individual with immunodeficiency, blood dyscrasia, leukemia, lymphomas, or malignant neoplasms	Vaccine provides immunization against measles (rubeola), mumps, and rubella (German measles). Keep epinephrine 1:1000 available for severe reactions. Store at 2°-8° C Protect solution from light. Reconstitute drug with supplied preservative-free diluent. Do not use if solution contains particulate matter. Vaccine is normally clear yellow. Discard reconstituted vaccine within 8 h. Do not administer concurrently with DPT or oral polio virus vaccine. Do not administer immune globulin concurrently with M-M-R. Do not administer less than 1 mo before or after administration of live vaccines. Do not administer to individuals with febrile respiratory illness, febrile infection, or active untreated tuberculosis. Administer with a 25-gauge, ⅝-inch needle. Administer vaccine into outer aspect of upper arm. Handle nasal and throat secretions with care; excretion of small amounts of live attenuated rubella virus has occurred 7-28 d after vaccination.
Measles Virus Vaccine Live (More attenuated Enders' strain) (Attenuvax) HOW SUPPLIED Powder for injection: ≥1000 TCID$_{50}$ per 0.5 ml dose DOSAGE 0.5 ml SC	**Undesired Clinical Responses** Burning and stinging at injection site Moderate fever for up to 1 mo after vaccination Fever and rash may appear between day 5 and day 12 after vaccination Cough, rhinitis, mild lymphadenopathy, diarrhea, and febrile seizures **Contraindications** See M-M-R	See M-M-R.
Measles and Rubella Virus Vaccine Live (M-R-Vax$_{II}$) HOW SUPPLIED Powder for injection: ≥1000 measles TCID$_{50}$ and ≥1000 rubella TCID$_{50}$ per 0.5 ml dose DOSAGE 0.5 ml SC	**Undesired Clinical Responses** See M-M-R **Contraindications** See M-M-R	See M-M-R.
Poliovirus Vaccine, Oral Live (Orimune) HOW SUPPLIED Oral liquid DOSAGE Primary series: three doses of 0.5 ml *Infants* Dose 1 at 2 mo Dose 2 at 4 mo Dose 3 at 15-18 mo Booster dose at elementary school entry (not necessary if dose 3 received after age 4)	**Undesired Clinical Responses** Paralytic disease after vaccination (rare) May be associated with Guillain-Barré syndrome; causal relationship does not exist **Contraindications** Individual with immunodeficiency disease Family with immunodeficient members Pregnancy (Pregnancy Category C drug)	Store frozen; thaw completely before use; can thaw-freeze-thaw up to 10 cycles, providing stored vaccine temperature never exceeds 8° C. Usual color of vaccine is pink; can normally appear red-pink or yellow. Assess family and close contacts for immunodeficient members. Teach recipients of vaccine to avoid close contact with all individuals with altered immune status for 6-8 wk. Vaccine can be administered to breast-feeding client.

*Tissue culture infection doses.

TABLE 52–5 *Continued*
Drugs Producing Active Immunity

Drug, How Supplied, Dosage, and Route of Administration	Undesired Clinical Responses and Contraindications	Nursing Considerations
Poliovirus Vaccine, Oral Live *Continued* *Older children, Adolescents, Adults* Two doses 6-8 wk apart Dose 3: 6-12 mo after dose 2 Children who are unimmunized should receive the needed number of doses to complete the series of three doses; if dosing schedule has been interrupted, series does not need reinitiation.		Vaccine can be administered concurrently with DPT, M-M-R, and *Haemophilus* b conjugated vaccine. Vaccine viruses are shed in the client's stool and pharyngeal secretions up to 6-8 wk. Teach caregiver to do good handwashing after diaper changes of immunized infant. Record on client's permanent record: date of administration; name, address, and title of individual administering the vaccine; manufacturer; lot number of vaccine administered; and vaccination reaction (requirements of the National Childhood Vaccine Injury Act).
Haemophilus *b* Conjugate Vaccine (HibTITER, Pedvax HIB) **HOW SUPPLIED** Injection solution: IM and SC **DOSAGE** 0.5 ml Infants 2-6 mo of age: three doses at 2-mo intervals Previously unvaccinated infants 7-11 mo of age: two doses at 2-mo intervals Previously unvaccinated children 12-60 mo of age: one dose Booster doses: all vaccinated children receive a single booster dose at 15 mo or older but not less than 2 mo after the previous dose	**Undesired Clinical Responses** Transient, mild fever; local erythema, warmth or swelling at injection site Rarely, irritability, sleepiness, prolonged crying, anorexia, vomiting, diarrhea, rash, convulsions, and Guillain-Barré syndrome **Contraindications** Hypersensitivity to the vaccine or diphtheria toxoid or thimerosal Individual with deficient production of antibody because of genetic defect or immunosuppressive therapy will not have expected immune response Pregnancy	Keep epinephrine 1:1000 available for potential anaphylactic or allergic reaction. Store at 2°-8° C. Do not freeze vaccine or diluent. Reconstitute only with supplied aluminum hydroxide diluent. Do not use if particulate matter or discoloration is present; vaccine is slightly opaque white suspension. Use reconstituted vaccine within 24 h. Delay vaccine administration in presence of febrile or acute infection except for mild upper respiratory infection. Administer deep SC or IM. Aspirate before injecting to avoid administering in a blood vessel. Use same conjugated vaccine throughout series. Vaccine can be administered concurrently with DPT, oral polio vaccine, and M-M-R. *Haemophilus* b disease primarily occurs in children <5 y of age and includes meningitis, cellulitis, epiglottitis, pericarditis, pneumonia, sepsis, and septic arthritis.
Hepatitis B Vaccine, Recombinant (Engerix-B, Recombivax HB) **HOW SUPPLIED** Injection suspension: 10, 20, and 40 μg/ml **DOSAGE** Dose 1 at selected date Dose 2 1 mo later Dose 3 6 mo after dose 1 *Recombivax HB* Birth-10 y of age: 2.5 μg 11-19 y of age: 5 μg >20 y of age: 10 μg *Engerix-B* Birth-10 y of age: 10 μg 11-19 y of age: 20 μg >20 y of age: 20 μg	**Undesired Clinical Responses** Generally well tolerated Soreness, pain, pruritis, erythema, ecchymosis, swelling, warmth, and nodule formation at injection site Fatigue, weakness, headache, fever, and malaise Nausea, diarrhea, pharyngitis, rhinitus, influenza, and cough **Contraindications** Any serious active infection Pregnancy (Pregnancy Category C drug) Hypersensitivity to yeast or any component of vaccine Hypersensitivity to thimerosol	Keep epinephrine 1:1000 available for potential anaphylactic or allergic reaction. Administer to individuals who are or will be at increased risk of infection with hepatitis B. Administer intramuscularly; deltoid muscle is preferred site in adults. Shake suspension well before withdrawal of drug. Inspect suspension for particulate matter and discoloration; vaccine is slightly opaque, white suspension after mixing. Store drug at 2°-8° C. Do not freeze drug. Do not dilute suspension; administer as supplied.

Table continued on following page.

TABLE 52–5 *Continued*
Drugs Producing Active Immunity

Drug, How Supplied, Dosage, and Route of Administration	Undesired Clinical Responses and Contraindications	Nursing Considerations
Influenza Virus Vaccine (Flu-Imune, Fluogen, Fluzone) HOW SUPPLIED 　Injection solution and suspension DOSAGE 　Intramuscularly only Children at 6-35 mo: 　0.25 ml of split virus only 　　Dose 1 on selected date 　　Dose 2 at least 4 wk later Children 3-8 y: 　0.5 ml of split virus only 　　Dose 1 on selected date 　　Dose 2 at least 4 wk later Children 9-12 y: 　0.5 ml of split virus only given in 　　one dose Clients 13 y of age and older: 0.5 ml 　of whole or split virus in one dose	**Undesired Clinical Responses** Slight tenderness or induration at injection site for 1-2 d Fever, malaise, myalgia lasting 6-12 h to 1-2 d after injection (occurs infrequently) **Contraindications** Allergy to neomycin or polymyxin Allergy to chicken eggs Pregnancy during first trimester Allergy to thimerosol Thrombocytopenia or any coagulation disorder that prevents IM injection	Purified surface antigen vaccine acts against influenza virus types A and B. Vaccine recommended for individuals 6 mo of age and older who have chronic illness, are at risk of complications from influenza, are health care providers, or are in close contact with high-risk individuals. Vaccines differ year to year; use only vaccines from current year. Store vaccine between 2° to 8° C. Do not use influenza virus vaccine that has been frozen. Shake solution or suspension well before withdrawing and administering. Vaccine may be administered concurrently with pneumococcal vaccine but at a different site. Antibody response may be decreased in HIV-infected individual or individual with impaired immune response. Delay administering vaccine to client with acute febrile illness. Avoid administering to individuals with active neurologic disorders. Vaccine may inhibit clearance of warfarin and theophylline. Report undesired clinical responses to U.S. Department of Health And Human Services (1-800-822-7967).
Pneumococcal Vaccine (Pneumovax 23, Pnu-Imune 23) HOW SUPPLIED 　Injection: 25 μg each of 23 polysaccharide isolates per 0.5 ml dose DOSAGE 　0.5 ml	**Undesired Clinical Responses** Local soreness at injection site, low-grade fever (37.8° C), mild myalgia, rash, and arthralgia Marked local swelling, urticaria, arthritis, fever >38.8° C, paresthesia, and acute radiculoneuropathy (occur rarely) **Contraindications** Hypersensitivity to vaccine, thimerosal, or phenol Acute febrile illness Child <2 y of age Pregnancy Individual with neurologic disorder or symptoms	Vaccine immunizes against infections caused by *Streptococcus pneumoniae.* Recommended for all adults 65 y or older in good health or for immunocompetent adults with chronic illnesses, splenic dysfunction, asplenia, Hodgkin's disease, lymphoma, multiple myeloma, chronic renal failure, or nephrotic syndrome. Recommended for children 2 y of age or older with chronic illness (e.g., asplenia, sickle cell disease, nephrotic syndrome, cerebrospinal fluid leaks, and conditions associated with immunosuppression). Have epinephrine 1:1000 available for allergic or anaphylactic reactions. Do not give if particulate matter or discoloration is present; vaccine is clear, colorless liquid. Store unopened and opened vials at 2° to 8° C. Administer SC or IM (preferably in deltoid muscle or lateral mid-thigh). Use with caution with lactating women; it is not known if vaccine is excreted in breast milk. Vaccine may be administered concurrently with influenza vaccine; use different site. Allow 2-wk interval between immunization and cancer chemotherapy or other immunosuppressive therapy.

🌿 NURSING RESEARCH

O'Mara, L., & Issacs, S. (1993). Evaluation of registered nurses follow up on the reported immunization status of children attending child care centres. *Canadian Journal of Public Health, 4*(2), 124-127.

The purpose of this study was to evaluate whether follow-up by nurses increased the reported rate of correctly immunized preschoolers in child care centers. Records from 14 randomly selected centers were assessed for the number of correctly immunized preschoolers. Nurses advised the centers about all incomplete records and reminded parents to update their child's immunization status.

Follow-up visits to the centers were made 2 to 5 weeks and 2 to 8 months after the initial contact. Review of records at that time revealed that the rates for all immunizations had increased significantly. The study suggests that monitoring records improves completeness of the records and compliance by the parents.

STUDENT ACTIVITIES

- Determine immunization requirements for admission to schools in your school district.
- Review available findings to determine degree of compliance with immunization requirements.
- Determine the consequences of incomplete immunization records.   🌿

TABLE 52–5 *Continued*
Drugs Producing Active Immunity

Drug, How Supplied, Dosage, and Route of Administration	Undesired Clinical Responses and Contraindications	Nursing Considerations
Typhoid Vaccine (Vivotif Berna) **HOW SUPPLIED** SC injection suspension: 8 U/ml **DOSAGE** *Primary Immunization* Adults and children 10 y of age: two doses of 0.5 ml each at an interval of 4 or more wk Children <10 y of age: two doses of 0.25 ml each at an interval of 4 or more wk *Booster Doses* Adults and children >10 y of age: 0.5 ml SC or 0.1 ml intradermally Children 6-10 y: 0.25 ml SC or 0.1 ml intradermally If insufficient time for regular two-dose schedule, three doses of the appropriate volume may be given at weekly intervals Under conditions of repeated exposure, a booster dose should be administered at least q3y	**Undesired Clinical Responses** Allergic reactions Local responses, including erythema, induration, and tenderness at injection site, especially with intradermal administration Systemic responses, including malaise, headache, myalgia, and elevated temperature **Contraindications** Postpone use in presence of acute respiratory or other active infection Prior severe systemic or allergic reaction to vaccine Use in pregnancy not contraindicated unless client had significant systemic or allergic reaction to previous dose.	Used for active immunization against typhoid fever. However, routine immunization is no longer recommended for individuals residing in the United States. Shake vial vigorously before withdrawing each dose.
Cholera Vaccine **HOW SUPPLIED** IM or SC injection suspension: 8 U/ml **DOSAGE** Two primary doses administered 1 wk-1 mo or more apart Booster dose q6mo in endemic areas Infants 6 mo-4 y: 0.2 ml SC or IM Children 5 y of age and older: 0.2 ml intradermal Children 5-10 y of age: 0.3 ml SC or IM Children 10 y to adults: 0.5 ml SC or IM	**Undesired Clinical Responses** Local reactions, including erythema, induration, pain, and tenderness at the site of injection, persist for a few days Systemic reactions, including malaise, headache, and mild-to-moderate temperature elevations, persist for 1-2 d **Contraindications** History of severe systemic or allergic reaction to prior cholera vaccine Postpone in the presence of any acute illness Pregnancy (Pregnancy Category C drug)	Vaccine used for active immunization; does not prevent transmission of infection. Do not freeze; store at 2 to 8° C. Cholera vaccine may be injected intradermally, subcutaneously, or intramuscularly. Have epinephrine 1:1000 available for potential systemic reactions. Shake vial vigorously before withdrawing each dose.

Table continued on following page.

TABLE 52–5 *Continued*
Drugs Producing Active Immunity

Drug, How Supplied, Dosage, and Route of Administration	Undesired Clinical Responses and Contraindications	Nursing Considerations
Rabies Vaccine (Imovax Rabies) **HOW SUPPLIED** IM injection solution **DOSAGE** Preexposure: three doses of 1 ml IM, one each on days 0, 7, and 21 or 28 Postexposure: six injections of 1 ml, each given on days 0, 3, 7, 14, 30, and 90 First dose should be accompanied by rabies immune globulin (RIG) or antirabies serum injected half into the wound (if possible) and half into another site (WHO) *or* One dose of RIG on day 0 and five 1-ml doses of rabies vaccine intramuscularly on days 0, 3, 7, 14, and 28 (CDC) Postexposure of previously immunized individual: two IM doses of 1 ml each, one immediately and one 3 d later; RIG should not be given	***Undesired Clinical Responses*** Local reactions such as pain, erythema, and swelling or itching at the injection site (uncommon) Mild systemic reactions such as headache, nausea, abdominal pain, muscle aches, and dizziness (also uncommon) Serious systemic anaphylactic or neuroparalytic reactions (rare) ***Contraindications*** Postexposure treatment: no known specific contraindications Preexposure treatment: developing febrile illness	Visually inspect the product for particulate matter or discoloration. Reconstitute the freeze-dried vaccine in its vial with the 1 ml of diluent supplied in the disposable syringe, using the longer of the two needles. Swirl contents until completely dissolved and withdraw all dissolved vaccine. Remove reconstitution needle and replace with smaller needle. Use reconstituted vaccine immediately. Administer vaccine in the deltoid muscle of adults and children; in infants and small children, the mid-lateral aspect of the thigh may be preferable. Store vaccine at 2° to 8° C. Preexposure immunization of immunosuppressed persons is not recommended.

Drugs Producing Passive Immunity

Protection against some diseases is achieved through **passive immunity.** In passive immunity, antibodies or sensitized lymphocytes produced by another individual or animal are administered to the client. These drugs are administered after an individual is exposed to an antigen. In some situations (i.e., with rabies and hepatitis) treatment requires the administration of both active and passive immunity drugs.

Pharmacotherapeutics   Passive immunity is used for diseases not commonly found in the general population. For example, passive immunity is used after exposure to rabies or hepatitis B. Additionally, individuals with conditions rendering them incapable of producing sufficient quantities of antibodies (i.e., hypogammaglobulinemia and agammaglobulinemia) are administered drugs that produce passive immunity as a means of protection against a variety of pathologic agents.[23]

Pharmacokinetics   These drugs produce immediate immunologic protection for the client. However, immunologic memory cells are not formed. Consequently, the immunization is short-lived, lasting only a few weeks or months.

Pharmaceutics   Drugs administered for passive immunity are usually administered parenterally. Table 52–6 contains additional information about drug dosage, route of administration, and recommended frequency of administration.

CONCEPT REVIEW

Active acquired immunity develops when immune bodies are actively formed by the host after exposure to modified pathogens or toxins.

Passive immunity develops when the host is administered antibodies or sensitized lymphocytes from another individual or animal.

SUMMARY

Two major types of drugs are discussed in this chapter, immunosuppressants and immunostimulants. Drugs used for immunosuppression are essential in the prevention of organ or tissue transplant rejection. Additionally, clients with certain autoimmune disorders benefit from drug therapy that suppresses an overactive or inappropriately responding immune system. Drugs that stimulate the immune system produce either active acquired or passive immunity. Administration of these drugs prevents the consequences of exposure to toxic substances and other antigens.

TABLE 52–6
Drugs Producing Passive Immunity

Drug, How Supplied, Dosage, and Route of Administration	Undesired Clinical Responses and Contraindications	Nursing Considerations
Hepatitis B Immune Globulin (H-BIG, Hep-B-Gammagee) **HOW SUPPLIED** IM solution **DOSAGE** Adult not previously vaccinated: Dose 1, 0.06 ml/kg IM within 24 h if possible or within 7 d of exposure. Dose 2 1 mo after dose 1 Dose 3 6 mo after dose 1 Adults previously vaccinated: check titer promptly after exposure; adequate antibody is 10 MIU/ml anti-HBs; if titer is not adequate, administer one dose of hepatitis B immune globulin and one dose of hepatitis B vaccine simultaneously at two different sites as soon as possible Infants born of HBsAg-positive mothers: 0.5 ml IM as soon after birth as possible, preferably within 12 h *or* Dose 1, 0.5 ml hepatitis B immune globulin at birth *and* 0.5 ml hepatitis B vaccine at birth (in opposite thigh) or within 7 d Dose 2, 0.5 ml hepatitis B vaccine at 1 mo of age Dose 3, 0.5 ml hepatitis B vaccine at 6 mo of age	**Undesired Clinical Responses** Local pain and tenderness at injection site Urticaria Angioedema Anaphylactic reaction **Contraindications** Hypersensitivity to any component of product Pregnancy Category C	Drug provides passive immunity for individuals exposed to hepatitis B virus. Circulating antibodies to hepatitis B persist for approximately 2 mo. Antibodies may interfere with immune response to live virus vaccines. Defer live virus vaccinations until approximately 3 mo after administering hepatitis B immune globulin. Store at 2°- 8° C; do not freeze.
Immune Serum Globulin (Human) (Gammar-IV, Gamastan, Gammagard) **HOW SUPPLIED** IV, IM solutions: variety of dosages available **DOSAGE** *Primary Immunodeficiency* Initial dose: 200-400 mg/kg Maintenance dose: at least 100 mg/kg/mo must be tailored to individual *Hypogammaglobulinemia or Recurrent Bacterial Infections due to B-cell Chronic Lymphocytic Leukemia* 400 mg/kg q3-4 wk *Idiopathic Thrombocytopenic Purpura* 1 g/kg, followed by two more doses on alternate days if needed	**Undesired Clinical Responses** **GAMMAR-IV** Headache, backache, myalgia, pyrexia, hypotension, chills, flushing, and nausea, usually beginning within 1 h of start of infusion; subsides in most cases within 30 min **IM GAMMAR** Local pain and tenderness at injection site, urticaria, and angioedema; anaphylactic reactions (rare) **Contraindications** History of anaphylactic or severe systemic response to immune globulin Pregnancy (Pregnancy Category C) Allergy to thimerosal **GAMMAR-IV** Contraindicated in isolated immunoglobulin A deficiency **IM GAMMAR** Contraindicated in severe thrombocytopenia	Gammar-IV is indicated for clients with agammaglobulinemia or hypogammaglobulinemia. IM Gammar is indicated for prophylactic value with hepatitis A, measles, immunoglobulin deficiency. Keep epinephrine available for treatment of acute allergic reactions. Read package insert carefully; reconstitute using diluent at room temperature. Do not shake vial. Mixing immune globulin with other drugs is not recommended. Administer IV solution by a separate infusion line. Administer IM doses >10 ml into several muscle sites. Do not administer IM Gammar at the same time as live viral vaccines such as measles, mumps, and rubella; defer these vaccines for 3 mo.

Table continued on following page.

TABLE 52–6 *Continued*
Drugs Producing Passive Immunity

Drug, How Supplied, Dosage, and Route of Administration	Undesired Clinical Responses and Contraindications	Nursing Considerations
Rabies Immune Globulin (Hyperab, Imogam) **HOW SUPPLIED** IM solution: 150 U/ml **DOSAGE** 20 IU/kg (0.133 ml/kg) given preferably at the time of the first vaccine dose; may also be given through the seventh day after the first dose of vaccine; half the dose should be thoroughly infiltrated into the wound area and the rest should be given IM in the upper, outer quadrant of the gluteal area, avoiding risk of injury to the sciatic nerve	**Undesired Clinical Responses** Soreness at site of injection and mild temperature elevations Angioneurotic edema, skin rash, nephrotic syndrome, and anaphylactic shock (rare) **Contraindications** None known Pregnancy (Pregnancy Category C drug) unless clearly needed	Administer immediately after exposure to rabies. Immune globulin is usually administered with rabies vaccine; thus active and passive immunization is produced. Repeated doses of immune globulin should not be administered once vaccine treatment has been initiated. Immunization with live vaccines such as measles, mumps, polio, or rubella should not be given within 3 mo after immune globulin.

REFERENCES

1. Winkelstein, A. (1992). Immunopharmacology. In C.M. Smith and A.M. Reynard (Eds.), *Textbook of pharmacology* (pp. 964-983). Philadelphia: W.B. Saunders.
2. Black, J.M., & Matassarin-Jacobs, E. (1993). *Luckmann and Sorensen's medical-surgical nursing: A psychophysiologic approach* (4th ed.). Philadelphia: W.B. Saunders.
3. Whedon, M. (Ed.). (1991). *Bone marrow transplantation: Principles, practice, and nursing insights.* Boston: Jones & Bartlett.
4. Morton, P.G. (1990). *Nurse's clinical guide: Health assessment.* Springhouse, PA: Springhouse.
5. Boyce, E. (1992). Pharmacology of antiarthritic drugs. *Clinics in Podiatric Medicine and Surgery, 9,* 327-348.
6. U.S. Pharmacopeial Convention. (1990). *United States pharmacopeia* (22nd rev.). Rockville, MD: Author.
7. Lake, K., & Kilkenny, J. (1992). The pharmacokinetics and pharmacodynamics of immunosuppressive agents. *Critical Care Nursing Clinics of North America, 4,* 205-215.
8. Payne, J. (1992). Immune modification and complications of immunosuppression. *Critical Care Nursing Clinics of North America, 4,* 43-61.
9. Dattwyler, R. (1991). Immunomodulation: Therapeutic manipulation of the immune system. In J. Dolan (Ed.), *Critical care nursing: Clinical management through the nursing process* (pp. 1181-1203). Philadelphia: F.A. Davis.
10. Salomon, D. (1991). The use of immunosuppressive drugs in kidney transplantation. *Pharmacotherapy, 11,* 153s-164s.
11. Shaefer, M., & Williams, L. (1991). Nursing implications of immunosuppression in transplantation. *Nursing Clinics of North America, 26,* 291-313.
12. Camitta, B., & Doney, K. (1990). Immunosuppressive therapy for aplastic anemia: Indications, agents, mechanism, and results. *American Journal of Pediatric Hematology/Oncology, 12,* 411-424.
13. Pezze, J., & Whiteman, K. (1991). Transplantation's newest weapon: FK 506. *American Journal of Nursing, 91*(10), 40-42.
14. Corwith, C. (1992). FK 506: An investigational immunosuppressant. *ANNA Journal, 19*(2), 180.
15. Thomson, A., & Starzl, T. (1993). New immunosuppressive drugs: Mechanistic insights and potential therapeutic advances. *Immunologic Review, 130,* 71-98.
16. Peter, G. (1992). Childhood immunizations. *New England Journal of Medicine, 327,* 1794-1800.
17. Centers for Disease Control. (1988). National Childhood Vaccine Injury Act: Requirements for permanent vaccination records and for reporting of selected events after vaccination. *Morbidity and Mortality Weekly Report, 37,* 197-200.
18. Betz, C., Hunsberger, M., & Wright, S. (1994). *Family-centered nursing care of children* (2nd ed.). Philadelphia: W.B. Saunders.
19. Campbell, H., & Carter, H. (1993). Rational use of *Haemophilus influenzae* type b vaccine. *Drugs, 40,* 370-373.
20. Vessey, J., & Ritchie, S. (1993, September). The who, what, and when of pediatric immunization. *RN Magazine,* pp. 42-48.
21. Wesche, H., & Overfield, T. (1992). Tetanus immunity in elder adults. *Public Health Nursing, 9*(2), 125-127.
22. Holt, D. (1992). Recommendations, usage and efficacy of immunizations for the elderly. *Nurse Practitioner: American Journal of Primary Health Care, 17*(3), 51-52, 58-59.
23. Workman, L. (1993). Antibody-mediated immunity. In L. Workman, J. Ellerhorst-Ryan, & V. Hargrave-Koertge (Eds.). *Nursing care of the immunocompromised patient* (pp. 32-51). Philadelphia: W.B. Saunders.

BIBLIOGRAPHY

Anderson, D., & Stiehm, E. (1992). Immunization. *JAMA, 268,* 2959-2963.
Cummins, A., Eglinton, D., Gonzalez, A., & Roberton D. (1994). Immune activation during infancy in healthy humans. *Journal of Clinical Immunology, 14*(2), 107-115.
Dressler, D. (1993). Transplantation in end stage heart failure. *Critical Care Nursing Clinics of North America, 5,* 35-40.
Kohler, G., & Milstein, C. (1975). Continuous cultures of fused cell secreting antibodies of predefined specificity. *Nature, 256,* 495-497.
Pezze, J. (1990). RATG: Implications for nursing care in organ transplantation. *Critical Care Nurse, 10*(9), 18-24.

Salaberry, P., Nickel, J.T., & Mitch, R. (1994). Immunization status of 2 year olds in middle/upper and lower income populations: A community survey. *Public Health Nursing, 11*(1), 17-23.

Salaberry, P., Nickel, J.T., & Mitch, R. (1993). Why aren't preschoolers immunized: A comparison of parents' and providers' perceptions of the barriers to immunizations. *Journal of Community Health Nursing, 10*(4), 213-224.

Treanor, J., et al. (1992). Protective efficacy of combined live intranasal and inactivated influenza A virus vaccines in the elderly. *Annals of Internal Medicine, 117,* 625-633.

Whitaker, J. (1994). Rationale for immunotherapy in multiple sclerosis. *Annals of Neurology* (Suppl. 30), S103-107.

White, W. (1993). Transplantation: A review of immunosuppressive agents. *Critical Care Nursing Quarterly, 15*(4), 13-22.

CHAPTER 53

HIV Therapy

ALAN W. HOPEFL • CYNTHIA MILLS SPIRO • ROBYN RICE

⊛ Acquired Immunodeficiency Syndrome

LEARNING OBJECTIVES:

Describe the pathophysiology of acquired immunodeficiency syndrome (AIDS).

Summarize the manifestations of AIDS.

Explain the primary mechanisms of transmission of AIDS.

Describe two complications associated with AIDS.

KEY TERMS:

Acquired immunodeficiency syndrome, human immunodeficiency virus, retrovirus

⊛ Drug Therapy for HIV and AIDS

LEARNING OBJECTIVES:

Develop a plan of care for the client receiving drugs for human immunodeficiency virus (HIV) or AIDS.

Summarize pharmacokinetic and pharmacodynamic properties of zidovudine, the prototype for retrovirus replication inhibitors.

Describe causative factors for major undesired clinical responses associated with retrovirus replication inhibitors.

Identify two additional drugs in this category.

⊛ Drug Therapy Associated with Opportunistic Infections

LEARNING OBJECTIVES:

Define the term *opportunistic infections.*

Describe two types of opportunistic infections.

Identify three drugs used in the treatment of *Pneumocystis carinii* pneumonia.

Discuss the pharmacokinetic and pharmacodynamic properties of one drug used in the treatment of cytomegalovirus infections.

Discuss the pharmacokinetic and pharmacodynamic properties of one drug used in the treatment of *Mycobacterium avium-intracellulare* complex infections.

KEY TERMS:

Macrolides, opportunistic infections

⊛ Drug Therapy for AIDS-Associated Neoplasms

LEARNING OBJECTIVES:

Identify common AIDS-associated neoplasms.

Discuss the pharmacokinetic and pharmacodynamic properties of the interferons used to treat AIDS-associated neoplasms.

CONCEPTS AND TERMS TO REVIEW

Review Chapter 49 for an overview of the body's defense mechanisms.

Reexamine the functions of the T-helper cells.

Read about HIV infection, AIDS, and opportunistic infections in an appropriate pathophysiology or medical textbook.

---

*A*cquired immunodeficiency syndrome (AIDS) was first reported in the United States in 1981. It is currently the best-known example of an acquired dysfunction of the immune system. AIDS has an extremely high mortality rate and can be transmitted by asymptomatic individuals who apparently incubate the disease over a period of years. AIDS, which is caused by the human immunodeficiency virus (HIV), predisposes the individual to various debilitating and life-threatening disorders.

Surveillance studies indicate that more than 1 million individuals in the United States are infected with HIV, with more than 60,000 to 70,000 new infections occurring each year. National projections for the United States indicate that approximately 120,000 individuals will be living with AIDS in 1995. (These projections do not take into account changes in the Centers for Disease Control [CDC] case definition of AIDS.)[1]

Since the pathophysiology of HIV infection and the manifestations of AIDS are the foundations of current study in pharmacologic therapy, this chapter provides a brief overview of these areas. It also presents information about drugs currently used in the treatment of HIV infections and AIDS.

ACQUIRED IMMUNODEFICIENCY SYNDROME

Infection with **human immunodeficiency virus (HIV)** causes progressive deterioration in cell-mediated immunity. In its most severe manifestations, it results in the disease syndrome known as **acquired immunodeficiency syndrome (AIDS).**

Etiology

Two strains of HIV have been identified, HIV-1 and HIV-2. HIV-1 is the prototype virus and is responsible for most cases of AIDS. HIV-2 is found mainly in West Africa. It is less easily transmitted and has a longer incubation period than HIV-1.[2]

Pathophysiology

HIV is a **retrovirus** containing RNA and reverse transcriptase that primarily infects $CD4^+$ T-helper cells. Pathology in the host results from the retrovirus' incorporating its genetic structure into the gene or DNA of the host cell. The virus enters the $CD4^+$ T cell after binding to a CD4 receptor protein on the cell's surface. Once inside the cell, the virus enters the cell cytoplasm. In the cytoplasm the virus is uncoated, and with the help of the enzyme reverse transcriptase, the viral RNA is transcribed into a complementary DNA. This viral DNA is incorporated into the genome of the $CD4^+$ T cell.[2–4] (The term *genome* refers to the complete set of hereditary factors contained in the haploid set of chromosomes.)

Once joined with the host DNA, the HIV genome may remain essentially quiet until the $CD4^+$ T cell is activated as part of the immune response. As long as the virus is dormant, clinical manifestations of AIDS do not occur. In some instances clinical manifestations do not appear for 5 years or longer after initial HIV infection.[3] However, if the $CD4^+$ T cell is activated or stimulated by exposure to other antigens (e.g., the common cold), viral replication occurs. When viral replication takes place, the helper cell is destroyed. This releases HIV, which infects more $CD4^+$ T cells, and the cycle continues.[2] When p24 antigen, one of the core proteins of HIV, is found in the serum of clients, it denotes active replication of the HIV.

HIV infection causes a wide range of immunologic abnormalities. The most important is a decrease in the number of $CD4^+$ T cells and a decrease in the functioning ability of the ones that remain. The extent of the damage to the immune system is measured by the client's absolute $CD4^+$ T-cell or lymphocyte count. According to recent CDC guidelines, an HIV-positive client is diagnosed as having AIDS if the absolute $CD4^+$ T-cell count is below $200/mm^3$ and recurrent opportunistic infections or AIDs-associated neoplasms exist.[5]

Other immunologic abnormalities that may occur include impaired delayed hypersensitivity responses, lymphopenia, decreased production of interleukin-2, impaired function of T-killer cells, increased production of some antibodies, and increased formation of immune complexes. These abnormalities leave the individual susceptible to a variety of opportunistic infections and neoplasms. Monocytes and macrophages can also be infected by HIV. This is probably the mechanism by which HIV is transported into the central nervous system (CNS). Once inside the CNS, damage to neural tissue occurs.[2,3,6]

Manifestations

HIV infection results in a variety of clinical manifestations that can be divided into four stages: acute infection stage, asymptomatic stage, transitional stage, and the stage marked by opportunistic infections or neoplasms.[7]

After the initial HIV infection, antibodies are usually detected within 3 to 6 weeks. The presence of HIV antibodies indicates that the individual has been exposed to the virus and that an immune response was initiated. At this point the individual is infectious and capable of infecting others.

Initial antibody conversion produces the acute infection stage. This stage is characterized by the sudden development of fever, fatigue, myalgias, sweats, photophobia, sore throat, nausea, vomiting, or headache. There may be generalized lymphadenopathy, an enlarged spleen, and a transient maculopapular rash. These symptoms develop 6 to 12 weeks after infection with HIV and usually resolve spontaneously in 2 to 3 weeks. Many clients become asymptomatic at this point. This asymptomatic stage may last from 2 months to 15 years and is characterized by continuous low-level viral replication and $CD4^+$ T-cell loss and, in some individuals, persistent generalized lymphadenopathy (PGL).[2,4,7]

As the HIV infection produces immunodeficiency, the client enters the transitional stage of symptomatic disease. During this stage the client may experience fevers, night sweats, severe malaise, fatigue, weight loss, oral or dermatologic disorders, PGL, and splenomegaly. Neutropenia, lymphopenia, thrombocytopenia, anemia, and a decreased number of $CD4^+$ T cells also occur. The final stage of HIV infection is AIDS and is characterized by severe immunodeficiency. The severe immunodeficiency results in the development of a variety of opportunistic infections or malignancies. Any body system or organ can be infected.[2,3,7] Figure 53–1 lists some of the frequent manifestations of the final stage.

Concurrent infections, congenital defects, stress, and use of recreational drugs and alcohol enhance HIV replication and disease manifestation. As the CD4 count drops, the client eventually becomes anergic; his or her immune system is unable to respond to antigens. In fact, anergic individuals often do not respond to purified protein derivative (PPD) tuberculin skin tests, even when they have active tuberculosis.

Mechanisms of Transmission

HIV is transmitted from one individual to another by body fluid that contains HIV. The probability of transmission increases with the concentration of HIV. HIV has been isolated from blood, semen, vaginal secretions, saliva, tears, breast milk, cerebrospinal fluid, amniotic fluid, alveolar fluid, and urine. However, body fluids shown to transmit the virus are limited to blood, cerebrospinal fluid, semen, vaginal secretions, and breast milk. The three routes of transmission are intimate sexual contact involving the exchange of body fluids;

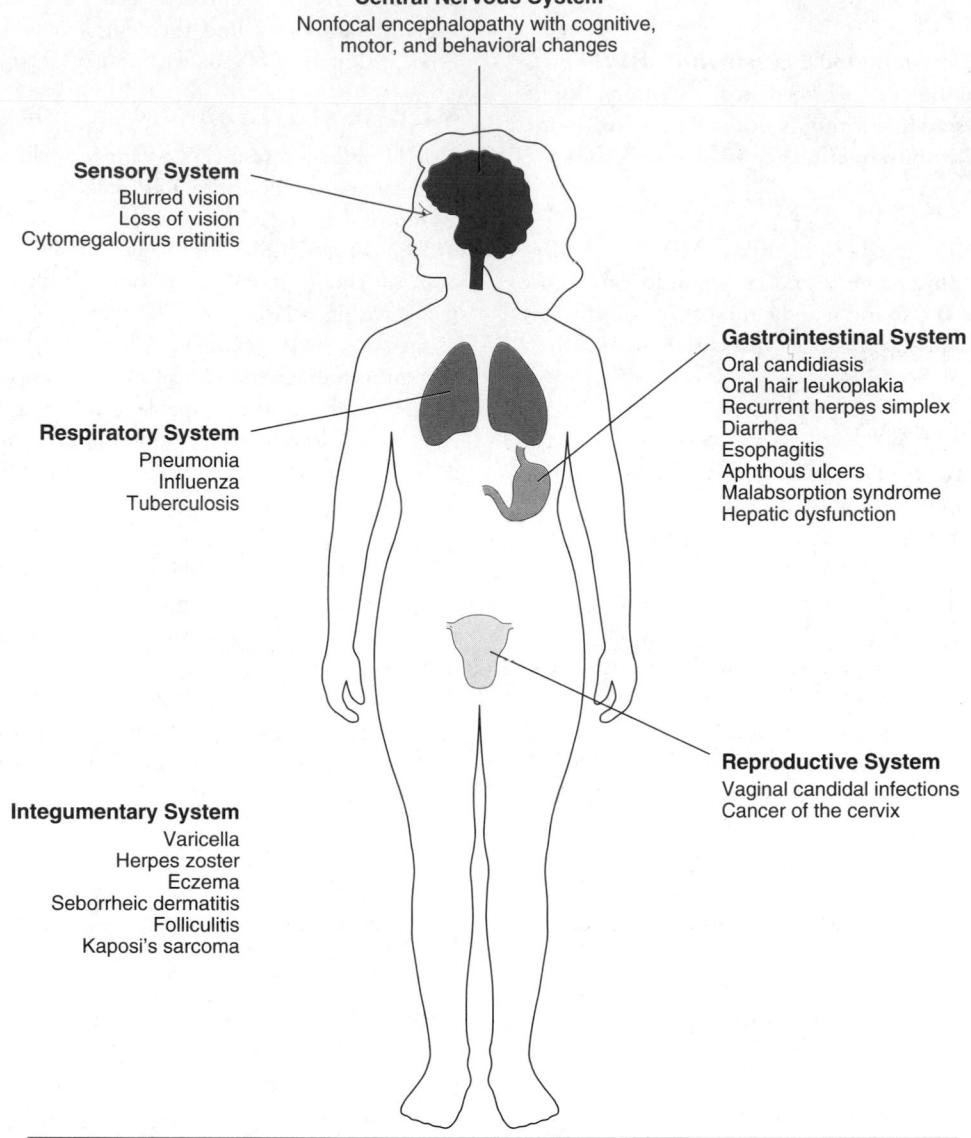

Central Nervous System
Nonfocal encephalopathy with cognitive, motor, and behavioral changes

Sensory System
Blurred vision
Loss of vision
Cytomegalovirus retinitis

Respiratory System
Pneumonia
Influenza
Tuberculosis

Gastrointestinal System
Oral candidiasis
Oral hair leukoplakia
Recurrent herpes simplex
Diarrhea
Esophagitis
Aphthous ulcers
Malabsorption syndrome
Hepatic dysfunction

Reproductive System
Vaginal candidal infections
Cancer of the cervix

Integumentary System
Varicella
Herpes zoster
Eczema
Seborrheic dermatitis
Folliculitis
Kaposi's sarcoma

FIGURE 53–1   Clinical manifestations associated with the final stage of HIV infection.

parenteral injection of infected blood, blood products, or body fluids; and from HIV-infected mother to fetus or infant.[2,8]

In the United States transmission of HIV most frequently occurs through intimate sexual activity. Although transmission of HIV occurs during both heterosexual and homosexual activity, homosexual and bisexual men have the highest rate of infection. Sexual practices such as anal, vaginal, and oral intercourse without the use of a latex barrier increase the risk of exposure to body fluids, thus increasing the chance of HIV infection. In addition, the risk of infection increases if there are breaks in the skin or mucous membrane of the active partner.[2,9]

Intravenous (IV) drug users have become the second largest group within the AIDS population. The mechanism of transmission in these individuals involves sharing used or dirty needles and syringes contaminated with HIV-infected blood. HIV

can also be transmitted through transfusion of blood and blood products that contain the virus and via organ transplantation from an infected donor. However, only a small proportion of the clients with AIDS have become infected by these routes.[1,2,9]

Women infected with HIV can transmit the virus to the fetus or newborn. During the perinatal period the route of transmission is maternal circulation to the fetus. Recent statistics from the CDC indicate that 1500 to 2000 new HIV infections occur each year among newborns as a result of perinatal HIV transmission. Transmission may also occur if the newborn is exposed to maternal blood and body fluids during labor and delivery or to infected breast milk.

Risk of acquiring HIV infection by occupational or casual transmission is statistically low. For health care workers, the primary route of exposure is by accidental needle sticks.

However, long-term studies indicate that the risk of HIV transmission from percutaneous exposure is approximately 0.3%. Cases of casual transmission in studies of family members are also statistically low, approximately 0.1%. Activities examined in these studies included kissing, embracing, and sharing common household items (i.e., dishes, linens, and toilet facilities), with the HIV-infected individual.[10]

Pharmacotherapeutics

At present, there is no cure for AIDS. It is a disease that eventually results in death. Therefore treatment is directed toward (1) slowing HIV replication; (2) decreasing the incidence of opportunistic infections and AIDS-associated neoplasms; and (3) increasing the client's sense of well-being by reducing disease symptomatology. Drugs used to treat HIV-infected clients are placed into four distinct categories based on their desired effect:

1. Drugs used to prevent replication of HIV
2. Drugs to treat or prevent opportunistic infections
3. Drugs to treat AIDS-associated neoplasms
4. Drugs with immunostimulant effects

CONCEPT REVIEW

Acquired immunodeficiency syndrome is the end result of a human immunodeficiency viral infection.

The HIV is a retrovirus that contains RNA and reverse transcriptase and primarily infects CD4+ T-helper cells.

Clinical manifestations of an HIV infection and AIDS depend on the stage of the illness. In the final stage of HIV disease, any body system or organ can be affected.

▨ NURSING CONSIDERATIONS

The nurse pla ys an important role in the therapy of clients with HIV infection.

Assessing   Nursing assessment of the client with an HIV infection involves physical, psychologic, and social components. During the **health history** include a review of present and past illness. Obtain a detailed description of current symptoms and their severity. Inquire about the presence of chest pain, coughing, and sputum production; about soreness of the mouth, bleeding gums, and difficulty chewing or swallowing; and about any weight loss, change in appetite, or diarrhea. If diarrhea is present, determine remedies that have been tried and their effectiveness. Obtain a dietary history to determine the adequacy of the client's nutritional intake and to determine if food sources are contributing to the diarrhea. Determine the client's ability to pay attention, concentrate, and follow commands. Assess memory, speech, judgment, and mood. Ask family or friends if changes have been observed in these areas.[2]

Since the client is immunosuppressed, determine potential sources of infections in the home environment. Ascertain the age of all household members. Does anyone living in the house have a chronic, low-grade infection (e.g., chronic bronchitis)? If young children live in the house, what is the status of their immunizations against childhood diseases (e.g., measles, mumps, pertussis)?

Assess the client's emotional status and coping ability. Explore the client's ability for self-care, including ability to follow the treatment regimen. Evaluate the client's understanding of the disease, including mode of transmission, infections that may develop, and prognosis. Determine existing relationships with family and friends. Since this is a chronic disease, effective support systems are important to help the client meet psychologic and physical needs. Determine if the client is aware of available community resources.

Since this disease can affect all body systems, perform a head-to-toe **physical assessment.** Be certain to weigh the client and assess for signs of dehydration, noting skin color and turgor. Because the client with HIV infection frequently has oral infections, assess his or her mouth carefully. Look for white patches, which are indicative of *Candida* infection or hairy leukoplakia, and herpes simplex lesions. Carefully assess the client's respiratory status since pulmonary infections are common in these individuals.

Diagnosing   Numerous nursing diagnoses are appropriate for the client with an HIV infection. However, only those related to drug therapy are included here:

- Activity intolerance related to fatigue and weakness associated with macrocytic anemia produced by drug therapy.
- Fluid volume deficit related to diarrhea or vomiting from drug therapy.
- High risk for altered health maintenance related to lack of knowledge of etiology and transmission of the disease, clinical course, and treatment plan.
- High risk for infection related to suppressed immune response (leukopenia) produced by drugs.
- Noncompliance related to adverse reactions of drug therapy.
- Nutrition, altered, less than body requirements related to inability to ingest adequate nutrients.

Planning   Once nursing diagnoses are established, interventions and expected outcomes are developed for each diagnosis. If needed, include in the plan an explanation of the etiology of the disease, how the disease affects the body, stages of disease progression, and available treatment possibilities. Also include information about how the disease is transmitted and precautions to take to avoid transmitting the disease to others.

Plan to provide the client information about his or her specific drug regimen. Develop a written plan that includes the name of each drug and its purpose. Incorporate information about undesired clinical responses, when to contact the primary care provider, and the importance of compliance. Include written information about follow-up care, including appointments with the primary care provider and required laboratory studies.

Expected outcomes for the plan of care might include the following:

- Client demonstrates a decrease in physiologic signs of activity intolerance.
- Client's fluid volume is maintained at a functional level as evidenced by adequate urinary output, stable vital signs, moist mucous membranes, and adequate skin turgor.
- Client demonstrates techniques and lifestyle changes that promote a safe environment.
- Client explains the etiology and course of HIV infection.
- Client identifies methods to reduce the risk of spreading the virus to others.
- Client states name, use, dosage, route, and reportable undesired clinical responses of all prescribed drugs.
- Client actively participates in treatment plan.
- Client remains free of signs and symptoms of infection.

Implementing You may not administer HIV therapy drugs as frequently as you administer those in other drug categories. Therefore be certain to familiarize yourself with the drug's pharmacokinetic and pharmacodynamic properties, method of administration, and recommended dosage schedule (e.g., administer HIV replication inhibitors on an empty stomach). Also keep yourself informed about new developments in the pharmacologic treatment of HIV and AIDS.

As you care for these clients, stress the importance of compliance. Once drug therapy reduces some of the symptoms of the disease, the client may find it difficult to follow the treatment plan. Explain to the client that the drug(s) will not produce a cure and that failure to comply with the prescribed drug regimen increases the risk of opportunistic infections and malignancies. Additionally, stress that the client is still infectious to others.

NURSING RESEARCH

Dutz, A., Hutton, N., Joyner, M., et al. (1993). HIV infected women and infants: Social and health factors impeding utilization of health care. *Journal of Nurse Midwifery, 30*(2), 103-109.

The purpose of this research was to study the use of health care by HIV-seropositive pregnant women and their infants. The study, which was conducted in an indigent urban population, included 90 HIV-seropositive women who delivered 99 HIV-exposed infants during the period studied.

Out of this group of subjects, repeat pregnancies occurred in 17 women. Of all the infants, 72.9% received primary immunization status by 9 months of age. However, only 45% of the women reported ever seeking HIV-related health care. Factors associated with maternal adherence with HIV-related health care included HIV status of the infant, maternal drug use, and incarceration.

STUDENT ACTIVITIES

- Interview an individual from the local health department. Determine the amount of follow-up care sought by women who have been identified as HIV seropositive.

- Determine the recommended health care for seropositive individuals.

Currently there is a tremendous push from health care providers to educate the public about routes of HIV transmission in an attempt to decrease the incidence of infection. As a nurse, you are at the forefront of this movement. When possible, become involved in your community's efforts toward public education (e.g., volunteer as a speaker or to distribute information).

DRUG THERAPY FOR HIV AND AIDS

The ideal goal of treatment for HIV-infected clients is a cure for their infection. However, this is not an achievable goal at present. Current therapy slows the progression of the disease by inhibiting replication of HIV. The net effect is preservation of the client's immune system. Along with therapy directed at inhibiting replication of the retrovirus, other measures such as pain control, hydration, and nutritional support are of equal importance.

Drugs That Inhibit Replication of HIV

Drugs that inhibit replication of HIV share some common characteristics. After therapy is initiated with antiretroviral nucleoside analogs, an increase in CD4$^+$ T cells and a fall in p24 antigen occur. Unfortunately, in most cases these positive laboratory parameters are of short duration, lasting only 4 to 6 months.[12,13] Treatment with antiretroviral drugs frequently enhances the client's sense of well-being. After therapy the client may experience an increase in weight, a reduction in fever or diarrhea, and overall improved physical and mental status. Much of this reaction is related to the alleviation of the symptomatology of the HIV infection.

HIV REPLICATION PROHIBITOR PROTOTYPE

ZIDOVUDINE

In the mid-1980s it was found that certain 2',3' dideoxynucleoside analogs could inhibit the reverse transcriptase enzyme of HIV. The first of these analogs and the most studied is 3'-azido-3'-deoythymidine, zidovudine (AZT, Retrovir).

Pharmacotherapeutics Zidovudine is used in the treatment of adult clients with HIV infection who have impaired immunity (CD4$^+$ T-cell count of 500/mm^3 or less). It is also used in the treatment of HIV-infected children over the age of 3 months.

Pharmacokinetics Zidovudine is rapidly absorbed from the gastrointestinal (GI) tract, and peak serum concentrations occur within $\frac{1}{2}$ to $1\frac{1}{2}$ hours. However, if the drug is administered with a high-fat meal, the time to peak serum level is delayed.[14] The serum half-life of zidovudine is approximately 1 hour. Based on this fact, the recommended dosing interval is every 4 hours. Cellular thymidine kinase converts zidovudine into zidovudine monophosphate, which is further converted into a triphosphate derivative. Since this derivative, triphosphate, has a longer half-life than zidovudine, current studies are examining the efficacy of more prolonged dosing intervals.

Zidovudine crosses the placenta, and therapeutic concentrations can be found in amniotic fluid and fetal plasma. The drug also readily crosses the blood-brain barrier and produces concentrations in the cerebrospinal fluid that reach approximately 25% of the plasma level. Zidovudine is rapidly metabolized in the liver to an inactive glucuronide, which is excreted in the urine. As a result of first-pass metabolism, the average oral dosage bioavailability is 65%.[15,16]

Pharmacodynamics As previously indicated, zidovudine is inactive and requires intracellular phosphorylation to its triphosphate form before it can inhibit the reverse transcriptase of HIV and other retroviruses. Zidovudine also becomes incorporated into the growing DNA strand where it prevents lengthening of the strand. Both retrovirus inhibition and DNA chain termination are required to inhibit viral replication fully.[17]

Pharmaceutics Zidovudine is available in capsule and syrup dosage forms for oral administration and in an IV solution.

Undesired Clinical Responses Initial treatment with zidovudine often causes symptoms such as headache, nausea, and insomnia. These symptoms tend to decrease in severity after 3 or 4 weeks of treatment. Macrocytic anemia commonly occurs with zidovudine therapy, especially when high doses of the drug are administered. Macrocytic anemia, which may develop after only 4 to 6 weeks of therapy, can be severe enough to require reduction in dosage, periodic transfusion, or treatment with erythropoietin injections. Neutropenia and thrombocytopenia also occur as a result of bone marrow suppression. Clients requiring long-term therapy with zidovudine may develop myopathy, usually of the proximal muscles of the legs or arms.[15–17]

Contraindications and Precautions Zidovudine should be administered with caution to clients with impaired renal or hepatic function.

Drug-Drug and Drug-Nutrient Interactions Although zidovudine has the potential for several drug-drug interactions, few have been studied systematically. It is known that any drug (e.g., pentamidine, amphotericin B, interferon, flucytosine) that has adverse effects on the bone marrow or renal function can enhance the toxicity of zidovudine. In addition, probenecid reduces the renal excretion of zidovudine and may inhibit glucoronidation. Methadone increases the serum levels of zidovudine and the risk for toxicity. Ganciclovir, which is contraindicated because of its additive effects on bone marrow suppression, also has an antagonistic effect on the antiretroviral effects of zidovudine.[15,18] Remember that a high-fat meal delays the peak serum concentration time.

Life-Span Considerations Zidovudine is classified as a Pregnancy Category C drug. It is not known if the drug is excreted in breast milk. However, mothers are instructed to discontinue nursing while receiving zidovudine. Although zidovudine is approved for use with children over the age of 3 months, the data are limited on its effectiveness in this age group.

Specific Drug-related Nursing Considerations Since high-fat meals affect serum levels, administer the drug on an empty stomach. Monitor the client carefully for indications of bone marrow suppression. A complete blood count (CBC) should be checked every 1 to 2 weeks.

MISCELLANEOUS DRUGS IN CATEGORY

Both didanosine and zalcitabine are inhibitors of retrovirus replication. **Didanosine** (ddI, dideoxyinosine, Videx) was approved by the Food and Drug Administration (FDA) in October 1991. This drug is indicated for the treatment of adult and pediatric clients over 6 months of age who have advanced HIV infection. It is recommended for use in clients who have demonstrated intolerance to zidovudine or are deteriorating while taking zidovudine. Didanosine has a serum half-life of 1.6 hours. The intracellular half-life of its active metabolite, dideoxyadenosine triphosphate, is approximately 8 to 24 hours, allowing twice-a-day dosing. Didanosine has a bioavailability of 40% and is rapidly degraded by acidic pH. Didanosine is distributed in all body tissues and is excreted through glomerular filtration. It crosses the placenta, but whether it is excreted in breast milk and removed by dialysis is unknown.[19,20]

Didanosine is available in solution, chewable tablets, and powder dosage forms for oral administration. Because the drug is affected by an acid environment, all oral formulations contain buffering agents designed to increase the pH of the gastric environment. The powder, which frequently is used with pediatric clients, is initially mixed with water and then brought to a final concentration of 10 mg per milliliter with Mylanta Double Strength or Maalox TC suspension to provide sufficient buffer. When chewable tablets are administered, each adult and pediatric dose must consist of two tablets to achieve adequate acid-neutralizing capacity. The only exception is for pediatric clients less than 1 year of age. For these individuals only one tablet is necessary to provide adequate acid-neutralizing capacity.

The most serious toxicity seen with didanosine is pancreatitis; therefore clients should be monitored for abdominal pain, nausea, and vomiting. Additionally, the drug must be used carefully in alcoholics, clients with a history of pancreatitis, or those taking other drugs known to cause pancreatitis (e.g., IV pentamidine). Peripheral neuropathy can also occur. Monitor the client for numbness, tingling, or pain in feet or hands. In addition, administer drugs requiring an acid gastric pH for absorption (e.g., ketoconazole, dapsone) at least 2 hours before administering didanosine.[19,20]

Since didanosine is acid labile, instruct the client to take the drug on an empty stomach. Advise the client to take the drug with water and to avoid fruit juices. Therapeutic drug levels depend on consistent drug administration; therefore caution the client about missing doses.

Zalcitabine (ddC, dideoxycytidine, HIVID) was approved by the FDA in mid-1992. Although zalcitabine is one of the most potent antiretroviral drugs available, it is recommended only for concurrent use with zidovudine. Like other nucleoside analogs, zalcitabine initially causes a decrease in p24 antigen levels and an increase in CD4+ T cells. After an oral dose the drug has a bioavailability of 87% and a plasma half-life of approximately 1 hour. It is converted to the active metabolite triphosphate, whose intracellular half-life is 2.6 hours. Zalcitabine is available in oral uncoated tablets. Since it is so potent, prescribed doses are extremely small compared to those of other agents.[15,21]

The most significant undesired clinical response associated with zalcitabine is peripheral neuropathy, which apparently is dose dependent. Neuropathy begins with numbness or burning in the upper extremities. It may progress to sharp, shooting pains or severe burning, possibly irreversible, if the drug is not discontinued. Risk of neuropathy may be greater in clients with low CD4$^+$ lymphocyte counts (<50/mm^3). Pancreatitis has also been reported. The drug manufacturer does not recommend using zalcitabine with didanosine since doing so increases the risk of pancreatitis. Avoid use of the drug with other medications that may cause peripheral neuropathy.

Instruct the client receiving zalcitabine to call his or her primary care provider if he or she notices numbness, tingling, or pain in the extremities. Inform the client that frequent laboratory studies (e.g., serum amylase, triglyceride, CBC) are necessary. Also instruct the client to take the drug on an empty stomach. Table 53–1 summarizes dosage information and nursing considerations associated with zidovudine, zalcitabine, and didanosine. Figure 53–2 provides a summary of common undesired clinical responses associated with these drugs.

Other nucleoside reverse transcriptase inhibitors are being developed (e.g., **D4T** [dideoxydidehydrothymidine] and

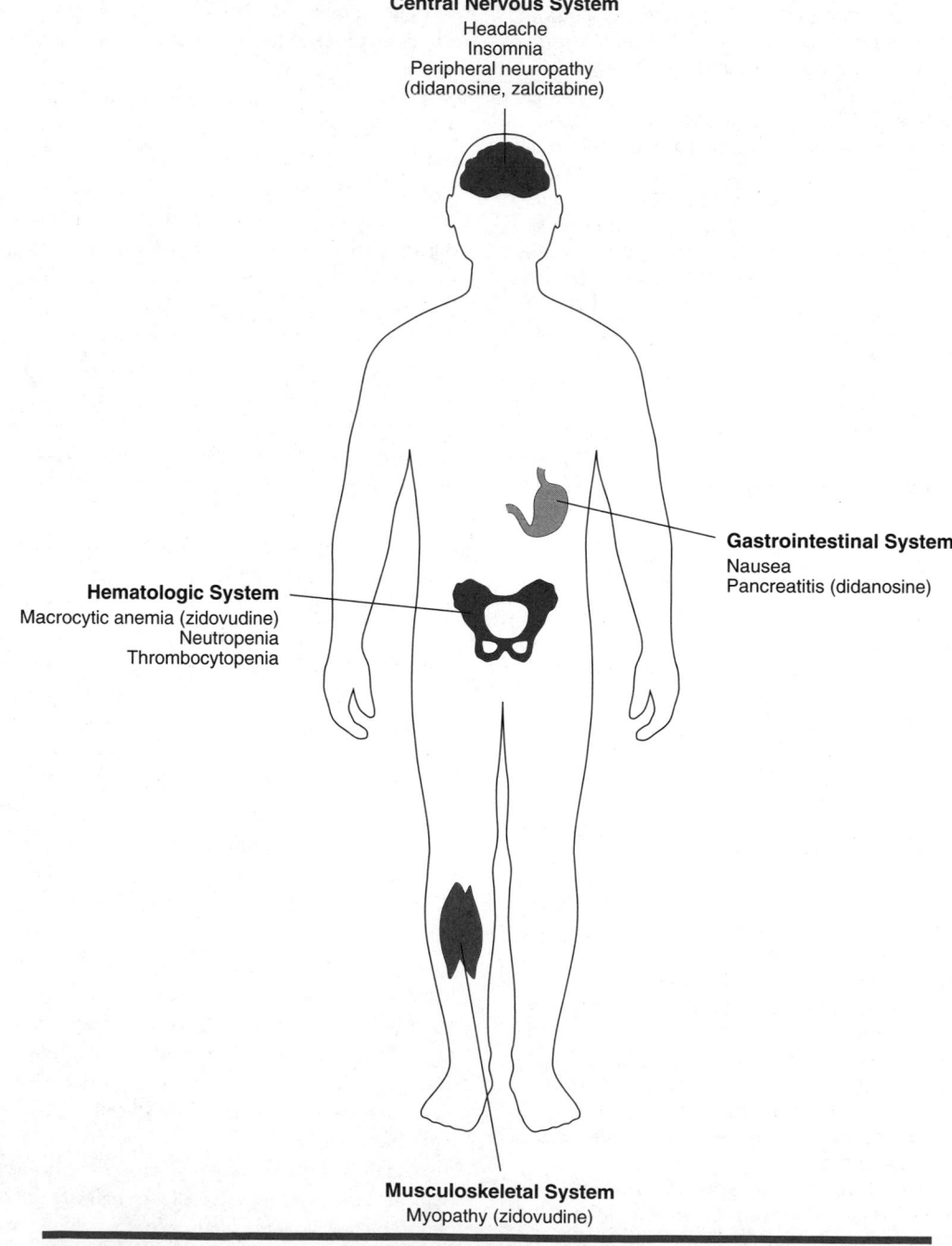

Central Nervous System
Headache
Insomnia
Peripheral neuropathy
(didanosine, zalcitabine)

Gastrointestinal System
Nausea
Pancreatitis (didanosine)

Hematologic System
Macrocytic anemia (zidovudine)
Neutropenia
Thrombocytopenia

Musculoskeletal System
Myopathy (zidovudine)

FIGURE 53–2 Common undesired clinical responses associated with retroviral replication inhibitors.

TABLE 53–1

Drugs That Inhibit Replication of HIV: Prototype and Major Drugs in Category

Drug Name	Dosage and Route of Administration	Nursing Considerations
ZIDOVUDINE (AZT, Retrovir) **HOW SUPPLIED** Capsule: 100 mg Syrup: 50 mg/5 ml IV: 10 mg/ml	**Symptomatic HIV** **ADULTS** Initial dose, 200 mg (two capsules or 20 ml syrup) q4h to total daily dose of 1200 mg After 1 mo may reduce dose to 100 mg q4h (600 mg total daily dose) **Asymptomatic HIV** **ADULTS** Oral: 100 mg q4h while awake (500 mg/d) **CHILDREN 3 MO-12 Y** Oral or IV: 180 mg/m² q6h (720 mg/m²/d), not to exceed 200 mg q6h IV: 1-2 mg/kg infused over 1 h; administer this dose q4h (six times daily). Use IV dosage form until oral form can be tolerated; if oral form cannot be tolerated after 1 mo of therapy, reduced IV dose would be 1 mg/kg IV q4h	**Assess** Determine if client has preexisting renal or hepatic dysfunction. Determine if client is pregnant; zidovudine is classified as Pregnancy Category C drug. **Implement** Remind client that drug is not a cure for HIV infection. Instruct client to report any significant changes in health status. Remind client that he or she is still infectious and can transmit HIV to others through sexual contact or blood contamination. Store oral syrup and vials at 15° to 25° C. Protect drug products from light. Mix IV drug with 5% dextrose solution to achieve proper concentration. Examine parenteral drug products for particulate matter and discoloration. If either is observed, discard solution. Diluted IV solution is physically and chemically stable for 24 h at room temperature. If refrigerated, solution is stable for 48 h. Administer diluted solution within 8 h if stored at 25° C or 24 hours if refrigerated at 2° to 8° C. Infuse IV at a constant rate over 1 h. **Monitor** Monitor hematologic indices frequently. Monitor for anemia and granulocytopenia. Monitor for undesired clinical responses, including anemia, severe headache, fever, anorexia, nausea, insomnia, and myalgia. **Evaluate** Assess for stabilization of physical condition.
Didanosine (ddI, dideoxyinosine, Videx) **HOW SUPPLIED** Packet: 100, 167, 250, and 375 mg Solution: 20 mg/ml Chewable tablet: 25, 50, 100, and 150 mg	**ADULTS** Client weighing 60 kg or more: 200 mg (tablets) bid or 250 mg (packet of buffered powder) q12h; when giving tablets, administer as two lower-dose tablets to provide sufficient buffering action Client weighing <60 kg: 125 mg (tablets) bid or 167 mg (packet of buffered powder) q12h Suspend dose if clinical signs of pancreatitis appear; resume dosage schedule when pancreatitis has been ruled out **CHILDREN** 1.1-1.4 m² body surface area (BSA): 100 mg tablets q12h *or* 125 mg powder with 12.5 ml admixture q12h 0.8-1.0 m² BSA: 75 mg tablets q12h *or* 94 mg powder with 9.5 ml admixture q12h 0.5-0.7 m² BSA: 50 mg tablets q12h *or* 62 mg powder with 6 ml admixture q12h 0.4 m² BSA or less: 25 mg tablet q12h *or* 31 mg powder with 3 ml admixture q12h With tablet regimen, give two tablets unless child is <1y	**Assess** Administer all oral dosage forms on an empty stomach. Administer drug with caution to clients receiving sodium-restricted diets, with renal impairment, with hepatic impairment, or with phenylketonuria. Instruct client receiving chewable tablets to chew thoroughly, crush, or disperse drug in at least 1 ounce water. Add packet drug content to 4 ounces of drinking water. Do not mix with fruit juice or other acid-containing liquid. For home use, drug should be dispensed in tint-glass bottles with child-resistant closures. Pediatric oral solution is stable for 30 d under refrigeration at 2° to 8° C. Instruct client to shake oral solution thoroughly before use. Use appropriate handling and disposal techniques. Inform client to report nausea, vomiting, or abdominal pain, which may indicate pancreatitis.

Table continued on following page.

TABLE 53–1 *Continued*

Drugs That Inhibit Replication of HIV: Prototype and Major Drugs in Category

Drug Name	Dosage and Route of Administration	Nursing Considerations
Didanosine Continued		***Monitor*** Monitor for clinical toxicities: pancreatitis and peripheral neuropathy. Monitor for undesired clinical responses, including hyperuricemia, diarrhea, and fluid retention. ***Evaluate*** Assess for stabilization of physical condition.
Zalcitabine (ddC, dideoxycytidine, HIVID) **HOW SUPPLIED** Tablet: 0.375, 0.75 mg	Not recommended for use as monotherapy. For client weighing 30 kg or more: 0.75 mg HIVID administered with 200 mg zidovudine q8h (total daily dose, 2.25 mg HIVID, 600 mg zidovudine) Suspend dose if signs of clinical toxicity appear and reintroduce at lower dosage; minimum effective dose has not been established	***Assess*** Determine if client is pregnant; zalcitabine is classified as a Pregnancy Category C drug. Determine if client is allergic to any of the excipients contained in tablets. Assess for preexisting renal or hepatic impairment. Review baseline test of serum amylase, triglyceride, CBC. ***Implement*** Store in tightly closed bottles at 15° to 30° C. Instruct client to report numbness, tingling, or pain in feet or ankles. Administer on an empty stomach. ***Monitor*** Monitor for clinical toxicity: peripheral neuropathy, pancreatitis, esophageal ulcers, cardiomyopathy, anaphylactic reaction. Monitor for undesired clinical responses: weight loss, chest pain, fever, myalgia, abdominal pain, fatigue, malaise. Review periodic CBC and serum amylase levels.

3-thiacytidine). In addition, a number of non–nucleoside inhibitors are under study (e.g., **nevirapine, pyridinone,** and the **TIBO compounds**). Some of these newer compounds have different toxicities than zidovudine or can be used against zidovudine-resistant HIV.[12]

Because the replication cycle of HIV is complex, other sites in the cycle are available for inhibition. For example, the gene for the CD4 receptor on T-helper cells has been cloned and formulated into a parenteral product. Since the CD4 receptor is the site of HIV attachment to cells before penetration by the virus, excess amounts of **recombinant soluble CD4** (rs CD4) may prevent binding of the virus to susceptible cells. Recombinant soluble CD4 has a short serum half-life and must be administered parenterally, which may limit its usefulness.[13]

Drugs are also being designed to inhibit other functions of the HIV retrovirus molecule that are related to the transcription of the HIV genome (i.e., as a ribonuclease or a protease). For example, synthetic nucleic acid chains (**antisense oligonucleotides**) are being synthesized that bind to the HIV genome or its messenger RNA transcript. These synthetic oligonucleotides interfere with normal gene function. However, at present, numerous technical problems are associated with the development of these drugs.

Other potential targets involve two regulatory genes of HIV, *tat* and *rev*. The protein products of these genes are important in amplifying and directing viral replication. Inhibitors of these genes or their protein products are under development.[13]

CONCEPT REVIEW

The primary drug therapy for HIV and AIDS involves retrovirus replication inhibitors. Zidovudine (azidothymidine) is the major drug in this group.

In the body zidovudine is converted to triphosphate, which is very active as a competitive inhibitor of the reverse transcriptase of HIV and other retroviruses.

Other drugs are being developed that inhibit other functions of the HIV retrovirus molecule or that inhibit other sites in the replication cycle.

DRUG THERAPY ASSOCIATED WITH OPPORTUNISTIC INFECTIONS

Opportunistic infections are caused by microorganisms (viruses, fungi, protozoans, or bacteria) that are ordinarily non-virulent and do not cause disease. However, under certain circumstances (e.g., in individuals with immunodeficiency), the microorganisms become pathogenic.

In general, the HIV-infected client or AIDS client is less responsive to conventional therapy for opportunistic infections. These individuals usually require a longer course of treatment. Additionally, immunodeficiency clients frequently recover from one infectious episode only to redevelop the infection or become infected with a new pathogen. Also it is not uncommon for the client to have several opportunistic infections at the same time.

Types of Opportunistic Infections

Infections from *Pneumocystis carinii,* cytomegalovirus (CMV), and herpesviruses are common in clients with AIDS. Recently, organisms such as *Cryptosporidium, Isospora belli,* and atypical mycobacteria (e.g., *Mycobacterium avium-intracellulare)* have also produced opportunistic infections in these clients. Table 53–2 summarizes information about opportunistic infections commonly seen in clients with AIDS.

Drug Therapy for *P. carinii* Pneumonia

Of the opportunistic infections, *P. carinii* pneumonia (PCP) is one of the most important. More than one half of the HIV-infected clients in the United States are diagnosed as hav-

ing AIDS on the basis of PCP, an AIDS-defining disease. Approximately 80% of AIDS clients have at least one occurrence of PCP during the course of their illness.[22]

A variety of drugs are used to treat PCP. Many of these drugs (e.g., trimethoprim-sulfamethoxazole, pyrimethamine, and the sulfonamides) have other primary uses. Both components of **trimethoprim-sulfamethoxazole** inhibit folic acid synthesis in microorganisms, but they each act at different sites in the synthetic pathway. It is unclear if this is the mechanism of action in the treatment of PCP. The dose of trimethoprim-sulfamethoxazole prescribed for PCP is approximately four times that used to treat ordinary infections (i.e., urinary tract infections, otitis media, chronic bronchitis). Because of this increased dose there is a higher incidence of GI intolerance. In general, the incidence of cutaneous reactions and bone marrow depression in clients with AIDS is higher.[22,23] (See Chapter 56 for additional information on trimethoprim-sulfamethoxazole.)

Pyrimethamine (Daraprim), an antimalarial agent, is similar in structure to trimethoprim. It functions as an inhibitor of dihydrofolate reductase (see Chapter 60). The **sulfonamides** (sulfadiazine, sulfamethoxazole, trisulfapyrimidines) all inhibit folic acid synthesis. Sulfonamides are used along with pyrimethamine in the treatment of toxoplasmosis and with trimethoprim for treatment of PCP. (See Chapter 55 for additional information about sulfonamides.)

Atovaquone Atovaquone (Mepron) was recently approved by the FDA for treatment of mild-to-moderate PCP in clients intolerant of trimethoprim-sulfamethoxazole or pentamidine isethionate. Atovaquone is believed to act as an inhibitor of mitochondrial electron transport. This action indirectly inhibits pyrimidine synthesis, which causes inhibition of nucleic acid synthesis. Pharmacokinetic data on atovaquone are limited, but it is known that the oral absorption is highly variable. Absorption of the drug is enhanced markedly by the presence of food, especially foods with a high-fat content.[23] Undesired clinical responses associated with atovaquone are minimal compared to those with alternative drugs. The most common adverse reactions are an innocuous rash, nausea, or vomiting. Currently, there is little information available on the use of atovaquone in children.[24,25]

Instruct the client to complete the entire 3-week course of treatment. Stress the importance of taking the drug at intervals as close to 8 hours as possible. Additionally, instruct the client to take the drug with food, particularly fatty foods, to enhance drug absorption.

Eflornithine hydrochloride Eflornithine (Ornidyl) is an antiprotozoal drug used primarily to treat parasitic infections in Third World countries. However, eflornithine may be useful in clients who cannot tolerate trimethoprim-sulfamethoxazole or pentamidine isethionate.

Eflornithine differs from other currently available antiprotozoal drugs in both structure and mode of action. It is a specific, enzyme-activated irreversible inhibitor of ornithine decarboxylase. This action causes the inhibition of polyamine synthesis, which affects both nucleic acid and protein synthesis. After IV administration of eflornithine, approximately

---

TABLE 53–2

Common Opportunistic Infections in HIV-Infected Clients

Mircroorganism	Usual Site of Infection
YEAST OR FUNGI	
Candida albicans	Oropharynx, lungs, liver, vagina
Coccidioides immitis	Disseminated (lungs, abdomen)
Cryptococcus neoformans	Central nervous system (CNS)
Histoplasma capsulatum	Disseminated (lungs, abdomen)
Pneumocystis carinii	Lungs
PROTOZOANS	
Cryptosporidium spp.	CNS
Isospora belli	Gastrointestinal (GI) tract
Microsporidium spp.	GI tract
Toxoplasma gondii	GI tract
VIRUSES	
Cytomegalovirus	Eye, CNS, GI tract, lungs
Herpes simplex	Mucous membranes, skin
Herpes zoster	Skin
BACTERIA	
Mycobacterium avium-intracellulare	Disseminated
Mycobacterium tuberculosis	Lungs, CNS, disseminated

80% of the dose is excreted unchanged in the urine within 24 hours. The drug has a half-life of 3.6 hours.[15]

Pentamidine isethionate   Pentamidine isethionate (Pentam 300) is another commonly used drug for PCP. The mode of action of pentamidine is not fully understood, but it probably interferes with nuclear metabolism. Information on the pharmacokinetic properties of pentamidine is also minimal, although recent studies do show a serum half-life of approximately 6 hours.

Since pentamidine is not absorbed orally, it must be administered parenterally for acute infections. It usually is administered intravenously every 24 hours. The diluted drug solution should be infused over a period of 60 minutes to prevent severe hypotensive episodes. In addition to severe hypotension, the drug has produced hypoglycemia and cardiac arrhythmias. Serum glucose levels should be monitored daily during therapy and for several months after therapy has been completed. Obtaining daily blood urea nitrogen and serum creatinine determinations is also recommended.

Pentamidine (Nebupent) is also administered by inhalation via a Respirgard II jet nebulizer. In this dosage form the drug is administered every 4 weeks to prevent PCP in high-risk, HIV-infected clients. Usually 300 mg of pentamidine is dissolved in 6 ml of sterile water (the drug precipitates in 0.9% sodium chloride) and is administered over a 30- to 45-minute period. If the client develops bronchospasm from pentamidine, he or she receives a β_2-agonist before the pentamidine aerosol treatment.[15,26] Since there are questions about the safety of health care workers exposed to aerosol pentamidine, the client usually administers the treatment to himself or herself in a closed room. (See Chapter 60 for additional information on pentamidine.)

Table 53–3 summarizes the drug therapy for PCP.

Drug Therapy for Cytomegalovirus Retinitis

CMV represents a group of highly host-specific herpesviruses that infect man, monkeys, and rodents. CMV is a common cause of infection in immunocompromised individuals, producing damage to the lung, intestines, and retina. CMV retinitis occurs in approximately 5% of the individuals with HIV infection. Indications of the disease include fever, fatigue, malaise, weight loss, blurred vision, and retinal hem-

TABLE 53–3
Drug Therapy for **Pneumocystis carinii** *Pneumonia*

Drug Name	Dosage and Route of Administration

Sulfamethoxazole-trimethoprim
(Bactrim, Septra, Trisulfam)
HOW SUPPLIED
IV solution: 80 mg/16 mg/ml
Oral suspension: 200 mg/40 mg/5 ml
Uncoated tablet: 400 mg/80 mg, 800
   mg/160 mg
	ADULTS
	Oral: 20 mg/kg trimethoprim and 100 mg/kg sulfamethoxazole per 24 h given in equally
	   divided doses q6h for 14 d
	CHILDREN
	Oral: Dosage amounts are given q6h for 14 d
	Weight 18 lb (8 kg): 5 ml (1 tsp)
	Weight 35 lb (16 kg): 10 ml (2 tsp) *or* 1 tablet
	Weight 53 lb (24 kg): 15 ml (3 tsp) *or* 1½ tablets
	Weight 70 lb (32 kg): 20 ml (4 tsp) *or* 2 tablets or 1 Septra DS tablet
	IV
	Children >2 mo of age to adult: total daily dose, 15-20 mg/kg (based on the trimetho-
	   prim component) given in three to four equally divided doses q6 or 8h for up to 14 d
	Dose diluted in 5% dextrose in water and infused slowly at separate site

Pentamidine Isethionate
(NebuPent, Pentam 300)
HOW SUPPLIED
IV, IM: 30 mg/ml (300-mg vial)
Inhalation nebulizer: 300 mg vial
	For Prevention
	NEBULIZER
	Adults
	300 mg once q4wk
	Children
	Safety and effectiveness not established
	IV
	Adults and Children
	4 mg/kg once a day for 14 d: first dissolve contents of one vial in 5 ml sterile water or 5%
	   dextrose solution; withdraw the calculated dose and dilute further in 50-250 ml of 5%
	   dextrose solution; infuse over 1 h
	IM
	Adults and Children
	4 mg/kg once a day for 14 d; dissolve one vial (300 mg) in 3 ml sterile water; withdraw
	   calculated daily dose and administer by deep IM injection

ATOVAQUONE (Mepron) **HOW SUPPLIED** Oral tablet: 250 mg	*Adults* 750 mg administered with food tid for 21 d (total daily dose, 2250 mg) *Children* Dose not established

orrhage.[2] Ganciclovir sodium and foscarnet sodium are used to treat CMV retinitis.

GANCICLOVIR SODIUM

Ganciclovir sodium is 9-guanine; the drug is sometimes referred to as *DHPG*.[15,18]

Pharmacotherapeutics   Because of its potential for causing serious undesired clinical responses, ganciclovir (Cytovene) is indicated only for life-threatening or sight-threatening infections caused by CMV.

Pharmacokinetics   Ganciclovir is widely distributed in tissues, including the brain. It has an elimination half-life of approximately 3 hours and a bioavailability of less than 10%. The drug is excreted unchanged by the kidneys in concentrations equaling 90% of the IV dose.

Pharmacodynamics   Ganciclovir is phosphorylated by the viral thymidine kinase of HSV-1 or HSV-2 to its monophosphate form within infected cells. Monophosphate is converted to the active triphosphate, which inhibits viral DNA polymerase, by activity of cellular enzymes. In addition, when incorporated into a growing DNA strand, triphosphate causes premature termination of the growing DNA chain.

Ganciclovir's antiviral effects on CMV are less certain since these viruses do not have viral thymidine kinases. The initial phosphorylation of ganciclovir is presumed to occur by the action of viral or cellular deoxyguanosine kinases. This activity allows the incorporation of ganciclovir into replicating CMV DNA. The triphosphate form of the drug accumulates in significantly higher concentrations in infected cells.

Pharmaceutics   Ganciclovir is available as an IV preparation.

Undesired clinical responses   Ganciclovir can produce dose-related bone marrow depression. Additional undesired clinical responses include fever, rash, abnormal hepatic and renal function, GI disturbances such as nausea, vomiting, and anorexia, granulocytopenia, and thrombocytopenia. In test animals ganciclovir has shown carcinogenic potential and has produced spermatogenesis.

Contraindications and precautions   Administration and dosages of the drug should be adjusted for clients with renal or hepatic impairment.

Drug-drug and drug-nutrient interactions   Ganciclovir is usually not used concurrently with zidovudine since the combination causes severe myelosuppression. Additionally, ganciclovir may antagonize the antiviral effect of zidovudine. It is also possible for probenecid to reduce the renal clearance of ganciclovir. Since excretion of the drug by the kidneys requires adequate hydration, the client's fluid intake must be maintained.

Life-span considerations   Administration of ganciclovir to pregnant and lactating women is contraindicated. Use in children requires extreme caution because of the probability of long-term carcinogenicity and reproductive toxicity.

Specific drug-related nursing considerations   You must assess for a history of renal impairment. You should also review baseline studies of hepatic and renal function and CBC with differential. This information helps identify early indications of drug intolerance when examining future laboratory studies.

Follow package directions for drug dilution carefully. Reconstitute the drug with bacteriostatic water and administer it with a controlled infusion device. Since ganciclovir is potentially carcinogenic, it should be handled, administered, and disposed of according to Occupational Safety and Health Administration (OSHA) guidelines. Monitor the infusion closely; phlebitis and pain at the infusion site are common.

FOSCARNET SODIUM

Foscarnet sodium (Foscavir) is an organic analog of inorganic pyrophosphate.[15,27]

Pharmacotherapeutics   Foscarnet is specifically indicated in the treatment of CMV retinitis in clients with AIDS.

Pharmacokinetics   Studies have shown that 14% to 17% of foscarnet is bound to plasma protein. In a client with normal renal function, the plasma half-life is 3 to 4 hours. Foscarnet crosses the blood-brain barrier. It is not known if it crosses the placental barrier or if it is excreted in breast milk. Approximately 90% of foscarnet is excreted unchanged via the kidneys.

Pharmacodynamics   Foscarnet exerts its antiviral activity by selective inhibition at the pyrophosphate-binding site on virus-specific DNA polymerase and reverse transcriptase.

Pharmaceutics   Foscarnet is available only as an IV solution.

Undesired clinical responses   Undesired clinical responses include fever, fatigue, malaise, headache, and GI disturbances. In addition, abnormal renal function, electrolyte disturbances of calcium, phosphorous, magnesium, and potassium, seizures, and anemia have been reported.

Contraindications and precautions   The high probability of nephrotoxicity requires that this drug be administered with adequate volumes of fluid. Additionally, concurrent administration of highly nephrotoxic drugs is contraindicated.

Life-span considerations   Foscarnet is classified as a Pregnancy Category C drug. Its safety and effectiveness in children have not been studied. Additionally, no studies of the efficacy or safety of foscarnet in individuals over age 65 have been conducted.

Specific drug-related nursing considerations   Before administering foscarnet, assess the client for a history of renal impairment. Baseline laboratory values for blood urea nitrogen, creatine clearance, and serum electrolytes should be examined as a basis for comparison after therapy is initiated.

Because of the risk of phlebitis at the infusion site, be certain to establish an adequate IV line. Administer the prepared drug solution over a period of 60 minutes, using an IV infusion device. Monitor the client's intake and output and assess laboratory values for renal function and electrolyte balance.

Table 53–4 summarizes the drug therapy for CMV retinitis.

TABLE 53–4
Drug Therapy for Cytomegalovirus Retinitis

Drug Name	Dosage and Route of Administration	Nursing Considerations
Foscarnet Sodium (Foscavir) **HOW SUPPLIED** IV solution: 24 mg/ml	**ADULTS** Initial dose: 60 mg/kg, adjusted for client's individual renal function, given intravenously at a constant rate over a minimum of 1 h q8h for 2-3 wk; infusion pump must be used to control the rate of infusion; adequate hydration is recommended to minimize renal toxicity Maintenance dose: 90-120 mg/kg/d given as an IV infusion over 2 h **CHILDREN** Not established	**Assess** Determine if client is pregnant; foscarnet is classified as a Pregnancy Category C drug. Determine if client has preexisting renal impairment. **Implement** Drug is deposited in teeth and bone; administer with caution in children. Administer either by central venous line or peripheral vein. Dilute with 5% dextrose in water when administered peripherally. Do not administer other drugs concurrently via same catheter. **Monitor** Monitor for major toxicity: renal impairment, neurotoxicity, seizures. Monitor laboratory studies: serum creatinine, serum electrolytes. Monitor for undesired clinical responses: fever, fatigue, rigors, malaise, infection, headache, dizziness, anorexia, nausea, vomiting. **Evaluate** Evaluate for diminished indication of CMV.
Ganciclovir Sodium (Cytovene) **HOW SUPPLIED** IV solution: 500 mg/vial	**ADULTS** Initial dose for client with normal renal function: 5 mg/kg (given IV at a constant rate over 1 h) q12h for 14-21 d Maintenance dose: 5 mg/kg (given as IV infusion over 1 h) once a day, 7 d a week *or* 6 mg/kg once a day on 5 d of each week	**Assess** Determine if client has preexisting renal impairment. Assess if client is nursing; nursing should not be resumed until at least 72 h after the last dose. **Implement** Reconstitute with 10 ml sterile water. Do not use bacteriostatic water. Shake vial to dissolve the drug. Inspect reconstituted solution for particulate matter and discoloration. Discard if either is present. Reconstituted solution in vial is stable at room temperature for 12h. Do not refrigerate. Infuse only into veins with adequate blood flow. Do not administer by rapid or bolus IV injection. Client should be informed that drug causes inhibition of spermatogenesis. Use with extreme caution in children. Infuse in 0.9% sodium chloride, 5% dextrose, Ringer's or lactated Ringer's solution. Use appropriate handling and disposal techniques. **Monitor** Monitor laboratory studies for granulocytosis and thrombocytopenia. Assess for undesired clinical responses: chills, edema, malaise, infections.

Drug Therapy for *Mycobacterium avium-intracellulare* Complex

Mycobacterium avium-intracellulare complex (MAC) bacteremia is a frequent late-occurring opportunistic infection in individuals with AIDS. Infections caused by this microorganism do not respond well to conventional antimycobacterial drugs such as isoniazid. In fact, at present no drug regimen has consistently controlled MAC bacteremia or changed the prognosis of the disease.

One drug group that has shown promise in the treatment of MAC bacteremia is the **macrolides.** These drugs are broad-spectrum antibiotics that act by inhibiting bacterial protein synthesis. Erythromycin is the oldest member of the group. **Clarithromycin** (Biaxin) and **azithromycin** (Zithromax), the newest macrolides, are derivatives of erythromycin. These drugs are more active against bacteria sensitive to erythromycin. In addition, they have a slightly broader spectrum of activity and a lower incidence of GI disturbances. Since both drugs have a longer serum half-life than erythromycin, they can be administered less frequently. In studies both drugs have been effective in the treatment of disseminated MAC.[27-29] (See Chapter 55 for additional information on the macrolides.)

Rifabutin (Mycobutin) is the first drug approved for the prevention of MAC. Rifabutin probably inhibits DNA-dependent RNA polymerase. Although administered orally, the drug is poorly absorbed by this route. Rifabutin is metabolized in the liver to three active metabolites. The drug has a serum half-life of 36 hours. A small percentage of rifabutin is excreted unchanged in the urine.

Rifabutin use is contraindicated in clients with active tuberculosis. There is a high potential for drug-drug interactions with rifabutin, but clinical information on them is lacking. Rifabutin is generally well tolerated. Neutropenia, GI disturbances, and drug rashes have been reported. Clients receiving rifabutin experience a brown-orange discoloration of the skin and body fluids (urine, feces, saliva, sputum, tears) similar to that caused by rifampin.[21]

DRUG THERAPY FOR AIDS-ASSOCIATED NEOPLASMS

Clients infected with HIV are prone to developing certain rare neoplastic diseases because of their immunosuppression. These neoplasms can be treated with antineoplastic drugs and interferons. However, the role of antineoplastic drug therapy is limited because of poor response rates. Interferon alfa-2a, which has antiviral and immunoregulatory properties, has been approved for treatment of Kaposi's sarcoma, which is a multifocal, metastasizing reticulosis involving primarily the skin. (It is an opportunistic neoplasm specifically associated with AIDS.) Interferon alfa-2a decreases circulating p24 antigen and blocks HIV assembly and release. (See Chapters 59 and 69 for additional information about interferons and antineoplastic drugs.)

CONCEPT REVIEW

Opportunistic infections and neoplasms occur as a result of the individual's immunosuppression.

Most of these disorders are treated with a variety of drugs in hopes that an effective combination can be achieved.

SUMMARY

AIDS is caused by the human immunodeficiency virus, a retrovirus containing RNA and reverse transcriptase. Once in the body, the HIV invades the host cells and infects CD4$^+$ T-helper cells. What follows is progressive viral replication and CD4$^+$ T-cell loss, eventually leading to severe immunodeficiency. As a result of the immunosuppressed state, the individual is at risk of opportunistic infections and neoplasms.

At present, there is no cure for AIDS. Treatment is directed at slowing the disease process and preventing complications. For the client with AIDS, the nurse's role includes providing supportive, sensitive care. The nurse has an important role in educating the HIV-negative population about AIDS and methods to prevent HIV infection.

REFERENCES

1. Centers for Disease Control. (1992). Projections of the number of persons diagnosed with AIDS and the number of immunosuppressed HIV-infected persons—United States, 1992-1994. *Morbidity and Mortality Weekly Report, 41*(RR-18), 1-14.
2. Monahan, F.D., Drake, T., & Neighbors, M. (1994). *Nursing care of adults.* Philadelphia: W.B. Saunders.
3. Lifson, A.R., Hessol, N.A., & Rutherford, G.W. (1992). Progression and clinical outcome of infection due to human immunodeficiency virus. *Clinics in Infectious Disease, 14,* 966-972.
4. McCance, K., & Huether, S. (1990). *Pathophysiology: The biologic basis for disease in adults and children.* St. Louis: C.V. Mosby.
5. Centers for Disease Control. (1992). 1993 revised classification system for HIV infection and expanded surveillance case definition for AIDS among adolescents and adults. *Morbidity and Mortality Weekly Report, 41*(RR-17), 1-14.
6. Centers for Disease Control. (1990). Update: Acquired immunodeficiency syndrome—United States 1989. *Morbidity and Mortality Weekly Report, 39*(5), 81.
7. Barrick, B. (1990). Light at the end of a decade. *American Journal of Nursing, 90*(11), 37.
8. Occupational Safety and Health Administration. (1991, December 7). *29CFR, Part 1910.1030 Occupational exposure to bloodborne pathogens: Final rule.* U.S. Department of Labor, Washington D.C..
9. Centers for Disease Control. (1991). Summary of notifiable diseases, United States—1990. *Morbidity and Mortality Weekly Report, 39*(53), 16.
10. Henderson, D., Fahey, B., Willy, M., et al. (1990). Risk for occupational transmission of human immunodeficiency virus Type 1 (HIV-1) associated with clinical exposures: A prospective evaluation. *Annals of Internal Medicine, 113,* 740-746.

11. Dutz, A., Hutton, N., Joyner, M., et al. (1993). HIV infected women and infants: Social and health factors impeding utilization of health care. *Journal of Nurse Midwifery, 30*(2), 103-109.
12. Connolly, K.J., & Hammer, S.M. (1992). Antiretroviral therapy: Reverse transcriptase inhibition. *Antimicrobial Agents and Chemotherapy, 36,* 245-254.
13. Connolly, K.J., & Hammer, S.M. (1992). Antiretroviral therapy: Strategies beyond single-agent reverse transcriptase inhibition. *Antimicrobial Agents and Chemotherapy, 36,* 509-520.
14. Unadkat, J.D., Collier, A.C., Crosby, S.S., et al. (1990). Pharmacokinetics of oral zidovudine (azidothymidine) in patients with AIDS when administered with and without a high-fat meal. *AIDS, 4,* 229-232.
15. U.S. Pharmacopeial Convention. (1990). *United States pharmacopeia* (22nd rev.). Rockville, MD: Author.
16. Wilde, M., & Langtry, M. (1992). Zidovudine. An update of its pharmacodynamic and pharmacokinetic properties, and therapeutic efficacy. *Drugs, 40,* 515-570.
17. McLeod, G., Hammer, S.M. (1992). Zidovudine: Five years later. *Annals of Internal Medicine, 117,* 487-501.
18. Arvin, A. (1992). Antiviral drugs. In C.M. Smith and A.M. Reynard (Eds.), *Textbook of pharmacology* (pp. 900-912). Philadelphia: W.B. Saunders.
19. Drusano, G.L., Yuen, G.J., Lambert, J.S., et al. (1992). Relationship between dideoxyinosine exposure, CD4 counts and p24 antigen levels in human immunodeficiency virus infection. *Annals of Internal Medicine, 116,* 562-566.
20. Anastasi, J., & Rivera, J. (1991). AIDS drug update: DDI and DDC. *Rn Magazine, 54*(11), 41-43.
21. Meyer, C. (1993). New drugs: A banner year for AIDS therapy. *American Journal of Nursing, 93*(5), 58-63.
22. Masur, H. (1992). Prevention and treatment of *Pneumocystis* pneumonia. *New England Journal of Medicine, 327,* 1853-1860.
23. Stein, D.S., Stevens, R.C., Terry, B., et al. (1991). Use of low-dose trimethoprim-sulfamethoxazole thrice weekly for primary and secondary prophylaxis of *Pneumocystis carinii* pneumonia in human immunodeficiency virus infected patients. *Antimicrobial Agents and Chemotherapy, 35,* 1705-1709.
24. Holdcraft, O. (1993). Atovaquone: A new oral treatment for pneumocystis. *Nurse Practitioner: American Journal of Primary Health Care, 18*(9), 22.
25. Artymowicz, R.J., & James, V.E. (1993). Atovaquone: A new antipneumocystis agent. *Clinical Pharmacokinetics, 12,* 563-570.
26. Smith, C.L. (1990). Nursing management of aerosolized pentamidine administration. *AIDS Patient Care, 4,* 13-17.
27. Polis, M.A., DeSmet, M., Baird, B.F., et al. (1993). Increased survival of a cohort of patients with acquired immunodeficiency syndrome and cytomegalovirus retinitis who receive sodium phosphonoformate (foscarnet). *American Journal of Medicine, 94,* 175-180.
28. Kemper, C.A., Meng, T.C., Nussbaum, J., et al. (1992). Treatment of *Mycobacterium avium* complex bacteremia in AIDS with a four-drug oral regimen. *Annals of Internal Medicine, 116,* 466-472.
29. Piscitelli, S.C., Danziger, L.H., & Rodvold, K.A. (1992). Clarithromycin and azithromycin: New macrolide antibiotics. *Clinical Pharmacokinetics, 11,* 137-152.

BIBLIOGRAPHY

Coleman, R., & Geletko, S. (1993). Avoiding drug interactions in HIV disease. *Patient Care, 27*(14), 152-165.

Fuerst, M. (1993). Current trends in the treatment and prevention of opportunistic infections. *AIDS Patient Care, 7*(1), 38-39.

Henry, S.B., & Holzemer, W. (1992). Critical care management of the patient with HIV infection who has *Pneumocystis carinii* pneumonia. *Heart and Lung, 21,* 243-249.

Kahn, J. (1991). Clinical issues in using didanosine (ddI). *AIDS Clinical Care, 3,* 89-96.

Rice, R. (1992). Caring for patients with AIDS. In R. Rice (Ed.), *Home health nursing: Concepts and application.* St. Louis: Mosby–Year Book.

Timby, B. (1992). Pneumocystosis in patients with Acquired Immunodeficiency Syndrome. *Critical Care Nurse, 12*(7), 64-71.

Workman, L., Ellerhorst-Ryan, J., & Hargrave-Koertge, V. (Eds.). (1993). *Nursing care of the immunocompromised patient.* Philadelphia: W.B. Saunders.

Antimicrobial Drugs

CHAPTER 54

PRINCIPLES OF
Antimicrobial Therapy

ANGELA M. ROSSINGTON

⊛ **Infectious Process**
LEARNING OBJECTIVES:
Summarize the chain of infection.
Describe each stage in the course of an infection.
KEY TERMS:
Incubation period, infection, microorganisms, pathogen, prodromal stage, reservoir

⊛ **History and Sources of Antimicrobials**
LEARNING OBJECTIVES:
Discuss the impact of antimicrobials on disease prevention and health restoration.
Identify two sources of antimicrobials.

⊛ **Classification of Antimicrobials**
LEARNING OBJECTIVES:
Describe three methods of classifying antimicrobials.
Explain the meaning of *spectrum of activity.*
KEY TERMS:
Broad spectrum, narrow spectrum

⊛ **Selection of Antimicrobials**
LEARNING OBJECTIVE: Summarize factors to consider when selecting antimicrobial drugs.

⊛ **Acquired Resistance to Antimicrobials**
LEARNING OBJECTIVE: Describe two ways resistance to antimicrobials is acquired.
KEY TERM: Acquired resistance

⊛ **Undesired Responses to Antimicrobials**
LEARNING OBJECTIVE: Identify common undesired responses to antimicrobials.

⊛ **Nursing Process**
LEARNING OBJECTIVE: Describe general nursing care of a client receiving antimicrobial drugs.

CONCEPTS AND TERMS TO REVIEW

Review content in Chapter 49 on nonspecific defense mechanisms.
Review the different types of pathogens (bacteria, viruses, fungi, and protozoa) in a microbiology textbook.

---

*I*nfectious diseases have featured prominently in the history of humans, causing epidemics and pandemics that have resulted at times in high mortality rates. During the Middle Ages, a pandemic of bubonic plague, the Black Death, and smallpox killed thousands in England and Europe. In the early Twentieth Century, yellow fever held up the completion of the Panama Canal. During the 1940s and 1950s, polio killed and crippled thousands in the United States and Europe. Influenza, pneumonia, and tuberculosis remain leading causes of death in the United States.[1,2]

Today thousands of drugs are used to treat the diseases produced by pathogenic organisms. Administration of these drugs becomes a routine part of nursing care. This chapter reviews the chain of infection and course of infection. It then focuses on the classification of antimicrobial drugs, drug selection, antimicrobial drug resistance, and undesired responses to antimicrobial drug therapy. Knowledge of this information enables the nurse to give safe, effective nursing care.

INFECTIOUS PROCESS

Infection is an invasion by and multiplication of an organism in body tissues. The process begins with transmission of the infectious organism and ends when symptoms disappear.

Chain of Infection

The spread of infection requires the presence of the following: an infectious agent or **pathogen;** a **reservoir** in which the pathogen flourishes; a portal of exit from the reservoir; a mode of transmission; a portal of entry; and a susceptible host[3] (Fig. 54–1). All elements in the chain of infection must remain intact to produce an infection. Conversely, a break in this chain at any point prevents the spread of infection. Interruption of this chain is the primary goal of antimicrobial therapy.

Infectious agents Pathogenic organisms include bacteria, viruses, fungi, and protozoa. The potential for these organisms to produce disease depends on their number, virulence, ability to enter the host, and susceptibility of the host.

Reservoir   Microorganisms need a reservoir in which to flourish. Most microorganisms have many sources or reservoirs for growth. One of the most common is the human body itself. Animals, plants, insects, inanimate objects, food, and water are also reservoirs for infectious organisms. The presence of food, oxygen, water, proper temperature, light, and proper pH determines the appropriateness of a reservoir.

Portal of exit   The portal of exit facilitates the microorganism's escape to another host. When the reservoir is a human, microorganisms can exit through the skin, mucous membranes, respiratory tract, urinary tract, gastrointestinal (GI) tract, reproductive tract, or blood.

Mode of transmission There are many vehicles for transmission of microorganisms from the reservoir to the host. Direct, indirect, and droplet contacts are involved in the transmission of many infections. Contaminated items and vectors (e.g., insects and animals) are also modes of transmission.

Portal of entry Organisms can enter the body through the same routes as portals of exit. Factors that reduce the body's defense mechanisms enhance the chances of pathogens' entering the body.

Susceptible host Whether an individual acquires an infection depends on his or her susceptibility. Susceptibility is the degree of resistance or immunity an individual has to pathogens. Resistance to infection by pathogenic organisms is a product of the host's defense mechanisms. These mechanisms include nonspecific resistance of intact barriers (e.g., skin and mucous membranes), an intact immune system, and factors such as nutrition, age, stress, emotional status, existing illness, and environment. (See Chapter 49 for an overview of the body's biologic defense mechanisms.)

Course of Infection

The infectious process can be divided into specific stages, which describe events occurring in the body at that time. The first stage, the **incubation period,** represents the interval between the entrance of the pathogenic organism into the body and the appearance of the first symptoms. Incubation periods vary from a few days to several months, depending on the causative organism and type of disease.

The second stage is the **prodromal stage.** This stage represents the interval from onset of nonspecific clinical manifestations to more specific ones. During the prodromal stage, the host is able to spread the disease to others, and the organism continues to grow and multiply. The **illness stage** is the third stage. During this interval, the host manifests the clinical signs and symptoms specific to the infection. **Convalescence** is the final stage. This interval represents the disappearance of acute symptoms of infection. Convalescence or recovery may take several days to months.

CONCEPT REVIEW

An infection can be caused by a variety of microorganisms.

The severity of the infection depends in part on the virulence of the organism and the susceptibility of the host.

Interruption of the chain of infection (i.e., infectious agent, reservoir, portal of exit, mode of transmission, portal of entry, and susceptible host) is a function of antimicrobial therapy.

HISTORY AND SOURCES OF ANTIMICROBIALS

The modern era of antimicrobial drug therapy began in the 1930s with the introduction of the first sulfonamides. In the 1940s penicillin was introduced into civilian hospitals. Penicillin was considered a miracle drug since it was effective against staphylococci, streptococci, and pneumococci, which were serious infectious pathogens at that time. Since the 1950s the number and variety of antimicrobial drugs have grown significantly. However, the range of opportunities for further discoveries is enormous.

Early antimicrobial drugs, with the exception of the sulfonamides, were obtained from natural sources such as fungi and bacteria. Today many of the drugs are synthetic or semisynthetic products.

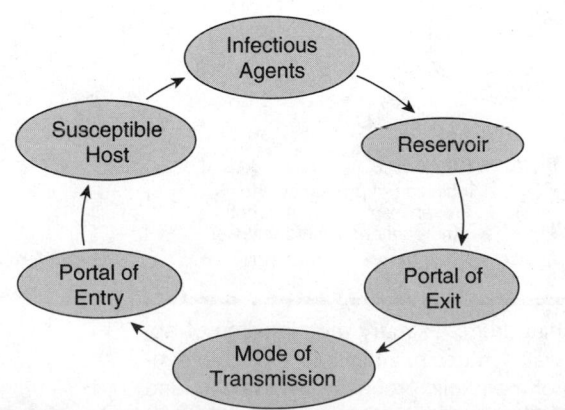

FIGURE 54–1   Chain of infection.

CLASSIFICATION OF ANTIMICROBIAL DRUGS

Several classification methods are used with antimicrobial drugs. These drugs may be classified according to the microorganisms affected, mechanism of action, and/or spectrum of activity. The following sections discuss each of these methods of classification.

Microorganisms Affected

A wide range of microorganisms is susceptible to drug therapy; some pathogens are easier to treat than others. Classifications of these drugs vary in different sources and reference books. For the purpose of this text, the following classifications are used: antibiotics, urinary tract anti-infectives, antimycobacterials, antifungals, antivirals, and antiparasitics.

Antibiotics comprise the largest group of drugs. They are used to treat infections caused by bacteria that are gram negative (e.g., *Escherichia coli, Haemophilus, Pseudomonas aeruginosa*) and gram positive (e.g., *Clostridium, Staphylococcus,* and *Streptococcus* species). These drugs are subclassified according to chemical class (e.g., β-lactam, cephalosporins, tetracyclines, aminoglycosides, sulfonamides). (Information on antibiotics is contained in Chapter 55.)

Urinary tract anti-infectives and antiseptics are used to treat urinary tract infections (UTIs). These infections are caused by a variety of microorganisms (e.g., *E. coli, Pseudomonas, Klebsiella*). Most urinary tract anti-infectives and antiseptics are limited to this specific problem. (Information on urinary tract anti-infectives and antiseptics is contained in Chapter 56.)

Antimycobacterial agents are used to treat infections caused by the bacterium *Mycobacterium.* Tuberculosis and leprosy are caused by this mycobacterium. (Information on antimycobacterial agents is contained in Chapter 57.)

Antifungal drugs are divided into two major groups: drugs that treat superficial mycoses and drugs that treat systemic mycoses. (Information on antifungal drugs is contained in Chapter 58.)

Antiviral drugs are active against a narrow range of viruses, and their clinical applications are limited to just a few viral infections. (Information on antiviral drugs is contained in Chapter 59.)

Antiparasitic drugs are used to treat diseases caused by helminths, protozoans, and ectoparasites. (Information on antiparasitic drugs is contained in Chapter 60.)

Mechanism of Action

Primary mechanisms of action of antimicrobial drugs are inhibition of cell wall synthesis; inhibition of protein synthesis; alteration of cell wall permeability; inhibition of metabolic processes in the cell; and inhibition of nucleic acid synthesis (Fig. 54–2). These actions either destroy or lyse the infecting organism (bactericidal) or inhibit the growth of the organism (bacteriostatic).

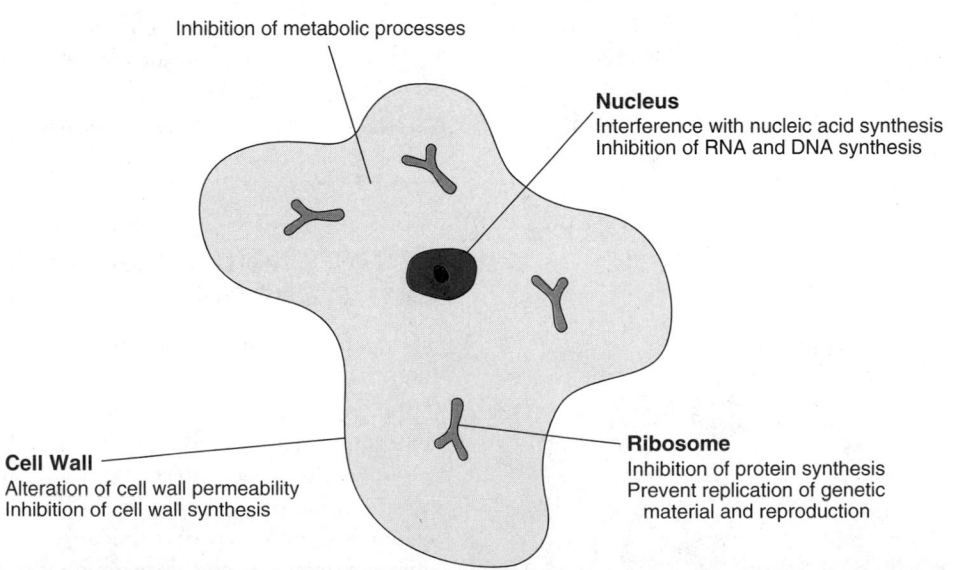

Inhibition of metabolic processes

Nucleus
Interference with nucleic acid synthesis
Inhibition of RNA and DNA synthesis

Cell Wall
Alteration of cell wall permeability
Inhibition of cell wall synthesis

Ribosome
Inhibition of protein synthesis
Prevent replication of genetic
material and reproduction

FIGURE 54–2   Mechanism of action of antimicrobial drugs. Primary mechanisms of action of antimicrobial drugs include inhibition of cell wall synthesis, inhibition of protein synthesis, alteration of cell wall permeability, inhibition of metabolic processes in the cell, and inhibition of nucleic acid synthesis. These actions either destroy or lyse the infecting organism or inhibit the growth of the organism.

Inhibition of cell wall synthesis Some antimicrobial drugs affect enzymes that are necessary for cell wall formation and integrity. This action results in lysis of the cell and destruction of the organism. Compounds that inhibit any step in the formation or maintenance of the cell wall are bactericidal. For example, penicillins inhibit the enzyme transpeptidase that resides on the outer surface of the cytoplasmic membrane.[4]

Inhibition of protein synthesis Some antimicrobial drugs cause the formation of abnormal proteins that impede translation of genetic material. Other drugs irreversibly bind to cellular ribosomes and prevent replication of genetic material and reproduction. These drugs can be either bactericidal or bacteriostatic. For example, aminoglycosides bind to proteins on the 30S ribosome of bacteria and inhibit protein synthesis. These drugs are considered bactericidal. With chloramphenicol and the tetracyclines, the binding is weak, and the end result is a bacteriostatic action.[4]

Alteration of cell wall permeability Antimicrobial drugs in this group bind to specific cell wall components. This alters the permeability of the cell wall, resulting in leakage of intracellular components. For example, amphotericin B, an antifungal agent, is incorporated into the fungal cell wall and causes leakage and cell death.[4]

Inhibition of cellular metabolic processes These antimicrobial drugs block or alter metabolic pathways that are essential to normal functioning of the cell. Sulfonamides, for example, inhibit folic acid synthesis.[4]

Inhibition of nucleic acid synthesis Drugs in this group inhibit RNA and DNA synthesis. Certain antiviral drugs act by inhibiting viral RNA and DNA synthesis.

Spectrum of Activity

The spectrum of an antimicrobial drug's activity refers to the number and type of organisms vulnerable to its effects. For example, bacteria are classified according to shape (i.e., bacilli, spirilla, cocci, rods) and reaction to laboratory staining procedure. The most common staining procedure is the Gram stain. The Gram stain distinguishes between bacteria with similar morphology and groups organisms into gram-positive or gram-negative organisms. Therefore the spectrum of an antimicrobial drug might be described as follows: *X* drug is effective against all gram-negative bacteria, whereas *Y* drug is effective against only bacilli.

Narrow-spectrum drugs affect a relatively limited number of microorganisms (e.g., penicillin G affects only gram-positive bacteria). These drugs act more specifically than most drugs and are less likely to destroy normal flora.

Broad-spectrum drugs, on the other hand, affect a wider range of organisms (e.g., both gram-negative and gram-positive bacteria, bacilli, and cocci). These drugs are useful in treating an infection for which the infecting organism has not been identified. However, the usefulness of these drugs is somewhat negated by their ability to destroy normal flora, diminishing one of the body's natural defense mechanisms.

Spectrum also refers to a drug's effect on microorganisms that are aerobic or anaerobic. *Aerobic* organisms exist in the presence of atmospheric oxygen, and *anaerobic* organisms cannot exist in the presence of oxygen in the atmosphere. These organisms obtain oxygen from oxygen-containing compounds (e.g., inorganic sulfates, nitrates).[5]

SELECTION OF ANTIMICROBIAL DRUGS

The goal of antimicrobial therapy is to control and effect a cure of the infection. To achieve this goal, agents must penetrate target tissues in adequate concentrations. Therefore the pharmacokinetics and pharmacodynamics of the drug, the suspected organism, and the site of infection must be considered. The choice of an appropriate antimicrobial is also based on careful assessment of the host; age and physical condition of the client; the most appropriate route of administration; cost of the drug regimen; and potential adverse reactions.

Infecting Pathogen

Since narrow-spectrum drugs are usually the most effective agents, it is important to identify the infecting organism as soon as possible. This is accomplished by establishing a culture of the infected material (e.g., sputum, drainage, blood, urine). Results of a culture for most microorganisms are available in 48 to 72 hours. Fungi and mycobacteria may require several weeks.[6] It is important to collect the infected specimen before starting antimicrobial therapy.

While awaiting the results of the culture or if the pathogenic organism cannot be identified, a broad-spectrum antimicrobial is usually prescribed. Selection of the broad-spectrum antimicrobial is based on the client's history and physical examination, site of infection, and presenting symptoms.

Combination therapy or the use of two or more antimicrobial drugs is necessary under certain circumstances. For example, combined therapy may be indicated when two different infectious organisms have been identified in the same host. Combination therapy is also used to prevent drug resistance, to treat resistant strains of bacteria, and to treat a serious infection whose causative agent has not been identified.

A few fixed-dose combinations such as trimethoprim-sulfamethoxazole (Bactrim, Septra) are available. However, fixed-dose combinations are rare and are prescribed only after careful assessment of the individual. Usually separate drugs are selected based on the specific microbes involved in the infection.

The administration of multiple drugs always carries the potential for adverse reactions and interactions that can harm the client. Careful monitoring of client reactions is necessary under any circumstances but particularly with combination treatment.

Site of Infection

Selection of the appropriate drug, route of administration, and dosage regimen is dependent in part on the site of infection. The pharmacokinetics of a drug, particularly its distribution to specific organs and tissues, must be considered. For example, a UTI is treated best with a drug that is concentrated in the urine such as nitrofurantoin (Macrodantin). Treatment of meningitis requires a drug that crosses the blood-brain barrier such as penicillin G (Pentids; Pfizerpen).

Route of administration is also a factor when considering the site of infection. For example, a *topical* antimicrobial preparation is appropriate for treating a mild skin infection, thus avoiding possible side effects from systemic therapy. The treatment of meningitis may require *intravenous* (IV) or *intrathecal* therapy.

Recipient of the Drug: The Client

Consideration must be given to physical, psychologic, social, cultural, and economic aspects of the client. A comprehensive physical assessment of the client is important. Factors to consider include the following: What is the status of the client's immune system? Does the client have impaired renal function that might impede the excretion of certain drugs? If renal impairment exists, are there nephrotoxic antimicrobial drugs that should be avoided? Does the client demonstrate manifestations of impaired liver function? If so, are there antimicrobial drugs that should be avoided? (Additional assessment factors are discussed in other chapters in this unit.)

The client's age is also an important consideration. Whenever possible, elderly clients should be prescribed oral drugs that are administered in the home environment. Treating the client in the home not only decreases the cost of drug therapy but diminishes the possibility of certain complications associated with hospitalization—nosocomial infection, disorientation, and deconditioning.[7]

Client compliance is also a factor in determining which drug to prescribe. Prescribing a drug that requires a complicated regimen might be contraindicated because of age or mental status of the client. Client education on correct administration of the drug, common side effects, and the necessity of completing the full course of therapy is essential to ensure successful treatment.

Another factor to consider when selecting an antimicrobial is the cost of a drug. Many clients cannot afford expensive antibiotics. Since generic antibiotics cost approximately one half to one third less than brand name drugs, they should be prescribed when appropriate. In addition, clients should be changed from IV to oral therapy as soon as possible to control cost.

New antimicrobial drugs are regularly introduced. Some of them are more expensive and more toxic than previously prescribed drugs. With some of them, research has not shown they are more effective. Therefore consideration should be given to using the older drugs if cost and potential undesired responses can be diminished.[8]

CONCEPT REVIEW

Fungi and bacteria are sources of antimicrobial preparations. Other antimicrobials are synthetic or semisynthetic.

Antimicrobials can be classified according to microorganism affected, mechanism of action, or spectrum of activity.

Many factors must be considered when selecting the most appropriate antimicrobial drug for a particular situation. Some of these factors include the type and virulence of the infecting organism, the site of the infection, and physical, social, economic, and psychologic condition of the client.

ACQUIRED RESISTANCE TO ANTIMICROBIALS

The term *strain* is used to describe a group of organisms within a species that are characterized by some particular quality. Strains of microorganisms with **acquired resistance** evolve through mutation, adaptation, or gene transfer and occur in one of the following ways:

- The microorganism develops a protective mechanism that prevents a drug from reaching its target site of action. *Pseudomonas,* for example, produces a protective membrane that keeps the drug from reaching the cell wall.
- The microorganism produces enzymes through chromosomal mutation that reduce or block the drug's effects. These strains of bacteria alter genetic material that code biochemical changes within their cells (e.g., aminotransferase inactivates gentamicin and chloramphenicol).
- Some bacteria develop methods of ejecting foreign molecules.[9]
- Normal flora may acquire and carry genes that confer resistance, transferring these genes to pathogenic organisms.[10]

Drug-resistant organisms first emerged in the early 1950s in the form of penicillin-resistant staphylococci. The widespread use of broad-spectrum antibiotics such as penicillins and tetracyclines in animal feed probably contributed to this situation.[10,11]

At present there are many strains of bacteria resistant to drugs. Methicillin-resistant *Staphylococcus aureus* (MRSA) was first reported in the United States in 1968. A newer strain of MRSA and a strain of bacteria resistant to aminoglycosides were reported in the 1970s. Resistant strains of *S. aureus* are common causes of nosocomial and community-acquired infections.[12,13] In addition, studies have shown that nursing staffs are being colonized with MRSA. This renders the staff carriers and endangers clients, especially those clients who are immunocompromised.[14]

Strains of *Neisseria gonorrhoeae* that are resistant to penicillin, tetracyline, cefoxitin, and spectinomycin have been found across the United States. Many strains of *Streptococcus pneumoniae,* which causes acute lower respiratory tract infections in children, have also developed. Vaccines are available against some but not all of these new strains. Virulent, drug-resistant strains of tuberculosis are threatening to produce epidemics in the United States, and *Haemophilus influenzae* is showing resistance in developing countries.[15–17]

Selecting alternative drugs is difficult. Cross-resistance to all drugs of similar chemical composition frequently occurs. As indicated previously, when combination therapy is used, the cost of drug therapy and the potential for allergic reaction increase.[10]

UNDESIRED RESPONSES TO ANTIMICROBIALS

Antimicrobial drugs affect biochemical processes that are essential to the life of a microbe. Theoretically, they do not affect the host cell. However, in reality antimicrobials are not purely selective. Therefore they cannot be regarded as benign or totally safe medications.

Antimicrobial agents produce a wide range of side and adverse effects. As indicated in Chapter 6, some undesired responses are predictable; others are considered idiosyncratic. Specific side effects associated with the various drug groups are discussed in more detail in later chapters in this unit. However, a general discussion of allergies and hypersensitivities, superinfections, organ toxicity, and GI effects is presented here since many of these responses are common to several antimicrobial classifications.

Allergies and Hypersensitivities

Allergic and hypersensitive reactions are the most common responses reported. They range from mild skin rashes to anaphylactic shock and death. Sensitivity can occur as the result of indirect exposure to the drugs (e.g., ingestion of food products from animals treated with antibiotics). Other responses result from direct exposure to internal or topical preparations of the drugs. Sensitivity can also occur across a class of antimicrobials that are related (e.g., between penicillins and cephalosporins). When allergic or hypersensitivity reactions occur, the drug is discontinued, and usually the primary care provider prescribes an antihistamine or epinephrine.

Superinfections

Normal flora protects the body against exogenous and endogenous pathogenic microorganisms. If normal flora is suppressed or destroyed, overgrowth of pathogenic microorganisms—a **superinfection**—can result. Superinfections are caused by broad-spectrum antimicrobials, combination therapy of antimicrobials, and administration of large doses of antimicrobials over a long period. Additional contributing factors include the client's age (the young and the elderly client are especially susceptible) and the status of the client's immune system. Recognition of the secondary infection and prompt response are critical since many of these infections are caused by resistant strains of microorganisms.

Organ Toxicity

Toxic effects from antimicrobials involve several organs or tissues, including the liver, the eighth cranial nerve (acoustic), the kidneys, and the nervous system. Bone marrow suppression with resulting blood dyscrasias and aplastic anemias and electrolyte imbalances also have been reported. In addition, teeth, nails and bones are sometimes affected.

Since most antimicrobials are excreted by the kidneys, clients with impaired renal function are at higher risk for complications. Performing renal function tests is recommended before and during treatment. Certain antimicrobials are known to be nephrotoxic (e.g., aminoglycosides) and should be used with extreme care in clients with impaired renal function.

Some potent antibiotics are used to treat cancerous tumors. These drugs kill cancer cells by interfering with DNA and RNA synthesis at various phases of the cell cycle. Although the action of these drugs is directed at cancer cells, their potency also makes them extremely toxic to normal cells. These drugs produce severe side effects, including nausea, vomiting, taste changes, stomatitis, anorexia, diarrhea, fever, alopecia, skin changes, phlebitis at the injection site, and vesication. In addition, they produce serious toxic effects to organs (e.g., the heart, lungs, and liver), cause severe blood dyscrasias, and affect the central nervous system.[18] (This topic is discussed more completely in Chapter 69.)

Gastrointestinal Effects

Many antimicrobials cause intestinal problems, and most have the potential to cause diarrhea, nausea, vomiting, and abdominal discomfort. This is especially true if the drugs are administered orally or in combinaton therapy.

Broad-spectrum antibiotics are more prone to produce GI problems than narrow-spectrum drugs. Some broad-spectrum drugs destroy normal flora that controls *Clostridium difficile* in the bowel. This allows the organism to proliferate and produce toxins, causing bowel inflammation and necrosis (colitis). Symptoms may occur within hours of the first dose or not until the client has taken many cycles of the same drug. Drugs most commonly associated with this problem are clindamycin, ampicillin, the cephalosporins, and certain aminoglycosides.[19]

CONCEPT REVIEW

Acquired resistance to antimicrobial therapy occurs when resistant strains of microorganisms develop.

When a strain of microorganisms develops resistance to a particular antimicrobial drug, cross-resistance usually develops in other closely related antimicrobial drugs.

Common undesired responses to antimicrobial therapy include allergies, hypersensitivity reactions, superinfections, organ toxicity, and GI problems.

▨ NURSING CONSIDERATIONS

The role of the nurse is crucial in all aspects of the infectious process—from preventing the spread of a pathogen to monitoring the therapy for an infected client. Effective nursing care begins with a thorough understanding of the infectious disease process. In addition, infection control measures and public education are imperative. To prevent the spread of the pathogen, you must use measures such as hand washing, gloves, and isolation procedures. It is also important that you participate in educating the public. Public education programs should contain information on personal and environmental hygiene, availability of immunizations, measures to prevent exposure to pathogens, and measures to prevent the spread of disease.

You are also responsible for monitoring the antimicrobial therapy. Obtaining a careful nursing history on admission is essential. Assess the client carefully for any history of drug allergies. If a history of allergies exists, carefully document your findings in the medical record. Follow the agency's procedure for marking charts and care plans of clients with allergies. In addition, most agencies have clients with allergies wear a special identification bracelet.

During the course of drug therapy, carefully monitor the client for allergic reactions and/or undesired responses. You must also educate the client about the drug. A principle that must be stressed with clients is that the full course of the antimicrobial regimen must be taken to ensure that all target organisms have been eliminated in the host. Microorganisms that are inhibited but not destroyed can develop resistance.[13]

The efficacy of some antimicrobials is evaluated by regular measurement of drug concentration levels in serum. The serum is usually drawn at times that coincide with the lowest concentration of drug in the serum *(trough level)* just before a dose is administered; with the highest concentrations *(peak level);* and at a point between doses *(mean level).* The timing of the blood draws is determined by the pharmacokinetics of a particular drug and by the route of administration. Documentation of all information is important because dosage adjustments depend on the values obtained. However, these laboratory studies do not take the place of subjective and objective assessment. Self-reporting by the client and observation of the client's condition are key components of the therapy.

SUMMARY

The advent of antimicrobial drugs has served the world's population well during much of this century. However, overuse and abuse of these drugs have resulted in the development of many resistant strains of microorganisms. Care must be taken by clinicians in the prescribing of antimicrobial drugs, and attention must be given to educating the client about proper drug administration.

REFERENCES

1. Kampmeir, R.H. (1989). From watchful waiting to antibiotics. *Journal of the American Medical Association, 262,* 2433-2436.
2. Krause, R.M. (1992). The origin of plagues old and new. *Science, 257,* 1073-1077.
3. Black, J., Matassarin-Jacobs, E. (1993). *Luckmann and Sorensen's medical-surgical nursing: A psychophysiologic approach* (4th ed.). Philadelphia: W.B. Saunders.
4. Smith, C., & Reynard, A. (1992). *Textbook of pharmacology.* Philadelphia: W.B. Saunders.
5. Styrt, B., & Gorbach, S.L. (1989). Recent developments in the understanding of pathogenesis and treatment of anaerobic infections. *New England Journal of Medicine, 321*(5), 298.
6. Chernecky, C., Krech, R., & Berger, B. (1993). *Laboratory tests and diagnostic procedures.* Philadelphia: W.B. Saunders.
7. McCue, J. (1992). Oral antibiotics: Practical prescribing rules for practitioners. *Geriatrics, 47*(7), 59-66.
8. Feder, H.M., Abrahamian, L.M., & Grant-Kels, J.M. (1991). Is penicillin still the drug of choice for non-bullous impetigo. *Lancet, 338,* 803-805.
9. Jacoby, G.A., & Archer, G.L. (1991). New mechanisms of bacterial resistance to antimicrobial agents. *New England Journal of Medicine, 324,* 601-611.
10. Wright, K. (1990). Bad new bacteria. *Science, 249,* 22-24.
11. Cohen, M.L. (1992). Epidemiology of drug resistance: Implications for a post-antimicrobial age. *Science, 257,* 1050-1055.
12. Kosmidis, J., et al. (1988). Staphylococcal infections in hospital: The Greek experience. *Journal of Hospital Infection, 11*(2), 109-115.
13. Shovein, J., & Young, M.S. (1992). MRSA: Pandora's box for hospitals. *American Journal of Nursing, 92*(2), 49-52.
14. Schwarcz, S.K., et al. (1990). National surveillance of antimicrobial resistance in *N. gonorrhea. Journal of the American Medical Association, 11,* 1413-1418.
15. Mastro, T.D., et al. (1991). Antimicrobial resistance of pneumococci in children with acute lower respiratory tract infection in Pakistan. *Lancet, 337,* 156-159.
16. Culliton, B.J. (1992). Drug resistant tuberculosis may bring epidemic. *Nature, 356,* 473.
17. Walters, P. (1990). Chemotherapy: A nurse's guide to action, administration and side effects. *RN Magazine, 53*(2), 52-63.
18. Rowland, M. (1989). When drug treatment causes diarrhea. *RN Magazine, 52*(12), 52-63.

BIBLIOGRAPHY

Becker, T.M., et al. (1990). Mortality from infectious diseases among New Mexico's American Indian, Hispanic Whites and other whites, 1958-87. *American Journal of Public Health, 80*(3), 320-324.

Denny, F.W. (1991). The streptococcus saga continues. *New England Journal of Medicine, 325*(2), 127-128.

Frieden, T.R., & Mangi, R.J. (1990). Inappropriate use of oral ciprofloxacin. *Journal of the American Medical Association, 264,* 1438-1440.

Neu, H.C. (1992). The crisis in antibiotic resistance. *Science, 257,* 1064-1073.

Schwartz, B., Faclam, R.R., & Breiman, R.F. (1990). Changing epidemiology of group A streptococcal infection in the U.S.A. *Lancet, 336,* 1167-1171.

Shovein, J. (1989). MRSA: An infection control crisis comes home. *RN Magazine, 52*(7), 42-47.

Wright, K. (1990). The policy response: In limbo. *Science, 249*(1), 24.

CHAPTER 55

Antibiotics

ROBERT J. KIZIOR • ANGELA M. ROSSINGTON • NORMA L. PINNELL

⊛ Nursing Considerations

LEARNING OBJECTIVES:

Develop a plan of care for a client requiring antibiotic therapy.

Identify factors that should be included in a teaching plan for the client receiving antibiotics.

⊛ Penicillins

LEARNING OBJECTIVES:

Describe the mechanism of action of the penicillins.

Discuss the differences in uses and undesired clinical responses among natural penicillins, penicillinase-resistant penicillins, aminopenicillins, and extended-spectrum penicillins.

KEY TERMS:

β-Lactam, β-lactamase, carbapenems, peptidoglycan

⊛ Cephalosporins

LEARNING OBJECTIVES:

Describe the mechanism of action of the cephalosporins.

Discuss the differences in uses, kinetics, undesired clinical responses, and spectrum of activity among first-, second-, and third-generation cephalosporins.

KEY TERMS:

Pseudolithiasis, pseudomembranous colitis

⊛ Aminoglycosides

LEARNING OBJECTIVES:

Describe the mechanism of action of aminoglycosides.

Discuss the differences in uses, kinetics, and spectrum of activity of the aminoglycosides.

Name the undesired clinical responses associated with aminoglycosides.

Discuss nursing considerations associated with aminoglycosides.

KEY TERMS:

Aminoglycoside, ototoxicity, nephrotoxicity

⊛ Quinolones

LEARNING OBJECTIVES:

Describe the mechanism of action of quinolones.

Explain the pharmacodynamic and pharmacotherapeutic properties of the quinolones.

⊛ Macrolides

LEARNING OBJECTIVES:

Describe the mechanism of action of macrolides.

Explain the pharmacodynamic and pharmacotherapeutic properties of the macrolides.

⊛ Sulfonamides

LEARNING OBJECTIVES:

Describe the mechanism of action of sulfonamides and trimethoprim.

Discuss the differences in uses and spectrum of activity among the sulfonamides.

Identify the adverse effects associated with the sulfonamides.

KEY TERMS:

Crystalluria, kernicterus

⊛ Tetracyclines

LEARNING OBJECTIVES:

Explain the mechanism of action of tetracyclines.

Discuss the differences in uses and kinetics of the tetracyclines.

Identify the adverse effects associated with the tetracyclines.

⊛ Miscellaneous Agents

LEARNING OBJECTIVES:

Describe the mechanism of action, uses, undesired clinical responses, and kinetics of clindamycin, chloramphenicol, and vancomycin.

Discuss nursing considerations specific to these antiinfectives.

CONCEPTS AND TERMS TO REVIEW

Review the different microorganisms responsible for infection, including gram-positive and gram-negative cocci and bacilli.
Review the concept of acquired resistance to antibiotics.
Review the host factors that modify the selection of an antibiotic, route of administration, and dosage.
Key terms to review: antibiotic, bactericidal, bacteriostatic, suprainfection.

Antibiotics are antimicrobial agents that act specifically against bacteria. Some are produced from microbes naturally; some are produced semisynthetically by modifying the natural compound; and others are produced totally synthetically. The search for new antibiotics continues. Scientists presently are developing theories to explain the emergence of antibiotics in the natural environment in the hope that new sources for these drugs can be found.

Chapter 54 provided general information on antiinfectives. This chapter addresses specific antibiotic drug categories: penicillins, cephalosporins, aminoglycosides, quinolones, macrolides, sulfonamides, tetracyclines, and miscellaneous agents. Initially pharmacologic properties common to the entire group are presented. Differences and drug-specific information are supplied when individual drugs are discussed.

NURSING CONSIDERATIONS

A thorough understanding of the pharmacodynamics and pharmacokinetics of antibiotics is essential to enable the nurse to administer them responsibly. The nurse's knowledge provides the basis of the plan of care.

Assessing While obtaining the **health history,** ask if the client has experienced any unusual reactions or problems with antiinfective drugs. Specifically ask about hives, rashes, or difficulty breathing. Check the medical history for contraindications specific for the class of antibiotics being prescribed. Collect a complete drug history to determine risk for drug-drug interactions.

During the **physical assessment** assess the client for indications of the infection. Assess temperature, blood pressure, pulse, and respiratory rate; review available laboratory results (e.g., complete blood count [CBC], urinalysis). When indicated, perform a complete head-to-toe examination. If the situation is not conducive to a complete examination, focus on specific body system(s) involved in the infection.

Diagnosing Based on the data collected, appropriate nursing diagnoses for the client may include the following:
• Anxiety related to change in health status.
• Ineffective breast-feeding related to interruption in breast-feeding during drug therapy.
• Fatigue related to altered body chemistry associated with drug therapy.

• Fear related to knowledge deficit of treatment plan.
• Fluid volume deficit related to diarrhea associated with drug therapy.

Planning As a part of the client's plan of care, identify teaching needs. Clients receiving antibiotics must be taught the following:
• To use antibiotics only under medical supervision
• The administration method and frequency schedule
• Signs and symptoms of side effects, adverse reactions, and toxic reactions
• To complete the recommended course of therapy
• To discard any drug remaining after the course of therapy has been completed
• Not to share prescription drugs with other individuals.

Develop teaching tools as needed; identify measures to increase the client's compliance with therapy. Determine the client's emotional and financial support systems. Antibiotics are frequently quite expensive, a factor that might diminish compliance.

With the client, establish expected outcomes. Possible outcomes follow:
• Client reports anxiety level is reduced.
• Client demonstrates healthy ways to deal with anxiety.
• Client reports improved sense of energy.
• Client participates in recommended treatment plan.
• Client uses resources effectively.
• Client demonstrates behaviors to monitor and correct deficit as indicated.

Implementing Report history of allergy to any antiinfective to the primary care provider. Conspicuously mark the client's record. Obtain diagnostic specimens for culture and sensitivity tests before administering the first antibiotic dose.

If the antibiotic is excreted mainly by the kidneys, anticipate using reduced dosages in clients with renal dysfunction. Schedule drug administration throughout the 24-hour period to maintain appropriate serum drug levels. (A drug administration schedule is determined in part by the half-life of the drug.) Encourage the client to maintain adequate hydration; ask the client to drink at least 2000 ml of water per day unless contraindicated.

Assess the client for superinfections, especially fungal infections characterized by black furred tongue, nausea, and diarrhea. Have the order for antibiotics reviewed at least every 5 to 7 days for renewal or discontinuance orders.

Evaluating Assess the client for therapeutic response such as reduction of fever, increased appetite, and increased sense of well being. Monitor serum drug levels throughout therapy to ensure the client is receiving the appropriate dosage. Review the expected outcomes with the client and determine changes needed in the plan of care.

PENICILLINS

Penicillins represent one of the most important groups of antibiotics. Penicillin was discovered by Alexander Fleming, a British scientist, in 1928. But it was not until World War II that the desperate need for a treatment for wound infections provided the motivation for the production of penicillin. The drug also proved itself useful in the successful treatment of many infectious diseases such as pneumonia, syphilis, and diphtheria. Presently the penicillins are the drugs of choice for treating a large variety of infections.[1]

The penicillins represent a group of antibiotics known as β-**lactam** antibiotics. These drugs all contain a β-lactam ring, a requirement for biologic activity. Penicillins can kill susceptible bacteria; thus they are termed *bactericidal.* They exert their effect by inhibiting cell wall synthesis, which is essential for normal growth and development of bacteria (Fig. 55–1).

A component of the cell wall, **peptidoglycan,** provides rigidity of the cell wall because of its cross-hatched lattice structure. Biosynthesis of peptidoglycan involves many enzymatic steps; it is the last step in the synthesis (completion of the cross-hatched structure) that is inhibited by the penicillins. The penicillins bind to a cellular receptor protein called *penicillin-binding protein (PBP).* All bacteria have PBPs, yet penicillins do not kill or even inhibit the growth of all bacteria.[2]

Possible mechanisms of bacterial resistance include mutations (structural differences in the PBPs that are targets of the antibiotic), inability of the antibiotic to penetrate to its site of action, and enzymatic changes (production of β-**lactamase,** which breaks down and inactivates the antibiotic). In an effort to minimize the activity of β-lactamase, antibiotic β-lactamase inhibitors have been developed. These inhibitors bind to and inactivate β-lactamase, thus preventing the destruction of the β-lactam antibiotic and extending the spectrum of activity of the antibiotic. Available β-lactamase inhibitors are clavulanic acid, sulbactam, and tazobactam. Clavulanic acid is combined

with amoxicillin (Augmentin) and ticarcillin (Timentin), sulbactam with ampicillin (Unasyn), and tazobactam with piperacillin (Zosyn).[2]

Penicillins can be classified into four subgroups based on their spectrum of activity:

- Natural penicillins (e.g., penicillin G) are highly active against gram-positive cocci but are readily inactivated by penicillinase, making them ineffective against most strains of *Staphylococcus aureus.*
- Penicillinase-resistant penicillins (e.g., methicillin) are less potent than the natural penicillins against gram-positive cocci but are effective against penicillinase-producing *S. aureus.*
- Aminopenicillins (e.g., ampicillin) extend their spectrum of activity to include some gram-negative organisms such as *Haemophilus influenzae, Escherichia coli,* and *Proteus mirabilis.*
- Extended-spectrum penicillins (e.g., ticarcillin) extend the spectrum of activity against gram-negative organisms, including *Pseudomonas, Enterobacter,* and *Klebsiella.*

Unfortunately, penicillins of the aminopenicillin and extended-spectrum group are readily hydrolyzed by β-lactamase. Many penicillins in these two groups are combined with β-lactamase inhibitors.[3]

The **pharmacokinetics** of penicillin vary. For example, penicillin G is poorly absorbed (15% to 30%) from the gastrointestinal (GI) tract as compared to penicillin V (60%) or amoxicillin (75% to 90%). Food generally decreases absorption of natural penicillin and the penicillinase-resistant penicillins, whereas the effect of food on absorption is minimal

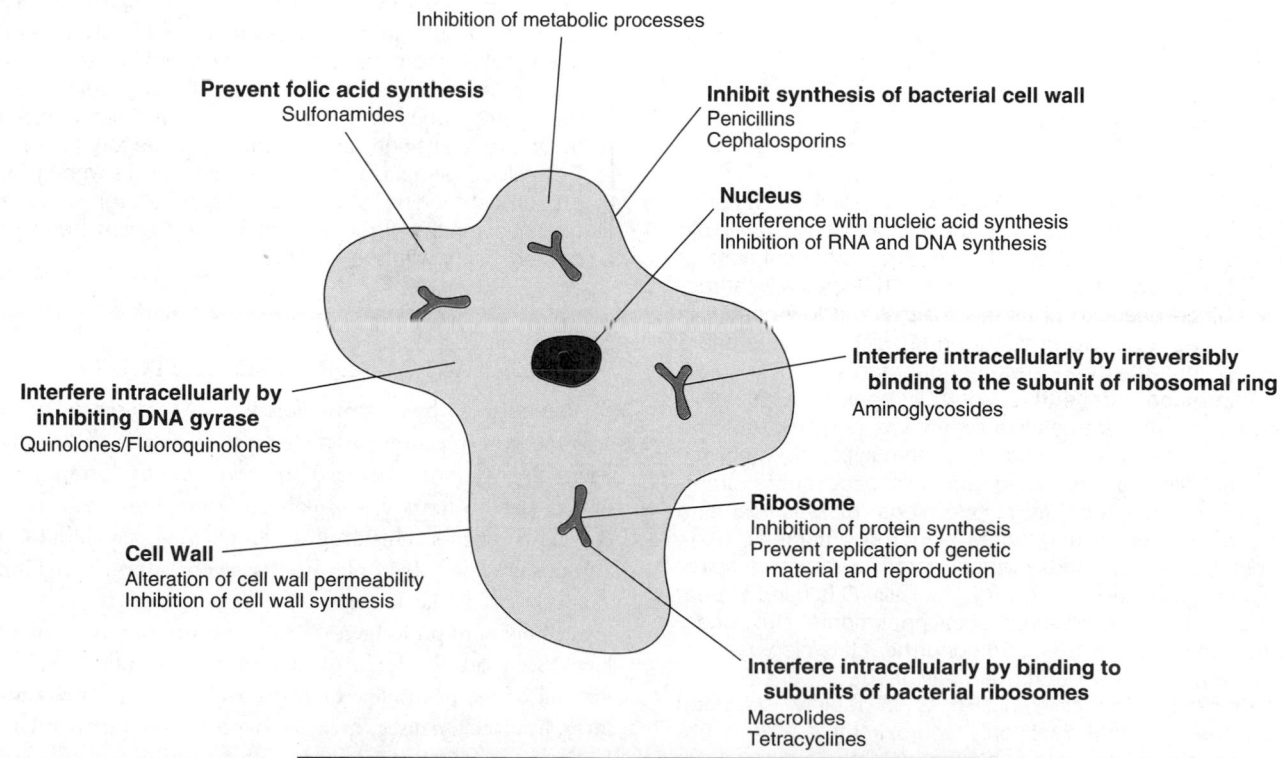

FIGURE 55–1   Mechanisms of action of major antibiotic groups.

with the aminopenicillins. Penicillins are low to moderately bound to plasma, primarily albumins, and are widely distributed throughout the body, including the kidneys, liver, lungs, heart, and intestines. Penetration into cerebrospinal fluid (CSF) occurs only with inflammation and usually does not exceed 5% of the peak serum concentration. Penicillins cross the placenta and appear in amniotic fluid and cord serum. Penicillins, except nafcillin and oxacillin, which are excreted via bile, are eliminated primarily unchanged in the urine.[2]

Hypersensitivity reactions are the most common undesired clinical responses occurring with penicillins and are the most common drug allergy. Allergic reactions to the penicillins include maculopapular rash, urticaria, fever, bronchospasm, vasculitis, serum sickness, exfoliative dermatitis, Stevens-Johnson syndrome, and anaphylaxis. Hypersensitivity reactions can occur with any dosage form of penicillin.[2]

Other undesired clinical responses associated with the penicillins include blood dyscrasias, pain and inflammation at injection sites, nausea with or without vomiting, and moderate to severe diarrhea. Lethargy, confusion, twitching, and localized or general epileptiform seizures may occur. Penicillins administered by any route change the composition of normal flora and in some instances can cause pseudomembranous colitis, which is due to overgrowth and production of *Clostridium difficile*. This disorder is characterized by watery diarrhea; it is frequently accompanied by fever, abdominal cramping, and leukocytosis.[2] (See Fig. 55–2.)

Natural Penicillins

Natural penicillins are considered narrow-spectrum antibiotics.

NATURAL PENICILLIN PROTOTYPE

PENICILLIN G

Penicillin G (Pfizerpen, Pentids, Crysticillin, Wycillin, Bicillin LA, Permapen) was the first penicillin available and is still the antibiotic of choice for the treatment of a wide variety of infections. It is an especially attractive choice because of its low toxicity and low cost. It is classed as a narrow-spectrum drug, although it is effective against a fairly wide variety of organisms.

Pharmacotherapeutics Clinically penicillin G is active against most gram-positive organisms (e.g., *Streptococcus pneumoniae*), group A β-hemolytic streptococci, nonpenicillinase producing staphylococci, some gram-negative organisms (e.g., *Neisseria meningitidis* and *N. gonorrhoeae*), and some anaerobic bacteria (e.g., *Clostridium* spp. and *Peptostreptococcus*), and spirochetes (*Treponema pallidum*). Penicillin G is used to treat infections such as pneumococcal pneumonia, streptococcal pharyngitis, syphilis, and gonorrhea. It is also used for long-term prophylaxis of rheumatic fever.[3]

Pharmacokinetics Penicillin G is rapidly absorbed from the intestinal tract; only approximately 30% is absorbed under favorable conditions. Gastric juice can destroy the antibiotic, and food decreases its absorption. After absorption, penicillin G reaches maximum serum concentrations within 1 to 2 hours. The drug is well absorbed after intramuscular (IM) administration. Penicillin G is moderately bound to plasma proteins (50% to 60%); it is widely distributed. Plasma half-life is 30 to 60 minutes but increases to $2\frac{1}{2}$ to 10 hours in clients with impaired renal function. The drug is minimally metabolized in the liver and is primarily excreted in the urine.[2,4,5]

Pharmaceutics Penicillin G is administered orally as tablets or suspension. It is administered IM as long-acting procaine penicillin G and benzathine penicillin G. By the intravenous (IV) route it is administered both by intermittent infusion and continuous infusion. Table 55–1 provides information on dosage forms, dosages, and routes of administration.

Undesired Clinical Responses Penicillin G shares the adverse reactions previously described, with hypersensitivity reactions most important. Seizures are more likely to occur in clients receiving more than 20 million units of penicillin G daily or in clients with renal impairment, localized central nervous system (CNS) lesions, or hyponatremia.[4]

Contraindications and Precautions Individuals allergic to penicillins should not receive penicillin G. It should be used with caution in clients with GI disease (e.g., ulcerative colitis, antibiotic-associated colitis) or impaired renal function.

Drug-Drug, Drug-Nutrient, Drug-Environment Interactions Angiotensin-converting enzyme (ACE) inhibitors (e.g., captopril), potassium-sparing diuretics, or potassium supplements may increase serum potassium levels when administered concurrently with parenteral potassium penicillin G. Cholestyramine may impair absorption of penicillin G; these drugs should be administered hours apart.

Penicillin G should be administered 30 minutes before or 2 hours after a meal to avoid interference with drug absorption.[6] Most parenteral dosage forms should be stored at controlled room temperature or should be refrigerated.

Life-Span Considerations Penicillin G should be used during pregnancy only if clearly indicated. Most preparations are classified as Pregnancy Category B drugs. Penicillin G should be used with caution in women who are breast-feeding since diarrhea or allergic response may occur in the nursing infant. Dosage adjustments may be necessary with the elderly.[7]

MISCELLANEOUS DRUGS IN CATEGORY

Penicillin G benzathine (Bicillin LA) is used to prevent streptococcal infections in clients with a history of rheumatic heart disease. It is also used to treat syphilis (primary, secondary, latent, tertiary, and congenital) and group A streptococcal pharyngitis. This drug is a long-acting penicillin G. It is administered deep IM only. It must *not* be administered intravenously or intraarticularly. After absorption, it produces a lower but more prolonged serum concentration. Clients who have been administered penicillin for syphilis should be warned of the possibility of **Jarisch-Herxheimer reaction**— fever, headache, nausea, myalgia, hypotension, tachycardia—6 to 12 hours after administration. This reaction probably is due

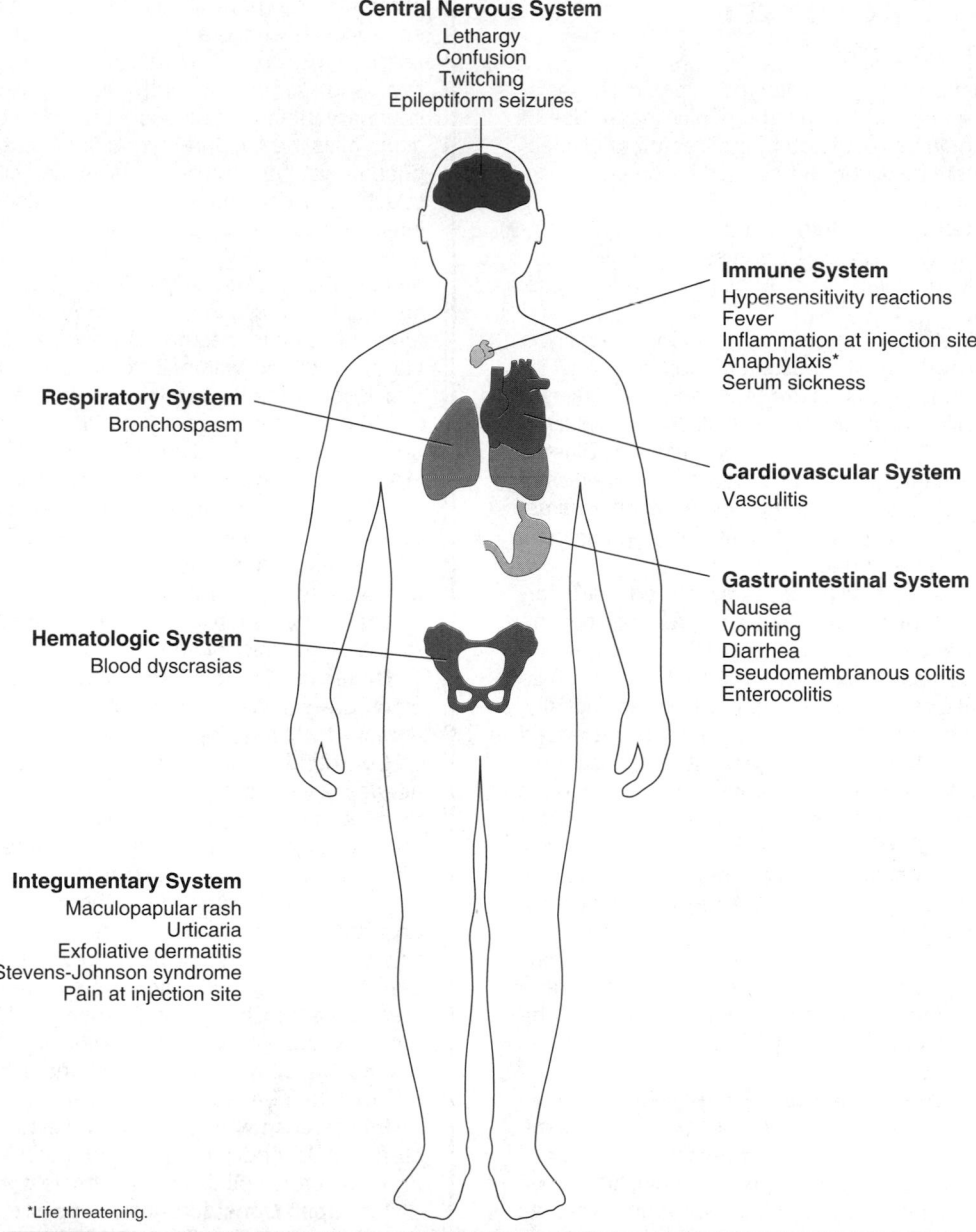

Central Nervous System
Lethargy
Confusion
Twitching
Epileptiform seizures

Immune System
Hypersensitivity reactions
Fever
Inflammation at injection site
Anaphylaxis*
Serum sickness

Respiratory System
Bronchospasm

Cardiovascular System
Vasculitis

Gastrointestinal System
Nausea
Vomiting
Diarrhea
Pseudomembranous colitis
Enterocolitis

Hematologic System
Blood dyscrasias

Integumentary System
Maculopapular rash
Urticaria
Exfoliative dermatitis
Stevens-Johnson syndrome
Pain at injection site

*Life threatening.

FIGURE 55–2   Common undesired clinical responses associated with penicillins and cephalosporins.

to the release of endotoxins by the spirochete and is only indirectly a result of the antibiotic therapy.[8]

Penicillin G procaine (Wycillin) is used to treat diphtheria, acute and chronic gonorrhea, and all forms of syphilis. It is also used to treat subacute bacterial endocarditis caused by group A streptococci and pharyngitis and pneumonia caused by pneumococci and group A streptococci. Like penicillin G benzathine, it must be administered IM.

Penicillin V potassium (V-Cillin-K, Betapen VK, Pen-Vee-K) is used in the prevention of bacterial endocarditis and streptococcal infection in clients with a history of rheumatic fever. It is also used to treat bacterial pharyngitis and skin and soft-tissue infections. Penicillin V potassium may be adminis-

tered without regard to food. Concurrent use with estrogen-containing oral contraceptives may decrease contraceptive effectiveness.

Penicillinase-Resistant Penicillins

Penicillinase-resistant penicillins are semisynthetic derivatives of penicillin G. They have similar properties but are resistant to the enzyme penicillinase. Penicillinase-resistant penicillins are used primarily to treat a narrow spectrum of penicillinase-producing microorganisms. Strains of staphylococcus are now resistant to methicillin (methicillin-resistant *S. aureus* [MRSA] strains). (See Chapter 54.)

PENICILLINASE-RESISTANT PENICILLIN PROTOTYPE

METHICILLIN SODIUM

Methicillin (Staphcillin) is the prototype of penicillins resistant to hydrolysis by staphylococcal penicillinase. Use of these drugs should be restricted to the treatment of infections known or suspected to be caused by staphylococci containing this enzyme.

Pharmacotherapeutic Methicillin is used in the treatment of pneumonia, skin and soft-tissue infections, sinusitis, septicemia, biliary tract infections, endocarditis, and meningitis.

Pharmacokinetics Methicillin is not absorbed orally. It is administered by deep IM injection or IV infusion. After IM injection, peak concentrations are reached within 30 to 60 minutes. Methicillin is approximately 40% bound to plasma proteins; it is widely distributed to body tissues. Plasma half-life is approximately 25 to 50 minutes but increases to 3 to 4 hours in clients with impaired renal function. Minimal metabolism of the drug occurs in the liver; it is primarily excreted unchanged in the urine.[2,4,9]

Pharmaceutics Methicillin is administered parenterally. Table 55–1 provides additional information on dosage forms, dosages, and routes of administration.

Undesired Clinical Responses Methicillin has a side effect profile similar to that of other penicillins. Additionally, interstitial nephritis with fever, rash, possible decreased urinary output, hematuria, and proteinuria may occur.

Contraindications and Precautions Methicillin shares the same precautions as other penicillins, but renal function determination may be needed during prolonged therapy because of possible interstitial nephritis. Since the drug contains sodium, caution must be used for clients with sodium restrictions.

Drug-Drug Interactions Administered concurrently, probenecid may increase the serum concentration and half-life of methicillin and decrease its excretion. Methicillin may interact with other nephrotoxic drugs such as aminoglycosides.

Interference with Laboratory Tests Methicillin may cause positive Coombs' test results and may increase aspartate aminotransferase (AST) test results.

Life-span Considerations Methicillin is classified as a Pregnancy Category B drug. Elderly clients may have an age-related decrease in renal function, requiring an adjustment in dosage.

Aminopenicillins

Aminopenicillins are effective against a broad range of gram-positive and gram-negative bacteria. Ampicillin was the first broad-spectrum penicillin available. This group is often used initially when identity of the infecting organism is inconclusive. Aminopenicillins are inactivated by the β-lactamase–producing organisms and are acid stable.

AMINOPENICILLIN PROTOTYPE

AMPICILLIN SODIUM

Ampicillin (Omnipen, Polycillin, Totacillin, Principen) is the prototype for the aminopenicillins.

Pharmacotherapeutics Clinically ampicillin is effective against gram-positive organisms (e.g., streptococci, pneumococci, penicillin-G–sensitive staphylococci, and enterococci) and gram-negative organisms (e.g., *H. influenzae*, *E. coli*, *P. mirabilis*, *N. gonorrhoeae*, *Shigella* spp., and *Salmonella* spp.). The drug is used to treat genitourinary tract infections, meningococcal meningitis, acute otitis media, parathyroid fever, bacterial pharyngitis, pneumonia, septicemia, sinusitis, and skin and soft-tissue infections. Additionally, ampicillin is used to treat GI tract infections caused by susceptible organisms.

Pharmacokinetics Ampicillin is moderately absorbed by the GI tract, with only 35% to 50% of an oral dose absorbed. It is stable in the acid medium of the GI tract, and food only slightly decreases absorption. Peak serum levels are attained within 2 hours after oral administration and 1 hour after IM administration. Ampicillin is only 15% to 20% bound to plasma protein. It is distributed throughout the body. Plasma half-life is 1 to 1½ hours, which increases to 10 to 15 hours in clients with renal impairment. Ampicillin is moderately metabolized in the liver and is variably excreted in the urine (25% to 60%).[2,4,9]

Pharmaceutics Ampicillin is administered orally and parenterally by IM and IV routes. Table 55–1 provides additional information on dosage forms, dosages, and routes of administration.

Undesired Clinical Responses Side effects with ampicillins are similar to those with other penicillins, with hypersensitivity reactions most important.

Contraindications and Precautions Special caution is needed when administering ampicillin to individuals with mononucleosis in that allergic rashes occur more frequently in them. Ampicillin has the same contraindications and precautions as other penicillins.

Drug-Drug Interactions Cholestyramine may impair absorption of ampicillin. If prescribed concurrently, the drugs must be administered several hours apart. Allopurinol administered concurrently may significantly increase the possibility of skin rash. Additionally, ampicillin may decrease the effectiveness of estrogen-containing oral contraceptives; thus an alternate form of contraception may be needed.

Interference with Diagnostic Tests Ampicillin may increase AST and alanine aminotransferase (ALT) levels and may cause positive Coombs' test results.

Life-Span Considerations Ampicillin is classified as a Pregnancy Category B drug. It is distributed in breast milk and may cause diarrhea, allergic sensitivity, and skin rash in infants.

MISCELLANEOUS DRUGS IN CATEGORY

Another form of the drug, **ampicillin-sulbactam sodium,** contains sulbactam, which inhibits bacterial β-lactamase. This drug is used in the treatment of genitourinary tract, intra-abdominal, and skin and soft-tissue infections caused by β-lactamase–producing strains of *Acinetobacter* spp., *Bacteroides* spp., *E. coli*, *Klebsiella* spp., *P. mirabilis,* and *S. aureus.*

Amoxicillin-clavulanate (Augmentin) is a combination of amoxicillin and clavulanate; clavulanate inhibits some β-lactamase enzymes. This drug is used to treat acute otitis media, sinusitis, pneumonia caused by *Branhamella catarrhalis* and *H. influenzae,* and skin and soft-tissue infection caused by *S. aureus, E. coli,* and *Klebsiella* spp. It is also used to treat urinary tract infections caused by *E. coli, Klebsiella* spp., and *Enterobacter* spp.

Extended-Spectrum Penicillins

Extended-spectrum penicillins are inactivated by penicillinase microorganisms.

EXTENDED-SPECTRUM PENICILLIN PROTOTYPE

TICARCILLIN

Ticarcillin (Ticar) is the prototype for the extended-spectrum penicillins.

Pharmacotherapeutics Clinically the antimicrobial activity of ticarcillin includes gram-negative organisms such as *Pseudomonas aeruginosa, Proteus* (both indole positive and indole negative), *E. coli, Enterobacter* spp., *Klebsiella* spp., *H. influenzae,* and *Serratia* spp. It is also effective against anaerobic bacteria (e.g., some *Bacteroides* spp.). Ticarcillin is used in the treatment of genitourinary and intraabdominal infections, infectious pneumonia, bacterial septicemia, skin and soft-tissue infections, and urinary tract infections.[3]

Pharmacokinetics Ticarcillin is administered either IM or IV. It is well absorbed after IM administration, reaching its peak concentration within 30 to 60 minutes. Ticarcillin is moderately bound to plasma proteins (50% to 60%) and is widely distributed throughout the body. The plasma half-life is 1 to 1.2 hours; it is markedly increased in clients with impaired hepatic and renal function. Ticarcillin is minimally metabolized in the liver; it is primarily eliminated in the urine, with a small amount excreted in bile.[4,5,9]

Pharmaceutics Ticarcillin is administered parenterally either by IM or IV routes. Table 55–1 provides additional information on dosage forms, dosages, and routes of administration.

Undesired Clinical Responses Undesired responses are similar to those of other penicillins, especially hypersensitivity reactions (see Fig. 55–2).

Contraindications and Precautions Ticarcillin use is contraindicated in clients with known allergies to penicillin. It should be administered with caution to clients with a history of GI disease or reduced renal function. Ticarcillin should also be used with caution in clients with a history of bleeding disorders since the drug may cause platelet dysfunction.[4,9]

Drug-Drug Interactions Use of anticoagulants or thrombolytic agents may increase the risk of hemorrhage when high doses of ticarcillin are administered. Similar interactions may occur with nonsteroidal antiinflammatory agents and salicylates.

Life-Span Considerations Ticarcillin is classified as a Pregnancy Category B drug. Elderly clients may require an adjustment in dosage.

MISCELLANEOUS DRUGS IN CATEGORY

Carbenicillin (Geocillin) is used in the treatment of prostatitis and urinary tract infections produced by susceptible organisms. It should be administered 1 hour before or 2 hours after meals.

Mezlocillin (Mezlin) may be used concurrently with an aminoglycoside for a synergistic effect against some microorganisms, including *P. aeruginosa* and Enterobacteriaceae. Approximately 20% of the drug is excreted in bile in clients with normal liver function. It may interact with other hepatotoxic drugs and should be used with caution in clients with impaired hepatic function.

Piperacillin (Pipracil) is used to treat bone and joint infections, urinary tract infections, and skin and soft-tissue infections. It can be used to treat anaerobic and gram-negative pneumonia, septicemia, and uncomplicated gonococcal urethritis. Like mezlocillin, it may be used concurrently with an aminoglycoside for a synergistic effect against susceptible microorganisms.

Piperacillin-tazobactam (Zosyn) and **ticarcillin-clavulanate** are combination drugs. Tazobactam and clavulanate inhibit some β-lactamase enzymes that inactivate penicillins and cephalosporins.

Related Drugs

IMIPENEM-CILASTATIN (PRIMAXIN)

Imipenem is the first of a class of β-lactam antibiotics known as **carbapenems.** It has a wider spectrum of activity, including activity against gram-positive, gram-negative, and anaerobic bacteria. Cilastatin has no antibacterial activity but blocks renal metabolism of imipenem, increasing its urinary recovery.

Pharmacotherapeutics Clinically imipenem is effective against gram-positive organisms, including most strains of staphylococci and streptococci and some enterococci. Resistance to *Streptococcus faecium,* MRSA, and coagulase-negative staphylococci has occurred. Gram-negative organisms susceptible to imipenem include *Enterobacter* spp., *Citrobacter* spp., *Acinetobacter* spp., *E. coli, H. influenzae, Klebsiella pneumoniae, P. mirabilis,* indole-positive *Proteus* spp., *Morganella morganii, Serratia marcescens,* and *P. aeruginosa.* Anaerobic species, including *Bacteroides* spp. and *Clostridium* spp. are inhibited. Imipenem is ineffective against many strains of *Pseudomonas cepacia* and virtually all strains of *Pseudomonas maltophilia.*

Imipenem is used in the treatment of bone and joint infections, bacterial endocarditis, intraabdominal infections, pelvic infections, bacterial pneumonia, septicemia, skin and soft-tissue infections, and bacterial urinary tract infections.

Pharmacokinetics Imipenem is given parenterally by either IM or IV administration. It is well absorbed after IM administration (95%), with its peak serum concentration occurring within 2 hours. Protein binding is low, approximately 20%. The drug is widely distributed to most tissues and fluids, including low concentrations in the CSF. Plasma half-life is 1 hour; it is increased in clients with impaired renal function. The drug is metabolized in the kidneys by hydrolysis of the β-lactam ring.

Pharmacodynamics Imipenem is bactericidal. Its mechanism of action is inhibition of bacterial cell wall synthesis by binding to PBPs, causing cell lysis and death.

Undesired clinical responses Side effects occurring frequently with use of imipenem include allergic reactions (skin rash, hives, itching, fever); CNS effects, including confusion, dizziness, seizures, or tremors; pain at the injection site; or GI effects, consisting of nausea, vomiting or diarrhea. Pseudo-

Text continued on page 723.

TABLE 55–1
Antibiotics: Penicillins

Drug Name	Dosage and Route of Administration	Nursing Considerations
PENICILLIN G POTASSIUM, PARENTERAL (Pfizerpen) HOW SUPPLIED 1-, 5-, 10-, 20-million U vials	ADULTS IM/IV: 1–5 million U q4-6h INFANTS AND CHILDREN IM/IV: 100,000–400,000 U/kg/d in divided doses q4-6h PREMATURE FULL-TERM NEONATES IM/IV: 50,000–100,000 U/kg/d in divided doses q12h	**Assess** Ask about sensitivity to penicillin and cephalosporins. Determine what drugs are being used concurrently. Obtain CBC and renal function test results. Identify any infectious process. Obtain specimens for culture and sensitivity testing before initiating therapy. Determine whether client is pregnant or breast-feeding. **Implement** Give oral dosage 1 h before or 2 h after meals. Give IM injections deep into upper outer quadrant of the gluteus maximus muscle. Check IM site for induration and tenderness. **Monitor** Monitor the CBC, urinalysis, and renal function test results. Observe for undesirable effects such as allergic reactions. Monitor intake and output (I&O). Monitor the infectious process. **Evaluate** Observe for resolution of signs and symptoms of infection.
Penicillin G Sodium, Parenteral (Generic) HOW SUPPLIED 5-million U vials	Same as penicillin G potassium, parenteral	Same as above.
Penicillin G Potassium, Oral (Pentids) HOW SUPPLIED Tablets: 200,000, 250,000, 400,000, 500,000, 800,000 U Powder for oral suspension: 400,000 U/5 ml when reconstituted	ADULTS 250,000–500,000 U q6-8h CHILDREN 25,000–90,000 U/kg/d in three to six divided doses	Same as above. Teach client to continue taking antibiotics for full length of treatment. Instruct client to space doses evenly.
Penicillin G Benzathine (Bicillin 1-A, Permapen) HOW SUPPLIED Injection: 300,000, 600,000, 1,200,000, 2,400,000 U	ADULTS IM: 1,200,000 U in one dose (some total doses, 2,400,000 U) CHILDREN > 27 KG IM: 900,000–1,200,000 U in one dose CHILDREN < 27 KG IM: 300,000–600,000 U in one dose NEONATES IM: 50,000 U/kg in one dose	**Assess** Same as penicillin G potassium. **Implement** Give deep IM injections only. **Monitor** Same as penicillin G potassium. **Evaluate** Same as penicillin G potassium.
Penicillin G Procaine (Crystacillin, Pfizerpen, Wycillin) HOW SUPPLIED Injection: 300,000, 600,000, 1,200,000, 2,400,000 U	ADULTS IM: 600,000–1,200,000 U daily CHILDREN IM: 25,000–50,000 U/kg/d given as single daily dose or divided dose q12h NEWBORN IM: 50,000 U/kg/d	Same as penicillin G benzathine.
Penicillin V Potassium (Beepen VK, Betapen VK, Ledercillin VK, Pen-Vee-K, V-Cillin K, Veetids) HOW SUPPLIED Tablets: 125, 250, 500 mg Powder for oral solutions: 125, 250 mg/5 ml when reconstituted	ADULTS 125–500 mg q6-8h CHILDREN 25–50 mg/kg/d in divided doses q6-8h	**Assess** Same as penicillin G potassium. **Implement** Drug may be given without regard to food. **Monitor** Same as penicillin G potassium. **Evaluate** Same as penicillin G potassium.

TABLE 55–1 *Continued*
Antibiotics: Penicillins

Drug Name	Dosage and Route of Administration	Nursing Considerations
Cloxacillin (Tegopen) HOW SUPPLIED Capsules: 250, 500 mg Powder for oral solution: 125 mg/5 ml when reconstituted	ADULTS 250–500 mg q6h CHILDREN > 20 KG 250–500 mg q6h CHILDREN < 20 KG 50–100 mg/kg/d in equally divided doses q6h	**Assess** Same as penicillin G potassium. **Implement** Give 1 h before or 2 h after meals. **Monitor** Same as penicillin G potassium. **Evaluate** Same as penicillin G potassium. Same as cloxacillin.
Dicloxacillin (Dycill, Dynapen, Pathocil) HOW SUPPLIED Capsules: 125, 250, 500 mg Powder for oral solution: 62.5 mg/5 ml when reconstituted	ADULTS 125–250 mg q6h CHILDREN > 40 KG 125–250 mg q6h CHILDREN < 40 KG 12.5–25 mg/kg/d in equally divided doses q6h	
METHICILLIN (Staphcillin) HOW SUPPLIED Injection: 1-, 4-, 6-, 10-g vials	ADULTS IM: 1 g q4-6h IV: 1–2 g q4h CHILDREN IM or IV: 100–400 mg/kg/d in divided doses q6h NEONATES IM or IV: 25–50 mg/kg/*dose* q6-12h	**Assess** Ask about sensitivity to penicillin or cephalosporins. Inquire about any concurrent drugs, especially nephrotoxic ones. Obtain CBC and renal function test results. Assess the infectious process and obtain specimen. Inquire about pregnancy and breast-feeding. **Implement** Administer by deep IM injection or IV injection. Assess IM injection sites for pain and induration. Evaluate IV site for phlebitis. **Monitor** Obtain CBC, urinalysis, and renal function test results. Monitor I&O. Observe for undesirable effects such as allergic reactions or interstitial nephritis. **Evaluate** Assess for resolution of signs and symptoms of infection.
Nafcillin (Nafcil, Nallpen, Unipen) HOW SUPPLIED Tablets: 500 mg Capsules: 250 mg Injection: 1, 2, 10 g	ADULTS Oral: 250 mg–1 g q4-6h IM: 500 mg q4-6h IV: 500–1500 mg q4h CHILDREN Oral: 50–100 mg/kg/d in divided doses q6h IM: 100–200 mg/kg/d in divided doses q12h IV: 100–200 mg/kg/d in divided doses q6h NEONATES IM or IV: 50–75 mg/kg/d in divided doses q6-12h	**Assess** Same as penicillin G. **Implement** Orally, give 1 h before or 2 h after meals. Parenterally, give by deep IM or IV administration. **Monitor** Same as penicillin G. **Evaluate** Same as penicillin G.
Oxacillin (Bactocill, Prostaphilin) HOW SUPPLIED Capsules: 250, 500 mg Powder for oral solutions: 250 mg/5 ml when reconstituted Injection: 250, 500 mg; 1, 2, 4, 10 g	ADULTS OR CHILDREN > 40 KG Oral: 500 mg–1 g q4-6h IM or IV: 1–2 g q4h CHILDREN < 40 KG Oral: 50–100 mg/kg/d in divided doses q6h IM: 100–200 mg/kg/d in divided doses q12h IV: 100–200 mg/kg/d in divided doses q6h	**Assess** Ask about sensitivity to penicillin or cephalosporins. Inquire about any concurrent drugs, especially nephrotoxic ones. Obtain CBC and renal function test results. Assess the infectious process and obtain specimen. Inquire about pregnancy and breast-feeding.

Table continued on following page.

TABLE 55–1 *Continued*
Antibiotics: Penicillins

Drug Name	Dosage and Route of Administration	Nursing Considerations
Oxacillin—Continued		**Implement** Orally, give 1 h before or 2 h after meals. Parenterally, give by deep IM or IV administration. **Monitor** Obtain results of CBC, urinalysis, and renal function tests. Observe for undesired effects such as allergic reaction. Monitor the infectious process. **Evaluate** Observe for resolution of signs and symptoms of infection.
Amoxicillin (Amoxil, Bromox, Polymox, Trimox, Wymox) HOW SUPPLIED Tablets (chewable): 125, 250 mg Capsules: 250, 500 mg Powder for oral suspension: 50 mg/ml, 125 mg/5 ml, 250 mg/5 ml when reconstituted	ADULTS 250–500 mg q8h CHILDREN > **40 KG** 250–500 mg q8h CHILDREN < **40 KG** 20–50 mg/kg/d in divided doses q8h	**Assess** Ask about sensitivity to penicillin and cephalosporins. Determine what drugs are being used concurrently, especially allopurinol and oral contraceptives. Use with caution in client with infectious mononucleosis. Obtain CBC and renal function test results. Identify the infectious process. Obtain specimens before initiating therapy. Determine whether client is pregnant or breast-feeding. **Implement** May give without regard to food. Parenterally, give by deep IM or IV administration. **Monitor** Same as penicillin G. **Evaluate** Same as penicillin G.
Amoxicillin-Clavulanate (Augmentin) HOW SUPPLIED Tablets: 250, 500 mg Tablets (chewable): 125, 250 mg Powder for oral suspension: 125 mg and 31.25 mg/5 ml; 250 mg and 62.5 mg/5 ml when reconstituted	ADULTS 250–500 mg q8h CHILDREN > **40 KG** 250–500 mg q8h CHILDREN < **40 KG** 20–40 mg/kg/d in divided doses q8h	**Assess** Same as amoxicillin. **Implement** Drug may be given without regard to food. **Monitor** Same as penicillin G. **Evaluate** Same as penicillin G.
AMPICILLIN SODIUM (Omnipen, Polycillin, Principen, Totacillin) HOW SUPPLIED Capsules: 250, 500 mg Powder for oral suspension: 100 mg/ml; 125, 250, 500 mg/5 ml after reconstitution Injection: 125, 250, 500 mg; 1, 2, 10 g	ADULTS Oral: 250–500 mg q6h IM or IV: 1–12 g/d in divided doses q4-6h CHILDREN Oral: 50–400 mg/kg/d in divided doses q4-6h IM or IV: 50–400 mg/kg/d in divided doses q4-6h NEONATES IM or IV: 50–200 mg/kg/d in divided doses q6-12h	**Assess** Same as penicillin G except must use with caution in client with infectious mononucleosis. **Implement** Drug may be given without regard to food. **Monitor** Same as penicillin G. **Evaluate** Same as penicillin G.
Ampicillin-Sulbactam (Unasyn) HOW SUPPLIED Injection: 1.5, 3 g	ADULTS IM or IV: 1.5–3 g q6h	**Assess** Ask about sensitivity to penicillin and cephalosporins. Determine what drugs are being used concurrently, especially allopurinol and oral contraceptives.

TABLE 55–1 *Continued*
Antibiotics: Penicillins

Drug Name	Dosage and Route of Administration	Nursing Considerations
Ampicillin-Sulbactam *Continued*		Use with caution in client with infectious mononucleosis. Obtain CBC and renal function test results. Identify the infectious process. Obtain specimens before initiating therapy. Determine whether client is pregnant or breast-feeding. **Implement** Administer by deep IM injection or IV injection. **Monitor** Same as penicillin G. **Evaluate** Same as penicillin G.
Bacampicillin (Spectrobid) HOW SUPPLIED Tablets: 400 mg Powder for oral suspension: 125 mg/5 ml after reconstitution	ADULTS 400–800 mg q12h CHILDREN > 25 KG 400–800 mg q12h CHILDREN < 25 KG 12.5–25 mg/kg q12h	**Assess** Ask about sensitivity to penicillin and cephalosporins. Determine what drugs are being used concurrently, especially allopurinol and oral contraceptives. Drug must be used with caution in client with infectious mononucleosis. Obtain CBC and renal function test results. Identify any infectious process. Obtain specimens before initiating therapy. Determine whether client is pregnant or breast-feeding. **Implement** Give 1 h before or 2 h after meals. **Monitor** Same as penicillin G. **Evaluate** Same as penicillin G.
Carbenicillin (Geocillin) HOW SUPPLIED Tablets: 382 mg	ADULTS 382–764 mg q6h	**Assess** Ask about sensitivity to penicillin and cephalosporins. Determine what drugs are being used concurrently. Obtain CBC and renal function test results. Identify any infectious process. Obtain specimens before initiating therapy. Determine whether client is pregnant or breast-feeding. **Implement** Give 1 h before or 2 h after meals. **Monitor** Same as penicillin G. **Evaluate** Same as penicillin G.
Mezlocillin (Mezlin) HOW SUPPLIED Injection: 1, 2, 3, 4, 20 g	ADULTS IM or IV: 3–4 g q4-6h CHILDREN 1 MO–12 Y IM or IV: 50–75 mg/kg q4h INFANTS 8–30 D IM or IV: 75 mg/kg q6-8h NEONATES < 8 D IM or IV: 75 mg/kg q12h	**Assess** Ask about sensitivity to penicillin and cephalosporins. Determine what drugs are being used concurrently, especially allopurinol and oral contraceptives. This drug may interact with hepatotoxic drugs. Use with caution in client with infectious mononucleosis. Obtain CBC and renal function test results.

Table continued on following page.

TABLE 55–1 *Continued*
Antibiotics: Penicillins

Drug Name	Dosage and Route of Administration	Nursing Considerations
Mezlocillin Continued		Identify the infectious process. Obtain specimens before initiating therapy. Determine whether client is pregnant or breast-feeding. **Implement** Administer by deep IM injection or IV injection. **Monitor** Same as penicillin G. **Evaluate** Same as penicillin G.
Piperacillin (Pipracil) HOW SUPPLIED Injection: 2, 3, 4, 40 g	ADULTS IM or IV: 3–4 g q4-6h (IM dose not to exceed 2 g at each injection site) CHILDREN > 12 Y IM or IV: 3–4 g q4-6h	**Assess** Same as mezlocillin. **Implement** Administer by deep IM injection or IV injection. **Monitor** Same as penicillin G. **Evaluate** Same as penicillin G.
Piperacillin-Tazobactam (Zosyn) HOW SUPPLIED Injection: 2/0.25; 3/0.375; 4/0.5	ADULTS IV infusion: 3.375 g q6h	**Assess** Same as mezlocillin. **Implement** Give as IV rider ("piggyback"). **Monitor** Same as penicillin G. **Evaluate** Same as penicillin G.
TICARCILLIN (Ticar) HOW SUPPLIED Injection: 1, 3, 6, 20, 30 g	ADULTS IV: 3 g q3h, q4h, or q6h IM: 1 g q4-6h (UTIs) CHILDREN > 40 KG IV: 3 g q3h, q4h, or q6h IM: 1 g q4-6h (UTIs) CHILD < 40 KG IV: 50–300 mg/kg/d in divided doses q4-8h IM: 50–100 mg/kg/d in divided doses q6-8h NEONATES > 2 KG IV or IM: 225–300 mg/kg/d in divided doses q8h NEONATES < 2 KG IM or IV: 150–225 mg/kg/d in divided doses q8-12h	**Assess** Ask about sensitivity to penicillin and cephalosporins. Determine what drugs are being used concurrently, especially anticoagulants. Obtain CBC and renal function test results. Identify any infectious process. Obtain specimens before initiating therapy. Determine whether client is pregnant or breast-feeding. **Implement** Administer by deep IM injection or IV injection. **Monitor** Same as penicillin G. **Evaluate** Same as penicillin G.
Ticarcillin-Clavulanate (Timentin) HOW SUPPLIED Injection: 3.1 g	ADULTS > 60 KG IV: 3.1 g q4-6h ADULTS < 60 KG IV 200–300 mg/kg/d in divided doses q4-6h	**Assess** Same as ticarcillin. **Implement** Give as IV rider ("piggyback"). **Monitor** Same as penicillin G. **Evaluate** Same as penicillin G.

TABLE 55–1 *Continued*
Antibiotics: Penicillins

Drug Name	Dosage and Route of Administration	Nursing Considerations
MISCELLANEOUS AGENTS *Aztreonam* (Azactam) **HOW SUPPLIED** Injection: 500 mg, 1, 2 g	ADULTS IM/IV: 1–8 g/d in divided doses q6-12h	**Assess** Identify sensitivity to aztreonam. Obtain results of baseline renal and liver function tests and CBC. Identify any infectious processes. Obtain specimens before initiating therapy. Determine if client is pregnant or breast-feeding. **Implement** Give IV infusion over 20–60 min. **Monitor** Monitor CBC, urinalysis, and renal and liver function test results. **Evaluate** Observe for resolution of signs and symptoms of infection.
Imipenem-Cilastatin (Primaxin) **HOW SUPPLIED** Injection (IM): 500, 750 mg Injection (IV): 250, 500 mg	ADULTS IV: 1–4 g/d in divided doses q6-8h IM: 1–1.5 g/d in divided doses q12h	**Assess** Identify sensitivity to imipenem-cilastatin, penicillin, cephalosporins. Obtain history of CNS disorders (e.g., seizures). Obtain results of baseline CBC and renal and liver function tests. Identify any infectious processes. Obtain specimens before initiating therapy. **Implement** Give IM or IV infusion over 20–60 min. **Monitor** Monitor CBC, urinalysis, and renal and liver function test results. Observe for undesired effects (especially CNS effects). Monitor the infectious process. **Evaluate** Observe for resolution of signs and symptoms of infection.

membranous colitis has been associated with imipenem only rarely.

Contraindications and precautions Imipenem should be used cautiously in clients allergic to other β-lactams or in clients with a history of a CNS disorder or impaired renal function.

Life-Span considerations Imipenem is administered during pregnancy only if the benefits of its use outweigh its risks. It is used cautiously in breast-feeding women since it is not known if imipenem is excreted in breast milk. Safety and efficacy in children less than 12 years of age have not been established.

Specific drug-related nursing considerations Assess for possible contraindications to imipenem. Review baseline CBC and renal and liver function test results. Administer IM preparations by deep IM injection into a large muscle mass (e.g., gluteal muscle). IV preparation (piggyback) should be infused over 20 to 60 minutes, depending on dosage.

AZTREONAM

Aztreonam (Azactam) is a narrow-spectrum antibiotic active only against aerobic, gram-negative organisms.

Pharmacotherapeutics Clinically aztreonam is effective against *Enterobacter* spp., *Citrobacter* spp., *Acinetobacter* spp., *E. coli*, *H. influenzae*, *K. pneumoniae*, *P. mirabilis*, *P. aeruginosa*, *S. marcescens*, *Salmonella* spp., and *Shigella* spp.

Aztreonam is used in the treatment of gram-negative bronchitis, pneumonia, skin and soft-tissue infections, cystitis, and bacterial urinary tract infections. It is also used to treat gynecologic infections (including endometritis), intra-abdominal infections, bacterial septicemia, and bone and joint infections.

Pharmacokinetics Aztreonam is completely absorbed after IM administration. Peak serum concentration occurs in less than 1.3 hours; protein binding is 56% to 60% and decreases to 36% to 43% in clients with impaired renal function. Aztreonam is widely distributed to body fluids and tissues, including CSF; it crosses the placenta and is excreted in breast milk. Plasma half-life is 1¼ to 2.2 hours; the half-life is increased in clients with impaired renal function. Aztreonam is partially metabolized by hydrolysis of the β-lactam bond and is excreted primarily unchanged in the kidney.

Pharmacodynamics Aztreonam, like the penicillins, is bactericidal. Its action is to inhibit bacterial cell wall synthesis by binding to PBPs, causing cell lysis and death.

Pharmaceutics Aztreonam may be administered by IM or IV routes. It may be administered concurrently with an aminoglycoside for synergistic effects with the aminoglycoside.

Undesired clinical responses Aztreonam is well tolerated. However, hypersensitivity reactions, including anaphylaxis, skin rash or redness, itching, and thrombophlebitis, may occur. Abdominal or stomach cramps, diarrhea, nausea, or vomiting may also occur.

Contraindications and precautions Aztreonam should be used with caution in clients with cirrhosis or impaired renal function. It should not to be used in clients with a previous allergic reaction to aztreonam. Although cross-sensitivity only rarely occurs with β-lactam antibiotics, caution should be used in clients with noted allergies to these drugs.

Interference with diagnostic tests Use of aztreonam produces a positive Coombs' test result. Its use may increase AST, ALT, lactate dehydrogenase (LDH), alkaline phosphatase, and creatinine levels.

Life-span considerations Aztreonam is classified as a Pregnancy Category B drug. It should be used during pregnancy only if the benefits of its use outweigh the risks. Aztreonam is excreted in breast milk, so nursing should be temporarily discontinued. Safety in infants and children has not been established.

Specific drug-related nursing considerations Assess for the presence or history of hepatic and renal impairment. Review baseline renal and hepatic function test results. Administer an IV infusion (piggyback) of aztreonam over 20 to 60 minutes.

CONCEPT REVIEW

The penicillins represent a large group of antibiotics. They are divided into four subgroups: natural penicillins, penicillinase-resistant penicillins, aminopenicillins, and extended-spectrum penicillins.

The mechanism of action for penicillins is inhibition of the bacterial wall synthesis. The most common undesired clinical responses are hyposensitivity reactions ranging from urticarial rash to anaphylaxis.

CEPHALOSPORINS

The cephalosporins are structurally related to the penicillins. They were first isolated in 1948 from a fungus, *Cephalosporium acremonium.*

The cephalosporins' mechanism of action is similar to that of the penicillins. They inhibit bacterial cell wall synthesis and are bactericidal. They are particularly effective against young, rapidly dividing bacteria in the process of cell wall formation. As with the penicillins, resistance to the cephalosporins can occur. Resistance may be due to the drug's inability to reach the site of action, changes in the antibiotic-binding proteins, or enzymes (β-lactamase) that can hydrolyze the β-lactam ring, thus inactivating the cephalosporin. Cephalosporins have variable susceptibility to β-lactamase. For example, cefazolin is more susceptible, whereas cefoxitin, cefuroxime, and the third-generation cephalosporins are most resistant to β-lactamase hydrolysis.

Cephalosporins may be classified according to their chemical structure, resistance to β-lactamase, or antimicrobial spectrum. The accepted system of classification is by "generations," a classification that, although very useful, is somewhat arbitrary.

First-generation cephalosporins are effective against gram-positive cocci, including β-lactamase–producing staphylococci. They have modest activity against gram-negative organisms. The spectrum of the **second-generation cephalosporins** is extended to gram-negative and anaerobic bacilli. The **third-generation cephalosporins** are more effective against gram-negative organisms than the previous two generations. They are more resistant to β-lactamase but less effective against gram-positive bacilli. A subset of that generation is active against *P. aeruginosa.* Cross-resistance to penicillins and cephalosporins has been demonstrated by some bacteria.[10]

Many cephalosporins have similar **pharmacokinetic properties.** Most cephalosporins that can be administered orally are well absorbed from the GI tract. However, cefixime and cefuroxime are only moderately absorbed. The presence of food in the stomach slows absorption of some cephalosporins. Protein binding is variable with these antibiotics. The cephalosporins are distributed extensively in tissue and in most body fluid. Only second-generation cefuroxime and all the third-generation products rapidly penetrate the CSF, especially, as with the penicillins, when fever and inflammation of the meninges occur. They all cross the placenta and enter breast milk. Most derivatives of this class are minimally metabolized in the liver except for cephalothin, cephapirin, cefoperazone, ceftriaxone, and cefotaxime, which appear in bile in varying degrees. Those cephalosporins not metabolized are eliminated unchanged in the urine. In clients with impaired renal function the half-life is increased, necessitating an adjustment in dosage. Action of the cephalosporins, like that of the penicillins, is prolonged with the concurrent administration of probenecid.[4,10]

Undesired clinical responses to cephalosporins are minimal. Hypersensitivity reactions identical to those of penicillins may occur. Immediate reactions such as anaphylaxis, bronchospasms, or urticaria have been reported, but maculopapular rash, with or without fever or eosinophilia, is more common. Because of similar structure between the cephalosporins and penicillins, cross-sensitivity may occur. In fact, 10% of the clients allergic to penicillin react to cephalosporins.

GI disturbances, which include enterocolitis and **pseudomembranous colitis,** nephrotoxicity, and blood dyscrasias may occur. Blood dyscrasias are dose related and have been reported with use of cefamandole, cefoperazone, and cefotetan. Figure 55–2 illustrates some of the common undesired clinical responses observed with penicillins and cephalosporins.

First-Generation Cephalosporins

As previously indicated, first-generation cephalosporins are effective against gram-positive cocci, including β-lactamase–producing staphylococci.

FIRST-GENERATION CEPHALOSPORIN PROTOTYPE
CEFAZOLIN

Cefazolin (Ancef, Kefzol, Zolicef) is the prototype for the first-generation cephalosporins.

Pharmacotherapeutics Clinically, cefazolin has a high degree of activity against most gram-positive organisms. Notable exceptions include methicillin-resistant staphylococci, penicillin-resistant *S. pneumoniae,* and *Enterococcus* spp. Activity is also found with gram-negative organisms, including *E. coli, Klebsiella* spp., and *P. mirabilis.*

Cefazolin is used in the treatment of septicemia, bone and joint infections, otitis media, pneumonia, skin and soft-tissue infections, and urinary tract infections caused by susceptible microorganisms. Cefazolin is not effective in the treatment of meningitis.[3,4,9]

Pharmacokinetics Cefazolin is administered parenterally, either by IM or IV injection or intermittent IV infusion. After IM administration, it is well absorbed, reaching a peak serum concentration within 1 to 2 hours. Cefazolin is highly bound to plasma proteins (85%). Like other cephalosporins, it is widely distributed throughout the body; however, it does not reach therapeutic concentrations in the CSF. Plasma half-life for cefazolin is 1.4 to 1.8 hours, increasing in clients with renal impairment.

Undesired Clinical Responses Cefazolin shares the same side effects as other cephalosporins, including allergic or hypersensitivity reactions. It also can cause pseudomembranous colitis, thrombophlebitis at the injection site, and GI effects.[4]

Contraindications and Precautions Individuals allergic to cephalosporins or having previous serious allergic reactions to penicillin should not receive cefazolin. Caution should be used in clients with a history of GI disease or impaired renal function.

Drug-Drug and Drug-Environment Interactions Probenecid decreases renal tubular secretion of cefazolin, prolonging its elimination half-life and increasing the risk of toxicity. Parenteral solutions of cefazolin appear light yellow to yellow. The IV infusion solution is stable for 24 hours at room temperature and for 96 hours if refrigerated.[11]

Life-Span Considerations Cefazolin is classified as a Pregnancy Category B drug. It readily crosses the placenta and is excreted in breast milk. Special caution must be used in administering it to the elderly since age-related renal impairment may occur.

Specific Drug-Related Nursing Considerations Monitor the IV site for phlebitis. Check IM injection sites for indurations. Reconstitute IM solutions with sterile water for injection, bacteriostatic water for injection, or 0.9% NaCl solution. Direct IV injections must be further diluted and administered over 3 to 5 minutes. Dilute intermittent IV infusion solutions further and infuse over 20 to 40 minutes.[11]

MISCELLANEOUS DRUGS IN CATEGORY

Several other first-generation cephalosporins are available, including **cephalexin** (Keflet, Keflex), **cefadroxil** (Duricef, Ultracef), **cephradine** (Velosef), **cephalothin** (Keflin), and **cephapirin** (Cefadyl). Cephradine, cephalothin, and cephapirin are rarely prescribed. Cephalexin is used to treat respiratory tract infections, otitis media, skin and soft-tissue infections, bone infections, and genitourinary tract infections. Cefadroxil is used in the treatment of group A β-hemolytic streptococcal pharyngitis, skin and soft-tissue infections, and urinary tract infections. Table 55–2 provides additional information on dosage forms, dosages, and routes of administration.

Second-Generation Cephalosporins

The spectrum of activity for second-generation cephalosporins is extended to gram-negative and anaerobic bacilli.

SECOND-GENERATION CEPHALOSPORIN PROTOTYPE
CEFUROXIME AXETIL AND CEFUROXIME SODIUM

Cefuroxime (Ceftin, Kefurox, Zinacef) is the prototype for the second-generation cephalosporins.

Pharmacotherapeutics Clinically, cefuroxime has increased activity against the gram-negative organisms *E. coli, Klebsiella* spp., and *P. mirabilis.* Additionally, gram-negative activity is increased to include *H. influenzae, N. meningitidis, N. gonorrhoeae,* and some *Serratia* and *Enterobacter* spp. Their activity against gram-positive cocci is slightly less than that of first-generation cephalosporins. Cefuroxime is not effective against methicillin-resistant staphylococci and enterococci. Cefuroxime shares some activity against anaerobes, including *Clostridium* spp. and *Bacteroides fragilis.*[3]

Cefuroxime is used in the treatment of septicemia, bone and joint infections, gram-negative pneumonia, skin and soft-tissue infections, and urinary tract infections caused by susceptible microorganisms. It is also used in the treatment of community-acquired pneumonia, meningitis, otitis media, sinusitis, and mild-to-moderate bronchitis.[4,12]

Pharmacokinetics Cefuroxime can be administered orally and parenterally. It is moderately absorbed from the GI tract, 52% with food consumption and 37% in the fasting state, and is well absorbed after IM administration. Peak serum concentrations are attained within 2 hours after oral dosage and approximately 45 minutes after IM dosage. It is moderately bound to plasma protein (50%) and is widely distributed throughout the body. Parenteral cefuroxime is the only second-generation cephalosporin to penetrate adequately into the CSF. Plasma half-life is 1 hour and may increase to 17 hours in clients with impaired renal function. Elimination of the drug occurs via the kidneys, primarily as unchanged drug.[4,9]

Undesired Clinical Responses Cefuroxime shares the same side effect profile as other cephalosporins (i.e., hypersensitivity reactions, possible development of pseudomembranous colitis, thrombophlebitis, and GI distress).

Contraindications and Precautions Cefuroxime use is contraindicated in clients allergic to cephalosporins or those who have had a severe allergic reaction to penicillin. It is used with caution in the presence of GI disease or impaired renal function.

Drug-Drug, Drug-Nutrient, Drug-Environment Interactions The oral dosage form of cefuroxime may be administered without regard to meals. If GI upset occurs, it may be administered with food or milk. Parenteral solutions appear light yellow to amber; the solution may darken, but this color change does not affect drug potency. The IV infusion solution is stable for 24 hours at room temperature or for 7 days if refrigerated.[11] Probenecid decreases renal tubular secretion of cefuroxime, causing increased concentrations and prolonged elimination half-life.

Interference with Diagnostic Tests Cefuroxime may cause positive direct or indirect Coombs' test results. Its use may increase AST, ALT, alkaline phosphatase, bilirubin, and LDH concentrations and may decrease hemoglobin and hematocrit concentrations.

Life-Span Considerations Cefuroxime is classified as a Pregnancy Category B drug. The drug readily crosses the placenta and is distributed in breast milk.

Specific Drug-Related Nursing Considerations Dilute IM and IV preparations before administering them. Check the drug insert for the proper dilution procedure. Administer the direct IV injection over 3 to 5 minutes. Infuse an intermittent IV infusion over 15 to 60 minutes. Evaluate the IV site for phlebitis, and check the IM site for tenderness and induration.

MISCELLANEOUS DRUGS IN CATEGORY

Cefaclor (Ceclor), **cefamandole** (Mandol), **cefoxitin** (Mefoxin), **cefonicid** (Monocid), **cefmetazole** (Zefazone), **cefotetan disodium** (Cefotan), **cefprozil** (Cefzil), **cefpodoxime proxetil** (Vantin), and **loracarbef** (Lorabid) are all second-generation cephalosporins. Cefamandole, cefmetazole, and cefotetan interact with alcohol, causing a disulfiram reaction. In addition, concurrent administration of anticoagulants or thrombolytic drugs increases the risk of bleeding. Cefmetazole and cefotetan possess good activity against anaerobic organisms. Cefonicid is administered parenterally. It has a long half-life (4½ hours), which allows dosing every 24 hours.[13,14] Table 55-2 provides additional information on second-generation cephalosporins.

Third-Generation Cephalosporins

Drugs in the third generation of cephalosporins are more effective against gram-negative organisms than the previous two generations. These drugs are more resistant to β-lactamase but less effective against gram-positive bacilli.

THIRD-GENERATION CEPHALOSPORIN PROTOTYPE

CEFTRIAXONE

Ceftriaxone (Rocephin) is the prototype for the third-generation cephalosporins.

Pharmacotherapeutics Clinically ceftriaxone has a wide spectrum of activity against gram-negative organisms because ceftriaxone has a high degree of stability in the presence of β-lactamase. Ceftriaxone is active against penicillinase-producing strains of *N. gonorrhoeae, H. influenzae,* and most Enterobacteriaceae. Activity also occurs with gram-positive organisms, but ceftriaxone is less active than first-generation cephalosporins. The gram-positive organisms include methicillin susceptible staphylococci, β-hemolytic streptococci, and *S. pneumoniae.* Ceftriaxone is not effective against enterococci. Ceftriaxone has shown some activity against anaerobes.[2,3]

Ceftriaxone is used in the treatment of serious gram-negative bacterial infections, including septicemia, bone and joint infections, female pelvic infections, intraabdominal infections, and complicated urinary tract infections. It also is used to treat meningitis.

Pharmacokinetics Ceftriaxone is well absorbed after IM administration, reaching peak serum concentration within 1 to 2 hours. Ceftriaxone is highly bound to plasma proteins (85% to 90%) and is widely distributed throughout the body, including the CSF. The plasma half-life is 4.3 to 8.7 hours; it is increased to 11.4 to 15.7 hours in clients with impaired renal function. This long half-life allows once-a-day dosing. Ceftriaxone is primarily eliminated unchanged in the urine.[4,9]

Pharmaceutics Ceftriaxone is administered parenterally by either IM or IV routes.

Undesired Clinical Responses Ceftriaxone shares the same undesired clinical responses as other cephalosporins, including hypersensitivity reactions, potential for developing pseudomembranous colitis, thrombophlebitis, and GI distress. Additionally, **pseudolithiasis,** or **biliary sludge,** with symptoms of epigastric pain, anorexia, nausea, and vomiting, may occur. Pseudolithiasis occurs especially if ceftriaxone is administered by IV injection over 3 to 5 minutes.

Contraindications and Precautions Ceftriaxone use is contraindicated in clients with known allergy to cephalosporins or serious reaction to penicillin.

Drug-Environment Interactions Ceftriaxone solutions appear light yellow to amber. The IV infusion solution is stable for 3 days at room temperature and 10 days if refrigerated. Ceftriaxone can interfere with the same diagnostic tests as cefuroxime.

Life-Span Considerations Ceftriaxone is classified as a Pregnancy Category B drug. The drug readily crosses the placenta and is excreted in breast milk.

Specific Drug-Related Nursing Considerations Dilute IM and IV preparations of ceftriaxone before their administration. Check the drug insert for proper dilution procedure. Administer the direct IV injection over 2 to 4 minutes. Infuse the intermittent IV infusion over 15 to 30 minutes for adults and 10 to 30 minutes for children and neonates. Evaluate the IV site for phlebitis, and check the IM site for tenderness and induration.

TABLE 55–2
Antibiotics: Cephalosporins

Drug Name	Dosage and Route of Administration	Nursing Considerations
FIRST GENERATION **Cefadroxil** (Dunicef, Ultracef) HOW SUPPLIED Capsules: 500 mg Tablets: 1 g Oral suspension: 125, 250, 500 mg/5 ml when reconstituted	ADULTS 1–2 g/d as single or divided doses q12h CHILDREN 30 mg/kg/d in divided doses q12h	**Assess** Inquire about sensitivity to cephalosporins or penicillin. Ask about concurrent drugs. Obtain history of other medical conditions (e.g., GI disease, renal or hepatic impairment). Obtain baseline values for liver and kidney function and CBC. Obtain specimens for cultures and sensitivities before initiating therapy. Inquire whether the client is pregnant or breast-feeding. **Implement** Give oral drug without regard to meals. **Monitor** Review CBC, urinalysis, and liver and renal function test results. Observe for undesired effects such as allergic reaction, GI effects (especially pseudomembranous colitis). **Evaluate** Watch for resolution of signs and symptoms of infection.
CEFAZOLIN (Ancef, Kefzol) HOW SUPPLIED Injection: 500 mg; 1, 5, 10, 20 g	ADULTS IV: 250 mg–1.5 g q6-8h CHILDREN > 1 MO IV: 25–100 mg/kg/d in divided doses q6-8h	**Assess** Same as cefadroxil. **Implement** Give parenterally by IV administration. Check package insert for proper dilution procedure. **Monitor** Same as cefadroxil. **Evaluate** Same as cefadroxil.
Cephalexin (Keflet, Keflex) HOW SUPPLIED Capsules: 250, 500 mg Tablets: 250, 500 mg, 1 g Oral suspensions: 100 mg/ml; 125, 250 mg/5 ml when reconstituted	ADULTS 250–500 mg q6h CHILDREN 25–100 mg/kg/d in divided doses q6-12h	Same as cefadroxil.
Cephalothin (Keflin) HOW SUPPLIED Injection: 1, 2, 20 g	ADULTS IV: 500 mg–2 g q4-6h CHILDREN IV: 20–40 mg/kg q6h (or 80–160 mg/kg/d in divided doses q6h)	**Assess** Inquire about sensitivity to cephalosporins or penicillin. Ask about concurrent drugs. Cephalothin is more likely to interact with nephrotoxic drugs. Obtain history of other medical conditions (e.g., GI disease, renal or hepatic impairment). Obtain baseline values for liver and kidney function and CBC. Obtain specimens for culture and sensitivities before initiating therapy. Inquire whether the client is pregnant or breast-feeding.

Table continued on following page.

TABLE 55-2 *Continued*
Antibiotics: Cephalosporins

Drug Name	Dosage and Route of Administration	Nursing Considerations
Cephalothin Continued		**Implement** Give parenterally by IV injection. Follow package insert directions for proper dilution procedure of parenteral solution. **Monitor** Same as cefadroxil. **Evaluate** Same as cefadroxil.
Cephapirin (Cefadyl) HOW SUPPLIED Injection: 500 mg; 1, 2, 4, 20 g	ADULTS IV or IM: 500 mg–1 g q4-6h CHILDREN > 3 MO IV or IM: 10–20 mg/kg q6h (or 40–80 mg/kg/d in divided doses q6h)	**Assess** Same as cefadroxil. **Implement** Give parenterally by deep IM injection or IV administration. Follow package insert directions for proper dilution procedure. **Monitor** Same as cefadroxil. **Evaluate** Same as cefadroxil.
Cephradine (Velosef) HOW SUPPLIED Capsules: 250, 500 mg Oral suspension: 125, 250 mg/5 ml when reconstituted	ADULTS 1–2 g/d in divided doses q6-12h CHILDREN 6.25–25 mg/kg q6h (or 25–50 mg/kg/d in divided doses q6-12h)	**Assess** Same as cefadroxil. **Implement** Give orally without regard to meals. **Monitor** Same as cefadroxil. **Evaluate** Same as cefadroxil.
SECOND GENERATION **CEFUROXIME** (Ceftin) HOW SUPPLIED Tablets: 125, 250, 500 mg Suspension: 125 mg/5 ml when reconstituted Injection: 750 mg; 1.5, 7.5 g	ADULTS Oral: 250–500 mg q12h IM or IV: 750 mg–1.5 g q8h CHILDREN > 3 MO Oral: 20–40 mg/kg/d in divided doses q12h IM or IV: 50–100 mg/kg/d in divided doses q6-8h	**Assess** Inquire about sensitivity to cephalosporins or penicillin. Ask about concurrent drugs. Obtain history of other medical conditions. Obtain baseline values for liver and kidney function and CBC. Assess the infectious process. Obtain specimens before initiating therapy. Inquire whether the client is pregnant or breast-feeding. **Implement** Give drug orally without regard to meals. **Monitor** Review CBC, urinalysis, and liver and renal function test results. Observe for undesired effects such as allergic reactions, GI effects (especially pseudomembranous colitis). **Evaluate** Watch for resolution of signs and symptoms of infection.
Cefaclor (Ceclor) HOW SUPPLIED Capsules: 250, 500 mg Powder for oral suspension: 125, 187, 250, 375 mg/5 ml when reconstituted	ADULTS 250–500 mg q8h CHILDREN > 1 MO 20–40 mg/kg/d in divided doses q8h	Same as cefadroxil.

TABLE 55–2 *Continued*
Antibiotics: Cephalosporins

729

Drug Name	Dosage and Route of Administration	Nursing Considerations
Cefamandole (Mandol) **HOW SUPPLIED** Injection: 500 mg; 1, 2, 10 g	ADULTS IM or IV: 2–12 g/d in divided doses q4-8h CHILDREN > 1 MO IV or IM: 50–150 mg/kg/d in divided doses q4-8h	**Assess** Inquire about sensitivity to cephalosporins or penicillin. Ask about concurrent drugs, including alcohol and anticoagulants. Obtain history of other medical conditions, especially history of bleeding disorders. Obtain baseline values for liver and kidney function and CBC. Obtain specimens for culture and sensitivities before initiating therapy. Inquire whether the client is pregnant or breast-feeding. **Implement** Give parenterally by deep IM injection or IV administration. Check package insert for proper dilution procedure. **Monitor** Obtain CBC, urinalysis, and liver and renal function test results. Monitor for undesired effects such as allergic reactions, GI effects (especially pseudomembranous colitis). Assess changes in the infectious process. **Evaluate** Observe for diminished signs and symptoms of infection.
Cefmetazole (Zefazone) **HOW SUPPLIED** Injection: 1, 2 g	ADULTS IV: 2 g q6-12h	**Assess** Same as cefamandole. **Implement** Give parenterally by IV administration. Follow package insert directions for proper dilution procedure. **Monitor** Same as cefamandole. **Evaluate** Observe for diminished signs and symptoms of infection.
Cefonicid (Monocid) **HOW SUPPLIED** Injection: 500-mg, 1-g vials	ADULTS IM or IV: 500 mg–2 g q24h	**Assess** Same as cefadroxil. **Implement** Give parenterally by deep IM injection or IV administration. Give IM doses of 2 g as divided doses in different sites. **Monitor** Same as cefadroxil. **Evaluate** Same as cefadroxil.
Cefotetan (Cefotan) **HOW SUPPLIED** Injection: 1, 2, 10 g	ADULTS IM or IV: 1–3 g q12h	**Assess** Same as cefadroxil. **Implement** Give parenterally by deep IM injection or IV administration. Give IM doses of 2 g as divided doses in different sites. **Monitor** Same as cefadroxil. **Evaluate** Same as cefadroxil.

Table continued on following page.

TABLE 55–2 *Continued*
Antibiotics: Cephalosporins

Drug Name	Dosage and Route of Administration	Nursing Considerations
Cefoxitin (Mefoxin) HOW SUPPLIED Injection: 1, 2, 10 g	ADULTS IV: 1–3 g q6h CHILDREN > 3 MO IM or IV: 20–40 mg/kg q6h (or 80–160 mg/kg/d in divided doses q6h) CHILDREN 1–3 MO IM or IV: 20–40 mg/kg q6–8h CHILDREN 1–4 WK IM or IV: 20–40 mg/kg q8h (or 60–120 mg/kg/d in divided doses q8h) CHILDREN < 1 WK IM or IV: 20–40 mg/kg q12h (or 40–80 mg/kg/d in divided doses q12h)	*Assess* Same as cefadroxil. *Implement* Give parenterally by deep IM injection or IV administration. *Monitor* Same as cefadroxil. *Evaluate* Same as cefadroxil.
Cefprozil (Cefzil) HOW SUPPLIED Tablets: 250, 500 mg Powder for suspension: 125, 250 mg/5 ml after reconstitution	ADULTS 500 mg–1 g as a single dose or in divided doses q12h CHILDREN > 6 MO 7.5–15 mg/kg q12h	Same as cefadroxil.
Cefpodoxime (Vantin) HOW SUPPLIED Tablets: 100, 200 mg Granules for suspension: 50, 100 mg/5 ml when reconstituted	ADULTS 200–800 mg/d in divided doses q12h CHILDREN > 6 MO 10 mg/kg/d in divided doses q12h	Same as cefadroxil.
Loracarbef (Lorabid) HOW SUPPLIED Capsules: 200 mg Powder for suspension: 100 mg/5 ml after reconstitution	ADULTS 400–800 mg/d in divided doses q12h CHILDREN > 6 MO 15–30 mg/kg/d in divided doses q12h	*Assess* Same as cefadroxil. *Implement* Drug is best given 1 h before or 2 h after meals. *Monitor* Same as cefadroxil. *Evaluate* Same as cefadroxil.

THIRD GENERATION

Drug Name	Dosage and Route of Administration	Nursing Considerations
Cefixime (Suprax) HOW SUPPLIED Tablets: 200, 400 mg Powder for oral suspension: 100 mg/5 ml after reconstitution	ADULTS 400 mg/d as a single dose or in divided doses q12h CHILDREN > 12 Y OR > 50 KG 400 mg/d as a single dose or in divided doses q12h CHILDREN 6 MO TO 12 Y 8 mg/kg/d as single dose or in divided doses q12h	Same as cefadroxil.
Cefoperazone (Cefobid) HOW SUPPLIED Injection: 1, 2 g	ADULTS IV: 2–12 g/d in divided doses q8-12h	*Assess* Inquire about sensitivity to cephalosporins or penicillin. Ask about concurrent drugs, including alcohol and anticoagulants. Obtain history of other medical conditions, especially history of bleeding disorders or severe liver and renal impairment. Obtain baseline values for liver and kidney function and CBC. Obtain specimens for culture and sensitivities before initiating therapy. Inquire whether the client is pregnant or breast-feeding. *Implement* Give parenterally by IV administration.

TABLE 55–2 *Continued*
Antibiotics: Cephalosporins

Drug Name	Dosage and Route of Administration	Nursing Considerations
Cefoperazone Continued		**Monitor** Same as cefadroxil. **Evaluate** Same as cefadroxil.
Cefotaxime (Claforan) HOW SUPPLIED Injection: 1, 2, 10 g	ADULTS IV: 1–2 g q4-12h IM: 1–6 g/d in divided doses q8-12h CHILDREN > 1 MO IM or IV: 50–200 mg/kg/d in divided doses q4-8h CHILDREN 1–4 WK IV: 50 mg/kg q6-8h CHILDREN < 1 WK IV: 50 mg/kg q12h	**Assess** Same as cefadroxil. **Implement** Give parenterally by IV administration. **Monitor** Same as cefadroxil. **Evaluate** Same as cefadroxil.
Ceftizoxime (Cefizox) HOW SUPPLIED Injection: 500 mg; 1, 2, 10 g	ADULTS IV: 2–12 g/d in divided doses q8-12h CHILDREN > 6 MO IV: 33–50 mg/kg q6-8h	**Assess** Same as cefadroxil. **Implement** Give parenterally by IV administration. **Monitor** Same as cefadroxil. **Evaluate** Same as cefadroxil.
Ceftazidime (Ceptaz, Fortaz, Tazidime) HOW SUPPLIED Injection: 500 mg; 1, 2, 6, 10 g	ADULTS IV: 1–6 g/d in divided doses q8-12h CHILDREN > 1 MO IV: 25–50 mg/kg q8h NEONATES 0–4 WK IV: 30 mg/kg q12h	**Assess** Same as cefadroxil. **Implement** Give parenterally by IV administration. **Monitor** Same as cefadroxil. **Evaluate** Same as cefadroxil.
CEFTRIAXONE (Rocephin) HOW SUPPLIED Injection: 250, 500 mg; 1, 2, 10 g	ADULTS IM or IV: 1–2 g/d as single dose or divided doses q12h CHILDREN > 45 KG IM or IV: 50–100 mg/kg/d as single dose or divided doses q12h CHILDREN < 45 KG IM or IV: 50 mg/kg as single daily dose INFANTS IM or IV: 25–50 mg/kg/d as single daily dose	**Assess** Same as cefadroxil. **Implement** Give parenterally by deep IM injection or IV administration. **Monitor** Same as cefadroxil. **Evaluate** Same as cefadroxil.

MISCELLANEOUS DRUGS IN CATEGORY

Cefixime (Suprax), **cefoperazone** (Cefobid), **cefotaxime** (Claforan), **ceftizoxime** (Cefizox), and **ceftazidime** (Fortaz) are all third-generation cephalosporins. Cefoperazone achieves high biliary concentrations. It must be used with caution in clients with severe hepatic or renal impairment. Cefoperazone interacts with alcohol, causing a disulfiram reaction. It also interacts with anticoagulants or thrombolytic drugs to increase the risk of bleeding.[3,5,15] Table 55–2 provides additional information on dosage forms, dosages, and routes of administration for third-generation cephalosporins.

CONCEPT REVIEW

The cephalosporins are widely used antibiotics. These drugs are classified as first-, second-, and third-generation cephalosporins. The spectrum of activity is generally against gram-positive organisms with the first generation, with increased effectiveness against gram-negative organisms with the third generation.

The cephalosporins' mechanism of action is to inhibit bacterial cell wall synthesis.

The most important undesired clinical responses to the cephalosporins are allergic reactions and the risk of pseudomembranous colitis. In addition, cross-sensitivity with the penicillins frequently occurs.

AMINOGLYCOSIDES

Aminoglycosides were first obtained in 1944 from a species of *Streptomyces*. Streptomycin was the first such drug available for clinical use, followed by neomycin in 1949 and kanamycin in 1957. Today these three drugs have limited use because of the development of resistance or the risk of toxic effects. Aminoglycosides in current use include gentamicin, tobramycin, amikacin, and netilmicin.

Aminoglycosides are broad-spectrum antibiotics that act by interfering with protein synthesis in susceptible microorganisms. Specifically, they are actively transported across the bacterial cell membrane, and they intracellularly, irreversibly bind to the 30S ribosomal ring. Aminoglycosides disrupt the normal cycle of ribosomal function by interfering with the initiation of protein synthesis. It is not known exactly how these drugs affect destruction of bacteria since other drugs that block protein synthesis do not cause bacterial death.[16]

The aminoglycosides are used primarily in the treatment of infections caused by gram-negative aerobic bacteria, including *P. aeruginosa*. Activity against most gram-positive bacteria is limited. For example, *S. pneumoniae* is highly resistant to aminoglycosides, but enterococci are sensitive when aminoglycosides are combined with a penicillin.[2-4]

As is the case with other antibiotics, bacteria may be resistant to the antimicrobial activity of the aminoglycosides. Resistance may occur because of failure of the antibiotic to permeate the bacterial cell membrane, low affinity of the antibiotic for bacterial ribosomes, or inactivation of the antibiotic by microbial enzymes.

Pharmacokinetic properties for aminoglycosides vary according to the dosage form. Since aminoglycosides are poorly absorbed after oral administration, they must be administered parenterally to treat systemic infections. The exceptions are neomycin, kanamycin, and paromomycin, which are administered orally preoperatively to decrease intestinal flora and to control intestinal disease caused by protozoa. Neomycin, gentamicin, and tobramycin are available for topical treatment of skin and eyes conditions because absorption is poor and resultant toxicity minimal.

Aminoglycosides are rapidly and completely absorbed after IM administration. They are poorly bound to plasma proteins (0% to 10%). Serum levels in the young and the elderly may be prolonged; they may be decreased in the febrile and severely burned client. Since aminoglycosides are lipid insoluble, they are poorly distributed in some tissues. Low concentrations are found in bile, breast milk, and CSF. They bind tightly to renal cortical tissue in which concentrations as much as 50% higher than in serum occur, hence the high potential for nephrotoxicity. Aminoglycosides cross the placental barrier and may adversely affect the fetus. Up to 98% of the drug dosage is excreted unchanged in urine. Half-life of aminoglycosides is 1 to 3 hours in clients with normal renal function. This time may be extended, sometimes to 80 to 100 hours, in clients with renal insufficiency.[2,4,9,16]

Undesired clinical responses are the major factors limiting the usefulness of the aminoglycosides. All aminoglycosides potentially can produce **ototoxicity** and **nephrotoxicity.**

Toxic effects on the ear can cause both vestibular and auditory dysfunction. Accumulation of aminoglycosides in otic tissue occurs predominantly when serum concentration levels are high and persistently elevated. Progressive destruction of vestibular or cochlear sensory cells occurs, with damage progressing from the base of the cochlea (high-frequency sounds) to the apex (low-frequency sounds). The degree of permanent dysfunction is correlated with the number of sensory cells destroyed or altered. Clients with renal insufficiency and the elderly are at higher risk for ototoxicity. Concomitant use of other ototoxic drugs such as ethacrynic acid or furosemide exacerbates the problem. Early signs of ototoxicity are tinnitus, vertigo, ataxia, and deafness.[7]

Approximately 8% to 26% of clients receiving aminoglycosides develop reversible mild renal impairment from nephrotoxicity. The toxicity apparently is due to accumulation and retention of the aminoglycoside in proximal tubular cells. The most common indication of kidney damage is a rise in serum creatinine levels. Total amount of aminoglycosides administered, concurrent administration of other drugs with nephrotoxic potential, and susceptible clients (e.g., the elderly), increase the risk for nephrotoxicity.

Aminoglycosides may also induce neuromuscular blockade by inhibiting nerve transmission. Skeletal weakness, respiratory depression, and paralysis may result. Concurrent use of neuromuscular blocking agents, preexistence of muscle weakness, and severe hypocalcemia are often predisposing factors. Common undesired clinical responses for aminoglycosides are illustrated in Figure 55–3.

Aminoglycosides can cause fetal harm when administered during pregnancy. All aminoglycosides cross the placenta. These drugs must be used with caution in premature infants and neonates since immature renal function results in prolonged half-life. The elderly, because of a possible age-related decrease in renal function, require monitoring of their renal function.[7]

AMINOGLYCOSIDE PROTOTYPE

GENTAMICIN SULFATE

Gentamicin (Garamycin, Genoptic, Jenamicin) is the prototype aminoglycoside. Gentamicin is similar in its properties to tobramycin, netilmicin, and amikacin. It is obtained from a species of *Actinomyces*.

Pharmacotherapeutics Clinically gentamicin is active against gram-negative microorganisms, including most Enterobacteriaceae. *Acinetobacter* and *Pseudo-monas* spp. are also susceptible. Gentamicin is active against gram-positive organisms such as *S. aureus* and *Enterococcus*.

Gentamicin is used for treatment of serious infections caused by susceptible gram-negative bacilli. It is used to treat infections of the biliary tract, bones and joints, skin and soft tissues, and urinary tract. Gentamicin is also used to treat pneumonia and septicemia.[5,16]

Pharmacokinetics Gentamicin is well absorbed after IM injection, with its peak serum concentration in ½ to 1½ hours. The drug is minimally bound to plasma proteins and is widely distributed in extracellular fluid. However, it

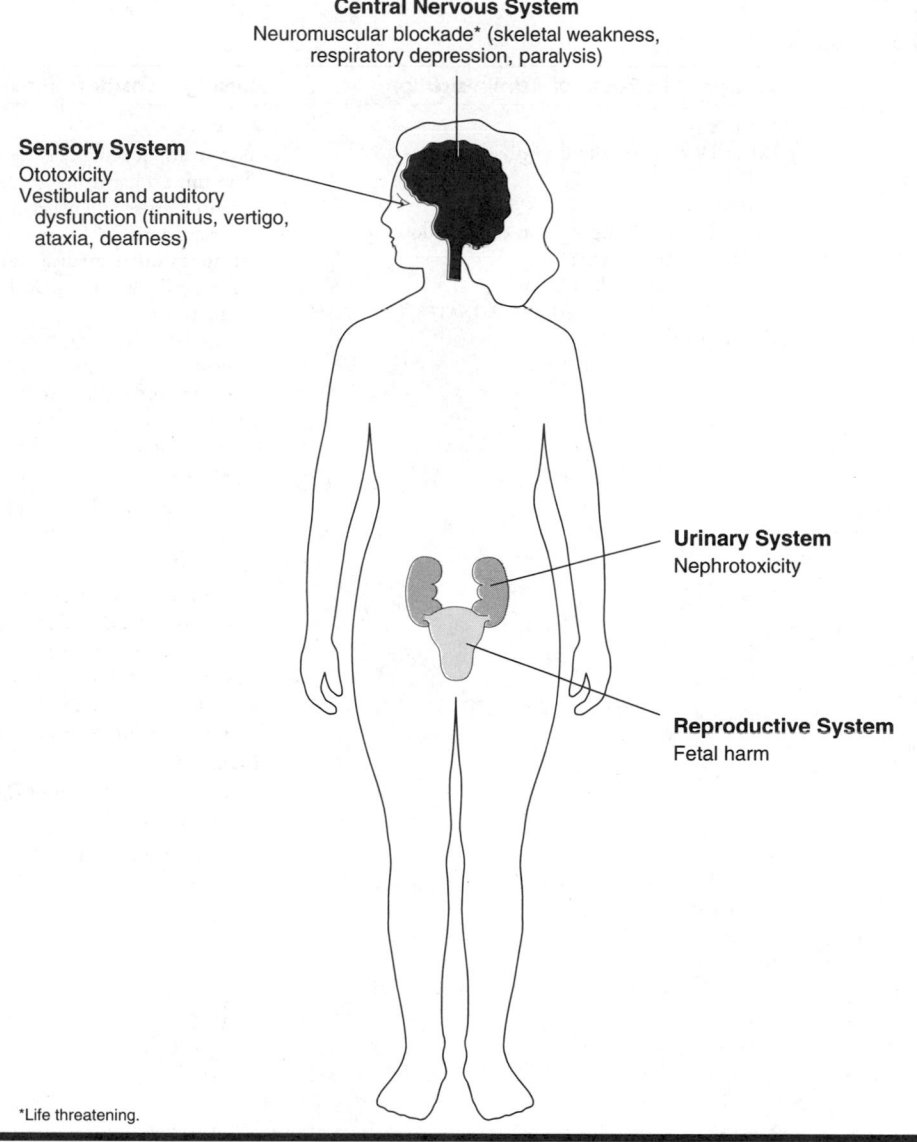

Central Nervous System
Neuromuscular blockade* (skeletal weakness,
respiratory depression, paralysis)

Sensory System
Ototoxicity
Vestibular and auditory
    dysfunction (tinnitus, vertigo,
    ataxia, deafness)

Urinary System
Nephrotoxicity

Reproductive System
Fetal harm

*Life threatening.

FIGURE 55–3   Common undesired clinical responses associated with aminoglycosides.

has poor CNS penetration. Its plasma half-life is 2 to 4 hours in adults and 5 to 8 hours in neonates. These times are greatly increased in clients with impaired renal function. Gentamicin is *not* metabolized and is primarily excreted in the urine.[4,9,17]

Pharmaceutics Gentamicin is administered IM, IV, topically, and intrathecally. It may also be administered by aerosol nebulization as an adjunct to parenteral therapy. Table 55–3 provides additional information about dosage forms, dosages, and routes of administration.[4,9,17]

Contraindications and Precautions Special precautions are needed in administering gentamicin to clients with myasthenia gravis or parkinsonism, impaired renal function, eighth cranial nerve impairment, or previous hypersensitivity reaction to the aminoglycosides.

Drug-Drug and Drug-Environment Interactions Other aminoglycosides and nephrotoxic- and ototoxic-producing drugs may increase the toxicity with gentamicin administration. Gentamicin may increase the effects of neuromuscular blocking agents.

Vials and ophthalmic and topical preparations are stored at room temperature. Solutions should appear clear or slightly yellow. The intermittent IV infusion solution is stable for 24 hours at room temperature.[10]

Interference with Diagnostic Tests Use of gentamicin may increase blood urea nitrogen (BUN), ALT, AST, bilirubin, creatinine, and LDH concentrations. It may decrease serum calcium, magnesium, potassium, and sodium concentrations.

Life-Span Considerations Gentamicin is classified as a Pregnancy Category C drug. It readily crosses the placenta and may produce fetal nephrotoxicity.

Specific Drug-Related Nursing Considerations It is strongly recommended that serum levels of gentamicin be measured to monitor therapy. Therapeutic peak levels 30 to 60 minutes after administration of IV injection should be 3 to 5 µg/ml in children and 4 to 6 µg/ml in adults. Trough levels just before administration of the next dose should not be greater than 2 µg/ml for both children and adults.

TABLE 55–3
Antibiotics: Aminoglycosides

Drug Name	Dosage and Route of Administration	Nursing Considerations
GENTAMICIN (Garamycin, Jenamicin) HOW SUPPLIED Injection: 40, 10 mg/ml Intrathecal: 2 mg/ml	ADULTS IM or IV: 3–5 mg/kg/d in divided doses q8-12h CHILDREN IM or IV: 6–7.5 mg/kg/d in divided doses q8h INFANTS AND NEONATES IM or IV: 2.5 mg/kg q8-16h PREMATURE AND FULL-TERM NEONATES IM or IV: 2.5 mg/kg q12-24h	*Assess* Inquire about sensitivity to aminoglycosides. Determine what drugs are being used concurrently, especially other nephrotoxic or ototoxic drugs. Ask about other medical conditions (myasthenia gravis, hearing defect, impaired kidney function). Obtain baseline renal function test and CBC results. Assess the infectious process. Obtain specimens before initiating therapy. Inquire whether the patient is pregnant. *Implement* Give parenterally by IM injection or IV administration. *Monitor* Determine aminoglycoside concentration. Review results from CBC, urinalysis, renal function test. Observe for undesired effects, especially nephrotoxicity and ototoxicity. Monitor the infectious process. *Evaluate* Observe for resolution of signs and symptoms of infection.
Amikacin (Amikin) HOW SUPPLIED Injection: 250, 50 mg/ml	ADULTS IM or IV: 5 mg/kg q8h or 7.5 mg/kg q12h CHILDREN IM or IV: 5 mg/kg q8h or 7.5 mg/kg q12h NEONATES IM or IV: 10 mg/kg initially, then 7.5 mg/kg q12h PREMATURE NEONATES IM or IV: 10 mg/kg initially, then 7.5 mg/kg q18-24h	Same as gentamicin.
Netilmicin (Netromycin) HOW SUPPLIED Injection: 100 mg/ml	ADULTS IM or IV: 3–6.5 mg/kg/d in divided doses q8-12h CHILDREN > 6 WK IM or IV: 5.5–8 mg/kg/d in divided doses q8-12h INFANTS < 6 WK IM or IV: 4–6.5 mg/kg/d in divided doses q12h	Same as gentamicin.
Tobramycin (Nebcin) HOW SUPPLIED Injection: 10, 40 mg/ml	ADULTS IM or IV: 3–5 mg/kg/d in divided doses q8-12h CHILDREN IM or IV: 6–7.5 mg/kg/d in divided doses q8h PREMATURE AND FULL-TERM NEONATES IM or IV: Up to 4 mg/kg/d in divided doses q12h	Same as gentamicin.

MISCELLANEOUS DRUGS IN CATEGORY

Other aminoglycosides include amikacin, netilmicin, streptomycin, and tobramycin. **Streptomycin** has a chemical structure different from that of other aminoglycosides. Use of streptomycin has greatly decreased because of its toxic effects. It is used to treat tuberculosis and is discussed briefly in Chapter 57. **Amikacin** (Amikin), **netilmicin** (Netromycin), and **tobramycin** (Nebcin) are administered parenterally IM or IV. They are used in the treatment of biliary tract infections, bone and joint infections, CNS infections, intraabdominal infections, skin and soft-tissue infections, and recurrent complicated urinary tract infections. They are also used to treat pneumonia and septicemia caused by gram-negative organisms. Tobramycin may also be administered in an aerosol nebulization. Table 55–3 contains information on dosage forms, dosages, and routes of administration.

CONCEPT REVIEW

The aminoglycosides are narrow-spectrum antibiotics primarily effective against aerobic gram-negative bacilli. These drugs are bactericidal and exert their action by inhibiting bacterial protein synthesis.

The most serious adverse effects of the aminoglycosides are ototoxicity and nephrotoxicity. Aminoglycoside serum concentrations are carefully monitored to minimize the occurrence of ototoxicity and nephrotoxicity.

QUINOLONES

The quinolones, or fluoroquinolones, represent an important therapeutic advance in treating infection. These agents have a broad spectrum of activity and are effective orally against a wide variety of infections. They produce relatively few side effects. The major quinolones in use are ciprofloxacin, norfloxacin, ofloxacin, and lomefloxacin.

The quinolones are bactericidal. They act intracellularly by inhibiting DNA gyrase, an essential bacterial enzyme that connects closed circular DNA into a supercoiled configuration. Without supercoiling, DNA replication cannot occur, and bacterial growth is inhibited.

Resistance to the quinolones can occur and has developed in some strains of *S. aureus, Serratia,* and *P. aeruginosa.* Possible mechanisms for resistance are alterations in DNA gyrase and decreased ability of the antibiotic to cross the bacterial membrane.

Pharmacokinetic properties are similar for all drugs in this group. The quinolones can be administered both orally and by IV infusion. They are well absorbed after oral administration and are moderately bound to plasma protein (10% to 40%). Quinolones are widely distributed to most body fluids and to tissues, with high concentrations in the kidneys, liver, lungs. Ciprofloxacin and ofloxacin also penetrate into CSF.

Peak serum concentrations after oral administration occur in 1 to 2 hours. The quinolones are partially metabolized in the liver and are primarily excreted in the urine, with some excretion via the biliary system. The elimination half-life ranges from 3 to 7 hours and is increased in clients with impaired renal function.[19,20]

The most common **undesired responses** are related to the GI tract and include abdominal pain or discomfort, diarrhea, nausea, or vomiting. CNS responses also occur and include dizziness or lightheadedness, headache, nervousness, drowsiness, or insomnia. Rashes, including photosensitivity reactions, occur less frequently. Rare side effects include CNS stimulation (e.g., agitation, confusion), hypersensitivity reaction (e.g., skin rash, itching, or redness), and phlebitis.[4,7]

Use of quinolones is not recommended during pregnancy. Also, because the quinolones are distributed in breast milk and can cause permanent lesions of cartilage on weight-bearing joints, use in women who are breast-feeding is not recommended. Use of quinolones is not recommended in children up to 18 years of age for the same reason. Special caution must be taken in the elderly because of an age-related decrease in renal function, which may require dosage adjustments.

Drug-drug interactions occur with several drugs. Quinolones, especially ciprofloxacin and enoxacin, can significantly reduce hepatic metabolism, thus increasing the serum concentration of aminophylline or theophylline. This increases the risk of toxicity associated with these bronchodilator agents. Antacids, ferrous sulfate, or sucralfate can decrease absorption of quinolones. Antacids inhibit GI absorption of quinolones, which chelate with aluminum, calcium, or magnesium to produce lower serum and urinary concentrations of the antibiotic. If antacids are required, they should be administered 2 to 4 hours before or after the quinolones. Quinolones, especially ciprofloxacin, may increase the anticoagulant effect of warfarin. The client's prothrombin time should be carefully monitored while he or she receives these drugs.[21,22]

QUINOLONE PROTOTYPE
CIPROFLOXACIN HYDROCHLORIDE

Ciprofloxacin (Cipro) is the prototype for the quinolones.

Pharmacotherapeutics Clinically ciprofloxacin has moderate activity against gram-positive organisms, including methicillin-susceptible *S. aureus*, coagulase-negative *Staphylococcus*, β-hemolytic streptococci, *S. pneumoniae*, and enterococci. Good activity is found against gram-negative organisms, including most Enterobacteriaceae (i.e., *Citrobacter* spp., *Enterobacter* spp., *E. coli, Klebsiella* spp., *M. morganii, Proteus* spp., *Salmonella, Shigella, B. catarrhalis, N. gonorrhoeae, N. meningitidis, H. influenzae,* and *Legionella pneumophila*). Ciprofloxacin is also the most active quinolone against *P. aeruginosa;* it has good activity against *Chlamydia trachomatis* and *Mycoplasma pneumoniae.*

Ciprofloxacin is used in the treatment of bone and joint infections, bronchitis, bacterial gastroenteritis, gonorrhea (endocervical and urethral), gram-negative and strepto-coccal pneumonia, bacterial prostatitis, skin and soft-tissue infections, and urinary tract infection caused by organisms susceptible to the antibiotic.

Pharmacokinetics Ciprofloxacin may be administered orally or by IV piggyback. It is well absorbed after oral administration (70% to 80%) and reaches its peak serum concentration within 1 to 2 hours. It is moderately bound to plasma proteins (20% to 40%) and is widely distributed to most body fluids and tissues, including the CSF. In the CSF ciprofloxacin reaches 10% of its peak serum concentration; this increases to 14% to 37% with inflamed meninges. Plasma half-life of the drug is 4 to 6 hours; this time is increased in clients with impaired renal function. Ciprofloxacin is minimally metabolized in the liver (20%) and is primarily excreted in the urine, with some elimination via the biliary system.

Pharmaceutics Ciprofloxacin is available for oral, IV, and ophthalmic administration. Table 55–4 provides additional information on dosage forms, dosages, and routes of administration.

Contraindications and Precautions Ciprofloxacin use is contraindicated in clients with a previous allergic reaction to the quinolones. It should be used with caution in clients with CNS disorder (e.g., epilepsy) because it can produce CNS stimulation or toxicity. Ciprofloxacin must be used with caution in individuals with impaired renal function.

Life-Span Considerations Ciprofloxacin should not be used during pregnancy; it is classified as a Pregnancy Category C drug. It also should not be used in breast-feeding women or children less than 18 years of age. It should be used with caution in elderly clients because of age-related impaired renal function.

Specific Drug-Related Nursing Considerations Oral ciprofloxacin may be administered without regard to meals; however, the preferred dosing time is 2 hours after meals. Advise the client to take the oral drug with a full glass of water and to drink several glasses of water between meals. Encourage the client to eat and drink high sources of ascorbic acid to prevent crystalluria. Instruct the client to avoid sunlight or ultraviolet exposure; and advise him or her to wear sunscreens and protective clothing if photosensitivity occurs.

Follow the instructions in the drug package insert about the dilution method for the IV infusion solution. Infuse the solution via a large vein to reduce venous irritation; infuse it slowly over an hour to minimize discomfort and the risk of venous irritation.

MISCELLANEOUS DRUGS IN CATEGORY

Other drugs in the category include enoxacin (Penetrex), lomefloxacin (Maxaquin), norfloxacin (Noroxin), and ofloxacin (Floxin). **Enoxacin** is used in the treatment of gonorrhea, gonococcal urethritis, and urinary tract infections. This drug produces the greatest risk of increasing theophylline levels and the toxicity of the quinolones. **Lomefloxacin** is used in the treatment of acute exacerbation of chronic bronchitis and urinary tract infections and as prophylaxis in transurethral surgery. It has a long half-life, allowing once-a-day dosing. It does not significantly interact with theophylline.[13]

Norfloxacin, which is best taken with full glass of water 1 hour before or 2 hours after meals, is used to treat urinary tract

infections, gonorrhea, and gonococcal urethritis. **Ofloxacin** is used in the treatment of lower respiratory tract infections, chlamydial infections, uncomplicated gonorrhea, skin and soft-tissue infections, prostatitis, and urinary tract infections. It produces a minimal risk of increasing theophylline levels. Table 55–4 provides additional information on dosages, dosage forms, and routes of administration.

CONCEPT REVIEW

The quinolones are bactericidal and have a broad spectrum of activity with relatively few side effects. Most common undesired clinical responses are related to the GI tract and CNS.

Quinolones act intracellularly by inhibiting DNA gyrase.

MACROLIDES

Erythromycin, the major macrolide antibiotic, was discovered in 1952. It was first isolated from a strain of *Streptomyces.* The macrolide antibiotics are either bacteriostatic or bactericidal; they are bactericidal when used in high concentrations or against highly susceptible organisms. The macrolides inhibit protein synthesis. They penetrate the bacterial cell membrane, reversibly binding to the 50S subunit of bacterial ribosomes. Translocation of peptides is prevented, with subsequent inhibition of protein synthesis. Activity of the macrolide antibiotics is only against dividing organisms (see Fig. 55–1).

Macrolides are most effective against gram-positive cocci (e.g., *Streptococcus pyogenes* and *S. pneumoniae*) and gram-negative cocci (e.g., *B. catarrhalis*). These antibiotics show good activity against strains of *Campylobacter jejuni, M. pneumoniae,* and the agent of legionnaires' disease, *L. pneumophila.* They have no activity against viruses, yeasts, or fungi. **Resistance** to macrolides occurs from at least three plasmid mediated alterations: (1) decreased permeability through the bacterial cell membrane; (2) modification of the target site on the ribosome; and (3) hydrolysis by an enzyme produced by Enterobacteriaceae.[3,4,19]

Pharmacokinetic properties of these drugs are important aspects of therapy. The macrolides are incompletely absorbed from the upper part of the small intestine. Some macrolides may be inactivated by gastric acid, with absorption decreased when administered with food. Macrolides are widely distributed into tissues and fluids throughout the body. It is poorly distributed into CSF but does cross the placenta and is excreted in breast milk. Macrolides are moderately bound to plasma protein. These antibiotics are metabolized in the liver. They are eliminated primarily by hepatic concentration and excretion with the bile.

Undesired clinical responses associated with macrolide antibiotics only rarely are serious. Hypersensitivity reactions occur less frequently and can include skin rash, redness, and itching. GI effects happen frequently, especially if large doses are administered. Abdominal or stomach cramping, nausea,

TABLE 55–4
Antibiotics: Quinolones

Drug Name	Dosage and Route of Administration	Nursing Considerations
CIPROFLOXACIN (Cipro) **HOW SUPPLIED** Tablets: 250, 500, 750 mg Injection: 200, 400 mg	ADULTS Oral: 250–750 mg q12h IV: 200–400 mg q12h	**Assess** Inquire about sensitivity to quinolones. Ask about concurrent drugs (including antacids, theophylline, warfarin). Obtain results of baseline liver and renal function tests and CBC. Assess the infectious process. Obtain specimens for culture and sensitivities before initiating therapy. Inquire whether client is pregnant or breast-feeding. If so, use of drug is not recommended. **Implement** Orally drug may be given without regard to food. Administer IV over at least 60 min. **Monitor** Review results of CBC, urinalysis, renal and liver function tests. **Evaluate** Assess for resolution of signs and symptoms of infection.
Enoxacin (Penetrex) **HOW SUPPLIED** Tablets: 200, 400 mg	ADULTS 400–800 mg/d as a single dose or divided doses q12h	**Assess** Same as ciprofloxacin. **Implement** Give on empty stomach with full glass of water. **Monitor** Same as iprofloxacin. **Evaluate** Same as ciprofloxacin.
Lomefloxacin (Maxaquin) **HOW SUPPLIED** Tablets: 400 mg	ADULTS 400 mg/d as single daily dose	**Assess** Same as ciprofloxacin. **Implement** May give drug without regard to food. **Monitor** Review results of CBC, urinalysis, renal and liver function tests. Observe for undesired effects, especially photosensitivity reaction. **Evaluate** Same as ciprofloxacin.
Norfloxacin (Noroxin) **HOW SUPPLIED** Tablets: 400 mg	ADULTS 800 mg/d as single dose or divided q12h	**Assess** Same as ciprofloxacin. **Implement** Give on empty stomach with full glass of water. **Monitor** Same as ciprofloxacin. **Evaluate** Same as ciprofloxacin.
Ofloxacin (Floxin) **HOW SUPPLIED** Tablets: 200, 300, 400 mg Injection: 200, 400 mg	ADULTS Oral: 200–400 mg q12h IV: 200–400 mg q12h	**Assess** Inquire about sensitivity to quinolones. Ask about concurrent medication (especially warfarin). Obtain results of baseline liver and renal function tests and CBC. Assess the infectious process. Obtain specimens before initiating therapy. Inquire whether client is pregnant or breast-feeding. If so, use of drug is not recommended. **Implement** Give oral form on empty stomach with full glass of water. Administer IV slowly over at least 60 min. **Monitor** Same as ciprofloxacin. **Evaluate** Same as ciprofloxacin.

vomiting, or diarrhea occur; these effects are more common in children and young adults. Oral candidiasis has also been reported with use of macrolides. Cholestatic jaundice evidenced by dark or amber urine, pale stools, stomach pain, unusual tiredness, weakness, and jaundiced skin or eyes can occur but is rare with most macrolides. (Cholestatic jaundice occurs most frequently with the estolate form of erythromycin.) All symptoms usually disappear within several days of stopping therapy and are rarely prolonged.

Several **drug-drug interactions** are common to the macrolide class. Macrolides can inhibit the metabolism of carbamazepine, warfarin, and cyclosporine, resulting in increased plasma concentrations of these drugs and increased risk of toxicity. Other drugs that are potentially hepatotoxic (e.g., amiodarone, fluconazole, or lovastatin) may increase the client's risk of hepatotoxicity. Concurrent administration of macrolides with terfenadine may increase the risk of cardiotoxicity, including torsades de pointes. Macrolides may decrease theophylline hepatic clearance, causing increased theophylline concentration or toxicity. This interaction is more likely to occur after 6 days of concurrent therapy.[4,9,23]

MACROLIDE PROTOTYPE
ERYTHROMYCIN

Erythromycin is the prototype for the macrolide antibiotics.

Pharmacotherapeutics Clinically erythromycin is effective against gram-positive cocci, including *S. aureus,* coagulase-negative staphylococci, β-hemolytic streptococci, and *S. pneumoniae.* Gram-negative organisms susceptible to erythromycin include *C. jejuni, L. pneumophila,* and *Pasteurella multocida. H. influenzae* is susceptible, but erythromycin is usually combined with a sulfonamide when this microorganism is treated. Erythromycin is effective against *C. trachomatis, M. pneumoniae,* and *T. palladium.* Low activity occurs against anaerobes (e.g., *Clostridium* spp., *B. fragilis*).[3,4,19]

Erythromycin or erythromycin combinations are used concurrently as a preoperative bowel preparation. Erythromycin is also used in the treatment of a wide range of infections, including chlamydial conjunctivitis, genitourinary tract infections, diphtheria, urethral or endocervical gonorrhea, legionnaires' disease, acute otitis media, pertussis, bacterial pharyngitis or sinusitis, *Mycoplasma* or pneumococcal pneumonia, skin and soft-tissue infections, syphilis, and nongonococcal urethritis. Erythromycin is also used in the treatment of acne vulgaris and enterocolitis caused by *C. jejuni.*

Pharmacokinetics Erythromycin is incompletely absorbed from the GI tract. Depending on the salt and dosage form, erythromycin may or may not be inactivated by gastric acid, or its absorption may be affected by food. For example, an erythromycin base, film-coated tablet is inactivated by gastric acid and its absorption decreased with food. Erythromycin estolate is unaffected by gastric acid, and food does not affect absorption. Peak serum concentration after oral administration occurs in 1 to 4 hours, and protein binding ranges from 70% to 96%. Erythromycin is readily distributed throughout the body. It crosses the placenta and is excreted in breast milk. Erythromycin does not penetrate the CSF to any appreciable amount. Plasma half-life is 1.4 to 2 hours; this time is increased to 4.8 to 6 hours in clients with impaired renal function. Erythromycin is partially metabolized in the liver and primarily excreted into the bile.[4,5,9,19]

Pharmaceutics Erythromycin may be administered orally or parenterally by IV administration. Erythromycin is also given topically or as an ophthalmic drug. A variety of compounds and preparations for this drug is available. For example, erythromycin base and erythromycin stearate are destroyed by gastric acid and are available in enteric-coated forms to avoid this problem. These dosage forms must be taken on an empty stomach. The estolate and ethylsuccinate forms are chemically altered; they are acid stable and absorbed in the presence of food. Erythromycin gluceptate and erythromycin lactobionate are available for parenteral injection, although absorption may be erratic and may cause pain, inflammation, or phlebitis at the site of injection. Table 55–5 provides additional information on dosage forms, dosages, and routes of administration.

Contraindications and Precautions Erythromycin should be used with caution in clients with impaired liver function, especially if using the estolate salt, and in clients hypersensitive to erythromycin.

Life-Span Considerations Erythromycin is classified as a Pregnancy Category B drug. It crosses the placenta and is excreted in breast milk.

Specific Drug-Related Nursing Considerations Remind the client not to swallow chewable tablets whole. Advise him or her to take the drug with 240 ml of water 1 hour before or 2 hours after food or beverage. Monitor hepatic function test results and assess for hepatotoxicity. Evaluate for superinfection: genital and anal pruritus, sore mouth or tongue, and moderate-to-severe diarrhea.[11] Pain at the injection site can be diminished by further diluting the drug.

MISCELLANEOUS DRUGS IN CATEGORY

Other macrolides include azithromycin (Zithromax), clarithromycin (Biaxin), and dirithromycin. **Azithromycin** is an azalide antibiotic. This drug apparently has a greater distribution into tissues, a longer elimination half-life, and a lower incidence of adverse effects than erythromycin.[24] Azithromycin is long acting and can be taken on a one-a-day regimen. It is absorbed rapidly by the GI tract, but its absorption is affected by food in the stomach. Rapid distribution also occurs in all body tissues and fluids, with low concentrations in CSF in noninflamed meninges. It is used in the treatment of exacerbation of bronchitis, chlamydial cervicitis, pharyngitis, pneumonia caused by *H. influenzae,* or *S. pneumoniae,* skin and soft-tissue infection, and chlamydial urethritis.

Clarithromycin is a semisynthetic macrolide. It is rapidly absorbed orally and peaks in 2 hours. Clarithromycin is used in the treatment of exacerbation of bronchitis, pharyngitis, pneumonia (*Mycoplasma,* streptococcal), sinusitis, and skin and soft-tissue infections. It is classified as a Pregnancy Category C drug; it is not known if the drug is distributed in

TABLE 55–5
Macrolides

Drug Name	Dosage and Route of Administration	Nursing Considerations
ERYTHROMYCIN ***Erythromycin Base*** (E-Mycin, Ery-Tab, PCE Disperstab) ***Erythromycin Estolate*** (Ilosone) ***Erythromycin Ethylsuccinate*** (EryPed, E.E.S.) ***Erythromycin Lactobionate*** (Erythrocin) ***Erythromycin Stearate*** (Erythrocin) HOW SUPPLIED *Erythromycin Base* Tablets, enteric coated: 250, 333, 500 mg Tablets with polymer-coated particles: 333, 500 mg Tablets, delayed release: 333 mg Tablets, film coated: 250, 500 mg Capsules, delayed release: 250 mg *Erythromycin Estolate* Tablets: 500 mg Capsules: 250 mg Suspension: 125, 250 mg/5 ml *Erythromycin Ethylsuccinate* Tablets: 200, 400 mg Suspension: 100 mg/2.5 ml, 200 or 400 mg/50 ml *Erythromycin Lactobionate* Injection: 500 mg, 1 g *Erythromycin Stearate* Tablets, film coated: 250, 500 mg	ADULTS Oral: 250 mg q6h (or 400 mg as ethylsuccinate q6h) or 500 mg q12h or 333 mg q8h IV: 250 mg–1 g q6h CHILDREN Oral: 30–100 mg/kg/d in divided doses q6h IV: 15–20 mg/kg/d q6h	***Assess*** Determine sensitivity to macrolides. Identify concurrent drugs (especially antacids, terfenadine, carbamazepine, chloramphenicol, warfarin, theophylline). Obtain baseline liver function test and CBC results. Identify infectious process. Obtain culture before initiating therapy. Determine if client is pregnant or breast-feeding. ***Implement*** Give at least 1 h before or 2 h after meals. If GI irritation occurs, drug may be given with food. ***Monitor*** Monitor liver function and CBC results. Observe for undesired effects (allergic reactions, GI disturbances). Monitor infectious process. ***Evaluate*** Observe for resolution of signs and symptoms of infection.
Azithromycin (Zithromax) HOW SUPPLIED Capsules: 250 mg	ADULTS 500 mg on day 1; then 250 mg on days 2–5 (1.5 g total dose) CHILDREN 10 mg/kg on day 1; then 5 mg/kg on days 2–5	Same as erythromycin. Identify concurrent drugs (especially antacids and terfenadine).
Clarithromycin (Biaxin) HOW SUPPLIED Tablets: 250, 500 mg Granules for oral suspension: 125, 250 mg/5 ml after reconstitution	ADULTS 250–500 mg q12h CHILDREN 15 mg/kg/d in divided doses q12h	***Assess*** Same as erythromycin. Ask about concurrent drugs (especially theophylline). ***Implement*** Give without regard to meals. ***Monitor*** Same as erythromycin. Observe for undesired clinical effects (abnormal taste, GI disturbances, headache). ***Evaluate*** Same as erythromycin.

breast milk. Clarithromycin can increase the the-ophylline serum concentration and cause toxicity. Clarithromycin can also cause an abnormal taste in the mouth, abdominal discomfort, diarrhea, and nausea. Clarithromycin may be administered without regard to food. Tablets should not be crushed or broken. Table 55–5 provides additional information on these drugs.

Dirithromycin is a relatively new macrolide. It has a spectrum and degree of antimicrobial activity similar to that of erythromycin, but it has a longer half-life, enabling once-daily administration. It also achieves a greater cellular-to-extracellular concentration ratio than erythromycin.[25]

CONCEPT REVIEW

Macrolides, with erythromycin the most common, are bacteriostatic. They are bactericidal when used in high concentrations or against highly susceptible organisms.

Macrolides are most effective against gram-positive cocci and *Campylobacter, Mycoplasma,* and *Legionella.*

These drugs act by penetrating the bacterial cell membrane and inhibiting protein synthesis.

SULFONAMIDES

The sulfonamides were the first drugs used systemically to prevent and treat infections. They were widely used before the advent of the penicillins and other antibiotics. Current resistance to sulfonamides is evident, especially by gonococci, β-hemolytic streptococci, and some coliforms; this reduces their usefulness. However, the sulfonamides remain of value, especially when used in combination with trimethoprim, to treat urinary tract infections and *Pneumocystois carinii.*

As a group, sulfonamides are active against both gram-positive and gram-negative bacteria. Sulfonamides, in general, exert a bacteriostatic effect. They are usually effective against *S. pyogenes, S. pneumoniae, H. influenzae, Actinomyces,* and *C. trachomatis.*

Sulfonamides are structural analogs of para-aminobenzoic acid (PABA) and exert their activity by competing with PABA. They prevent bacteria from using PABA for synthesis of folic acid. Bacteria that synthesize their own folic acid are sensitive, whereas bacteria that use preformed folic acid are not affected by sulfonamides.

Pharmacokinetic properties of the sulfonamides influence drug selection. As a class, oral sulfonamides are rapidly absorbed from the GI tract, with the small intestine the major site of absorption. Approximately 70% to 97% of an oral dose is absorbed. An exception is sulfasalazine, which is administered primarily for its local effect. Sulfonamides are bound to plasma protein, especially albumin, and are widely distributed throughout the body. They readily pass through the placenta to reach fetal circulation. Metabolism of the sulfonamides oc-

curs primarily in the liver by acetylation, and excretion mainly occurs in the urine. Because excretion is primarily renal, the half-life may be prolonged in clients with renal dysfunction.

Sulfonamides are classified into four groups based on absorption and excretion:

- Agents rapidly absorbed and rapidly excreted (e.g., sulfisoxazole [Gantrisin])
- Agents poorly absorbed and thus active in the bowel (e.g., sulfasalazine)
- Agents primarily used for topical use (e.g., sulfacetamide, silver sulfadiazine)
- Agents rapidly absorbed and slowly excreted

Undesired clinical responses occurring with sulfonamides are numerous, with the overall incidence approximately 5%. **Crystalluria,** although high with less soluble sulfonamides, is less of a problem with more soluble sulfonamides. Fluid intake of at least 1200 ml daily in adults and alkalinization of the urine decrease the incidence of crystalluria. Disorders of the hematopoietic system include acute hemolytic anemia, agranulocytosis, and aplastic anemia, which occurs rarely.

Hypersensitivity reactions may occur, affecting the skin and mucous membranes. Examples of these reactions include morbilliform (resembling measles), urticarial, purpuric, and petechial rashes; exfoliative dermatitis; Stevens-Johnson syndrome; and photosensitivity. Reactions usually occur within the first week of therapy. Drug fever is also a common effect of sulfonamide therapy. Necrosis of the liver may also occur, causing headache, nausea, vomiting, fever, hepatomegaly, and increased liver function test results. Other effects include anorexia, nausea, and vomiting.[4,9,26] Figure 55–4 illustrates common undesired clinical responses associated with sulfonamides.

SULFONAMIDE PROTOTYPE
TRIMETHOPRIM AND SULFAMETHOXAZOLE

Since compounds of sulfonamide drugs are currently used more frequently than single drug preparations, the trimethoprim-sulfamethoxazole compound, also known as *co-trimoxazole* or *TMP-SMX,* has been selected as the prototype.

Pharmacotherapeutics TMP-SMX (Bactrim, Septra) is active against a wide range of sensitive gram-positive and gram-negative microorganisms: *E. coli, K. pneumoniae, P. mirabilis, Str. pneumoniae, S. aureus,* coagulase-negative staphylococci, *B. catarrhalis,* and *H. influenzae.* Use of TMP-SMX is indicated in the treatment of acute exacerbations of chronic bronchitis, enterocolitis, acute otitis media, *P. carinii* pneumonia, and bacterial urinary tract infections.[3,26-28]

Pharmacokinetics TMP-SMX is rapidly and completely absorbed from the GI tract. Once absorbed, it is 40% to 70% bound to plasma protein. It is widely distributed throughout the body, with peak plasma concentrations occurring within 1 to 4 hours. TMP-SMX is metabolized in the liver, with primary elimination in the urine. The elimination half-life of TMP is approximately 8 to 10 hours,

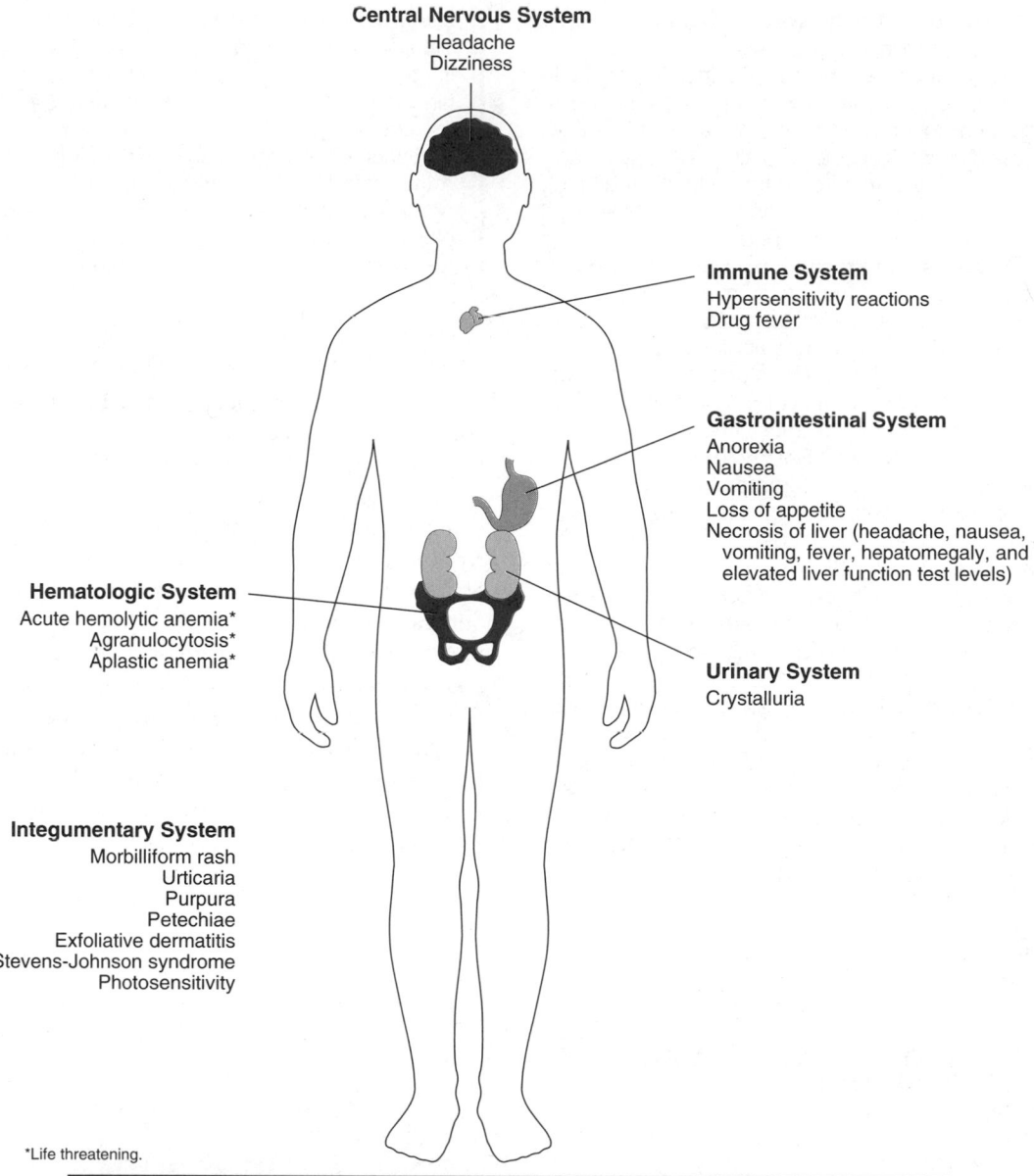

Central Nervous System
Headache
Dizziness

Immune System
Hypersensitivity reactions
Drug fever

Gastrointestinal System
Anorexia
Nausea
Vomiting
Loss of appetite
Necrosis of liver (headache, nausea,
    vomiting, fever, hepatomegaly, and
    elevated liver function test levels)

Hematologic System
Acute hemolytic anemia*
Agranulocytosis*
Aplastic anemia*

Urinary System
Crystalluria

Integumentary System
Morbilliform rash
Urticaria
Purpura
Petechiae
Exfoliative dermatitis
Stevens-Johnson syndrome
Photosensitivity

*Life threatening.

FIGURE 66–1   Common undesired clinical responses associated with sulfonamides.

and that of SMX is 6 to 12 hours. Half-life of the drug is increased in clients with renal impairment.[1,8]

Pharmacodynamics TMP-SMX exerts its antimicrobial effect by virtue of its action on two steps in the synthesis of tetrahydrofolic acid. TMP prevents the reduction of dihydrofolate to tetrahydrofolate, and SMX inhibits incorporation of PABA into folic acid. The drug is selective for microbes because (1) mammalian cells do not synthesize folic acid but use preformed folic acid from the diet and (2) mammalian cells are virtually insensitive to the inhibitory activity of TMP.

Pharmaceutics TMP-SMX usually is administered orally as tablets or a suspension every 12 hours for 10 to 14 days. It can also be administered as an IV infusion in two to four equally divided doses per day. When administered IV, it is diluted in 5% dextrose solution. Use of NaCl solution should be avoided because it may cause a precipitate.

Undesired Clinical Responses TMP-SMX is generally well tolerated. Common side effects associated with TMP-SMX include hypersensitivity reactions (fever, itching, skin rash), photosensitivity, dizziness, headache, and GI disturbances such as nausea, vomiting, diarrhea, or loss of appetite. Although the overall incidence of side effects is less than 5%, in clients with acquired immunodeficiency syndrome (AIDS), the incidence of side effects (especially fever, malaise, rash, or pancytopenia) increases dramatically to more than 50%.

Less common reactions with TMP-SMX are blood dyscrasias (e.g., agranulocytosis, hemolytic anemia, aplastic anemia) and hepatitis, with evidence of liver toxicity occurring within 3 to 5 days after initiation of therapy. Stevens-Johnson syndrome occurs rarely, but the syndrome consists of aching joints and muscles, redness, blistering, peeling of skin, and unusual tiredness or weakness. Another rare reaction is toxic epidermal necrolysis; along with the skin reaction, difficulty swallowing may occur.

Other reactions occurring rarely include crystalluria or hematuria characterized by blood in urine, lower back pain, and pain or burning on urination; interstitial nephritis with change in frequency of urination and amount of urine, increased thirst, nausea, vomiting, or loss of appetite; bluish fingernails, lips, or skin; difficult breathing; sore throat; fever; and unusual bruising or bleeding, which may be characteristic of methemoglobinemia.

Contraindications and Precautions Use of TMP-SMX is contraindicated in individuals with hypersensitivity to the drug or sulfonamides. Caution should be followed in clients with blood dyscrasias, megaloblastic anemia resulting from folic acid deficiency, glucose-6-phosphate dehydrogenase deficiency, and liver or renal impairment.

Drug-Drug Interactions The most important drug interactions occur between TMP-SMX and anticoagulants, oral antidiabetic agents (e.g., chlorpropamide, glyburide), hydantoin anticonvulsants (e.g., phenytoin), and methotrexate. Displacement from protein-binding sites or inhibition of metabolism by SMX increases the effect or toxicity of these drugs. Additionally, drugs that may cause hemolytic anemia or are hepatotoxic may increase the incidence of anemia or liver toxicity when combined with TMP-SMX.

Life-Span Considerations TMP-SMX crosses the placenta, although studies in humans have not been done. The drug may interfere with folic acid metabolism in the fetus. It is excreted in breast milk; its use in nursing women is not recommended because it may cause **kernicterus** in nursing infants. Additionally, TMP-SMX may cause hemolytic anemia or interfere with folic acid metabolism in the nursing infant. Except for treating congenital toxoplasmosis or as prophylaxis of *P. carinii* pneumonia, use of the drug is contraindicated in infants up to 2 months of age.[4,9,26]

Specific Drug-Related Nursing Considerations Administer TMP-SMX with 240 ml of water 1 hour before or 2 hours after meals. Instruct the client to drink several glasses of water between meals. Monitor client carefully for possible undesired clinical responses.

MISCELLANEOUS DRUGS IN CATEGORY

Examples of other drugs belonging to the sulfonamide category include sulfadiazine, sulfamethoxazole, sulfisoxazole, mafenide, and silver sulfadiazine. **Sulfadiazine** (Sulfadiazine) is used in combination with pyrimethamine in the treatment of toxoplasmosis and malaria resistant to chloroquine. It is not recommended for treatment of urinary tract infections because of low solubility and increased risk of crystalluria. **Sulfamethoxazole** (Gantanol) is used in the treatment of acute, uncomplicated urinary tract infections and *C. trachomatis* infections. It has slower absorption and excretion than sulfisoxazole, resulting in a greater tendency to cause crystalluria. **Sulfisoxazole** (Gantrisin) is used to treat acute, uncomplicated urinary tract infections and infections caused by *C. trachomatis*. It is highly soluble, making it less likely to cause crystalluria (Table 55–6).

TABLE 55–6
Sulfonamides

Drug Name	Dosage and Route of Administration
TRIMETHOPRIM AND SULFAMETHOXAZOLE; TMP-SMX; CO-TRIMOXAZOLE (Bactrim, Septra) **HOW SUPPLIED** Tablets: 80/400, 160/800 mg Suspension: 40/200 mg/5 ml Injection: 80/400 mg/5 ml	**ADULTS** Oral: 160 mg q12h IV: 8–10 mg/kg/d in divided doses q6-12h **CHILDREN > 2 MO** IV: 8–10 mg/kg/d in divided doses q6-12h Oral (> 40 kg): 160 mg q12h Oral (< 40 kg): 8–12 mg/kg/d in divided doses q12h **For Pneumocystis carinii *Pneumonia*** **ADULTS** 15–20 mg/kg/d orally in divided doses q6h **CHILDREN** 20 mg/kg/d orally in divided doses q6h
Sulfadiazine **HOW SUPPLIED** Tablets: 500 mg	**ADULTS** 2–4 g initially, then 1 g q4-6h **CHILDREN > 2 MO** 75 mg/kg initially, then 120–150 mg/kg in four to six divided doses
Sulfamethoxazole (Gantanol) **HOW SUPPLIED** Tablets: 500 mg Suspension: 500 mg/5 ml	**ADULTS** 2 g initially, then 1 g q8-12h **CHILDREN > 2 MO** 50–60 mg/kg initially, then 25–30 mg/kg q12h
Sulfisoxazole (Gantrisin) **HOW SUPPLIED** Tablets: 500 mg Suspension: 500 mg/5 ml	**ADULTS** 2–4 g initially, then 4–9 g/d in divided doses q4-6h **CHILDREN > 2 MO** 75 mg/kg initially, then 120–150 mg/kg/d in divided doses q4-6h

Mafenide acetate (Sulfamylon) is used topically for prophylaxis and treatment of burn wound infections. Common side effects associated with mafenide are pain or burning sensation on treated areas. After application of a thin layer of mafenide, the area may be covered with a dressing or left uncovered. **Silver sulfadiazine** (SSD, Silvadene) is also used topically for prophylaxis and treatment of burn wound infections.

CONCEPT REVIEW

Sulfonamides generally are bacteriostatic and are active against both gram-positive and gram-negative bacteria.

Sulfonamide activity is based on competition with PABA, which is necessary for bacteria to synthesize folic acid.

Undesired clinical responses associated with sulfonamides include crystalluria, disorders of the hematopoietic system, and hypersensitivity reactions.

TETRACYCLINES

The tetracyclines were first introduced in 1948 with the compound chlortetracycline. Soon after, they were found effective against rickettsiae, a number of gram-positive and gram-negative bacteria, and *Chlamydia* spp. As a result, they became widely used in therapy.

Because of increased resistance to the drugs and the development of new, less toxic antibiotics, use of tetracyclines has declined. In general, the tetracyclines are used in clients with diseases caused by *Rickettsia, Mycoplasma,* and *Chlamydia.* They can also be used in the treatment of nonspecific urethritis, sexually transmitted diseases, and bacillary infections. Additionally, the tetracyclines have been used to treat acne.

The tetracyclines are bacteriostatic. They act intracellularly by inhibiting protein synthesis. Once in the bacterial cell, tetracyclines bind primarily to the 30S subunits of the bacterial ribosomes. Bacterial cell wall synthesis is not inhibited.

Pharmacokinetic properties vary slightly within this group. The tetracyclines are adequately, but incompletely, absorbed from the GI tract. Absorption is impaired by concurrent ingestion of dairy products and antacids. Protein binding is variable, high with doxycycline and demeclocycline and moderate with tetracycline and minocycline. The drugs are readily distributed to most body fluids; CSF concentrations may achieve 10% to 25% of plasma concentration after parenteral administration. All tetracyclines are concentrated in the liver, cross the placenta, and enter fetal circulation and amniotic fluid. Tetracyclines also achieve high concentrations in breast milk. The drugs are eliminated primarily unchanged via glomerular filtration and biliary secretion.[3,9,29]

Undesired clinical responses associated with the tetracyclines include GI symptoms (epigastric burning, abdominal discomfort, nausea, and vomiting). The likelihood of these reactions increases with larger doses.

Increased sensitivity of the skin to sunlight, a phototoxic reaction, may occur. Liver toxicity, characterized by abdominal pain, nausea, vomiting, and jaundice, occurs rarely, with most reactions occurring in clients receiving more than 2 g daily parenterally. Pregnant women appear more susceptible than other individuals.

Children who receive tetracycline may develop permanent brown discoloration of the teeth; the greater the dose, the more intense the discoloration of the enamel. The risk is highest when the drug is administered to neonates. However, children up to 8 years of age are susceptible to this complication. In addition, treatment of pregnant women may produce discoloration of teeth, enamel hypoplasia, and decreased linear skeletal bone length in their children.[4,9,29] (See Fig. 55–5.)

TETRACYCLINE PROTOTYPE
DOXYCYCLINE

Doxycycline (Doryx, Vibramycin) is the prototype for the tetracyclines.

Pharmacotherapeutics Clinically doxycycline shows moderate activity against a wide spectrum of microorganisms. Activity occurs against the gram-positive organism *S. aureus,* coagulase-negative staphylococci, β-hemolytic streptococci, *S. pneumoniae,* and *Enterococcus* spp. Gram-negative activity affects *B. catarrhalis, Neisseria* spp., *Citrobacter, Enterobacter, E. coli, K. pneumoniae, P. mirabilis, Serratia* spp., *Shigella, C. jejuni, H. influenzae, P. aeruginosa,* and *P. maltophilia.* Low activity occurs with anaerobes.

Doxycycline is used in the treatment of bronchitis, brucellosis, inclusion conjunctivitis, and genitourinary tract infections caused by *N. gonorrhoeae* and *C. trachomatis.* It is also used to treat acute otitis media, pharyngitis, pneumonia, sinusitis, syphilis, trachoma, Rocky Mountain spotted fever, nongonococcal urethritis, and urinary tract infections caused by organisms susceptible to doxycycline.

Pharmacokinetics Doxycycline is well absorbed (90% to 100%) after oral administration. It may be administered without regard to food. Peak serum concentration after oral administration is attained in 2 to 4 hours. Protein binding is approximately 93%. The drug is widely distributed to most body fluids. Plasma half-life is 11 to 23 hours and is unaffected in clients with renal impairment. Doxycycline is partially inactivated in the liver and is excreted in urine and bile. In clients with renal impairment, biliary secretion via the feces becomes an important route of excretion.

Pharmacodynamics Doxycycline inhibits protein synthesis but does not affect bacterial cell wall synthesis.

Pharmaceutics Doxycycline is administered orally or by IV piggyback infusion. It is not administered by the IM or SC routes. Table 55–7 provides additional information on dosage forms, dosages, and routes of administration.

Undesired Clinical Responses Undesired clinical responses are the same as those previously described for all tetracyclines. GI symptoms and photosensitivity reactions occur most frequently.

Contraindications and Precautions Doxycycline should be used with caution in clients with impaired liver function and in clients hypersensitive to tetracyclines.

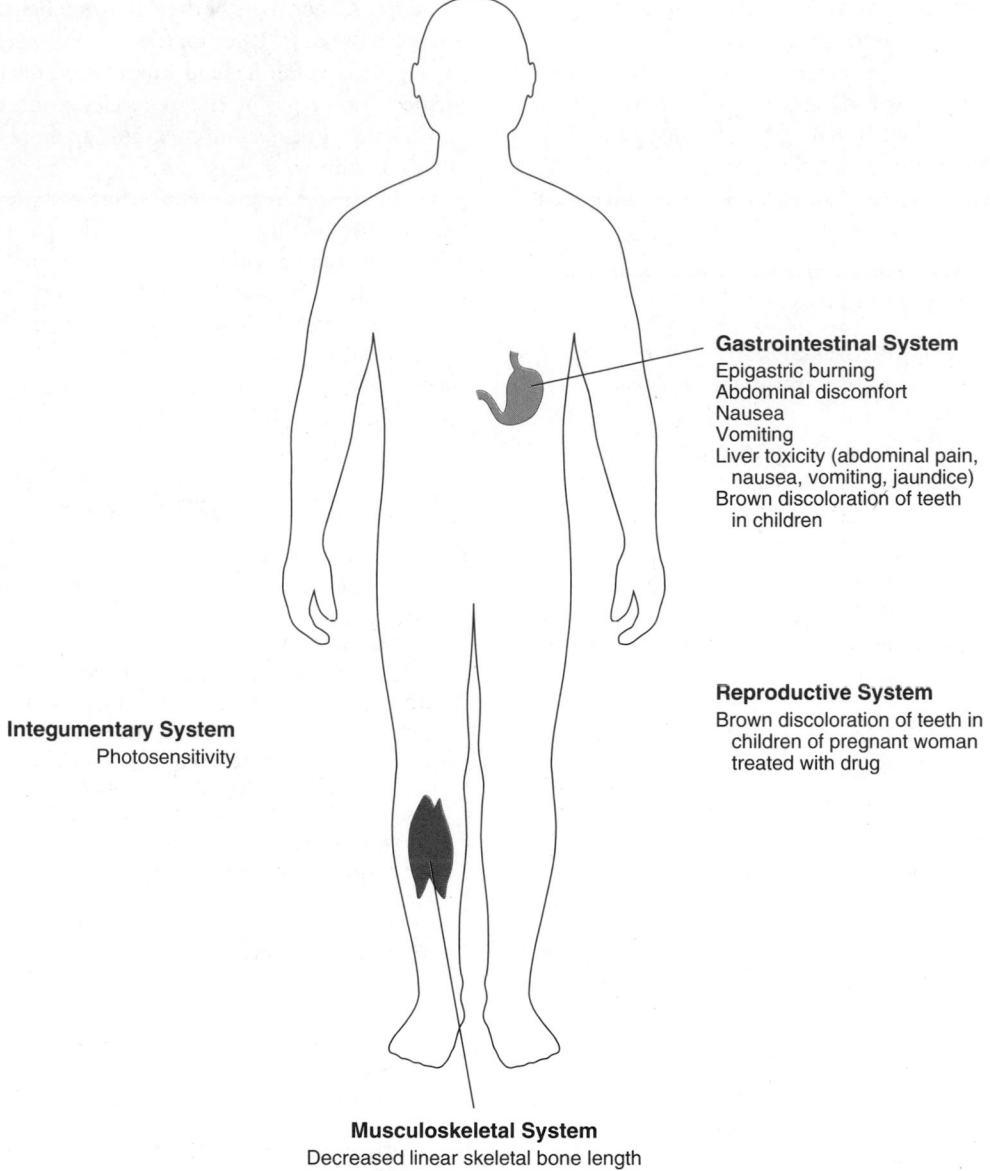

Gastrointestinal System
Epigastric burning
Abdominal discomfort
Nausea
Vomiting
Liver toxicity (abdominal pain,
    nausea, vomiting, jaundice)
Brown discoloration of teeth
    in children

Reproductive System
Brown discoloration of teeth in
    children of pregnant woman
    treated with drug

Integumentary System
Photosensitivity

Musculoskeletal System
Decreased linear skeletal bone length

FIGURE 55–5   Common undesired clinical responses associated with tetracyclines.

Drug-Drug, Drug-Nutrient, and Drug-Environment Interactions Clients taking doxycycline may experience increased skin sensitivity to sunlight. Dairy products may form a complex with tetracyclines, decreasing their absorption. Aluminum, calcium, or magnesium in antacids chelate with tetracyclines and inhibit absorption. Sodium bicarbonate interferes with absorption by increasing gastric pH and decreasing gastric breakdown of some dosage forms of tetracycline.[21,22]

Concurrent administration of cholestyramine may cause binding of the tetracyclines, thus impairing drug absorption. Estrogen-containing oral contraceptives given concurrently with long-term tetracycline therapy may reduce contraceptive reliability and increase breakthrough bleeding.

Life-Span Considerations Doxycycline is classified as a Pregnancy Category D drug. Its use should be avoided during the last half of pregnancy and by breast-feeding women.

Specific Drug-Related Nursing Considerations If antacid therapy is needed, counsel clients to take antacids at least 1 to 3 hours after taking a tetracycline drug. Instruct the client to take the drug 1 hour before or 2 hours after meals. Remind him or her to take the drug with a full glass of water. Advise the client to protect his or her skin from the sun and ultraviolet light exposure.

TABLE 55–7
Tetracyclines

Drug Name	Dosage and Route of Administration	Nursing Considerations
DOXYCYCLINE (Doryx, Vibramycin) HOW SUPPLIED Capsules: 50, 100 mg Capsules (coated pellets): 100 mg Tablets: 50, 100 mg Powder for oral suspension: 25 mg/5 ml when reconstituted Syrup: 50 mg/5 ml Injection: 100, 200 mg	ADULTS Oral: 200 mg day 1, then 100–200 mg/d as single daily dose or divided doses q12h IV: 200 mg initially, then 100–200 mg/d as single daily dose or divided doses q12h CHILDREN > 8 Y, > 45 KG Oral or IV: same as adult CHILDREN > 8 Y, < 45 KG Oral or IV: 4.4 mg/kg day 1, then 2.2–4.4 mg/kg/d as single daily dose or divided doses q12h	***Assess*** Determine sensitivity to tetracyclines. Identify concurrent drugs (especially antacids, iron, cholestyramine, carbamazepine, barbiturates, phenytoin). Obtain results of baseline renal and liver function tests and CBC. Identify any infectious processes. Obtain specimen for culture and sensitivity before initiating therapy. Determine if client is pregnant or breast-feeding. ***Implement*** Give orally without regard to food or dairy products. Administer IV slowly over at least 60 min. Do not give to child 8 y of age or less. ***Monitor*** Monitor CBC, urinalysis, and renal and liver function test results. Observe for undesired effects (especially CNS effects, GI disturbances, photosensitivity reactions). Monitor the infectious process. ***Evaluate*** Observe for resolution of signs and symptoms of infection.
Demeclocycline (Declomycin) HOW SUPPLIED Capsules: 150 mg Tablets: 150, 300 mg	ADULTS 150–300 mg q12h CHILDREN > 8 Y 6–12 mg/kg/d in divided doses q6-12h	***Assess*** Same as doxycycline. Identify concurrent drugs (especially antacids, iron, cholestyramine). ***Implement*** Do not give concurrently with food or dairy products. Give with full glass of water. ***Monitor*** Same as for doxycycline. ***Evaluate*** Same as for doxycycline.
Minocycline (Minocin) HOW SUPPLIED Capsules: 50, 100 mg Tablets: 50, 100 mg Oral suspension: 50 mg/5 ml Injection: 100 mg	ADULTS Oral: 100–200 mg initially, then 200 mg/d in divided doses q6-12h IV: 200 mg initially, then 100 mg q12h CHILDREN > 8 Y Oral or IV: 4 mg/kg initially, then 2 mg/kg q12h	***Assess*** Same as for demeclocycline. ***Implement*** Same as for doxycycline. ***Monitor*** Same as for demeclocycline. ***Evaluate*** Same as for demeclocycline.
Tetracycline (Achromycin, Sumycin) HOW SUPPLIED Capsules: 250, 500 mg Tablets: 250, 500 mg Oral suspension: 125 mg/5 ml	ADULTS 1–2 g/d in divided doses q6-12h CHILDREN > 8 Y 25–50 mg/kg/d in divided doses q6-12h	Same as for demeclocycline.

MISCELLANEOUS DRUGS IN CATEGORY

Other commonly prescribed tetracylines include **demeclocycline** (Declomycin), **minocycline** (Minocin), and **tetracycline** (Achromycin, Sumycin). One significant difference among these drugs is that minocycline may be administered without regard to food or milk.

CONCEPT REVIEW

The tetracyclines are bacteriostatic and act intracellularly by inhibiting protein synthesis.

Undesired clinical responses associated with tetracyclines include GI disorders and increased sensitivity to light.

Use of tetracyclines should be avoided during pregnancy and in children less than 8 years of age, for the drugs may discolor teeth and retard linear skeletal bone length.

MISCELLANEOUS AGENTS

Chloramphenicol, clindamycin, and vancomycin are also important antiinfective drugs.

Chloramphenicol

Pharmacotherapeutics   Chloramphenicol (Chloromycetin) has in vitro activity against gram-positive, gram-negative, and anaerobic bacteria, rickettsiae, spirochetes, and chlamydia. It is highly effective and is considered bactericidal against the gram-positive organism *Str. pneumoniae* and the gram-negative organisms *H. influenzae* and *N. meningitidis.*

Chloramphenicol is less effective and is considered bacteriostatic against the gram-positive organisms *S. aureus, Str. pyogenes,* and group B streptococci; the gram-negative organisms *E. coli, K. pneumoniae, P. mirabilis, Salmonella* spp., and *Shigella* spp.; and the anaerobes, including *B. fragilis.* Chloramphenicol is considered resistant to MRSA, *Enterococcus* spp., and the gram-negative organism *P. aeruginosa.*

Use of chloramphenicol is indicated for treatment of serious infections in which use of less toxic antibacterials is ineffective or contraindicated. It is used in clients with meningitis caused by *H. influenzae, Str. pneumoniae,* and *N. meningitidis.* Chloramphenicol is also used to treat acute typhoid fever, parathyroid fever, brain abscess, and rickettsial infections.

Pharmacokinetics   Chloramphenicol is rapidly and completely absorbed from the GI tract and after IM administration. Peak serum concentration occurs within 1 to 3 hours after oral administration and 1 to 1½ hours after IM administration. Protein binding is moderate (50% to 60%). The drug is widely distributed, with its highest concentration in the liver and kidneys. Chloramphenicol achieves a concentration in the CSF of 49% to 89% of the serum concentration if meninges are inflamed. The drug crosses the placenta and is excreted in breast milk. Chloramphenicol is metabolized in the liver to the metabolite glucuronide and is primarily excreted by the kidneys.

Pharmacodynamics   Chloramphenicol inhibits bacterial peptide bond formation and subsequent protein synthesis. After diffusing through the bacterial cell membrane, the drug reversibly binds to the 50S subunits of bacterial ribosomes.

Pharmaceutics   Chloramphenicol is given orally or by IV or IM administration. It is also available for topical, ophthalmic, or otic administration. Table 55–8 contains additional information about chloramphenicol.

Undesired clinical responses   Serious toxicity with chloramphenicol has limited its usefulness as an antibacterial agent. Serious and fatal blood dyscrasias are manifested as either reversible bone marrow depression or aplastic anemia. Bone marrow depression is dose related; it is common when the serum concentration exceeds 25 µg/ml. Aplastic anemia occurs in 1 of every 25,000 to 40,000 treatment courses; its occurrence is not related to dose or duration of therapy. The onset of aplasia may not occur until weeks or months after discontinuing chloramphenicol therapy. Symptoms of blood dyscrasias include pale skin, sore throat, fever, unusual bruising or bleeding, and unusual tiredness or weakness.

Other less frequent effects are GI reactions (nausea, vomiting, or diarrhea). Rarely allergic reactions (skin rash, fever, shortness of breath), optic neuritis (eye pain, blurred vision), peripheral neuritis (numbness, tingling, burning pain, or weakness in hands or feet) occur. Gray syndrome may occur in newborn infants with use of inappropriately high doses. Symptoms include abdominal distention, blue-gray skin color, low body temperature, uneven breathing, unresponsiveness, or cardiovascular collapse. This reaction occurs rarely.

Contraindications and precautions   Chloramphenicol use is contraindicated in clients with a previous allergic or toxic reaction to chloramphenicol. Caution should be used in clients with bone marrow depression or impaired liver function or in clients who have had previous cytotoxic drug therapy or radiation therapy.

Drug-drug interactions   Concurrent use of hydantoin anticonvulsants (e.g., phenytoin), other bone marrow depressants (e.g., antineoplastic agents), or radiation therapy may increase bone marrow depression. Chloramphenicol may antagonize the effects of erythromycin or clindamycin by competing for the same binding site of bacterial ribosomes. It may inhibit metabolism and increase blood concentrations of phenobarbital, phenytoin, or oral anticoagulants.

Life-span considerations   Chloramphenicol should not be used in pregnant women at term or during labor with either premature or full-term infants because of the potential for gray syndrome. It is classified as a Pregnancy Category C drug and is not recommended for use in nursing mothers.

Specific drug-related nursing considerations   Monitor hematology reports carefully and coordinate with laboratory personnel for drawing specimens to determine chloramphenicol plasma levels. Administer oral dosages on an empty stomach 1 hour before or 2 hours after meals. Chloramphenicol may be administered with food if GI upset occurs. Notify the primary care provider if bleeding or bruising, blurred vision, tiredness, or other new symptoms occur.[10]

Clindamycin

Clindamycin (Cleocin) is produced by a *Streptomyces* strain of bacteria. It is similar to the erythromycins in its antibacterial activity.

Pharmacotherapeutics   Clindamycin is generally bacteriostatic but is bactericidal against susceptible bacteria such as *Clostridium perfringens.* The spectrum of activity of clindamycin is broad, being active against most gram-positive and gram-negative bacteria, including enterococci, and against some anaerobes. The antibacterial activity and absorption rate of clindamycin are excellent. Its use, however, is severely limited because of its potential for causing pseudomembranous colitis. The use of this drug is recommended only for treatment of severe infections in clients unable to tolerate other antibiotics.

Pharmacokinetics   Clindamycin is well absorbed after oral or IM administration. Peak serum concentration occurs within 0.75 to 1 hour after oral administration and 1 to 3 hours after IM administration. The drug is unaffected by food in the stomach. Clindamycin is widely distributed to most body fluids and tissues except the CSF. It crosses the placenta and is excreted in breast milk. Clindamycin is metabolized in the liver, with only approximately 10% to 15% excreted in the urine.[4,9]

Pharmacodynamics   Clindamycin inhibits protein synthesis in susceptible bacteria by binding to the 50S subunits of bacterial ribosomes, thereby inhibiting protein synthesis.

Pharmaceutics   Clindamycin is available as oral capsules, as granules for pediatric oral solution, in a parenteral form for IM or IV administration, and as topical gel and lotion. Table 55–8 contains additional information on dosage forms, dosages, and routes of administration.

Undesired clinical responses   Most common undesired clinical responses to clindamycin are GI related; nausea and vomiting, diarrhea, or severe colitis is experienced in 10% of clients who take the drug orally. In mild cases discontinuance of the drug reverses the condition, but it may be necessary in more severe cases to replace fluids and electrolytes and to administer protein supplements and rectal corticosteroid drugs. Treatment with metronidazole or vancomycin may also be necessary because the *C. difficile* pathogen, the causative agent in most cases of severe colitis, responds well to these antibiotics. Treatment with antidiarrheal agents is *not* recommended.

Hematologic responses include leukopenia, eosinophilia, agranulocytosis, and thrombocytopenia. Increases in liver enzymes, bilirubin, and alkaline phosphatase, jaundice, vaginitis, and urinary frequency may occur. Allergic reactions include rash, urticaria, pruritus, and erythema.

Contraindications and precautions   Clindamycin should be used with caution in clients with a history of GI disease such as ulcerative colitis. Its use is also not recommended in clients with serious liver function impairment; the liver dysfunction may prolong the drug's half-life, requiring a dosage adjustment.

Drug-drug interactions   Concurrent use of neuromuscular blocking agents may result in skeletal muscle weakness and respiratory depression. Adsorbent antidiarrheals (e.g., kaolin-pectin) may significantly delay absorption. Clindamycin's action may be antagonized by chloramphenicol or erythromycin.

Life-span considerations   Clindamycin is classified as a Pregnancy Category B drug and is excreted in breast milk. The parenteral dosage form should be used with caution in infants up to 1 month of age since it contains benzyl alcohol, which may cause fatal gasping syndrome.

Specific drug-related nursing considerations   Administer IM doses of clindamycin deep in a large muscle mass. The IV infusion should be administered over 10 to 30 minutes, depending on the dosage. Administer the oral dose with 240 ml of water to avoid esophageal irritation. Encourage intake of 2000 ml of fluid daily, especially during diarrheal episodes.

Vancomycin Hydrochloride

Vancomycin (Vancocin) is a tricyclic glycopeptide antibiotic produced by *Streptomyces orientalis.*

Pharmacotherapeutics   Vancomycin is a narrow-spectrum antibiotic. It is primarily effective against gram-positive bacteria, including methicillin-sensitive and methicillin-resistant *S. aureus,* β-hemolytic streptococci, *Str. pneumoniae,* and *Enterococcus* spp. Vancomycin is also effective against *C. difficile.*

IV vancomycin is used in the treatment of bone and joint infections, bacterial septicemia, and endocarditis. It is also used to treat potential life-threatening staphylococcal infections that have failed to respond to penicillin or cephalosporin therapy. Orally vancomycin is used in the treatment of antibiotic-associated pseudomembranous colitis caused by *C. difficile* and staphylococcal enterocolitis.[2–4]

Pharmacokinetics   Vancomycin is poorly absorbed from the GI tract. High concentrations of the oral dosage form are eliminated in feces. After IV administration, vancomycin is widely distributed to most tissues and body fluids. However, it does not readily cross the blood-brain barrier; when the meninges are inflamed, the CSF may achieve therapeutic concentrations. Vancomycin does cross the placenta. Protein binding is moderate, 50% to 55%. Drugs administered IV reach a peak within 5 minutes. The IV dosage is primarily eliminated unchanged in the urine. Elimination half-life is 4 to 11 hours, but in clients with oliguria or anuria, the half-life may increase to 6 to 10 days. IM administration is not recommended because it causes tissue irritation and necrosis in muscle.[4,9]

Pharmacodynamics   Vancomycin is bactericidal. It inhibits bacterial cell wall synthesis by binding to a site different from that of penicillins and cephalosporins. It binds to the D-alanyl–D-alanine portion of the cell wall precursor, causing lysis of the bacterial wall. Other possible mechanisms include

TABLE 55–8
Miscellaneous Agents

Drug Name	Dosage and Route of Administration	Nursing Considerations
Chloramphenicol (Chloromycetin) **HOW SUPPLIED** Capsules: 250 mg Oral suspension: 150 mg/5 ml Injection: 100 mg/ml	ADULTS Oral or IV: 50–100 mg/kg/d in divided doses q6h CHILDREN > 2 WK Oral or IV: 50–100 mg/kg/d in divided doses q6-12h CHILDREN < 2 WK Oral or IV: 25–50 mg/kg/d as single daily dose or q12h	**Assess** Identify sensitivity or toxicity to chloramphenicol. Determine what drugs are being used concurrently (especially anticonvulsants, bone marrow depressants). Obtain baseline CBC and renal and liver function test results. Identify any infectious processes. Obtain specimen for culture and sensitivity testing before initiating therapy. Determine if client is pregnant or breast-feeding. **Implement** Give orally on empty stomach. Give IM or IV push or infusion over 20–30 min. **Monitor** Monitor CBC, urinalysis, and renal and liver function test results. Observe for undesired effects (especially blood dyscrasias). Monitor the infectious process. **Evaluate** Observe for resolution of signs and symptoms of infection.
Clindamycin (Cleocin) **HOW SUPPLIED** Capsules: 75, 150, 500 mg Granules for oral solution: 75 mg/5 ml Injection: 150 mg/ml	ADULTS Oral: 150–300 mg q6h IM or IV: 900–2700 mg/d in divided doses q6-8h CHILDREN > 1 MO Oral: 8–20 mg/kg/d in divided doses q6-8h IM or IV: 20–40 mg/kg/d in divided doses q6-8h CHILDREN < 1 MO IM or IV: 15–40 mg/kg/d in divided doses q6-8h	**Assess** Identify sensitivity or toxicity to clindamycin. Identify other medical conditions (especially GI disease). Obtain baseline CBC and renal and liver function test results. Identify any infectious processes. Obtain specimen for culture and sensitivity testing before initiating therapy. Determine if client is pregnant or breast-feeding. **Implement** Give without regard to food. Give IM or IV push or infusion over 10–30 min. **Monitor** Monitor CBC, urinalysis, and renal and liver function tests. Observe for side effects (especially pseudomembranous colitis). Monitor the infectious process. **Evaluate** Observe for resolution of signs and symptoms of infection.
Vancomycin (Vancocin, Vancoled) **HOW SUPPLIED** Capsules: 125, 250 mg Powder for oral solution: 1, 10 g Injection: 500 mg; 1, 5, 10 mg	ADULTS Oral: 125–500 mg q6h IV: 15 mg/kg (or 1 g) q12h CHILDREN > 1 MO Oral: 40–50 mg/kg/d in divided doses q6h IV: 30–45 mg/kg/d in divided doses q8h CHILDREN 1 WK TO 1 MO IV: 15 mg/kg initially, then 10 mg/kg q8-18h NEONATE < 1 WK IV: 15 mg/kg initially, then 10 mg/kg q12-24h	**Assess** Identify sensitivity to vancomycin. Determine what drugs are being used concurrently (especially ototoxic, nephrotoxic ones). Identify other medical conditions (especially impaired renal function). Obtain baseline CBC, urinalysis, and renal function values. Identify any infectious processes. Obtain specimen for culture and sensitivity testing before initiating therapy. Determine if client is pregnant or breast-feeding. **Implement** Give drug orally without regard to food. Give IV infusion over 60–90 min. **Monitor** Monitor CBC, urinalysis, and renal function values. Monitor stools (when treating pseudomembranous colitis). Monitor vancomycin serum concentration when given parenterally. Observe for undesired effects, including "red-neck syndrome," ototoxicity, nephrotoxicity. Monitor the infectious process. **Evaluate** Observe for resolution of signs and symptoms of infection.

altering the cell wall permeability and selectively inhibiting RNA synthesis.

Undesired clinical responses Vancomycin, when administered orally, may cause a bitter or unpleasant taste, nausea, or vomiting. Parenterally, vancomycin may cause ototoxicity; this problem occurs more frequently with large doses and with long-term therapy. Tinnitus and high-frequency hearing loss are early indications of hearing loss and occur with high serum concentrations. Additionally, vancomycin may cause nephrotoxicity characterized by a change in the frequency or amount of urine, increased thirst, decreased appetite, or nausea and vomiting.

More common is "red-neck syndrome" or "red-man syndrome," which may occur with too-rapid infusion of the drug. This syndrome is characterized by hypotension, chills, fever, and a maculopapular rash on the neck and upper torso. Antihistamine or corticosteroid therapy may be necessary, although the reaction is usually self-limiting, resolving with discontinuance of the infusion.

Contraindications and precautions Vancomycin should be used with caution in clients hypersensitive to the drug. Caution should also be used in clients with a history of hearing loss or impaired renal function.

Drug-drug, drug-nutrient, drug-environment interactions Vancomycin powder for oral solution may be reconstituted and administered by mouth or nasogastric tube. This mixture may be kept for 2 weeks in a refrigerator without significant loss of potency. Once IV dosage forms are reconstituted, they may also be stored in the refrigerator without significant loss of potency.

When administered concurrently with cholestyramine, the effectiveness of oral vancomycin is decreased. Cholestyramine binds oral vancomycin, reducing its antibacterial effect. Aminoglycosides, amphotericin, aspirin, cyclosporine, ethacrynic acid, and streptomycin may increase vancomycin's potential for causing ototoxicity and nephrotoxicity.

Life-span considerations Vancomycin is classified as a Pregnancy Category C drug. Since it is not known if the drug is distributed in breast milk, caution should be used in breast-feeding women. Elderly clients may require dosage adjustments since they have increased risk for ototoxicity and nephrotoxicity.

Specific drug-related nursing considerations Follow dilution instructions carefully for intermittent IV infusion of vancomycin. Alternate IV sites every 2 to 3 days to reduce the risk of phlebitis. Monitor the client's blood pressure closely during the infusion. Keep the client well hydrated, administering at least 2000 ml of fluids daily.

SUMMARY

Antibiotics are used to prevent or treat infections. Rational use of antibiotics to treat infections generally requires the identification of the causative organisms before selecting the appropriate therapy. In some situations the identity of the organism can be deduced by observing the client's symptoms. In other cases, diagnostic testing through culture and sensitivity tests must be completed before specific therapy is initiated.

Several drug groups are discussed in this chapter (e.g., tetracyclines, penicillins, cephalosporins). These groups are described as narrow- or broad-spectrum antibiotics or as bactericidal or bacteriostatic. In addition, specific susceptible organisms are identified in regard to each drug's spectrum of activity. Knowledge of this information helps the nurse anticipate what drugs will be prescribed for the client.

REFERENCES

1. Snider, S. (1990). Penicillins. *FDA Consumer, 24*(6), 28–31.
2. Reynard, A.M. (1992). The penicillins, vancomycin, and bacitracin. In C.M. Smith & A.M. Reynard (Eds.), *Textbook of pharmacology* (pp. 817–828). Philadelphia: W.B. Saunders.
3. Abramowicz, M. (Ed.). (1994). The choice of antibacterial drugs. *Medical Letter on Drugs and Therapeutics, 36*(925), 53–60.
4. Data Pharmaceutica, Inc. (1993). *1993 physicians' genrx.* Smithtown, NY: Author.
5. Reese, R.E. (1993). *Handbook of antibiotics.* Boston: Little, Brown.
6. Trovato, A., Nuhlicek, D., & Midtling, J. (1991). Drug-nutrient interactions. *American Family Physician, 44,* 1651–1657.
7. Esposito, A., Jones, S., & Yoshikawa, T. (1990). Antibiotic choices in the elderly. *Patient Care, 24*(8), 51–71.
8. Nettina, S.I. (1990). A new look at an old killer. *American Journal of Nursing, 90*(4), 68–70.
9. U.S. Pharmacopeial Convention. (1990). *The United States pharmacopeia* (22nd rev.). Rockville, MD: Author.
10. Beam, T. (1992). Cephalosporins. In C.M. Smith & A.M. Reynard (Eds.), *Textbook of pharmacology* (pp. 829–843). Philadelphia: W.B. Saunders.
11. Hodgson, B., Kizior, R., & Kingdon, R. (1995). *1995 nurse's drug handbook.* Philadelphia: W.B. Saunders.
12. Schaad, U.B., et al. (1990). A comparison of ceftriaxone and cefuroxime for the treatment of bacterial meningitis in children. *New England Journal of Medicine, 322*(3), 141–147.
13. Meyer, C. (1993). Four against infection. *American Journal of Nursing, 93*(4), 68–72.
14. Stutman, H.R. (1993). Cefprozil. *Pediatric Annals, 22*(3), 167–168, 171–176.
15. Sirgo, M.A., & Norris, S. (1991). Ceftazidime in the elderly: Appropriateness of twice-daily dosing. *DICP, 25*(3), 284–288.
16. Reynard, A.M. (1992). Aminoglycosides. In C.M. Smith & A.M. Reynard (Eds.), *Textbook of pharmacology* (pp. 844–847). Philadelphia: W.B. Saunders.
17. Fisk, K. (1993). A review of gentamicin use in neonates. *Neonatal Network: Journal of Neonatal Nursing, 12*(7), 19–28.
18. Prins, J., et al. (1993). Once versus daily gentamicin in patients with serious infections. *Lancet, 341,* 335–339.
19. Bean, T. (1992). Miscellaneous antimicrobial drugs. In C.M. Smith & A.M. Reynard (Eds.), *Textbook of pharmacology* (pp. 876–878). Philadelphia: W.B. Saunders.
20. Neu, H. (1992). Pharmacokinetics, microbiology, cost: Interrelated problems for the 1990s that impact on the use of fluoroquinolone antimicrobial agents. *American Journal of Medicine, 92*(4A), 25–75.
21. Chase, S. (1993). OTC interactions: Antacids. *RN Magazine,* August, 46–50.
22. Gugler, R., & Allgayer, H. (1990). Effects of antacids on the clinical pharmacokinetics of drugs: An update. *Clinical Pharmacokinetics, 18,* 210–219.
23. Tatro, D.S. (Ed.). (1990). *Drug interaction facts* (2nd ed.). St. Louis: J.B. Lippincott.
24. Nahata, M.C., Koranyl, K.I., Gadgil, S.D., Hilligoss, D.M., et al. (1993). Pharmacokinetics of azithromycin in pediatric pa-

tients after oral administration of multiple doses of suspension. *Antimicrobial Agents Chemotherapy, 37,* 314–316.

25. Brogden, R.N., & Peters, D.H. (1994). Dirithromycin: A review of its antimicrobial activity, pharmacokinetic properties and therapeutic efficacy. *Drugs, 48,* 599–616.

26. Bean, T. (1992). Sulfonamides, trimethoprim, and their combination. In C.M. Smith & A.M. Reynard (Eds.), *Textbook of pharmacology* (pp. 848–860). Philadelphia: W.B. Saunders.

27. Sattler, F., & Feinberg, J. (1992). New developments in the treatment of Pneumocystis carinii pneumonia. *Chest: The Cardiopulmonary Journal, 101,* 451–457.

28. Stamm, W.E., & Hooten, T.M. (1993). Management of urinary tract infections in adults. *New England Journal of Medicine, 329,* 1328–1334.

29. Reynard, A.M. (1992). Tetracyclines and chloramphenicol. In C.M. Smith & A.M. Reynard (Eds.), *Textbook of pharmacology* (pp. 856–860). Philadelphia: W.B. Saunders.

BIBLIOGRAPHY

Becker, T.M., et al. (1990). Mortality from infectious diseases among New Mexico's American Indian, Hispanic Whites and other whites, 1958–87. *American Journal of Public Health, 80,* 320–324.

Cohen, M.L. (1992). Epidemiology of drug resistance: Implications for a post-antimicrobial age. *Science, 257,* 1050–1055.

Cunha, B.A. (1992). The urologic uses of aminoglycosides. *Emergency Medicine, 24,* 299–300, 303–304, 307–308.

Denny, F.W. (1991). The streptococcus saga continues. *New England Journal of Medicine, 325,* 127–128.

Jacoby, G.A., & Archer, G.L. (1991). New mechanisms of bacterial resistance to antimicrobial agents. *New England Journal of Medicine, 324,* 601–611.

McCue, J. (1992). Oral antibiotics: Practical prescribing rules for practitioners. *Geriatrics, 47*(7), 59–66.

Neu, H.C. (1992). The crisis in antibiotic resistance. *Science, 257,* 1064–1073.

Schwartz, B., Faclam, R.R., & Breiman, R.F. (1990). Changing epidemiology of group A streptococcal infection in the U.S.A. *Lancet, 336,* 1167–1171.

Shovein, J., & Young, M.S. (1992). MRSA: Pandora's box for hospitals. *American Journal of Nursing, 92*(2), 49–52.

Walsh, M.L., & Johnson, C.C. (1991). Update on antimicrobial agents. *Nursing Clinics of North America, 26,* 341–360.

CHAPTER 56

Urinary Tract Antiseptics

LINDA RUHOLL

⊛ **Urinary Tract Infections**

LEARNING OBJECTIVE: Define four different types of urinary tract infections (UTIs).

KEY TERMS:
Cystitis, glomerulonephritis, pyelonephritis, urethritis

⊛ **Urinary Tract Antiseptics**

LEARNING OBJECTIVES:
Describe the therapeutic use of urinary tract antiseptics.
Discuss general characteristics of common urinary tract antiseptics.
Develop a plan of care for the client receiving urinary tract antiseptics.

KEY TERM: Antiseptic

⊛ **Urinary Tract Antiseptics: The Quinolones**

LEARNING OBJECTIVES:
Summarize essential information about the prototype drug nalidixic acid.
Outline a plan of care for a client receiving a quinolone drug.

KEY TERM: Quinolone

⊛ **Fluoroquinolones**

LEARNING OBJECTIVE: Identify the role of fluoroquinolones in the treatment of UTIs.

⊛ **Urinary Antiseptics: Nitrofuran Compounds**

LEARNING OBJECTIVES:
Summarize essential information about the pharmacokinetic and pharmacodynamic properties of nitrofurantoin.
List major undesired clinical responses associated with nitrofurantoin.
Develop a plan of care for the client receiving nitrofurantoin.

KEY TERM: Nitrofurantoin

⊛ **Urinary Antiseptic: Methenamine**

LEARNING OBJECTIVES:
Summarize essential information about the pharmacokinetic and pharmacodynamic properties of methenamine.
Develop a plan of care for the client receiving methenamine.

KEY TERM: Methenamine

⊛ **Other Drugs Used to Treat UTIs**

LEARNING OBJECTIVE: Identify two other drugs used to treat UTIs.

CONCEPTS AND TERMS TO REVIEW

Review Chapter 54 for general principles of antimicrobial therapy.
Review Chapter 49 for an overview of normal biologic defense mechanisms.

---

*T*he most common urologic disorders are infections and inflammations of the urinary tract. In the United States symptomatic urinary tract infections (UTIs) account for 6 million outpatient visits yearly. In addition, UTIs hospitalize an-other 300,000 individuals yearly, many of them elderly.[1] Prevention and control of these infections are important. The nursing role includes holistic assessment of the client, client education, administration of antiseptics and other agents as or-dered by the primary care provider, and evaluation of the client's response to therapy.

URINARY TRACT INFECTIONS

Urine, which normally is sterile, contains fluid, wastes, and salts but is free of bacteria and other microorganisms. Infec-tions in the urinary tract frequently begin in the urethra. From the urethra, the organisms may ascend to the urinary bladder.

If left untreated, pathogens may ascend the ureters to the kidneys, producing infection in the renal structures.[2] Confirmation of a UTI occurs when specific microorganisms are identified through a urine culture. To be classified as a UTI, there must be more than 100,000 organisms per milliliter in a clean-catch urine specimen.[3]

Urethritis, inflammation of the urethra, occurs in both males and females. Organisms commonly associated with urethritis are *Ureaplasma, Chlamydia,* and *Trichomonas vaginalis.* Irritants such as soap, perfumed toilet paper, and bubble baths can cause urethritis. Clients with urethritis experience burning during urination, frequency, and nocturia. Males usually have a discharge from the urethral meatus. Clients may complain of difficulty urinating and discomfort in the lower abdomen.[3]

Cystitis, inflammation of the urinary bladder, is more common in women. Bacteria that originate in either the rectum or vagina may ascend to the bladder via the female's relatively short urethra. In men, especially those over the age of 50 years, cystitis usually is the result of prostatitis or prostatic enlargement with accompanying urinary stasis. Not everyone who develops cystitis has symptoms. However, common symptoms include dysuria, urgency, nocturia, nocturnal enuresis, incontinence, urethral pain, low back pain, suprapubic pain, and fever accompanied by cloudy, foul-smelling urine. In addition, hematuria is not uncommon.[3] Most clients also experience the urge to urinate frequently (frequency) and pain in the bladder and urethra during urination. Despite the constant urge to urinate, only small amounts of urine are passed. Some males complain of fullness in the rectum.[2]

Pyelonephritis, an infection of the upper urinary tract, produces pain and edema in the kidney, renal pelvis, and surrounding structures. The most common cause of pyelonephritis is reflux of infected urine from the bladder to the upper urinary tract. The source of bacterial contamination of the urinary tract is usually fecal flora. Organisms causing pyelonephritis include *Escherichia coli, Proteus, Pseudomonas, Enterobacter, Klebsiella, Staphylococcus,* and enterococcus. The client with acute pyelonephritis experiences persistent ache in the flank or back, cystitis-like symptoms, fever with chills, general malaise, nausea, vomiting, and diarrhea. There also may be tenderness in the area of the costovertebral angle and pus, bacteria, and white cells in the urine.[2–4]

Glomerulonephritis, an inflammation of the kidney, affects the capillary loops in the glomeruli. Although the onset of glomerulonephritis is usually secondary to an infection of the upper respiratory tract, it can result from a primary infection elsewhere in the body. Drugs used to treat glomerulonephritis (e.g., penicillin) are discussed in Chapter 55.

URINARY TRACT ANTISEPTICS

Several compounds exert their only antibacterial effect in the urinary tract. Most urinary tract **antiseptics** are members of one of three families: the quinolones, the nitrofurantoins, and the methenamines. A new group, fluroquinolones, is widely distributed in the body and currently is the most actively investigated group of antimicrobial drugs.

Pharmacotherapeutics

Urinary tract antiseptics are used primarily for the prevention and treatment of urethritis and cystitis. Since most of these drugs inhibit the growth of bacteria and do not destroy the microorganism, they are not the drugs of choice for acute infections of the ureters or kidneys.

Urinary tract antiseptics are used in the treatment of both chronic or recurrent infections. With a chronic infection, the client harbors the same organism for months or even years, with relapses occurring after treatment is terminated. Recurrent infection is the result of an infection with the same organism or a reinfection with a different microorganism. Recurrent infection often is associated with an enlarged prostate, urethral strictures, long-term catheterization, or neurogenic bladder. In women, most recurrent infections are caused by different strains of bacteria. In the presence of structural anomalies or chronic medical problems such as cancer or diabetes, long-term therapy with urinary tract antiseptics may be indicated to prevent pyelonephritis.[5,6]

General Characteristics of Urinary Tract Antiseptics

Most urinary tract antiseptics are administered orally, and their desired effects are confined to the urinary tract. Absorbed well after oral administration, these drugs concentrate in the kidneys and achieve antibacterial status only within the urinary tract. Additionally, most urinary tract antiseptics cannot be given in doses large enough to achieve a therapeutic effect in the rest of the body. However, the newer fluoroquinolones do achieve serum concentration levels that approach those of an intravenous infusion.[7]

✖ NURSING CONSIDERATIONS

Even though many clients with UTIs are treated outside the hospital, the role of the nurse remains important. In addition, the nurse plays a major role in preventing the development of UTIs in hospitalized clients.

Assessing Begin the assessment with a **health history** that considers the age, gender, and level of sexual activity of the client. Remember that UTIs are 10 times more common in females than in males. In addition, recurrent UTIs often begin about the same time a young woman becomes sexually active. Inquire if the client has any allergies, and determine if the client has previously received urinary tract antiseptics. As you talk to the client, clarify his or her misconceptions. Clients may believe that symptoms associated with the UTI represent a sexually transmitted disease. Men frequently fear that any alteration in the urinary tract impairs sexual functioning.[4]

Determine if the client experiences difficulty starting or maintaining the stream of urine or if the client has noted any narrowing or diminished force in the urine stream. These manifestations can be signs of urinary tract obstruction. Ask if voiding is occurring more often than usual and obtain a description of the appearance and odor of the urine. Determine whether the client has experienced burning with urination, urgency, or back discomfort and whether fever or chilling has occurred.

Inquire about risk factors such as prior UTIs. Assess for chronic health problems such as diabetes mellitus, prostatic cancer, kidney stones, or a compromised immune system. These and other chronic diseases increase the likelihood of infection.

Begin the **physical assessment** with a general inspection of the client. Note the client's fluid status by checking skin turgor and status of mucous membranes. Determine if signs of edema are present. Weigh the client and compare the findings with the client's stated weight. Analyze the client's daily fluid intake and output.

Have the client void before palpating the bladder. Then inspect and palpate the lower abdomen for tenderness and bladder distention. Begin palpation at the level of the umbilicus and move downward toward the symphysis pubis. Wearing gloves, inspect the urinary meatus to determine whether surrounding tissues are inflamed. Perform a rectal examination on males since prostate enlargement can be detected with this technique. In addition, males with infections that extend into urethral tissue may have a purulent white discharge from the penis.

In most instances a urine specimen is collected and sent to the laboratory for culture and sensitivity. Cultures may also be repeated periodically during long-term drug therapy. Check the procedure manual of the agency to determine the specific technique to follow when collecting the urine. Remember that contamination of the specimen renders the results meaningless. If the urine specimen cannot be examined in 30 minutes, a preservative should be added and the urine refrigerated. Refrigeration prevents bacterial multiplication, and the preservative keeps other cells from deteriorating.[8]

Before sending the specimen to the laboratory, note the color of the urine. A change in the color is often an early sign of infection. For example, lime-green urine may indicate a *Pseudomonas* infection.[9] Since urine color is a subjective value difficult to describe, posting a carefully selected chart of paint chips in the utility room can provide a common standard. You also must inspect the urine for blood.

As a screen to detect the presence of a UTI, an on-unit or in-home dipstick test for nitrates may be performed. This test is especially useful when the client cannot cooperate in providing an uncontaminated urine specimen. Using nitrate dipsticks is more economical than using cultures. However, they are not sensitive to gram-positive organisms; thus their use is limited.[10]

🌿 NURSING RESEARCH

Pritchard, V., & Leverneir, J. (1991). Multistix versus laboratory urinalysis in the detection of urinary tract infections. *Journal of Gerontological Nursing, 17*(8), 39–42.

The object of this study was to determine if multidipstick testing compared favorably with laboratory tests in detecting active UTIs. The sample consisted of 37 males

in three extended care units of a Veterans Administration Medical Center.

A clean-catch urine specimen was obtained from 26 subjects by six nurse researchers. The same nurses collected needle-aspirated samples from 11 catheterized subjects. These specimens were subjected to a nurse-prepared nitrate test, a nurse-prepared leukocyte esterase test, and a laboratory culture. In this clinical setting a laboratory urinalysis cost $15.00 and the dipstick test 17 cents per subject. A urine culture fee was not mentioned.

A positive correlation (0.88 at the 1.0 level) existed between the nurse-prepared nitrate test and laboratory culture. Correlation between laboratory culture and the nurse-prepared leukocyte esterase test was less favorable at 0.62.

Based on these results, it is tentatively concluded that the nurse-prepared nitrate test may be of some use in assisting long-term care facilities to detect UTIs early. Additional studies with larger samples and with female subjects are needed to confirm preliminary findings with a higher level of significance. Caution also is needed when using nitrate sticks because gram-positive organisms yield false-negative results for the presence of bacteria. In addition, a highly acid diet or oral ascorbic acid affects the results.

STUDENT ACTIVITIES

- Contact three long-term care facilities in your area and determine the tests used to diagnose UTIs. Ascertain whether the agencies are familiar with nurse-prepared nitrate tests.
- Interview the laboratory supervisor in your assigned agency and determine his or her opinion of nurse-prepared nitrate tests. 🌿

Diagnosing After the assessment, analyze the information and develop individualized nursing diagnoses. Appropriate diagnoses for the client receiving urinary tract antiseptics include the following:

- Activity intolerance related to discomfort, fatigue, and weakness caused by the infectious processes.
- Altered patterns of urinary elimination related to inflammation of the lower urinary tract.
- Body image disturbance related to incontinence.
- Knowledge deficit regarding the use of urinary tract antiseptic drugs.
- High risk for noncompliance related to difficulty obtaining, storing, or self-administering the drugs.
- Anxiety related to changes in appearance of urine associated with drug therapy.
- Ineffective individual coping related to chronicity of recurrent infections.
- High risk for poisoning related to accessibility of drugs to children.

Planning During this phase, expected outcomes and the plan of care are developed. Client education is essential for these clients. Plan to review the specifics of good personal hygiene with the client. Teach female clients to cleanse the perineum from the front of the labia toward the anal region. Perineal pads must also be moved front to back. Recommend that female clients avoid the use of colored or scented toilet paper and bubble baths and bath salts, which allow bath water to penetrate the urethra. Females with recurrent UTIs may need to avoid tub baths altogether. Both males and females benefit from wearing cotton underwear, which offers ventilation and reduction of moisture. Instruct clients that careful perineal hygiene before and after intercourse reduces the mechanical introduction of microbes into the urinary meatus. Advise the client that the penis should be cleansed between anal sex and vaginal penetration. Voiding immediately after intercourse is also helpful.

Provide information in the teaching plan about recommended dietary changes. Since an increased urinary output flushes pathogens out of the urinary tract and reduces the resident population, the client must increase the oral intake of liquids, especially water. Plan to help the client develop a schedule for fluid intake (e.g., drink an 8-ounce glass of fluid hourly during waking hours).

Maintaining a urine pH of 5.5 or less is recommended with use of some urinary tract antiseptics. If needed, provide the client information about the acid-ash diet (see box). This diet regulates the urine pH by controlling the client's food choices. Plan to send a diet sheet home with the client and, if possible, arrange a dietary consultation. Since maintenance of a urine pH of 5.5 by diet alone is difficult, oral ascorbic acid or other acidifiers may be ordered in conjunction with the urinary tract antiseptics.

Be certain to provide information about the prescribed drug. Advise the client to take the urinary tract antiseptic exactly as ordered. Urge the client to take the full course of therapy, even if symptoms subside. Warn the client if the drug causes color changes in the urine. Provide information about undesired clinical responses and what actions to take if they occur. Drug information handouts provide good backup information if the client has adequate reading and comprehension skills.[2]

The ideal overall goal of the drug therapy is that the client's infection will be eradicated or controlled. The following expected outcome criteria may be applicable:

- Client identifies interventions to reduce risk of infection.
- Client participates in recommended treatment plan.
- Client maintains fluid volume at a functional level.
- Client reestablishes normal pattern of urinary functioning.
- Client's urine becomes clear and free of significant amounts of nitrates or white blood cells (WBCs).
- Client reports absence of urinary urgency, frequency, and burning.
- Client verbalizes major points included in teaching plan (e.g., components of an acid-ash diet, technique for proper perineal hygiene).

Implementing   You have an important role in preventing UTIs in the hospitalized client. Assist the client on bedrest with perineal hygiene each shift and after every bowel move-

---

ACID-ASH DIET

The purposes of an acid-ash diet are to furnish a balanced diet and to provide a diet higher in total acid ash than total alkaline ash.

Foods to Eliminate
Carbonated beverages
Cakes and cookies made with soda or baking powder
Fruits such as bananas, dried apricots, dates, figs, raisins, rhubarb
Vegetables: dried beans, carrots, lima beans
Sweets, chocolates

Foods to Restrict
Milk: no more than two servings daily
Vegetables (other than above): no more than two servings daily
Fruits: one serving daily of fruits not included in "Foods to Eliminate" or "Unrestricted Foods" lists

Unrestricted Foods
Whole grain bread, cereal, crackers, and rolls
Certain desserts (e.g., angel food cake, cookies made without baking powder or soda)
Gelatin desserts, rice or tapioca pudding
Sweets: plain sugar candy
Fats
Fruits: cranberries, plums, prunes
Meat, eggs, cheese, fish, fowl, peanut butter
Potato substitutes: corn, lentils, noodles, macaroni, rice
Popcorn
Nuts: peanuts, walnuts

---

ment. When bathing the genitals of a dependent client, cleanse the urinary meatus with a fresh washcloth and then cleanse outward from the meatus. Be certain to rinse and dry the area thoroughly.

Use of a Foley catheter introduces additional risk factors that promote UTIs. Manipulation of the catheter, tension on the catheter, and blocked catheters damage the uroepithelial lining of the bladder. Bacteria favor this damaged mucosa. Secure Foley catheters to minimize trauma to the meatus. Maintain sterile technique during catheter insertions, and cleanse the urinary meatus daily. Always keep the urine collection bag below the level of the bladder to prevent reflux or stasis, and do not disconnect the catheter from the drainage tube needlessly.

Unless medically contraindicated, encourage a fluid intake of 2000 to 3000 ml daily for adult clients. Cranberry juice and prune juice form an acid ash, whereas other fruit juices and milk may raise the pH of the urine. A healthy choice of liquids for most clients is plain water. If the client does not like the taste of tap water, add a little lemon. In addition, if economically feasible, bottled water can be substituted.[3,4]

Before he or she is discharged from the agency, determine if the client has the means to get a prescription filled; seek assistance for the client if necessary. Most clients need a follow-up appointment 10 to 14 days after completion of the drug regimen. Usually a urine sample is analyzed for the presence of bacteria at that time.

Evaluating When evaluating the client's response to urinary tract antiseptics, compare the client's present condition with the expected outcomes. Decreased severity or disappearance of UTI symptoms indicates a positive response to drug therapy. Include in your documentation the client's description of the ongoing comfort level in the bladder area and during urination. Odor and appearance of the urine and vital signs, especially temperature, should be recorded. (Resolution of hyperthermia is another positive indicator of successful therapy.) Urinalysis and urine culture and sensitivity are used to track the effectiveness of the drug.

Ascertain that the ambulatory client has obtained and taken the prescribed drug as ordered. In all clinical settings determine if the client can describe the purpose and limitations of urinary tract antiseptic therapy. Monitor the client for undesired clinical responses to the drug. Since some urinary tract antiseptics can produce blood dyscrasias, obtaining complete blood counts may be indicated.[12]

CONCEPT REVIEW

The most common urologic disorders are infections and inflammations of the urinary tract. The infections include urethritis, cystitis, pyelonephritis, and glomerulonephritis. Urinary tract antiseptics are prescribed primarily in the treatment of urethritis and cystitis.

Most urinary tract antiseptics are members of one of three families: the quinolones, the nitrofurantoins, and the methenamines.

Even though many clients with UTIs are treated outside the hospital, the role of the nurse remains important. In addition, the nurse plays a major role in preventing the development of UTIs in hospitalized clients.

URINARY TRACT ANTISEPTICS: THE QUINOLONES

Cinoxacin and nalidixic acid are both classified as **quinolones.**

QUINOLONE PROTOTYPE

NALIDIXIC ACID

Nalidixic acid (NegGram) was introduced in 1964; it is the oldest of the quinolones and is the precursor of the fluoroquinolones.

Pharmacotherapeutics Nalidixic acid is effective for the prevention and treatment of uncomplicated cystitis and against many urinary tract pathogens. It is specifically recommended for the treatment of UTIs caused by the *E.*

coli species, which are the cause of approximately 90% of all initial UTIs. Nalidixic acid is effective against most strains of *Klebsiella, Enterobacter,* and *Proteus.* However, these organisms develop resistance rapidly, usually within 48 hours after the start of therapy. Nalidixic acid is ineffective against *Staphylococcus* and the *Pseudomonas* species.[7,13]

Pharmacokinetics Nalidixic acid is absorbed rapidly after oral administration. Although food delays absorption of the drug, it does not decrease the amount absorbed. The serum half-life of nalidixic acid is 6 to 7 hours; the half-life is increased in individuals with poor renal function. Peak serum concentration is reached in 1 to 2 hours and peak urine concentration in 3 to 4 hours. Nalidixic acid is 93% protein bound. High concentrations of the drug are found in bladder and renal tissues. However, it does not accumulate outside the urinary tract. Nalidixic acid is rapidly metabolized by the liver, and approximately one third of the drug is converted to an active metabolite, hydroxynalidixic acid, which is 16 times more active than its original form. Nalidixic acid continues to clear the kidneys in clients with mild to moderate renal failure. In those with marked renal dysfunction, serum half-life is prolonged up to 21 hours.[13]

Pharmacodynamics Nalidixic acid binds to DNA and interferes with the A subunit of DNA gyrase, an enzyme that introduces negative twists in DNA and separates interlocked DNA molecules. This inhibition prevents duplication of bacterial DNA[7] (Fig. 56–1).

Pharmaceutics Nalidixic acid is available in capsule, caplet, tablet, and suspension dosage forms for oral administration. Note that an underdose during initial therapy (less than 4 g/day) predisposes the client to the development of bacterial resistance. See Table 56–1 for information about recommended doses for adults and children.

Undesired Clinical Responses Gastrointestinal (GI) side effects, including nausea, vomiting, and diarrhea, are the most common unwanted responses to nalidixic acid (Fig. 56–2). Skin-related problems, including an itchy rash and increased sun sensitivity, are also fairly common. Some clients may experience central nervous system (CNS) symptoms such as headaches, dizziness, drowsiness, and visual disturbances. Potentially serious adverse reactions include liver damage, blood dyscrasias, and hemolytic anemia. If liver damage is present, the client may experience jaundice, abdominal pain, pale stools, dark urine, and elevated liver enzymes. Blood dyscrasias are evidenced by pallor, weakness, bleeding problems, fever, and sore throat. Hemolytic anemia is more likely to develop in clients with glucose-6-phosphate dehydrogenase (G-6-PD) deficiency.

Anaphylactic reactions are rare. However, at high doses nalidixic acid can be toxic to the CNS, causing hallucinations, confusion, and seizures. Neurologic undesired responses are more common in children and in adults with a history of epilepsy, parkinsonism, or cerebral arteriosclerosis.[7,13,14]

Contraindications and Precautions Nalidixic acid should not be used by clients with severe liver or kidney damage or by clients with a history of convulsive disorders.

Drug-Drug and Drug-Environment Interactions Nalidixic acid interacts with oral anticoagulants, displacing them from their protein-binding sites. This allows more unbound anticoagulant to circulate, putting the client at

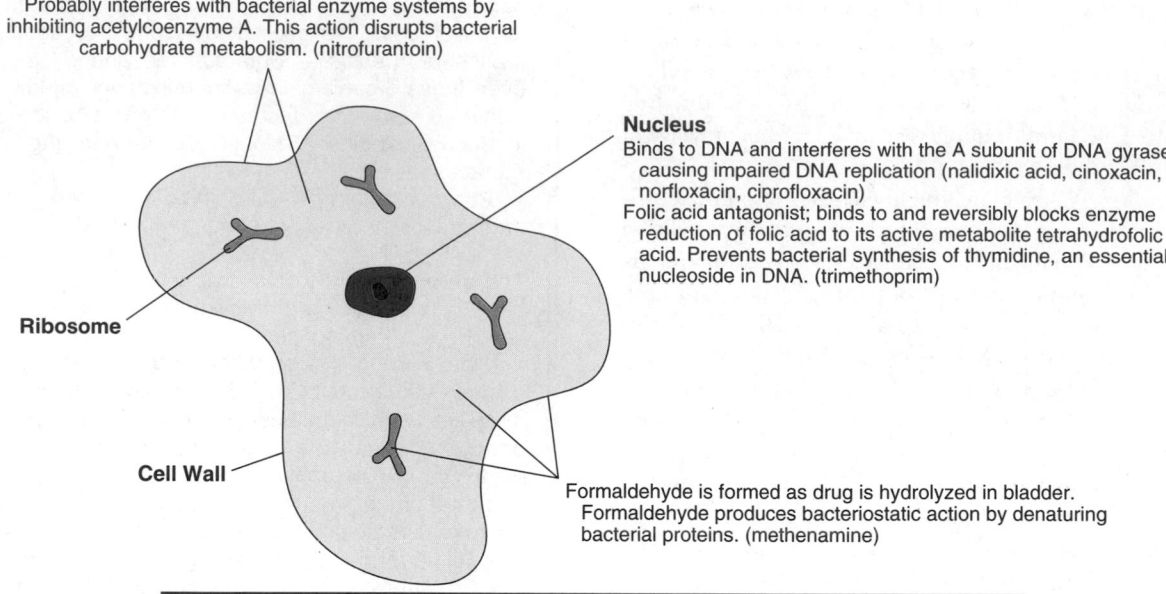

Probably interferes with bacterial enzyme systems by inhibiting acetylcoenzyme A. This action disrupts bacterial carbohydrate metabolism. (nitrofurantoin)

Nucleus
Binds to DNA and interferes with the A subunit of DNA gyrase, causing impaired DNA replication (nalidixic acid, cinoxacin, norfloxacin, ciprofloxacin)
Folic acid antagonist; binds to and reversibly blocks enzyme reduction of folic acid to its active metabolite tetrahydrofolic acid. Prevents bacterial synthesis of thymidine, an essential nucleoside in DNA. (trimethoprim)

Ribosome

Cell Wall

Formaldehyde is formed as drug is hydrolyzed in bladder. Formaldehyde produces bacteriostatic action by denaturing bacterial proteins. (methenamine)

FIGURE 56–1   Pharmacodynamic mechanism of major urinary tract antiseptics.

risk for hemorrhage. If nalidixic acid and an oral anticoagulant must be administered concurrently, the anticoagulant dosage may need to be reduced. In addition, the prothrombin time used to monitor anticoagulant effectiveness should be checked more frequently than usual during the duration of nalidixic acid use.[13]

Increased photosensitivity during nalidixic acid therapy places the client at risk for serious sunburn. This reaction can be triggered by 15 minutes in the sun and may develop into painful bullae that takes months to resolve. Repeated episodes of sun exposure exacerbate the condition. The increased risk for serious burns persists for 3 months after nalidixic acid has been discontinued.

Interference with Laboratory Tests When Benedict's or Fehling's solution or Clinitest reagent tablets are used to test the urine of clients with diabetes mellitus, a false-positive reaction for glucose may be obtained.

Incorrect values may be obtained for urinary 17-ketosteroids and ketogenic steroids if the m-dinitrobenzene is used.[13,14]

Life-Span Considerations Nalidixic acid should not be prescribed for children younger than 3 months, since its use is associated with increased intracranial pressure in this age group. It is also not recommended for children who have not entered puberty. Although joint damage in children has not been reported, animal studies have shown that nalidixic acid can cause erosion of immature joints. Safe use in the first trimester of pregnancy has not been established. However, the drug has been used during the last two trimesters without producing ill effects to mother or child. Clients using nalidixic acid during pregnancy should discontinue the drug at the first sign of labor to avoid significant blood levels of the drug in the neonate. In addition, small amounts of nalidixic acid appear in breast milk, which may pose a risk for hemolytic anemia in the infant with G-6-PD deficiency.[13,14]

Specific Drug-Related Nursing Considerations Caution clients to avoid operating power machinery or motor vehicles immediately after starting the course of therapy.

If dizziness or other CNS symptoms do not develop after the first couple of days, the client can resume driving and working with power tools. Advise using sunglasses and window shades to manage photophobic reactions. Subdued indoor lighting is appropriate. A sunscreen with a high sun protection factor (SPF) can ward off burns. Remind the client that sunscreen is needed on overcast days as well as in bright sunlight. Sunlamps, sunbathing, and tanning beds should be avoided. Instruct the client to contact the health care provider if UTI symptoms do not begin to subside after 1 week of nalidixic acid therapy.

If nalidixic acid is continued for more than 2 weeks, the complete blood count, serum creatinine levels, and liver enzyme levels are usually monitored to detect early signs of blood dyscrasias or liver damage. Diabetic clients who monitor urine glucose should use a colorimetric test based on an enzyme reaction (e.g., Clinistix reagent strips or Tes-Tape). Table 56–1 summarizes additional nursing considerations.

MISCELLANEOUS DRUGS IN CATEGORY

Cinoxacin (Cinobac) is a quinolone with antimicrobial properties very similar to those of nalidixic acid. Cinoxacin can be used for the treatment of uncomplicated cystitis. When compared to nalidixic acid, cinoxacin requires less frequent administration and does not cause as many undesired reactions. However, with the availability of the new potent fluroquinolones, the role of cinoxacin has become very limited.[15]

Cinoxacin is well absorbed after oral administration. Approximately 70% of the drug is bound to plasma proteins, with a serum half-life of $1\frac{1}{2}$ hours. Cinoxacin is concentrated in the urine, and 95% is excreted within 24 hours. The half-life is longer in clients with poor renal function. The usual dose is 500 mg every 12 hours continued for 7 to 14 days. For maintenance, 500 mg can be given daily at bedtime. In clients with impaired renal function, the dose is reduced and based on

TABLE 56–1
Major Urinary Tract Antiseptics: Prototypes and Other Drugs in Category

Drug Name	Dosage and Route of Administration	Nursing Considerations
NITROFURAN COMPOUNDS: **NITROFURANTOIN** (Furadantin, Furalan, Macrodantin) HOW SUPPLIED Capsule: 25, 50, 100 mg Oral suspension: 25 mg/5 ml	*Therapeutic Use* Bactericidal and bacteriostatic against some *Klebsiella, Staphylococcus aureus, Escherichia coli,* some *Enterobacter, Enterococcus, Proteus* **Treatment of Acute UTIs** *Adult:* 50–100 mg q6h, not to exceed 600 mg in 24 h *Child: >1 mo of age;* 5–7 mg/kg/d in four divided doses **Prophylaxis** *Adult:* 50–100 mg hs *Child:* 1 mg/kg/d in one or two divided doses	**Assess** Determine if client is pregnant; some preparations are classified as Pregnancy Category B drugs, whereas others have not been sufficiently tested for use during pregnancy. **Implement** Administer with food or milk. Avoid crushing tablets or opening capsules. Shake suspensions well. Oral suspensions may be mixed with water, juice, or formula. Have client rinse mouth well with water after taking suspension. Warn client about possible staining of teeth. Administer drug at equally spaced intervals around the clock. Store in dark container with tight cap. Instruct client not to take antacids with magnesium trisilicate while receiving this drug. Inform client that drug may turn urine brown or rust color. **Monitor** Monitor for undesired clinical responses (e.g., chest pain, cough, fever with chills, dizziness, nausea, vomiting, anorexia, diarrhea). Monitor intake and output (I&O). Report oliguria and any changes in I&O ratio. Evaluate CBC periodically during long-term drug therapy. **Evaluate** Evaluate response to therapy (e.g., decreased indications of UTI).
QUINOLONES: **NALIDIXIC ACID** (NegGram) HOW SUPPLIED Uncoated tablet: 250, 500 mg, 1 g Oral suspension: 250 mg/5 ml	*Therapeutic Use* Bacteriostatic and bactericidal against *E. coli, Klebsiella, Enterobacter, Proteus mirabilis, P. vulgaris, Morganella morganii* **RECURRENT UTIs** *Adult:* 1 g qid for 1–2 wk for short-term therapy *Child: 3 mo–12 y:* 55 mg/kg/d in four divided doses for short-term therapy **Prophylaxis** *Adult:* 2 g/d in divided doses for prolonged therapy *Child:* 33 mg/kg/d in divided doses for maintenance	**Assess** Collect urine specimen for culture and sensitivity before starting therapy. Determine if client is pregnant; nalidixic acid is classified as a Pregnancy Category B drug. Assess drug history; nalidixic acid interacts with oral anticoagulants and requires frequent monitoring of prothrombin time. **Implement** Administer 1 h before meals. If client complains of GI distress, administer with milk or food. Shake suspension thoroughly. Store in tight container at 15° to 30° C. Teach client to take drug at regular intervals during 24 h and to complete course of therapy. Caution client not to omit doses, especially in early days of therapy. Such omission may promote bacterial resistance. Advise client to avoid direct sunlight or ultraviolet light while receiving drug. Encourage client to drink 2000–3000 ml/d if tolerated.

Table continued on following page.

TABLE 56–1 *Continued*
Major Urinary Tract Antiseptics: Prototypes and Other Drugs in Category

Drug Name	Dosage and Route of Administration	Nursing Considerations
QUINOLONES—CONT'D		**Monitor**
		Assess client periodically for signs of infection. Bacterial resistance may develop within 48 h.
		Monitor blood counts and renal and hepatic function tests if therapy is continued longer than 2 wk.
		Monitor carefully for undesired clinical response (e.g., drowiness, headache, dizziness, vertigo, papilledema, visual disturbance, nausea, vomiting, photosensitivity).
Cinoxacin	**Simple Cystitis**	**Evaluate**
(Cinobac)	*Adult:* 250 mg q6h or 500 mg q12h for 7–14 d	Evaluate response to therapy (e.g., decreased WBCs in urine).
HOW SUPPLIED	Particularly effective in a 250-mg dose when combined with post-coital voiding in premenopausal women.	
Gelatin capsules: 250, 500 mg		See nalidixic acid with following exceptions:
	MAINTENANCE	Cinoxacin is classified as a Pregnancy Category C drug.
	Adult: 500 mg daily hs	Drug may be taken with food. However, presence of food in stomach may reduce peak serum concentrations.
		Effectiveness of drug is enhanced by administering drug at evenly spaced intervals throughout 24 h.
METHENAMINES:		**Assess**
Methenamine Hippurate	*Adults:* 1 g bid	Assess for preexisting renal insufficiency.
(Hiprex, Urex)	*Children 6 to 12 y:* 500 mg to 1 g bid	Determine if client is pregnant: methenamine is classified as Pregnancy Category C drug.
HOW SUPPLIED	*Children <6 y:* None	Assess client's hydration status: drug is contraindicated with dehydration.
Uncoated tablets: 1 g		
Methenamine Mandelate	*Adults:* 1 g qid	**Implement**
(Mandelamine, Mandameth, etc.)	*Children 6 to 12 y:* 500 mg qid	Shake suspensions well before using.
HOW SUPPLIED	*Children <6 y:* 18.4 mg/kg qid	Teach client to avoid alkaline foods.
Oral suspension: 250, 500 mg/5 ml		Advise client to maintain a fluid intake of 1500 to 200 ml/d.
Granule for reconstitution: 1 g/pkg for oral administration		Teach client how to read dipstick tests for pH and specific gravity.
Enteric coated tablet: 0.5, 1 g		**Monitor**
		Monitor for undesired clinical responses, e.g., nausea, vomiting, diarrhea, anorexia, bladder discomfort.
		Monitor I&O.
		Evaluate
		Assess for diminished indications of infection.

creatinine clearance results. Undesired clinical responses are similar to those of nalidixic acid. Cinoxacin use is contraindicated in clients with a history of hypersensitivity to cinoxacin or other quinolones.[13,14]

FLUOROQUINOLONES

As previously indicated, the quinolones are the precursors of fluoroquinolones. The fluoroquinolones have a broad spectrum of antimicrobial activity. They are widely distributed through extravascular tissue sites and have a long serum half-life. Because fluoroquinolones are used in the treatment of other infections in addition to UTIs, they are discussed in Chapter 55. Dosage and routes of administration for UTIs are summarized in Table 56–2.

CONCEPT REVIEW

Nalidixic acid is the original compound of the quinolone group. Nalidixic acid and its derivatives inhibit DNA supercoiling and ultimately kill the bacterial cell wall.

GI disturbances, photosensitivity reactions, and CNS side effects are common undesired responses associated with nalidixic acid.

Nalidixic acid is the precursor for the fluoroquinolones, which have a broad spectrum of antimicrobial activity, wide distribution through extravascular tissue, and a long serum half-life.

The mechanism of action for the fluoroquinolones is the same as for nalidixic acid.

TABLE 56–2

Prearations and Dosages of Fluoroquinolone Drugs

Drug Name	Dosage and Route of Administration
Norfloxacin (Noroxin) HOW SUPPLIED Tablet: 400 mg	Oral: 400 mg bid for 3–21 d depending on causative organism Administer 1 h before or 2 h after meals with full glass of water at same time each day If client is receiving an antacid, administer antacid at least 2 h after norfloxacin.
Ciprofloxacin Hydrochloride (e.g., Ciloxan, Cipro) HOW SUPPLIED IV solution: 200, 400 mg Uncoated tablet: 250, 500, 750 mg	Oral: 250–500 mg q12h for 7–14 d IV: 200–400 mg q12h infused slowly over a period of 60 min

URINARY TRACT ANTISEPTICS: NITROFURAN COMPOUNDS

Nitrofuran compounds are characterized by a ring containing one oxygen and four carbon atoms.

NITROFURAN COMPOUND PROTOTYPE

NITROFURANTOIN

Nitrofurantoin (Furadantin, Furalan, Macrodantin) became available for clinical use in 1953.[7]

Pharmacotherapeutics Nitrofurantoin is indicated in the treatment of UTIs caused by susceptible organisms. Although effective in the management of urethritis, prostatitis, cystitis, and pyelonephritis, its usefulness is limited by undesired clinical responses.

Most strains of *E. coli* are susceptible to nitrofurantoin, as are most gram-negative bacilli and gram-positive cocci commonly associated with UTIs. They include the *Klebsiella* and *Enterobacter* species and *Staphylococcus aureus*. Some *Klebsiella* and *Enterobacter* strains have developed resistance, and most *Proteus, Serratia,* and *Acinetobacter* strains are resistant. Nitrofurantoin has no

effect against *Pseudomonas.* Organisms sensitive at the beginning of therapy usually do not develop resistance later.[13,14]

Pharmacokinetics Nitrofurantoin is well absorbed from the small intestine after oral administration. The presence of food delays absorption, increases the amount absorbed, increases peak concentration, and prolongs the drug's stay in the urine. Nitrofurantoin is irritating to the GI tract during absorption. A macrocrystalline form (Macrodantin) was developed in 1967 in an attempt to reduce the GI irritation. Nitrofurantoin macrocrystals have a controlled crystal size that regulates the rate of drug absorption, thus reducing gastric side effects.[7]

Sixty percent of the absorbed drug is protein bound. The serum half-life is only 20 minutes in clients with normal renal function but increases to 60 minutes in those with severe renal disease. Nitrofurantoin crosses the placenta and enters breast milk and bile. The drug is rapidly broken down in tissues; 30% to 50% of the drug is excreted unchanged in the urine. Acidification of the urine increases renal parenchymal concentrations. Clients with impaired renal function do not obtain therapeutic urine concentrations of the drug.[7,13,14]

Pharmacodynamics Nitrofurantoin is bacteriostatic in low concentrations and is considered bactericidal in higher concentrations. The drug probably interferes with bacterial enzyme systems by inhibiting acetylcoenzyme A, thus disrupting bacterial carbohydrate metabolism. Nitrofurantoin is reduced by bacterial flavoproteins to reactive intermediates, which inactivate or alter bacterial ribosomal proteins and other macromolecules. As a result, vital biochemical processes such as protein synthesis, aerobic energy metabolism, DNA synthesis, RNA synthesis, and cell wall synthesis are inhibited.[13]

Pharmaceutics Nitrofurantoin is available in capsule, tablet, and suspension dosage forms for oral administration. See Table 56–1 for information about recommended doses for adults and children.

Undesired Clinical Responses GI symptoms, including loss of appetite, nausea, vomiting, and diarrhea, are the most common undesired clinical responses associated with nitrofurantoin. These symptoms are less common when the client receives the macrocrystalline version of the drug.[7,16] Although rare, hepatitis does develop in some clients. (See Fig. 56–2 for an illustration of common undesired clinical responses associated with nitrofurantoin.)

Although less common, skin reactions such as itching and rashes occur. Occasionally hives are noted, and there are rare reports of angioedema and a lupus erythematosus-like condition. Like nalidixic acid, nitrofurantoin can produce CNS effects, including headaches, dizziness, and visual disturbances. Progressive peripheral polyneuropathy is another serious adverse response to nitrofurantoin therapy. This condition is more common in clients with anemia and those with electrolyte imbalances or renal failure. The neuropathy may become irreversible.[13,14]

Nitrofurantoin can also trigger blood dyscrasias. Acute hemolytic anemia is possible in the client with G-6-PD deficiency. Hemolysis usually stops when the drug is discontinued. Although usual doses do not affect spermatogenesis, large doses of nitrofurantoin can depress sperm formation. Nitrofurantoin may also turn urine brown.

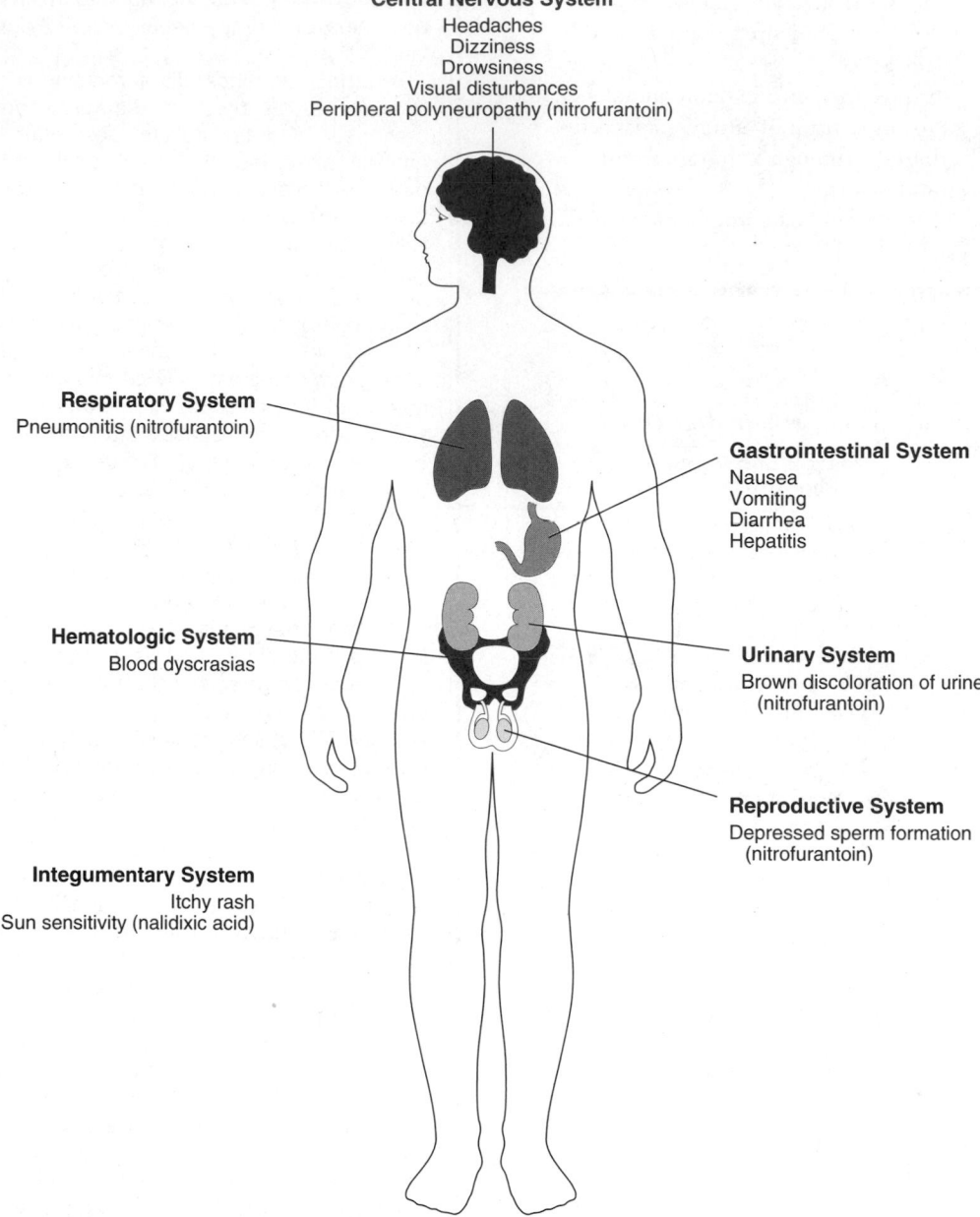

Central Nervous System
Headaches
Dizziness
Drowsiness
Visual disturbances
Peripheral polyneuropathy (nitrofurantoin)

Respiratory System
Pneumonitis (nitrofurantoin)

Gastrointestinal System
Nausea
Vomiting
Diarrhea
Hepatitis

Hematologic System
Blood dyscrasias

Urinary System
Brown discoloration of urine
(nitrofurantoin)

Reproductive System
Depressed sperm formation
(nitrofurantoin)

Integumentary System
Itchy rash
Sun sensitivity (nalidixic acid)

FIGURE 56–2   Common undesired clinical responses associated with quinolones and nitrofuran compounds.

Acute, subacute, and chronic pulmonary hypersensitivity reactions may occur. Acute pulmonary reactions are commonly manifested by fever, chills, cough, chest pain, dyspnea, pulmonary effusion or infiltration, and eosinophilia. These reactions usually occur within the first week of therapy and are reversible with cessation of the drug. Fever and eosinophilia occur less often with subacute pulmonary reactions. After discontinuation of the drug, recovery may require several months. Chronic pulmonary reactions generally occur in clients who have received continuous therapy for 6 months or longer. Malaise, dyspnea on exertion, cough, and altered pulmonary function are common manifestations. The risk of permanently impaired pulmonary function increases if chronic pulmonary reactions are not recognized and treated early.[13,17]

Contraindications and Precautions Nitrofurantoin use is contraindicated for clients with oliguria, a history of hypersensitivity to nitrofurantoin, or with a G-6-PD deficiency. The drug is not recommended for pregnant clients near term or for infants less than 4 weeks old. In addition, nitrofurantoin should be given with caution to debilitated or diabetic clients.

Drug-Drug Interactions Nitrofurantoin interacts with several drugs. For example, nitrofurantoin antagonizes the antimicrobial effects of nalidixic acid. When administered concomitantly with nitrofurantoin, antacids containing magnesium trisilicate reduce both the rate and extent of absorption. Uricosuric drugs such as probenecid and sulfinpyrazone can inhibit renal tubular secretion of nitrofurantoin; this increases serum nitrofurantoin levels but decreases urinary levels. In addition, drugs that delay gastric emptying, such as anticholinergics, increase the absorption and bioavailability of nitrofurantoin.

Interference with Laboratory Tests Nitrofurantoin can decrease serum glucose levels and elevate serum bilirubin, alkaline phosphatase, and urine creatinine levels.

False-positive urine glucose test results may occur if the client uses a copper sulfate testing material such as Benedict's solution.[13,14]

Life-Span Considerations As indicated previously, nitrofurantoin should not be administered to infants less than 1 month of age because of the danger of hemolytic anemia. Nitrofurantoin is classified as a Pregnancy Category B drug. Even though there are no adequate studies in pregnant women, the drug is contraindicated in near-term pregnancies because of the risk for hemolytic anemia. Nitrofurantoin use is not recommended in nursing mothers since it has been detected in human breast milk. The risk of serious neuropathy is higher in elderly clients.[13,14]

Specific Drug-Related Nursing Considerations Administer the drug with food (ideally breakfast and dinner) to enhance drug tolerance and improve drug absorption. Since suspensions of nitrofurantoin can stain teeth, have the client rinse the mouth well after swallowing the drug. Monitor the client's intake and output and notify the primary care provider of significant discrepancies in 24-hour totals.

Teach the client to avoid operating power tools or heavy machinery until it is known if the drug causes dizziness. Inform the client that the drug may change urine to a brown or rust color. Advise the client that the color change is harmless. Advise the client to notify the health care provider immediately if chest pain, cough, and fever with chills develop. This cluster of symptoms could signal the onset of pulmonary toxicity.

CONCEPT REVIEW

Although nitrofurantoin is effective in managing UTIs, its use is limited by undesired clinical responses.

Nitrofurantoin probably interferes with bacterial enzyme systems by inhibiting acetylcoenzyme A. This action disrupts bacterial carbohydrate metabolism.

Common undesired clinical responses include loss of appetite, nausea, vomiting, diarrhea, headaches, dizziness, and visual disturbances. Nitrofurantoin can produce serious responses such as blood dyscrasias and pulmonary toxicity.

URINARY TRACT ANTISEPTIC: METHENAMINE

Methenamine was introduced in 1895 for the treatment of UTIs.

Pharmacotherapeutics The only indications for using methenamine are to treat acute UTIs or suppress recurrent ones. It is particularly well suited for long-term treatment of UTIs because susceptible bacteria and fungi cannot develop resistance. Methenamine is effective against fungi and many gram-positive and gram-negative organisms, including *E. coli*, staphylococci, and enterococci. *Enterobacter* and *Proteus vulgaris* are among the few organisms displaying resistance to methenamine.[13,14]

Pharmacokinetics Methenamine and its salts are readily absorbed in the GI tract after oral administration. However, up to 30% of a dose may be hydrolyzed in the gastric juices. In this acid medium, hydrolysis of methenamine produces ammonia and formaldehyde. Enteric-coated methenamine is less likely to convert to formaldehyde in the stomach.

Peak serum concentration of methenamine is achieved 1 hour after a 1-g dose. Drug molecules enter red blood cells and are widely distributed in body fluids, including fluids that surround the brain, heart, and joints and fluids in the eye. However, the drug has no antibacterial action in these fluids. Between 10% and 25% of the methenamine is metabolized by the liver.

Excretion of methenamine is achieved by glomerular filtration and tubular secretion. At least 90% of each dose is excreted by the kidneys within 24 hours. Approximately 20% of each dose is hydrolyzed to formaldehyde. However, the drug passes through the kidneys so rapidly that little formaldehyde is created. Most of the formaldehyde formation takes place in the bladder.[7,13,14]

Pharmacodynamics Formaldehyde is formed as methenamine is hydrolyzed in the bladder. The formaldehyde produces a bacteriostatic action by denaturing bacterial proteins (see Fig. 56-1). At a urine pH of 6, only 6% of the methenamine is converted to formaldehyde. If the urine pH is between 5.0 and 5.5, it takes approximately 2 to 3 hours to create enough formaldehyde to be bacteriostatic. A formaldehyde concentration of more than 25 μg/ml of urine is needed to destroy organisms. The formaldehyde continues to kill organisms for 6 hours or until the client empties the bladder. A steady-state urinary formaldehyde level can be achieved after 2 to 3 days of drug administration.[7,13,14]

Since acidification of the urine is necessary to convert methenamine to formaldehyde, methenamine has been combined with either mandelic acid or hippuric acid in an attempt to acidify the urine. However, current opinions vary about the benefit of these weak acids or dietary supplements in generating additional formaldehyde from the methenamine.[7]

Pharmaceutics All methenamine dosage forms are intended for the oral route. These forms include tablets, enteric-coated tablets, granules, and suspensions. The prescribed dosages vary depending on the methenamine formulation used. Table 56-1 has information about recommended doses for adults and children.

Undesired clinical responses Undesired clinical responses with methenamine occur less frequently than those associated with other urinary tract antiseptics. GI discomfort, including nausea, vomiting, and diarrhea, is the most common. A sore mouth and loss of appetite may accompany the GI symptoms. In large doses the client may experience bladder discomfort (e.g., frequency, urgency, and presence of protein, blood, or crystals in the urine).

One form of methenamine (Hiprex) contains tartrazine,

which can trigger asthma attacks in susceptible individuals. This response occurs most frequently among clients who also suffer from aspirin hypersensitivity.[7,13,14]

Contraindications and precautions Hypersensitivity to methenamine contraindicates its use. Methenamine use is also contraindicated in clients with dehydration, renal insufficiency, gout, and hepatic disease. When administered to clients with gout, the drug may cause precipitation of urate crystals. In addition, oral suspensions of methenamine contain a vegetable oil. This dosage form should be used with caution in clients susceptible to lipoid pneumonia (e.g., elderly, debilitated individuals).[7,13]

Drug-drug interactions Methenamine should not be prescribed in combination with sulfa antimicrobials because the drug chemically combines with the sulfa preparation, resulting in mutual antagonism. Drugs that alkalinize the urine inhibit the effectiveness of methenamine because the increase in pH stops the conversion of methenamine to formaldehyde. Specific alkalinizing agents to avoid are sodium bicarbonate and the diuretic acetazolamide (Diamox).[7,18]

Interference with laboratory tests Methenamine's breakdown product, formaldehyde, may increase catecholamines and vanillylmandelic acid (VMA), decrease estriol, increase 17-hydroxycorticosteroid, and decrease 5-hydroxyindoleacetic acid (5-HIAA).

Life-span considerations Methenamine is classified as Pregnancy Category C drug; the drug crosses the placenta and passes to the fetus. However, there have been no reports of fetal abnormalities. Methenamine also enters breast milk. An infant receives an estimated 0.15 to 0.4 mg of methenamine in a feeding. There have been no reports of harm to nursing infants.

Specific drug-related nursing considerations Since methenamine is most effective at a urine pH below 5.5, teach the client to avoid alkaline foods. Provide information on the acid-ash diet and assist with meal planning. (Review the box on p. 754.) Drugs that acidify the urine (e.g., ascorbic acid,

ammonion chloride, sodium biphosphate) may also be prescribed for the client. Make certain the client understands the reason for taking these drugs.

Advise the client to maintain a fluid intake of 1500 to 2000 ml per day since excess fluids may increase diuresis and dilute the formaldehyde concentration. Teach the client how to read dipstick tests for pH and specific gravity. If the specific gravity falls below 1.015 or the pH rises, the client should notify the primary care provider. Also teach the client to monitor the appearance of the urine carefully since hematuria may indicate the accumulation of mandelate salts.

MISCELLANEOUS DRUGS IN CATEGORY

Methenamine hippurate and **methenamine mandelate** are examples of acid salts sometimes added to methenamine to enhance formaldehyde formation. (See Table 56–1 for additional information about these two preparations.) In addition, a number of drugs are available that combine methenamine with other drugs. For example, salicylamide, sodium salicylate, and phenyl salicylate are added for pain relief. Atropine sulfate, hyoscyamine, or belladonna is intended to relax the bladder smooth muscle and thus add to the analgesic effect. Benzoic acid and methylene blue are used as weak germicides. These methenamine combinations are rarely prescribed today.[13]

OTHER DRUGS USED TO TREAT UTIS

In addition to nitrofurantoins, quinolones, fluoroquinolones, and methenamines, a few other agents are used to treat UTIs. In addition, with complicated UTIs the primary care provider may resort to using antimicrobial drugs that have systematic effects. These drugs are discussed in Chapter 55.

Trimethoprim

Trimethoprim is used to treat initial episodes of acute uncomplicated lower UTI and to treat and prevent chronic and

---

TABLE 56–3
Miscellaneous Drugs Used to Treat UTIs

Drug Name	Dosage and Route of Administration	Nursing Considerations
TRIMETHOPRIM (Proloprim, Trimpex) HOW SUPPLIED Uncoated tablet: 100, 200 mg	*Adult:* 100 mg q12h for 10 d or 200 mg q24h for 10 d Effectiveness in children less than 12 y of age has not been established	Drug is not recommended for client with creatinine clearance of less than 15 ml/min. Administer on an empty stomach or at least 2 h after meals. If GI upset occurs, administer with food. Encourage fluid intake sufficient to maintain urinary volume at 1500 ml/d.
Methenamine Combination Drugs: Atropine Sulfate, Hyoscyamine, Methylene Blue, Phenyl Salicylate (Atrosept, Hexalol, Urised, Uriseptic) HOW SUPPLIED Coated tablets Uncoated tablets	*Adult:* two tablets qid	Administer with full glass of water after meals. Advise client that urine may become blue to blue-green and that feces may be discolored. Encourage fluid intake sufficient to maintain urinary volume at 1000–1500 ml/d. Store in tight, light-resistant container. This is a Pregnancy Category C drug.

recurrent UTIs. Trimethoprim is effective against most common UTI pathogens, including *E. coli, Enterobacter* species, and *Proteus mirabilis.* It is not effective against *Pseudomonas aeruginosa.*

Trimethoprim is a folic acid antagonist with slow bactericidal action. It binds to and reversibly blocks enzyme reduction of folic acid to its active metabolite, tetrahydrofolic acid. This prevents bacterial synthesis of thymidine, an essential nucleoside in DNA.

Trimethoprim is well absorbed after oral administration and peaks within 1 to 4 hours. The drug is widely distributed in the body. Trimethoprim is metabolized in the liver and has a half-life of 8 to 11 hours. Approximately 80% of the drug is excreted unchanged in the urine. Uncomplicated infections in adults are managed with 100 mg of trimethoprim every 12 hours. A low dose of trimethoprim (20 mg) is sufficient to treat UTIs in most pediatric clients with an unobstructed urinary tract. Full-dose trimethoprim often is given routinely to children undergoing micturating cystograms.[19] (See Table 56–3 for additional dosage information.)

The most common undesired responses associated with trimethoprim are rash, pruritus, and GI tract symptoms, including sore mouth, altered taste, nausea, vomiting, and epigastric pain. Hematologic responses, including anemia, neutropenia, and thrombocytopenia, occur but are rare.[20]

Trimethoprim may inhibit the hepatic metabolism of phenytoin, causing increased levels of the anticonvulsant. In addition, concurrent administration of trimethoprim with the antitubercular drug rifampin increases the elimination of trimethoprim. Trimethoprim can interfere with some methotrexate assays and falsely elevate serum creatinine levels.

Trimethoprim use is contraindicated for individuals with known hypersensitivity or megaloblastic anemia caused by folate deficiency. It is classified as a Pregnancy Category C drug, and its use is not recommended during pregnancy and lactation. Treatment of elderly debilitated clients with trimethoprim should be attempted only under very close supervision.

During the period of drug therapy, fluid intake should be sufficient to maintain a daily urine output of at least 1500 ml. Symptoms of a hematologic disorder—fever, sore throat, pallor, purpura, ecchymosis—should be reported immediately.[7,13,14,18] (See Table 56–3 for additional information on trimethoprim.)

Methylene Blue

Methylene blue, a weakly germicidal blue dye, is infrequently prescribed alone as a urinary tract antiseptic. However, in some dosage forms it is combined with other drugs (e.g., atropine sulfate, hyoscyamine, methenamine, phenyl salicylate) for that purpose. When prescribed in this manner, the drug should be administered with a full glass of water. In addition, advise the client that the urine and possibly stools may turn blue or blue-green. Use of methylene blue or methylene blue combinations is contraindicated when the client is in renal failure.

CONCEPT REVIEW

Methenamine is the oldest of the urinary tract antiseptics. It is effective because one of its by-products, formaldehyde, denatures bacterial protein. Since formaldehyde is formed more readily in acidic urine, acid salts (e.g., hippuric acid, mandelate acid) are combined with methenamine to help lower urinary pH.

Trimethoprim sometimes is used to treat uncomplicated UTIs and chronic recurrent UTIs. It works by interfering with folic acid synthesis in sensitive microorganisms.

SUMMARY

Symptoms of UTIs send many clients to health care providers yearly. Although UTIs affect all age groups, their incidence increases with age. Because the risk for kidney damage exists even with asymptomatic UTIs, these disorders require vigorous treatment. Urinary tract antiseptics are part of the classic medical protocol to prevent or treat UTIs. These drugs are effective in the treatment of urethritis and cystitis and in the prevention of pyelonephritis.

A careful nursing health history and physical assessment of the client establishes a baseline for later evaluation of the effectiveness of the therapy. Appropriate administration of these drugs must be coupled with education of the client, especially when long-term treatment is planned. Evaluation of the outcomes of urinary tract antiseptic therapy includes assessment of symptomatic relief, laboratory value comparisons, and monitoring for undesired clinical responses.

REFERENCES

1. U.S. Preventive Services Task Force. (1990). Screening for asymptomatic bacteriuria, hematuria, and proteinuria. *American Family Physician, 42,* 389–395.
2. National Institutes of Health. (1991). *Urinary tract infections in adults.* Bethesda, MD: Author.
3. Monahan, F., Drake, T., & Neighbors, M. (1994). *Nursing Care of adults* (pp. 1086–1089). Philadelphia: W.B. Saunders.
4. Ignativicius, D.D., & Bayne, M.V. (1991). *Medical-surgical nursing: A nursing process approach* (pp. 1833–1850). Philadelphia: W.B. Saunders.
5. Sobel, J., & Kay, D. (1991). *Adult and pediatric urology* (2nd ed.). St. Louis: C.V. Mosby.
6. Krieger, J. (1990). Urinary tract infections in women: Causes, classification, and differential diagnoses. *Urology, 35*(1), Suppl. 4.
7. Beam, T.R. (1992). Miscellaneous antimicrobial drugs. In C.M. Smith & A.M. Reynard (Eds.), *Textbook of pharmacology* (pp. 871–899). Philadelphia: W.B. Saunders.
8. Wilson, L.M. (1992). Diagnostic procedures in renal disease. In S. A. Price & L. M. Wilson (Eds.), *Pathophysiology: Clinical concepts of disease processes* (pp. 634–646). St. Louis: C.V. Mosby.
9. Cooper, C. (1993). What color is that urine specimen? *American Journal of Nursing, 93*(8), 37.
10. Pritchard, V., & Levernier, J. (1991). Multistix versus laboratory analysis in the detection of urinary tract infections. *Journal of Gerontological Nursing, 17*(8), 39–42.

11. Davis, J.R., & Sherer, K. (1994). *Applied nutrition and diet therapy for nurses* (2nd ed.). Philadelphia: W.B. Saunders.

12. Harvey, S.C. (1990). Antimicrobial drugs. In A.R. Gennaro (Ed.), *Remington's pharmaceutical sciences* (18th ed.) (pp. 1163–1173). Easton, PA: Mack Publishing.

13. Data Pharmaceutica, Inc. (1993). *1993 physicians' genRx.* Smithtown, NY: Author.

14. United States Pharmacopeial Convention, Inc. (1994). *USP DI* (14th ed.) (Vol. 1). Taunton, MA: Author.

15. Hoope, D.C., & Wolfson, J.S. (1991). Fluoroquinolone antimicrobial agents. *New England Journal of Medicine, 324,* 384–392.

16. Guelen, P.J., et al. (1988). Comparative bioavailability study of macrocrystalline nitrofurantoin and two prolonged-action hydroxymethylnitrofurantoin preparations. *Drug Intelligences and Clinical Pharmacy, 22,* 959–963.

17. Witten, C.M. (1989). Pulmonary toxicity of nitrofurantoin. *Archives of Physical Medicine and Rehabilitation, 70,* 55–57.

18. Tatro, D. (1990). *Drug interaction facts.* St. Louis: Facts and Comparisons Division, J.B. Lippincott.

19. Jones, K.V. (1990). Antimicrobial treatment of urinary tract infections. *Diseases in Childhood, 65,* 327–330.

20. United States Pharmacopeial Convention, Inc. (1993). *USP DI* (14th ed.) (Vol. 2). Taunton, MA: Author.

BIBLIOGRAPHY

Emmanouilides, C.E., et al. (1990). Trimethoprim, sulfamethoxazole, bacterial adhesion, and polymorphonuclear leukocyte function. *Journal of Antimicrobial Chemotherapy, 26,* 803–812.

Fantl, J.A., Wyman, J.F., McClish, D.K., & Bump, R.C. (1990). Urinary incontinence in community dwelling women: Clinical, urodynamic, and severity characteristics. *American Journal of Obstetrics and Gynecology, 16,* 946–951.

Gray, M. (1992). *Genitourinary disorders.* St. Louis: C.V. Mosby.

Johnson, M.A.G. (1990). Urinary tract infections in women. *American Family Physician, 41,* 565–571.

Kemper, K.J., & Avner, E.D. (1992). The case against screening urinalysis for asymptomatic bacteriuria in children. *American Journal of Diseases in Children, 146,* 343–345.

Martens, M.G. (1991). Cystitis: Improving patient compliance. *Contemporary OB/GYN, 36*(6), 65–66.

Mitagawa, C.I. (1993). Drug-nutrient interactions in critically-ill patients. *Critical Care Nurse, 13*(5), 69–90.

National Kidney Foundation. (1990). *Urinary tract infections.* New York: Author.

Pearlstein, G. (1990). Renal system complication in HIV infection. *Critical Care Nursing Clinics of North America, 2*(1), 79.

Raz, R., Rottensterich, E., Leshem, Y., et al. (1994). Double-blind study comparing 3-day regimens of cefixime and of cinoxacin in treatment of uncomplicated urinary tract infections in women. *Antimicrobial Agents and Chemotherapy, 38,* 1176–1177.

Sherbotie, J.R., & Cornfeld, D. (1991). Management of urinary tract infections in children. *Medical Clinics of North America, 75,* 327–337.

Todd, B. (1990). Treating UTIs. *Geriatric Nursing, 11*(2), 95–96.

Willis, D. (1992). Taming the overgrown prostate. *American Journal of Nursing, 92*(2), 34–40.

 Antimycobacterial Drugs

DOTTYE AKERSON • CYNTHIA MILLS SPIRO

⊛ **Mycobacterial Infections**

LEARNING OBJECTIVE: Identify the two most common species of *Mycobacterium.*
KEY TERMS:
Mycobacterium leprae, Mycobacterium tuberculosis

⊛ **Nursing Considerations**

LEARNING OBJECTIVE: Describe the basic nursing care for a client receiving antimycobacterial drugs.

⊛ **Drug Therapy for Tuberculosis**

LEARNING OBJECTIVES:
Distinguish between first-line and second-line antitubercular drugs.

Describe the pharmacodynamics of three major antitubercular drugs.
Summarize essential information about the prototype drug, isoniazid.
KEY TERM: Tubercles

⊛ **Drug Therapy for Leprosy**

LEARNING OBJECTIVES:
Describe the pharmacodynamics of antileprotic drugs.
Summarize essential information about the prototype drug, dapsone.

CONCEPTS AND TERMS TO REVIEW

Review Chapter 54 for general principles of antimicrobial therapy.
Review Chapter 49 for an overview of normal biologic defense mechanisms.

---

*D*rugs presented in this chapter are used to treat mycobacterial infections, specifically tuberculosis and leprosy. Both diseases were once believed to be controlled but recently have reemerged, thus providing a new challenge for nurses today. Since mycobacteria are slow-growing microorganisms, the resulting infections usually require prolonged drug therapy. This prolonged drug therapy is accompanied by several problems, including increased risk for drug toxicity, lack of compliance by the client, and emergence of drug-resistant bacteria.

This chapter presents an overview of the pathogenesis of tuberculosis and leprosy. It also discusses the nurse's role in administering antitubercular and antileprotic drugs and describes commonly used drug regimens.

MYCOBACTERIAL INFECTIONS

Mycobacterium is a genus of gram-positive, aerobic, acid-fast bacteria. These microorganisms are slightly curved or straight rods. The genus contains many species, including the pathogenic organisms that cause tuberculosis, **Mycobacterium tuberculosis,** and leprosy, **Mycobacterium leprae.**

⊞ NURSING CONSIDERATIONS

As with all drug therapy, the nurse's role follows the format established by the steps in the nursing process: assessing, diagnosing, planning, implementing, and evaluating.

Assessing Initial treatment of a mycobacterial infection usually takes place in an acute care setting. The client is generally isolated until the sputum or, in the case of leprosy, skin-scrape cultures indicate that the individual is no longer infectious. The prolonged hospital stay allows time for assessment and planning for client discharge and for taking steps to improve the client's compliance with therapy.

Before treatment is begun, perform a complete **health history** and physical assessment. Assess the client's history of fever, cough, sputum production, and central nervous system

(CNS) and respiratory difficulties. Past treatment for respiratory problems, including drug therapies and client response, is considered. For nonmenopausal female clients, collect a reproductive history.

Note any contraindications to the specific drug to be administered. Consider the client's compliance with previous treatment regimens. Assess the client's use of other drugs, including social drugs, alcohol, and nicotine. Since alcohol impairs liver function, it can intensify the hepatotoxic and neurotoxic effects of antimycobacterial drugs. Smoking, because of its influence on the lungs and circulatory system, is also harmful to the client.

Examine the client's understanding of the disease process and the need for a lengthy treatment period. To tailor the teaching to the client's ability to learn, assess the client's developmental level. Also gather a **social history** of the client. Ethnic origin, poor living conditions, impaired nutrition, poverty, and lack of emotional support influence a client's acceptance of and response to therapy. Include members of the client's support system in the assessment when possible.

A **physical assessment** to establish baseline data is also completed before initiating treatment. Hepatic and renal function tests, including aspartate transaminase (AST), alanine transaminase (ALT), blood urea nitrogen (BUN), and bilirubin levels, are done. In addition, serum uric acids levels are determined. For nonmenopausal females, a pregnancy test is performed.

Assess the client for cardiovascular, CNS, neuromuscular, or gastrointestinal (GI) disorders. Inspect the color of the skin. Is there evidence of jaundice? Palpate the abdomen for tenderness in the liver region. Note the characteristics of the urine— amount, color, odor, and general appearance. Also assess the client's visual and hearing acuity.

Diagnosing Nursing diagnoses for a client receiving antimycobacterial therapy can pertain to the physical or emotional aspects of treatment. Diagnoses appropriate for these clients include the following:

• Altered nutrition: less than body requirement related to undesired clinical responses to drugs (anorexia, nausea, vomiting).
• Altered sensory perception (visual and hearing changes) related to drug action.
• Altered body image related to dependence on long-term drug therapy.
• Impaired social interactions related to therapeutic isolation.
• Anxiety related to change in health status.
• Noncompliance related to lack of knowledge concerning drug therapy.

Planning Initially the plan of care is directed at supporting the client during the treatment regimen. However, this phase also involves teaching the client to perform required therapies accurately. Planning for discharge and preparing the client to assume responsibility for his or her health care must start immediately; therefore client education begins as soon as the client is admitted into the health care system.

Provide the client with detailed instruction on the drug regimen, including how and when to take the drugs, undesired clinical responses, and techniques for managing these responses. Safety factors such as proper storage of drugs in homes with small children should be stressed. Based on the type of drug therapy, supply the client appropriate dietary instructions. Also include information on basic health-promotion measures such as hygiene and sanitation practices, hand-washing techniques, and anxiety and stress reduction techniques.

Develop a drug calendar for the client, with drug doses and frequency of administration clearly marked. Since most clients benefit from both verbal and written instructions, provide pamphlets when possible. Include members of the client's support system in the teaching sessions.

Expected outcomes for the plan of care must be addressed. Appropriate outcomes for a client receiving antimycobacterial therapy include the following:

• Client reports anxiety is reduced to a manageable level.
• Client verbalizes acceptance of self.
• Client verbalizes understanding of vitamin B_6 and B_{12} deficiencies.
• Client develops effective social support system.
• Client verbalizes accurate knowledge of disease and treatment regimen.
• Client follows prescribed drug regimen.

Implementing Use proper techniques when administering the drugs. For oral dosage forms, follow guidelines for administering with food or between meals. Ensure that adequate vitamin, mineral, and fluid intake is maintained to reduce undesired clinical responses. With intravenous (IV) dosage forms, monitor the rate of infusion and patency of the line to prevent too rapid infusion or infiltration. Since intramuscular (IM) injections of these drugs cause pain, select the proper needle size and injection site. In addition, follow-up positioning of the client may reduce the individual's discomfort. Response to the medication regimen must be monitored frequently, and means of reducing side effects should be offered.

Emotional support for the client and his or her support system should be ongoing throughout the treatment regimen. In the case of clients with leprosy, emotional support and acceptance are especially important. Encouragement throughout the extended treatment period can mean the difference between compliance and noncompliance. Also consider referring the client to a social worker or agency to ensure he or she has proper nutrition, shelter, medication, and support.

Evaluating Evaluation of the client's progress is based on assessment of the status of the infection, presence or absence of undesired clinical responses, client compliance, and client's emotional state. The results of laboratory tests and a physical assessment provide information about the nutritional and drug status of the client. Interviews with the client and members of the support system can offer insight into compliance and emotional state and into areas in which more teaching or reinforcement are needed. Review the expected outcomes with the client and determine the status of each.

DRUG THERAPY FOR TUBERCULOSIS

Initially several agents were used to treat tuberculosis, including various heavy metals, garlic extract, aniline dyes, chaulmoogra oil, tuberculin, vitamins, sulfones, and sulfonamides. Not until the 1940s was an effective treatment discovered.[1]

Historical Perspectives

Tuberculosis is not a new disease. Signs of the disease have been found in Stone Age skeletons and mummies from the Old Kingdom of Egypt. Records reveal that it continued as a problem during the Middle Ages and flourished during the eighteenth and nineteenth centuries as urbanization occurred in Western Europe.[2] In the United States, crowded living conditions, poor sanitation, inadequate nutrition, and lack of access to health care combined to make tuberculosis a common cause of death during the early 1900s.

Although many treatments were tried, it was not until 1945 that an effective drug was introduced—the antibiotic streptomycin. With the advent of an effective antimicrobial therapy, the number of cases of tuberculosis declined. It appeared that tuberculosis had been controlled, and efforts to control transmission were relaxed. Sanatoriums designed to care for the tubercular client were closed, and funds were diverted to other causes. But the war on tuberculosis was declared over before the enemy was vanquished. Since 1986, cases of tuberculosis have increased every year. Poverty, homelessness, the influx of refugees from underdeveloped countries, and the increasing numbers of individuals with acquired immunodeficiency syndrome (AIDS) have fostered the resurgence of the disease.[2]

Epidemiology

Organisms of the genus *Mycobacterium* are slender aerobic bacilli that retain staining dyes despite exposure to decolorizing acids. This quality gives them the designation *acid-fast bacilli.* More than 50 species of mycobacteria are present in the environment. The one most commonly associated with human disease is *M. tuberculosis.*[3]

Tuberculosis is transmitted by respiratory droplets, which become airborne when an infected individual coughs, sneezes, or speaks. In individuals with healthy immune systems the bacteria are enclosed in capsules known as **tubercles,** and no symptoms occur. However, some individuals are especially susceptible to the disease, including children, the elderly, and those with compromised immune systems.[4] Multiple, long-term exposure to the bacillus is necessary for transmission. Sharing close living quarters with someone with active tuberculosis is the most common means of acquiring the disease.

The advent of AIDS has further complicated the spread of tuberculosis. Very susceptible to *M. tuberculosis* because of their compromised immune systems, clients with AIDS are presenting with tuberculosis at hospitals and clinics in increasing numbers. In clients with AIDS the presenting symptoms may be nonspecific and include extrapulmonary disease, hilar adenopathy, and multiple brain abscesses. The atypical presentation of symptoms of tuberculosis, especially in later-stage human immunodeficiency virus (HIV) disease, results in mistaken diagnoses, delay in treatment, and potential infection of health care workers who are unwittingly exposed.[5,6]

Pharmacotherapeutics

Antitubercular drugs are considered either first-line or second-line drugs. **First-line drugs** provide the most effective antituberculosis activity with an acceptable degree of toxicity. **Second-line drugs** provide adequate antimicrobial activity but have excessive toxicities.

Current infecting organisms are proving resistant to standard first-line drug therapy. Resistant organisms develop because individuals with the disease fail to complete the course of treatment. Surviving bacteria adapt to the drug and become resistant. For this reason, multidrug therapies are instituted.

However, tuberculosis therapy has also been hampered by an increase in multidrug-resistant tuberculosis (MDR TB). It occurs when a client receiving two drugs (first-line and second-line drugs) discontinues one of the drugs without the knowledge of the primary care provider. The client briefly experiences some response from the single-drug therapy, but then large numbers of resistant organisms begin to grow. The client, infectious again, transmits the drug-resistant organism to other individuals. As this event is repeated, an organism develops that is resistant to many of the first-line tuberculosis therapies.[7]

Pharmacodynamics

Pharmacodynamic mechanisms vary with each drug. Most of the drugs suppress or interfere with the synthesis of essential cellular components (i.e., RNA, metabolites, folic acid, and peptide). Some drugs disrupt the cell membrane or inhibit cell wall synthesis.

Antitubercular Drugs

Although isoniazid (INH) is not the first drug developed for use in the treatment of tuberculosis, it is the prototype for first-line drugs (Fig. 57–1).

ANTITUBERCULAR PROTOTYPE
ISONIAZID

Pharmacotherapeutics INH (isonicotinic acid hydrazide) is highly effective as a first-line drug in the treatment of *M. tuberculosis.* It is also used alone as preventive treatment for vulnerable individuals.

Pharmacokinetics INH is rapidly absorbed when administered by either the oral or IM route. Peak serum levels are achieved within 1 to 2 hours. If given orally with food, it takes longer for peak levels to occur. INH is also vulnerable to significant first-pass metabolism by the liver.

INH is distributed to all body fluids. The drug has a large volume of distribution including cerebrospinal fluid (CSF). The drug is also found in tissues, organs, pleural and ascitic fluids, feces, saliva, and sputum. It readily crosses the placenta and is present in breast milk.[8]

INH is metabolized in the liver by acetylation and hydroxylation. Acetylation is genetically controlled. Approximately half of the population of the United States acetylate this drug rapidly. Individuals who are rapid or fast acetylators metabolize the drugs at roughly five to six times the rate of slow acetylators. Eskimos, Asians, and approximately 50% of the African-American and

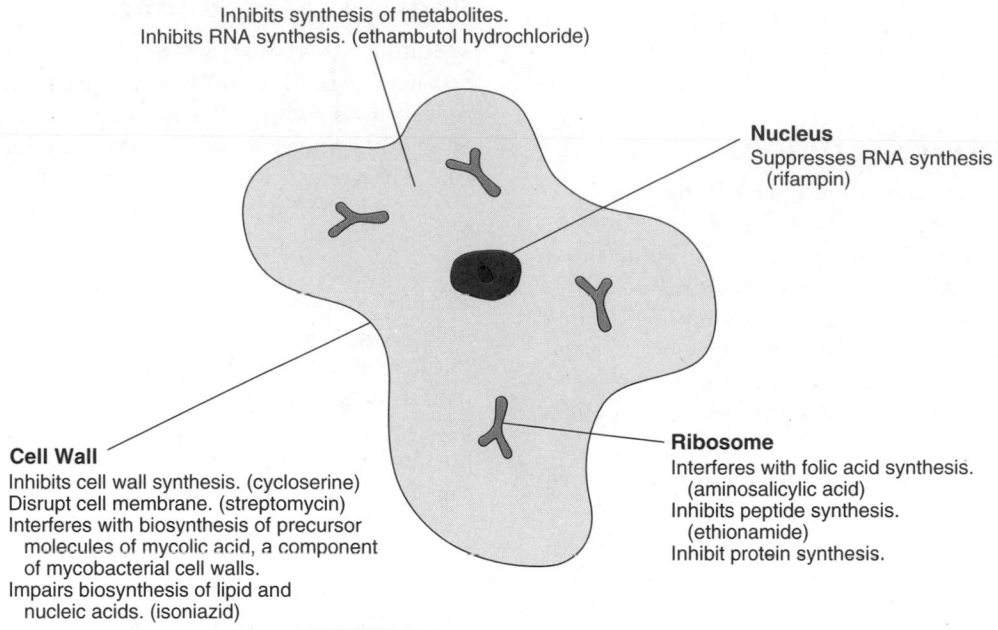

Inhibits synthesis of metabolites.
Inhibits RNA synthesis. (ethambutol hydrochloride)

Nucleus
Suppresses RNA synthesis
(rifampin)

Cell Wall
Inhibits cell wall synthesis. (cycloserine)
Disrupt cell membrane. (streptomycin)
Interferes with biosynthesis of precursor
molecules of mycolic acid, a component
of mycobacterial cell walls.
Impairs biosynthesis of lipid and
nucleic acids. (isoniazid)

Ribosome
Interferes with folic acid synthesis.
(aminosalicylic acid)
Inhibits peptide synthesis.
(ethionamide)
Inhibit protein synthesis.

FIGURE 57–1   Pharmacodynamic mechanisms of antitubercular drugs.

Caucasian populations in North America are fast acetylators. The remaining African-Americans and Caucasians, most Scandinavians, Jews, and Arabs are slow acetylators.

This phenomenon does not affect the efficacy of the drug; however, slow acetylation can result in increased blood levels of the drug and more toxic reactions. In addition, fast acetylators are more prone to liver toxicity reactions. The drug is excreted in the urine where approximately 50% to 70% of a dose appears unchanged with metabolites within 24 hours.[8–10]

Pharmacodynamics INH is bactericidal against tubercle bacilli undergoing division and is bacteriostatic against latent *M. tuberculosis* organisms. The drug is thought to exert its effect by interfering with biosynthesis of precursor molecules that make up mycolic acid, a component of mycobacterial cell walls. It also impairs biosynthesis of lipid and nucleic acids and acts as an antagonist to pyridoxine (vitamin B_6), leading to B_6 deficiency.[8]

Pharmaceutics INH is available as tablets or syrup for oral administration and in a sterile solution for IM injection.

Undesired Clinical Responses Undesired clinical responses are usually dose related and primarily involve the nervous system and the liver (Fig. 57–2). The most common effect is peripheral neuropathy, characterized by numbness and tingling of the extremities. This effect is related to the vitamin B_6 deficiency produced by INH. Peripheral neuropathy occurs more frequently in slow acetylators, diabetics, alcoholics, the malnourished, the elderly, and those with chronic liver disease.[11] Other neurologic effects such as convulsions, encephalopathy, optic neuritis, stupor, ataxia, tinnitus, memory impairment, dizziness, and psychosis occur infrequently at recommended dosages. Mild hepatic dysfunctions, indicated by elevated AST and ALT levels and bilirubinemia, bilirubinuria, and jaundice, can occur. More severe reactions such as potentially fatal hepatitis have been reported. Up

to 10% of the clients die if they do not discontinue INH after the onset of jaundice.[11] Using alcohol appears to increase the risk of hepatitis.

Blood dyscrasias such as agranulocytosis, aplastic anemia, and thrombocytopenia have been noted. Hypersensitivity reactions, including fever, chills, skin eruptions, lymphadenopathy, and vascularities, also may occur. These reactions most commonly occur in the fourth or fifth week of treatment.[8,10]

Contraindications and Precautions INH use is contraindicated in clients with preexisting hepatic or renal dysfunction.

Drug-Drug, Drug-Nutrient, Drug-Environment Interactions If INH is taken concurrently with alcohol, the risk of hepatitis increases. The drug also interacts with tyramine-containing and histamine-containing foods. Foods containing tyramine such as smoked fish and aged cheese may cause flushing, palpitations, and elevated blood pressure. Foods containing histamine, such as tuna, sauerkraut, and yeast extracts, may cause hypotension, sweating, diarrhea, and flushing.

There are several drug-drug interactions. Antacids and laxatives containing aluminum decrease absorption of INH. In addition, the combination of INH and disulfiram (Antabuse) may cause neurologic symptoms. INH decreases the metabolism of phenytoin (Dilantin), carbamazepine (Tegretol), benzodiazepines, and anticoagulants and results in higher-than-expected levels of these drugs.

Life-Span Considerations The risk of administering INH to pregnant women must be weighed against the benefits of taking the drug. Although no studies to date indicate harm to the fetus, therapy should begin after the first trimester since the drug does cross the placental barrier. In addition, since the drug is excreted in breast milk, infants who are breast-fed should be monitored for INH side effects. Children should be closely monitored, especially for the first 3 months of therapy when liver damage

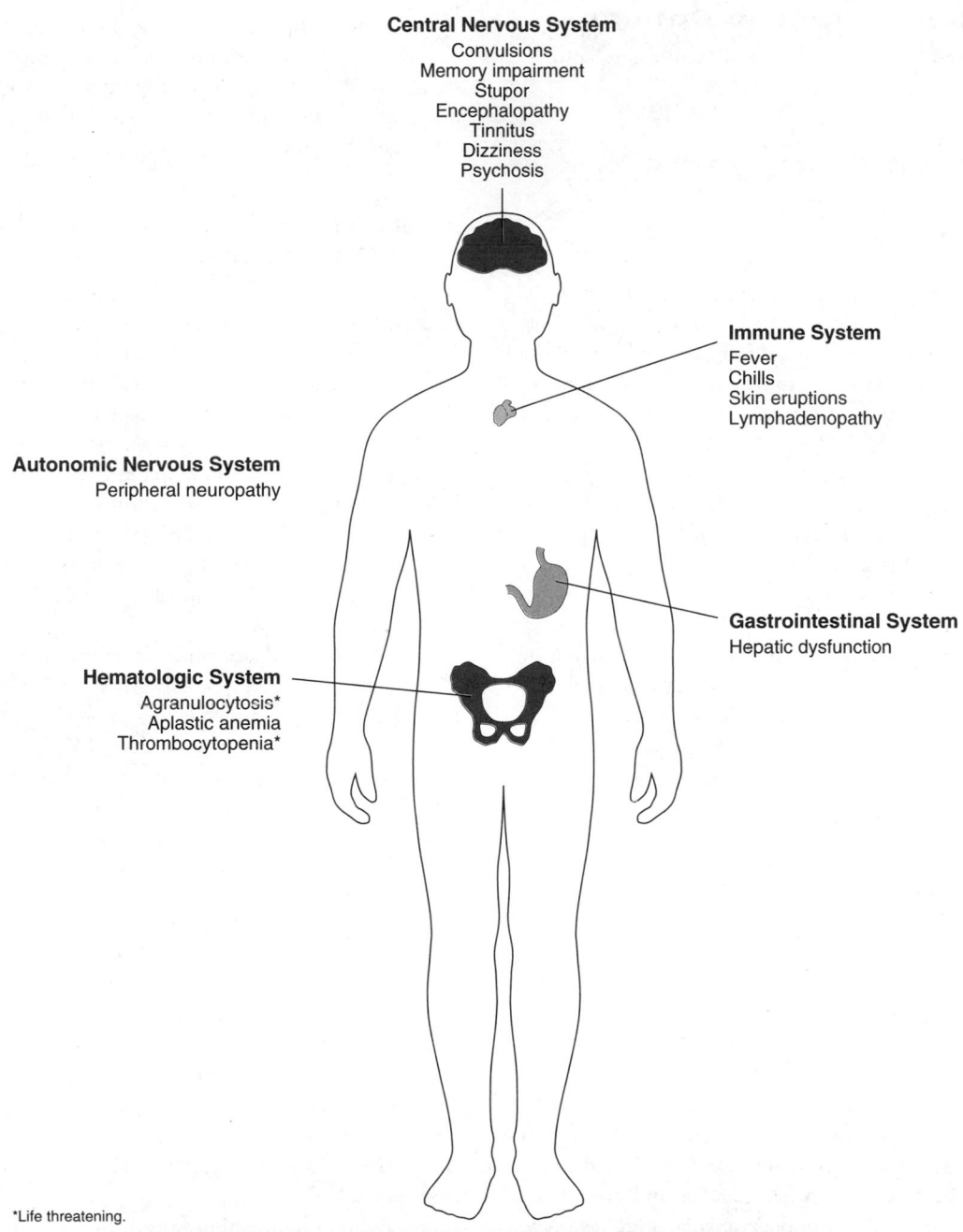

Central Nervous System
Convulsions
Memory impairment
Stupor
Encephalopathy
Tinnitus
Dizziness
Psychosis

Immune System
Fever
Chills
Skin eruptions
Lymphadenopathy

Autonomic Nervous System
Peripheral neuropathy

Gastrointestinal System
Hepatic dysfunction

Hematologic System
Agranulocytosis*
Aplastic anemia
Thrombocytopenia*

*Life threatening.

FIGURE 57–2   Undesired clinical responses associated with INH.

is most likely to occur. After this period there is a low incidence of liver damage in children. Clients over 50 years of age should be watched closely for adverse effects, particularly hepatitis.[10,12]

Specific Drug-Related Nursing Considerations (Table 57–1) Visual acuity, renal and hepatic function, and red blood cell (RBC) and white blood cell (WBC) levels should be monitored at the start of therapy and frequently thereafter. If GI distress occurs, administer the drug with food. The drug may also be administered 1 hour before or 2 hours after meals. CNS effects such as dizziness and stupor are decreased if the drug is administered at bedtime.

Teach diabetic clients who check their urine for glucose to use Clinitest strips. This brand of test strips apparently is not influenced by INH. Instruct the client to maintain contact with health care team members so that adverse effects can be detected early and response to therapy monitored. Caution the client not to discontinue the drug without checking with the primary care provider. During conversations with the client and members of the support system, observe for behavioral changes, complaints of side effects, and symptoms of renal or hepatic toxicity.

Miscellaneous Drugs in Category

There are several other first-line and second-line antimycobacterial drugs.

FIRST-LINE ANTITUBERCULAR DRUG: RIFAMPIN

Rifampin (Rimactane, Rifadin) is a semisynthetic, first-line antitubercular drug. In combination with INH, it is considered the therapy of choice for treatment of tuberculosis. Rifampin is never used as the sole therapeutic drug for treatment of any infectious disease because of the rapid emergence of resistant strains. It is also used to treat staphylococcal infections and for prophylaxis against *Neisseria meningitidis* and *Haemophilus influenzae.*[8]

Rifampin is most active against rapidly replicating organisms. It is both bacteriostatic and bactericidal, depending on the concentration and the susceptibility of the infecting organism. Rifampin inhibits the DNA-dependent RNA polymerase; inhibition of this enzyme suppresses RNA synthesis.[11,12]

Rifampin is administered orally on an empty stomach or by IV infusion (Table 57–1). It is well absorbed after an oral dose and is widely dispersed into body tissue and fluids because of its high degree of lipid solubility.[11] Plasma-protein binding is 80%. The drug is metabolized in the liver and is excreted in the bile. It reenters the portal venous circulation and participates in the enterohepatic cycle. Eventually 60% of the administered dose is excreted in the stool, and 25% is cleared through the kidneys.[8]

The major undesired clinical response involves the liver (Fig. 57–3). Mild disturbances in liver enzymes are common but usually do not require discontinuation of the drug. Alcoholics with preexisting liver disease are most prone to serious hepatotoxicity. Other reactions to rifampin are infrequent, with GI disturbances, headache, skin eruptions, drowsiness, dizziness, and visual disturbances the most common. An unusual adverse reaction is the "flu syndrome," which is most common among clients receiving intermittent therapy. Symptoms include fever, headache, malaise, and arthralgias. Occasionally dose-related thrombocytopenia and hemolytic anemia occur.[8,11]

Rifampin can stimulate the liver's microsomal drug-metabolizing enzymes. This stimulation results in diminished blood levels and activities of other drugs. Because of this action, rifampin can produce clinically important interactions when used with drugs excreted or metabolized by the liver.[8,11]

Tell the client to expect orange-red discoloration of body secretions, including urine, feces, sputum, tears, and sweat. Warn him or her that soft contact lenses may become permanently discolored. In addition, tell the client that drug-related symptoms such as headache, drowsiness, confusion, fever, and muscle and joint aching may occur during the first few weeks of therapy. Instruct the client to notify the primary care provider if symptoms worsen in intensity or are persistent.[8,12]

Interference with diagnostic studies. Rifampin inhibits standard assays for serum folate and vitamin B$_{12}$.

It causes transient abnormalities in liver function tests (e.g., elevation in serum bilirubin, alkaline phosphatase, and serum transaminase levels); and the drug interferes with contrast media used for gallbladder study; tests should precede administration of the daily dose.

FIRST-LINE ANTITUBERCULAR DRUG: ETHAMBUTOL HYDROCHLORIDE

Ethambutol hydrochloride (Myambutol) is a first-line antitubercular drug currently used as an alternative for clients unable to tolerate INH or rifampin. It is also used when there is primary or acquired resistance to one of the other drugs. Ethambutol hydrochloride is recommended as part of the combination therapy of mycobacterial infections due to *M. kansasii* and *M. avium-intracellulare.*[8]

Ethambutol hydrochloride diffuses to actively growing *Mycobacterium* cells and inhibits the transfer of mycolic acids into the cell wall of the tubercle bacillus. The drug is bactericidal and causes impairment of cell multiplication and eventual cell death.[8,12]

Ethambutol hydrochloride is administered orally, with 75% to 80% of the drug rapidly absorbed. Protein binding averages 40%. The drug is widely dispersed in body tissue except the CSF. Peak serum concentration of 2 to 5 μg/ml occurs 2 to 4 hours after administration. Approximately 15% of the drug is converted to inactive metabolites; 50% is excreted unchanged in the urine; and 22% is excreted unchanged in the feces. Dose modification is necessary if renal dysfunction exists.[8,12]

The most serious undesired clinical response to ethambutol hydrochloride is optic neuritis. Symptoms include decreased visual acuity, constriction of visual fields, central and peripheral scotomas, and loss of red-green color discrimination. The extent and frequency of optic neuritis are directly related to the dose and duration of therapy. The visual effects of ocular toxicity are usually reversible over a period of weeks or months if symptoms are detected early and the drug is discontinued. Instruct the client to report any changes in visual acuity or color perception.[11]

Ethambutol hydrochloride is not recommended for use in children less than 13 years of age since safety has not yet been established. The same is true regarding use of the drug with pregnant women or women of childbearing age.[12]

SECOND-LINE ANTITUBERCULAR DRUG: STREPTOMYCIN

Streptomycin is an aminoglycoside antibiotic that interferes with normal protein synthesis. It is a second-line antitubercular drug used when *M. tuberculosis* is resistant to first-line drugs or the disease process is severe. Streptomycin should always be used in combination with other antituberculosis drugs.[11,12]

Streptomycin is administered by IM injection two to three times a week, with the dose dependent on age and renal function. Ototoxicity and nephrotoxicity are frequent adverse effects. If possible, treatment with streptomycin should be

Text continued on p. 776.

TABLE 57–1

Antitubercular Drugs: Prototype and Major Drugs in Category

Drug Name	Dosage and Route of Administration	Nursing Considerations
ISONIAZID (INH, Laniazid, Nydrazid) **HOW SUPPLIED** Syrup: 50 mg/ml Uncoated tablets: 100 mg, 300 mg IM: 100 mg/ml	**ADULTS** *Treatment* Oral and IM: 5 mg/kg up to 300 mg/d *Prevention* Oral: 300 mg/d **CHILDREN** *Treatment* Oral and IM: 10-20 mg/kg up to 300-500 mg/d *Prevention* Oral: 10 mg/kg up to 300 mg/d or 15 mg/kg three times per week	**Assess** Assess level of visual and hearing acuity. Obtain baseline liver and renal function tests. Assess client for preexisting hepatic or renal dysfunction. **Implement** Instruct client to take on an empty stomach at least 1 h before or 2 h after meals to prevent GI upset. Transient pain may occur at IM injection site. Instruct client to avoid alcohol ingestion because of increased risk of hepatitis. Monitor clients with active chronic liver disease or severe renal dysfunction. Administer with caution in clients with a history of convulsive disorders. Administer with caution to client receiving phenytoin (Dilantin). Anticipate that pyridoxine (vitamin B_6) may be administered concomitantly to decrease CNS effects. Client may experience hypotension during dosage changes. Monitor for orthostatic hypotension. **Monitor** Monitor for undesired clinical responses such as numbness and tingling of extremities, convulsions, tinnitus, dizziness, optic neuritis, and ataxia. Monitor vision and hearing acuity and liver and renal function tests periodically throughout therapy. Serum transaminase concentration becomes elevated in approximately 10% to 20% of clients. Monitor intake and output (I and O) to ascertain that renal output is adequate to prevent systemic accumulation of the drug. Monitor CBC and RBC results. Monitor prothrombin time (PT) and partial thromboplastin time (PTT) levels since anticoagulant activity may be enhanced. **Evaluate** Evaluate for absence of infectious process.
Rifampin (Rifadin, Rimactane) **HOW SUPPLIED** Gelatin capsules: 150 mg, 300 mg IV: 600 mg/vial	**Pulmonary Tuberculosis** **ADULTS** Oral or IV: 600 mg once daily in conjunction with other antituberculosis agent **CHILDREN** Oral: 10-20 mg/kg/d (600 mg/d) **Meningococcal Carriers** **ADULTS** Oral: 600 mg bid for 2 consecutive days **CHILDREN** Oral: 10-20 mg/kg/d for 2 consecutive days (maximum, 600 mg/d)	**Assess** Assess client for preexisting hepatic disease, GI disturbance, or auditory nerve impairment. Determine if client is pregnant; rifampin is classified as Pregnancy Category C drug. Assess if client is receiving anticoagulants, corticosteroids, quinidine, cardiac glycoside, or oral hypoglycemic drugs. **Implement** Administer 1 h before or 2 h after meals. Peak serum levels are delayed and may be lower when given with food. Oral suspension can be prepared from capsules for adults or children who have difficulty swallowing capsules. Consult pharmacist for preparation directions. Capsule may be emptied and content swallowed with fluid or mixed with food.

Table continued on following page.

TABLE 57–1 *Continued*
Antitubercular Drugs: Prototype and Major Drugs in Category

Drug Name	Dosage and Route of Administration	Nursing Considerations
Rifampin Continued	**Prophylaxis for Haemophilus influenzae type b** **ADULTS** Oral: 20 mg/kg/d for 4 d **CHILDREN** Oral: 10-20 mg/kg/d for 4 d (maximum, 600 mg/d) **Dapsone-Sensitive Multibacillary Leprosy** **ADULTS** Oral: 600 mg once a month with clofazimine and dapsone for a minimum of 2 y Data not available to determine dosage for children <5 y of age	IV rifampin is reconstituted with 10 ml of sterile water to each 600 mg of drug. The resultant solution contains 60 mg/ml and is stable at room temperature for 24 h. The ordered dose is further diluted in 100-500 ml D$_5$W. Infuse over 30 min to 3 h, depending on volume. Drug must not be administered by IM or subcutaneous (SC) route. Instruct client that drug may turn urine, feces, saliva, sputum, sweat, and tears red-orange. Permanent discoloration of soft contact lenses may occur. Instruct female clients that reliability of oral contraceptives may be affected. Instruct client to take on regular basis and avoid missing a dose. If used in conjunction with at least one other antituberculous agent, continue therapy for 6 to 9 mo or until at least 6 mo have elapsed from conversion of sputum to culture negativity. **Monitor** Monitor results of hepatic functions tests. Monitor client for undesired clinical responses such as rash, pruritus, headache, drowsiness, blood dycrasias, muscular weakness, visual disturbances, and hepatic and renal dysfunction. **Evaluate** Evaluate absence of infectious process.
Pyrazinamide (Tebrazid) HOW SUPPLIED Uncoated tablet: 500 mg	**Tuberculosis** **ADULTS** Oral: 20-35 mg/kg/d in three or four divided doses; not to exceed 3 g/d	**Assess** Assess client for preexisting acute intermittent porphyria, diabetes mellitus, gout, and impaired renal function. Obtain baseline CBC, uric acid level, and renal and liver function studies. **Implement** Client should receive at least one other effective antituberculosis agent concurrently. Anticipate that hepatic reactions occur more frequently in clients receiving high doses. **Monitor** Examine clients at regular intervals for signs of toxicity: liver enlargement or tenderness, jaundice, fever, anorexia, malaise, impaired vascular integrity (ecchymoses, petechiae, abnormal bleeding). Monitor liver function tests (AST, ALT, serum bilirubin) at 2-4–wk intervals during therapy. Obtain blood uric acid determinations during therapy. **Evaluate** Evaluate absence of infectious process.
Ethambutol hydrochloride (Myambutol) HOW SUPPLIED Uncoated tablet: 100 mg, 400 mg	**Tuberculosis** **ADULTS** Oral: 15 mg/kg q24h; for treatment, start with 25 mg/kg/d for 60 d, then decrease to 15 mg/kg/d **CHILDREN 6-12 Y** Oral: 10-15 mg/kg/d	**Assess** Perform culture and susceptibility tests before initiation of therapy. Perform visual acuity testing before therapy. Assess client for preexisting gout, impaired renal function, optic neuritis, or diabetic retinopathy.

TABLE 57–1 *Continued*
Antitubercular Drugs: Prototype and Major Drugs in Category

Drug Name	Dosage and Route of Administration	Nursing Considerations
Ethambutol hydrochloride **Continued**		**Implement** Inform client of importance of following drug regimen and of keeping follow-up appointments. Anticipate reduced doses for clients with renal insufficiency. Instruct client to take drug with food. Instruct client to notify primary care provider if changes in vision or color perception occur. Report oliguria or any significant changes in renal function. Protect drug from light, moisture, and excessive heat. Store in tightly closed container at 15° to 30° C. **Monitor** Monitor I and O in clients with renal impairment. Perform visual acuity testing every 2 wk. Anticipate serum drug level testing 2-4 h after administration. Monitor hepatic and renal function tests, CBC, and serum uric acid levels at regular intervals. Monitor client for undesired clinical responses such as optic neuritis, visual changes, allergic reactions, nausea, anorexia, and CNS involvement. **Evaluate** Evaluate for absence of infectious process.
Aminosalicylate sodium (Parasal Sodium, Sodium P.A.S., Teebacin) HOW SUPPLIED Coated tablet: 0.5 g Uncoated tablet: 0.5 g	**Tuberculosis** ADULTS Oral: 14-16 g/d in two or three divided doses CHILDREN Oral: 275-420 mg/kg/d in three or four divided doses	**Assess** Assess client for preexisting hepatic or renal dysfunction, congestive heart failure, gastric ulcer, or goiter. Assess client for hypersensitivity to aminosalicylates, salicylates, or compounds containing para-aminophenyl group. **Implement** Offer client clear water to rinse mouth, chewing gum, or hard candy since drug leaves a bitter taste in mouth. Monitor I and O and encourage fluid intake. High concentrations of drug are excreted in urine and can cause crystalluria and hematuria. Inform client that urine may turn red on contact with hypochlorite bleach used to clean commercial toilets. Instruct client not to take aspirin or OTC drugs without approval. Inform client that drug can produce false-positive results in urinary glucose monitoring. Instruct client to store drug in dry, light-resistant container at 15° to 30° C. Teach client to discard drug after 24 h or if purplish-brown discoloration occurs. Administer drug with meals to minimize GI upset. Anticipate concurrent administration of drugs that keep urinary pH neutral or alkaline. Instruct client to report indications of blood dyscrasia: sore throat or mouth, malaise, unusual fatigue, bleeding, or bruising.

Table continued on following page.

TABLE 57–1 *Continued*
Antitubercular Drugs: Prototype and Major Drugs in Category

Drug Name	Dosage and Route of Administration	Nursing Considerations
Aminosalicylate sodium **Continued**		**Monitor** Monitor for undesired clinical responses such as nausea, vomiting, abdominal pain, or allergic reactions. **Evaluate** Evaluate for absence of infectious process.
Capreomycin sulfate (Capastat Sulfate) HOW SUPPLIED IM: 1 g/5 ml	**Tuberculosis** ADULTS IM: 1 g/d (not to exceed 20 mg/kg/d) for 60-120 d; then 1 g two or three times per week	**Assess** Perform susceptibility studies to determine presence of capreomycin-susceptible strain of mycobacterium tuberculosis. Perform audiometric measurements, CBC, renal and hepatic function tests, and serum potassium level determinations before beginning drug therapy. Assess for preexisting renal insufficiency, acoustic nerve impairment, hepatic disorder, myasthenia gravis, and parkinsonism. Assess for concurrent administration of other antimicrobial drugs. **Implement** Administer intramuscularly since not absorbed in significant quantities in GI tract. Reconstitute by adding 2 ml of 0.9% isotonic NaCl injection or sterile water for injection to each gram vial. Allow 2-3 min for drug to dissolve completely. Reconstituted solutions may be stored for 48 h at room temperature. Store up to 14 days at 15° to 30° C temperatures. Administer deep IM injection in large muscle mass. Superficial injections tend to cause increased pain and are associated with sterile abscesses. Rotate injection sites. Observe injection site for redness, excessive bleeding, and inflammation. Instruct client not to perform tasks that require mental alertness. Instruct client to report any change in hearing or disturbance of balance. Anticipate administration of at least one other antitubercular drug. Inform client that therapy may last 12-24 mo. Anticipate using reduced doses in clients with impaired renal function. Report immediately any changes in I and O ratio or unusual appearance of urine. Do not administer to client receiving streptomycin. **Monitor** Monitor audiometric measurements weekly or biweekly. Monitor renal function studies weekly. Monitor potassium levels monthly. Monitor liver function tests periodically. Assess client for undesired clinical responses such as respiratory depression, skeletal muscle weakness, hypersensitivity reactions, renal changes, eighth cranial nerve damage, or electrolyte imbalance. **Evaluate** Evaluate for absence of infectious process.

TABLE 57–1 *Continued*

Antitubercular Drugs: Prototype and Major Drugs in Category

Drug Name	Dosage and Route of Administration	Nursing Considerations
Cycloserine (Seromycin) HOW SUPPLIED Gelatin capsule: 250 mg	**Tuberculosis** ADULTS Oral: 250 mg q12h for 2 wk; may increase to 500 mg q12h, not to exceed 1 g/d	**Assess** Perform culture and susceptibility tests before initiation of therapy. Assess client for preexisting epilepsy, depression, severe anxiety, psychosis, renal insufficiency, or excessive concurrent use of alcohol. **Implement** Teach client to take drug after meals to prevent GI irritation. Instruct client to notify primary care provider immediately if skin rash or early signs of CNS toxicity are noted. Instruct client to avoid driving or tasks requiring alertness until reaction to drug has been determined. Instruct client to take drug precisely as prescribed and to keep follow-up appointments. Inform client that alcohol intake increases risk of seizure activity. Store in tightly closed container at 15° to 30° C. Anticipate that pyridoxine may be administered concurrently. **Monitor** Monitor culture and susceptibility tests periodically to monitor bacterial resistance. Anticipate determining serum drug levels weekly. (Serum drug level <30 mg/ml reduces incidence of neurotoxicity.) Monitor renal and hepatic function at regular intervals. Assess for undesired clinical responses such as congestive heart failure, allergic reactions, and CNS disturbance—seizures, drowsiness, headache, vertigo, altered level of consciousness. **Evaluate** Evaluate for absence of infectious process.
Ethionamide (Trecator-SC) HOW SUPPLIED Sugar-coated tablet: 250 mg	**Tuberculosis** ADULTS Oral: 0.5-1 g/d divided q8-12h CHILDREN Oral: 12-15 mg/kg/d in three or four equally divided doses (not to exceed 1 g/d)	**Assess** Perform culture and susceptibility tests before start of therapy. Review results of liver function tests (AST and ALT), CBC, and renal function tests, including urinalysis, before initiating therapy. Assess client for preexisting diabetes mellitus or renal dysfunction. **Implement** Instruct client to report onset of skin rash. Rash can progress to exfoliative dermatitis if drug is not discontinued promptly. Perform glucose monitoring for diabetic clients more frequently than usual. Drug may make blood glucose levels difficult to manage. Instruct client to decrease or eliminate alcohol ingestion. Anticipate concurrent administration of pyridoxine to prevent peripheral neuritis. Instruct client to take drug with food or after meals to minimize GI effects.

Table continued on following page.

TABLE 57–1 *Continued*
Antitubercular Drugs: Prototype and Major Drugs in Category

Drug Name	Dosage and Route of Administration	Nursing Considerations
Ethionamide Continued		**Implement—Continued**
		Store in cool, dry place at 8° to 15° C in tightly closed container.
		Instruct client to change positions slowly since drug causes postural hypotension.
		Monitor
		Monitor hepatic and renal function tests every 2-4 wk.
		Monitor visual acuity.
		Monitor for undesired clinical responses such as nausea, vomiting, metallic taste, neurotoxicity, and allergic reactions.
		Evaluate
		Evaluate for absence of infectious process.

avoided in older individuals because of their greater risk of impaired renal function.[11] (Chapter 55 contains additional information about streptomycin.)

SECOND-LINE ANTITUBERCULAR DRUG: PYRAZINAMIDE

Pyrazinamide is a second-line antitubercular agent used in combination with at least one other antitubercular drug. Treatment with pyrazinamide is initiated when first-line drugs have failed or when the causative organism proves highly resistant. Pyrazinamide is one of the older antimycobacterial drugs; it is too toxic for routine use.[8,11]

The antibacterial activity of pyrazinamide is restricted to *M. tuberculosis.* The drug is bacteriostatic and bactericidal. Although the exact mechanism of action is unknown, it is known that organisms must be actively growing for the drug to exert its effect.[8]

Given orally, pyrazinamide is well absorbed in the GI tract. After absorption, the drug is widely dispersed. It passes freely into body tissues and fluids, including the lungs, liver, and CSF. Dose-related hepatotoxicity is the major adverse side effect of pyrazinamide; therefore the use of this drug is contraindicated in the presence of liver damage. Even in the absence of liver disease, nausea, vomiting, and diarrhea frequently occur. Other adverse effects include gout, defects in blood clotting, sideroblastic anemia, joint pain, skin rashes, photosensitivity, and splenomegaly.[10,12]

Before pyrazinamide is administered, baseline CBC and renal and liver function studies are obtained. These same studies are monitored at frequent intervals throughout therapy.[11] Client and family teaching should focus on the early warning signs of liver damage, which include fever, malaise, nausea, or jaundice.

Interference with diagnostic studies Pyrazinamide may produce a temporary decrease in 17-ketosteroids. It may cause an increase in proteinbound iodine.

SECOND-LINE ANTITUBERCULAR DRUG: AMINOSALICYLIC ACID

Aminosalicylic acid is a second-line antitubercular drug used in cases of known drug resistance or when other agents are contraindicated. It is a highly specific agent active only against *M. tuberculosis.* It is bacteriostatic in action and interferes with folic acid synthesis.[10,12]

Administered in powder or tablet forms, aminosalicylic acid is rapidly absorbed in the GI tract and is widely distributed into body tissue and fluids. Aminosalicylic acid may interfere with absorption of other antitubercular drugs. Malabsorption of vitamin B, folic acid, iron, and lipids during therapy is possible. If malabsorption occurs, replacement therapy is required.[11,12]

GI disturbance is the most common adverse effect. Nausea, vomiting, abdominal pain, diarrhea, and anorexia are frequently experienced. Peptic ulcers and gastric hemorrhage have also been reported. Allergic reactions (fever, urticaria, and pruritus), hypothyroidism, and goiters have been noted. Aminosalicylic acid is used with caution in clients with a history of impaired renal or hepatic function, congestive heart failure, or gastric ulcers.[10,12]

Aminosalicylic acid can produce several important drug-drug interactions (e.g., increased effects of oral anticoagulants, decreased absorption of digoxin, altered phenytoin [Dilantin] levels). Therefore all the drugs the client is receiving must be determined. To minimize GI disturbance, the drug is administered with meals. In addition, aluminum hydroxide (5 to 10 ml) may be prescribed to lessen adverse GI effects. Inform the client that aminosalicylic acid may turn the urine dark in color and cause false-positive results for urinary glucose monitoring.[10,12]

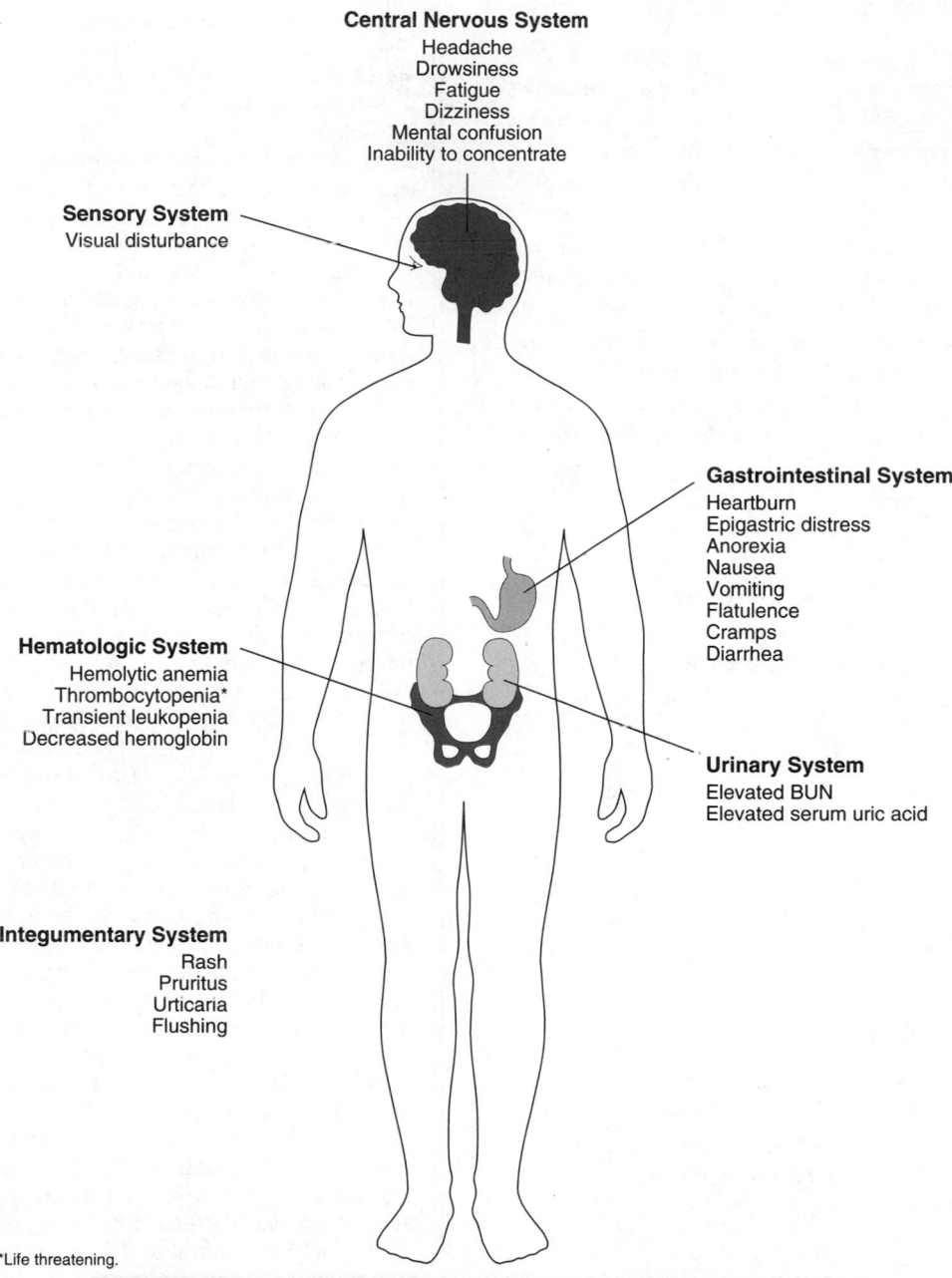

Central Nervous System
Headache
Drowsiness
Fatigue
Dizziness
Mental confusion
Inability to concentrate

Sensory System
Visual disturbance

Gastrointestinal System
Heartburn
Epigastric distress
Anorexia
Nausea
Vomiting
Flatulence
Cramps
Diarrhea

Hematologic System
Hemolytic anemia
Thrombocytopenia*
Transient leukopenia
Decreased hemoglobin

Urinary System
Elevated BUN
Elevated serum uric acid

Integumentary System
Rash
Pruritus
Urticaria
Flushing

*Life threatening.

FIGURE 57–3   Undesired clinical responses associated with rifampin.

CONCEPT REVIEW

Cases of *M. tuberculosis* in the United States have increased annually since 1986 because of poverty, homelessness, the influx of refugees, and the increase in the numbers of individuals with AIDS.

Nursing responsibilities in the treatment of *M. tuberculosis* are complicated by the need for long-term therapy, sometimes using both first-line and second-line drugs. Failure to complete the lengthy course of treatment results in drug-resistant organisms and recurrence of disease.

Client teaching should be initiated when the client is admitted to the health care system. The client's support system should be involved in learning proper hygiene, storage, administration techniques, and stress-reducing measures.

DRUG THERAPY FOR LEPROSY

Another *Mycobacterium* associated with human disease is *M. leprae.* This pathogen causes Hansen's disease, otherwise known as *leprosy.* Leprosy is a chronic granulomatous disease characterized by progressive anesthetic skin lesions and peripheral neuropathy. It is found predominantly in tropical countries.

Leprosy was once treated by banishing the leper to a cave or community well outside the city limits. The earliest recorded medicinal treatment was the Indian remedy, chaulmoogra oil, which was administered orally and topically. In the 1930s, sulfones were used to treat leprosy. The sulfone drug dapsone was first used in 1947. It remains the primary drug for treatment of *M. leprae* infection. However, an increased incidence of dapsone-resistant strains has led to the use of a multidrug regimen in treatment of the disease.[13]

Pathogenesis

M. leprae is a slow-growing intracellular parasite that causes leprosy in individuals with a defective cell-mediated response to the organism. Approximately 5% of the world's population have this defect and are susceptible to the disease. In three quarters of those cases the individual has enough immune response to localize the infection as tuberculoid leprosy. Individuals with the poorest immune response develop lepromatous leprosy, with skin lesions and sensory loss.[14–16]

Leprosy is transmitted by droplet; the probable portal of entry is the nasal mucosa. The disease has a long incubation period and a slow, chronic spread. Hansen's disease is most prevalent in Africa and Asia, with approximately 6000 cases in the United States.[17]

Antileprotic Drugs

Drug therapy for clients with lepromatous leprosy continues until skin and mucosal lesions have healed and acid-fast bacilli are no longer cultured. This treatment may require as long as 10 years. In some instances, drug therapy is necessary for the rest of the client's life. Dapsone is the prototype for antileprotic drugs.

ANTILEPROTIC PROTOTYPE
DAPSONE

Pharmacokinetics Dapsone is rapidly and almost completely absorbed from the GI tract. Approximately 70% to 90% of the drug is plasma-protein bound. Peak plasma concentrations occur in 2 to 8 hours. Plasma half-life is 10 to 50 hours, with the average being 28 hours. Dapsone is distributed to all body tissues, with high concentrations found in kidneys, liver, muscles, and skin. Approximately 70% to 85% of the drug is excreted in the urine. Enterohepatic circulation of dapsone is responsible for traces of the drug in tissues up to 3 weeks after discontinuation of therapy.[10]

Pharmacodynamics Dapsone is a sulfone-derivative chemically related to sulfonamides. It has bactericidal and bacteriostatic effects similar to those of the sulfonamide group. The drug is effective against *M. leprae, M. tuberculosis,* and, to a lesser extent, *Pneumocystis carinii* and *Plasmodium.* Dapsone interferes with bacterial cell growth by competitively inhibiting folic acid synthesis.

Pharmaceutics Dapsone is available in 25-mg and 100-mg tablets.

Undesired Clinical Responses Side effects associated with dapsone involve the hematologic, dermatologic, GI, urinary, and central nervous systems. The most common undesired response is dose-related hemolysis. Peripheral neuropathy and drug-induced lupus erythematosus can also occur. In addition, the client may experience sulfone syndrome, which consists of fever, malaise, exfoliative dermatitis, hepatic necrosis with jaundice, methemoglobinemia, and anemia.

Contraindications and Precautions Dapsone should be used with caution in clients with chronic renal, hepatic, pulmonary or cardiovascular disease, albuminuria, or refractory anemias. Dapsone use is contraindicated in clients with sulfone hypersensitivity.

Drug-Drug, Drug-Nutrient, Drug-Environment Interactions Because of increased plasma clearance, serum levels of dapsone are drastically decreased when the drug is taken in conjunction with rifampin. However, inhibitory drug concentrations in the serum remain high enough to be effective. When dapsone is administered with folic acid antagonists such as pyrimethamine, hematologic reactions increase. If dapsone is administered with *p*-aminobenzoic acid (PABA), the bactericidal action of dapsone is decreased.[18]

Life-Span Considerations Dapsone is classified as a Pregnancy Category C drug. No controlled studies indicate an increase in fetal abnormalities if the drug is taken during all trimesters. Dapsone is excreted in breast milk and can cause hemolytic reactions in newborns.

Specific Drug-Related Nursing Considerations (Table 57–2) Before drug therapy with dapsone is begun a thorough health history and physical assessment are completed. The stigma attached to the diagnosis of leprosy usually has an adverse effect on the client's acceptance of and compliance with the medication regimen required. Assess the client's emotional health and access to supportive individuals or facilities. Note any preexisting liver, renal, cardiovascular, or hematologic conditions. Also anticipate that hearing and vision screening tests, CBC, and renal and liver function studies will be performed.

During early phases of drug therapy, monitor the temperature and pulse rate at frequent intervals. Also inspect mucous membranes for color changes (i.e., cyanosis or brownish discoloration), which are suggestive of methemoglobinemia.

Miscellaneous Drug in Category

Other drugs used in conjunction with dapsone in the treatment of leprosy include rifampin, ethionamide, and clofazimine.[16] **Clofazimine** (Lamprene) is a phenazine dye that exerts a slow bactericidal effect on *M. leprae.* The drug inhibits bacterial growth by binding to mycobacterial DNA. Clofazimine also possesses an anti-inflammatory effect that helps in management of reactions. It is especially effective in treating dapsone-resistant disease. Adult dosage is 100 to 300 mg/d in combination with at least one other antileprotic for at least 3 years, then 100 mg/d alone.

TABLE 57–2
Antileprotic Drugs: Prototype and Major Drug in Category

Drug Name	Dosage and Route of Administration	Nursing Considerations

DAPSONE
(Dapsone USP)
HOW SUPPLIED
    Scored tablets: 25 mg, 100 mg
	Treatment
	ADULTS
	Oral: 100 mg daily for at least 3 y (plus ri-
	    fampin, 600 mg/d, for 6 mo)
	CHILDREN
	Oral: 1.4 mg/kg/d
	Prophylaxis
	ADULTS
	Oral: 50 mg daily
	CHILDREN
	6-12 y: 25 mg daily
	2-5 y: 25 mg three times weekly
	6-23 mo: 12 mg three times weekly
	<6 mo: 6 mg three times weekly
		Assess
		Assess client for preexisting chronic renal, he-
		    patic, pulmonary, or cardiovascular disease.
		Determine if client is pregnant; dapsone is
		    classified as Pregnancy Category C drug.
		Assess vision, hearing, and pulse rate before
		    beginning therapy.
		Implement
		Administer with food to prevent GI upset.
		Monitor temperature for first few weeks of
		    treatment.
		Educate client about therapy and outcomes.
		Provide skin care for dryness.
		Check hands and feet frequently for soreness
		    if anesthesia is present.
		Store drug at controlled room temperature.
		Protect drug from light.
		Anticipate administering ascorbic acid, folate,
		    and iron to prevent deficiencies associated
		    with drug.
		Monitor I and O.
		Monitor
		Monitor compliance to therapy by determin-
		    ing periodic urinary dapsone levels.
		Monitor for undesired clinical responses such
		    as hepatitis, peripheral neuropathy, albu-
		    minuria, and hematologic changes.
		Monitor CBC weekly for 1 mo, monthly for
		    6 mo, and then semiannually.
		Monitor liver function tests: AST, lactate de-
		    hydrogenase (LDH), ALT.
		Monitor renal function tests.

Clofazamine
(Lamprene)
HOW SUPPLIED
    Capsules: 50 mg, 100 mg
	Dapsone-resistant Leprosy
	ADULTS
	Oral: 100 mg/d in combination with one
	    or more antileprosy drugs for 3 y; then
	    100 mg/d as monotherapy
	Erythema Nodosum Leprosum
	ADULTS
	Oral: 100-300 mg/d for up to 3 mo; taper
	    dose to 100 mg/d as soon as possible
	M. avium-Intracellulare
	ADULTS
	Oral: 100 mg one to three times per day.
		Implement
		Instruct client to take as ordered with meals.
		Instruct client that drug may discolor the
		    skin, the conjunctivae, lacrimal fluid,
		    sweat, sputum, urine, and feces (all body
		    fluids) from red to brownish black.
		Instruct client to adhere strictly to established
		    drug regimen. No drug dosage should be
		    adjusted without advice of physician.
		Instruct client to report bone and joint pain,
		    GI bleeding, colicky abdominal pain, nau-
		    sea, vomiting, diarrhea, and diminished vi-
		    sion immediately.
		Instruct client that oil baths and frequent ap-
		    plications of lotion can help decrease itch-
		    ing and dry skin and to minimize use of
		    soap and rinse it off thoroughly.
		Instruct client to avoid driving or operating
		    hazardous equipment if episodes of dizzi-
		    ness, drowsiness, or visual impairment are
		    experienced.
		Evaluate
		Evaluate for absence of skin and mucosal le-
		    sions and acid-fast bacilli.

Clofazimine is incompletely and slowly absorbed when taken orally. It is highly lipophilic and is predominantly deposited in fatty tissue and the reticuloendothelial system (RES). In the RES it is taken up by macrophages.

Undesired clinical responses include a pinkish-brown discoloration of the skin in 75% to 100% of the clients. Body fluids also have a reddish tinge. The skin discoloration is reversible but may take several years for all changes to disappear. Other undesired responses include ecchymoses, skin dryness, pruritus, conjunctival discoloration, GI disturbances, hepatitis, jaundice, elevated blood sugar, decreased visual acuity, and lymphadenopathy. Albumin, bilirubin, and AST levels may also be elevated.[1,12,14,17]

CONCEPT REVIEW

Hansen's disease (leprosy) requires supportive nursing care because of the social stigma attached to infection with *M. leprae*. Compliance often depends on access to supportive individuals and facilities.

Therapy may take 10 years to clear the lesions of the acid-fast bacilli, and drug therapy may be necessary for the rest of the client's life.

SUMMARY

Because of the increasing incidence of multidrug-resistant pathogens, nurses must be alert to signs and symptoms of mycobacterial infections in the populations they serve. Obtaining thorough health histories and assessments, use of appropriate body-substance isolation techniques, and client education are important nursing interventions. In addition, careful monitoring of compliance to the drug regimen, whether in a hospital, home care, or clinic setting, is crucial.

REFERENCES

1. Wolinsky, E. (1992). Antimycobacterial Drugs. In S.L. Gorbach, J. Bartlett, & N. Blacklow (Eds.), *Infectious Diseases*. Philadelphia: W.B. Saunders.
2. Bates, B. (1992). *Bargaining for life: A social history of tuberculosis, 1876-1938*. Philadelphia: University of Philadelphia Press.
3. Griffith, D.E., & Wallace, R.J. (1992). Environmental (nontuberculosis) mycobacterial disease. In W. Kelley (Ed.), *Textbook of Internal Medicine* (2nd ed.). Philadelphia: J.B. Lippincott.
4. O'Brien, L.M., & Bartlett, K.A. (1992). Tuberculosis plus HIV spells trouble. *American Journal of Nursing, 92,* 28-34.
5. Nolan, C.M. (1992). Human immunodeficiency syndrome—Associated tuberculosis: A review with an emphasis on infection control issues. *American Journal of Infection Control, 20*(1), 30-34.
6. Pierce, J.R., et al. (1992). Transmission of tuberculosis to hospital workers by a patient with AIDS. *Chest, 101,* 581-582.
7. Iseman, M.D., & Madsen, L.A. (1989). Drug-resistant tuberculosis. *Clinics in Chest Medicine, 10,* 341-353.
8. Smith, C.M., & Reynard, A. (1992). *Textbook of pharmacology*. Philadelphia: W.B. Saunders.
9. Goddard, H. (1990). Treating differences: How race affects drug therapy. *Canadian Pharmaceutical Journal, 123,* 314-315.
10. U.S. Pharmacopeial convention. (1990). *United States pharmacopeia* (22nd rev.). Rockville, MD: Author.
11. Perez-Stable, E.U., & Hopewell, P.C. (1989). Current tuberculosis treatment regimens. *Clinics in Chest Medicine, 10,* 323-339.
12. Data Pharmaceutica, Inc. (1993). *1993 physicians' genRx*. Smithtown, NY: Author.
13. Lockwood, D., & McAdam, K. (1992). Leprosy. In S.L. Gorbach, J. Bartlett, & N. Blacklow (Eds.), *Infectious Diseases*. Philadelphia: W.B. Saunders.
14. Iseman, M.D. (1992). Nontuberculous mycobacterial infections. In S.L. Gorbach, J. Bartlett, & N. Blacklow (Eds.), *Infectious Diseases*. Philadelphia: W.B. Saunders.
15. Jacobsen, R.R. (1992). Leprosy. In W. Kelley (Ed.), *Textbook of Internal Medicine* (2nd ed.). Philadelphia: J.B. Lippincott.
16. Venkatesan, K. (1992). Pharmacokinetic drug interactions with rifampicin. *Clinical Pharmacokinetics, 22*(1), 47-65.
17. Cynamon, M.H., & Klemens, S.P. (1989). New antimycobacterial agents. *Clinics in Chest Medicine, 10,* 355-364.
18. Tatro, D. (1990). *Drug interaction facts*. St. Louis: Facts and Comparisons Division, J.B. Lippincott.

BIBLIOGRAPHY

Cuneo, W.D., & Snider, D.E. (1989). Enhancing patient compliance with tuberculosis therapy. *Clinics in Chest Medicine, 10,* 375-380.
DeCoch, K.M., et al. (1992). Tuberculosis and HIV infection in Subsaharan Africa. *Journal of American Medical Association, 268,* 1581-1587.
Jackson, M.M. (1993). Tuberculosis in infants, children, and adolescents: New dilemmas with an old disease. *Pediatric Nursing, 19,* 437-442.
Smith, M., et al. (1992). Tuberculosis and opportunistic mycobacterial infections. In R.D. Feigen & J.D. Cherry (Eds.), *Textbook of Pediatric Infectious Disease* (3rd ed.). Philadelphia: W.B. Saunders.
Underwood, M.A., et al. (1992). Commentary from the APIC guidelines committee on the Centers for Disease Control "Guidelines for preventing the transmission of tuberculosis in health care settings, with special focus on HIV-related issues." *American Journal of Infection Control, 20*(1), 27-29.

CHAPTER 58

Antifungal Drugs

KATHY M. KETCHUM • DAVID J. RITCHIE

⊛ **Fungal Infections**
LEARNING OBJECTIVE: Differentiate between superficial and systemic fungal infections.
KEY TERMS:
Candida, dermatophyte, mycoses, tinea

⊛ **Classification of Antifungal Drugs**
LEARNING OBJECTIVES:
Identify the three major groups of antifungal drugs.
Describe three pharmacodynamic mechanisms involved in the action of antifungal drugs.
KEY TERMS:
Azole, fluorinated pyrimidine, polyene

⊛ **Nursing Process**
LEARNING OBJECTIVES:
Outline a plan of care for a client receiving a systemic antifungal drug.
Describe items to incorporate into the teaching plan of a client receiving a topical antifungal drug.

⊛ **Polyenes**
LEARNING OBJECTIVES:
Describe the pharmacodynamics of amphotericin B.
Describe three important nursing considerations for the administration of amphotericin B.

⊛ **Fluorinated Pyrimidine**
LEARNING OBJECTIVES:
Describe the pharmacodynamics of flucytosine.
Identify two important nursing considerations for the administration of flucytosine.

⊛ **Azoles**
LEARNING OBJECTIVES:
Summarize essential information about one major drug from each subcategory: imidazole and triazole.
List five over-the-counter preparations that contain an azole as a key ingredient.
KEY TERMS:
Imidazole, triazole

⊛ **Miscellaneous Antifungal Drugs**
LEARNING OBJECTIVE: Summarize important information about griseofulvin.

⊛ **Life-Span Considerations**
LEARNING OBJECTIVE: Describe life-span considerations involved in antifungal drug therapy.

CONCEPTS AND TERMS TO REVIEW

Review Chapter 54 for general principles of antimicrobial therapy.
Review Chapter 49 for an overview of normal biologic defense mechanisms.

O ver the last decade, the incidence of fungal infections has increased, probably because of the ongoing acquired immunodeficiency syndrome (AIDS) epidemic, immunosuppressant drug use, bone marrow and solid organ transplantations, intravenous (IV) hyperalimentation treatments, and increased broad-spectrum antibiotic use.

All nursing professionals, regardless of their areas of expertise, are likely to encounter clients requiring antifungal therapy. This chapter provides a brief review of fungal infections **(mycoses),** nursing care specific for clients receiving antifungal drugs, and a description of major antifungal drugs.

FUNGAL INFECTIONS

The severity of fungal infections varies widely from superficial (topical or subcutaneous) infections to systemic, life-threatening, or disseminated infections. Superficial mycoses are caused primarily by the **Candida** species and dermatophytes. *Candida* causes oral, esophageal, vaginal, urinary tract, and dermatologic infections. Dermatophytes typically infect the skin, hair, and nails.[1] Systemic or disseminated mycoses are generally more difficult to treat and include candidiasis, aspergillosis, cryptococcosis, blastomycosis, and coccidioidomycosis.[2] Treatment approaches for both superficial and systemic fungal infections vary widely, depending on the client population and severity of infection.

It is not always possible to make a definitive diagnosis of a fungal infection. In such a situation, clients with fevers of unknown cause become candidates for antifungal treatment when antibacterial therapy has proved inadequate.[3]

Superficial Mycosis

Superficial candidiasis is caused by an overgrowth of *Candida albicans,* a yeast normally found on the skin and in the gastrointestinal (GI) and vaginal tracts. Overgrowth of normal colonization develops into a superficial infection. This type of infection occurs most commonly in the oral cavity (thrush), GI tract, esophagus, vagina, and perineal area, including the diaper area. Superficial candidiasis is generally treated with topical antifungal agents (e.g., nystatin [Mycostatin, Nilstat], clotrimazole [Gyne-Lotrimin, Lotrimin, Mycelex, FemCare], and miconazole [Monistat]).

Superficial fungal infections may also be caused by a fungal parasite, a **dermatophyte.** These infections are called **tinea infections.** Tinea capitis (scalp), tinea barbae (beard), tinea unguium (nail), tinea cruris (groin), tinea pedis (athlete's foot), tinea corporis (ringworm), and tinea versicolor (dermal skin layers) are examples of superficial dermatophyte fungal infections. As with superficial candidiasis, treatment of dermatophyte infections frequently consists of the use of topical agents. However, systemic therapy with azole antifungal agents or griseofulvin (Fulvicin, Grisactin, Gris-Peg) may be warranted in more severe cases.

Systemic Mycosis

Systemic mycosis is either a primary infection or occurs secondarily to precipitating factors. Systemic infections can involve the lungs, central nervous system, liver, spleen, kidney, eyes, skin, bone, or joints.

Histoplasmosis *(Histoplasma capsulatum),* coccidioidomycosis *(Coccidioides immitis),* and blastomycosis *(Blastomyces dermatitidis)* are examples of fungal infections usually acquired in areas of the country where the organisms are endemic. Histoplasmosis occurs commonly in the Mississippi River Valley, and coccidioidomycosis generally is found in western areas of the United States. Blastomycosis commonly is reported in central, north central, and eastern parts of the United States and central Canada.[1]

Candidiasis, aspergillosis *(Aspergillus* spp.), and cryptococcosis *(Cryptococcus neoformans)* are examples of fungal infections occurring as opportunistic (secondary) infections generally found in immunocompromised hosts. Clients having AIDS, those receiving immunosuppressive drug therapy or total parenteral nutrition, and those with intravascular devices are predisposed to the development of opportunistic fungal infections.

CLASSIFICATION AND PHARMACODYNAMICS OF ANTIFUNGAL DRUGS

There are three major groups of antifungal drugs: **polyenes, fluorinated pyrimidines,** and **azoles.** In addition, some miscellaneous drugs are used to treat fungal infections. Many of them are in over-the-counter (OTC) preparations.

Various pharmacodynamic mechanisms are involved with these drugs (Fig. 58–1). Most antifungal drugs suppress or in-

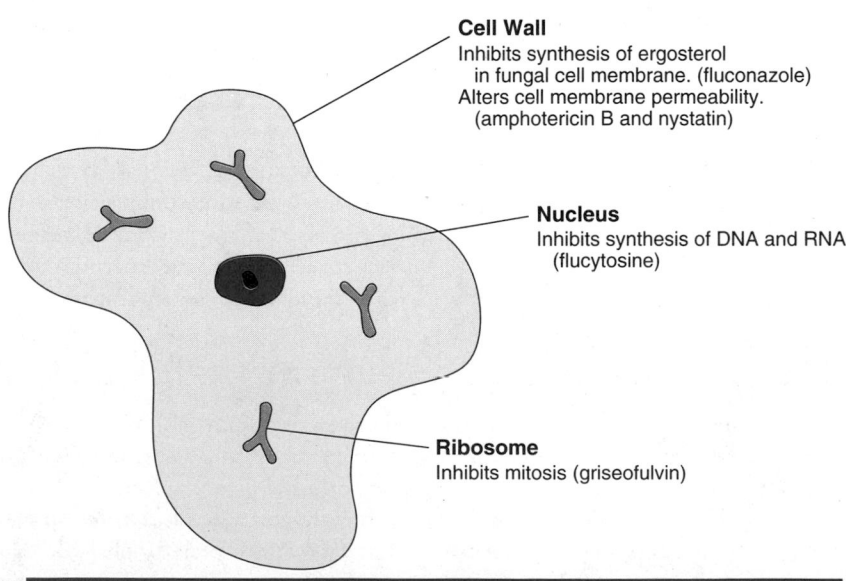

Cell Wall
Inhibits synthesis of ergosterol in fungal cell membrane. (fluconazole)
Alters cell membrane permeability. (amphotericin B and nystatin)

Nucleus
Inhibits synthesis of DNA and RNA. (flucytosine)

Ribosome
Inhibits mitosis (griseofulvin)

FIGURE 58–1   Pharmacodynamic mechanism of major antifungal drugs.

terfere with the synthesis of essential cellular components (i.e., RNA metabolites, folic acid, and peptide). Some disrupt the cell membrane or inhibit cell wall synthesis.

☒ NURSING CONSIDERATIONS

Administration of antifungal drugs can be accomplished safely by following the steps of the nursing process.

Assessing   You must complete a health history and physical assessment before the onset of drug therapy. These data help determine if subsequent client responses are related to the underlying illness or are adverse reactions to the drug treatment regimen.

During the **health history,** obtain information about the client's past medical history. Clients with impaired immune systems such as those with AIDS, cancer, diabetes mellitus, and transplant recipients are more prone to fungal infections. Determine the client's knowledge of fungal infections and the proposed drug treatment.

Obtain a thorough nutritional assessment, including information on the client's fluid and electrolyte status. Also collect a complete drug history, including whether the client has experienced allergic reactions to any drugs in the past. Review all of the client's drugs, and determine if potential risks of interactions exist. Ask the client if previous medical treatment was sought, and determine if the client used OTC drugs in an attempt to relieve signs and symptoms of the infection.

If a systemic fungal infection is suspected, question the client about the presence of fever, weakness, malaise, or weight loss. Determine if the client has any pulmonary involvement. Ask about shortness of breath, cough, sputum production, hemoptysis, or aching chest pain. Also ask the client if symptoms of a urinary tract infection (UTI) such as urgency, frequency, or burning during urination are present. Clients, especially the elderly, with chronic UTIs that do not improve with antibiotic therapy may have urinary candidiasis.

Review the results of any diagnostic tests (e.g., culture and sensitivity, urinalysis, biopsy). Since antifungal drugs may affect renal, hepatic, and hematologic functions, examine the results of baseline electrolyte studies, complete blood cell count, and renal and hepatic function tests.

During the **physical assessment,** carefully examine any areas of the body where a dermatophyte infection or candidiasis would be suspected. Note areas of redness, scaling, warmth, or tenderness on the skin. Examine the oral cavity for white patchy areas if oral candidiasis is suspected. If vulvovaginal candidiasis is suspected, examine the client for a white, cheesy vaginal discharge.

Auscultate the client's lungs. Determine the client's baseline blood pressure, pulse, respirations, and temperature. If he or she has a UTI, examine the urine carefully. Note the color, amount, odor, and presence of sediment in the urine.

Diagnosing   After completing the client assessment, analyze the data and identify specific nursing diagnoses. Examples of nursing diagnoses appropriate for clients receiving antifungal drugs include the following:

- Body image disturbance related to presence of skin rashes and lesions.
- Impaired skin integrity related to scratching of rashes or lesions.
- High risk for infection related to impaired skin integrity.
- Altered nutrition: less than body requirements related to anorexia, nausea, or vomiting associated with systemic drug therapy.
- Fluid volume deficit related to anorexia, nausea, and vomiting associated with systemic drug therapy.
- Diarrhea related to administration of antifungal drugs.
- Anxiety related to lack of knowledge about antifungal drug therapy.

Planning   During the planning phase, develop a plan of care that incorporates the identified nursing diagnoses and relevant goals of therapy. In addition, develop a discharge or teaching plan.

Include in the discharge or teaching plan information about drug actions, drug response, administration techniques, and undesired clinical responses (Fig. 58–2). If the client has impaired skin integrity (e.g., that caused by dermatophyte fungal infections or superficial candidiasis), a lotion or ointment preparation may be prescribed. Include in the teaching plan directions for proper hand washing: hands should be washed before and after application of the drug. Demonstrate proper cleaning of skin lesions and application of the drug preparation. Teach the client that residual ointments or creams affect absorption of the newly applied medicine. Teach the client to look for changes in skin color or condition during the period of drug therapy and to use the drug for the entire time prescribed. If skin changes occur or symptoms are not relieved, instruct the client to contact the primary care provider.

If the client has oral candidiasis, a suspension is usually prescribed. For this client, include information such as the length of time to hold the suspension in the mouth and whether the suspension is swallowed or expectorated. A cream or vaginal suppository is prescribed for the client with vaginal candidiasis. For her, include the proper method for inserting the drug into the vagina. Instruct the client with recurrent vulvovaginitis to avoid the use of bubble baths, colored toilet paper with fragrances, and tight-fitting undergarments.

The ideal overall goal of antifungal drug therapy is the client's fungal infection will be eradicated or controlled. The following expected outcome criteria may be applicable:

- Client has intact skin, free of lesions.
- Client identifies interventions to reduce risk of infection.
- Client demonstrates techniques to reduce risk of infection.
- Client participates in recommended treatment plan.
- Client reports improved sense of energy.
- Client maintains body weight.
- Client maintains body fluid volume at a functional level.
- Client reestablishes normal pattern of bowel functioning.
- Client reports anxiety is reduced.

Implementing   The type of fungal infection and the drug preparation prescribed dictate what interventions are required. Familiarize yourself with diagnostic tests ordered for clients with fungal infections. These tests include culture and sensi-

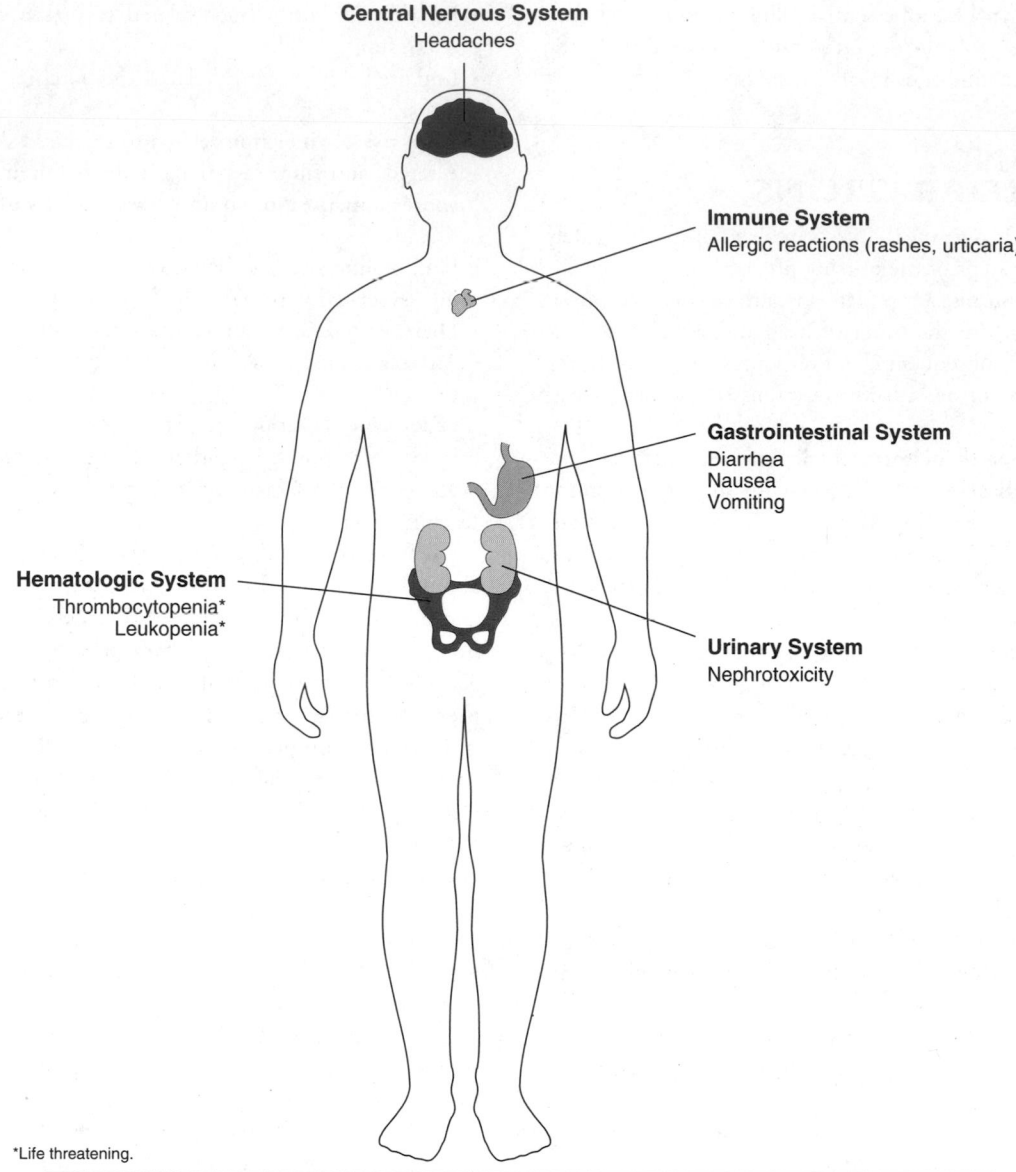

Central Nervous System
Headaches

Immune System
Allergic reactions (rashes, urticaria)

Gastrointestinal System
Diarrhea
Nausea
Vomiting

Hematologic System
Thrombocytopenia*
Leukopenia*

Urinary System
Nephrotoxicity

*Life threatening.

FIGURE 58–2   Common undesired clinical responses to systemic antifungal therapy.

tivity, urinalysis, potassium hydroxide (KOH) smear, Wood's light examination, biopsy, or radiologic studies. Also familiarize yourself with proper drug administration techniques.

To prevent spread of these infections, orient yourself to the infectious process involved in the particular infection being treated: What is the infectious agent? The reservoir? The portal of exit? The portal of entry? The susceptible host? Practice proper hygiene techniques and universal precautions.

The client with a superficial fungal infection may experience extreme discomfort from the itching that occurs. Apply the prescribed drug preparation as frequently as possible within the manufacturer's guidelines. The client with a systemic fungal infection may experience fever, pulmonary complications, fatigue, and/or malaise. Administration of antipyretics may be necessary to reduce the fever. In addition, use

other cooling measures that are appropriate (e.g., reduce environmental temperature, decrease bed coverings, and promote air circulation).

Clients receiving oral or IV antifungals frequently experience anorexia, nausea, vomiting, and/or diarrhea. If this occurs, an order for an antiemetic or antidiarrheal drug may be required. If these symptoms are not relieved, the prescribed antifungal drug or dosage must be adjusted.

To guarantee the client is receiving adequate caloric intake, consult with the dietician. In some instances, supplemental vitamins or protein may be required. To assess fluid volume loss, maintain an accurate measurement of intake and output.

Evaluating   Ongoing evaluations are an integral part of the nursing care of the client with a fungal infection. Examine the outcome criteria identified in the planning stage to see if they have been accomplished. In addition, evaluate the individualized response of the client to the infection and to the antifungal agents.

POLYENES

Amphotericin B and nystatin are the two polyene drugs currently in clinical use (Table 58–1).

POLYENE PROTOTYPE

AMPHOTERICIN B

Amphotericin B (Fungizone), available and used clinically since the mid-1950s, has been and remains the gold standard of therapy for treatment of systemic fungal infections.[2]

Pharmacotherapeutics Amphotericin B is used for the treatment of invasive systemic fungal infections, including candidiasis, aspergillosis, cryptococcosis, blastomycosis, and coccidioidomycosis.

Pharmacokinetics Amphotericin B is poorly absorbed from the GI tract and must be administered intravenously for treatment of systemic fungal infections. An IV infusion of amphotericin B circulates in the plasma in a highly (>90%) protein-bound state. It is distributed widely in the body, with approximately two thirds of the plasma concentration detected in fluids from inflamed pleura, peritoneum, synovium, and aqueous humor. Concentrations in the cerebrospinal fluid seldom exceed 2.5% of the plasma concentration.[4]

Details of possible metabolic pathways are not known. However, amphotericin B is excreted slowly (over weeks and months) by the kidneys; the elimination half-life is approximately 15 days. Two to 5% of a given dose is excreted in the active form. After treatment has been discontinued, the drug can be detected in the urine for at least 7 days.[4–6]

Pharmacodynamics Amphotericin B is fungistatic or fungicidal, depending on its concentration in body fluids and the susceptibility of the fungus. The drug binds to sterols in the fungal cell membrane, altering membrane permeability and allowing leakage of intracellular components.[4,5]

Pharmaceutics Amphotericin B is available in sterile solution for IV infusion. The drug is also available as a topical cream, lotion, or ointment for superficial use.

Undesired Clinical Responses Infusion-related undesired clinical responses are common with the administration of amphotericin B. These responses include chills and rigor (muscle rigidity associated with chills), fever, headaches, diarrhea, cramping epigastric pain, nausea, and vomiting. Other possible responses include hypotension, tachypnea, generalized muscle and joint pain, and allergic reactions. In addition, the client may experience nephrotoxicity, distal tubular acidosis, hypokalemia, hypomagnesemia, bone marrow suppression, and normochromic, normocytic anemia.[4,7]

Contraindications and Precautions Amphotericin B must be administered with extreme caution to clients with renal impairment or electrolyte abnormalities. Amphotericin B therapy is contraindicated in clients hypersensitive to the drug.[4]

Drug-Drug, Drug-Nutrient, Drug-Environment Interactions When administered concurrently, the following drugs may interact with amphotericin B: antineoplastic drugs, corticosteroids, cardiac glycosides, skeletal muscle relaxants, and other antifungal drugs. When some antineoplastic drugs are administered concomitantly with amphotericin B, the risks for renal toxicity, bronchospasm, and hypotension are enhanced. Corticosteroids may potentiate the drug-induced hypokalemic state produced by amphotericin B. In turn, the hypokalemia may potentiate digitalis toxicity and enhance the curariform effect of skeletal muscle relaxants.[4]

Life-Span Considerations Amphotericin B is classified as a Pregnancy Category B drug. This drug should be used during pregnancy only if clearly indicated. If it is administered to nursing mothers, they should be advised to discontinue nursing since it is not known if amphotericin B is excreted in human milk. Drug safety and effectiveness in pediatric and elderly clients have not been established. Amphotericin B should be used with caution in these individuals. Elderly clients appear to be at greater risk for nephrotoxicity when receiving amphotericin B. In addition, serum electrolyte values should be followed closely in elderly clients receiving diuretics.[4]

Specific Drug-Related Nursing Considerations Reconstitute amphotericin B with sterile water without a bacteriostatic agent. Do not use saline diluents since saline solutions produce a precipitate. Assess the client's vital signs before initiating the infusion and every 15 minutes during the first dose. A test dose of 1 mg in 20 to 50 ml of D_5W should be given over 30 minutes to determine sensitivity to the drug. Monitor the infusion carefully. If the client experiences a hypersensitivity reaction to the drug (e.g., respiratory distress, hypotension), discontinue the drug and notify the primary care provider.

As previously indicated, IV administration of amphotericin B may produce severe side effects such as fever, chills, and rigor. Chills and muscle rigidity associated with amphotericin B increase the client's metabolic needs, a situation detrimental to the individual with a fungal infection. To prevent these responses, nonsteroidal anti-inflammatory drugs, acetaminophen, antihistamines, narcotics, or antipyretics sometimes are administered before the infusion.[8] Providing extra blankets, increasing room temperature, offering warm oral fluids, using relaxation techniques, or using extremity wraps may be helpful in preventing infusion-related complications.[9–12] The febrile reaction usually subsides within 4 hours after the IV infusion has been completed.

Examine the IV site frequently for indications of leakage or thrombophlebitis. Amphotericin B is extremely irritating to tissue. Using central venous catheters or frequent site rotations decreases the incidence of thrombophlebitis. If thrombophlebitis does occur at the IV site, application of warm moist packs is helpful.

During therapy, monitor serum levels of blood urea nitrogen (BUN), creatinine, and electrolytes carefully. Weigh the client daily, and assess intake and output to identify any changes in renal function. Offer the client fluids frequently; adequate hydration (2000 to 3000 ml/d) may minimize nephrotoxicity.

🦚 NURSING RESEARCH

Holtzclaw, B.J. (1990). Control of febrile shivering during amphotericin B therapy. *Oncology Nursing Forum, 17,* 521-524.

Intravenous infusion of amphotericin B often produces fever and severe shivering or "rigors." These responses increase heart rate, respiratory rate, blood pressure, metabolism, and oxygen consumption. Concomitant drug therapy to prevent shivering is not always effective.

The purpose of this study was to determine if wrapping extremities with terry cloth toweling would prevent heat loss. The sample consisted of 20 hospitalized clients with cancer. Each extremity, including the feet and hands, of the experimental group was wrapped. The experimental and control groups wore pajamas and used light coverings as needed. Measures of shivering included electromyograph (EMG) signals from the pectoral muscles and visual observation of rigors by the data collector. Heart rates, blood pressure, and meperidine requirements were also examined.

Shivering was recorded in 75% of the subjects. Duration of shivering in the experimental group was significantly less according to independent t tests (p <0.04). The subjects also required less meperidine ($p = 0.04$).

STUDENT ACTIVITIES

- Check the procedure manual at your assigned agency and determine the procedure for administering amphotericin B. Focus on techniques used to reduce and/or prevent shivering.
- Share the research findings with the nursing staff responsible for administering the drug.   🦚

Nystatin

The antifungal drug nystatin (Mycostatin, Nilstat) can be both fungistatic and fungicidal. It acts by binding to sterols in the cell membrane of the fungus. This results in a change in the membrane permeability, allowing leakage of intracellular components.

After oral administration, nystatin is minimally absorbed, with no detectable blood levels. Most of the orally administered drug is eliminated unchanged in the feces. Oral tablets of the drug are used to treat intestinal candidiasis. Oral suspensions and troches are used for the treatment of candidiasis in the oral cavity. Topical dosage forms (i.e., powders, creams, and ointments) are indicated in the treatment of cutaneous or mucocutaneous infections caused by *C. albicans.* Nystatin vaginal tablets are effective for the local treatment of vulvovaginal candidiasis.[4]

Nystatin is generally well tolerated by all age groups. Large oral doses occasionally have produced diarrhea, nausea, and vomiting.

CONCEPT REVIEW

Fungal infections vary from superficial to systemic and life threatening.

Amphotericin B is used for the treatment of invasive systemic fungal infections. It can produce many undesired clinical responses, must be used with caution in clients with renal impairment or electrolyte abnormalities, and interacts with numerous drugs.

Amphotericin B and nystatin are the two polyenes currently in clinical use.

FLUORINATED PYRIMIDINE

Only one drug—flucytosine (Ancobon)—is categorized as a fluorinated pyrimidine. It is rarely administered without amphotericin B because of the risk for developing resistant species.

FLUORINATED PYRIMIDINE PROTOTYPE

FLUCYTOSINE

Flucytosine (Ancobon) was synthesized in 1957 as part of a screening program for antitumor agents in the treatment of leukemia. It is relatively noncytotoxic but does produce antifungal effects.[13]

Pharmacotherapeutics Flucytosine is used in combination with amphotericin B for treatment of selected invasive mycoses such as *C. neoformans.*

Pharmacokinetics Flucytosine is rapidly and almost completely absorbed after oral administration and is widely distributed in the body. It penetrates the blood-brain barrier, achieving clinically significant concentrations in the cerebrospinal fluid. The drug's half-life is 3 to 6 hours in clients with normal renal function but is increased in patients with renal failure. Flucytosine is excreted by the kidneys through glomerular filtration without significant tubular reabsorption.[4,14]

Pharmacodynamics Flucytosine is converted to 5-fluorouracil (5-FU) within the fungal cell. The 5-FU is incorporated into fungal RNA and inhibits synthesis of DNA and RNA.[4]

Pharmaceutics Flucytosine is available in 250- and 500-mg gelatin capsules.

Undesired Clinical Responses Flucytosine can cause bone marrow suppression (anemia, leukopenia, and thrombocytopenia), particularly when serum levels exceed 100 μg/ml.[14] Liver dysfunction and GI disturbances (nausea, vomiting, diarrhea) may also occur. In rare cases clients experience headache, dizziness, or confusion.

Contraindications and Precautions Flucytosine is contraindicated for clients hypersensitive to the drug. It must be used with extreme caution in individuals with impaired renal or hepatic function or bone marrow depression.

Drug-Drug, Drug-Nutrient, Drug-Environment Interactions Flucytosine has no major drug, nutrient, or environmental interactions. When flucytosine is administered with the antineoplastic cytarabine (cytosine arabinoside, Cytosar-U), antifungal activity may be inactivated.

Interference with Diagnostic Studies Serum creatinine levels should be determined by the Jaffé method, since flucytosine interferes with other testing methods.

Life-Span Considerations Flucytosine is classified as a Pregnancy Category C drug; it should be used during pregnancy only if the potential benefits outweigh the risks. Safety and effectiveness in children have not been established; however, the dose should be adjusted for pediatric clients according to the pediatric dose schedule.

Specific Drug-Related Nursing Considerations Anticipate that the client's hematologic status and renal and hepatic function will be monitored during therapy. In addition, watch serum levels for flucytosine concentrations. Therapeutic serum levels of flucytosine range from 25 to 100 µg/ml.[14]

If the client experiences any mental status changes, bleeding episodes, or dizziness, the primary care provider should be notified. If the client must take more than one capsule at a time, instruct him or her to take the capsules over a 15-minute period to reduce GI complications.

Table 58–1 summarizes information about flucytosine.

AZOLES

The azole category of antifungal drugs includes two subcategories: the **imidazoles** and **triazoles.** Although the subcategories include drugs that have slightly different pharmacokinetics and pharmacotherapeutic uses, their mechanism of action, side effects, and nursing considerations are similar.

AZOLE PROTOTYPE

FLUCONAZOLE

Fluconazole (Diflucan) was the first commercially available triazole systemic antifungal agent.

Pharmacotherapeutics Fluconazole is effective in the treatment of oral and esophageal candidiasis, especially in clients with AIDS.[15] It is also used for treatment of systemic *Candida* infections (e.g., pneumonia and peritonitis) and for treatment of acute and chronic *Cryptococcus* meningitis. Because it is predominantly eliminated unchanged by the kidneys, it is useful for the treatment of urinary tract candidiasis.[16]

Pharmacokinetics The pharmacokinetics of orally and IV administered fluconazole are similar. Oral fluconazole is extremely well absorbed from the GI tract. Protein binding after an oral or IV dose averages 12%. The drug is widely distributed in the body and achieves high levels in the cerebrospinal fluid and urinary tract. Fluconazole's half-life is approximately 30 hours. Approximately 80% of an administered dose of fluconazole appears unchanged in the urine. Another 10% is excreted by the kidney as inactive metabolites.[4,17]

Pharmacodynamics Fluconazole inhibits the synthesis of ergosterol, a primary constituent of the fungal cell membrane, thus inhibiting fungal growth.

Pharmaceutics Fluconazole is available in 50-, 100-, 150-, and 200-mg oral tablets and in sterile solution for IV infusion.

Undesired Clinical Responses The most common undesired responses associated with fluconazole administration are nausea, vomiting, diarrhea, headache, abdominal pain, and skin rash. Hepatocellular dysfunction has also been reported.[4,13]

Contraindications and Precautions Fluconazole is contraindicated for clients hypersensitive to the drug. The drug should be used with caution in clients with hypersensitivity to other azoles.

Drug-Drug, Drug-Nutrient, Drug-Environment Interactions Fluconazole interacts with several major drugs including warfarin (Coumadin), phenytoin (Dilantin), sulfonylurea (oral hypoglycemic) drugs, and rifampin. Fluconazole increases the plasma concentrations of phenytoin. Serum levels of phenytoin should be monitored carefully if these drugs are given concomitantly. Fluconazole also increases the prothrombin time after the administration of warfarin. The plasma level of oral sulfonylurea hypoglycemic drugs is increased and metabolism of the drugs reduced by the administration of fluconazole. Therefore blood glucose levels must be carefully monitored and the dose of sulfonylurea adjusted if necessary.[18,19]

Life-Span Considerations Fluconazole is classified as a Pregnancy Category C drug. It is also secreted in human milk at concentrations similar to plasma levels; therefore the use of fluconazole in nursing mothers is not recommended. The efficacy of fluconazole has not been established in children. However, a pediatric dosage schedule is available. Elderly clients should be assessed for signs of hepatic impairment during fluconazole therapy.[4]

Specific Drug-Related Nursing Considerations Liver function tests should be monitored during the course of therapy with fluconazole. In addition, the client should be assessed for symptoms of hepatic impairment such as jaundice, right upper abdominal pain, pale stools, or extreme fatigue. Explain to the client the importance of taking the drug for the entire time that it is prescribed. Since long-term therapy over several months may be necessary, instruct the client about the importance of keeping follow-up appointments with the primary care provider.

Miscellaneous Drugs in Category

Itraconazole (Sporanox) is also a triazole antifungal agent with some significant antifungal-spectrum advantages over fluconazole. Itraconazole appears to possess superior activity against *H. capsulatum* (histoplasmosis) and *Aspergillus* spp. (aspergillosis). Although currently indicated only for treatment of histoplasmosis and blastomycosis, the drug appears effective for treatment of oral candidiasis, *Cryptococcus* meningitis, and vaginal candidiasis.[17]

Miconazole and **ketoconazole** are the primary drugs in the subcategory *imidazoles*. Miconazole was the first systemically administered azole agent available for clinical use. Because of numerous toxicities associated with IV administration of this drug, it is rarely used systemically any longer. However, it is

TABLE 58–1
Antifungal Drugs/Prototypes and Major Drugs in Category

Drug Name	Dosage and Route of Administration	Nursing Considerations
POLYENES: AMPHOTERICIN B (Fungizone) **HOW SUPPLIED** IV: 50 mg/vial Cream: 3% Lotion: 3% Ointment: 3%	*Treatment* **ADULTS** IV: 1 mg/50 ml D₅W test dose over 30 min to evaluate tolerance; increase gradually up to 0.5 mg/kg/d Topical: apply to skin bid to qid. **CHILDREN** IV: 0.25-0.5 mg/kg/d	*Assess* Assess if client is receiving aminoglycosides, vancomycin, steroids, diuretics, or digoxin. Assess client for preexisting renal dysfunction and electrolyte imbalance. *Implement* Reconstitute with nonsaline diluents to avoid precipitation of drug. Assess vial for foreign particles; discard if any are present. Use an in-line filter when administering IV infusion. Administer through central venous line if possible. Record vital signs before IV administration and every 15-30 min during first dose. Infuse IV solution slowly over 4-6 h. Observe infusion site for signs of phlebitis. Keep room warm; provide warm clothing; and wrap extremities if client develops chills and rigors. Instruct client to report undesired response (i.e., irritation at site) to topical preparations. *Monitor* Review renal function test results and serum electrolyte levels regularly. Monitor client for indications of undesired clinical responses: chills, fever, nausea, vomiting, hypokalemia. Monitor I and O and report any change in fluid status. *Evaluate* Evaluate absence of infectious process. Evaluate healing status of skin lesions.
Nystatin (Mycostatin, Nadostine, Nilstat) **HOW SUPPLIED** Tablets: 500,000 U Suspension: 100,000 U/ml Vaginal tablets: 100,000 U Ointment and powder: 100,000 U/g	**ADULTS** Oral: 500,000 U q6h Vaginal: insert cream at bedtime for 7 d Topical: apply bid to tid **CHILDREN** Same as adult **INFANT** Oral: 200,000 U q6h	*Assess* Assess for signs and symptoms of fungal infection. *Implement* Advise client to use cream, lotion, or ointment exactly as prescribed. Teach client proper use of oral suspension (swish and expectorate or gargle and then swallow). Avoid use of alcohol-containing mouthwashes if client has thrush. Teach to insert vaginal cream high into vagina. Do not apply occlusive dressings over areas of candidiasis. *Monitor* Assess client for undesired clinical responses: epigastric distress, nausea, vomiting, and diarrhea. *Evaluate* Evaluate status of skin and mucous membranes.

TABLE 58–1 *Continued*
Antifungal Drugs/Prototypes and Major Drugs in Category

Drug Name	Dosage and Route of Administration	Nursing Considerations
FLUORINATED PYRIMIDINE: FLUCYTOSINE (Ancobon) HOW SUPPLIED Capsules: 250 and 500 mg	ADULTS Oral: 37.5 mg/kg q6h; keep serum level below 100 μg/ml to minimize hematologic toxicity CHILDREN Oral: 50-150 mg/kg/d; 1.5-4.5 g/m^2/d for those weighing <50 kg	**Assess** Determine if client is receiving bone marrow suppressants or other antifungal drugs. Assess for preexisting renal, hepatic, and hematologic dysfunction. **Implement** Teach client to take capsules one at a time over 15 min to decrease GI effects. Report any episodes of bleeding. Provide an antiemetic if client experiences nausea or vomiting. **Monitor** Monitor renal, hepatic, and hematologic function during therapy. Monitor for indications of undesired clinical responses: nausea, vomiting, diarrhea, headache, dizziness, anemia, leukopenia, or thrombocytopenia. **Evaluate** Evaluate for absence of infectious process.
AZOLES: FLUCONAZOLE (Diflucan) HOW SUPPLIED Coated tablets: 50, 100, and 200 mg IV: 2 mg/ml Powder for oral suspension: 10 and 40 mg/ml	ADULTS Oral or IV: 100-400 mg/d CHILDREN 3-6 mg/kg/d (investigational)	**Assess** Assess client for possible drug-drug interactions. Assess for preexisting hepatic dysfunction. Interview client about preexisting hypersensitivity to azole drug. **Implement** Avoid mixing drug with other IV drugs. Discard solution if precipitate is present. Encourage client to maintain fluid intake. **Monitor** Monitor client for undesired clinical responses: nausea, vomiting, diarrhea, and abdominal pain. Assess for indications of hepatotoxicity (jaundice, pale stools, right upper quadrant pain, fatigue). **Evaluate** Evaluate for absence of infectious process.
Ketoconazole (Nizoral) HOW SUPPLIED Uncoated tablet: 200 mg Cream: 20 mg/g Shampoo: 2%	ADULTS Oral: 200-400 mg/d Topical: apply one or two times daily CHILDREN >2 Y Oral: 3.3-6.6 mg/kg/d	**Assess** See fluconazole. **Implement** Avoid concomitant administration of drugs that increase gastric pH. Assess for unusual bleeding if client is taking warfarin. Instruct client to take drug for duration of prescribed time. **Monitor** Assess levels of serum electrolytes regularly. Monitor for indications of undesired clinical responses: abdominal pain, nausea, vomiting, diarrhea, headache, dizziness, leukopenia, and anemia. Monitor hepatic function during therapy. **Evaluate** Evaluate for absence of infectious process.

Table continued on following page.

TABLE 58–1 *Continued*
Antifungal Drugs/Prototypes and Major Drugs in Category

Drug Name	Dosage and Route of Administration	Nursing Considerations
Miconazole Nitrate (Monistat) **HOW SUPPLIED** IV, IT: 10 mg/ml Cream: 2% Vaginal cream Vaginal suppository	**ADULTS** IV: 200-3600 mg/d Topical: apply cream bid for 2-4 wk Vaginal cream or suppository: insert at bedtime for 3-7 d **CHILDREN** IV: 20-40 mg/kg/d	**Assess** See fluconazole. **Implement** Dilute drug in 200 ml of 0.9% NaCl or D₅W for IV infusion. Administer slowly (over 30-60 min) if given IV. Provide adequate fluids to clients receiving drug IV. Instruct client to avoid sexual intercourse during course of vaginal therapy. Instruct client to continue use of drug during menses. **Monitor** Monitor I and O if drug is administered IV. Monitor client for indications of undesired clinical responses associated with IV infusion: tachycardia, arrhythmias, phlebitis at IV site, nausea, vomiting, diarrhea, and hematologic dysfunction. **Evaluate** Evaluate for absence of infectious process.
Clotrimazole (Gyne-Lotrimin, Lotrimin, Mycelex) **HOW SUPPLIED** Buccal troche: 10 mg Cream: 10 mg/g Lotion 10% Solution 1% *Vaginal* Uncoated tablet: 100 mg Uncoated sustained action tablet: 10 and 500 mg Cream: 50 mg per tube	**ADULTS** Oral: 1 troche five times daily Topical: apply two times daily Vaginal: insert at bedtime. **CHILDREN** <2 y: avoid use of topical cream <3 y: avoid use of lozenges <12 y: avoid use of vaginal cream	**Assess** See fluconazole. **Implement** Instruct client not to wear tight-fitting underclothing if receiving treatment for vaginal infection. Instruct client to avoid sexual intercourse during drug therapy for vaginal infection. Teach client to continue use of drug during menses. **Monitor** Monitor client for indications of undesired clinical responses: irritation at site with topical therapy; nausea, vomiting, and hepatic dysfunction with oral troche. **Evaluate** Evaluate for absence of infectious process.
Itraconazole (Sporanox) **HOW SUPPLIED** Gelatin capsule: 100 mg	**ADULTS** Oral: 200 to 400 mg/d **CHILDREN** Oral: 100 mg/d (investigational)	**Assess** See fluconazole. **Implement** Administer with food to increase absorption. Avoid concomitant administration with drugs that increase gastric pH. **Monitor** See fluconazole. **Evaluate** Evaluate for absence of infectious process.

still a key ingredient in many OTC preparations used to treat vaginal candidiasis and other superficial fungal infections (Table 58–2). **Clotrimazole** is another imidazole used to treat oral, vaginal or cutaneous candidiasis. Additional azole agents used to treat vaginal candidiasis that are similar to clotrimazole include **terconazole** and **butoconazole.** Other topical agents

used to treat dermatophyte infections and candidiasis include **econazole** and **oxiconazole.**

Ketoconazole (Nizoral) was the first orally available systemic azole antifungal agent. Currently it is used primarily for treatment of candidiasis, blastomycosis, and dermatophyte fungal infections. However, ketoconazole is associated with a

TABLE 58–1 *Continued*

Antifungal Drugs/Prototypes and Major Drugs in Category

Drug Name	Dosage and Route of Administration	Nursing Considerations
MISCELLANEOUS AGENTS: GRISEOFULVIN (Fulvicin-U/F, Fulvicin P/G, Grisactin, Gris-PEG) HOW SUPPLIED *Microcrystalline* Uncoated tablets: 250 and 500 mg Gelatin capsules: 125 and 250 mg Suspension: 125 mg/5 ml *Ultramicrocrystalline* Uncoated tablets: 125, 165, 250, and 330 mg	ADULTS *Microsize* Oral: 125-250 mg q6h *Ultramicrosize* Oral: 250-500 mg/d CHILDREN >2 Y Oral: 7.3 mg/kg/d	**Assess** Determine if client is concurrently receiving phenobarbital, oral contraceptives, or warfarin. Assess alcohol intake of client. Assess for preexisting hepatic failure or porphyria. Assess for hypersensitivity to drug. **Implement** Advise client that alternate methods of birth control may be needed. Instruct client to administer with fatty foods to increase absorption. Stress importance of daily hygiene to affected areas. Teach client that exposure to direct sunlight should be avoided. Instruct client to avoid ingesting alcohol during drug therapy; alcohol may precipitate tachycardia, flushing, or diaphoresis. **Monitor** Schedule regular prothrombin time checks if client is receiving warfarin. Assess for indications of undesired clinical responses: headache, nausea, vomiting, diarrhea, urticaria, rash, photosensitivity, and oral thrush. Monitor hepatic, renal, and hematologic functioning. **Evaluate** Evaluate for absence of infectious process.

TABLE 58–2

Examples of OTC Topical Antifungal Preparations

Key Ingredient	Product	Dosage Form	Therapeutic Use
Undecylenic acid	Caldesene	Powder, ointment	Diaper rash, prickly heat, chafing
	Cruex	Cream, powder, spray powder	Tinea cruris (jock itch), itching, chafing, irritation in groin area
	Desenex	Foam, cream, liquid, powder, ointment	Tinea pedis (athlete's foot)
Miconazole nitrate	Micatin	Cream, powder, spray	Tinea cruris
	Monistat 7	Cream, suppositories	Vulvovaginal candidiasis
Clotrimazole	Gyne-Lotrimin	Vaginal inserts and cream	Vaginal yeast (*Candida*)
	Lotrimin-AF	Cream, lotion, solution	Vaginal yeast (*Candida*)
	Mycelex OTC	Cream, lotion	Tinea cruris, tinea pedis, tinea corporis (ringworm)
Tolnaftate	Aftate	Liquid, gel, powder, aerosol powder	Tinea cruris, tinea pedis
	NP•27	Cream, solution, spray powder, powder	Tinea cruris, tinea pedis
	Tinactin	Aerosol liquid, aerosol powder, cream, powder, solution	Tinea cruris, tinea pedis, tinea corporis

number of significant drug interactions that have limited its use. For example, ketoconazole should not be administered concomitantly with drugs that decrease gastric acidity such as antacids, H₂-blockers, and omeprazole (Prilosec). Keto-conazole also may inhibit cisapride metabolism, prolonging the QT interval on EGGs. Administration of the drug with food may decrease GI disturbances. Liver function tests should be monitored during the course of therapy. In addition, the client should be assessed for symptoms of hepatic impairment such as jaundice, right upper abdominal pain, pale stools, or extreme fatigue.

Table 58–1 summarizes information about the azoles.

CONCEPT REVIEW

Flucytosine, the only fluorinated pyrimidine, is used in combination with amphotericin B for treatment of selected invasive mycoses. It can have some serious undesired clinical responses and must be used with extreme caution in individuals with impaired renal or hepatic function or bone marrow suppression.

Imidazoles and triazoles are the two subcategories of azoles. They are used to treat a variety of fungal infections. They have some undesired clinical responses and interactions with other drugs.

MISCELLANEOUS ANTIFUNGAL DRUGS

This category of agents contains many different oral and topical drugs. Most of these drugs are administered over the counter. However, griseofulvin requires a prescription and is the prototype drug in this category.

MISCELLANEOUS ANTIFUNGAL PROTOTYPE

GRISEOFULVIN

Griseofulvin (Fulvicin P/G, Gris-PEG, Grisactin) is an oral fungistatic antibiotic derived from a species of *Penicillium*.

Pharmacotherapeutics Griseofulvin is indicated for treatment of superficial dermatophyte fungal infections.

Pharmacokinetics After oral administration, GI absorption of ultramicrocrystalline griseofulvin is approximately one and one-half times that of the conventional microsize griseofulvin. The drug is widely distributed; it concentrates in hair, nails, liver, fat, skin, and muscle. The drug has a half-life of 9 to 24 hours and is primarily eliminated by the liver.[4,18]

Pharmacodynamics Griseofulvin inhibits fungal cell division by inhibiting mitosis.

Pharmaceutics Griseofulvin is available in microsize and ultramicrosize tablets, as microsize capsules, and as a microsize suspension.

Undesired Clinical Responses The most common undesired responses to griseofulvin are hypersensitivity reactions—skin rashes and urticaria. Occasionally

headache, mental status changes, GI disturbances, photosensitivity, and oral thrush are reported.

Contraindications and Precautions Griseofulvin use is contraindicated in clients with porphyria or hepatic failure and those exhibiting hypersensitivity to the drug. Since griseofulvin is derived from species of *Penicillium*, cross-sensitivity with penicillin is possible.[4]

Drug-Drug, Drug-Nutrient, Drug-Environment Interactions The action of griseofulvin is enhanced when fatty foods are ingested simultaneously.[20] Griseofulvin also may cause photosensitivity. Clients should be advised to use sunscreen when out in the direct sunlight.

Griseofulvin decreases the activity of warfarin-type anticoagulants. Clients receiving these drugs concomitantly with griseofulvin may require dosage changes. Barbiturates usually decrease the activity of griseofulvin, whereas alcohol may potentiate its effects.[4]

Specific Drug-Related Nursing Considerations Since griseofulvin is absorbed better in the presence of fatty foods, it should be administered with meals. This will also decrease the risk of GI disturbances. Teach the client to avoid direct sunlight and to apply sunscreens when outside. Instruct the client that alcohol should be avoided while taking griseofulvin. If the client ingests alcohol, tachycardia, flushing, or diaphoresis may occur.

The course of therapy may be long, and regular follow-up visits are necessary to monitor the response of the infection. Advise the client to keep affected areas clean and dry. Teach the client indications of undesired clinical responses (i.e., lesions in the mouth, skin rashes, and urticaria). Instruct the client that studies to monitor hepatic, renal, and hematologic functions will continue throughout therapy.

Table 58–1 summarizes information about griseofulvin.

LIFE-SPAN CONSIDERATIONS

Fungal infections can occur in both women and men at any age. Clients can experience primary infection by contact with specific organisms, or they can experience infections secondary to other disease states.

Infants and Children

Candidiasis occurs throughout the life span. The perineal area of infants provides a moist environment for the growth of a fungal infection. Children with dental braces may develop sores in the corner of their mouths. These lesions can develop candidiasis, commonly termed *perlèche*, which is treated topically with nystatin, clotrimazole, or miconazole.[20]

Dermatophyte infections also occur in young children. **Tinea capitis,** an invasion of the hair shaft by dermatophytes, occurs mainly in children 3 to 9 years of age. Treatment, which may take 1 to 2 months, consists of griseofulvin or ketoconazole in conjunction with selenium sulfide shampoos. **Tinea versicolor,** a rash commonly seen on the face, head or neck, is also found in children. Treatment methods include use of selenium sulfide shampoos, tolnaftate, haloprogin, miconazole, clotrimazole, or, in severe cases, ketoconazole.

Whenever rashes occur, treatment may cure the infection, but changes in the skin may take several weeks to disappear completely.[20]

Young Women and Men

Certain types of dermatophyte infections are common in this age group. **Tinea cruris,** an infection of the groin and thighs, is more common in males. It is complicated by obesity, tight-fitting clothes, athletic supports, and wet swimsuits. Diagnosis is made by culture, and the infection is treated with topical miconazole, clotrimazole, or oral griseofulvin. **Tinea barbae** is a dermatophyte infection that occurs in men who have beards. It can be treated with griseofulvin or ketoconazole.

Another type of dermatophyte infection seen as early as adolescence is **tinea pedis** (athlete's foot). Topical treatment with clotrimazole, miconazole, haloprogin, or econazole is helpful. In severe cases griseofulvin is administered. Nursing interventions include teaching the client about proper hygiene practices.

Women are prone to vulvovaginitis, which is a common occurrence after antibiotic administration. This candidiasis is easily diagnosed by doing a potassium hydroxide smear. Treatment is usually successful with application of OTC topical azoles. However, recurrences of the infection may happen. Should women continue to have vulvovaginal candidiasis, they should contact their health care provider for further follow-up.[20,21]

Elderly Clients

Because cell-mediated immunity is decreased in the elderly, fungal infections in this age group may be more severe. For example, progressive disseminated histoplasmosis is common in adults over the age of 54. Although the disease occurs at any age, it may be fatal in the elderly. Coccidioidomycosis, a systemic fungal infection common in hot, dry geographic locations, is also more severe in the elderly.[22]

In addition to changes in immunocompetence, the elderly are more prone to renal and hepatic dysfunction. Careful monitoring of renal and liver function tests is essential when antifungal drugs are administered to this age group. Elderly clients may also be taking a variety of other medications. The health care provider must be alert for possible drug-drug interactions.

SUMMARY

The population of clients susceptible to fungal infections is increasing with the development of drugs that affect the immune system, the rise in the AIDS population, and new invasive high technology procedures. Although researchers are trying to develop safer antifungal drugs, parenteral administration of amphotericin B remains the gold standard for treatment of systemic mycoses. Newer preparations of oral azole drugs are helpful in treating many systemic infections. Superficial mycoses such as candidiasis and dermatophyte infections are treated with oral or topical drugs. Treatment with antifungal drugs is usually long term; thus client compliance often is affected.

REFERENCES

1. Medoff, G., & Kobayashi, G.S. (1991). Systemic fungal infections: An overview. *Hospital Practice, 15,* 41-52.
2. Hoeprich, P.D. (1992). Clinical use of amphotericin B and derivatives: Lore, mystique, and fact. *Clinical Infectious Disease, 14*(Suppl. 1), S114-S119.
3. Rutledge, D.N., & Holtzclaw, B.J. (1990). Use of amphotericin B in immunosuppressed patients with cancer. Part 1: Pharmacology and toxicities. *Oncology Nursing Forum, 17,* 731-736.
4. Data Pharmaceutica, Inc. (1993). *1993 physicians' genRx.* Smithtown, NY: Author.
5. Lyman, C.A., & Walsh, T.J. (1992). Systemically administered antifungal agents: A review of their clinical pharmacology and therapeutic applications. *Drugs, 44*(1), 9-35.
6. Janknegt, R., de Marie, S., Bakker-Woudenberg, I., & Crommelin, D. (1992). Liposomal and lipid formulations of amphotericin B; Clinical pharmacokinetics. *Clinical Pharmacokinetics, 23,* 279-291.
7. Maddux, M.S., & Barriere, S.L. (1980). A review of complications of amphotericin B therapy: Recommendations for prevention and management. *Drug Intelligence and Clinical Pharmacy, 14,* 177-181.
8. Burks, L.C., Aisner, J., Fortner, C.L., & Wiernick, P.H. (1980). Meperidine for treatment of shaking chills and fever. *Archives of Internal Medicine, 140,* 483-484.
9. Rutledge, D.N., & Holtzclaw, B.J. (1988). Amphotericin B–induced shivering in patients with cancer: A nursing approach. *Heart and Lung, 17,* 432-440.
10. Holtzclaw, B.J., & Rutledge, D.N. (1990). Use of amphotericin B in immunosuppressed patients with cancer. Part 2: Pharmacodynamics and nursing implications. *Oncology Nursing Forum, 17,* 737-742.
11. Holtzclaw, B.J. (1990). Control of febrile shivering during amphotericin B therapy. *Oncology Nursing Forum, 17,* 521-524.
12. Holtzclaw, B.J. (1990). Effects of extremity wraps to control drug-induced shivering: A pilot study. *Nursing Research, 39,* 280-283.
13. Smith, C.M., & Reynard, A.M. (Eds.) (1992). *Textbook of pharmacology.* Philadelphia: W.B. Saunders.
14. Francis, P., & Walsh, T.J. (1992). Evolving role of flucytosine in immunocompromised patients: New insights into safety, pharmacokinetics, and antifungal therapy. *Clinical Infectious Diseases, 15,* 1003-1018.
15. Laine, L., Dretler, R.H., Conteas, C.N., Tuazon, C., Koster, F.M., Sattler, F., Squires, K., & Islam, M.Z. (1992). Fluconazole compared with ketoconazole for the treatment of candida esophagitis in AIDS. *Annals of Internal Medicine, 117,* 655-660.
16. Corbella, X., Carratala, J., Castells, M., & Berlanga, B. (1992). Fluconazole treatment in *Torulopsis glabrata* upper tract infection causing ureteral obstruction. *Journal of Urology, 147,* 1116-1117.
17. Dudley, M.N. (1990). Clinical pharmacology of fluconazole. *Pharmacotherapy, 10*(Suppl6), 141S-145S.
18. Perfect, J.R., Lindsay, M.H., & Drew, R.H. (1992). Adverse drug reactions to systemic antifungals: Prevention and management. *Drug Safety, 7,* 323-363.
19. Lazar, J.D., & Wilner, K.D. (1990). Drug interactions with fluconazole. *Review of Infectious Diseases, 12*(Suppl 3), S327-S333.
20. Rezabek, G.H., & Friedman, A.D. (1992). Superficial fungal infections of the skin: Diagnosis and current treatment recommendations. *Drugs, 43,* 674-682.

21. Summers, P.R., Biswas, M.K., Herrera, E.H., Wheeler, C., & O'Quinn, A.G. (1990). Management of difficult cases of vulvo-vaginitis. *Journal of the American Academy of Physician Assistants, 3,* 540-544.
22. Anonymous. (1988). Fungal infections late in life. *Emergency Medicine, 20*(19), 28-45.

BIBLIOGRAPHY

Baciewicz, A.M., & Baciewicz, F.A. (1993). Ketoconazole and fluconazole drug interactions. *Archives of Internal Medicine, 153,* 1970-1976.

Beck-Sague, C.M., Jarvis, W.R., & National Nosocomial Infections Surveillance System (1993). Secular trends in the epidemiology of nosocomial fungal infections in the United States, 1980-1990. *Journal of Infectious Diseases, 167,* 1247-1251.

Carney-Gersten, P., Giuffre, M., & Levy, D. (1991). Factors related to amphotericin-B–induced rigors (shivering). *Oncology Nursing Forum, 18,* 745-750.

Denning, D.W., Tucker, R.M., Hanson, L.H., Hamilton, J., & Stevens, D.A. (1989). Itraconazole therapy for cryptoccal meningitis and cryptococcosis. *Archives of Internal Medicine, 149,* 2301-2308.

Grant, S.M., & Clissold, S.P. (1989). Itraconazole: A review of its pharmacodynamic and pharmacokinetic properties, and therapeutic use in superficial and systemic mycoses. *Drugs, 37,* 310-344.

Jacobs, P.H. (1990). Antifungal therapy. In P.H. Jacob & L. Nall (Eds.), *Antifungal drug therapy: A complete guide for the practitioner* (pp. 1-4). New York: Marcel Dekker.

Lynn, M.M., & Holdcroft, C. (1989). Treatment for fungal skin infections: An update. *Nurse Practitioner, 14*(8), 64-72.

Podrasky, D.L. (1989). Amphotericin B: The nurse's role in controlling adverse reactions. *Focus on Critical Care, 16*(3), 194-198.

Terrell, C.L., & Hughes, C.E. (1992). Antifungal agents used for deep-seated mycotic infections. *Mayo Clinic Proceedings, 67,* 69-91.

Weiss, S.J., Schoch, P.E., & Cunha, B.A. (1991). *Malassezia furfur* fungemia associated with central venous catheter lipid emulsion infusion. *Heart and Lung, 20*(1), 87-89.

CHAPTER 59

Antiviral Drugs

SUSAN GRINSLADE • NORMA L. PINNELL

⊛ Viral Infections

LEARNING OBJECTIVE: Describe the two phases of viral infection of a host cell.

KEY TERMS:

Infection phase, integration phase, virion

⊛ Antiviral Drugs

LEARNING OBJECTIVE: Explain the pharmacodynamic properties of most antiviral drugs.

⊛ General Nursing Considerations

LEARNING OBJECTIVE: Develop a plan of care for a client receiving antiviral drugs.

⊛ Nucleoside Analogs

LEARNING OBJECTIVE: Discuss the therapeutic uses and pharmacokinetic and pharmacodynamic properties of vidarabine, acyclovir, and ribavirin.

⊛ Interferons

LEARNING OBJECTIVE: Explain the use of interferons in the treatment of viral diseases.

⊛ Amantadine Hydrochloride

LEARNING OBJECTIVE: Describe the pharmacodynamic properties of amantadine hydrochloride.

⊛ Ophthalmic Antiviral Drugs

LEARNING OBJECTIVE: Identify two drugs used to treat ocular viral infections.

CONCEPTS AND TERMS TO REVIEW

Review Chapter 54 for general principles of antimicrobial therapy.

Review Chapter 49 for an overview of normal biologic defense mechanisms.

Read appropriate sections of Chapter 53 for additional information about antiviral drugs.

Read appropriate sections of Chapter 69 for additional information about interferons.

Viruses produce some of the most common diseases affecting humans. Yet drug therapy for viral diseases is more limited than drug therapy for bacterial diseases. Most antiviral drugs work by interfering with viral replication. Viruses reproduce or replicate within the cells of the host and depend on the metabolic processes of the host cell to survive. It is this association with the host cell that makes drug therapy difficult. Drugs must target the virus and not destroy the host cell.

This chapter provides material about viruses and viral infections. Information on five specific antiviral drugs—vidarabine, acyclovir, ribavirin, idoxuridine, and trifluridine—is presented. In addition, the antiviral actions of interferons and amantadine hydrochloride are discussed. For the most part, these drugs are effective against herpesviruses (herpes simplex and herpes zoster), papovaviruses, and influenza A virus. Drugs used specifically to treat the human immunodeficiency virus (HIV)—zidovudine, zalcitabine, didanosine, foscarnet sodium, and ganciclovir—are discussed in Chapter 53.

VIRAL INFECTIONS

Viruses are intracellular parasites that take over the metabolic processes of the host cell. **Virions,** or viral particles, do not possess any metabolic organelles; therefore viruses have no metabolism. Unlike bacteria, viruses cannot reproduce independently. Their replication depends on their ability to infect a host cell.

The replication cycle of most viruses is divided into two phases: infection and integration. **Infection phase** begins when a virion binds to a receptor site on the plasma membrane of a host cell. Once bound, the virion penetrates the plasma membrane. Inside the host cell, the outer coats of the virus dissolve, releasing viral genetic material, either DNA or RNA.

After uncoating, viral DNA enters the cell's nucleus and becomes incorporated into the host cell's chromosomal DNA. This is the **integration phase.** During this phase the viral genome regulates the metabolic activities of the host cell by directing its own replication. New virions are then released from the cell for transmission of the viral infection to other host cells. Replication of viruses containing RNA is essentially the same as for DNA viruses. The infection and integration phases are illustrated in Figure 59–1.[1]

In addition to taking over the host cell's metabolic processes, viral infections can injure cellular structures. With some viral infections, the plasma membrane is damaged when a virion binds with the receptor site. Once inside the host cell, virions produce other cytopathic effects, including the following:

- Cessation of protein synthesis
- Disruption of lysosomal membranes
- Fusion of host cells, producing multinucleated giant cells
- Alteration of antigenic properties
- Transformation of host cells into cancerous cells[1]

Viruses affect multiple target organs and systems, including the respiratory tract, skin, blood, liver, immune system, and nervous system. Viral infections are acquired by direct contact with the targeted cell (e.g., cold or influenza) or through entrance via the bloodstream (e.g., hepatitis B). Viruses that are treated with antiviral agents include HIV, herpesviruses, varicella-zoster virus (VZV), cytomegalovirus (CMV), Epstein-Barr virus, hepatitis A virus, hepatitis B virus, influenza, papovavirus, and respiratory syncytial virus (RSV).

ANTIVIRAL DRUGS

As illustrated in Figure 59–1, the virus follows a specific growth cycle during replication. At present, there are no clini-

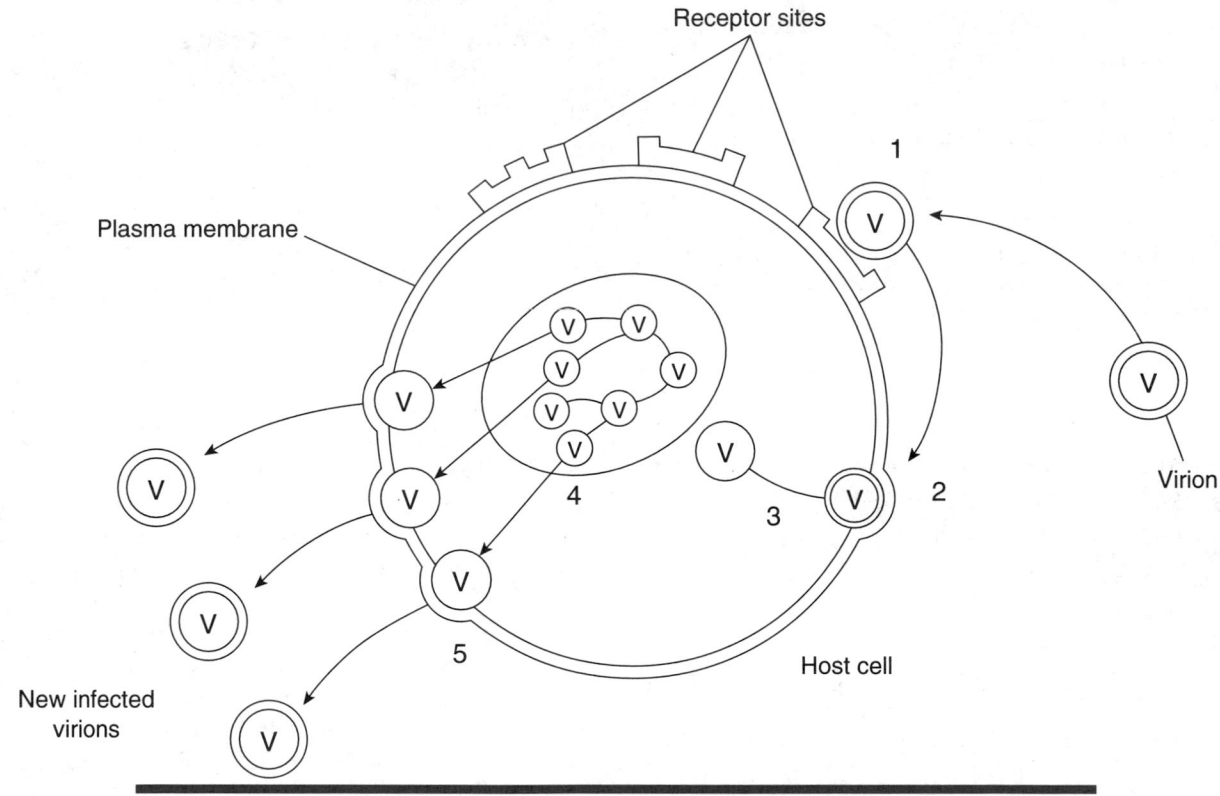

FIGURE 59–1   Infection and integration phases of viral infection:
1. **Adsorption:** Virus attaches itself to receptor sites on the cell surface.
2. **Enzyme release and penetration:** Once attached to the surface of the host cell, virus releases enzymes that weaken the plasma membrane and allow the virus to penetrate the cell.
3. **Uncoating:** After the viral particles enter the cell, the outer coats of the virus dissolve, releasing viral genetic material.
4. **Replication and transcription:** Virus synthesizes new messenger RNA, using host ribosomes. Viral proteins are also synthesized.
5. **Budding and release:** Once the viral nucleic acids and proteins are assembled to form mature viruses, the mature viruses are released from the infected host cell by budding. The infection can now spread to other host cells.

cally useful drugs that block the attachment of the virus to the receptor sites on the cell wall. Amantadine hydrochloride is the only drug believed capable of interrupting the penetration and coating phases of viral replication. Acyclovir, zidovudine, didanosine, ganciclovir, foscarnet, vidarabine, idoxuridine, and trifluridine inhibit the replication and transcription phase of viral reproduction. These drugs are administered systemically or topically.

NURSING CONSIDERATIONS

Since viral diseases are so common, prevention and treatment of these disorders are important nursing responsibilities. Clients with viral diseases require a variety of nursing interventions, which range from simple to complex and must be adapted to meet a diversity of problems.

Assessing   Focus the **health history** on the chief complaint, past medical history, drug history, family history, psychosocial history, including lifestyle, and review of systems. Since the type and severity of symptoms depend on the nature of the viral disease and the client's individual susceptibility, collect subjective data about each reported symptom. For each symptom, determine onset, location, duration, aggravating and relieving factors, medical intervention, self-treatment, and compliance factors. Ask the client about past episodes of viral infections. Determine the symptoms that developed, treatment, and effectiveness of treatment.

Ask the client about fatigue, malaise, fever, lassitude, chills, or sweating. Determine if the client has noted any localized swelling, pain, or tenderness in lymph node regions. Specifically inquire about skin changes. Determine if the client has ever experienced itching, dryness, rashes, ecchymoses, masses, lesions, or color changes. Information on recent exposure to infectious diseases is helpful, as is knowing the client's immunization status. All women of childbearing age must be assessed for pregnancy and lactation.

Extreme caution is needed during **physical assessment** of all clients but is especially important in individuals with viral diseases. Wear gloves when appropriate and follow universal precautions in regard to body fluids and secretions. During the head-to-toe physical assessment, examine the skin, hair, scalp, nails, and mucous membranes thoroughly. Changes such as altered total body skin color, turgor, temperature, and vascularity should be noted. If skin lesions are present, describe location, distribution, size, arrangement, color, configuration, and presence of drainage. Palpate lesions to determine characteristics of contour (e.g., flat, raised, or depressed), size, consistency (e.g., firm, soft), mobility, and tenderness.

Inspect the client's abdomen for ascites and prominent venous collateral networks. Palpate the abdomen, especially in the areas of the liver and spleen; note any tenderness. Percuss the abdomen to determine the size of the liver and spleen and the presence of ascites.

Diagnosing   Analysis of the data provides the basis of nursing diagnoses. Nursing diagnoses appropriate for the client receiving antiviral drugs with systemic actions follow:

- Anxiety related to uncertainty of effectiveness of drug therapy.
- Fluid volume excess related to decreased urinary output associated with drug therapy.
- High risk for injury related to dizziness and lightheadedness caused by some antiviral drugs.
- Knowledge deficit regarding expected therapeutic drug effects, undesired clinical responses, and drug administration procedure.
- Altered nutrition, less than body requirements, related to nausea produced by drug therapy.
- Sleep pattern disturbance related to restlessness, headache, and flulike symptoms produced by antiviral drugs.

Planning   During the planning phase expected outcomes specific for the client are established. In addition, teaching and discharge plans are developed. Expected outcomes appropriate for the client receiving antiviral drugs include the following:

- Client appears relaxed and reports anxiety is reduced.
- Client demonstrates measures to monitor fluid status.
- Client verbalizes factors that contribute to injury risk.
- Client verbalizes understanding of disease process and treatment plan.
- Client's ingestion of food is adequate to maintain appropriate weight.
- Client reports improvement in sleep and rest patterns.

Teaching plans should include information about the importance of immunizations for small children and adults at high risk for acquiring influenza. Additionally, the increasing incidence of hepatitis should be addressed in the plans of at-risk populations and communities.

Implementing   You must understand how viruses are transmitted, measures to initiate to prevent transmission, and clinical manifestations of viral diseases. Additionally, remember that nursing measures that promote health and hygiene contribute to the integrity of the host and increase viral resistance.

Monitor the client closely for undesired clinical responses and toxicity associated with antiviral drugs. Monitor renal function, including intake and output. Review results from laboratory studies directed at assessing renal and hepatic function and the integrity of the hemopoietic system. Since many antiviral drugs are metabolized and excreted through the kidneys, adequate fluid intake is essential for preventing renal tubular damage. Intravenous (IV) infusion of antiviral drugs must be monitored closely. Most IV infusions are administered with an infusion pump. Inspect the infusion site carefully for indications of phlebitis and question the client about pain at the injection site.

Evaluating   Evaluation of the plan of care is based on the client's response to therapy, including decreased signs and symptoms of the viral disease and a lack of undesired clinical responses. Discuss with the client and family their perception of the plan and compare the outcome of care with the previously established expected outcomes.

CONCEPT REVIEW

Viruses are major contributors to illness. The severity of viral diseases varies from the common cold to viral encephalitis.

Viral diseases are difficult to treat because viruses become integrated into the host cell. Thus the efficacy of an antiviral drug is determined by its ability to target the virus without damaging the host cell.

NUCLEOSIDE ANALOGS

Nucleoside analogs originally were used as antitumor agents. However, during the 1950s and 1960s their use as antiviral drugs was established. Systemic administration of early nucleoside analogs was associated with significant toxicity because of damage to rapidly dividing host cells. Because of these toxic effects, most original nucleoside analogs have been replaced by alternative antiviral drugs that produce limited interference with host cell DNA metabolism.

Vidarabine

Vidarabine, also known as adenine arabinoside, is one of the oldest antiviral drugs still available. Vidarabine (Vira-A) is a fermentation product of *Streptomyces antibioticus;* it also has been synthesized.[2]

Pharmacotherapeutics Vidarabine is effective in the treatment of herpes simplex virus (HSV-1) encephalitis, neonatal HSV infections, and herpes zoster or varicella in the immunocompromised client. It also is effective as an ophthalmic ointment for acute HSV keratoconjunctivitis. Vidarabine is used less frequently now, for it has been almost exclusively replaced by acyclovir.

Pharmacokinetics After IV administration vidarabine is rapidly changed into arabinosyl hypoxanthine (Ara-Hx), its principal metabolite. This metabolite is quickly distributed into body tissues. Ara-Hx penetrates the cerebrospinal fluid (CSF) to produce a CSF-plasma ratio of approximately 1:3. ARA-Hx has a mean half-life of 3.3 hours. Excretion of the drug is primarily via the kidneys, with 41% to 53% of the daily doses recovered in the urine.[4]

Pharmacodynamics The drug is taken up by mammalian cell in its intact form. It is then phosphorylated intracellularly by cellular enzymes to triphosphate, its active form. Triphosphate inhibits the DNA polymerase of HSV and other herpesviruses and acts as a chain terminator when incorporated into HSV DNA.[4,5]

Pharmaceutics Vidarabine is available in an IV preparation and as a 3% ophthalmic ointment for the treatment of neonatal herpes keratitis.

Undesired clinical responses Common undesired clinical responses associated with IV administration of vidarabine include nausea, vomiting, and diarrhea. Its most serious effect is encephalopathy, which produces headaches, dizziness, confusion, hallucinations, and tremors. Hematologic suppression also occurs, resulting in decreased hemoglobin, granulocyte, and platelet counts. In addition, the results of liver function studies (e.g., serum glutamic-oxaloacetic transaminase) may become elevated.[2,5] Adverse effects to the ophthalmic ointment include itching, redness, swelling, photosensitivity, and burning. Figure 59–2 illustrates undesired clinical responses associated with vidarabine and acyclovir.

Contraindications and precautions IV vidarabine is not recommended for use in clients with preexisting renal or hepatic impairment. It should be administered with care to clients susceptible to fluid overloading or cerebral edema.

Drug-drug interactions Allopurinol may interfere with vidarabine metabolism.

Life-span considerations Vidarabine administered parenterally is classified as a Pregnancy Category C drug. It is not known whether vidarabine is excreted in human milk.

Specific drug-related nursing considerations If the ophthalmic ointment is prescribed, teach the client how to instill the ointment. Instruct the client to wash his or her hands before and after administration of the drug. Also inform the client to expect some hazing of vision until the ointment is distributed and absorbed.[6] Table 59–1 summarizes information about dosage, route of administration, and nursing considerations for vidarabine.

Acyclovir

Acyclovir (Zovirax) is a synthetic acyclic purine nucleoside; it was approved for use in 1982.

Pharmacotherapeutics Acyclovir is recommended for treatment and prevention of HSV-1 and HSV-2. IV acyclovir is indicated for HSV encephalitis, neonatal HSV, and life-threatening HSV and VZV infections in immunocompromised clients.[7,8] Acyclovir has also been used in the treatment of VZV in children and adults.[9]

Oral acyclovir is indicated in the treatment of primary and recurrent genital herpes. Topical acyclovir reduces the duration of primary genital herpes but is not effective against recurrence.[2]

Pharmacokinetics Acyclovir is well absorbed and is distributed to all body tissues. It crosses the placenta and is secreted in breast milk. Plasma concentrations at steady state after oral administration are 0.5 μg/ml at the 200-mg dose and 1.3 μg/ml at the 600-mg dose. The plasma half-life of acyclovir after an oral dose to adults is 3 to 4 hours. More than 80% of the drug dose is eliminated by renal excretion through glomerular filtration and to a lesser extent by tubular secretion. Acyclovir is significantly removed by hemodialysis but is unaffected by peritoneal dialysis.[2,5]

Pharmacodynamics Acyclovir is taken up selectively by cells infected with herpesviruses. Like vidarabine, its activity depends on conversion to the triphosphate form, which interferes with herpesviruses DNA polymerase. In addition, incorporation of the compound into viral DNA results in chain termination. The antiviral specificity of acyclovir for HSV and VZV is enhanced because its phosphorylation is mediated by the viral thymidine kinase of these viruses. Thus phosphoryla-

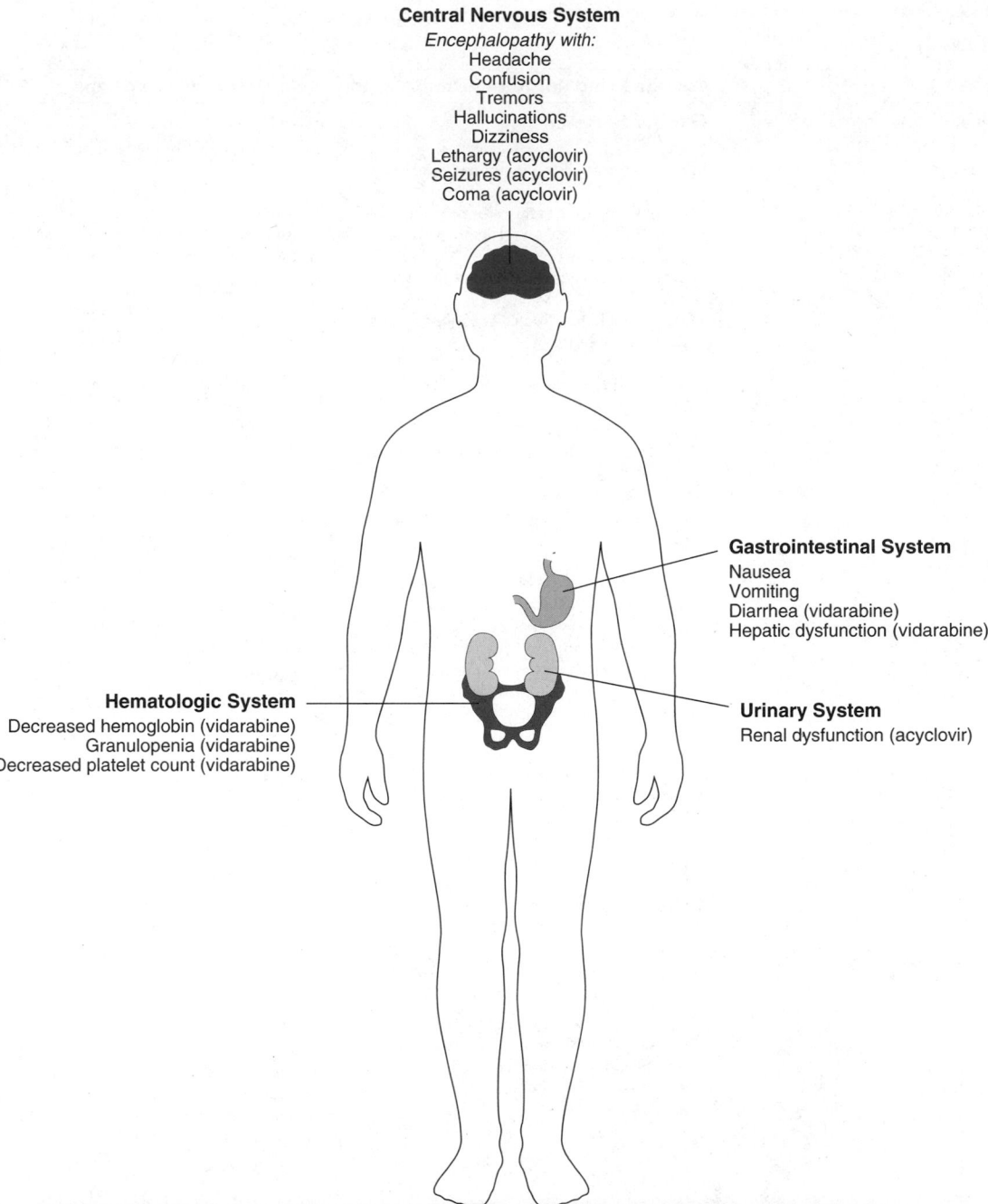

Central Nervous System
Encephalopathy with:
Headache
Confusion
Tremors
Hallucinations
Dizziness
Lethargy (acyclovir)
Seizures (acyclovir)
Coma (acyclovir)

Gastrointestinal System
Nausea
Vomiting
Diarrhea (vidarabine)
Hepatic dysfunction (vidarabine)

Hematologic System
Decreased hemoglobin (vidarabine)
Granulopenia (vidarabine)
Decreased platelet count (vidarabine)

Urinary System
Renal dysfunction (acyclovir)

FIGURE 59–2   Undesired clinical responses associated with vidarabine and acyclovir.

tion of acyclovir occurs mainly in virus-infected cells, sparing cells not infected with the virus.[2]

Pharmaceutics   Acyclovir is available as a capsule, uncoated tablet, or suspension for oral administration. It is also available as an IV preparation and in a 5% topical ointment.

Undesired clinical responses   Common undesired clinical responses include nausea, vomiting, and headache. If administered in excessive dosages or infused rapidly, acyclovir can precipitate in the renal tubules. An increase in serum creatinine levels and a decrease in creatinine clearance reflects impaired renal function. A few cases of encephalopathy, with signs of lethargy, tremors, hallucination, seizures, and coma, have been reported in clients with deficient renal clearance. Extravasation of the drug into soft tissues can produce severe cutaneous lesions.[2,10] Figure 59–2 illustrates undesired clinical responses associated with vidarabine and acyclovir.

Contraindications and precautions   Acyclovir is not recommended for clients with preexisting renal impairment. Additionally, it must be used with caution in clients susceptible to fluid overloading.

Drug-drug and drug-environment interactions   Concurrent administration of acyclovir with drugs that reduce re-

TABLE 59–1
Antiviral Drugs

Drug Name	Dosage* and Route of Administration	Nursing Considerations
ACYCLOVIR (Zovirax) **HOW SUPPLIED** Capsule: 200 mg Uncoated tablet: 800 mg Oral suspension: 200 mg/5 ml Topical ointment: 5% IV: 1000 mg/vial, 500 mg	**Genital Herpes** ORAL Initial treatment: 200 mg q4h five times daily for 10 d Chronic suppressive therapy for recurrent disease: 400 mg two times daily for up to 12 mo, followed by re-evaluation Intermittent therapy: 200 mg q4h five times daily for 5 d Therapy should be initiated at earliest sign or symptom of recurrence IV Severe initial clinical episode *Adults* 5 mg/kg infused at a constant rate over 1h q8h (15 mg/kg/d) for 5 d in clients with normal renal function *Children 12 y or younger* 250 mg/m² at a constant rate over 1h q8h (750 mg/m²/d) for 5 d TOPICAL Approximately ½-in ribbon of ointment per 4 square inches of surface area, applied to cover all lesions q3h six times a day for 7 d; ointment must be applied with a finger cot or rubber glove to prevent autoinoculation of other body sites or transmission of disease **Herpes Zoster** ORAL 800 mg q4h five times daily for 7-10 d IV IN IMMUNOCOMPROMISED CLIENTS *Adult with normal renal function* 10 mg/kg infused at a constant rate over 1 h q8h for 7 d (obese patients dosed by ideal body weight) *Children 12 y or younger* 500 mg/m² at a constant rate over at least 1 h q8h for 7 d Do not exceed a maximum dose equivalent to 500 mg/m² q8h for any client	**Assess** Review results from renal function and electrolyte studies. Determine if client is pregnant; acyclovir is classified as a Pregnancy Category C drug. Assess for concomitant use of other nephrotoxic drugs, preexisting renal disease, and dehydration. **Implement** Reconstitute acyclovir sodium for injection with sterile water for injection. Once reconstituted, use drug within 12 h. Add calculated IV dose to any appropriate IV solution. Infusion concentrations of approximately 7 mg/ml or lower are recommended. Once diluted for administration, use within 24 h. Administer IV infusion over a period of 60 min. Monitor urinary output carefully for first 2 h after infusion. Recommended output is >500 mg/g of drug infused. Assess infusion site for inflammation and phlebitis. Teach client the importance of adequate fluid intake. Teach client to apply ointment with rubber glove or finger cot. **Monitor** Monitor results of laboratory studies. Monitor for undesired clinical responses: transient elevation of creatinine clearance, nausea, vomiting, itching, rash, hives, lethargy, confusion, hallucinations. **Evaluate** Assess for diminished clinical manifestations of herpes infection.
Ribavirin (Virazole) **HOW SUPPLIED** Solution: 6 g/dl vial	20 mg/ml as starting solution in the drug reservoir of the SPAG-2 unit, with continuous aerosol administration for 12-18 h/d for 3-7 d (approximately 190 μg/L of air for a 12-h delivery period)	**Assess** Determine if client is pregnant or may become pregnant during exposure to drug. Ribavirin is classified as a Pregnancy Category X drug and is not completely cleared from human blood even 4 wk after administration. **Implement** Mix drug with sterile water for injection or inhalation. Administer aerosol via oxygen hood, face mask, or oxygen tent. Administer only with Viratek Small Particle Aerosol Generator. Do not administer ribavirin aerosol with any other aerosol generating device or with other aerosolized drugs. **Monitor** Monitor for undesired clinical responses: worsening of respiratory status, hypotension, pneumothorax. **Evaluate** Assess for improved respiratory status.

*Dosages are adjusted for clients with renal dysfunction. Dosage based on creatinine clearance.

TABLE 59–1 *Continued*
Antiviral Drugs

Drug Name	Dosage* and Route of Administration	Nursing Considerations
Vidarabine (Vira-A) **HOW SUPPLIED** IV: 200 mg/ml Ophthalmic ointment: 3%	**Herpes Simplex Encephalitis** IV: 15 mg/kg/d for 15 d; dose is administered slowly (over 12-24 h) **Herpes Zoster** IV: 10 mg/kg/d for 5 d administered slowly (over 12-24 h) **Ophthalmic Ointment** Administer approximately ½ in of 3% ointment into lower conjunctival sac five times daily at 3-h intervals	**Assess** Determine if client has preexisting renal or hepatic impairment. Determine if client is receiving allopurinol, which may interfere with vidarabine metabolism. Determine if client is pregnant; vidarabine is classified as a Pregnancy Category C drug. **Implement** Dilute drug solution with an appropriate IV solution. Prewarm IV infusion fluid to 35° to 40° C before mixing with drug. Drug dilution should be made just before administration and used at least within 48 h. *Do not refrigerate dilution.* Slowly infuse total daily dose at a constant rate over a 12- to 24-h period. **Monitor** Carefully monitor clients susceptible to fluid overloading or cerebral edema. Monitor results of laboratory studies: hematocrit, hemoglobin, white blood cell count, and platelet count. Monitor client for undesired clinical responses associated with parenteral drug: anorexia, nausea, vomiting, diarrhea, tremor, dizziness, confusion. Monitor client for undesired clinical responses associated with ophthalmic ointment: burning.

nal clearance (e.g., amphotericin) may raise the plasma and renal concentrations of acyclovir. Probenecid reduces the excretion of acyclovir.[2] Acyclovir must be protected from light and moisture and stored at 15° to 25° C.

Life-span considerations Acyclovir is classified as a Pregnancy Category C drug. Concentrations of the drug have been found in breast milk; therefore it should be used with caution in nursing women. Additionally, elderly clients are more susceptible to the renal impairment produced by acyclovir.

Specific drug-related nursing considerations Maximum urinary concentration of acyclovir occurs within the first 2 hours after IV infusion. During this time it is recommended that urinary output be >500 ml per gram of drug infused. Consequently, you must encourage the client to consume an adequate oral intake of fluids. Monitor the client's pattern of urinary elimination and intake and output. Report changes in urinary output or pattern to the primary care provider. In addition, since some clients develop encephalopathy, assess the client frequently for changes in his or her mental status. Note complaints of headache, dizziness, and lethargy.

Acyclovir parenteral solution must not be administered IM or SC; it must be administered only intravenously. IV infusions must be administered over a period of at least 1 hour to reduce the risk of renal tubular damage. When possible, use an infusion pump to prevent too rapid infusion of the drug. Assess the infusion site carefully for indications of phlebitis or irritation.

Instruct the client receiving acyclovir for herpesvirus lesions to complete the entire course of the drug and to avoid missing doses. Provide female clients being treated for genital herpes information about the possible link between genital herpes and cervical cancer. Inform these clients of the importance of annual Papanicolaou testing. Teach the client to wear a latex glove or finger cot when applying topical acyclovir. This technique prevents contact spread of the virus to unaffected skin areas. Instruct the client to wear loose-fitting clothes to avoid irritation of skin or mucocutaneous lesions.[11] Table 59–1 summarizes information about dosage, route of administration, and nursing considerations for acyclovir.

Ribavirin

Ribavirin (Virazole) is a synthesized nucleoside analog.

Pharmacotherapeutics Ribavirin is recommended for the aerosolized treatment of lower respiratory tract disease caused by RSV. Multiple clinical trials have reported significant improvement in the client's respiratory status, including decreased ventilatory support time and reduced morbidity and mortality.[12–14] Ribavirin is not approved for use in infants with RSV pneumonia who require assisted ventilation. Given systemically, it is highly effective for the treatment of Lassa fever, a rare arenavirus infection. Other reported uses include the treatment of influenza A and influenza B.[2,5]

Pharmacokinetics When administered orally, ribavirin is quickly absorbed via the gastrointestinal (GI) tract, with peak plasma concentrations occurring in 1 to 2 hours. Ribavirin is actively taken up by erythrocytes when administered orally or IV, with the half-life in these cells 40 days. The drug is found in plasma after 3 or more days of aerosol treatment. Concentration levels in the plasma depend on method of administration and number of hours of treatment. However, plasma concentrations are usually 1000-fold lower than concentrations in respiratory secretions. Most ribavirin is excreted unchanged in the urine regardless of the route of administration.[2,5]

Pharmacodynamics Ribavirin has broad activity against both RNA and DNA viruses. However, RNA viruses are generally more susceptible to ribavirin.[2] The drug is phosphorylated intracellularly by cellular enzymes into the triphosphate form and other active antiviral forms. The active forms of ribavirin interfere with RNA and DNA synthesis, prohibiting viral replication.[4,15,16]

Pharmaceutics Ribavirin is prepared as oral, IV, and aerosol dosage forms. Only the aerosol dosage form is currently available in the United States.[2] Aerosol treatment is provided via a small-particle aerosol generator attached to an oxygen hood, mask, or tent.[15] When used with a mechanical ventilator, ribavirin has produced serious mechanical interference because the drug precipitates in the ventilator.

Undesired clinical responses Few undesired clinical responses have been attributed to ribavirin aerosol treatments. Some clients have experienced rashes and conjunctivitis. Additionally, deterioration of respiratory function has been documented in some infants and adults.

Contraindications and precautions Ribavirin is contraindicated in females who are or may become pregnant.

Drug-drug and drug-environment interactions Minimal evaluation of drug-drug interactions involving ribavirin has been conducted. However, when administered by aerosol, ribavirin produces an occupational hazard for health care personnel. Individuals responsible for administering the drug have reported eye irritation, headache, sneezing, and precipitation and damage to contact lenses.[15-17]

Life-span considerations Ribavirin is classified as a Pregnancy Category X drug. Use of ribavirin in nursing mothers is not indicated because RSV infection is self-limiting in this population.[5]

Specific drug-related nursing considerations Nursing actions are directed toward safe administration of ribavirin and protection of self and others from unnecessary exposure. Monitor the client continuously to determine the effectiveness of treatment. Assess the client's respiratory and cardiovascular status and examine the eyes for evidence of irritation.

Adhere strictly to manufacturer's guidelines for the use of aerosol devices and hoods. In addition, initiate measures to minimize the exposure of health care workers and visitors to the aerosolized drug. The use of a high-efficiency respiratory mask, goggles for contact lens wearers, signs alerting visitors, and specific cautions for children and pregnant women not to enter a room where ribavirin is being administered are some recommended measures.[16] Table 59–1 summarizes information about dosage, route of administration, and nursing considerations for ribavirin.

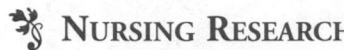

NURSING RESEARCH

Arnold, S.D., & Alonso, R. (1993). Ribavirin aerosol: Methods for reducing employee exposure. *American Association of Occupational Health Nursing Journal, 41,* 382-392.

The purpose of this study was to investigate the effectiveness of two different exhaust-control methods for removing excess ribavirin from treatment rooms. The two hoods evaluated were the Matlock reusable double hood and the Torres enclosure tent. Three air samples were obtained in each 8-hour period of ribavirin therapy. The air samples were obtained from the head of the bed, the foot of the bed, and the breathing area of the client receiving therapy.

Data analysis revealed that both devices were effective in reducing room air concentrations. Furthermore, employees involved in the study found both methods easy to handle. However, they voiced a preference for the Matlock double hood.

STUDENT ACTIVITIES

- Determine what health care providers administer ribavirin at your assigned agency.
- Investigate precautions taken to diminish the danger of accidental exposure to the aerosolized drug.
- Research the topic of employee exposure to ribavirin and develop a list of protective measures to share with your agency.

CONCEPT REVIEW

The nucleoside analogs presented in this chapter—vidarabine, acyclovir, and ribavirin—inhibit viral replication.

The triphosphate form is the active compound in vidarabine. Vidarabine use is being replaced by that of acyclovir, which has less severe undesired clinical responses.

Acyclovir is taken up selectively by cells infected with herpesvirus. Its activity depends on conversion to the triphosphate form. Acyclovir can precipitate in the renal tubules.

Ribavirin is indicated in the treatment of RSV pneumonia. In contrast to vidarabine and acyclovir, ribavirin has broad activity against both RNA and DNA viruses.

INTERFERONS

Interferons constitute a family of glycoproteins made by mammalian cells exposed to viruses, double-stranded RNA, and other compounds. The interferons, classified as **interferon alfa-2a** (Roferon-A), **interferon alfa-2b** (Intron A), and **in-**

terferon **alfa-N3** (Alferon N), possess antiviral and immunoregulatory properties.[2,18]

Although they have similar pharmacologic properties, each group of interferons is unique in given situations. Like many of the other antiviral drugs, the interferon's primary mode of action is to inhibit viral replication. Approved uses for the interferons include the treatment of hairy cell leukemia (alfa-2a and alfa-2b), Kaposi's sarcoma (alfa-2a and alfa-2b), condylomata acuminata (alfa-2b and alfa-N3), and chronic hepatitis non-A, non-B hepatitis, or hepatitis C (alfa-2b).[19]

Interferons are administered parenterally, through either the SC or IM routes, or intralesionally. With SC or IM routes, plasma levels are achieved after approximately 4 hours. Administered by these routes, interferons are filtered and reabsorbed in the renal tubules, leading to systemic circulation of intact interferons. Intralesional use produces minor systemic effects. Dosage for all three classifications of interferons is determined by the underlying pathology.

Interferon alfa-2a and interferon alfa-2b, which are effective against hairy cell leukemia and Kaposi's sarcoma, are discussed further in Chapter 69. Since interferon alfa-N3 is derived from human leukocytes, it is designated a *natural interferon.* It is indicated in the treatment of refractory or recurring external condylomata acuminata—genital or venereal warts. These warts, associated with human papilloma virus infection, are highly contagious.

Even though genital warts usually begin to disappear after several weeks of treatment, treatment should continue for a maximum of 8 weeks. Some clients experience improvement after cessation of treatment; therefore repeat treatment is usually not started for 3 months after the last treatment session.

Common undesired clinical responses associated with interferon alfa-N3 include flulike symptoms (i.e., fever, myalgias, headache, and dizziness). Back pain, insomnia, sensitivity to allergens, disruptions in menstrual cycle, decreased serum estradiol and progesterone levels, depression, GI disturbances, leukopenia, and thrombocytopenia have also been reported.[20] Interferon alfa-N3 should be used with caution in individuals with debilitating medical conditions or coagulation disorders. It is not recommended during pregnancy; very high doses can cause abortion.

Interferon alfa-N3 is injected into the base of each wart. Care should be taken to select injection sites without previous trauma and to assess sites for signs of irritation. (See Table 59–2 for information on administration of interferon alfa-2b and interferon alfa-N3.) In some situations, clients are taught to self-administer the injections. If so, provide instructions about the procedure for preparation and administration of an injection and about safe disposal of needles and syringes. In addition, advise the client that a temporary loss of hair may accompany therapy. Normal hair growth is expected after the drug is discontinued.[11]

AMANTADINE HYDROCHLORIDE

Amantadine (Symmetrel) is an antiviral drug also known for its therapeutic effectiveness in the treatment of Parkinson's disease. (For information on amantadine's pharmacokinetic properties, contraindications and precautions, and drug interactions, refer to Chapter 23.)

Pharmacotherapeutics Amantadine shortens the course of the fever, cough, and sore throat that accompany influenza.

TABLE 59–2
Administration of Interferon Alfa-2b and Interferon Alfa-N3

Drug and Clinical Indications	Nursing Considerations
Interferon alfa-2b, recombinant (Intron-A)	Store drug at 2° to 8° C before and after reconstitution.
Treatment of condylomata acuminata involving external surfaces of genital and perianal areas	Dilute drug with bacteriostatic water; agitate gently to dissolve powder completely.
	Reconstitute 10 million IU vial with 1 ml diluent.
	Inject 1 million IU (0.1 ml of reconstituted drug) into each lesion three times per week on alternate days for 3 wk.
	Injection is intralesional, using tuberculin or similar syringe with a 25- to 30-gauge needle. Direct needle at center of base of lesion and at an angle almost parallel to plane of skin.
Treatment of chronic hepatitis non-A, non-B (hepatitis C)	Use 3 million IU vial and dilute with 1 ml diluent.
	Inject 3 million IU three times per week SC or IM.
	Usually treatment lasts for 6 mo.
Interferon alfa-N3 (Alferon N)	Before client receives first dose, check for previous reactions to human interferon alfa, mouse immunoglobulin, eggs, and neomycin.
Treatment of external condylomata in clients >18 y old	Teach client signs and symptoms of hypersensitivity reactions (hives, itching, difficulty breathing). Tell client to go to emergency room or contact primary care provider if they occur.
	Use injectable solution containing 5 million IU per vial.
	Inject 0.05 ml (250,000 IU) into base of wart. Admiister two times per week for up to 8 wk. Maximum recommended dose per treatment session is 0.5 ml.
	Use same injection technique as described for interferon alfa-2b.

It is also recommended as a prophylactic drug for clinical populations at high risk for pulmonary complications of influenza: nursing home residents, individuals with chronic pulmonary or cardiovascular disease, and individuals who did not receive the influenza vaccination.[10,21,22] Amantadine is also recommended for health care workers in chronic care and nursing home facilities.

Pharmacodynamics The exact mechanism of amantadine's antiviral activity is not well understood. It is believed to interfere with the uncoating of the influenza A virus and therefore its replication.[5]

Pharmaceutics Amantadine is administered orally in capsule or syrup form. The dosages for individuals with renal insufficiency and the elderly should be adjusted according to creatine clearance values to prevent renal compromise. The drug should be initiated within 24 to 48 hours after the onset of flulike symptoms and continued for the same period after symptoms have dissipated. Dosages for prophylaxis and symptomatic relief are as follows:

- Adults and children 9 to 12 years: 100 mg bid
- Children 1 to 9 years: 4.4 to 8.8 mg/kg/d

Undesired clinical responses Undesired clinical responses include nausea, dizziness, lightheadedness, unsteady gait, and insomnia.[5,22]

Life-span considerations Amantadine can cross the placenta and can be secreted in breast milk.[5]

Specific drug-related nursing considerations Before initiating amantadine therapy, determine if the client has a history of seizures or renal dysfunction. A positive history for either one may preclude safe administration of the drug. In addition, a recent evaluation of renal function in the elderly is recommended.

Caution the client about the concurrent use of alcohol; this combination may increase the side effects of dizziness and lightheadedness. Instruct the client to change positions slowly to avoid falls precipitated by the lightheadedness. If the client complains of dry mouth or throat, suggest increased ingestion of oral fluids and the use of hard candies or gum. The client who experiences a decrease in concentration should be cautioned about operating a motor vehicle while taking this drug.[11]

🌿 NURSING RESEARCH

Flaherty, E. (1990). Amantadine attack on influenza A. *Geriatric Nursing, 11,* 253-254.

During an influenza outbreak at a Jewish Home and Hospital for Aged, prophylactic use of amantadine hydrochloride, 100 mg once daily, was initiated. Although the initial treatment was limited to residents in one ward, the subsequent spread of the epidemic resulted in the treatment of 423 of 514 residents with amantadine. Subjects with a previous history of seizure disorders or renal disease were excluded from the treatment protocol.

After 14 days of treatment, 9% of the subjects had to discontinue the drug because of undesired clinical responses. The drug was discontinued for other reasons in an additional 29 subjects. Data analysis after the epidemic indicated that 18% of those who received the drug developed pulmonary complications from the influenza. In contrast, a total of 44% of the subjects who did not receive the drug developed significant flulike syndromes.

STUDENT ACTIVITIES

- Contact four local nursing homes and determine prophylactic measures used against influenza A.
- Contact the local health department and determine recommendations regarding influenza A. 🌿

CONCEPT REVIEW

Interferons possess antiviral and immunoregulatory properties. Their primary mode of action is to inhibit viral replication.

Amantadine hydrochloride is used to shorten the course of the fever, cough, and sore throat that accompany influenza.

OPHTHALMIC ANTIVIRAL DRUGS

Idoxuridine and trifluridine are antiviral drugs used for ocular infections.

Idoxuridine

Idoxuridine (Herplex) is indicated only in the treatment of herpes simplex keratitis. It inhibits replication of HSV by irreversibly inhibiting the incorporation of thymidine into the viral DNA. Idoxuridine is available as an ophthalmic solution.

Idoxuridine should be administered with caution in pregnancy or in women of childbearing age. It is not known if the drug is secreted in human milk. Occasionally irritation, pain, pruritus, inflammation, or edema is experienced in the eye or

---

IDOXURIDINE DOSAGE AND ADMINISTRATION

Ophthalmic 0.1% Solution
Initially instill 1 drop in infected eye every hour during the day and q2h at night. Continue this dosage until improvement has occurred. Then reduce dosage to 1 drop q2h during the day and q4h at night. Therapy should be continued at this reduced dosage for 3 to 5 days after healing apparently is complete.

lid. Allergic reactions are rare, but photophobia has been reported.

Instruct the client in proper administration of the drug, stressing the importance of medical asepsis. Advise the client that gentle closing of the eye for 1 to 2 minutes after instillation improves the drug's effectiveness. Teach the client how to assess for signs of irritation and healing. Caution the client that concurrent administration of other ophthalmic drugs is not advised without approval from the primary care provider. Tell the client to store the ophthalmic solution in the refrigerator.

Trifluridine

Trifluridine (Viroptic) is a pyrimidine nucleoside antiviral ophthalmic solution. It interferes with DNA synthesis in cultured mammalian cells. However, its antiviral mechanism of action is not completely known. Trifluridine is indicated for the treatment of primary keratoconjunctivitis and recurrent epithelial keratitis caused by HSV-1 and HSV-2.[3]

Trifluridine is well tolerated, with few undesired clinical responses. The most frequent responses are mild transient burning or stinging upon instillation and palpebral édema. Trifluridine should be used with caution in pregnant and lactating women.[3]

TRIFLURIDINE DOSAGE AND ADMINISTRATION

Ophthalmic 1% Solution
Instill 1 drop onto cornea of infected eye q2h while awake for a maximum daily dosage of 9 drops. When corneal ulcer has completely reepithelialized, treat for another 7 days with 1 drop q4h while awake for a maximum daily dosage of 5 drops.

SUMMARY

Viruses produce many of the common diseases that affect humans. Even though viral diseases are common, the number of antiviral drugs is limited. Most antiviral drugs prevent replication of the virus by inhibiting DNA or RNA material or both. These same drugs are also capable of altering host-cell DNA metabolism.

REFERENCES

1. McCance, K., & Huether, S. (1993). *Pathophysiology: The biologic basis for disease in adults and children* (2nd ed.). St. Louis: Mosby.
2. Arvin, A. (1992). Antiviral Drugs. In C.M. Smith and A.M. Reynard (Eds.), *Textbook of pharmacology* (pp. 900-912). Philadelphia: W.B. Saunders.
3. Data Pharmaceutica, Inc. (1993). *1993 physicians' genRx*. Smithtown, NY: Author.
4. Arvin, A., Corey, L., & Hirschman, S. (1992). Using today's antivirals. *Patient Care, 26*(19), 28-30, 35-36, 40-42.
5. United States Pharmacopeial Convention, Inc. (1994). *USP DI* (14th ed.). *Vol. 1. Drug Information for the Health Care Professional.* Taunton, MA: Author.
6. Micromedex Inc. (1993). *Drug Evaluation Monographs, 76,* Author.
7. Dominquez, H.A., & Keitel, W.A. (1991). Management guidelines for primary and recurrent episodes. *Consultant, 31*(10), 21-30.
8. Whitley, R.J., & Gnann, J.W. (1992). Acyclovir: A decade later. *New England Journal of Medicine, 327,* 782-789.
9. Dunkle, L.M., Arvin, A.M., Whitley, R., & McGuirt, P.V. (1991). A controlled trial of acyclovir for chickenpox in normal children. *New England Journal of Medicine, 325,* 1539-1544.
10. Postic, B. (1990). Reviewing the use of amantadine, acyclovir, ganciclovir, and zidovudine. *Consultant, 30*(6), 43-50.
11. United States Pharmacopeial Convention, Inc. (1993). *USP DI* (4th ed.). *Vol. 2. Advice for the Patient: Drug Information in Lay Language.* Taunton, MA: Author.
12. Groothuis, J.R., Woodin, K.A., Katz, R., Robertson, A.D., McBride, J.T., Hall, C.B., McWilliams, B.C., & Lauer, B.A. (1990). Early ribavirin treatment of respiratory syncytial viral infections in high-risk children. *Journal of Pediatrics, 117,* 792-798.
13. Sanchez, J.L., Kacica, M.A., Walsh, R.F., & Leprow, M.L. (1992). *Thirty-Second Interscience Conference on Antimicrobial Agents and Chemotherapy (ICAAC).* Unpublished Research.
14. Smith, D.W., Frankel, L.R., Mathers, L.H., Tang, A.T., Ariagno, R.L., & Prober, C.G. (1991). A controlled trial of aerosolized ribavirin in infants receiving mechanical ventilation for severe respiratory syncytial virus infection. *New England Journal of Medicine, 325,* 24-29.
15. Cohen, B.A., & Brady, M. (1992). Practices surrounding ribavirin administration. *Pediatric Nursing, 18,* 253-257.
16. Jury, D.L. (1993). More on RSV and ribavirin. *Pediatric Nursing, 19,* 89-92.
17. Arnold, S.D., & Alonso, R. (1993). Ribavirin aerosol: Methods for reducing employee exposure. *American Association of Occupational Health Nursing Journal, 41,* 382-392.
18. Vitale, M.K., Willwerth-Fortin, J., & Robbins, K. (1993). Management of children on interferon therapy. *Pediatric Nursing, 19,* 230-234.
19. Medical Letter, Inc. (1992). *The medical letter: On drugs and therapeutics, 34*(867), 31-36.
20. Kaplan, M.M. (1993). Twelve questions physicians often ask. *Consultant, 33*(3), 145-152.
21. Blake, G.J. (1990). Amantadine for influenza A. *Nursing '90, 20*(12), 21.
22. Flaherty, E. (1990). Amantadine attack on influenza A. *Geriatric Nursing, 11,* 253-254.

BIBLIOGRAPHY

Anselmo, A.M. (1992). Ganciclovir: Handle with care. *American Journal of Nursing, 92*(5), 16.
Dudak, L.A. (1992). New roles for interferon-alpha? *American Journal of Nursing, 92*(2), 16.
Lietman, P. (1992). Clinical pharmacology: Foscarnet. *American Journal of Medicine, 92*(2A), 85-115.
Plona, R.P., & Schremp, P.S. (1992). Nursing care of patients with ocular manifestations of human immunodeficiency virus infection. *Nursing Clinics of North America, 27,* 793-805.
Ward, C. (1992). Influenza: The unwanted visitor. *Geriatric Nursing, 13,* 329-331.

CHAPTER 60

Antiparasitic Drugs

NORMA L. PINNELL • JUNE HERTELL

⊛ **Parasitic Infections**

LEARNING OBJECTIVE: Identify major organisms that cause parasitic infections.

⊛ **Helminth Infections**

LEARNING OBJECTIVES:

Discuss the three groups of helminth organisms.

Develop a plan of care for a client requiring anthelmintic drugs.

Describe the pharmacodynamic properties of major drugs used to treat intestinal nematode infections.

Describe the pharmacodynamic properties of major drugs used to treat blood and tissue nematode infections.

Discuss the pharmacodynamic properties of drugs used to treat cestode infections.

Explain the pharmacodynamic properties of drugs used to treat trematode infections.

KEY TERMS:

Cestode, nematode, trematode

⊛ **Protozoan Infections**

LEARNING OBJECTIVES:

Identify nursing diagnoses appropriate for the client requiring antiprotozoan drugs.

Describe the pharmacodynamic properties of major drugs used to treat protozoan infections.

Match the drug of choice with each protozoan infection.

CONCEPTS AND TERMS TO REVIEW

Review Chapter 49, Overview of Biologic Defense Mechanisms.

Read Chapter 54, Principles of Antimicrobial Therapy.

Read section on parasites in a general biology textbook.

---

*P*arasites are representative of four phyla: the Protozoa, or single-celled organisms; the Nematoda, or roundworms; the Platyhelminthes, or flatworms; and the Arthropoda, or invertebrate animals with jointed appendages. Parasites live on or in the human body during some part of their life cycle and depend on the human host for shelter and sustenance. Human infections caused by some parasites are serious health problems, particularly in the underdeveloped countries of the world.

PARASITIC INFECTIONS

Multiple environmental factors affect the prevalence of parasitic infections (e.g., hot and humid climatic conditions, over-

crowded living conditions, improper sewage disposal, lack of clean water, and consumption of contaminated raw meat or vegetables).[1] Symptoms of parasitic infection depend on the area in which infestation develops. For example, protozoan infestation of the gastrointestinal (GI) tract produces cramping, abdominal pain, and bloody diarrhea. Infestation of the blood produces fever, chills, rigor, and eventually anemia. The nutritional and immune status of the host also affects the symptoms and aggressiveness of the parasitic infection. Identification of the infectious agent is usually accomplished by visualizing either the adult parasite or its ova. This is done by direct observation or by microscopic examination.[1] Table 60–1 summarizes various parasitic infections of humans.

HELMINTH INFECTIONS

Infections caused by helminths can be located in small intestine, lungs, cecum, eye, muscles, lymphatics, liver, urinary tract, or blood vessels of the gut. In addition, the skin is a common site for helminth infection.

Classification of Helminths

Helminths that cause human infections are divided into three general groups: nematodes (roundworms), trematodes (flukes), and cestodes (tapeworms). **Nematodes** are members of the class Nematoda and include true roundworms or threadworms. Nematodes are cylindrical or spindle shaped. Most nematodes exist as separate male and female sexes.

Trematodes (flukes) are parasitic worms that belong to the class Trematoda. In humans they can infect the blood, intestinal tract, liver, or lungs. There are two types of trematodes; one is external or semiexternal, and the other is internal. Both types develop asexually. Blood flukes are called *schistosoma*.

Cestodes comprise a subclass of the class Cestoidea. These worms have a scolex (head) and a chain of segments. They are hermaphroditic, containing both male and female sex organs.

▨ NURSING CONSIDERATIONS

Much of the care of individuals with parasitic infections focuses on education—teaching the individual how to avoid future infections and how to prevent spread of the current infection.

Assessing You must complete a health history and physical assessment before the onset of drug therapy administration. The data help determine if subsequent client responses are related to the underlying illness or are adverse reactions to the drug treatment regimen.

While obtaining the **health history**, obtain information about the client's past medical history. Determine the client's knowledge of parasitic infections and the proposed drug treatment.

Obtain a thorough nutritional assessment, including information on the client's fluid and electrolyte status. Also collect a complete drug history. Ask if the client has experienced allergic reactions to any drugs in the past. Review all of the client's drugs. Determine if potential risks of interactions exist. Ask the client if previous medical treatment was sought, and determine if the client used over-the-counter (OTC) drugs in an attempt to relieve signs and symptoms of the infection.

Question the client about the presence of fever, weakness, malaise, or weight loss. Determine if the client has any pulmonary involvement. Ask about shortness of breath, cough, sputum production, hemoptysis, or aching chest pain. Also ask the client if GI symptoms such as nausea, vomiting, abdominal cramping, anorexia, diarrhea, or constipation exist.

Review the results of any diagnostic tests that are conducted (e.g., culture and sensitivity, urinalysis, biopsy). Since some drugs affect renal, hepatic, and hematologic functions, examine the results of baseline electrolyte studies, complete blood count (CBC), and renal and hepatic function tests.

During the physical assessment carefully examine any areas of the body where an infection would be suspected. Note areas of redness, scaling, warmth, or tenderness on the skin. Auscultate the client's lungs. Obtain baseline blood pressure, pulse, respirations, and temperature.

Diagnosing After completing the client assessment, analyze the data and identify specific nursing diagnoses. Examples of nursing diagnoses appropriate for clients receiving antifungal drugs follow:
- Body image disturbance related to presence of skin rashes.
- Impaired skin integrity related to scratching of rashes.
- High risk for infection related to impaired skin integrity.
- Altered nutrition: less than body requirements related to anorexia, nausea, or vomiting associated with drug therapy.
- Fluid volume deficit related to anorexia, nausea, and vomiting associated with drug therapy or infectious process.
- Anxiety related to lack of knowledge regarding antiparasitic drug therapy.

Planning During the planning phase develop a plan of care that incorporates the identified nursing diagnoses and relevant goals of therapy. In addition, develop a discharge or teaching plan. Teaching should include basic hygienic measures. In addition, advise the client to launder bed linens, towels, washcloths, underwear, and nightclothes daily and to disinfect toilet bowls daily.

The ideal overall goal of antiparasitic drug therapy is that the fungal infection will be eradicated or controlled. The following expected outcome criteria may be applicable:
- Client has intact skin, free of lesions.
- Client identifies interventions to reduce risk of infection.
- Client demonstrates techniques to reduce risk of infection.
- Client participates in recommended treatment plan.
- Client reports improved sense of energy.
- Client maintains body weight.
- Client maintains fluid volume at a functional level.
- Client reestablishes normal pattern of bowel functioning.
- Client reports anxiety is reduced.

Implementing The type of infection and the drug preparation prescribed dictate what interventions are required. Familiarize yourself with diagnostic tests ordered for clients with parasitic infections. Also familiarize yourself with proper drug administration techniques.

To prevent spread of these infections, orient yourself to the infectious process involved in the particular infection being treated. What is the infectious agent? The reservoir? The portal of exit? The portal of entry? The susceptible host? Practice proper hygiene techniques and universal precautions.

The client with a superficial infection may experience extreme discomfort related to the itching that occurs. Apply the prescribed drug preparation as frequently as possible. The client with a systemic infection usually experiences fever, pulmonary complications, fatigue, or malaise. You may need to administer antipyretics to reduce the fever. In addition, use other appropriate cooling measures (e.g., reduce environmental temperature, decrease bed coverings, and promote air circulation).

Evaluating Ongoing evaluations are an integral part of the nursing care of the client with a parasitic infection. Examine the outcome criteria identified in the planning stage to see if they have been accomplished. In addition, evaluate the individualized response of the client to the infection and to the antiparasitic agents.

TABLE 60–1
Parasitic Infections

Parasitic Agent	Common Name of Disease	Location of Infection	Symptoms	Mode of Transmission
HELMINTHS (WORMS)				
Nematodes (Roundworms)				
Ancylostoma duodenale	Hookworm	Blood vessels of gut	Anemia	Skin penetration
Ascaris lumbricoides	Giant roundworm	Small intestine, lungs	Pneumonitis (rare), intestinal obstruction (rare)	Oral (fecal contamination), auto-infection
Enterobius vermicularis	Pinworm	Cecum	Anal pruritus	Oral
Onchocerca volvulus	River blindness	Skin, eye	Blindness	Insect inoculation
Strongyloides stercoralis	Strongyloidiasis	Small intestine, lungs	Eosinophilia, urticaria, rash, abdominal pain, pneumonitis	Skin penetration, auto-infection
Trichinella spiralis	Trichinosis	Muscles	Muscular pain, eosinophilia, fever, periorbital edema	Oral (infected meat)
Trichuris trichiura	Whipworm	Intestine	Rectal prolapse	Oral (fecal contamination)
Wuchereria bancrofti	Filariasis	Lymphatics	Elephantiasis	Insect (mosquito)
Trematodes				
Clonorchis sinensis	Liver fluke	Liver	Biliary obstruction (rare)	Oral—raw fish
Fasciola hepatica	Liver fluke	Liver	Fever, right upper quadrant abdominal pain, eosinophilia	Oral
Fasciolopsis buski	Intestinal fluke	Liver	Abdominal pain, diarrhea	Oral
Paragonimus westermani	Lung fluke	Lung, intestine	Eosinophilia, cough, chest pain, bronchitis	Oral—poorly cooked freshwater crab or crayfish
Schistosoma haematobium	Blood fluke	Urinary tract	Acute: rash, fever, cough, chills	Skin inoculation
Schistosoma japonicum	Blood fluke	Mesenteric blood vessels	Hepatomegaly, splenomegaly	Skin inoculation
Schistosoma mansoni	Blood fluke	Mesenteric blood vessels	Lymphadenopathy, eosinophilia	Skin inoculation
Cestodes (Tapeworms)				
Diphyllobothrium latum	Fish tapeworm	Intestine	Megaloblastic anemia	Oral—poorly cooked fish
Taenia saginata	Beef tapeworm	Intestine	Mild abdominal pain	Oral—poorly cooked beef
Taenia solium	Pork tapeworm	Intestine	Mild abdominal pain	Oral—poorly cooked pork
Echinococcus granulosus	Hydatid cyst	Lungs, liver	Cholestasis, liver congestion and atrophy, biliary obstruction	Oral—inoculation with sheep, cattle, or dog feces
PROTOZOA				
Entamoeba histolytica	Amebic dysentery	Intestine	Bloody, mucoid diarrhea; colicky abdominal pain	Contaminated water, raw vegetables
Plamodium spp.	Malaria	Liver, erythrocytes	High fever, chills, rigor, anemia, headache, malaise, chest pain, abdominal pain	Female *Anopheles* mosquito
Leishmania spp.	Kala-azar; cutaneous and mucocutaneous leishmaniasis	Reticuloendothelial cells of the body; disseminates to spleen, liver, bone marrow, lymph glands	Chronic: abdominal discomfort, ascites, fever, weakness, pallor, weight loss, cough Acute: sudden fever, chills	All transmission accomplished through bite of sandflies after biting specific infected mammals
Trypanosoma spp. *T. cruzi*	 Chagas' disease	Bloodstream	Local inflammation, lymphadenopathy, muscular necrosis, including myocardium (heart failure), esophagus, and colon (dilation); fever, malaise, anorexia, edema of face	Insects—hematophagous (blood-drinking) *Triatoma*
T. brucei	African sleeping sickness	Bloodstream	Fever, malaise, headache, rash, CNS disturbances	*Glossina* flies (tsetse flies)

TABLE 60–1 *Continued*
Parasitic Infections

Parasitic Agent	Common Name of Disease	Location of Infection	Symptoms	Mode of Transmission
PROTOZOA—CONTINUED				
Toxoplasma gondii	Toxoplasmosis	Throughout body	Acute: usually asymptomatic; Immunosuppressed: encephalitis, myocarditis, pneumonitis; Newborn: impaired vision, neurologic disorders	Eating raw or undercooked meat, poultry, or dairy foods; oral inoculation with cat feces
Pneumocystis carinii	Pneumonitis	Lungs	Fever, cough, tachypnea, costal retractions, cyanosis	Inhalation
Giardia lamblia	Epidemic diarrhea	Intestine	Acute, self-limited diarrhea; occasionally malabsorption with weight loss	Fecal contamination of water; person-to-person
Trichomonas vaginalis	Trichomoniasis (vaginitis)	Vagina	Irritation, discharge	Venereal
ECTOPARASITES				
Pediculus humanus var. *corporis*	Body louse	All hair-covered parts of body	Pruritus; Nits at base of hair shaft	Person-to-person, via fomites
var. *capitis*	Head louse	Head area		
Pediculus pubis	Pubic louse	Pubic area		
Sarcoptes scabiei var. *hominis*	Scabies	Skin	Pruritus, worse at night; linear burrows in folds of fingers, elbows, knees, axillae, pelvic girdle	Person-to-person
Maggots (larvae of dipterous flies	Myiasis	Necrotic tissue	Depends on location of infestation	Dipterous flies
Chiggers (mites)		Skin	Intense pruritus, hemorrhagic papules	Inhabit dogs, rabbits, cats, rats; foul cheese, flour, house dust
Ticks		Skin	Can transmit tick paralysis, Lyme disease	Reside in wooded and grassy areas

From Copstead L.E. (1995). *Perspectives on pathophysiology.* Philadelphia: W.B. Saunders.

Drug Therapy of Helminth Infections

Drugs used to treat helminth infections are usually specific. Treatment with anthelmintic drugs is targeted at one of three biochemical functions in the adult helminth: neuromuscular coordination; carbohydrate metabolism for energy supply; and microtubular integrity. Microtubular integrity must remain intact for the organism to accomplish egg laying and hatching, larval development, transportation of glucose, and secretion and use of enzymes.[2] (Table 60–2 provides information on various anthelmintic drugs.)

CONCEPT REVIEW

- Parasitic disease is one of the most pressing and serious public health problems. Improved hygiene, vector control, vaccines, and chemotherapy are approaches to the management of parasitic disease.
- Chemotherapy can control the infection and reduce the rate of transmission of parasitic infection within the community.

Drugs Used to Treat Intestinal Nematode Infections

Mebendazole, thiabendazole, and pyrantel pamoate are primary drugs used to treat intestinal nematode infections.

MEBENDAZOLE

Mebendazole (Vermox) belongs to the benzimidazole group of compounds.

Pharmacotherapeutics Mebendazole is used to treat intestinal and tissue nematodes. Parasites treatable with this drug include pinworm, roundworm, common hookworm or American hookworm, and whipworm.[3] Mebendazole is the drug of choice for treating ascariasis.

Pharmacokinetics Mebendazole is poorly absorbed; it is estimated that only 5% to 10% of the drug is absorbed after oral administration. Within 2 to 4 hours, peak plasma levels are reached. Protein bonding is approximately 90% to 95%. The half-life of the drug is 2½ to 9 hours. Approximately 2% of the drug is excreted in the urine within 24 to 48 hours as unchanged drug or its primary metabolites. Most of the administered dose is excreted in the feces.[4]

Pharmacodynamics Mebendazole irreversibly blocks glucose uptake by susceptible parasites, thus depleting stores of glycogen within the organism without affecting the glucose level in the host. Without the necessary glucose, the parasite's ability to reproduce is precluded.

Pharmaceutics Mebendazole is available in chewable tablets. The recommended dose is 100 mg orally twice daily for 3 days. Table 60–2 provides additional information about anthelmintic drugs.

Undesired clinical responses Transient symptoms of abdominal pain and diarrhea with administration of mebendazole have occurred in clients with massive infection. Some clients have experienced nausea, vomiting, rashes, dizziness, and lightheadedness.

Contraindications and precautions Mebendazole use is contraindicated in individuals who have shown hypersensitivity to the drug.

Drug-drug and drug-environment interactions Mebendazole should be stored at room temperature, 15° to 30° C. Carbamazepine may decrease concentrations of mebendazole.

Interference with diagnostic studies Mebendazole use may increase aspartate aminotransferase (AST), alanine aminotransferase (ALT), alkaline phosphatase, and blood urea nitrogen (BUN) test results. Its use may decrease the hemoglobin level.

Life-span considerations Mebendazole is classified as a Pregnancy Category C drug. It is not known if it is excreted in human milk. Mebendazole has not been extensively studied in children less than 2 years of age.[3]

Specific drug-related nursing considerations Explain to the client that the tablet may be chewed, swallowed, or crushed and mixed with food. Instruct client to complete the full course of therapy. Teach him or her the proper handling of bedclothing, toilet facilities, and laundry.

Encourage intake of fruit and vegetables to avoid constipation since parasites are expelled by normal peristalsis. Collect stool or perianal specimens as needed to confirm diagnosis or cure. Monitor the client for neutropenia with high doses.

THIABENDAZOLE

Thiabendazole (Mintezol) also belongs to the benzimidazole group of compounds.

Pharmacotherapeutics Thiabendazole is used to treat pinworm, threadworm, roundworm, hookworm, whipworm, and cutaneous larvae. It is also used to alleviate the symptoms of trichinosis (pork roundworm) during its invasive stage. Thiabendazole is the drug of choice for treating strongyloidiasis.

Pharmacokinetics Thiabendazole is rapidly absorbed, and peak plasma concentrations occur in 1 to 2 hours. It is metabolized almost completely to 5-hydroxythiabendazole. Within 48 hours, approximately 5% of the dose is recovered from the stool and approximately 90% from the urine. Most of the drug is excreted within 24 hours.[3,5]

Pharmacodynamics Thiabendazole suppresses egg or larval production and probably inhibits the development of eggs and larvae. Although the exact mechanism of action is not known, it is known that thiabendazole inhibits a specific helminth enzyme, fumarate reductase.[3]

Pharmaceutics Thiabendazole is available as a suspension and as a chewable tablet for oral administration. Table 60–2 contains additional information on dosing.

Undesired clinical responses Undesired responses to thiabendazole include anorexia, epigastric distress, nausea, vomiting, and diarrhea. The central nervous system (CNS) may be adversely affected, and the client may experience giddiness, dizziness, drowsiness, or headaches. The client may also report flushing, rashes, erythema, or angioedema.[3,6]

Contraindications and precautions Thiabendazole use is contraindicated in individuals with known hypersensitivity to the drug.

Drug-drug interactions Thiabendazole may compete with other drugs such as theophylline for sites of metabolism in the liver. This action may elevate serum levels of the other drugs to toxic levels.

Life-span considerations Thiabendazole is classified as a Pregnancy Category C drug. It is not known if it is excreted in human milk. Safety and effectiveness in children weighing less than 16 kg have not been established.

Specific drug-related nursing considerations Monitor laboratory values carefully, including blood counts, liver function tests, and glucose levels. Assess for adverse reactions, especially hypersensitivity reactions.

Instruct the client to chew the tablet before swallowing and to take the drug with food. (Even the oral suspension should be administered with food.) Since the drug may cause dizziness or drowsiness, extreme caution must be taken when performing tasks that require alertness.

MISCELLANEOUS DRUG

Pyrantel pamoate (Antiminth) is also effective against intestinal nematodes. It is used to treat roundworm and pinworm infections. Pyrantel is a depolarizing neuromuscular blocking agent that produces spastic paralysis of the parasite. It also inhibits cholinesterases.

Pyrantel is poorly absorbed by the GI tract, and plasma levels of unaltered drug are low. Peak plasma levels are reached in approximately 1 to 3 hours. More than 50% of the dosage is excreted in the feces before being changed. Approximately 7% of the dosage is found in the urine as the parent drug or one of its metabolites.

Its most common undesired clinical responses are anorexia, nausea, vomiting, gastralgia, abdominal cramps, and diarrhea. Less frequent side effects include headache, dizziness, drowsiness, insomnia, or rash. Pyrantel should be used with caution when the client has an existing hepatic disease.[7,8]

Drugs Used to Treat Blood and Tissue Nematodes

Diethylcarbamazine is a piperazine derivative. It is rapidly absorbed after oral administration, and peak plasma concen-

TABLE 60–2
Anthelmintic Drugs

Drug Name	Indications and Dosage
Mebendazole (Vermox)	**Angiostrongyliasis** 100 mg bid for 5 d **Ascariasis** 100 mg bid for 3 d **Enterobius vermicularis (Pinworm)** Single dose, 100 mg; repeat after 2 wk **Hookworm** 100 mg bid for 3 d **Trichinosis** (Steroids for severe symptoms plus mebendazole) 200–400 mg tid for 3 d, then 400–500 mg tid for 10 d
Thiabendazole (Mintezol)	**Angiostrongyliasis** 75 mg/kg/d in three doses for 3 d to a maximum of 3 g/d
Pyrantel pamoate (Antiminth)	**Ascariasis** 11 mg/kg once (maximum, 1 g) **E. vermicularis (Pinworm)** 11 mg/kg once (maximum 1 g); repeat after 2 wk **Hookworm Infection** 11 mg/kg (maximum, 1 g) for 3 d
Diethylcarbamazine (Hetrazan)	**Filariasis** ADULTS Day 1, 50 mg; day 2, 50 mg tid; day 3, 100 mg tid; days 4–21, 6 mg/kg/d in three doses CHILDREN Day 1, 1 mg/kg; day 2, 1 mg/kg tid; day 3, 1–2 mg/kg tid; days 4–21, 6 mg/kg/d in three doses
Praziquantel (Biltricide)	**All Fluke Infections Except Nanophyetus salmincola** 75 mg/kg/d in three doses for 1 d **N. salmincola Fluke Infection** 60 mg/kg/d in three doses for 1 d **Schistosomiasis due to Schistosoma japonicum or S. mekongi** 60 mg/kg/d in three doses for 2 d **Schistosomiasis due to S. haematobium** 40 mg/kg/d in two doses for 1 d **Schistosomiasis due to S. mansoni** 40 mg/kg/d in two doses for 1 d **Tapeworm (Adult; of Fish, Beef, Pork, Dog)** 5–10 mg/kg once **Tapeworm (Tissue Stage)** 50 mg/kg/d in three doses for 15 d
Niclosamide (Nicloside)	**Fluke Infection** One dose of four tablets (2 g) chewed thoroughly **Tapeworm, Adult (Fish, Beef, Pork, Dog)** One dose of four tablets (2 g) chewed thoroughly **Dwarf Tapeworm** One dose of four tablets (2 g) chewed thoroughly daily for 7 d
Oxamniquine (Vansil)	**Schistosomiasis due to S. mansoni** 15 mg/kg once

trations occur within 1 to 2 hours. The drug's renal clearance depends on the urinary pH. Under acidic conditions, more than 50% of the unchanged drug appears in urine, with a half-life of 2 to 3 hours. Alkalinization of the urine prolongs the plasma half-life to 10 to 12 hours and decreases renal clearance.

Undesired clinical responses associated with the drug include transient anorexia, nausea, headache, joint pain, and vomiting. Other side effects, including papular rash, severe itching, tachycardia, and intense headache, result from allergic reactions to dead and dying microfilariae.[5,9]

CONCEPT REVIEW

Although active against a variety of nematodes, mebendazole is the drug of choice for treating ascariasis. It is always administered orally.

Thiabendazole is the drug of choice for treating strongyloidiasis. In most cases it is administered as an oral suspension or chewable tablet.

Pyrantel is well tolerated in adults and children over the age of 2 years. It is the drug of choice after benzimidazoles for treating ascariasis, hookworm, and pinworm infections.

Diethylcarbamazine, a piperazine derivative, is used to treat blood and tissue nematodes.

Drugs Used to Treat Cestode Infections

Cestode infections are treated with several drugs, including niclosamide and praziquantel.

NICLOSAMIDE

Niclosamide (Niclocide) is a halogenated salicylanilide derivative.

Pharmacotherapeutics   Niclosamide is effective against beef, fish, and dwarf tapeworms. It is used to treat intestinal cestodes only.

Pharmacokinetics   Niclosamide is poorly absorbed from the GI tract. It is excreted in the feces.

Pharmacodynamics   The primary action of niclosamide involves inhibition of energy production in parasite mitochondria through inhibition of anaerobic phosphorylation of adenosine diphosphate.[9]

Pharmaceutics   Niclosamide is available in chewable tablets.

Undesired clinical responses   Nausea, vomiting, abdominal discomfort, anorexia, and diarrhea have been reported with niclosamide use. In addition, headaches, dizziness, and drowsiness have occurred.

Contraindications and precautions   Use of niclosamide is contraindicated in individuals with known hypersensitivity to the drug.

Life-span considerations   Niclosamide is classified as a Pregnancy Category B drug. Safety of the drug has not been established in children under the age of 2 years.

Specific drug-related nursing considerations   Monitor all laboratory values, especially from liver function studies. Instruct the client to chew the tablet thoroughly or to crush it for children. The drug may be administered with food if necessary. Follow-up care is necessary; the presence of segments of ova in the feces 7 days after therapy indicates unsuccessful treatment. The client is not considered cured until stool test results have been negative for at least 3 days.

Drugs Used to Treat Trematode Infections

A variety of drugs, including praziquantel and oxamniquine, are used in the treatment of trematode infections.

PRAZIQUANTEL

Praziquantel (Biltricide) is a pyrazinoisoquinoline derivative.

Pharmacotherapeutics   Praziquantel is the drug of choice for treating all species of human schistosomiasis.[9]

Pharmacokinetics   Approximately 80% of praziquantel is absorbed very rapidly after oral ingestion. The drug reaches maximum serum concentrations in approximately 1 to 3 hours. Metabolites of the drug are excreted mainly by the kidneys.

Pharmacodynamics   Praziquantel produces an increase in cell membrane permeability in susceptible parasitic worms. The change in membrane permeability allows leakage of intracellular calcium, which is followed by muscular contraction and paralysis of the parasite. The drug also damages the body covering of the parasite, which permits phagocytes to attach to the organism and destroy it.

Pharmaceutics   Praziquantel is available in plain-coated tablets for oral administration.

Undesired clinical responses   In general, praziquantel is well tolerated. Malaise, headache, dizziness, and abdominal discomfort have been reported.

Contraindications and precautions   Since praziquantel can cause dizziness, the client should be warned of the danger involved in driving a car or operating machinery on the day of the treatment.

Life-span considerations   Praziquantel is classified as a Pregnancy Category B drug. Since the drug is excreted in human milk, women should not breast-feed the day of therapy and during the subsequent 72 hours.[3]

Specific drug-related nursing considerations   Instruct the client to swallow the tablet whole at bedtime with liquids. Teach the client to swallow the tablet immediately and not hold it in the mouth.

MISCELLANEOUS DRUGS

Oxamniquine (Vansil) is effective against male schistosomas. The drug is well absorbed, and plasma concentrations peak within 1 to 1½ hours. Extensive metabolism occurs, and inactive acidic metabolites are excreted in the urine. Undesired clinical responses include nausea, vomiting, abdominal anorexia, transient dizziness or drowsiness, and headaches.

CONCEPT REVIEW

Praziquantel possesses a broad spectrum of anthelmintic activity. It is the drug of choice to treat tapeworm if a definitive diagnosis cannot be obtained.

Niclosamide is effective against adult tapeworms but not against ova.

PROTOZOAN INFECTIONS

Protozoan parasites can be found in the United States but are more prevalent in tropical climates. Increasing international travel and immigration from other countries to the United States have resulted in an increased risk from these diseases in the United States.

The most significant protozoan disease in relation to morbidity and mortality is malaria. In addition, other parasites cause a variety of health problems, including leishmaniasis, trypanosomiasis, amebiasis, giardiasis, trichomoniasis, and toxoplasmosis.

Classifications of Protozoa

Protozoa belong to the kingdom Protista. Some biologists believe there is a single phylum of protozoa; others divide the single phylum into four major phyla.

▨ NURSING CONSIDERATIONS

Since protozoan diseases are common, prevention and treatment of these disorders are important nursing responsibilities.

Assessing Focus the health history on the chief complaint, past medical history, drug history, family history, psychosocial history, including lifestyle, and review of systems. Since the type and severity of symptoms depend on the nature of the disease and the client's individual susceptibility, collect subjective data about each reported symptom. For each symptom, determine onset, location, duration, aggravating and relieving factors, medical intervention, self-treatment, and compliance factors. Ask the client about past episodes of protozoan infections. Determine the symptoms that developed, treatment, and effectiveness of treatment.

Ask the client about fatigue, malaise, fever, lassitude, chills, or sweating. Specifically inquire about skin changes. Determine if the client has ever experienced itching, dryness, rashes, ecchymoses, masses, lesions, or color changes. Information about recent exposure to infectious diseases is helpful, as is knowing the client's immunization status. All women of childbearing age must be assessed for pregnancy and lactation.

Use extreme caution during the physical assessment of all clients but especially for individuals with infectious diseases.

Be certain to wear gloves when appropriate and to follow universal precautions in regard to body fluids and secretions. During the head-to-toe physical assessment examine the skin, hair, scalp, nails, and mucous membranes thoroughly. Note changes such as altered total body skin color, turgor, temperature, and vascularity. If skin lesions are present, describe their location, distribution, size, arrangement, color, and configuration and the presence of drainage. Palpate lesions to determine characteristics of contour (e.g., flat, raised, or depressed), size, consistency (e.g., firm, soft), mobility, and tenderness.

Inspect the client's abdomen for ascites and prominent venous collateral networks. Palpate the abdomen, especially in the areas of the liver and spleen; note any tenderness. Percuss the abdomen to determine the size of the liver and spleen and the presence of ascites.

Diagnosing Analysis of the data provides the basis of nursing diagnoses. Nursing diagnoses appropriate for the client receiving antiviral drugs with systemic actions follow:
- Anxiety related to uncertainty of effectiveness of drug therapy.
- High risk for injury related to dizziness and lightheadedness caused by some antiprotozoan drugs.
- Knowledge deficit regarding expected therapeutic drug effects, undesired clinical responses, and drug administration procedure.
- Altered nutrition: less than body requirements related to nausea produced by drug therapy.

Planning During the planning phase expected outcomes specific for the client are established. In addition, teaching or discharge plans are developed. Expected outcomes appropriate for the client include the following:
- Client appears relaxed and reports anxiety is reduced.
- Client verbalizes factors that contribute to injury risk.
- Client verbalizes understanding of disease process and treatment plan.
- Client's ingestion of food is adequate to maintain appropriate weight.
- Client reports improvement in sleep-rest patterns.

Implementing You must understand how protozoan infections are transmitted, measures to initiate to prevent transmission, and clinical manifestations of the diseases. Additionally, remember that nursing measures that promote health and hygiene contribute to the integrity of the host and increase resistance.

Monitor the client closely for undesired clinical responses and toxicity associated with use of antiprotozoan drugs. Monitor renal function, including intake and output. Review results from laboratory studies directed at assessing renal and hepatic function and the integrity of the hematopoietic system. Since many drugs are metabolized and excreted through the kidneys, adequate fluid intake is essential for preventing renal tubular damage.

Evaluating Evaluation of the plan of care is based on the client's response to therapy, including decreased signs and symptoms of the disease and a lack of undesired clinical responses. Discuss with the client and family their perception of the plan and compare the outcome of care with the previously established expected outcomes.

Drug Therapy for Protozoan Infections

Drug therapy for protozoan infections is complex, with both the drug of choice and alternative drugs identified. Drug choice for some infections is based on the stage of the disease or the presenting symptoms. Because of the complexity of therapy, only major drugs are presented; information on additional drugs is available in Table 60–3.

CHLOROQUINE PHOSPHATE

Chloroquine phosphate (Aralen) is the prototype of a class of antimalarial aminoquinoline derivatives. It was developed during World War II and has become the main weapon against human malaria.

Pharmacotherapeutics Chloroquine is used to treat the *erythrocytic* forms of the malarial parasite. It is the drug of choice for treating malarial attacks caused by *Plasmodium vivax* and chloroquine-sensitive strains of *P. falciparum*.[7,8,10]

Pharmacokinetics Chloroquine is rapidly and completely absorbed from the GI tract. Only 50% of the drug is bound to plasma proteins. Some of the drug is absorbed and deposited in certain tissues (e.g., lung, spleen, liver, kidney). Slow release from these sites maintains therapeutic levels of the drug. Approximately half of the absorbed drug is excreted unchanged in urine.[8,9]

Pharmacodynamics Chloroquine may bind to DNA, inhibiting replication of DNA and synthesis of RNA. However, current studies suggest that other mechanisms are involved.

Pharmaceutics Chloroquine phosphate is available as uncoated tablets for oral administration. Chloroquine hydrochloride is available in a parenteral solution for intramuscular (IM) administration.[3]

Undesired clinical responses Chloroquine generally is well tolerated by clients. GI upset, pruritus, transient headaches, and visual disturbances are noted at therapeutic dosages. Acute chloroquine toxicity at high doses can produce hypotension, lowered myocardial function, vasodilation, and abnormal electrocardiogram (ECG) patterns. Long-term therapy with chloroquine can cause retinopathy.[6,9]

Contraindications and precautions Chloroquine should be administered with caution to clients with impaired renal or hepatic function. Chloroquine use is contraindicated in clients with retinal or visual field changes.[3,10]

Drug-drug interactions Chloroquine may increase the concentration of penicillamine.

Life-span considerations Children and infants are extremely susceptible to adverse effects from an overdose of the parenteral form of chloroquine. The drug is classified in Pregnancy Category C.

Specific drug-related nursing considerations Administer the oral dosage of chloroquine with food. Advise the client that the IM injection may produce local pain. Monitor hepatic function tests and CBC for adverse hematologic effects.

MEFLOQUINE HYDROCHLORIDE

Mefloquine hydrochloride (Lariam) was approved by the Food and Drug Administration (FDA) in 1989.

Pharmacotherapeutics Mefloquine is used to treat and prevent chloroquine-resistant falciparum malaria.

Pharmacokinetics Mefloquine is well absorbed after oral administration and is extensively bound to plasma proteins. Peak plasma concentrations are reached within hours; the drugs' half-life is 17 days. Mefloquine is concentrated in the liver and lungs. It undergoes some biotransformation; its major route of elimination is in bile.[3,9]

Pharmacodynamics The exact mechanism of action for mefloquine is not known.

Pharmaceutics Mefloquine is available in uncoated tablets for oral administration.

Undesired clinical responses Mefloquine is well tolerated. Dose-related side effects include mild nausea, vomiting, diarrhea, abdominal pain, skin rash, anorexia, tinnitus, and dizziness.

Contraindications and precautions Mefloquine use is contraindicated in individuals with known hypersensitivities to the drug. It has not been administered for long-term therapy. If the drug is used for a prolonged period, periodic evaluation of hepatic function is needed.[3]

Drug-drug interactions Mefloquine can slow cardiac conduction. Therefore it should not be used concurrently with other cardiosuppressants, including β-blockers and calcium channel blockers.

Life-span considerations Mefloquine is classified as a Pregnancy Category C drug. Low concentrations of the drug are excreted in human milk; therefore caution must be used when administering the drug to nursing mothers. Safety and effectiveness in children have not been established.

QUININE SULFATE

Quinine (Quin-260, Quinamm) is an alkaloid derived from the bark of the cinchona tree.

Pharmacotherapeutics Quinine is used to treat chloroquine-resistant falciparum malaria. The drug is seldom used alone, but it is frequently administered with pyrimethamine and a sulfonamide.

Pharmacokinetics Quinine is well absorbed when administered orally. Peak plasma concentrations occur within 1 to 3 hours; the plasma half-life is approximately 12 hours. Approximately 70% of the drug is bound to plasma protein. Although only small amounts of the drug reach the cerebrospinal fluid, it rapidly crosses the placenta. Quinine is extensively metabolized in the liver.[9,11]

Pharmacodynamics Quinine's action on malarial parasites is not clearly understood. It probably interferes with the function of plasmodial DNA. Quinine also depresses oxygen uptake and carbohydrate metabolism by the organism.[4]

Pharmaceutics Quinine is available in tablets for oral administration.

Undesired clinical responses At therapeutic dosages, quinine produces a group of side effects called *cinchonism*. These symptoms include tinnitus, vertigo, headache, nausea, and

TABLE 60–3
*Antiprotozoan Drugs**

Drug Name	Indications and Dosage
Iodoquinol	**Amebiasis** ADULTS 650 mg tid for 20 d CHILDREN 30–40 mg/kg/d in three doses for 20 d
Paromomycin	**Amebiasis** 25–30 mg/kg/d in three doses for 7 d **Giardiasis** 25–30 mg/kg/d in three doses for 7 d
Diloxanide furoate	**Amebiasis** ADULTS 500 mg tid for 10 d CHILDREN 20 mg/kg/d in three doses for 10 d
Metronidazole	**Amebiasis** ADULTS 750 mg tid for 10 d CHILDREN 35–50 mg/kg/d in three doses for 10 d **Giardiasis** ADULTS 250 mg tid for 5 d CHILDREN 15 mg/kg/d in three doses for 5 d **Trichomoniasis** ADULTS 2 g once or 250 mg tid orally CHILDREN 15 mg/kg/d orally in three doses for 7 d
Tinidazole	**Amebiasis** ADULTS (MILD TO MODERATE) 2 g/d for 3 d ADULTS (SEVERE) 600 mg bid for 5 d CHILDREN 50 mg/kg (maximum, 2 g)/d for 3 d **Giardiasis** ADULTS 2 g once CHILDREN 50 mg/kg once (maximum, 2 g) **Trichomoniasis** ADULTS 2 g once CHILDREN 50 mg/kg once (maximum, 2 g)
Dehydroemetine	**Amebiasis** ADULTS 1–1.5 mg/kg/d (maximum, 90 mg/d) IM for up to 5 d CHILDREN 1–1.5 mg/kg/d (maximum, 90 mg/d) IM in two doses for up to 5 d
Quinacrine hydrochloride	**Giardiasis** ADULTS 100 mg tid pc for 5 d CHILDREN 6 mg/kg/d in three doses pc for 5 d (maximum, 300 mg/d)
Sodium stibogluconate	**Leishmaniasis** 20 mg Sb/kg/d IV or IM for 20–28 d

* Some of these drugs are classified as investigational in the United States.   *Table continued on following page.*

TABLE 60–3 *Continued*
Antiprotozoan Drugs

Drug Name	Indications and Dosage
Meglumine antimonate	**Leishmaniasis** 20 mg Sb/kg/d for 20–28 d
Amphotericin B	**Leishmaniasis** 0.25–1 mg/kg by slow infusion daily or q2d for up to 8 wk
Pentamidine isethionate	**Leishmaniasis** 2–4 mg/kg daily or q2d IM for up to 15 doses; may repeat

Quinine sulfate plus pyrimethamine-sulfadoxine, tetracycline, and clindamycin	**Malaria**
	ADULTS
	650 mg q8h for 3–7 d; three tablets at once on last day
	CHILDREN
	25 mg/kg/d in three doses for 3–7 d
	   <1 y: ¼ tablet
	   1–3 y: ½ tablet
	   4–8 y: 1 tablet
	   9–14 y: 2 tablets

Mefloquine	**Treatment of Malaria** ADULTS 1250 mg once CHILDREN 25 mg/kg once (<45 kg) **Prevention of Malaria** ADULTS 250 mg orally once per week CHILDREN 15–19 kg: ¼ tablet 20–30 kg: ½ tablet 31–45 kg: ¾ tablet <45 kg: 1 tablet
Halofantrine	**Malaria** ADULTS 500 mg q6h for three doses; repeat in 1 wk CHILDREN 8 mg/kg q6h for three doses (<40 kg); repeat in 1 wk
Quinidine gluconate	**Malaria** 10 mg/kg loading dose (maximum, 600 mg) in normal saline solution slowly over 1–2 h, followed by continuous infusion of 0.02 mg/kg/min until oral therapy can be started
Quinine dihydrochloride	**Malaria** 20 mg salt/kg loading dose in 10 ml/kg 5% dextrose solution over 4 h, followed by 10 mg salt/kg over 2–4 h q8h (maximum, 1800 mg/d) until oral therapy can be started
Chloroquine phosphate	**Treatment of Malaria** ADULTS 600 mg base (1 g), then 300 mg base (500 mg) 6 h later; then 300 mg base (500 mg) at 24 and 48 h CHILDREN 10 mg base/kg (maximum, 600 mg base), then 5 mg base/kg 6 h later; then 5 mg base/kg at 24 and 48 h **Prevention of Malaria** ADULTS 300 mg base (500 mg salt) orally once per week CHILDREN 5 mg/kg base (8.3 mg/kg salt) once per week up to adult dose of 300 mg base

visual impairment. At higher doses, a number of organ systems, including the cardiovascular system, skeletal system, and the GI tract, are affected.[9,12]

Contraindications and precautions Quinine use is contraindicated in individuals with known hypersensitivities to the drug. It should not be administered to individuals with glucose-6-phosphate dehydrogenase deficiency. It is also not recommended for use in clients with tinnitus, optic neuritis, or a history of thrombocytopenia.[4]

Drug-drug interactions Quinine may increase the concentration of digoxin.

Life-span considerations Quinine is classified as a Pregnancy Category X drug. Since it is excreted in breast milk, it is not recommended for use during lactation.

TABLE 60–3 *Continued*
Antiprotozoan Drugs

Drug Name	Indications and Dosage
Chloroquine phosphate plus pyrimethamine-sulfadoxine	**Prevention of Malaria** Same as chloroquine phosphate Carry a single dose for self-treatment **ADULTS** Three tablets **CHILDREN** <1 y: $\frac{1}{4}$ tablet 1–3 y: $\frac{1}{2}$ tablet 4–8 y: 1 tablet 9–14 y: 2 tablets
Nifurtimox	**Trypanosomiasis** **ADULTS** 8–10 mg/kg/d orally in four doses for 120 d **CHILDREN** 1–10 y: 15–20 mg/kg/d in four doses for 90 d 11–16 y: 12.5–15 mg/kg/d in four doses for 90 d
Benzimidazole	5–7 mg/kg/d for 30–120 days
Sura-min	**African Trypanosomiasis, Sleeping Sickness** **ADULTS** 100–200 mg (test dose) IV, then 1 g IV on days 1, 3, 7, 14, and 21 **CHILDREN** 20 mg/kg on days 1, 3, 7, 14, and 21
Pentamidine isethionate	**African Trypanosomiasis, Sleeping Sickness** 4 mg/kg/day IM for 10 d
Melarsoprol	**Late-Stage Trypanosomiasis with CNS Involvement** **ADULTS** 2–3.6 mg/kg/d IV for 3 d; after 1 wk, 3.6 mg/kg/d IV for 3 d; repeat again after 10–21 d **CHILDREN** 18–25 mg/kg total over 1 mo; initial dose, 0.36 mg/kg/IV, increasing gradually to maximum of 3.6 mg/kg at intervals of 1–5 d for total of 9–10 doses
Tryparsamide	**Late-Stage Trypanosomiasis with CNS Involvement** **ADULTS** One injection of 30 mg/kg (maximum, 2 g) IV q5d to total of 12 injections; may repeat after 1 mo

Specific drug-related nursing considerations Observe for hypersensitivity to the drug (e.g., flushing, rash, urticaria, itching, wheezing). If symptoms occur, stop the drug administration and contact the primary care provider. Assess the client's level of hearing and visual acuity regularly. Monitor his or her CBC for blood dyscrasias.

PRIMAQUINE PHOSPHATE

Primaquine phosphate (Primaquine) is a synthetic compound similar to chloroquine in structure.

Pharmacotherapeutics Primaquine is used to treat *hepatic* forms of vivax malaria.

Pharmacokinetics Primaquine is readily absorbed and rapidly metabolized after ingestion. Only a small portion of the dosage is excreted as the parent drug. Plasma concentrations peak in 1 to 2 hours.[3] Pharmacokinetic studies have shown wide individual variability.[9]

Pharmacodynamics The exact mechanism of action of primaquine is not known. However, it may act by inhibiting DNA and RNA synthesis.

Pharmaceutics Primaquine is available as an uncoated tablet for oral administration.

Undesired clinical responses Common undesired responses include nausea, vomiting, epigastric distress, and abdominal cramps. The most serious and frequent response to primaquine is hemolysis in clients with glucose-6-phosphate dehydrogenase deficiency. This occurs more frequently in ethnic groups of the Eastern Mediterranean region. During therapy periodic blood counts should be obtained.[9,12]

Contraindications and precautions Primaquine use is contraindicated in acutely ill clients with systemic disease manifested by a tendency to granulocytopenia.

Drug-drug interactions Primaquine should not be administered concurrently with other potentially hemolytic drugs or bone marrow depressants.

Life-span considerations Safety and effectiveness of primaquine in children have not been established.

METRONIDAZOLE

Metronidazole (Flagyl) is the drug of choice in the treatment of trichomoniasis. It is also used to treat amebiasis, a protozoan GI infection.

Metronidazole is a nitroimidazole that exerts direct trichomonacidal action. It is rapidly and completely absorbed after oral administration. The drug is well distributed to various tissues, reaching therapeutic concentrations in vaginal secretions, semen, saliva, breast milk, and cerebrospinal fluid. Peak serum levels are reached within 1 hour when the drug is administered orally, 4 hours after rectal administration, and 8 to 24 hours after a vaginal dose. The major route of elimination from the body is via the urinary tract. Approximately 6% to 15% is excreted via the feces.[3,10]

CONCEPT REVIEW

Chloroquine is the prototype of a class of antimalarial aminoquinoline derivatives. Its mechanism of action has not been established, but it may interfere with replication. Chloroquine does not prevent malaria but does suppress the clinical disease.

Quinine is the first known antimalarial drug. It is significantly more toxic than chloroquine and produces a variety of side effects.

Mefloquine is a relatively new drug that is structurally related to quinine. This drug is used to treat and prevent chloroquine-resistant falciparum malaria.

Primaquine is the only tissue schizonticide available for the treatment of *P. vivax* and *P. ovale* infections. Its mechanism of antimalarial action is unknown.

Metronidazole is the drug of choice for treating trichomoniasis. It may also be used to treat amebiasis, giardiasis, and a variety of bacterial infections.

SUMMARY

Parasites live on or in the human body during some part of their life cycle and depend on the human host for shelter and sustenance. Multiple environmental factors affect the prevalence of parasitic infections. Symptoms of parasitic infection depend on the area of the body in which infestation develops. Chemotherapy can control most parasitic infections.

REFERENCES

1. Copstead, L.C. (1995). *Perspectives on pathophysiology.* Philadelphia: W.B. Saunders.
2. Wingard, L., et al. (1991). *Human pharmacology molecular to clinical.* St. Louis: Mosby–Year Book.
3. Data Pharmaceutica, Inc. (1993). *1993 physicians' genRx.* Smithtown, NY: Author.
4. Hodgson, B., Kizior, R., & Kingdon, R. (1995). *1995 nurse's drug handbook.* Philadelphia: W.B. Saunders.
5. United States Pharmacopeial Convention, Inc. (1994). *USP DI* (14th ed.). (Vol. I: Drug Information for the Health Care Professional). Taunton, MA: Author.
6. DiPiro, J.T., et al. (1992). *Pharmacotherapy: A pathophysiologic approach* (2nd ed.). New York: Elsevier.
7. Abramowicz, M. (Ed.). (1993). Drugs for parasitic infections. *Medical Letter on Drugs and Therapeutics, 35*(911), 111–122.
8. Lehne, R. (1994). *Pharmacology for nursing care* (2nd ed.). Philadelphia: W.B. Saunders.
9. Vande Waa, E.A., & Tracy, J. (1992). Antiparasitic agents. In C.M. Smith & A.M. Reynard (Eds.), *Textbook of pharmacology* (pp. 913-938). Philadelphia: W.B. Saunders.
10. Towle, A. (1993). *Modern Biology* (8th ed.). Austin, TX: Holt, Rinehart & Winston.
11. Goodman, A., Gilman, A., Rall, T., Niles, A., & Taylor, P. (Eds.). (1990). *Goodman and Gilman's The pharmacological basis of therapeutics* (8th ed.). New York: Pergamon Press.
12. Katzung, B. (Ed.). (1992). Basic and clinical pharmacology. Norwalk, CT: Appleton & Lange.

Drugs Affecting the Reproductive System

CHAPTER 61

OVERVIEW OF

Female and Male Reproductive Systems

CAROL M. VIAMONTES • WILLIAM R. GERBER

⊛ Female Reproductive System

LEARNING OBJECTIVES:

Describe the functions of the primary sex organs of a female.

Identify the internal and external accessory organs.

Describe the functions of each internal and external accessory organ.

Summarize the physiologic changes that occur during the female sexual response.

Explain the functions of the female sex hormones.

Summarize the events of the female reproductive cycle.

KEY TERMS:

Bartholin's glands, clitoris, endometrium, estrogen, follicle-stimulating hormone, gonadotropin releasing hormone, luteinizing hormone, menarche, menopause, menstruation, orgasm, ovulation, progesterone

⊛ Male Reproductive System

LEARNING OBJECTIVES:

Describe the functions of the internal and external male reproductive organs.

Explain the functions of the internal male accessory organs.

Describe the process of spermatogenesis.

Summarize the physiologic changes that occur during the male sexual response.

Discuss the influence of hormones on male reproductive functions.

KEY TERMS:

Capacitation, Cowper's glands, ejaculation, emission, epididymis, erection, fertilization, meiotic division, semen, seminiferous tubules, spermatogenesis, testosterone

⊛ Pharmacologic Impact on the Reproductive System

LEARNING OBJECTIVE: Describe the influence of drugs on the reproductive system.

CONCEPTS AND TERMS TO REVIEW

Review in an anatomy and physiology textbook the male and female reproductive systems.

Study the actions of the pituitary and hypothalamic hormones that affect the male and female reproductive systems. (See Chapters 38 and 40.)

Review the autonomic regulation of the reproductive structures.

Reexamine meiotic cell division.

*R*eproduction is the process by which a living entity or organism produces a new individual of the same species. The organs of the male and female reproductive systems are adapted to perform the specialized tasks involved in the reproductive process.

Organs of the female and male reproductive systems can be grouped according to function. The testes and ovaries, also called the *gonads,* produce gametes—sperm cells and ova, respectively. Accessory sex glands produce materials that support gametes. Ducts within the reproductive systems transport, receive, and store the sperm cells and ova. Because the gonads produce gametes and discharge them into ducts, they are classified as exocrine glands. They are also classified as endocrine glands since they secrete hormones.

To administer drugs that affect the female and male reproductive systems safely, a solid knowledge base of the normal anatomy and physiology of these systems is needed. This knowledge provides a basis for understanding pathologic states and the relationship of pharmacologic treatment.

FEMALE REPRODUCTIVE SYSTEM

Organs in the female reproductive system produce and maintain egg cells; transport these cells to the site of fertilization; provide an environment favorable for a developing fetus; and produce female sex hormones. Functions of the female reproductive system are divided into two phases: (1) preparation for conception and gestation and (2) gestation. This chapter focuses on preparation for conception and gestation.

Organs of Female Reproductive System

The primary sex organs or gonads of the female reproductive system are the ovaries. Internal and external accessory organs make up the other parts of the system.

PRIMARY SEX ORGANS: OVARIES

The **ovaries** are the paired female gonads that release the female hormones estrogen and progesterone and also release the ovum at ovulation. They are located, one on each side, in the lateral wall of the pelvic cavity and are held in position by several ligaments.

Each ovary is divided into a medulla and cortex. The medulla is composed of connective tissue, blood vessels, lymphatic vessels, and nerves. Ovarian follicles make up the cortex.[1,2]

INTERNAL ACCESSORY REPRODUCTIVE ORGANS

Internal female accessory reproductive organs include the vagina, cervix, uterus, and uterine or fallopian tubes. Paired **uterine** or **fallopian tubes** (oviducts) extend from the fundus of the uterus bilaterally. These tubes connect the endometrial cavity of the uterus to the peritoneal cavity. They play a major role in conception by allowing passage of sperm traveling upward in search of an ovum to fertilize. Fertilization occurs within the tube where the upward-traveling sperm meets the downward-traveling ovum. The fertilized egg then travels down the tube to reach the endometrial cavity and implants in the endometrim approximately 10 days after ovulation.[3]

The **uterus** is a fibromuscular organ that expands in pregnancy to house and nourish the fetus. Glandular tissue called **endometrium** lines the uterine cavity. This tissue responds to hormonal stimulation from the ovary to produce the proper environment for implantation and growth of the fertilized ovum. The endometrium is also the source of menstrual discharge when conception has not occurred. The **cervix** is the lower part of the uterus that extends into the vagina.

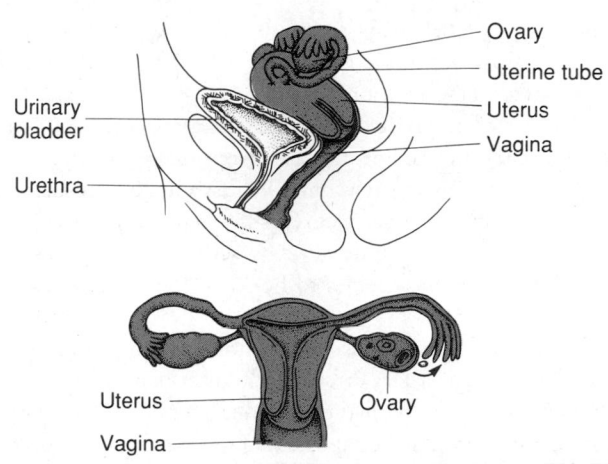

FIGURE 61-1 Female reproductive organs. (From Guyton, A.C. [1991]. *Textbook of medical physiology* [8th ed.]. Philadelphia: W.B. Saunders.)

A fibromuscular tube, the **vagina,** extends from the uterus to the outside of the body. Usually a thin membrane called the *hymen* partially closes the vaginal orifice. The vagina carries uterine secretions, receives the erect penis during sexual intercourse, and transports the fetus during the birth process.

A lateral view of the female pelvis (Fig. 61-1) demonstrates the relationships between the female genital system and the terminal end of the urinary and gastrointestinal (GI) systems. The terminal end of the urinary system (urinary bladder and urethra) is located immediately anterior to the female genital system. Posterior to the vagina is the terminal end of the GI system (rectum and anal orifice).[1,4]

EXTERNAL ACCESSORY REPRODUCTIVE ORGANS

External female accessory reproductive organs include the labia majora, labia minora, clitoris, and vestibular glands. Paired **labia majora** enclose and protect the other external organs. These structures are composed primarily of folds of adipose tissue. The outer skin covering of the labia major contains numerous hairs, sweat glands, and sebaceous glands. Between the labia majora are flattened, longitudinal folds of tissue called the **labia minora;** anterior ends of the labia minora fuse at the clitoris. The externally visible reproductive structures, paired labia majora and labia minora, make up the vulva.

At the anterior end of the vulva is a small projection, the **clitoris.** The clitoris corresponds to the male penis and is composed of erectile tissue. The vestibule of the vulva is the space between the labia minora into which the urethra and vagina open. Located on either side of the vaginal opening are the vestibular glands **(Bartholin's glands).** These glands secrete fluid that moistens and lubricates the vestibule.[1,2,5]

Sexual Response in the Female

There is a saying that the primary sex organ is the brain. The rationale behind this statement is that ultimately the central nervous system (CNS) is the center in which sexual pleasure is perceived. Having stated that the end point is perception in the brain, this section begins at the other end—the initiation of sexual excitation.

Sources of sexual excitation   There are three sources of sexual excitation. Any of the three—optimally all three—may be present in a given situation. The first source of sexual excitation is fantasy, which occurs in the cerebral cortex. (Thus arousal starts in the brain and ends with its perception in the brain.) Sexual fantasy serves to heighten the desire for sexual activity.

The second source of sexual excitation is nongenital sensory stimulation (e.g., a kiss, a caress, holding hands, or stroking the hair). But even with these actions, the brain's interpretation of that stimulus is important. For example, the stroking of a woman's ear by her lover may elicit a far different response from that same sensation produced by a bug's crawling on her ear.

The third source of sexual stimulation is direct genital stimulation. The main difference neurologically between it and the nongenital stimulus is that the genital area is richly innervated. Therefore stimulation of the vulva, vagina, or clitoris can provide massive sensory input. This input runs from the point of the stimulus along the pudendal nerve and sacral plexus to the sacral segments of the spinal cord and ultimately to the cerebral cortex where the sensation is perceived.

Erection, lubrication, and orgasm   The above-mentioned stimuli result in a series of physiologic changes referred to as the *sexual response.* Erectile tissue in the clitoris is almost identical to that of the penis. Efferent nervous impulses flowing to the clitoris through parasympathetic nerves of the sacral plexus result in vascular engorgement and erection of this tissue. This same parasympathetic outflow triggers the paired vestibular glands at the vaginal introitus to produce mucous lubrication. (There is also lubrication from the vaginal walls and cervix.) Absence of lubrication during intercourse can result in dryness and discomfort for both partners.

As the stimulation continues, additional physiologic changes occur, including increased heart rate (tachycardia) and respiratory rate (tachypnea). Continued stimulation causes an increased muscular tension throughout the body. At **orgasm,** there is an intense, pleasurable, neuromuscular release. After it is an interval of physical and psychic relaxation referred to as *resolution.*[1,4]

Hormonal Control of Female Reproductive Functions

Female reproductive functions are controlled largely by hormones secreted by the hypothalamus, the anterior pituitary gland, and the ovaries. These hormones are responsible for the development and maintenance of female secondary sex characteristics, the maturation of the sex cells, and the monthly reproductive cycle.

FEMALE SEX HORMONES

The most important female sex hormones are estrogen and progesterone. In a nonpregnant female the primary source of **estrogen** is the ovaries. At puberty, under the influence of the anterior pituitary gland, the ovaries secrete increasing amounts of this hormone, which stimulates enlargement of various accessory organs and the external reproductive organs. In addition, estrogen is responsible for the development and maintenance of most female secondary sexual characteristics.

The ovaries are also the primary source of **progesterone** in the nonpregnant female. Progesterone causes changes in the uterus during the female reproductive cycle. In addition, it affects the mammary glands and regulates the secretions of gonadotropins from the anterior pituitary.[2,5,6]

FEMALE REPRODUCTIVE CYCLE

The first female reproductive cycle or menstrual cycle **(menarche)** occurs after the ovaries and other reproductive organs have reached maturity. In healthy and well-nourished women in the United States, the average age for menarche is near the twelfth year. Menstrual cycles usually continue into middle age at which time the cycles cease **(menopause).** *Premature menopause* is arbitrarily defined as menopause with onset at or before age 35 years.

There are three levels of hormonal control in the normal reproductive cycle. Each level occurs in an anatomically distinct area of the body. The first level is in the hypothalamus where **gonadotropin releasing hormone (Gn-RH)** is produced. This hormone acts on the anterior pituitary gland, the second anatomic level, to control the secretion of **follicle-stimulating hormone (FSH)** and **luteinizing hormone (LH).** FSH and LH then control the production of the ovarian hormones, estrogen and progesterone, at the third anatomic level.

Research has not yet fully determined the monthly variation in the release of Gn-RH from the hypothalamus. However, the monthly variation in the other hormones is well established. Figure 61–2 depicts these cyclic changes for both FSH and LH from the anterior pituitary gland and for estradiol and progesterone from the ovaries.

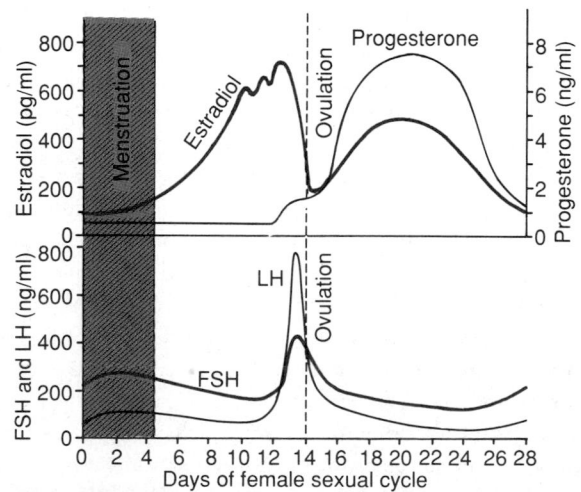

FIGURE 61–2   Serum hormonal levels during the menstrual cycle. (From Guyton, A.C. [1991]. *Textbook of medical physiology* [8th ed.]. Philadelphia: W.B. Saunders.)

In the first half of the menstrual cycle, under the influence of FSH and LH, the ovaries are in a follicular phase. During this phase, several follicles, each containing an ovum, grow and mature. Typically only one follicle matures beyond a certain stage; the others regress. During the maturation process, the follicle secretes estrogen and progesterone. The estrogen causes the uterine lining to thicken **(proliferative phase).** Near the fourteenth day of follicular development is a surge in LH concentration (and to a lesser extent, one of FSH). As a result, the follicle ruptures, releasing the ovum into the peritoneal cavity. This process is called **ovulation.** Ovulation usually occurs on approximately day 14 of a 28-day cycle, with day 1 considered the first day of menses.

After ovulation, a yellow glandular mass **(corpus luteum)** is formed by the ovarian follicle that has matured and discharged its ovum. Corpus luteum cells secrete large quantities of progesterone and estrogen during the last half of the reproductive cycle. Progesterone acts on the uterine lining, causing it to become more vascular and glandular. It also stimulates uterine glands to secrete increased quantities of glycogen and lipids **(secretory phase).** These changes prepare the endometrial tissues for the development of an embryo.

If the oocyte is not fertilized by a sperm cell, the corpus luteum begins to degenerate near the twenty-fourth day of the cycle. Concentration levels of estrogen and progesterone decline rapidly after the deterioration of the corpus luteum. As a result, the blood vessels in the endometrium constrict, reducing the supply of oxygen and nutrients to the uterine lining. These lining tissues disintegrate and slough off. At the same time, blood that escaped from damaged capillaries passes through the vagina **(menstruation).** The combined cellular debris and blood loss create the menstrual flow. This flow usually begins near the twenty-eighth day of the cycle and continues for 3 to 5 days.[1,2,4,7]

CONCEPT REVIEW

Estrogen is responsible for the development and maintenance of secondary sex characteristics.

Progesterone and estrogen prepare the uterine lining each month for possible conception.

Events of the female reproductive cycle are coordinated by the interaction of gonadotropic and ovarian hormones.

MALE REPRODUCTIVE SYSTEM

The organs of the male reproductive system are specialized to produce and maintain sperm cells and to transport these cells to the female reproductive tract. Male reproductive organs also secrete male sex hormones. This section presents an overview of the male reproductive system and includes information on spermatogenesis, the male sexual response, and hormonal regulation of male reproductive functions.

Organs of Male Reproductive System

The organs of the male reproductive system consist of the primary sex organs (testes), internal accessory organs, and external reproductive organs.

PRIMARY SEX ORGANS: TESTES

Primary sex organs in the male are the two testes in which sperm cells and the male sex hormones are formed. The **testes** are ovoid organs suspended by a spermatic cord within the scrotum. Each testis is approximately 4 to 5 cm long and is divided into approximately 250 to 300 cone-shaped lobules. Within each lobule are one to four coiled **seminiferous tubules** (Fig. 61–3). These tubules are lined with specialized stratified epithelium, which includes spermatogenic cells. Other specialized cells in the testes are **interstitial cells,** or **cells of Leydig,** which produce and secrete the male sex hormones.[1,2]

Spermatogenesis, the production of mature sperm cells, begins in adolescence in response to hormonal influence. Spermatogenesis occurs in the seminiferous tubules, specifically in **spermatogonia cells** (undifferentiated male germ cells) that lie along the outer border of the tubular epithelium. These primitive spermatogonia, called *type A spermatogonia,* divide into more differentiated cells called *type B spermatogonia.* Type B spermatogonia move away from the tubular epithelium and become enveloped by Sertoli's cells, which contain nutrients needed for sperm maturation.

For the next 24 days, the spermatogonia enlarge to become primary spermatocytes. Each spermatocyte contains 23 pairs of chromosomes. One of the pairs has the sex-determining chromosomes: an X (female) chromosome and a Y (male) chromosome. At the end of 24 days, the primary spermatocytes divide to form secondary spermatocytes. This **meiotic division** results in 23 chromosomes going to one secondary sper-

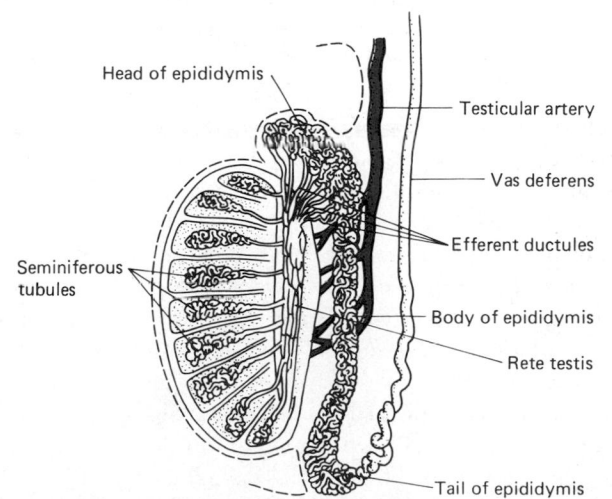

FIGURE 61–3   Cross section of the testicle. (From Guyton, A.C. [1991]. *Textbook of medical physiology* [8th ed.]. Philadelphia: W.B. Saunders.)

matocyte and 23 chromosomes going to the other spermatocyte. The XY chromosomal pair also splits so that one spermatocyte receives the X chromosome and the other receives the Y chromosome.

Within the next 2 to 3 days, the secondary spermatocytes undergo further meiotic division to form spermatids. Each spermatid contains 23 chromosomes. During the next few weeks of spermatogenesis, the spermatids continue to develop, losing most of their cytoplasm and elongating into the shape of mature sperm. A mature sperm consists of a head and a tail. The head contains the genetic material. The anterior two thirds of the head is covered by a cap called the *acrosome,* which contains enzymes used to penetrate the ovum. The tail of the sperm is called the *flagellum.* It consists of a body containing mitochondria (provides energy for movement) and an axoneme. The flagellar (to-and-fro) movement allows the sperm to travel in a straight line.

Spermatogenesis is completed in approximately 74 days. However, the sperms are incapable of fertilization at this point. The maturation process is completed as the sperms pass through the epididymis. The sperms cells then are capable of motility and fertilization. They are stored in the vas deferens and ampulla of the vas deferens where they maintain fertility for 1 month.[1,2,7]

Spermatogenesis occurs most ideally at temperatures lower than core body temperature. For this reason the testes are located in the scrotum. A spinal reflex mechanism controls contraction and relaxation of the scrotal muscles. When testicular temperature rises, muscles relax and the scrotum becomes more pendulous, thus drawing the testes away from the body and lowering their temperature. When testicular temperature drops, scrotal muscles contract, causing the testes to pull closer to the body and increasing their temperature.[1,4]

INTERNAL ACCESSORY ORGANS

The internal accessory organs include the epididymides, vas deferens, ejaculatory ducts, urethra, seminal vesicles, prostate gland, and bulbourethral glands. Each **epididymis** is a tightly coiled, thin tube. This tube is connected to ducts within a testis. The epididymis emerges from the top of the testis and descends along the posterior surface of the testis. The epididymis eventually becomes the **vas deferens,** a muscular tube that begins at the lower end of the epididymis, passes along the medial side of a testis, and becomes a part of the spermatic cord. Each vas deferens enters the abdominal cavity by passing through an inguinal canal. Near its point of termination, the vas deferens becomes dilated, forming the *ampulla.* The ampulla joins the duct of a seminal vesicle to form an **ejaculatory duct,** which passes through the prostate gland and becomes the internal urethra.

The **seminal vesicle** is a contorted tube that secretes a slightly alkaline fluid that contains nutrients and prostaglandins. The fluid helps regulate the pH of the tubular contents and nourish the sperm until fertilization occurs. In addition, prostaglandins make the cervix more receptive to sperm and cause reverse peristaltic contractions in the uterus and fallopian tubes, which aid the movement of the sperm.

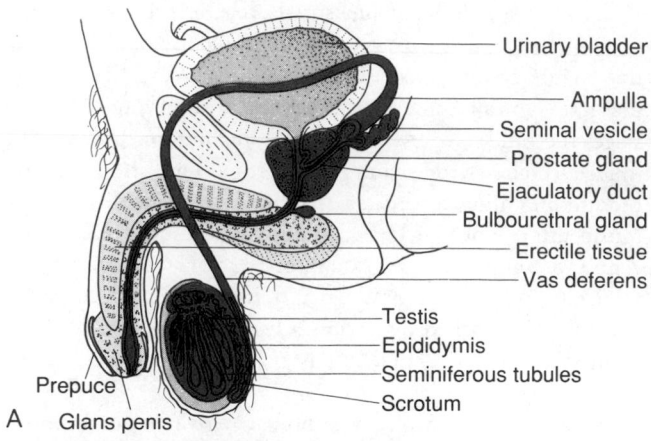

FIGURE 61–4   Cross section of the male reproductive system. (From Guyton, A.C. [1991]. *Text-book of medical physiology* [8th ed.]. Philadelphia: W.B. Saunders.)

The **prostate gland** surrounds the beginning of the urethra just below the urinary bladder. This gland secretes a thin, milky alkaline fluid that empties into the ejaculatory duct. The fluid neutralizes the slightly acidic fluid from the vas deferens. It also helps neutralize the acidic environment of the female genital tract, thus enhancing the motility and fertility of the sperm.

Bulbourethral (Cowper's) glands are located below the prostate gland and lateral to the internal urethra. These glands secrete a mucouslike fluid in response to sexual stimulation. The fluid provides some lubrication to the end of the penis in preparation for sexual intercourse.

Semen is the fluid ejaculated from the penis during the male sexual act. It consists of sperm and fluid from the vas deferens, seminal vesicles, and prostate gland and mucus from the bulbourethral and urethral glands. Semen has a pH of 7.5 and is milky in color with a mucoid consistency. In a normal ejaculate are 2.5 to 6 ml of semen, with 35 to 200 million sperm per milliliter. Figure 61–4 provides a cross-sectional view of the various parts of the male reproductive system.[1,2,5,8]

EXTERNAL REPRODUCTIVE ORGANS

The male external reproductive organs are the penis and the scrotum. The **penis** is designed to allow passage of urine from the bladder and semen from the internal reproductive organs. It consists of a shaft with an expanded tip, the *glans.* Part of the loose-fitting skin of the penis folds over the glans to form the *prepuce,* or foreskin. This cuff of skin can be removed in a surgical procedure called *circumcision.*

The body or shaft of the penis contains two cylinders of erectile tissue called *corpora cavernosa* and one cylinder of erectile tissue called the *corpus spongiosum.* The urethra is contained within this third cylinder. The three columns or cylinders of erectile tissue allow the penis to become enlarged and stiffened, an **erection,** during sexual intercourse.[8]

A pouch of skin and subcutaneous tissue, the **scrotum,**

hangs from the lower abdominal region behind the penis. The testes are housed within the scrotum.

Sexual Response in the Male

There are two stages in the male sexual response. The first is erection of the penis. An erection occurs in response to parasympathetic nerve impulses. These impulses cause the arterioles within the erectile tissues of the penis to dilate and fill with blood.

The second stage in the sexual response is orgasm, which consists of emission and ejaculation. Spinal reflexes at L1 and L2 emit sympathetic impulses to the smooth muscles within the walls of the testicular ducts, epididymides, vas deferens, and ejaculatory ducts. In addition, other sympathetic impulses stimulate rhythmic contractions of the seminal vesicles and prostate gland. These impulses cause rhythmic contractions of the genital ducts, forcing sperm and seminal and prostatic fluids into the internal urethra where they are mixed to form semen. This is known as **emission.** As the urethra fills with semen, sensory impulses are stimulated. In response, motor impulses are transmitted to skeletal muscles at the base of the penis, causing a series of wavelike muscular contractions. Semen is forced through the urethra to the outside, a process called **ejaculation.**

Immediately after ejaculation, sympathetic impulses cause vasoconstriction of the penile arterioles. Vasoconstriction causes a slowing of blood inflow and results in cessation of the erection. A latent period follows in which a second erection cannot occur. This period varies, lasting from 10 minutes to a few hours in a healthy male.[1,2,8,9]

Capacitation and Fertilization

Capacitation denotes changes spermatozoa undergo after ejaculation. These changes include removal of certain inhibitory factors and weakening of the acrosome to enhance motility and fertility capabilities.

Fertilization is the penetration of one sperm into one ovum. The acrosomal cap on the head of the sperm contains enzymes that can penetrate the granulosa and zona pellucida layers of the ovum. Once one sperm has penetrated the zona pellucida, chemical changes occur that cause other sperm to fall off the ovum. In addition, electric depolarization of the oocyte membrane occurs that may also inhibit further sperm penetration.

When fertilization takes place, the 23 chromosomes contained in the sperm combine with the 23 chromosomes in the ovum to provide the genetic material needed to produce offspring. The sex of the offspring is determined by which sperm fertilized the ovum, either a female (X-containing) sperm or a male (Y-containing) sperm.[1,8]

Hormonal Control of Male Reproductive Functions

A number of hormones either directly or indirectly influence the male reproductive system. These hormones include testosterone, Gn-RH, LH, and FSH.

HYPOTHALAMIC AND PITUITARY HORMONES

Gn-RH is secreted by the hypothalamus. It stimulates the anterior pituitary gland to secrete LH and FSH. LH stimulates the interstitial cells of Leydig to secrete testosterone. FSH causes the Sertoli cells in the seminiferous tubules to grow and secrete substances needed for spermatogenesis.

Secretion of these hormones is regulated by negative-feedback control. Increased testosterone production inhibits Gn-RH secretion, which decreases the secretion of LH and FSH. Too little testosterone causes the opposite effect. A similar negative-feedback control is present in spermatogenesis. A hormone known as *inhibin* is secreted by the Sertoli cells during spermatogenesis. When spermatogenesis occurs too quickly, inhibin is secreted. This inhibits the secretion of FSH. When spermatogenesis is decreased, inhibin levels drop, and FSH levels rise to stimulate spermatogenesis.[1]

MALE SEX HORMONES

Testosterone, an androgen, has a variety of effects on the testes, accessory reproductive organs, secondary sex characteristics, sexual behavior, and metabolism in the male. It is secreted by the interstitial cells of Leydig in the testes. During fetal growth, testosterone causes development of the external genitalia and internal reproductive organs and descent of the testes into the scrotum. From approximately 10 weeks after birth until adolescence, testosterone production stops. When it resumes, it causes further growth of the penis, scrotum, and testes and appearance of secondary sex characteristics. Secondary sex characteristics include growth of facial, pubic, and other body hair; deepening of the voice; changes in skin texture; thickening of secretions from sebaceous glands; and the masculine pattern of fat and muscle distribution. In spermatogenesis testosterone is needed for the development of spermatogonia into mature sperm.[1,10]

CONCEPT REVIEW

Testosterone is responsible for the development of reproductive structures and the development and maintenance of secondary sex characteristics.

Hormonal control of the male reproductive system involves the release of FSH and LH from the anterior lobe of the pituitary gland.

PHARMACOLOGIC IMPACT ON REPRODUCTIVE SYSTEM

The reproductive process in both females and males is highly sophisticated and complex. Hormonal secretion provides a delicate balance in reproductive functions. Many drugs, particularly synthetic hormones, are intended to replace or enhance normal hormone production. However, these drugs can disrupt that balance. A thorough understanding of the normal anatomy, physiology, and pathophysiology of the reproductive system is needed to administer drugs affecting this system safely and to provide quality care to the patient receiving the drugs.

SUMMARY

The normal female reproductive system functions to prepare a woman for conception and gestation and to support the fetus during its development. The average woman in the United States experiences menarche at age 12 years and menopause at age 50. In the years between these two points, reproductive functions are governed by a menstrual cycle. This cycle is hormonally controlled at three levels: the hypothalamus, which secretes Gn-RH; the anterior pituitary, which secretes LH and FSH; and the ovaries, which secrete estrogens and progesterone. Changes in these hormonal levels during the menstrual cycle help provide the proper medium for conception. In the absence of conception, the woman experiences menses. The sexual response in a woman is usually governed by the CNS.

The normal male reproductive system has three functions: spermatogenesis, the male sexual response, and hormonal regulation. As with the female, hormonal control occurs at three levels: the hypothalamus, which secretes Gn-RH; the anterior pituitary, which secretes LH and FSH; and the testes, which secrete testosterone. Testosterone is needed for development of the secondary sex characteristics and spermatogenesis. There are two stages in the male sexual response: erection of the penis and orgasm. As in a female, the sexual response is mediated by the CNS.

REFERENCES

1. Guyton, A. (1991). *Textbook of medical physiology* (8th ed.). Philadelphia: W.B. Saunders.
2. Hole, J. (1993). *Human anatomy and physiology* (6th ed.). Dubuque, IA: Wm. C. Brown.
3. Chard, T., & Lilford, R. (1990). *Basic sciences for obstetrics and gynaecology* (3rd ed.). New York: Springer-Verlag.
4. Guyton, A.C. (1992). *Human physiology and mechanisms of disease* (5th ed.). Philadelphia: W.B. Saunders.
5. Tortora, G., & Grabowski, S. (1993). *Principles of anatomy and physiology* (7th ed.). New York: Harper Collins.
6. Yen, S., & Jaffe, R. (Eds.). (1991). *Reproductive endocrinology: Physiology, pathophysiology, and clinical management* (3rd ed.). Philadelphia: W.B. Saunders.
7. Seeley, R., Stephens, T., & Tate, P. (1992). *Anatomy and physiology* (2nd ed.). St. Louis: Mosby–Year Book.
8. Hall-Craggs, E.C.B. (1990). *Anatomy as a basis for clinical medicine* (2nd ed.). Baltimore: Urban & Schwarzenberg.
9. Creager, J. (1992). *Human anatomy and physiology*. Dubuque, IA: Wm. C. Brown.
10. Soloman, E., & Phillips, G. (1987). *Understanding human anatomy and physiology*. Philadelphia: W.B. Saunders.

BIBLIOGRAPHY

Boeke, A. (1991). Beyond reproduction: A paradigm shift in women's health. *Journal of Obstetric, Gynecologic, and Neonatal Nursing, 12*(1), 12-13.

Dennis, R. (1992). Cultural change and the reproductive cycle. *Social Science and Medicine, 34,* 485-489.

Hunt, P. (1992). Reproductive health issues: Workplace perspectives. *AAOHN Journal, 40*(2), 72-77.

Klitsch, M. (1991). Hispanic ethnic groups face variety of serious health, social problems. *Family Planning Perspectives, 23,* 186-188.

Lamb, J., & Foster, P. (Eds.) (1988). *Physiology and toxicology of male reproduction.* San Diego: Academic Press.

Mishell, D.R., et al. (Eds.) (1991). *Infertility, contraception, and reproductive endocrinology* (3rd ed.). Boston: Blackwell Scientific.

Roberts, A. (1991). Reproductive system: Part 1. *Nursing Times, 87*(37), 49-52.

Roberts, A. (1991). Reproductive system: Part 2. *Nursing Times, 87*(41), 45-48.

Roberts, A. (1991). Reproductive system: Part 3. *Nursing Times, 87*(46), 53-56.

Sweezy, S.R. (1992). Contraception for the postpartum woman. *NAACOG's Clinical Issues in Perinatal and Women's Health Nursing, 3,* 209-226.

CHAPTER 62

DRUGS AFFECTING THE
Female Reproductive System

CAROL M. VIAMONTES • WILLIAM R. GERBER • MICHAEL F. THOMURE

◉ **Nursing Process**

LEARNING OBJECTIVES:

List the six categories of drugs that affect the female reproductive system.

Summarize information to obtain in the health history of the client receiving these drugs.

Describe nursing management of clients taking drugs affecting the female reproductive system.

KEY TERM: Basal body temperature

◉ **Hypothalamic Stimulants**

LEARNING OBJECTIVES:

Describe the action and therapeutic uses of hypothalamic stimulants.

Describe undesired clinical responses associated with hypothalamic stimulants.

◉ **Ovulatory Stimulants**

LEARNING OBJECTIVES:

Describe the action and therapeutic uses of ovulatory stimulants.

Describe undesired clinical responses associated with ovulatory stimulants.

KEY TERMS:

Anovulation, endogenous

◉ **Hypothalamic Inhibitors**

LEARNING OBJECTIVES:

Describe the action and therapeutic uses of hypothalamic inhibitors.

Describe undesired clinical responses associated with hypothalamic inhibitors.

KEY TERM: Endometriosis

◉ **Female Sex Hormones**

LEARNING OBJECTIVES:

Describe the actions and therapeutic uses of estrogens and progesterone or progestins.

List specific estrogens and progestins.

Describe undesired clinical responses associated with estrogens and progestins.

Compare monophasic, biphasic, and triphasic oral contraceptives.

KEY TERMS:

Biphasic, estrogen, exogenous, hypoestrogenic, monophasic, progesterone, progestin, triphasic

◉ **Uterine Stimulants**

LEARNING OBJECTIVES:

Describe the actions and therapeutic uses of uterine stimulants.

Describe undesired clinical responses associated with uterine stimulants.

◉ **Uterine Inhibitors**

LEARNING OBJECTIVES:

Describe the actions and therapeutic uses of uterine inhibitors.

Describe undesired clinical responses associated with uterine inhibitors.

◉ **Lactation Inhibitors**

LEARNING OBJECTIVE: Describe the actions and therapeutic uses of lactation inhibitors.

When a female reaches adolescence, a number of physical changes occur that are brought on by the increased
secretion of various hormones. The physical changes prepare
the reproductive system for fertilization and gestation. As described in Chapter 61, the changes are cyclical and usually occur monthly unless interrupted by pregnancy or altered by factors such as illness or stress. The cycles cease at menopause.

During a woman's reproductive years, conditions may arise
that require drug therapy. Six general categories of drugs affect
the female reproductive system: (1) hypothalamic and ovulatory stimulants, (2) hypothalamic inhibitors, (3) female sex
hormones, (4) uterine stimulants, (5) uterine inhibitors, and
(6) lactation inhibitors. Hypothalamic and ovulatory stimulants are generally used in the diagnosis and treatment of infertility. Hypothalamic inhibitors are used to treat endometriosis and uterine fibroids. The female sex hormones, estrogen and progesterone, are used both as a means of
contraception and as a replacement in hypoestrogenic states
such as menopause. Uterine stimulants are effective in initiating or augmenting the labor process, whereas uterine inhibitors are used in the treatment of preterm labor. For the
woman who does not wish to breast-feed, lactation inhibitors
may be prescribed.

▨ NURSING CONSIDERATIONS

Women's health care is an important issue. Women with reproductive concerns such as contraception, infertility, premenstrual syndrome (PMS), and menopause are commonly
treated outside the hospital. The nurse plays an important role
in the care of these individuals.

Assessing   Before administering drugs that affect reproduction, it is important to obtain a thorough **health history.**
Identifying information should include age, race, occupation,
and name of significant other. Medical history should include
a drug history, history of allergies, past surgical procedures,
and previous medical problems such as hypertension, diabetes,
or cancer. Also determine if the client smokes, drinks alcohol,
or uses recreational drugs. A family history is taken to determine if family members have been treated for any type of illness. Note especially if any family members have been born
with structural anomalies, mental retardation, or musculoskeletal or neuromuscular disorders.

More detailed information is taken about menstrual history
(e.g., age of menarche and menstrual patterns). Following are
examples of important questions:

- When was the first day of your last menstrual period
  (LMP)?
- How often do your periods occur?
- How long do your periods normally last?
- How many pads or tampons do you use on each day of
  your period?

Note the date and results of the client's last Papanicolaou
(Pap) test. Ask if there has been treatment for abnormal test results. If the client is sexually active, identify the method of
birth control used. In addition, the client should be questioned about her history of and treatment for sexually transmitted diseases. If indicated, an obstetric history is taken to determine the number of pregnancies and their outcomes.
Document gravida (number of conceptions), parity (number
of deliveries of 20 weeks or greater), and abortions (number of
terminations, spontaneous or elective, earlier than 20 weeks)
(e.g., 26 year old, $G_4 P_3 A_1$).

Physical assessment includes a head-to-toe examination,
with particular emphasis on the female reproductive system.
This includes examination of the external and internal genitalia, obtaining a Pap smear, and bimanual examination. In
addition, blood pressure, height, and weight are noted.

Diagnosing   Nursing diagnoses are developed for the
client based on analysis of the assessed data. Appropriate diagnoses include the following:

- Anxiety related to change in health status.
- Disturbance in body image related to physical changes
  caused by drug therapy.
- Altered family processes related to addition of a family mem-
  ber (the newborn).
- Fatigue related to drug therapy.
- Fluid volume excess related to drug therapy.
- Noncompliance with drug therapy related to lack of knowl-
  edge.

Planning   Since most clients are seen in ambulatory care
settings, planning primarily involves client education.
Teaching plans can be developed that address knowledge
deficit of specific drugs, methods of administration, mechanisms of drug action, and undesired clinical responses. The
client may also need instruction in normal female anatomy
and physiology, particularly hormonal regulation.

Planning also includes development of expected outcomes.
The outcomes are based on the nursing diagnoses and are developed with the client when possible. Appropriate expected
outcomes might include the following:

- Client reports anxiety is reduced.
- Client verbalizes understanding of body changes.
- Client demonstrates involvement in problem-solving pro-
  cesses.
- Client reports improved sense of energy.
- Client lists signs that require notification of primary care
  provider.
- Client verbalizes accurate knowledge about treatment regi-
  men.

Implementing   Drugs affecting the female reproductive
system are administered through a variety of routes: oral, intramuscular (IM), intravenous (IV), transdermal, and intravaginal and intracervical instillation. Specific nursing consider-

ations for each drug group are discussed in detail throughout the chapter.

Evaluating   A number of methods are used to determine clinical response to drug therapy. They include diagnostic tests such as determining serum hormone levels and ultrasounds. Another method of evaluation is review of the records kept by the client (e.g., basal body temperature charts and menstrual records). (**Basal body temperature** is the oral temperature customarily taken daily just before getting out of bed. Recorded on a graph, it is helpful in determining when ovulation occurs.) Client reports of control of symptoms such as hot flashes and of the absence of clinical signs such as vaginal bleeding, pain, and uterine contractions are also noted. In addition, review the status of the expected outcomes with the client.

HYPOTHALAMIC STIMULANTS

The neuroendocrinologic control of the female reproductive system involves complex hormonal interactions between the hypothalamus, the pituitary gland, and the ovaries. This hormonal cascade begins with the hypothalamus. Specific loci in the hypothalamus produce a substance called gonadotropin releasing hormone (Gn-RH), which is released in an episodic and pulsatile fashion. The role of the releasing hormone is to stimulate the production of gonadotropin follicle-stimulating hormone (FSH) and luteinizing hormone (LH) from the pituitary gland. The timing of the Gn-RH pulses determines the predominance of FSH or LH.

Gonadotropins are released into the bloodstream and act on the ovarian follicles. Both of these hormones, along with estrogen, are required for the successful development and ultimate ovulation of the oocytes contained within the follicles. Alterations in the hypothalamic-pituitary-ovarian axis are responsible for a large proportion of the infertility disorders seen clinically. Recent advances in reproductive drug therapy have allowed practitioners to modify the axis at the three different levels mentioned above. Pharmacologic treatment allows a couple to conceive successfully in cases that otherwise have a poor prognosis. The following section describes the latest pharmacologic armamentarium used in the treatment of infertility.[1]

Gonadorelin acetate (Lutrepulse) and gonadorelin hydrochloride (Factrel) are two very similar drugs used in the diagnosis and treatment of infertility. Both are identical to the decapeptide-structure Gn-RH produced in the hypothalamus. Although the chemical structures are identical, gonadorelin acetate is marketed as an ovulation-induction agent, whereas gonadorelin hydrochloride is labeled as a diagnostic agent.

HYPOTHALAMIC STIMULANT PROTOTYPE

GONADORELIN ACETATE

Gonadorelin acetate is a relatively new drug, receiving Food and Drug Administration (FDA) approval in 1989.

Pharmacotherapeutics   Gonadorelin acetate is indicated in the treatment of conditions of infertility caused by a defect in the secretion of Gn-RH from the hypothalamus.

Pharmacokinetics   After IV injection, gonadorelin acetate has an initial half-life of 2 to 10 minutes and a terminal half-life of 10 to 40 minutes. It is rapidly metabolized to inactive peptide fragments and is excreted in the urine. Renal failure can prolong the half-life and excretion of the drug.[2,3]

Pharmacodynamics   Gonadorelin acetate is a synthetic decapeptide hormone that stimulates the release of FSH and LH in the anterior pituitary gland.[2]

Pharmaceutics   Gonadorelin acetate is administered by pulsatile IV doses to mimic the normal secretory patterns of the hypothalamus. This action in turn stimulates the pulsatile release of FSH and LH from the anterior pituitary.

The usual dosage is 5 μg every 90 minutes, delivered by the Lutrepulse pump. The pump is filled with 0.8-mg solution that delivers 50 μl per pulse. The pump can also be adjusted to deliver 2.5, 10, or 20 μg of the drug, depending on the needs of the individual client.

The recommended course of treatment is 21 days. When ovulation occurs, the drug is usually continued for an additional 2 weeks to maintain the corpus luteum. If there is no response (i.e., no ovulation), treatment cycles may be repeated two additional times. Dosage may be increased slowly in a stepwise fashion if there is no response after three cycles.[2,4]

Undesired Clinical Responses   Undesired clinical responses from gonadorelin acetate include multiple follicle development, multiple pregnancies, and ovarian hyperstimulation as manifested by ovarian enlargement, increased abdominal girth secondary to ascites, and abdominal pain. Adverse reactions include urticaria and anaphylaxis (bronchospasm, tachycardia, and flushing). Other reported undesired clinical responses include induration, inflammation, infection, thrombophlebitis, hematoma, and pruritus at the injection site.[2,3]

Contraindications and Precautions   Gonadorelin acetate use is contraindicated in women who have conditions that may be exacerbated by pregnancy—pituitary prolactinoma and ovulatory disorders other than those of the hypothalamus. Gonadorelin acetate use is also contraindicated in the presence of tumors dependent on reproductive hormones such as estrogen-dependent carcinomas of the breast. Women with a known sensitivity to gonadorelin acetate should not receive the drug.

Drug-Drug Interactions   No drug-drug interactions have been documented. However, gonadorelin acetate should not be administered concomitantly with other ovarian-stimulating drugs. Gonadorelin acetate has not been shown to interfere with laboratory tests.

Life-Span Considerations   Gonadorelin acetate is classified as a Pregnancy Category B drug. It does not appear to increase the risk of abnormalities if administered in the first trimester of pregnancy. It is not known if this drug is excreted in human milk, but there is no indication for administration in lactating women. Safety and efficacy of administering this drug to women under the age of 18 years have not been established.[2]

Specific Drug-Related Nursing Considerations   Before initiation of treatment, baseline ovarian ultrasound and hormonal levels are obtained. A pelvic examination is also done.

Inside the opened Lutrepulse pump kit are powder for injection, diluent, sterile catheter tubing, sterile reserve catheter, IV cannula units, syringe and needle, alcohol swabs, the Lutrepulse pump, batteries, elastic belt, pump manual, package insert, and client information. The reconstituted solution is placed in the reservoir bag, and the pump is set to deliver 25 or 50 μl over a pulse period of 1 minute, with pulse intervals set at every 90 minutes. The 8 ml of solution lasts 7 days.[4]

The cannula and IV site are changed every 48 hours. Instruct the client on the care of the infusion site, including aseptic technique. Teach the client to observe the injection site for inflammation, phlebitis, and hematoma, and tell her to notify the primary care provider if they occur.

During therapy, the client must continue to monitor basal body temperature, menstrual cycle patterns, and weight. Any side effects or adverse reactions should be reported to the health care provider immediately. In addition, encourage the client to keep appointments for regularly scheduled clinical examinations so that response to therapy can be monitored. A serum progesterone level is determined in the midluteal phase, around day 22, to help determine if ovulation has occurred. Ovarian ultrasounds are repeated as needed, depending on client response.

MISCELLANEOUS DRUGS IN CATEGORY

Gonadorelin hydrochloride, the other major drug in this category, is chemically identical to gonadorelin acetate. Thus their pharmacodynamics, pharmacokinetics, and undesired clinical responses are the same. Gonadorelin hydrochloride is marketed as a diagnostic agent used in both males and females to evaluate hypothalamic-pituitary-gonadotropic function. It stimulates the release of LH from the anterior pituitary and is useful in determining hypothalamic deficiency and pituitary failure. It can also be used to determine reserve pituitary function in clients who have had pituitary tumors either surgically removed or irradiated.

Gonadorelin hydrochloride is administered either subcutaneously or intravenously in a single injection dose of 100 μg. For women who have a well-documented menstrual cycle the drug is administered in the early follicular phase. The recommended protocol for testing gonadotropin function is summarized in the box. Test results are interpreted based on the clinical status of the individual client. These results allow the health care provider to determine the responsiveness of the hypothalamic-pituitary axis to hormonal stimulation.

> *PROTOCOL FOR TESTING GONADOTROPIN FUNCTION*
>
> Draw serum LH levels 15 minutes before and immediately before administration of gonadorelin hydrochloride. The LH baseline is the average of the two values. Administer 100 μg of gonadorelin hydrochloride subcutaneously or intravenously. Serum LH levels are then drawn at 15, 30, 45, 60, and 120 minutes after administration.

Gonadotropin hydrochloride should not be administered concomitantly with other drugs that would affect pituitary secretion of gonadotropins. They include androgens, estrogens, progestins, and glucocorticosteroids.[3] Table 62–1 summarizes dosage information and additional nursing considerations about hypothalamic stimulants.

OVULATORY STIMULANTS

A couple can be characterized as infertile if there has been failure to conceive despite sexual activity without contraception for a period of 1 year. Infertility affects 15% of couples. The most common cause of female infertility is **anovulation,** the failure of the ovary to release an egg.

For various physiologic reasons, a large number of women in the general population do not have a cyclic ovulatory pattern and thus can be treated by intermittent progestin withdrawal to induce regular menses. For those women wishing to conceive, ovulation-induction agents can create a more regular ovulatory menstrual pattern, thus affording an increased chance of conceiving per cycle than would otherwise be present. Ovulatory agents work at the hypothalamic level in clients who have normal pituitary and ovarian function or at the level of the ovary in women who do not have normal pituitary function. Their role is to enhance an otherwise normal pituitary-ovarian axis.

OVULATORY STIMULANT PROTOTYPE

CLOMIPHENE CITRATE

A number of ovulatory stimulants are available in the treatment of infertility. The most common and usual first drug of choice is clomiphene citrate (Clomid, Serophene).

Pharmacotherapeutics Clomiphene citrate is indicated for the induction of ovulation in a woman who is anovulatory and wishes to conceive. The client must have normal production of **endogenous** estrogen. Since the drug is not effective when anovulation is due to primary ovarian failure or hypothalamic failure, other causes of infertility should be excluded before its administration.

Pharmacokinetics Clomiphene citrate is readily absorbed from the gastrointestinal (GI) tract. It is gradually excreted, primarily in the feces. After a single 50-mg dose, serum levels of the drug exist 4 to 6 weeks.[3,4]

Pharmacodynamics Clomiphene citrate is an orally active synthetic hormone, nonsteroidal in structure, with both estrogenic and nonestrogenic properties. When clomiphene molecules bind to estrogen receptors, the hypothalamic-pituitary axis responds as if there were a serious estrogen deficit. This hypothalamic-pituitary response stimulates the release of LH and FSH, which leads to ovulation.[3,4]

Pharmaceutics Clomiphene citrate is available in 50-mg tablets.[4]

Undesired Clinical Responses Side effects of clomiphene citrate occur infrequently. The most common side effects are ovarian enlargement, which occurs in approximately 14% of clients, hot flashes (10%), and pelvic discomfort (7%). Ovarian hyperstimulation syndrome

TABLE 62–1

Hypothalamic Stimulants: Prototype and Major Drug in Category

Drug Name	Dosage and Route of Administration	Nursing Considerations
GONADORELIN ACETATE (Lutrepulse) HOW SUPPLIED IV: 0.8 and 3.2 mg	ADULTS Usual IV dose: 5 μg q90min Delivered as 50 μl per pulse	*Assess* Review baseline ovarian ultrasound and hormone level results. Assess client for preexisting pituitary prolactinoma and ovulatory disorders. Determine if client is pregnant; gonadorelin acetate is classified as Pregnancy Category B drug. *Implement* Reconstitute powder with 8 ml of diluent. Check solution for odor, discoloration, or particles. Instruct client on care of infusion pump. Teach client to monitor basal body temperature, body weight, and menstrual cycle patterns. *Monitor* Monitor client for undesired clinical responses: urticaria, pruritus, or infection, thrombophlebitis, hematoma, or inflammation at injection site. *Evaluate* Serum progesterone level is determined mid-luteal phase.
Gonadorelin Hydrochloride Factrel HOW SUPPLIED IV, SC: 100, 500 μg vials	ADULTS SC, IV: single injection of 100 μg	*Assess* See gonadorelin acetate. *Implement* Administer drug in early follicular phase for women with well-documented menstrual cycle. *Evaluate* Determine serum LH levels at 15, 30, 45, 60, and 120 min after administration.

(OHSS) sometimes occurs and is characterized by severe abdominal pain and enlargement of one or both ovaries. A small number of clients complain of visual disturbance such as blurred vision, which usually resolves within a few days to a few weeks. Breast tenderness, nausea and vomiting, nervousness, mood swings, and insomnia have also been reported. Less than 1% of clients have reported other symptoms such as dizziness, abnormal uterine bleeding, depression, fatigue, weight gain, and reversible hair loss.

In some clients, clomiphene citrate causes cervical mucus to become thick and tenacious, thus interfering with sperm survival. This change in cervical mucus is due to the antiestrogenic properties of clomiphene.[5]

Contraindications and Precautions Clomiphene citrate use is contraindicated in clients with thyroid and adrenal diseases, pituitary tumors, hepatic dysfunction, and undiagnosed abnormal uterine bleeding. It is also contraindicated in the presence of ovarian enlargement other than with polycystic ovarian (PCO) syndrome.

Life-Span Considerations Pregnancy safety has not been established by the FDA. There are insufficient data on the teratogenic effect on humans when used for ovulation induction. If there is a possibility of pregnancy, clomiphene should not be administered.

Specific Drug-Related Nursing Considerations A thorough assessment is necessary to determine if the client is an appropriate candidate for therapy. She should have normal hepatic function and normal production of endogenous estrogen. The potential father must have a normal result of semen analysis. Preexisting conditions such as undiagnosed, abnormal vaginal bleeding, ovarian cysts, uterine fibroids, and endometriosis should be evaluated.

Intervention focuses on education and monitoring. The client must understand normal reproductive function and factors that contribute to infertility. Explain the treatment plan in detail.

The client should also understand the schedule of drug administration. Instruct her to continue monitoring her basal body temperature daily to determine if ovulation takes place. A temperature rise of 0.5° C or 1° F that occurs 3 to 10 days after the last dose of clomiphene and lasts 12 to 16 days is suggestive of ovulation.

Review with the client possible undesired clinical responses. Teach the client responses that should be re-

TABLE 62–2
Ovulatory Stimulants: Prototype and Major Drugs in Category

Drug Name	Dosage and Route of Administration	Nursing Considerations
CLOMIPHENE CITRATE (Clomid, Serophene) HOW SUPPLIED Tablet: 50 mg	ADULTS Oral: 50 mg/d for 5 d from day 5 through day 9 of menstrual cycle If client does not ovulate, increase dose to 100 mg/d for 5 d; to achieve ovulation, dosage may be increased in 50-mg increments to a maximum of 250 mg/d.	**Assess** Assess client for preexisting thyroid and adrenal diseases, hepatic dysfunction, pituitary tumors, and undiagnosed abnormal uterine bleeding. **Implement** Teach client to monitor basal body temperature to determine when ovulation occurs. Instruct client about the schedule of drug administration. **Monitor** Monitor client for undesired clinical responses such as hot flashes, pelvic discomfort, and severe abdominal pain. **Evaluate** Evaluate effectiveness of drug, based on increase in body basal temperature, increased serum LH, a progesterone level >15 ng/ml in midluteal phase, and follicular development as shown on ultrasound.
Human Menotropins (Pergonal) HOW SUPPLIED Mixture of FSH and LH in a 1:1 ratio packaged in glass ampule; available as 75 IU and 150 IU	**Stimulation of Follicular Growth** ADULTS IM: 75 IU/d for 9-12 d; usually start day 3 of cycle Increase if there is no increase in serum estradiol or follicular growth	**Assess** See clomiphene. **Implement** Reconstitute with sterile saline solution provided by manufacturer. Administer immediately after reconstitution. Inspect solution for discoloration and particles. Anticipate administration of human chorionic gonadotropin (hCG) 24 h after last dose of human menotropins to trigger ovulation. Administer drug at same time every day, usually in afternoon after receiving results of estradiol level check. Instruct client to record weight daily. Teach client parenteral administration technique. **Monitor** Monitor serum estradiol levels as required starting 4-5 d after therapy begins. **Evaluate** Monitor serum estradiol level 12-18 h after last dose of human menotropins. Perform ultrasound when estradiol level reaches 150 pg/ml to monitor follicle development.
Human Chorionic Gonadotropin (Profasi) HOW SUPPLIED Powder: 10-ml multidose vial Available as 5000 or 10,000 USP U/vial	Drug is used in conjunction with human menotropins to stimulate ovulation. ADULTS IM: 5000-10,000 U/24 h after last dose of human menotropins (serum estradiol level of 600-1500 pg/ml indicates correct time to administer hCG)	**Implement** Reconstitute with 10 ml of bacteriostatic water provided by manufacturer. Reconstituted solution is good for 60 d. Inspect solution for discoloration and particles. Instruct client to have intercourse daily from day before administration of hCG. Do not administer if serum estradiol levels are greater than 1500 pg/ml.

TABLE 62–2 *Continued*
Ovulatory Stimulants: Prototype and Major Drugs in Category

Drug Name	Dosage and Route of Administration	Nursing Considerations
Human Chorionic Gonadotropin Continued		**Evaluate**
		Monitor serum estradiol levels and ultrasound
Urofollitropin (Metrodin)	Drug is often used to treat anovulation in women with polycystic ovarian syndrome.	**Implement** Anticipate administration of hCG 24 h after last dose of urofollitropin.
How Supplied Lyophilized powder or pellet: Packaged in glass ampules containing 75 IU	**ADULTS** IM: 75 IU/d starting day 2 or 3 of cycle for 7–12 d	Reconstitute with sterile saline solution provided by manufacturer. Administer immediately after reconstitution.
	Increase to 150 IU in subsequent cycles if serum estradiol levels remain low	Inspect solution for discoloration and particles.

ported to the health care provider immediately such as sharp abdominal or pelvic pain or abdominal bloating. If dizziness, visual disturbances, or lightheadedness occurs, instruct the client to avoid tasks that require concentration or coordination. Tell her to discontinue therapy immediately if pregnancy is suspected.

Evaluation of therapy is carried out by monitoring basal body temperatures, hormonal blood tests, and ultrasounds. A pelvic examination is done during the midluteal phase to ascertain that there is no ovarian enlargement. Ovulation is reflected by a rise in basal body temperature and progesterone levels greater than 15 ng/ml during the midluteal phase. Ultrasound findings that indicate ovulation include follicular development initially and a collapsed follicle and fluid in the cul-de-sac later. Instruct the client to observe her cervical mucus for changes. A postcoital test can be done at midcycle to evaluate antiestrogenic effects.

Approximately 70% to 80% of clients receiving clomiphene therapy achieve ovulation and 35% to 50% conceive. For those clients who do not respond to or who are not candidates for clomiphene, other types of ovulatory stimulants are available.[5] Table 62–2 summarizes dosage information and additional nursing considerations about ovulatory stimulants.

🌿 NURSING RESEARCH

Blenner, J.L. (1991). Clomiphene induced mood swings. *Journal of Gynecologic and Neonatal Nursing, 20* 321-327.

The purpose of this qualitative research was to study couples' perceptions of mood swings in women receiving clomiphene for infertility treatment. During the review of literature, the researchers found limited reference to mood swings as a side effect of clomiphene. However, their study revealed three phases of mood-swing response: (1) a lack of awareness of the relationship of the mood swing to the drug; (2) a gain in awareness of the relationship; and (3) management of the mood swings. The results of the study provide important information for nurses counseling couples experiencing clomiphene-induced mood swings.

STUDENT ACTIVITIES

- Review recent research literature to determine if further research has been completed on this topic.
- Interview nurses who care for clients receiving clomiphene and determine the prevalence of mood swings. 🌿

HYPOTHALAMIC INHIBITORS

Hypothalamic inhibitors are more commonly referred to as Gn-RH agonists. As previously mentioned, Gn-RH is secreted by the hypothalamus in a pulsatile fashion, intermittently stimulating the anterior pituitary gland to secrete FSH and LH. Gn-RH agonists produce a constant stimulation of the pituitary that causes the pituitary gland to become desensitized to Gn-RH. As a result, FSH and LH secretion drops, causing a drop in estrogen in women and testosterone in men.

Gn-RH agonists are used in the treatment of benign and malignant diseases sensitive to sex hormones. Thus far they have been approved for use in clients with endometriosis or precocious puberty and as palliative treatment of clients with advanced prostate cancer. In addition, they are used in the treatment of uterine fibroids, infertility, breast cancer, PCO syndrome, and benign prostatic hypertrophy.

Gn-RH agonists are poorly absorbed in the GI tract because of the high peptidase activity of the gut. They are administered only by intranasal spray or subcutaneous (SC), IM, or IV injection.[6–8] Only two hypothalamic inhibitors, leuprolide acetate and nafarelin acetate, are discussed in this section.

HYPOTHALAMIC INHIBITOR PROTOTYPE
LEUPROLIDE ACETATE

Leuprolide acetate (Lupron Depot) was approved by the FDA in 1985.

Pharmacotherapeutics Leuprolide acetate is indicated for the treatment of endometriosis and uterine fibroids. **Endometriosis** is the presence of endometrial tissue outside the uterus. Most common locations are the ovaries, posterior cul-de-sac, uterine ligaments, fallopian tubes, vagina, colon, and appendix. Endometriosis affects 10% to 20% of women and can result in infertility, dysmenorrhea, dyspareunia, chronic pelvic pain, abnormal menstrual patterns, and changes in bowel and bladder habits.

Pharmacokinetics In the treatment of endometriosis, leuprolide acetate for depot suspension is recommended. Plasma concentrations of this form of the drug are maintained for 1 month. Metabolism, distribution, and excretion in humans have not been fully determined.[9,10]

Pharmacodynamics Leuprolide acetate constantly stimulates the anterior pituitary gland to secrete FSH and LH. With prolonged administration, pituitary receptors become desensitized, and subsequently FSH and LH secretion is suppressed. Estrogen production is diminished.

Pharmaceutics Since leuprolide acetate is not active when administered orally, it must be administered subcutaneously or intramuscularly. The leuprolide acetate for depot suspension used for treating endometriosis is supplied in a single-dose vial. The recommended dosage is administered monthly in an IM injection; treatment should not exceed 6 months.

Undesired Clinical Responses Common side effects are those seen in menopause, including hot flashes (90% incidence), vaginal dryness, headaches, dyspareunia, decreased libido, and emotional lability. Leuprolide acetate also causes minimal but reversible loss in bone density. Some women experience an initial worsening of symptoms of endometriosis as a result of a transient increase in estrogen production during the first few weeks of therapy.[9,10]

Contraindications and Precautions Leuprolide acetate use is contraindicated in women who are hypersensitive to Gn-RH analogs or agonists or who have had an anaphylactic reaction to gonadorelin hydrochloride. It is also contraindicated in women with undiagnosed vaginal bleeding, during pregnancy, and during lactation.

Drug-Drug Interactions No drug interaction studies have been done. Because leuprolide acetate suppresses the pituitary-gonadal axis, laboratory tests measuring pituitary or ovarian function would give inaccurate results.

Life-Span Considerations Leuprolide acetate is classified as Pregnancy Category X. Studies done on rabbits showed a dose-related increase in fetal abnormalities. It is not known if leuprolide acetate is excreted in human breast milk, and studies on breast-fed babies have not been done. Safety and efficacy in children also have not been determined.[9,10]

Specific Drug-Related Nursing Considerations Client education is essential with leuprolide acetate. Review the course of therapy, expected results, and undesired clinical responses with the client. Explain to the client that most women stop having menstrual periods, although some have light bleeding around the expected time of menses during the first month of therapy. If normal menstruation persists after the second month, instruct the client to notify the primary care provider. Explain to the client that doses cannot be skipped or administered later than every 33 days. If this occurs, the effectiveness of the therapy is decreased, and the client may experience breakthrough bleeding.

Explain to the client that relief of symptoms is usually experienced after the first month of therapy. However, some exacerbation of symptoms may be experienced in the first few weeks because of initial increases in estrogen production. Although ovulation ceases in most women, there is a possibility of conceiving while receiving leuprolide acetate therapy. If the client is sexually active, instruct her to use a barrier method of contraception during therapy and for 2 months after therapy has been completed. Explain to the client that menstrual periods usually resume 2 months after completion of therapy. If the client has not had a menstrual period by the third month, she should notify her primary care provider.

This client also requires additional emotional support. Coping strategies should be identified to help her during periods of emotional lability and depression. Reassure her that hypoestrogenic effects are reversible, usually within 2 months of completion of therapy.

MISCELLANEOUS DRUGS IN CATEGORY

Nafarelin acetate (Synarel) is similar to leuprolide acetate. Therefore only the differences between the two drugs are presented.

Pharmacokinetics Nafarelin acetate is rapidly absorbed across the mucous membranes of the nasal passages into systemic circulation. Peak serum levels are obtained within 10 to 40 minutes, and the average serum half-life is 3 hours. Eighty percent of the drug is bound to plasma proteins. It is metabolized in the liver and excreted in the urine and feces.[10]

Pharmaceutics Nafarelin acetate is available as a nasal spray.[10]

Undesired clinical response Nasal irritation has been documented. Adverse reactions are rare and include hypersensitivity, palpitations, myalgias, breast enlargement, lactation, chloasma, and maculopapular rash.

Drug-drug interactions No drug-drug interactions have been documented. Nafarelin acetate increases triglyceride, cholesterol, and plasma phosphorus levels, increases eosinophil counts, and decreases serum calcium levels and white blood cell (WBC) counts.[10]

Specific drug-related nursing considerations Provide the client specific instructions about drug administration. Instruct the client to administer the spray only as directed (i.e., each morning and at bedtime). Teach her to clear the nasal passages by blowing the nose before administration. Have the client insert the tip of the container into one nostril, tip her head slightly forward, and close the opposite nostril. Instruct the client to squeeze the container gently, inhaling as the spray enters the nasal passage. The client should be told to exhale through her mouth. Emphasize to the client the importance of alternating nostrils to minimize nasal irritation.

Explain to the client that she may experience some nasal stinging; this usually diminishes over the course of therapy. If a nasal decongestant is required because of nasal rhinitis, it should be administered at least 30 minutes after using the spray to ensure maximum absorption of naforelin.

Table 62–3 summarizes dosage information and additional nursing considerations about hypothalamic inhibitors.

TABLE 62–3
Hypothalamic Inhibitors: Prototype and Major Drug in Category

Drug Name	Dosage and Route of Administration	Nursing Considerations
LEUPROLIDE ACETATE (Lupron, Lupron Depot) **HOW SUPPLIED** SC: 1 mg/0.2 ml IM: 3.75 and 7.5 mg/vial (depot formation)	**Endometriosis** Lupron Depot: 3.75 mg IM once a month, not to exceed 6 mo	**Assess** Assess client for preexisting undiagnosed vaginal bleeding. Determine if client is pregnant. Leuprolide is classified as Pregnancy Category X drug. **Implement** Administer depot formulation IM. Reconstitute drug with diluent provided by manufacturer. Shake suspension thoroughly; it should appear milky white. Rotate site monthly. **Monitor** Monitor client for undesired clinical responses such as hot flashes, vaginal dryness, headaches, dyspareunia, decreased libido, and emotional lability. **Evaluate** Evaluate absence of menstrual cycle.
Nafarelin Acetate (Synarel) **HOW SUPPLIED** Nasal solution: 2 mg/ml	**Endometriosis** **ADULTS** Nasal spray: one spray (200 µg) into one nostril in the morning and one spray into the other nostril in the evening; if amenorrhea does not occur, dose may be increased to 800 µg/d; treatment limited to 6 mo	**Assess** See leuprolide acetate. **Implement** Anticipate that therapy will begin between day 2 and day 4 of menstrual cycle. Instruct client in nonhormonal method of contraception. **Evaluate** Evaluate absence of menstrual cycle.

CONCEPT REVIEW

Alterations in the hypothalamic-pituitary-ovarian axis are responsible for a large proportion of infertility disorders.

Drug therapy can modify the axis that controls Gn-RH, FSH, and LH.

Gn-RH agonists can benefit clients with benign and malignant diseases that are sensitive to sex hormones.

FEMALE SEX HORMONES

The ovaries secrete a number of sex hormones in response to stimulation by the anterior pituitary gland. Estrogen and progesterone are considered the primary female sex hormones. **Estrogen** refers to a group of chemically similar hormones that include estrone, estradiol, and estriol. Estrogen is primarily produced by the developing graafian follicle during the follicular phase of the menstrual cycle. Some estrogen is derived from the adrenal glands and is secreted by the placenta and testes. **Progesterone** is secreted by the developing corpus luteum during the luteal phase. Although estrogen and proges-

terone are both female sex hormones, in many aspects these two steroid compounds have opposing roles on individual organ systems.

Estrogen

The onset of estrogen production at menarche leads to a growth spurt and the subsequent closure of the epiphyses of the long bones, which halts further increase in height. It also stimulates enlargement of various accessory organs and the external reproductive organs. For example, estrogen stimulates the growth and development of the fallopian tubes, uterus, and vagina.

During the normal menstrual cycle, rising estrogen levels during the follicular phase result in proliferation of uterine glandular tissue (endometrium), an increase in cervical mucous production, and an increase in breast size. After ovulation, if no conception has occurred, falling estrogen levels during the luteal phase lead to reversal of these effects. If conception occurs, high levels of estrogen help nourish and support the gestation.

Estrogen also plays a role in bone metabolism and mineral balance. Cessation of estrogen production at menopause leads to **osteoporosis,** thinning of bone matrix and brittle bones. In greater than physiologic doses, estrogen can lead to water and sodium retention. Estrogen also affects serum lipid levels. The hormone decreases low-density lipoprotein (LDL) and increases high-density lipoprotein (HDL), resulting in a protective effect on the cardiovascular system.[11]

Exogenous estrogens (originating outside the body) are either steroidal or nonsteroidal. All natural estrogen is steroidal and is either obtained from the urine of pregnant mares or prepared synthetically. Examples of natural estrogen include estradiol, estrone, and estriol. Conjugated estrogens such as Premarin are mixtures of natural estrogenic substances. Nonsteroidal estrogens are synthetically prepared and include diethylstilbestrol (DES) and chlorotrianisene (Tace).[12]

ESTROGEN PROTOTYPE
CONJUGATED ESTROGENS

Conjugated estrogens (Estrone Suspen, Lanestrin, Premarin) contain a mixture of estrogens obtained exclusively from natural sources, consisting mostly of sodium estrone sulfate and sodium equilin sulfate. The pharmacologic effects of conjugated estrogens are similar to those of endogenous estrogen.[3,4]

Pharmacotherapeutics The most common indication for estrogen administration is as a hormone replacement in **hypoestrogenic** states such as menopause or surgical castration (bilateral oophorectomy). Menopausal symptoms, including vasomotor instability (hot flashes), vaginal dryness and atrophy, mood swings and irritability, and bladder dysfunction, are usually corrected by appropriate replacement of estrogen. Additionally, estrogen replacement in the postmenopausal woman reduces the tendency toward osteoporosis by normalizing bone mineral metabolism and reduces the risk of cardiovascular disease. Estrogen is also used in the palliative treatment of inoperable advanced breast cancer in selected postmenopausal women. It is used in men for palliation of advanced prostatic cancer.[3,11]

Pharmacokinetics Metabolism and inactivation of the exogenous estrogens occurs primarily in the liver. Some forms of estrogens are excreted into the bile. However, they are reabsorbed from the intestine and returned to the liver through the portal venous system. Water-soluble estrogen conjugates are strongly acidic. This form of estrogen is ionized in body fluids and is excreted through the kidneys.[3] Peak serum levels and the half-life of exogenous estrogen are determined by the dosage form. For example, oral preparations of Premarin are absorbed and metabolized rapidly. Serum peak levels of Premarin occur at 4 hours, and the half-life is approximately 12 hours.

Pharmacodynamics In responsive tissue estrogens enter the cell and are transported into the nucleus. As a result of estrogen action, specific RNA and protein synthesis occurs.[3]

Pharmaceutics Oral, IM, topical, SC, IV, and intravaginal dosage forms of estrogen are available. Parenteral preparations come in oil solutions or aqueous solutions. Topical preparations are available for transdermal application.

Undesired Clinical Responses Undesired clinical responses are usually dose dependent and occur in almost every organ system in the body. Some of the more common responses include nausea, changes in menstrual patterns, breakthrough bleeding, breast enlargement or tenderness, edema, and weight gain. Undesired clinical responses associated with exogenous estrogen therapy are summarized in Figure 62–1.[3,4]

Contraindications and Precautions The use of **unopposed estrogen** (i.e., not offset by progesterone) is contraindicated in any woman who still has her uterus. Estrogen causes endometrial proliferation and, in the extreme, endometrial hyperplasia and endometrial cancer. This effect can be offset by the concomitant cyclic administration of progesterone.[12]

Estrogen therapy is usually contraindicated in a woman who has been diagnosed with breast cancer. However, in isolated cases in which the tumor has been demonstrated as estrogen- and progesterone-receptor negative and the client has severe symptomatology, it may be acceptable to treat with hormone replacement.

Estrogen therapy is also contraindicated in nursing mothers because it is excreted in breast milk, thus exposing the neonate to the hormone. It can also inhibit lactation. Other contraindications for estrogen therapy are undiagnosed breast mass or vaginal bleeding and active thrombophlebitis or thromboembolic disorders. Estrogen is used with caution in clients with a history of deep-vein thrombosis or pulmonary embolism, hyperlipidemia, hypertension, cardiovascular disease, and blood dyscrasias. Caution is also taken in clients with migraines, epilepsy, asthma, thyroid dysfunction, hepatic or renal disease, and diseases involving calcium or phosphorus metabolism.[3,12]

Drug-Drug, Drug-Nutrient, Drug-Environment Interactions One important drug-environment interaction is that with sunlight. When exposed to excessive sunlight, women receiving estrogen therapy can develop a blotchy discoloration of the skin. This discoloration is not always reversible when drug therapy is discontinued. Tanning should be avoided and sunscreens applied before any outdoor activity. No specific drug-nutrient interactions have been identified. In fact, most oral preparations of estrogen are taken with food to lessen any GI irritation.

Significant drug-drug interactions do occur with estrogen. For example, the concomitant use of estrogen and oral anticoagulants can decrease anticoagulant response. Estrogen therapy enhances the effect of certain clotting factors (e.g., prothrombin, factors VII, VIII, IX, and X). Estrogen potentiates the anticonvulsant effect of anticonvulsant drugs. Estrogen also increases the risk of hepatotoxicity when given with hepatotoxic drugs. Diabetics receiving exogenous estrogens may have increased insulin requirements.

Interferences with Diagnostic Studies Following are the effects of estrogen on four diagnostic studies:
1. Reduces serum folate concentration
2. Impairs glucose tolerance
3. Increases circulating total thyroid hormone as measured by T_4 levels
4. Increases thyroxine-binding globulin (TBG)

Life-Span Considerations Estrogens are classified as Pregnancy Category X drugs and are contraindicated in pregnancy. There is no benefit to such therapy during pregnancy, and there is a potential for teratogenic effects on the developing fetus. A woman planning to conceive should not take estrogen.

The safety and efficacy of estrogen therapy in children

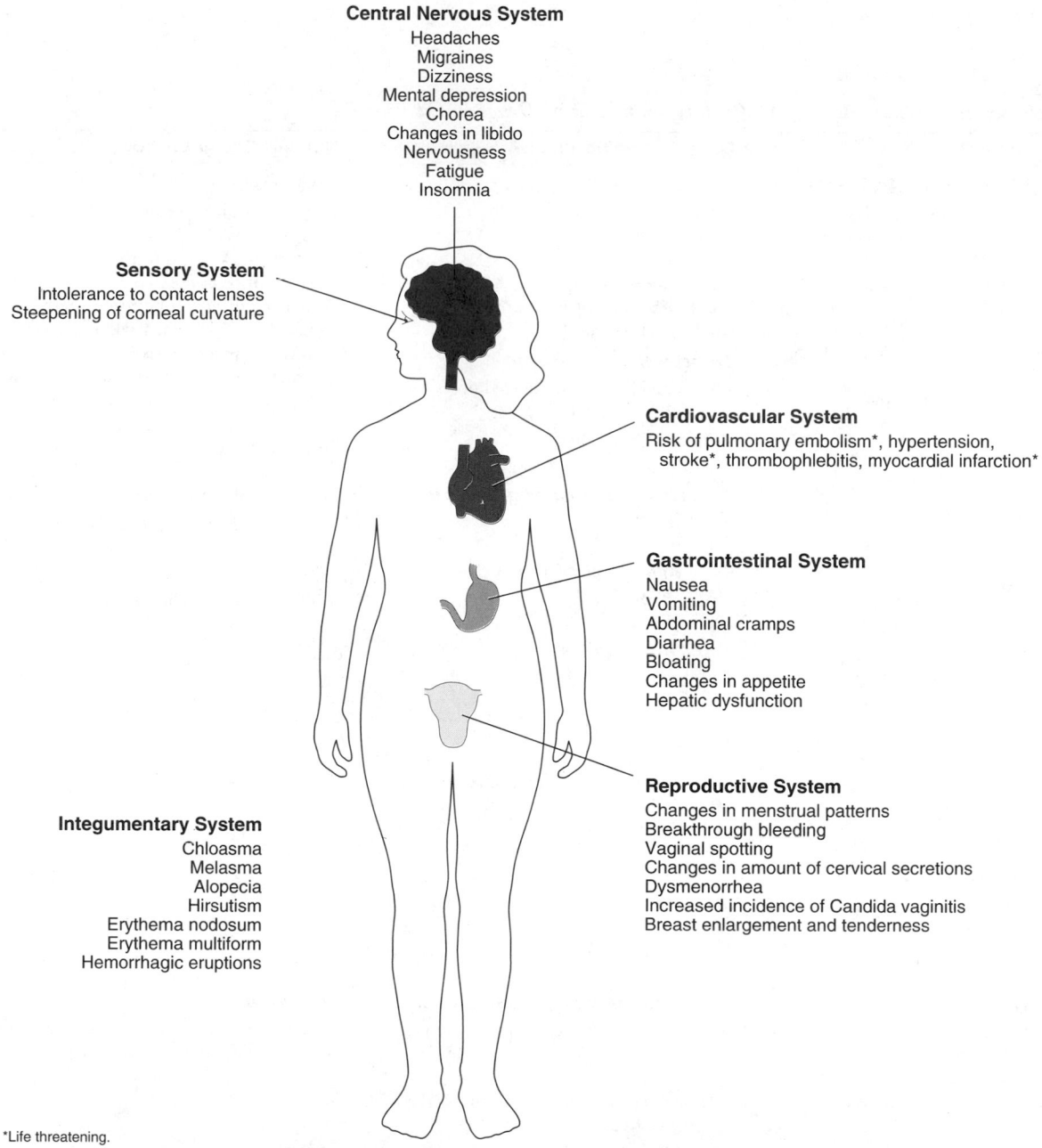

Central Nervous System
Headaches
Migraines
Dizziness
Mental depression
Chorea
Changes in libido
Nervousness
Fatigue
Insomnia

Sensory System
Intolerance to contact lenses
Steepening of corneal curvature

Cardiovascular System
Risk of pulmonary embolism*, hypertension,
stroke*, thrombophlebitis, myocardial infarction*

Gastrointestinal System
Nausea
Vomiting
Abdominal cramps
Diarrhea
Bloating
Changes in appetite
Hepatic dysfunction

Integumentary System
Chloasma
Melasma
Alopecia
Hirsutism
Erythema nodosum
Erythema multiform
Hemorrhagic eruptions

Reproductive System
Changes in menstrual patterns
Breakthrough bleeding
Vaginal spotting
Changes in amount of cervical secretions
Dysmenorrhea
Increased incidence of Candida vaginitis
Breast enlargement and tenderness

*Life threatening.

FIGURE 62–1   Undesired clinical responses associated with exogenous estrogen therapy.

have not been determined. In addition, estrogen should be used with caution in adolescents in whom bone growth is not yet complete.[3]

Specific Drug-Related Nursing Considerations
Obtain a thorough health history before the client begins estrogen therapy. Note if the client has a history of thromboembolic disease, diabetes, liver disease, migraine headaches, cardiovascular disease (hypertension or myocardial infarction), stroke, or psychiatric illness (e.g., depression).

Client education is important. As mentioned previously, a number of estrogen preparations are available. The type of drug used depends on the condition to be treated. Therefore teaching must be adjusted to the specific client, diagnosis, drug preparation, and dosage form.

Review with the client the expected drug actions and the desired responses to drug therapy. Instruct her about the proper dosing schedule and administration techniques. Teach the client using intravaginal instillations that vaginal creams are instilled at bedtime. Explain to the client that she might be more comfortable if she wears a sanitary pad during the day and that tampon use and douching are not recommended. For clients using the transdermal system, provide information on correct application of the patch and rotation of sites. Instruct the client not to apply the patch to breasts or waistline.

TABLE 62–4

Female Sex Hormones—Estrogens: Prototype and Major Drugs in Category

Drug Name	Dosage and Route of Administration	Nursing Considerations
CONJUGATED ESTROGENS (Menopak-E, Ovest-0.3, Ovest-0.625, Ovest-1.25, Premarin) **HOW SUPPLIED** Vaginal cream: 0.625 mg/g IM, IV: 25 mg/5 ml IM: 2 mg/ml and 20,000 U/ml Coated tablet: 0.3, 0.625, 0.9, 1.25, and 2.5 mg Uncoated tablet: 0.625 mg	Dosages are individualized, depending on diagnosis and client response. Lowest possible dose is used. Reevaluate every 6-12 mo. **Vasomotor Symptoms, Atrophic Vaginitis, Atrophic Urethritis** Oral: 0.3-1.25 mg/d **Female Hypogonadism** Oral: 2.5-7.5 mg/d in divided doses for 20 d, followed by 10 d of rest **Female Castration** Oral: initial dose—1.25 mg/d **Prevention and Management of Osteoporosis** Oral: 0.625 mg/d **Palliative Treatment of Advanced Breast Cancer** Oral: 10 mg tid **Atrophic Vaginitis** Intravaginal: 2-4 g (one half to one applicator) **Acute Bleeding** IV: 25 mg q6h	**Implement** Administer oil solutions slowly into large muscle mass. Administer IV solution to minimize acute vasomotor response. Anticipate drug will be administered on cyclic schedule (3 wk on, 1 wk off) in women with an intact uterus. Instruct client that drug can be taken with food or at bedtime to minimize associated nausea and vomiting. Instruct client to do monthly self-breast examination. Instruct diabetic client to monitor blood and urine closely for signs of hyperglycemia and glycosuria. **Monitor** Monitor liver function studies.
Estradiol (Estrace) **HOW SUPPLIED** Tablets: 1 and 2 mg Vaginal cream: 42.5-g tube (0.01%) with plastic calibrated applicator	**Vasomotor Symptoms, Atrophic Vaginitis, Kraurosis Vulvae, Female Hypogonadism, Female Castration, Primary Ovarian Failure** Oral: 1-2 mg/d **Atrophic Vaginitis** Vaginal cream (0.01%): 2-4 g/d for 2 wk; then reduce to half initial dose for 2 wk *Maintenance:* 1 g three times a week	See conjugated estrogens.
Dienestrol (Ortho Dienestrol) **HOW SUPPLIED** Vaginal cream: 2.75-oz (78 g) tube with or without applicator	**Atrophic Vaginitis, Kraurosis Vulvae** Vaginal cream: one to two applicators full daily for 1-2 wk; then half of initial dose for 1-2 wk *Maintenance:* one applicator one to three times a week	**Implement** Teach client to administer cream at bedtime. Instruct client to wear sanitary pads; tampon use is contraindicated.
Diethylstilbestrol (DES, Stilbestrol) **HOW SUPPLIED** Tablets: 1 and 5 mg	**Palliative Treatment in Inoperable Breast Cancer in Postmenopausal Women** Oral: 15 mg/d **Palliative Treatment in Inoperable Prostatic Carcinoma** Oral: 1-3 mg/d	**Assess** Determine if client is pregnant. Drug is not for use during pregnancy because of risk of vaginal cancer in female offspring. See conjugated estrogens.
Quinestrol (Estrovis) **HOW SUPPLIED** Tablets: 100 μg	**Vasomotor Symptoms, Atrophic Vaginitis, Kraurosis Vulvae, Female Hypogonadism, Female Castration, Primary Ovarian Failure** Oral: 100-μg/d for 7 d *Maintenance:* 100 μg/wk starting 2 wk after beginning treatment; may increase dose to 200 μg/wk to achieve therapeutic response	See conjugated estrogens.

TABLE 62–4 *Continued*
Female Sex Hormones—Estrogens: Prototype and Major Drugs in Category

Drug Name	Dosage and Route of Administration	Nursing Considerations
Estradiol (Estraderm) **How Supplied** Estraderm 0.05: 10-cm² system in calendar packs of 8 or 24 systems Estraderm 0.1: 20-cm² system in calendar packs of 8 or 24 systems	Drug has variety of therapeutic uses. Dosage is adjusted to control symptoms.	**Implement** Teach client to apply Estraderm system to clean, dry skin on body trunk. Instruct client not to apply to breasts. Teach client to rotate sites with at least 1-wk interval before reapplying to same site. Teach client to apply system immediately after removing protective liner and hold in place 10 s to ensure good contact with skin. Tell client to contact primary care provider if skin becomes reddened or irritated.

For a woman with an intact uterus, a cyclic dosing schedule of 3 weeks of estrogen with progestin added for the last 10 days of the estrogen therapy is most frequently recommended. No medication is taken for the last 7 days of the 28-day cycle. This most closely approximates the natural female hormonal schedule. This type of dosing schedule avoids continuous stimulation of estrogen-receptive tissues. The progesterone component of treatment is not necessary in women who have had a hysterectomy.[12]

Teach the client the undesired clinical responses associated with estrogen therapy. Inform the client that nausea, vomiting, headaches, and fatigue can occur early in therapy; they usually disappear after a few weeks. If fluid retention develops, it can be minimized by a low-sodium diet. Instruct the client to notify the primary care provider if any of the following occur: sudden chest pain, sudden leg pain, shortness of breath, sudden weight gain, weakness of arms or legs, abnormal vaginal bleeding, or sudden headaches or dizziness. Any changes in emotional status such as depression, withdrawal, lack of interest in self, or anorexia should also be reported.

Encourage the client to make regular visits to the primary care provider for follow-up care. The client's blood pressure should be monitored regularly, and breast and pelvic examinations are recommended every 6 to 12 months. In addition, a Pap test should be done once a year. If the client suspects she is pregnant, she should discontinue estrogen therapy immediately and contact her health care provider.

If estrogen is prescribed for the prevention or management of osteoporosis, instruct the client to exercise regularly and to maintain an intake of 1000 to 1500 mg of elemental calcium daily. Diabetics should be instructed to monitor their blood and urine closely for hyperglycemia and glycosuria. Any changes should be reported to the primary care provider. If the client smokes, she should be advised to stop smoking because smoking increases the risk of side effects. This is especially true in women over the age of 35 years.

MISCELLANEOUS DRUGS IN CATEGORY

Some of the numerous exogenous estrogen preparations are summarized in Table 62–4.

Progesterone

Progesterone is a female sex hormone secreted by the ovary, primarily the corpus luteum, during the luteal phase of the menstrual cycle. Its synthesis and secretion are stimulated by LH. Usually by the second month of pregnancy, the placenta is secreting progesterone and estrogen.

Progestin is the term used for certain synthetic and natural progestational drugs. As implied by the name, progestin compounds are capable of sustaining pregnancy. Progesterone is the only naturally occurring progestin. Synthetic progestins are derived either from progesterone or testosterone.

PROGESTERONE PROTOTYPE
MEDROXYPROGESTERONE ACETATE

Medroxyprogesterone acetate (Depo-Provera, Med-Pro, Provera) is a derivative of progesterone.

Pharmacotherapeutics Oral synthetic progestins are primarily used either alone or in combination with estrogens for contraception. Other uses for progestins include inhibiting the effects of estrogen on the endometrium in treatment of menopausal symptoms; regulation of menstrual cycles in clients with dysfunctional uterine bleeding; regression of ectopic endometrial lesions in clients with endometriosis; and treatment of symptoms associated with premenstrual syndrome. Progestins have also been used in the palliative treatment of renal, breast, and endometrial carcinomas.[12]

Pharmacokinetics The absorption of most oral progesterone preparations is inefficient and subject to first-pass hepatic metabolism. However, oral delivery systems of progesterone that involve micronization have recently been developed. This system enhances absorption. The absorption of oral progestins is variable. Progesterone is absorbed well from the vaginal, rectal, and IM routes of administration. Progesterone and progestins are metabolized in the liver and excreted in the urine.[3,12]

Pharmacodynamics Progesterone acts by binding to an intranuclear protein receptor that is specific for the progestins. The progestin-receptor complex binds to DNA and activates specific mRNA synthesis, ultimately resulting in the production of proteins.

Progestins stimulate the development of the endometrium, preparing it for implantation of a fertilized ovum. Progestins affect the cervical mucus, changing it from copious, thin, and watery to a more scant, viscous material. If fertilization occurs, progestins suppress ovulation and cause relaxation of the smooth muscles in the uterus, GI tract, gallbladder, and ureter. If fertilization does not occur, the elevated estrogen and progesterone levels stimulate the anterior pituitary to stop secretion of FSH and LH, the result of which is to shut down secretion of estrogen and progesterone. As a result, menstruation occurs.

Progestins also stimulate the growth of acini in the mammary glands during the luteal phase and cause thinning of the vaginal wall. These hormones have a thermo-genic effect on the body, causing the body temperature to rise approximately 1° F, starting at midcycle.[12]

Pharmaceutics As with estrogen, dosage and method of administration of synthetic and natural progestins are individualized, based on diagnosis and client response. The lowest possible dose is administered to control symptoms. Natural progestins (progesterone) are available in a parenteral preparation and in a intrauterine contraceptive device (IUD). Synthetic progestins are available in oral and parenteral forms.

Progestasert IUD is inserted into the uterine cavity for the purpose of contraception. The device is composed of a plastic polymer embedded with 38 mg of progesterone. The IUD acts locally to create a hostile endometrium that inhibits serum capacitation and implantation. The addition

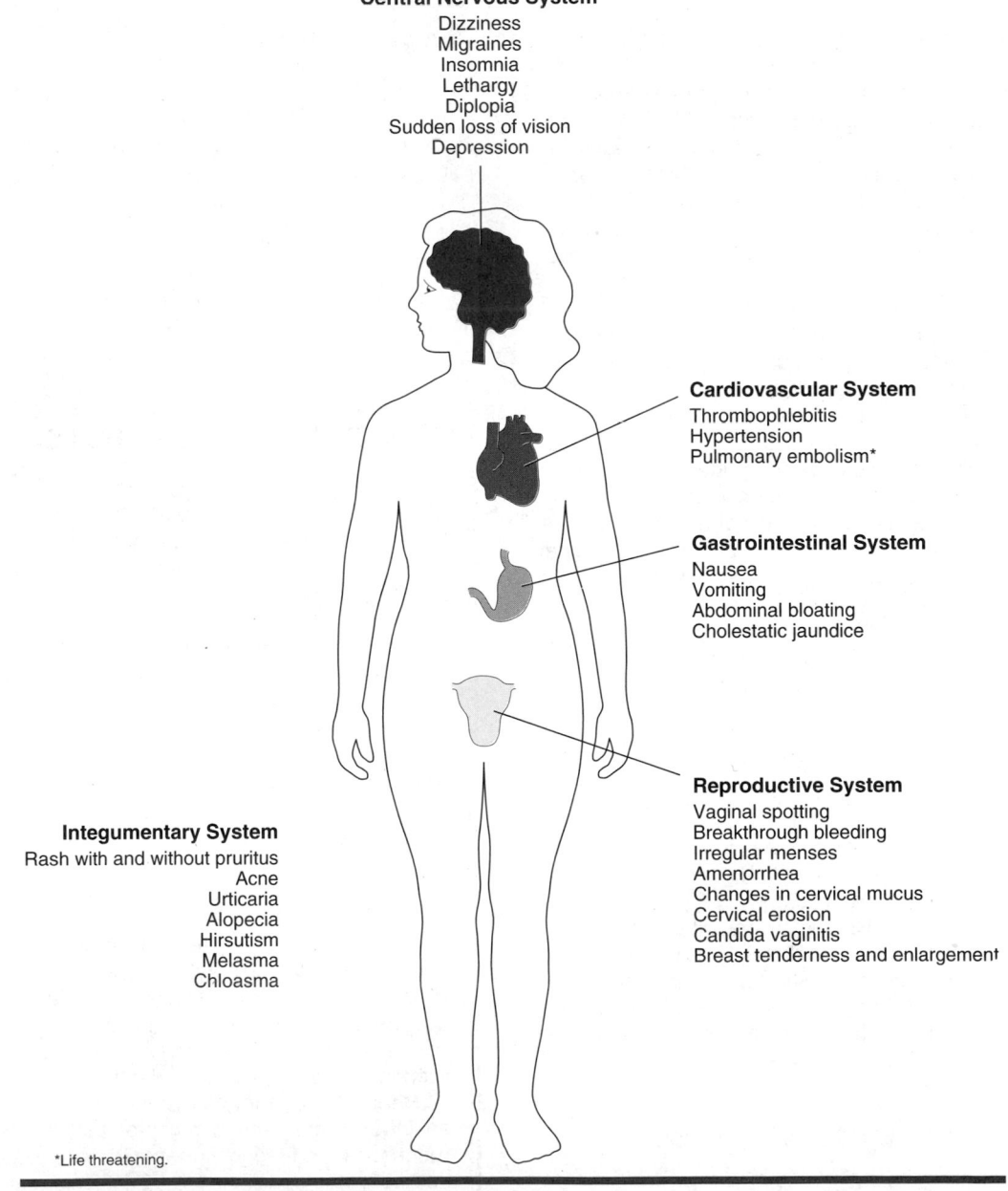

Central Nervous System
Dizziness
Migraines
Insomnia
Lethargy
Diplopia
Sudden loss of vision
Depression

Cardiovascular System
Thrombophlebitis
Hypertension
Pulmonary embolism*

Gastrointestinal System
Nausea
Vomiting
Abdominal bloating
Cholestatic jaundice

Reproductive System
Vaginal spotting
Breakthrough bleeding
Irregular menses
Amenorrhea
Changes in cervical mucus
Cervical erosion
Candida vaginitis
Breast tenderness and enlargement

Integumentary System
Rash with and without pruritus
Acne
Urticaria
Alopecia
Hirsutism
Melasma
Chloasma

*Life threatening.

FIGURE 62–2 Undesired clinical responses associated with exogenous progesterone therapy.

of progesterone thickens the cervical mucus, producing a barrier to sperm penetration.[13]

Undesired Clinical Responses As with estrogen, undesired clinical responses to progestins are dose dependent and affect almost every major organ system in the body. The most common response is withdrawal bleeding. Other responses include breast tenderness, edema, bloating, headaches, irritability, and depression. Undesired clinical responses are depicted in Figure 62–2.

Contraindications and Precautions Contraindications for progestin therapy include a history of or active thromboembolic disease, thrombophlebitis, undiagnosed uterine bleeding, breast cancer, missed abortion, liver disease, and genital malignancies. Use of progesterone intrauterine contraceptive systems is contraindicated in women with a history of pelvic inflammatory disease, venereal disease, and previous pelvic surgery. The IUD also should be used with caution in clients receiving anticoagulants.

Drug-Drug Interactions Rifampin (Rifadin), phenytoin (Dilantin), phenobarbital, and carbamazepine (Tegretol) decrease the effectiveness of progesterone by increasing its metabolism in the liver. In addition, aminoglutethimide (Cytadren) can depress the bioavailability of progestins.

Life-Span Considerations Natural progestin (progesterone) is classifed by the FDA as a Pregnancy Category D drug. Synthetic progestins are classified as Pregnancy Category X drugs or are unclassified. With use of synthetic progestins, congenital fetal anomalies have been reported during the first 4 months of pregnancy. In addition, synthetic progestins are excreted in the breast milk and can interfere with lactation. Therefore they should not be taken by women who are breast-feeding.

Specific Drug-Related Nursing Considerations Obtain a health history to determine that the client does not have preexisting thromboembolic disease, thrombophlebitis, breast cancer, liver disease, or undiagnosed abnormal vaginal bleeding. Since progestins can exacerbate fluid retention, determine if the client has a history of asthma, cardiac insufficiency, renal disease, active depression, or epilepsy. Obtain a baseline weight, blood pressure, and pulse. A gynecologic examination including a Pap test is performed. If there is a question of pregnancy, a pregnancy test is performed.

As with other drugs that affect the female reproductive system, client education is essential. Instruct the client about drug action, undesired clinical responses, and the action to take if these responses occur. Encourage the client to use a menstrual record to monitor bleeding patterns. Teach the client that routine monitoring of blood pressure and weight is important. If fluid retention develops, instruct the client about a low-sodium diet. If nausea occurs, instruct the client to take the prescribed drug with a light snack at bedtime.

MISCELLANEOUS DRUGS IN CATEGORY

There are many preparations of progestins. Information about some of these drugs is summarized in Table 62–5. Levonorgestrel is discussed in more depth.

Levonorgestrel (Norplant system) is considered a long-acting, low-dose, reversible method of contraception. It was approved for marketing in the United States in 1990. It had previously undergone extensive clinical trials outside the United States.

Pharmacotherapeutics The implant system is ideal for women who have difficulty remembering to take birth control pills or who have experienced undesired clinical responses with estrogen-containing oral contraceptives. The implant provides an alternative to IUDs or barrier methods of contraception. It is also convenient for women who do not want sterilization or who want a long interval before the next pregnancy. Implants have also been used in women with chronic illness.

Pharmacokinetics Levonorgestrel is considered to have almost 100% bioavailability. Plasma concentration levels reach their maximum within 24 hours of insertion and average approximately 0.3 ng/ml over 5 years. Levonorgestrel is metabolized in the liver and is excreted in the urine.[14]

Pharmacodynamics Levonorgestrel acts in the same way as other progestins. It suppresses LH secretion from the anterior pituitary, thus preventing ovulation. It causes thickening of cervical mucus, which serves as a barrier to sperm penetration. It also suppresses cyclic maturation of the endometrium, eventually causing atrophy.[14]

Pharmaceutics The implant system usually consists of six Silastic capsules, each containing 36 mg of levonorgestrel.[3,14]

Undesired clinical responses Undesired clinical responses in the immediate postinsertion period include bruising, reaction to local anesthetic, infection, phlebitis, and expulsion of one or more capsules. Other side effects related to levonorgestrel are minor but can be annoying enough to the client that she would want the capsules removed. They include irregular bleeding patterns (usually corrected spontaneously in 6 to 12 months), weight gain, headaches, breast tenderness, acne, galactorrhea, and ovarian cysts. Unless side effects become severe, they can be controlled with simple therapies.

Contraindications and precautions As with other progestins, levonorgestrel use is contraindicated in women with a history of or active thromboembolic disease or thrombophlebitis, liver disease, undiagnosed uterine bleeding, or breast cancer. Levonorgestrel is used with caution in women who are heavy smokers and older than 35 years or have a history of ectopic pregnancy, cardiovascular disease, migraine headaches, depression, or severe acne.[14]

Drug-drug interactions The effectiveness of levonorgestrel is decreased in clients who are taking phenytoin, phenobarbital, carbamazepine, and rifampin. When administered concomitantly with these drugs, the risk of pregnancy increases.

Life-span considerations Levonorgestrel is classified as Pregnancy Category X drug. Its use during lactation is not recommended, although studies have demonstrated no significant effects on the growth and health of infants nursed by women starting levonorgestrel 6 weeks postpartum. No data are available on infants nursed earlier than 6 weeks postpartum.

Specific drug-related nursing considerations The implant should be inserted during menses or in the postpartum period. Before the procedure, obtain a complete health history and physical assessment to determine if the client is a suitable candidate for the implant system. Provide the individual a de-

TABLE 62–5
Female Sex Hormones: Prototype and Major Drugs in Category

Drug Name	Dosage and Route of Administration	Nursing Considerations
MEDROXYPROGESTERONE ACETATE (Provera, Depo-Provera, Med-Pro) **HOW SUPPLIED** Uncoated tablets: 2.5, 5, and 10 mg IM: 100 and 400 mg/ml	***Secondary Amenorrhea*** Oral: 5-10 mg/d for 5-10 d; if endometrium has been primed with estrogen: 10 mg/d for 10 d beginning day 16 of menstrual cycle ***Abnormal Uterine Bleeding Due to Hormonal Imbalance*** Oral: 5-10 mg/d beginning on day 16 or 21 of cycle for 5-10 d; if endometrium has been primed with estrogen: 10 mg/d for 10 d. ***Contraception*** IM: 150 mg as single injection q3mo	***Assess*** Assess client for preexisting active thromboembolitic disease, thrombophlebitis, undiagnosed uterine bleeding, breast cancer, and liver disease. Determine if client is pregnant; medroxyprogesterone acetate is classified as a Pregnancy Category D drug. ***Implement*** Administer IM injection in large muscle mass to decrease discomfort at injection site. Provide client a thorough explanation of drug, including dosing schedule. Tell client to take oral drug with light snack at bedtime to minimize undesired symptoms. Instruct diabetic clients to monitor serum and urine closely for abnormal glucose levels. Instruct client about a low-sodium diet to help control edema. Instruct client to discontinue drug immediately if pregnancy is suspected. Instruct client to perform monthly self-breast examination. Encourage client to have routine gynecologic examinations q6-12mo. ***Monitor*** Monitor client for undesired clinical responses: withdrawal bleeding, breast tenderness, edema, bloating, headaches, irritability, and depression. Monitor blood pressure and weight. ***Evaluate*** Evaluate for absence of symptoms: amenorrhea, abnormal uterine bleeding.
Levonorgestrel (Norplant System) **HOW SUPPLIED** Silastic capsules: each capsule contains 36 mg of levonorgestrel	***Contraception*** Subdermal implant system: six Silastic capsules implanted subdermally, which initially release about 85 μg/d, decreasing to about 50 μg/d at 9 mo and eventually to 30 μg/d	***Assess*** Assess client for known contraindications (see medroxyprogesterone). ***Implement*** Teach client to keep gauze dressing clean, dry, and in place for 24 h. Instruct client to avoid heavy lifting for a few days but to resume other normal activities after 24 h. Encourage client to keep menstrual record. ***Monitor*** Monitor client for undesired clinical responses such as weight gain, irregular bleeding patterns, headaches, breast tenderness, and acne. ***Evaluate*** Check for plasma concentration level of 0.3 ng/ml.

TABLE 62–5 *Continued*

Female Sex Hormones: Prototype and Major Drugs in Category

Drug Name	Dosage and Route of Administration	Nursing Considerations
Progesterone (Progesterone in oil, Progestaject, Progestasert) **HOW SUPPLIED** IM: 50 mg/ml Intrauterine sustained-action insert: 38 mg	**Intrauterine Contraception** Progestasert System: inserted into uterine cavity; releases 65 µg of progesterone daily for 1 y.	**Implement** Anticipate that system will be inserted during menstruation. Instruct client to read package insert. Explain to client that cramps may occur for a few days after insertion. Inform client that menses may be heavier for first few cycles after insertion. Teach client to check placement of IUD after each menses (IUD threads should protrude from cervix.) Instruct client to report unusual cramping pain or bleeding, delayed menses, pelvic pain, fever, or vaginal discharge. Instruct client that device must be replaced in 1 y.

PROCEDURE FOR INSERTION AND REMOVAL OF NORPLANT SYSTEM

Insertion

Time required for insertion of the Norplant system is approximately 10 to 15 minutes. The implant is placed in the upper, inner aspect of the nondominant arm. The site is usually 8 to 12 cm superior and lateral to the medial epicondyle of the humerus. At the site, six lines are drawn in a fanlike configuration on the skin. The area is prepared and draped, using sterile aseptic technique. Local anesthesia (1% lidocaine) is injected subdermally at the base of the fan and along each of the six lines marked on the skin. A small incision is made at the base of the fan. A trocar with obturator is inserted, bevel up, through the incision. It is advanced along the line on the skin at a shallow subdermal angle. When properly located, the obturator is removed, and a capsule is loaded into the trocar. The obturator is used to advance the capsule. The trocar is then retracted, leaving the capsule in place. The procedure is repeated until all six capsules are inserted. The site is then palpated to determine correct positioning of the capsules. Pressure is applied to the incision site. The incision is closed with skin closure strips, and a gauze dressing is applied. No suturing is required.

Removal

Removal of the implant can be done at any time. An informed, written consent is required. Location of the capsules is identified, and the area is prepared and draped, using sterile technique. A local anesthetic with epinephrine is injected immediately distal to the capsule tips. A small incision is made, and capsules are removed one at a time. After the last capsule is removed, pressure is applied to the site, and the incision is closed with skin closure strips. A dressing is applied. The removal procedure can take 10 to 60 minutes.

---

tailed explanation, including effectiveness, risks, benefits, undesired clinical responses, and description of the insertion and removal procedures. If there is a question of pregnancy, a pregnancy test is performed. Informed written consent is also obtained. The procedure, which is summarized in the box, must be done by a primary care provider trained in the technique.

After the procedure, a gauze dressing is placed over the incision site. This dressing is left in place for 24 hours; the skin closure strips are kept on an additional 2 days. Explain to the client that some tenderness and bruising over the operative site may exist for a few days. Instruct the client to report any unusual arm pain, discharge, or bleeding from the operative site or expulsion of a capsule. Yearly gynecologic examinations with inspection of the insertion site are encouraged.

Explain to the client that, although the implant system is a contraceptive device, it does not provide protection from sexually transmitted diseases, including acquired immunodeficiency syndrome (AIDS). For a woman at risk, the additional use of condoms is recommended.

Combination Oral Contraceptive Pills

Combination oral contraceptive pills (OCPs) consist of both an estrogen and a progestin combined in one pill. As such, they have been on the market in the United States since the 1960s, with the most notable change since their introduction a significant reduction in dosage strength. Another more recent change has been a variation in dosage at different times of the month. A **monophasic OCP** has the same dose of estrogen and progestin each day for 21 days per cycle. A **biphasic OCP** has the same dose of estrogen in each pill, but the progestin is lower for 10 days and reaches a second, higher dose for the next 11 days. A **triphasic OCP** has the 21 days of medication subdivided into three intervals, each having a certain dosage of estrogen and progestin. This variation allegedly mimics the normal cycle, thereby reducing breakthrough bleeding.[15]

Pharmacotherapeutics   The most obvious and the most common use of OCP is contraception, the prevention of unplanned pregnancy. The effectiveness of OCPs for contraception has been extensively studied. The unplanned pregnancy rate for women who are sexually active and who are compliant in taking their OCP is near 0.1% per year for combination OCPs and 0.5% for the progesterone-only (minipill) pill.[15]

There are additional benefits of the OCP that allow its use for other purposes. OCPs provide close control and regimentation of the entire menstrual cycle. Therefore they can be used to control dysfunctional uterine bleeding, regulate irregular cycles, reduce blood loss with menses, suppress functional ovarian cysts, and suppress endometriosis.

Another benefit of long-term use of OCPs is reduction in the incidence of benign breast disease, including fibroadenoma and fibrocystic breast changes. In addition, since the uterus is subjected to an appropriate balance of estrogen and progestin, regular monthly cycling occurs. It reduces the incidence of endometrial cancer. Studies also find a reduction in the incidence of ovarian cancer among OCP users compared to nonusers.[15]

Pharmacodynamics   Combination OCPs act by suppression of gonadotropins. The result of this suppression is the elimination of the midcycle surge in LH and FSH and thus the suppression of ovulation. Additional effects include altered cervical mucus, which provides a barrier to sperm penetration. There are also modifications in the endometrium, which becomes unfavorable for implantation.[16]

Pharmaceutics   There are many options in the selection of OCPs. Most of them are available in the United States. Typically the dosing schedule consists of taking one pill daily, at approximately the same time each day, for 21 days. Then no medication is taken for 7 days. During this 7-day interval, a light menstrual period should occur. After the 7-day hiatus, a new package of pills is again begun as indicated above.[3,13]

As an alternative, a placebo may be taken during the 7-day hormonefree interval. This aids the client in keeping the correct timing in her medication schedule. If the placebo includes an iron supplement, preventing iron deficiency anemia is an added benefit.

Undesired clinical responses   Since OCPs are a combination of estrogen and progestin, the undesired clinical responses are the sum of those noted in the sections on estrogen and progesterone. In summary, they include breakthrough bleeding, amenorrhea, weight gain, acne, headaches, nausea, and changes in libido.

Contraindications and precautions   Since OCPs are a combination of estrogen and progestin, the contraindications to OCPs are the contraindications already listed for estrogen and progesterone. They include the following: history of or active thrombophlebitis or thromboembolic disease, breast cancer or undiagnosed breast mass, endometrial carcinoma, coronary artery or cerebrovascular disease, liver disease, and undiagnosed vaginal bleeding. OCPs should be prescribed with caution to clients with diabetes, hypertension, gallbladder disease, hyperlipidemia, blood dyscrasia, migraines, epilepsy, asthma, thyroid dysfunction, renal disease, and disease involving calcium or phosphorus metabolism.

Drug-drug interactions   Many interactions have been reported between other drugs and OCPs. When antibiotics such as tetracycline, ampicillin, and griseofulvin are administered concurrently with OCPs, the effectiveness of the oral contraceptives is reduced. Therefore these clients must use a barrier method of contraception until antibiotic therapy is complete. The actions of tricyclic antidepressants, theophylline, and diazepam are potentiated by OCPS. Consequently, it is important to monitor closely for undesired clinical responses and/or toxicity. Some drugs such as barbiturates and phenytoin stimulate liver metabolism and decrease the effectiveness of OCPs.[3,15]

Life-span considerations   Because of potential teratogenic effects, OCP use should be avoided in clients with known or suspected pregnancy. OCPs are classified as Pregnancy Category X drugs. Similarly, OCPs should not be taken by women that are breast-feeding.

Specific drug-related nursing considerations   In assessing the client, determine if OCPs provide the most appropriate form of contraception. Compliance and an understanding of the dosage schedule are important. Screen the client for the risk factors previously described in the contraindication and precaution section.

Interventions focus primarily on client education. Teach the client to take her medication at the same time every day. If nausea occurs, pills can be taken at bedtime or with food. For the first cycle of OCP, the client starts the pack on either day 5 of the cycle or on the Sunday after menses starts. (Review the product inserts with the client for specific information on starting dates.)

Pills are taken in the same sequence that they are packaged. If the client misses one pill, she should take two the next day. If two pills are missed, the client must take two a day for 2 days and use a barrier method of contraception for the rest of the month. If three pills are missed, instruct the client to discard the package, use a barrier method of contraception for the rest of the cycle, and resume the OCP after the next menses.

For the first cycle of OCP only, a barrier method of contraception is used in addition to the pills during the first week of the cycle. Strongly emphasize that OCPs do not prevent sexually transmitted diseases. If the client is not in a monogamous relationship, condoms should be used.

Instruct the client to report side effects such as breakthrough bleeding, nausea, and edema that persist for more than three cycles to the primary care provider. A dosage adjustment or change in medication may be required. Tell the client to report sudden chest or leg pain, shortness of breath, visual changes, dizziness, or severe headaches immediately.

OCPs increase a client's susceptibility to vaginal infections because of changes in cervical mucus. Vaginal itching and/or discharge should be reported to the health care provider. Androgenic effects such as oily skin, hirsutism, and weight gain should also be reported. These signs may necessitate a dosage adjustment or change in medication.

CONCEPT REVIEW

Estrogen and progesterone are the primary female sex hormones. In many aspects they act in opposing roles on individual organ systems.

Although they have many potential benefits for clients, there are numerous contraindications to their use.

UTERINE STIMULANTS

Normally spontaneous labor begins as a result of hormonal changes in the body. One of these hormones is **oxytocin**, which is synthesized in the hypothalamus and transported via neural tracts to the posterior pituitary. Oxytocin is secreted by the posterior pituitary throughout pregnancy, but uterine sensitivity to it increases at the end of pregnancy as myometrial receptors increase.

Situations arise in which the labor process must be initiated even though spontaneous labor has not begun. These situations include pregnancy-induced hypertension, premature rupture of membranes, chorioamnionitis, intrauterine fetal demise, postterm gestation, and maternal medical conditions such as diabetes mellitus or renal disease. In these situations exogenous oxytocin is administered to stimulate uterine contractions. This procedure is referred to as *induction of labor*. Small amounts of oxytocin are also administered during abnormally prolonged or arrested spontaneous labor. This is called *augmentation of labor*.[17]

UTERINE STIMULANT PROTOTYPE

OXYTOCIN

Exogenous oxytocin (Pitocin, Syntocinon) is currently the only drug approved for use in induction and augmentation of labor.

Pharmacotherapeutics Exogenous oxytocin is indicated for induction of labor when delivery would clearly be the best for mother and baby. It is also indicated when augmentation of existing labor is necessary because of weak and ineffective contractions. The decision of when to start oxytocin is based, in part, on a **Bishop score.** This score is determined after an evaluation of cervical dilation, effacement, station of the fetal head, consistency of the cervix, and cervical position. A score of 5 or more indicates that the cervix is favorable for oxytocin induction.

Oxytocin can also be given to facilitate the emptying of the uterus in spontaneous abortion, but the uterus is less responsive to oxytocin in early pregnancy. Another indication is administration in the postpartum period to aid the uterus in contracting, thus preventing or controlling postpartum hemorrhage.[17,18]

Pharmacokinetics After IV administration of oxytocin to a pregnant woman at or near term, uterine response occurs within 3 to 5 minutes unless the dosage is insufficient. The plasma half-life is 1 to 6 minutes; the interval to reach a steady-state concentration is 40 to 60 minutes. After cessation of administration, uterine contractions subside within approximately 60 minutes. Its rapid removal from the plasma is accomplished largely by the kidney and liver. Only small amounts of oxytocin are excreted unchanged in the urine.[3,17,18]

Pharmacodynamics During pregnancy, the myometrium increases its sensitivity to oxytocin by increasing the number of oxytocin receptors. Thus the administration of exogenous oxytocin to a pregnant woman at or near term can result in uterine contractions indistinguishable from spontaneous labor. Oxytocin also causes contraction of the myoepithelial cells in the breasts to effect the ejection of breast milk for lactation.

Pharmaceutics Exogenous oxytocin is prepared synthetically from pituitary extracts of mammals. It is available as a sterile, clear, colorless aqueous solution for IV and IM injection. Oxytocin is packaged in both single-dose ampules and multidose vials in a concentration of 10 U/ml. Oxytocin is also dispensed as a spray (40 U/ml) for intranasal application.[19]

Undesired Clinical Responses Oxytocin has a chemical structure similar to that of vasopressin, which is also from the posterior pituitary. Therefore it has many vasopressin-like effects. These effects include fluid retention and a risk of electrolyte imbalance and water intoxication, which can result in seizures, coma, and death. Other untoward effects include hypertension.

Excessive or inappropriate dosage of exogenous oxytocin can result in uterine hyperstimulation, which can be very dangerous for both mother and fetus. Excessively strong contractions can cause fetal distress, resulting in hypoxic brain damage or death to the fetus. In the extreme, hyperstimulation can result in rupture of the uterus, which is imminently life-threatening to both mother and fetus.[17,19]

Contraindications and Precautions Exogenous oxytocin use is contraindicated in the presence of hypersensitivity to the drug. It is also contraindicated in any situation in which its effect would be adverse for mother or fetus. These situations include but are not limited to placenta previa, abnormal fetal lie, cord prolapse, fetal distress when delivery is not imminent, and deformities of the maternal pelvic structures.

Drug-Drug Interactions Administration of exogenous oxytocin after administration of a vasoconstrictor with caudal block anesthesia can cause severe hypertension. Cyclopropane anesthesia can produce cardiovascular effects such as maternal hypotension and maternal sinus bradycardia with abnormal atrioventricular rhythms.

Specific Drug-Related Nursing Implications Before initiating therapy for induction or augmentation of labor, assess the client for risk factors such as hypersensitivity to oxytocic drugs, history of multiparity (several prior births), and history of major surgery of the cervix or uterus. Check the client for the degree of cervical dilation and the frequency and length of contractions. Also determine baseline vital signs and the fetal heart rate.

Exogenous oxytocin is administered under specific institutional guidelines. However, there are some general principles that should be followed. Because of the risks associated with the drug, the dosage must be carefully titrated to the client's response. The goal is to achieve an adequate contraction pattern. Usually this pattern consists of a maxium of three contractions in 10 minutes with each contraction lasting 40 to 90 seconds. The intensity of the intrauterine pressure should be 40 to 90 mmHg.[3,18,19]

Exogenous oxytocin is administered via a dilute IV solution (10 U of oxytocin in 1000 ml normal saline solution). Connect the oxytocin solution by a Y connection so that the drug can be discontinued at any time while access to the vein is kept open. The infusion rate of the solution is controlled by an infusion pump. During infusion, monitor maternal blood pressure, pulse rate, frequency and length of contractions, and resting uterine tone. Continuous electronic monitoring of the fetal heart rate patterns is done. Also monitor the client for water intoxication, changes in mental status, and neuromuscular excitability.

Be prepared to discontinue the oxytocin infusion if there are signs of fetal distress such as nonreassuring fetal heart rate patterns. The solution is also discontinued if signs of uterine hyperstimulation occur (i.e., contractions occur more frequently than every 2 minutes; contractions last longer than 90 seconds; or baseline uterine pressure is greater than 15 to 20 mm Hg).[18,19]

When oxytocin is administered to prevent or control postpartum hemorrhage, palpate the uterus to determine size, firmness, and location. Report evidence of uterine displacement. Also assess the vaginal discharge (lochia) and report bright red discharge, excessive amounts of discharge, or passage of clots.

Throughout oxytocin therapy, provide emotional support to the client and her partner. Keep the couple informed about why labor is being induced or augmented, the monitoring process, the effects of oxytocin on the labor process, and progress being made in terms of cervical change. A nurturing, supportive approach can enhance therapy.

MISCELLANEOUS DRUGS IN CATEGORY

Two additional uterine stimulants, methylergonovine maleate and dinoprostone, are discussed.

Methylergonovine maleate (Methergine) is a synthetic ergot alkaloid that acts directly on myometrial cells to cause sustained uterine tetany. It is indicated for the prevention or treatment of postpartum hemorrhage. The onset of action for methylergonovine maleate is very rapid. It occurs almost immediately after IV administration, 2 to 5 minutes after IM injection, and 5 to 10 minutes after oral administration. The half-life of the drug is approximately 30 minutes, and excretion occurs rapidly via the kidneys and liver.

Hypertension is a common undesired clinical response that can lead to headaches, seizures, and stroke. This response occurs most frequently with the IV route. Other undesired responses involving the cardiovascular, GI, and central nervous systems have been reported. Because of the danger of hyper-tension, methylergonovine maleate use is contraindicated in clients with hypertension and toxemia. It should be used with caution in clients receiving other ergot alkaloids or vasocon-strictors. Methylergonovine is classified as a Pregnancy Category C drug. However, since there is a risk of a tetanic contraction of the uterus with resultant fetal distress or fetal entrapment, the drug should never be used while the fetus is still in the uterus.[20]

Dinoprostone and low doses of oxytocin are used to "ripen" or prepare the cervix so that oxytocin induction is more successful. Dinoprostone is a naturally occurring form of prostaglandin E_2 that may directly stimulate the myometrium to contract. Evidence also suggests that dinoprostone affects the cervix locally, causing it to soften and begin to efface and dilate.[19]

A dinoprostone gel preparation is used to prepare the cervix for oxytocin induction. The gel is instilled into the cervical canal just below the level of the internal os. Once instilled, it is rapidly absorbed into the tissue within 30 to 45 minutes. Dinoprostone is extensively metabolized in the lungs; resulting metabolites are further metabolized in the liver and kidneys. The drug is excreted in the kidneys.[19] The gel preparation should not be used concomitantly with oxytocic drugs. A 6- to 12-hour interval should elapse between the administration of the gel and the initiation of oxytocin induction or augmentation.

Undesired clinical responses in the mother include abnormal uterine contractility, GI disturbance, back pain, a warm sensation in the vagina, and fever. Overdose may result in uterine hypercontractility and hypertonia. An undesired clinical response in the fetus is bradycardia. Dinoprosterone use is contraindicated in any situation in which oxytocic drugs are contraindicated (e.g., hypertonic uterine contractions, cephalopelvic disproportion, nonvertex presentation). It is not used in the presence of ruptured membranes or placenta previa or when a vaginal delivery is contraindicated. Dinoprostone use is also contraindicated in clients hypersensitive to prostaglandins, and it is used with caution in clients with a history of asthma, glaucoma, or raised intraocular pressure. Dinoprostone is classified as a Pregnancy Category C drug since it is administered at term.

Sterile technique must be used when preparing and administering the gel. Use caution when handling the drug. If any of the gel comes in contact with the skin, wash the area thoroughly with soap and water. The gel should be at room temperature before instillation.

After administration, ask the client to remain lying in a supine position for 15 to 30 minutes to minimize leakage of the gel from the cervix. Provide support, reassurance, and information on the progress of the labor process. Instruct the client on possible side effects and the length of time expected before cervical changes may occur. As with the oxytocic drugs, monitor the pattern of uterine contractions, blood pressure, and body temperature. Maintain continuous fetal heart monitoring and observe for abnormalities in heart rate such as bradycardia and late or variable decelerations. Table 62–6 summarizes information on uterine stimulants.

TABLE 62–6
Uterine Stimulants and Inhibitors: Prototypes and Major Drugs in Categories

Drug Name	Dosage and Route of Administration	Nursing Considerations
UTERINE STIMULANTS		
OXYTOCIN (Pitocin, Syntocinon) HOW SUPPLIED IM, IV: 10 U/ml Nasal solution: 40 U/ml	***Induction or Stimulation of Labor*** IV: 1-2 mU/min; increase gradually in increments of 1-2 mU/min until contraction pattern has been established (dilute solution of 10 U oxytocin to 1000 ml nonhydrating diluent equals 10 mU/ml) ***Control of Postpartum Uterine Bleeding*** IM: 1 ml after delivery of placenta IV: 10-40 U in 1000 ml diluent; rate adjusted to control uterine tone	***Assess*** Assess client for contraindications associated with drug (e.g., placenta previa, cord prolapse, fetal distress) when delivery is not imminent. Assess for degree of cervical dilation, frequency and duration of contractions, baseline vital signs, and fetal heart rate. ***Implement*** Dilute IV solution is administered via infusion pump. Monitor infusion rate frequently. Anticipate that IV infusion of nonoxytocin-containing solution will be used to keep vein open. Provide emotional support. ***Monitor*** During infusion, monitor maternal blood pressure and pulse and fetal heart rate. Monitor frequency and duration of contractions and resting uterine tone. ***Evaluate*** Monitor for maximum of three contractions in 10 min, with each contraction lasting 40-90 s and intensity of intrauterine pressure at 40-90 mm Hg.
Methylergonovine Maleate (Methergine) HOW SUPPLIED Tablets: 0.2 mg IM: 0.2-mg vials	***Postpartum Hemorrhage*** Oral: 0.2 mg tid or qid up to 1 wk IM: 0.2 mg	***Assess*** Assess for contraindications such as hypertension, cardiac, hepatic, or renal disease and hypersensitivity to ergot derivatives. Assess baseline vital signs, height and consistency of uterine fundus, and characteristics of lochia. ***Implement*** Do not administer drug while fetus is still in uterus. ***Monitor*** Monitor blood pressure and pulse continuously during infusion. ***Evaluate*** Monitor fundal tone and placement.
Dinoprostone (Prepidil) HOW SUPPLIED Prefilled 2.5-ml syringe containing 0.5 mg of PGE$_2$/3 g gel	Usual dose: one syringe (2.5 ml) instilled into cervical canal Dose repeated if needed in 6 h Maximum dose for 24-h period: 1.5 mg (7.5 ml)	***Assess*** See oxytocin. ***Implement*** Anticipate that each package contains a 10-mm and 20-mm shielded catheter. Drug preparation: remove protective seal from end of barrel; remove protective cap from top of syringe and insert it into barrel to serve as plunger; attach catheter to tip of barrel (20-mm catheter if no effacement and 10-mm catheter if 50% effacement). Drug administration: place client in dorsal-recumbent position; sterile speculum is inserted to visualize cervix; catheter is gently inserted into cervix; and gel is instilled.

Continued on following page.

TABLE 62–6 *Continued*
Uterine Stimulants and Inhibitors: Prototypes and Major Drugs in Categories

Drug Name	Dosage and Route of Administration	Nursing Considerations
Dinoprostone Continued		**Monitor** Assess client for undesired clinical responses such as GI disturbances, back pain, abnormal uterine contractility, and fever. Monitor blood pressure, temperature, and pattern of uterine contractions. **Evaluate** Cervix softens and begins to efface and dilate.
UTERINE INHIBITORS		
RITODRINE HYDROCHLORIDE (Yutopar) HOW SUPPLIED IV: 0.3, 10, and 15 mg/ml; 150 mg/syringe; 150 mg/vial Uncoated tablet: 10 mg	IV dilution of 150 mg in 500 ml of D₅W solution *Initial dose* IV: 0.1 mg/min (20 microdrops/min) Increase by 0.05 mg/min (10 microdrops/min) q10min until contractions stop *Maintenance* IV: 30-70 microdrops/min Oral:—started 30 min before IV therapy discontinued: 10-mg q2h for first 24 h; then 10-20 mg q4-6h Oral dose not to exceed 120 mg/d	**Assess** Determine gestational age of fetus. Assess for contraindications such as hypertension, maternal hyperthyroidism, hemorrhage, and maternal cardiac disease. Determine if client is sensitive to sulfites; solution for injection contains sodium metabisulfite. **Implement** Inspect solution for discoloration or presence of precipitate. Anticipate that IV therapy will be continued for at least 12 h after cessation of contractions. Provide emotional support. **Monitor** Monitor maternal vital signs, fetal heart rate and rhythm, and uterine contraction frequency and duration. Report maternal pulse rate >120 bpm and fetal heart rate >180 bpm. **Evaluate** Contractions are absent or reduced to less than one contraction q15min.
Terbutaline Sulfate (Brethine) HOW SUPPLIED SC: 1 mg/ml Uncoated tablets: 2.5 and 5 mg	SC: 0.25 mg q20min for a total of three bolus injections Oral: 2.5 or 5 mg q2-6h	**Assess** See ritodrine. **Implement** Anticipate parenteral drug administration via portable SC infusion pump. Teach client self-administration technique. **Monitor** See ritodrine. **Evaluate** See ritodrine.

UTERINE INHIBITORS

Preterm labor refers to the onset of labor before 37 weeks' gestation. Preterm deliveries account for more than 75% of all perinatal morbidity and mortality.[21] Many different therapies are used to prevent or treat preterm labor, including bed rest, hydration, and tocolysis (administration of drugs that inhibit uterine contractions).

Several drugs are used to inhibit uterine contractions, including magnesium sulfate and indomethacin. **Magnesium sulfate** relaxes the myometrium by antagonizing calcium, and **indomethacin** (Indocin), a nonsteroidal anti-inflammatory agent, inhibits prostaglandin synthase. Although these two drugs are commonly used, they are not approved by the FDA for tocolysis. The most common tocolytic agents used are β-adrenergic agonists.

β-Adrenergic agonists cause smooth-muscle relaxation. (See Chapters 30 and 33 for additional information on β-adrenergic agonists.) Their use in the prevention and treatment of preterm labor began in the 1970s in the United States. Both ritodrine hydrochloride and terbutaline sulfate are used by clinicians for achieving labor tocolysis. Ritodrine hydrochloride has been approved by the FDA for tocolysis, but terbutaline sulfate (Brethine) has not.[22]

Uterine Inhibitor Prototype

RITODRINE HYDROCHLORIDE

Ritodrine hydrochloride (Yutopar) was approved by FDA as an autonomic drug before 1982.

Pharmacotherapeutics Ritodrine hydrochloride is indicated in the management of preterm labor.

Pharmacokinetics Limited kinetic results with ritodrine have been documented for pregnant females; males and nonpregnant females have been used in most studies. After oral administration in men, therapeutic serum levels are achieved within 30 to 60 minutes. Oral half-life is 12 to 20 hours. In nonpregnant females therapeutic levels are reached within 5 minutes after IV administration. The distribution half-life is 6 to 9 minutes, and the effective half-life is 1 to 3 hours. Ritodrine is metabolized in the liver, and 90% is excreted in 24 hours after administration.[4,22]

Pharmacodynamics Ritodrine stimulates the β_2-adrenergic receptors in the uterine smooth muscle, inhibiting contractility of the uterine smooth muscles.

Pharmaceutics Ritodrine is available in oral uncoated tablets and sterile solution for IV infusion.

Undesired Clinical Responses Cardiovascular side effects include increased maternal and fetal heart rate, widening maternal pulse pressure, tachycardia, palpitation, arrhythmias, angina, heart murmur, and myocardial ischemia. Effects on the GI tract include nausea, vomiting, bloating, paralytic ileus, diarrhea, and constipation. In addition, the client may experience central nervous system (CNS) effects such as headaches, malaise, tremors, nervousness, restlessness, anxiety, emotional upset, and drowsiness. Ritodrine can also cause dyspnea and hyperventilation. Metabolic effects on the mother include changes in serum glucose and insulin levels, decrease in the potassium level, and lactic acidosis. Fetal metabolic effects include hypoglycemia and hypocalcemia.[4]

Contraindications and Precautions Ritodrine is contraindicated before week 20 of gestation and in any condition in which continuation of the pregnancy may be hazardous to the mother or fetus. These conditions include pregnancy-induced hypertension, chorioamnionitis, hemorrhage, intrauterine fetal demise, maternal cardiac disease, maternal hyperthyroidism, and uncontrolled diabetes mellitus. It should not be administered to anyone with known hypersensitivity to any component of the drug.

Drug-Drug Interactions If ritodrine is administered with general anesthetics, magnesium sulfate, or meperidine (Demerol), the hypotensive and cardiac arrhythmic effects are potentiated. Administration of ritodrine concomitantly with sympathomimetic amines potentiates the effects of the amines. In addition, the combination of ritodrine and corticosteroids can lead to pulmonary edema.

Life-Span Considerations Ritodrine hydrochloride is classifed as Pregnancy Category B drug.

Specific Drug-Related Nursing Considerations Before initiating therapy, assess the client for the gestational age of the fetus and a history of hypertension or cardiac arrhythmias, pregnancy-induced hypertension, diabetes mellitus, asthma, or sensitivity to sulfite preparations. Obtain baseline maternal vital signs, fetal heart rate, and uterine contraction frequency and duration.

A controlled infusion pump is used to administer ritodrine intravenously. Position the client on her left side to minimize hypotension. (Once the client's blood pressure stabilizes, other positions may be assumed to maximize comfort levels.) Monitor intake and output and auscultate lung sounds to assess fluid volume status. Monitor and record maternal vital signs, fetal heart rate and rhythm, and uterine contraction frequency and duration every 15 to 30 minutes. Report a maternal pulse rate over 120 and fetal heart rate over 180 to the primary care provider immediately.

The goal of IV therapy is control of contractions. The infusion is usually continued for at least 12 hours after uterine contractions cease. The client is gradually weaned from the IV infusion; the infusion rate is reduced by 10 microdrops per minute at half-hour intervals. Oral administration of ritodrine is initiated 30 minutes before discontinuing IV administration.[4,22]

The client may be discharged home while receiving oral ritodrine. Instruct the client to monitor for contractions and to report any increase in frequency. Teach the client to take her pulse daily and to notify the health care provider if the rate is above 120 beats per minute.

Women who experience preterm labor may feel guilty about something they did or did not do during the pregnancy. They are fearful and anxious about potential danger to the baby. In addition, they may experience chronic fatigue from interrupted sleep because of the drug schedule and depression because of forced limitations in activity level; therefore it is important to provide counseling and emotional support.

MISCELLANEOUS DRUG IN CATEGORY

As indicated previously, **terbutaline sulfate** (Brethine) is commonly used for the treatment of preterm labor, even though it has not been approved by the FDA for tocolysis. Pharmacologic actions, undesired clinical responses, and nursing considerations are the same as for ritodrine.

Terbutaline is administered orally or via a portable SC infusion pump. The infusion pump is useful for clients who are not well controlled when taking oral terbutaline. Criteria for client selection include fetal gestational age between 20 and 34 weeks; a viable fetus with an estimated weight less than 2500 g; cervical dilation less than 4 cm; confirmed diagnosis of preterm labor; intact amnion with no bulging through the cervical os; and no maternal medical contraindications for receiving terbutaline.

The client initially is hospitalized to stabilize uterine contractions. Discharge planning includes instruction on self-administration of terbutaline using the pump and home uterine monitoring. Many home health agencies have a program on home terbutaline therapy and will follow clients closely after discharge. Table 62–6 summarizes information on uterine inhibitors.

LACTATION INHIBITORS

Under the influence of a postpartum elevation of prolactin, a woman's breasts engorge in preparation for lactation. For the woman planning to bottle-feed, this can cause variable degrees of discomfort and unwanted nipple discharge. These symptoms can be prevented by a lactation inhibitor.

For years the drug of choice was **chlorotrianisene** (Tace), a synthetic estrogen. Its major drawback was an increased risk of thromboembolism. More recently, bromocriptine, an ergot alkaloid, has been used. Although bromocriptine is more effective, it has been associated with an increased risk of stroke and is no longer approved by the FDA for lactation inhibition. Since engorgement is a normal physiologic process, many clinicians prefer to avoid these risks by conservative management consisting only of mild analgesics and mechanical breast support (a tight bra or breast binder). In addition, the American College of Obstetricians and Gynecologists (ACOG) recommends using this approach to avoid drug risks.

CONCEPT REVIEW

Uterine stimulators are used for induction or augmentation of labor and for passing the placenta and prevention or control of postpartum hemorrhage.

Uterine inhibitors are used to prevent preterm labor.

Lactation inhibitors prevent discomfort and unwanted nipple discharge after labor in a mother who is not planning to breast-feed.

SUMMARY

Drugs affecting the female reproductive system include hypothalamic and ovulatory stimulants, hypothalamic inhibitors, female sex hormones, uterine stimulants, uterine inhibitors, and lactation inhibitors. These drugs are used for a variety of reasons, including gynecologic disorders, contraception, and diagnostic testing. For most of the drugs, nursing management focuses on client education for accurate drug administration and recognition of undesired clinical responses. In addition, drugs used during the birthing process require close monitoring of the physiologic status of both the mother and the fetus.

Because these drugs affect reproductive function, the client may experience changes in both body image and self-concept. You must be aware of the impact these changes can have on the client and explore with her various coping strategies and other mechanisms of support.

REFERENCES

1. Speroff, L., Glass, R.H., & Kase, N.G. (1989). *Clinical gynecologic endocrinology and infertility* (4th ed.). Baltimore: Williams & Wilkins.
2. Yen, S., & Jaffe, R. (1991). *Reproductive endocrinology* (3rd ed.). Philadelphia: W.B. Saunders.
3. Data Pharmaceutica, Inc. (1993). *1993 physicians' genRx.* Smithtown, NY: Author.
4. U.S. Pharmacopeia Convention. (1990). *The United States pharmacopeia* (22nd rev.). Rockville, MD: Author.
5. Blenner, J.L. (1991). Clomiphene-induced mood swings. *Journal of Obstetrics, Gynecologic, and Neonatal Nursing, 20,* 321-327.
6. Schmidt, C. (1991). Applications of GnRH agonists for GYN patients. *Contemporary OB/GYN, 36*(10), 50-63.
7. Barbieri, R.L., & Friedman, A.J. (Eds.) (1991). *Gonadotropin-releasing hormone analogs: Applications in gynecology.* New York: Elsevier Science Publishers.
8. Adamson, G.D. (1991). Treating endometriosis. *Contemporary OB/GYN, 36*(7), 48-63.
9. Wheeler, J.M., Knittle, J.D., & Miller, J.D. (1992). Depot leuprolide versus danazol in treatment of women with symptomatic endometriosis. *American Journal of Obstetrics and Gynecology, 167,* 1367-1371.
10. Saltiel, E. (1993). GnRH agonists and sex hormone disorders. *US Pharmacist.*
11. Ravnikar, V.A. (1992). Hormonal management of osteoporosis. *Clinical Obstetrics and Gynecology, 35,* 913-922.
12. Jones, K.P. (1992). Estrogens and progestins: What to use and how to use it. *Clinical Obstetrics and Gynecology, 35,* 871-883.
13. Smith, C.M., & Reynard, A.M. (Eds.) (1992). *Textbook of pharmacology.* Philadelphia: W.B. Saunders.
14. Sharts-Engel, N.C. (1991). Levonorgestrel subdermal implants (Norplant) for long-term contraception. *MCN: American Journal of Maternal-Child Nursing, 16,* 232.
15. Harris, C.D. (1992). The birth control pill revisited. *NAACOG's clinical issues in perinatal and women's health nursing, 3,* 246-252.
16. Franklin, M. (1990). Reassessment of the metabolic effects of oral contraceptives. *Journal of Nurse Midwifery, 35,* 358-363.
17. Petrie, R.H., & Williams, A.M. (1993). Induction of labor. In R.A. Knuppel & J.E. Drukker (Eds.). *High-risk pregnancy: A team approach* (2nd ed.). Philadelphia: W.B. Saunders.
18. Owen, J., & Hauth, J.C. (1992). Oxytocin for the induction or augmentation of labor. *Clinical Obstetrics and Gynecology, 35,* 464-475.
19. Brodsky, P.L., & Pelzar, E.M. (1991). Rationale for the revision of oxytocin administration protocols. *Journal of Obstetrics, Gynecologic and Neonatal Nursing, 20,* 440-444.
20. Gilman, A.G., Rall, T.W., Nies, A.S., & Taylor, P. (Eds.) (1990). *Goodman and Gilman's: The pharmacological basis of therapeutics* (8th ed.). New York: Pergamon Press.
21. Lipshitz, J., Pierre, P.M., & Arntz, M. (1993). Preterm labor. In R.A. Knuppel & J.E. Drukker, (Eds.), *High risk pregnancy: A team approach* (2nd ed.). Philadelphia: W.B. Saunders.
22. Graf, R.A., & Perez-Woods, R. (1992). Trends in pre-term labor. *Journal of Perinatology, 12*(1), 51-58.
23. Sala, D.J., & Moise, K. (1990). The treatment of preterm labor using a portable subcutaneous terbutaline pump. *Journal of Obstetrics, Gynecologic and Neonatal Nursing, 19*(2), 108-115.

BIBLIOGRAPHY

Cowan, M. (1993). Home care of the pregnant woman using terbutaline. *MCN: American Journal of Maternal-Child Nursing, 18*(2), 99-105.

Davis, D.C., & Dearman, C.M. (1991). Coping strategies of infertile women. *Journal of Obstetrics, Gynecologic and Neonatal Nursing, 20,* 221-228.

Kaunitz, A.M. (1993), DMPA: A new contraception option. *Contemporary OB/GYN, 38*(1), 19-34.

Knowlden, H. (1990). The pill and cancer: A review of the literature. A case of swings and roundabouts? *Journal of Advanced Nursing, 15,* 1016-1020.

Lindell, M., & Olsson, H. (1991). Can combined oral contraceptives be made more effective by means of a nursing care model? *Journal of Advanced Nursing, 16,* 475-479.

MacPherson, K.I. (1992). Cardiovascular disease in women and non-contraceptive use of hormones: A feminist analysis. *Advances in Nursing Science, 14*(4), 34-49.

Maddox, M.A. (1992). Women at midlife: Hormone replacement therapy. *Nursing Clinics of North America, 27,* 959-969.

Muse, K. (1992). Hormonal manipulation in the treatment of pre-menstrual syndrome. *Clinical Obstetrics and Gynecology, 35,* 658-664.

Root, W.B. (1992). Contraception for midlife women. *NAACOG's Clinical Issues in Perinatal and Women's Health Nursing, 3,* 227-235.

Sharts-Hopko, N.C. (1993). Depo-provera. *MCN: American Journal of Maternal-Child Nursing, 18*(2), 108.

Sweezy, S.R. (1992). Contraception for the postpartum woman. *NAACOG's Clinical Issues in Perinatal and Women's Health Nursing, 3,* 209-226.

CHAPTER 63

DRUGS AFFECTING THE
Male Reproductive System

PAMALA D. LARSEN

⊛ **Nursing Considerations**

LEARNING OBJECTIVES:

Outline a plan of care for a client receiving androgen drug therapy.

Develop a teaching plan for the client receiving androgen drug therapy.

⊛ **Androgens**

LEARNING OBJECTIVES:

Describe the physiologic response of the body to androgens.

List four therapeutic uses for androgens.

Distinguish between the three subcategories of androgens.

Summarize essential information about the prototype drug for each subcategory.

KEY TERMS:

Anabolism, androgens, anabolic steroids, catabolism, testosterone

⊛ **Anabolic Steroid Abuse**

LEARNING OBJECTIVE: Describe three of the major undesired responses associated with anabolic steroid abuse.

⊛ **Miscellaneous Drugs**

LEARNING OBJECTIVE: Describe the use of antiandrogens and androgen-suppressive drugs.

CONCEPTS AND TERMS TO REVIEW

Read Chapter 61 for an overview of the anatomy and physiology of the male reproductive system.

Study the actions of the hormone testosterone.

Review the chemical process of esterification.

---

*T*he 1930s produced some important findings that led to the development of drugs that affect the male reproductive system. Initially androgenic substances were extracted from urine. Eventually testosterone was isolated from the testes, and finally, synthesis of testosterone was accomplished in 1935.[1]

In the past drugs affecting the male reproductive system have been termed *androgens* and *anabolic steroids*. **Androgens** stimulate the growth of the male accessory sex organs and produce masculinizing effects. **Anabolic steroids** produce a positive nitrogen balance that in turn stimulates tissue building. However, current knowledge indicates an overlap of ac-

tion of androgens and anabolic steroids. There are no purely androgenic drugs or anabolic steroids; each drug group has properties of the other. In fact, testosterone is the base structure of anabolic steroids.[2]

To provide care to the individual receiving these drugs, it is important to understand the actions they produce in the body. This chapter reviews the normal functions of androgens in the body and describes the primary drug categories. Additionally, antiandrogens, androgen-suppressant drugs, and a prototype of a new drug described as a 5-α-reductase inhibitor are discussed.

▦ NURSING CONSIDERATIONS

Reproductive concerns such as impotence, male contraception, male infertility, testicular failure, and delay of puberty are commonly treated outside the hospital. Therefore the nurse's time with the client must be used effectively.

Assessing   Assessing the male reproductive system is an essential part of a complete health assessment. Careful assessment may detect actual or potential problems or concerns that the client may not readily volunteer. Many common disorders of the male reproductive system have the potential for serious psychologic or physiologic consequences.

Interviewing a male client about his reproductive system requires sensitivity and tact. Initially it is important to establish rapport with the client so that he relaxes and has confidence in you. Once this has been achieved, ask questions about the client's health and illness patterns. For example, determine the answer to questions such as "Have you noticed any discharge or bleeding from the urethral opening?" "Have you felt a lump or tenderness in the groin?" "Do you get up during the night to urinate?" "Have you fathered any children?"

Assess the client's health promotion and protection practices. Ask questions such as "Do you examine your testes periodically?" "Have you been taught the proper procedure for testicular examination?" "If you are sexually active, do you have more than one partner?" "Does your work expose you to toxic chemicals?"

The client may range in age from infancy to older adult. Therefore the health history must be adjusted to meet the client's particular developmental stage. For example, determine if a pediatric client's mother used hormones during pregnancy; ask about hygienic measures used if the child is uncircumcised; and determine if the child had any genitourinary abnormalities at birth. Questions for the adolescent male should be appropriate for his age. Use a direct, matter-of-fact approach; do not be judgmental. Questions such as "Has your body changed physically during the last 2 years?" or "Often boys your age have questions about sexual activity; what questions do you have?" are usually not threatening to the adolescent. Questions for the elderly adult male should focus on sexual performance and the urinary system; ask, for example, "Have you experienced any change in your frequency of sex?" or "Do you need to get up at night to urinate?"[3]

In addition, determine the client's past medical history. Administration of androgenic drugs to male clients with a history of breast or prostate cancer is contraindicated. Additionally, caution is exercised when prescribing these agents to clients with severe cardiac or renal disease, prostatic hypertrophy, liver disease, or hypercalcemia. Drug-induced sodium and fluid retention can cause complications of these chronic conditions.

Diagnosing   After the data base is complete, analyze the data to determine nursing diagnoses. Appropriate nursing diagnoses for clients receiving these drugs include the following:
- Anxiety related to change in health status.
- Body image disturbance related to physical changes caused by drug therapy.
- Fluid volume excess related to drug therapy.
- Noncompliance with drug therapy related to lack of knowledge.

Planning   Since most clients are seen in ambulatory care settings, planning primarily involves client education. Teaching plans can be developed that address a knowledge deficit about specific drugs, methods of administration, mechanisms of drug action, and undesired clinical responses. The client may also need instruction in normal male anatomy and physiology, particularly hormonal regulation.

Since these agents cause changes in secondary sex characteristics of both males and females, inform the client about these potential changes. Changes in the female client may include unnatural hair growth patterns (i.e., facial hair growth), clitoromegaly, altered libido, menstrual irregularities, and hoarseness or deepening of the voice. Such changes, if detected and reported early, may be reversible. The male client needs information about potential voice changes, change in size of sex organs, altered hair growth patterns, and persistent abnormal erection of the penis. Advise the client to report these changes promptly to his primary health care provider.

Since fluid retention usually occurs with drug therapy, instruct the client to monitor his or her weight on a regular basis. Inform the client that a weight gain greater than 2 pounds per week should be reported to the client's primary care provider.

Planning also includes development of expected outcomes. The outcomes are based on the nursing diagnoses and are developed with the client when possible. Appropriate expected outcomes might include the following:
- Client reports that anxiety is reduced.
- Client verbalizes understanding of body changes.
- Client demonstrates involvement in problem-solving processes.
- Client lists signs that require notification of primary care provider.
- Client verbalizes accurate knowledge about treatment regimen.

Implementing   Drugs affecting the male reproductive system are usually administered orally or intramuscularly. Oral preparations are given with food to decrease the potential for gastric distress. Intramuscular (IM) preparations are administered deep into the gluteal muscle for less irritation and better absorption.

Advise clients to maintain contact with their primary health care provider because laboratory tests must be obtained periodically. Providing emotional support is important for these clients. Both male and female clients are attempting to cope with the disease process requiring the drug therapy and with the changes produced by the drugs.

Evaluating   A number of serum laboratory tests should be obtained on a regular basis. Androgenic drugs can mobilize calcium from the bone and elevate serum cholesterol levels; therefore serum calcium and cholesterol levels should be monitored frequently. Polycythemia is a potential side effect; consequently, hemoglobin and hematocrit levels must be evaluated regularly. In addition, since some androgenic drugs cause liver dysfunction, liver function tests should be performed on a regular basis.

As with all drugs, risks and benefits to the client are determinants of continued use or discontinuance. Review the status of the expected outcomes with the client.

ANDROGENS

Androgens produce both their androgenic and anabolic effects by binding to androgen receptors in the target organs of skeletal muscles, the prostate gland, and bone marrow. This binding stimulates development in those organs and also increases protein synthesis. Effects of the androgens are evident in masculinization of male sex accessory tissues. These masculinization effects include gonadotropin regulation, spermatogenesis, and sexual restoration and development.

Androgens also cause retention of nitrogen, sodium, potassium, and phosphorus. They decrease the urinary excretion of calcium, thus elevating serum calcium levels. Androgens increase protein anabolism and decrease protein catabolism. Protein anabolic effects produced by androgens include increased bone density, increased muscle mass, and increased red blood cell mass[2,3] (Table 63–1).

Pharmacotherapeutics

The primary use of androgens in males is as a hormone replacement for hypogonadism. If for some reason (e.g., pituitary failure, primary testicular failure, or hypothalamic failure) the testes fail to produce adequate amounts of testosterone, replacement therapy is required. Androgens also can be used for male contraception. These drugs inhibit spermatogenesis by suppression of the hypothalamus and pituitary, which in turn suppresses the luteinizing hormone (LH) and follicle-stimulating hormone (FSH). Micropenis in children and delay of puberty in adolescence are also treated with androgens. Androgens may be prescribed for the older adult male with evidence of androgen deficiency to restore libido, increase ejaculate volume, and enhance expression of secondary sex characteristics.[2]

Some androgens are used in high doses for palliation of advanced or metastatic breast cancer in women. The mechanism for palliative action is not known.[4] Hereditary angioedema is another condition for which androgens may be prescribed. In a client with hereditary angioedema an inhibitor of the complement system is deficient. Without this inhibitor, there is uncontrolled activation of the complement cascade, resulting in increased vascular permeability and angioedema. Androgens are administered to increase plasma levels of the deficient inhibitor.[2,4]

General Characteristics

If unmodified testosterone is administered orally, it is rapidly absorbed in the portal blood. After first-pass metabolism by the liver, only small amounts of the drug reach the systemic circulation. When testosterone is administered parenterally, it is also rapidly absorbed from the injection site and degraded. For this reason, testosterone is chemically modified to retard the rate of absorption and catabolism. Common modifications of the chemical structure of testosterone include (1) esterification of the 17-β-hydroxyl group; (2) alkylation at the 17-α-position; and (3) changes in the ring structure of testosterone.[2]

TABLE 63–1
Androgen Target Tissues and Biologic Actions

Target Tissues	Biologic Actions
Hypothalamus	Negative feedback on gonadotropin-releasing hormone secretion
Pituitary	Negative feedback on LH and follicle-stimulating hormone secretion
Reproductive tissues	
Seminiferous tubules ⎫	Initiation and maintenance of spermatogenesis
Seminal vesicles ⎬ (Testosterone dependent)	
Epididymis ⎪	
Vas deferens ⎭	
Prostate ⎫	Differentiation and development of the male accessory ducts and external genitalia
Penis ⎬ (Dihydrotestosterone dependent)	
Scrotum ⎭	
Nonreproductive tissues	
Liver (enzymes/lipoprotein)	Stimulation or suppression of protein synthesis
Kidney	Stimulation of erythropoietin, which indirectly increases hematopoiesis
Hematopoietic system	Direct stimulation of growth of stem cells; indirect stimulation of erythropoietin
Central nervous system	Facilitation of libido and sexual function; male aggressive behavior
Muscle	Development of muscle mass and strength
Skin, sebaceous gland, and hair (dihydrotestosterone dependent)	Stimulation of growth of beard, axillary, and pubic hair; increase in temporal hair recession and balding; increase in sebum secretion
Bone/cartilage	Promotion of epiphyseal fusion Maintenance of bone mass
Larynx and vocal cords	Enlargement of larynx and thickening of vocal cords; deepening of voice
Mammary glands (estrogen dependent)	Development of gynecomastia affected by ratio of androgen to estrogen

From Smith, C.M., & Reynard, A.M. (1992). *Textbook of pharmacology*. Philadelphia: W.B. Saunders.

All androgens are classified as Pregnancy Category X drugs. Use during lactation is not recommended since it is not known if androgens are excreted in human milk. Androgens are also controlled substances under the Anabolic Steroids Control Act of 1990. These drugs are classified as Schedule III drugs.[5,6]

TESTOSTERONE AND TESTOSTERONE ESTER PROTOTYPE

TESTOSTERONE

Testosterone is the major androgen in males. Nearly all of the androgens, including testosterone, are produced by the cells of Leydig, which are interstitial cells between the seminiferous tubules of the testes. **Testosterone** causes the development of male secondary sexual characteristics and stimulates the accessory sex organs. The hormone is necessary for spermatogenesis and is required for the descent of the testes near the end of fetal development.

Pharmacotherapeutics Testosterone is used to treat all of the conditions discussed in the previous section on pharmacotherapeutics.

Pharmacokinetics Testosterone in plasma is 98% bound to a specific testosterone-estradiol binding globulin, with approximately 2% free. Generally the amount of this sex hormone–binding globulin in the plasma determines the distribution of testosterone between free and bound forms. The free testosterone concentrations determine its half-life. The half-life of oral versus IM testosterone varies considerably. Oral preparations' half-life is 10 to 100 minutes, whereas IM preparations have a half-life of several days.

Inactivation of testosterone occurs primarily in the liver. Nearly 90% of testosterone is excreted in the urine as glucuronic and sulfuric acid conjugates of testosterone and its metabolites. Approximately 6% is excreted in feces.[5,6]

Pharmacodynamics Testosterone is a natural androgen. The effects of testosterone on its target tissues—primarily skeletal muscle, the prostate gland, and bone marrow—are mediated by specific androgen receptors located within the cell. The binding of testosterone with its receptor acts on DNA to promote synthesis of specific messenger RNA molecules. In some tissues, testosterone is converted into dihydrotestosterone (DHT) first to permit binding to the androgen receptors. These hormone-receptor pairs serve as models for production of specific proteins. The effects of testosterone are evidenced through these proteins.[2,4,7]

Pharmaceutics Testosterone is available in a sterile solution for IM injections.

Undesired Clinical Responses Testosterone and its esters have fewer side effects than the 17-α-alkylated androgens. Acne and oily skin are frequently experienced by clients undergoing androgen therapy. Gynecomastia, weight gain, suppression of spermatogenesis, decrease in testicular size, and too frequent or persistent erections of the penis also occur. Weight gain is related to sodium and water retention, increased blood volume, and increased lean body mass. Androgens also cause slight increases in hemoglobin and hematocrit levels and in total red blood cell (RBC) count. Prepubertal children may experience masculinization while receiving androgens. In addition, these drugs promote premature epiphyseal closure in children. When administered to women, voice hoarseness, acne, changes in menstrual periods, and facial hair may occur[2,5,7] (Fig. 63–1).

Contraindications and Precautions Androgen administration is not recommended in women and in children of either sex unless for specific indications. Testosterone use is contraindicated in males with carcinoma of the breast or carcinoma of the prostate gland. Because of sodium and water retention, edema with or without congestive heart failure may occur. Therefore clients with serious cardiac, hepatic, or renal disease should not receive testosterone. Caution must be used if it is administered to an individual with a history of drug abuse.[5]

Drug-Drug Interactions Concurrent administration of androgens and oral anticoagulants may intensify the effects of the anticoagulant, requiring a reduction in the anticoagulant dosage. In diabetic clients the metabolic effects of androgens may decrease blood glucose levels, resulting in a reduction of the insulin requirements. Androgens should not be administered concurrently with adrenocorticotropic hormone (ACTH) and corticosteroids. This combination enhances the tendency toward edema.[5]

Interference with Diagnostic Studies Androgens decrease the level of thyroxine-binding globulin, resulting in decreased total T_4 serum levels, and increased resin uptake of T_3 and T_4

Life-Span Considerations Androgens are administered to individuals of varying ages, but there are special considerations for each age group. When given to children with hypogonadism or for stimulation of puberty, care must be exercised because the androgens accelerate epiphyseal closure and may compromise linear growth. To avoid decreasing the child's attainable adult height, radiologic studies of the hand and wrist area that focus on the epiphyseal area should be performed on a regular basis. Decreased cardiac, hepatic, and renal functions are associated with the aging process. Therefore androgen administration in the older adult requires caution.

MISCELLANEOUS DRUGS IN CATEGORY

As indicated previously, androgens contain a 17-α-hydroxyl group. Esterification of this group increases the duration of action of the drug preparation. (**Esterification** is the conversion of an acid into an ester by combining the acid with an alcohol and removing a molecule of water.) **Testosterone cypionate** is an oil-soluble ester of testosterone that is available for IM injection. The sterile solution of testosterone cypionate contains cottonseed oil, which increases the drug's solubility and delays its absorption. **Testosterone enanthate** is also a testosterone ester. This drug preparation is also administered intramuscularly; the vehicle for testosterone enanthate is sesame oil. Another testosterone ester is **testosterone propionate.** Testosterone propionate is insoluble in water but is freely soluble in alcohol, ether, or vegetable oils. This drug preparation contains sesame oil and must be administered intramuscularly.[5,6] Table 63–2 summarizes information on some of the common testosterone and testosterone ester preparations.

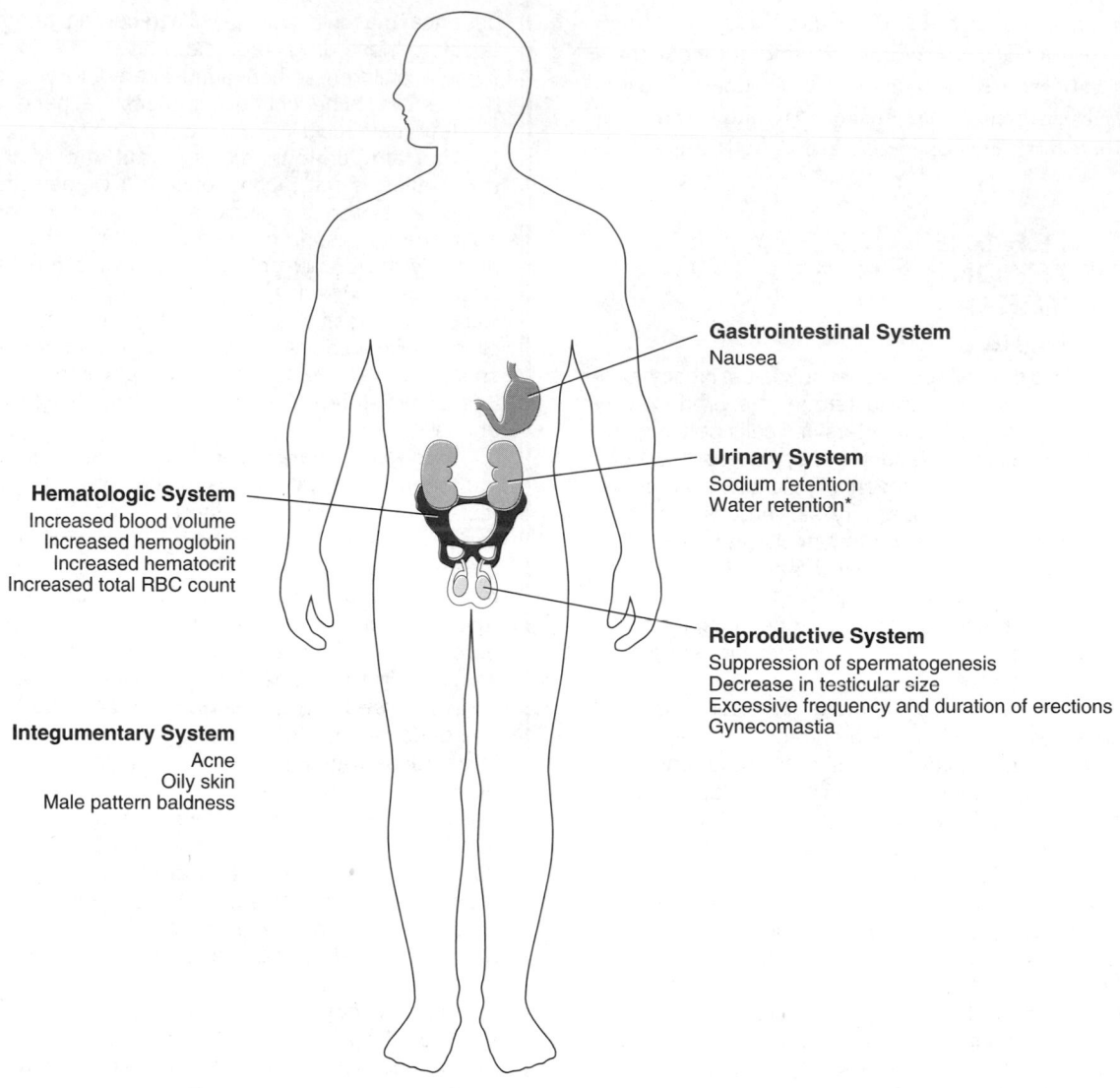

Gastrointestinal System
Nausea

Urinary System
Sodium retention
Water retention*

Hematologic System
Increased blood volume
Increased hemoglobin
Increased hematocrit
Increased total RBC count

Reproductive System
Suppression of spermatogenesis
Decrease in testicular size
Excessive frequency and duration of erections
Gynecomastia

Integumentary System
Acne
Oily skin
Male pattern baldness

*Weight gain associated with fluid retention, increased blood volume, and increased lean muscle mass.

FIGURE 63-1 Undesired clinical responses associated with testosterone and testosterone ester therapy in males.

α-ALKYLATED ANDROGEN PROTOTYPE

METHYLTESTOSTERONE

Methyltestosterone is a synthetic derivative of testosterone. It is used clinically for its androgenic and anabolic action. Because of its similarity to testosterone, only the major differences between the drug groups are discussed.

Pharmacotherapeutics Methyltestosterone is prescribed for replacement therapy in clients with deficient or absent endogenous testosterone, in females 1 to 5 years postmenopausal with metastatic breast cancer, and in females with postpartum breast engorgement. It is also used to treat delayed puberty.

Pharmacokinetics Methyltestosterone is well absorbed. The rate of absorption depends on the route of administration. The peak serum concentration level is reached 2 hours after oral administration of the drug. Methyltestosterone is extensively metabolized in the liver. It has a half-life of 1 hour initially. This changes to $3\frac{1}{2}$ hours within 3 to 4 hours of receiving the dose. Approximately 10% of the dose is recovered in feces. Buccal administration allows direct absorption and has almost twice the potency of oral administration. Peak serum concentrations, when given buccally, are reached 1 hour after administration.[5,6]

Pharmacodynamics The action of methyltestosterone depends on its reduction to dihydrotestosterone, which binds to cytosol-receptor proteins. The androgen-receptor complex is transported to the nucleus where it initiates cellular changes related to androgen action.

Pharmaceutics Oral preparations are available as uncoated tablets, capsules, and sublingual and buccal dosage forms.

TABLE 63–2
Androgens: Prototype and Major Drugs in Category

Drug Name	Dosage and Route of Administration	Nursing Considerations
TESTOSTERONE (Numerous brand names are available) **HOW SUPPLIED** Sterile aqueous suspension for IM injection: 25, 50, and 100 mg/ml	Dosages individualized for all androgens **Replacement Therapy** 10-50 mg two to three times weekly **Delayed Puberty** 40-50 mg/m² dose monthly for 4-6 mo **Palliation of Advanced Breast Cancer in Females** 50-100 mg three times weekly	**Assess** Determine if client has preexisting cardiac, renal, or hepatic disease or has diabetes mellitus. Determine if client is pregnant; androgens are classified as Pregnancy Category X. Review laboratory studies for hepatic function, complete blood count, and serum electrolytes before beginning therapy.
TESTOSTERONE ESTERS **Testosterone Propionate** **HOW SUPPLIED** Sterile sesame oil solution for IM injection: 25, 50, and 100 mg/ml	**Replacement Therapy** 25-50 mg two or three times weekly **Palliation in Breast Cancer in Females** 50-100 mg three times weekly	**Implement** Store solutions at controlled room temperature. Inspect solution for particulate matter and discoloration. Warm and rotate drug container in hand if crystals exist in solution. Administer all oil preparations deep in gluteal muscle. Educate client about need to have contact with primary health care provider on a regular basis. Advise females to report any masculinizing effects.
Testosterone Cypionate **HOW SUPPLIED** Sterile cottonseed oil solution for IM injection: 100 and 200 mg/ml **Testosterone Enanthate** **HOW SUPPLIED** Sterile sesame oil solution for IM injection: 100 and 200 mg/ml	**Replacement Therapy** 50-400 mg q2-4wk **Hypergonadism** 50-400 mg q2-4wk **Delayed Puberty** Highly individualized—50-200 mg q2-4wk for limited duration (e.g., 4-6 mo) **Palliation with Breast Cancer in Females** 200-400 mg q2-4wk	Educate client to report nausea, vomiting, changes in skin color, and/or ankle swelling. Advise male clients to report too frequent or persistent erections of the penis. Provide emotional support to client. Monitor clients with diabetes closely for alterations in blood glucose levels. Observe elderly male clients for signs of prostatic hypertrophy. Observe clients receiving anticoagulant therapy for signs of increased prothrombin time.
Testosterone Transdermal 4,6 mg	**Replacement Therapy** Topical: 6 mg/d	**Monitor** Monitor laboratory studies for hepatic function, hemoglobin, and hematocrit during therapy. Monitor radiologic studies of male adolescent receiving treatment for delayed puberty. Monitor urine and serum calcium levels for females receiving treatment for disseminated breast cancer. Monitor the client's weight regularly. **Evaluate** Evaluate client for diminished symptoms.
17-α-ALKYLATED ANDROGENS	Doses vary depending on age, sex, and diagnosis	See testosterone with the following additions or exceptions: **Assess** Perform a complete assessment of the client's physical and nutritional status before beginning therapy.
METHYLTESTOSTERONE (Android, Metestone, Oreton) **HOW SUPPLIED** Uncoated tablets: 10 and 25 mg Gelatin capsules: 10 mg Sublingual tablets: 10 mg Buccal uncoated tablets: 10 mg	**Hypogonadism** Oral: 10 to 40 mg/d **Androgen Deficiency** Oral: 10-50 mg/d Buccal: 5-25 mg/d **Cryptorchidism** Oral: 30 mg/d **Breast Cancer** Oral: 200 mg/d	**Implement** Do not store drug above 30° C. Store in tight, light-resistant container. Instruct client to report any weight gain >2 lb/wk. Assess sclera and skin for signs of jaundice.

Table continued on following page.

TABLE 63–2 *Continued*
Androgens: Prototype and Major Drugs in Category

Drug Name	Dosage and Route of Administration	Nursing Considerations
Fluoxymesterone (Android-F, Halotestin) **How Supplied** Uncoated tablets: 2, 5, and 10 mg	**Hypogonadism** Oral: 5-20 mg/d **Breast Cancer** Oral: 10-40 mg/d in divided doses	**Monitor** Monitor liver function tests periodically. Monitor serum lipid and high-density lipoprotein levels. Monitor cholesterol levels. Monitor prothrombin level for clients receiving oxymetholone.
Stanozolol (Winstrol) **How Supplied** Uncoated tablets: 2 mg	**Hereditary Angioedema** Oral: initial dose of 2 mg tid; maintenance dose determined by individual client	
Oxymetholone (Anadrol-50) **How Supplied** Uncoated tablets: 50 mg	**Red Blood Cell Production** **ADULTS AND CHILDREN** Oral: 1-5 mg/kg/d; usual effective dose: 1-2 mg/kg/d	
Oxandrolone (Oxandrin) **How Supplied** Uncoated tablets: 2.5 mg	**Weight Gain or Bone Pain in Osteoporosis** **ADULTS** Oral: 2.5 mg bid or qid; range is 2.5-20 mg/d **CHILDREN** Oral: ≤0.1 mg/kg; repeat as indicated	

MODIFIED RING STRUCTURE ANDROGENS

Drug Name	Dosage and Route of Administration	Nursing Considerations
NANDROLONE PHENPROPIONATE (Anabolin, Durabolin, Nandrobolic) **How Supplied** Sterile sesame oil solution for IM injections: 25 and 50 mg/ml; 50 mg/2 ml	**Palliation of Metastatic Breast Cancer** IM: 50-100 mg/wk based on therapeutic response	See testosterone with the following additions or exceptions: **Implement** Store solution at 15° to 30° C. Administer deep IM in gluteal muscle.
Nandrolone Decanoate (Androlone D, Hybolin, Deca-Durabolin, Neo-Durabolic) **How Supplied** Sterile sesame oil solution for IM injection: 50, 100, and 200 mg/ml	**Anemia Associated with Renal Insufficiency** **ADULTS** IM: 50-100 mg/wk for females; 100-200 mg/wk for males **CHILDREN** 2-13 y IM: 25-50 mg q3-4wk	

MISCELLANEOUS ANDROGENS

Drug Name	Dosage and Route of Administration	Nursing Considerations
DANAZOL (Danocrine) **How Supplied** Gelatin capsules: 50, 100, and 200 mg	**Endometriosis** Oral: 800 mg/d in two divided doses for moderate-to-severe disease; 200-400 mg/d in two divided doses for mild cases **Fibrocystic Breast Disease** Oral: 100-400 mg/d in two divided doses **Hereditary Angioedema** Oral: initial dose 200 mg bid or tid; individualized based on response	See testosterone with the following additions or exceptions: **Assess** Determine if client has preexisting conditions such as migraine or epilepsy. Fluid retention may influence these conditions. **Implement** Observe for indications of increased intracranial pressure: headache, nausea, vomiting, visual disturbance. Review laboratory studies carefully. Abnormalities may occur in creatine kinase, glucose tolerance, glucagon, thyroid-binding globulin, sex hormones, and other plasma protein studies.

Undesired Clinical Responses Methyltestosterone produces the same undesired clinical responses as testosterone and testosterone esters. In addition, it decreases the production and serum level of high-density lipids and elevates the level of low-density lipids, resulting in an increase in the individual's risk of atherosclerosis.

Methyltestosterone also produces cholestatic hepatitis and jaundice. The drug-induced jaundice is reversible when drug therapy is terminated. Peliosis hepatitis can occur as a result of any androgen drug therapy; however, it is more common with the α-alkylated androgens. With this disease, the liver tissue is replaced with blood-filled cysts. The condition can produce minimal to life-threatening hepatic dysfunction. Liver cell tumors have also been reported with methyltestosterone use.[5,7]

Interferences with Diagnostic Studies Following are ways methyltestosterone may interfere with diagnostic studies:

- Increases levels of protein-bound iodine (PBI) in thyroxine-binding capacity and radioactive iodine uptake tests.
- Alters glucose tolerance test results.
- Alters metyrapone test.

MISCELLANEOUS DRUGS IN CATEGORY

Several other drugs are in this category, including fluoxymesterone, oxymetholone, oxandrolone, and stanozolol. **Fluoxymesterone** is similar to methyltestosterone. It is administered orally to treat hypogonadism and breast cancer. **Oxymetholone** is used to treat anemias caused by deficient RBC production, including acquired and congenital aplastic anemia, myelofibrosis, and hypoplastic anemia. **Oxandrolone** is used to promote weight gain after weight loss associated with extensive surgery, chronic infections, or severe trauma. Additional undesired clinical responses associated with oxandrolone therapy include suppression of clotting factors II, V, VII, and X, iron deficiency anemia, excitation, and insomnia. **Stanozolol** is used for prophylactic treatment of hereditary angioedema. Hereditary angioedema is an autosomal dominant disorder caused by deficient or nonfunctional C1 esterase inhibitor. Symptoms produced by this disease include swelling of the face, extremities, genitalia, and bowel wall and frequent upper respiratory tract infections.

See Table 63–2 for a summary of information on the 17-α-alkylated androgens.

MODIFIED RING STRUCTURE PROTOTYPE

NANDROLONE PHENPROPIONATE

Because of nandrolone phenpropionate's similarity to testosterone, only the major differences between the drug groups are discussed. The primary use for this drug is the control of metastatic breast cancer. This drug preparation has been modified so that the CH3 group has been deleted. This modification decreases the drug's androgenic properties and retains and increases the anabolic properties.[5,8]

OTHER DRUGS IN CATEGORY

Nandrolone decanoate is another drug in this category. It is prepared in a manner similar to that for nandrolone phenpropionate. It is used primarily to treat anemia associated with renal insufficiency.

See Table 63–2 for a summary of information on the modified ring structure androgens.

Other Androgens

Danazol (Danocrine) is an androgen that suppresses the pituitary-ovarian axis. This suppression probably results from a combination of depressed hypothalamic-pituitary response to lowered estrogen production and altered sex steroid metabolism. The drug has a weak androgenic effect.

Danazol is used to treat endometriosis, fibrocystic breast disease, and hereditary angioedema. It causes some degree of fluid retention, so it must be used with caution in clients with hepatic, renal, or cardiac dysfunction. Therapy should begin during menstruation to ensure that the client receiving treatment for endometriosis or fibrocystic breast disease is not pregnant. Undesired clinical responses associated with this drug include weight gain, acne, seborrhea, and menstrual disturbance. Flushing, sweating, and vaginal dryness have also been reported. Danazol therapy may interfere with the laboratory determination of testosterone.[2,5,6,8]

CONCEPT REVIEW

The action of androgens and anabolic steroids does overlap, but androgens primarily stimulate the growth of male accessory organs and produce masculinizing effects.

Some of the major uses of androgens are hormone replacement for hypogonadism in males, palliation of advanced or metastatic breast cancer in females, and treatment of hereditary angioedema.

Esterification, alkylation, and change in the ring structure can prolong action of these drugs, which otherwise are rapidly absorbed and degraded.

ANABOLIC STEROID ABUSE

As indicated previously, all androgens possess an anabolic quality. However, some androgens have high anabolic and low androgenic activity. The abuse of these androgens precipitated their inclusion as controlled substances.

General Characteristics

Androgens with high anabolic activity (anabolic steroids) increase body tissue-building processes and reverse catabolic action. Anabolic effects occur because the uptake of cortisol in muscle and liver cells is blocked. Normally cortisol acts as a catabolic agent, but anabolic steroids block this action in the muscle cells and reduce muscle breakdown while increasing muscle mass. In liver cells when cortisol uptake is blocked, cortisol's action on body stress reactions is affected. Additionally, these drugs decrease plasma protein synthesis in the liver and thus enhance their effects by increasing the amount of free drug in the plasma.[1,7,8]

Anabolic Steroid Use

To increase athletic performance, some professional and nonprofessional athletes use anabolic steroids. These athletes use steroids to increase muscle mass and strength, decrease muscle recovery time, decrease healing time after muscle injury, and increase aggressiveness. However, studies in male athletes have indicated that these drugs have done very little to enhance strength or performance.[1,9–12] The effect of these drugs on female performance is unclear. Although the use of anabolic steroids in athletic competition is banned, usage continues to exist.

In addition to questionable benefits, health risks and side effects are common with the use of these drugs. Adverse effects among men include lowered sperm count, with a decrease in volume and motility of sperm; decrease in size of testicles; priapism (painful, sustained erection of the penis); lowered endogenous testosterone levels; and gynecomastia. Among women, the most common effects are increased facial hair, acne, abnormal darkening of the skin, voice change, altered menstrual cycle, and clitoromegaly. Some effects are permanent even after a client discontinues taking anabolic steroids.[1,7,10]

Severe effects are impaired liver function (i.e., cholestatic hepatitis, hepatic cysts, benign hepatomas, malignant hepatic tumors) and increased cardiovascular risk due to change in lipid parameters. Other cardiovascular effects include secondary polycythemia, hypertension, hypertrophy of the left ventricle, and cardiac muscle lesions. In addition, myocardial infarction and cerebral vascular accident have been associated with the use of anabolic steroids.[1] A psychotic-like syndrome has also been described in response to anabolic steroid use. Symptoms include auditory hallucinations, paranoid delusions, and manic episodes. These symptoms are usually associated with long-term use of the drugs.[2]

CONCEPT REVIEW

Anabolic steroids produce a positive nitrogen balance that in turn stimulates tissue building; the base structure of anabolic steroids is testosterone.

Their value in enhancing athletic strength and performance is unclear, but their abuse in this area continues.

MISCELLANEOUS DRUGS

Other drugs in addition to androgens affect the male reproductive system. They include antiandrogens and androgen-suppressant drugs.

Antiandrogens or Androgen Inhibitors

Androgen inhibitors comprise a chemically diverse class of drugs that inhibit the uptake or binding of DHT. The result is blockage of androgen-mediated action in all androgen-sensitive target cells. Antiandrogen drugs are used to treat prostatic neoplasms since these tumors are androgen dependent.

Flutamide (Eulexin) is a nonsteroidal androgen inhibitor that inhibits the uptake or binding of testosterone or DHT to target cell receptors, thus interfering with androgen action. Flutamide is absorbed well in humans, with maximal plasma concentrations occurring 2 to 4 hours after a single 200-mg oral dose. The drug is rapidly metabolized. One hour after administration, only 2.5% of the plasma level contains unchanged flutamide. Excretion is mainly through the urine.

Flutamide is often used in combination with a luteinizing hormone releasing hormone (LH-RH) agonist analog for treatment of metastatic prostatic cancer (stage D_2). The recommended dosage of flutamide is two 125-mg capsules three times a day at 8-hour intervals for a total daily dose of 750 mg. Adverse effects include hypertension, central nervous system reactions, anorexia, anemia, leukopenia, thrombocytopenia, hepatic toxicity, gynecomastia, jaundice, and edema.[5,6]

Androgen Suppression

Leuprolide acetate (Lupron) is an LH-RH agonist. It acts as an inhibitor of gonadotropin secretion when given continuously. It is indicated for palliative treatment of advanced prostatic cancer. It offers an alternative treatment to orchiectomy or estrogen administration. Leuprolide acetate is described in detail in Chapter 62.

Other Drugs

Finasteride (Proscar) is a new drug used in the treatment of benign prostatic hyperplasia. It is classified by the Food and Drug Administration (FDA) as an α-reductase inhibitor. Its action inhibits the enzyme 5-α-reductase, which is needed to metabolize testosterone to DHT. Since the development of the prostate gland is dependent on DHT, finasteride interferes with prostatic activity.

Finasteride is 90% bound to plasma proteins. Maximum plasma concentrations are reached within 1 to 2 hours after oral administration. After an oral dose, approximately 39% is excreted in the urine and 57%, in the form of metabolites, in the feces. The elimination rate is decreased in the elderly, but no dosage adjustment is necessary. Past studies reveal a mean half-life of 8 hours for clients greater than 70 years of age. The mean half-life is 6 hours in clients 45 to 60 years of age.

Finasteride is administered orally. The recommended dose is 5 mg daily. Initial studies have shown finasteride is tolerated well. Side effects, usually mild and transient, include impotence, decreased libido, and decreased volume of ejaculate. In addition, finasteride causes a decrease in serum prostate specific antigen (PSA) levels, even in the presence of prostatic cancer. Because serum PSA is used as a screening tool for prostatic cancer, caution must be exercised in the use of the PSA level in diagnosing prostatic cancer in clients taking finasteride.[5,6]

CONCEPT REVIEW

Antiandrogens or androgen inhibitors block androgen-mediated action in all androgen-sensitive target cells. They are used to treat androgen-dependent prostatic neoplasms.

Finasteride, a new drug used to treat benign prostatic hyperplasia, causes a decrease in serum PSA levels and can interfere with accurate diagnosis of prostatic cancer.

SUMMARY

Drugs affecting the male reproductive system include androgens, androgen inhibitors, androgen suppression drugs, and α-reductase inhibitors. These drugs are used for a variety of reasons, including hypogonadism, male contraception, delayed puberty, and palliation for female breast cancer. For most of the drugs, nursing management focuses on client education for accurate drug administration and recognition of undesired clinical responses. Because these drugs affect reproductive function, the client may experience changes in both body image and self-concept. The nurse must be aware of the impact these changes can have on the client and explore with the client various coping strategies and other mechanisms of support.

REFERENCES

1. Joyce, J.A. (1991). Anesthesia for athletes using performance-enhancing drugs. *Journal of the American Association of Nurse Anesthetists, 59*(2), 139-144.
2. Smith, C.M., & Reynard, A.M. (1992). *Textbook of pharmacology.* Philadelphia: W.B. Saunders.
3. Jarvis, C. (1992). *Physical examination and health assessment.* Philadelphia: W.B. Saunders.
4. Lehne, R. (1994). *Pharmacology for nursing care* (2nd ed.). Philadelphia: W.B. Saunders.
5. U.S. Pharmacopeial Convention. (1990). *The United States pharmacopeia* (22nd rev.). Rockville, MD: Author.
6. Data Pharmaceutica, Inc. (1993). *1993 physicians' genRx.* Smithtown, NY: Author.
7. Cheever, K., & House, M.A. (1992). Cardiovascular implications of anabolic steroid abuse. *Journal of Cardiovascular Nursing, 6*(2), 19-30.
8. Council on Scientific Affairs. (1990). Medical and nonmedical uses of anabolic-androgenic steroids. *Journal of American Medical Association, 264,* 2923-2927.
9. Porterfield, L.M. (1991). Steroid abuse. *Advancing Clinical Care, 6*(2), 44.
10. Hough, D., & Voy, R. (1990). When to suspect steroid abuse. *Patient Care, 24*(13), 129-132, 134, 136.
11. Johnson, M.D. (1990). Anabolic steroid use in adolescent athletes. *Pediatric Clinics of North America, 37,* 1111-1123.
12. Woolley, B.H. (1991). The latest fads to increase muscle mass and energy: A look at what some athletes are using. *Postgraduate Medicine, 89,* 195-198, 201-205, 221-223.

BIBLIOGRAPHY

Collin, L.H. (1993). Doping in sports. *Journal of the American Academy of Physician Assistants, 6,* 465-477.

Engel, N.S. (1989). Anabolic steroid use among high school athletes. *MCN: American Journal of Maternal Child Nursing, 14,* 417.

Matzkin, H., & Braf, Z. (1991). Endocrine treatment of benign prostatic hypertrophy: Current concepts. *Urology, 37*(1), 1-16.

Miller, C. (1993). New medication for the treatment of benign prostatic hyperplasia. *Geriatric Nursing, 14*(2), 111-112.

Nemechek, P.M. (1991). Anabolic steroid users—Another potential risk group for HIV infection. *New England Journal of Medicine, 325,* 357.

Omeprazole/warfarin interaction. (1991). *Nurse's Drug Alert, 15*(19), 65.

Drugs Affecting the Sensory System

CHAPTER 64

DRUGS USED IN
Ocular Disorders

LASCA BECK • NORMA L. PINNELL

⊛ Anatomy and Functions of the Eye
LEARNING OBJECTIVES:
Identify common anatomic eye structures.
Describe how the function of different eye structures can be influenced by drugs.
KEY TERM: Intraocular pressure

⊛ Disorders of the Eye
LEARNING OBJECTIVE: Describe pathologic changes that occur with common eye disorders.
KEY TERMS:
Glaucoma, allergic conjunctivitis, blepharitis, chalazion, conjunctivitis, keratitis, keratocon junctivitis sicca, hordeolum

⊛ Nursing Considerations
LEARNING OBJECTIVES:
Discuss assessment measures for the eye.
Identify possible nursing diagnoses for eye disorders.
Identify important topics for client education.
Prepare a teaching and discharge plan for a client with an ophthalmic disorder.
Describe the administration of eyedrops and ointments.

⊛ Ophthalmic Preparations
LEARNING OBJECTIVES:
Discuss the problems related to bioavailability of topical ocular agents.
Explain the differences between eyedrops and eye ointments.

⊛ Ocular Drugs Affecting the Autonomic Nervous System
LEARNING OBJECTIVE: Describe the purpose and function of the different autonomic drugs.
KEY TERMS:
Cycloplegia, miosis, mydriasis

⊛ Diuretics
LEARNING OBJECTIVE: Discuss the purpose and function of diuretics in treating ocular disorders.

⊛ Antiinfective Drugs
LEARNING OBJECTIVE: Discuss the purpose and function of major ocular antiinfective drugs.
KEY TERMS:
Endophthalmitis, fungal keratitis

⊛ Antiinflammatory Drugs
LEARNING OBJECTIVE: Explain the purpose and function of major ocular antiinflammatory drugs.

⊛ Miscellaneous Ocular Drugs
LEARNING OBJECTIVES:
Describe the pharmacotherapeutic properties of ocular anesthetics.
Explain the pharmacodynamic properties of ocular antiallergic drugs.
Discuss the pharmacotherapeutic properties of ocular antihistamine-decongestant drugs.
Discuss the pharmacotherapeutic properties of ocular irrigation solutions and lubricants.
KEY TERMS:
Artificial tear inserts, epitheliopathy

⊛ Agents Used to Diagnose Ocular Disorders
LEARNING OBJECTIVES:
Identify categories of drugs used to diagnose ocular disorders.
Discuss the pharmacodynamic properties of fluorescein and rose bengal.

*T*he visual system includes the eyes, the accessory structures (eyebrows, eyelids, conjunctivae, lacrimal glands), and the optic nerves, tracts, and pathways. Much of human education depends on functioning of the visual system; when this system fails, other systems adapt to compensate.

ANATOMY AND FUNCTIONS OF THE EYE

The function of the eye is to convey surrounding light rays through the optic nerve to the brain where they are interpreted into meaningful images. The eye is composed of three coats or tunics: fibrous, vascular, and nervous.

The outer, or fibrous, tunic consists of the sclera and cornea. The **sclera** is the white outermost lining over the eyeball that protects the eye from foreign matter and supports inner eye structures. The **cornea,** the transparent portion of the outer coat of the eyeball, lies behind the conjunctiva. It serves as the window through which light rays are refracted for vision. It is avascular so that it is free of antibodies, but it is filled with nerves.

The middle, vascular tunic, or uveal tract, consists of the choroid, ciliary body, and iris. The **iris** lies behind the cornea and in front of the lens. It contracts and expands to regulate the amount of light that enters the eye, thus determining whether the pupil is dilated or constricted. The **pupil** is the space where the iris does not meet. The pupil does not reflect light through it and normally appears round and black.

The inner, or nervous, tunic consists of the **retina**. Specific nerve fibers from the retina form together into the optic nerve, which conveys light image messages to the cerebral cortex for interpretation. Another important function of the retina is the interpretation of colors; this is accomplished by photoreceptor cells known as *rods* and *cones*.[1-4] The **fundus** is the area where the macula and optic nerve are located on the retina.

Many other important eye structures are intermingled through the three tunics. In addition, there are several accessory structures external to the eye. A brief description of some of these parts follows.

The **canthus** is the angle at each side of the junction of the eyelids. The inner nasal angle is referred to as the *inner canthus* and the outer brow angle is referred to as the *outer canthus*. Within the upper and lower inner canthi lie inlets to the **lacrimal canaliculi** through which tears drain.[1, 3]

The **conjunctiva** is the transparent thin mucous membrane that is a continuous covering of the inner surface of the eyelid and the front of the eye. The function of the conjunctiva is to prevent foreign objects' getting behind the eye.

Two major compartments exist within the eye: a large cavity posterior to the lens and a much smaller cavity anterior to the lens. The anterior cavity is divided into two chambers. The **anterior chamber** lies between the cornea and the iris, and a smaller **posterior chamber** lies between the iris and the lens. Both of these chambers are filled with **aqueous humor** (also called *aqueous*), a watery, plasma-like substance that nourishes the cornea and lens and removes waste products from them. Aqueous is constantly formed by the ciliary body and is secreted into the posterior chamber. From there, aqueous moves into the anterior chamber where it drains through spaces in the trabecular meshwork into **Schlemm's canal**. After reaching Schlemm's canal, aqueous drains into the venous blood supply. Secretion and outflow of aqueous normally are balanced, with the degree of balance governing the **intraocular pressure (IOP).** Normal IOP ranges from 12 to 20 mmHg.[1-4]

The posterior cavity of the eye is surrounded almost completely by the retina and is filled with a transparent jellylike substance, the **vitreous humor**. Vitreous humor is not produced on a regular basis; the vitreous humor helps maintain IOP and holds the lens and retina in place. It also functions in the refraction of light in the eye.

The **lens,** which is a clear biconvex-shaped structure located behind the iris, is responsible for **accommodation.** Accommodation is the refraction of light rays so that they focus the retina.[3] (See Fig. 64–1 for an illustration of the structure of the eye.)

DISORDERS OF THE EYE

Because vision is one of the most treasured of all the senses, visual disorders can represent a threat to the individual. Eye disorders, which can occur throughout life, are due to a wide variety of causes. In general practice settings, some of the disorders are rarely seen; however, others may be seen singularly or in combination with other body dysfunctions. Use of medications is one of the major approaches to the treatment of eye disorders. Therefore knowledge of ocular disorders and drugs used for ophthalmic treatment is important. An overview of some of the most common ophthalmic disorders treatable with drugs is presented to serve as a basis to the study of ophthalmic pharmacotherapeutic agents.

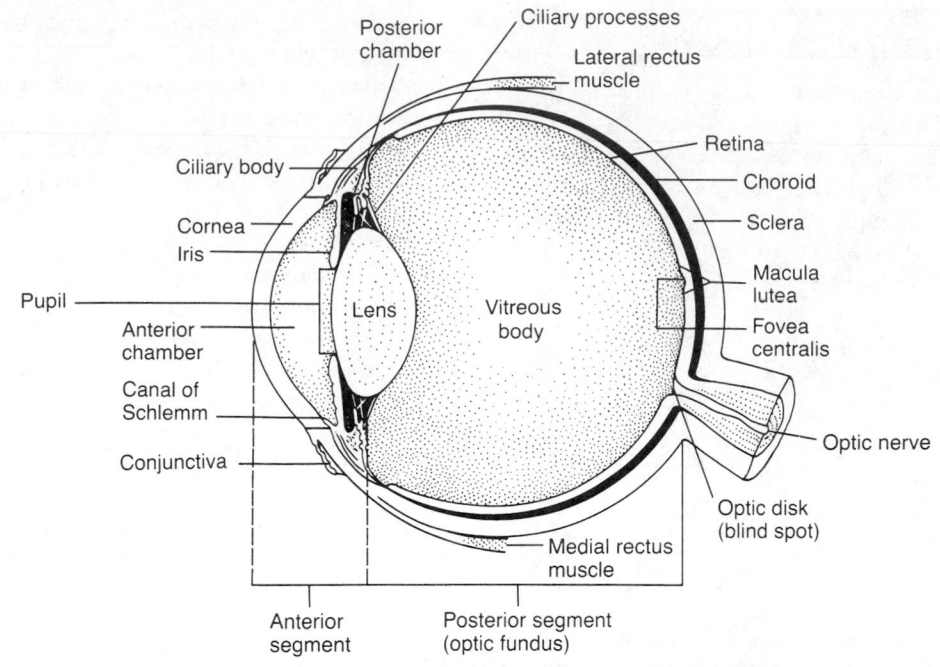

FIGURE 64–1   Structure of the eye. (From Ignatavicius, D.D., & Bayne, M.V. [1991]. *Medical-surgical nursing: A nursing process approach* [p. 994]. Philadelphia: W.B. Saunders.)

Glaucoma

Glaucoma, which is one of the leading causes of blindness, is a disorder resulting from increased IOP within the eye. The increased IOP can damage the optic disc and ultimately lead to blindness.

Inflammatory Conditions

Allergic conjunctivitis often occurs during the hay fever seasons in warm and hot weather. The allergic reaction typically causes pruritus and a watery mucinoid eye discharge.

Foreign objects in the conjunctiva are especially common but are usually easily removed, with resultant immediate relief from the eye discomfort. When foreign objects cause corneal irritation, corneal erosion can occur. Foreign matter in the cornea typically causes tearing, pain, and photophobia.

Keratoconjunctivitis sicca (dry eye) is a bilateral partial or total deficiency in aqueous tear production. It can occur in men and in young women, but it is common in menopausal and postmenopausal women. The usual complaints of discomfort include burning and a foreign body or scratchy sensation in the eyes.

Infectious Conditions

Blepharitis is an inflammation that can progress to an infection of eyelid margins. Initially lid margins become red, thickened, painful, and scaly. When infected, a purulent discharge is present.

Hordeolum (stye) is an infected gland on the external eyelid near the lid margin. It appears as a reddened raised bump often pointing toward the lid margin.

Chalazion (meibomian cyst) is an infected gland on the internal eyelid, which causes a reddened edematous lid. In addition, a sticky discharge may be present.

Conjunctivitis, commonly known as *pinkeye*, may be caused by viruses, bacteria, fungi, parasites, toxins, chemicals, or a foreign body. The eye reacts with the characteristic redness (**hyperemia**) and discomfort in the form of a burning sensation. A discharge, which can vary from frequent watering to purulent matter, causes the lids to stick together. Often both eyes are affected.

Keratitis is inflammation of the cornea that can result from a variety of causes, including viruses, bacteria, fungi, and injury. Symptoms of keratitis are photophobia, pain, and lacrimation.

▨ NURSING CONSIDERATIONS

Nurses in current day acute care and outpatient settings are responsible for the management of eye disorders, which are often secondary to primary disorders. Because ophthalmology is a specialty, maintaining a readily recalled knowledge base of the varied ocular disorders and their treatment can be a challenge. Ideally, preprinted standardized plans of care that can be individualized and printed teaching materials will be available. Nursing management of clients with ocular disorders includes performance of ocular procedures, administration of drugs, and evaluation of the outcome of care.

Assessing   During the **health history** question the client about past and present medical problems that could cause visual impairment. Inquire about past and present occupations; assess for a possible relationship between occupation and visual or eye disorder. Ask the client about eye disorders of parents and grandparents. Ask about past eye disorders, how they were treated, and the degree of success with treatment. Determine the frequency of eye examinations.

Once general information is collected, focus on the chief complaint. Determine the duration of the problem. If it is an injury, determine when and how the injury occurred and what measures were taken before medical attention was received.

Obtain a drug history from the client. Focus on all prescribed and over-the-counter (OTC) drugs, not just ophthalmic preparations. Determine the client's level of knowledge about the drugs (e.g., drug action, dosage, major side effects).

Talk with the client about his or her usual daily routine. Has it been affected by the present eye condition? Are there aspects in the routine that may precipitate visual changes or eye problems? Ask the client about the presence of pain or discomfort such as lacrimation, photophobia, itching, or foreign body sensation.

After collecting the health history, perform a **physical assessment.** Test visual function, including near and distance visual acuity, color perception, and peripheral vision. Perform these tests in a room that is well lit. The Snellen eye chart can be used to test near and distance vision. Inspect the eyelids for edema, exudate, scaling, or ptosis. Assess the nasolacrimal area for signs of inflammation, erythema, or edema. Inspect the cornea; it is normally clear.

Extraocular muscle function is tested by use of the gaze test, cover-uncover test, and corneal light reflex test. (See a health assessment text for additional information on these tests.) Examine the pupil of each eye for equality of size, shape, reaction to light, and accommodation. If abnormalities are detected, perform additional assessment measures such as ophthalmoscopic examination.

Diagnosing After analysis of the data base, formulate nursing diagnoses. Appropriate diagnoses for the client might include the following:

- Noncompliance with drug therapy related to lack of understanding of desired action.
- Knowledge deficit regarding purpose and correct usage of ophthalmic drug.
- Ineffective individual coping related to lack of acceptance of long-term chronic eye disorder.
- Altered health maintenance related to lack of material resources or complete or partial lack of gross or fine motor skills.
- Fear related to perceived inability to control the eye disorder.

Planning During the planning phase develop, as a part of the overall plan of care, individualized teaching and discharge plans. Identify family members or other individuals available as a support system to the client. Include these individuals in the teaching sessions. Also identify individuals who have effectively adapted to the same disorder as the client; these individuals can be used as support resources. Determine the appropriate methods to correct knowledge deficits.

Expected outcomes should be developed with the client. They include the following:

- Client participates in treatment plan.
- Client verbalizes purpose and correct usage of ophthalmic drug.
- Client indicates acceptance of long-term chronic eye disorder.
- Client demonstrates methods of drug self-administration.

Implementing Before administering ophthalmic drugs, you must learn the terms and abbreviations specific to the treatment of the eye:

- **OS** (oculus sinister): abbreviation for *left eye*
- **OD** (oculus dexter): abbreviation for *right eye*
- **OU** (oculus uterque): abbreviation for *each eye*
- **Miosis**: constriction of the pupil due to expansion of pupillary muscles
- **Mydriasis**: enlargement of the pupil due to contraction of pupillary muscles
- **Photophobia**: sensitivity to light characterized by frequent blinking or keeping an eyelid closed

There are several methods for administering topical ophthalmic preparations, including the use of drops, ointments, sprays, gels, and membrane-bound inserts. Most of the drugs described in this chapter are instilled as drops or ointments.

Eyedrops are available in solutions and suspensions. Solutions are the most commonly used of all ophthalmic medications. Both solutions and suspensions are easily instilled, interfere less with vision, and have fewer potential complications than other methods. Their disadvantages include short contact time with ocular tissues, incorrect timing and technique of instillation, and frequent contamination of the drug. In addition, aqueous suspensions may precipitate, and although shaken well, the degree of resuspension is never consistent.

The standard size of a drop from a dropper bottle, which is 1 μl, is used to achieve the desired contact time of the drug with eye structures. When drops larger than the standard are used, excessive tearing and dilution of the drug occur. After instillation of one eyedrop, 5 minutes are required for the reflex tearing response to subside. Therefore a second drop should not be instilled until 5 minutes after the first drop; otherwise a portion or all of the second drop is diluted and lost through spillage over the lid margin or washed with tears through the lacrimal system into the nasopharynx.[5]

Because there are several types of eyedrop medications, some manufacturers color code drug labels and caps to assist with accurate identification. Standard colors are red for mydriatics and cycloplegics; green for miotics; gray for nonsteroidal antiinflammatory drugs (NSAIDs); brown or tan for antiinfective drugs; and yellow, blue, or both for β-blockers.[6]

Eye ointments are available for a variety of purposes and many have an action identical or similar to that of ocular drops. Generally an ointment is used when a lubricating effect is desired or when a longer contact time with external eye structures is indicated. Ointments have a turnover or loss rate of approximately 0.5% per minute, in contrast to eyedrops, which have a turnover rate of approximately 16% per minute, the same rate as tears.[5] Ointments are cleared from the eye through the lacrimal drainage system, the same as for eyedrops, only at a slower rate. After application, ointments melt quickly and spread to lid margins, lashes, and the skin of the lids. Ointment that reaches lid margins acts as a reservoir and prolongs drug contact time with eye tissues; thus ointments have an advantage of requiring less frequent instillation. Also ointments have less systemic effect than eyedrops.

A disadvantage of using ointments is that the same degree of drug concentration cannot be reached as with eyedrops. Another undesirable temporary effect is that ointments tend to blur vision. When an ointment is cool or cold, it tends to curl upon itself during instillation. This can be avoided by warming the ointment before instillation. When both ointments and eyedrops will be instilled, administer the eyedrops first. If an ointment is instilled first, it can block distribution of an eyedrop.

Before administering eye medications, wash your hands carefully. Then cleanse any discharge from the eye with a warm, moist cloth. Make certain that the solution or ointment is at room temperature. Eyedrops or ointments are most easily administered when the individual lies supine and the head is hyperextended. Since individuals are usually quite sensitive to having another individual manipulate their eyelids, they may not be able to keep their eyes open for drops without your holding them open.

Eyedrops are most easily instilled into the eye by resting the hand that holds the medicine bottle on the client's forehead so that the hand moves with the head whenever it moves. Place the other hand on the client's cheekbone below the eye, and use the index finger to pull down the lower lid and expose the conjunctival sac where the drop is released. Allow the lids to close slowly so they will not squeeze out the medication. After

the administration of most eyedrops, apply gentle finger pressure to the lacrimal sac for 1 to 2 minutes (Fig. 64–2). Remove excess solution around the eye with a tissue and wash your hands immediately to remove the drug on your skin. Do not rinse the dropper. (See box on p. 869 for suggested modifications based on the age of the child.) The technique for administering ophthalmic ointment is described and illustrated in the box on p. 869 and the illustration below the box.

Evaluating During the evaluation phase, determine the effectiveness of the plan of care and treatment plan. If the client is having difficulty managing the ocular problem, determine with the client what changes are needed.

OPHTHALMIC PREPARATIONS

Topical administration is the most common route used for treating eye disorders with drugs. Systemic administration is used to achieve adequate drug levels in specific eye tissue, when a drug is available only in systemic form, or when a drug is only effective by the systemic route. This chapter focuses mainly on topically administered agents.

Topical administration is a safe, convenient, and noninvasive method of medicating eyes. Most topical ocular drugs contain a preservative and an agent that provides proper tonicity, buffering, and viscosity. A preservative is added to give ocular drugs antimicrobial properties and thus provide sufficient shelf life. An agent is added to delay washout from the tear film covering the cornea and to increase the bioavailability of the drug to ocular tissue.

Bioavailability is affected by two sources of drug loss from topical administration: (1) diffusion into the circulating blood, and (2) drainage through the aqueous humor into the canal of

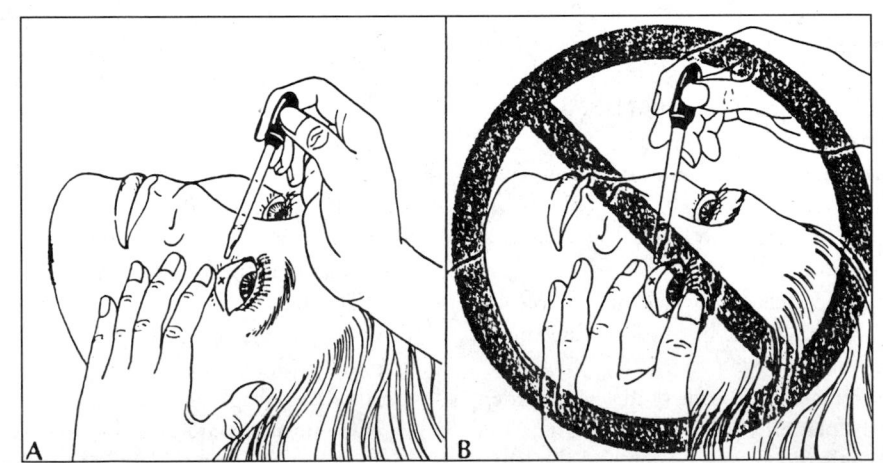

FIGURE 64–2 Administering eye drops. **A,** shows correct method. Note that nurse's hand rests on forehead. If the person moves, the nurse's hand will tend to move also, thereby diminishing the chance that the dropper might strike the eye. Incorrect method **(B)** could result in injury to a person's eye with a sudden head movement. (From Bolander, V.B. [1994]. Sorensen and Luckmann's Basic Nursing: A psychophysiologic approach [3rd Ed.]. Philadelphia: W.B. Saunders.)

Administration Techniques for Infants and Toddlers

Young Infants
Instilling medication in the eyes of young infants is difficult because they often clench the lids tightly closed. One strategy is to hold the medication bottle poised above the infant's eye; when the infant opens the eye, quickly squeeze the container, releasing the drop of medication into the eye.

Older Infants and Toddlers
Older infants and toddlers resist administration of eye medications. It is not unusual for them to flail their arms, kick, scream, and hold their eyes closed. It may help to have the parent or another nurse hold the child securely and talk soothingly to him or her. At times it may be necessary to "mummy" the child. Once the movement of the child is minimized, rest the left hand on the forehead and use the thumb to retract the upper eyelid. At the same time, rest the right hand on the cheek and retract the lower lid with the small finger; using the thumb and index finger to hold the medicine bottle, squeeze the medication into the conjunctival sac.

Ointments
Ointments can be applied while the child sleeps by pulling down the lower lid and placing the ointment in the lower conjunctival sac.

Instillation of Eye Ointment

1. Open the eye and tilt the head backward toward the ceiling.
2. Gently pull down the lower lid to form a pouch.
3. Squeeze the ointment from the tube along the pouch, but do not touch the eye or eyelid with the tube.
4. Close the eye (do not rub the eyes) and blink several times.
5. Vision may be blurred for a few minutes after applying this medication. Do not drive a car or operate machinery until vision has cleared.
6. If possible, have someone administer the eye ointment for you.

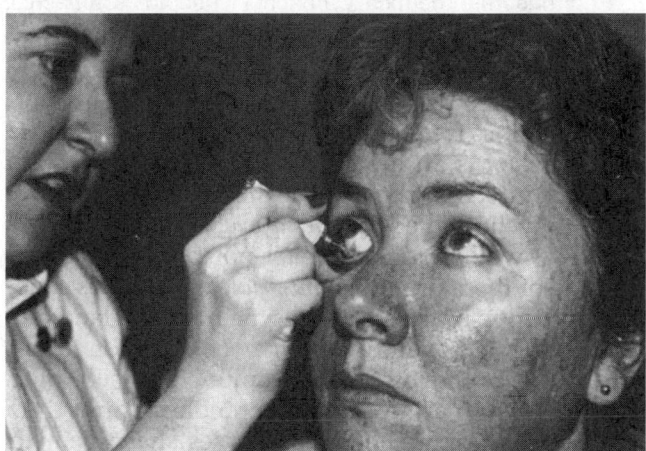

Illustration from Ignatavicius, D.D., & Bayne, M.V. (1991). *Medical-surgical nursing: A nursing process approach* (p. 1013). Philadelphia: W.B. Saunders.

Schlemm. Drugs instilled topically are generally of benefit only to anterior eye structures. Therefore topical administration is not indicated for treatment of posterior eye disorders.[6]

CONCEPT REVIEW

- The eye is composed of three coats or tunics: fibrous, vascular, and nervous. The outer, or fibrous, tunic consists of the sclera and cornea. The middle, vascular tunic, or uveal tract, consists of the choroid, ciliary body, and iris. The inner, or nervous, tunic consists of the retina.
- Specific nerve fibers from the retina form together into the optic nerve, which conveys light image messages to the cerebral cortex of the brain.
- The photoreceptors of the retina (rods and cones) interpret color.
- Aqueous humor fills the anterior and posterior chambers between the cornea and the iris.
- Vitreous humor fills the eyeball behind the lens.
- Glaucoma, inflammatory conditions, and infections are all treatable with drug therapy.

- Ophthalmic preparations are normally administered topically, most commonly as eyedrops or ointments. Ointments provide longer contact time with the external eye structures than do drops, but they are not as concentrated and may blur vision.
- Client teaching for self-administration of ophthalmic drugs is a major part of nursing care in this area.

OCULAR DRUGS AFFECTING THE AUTONOMIC NERVOUS SYSTEM

A large number of ophthalmic drugs widely used to diagnose and treat eye disorders affect the autonomic nervous system. Their actions affect pupil size, IOP, and accommodation. (See Chapter 25 for an overview of the autonomic nervous system.) Even when applied locally to the eye, most autonomic drugs do not act on a single, direct site. Topically applied ocular drugs can penetrate to secondary eye structures and to the systemic circulation, with distant sites influenced by the drugs.

Cholinergic Agonists

Cholinergic agonists are also known as *parasympathomimetics, cholinomimetics,* or *miotics*. Drugs in this category produce effects similar to those of acetylcholine. There are two subgroups of drugs in this category: direct-acting cholinergic agonists and cholinesterase inhibitors. These classifications denote whether the drug acts directly on the intended site or acts indirectly, interacting with several sites.

DIRECT-ACTING CHOLINERGIC AGONISTS

The prototype for this group is carbachol.

DIRECT-ACTING CHOLINERGIC AGONIST PROTOTYPE

CARBACHOL

Pharmacotherapeutics Carbachol (Isopto Carbachol, Miostat) is used to control IOP in clients with glaucoma.

Pharmacokinetics With carbachol, mydriasis is maximal in 2 to 5 minutes and persists for 24 hours. Several of the cholinergic agonist drugs have a short duration (10 to 30 minutes) of action.

Pharmacodynamics Cholinergic agonist drugs exert their influence directly at the receptor sites of the iridic sphincter muscle, the ciliary body, and the lacrimal gland. Carbachol directly stimulates cholinergic receptors; it may also stimulate autonomic effector cells to release acetylcholine. These actions cause the iridic sphincter to contract **(miosis)** and decrease IOP. The action of the released acetylcholine is terminated through hydrolysis by cholinesterases in varying degrees of speed. Once hydrolysis is complete, the pupil returns to the premedicated state.[7] Figure 64–3 illustrates common ocular and systemic physiologic responses to cholinergic agonists.

Pharmaceutics Carbachol ophthalmic solution is available in a variety of concentrations. Table 64–1 provides additional information about dosage forms, dosages, and routes of administration.

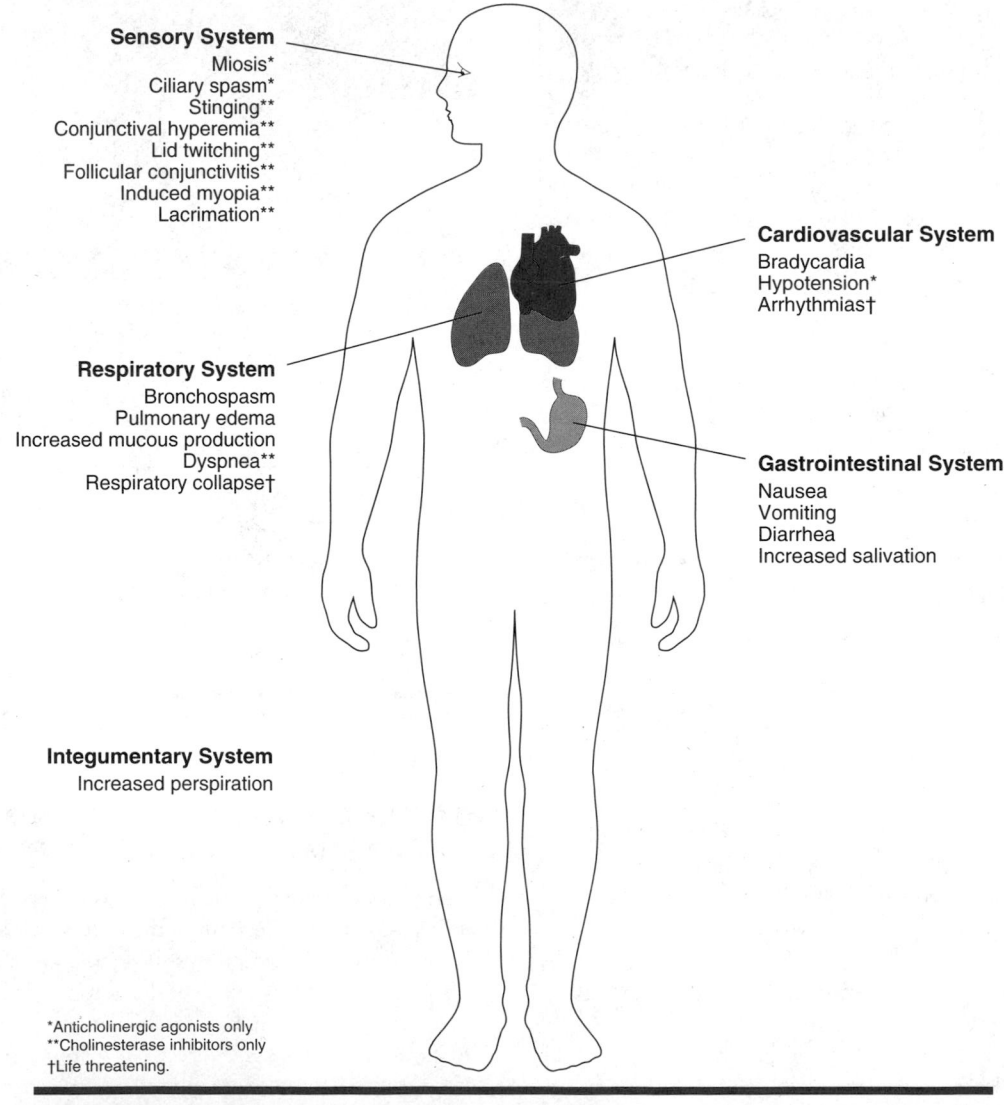

Sensory System
Miosis*
Ciliary spasm*
Stinging**
Conjunctival hyperemia**
Lid twitching**
Follicular conjunctivitis**
Induced myopia**
Lacrimation**

Cardiovascular System
Bradycardia
Hypotension*
Arrhythmias†

Respiratory System
Bronchospasm
Pulmonary edema
Increased mucous production
Dyspnea**
Respiratory collapse†

Gastrointestinal System
Nausea
Vomiting
Diarrhea
Increased salivation

Integumentary System
Increased perspiration

*Anticholinergic agonists only
**Cholinesterase inhibitors only
†Life threatening.

FIGURE 64–3   Common ocular and systemic physiologic responses to cholinergic agonists and cholinesterase inhibitors.

TABLE 64–1
Cholinergic Agonists and Cholinesterase Inhibitors

Drug Name	Dosage and Route of Administration	Nursing Considerations
CHOLINERGIC AGONISTS **CARBACHOL** (Miostat, Isopto, Carbachol) HOW SUPPLIED Miostat: 0.01% solution Isopto Carbachol: 0.75%–3% solution	*Glaucoma* *Adults or Elderly* 1–2 gtt up to four times/d ***Pupillary Miosis During Ophthalmic Surgery*** *Adults or Elderly* Up to 0.5 ml into anterior chamber before or after securing sutures	***Assess*** Ask whether client is sensitive to carbachol or any of its components. Take baseline pulse and blood pressure. Assess appearance of the eye and client's perception of vision. Inquire about other conditions. Drug must be used with caution in clients with asthma, cardiac failure, peptic ulcer disease, Parkinson's disease, and hyperthyroidism. Ask if client is pregnant; carbachol is Pregnancy Category C drug. ***Implement*** Check solution; do not use if discolored. Have client lie down, tilt head back, and look up. Instill drug in pouch of lower lid without touching tip of applicator to any surface. Apply gentle pressure to inside corner of the eye for 1–2 min and have client keep eye open without blinking for at least 30 sec. Blot excess solution with tissue and wash hands. Do not rinse dropper. Instruct client not to close eyes tightly or blink more than necessary. Tell client not to drive for several hours and to avoid night driving or performing dangerous tasks in poor light. Teach that drug use may be necessary for rest of life and that client should remain under care of primary care provider. ***Monitor*** Observe for systemic reaction (e.g., sweating, flushing, increased salivation). Check client's blood pressure, pulse, and respiration. ***Evaluate*** Observe for therapeutic response.
Acetylcholine Chloride (Miochol) HOW SUPPLIED Powder to reconstitute for solution	***Pupillary Miosis During Ophthalmic Surgery*** See package insert	***Implement*** Drug is not indicated for diagnostic procedures and treatment of glaucoma because of its short duration of action. Drug is not applied topically to the eye (Drug is applied directly to the exposed iris during surgery.)
Pilocarpine Hydrochloride (Isopto-Carpine, Pilocar, Ocusert-20) HOW SUPPLIED 1%–6% concentration: in combination with 1% epinephrine bitartrate; 2% concentration in combination with physostigmine Ocusert Wafers: sustained system lasting approximately 7 d Pilopine HS Gel: 4%, ½ in (1.25 cm) ribbon instilled on conjunctiva cul-de-sac hs	*Glaucoma* SOLUTION *Adults and Elderly* 1–2 gtt up to six times/d OCUSERT Initially insert 20-μg system (releases 20 μg/h7d); may increase to 40-μg system *Xeroma* *Adults* Initial dose: 5 mg tid; may increase to 10 mg tid	***Assess*** See carbachol. Use is contraindicated in clients with cataracts because the miotic and spasmatic effects greatly reduce vision and may speed the development of cataracts. Drug is generally not used in individuals <40 y old because of blurring of vision caused by accommodative spasm and miosis. Drug usually is not used in clients with asthma. Drug use is not indicated in clients with history of poor administration compliance because at least 4 gtt daily are required.

Table continued on following page.

TABLE 64–1 *Continued*
Cholinergic Agonists and Cholinesterase Inhibitors

Drug Name	Dosage and Route of Administration	Nursing Considerations
Pilocarpine Hydrochloride Continued		**Implement** See carbachol for drop instillation. If drops and gel are both prescribed, use drops, wait 5 min, then use gel. Apply gel as a ribbon in the lower conjunctival sac at bedtime. Place Ocusert in lower conjunctival sac at bedtime. Move to upper conjunctival sac by gentle pressure through closed lids while client rolls eyes. Do not move over colored part of eye. Advise the client at start of therapy that ocular and systemic effects may disappear or become tolerable after 7–10 d.
CHOLINESTERASE INHIBITORS: REVERSIBLE DEMECARIUM BROMIDE (Humorsol) HOW SUPPLIED 0.125%, 0.25% solution	**Primary and Secondary Open-Angle Glaucoma** 1–2 gtt bid	**Implement** Apply pressure to puncta for at least 1 min after application. Wash hands immediately after instillation to prevent absorption through the skin and accidental oral ingestion. Measure IOP hourly for 3–4 h after first instillation because transient paradoxical increase in IOP can occur. Advise client to report redness or irritation of conjunctivae.
Physostigmine Sulfate (Eserine Sulfate Ointment, Isopto-Eserine Solution) HOW SUPPLIED 0.25%, 0.5% solution 0.25% ointment	**Primary and Secondary Glaucoma** 1–3 gtt tid or ¼-in strip to lid margins one to three times/d	**Implement** Apply pressure to puncta after instillation of drops to decrease systemic effects. Advise client to contact primary care provider if conjunctival redness or irritation occurs. Solutions are generally stable, effective, and safe for 1 y. Discard if solution turns pink.
CHOLINESTERASE INHIBITORS: IRREVERSIBLE ECHOTHIOPHATE IODIDE (Phospholine Iodide) HOW SUPPLIED 0.03%, 0.25% solution	**Primary and Secondary Glaucoma** 1 gtt daily	**Implement** Apply pressure to puncta for at least 1 min after application. Clients receiving anticholinesterase drug treatment for myasthenia gravis or who have been exposed to insecticides or fertilizers containing organophosphate may experience systemic effects of anticholinesterase. Do not use in clients who will have surgery while under succinylcholine-type anesthesia within several weeks.
Diisopropyl Phosphorofluoridate (DFP, Isoflurophate, Floropryl Ointment) HOW SUPPLIED DFP ointment: 0.025%	**Primary Open-Angle Glaucoma** ¼-in strip to lid margin q8-12h	**Implement** When reversible cholinesterase inhibitors have been used previously, they may antagonize effects of DFP.

Undesired Clinical Responses A frequent side effect of carbachol is difficulty in dark adaptation. In addition, the client may experience headaches and decreased visual acuity.

Contraindications and Precautions Carbachol use is contraindicated in a client with any condition in which miosis is undesirable (e.g., acute iritis, some forms of secondary glaucoma). The drug should be used with caution in clients with corneal abrasions, bronchial asthma, spastic gastrointestinal (GI) conditions, peptic ulcer disease, urinary tract obstruction, hypotension, bradycardia, epilepsy, or hyperthyroidism.[8]

Drug-Drug Interactions Carbachol may be ineffective after flurbiprofen use.

Life-Span Considerations Carbachol is classified as a Pregnancy Category C drug.

Specific Drug-Related Nursing Considerations When possible, administer cholinergic agonists at bedtime to decrease blurring of vision. Instruct the client to remove soft contact lens before instilling a miotic.

Miscellaneous Drugs in Category

Information on other direct-acting cholinergic agonists is summarized in Table 64–1.

INDIRECT-ACTING DRUG: CHOLINESTERASE INHIBITORS

Cholinesterase inhibitors are subclassified into two groups, depending on whether their action is reversible or irreversible. Both groups mimic the effects of parasympathetic nerve stimulation by inhibiting cholinesterase and causing accumulation of acetylcholine, which results in miosis. Figure 64–3 illustrates common ocular and systemic physiologic responses to cholinesterase inhibitors.

Reversible inhibitors halt activity of cholinesterase. These drugs halt the activity of the enzyme for varying time periods (i.e., 12 to 36 hours). Then the enzyme is hydrolyzed and regenerated. **Demecarium** (Humorsol) is an example of a reversible inhibitor.

Irreversible inhibitors form a covalent bond at the site of the enzyme so that the inactivation of the cholinesterase is irreversible. The effect of irreversible inhibitors may last several days or weeks. **Echothiophate iodide** (Phospholine Iodide) is an example of an irreversible cholinesterase inhibitor. Information on indirect-acting cholinesterase inhibitors is summarized in Table 64–1.

🌱 NURSING RESEARCH

Gurwitz, J. H., Glynn, R. J., Monane, M., Everitt, D. E., Avorn, J., et al (1993). Treatment for glaucoma: Adherence by the elderly. *American Journal of Public Health, 83,* 711–716.

The purpose of the study was to examine the compliance of 2440 elderly clients with a new topical therapy for glaucoma. Of the 2440 clients, 569 did not adhere to therapy. Factors associated with nonadherence included the requirement of more than two administrations per day and use of several other medications. Results showed that clients who received multiple glaucoma medications from the beginning were more adherent than those who began with one agent. Age and sex were not significant factors. The study concluded that substantial nonadherence with therapy was common in these elderly clients receiving topical glaucoma therapy.

STUDENT ACTIVITIES

- From charts of 10 elderly clients receiving glaucoma therapy, list the number of times a glaucoma drug will be administered. List concurrent medications and the number of times each will be administered per day.
- Make a chart of one client's day, showing time and dose of each drug that will be taken. 🌿

β-Adrenergic Blocking Drugs

β-Adrenergic blocking drugs, which are used widely to treat other systemic disorders, are used in ophthalmology to inhibit the action of catecholamines and other sympathomimetic agents at β_2-receptor sites. The pharmacologic treatment of all types of glaucoma has been influenced greatly by topically administered β-blockers. Both normal and glaucomatous eyes respond to β-blocker systemic or topical ocular drug administration with a decrease in IOP. The decreased IOP results from inhibition of aqueous humor formation.[6]

β-ADRENERGIC BLOCKING DRUG PROTOTYPE

TIMOLOL MALEATE

Timolol maleate (Timoptic), which was approved by the Food and Drug Administration (FDA) in 1978 as an ophthalmic preparation, has become the standard for all ophthalmic β-blockers.

Pharmacotherapeutics Timolol ophthalmic solution lowers IOP. It is used in the treatment of chronic open-angle glaucoma, aphakic glaucoma, and some secondary glaucomas.

Pharmacokinetics Onset of reduction in IOP occurs within $\frac{1}{2}$ hour of drop administration of timolol. The maximal effect usually occurs in 1 to 2 hours, and significant lowering of IOP is maintained for as long as 24 hours.[10]

Pharmacodynamics Timolol is a β_1- and β_2-adrenergic blocking agent. It does not have significant systemic sympathomimetic activity. The precise mechanism of ocular hypotensive action has not clearly been established. It is probably due to reduced aqueous formation.[10]

Pharmaceutics For ocular use, timolol is available in 0.25% and 0.5% solutions. Table 64–2 provides additional information on dosage, dosage forms, and routes of administration. An oral tablet, used to treat hypertension, is also available.

Undesired Clinical Responses Although timolol ophthalmic solution is usually well tolerated, some undesired responses have been reported, including headache, asthenia, and chest pain. Other adverse reactions include hypotension, bradycardia, arrhythmia, dizziness, bronchospasm, ocular irritation, conjunctivitis, keratitis, decreased corneal sensitivity, and visual disturbances. Table 64–3 summarizes undesired responses associated with timolol.

Contraindications and Precautions Timolol use is contraindicated in clients with, or with a history of, bronchial asthma, severe chronic obstructive pulmonary disease (COPD), sinus bradycardia, second- and third-degree atrioventricular block, or overt cardiac failure. The drug should be used with caution in clients receiving β-blockers orally.[10] (See Table 64–3.)

Drug-Drug Interactions Close observation of the client is needed when administering timolol concurrently with catecholamine-depleting drugs such as reserpine.

Life-span Considerations Timolol is classified as a Pregnancy Category C drug.

Specific Drug-related Nursing Considerations Store the timolol ophthalmic solution at room temperature. Assess baseline blood pressure and pulse rate since timolol can affect these parameters. Continue to monitor pulse and blood pressure regularly. Teach client how to instill drops correctly and how to take his or her radial pulse.

TABLE 64–2
β-Adrenergic Blocking Drugs

Drug Name	Dosage and Route of Administration
TIMOLOL MALEATE (Timoptic) HOW SUPPLIED 0.25%, 0.5% solution	***Primary Open-Angle Glaucoma, Aphakic Glaucoma, Ocular Hypertension, Closed-Angle Glaucoma, Secondary Glaucoma, Congenital Glaucoma*** 1 gtt bid
Levobunolol (Betagan) HOW SUPPLIED 0.5% solution	1 gtt daily or bid
Betaxolol Hydrochloride (Betoptic) HOW SUPPLIED 0.5% solution	1 gtt bid
Carteolol (Ocupress) HOW SUPPLIED 1% solution	***Open-Angle Glaucoma, Ocular Hypertension*** 1 gtt bid
Metipranolol (OptiPranolol) HOW SUPPLIED 0.3% solution	1 gtt bid

TABLE 64–3
β-Adrenergic Blocking Drugs: Undesired Clinical Responses, Contraindications, and Nursing Considerations

Drug Name	Undesired Clinical Responses	Contraindications	Nursing Considerations
TIMOLOL MALEATE (Timoptic, Blocadren)	***Ocular Responses*** Minimal responses compared to those of pilocarpine and epinephrine Orbital pain, photophobia, blurred vision, itching, diplopia, allergic conjunctivitis, corneal anesthesia, blepharoptosis (ocular myasthenia gravis), dry eyes, decreased tear flow, and superficial keratitis ***Systemic Responses*** Headache, mental depression, hypotension, bradycardia, and heart block (in clients receiving the drug topically and orally); asthmatic attacks; lightheadedness; memory loss; decreased libido and impotence; alopecia; skin rash; vomiting; diarrhea; cramps; nausea	May be contraindicated in high-risk clients with dyspnea, asthma, chronic bronchitis, and cardiovascular disease Contraindicated in individuals with congenital glaucoma, narrow angles, labile diabetes, chronic obstructive lung disease (COPD), heart block	Side effects are most noticeable during the first 1–2 wk of treatment; they then diminish to a tolerable level. Because there is no pupillary constriction, timolol is very useful for treatment of clients with cataracts. Drug can be used in combination with an oral β-blocker to achieve desired systemic effects and to control IOP. Side effects are not as predictable as they are with pilocarpine and other antiglaucoma drugs. Drug can produce side effects unlike those common to other antiglaucoma drugs. Monitor clients with decreased tear film closely. Instruct client to occlude the puncta after administration to discourage serious side effects of systemic absorption.

TABLE 64–3 *Continued*

β-*Adrenergic Blocking Drugs: Undesired Clinical Responses, Contraindications, and Nursing Considerations*

Drug Name	Undesired Clinical Responses	Contraindications	Nursing Considerations
Levobunolol (Betagan)	**Ocular Responses** Transient ocular stinging and burning; occasional mild reduction in visual acuity; change in pupil size; blepharitis **Systemic Responses** Similar to those with timolol	Same as for timolol Used with caution in diabetic clients because can mask symptoms of hypoglycemia	Administration in one eye results in contralateral pressure reduction in the untreated eye. Other implications for timolol apply to levobunolol. Clients who have been using β-blocking agents can experience severe hypotension during anesthesia. Instruct client to apply pressure to puncta after administration.
Betaxolol Hydrochloride (Betopic)	**Ocular Responses** Mild to moderate burning or stinging **Systemic Responses** Severe depression; disorientation; vertigo; rhinitis; dysuria; prolonged prothrombin time; bradycardia; sinus arrest	Same as for timolol and levobunolol but is safer for use in clients with COPD	Approximately 2 wk of therapy are required for maximal ocular effect. Pulmonary function tests can be done to identify high-risk clients for systemic β-blocker administration when an ocular β-blocker is being used to control IOP.
Carteolol (Cartrol)	**Ocular Responses** Conjunctival hyperemia; blepharoconjunctivitis; edema; droopy upper eyelid; corneal staining; blurred vision **Systemic Responses** Skin rash; hives; itching; change in taste; coughing, wheezing, dyspnea; dizziness, faintness; headache; insomnia; irregular slow, pounding heartbeat; rhinitis; sinusitis; unusual tiredness; weakness	Use contraindicated in clients with history of bronchial asthma, severe COPD, overt cardiac failure, second- or third-degree atrioventricular block, sinus bradycardia, previous allergic reaction to ophthalmic β-blocker Used with caution in clients with bronchitis, emphysema, other pulmonary impairments, congestive heart failure, diabetes mellitus, hyperthyroidism, myasthenia gravis	Same as for timolol
Metipranolol (OptiPranolol)	**Ocular Responses** Blepharitis, conjunctivitis, dermatitis of eyelid, edema, visual disturbances (e.g., blurred vision), stinging of the eye, eye irritation **Systemic Responses** Allergic reaction, anxiety, nervousness, arthritis, myalgia, confusion, coughing, wheezing, dyspnea, dizziness, faintness, drowsiness, epistaxis, headache, increased blood pressure, irregular heartbeat, rhinitis, sinusitis, unusual tiredness or weakness	Same as for carteolol	Same as for timolol

MISCELLANEOUS DRUGS IN CATEGORY

Along with timolol, other topical β-blocking drugs are levobunolol, betaxolol, carteolol, and metipranolol. Basically these drugs have pharmacodynamic and pharmacotherapeutic properties similar to those of timolol. Tables 64–2 and 64–3 summarize information on these β-adrenergic blocking drugs.

Sympathomimetic Mydriatics

Sympathomimetic mydriatics are also known as *adrenergics* because they induce physiologic responses similar to those of the sympathetic nervous system. Epinephrine, epinephrine preparations, and dipivefrin are the major drugs in this group.

Epinephrine is an adrenergic agonist that acts at α-adrenergic and β-adrenergic receptors. The basic pharmacology of the drug is discussed in Chapter 27. Discussion in this chapter is limited to its use as an ocular drug. **Dipivefrin** (Propine) is a prodrug form of epinephrine. Dipivefrin penetrates the cornea more readily than epinephrine because of its high lipid solubility. Once in the eye, the drug is converted to its active form—epinephrine—by ocular enzymes.[10–12]

Pharmacotherapeutics Epinephrine is used to treat open-angle glaucoma. Adrenergics are also used to dilate the pupil for examination of the fundus, to vasoconstrict small ocular vessels to prevent hemorrhage, and to act as an ocular decongestant during allergic reactions.

Pharmacodynamics Epinephrine preparations mimic the action of natural norepinephrine or epinephrine. Adrenergic stimulation includes the following ocular effects:
- Mydriasis due to contraction of the iridic dilator muscle
- Ciliary muscle relaxation
- Increased outflow of aqueous humor
- Vasoconstriction of conjunctival blood vessels

Pharmaceutics Ophthalmic preparations of epinephrine contain a salt, either epinephrine borate (Epinal, Eppy/N) or epinephrine hydrochloride (Epifrin, Glaucon). These preparations and dipivefrin are available in ophthalmic solutions. Table 64–4 summarizes additional information on sympathomimetic mydriatics.

Undesired clinical responses Headache, brow ache, blurred vision, and ocular irritation are relatively common with use of epinephrine preparations. Systemic absorption can cause tachycardia and hypertension.

TABLE 64–4
Sympathomimetic Mydriatics

Drug Name	Dosage and Route of Administration	Nursing Considerations
EPINEPHRINE BORATE (Epinal, EpiPen) HOW SUPPLIED Epinal: 0.5%–1% solution EpiPen: 0.5%, 1%, 2% solution	***Primary and Secondary Open-Angle Glaucoma; Some Chronic Closed-Angle Glaucoma in Combination with Miotics; Some Inflammatory Glaucomas*** 1 gtt bid	**Assess** Use epinephrine solutions with caution in clients with cardiac disease or hyperthyroidism or in combination with monoamine oxidase (MAO) inhibitors or tricyclic antidepressants. **Implement** Epinephrine solutions can become unstable because of oxidation from exposure to the atmosphere or to light. Instruct clients to close cap of the bottle securely after administration and to discard solutions that become discolored or contain a precipitate. Do not use epinephrine solutions when clients are wearing soft contact lenses because the solution discolors the lenses. **Monitor** Undesired clinical responses follow: Ocular: stinging and lacrimation, conjunctival hyperemia, staining of contact lenses, eye ache. Systemic: severe headache, palpitations, tachycardia, premature ventricular contractions, hypertensive crisis, anxiety.
Epinephrine Hydrochloride (Epifrin, Glaucon) HOW SUPPLIED 0.25%–2% solution	1 gtt bid	See epinephrine borate.
Epinephrine Bitartrate (Epitrate) HOW SUPPLIED 2% solution	1 gtt bid	See epinephrine borate.

TABLE *64–4 Continued*
Sympathomimetic Mydriatics

Drug Name	Dosage and Route of Administration	Nursing Considerations
Dipivefrin (Propine) HOW SUPPLIED 0.1% solution	***Alternative Treatment for Glaucoma When Client Does Not Tolerate Epinephrine Preparations*** 1 gtt bid	**Implement** Drug may be used in clients who wear soft contact lenses without risk of staining. **Monitor** Ocular and systemic side effects are the same as with epinephrine but are less severe and less common.
Phenylephrine Hydrochloride (Neo-Synephrine, AK-Dilate, Mydfrin, Ocr-Phrin) HOW SUPPLIED 2.5%–10% solutions OTC products: 0.12% solution as ocular decongestant	***Dilation of Eye for Examination; Improvement of Vision in Individuals With Lens Opacities; Reduction of Redness of Eye by Vasoconstriction*** Dosage dependent on intended use (i.e., 1–2 gtt of 2.5% solution instilled for routine fundal examination)	**Assess** Use with caution in clients taking MAO inhibitors, tricyclic antidepressants, reserpine, guanethidine, and methyldopa. Avoid use in clients with shallow or narrow anterior angles. Concurrent use is not recommended in clients taking atropine preparations because tachycardia and hypertension can occur. **Implement** Normally phenylephrine solutions are clear and colorless to slightly yellow. Like epinephrine, these solutions are subject to changes from oxidation that may cause them to darken in color or form a precipitate. Instruct clients to follow the manufacturer's directions for expiration date and storage. These solutions can lose their action without visible change in appearance. **Monitor** Only 2.5% solution is recommended for routine use, especially for infants and the elderly. Risks are greatly increased with use of 10% solution. Undesired clinical responses follow: Ocular: lacrimation, transient pain, keratitis, pigmented iridic floaters in the aqueous humor, rebound miosis (especially in individuals >50 y old). Systemic: headache, hypertension, subarachnoid hemorrhage, ventricular arrhythmia, tachycardia, blanching or skin.
Hydroxyamphetamine Hydrobromide (Paredrine) HOW SUPPLIED 1% solution	***Mydriatic for Ocular Examination*** 1–2 gtt instilled in conjunctival sac: produces pupil dilation for 2–3 h	**Assess** Drug is safe for use in eyes with shallow or narrow anterior chambers. Use is contraindicated in clients with narrow-angle glaucoma. **Monitor** Undesired clinical responses follow: Ocular—little or no irritation; can cause blurred vision, lacrimation, and photophobia. Systemic—rare hypertension. NOTE: Lack of reported systemic effects from ocular administration may be due to limited usage of this drug.

Anticholinergic Mydriatics

Anticholinergic mydriatics, also commonly known as *cycloplegics*, block the actions of parasympathetic innervation. When present, they also block the actions of cholinergic drugs on the muscles and vasculature of the ciliary body and iris.[5] Paralysis of the ciliary muscle and relaxation of the circular muscle of the iris result in pupil dilation (mydriasis) and loss of accommodation **(cycloplegia).** Whereas the cycloplegic drug dilates the pupil and paralyzes accommodation, a mydriatic drug dilates the pupil without affecting accommodation. Cycloplegic drugs listed in order of potency are **atropine, scopolamine, homatropine, cyclopentolate,** and **tropicamide.**[5] Atropine and scopolamine are discussed in Chapter 26 with other muscarinic antagonists; only ocular considerations are discussed in this chapter.

Pharmacotherpeutics Cycloplegics are used to dilate the pupil for ocular examination, for measuring refraction, and for treatment of anterior eye disorders such as corneal ulceration, anterior uveitis, and keratitis. They are also used to facilitate ocular surgery and to reduce postoperative complications.

Pharmacodynamics Cycloplegics block the muscarinic receptors that promote contraction of the iridic sphincter.

Pharmaceutics Cycloplegics are available in a variety of ophthalmic solutions. Table 64–5 summarizes additional information on dosage forms, dosages, and routes of administration.

Undesired clinical responses Side effects, including toxic reactions, after ocular instillation of cycloplegics can occur as a result of systemic absorption through the nasolacrimal ducts, the episcleral blood vessels, and the GI mucosa. Children and the elderly are particularly vulnerable to side effects and toxicity. Ocular responses include blurred vision, photophobia, and precipitation of angle-closure glaucoma. Systemic effects include dry mouth, constipation, fever, tachycardia, and central nervous system effects.

CONCEPT REVIEW

Ocular drugs that affect the autonomic nervous system alter pupil size, IOP, and accommodation.

Cholinergic agonists or miotics act directly or indirectly to dilate the pupil; their action may be reversible or irreversible. β-Adrenergic blocking drugs are used primarily to treat glaucoma.

Sympathomimetic mydriatics mimic the action of norepinephrine or epinephrine. They cause mydriasis, ciliary muscle relaxation, increased outflow of aqueous humor, and vasoconstriction of conjunctival blood vessels. These drugs are used to dilate the pupil during fundal examination, to reduce IOP in clients with glaucoma, to vasoconstrict small ocular vessels, and to act as a decongestant during allergic reactions.

Anticholinergic mydriatics, or cycloplegics, relax the circular muscle of the iris and paralyze the ciliary muscle, causing loss of accommodation. Cycloplegics are used to dilate the pupil for ocular examination, to measure refraction, and to treat anterior eye disorders.

DIURETICS

Two categories of drugs used in ophthalmology for their diuretic effect are carbonic anhydrase inhibitors and hyperosmotic agents. Both categories are ocular hypotensives used to lower IOP in clients with glaucoma and used preoperatively and postoperatively for eye surgery.

Carbonic Anhydrase Inhibitors

Carbonic anhydrase inhibitors are sulfonamide derivatives. Three carbonic anhydrase inhibitors are available to treat glaucoma: acetazolamide, dichlorphenamide, and methazolamide. Acetazolamide is prescribed most frequently.

CARBONIC ANHYDRASE INHIBITORS PROTOTYPE
ACETAZOLAMIDE

Because of acetazolamide's diverse actions, it is used for other purposes than as an ocular diuretic. In Chapter 36 acetazolamide (Diamox) is presented as the prototype drug for carbonic anhydrase inhibitors; thus in this chapter only its role in the treatment of ocular disorders is considered.

Pharmacotherapeutics Acetazolamide is used to treat chronic simple glaucoma, secondary glaucoma, and acute angle-closure glaucoma in the preoperative state.

Pharmacokinetics Most tissues in the body contain carbonic anhydrase in greater quantities than are physiologically necessary. Approximately 99% of carbonic activity must be inhibited to reduce aqueous formation significantly. Onset of action occurs in 60 to 90 minutes with tablets; the peak occurs within 2 to 4 hours; and duration of action is 8 to 12 hours. With sustained-release capsules, onset of action occurs in 2 hours, and peak action occurs in 8 to 18 hours. The duration of action with sustained-release capsules is 18 to 24 hours.[8]

Pharmacodynamics Acetazolamide is an enzyme inhibitor that acts specifically on carbonic anhydrase, the enzyme that catalyzes the reversible action involving the hydration of CO_2 and dehydration of carbonic acid. In the eye this inhibitory action decreases the secretion of aqueous humor and results in a drop in IOP.[10]

Pharmaceutics Acetazolamide is available in tablets and sustained-release capsules for oral administration. It is available in parenteral solutions for intramuscular and intravenous administration. Table 64–6 summarizes information on dosage forms, dosages, and routes of administration.

Undesired Clinical Responses Undesired clinical responses to this drug include paresthesias, hearing dysfunction, tinnitus, anorexia, taste alteration, and GI disturbance. Transient myopia has also been reported.[10]

Contraindications and Precautions Acetazolamide use is contraindicated in clients with depressed sodium or

TABLE 64–5
Anticholinergic Mydriatics (Cycloplegics)

Drug Name	Dosage and Route of Administration	Nursing Considerations
Atropine Sulfate (Atropisol, Isopto-Atropine, Atropine Care Ophthalmic, Atropine Sulfate S.O.P.) HOW SUPPLIED Solutions: Atropisol—0.5%, 1%, 2%; Isopto-Atropine—0.5%, 1%, 3%; Atropine Care Ophthalmic—1% Ointments: Atropine Sulfate Ophthalmic—1%; Atropine Sulfate S.O.P.—0.5%, 1%	**Mydriatic Examination** 1 gtt 15–30 min before examination **Cycloplegic Refraction** SOLUTION *Adults and Elderly* 1 gtt 1% solution for 1–3 d and 1 h before procedure *Children* 1–2 gtt 0.5% solution bid for 1–3 d before and 1 h before procedure OINTMENT *Adults and Elderly* 0.3–0.5 cm one to three times/d for 1–3 d before procedure *Children* 0.3 cm tid for 1–3 d before procedure **Inflammatory Disorders** *Adults and Elderly* 1–2 gtt of 0.5% to 1% solution up to three to four times/d *Children* 1–2 gtt 0.5% solution up to three to four times/d	**Assess** Atropine is not recommended for cycloplegic refraction in adults because of visual impairment caused by long-term paralysis of accommodation muscles (up to 7–10 d). **Implement** Atropine is the most potent mydriatic and cycloplegic currently available. Apply digital pressure to puncta after administration to discourage systemic absorption via lacrimal drainage ducts. Atropine and other anticholinergic drugs can induce acute closed-angle glaucoma when used in client with narrow anterior angles. Strength of solution and dosage used depend on the color of the iris.
Homatropine Hydrobromide (Homatropine HBr, Isopto Homatropine, AK-Homatropine) HOW SUPPLIED Solution: 2%, 5%	**Treatment of Iridocyclitis and as Alternative to Treatment With Atropine** Usual dose: 1 gtt bid **Eye Examination** 1–2 gtt 30 min before examination	**Implement** This is not a drug of choice for ocular examination because of the prolonged mydriasis and weak cycloplegic action. Color of eye affects strength of drug needed. Apply pressure over puncta after instillation (see Fig. 64-2).
Scopolamine Hydrobromide (Isopto Hyoscine) HOW SUPPLIED Solution: 0.25%	**Alternative to Atropine** Used only in clients with sensitivity to that drug **Eye Examination** 1 gtt 30 min before examination **Inflammation** 1 gtt one to four times/d	**Implement** Side effects are similar to those of atropine, but CNS toxicity is also possible. Apply pressure over puncta after instillation (see Fig. 64–2).
Cyclopentolate Hydrochloride (Cyclogyl, AK-Pentolate) HOW SUPPLIED Solution: 0.5%, 1%, 2%	**Cycloplegic Agent for Refractive Procedures** *All Ages* 1 gtt at 15-min intervals 30 min before examination **Iridocyclitis** 1 gtt one to three times/d	**Implement** Drug has cycloplegic effect equal to that of atropine and greater than that of homatropine. Pupils dilated by cyclopentolate do not constrict when exposed to intense light. Color of iris influences strength of drug needed.
Tropicamide (Mydriacyl Ophthalmic, Tropicacyl) HOW SUPPLIED Solution: 0.5%, 1%	**Mydriasis Before Ocular Examination** 1 gtt one to two times over a 10- to 15-min period, depending on purpose	**Implement** Tropicamide is drug of choice for achieving mydriasis before ocular examination. Drug has fast onset, with a stronger concentration of drug reaching receptor sites than with other drugs in category. Short duration of action eliminates long-term visual impairment from mydriasis. Color of iris does not influence strength of drug. Advise client to wear dark glasses while sensitive to light.

TABLE 64-6
Drugs Used as Ocular Diuretics

Drug Name	Dosage and Route of Administration	Onset of Action	Peak Action	Duration of Action	Desired Action and Clinical Uses
CARBONIC ANHYDRASE INHIBITORS					
ACETAZOLAMIDE (Diamox)	Tablets: 125, 250 mg Usual dose: 250 mg PO q6h	½–1 h	2–4 h	4–6 h	Most commonly used carbonic anhydrase inhibitor for all types of glaucoma to reduce IOP; not usually used as initial treatment of glaucoma but is added to treatment regimen after other topical drugs (e.g., β-blockers, sympathomimetics, cholinergics) alone or in combination do not control IOP
	Capsule (sustained release): 500 mg Usual dose: 500 mg bid	1–2 h	8–12 h	10–18 h	
	Vial: 500 mg Usual dose: 500 mg IV Children's dose: 5–10 mg/kg q4-6h	1 min	20–30 min	4 h	
Methazolamide (Neptazane)	Tablets: 25, 50 mg Usual adult dose: 25–100 mg tid PO	1 h	7–8 h	10–14 h	Same as acetazolamide; because it alters acid-base balance less, is safer to use with clients with chronic obstructive pulmonary disease or renal calculi
Dichlorphenamide (Daranide)	Tablets: 50 mg Usual adult dose: 25–100 mg tid PO	½ h	2–4 h	6–12 h	A very strong carbonic anhydrase inhibitor mainly used in treatment of open-angle glaucoma and some secondary glaucomas; usually added to treatment program when other antiglaucoma drugs alone or in combination do not control IOP
Dorzolamide (TruSopt)	Ophthalmic solution: 1 gtt tid	—	—	—	Used in clients with ocular hypertension or open-angle glaucoma; reduces IOP

HYPEROSMOTIC AGENTS

Topically Administered

Drug	Dosage	Onset	Peak	Duration	Remarks
Glycerin (Ophthalgan)	1–2 gtt	1–2 min	—	Transient	Mainly for diagnostic purposes before ophthalmoscopic and fundoscopic examination for eyes with acute closed-angle glaucoma or bullous keratopathy
Sodium chloride					
Adsorbonac Solution: 2%, 5%	1–2 gtt q3–4h	—	—	3–4 h	Useful for corneal dehydration when epithelium is intact
Muro 128 Solution	Same as above	—	—	Same as above	Same as above
Muro 128 Ointment	Apply hs	—	—	Overnight	Same as above
AK-NACl Ointment	Same as above	—	—	Same as above	Same as above

Systemically Administered

Drug	Dosage	Onset	Peak	Duration	Remarks
Glycerin Osmoglyn: 50% lime-flavored solution	2–3 ml/kg or 4–6 oz per client; serve over ice with a straw 1–1½ h preoperatively or q8–10 h prn	10–30 min	—	4–5 h	For short-term reduction of IOP preoperatively and postoperatively
Glyrol: 75% solution	1–2 ml/kg or 3–5 oz per client; can flavor with orange juice and serve over ice	Same as above	—	Same as above	Same as above
Mannitol (Osmitrol 20% solution) Solution should be warm (38°–39° C) to dissolve any crystals	2.5–10 ml/kg IV; give over 45–60 min in IV solution	20–30 min	1 h	4–10 h	Hyperosmotic agent of choice for IV administration; used to reduce IOP preoperatively and to treat open-angle glaucoma and acute closed-angle glaucoma; can be stored without deterioration
Urea (Ureaphil 30% IV solution; Urevert 30% IV solution) Both are administered in 10% invert sugar solution to prevent hemolysis of red blood cells	2–7 ml/kg administer over 1–2½ h	30–45 min	1 h	5–6 h	Rarely used currently to reduce IOP; solution must be freshly prepared because drug decomposes on standing
Isosorbide (Ismotic 45% solution in vanilla-mint–flavored solution)	1.5 g/kg; administer 100 g/220 ml po	Approximately 30 min	1–1½ h	5–6 h	For short-term reduction of IOP

potassium serum levels. It is also contraindicated in clients with hepatic and renal disease, suprarenal gland failure, and hyperchloremic acidosis.

Drug-Drug and Drug-Environment Interactions Store tablets and capsules at room temperature. Acetazolamide may increase excretion of lithium, and it may decrease excretion of quinidine, procainamide, and methenamine.[13]

Life-span Considerations Acetazolamide is classified as a Pregnancy Category D drug. Safety and effectiveness in children have not been established.

Specific Drug-Related Nursing Considerations When oral liquid is needed, crush the acetazolamide tablets and mix them with a highly flavored carbohydrate syrup (e.g., cherry, chocolate, raspberry). Tablets may also be softened with hot water and added to honey or syrup. Do not crush or break sustained-release capsules.[8]

MISCELLANEOUS DRUGS IN CATEGORY

Additional drugs in this category include methazolamide and dichlorphenamide. A relative new carbonic anhydrase inhibitor, dorzolamide hydrochloride, is also available.

Hyperosmotic Drugs

Hyperosmotic drugs make the plasma hypertonic to intraocular fluid; this draws fluid from the corneal epithelium to the tear film and eliminates it from the eye by the usual drainage mechanism. Hyperosmotic drugs serve as short-term ocular hypotensives. They are used to treat glaucoma and corneal edema and to manage corneoscleral lacerations. In addition, they are administered preoperatively and postoperatively for surgery to repair a detached retina, cataract extraction, and keratoplasty.

Effects of these drugs can be achieved from topical or systemic administration. Mannitol, urea, glycerin, and isosorbide are examples of hyperosmotic drugs used to treat ocular conditions. Osmotic diuretics are discussed in more detail in Chapter 36. In addition, Table 64–6 summarizes information on dosage forms, dosages, and routes of administration.

CONCEPT REVIEW

Diuretics used in ophthalmology are carbonic anhydrase inhibitors and hyperosmotic drugs. These drugs lower IOP in clients with glaucoma and are used preoperatively and postoperatively for eye surgery.

Carbonic anhydrase inhibitors decrease aqueous humor production by the ciliary body, thus lowering IOP.

Hyperosmotic drugs produce hypertonic plasma, which draws fluid from the corneal epithelium to the tear film, from which it is eliminated by the usual drainage mechanism of the eye.

ANTIINFECTIVE DRUGS

When an ocular infection exists, the anatomic part of the eye affected determines the route of administration of the drug. The most common route is topical instillation. Other routes are oral, subconjunctival injection, and intravitreal injection.

Three categories of microorganisms cause eye infections: bacteria, viruses, and fungi. Microorganisms within each category have unique physical structures and metabolism. A culture and sensitivity of ocular fluid, exudate, or tissue can be done to identify specific microorganisms, but often treatment is initiated before results are known.

Drugs used to treat ocular infections are available as drops or ointment. Solutions are commonly used for topical instillation in adults because ointments cause visual blurring. However, ointments may be preferred for topical instillation in infants and children because of the prolonged contact time of the drug to the eye and the resistance of ointments to tear washout.

Topically administered drugs enter the eye primarily through the cornea. Penetration of the drug depends on the chemical properties of the drug, drug concentration, frequency of administration, and the presence or absence of inflammation. Drugs administered by injection into the subconjunctival space enter the eye by direct penetration through the cornea and sclera and through leakage into the precorneal tear film. High drug concentrations are achieved from this method, but the drugs have a short duration of action, approximately 3 to 6 hours.

Intravitreal injection is the administration of a drug by injection into the vitreous humor. It is used to treat conditions such as endophthalmitis. Water-soluble drugs diffuse within the aqueous and exit the eye by the trabecular meshwork. The duration of action varies from 10 to 48 hours according to the drug used.

Antibacterial drugs are often administered systemically and topically to treat ocular infections. Systemic antibacterial drugs are used to treat eye disorders such as corneal ulcers, blepharitis, endophthalmitis, trachoma, and retinitis due to acquired immunodeficiency syndrome (AIDS). (Systemic antibacterial drugs are discussed in Chapter 55.) Some of the common topical antibacterial drugs include bacitracin, cephalosporin, chloramphenicol, and gentamicin. Dosage form, dosage, desired action, and undesired clinical responses for common topical antibacterial drugs are summarized in Table 64–7.

Three standard **antiviral ocular drugs** are idoxuridine, vidarabine, and trifluridine. Newer antiviral drugs have emerged in recent years for treatment of the ocular effects of AIDS. These drugs are used to treat the cytomegalovirus (CMV) that causes retinitis. Zidovudine (Azidothymidine, AZT, Retrovir), which has been approved by the FDA to treat individuals with AIDS, is effective in treating CMV retinitis, human immunodeficiency virus (HIV)-induced iridocyclitis, and anterior uveitis. However, zidovudine is very toxic; its use results in bone marrow hypoplasia, which makes the client vulnerable to systemic bacterial infections. Dosage form, dosage, desired action, and undesired clinical responses for common topical antiviral drugs are summarized in Table 64–7.

Antifungal ocular drugs are used to treat fungal infections such as fungal keratitis and endophthalmitis. These infections frequently occur after an injury or surgery. Fungal corneal ulcers also occur and have increased in frequency in recent years. This increase probably is associated with increased use of cor-

TABLE 64–7
Antiinfective Drugs

Drug Name	Dosage and Route of Administration	Desired Action and Clinical Uses
ANTIBACTERIAL DRUGS *Bacitracin Ointment (500 U/g)* (AK-Tracin, Polysporin)	When indicated, first clean lid margin with warm compresses and lid scrub Apply ½ in of ointment in conjunctival cul-de-sac or place ointment on a sterile cotton-tipped applicator and rub along base of lashes Apply q3-4h according to severity of condition	Antibiotic that penetrates the cornea and conjunctiva after administration Used for superficial infections, especially those caused by staphylococci
Cephalosporin (Cefazolin, cephaloridine, cefoxitin, cefoperazone, ceftazidine solutions)	See package insert	A parent compound that affects bacterial cell wall synthesis, acting as a bactericidal A number of subdrugs have been developed by modifying their chemical structure so that their spectra of activity and clinical uses are similar but vary Used for surgical prophylaxis and varied anterior eye infections
Chloramphenicol (AK-Chlor solution, Chlorofair Solution and Ointment, Chloromycetin Solution and Ointment, Chloroptic Solution and Ointment)	1 gtt q5 min for 1 h then q30-60 min *or* ½ in ointment instilled in cul-de-sac	Bacteriostatic action effective against most gram-positive and gram-negative bacterial infections of anterior eye Must be refrigerated
Erythromycin Ointment (0.5%) (Ocu-Mycin, Ilotycin)	½ in ribbon into conjunctival cul-de-sac instilled one to two times/d, depending on severity of infection	Kills gram-positive bacteria Drug of choice to treat trachoma Erythromycin and tetracycline ointments recommended by the Centers for Disease Control as effective alternatives to silver nitrate for prophylaxis of ophthalmia neonatorum
Gentamicin Solution and Ointment (0.3%) (Gentak, Genoptic, Gentaciden, Gentasul, Garamycin)	Solution: 1–2 gtt q4h Ointment: ¼ in strip to conjunctival cul-de-sac two to three times/d for 7–10 d	An aminoglycoside that kills gram-negative bacteria Used to treat variety of external eye infections such as conjunctivitis Most commonly used for treatment of infected burns Also commonly used as initial treatment of bacterial corneal ulcers
Tobramycin (Tobrex 0.3% Solution and Ointment; Tobradex 0.3% solution and ointment—contains 0.1% dexamethasone)	Solution: 1–2 gtt q4h Ointment: ¼ in strip to cul-de-sac two to three times/d	Tobramycin alone effective in treating superficial infections of the eye (e.g., blepharitis, conjunctivitis, and keratitis) caused by susceptible bacteria May be used in combination with a corticosteroid in some bacterial ocular infections Action is against many gram-negative aerobic bacteria and some gram-positive aerobic bacteria
Tetracycline Suspension and Ointment (Achromycin 1%)	Suspension: 2 gtt two to four times/d Ointment: ½ in strip in cul-de-sac q2h, depending on severity of infection	A broad-spectrum antibiotic usually bacteriostatic in action; may be bacteriocidal in high concentrations or against highly susceptible organisms Active against many gram-negative and gram-positive bacteria and against most *Rickettsia, Chlamydia, Mycoplasma,* and spirochetes Used alone to treat superficial infections of the eye such as blepharitis, conjunctivitis and keratitis May be used topically as an adjunct to oral antiinfective therapy for treatment of trachoma May be used for prophylaxis of gonococcal ophthalmia neonatorum

Table continued on following page.

TABLE 64–7 *Continued*
Antiinfective Drugs

Drug Name	Dosage and Route of Administration	Desired Action and Clinical Uses
Sulfonamides Sulfacetamide sodium ophthalmic solution and ointment 10% solutions: Bleph 10, Sodium Sulamyd 30% solution: Sodium Sulamyd 10% ointment: Cetamide, Bleph-10 S.O.P. Sulfisoxazole Solution and ointment 4% (Gantrisin)	Solution: 1 gtt q2h for severe infections or three to four times/d for chronic conditions Ointment: ½ in strip in cul-de-sac usually hs but can be instilled several times during the day	A broad-spectrum antibiotic effective against gram-negative and gram-positive bacteria and against *Actinomyces, Chlamydia,* plasmodia, and *Toxoplasma* 10% solution: most common preparation used for the treatment of routine bacterial conjunctivitis 30% solution: characterized by burning on instillation Combinations of sulfacetamide and prednisolone used to treat chronic blepharitis Other use: after removal of foreign bodies as prophylaxis against infection
ANTIVIRAL DRUGS *Idoxuridine solution* (Herplex 0.1% solution)	Solution: 1 gtt in cul-de-sac qh during day and q2h at night until improvement seen; then 1 gtt q2h during the day and q4h at night for 3–5 d after corneal healing is complete Ointment: ½ in strip q4h during the day and once hs	Attacks herpes simplex virus (HSV) infection of the cornea (herpes simplex keratitis) Relatively insoluble in water so does not penetrate into or through the cornea Cures approximately 75% of clients with epithelial herpes after 2 wk of treatment with idoxuridine Does not eradicate the virus in the trigeminal ganglion, so herpetic keratitis recurs in some individuals
Vidarabine Ointment (Vira-A 3%)	½ in strip five times/d for 21 d; continue treatment for 3–5 d after corneal healing	Active against HSV, cytomegalovirus (CMV), and varicella-zoster virus (VZV) Primary clinical use: treatment of herpes simplex keratitis Reported as effective as idoxuridine for treatment of HSV keratitis
Trifluridine solution (Viroptic 1%)	1–2 gtt nine times/d for 14 d or until re-epithelialization has occurred; then decrease to 1 gtt q4h during waking hours for 7d Avoid more than 21 d of continuous use because of ocular toxicity	Effective agent in treatment of HSV keratitis Present drug of choice for treatment of HSV keratitis
ANTIFUNGAL DRUGS *Natamycin* (Natacyn 5% solution)	1 gtt into the cul-de-sac q1-2h for the first 3–4d; then may reduce to 1 gtt six to eight times/d Continue treatment for 14–21d or until the infection resolves	Drug of choice for initial treatment of fungal keratitis because of its broad spectrum of activity against fungi Also effective in topical treatment of blepharitis and conjunctivitis
Amphotericin B (Fungizone) 0.10%–0.25% solution is prepared in the pharmacy from the commercial preparation intended for systemic use	1 gtt qh during day and q2-4h at night; can taper dosage over several weeks of therapy Can be injected subconjunctivally but can result in permanent yellowing of the cornea	Effective in treatment of corneal ulcers caused by *Fusarium, Candida, Aspergillus,* and *Alternaria*
Miconazole (Monistat) Diluted parenteral preparation: 1% or 10 mg/ml	1 gtt qh around the clock for several days; then taper to 1 gtt six times/d, depending on clinical response Treatment with drops may extend over 6–8 wk May use subconjunctival and oral administration in combination with topical instillation	A broad-spectrum antifungal drug used to treat corneal infections caused by several fungi

ticosteroids (with resultant depression of the immune system) and with use of broad-spectrum antibiotics. Most antifungal drugs penetrate the eye poorly whether administered topically or systemically. Therefore fungal eye infections are a challenge to treat. **Natamycin** (Natacyn) is the only topical ophthalmic antifungal drug commercially available in the United States. Some parenteral antifungal drugs can be diluted for topical use. Dosage form, dosage, desired action, and undesired clinical responses for common topical antibacterial drugs are summarized in Table 64–7.

CONCEPT REVIEW

Antiinfective drugs for the eye are administered topically, orally, by subconjunctival injection, or by intravitreal injection, depending of the structure of the eye affected.

These drugs are often administered by two routes simultaneously to enhance antiinfective effect.

ANTIINFLAMMATORY DRUGS

Eye structures threatened by foreign particles or antigens respond through the immune system with inflammatory reactions just as other body parts do. Drugs used to counter inflammatory reactions (i.e., corticosteroids and NSAIDs) suppress the inflammatory response, causing symptoms to decrease or disappear. (Corticosteroids as a primary drug category are discussed in Chapter 42; NSAIDs are presented in Chapter 51.)

Corticosteroid drugs have been the mainstay for treatment of ocular inflammatory disorders since the 1950s.[5] Corticosteroids protect eye structures from the harmful effects of inflammation, particularly scarring and neovascularization. These drugs are more effective for acute than chronic conditions. Their use to treat ocular infections is generally contraindicated because they are not bactericidal and they mask signs of infection. When corticosteroids are used to treat ocular infections, their use is in combination with appropriate antiinfective drugs.

The **pharmacodynamic properties** of corticosteroid drugs are the same whether the inflammation results from an allergy, trauma, or infection. Corticosteroids reduce capillary permeability and cellular exudation. In addition, migration of poly-

TABLE 64–8
Antiinflammatory Drugs

Drug Name	Dosage and Route of Administration	Clinical Uses
Dexamethasone Alcohol Suspension: 0.1% (Maxidex) Sodium phosphate solution: 0.1% (Decadron Phosphate/MSD) Sodium phosphate ointment: 0.05% (Decadron Phosphate)	1 gtt of solution or suspension q1-2h for first 24–48 h, then two to four times/d until disease process controlled Taper dosage over several days or weeks before stopping treatment	Dexamethasone phosphate is the most potent of all topical ocular steroid preparations.
Prednisolone Acetate Suspension: 0.125% (Econopred, Pred Mild); 1.0% (Econopred Plus, Pred-Forte, and AK-Tate)	Same as dexamethasone	In higher concentrations prednisolone is one of the most potent ocular steroids. It is indicated for moderate to severe external and anterior eye inflammation.
Prednisolone Sodium Phosphate Solution: 0.125% (Inflamase, AK-Pred); 0.5% (Metreton); 1% (Inflamase Forte, AK-Pred)	Same as dexamethasone	See dexamethasone.
Fluorometholone Suspension: 0.25% (FML Forte); 0.1% (FML) Ointment: 0.1% (FML)	Instilled one to three times/d	Drug is indicated for treatment of milder, superficial ocular inflammation and allergy. It has lower potency and less intraocular penetration than all other steroids except medrysone.
Medrysone Suspension: 1.0% (HMS)	1 gtt/d or up to four times/d as indicated	A weaker antiinflammatory drug indicated for minor external inflammatory conditions. The reduced action is due to the drug's inability to penetrate the cornea like other corticosteroids except fluorometholone. Drug is less likely to produce increased IOP.
NSAIDS **Flubiprofen Sodium** Solution: 0.03% (Ocufen)	1 gtt q ½ h four times beginning 2 h before surgery	Drug is indicated for inhibition of intraoperative miosis for surgical procedures such as cataract extraction and intraocular lens implantation.
Suprofen Solution 1% (Syntex)	2 gtt qh for three doses before surgery	See flubiprofen.
Diclofenac Solution (Voltaren, Cataflam)	1 gtt qid	Treats postoperative inflammation after cataract surgery.
Ketorolac (Toradol, Acular)	1 gtt qid	Drug relieves ocular itching caused by seasonal allergic conjunctivitis.

morphonuclear leukocytes to the invasion site is suppressed. Fibroblast growth and release of hydrolytic enzymes from inflamed cells are inhibited, and the stimulus or antigen that attracts inflammatory cells to the invasion site is inhibited.[14]

Corticosteroid preparations differ in their ability to penetrate the eye and to exert antiinflammatory effectiveness. The lowest concentration of a corticosteroid drug in the cornea can have the greatest antiinflammatory effect. Corticosteroid levels in aqueous and vitreous humor are increased after both topical instillation and systemic administration of a steroid drug. Corticosteroid treatment reduces the outflow of aqueous in some clients. Certain individuals, particularly those with genetic predisposition for conditions such as glaucoma, have increased IOP after treatment with corticosteroids.[6] Table 64–8 provides additional information about corticosteroids.

NSAIDs are administered orally or topically for ocular inflammatory disorders. Pharmacodynamic properties of NSAIDs include inhibition of cyclooxygenase, an enzyme involved in the conversion of arachidonic acid to inflammatory mediators, including the prostaglandins. Table 64–8 provides additional information about some NSAIDs used in the treatment of ocular disorders.

CONCEPT REVIEW

Two groups of antiinflammatory drugs used to treat eye disorders are corticosteroids and NSAIDs. Corticosteroids protect the eye from harmful effects of inflammation, especially scarring and neovascularization. These drugs are more effective in the treatment of acute disorders than chronic conditions. They are not bactericidal but may be administered in combination with antiinfective drugs.

NSAIDs can be administered either orally or topically. These drugs are used preoperatively to inhibit intraoperative miosis. They are also administered in conjunction with topical steroids for long-term treatment of recurrent anterior uveitis.

MISCELLANEOUS OCULAR DRUGS

Additional groups of ocular preparations include local anesthetics, antiallergic drugs, irrigation solutions, and lubricants.

Local Anesthetics

Local anesthetics block initiation and conduction of nerve impulses, causing loss of ocular sensation without loss of consciousness. The duration of the anesthesia is proportional to the contact time of the drug with nerve tissue. After the local anesthesia, nerve tissue recovers completely with no evidence of damage to nerve fibers or cells.[6]

Local anesthesia of eye structures is accomplished by two routes of administration: topical instillation and injection. The effectiveness of topically instilled agents depends on their ability to suppress corneal sensitivity. The usual onset of action for

topical anesthetic agents is rapid, usually within 30 seconds; duration of action is approximately 20 minutes. Topically administered anesthetic drugs are used successfully for procedures such as removal of foreign bodies from the cornea, suture removal, tonometry, minor surgical procedures, laser therapy, and irrigation for chemical burns. Some drugs used for topical anesthesia are tetracaine hydrochloride (Pontocaine), proparacaine hydrochloride (AK-Taine, Alcaine, Ophthaine, and Ophthetic), benoxinate hydrochloride with sodium fluorescein (Fluress), and proparacaine hydrochloride with sodium fluorescein (Fluoracaine). The latter two agents contain fluorescein so that both staining of the conjunctival tissue and local anesthesia are accomplished. Use of drugs containing dyes such as fluorescein is indicated when the eye must be relaxed and stained for diagnostic study.

Anesthetics are injected into ocular areas such as subconjunctival and retrobulbar regions. Injected anesthetics are used in the treatment of severe corneal disease and to anesthetize the globe for surgery. Some drugs used for injectable ocular anesthesia are procaine hydrochloride (Novocain), lidocaine hydrochloride (Xylocaine), mepivacaine hydrochloride (Carbocaine), bupivacaine hydrochloride (Marcaine), and etidocaine hydrochloride (Duranest). The onset of action for these drugs ranges from 4 to 11 minutes, and the duration of action ranges from 30 minutes to 12 hours. Some of these drugs are combined with epinephrine, a vasoconstrictor, which decreases the rate of systemic absorption and the risk of systemic toxicity.[6,14]

Nursing responsibilities include instructing clients not to rub the anesthetized eye. Rubbing a desensitized eye can result in corneal injury. Prolonged use of local anesthetics is not indicated for ocular pain relief because such use can lead to severe keratitis; thus clients should not be given local anesthetics for self-administration. Table 64–9 provides additional information on local anesthetic drugs.

Antiallergic Agents

Drugs used to treat ocular allergy include cromolyn sodium (Opticrom), antihistamine decongestants, single decongestants, steroidal and nonsteroidal antiinflammatory drugs, and systemic antihistamines.

Cromolyn sodium (Opticrom), a mast cell stabilizer, inhibits the release of mediators from mast cells, thus preventing the rise of intracellular calcium necessary for degranulation. The drug acts only on ocular, nasal, and bronchial mucosa and is poorly absorbed from the GI tract; therefore it must be administered topically to the eye or as an inhalant. Cromolyn is indicated for treatment of ocular allergic conditions such as vernal conjunctivitis and keratitis, allergic keratoconjunctivitis, and giant papillary conjunctivitis, which often occurs in individuals who wear contact lenses.

Cromolyn should be used daily until symptomatic improvement has occurred. Reduced itching, tearing, redness, and discharge usually occur within a few days after initiation of cromolyn therapy. Because of the risk of staining, soft contact lenses should not be worn during the treatment period; they can be worn several hours after discontinuing the drug.[5] Cromolyn can be used in combination with other antiallergic treatments such as antihistamine and corticosteroid drugs. (For additional information on cromolyn, refer to Chapter 45.)

Antihistamine-decongestant combination drugs are also classified as antihistamine-vasoconstrictor agents. The action of the antihistamine is to block histamine receptor sites so that released histamine from inflamed cells cannot act on the target sites. Decongestant drugs are sympathomimetics that produce vasoconstriction, resulting in whitening of the eye and relief of discomfort. These drugs are indicated for symptomatic control of mild to moderate ocular allergy such as hay fever or mild vernal conjunctivitis. Antihistamine-decongestant combination drugs may be used in conjunction with mast cell stabiliz-

ers, corticosteroids, NSAIDs, and oral antihistamines to treat more severe allergic disorders.

Use of these drugs is contraindicated in clients with hypersensitivity to any component of the drug combination. The drugs should not be used in individuals with narrow-angle glaucoma because of the risk of mydriasis. Because of the possible systemic vasoconstriction, caution should be used in topically administering these drugs to older individuals with cardiovascular disease, poorly controlled hypertension, and brittle diabetes mellitus. The drugs have not been proved safe for use during pregnancy or for nursing mothers. (For additional information on antihistamines, refer to Chapter 50. For more information on decongestants, refer to Chapter 44.) See Table 64–9 for additional information on antiallergic drugs.

TABLE 64–9
Miscellaneous Ocular Drugs

Drug Name	Dosage	Undesired Clinical Response
ANESTHETICS (LOCAL)		
Tetracaine Hydrochloride 0.5% solution and ointment (Pontocaine)	1–5 gtt topically 1–2 min apart *or* ¾ in strip of ointment	Brief, moderate stinging or burning sensation after instillation Allergic reaction possible
Proparacaine Hydrochloride 0.5% solution (AK-Taine, Alcaine, Ophthaine, Ophthetic)	1 gtt q1-2 min; may repeat in 20 min for three to four times	Side effects (rare and usually mild): less common than with tetracaine Hypersensitivity reactions: rare
Benoxinate Hydrochloride 0.4% with sodium fluorescein: 0.25 (Fluress)	1–3 gtt before tonometry (has combination anesthetic and dye action)	Brief stinging or burning sensation after instillation that is greater than that produced by proparacaine and less than that caused by tetracaine Low potential for allergic response
Proparacaine Hydrochloride 0.5% solution with sodium fluorescein 0.25% (Fluoracaine)	1 gtt q1-2 min	See proparacaine
ANTIALLERGIC DRUGS		
Cromolyn Sodium 4% solution (Opticrom)	1 gtt four to six times/d; may be needed for as long as 6 wk or until symptoms controlled	Transient ocular stinging or burning after instillation Infrequent adverse responses: conjunctival injection, watery or itchy eyes, dryness of the eyes, styes
Antihistamine Decongestant Combination Drugs Antazoline phosphate 0.5% with naphazoline HCl 0.05% solution (Albalon-A) Antazoline phosphate 0.5% with naphazoline HCl 0.05% solution (Vasocon-A) Pheniramine maleate 0.3% with naphazoline HCl 0.025% solution (Naphcon A) Pyrilamine maleate 0.3% with phenylephrine HCl 0.12% solution (Prefrin-A) Pheniramine maleate 0.5% with phenylephrine HCl 0.125% solution (AK-Vernacon) Pheniramine maleate 0.3% with naphazoline HCl 0.025% solution (AK-Con-A) Pheniramine maleate 0.3% with naphazoline HCl 0.025% (Muro's Opcon A)	1–2 gtt q3-4h until symptoms relieved; apply digital pressure to puncta after instillation	Pupillary dilation, increased or decreased IOP, transient mild stinging or burning, tearing, and altered accommodation with decreased vision Rare systemic effects: lightheadedness, hyperglycemia, hypothermia, weakness, nausea, nervousness, drowsiness, anaphylaxis

Topical antihistamines are commercially available in combination with sympathomimetic decongestants. In addition, several single-agent decongestants are available OTC for ocular instillation. These OTC products are indicated for treatment of mild, nonspecific eye irritation or allergy. Because the drugs are sympathomimetic vasoconstrictors, the same precautions apply as described previously for antihistamine-decongestant combinations. Some of the decongestant drug preparations are naphazoline (Albalon, Clear Eyes, Degest, Muro's Opcon, Naphcon, VasoClear), phenylephrine (AK-Nephrin, Prefrin, Relief), and tetrahydrozoline (Collyrium, Murine Plus, Visine).[5, 15]

Irrigating Solutions

Irrigating solutions include any aqueous solution used to cleanse the eye of foreign matter. Sterile solutions are commercially available with the desired osmolarity, pH, preservatives, and buffers. They contain no active ingredient. The ideal irrigating solution should be isotonic, with a pH of 7.4.

OTC extraocular solutions are used to remove foreign material and liquid from the external eye. In the clinical setting they are used to remove foreign material and dyes after ophthalmic examinations and to cleanse eyes of mucus or purulent drainage before instillation of medications and between dressing changes. Some common solutions used for extraocular irrigation include normal saline, Eye-Stream, Collyrium Eye Lotion, and Trisol Eye Wash.[16]

Normal saline solution is not satisfactory for intraocular irrigation or perfusion because of its physiologic effect on the cornea and intraocular structures. Currently a balanced salt solution for short-term perfusion during surgery and a balanced salt solution plus bicarbonate, glucose, and glutathione for long-term surgical perfusion are commonly used preparations.

Lubricants

Lubricants are used to treat dryness of the eyes, a common eye disorder, especially in older persons. They also are used by soft and hard contact lens wearers. Dryness of the eye can be caused by a tear film abnormality or a disorder of an ocular surface. Conditions that cause dry eye states are aqueous deficiency, mucin deficiency, lipid abnormality, lid function impairment, and epitheliopathy.

Lubricants are commercially available as solutions, ointments, and artificial tear inserts. In addition, there are a large number of artificial tear solutions available. Artificial tears are used as substitutes for natural tears. Most of these preparations contain polyvinyl alcohol, cellulose esters, or both. Artificial tears do not produce adverse effects and can be administered as frequently as desired. **Artificial tear inserts** are small rods that are placed in the inferior cul-de-sac. The insert swells and dissolves, releasing its lubricating contents. Inserts are designed to be replaced every 24 hours but can be replaced more often if needed. Lubricating solutions are usually administered three to four times daily, and lubricating ointments are usually administered twice daily.[12, 16]

CONCEPT REVIEW

Local anesthetics are administered topically or by injection. They suppress corneal sensitivity without causing loss of consciousness. These drugs are used in procedures such as foreign body extraction, suture removal, laser therapy, and irrigation for chemical burns.

The prototype of antiallergic drugs is cromolyn sodium, which inhibits the release of mediators from mast cells and prevents the rise of intracellular calcium that must exist for degranulation to occur. Cromolyn must be administered topically or as an inhalant. Antihistamine-decongestant combination drugs block histamine receptor sites and produce vasoconstriction, thus whitening eyes and relieving discomfort. These drugs are useful in treating moderate ocular allergy such as hay fever but carry some precautions for those with glaucoma, hypertension, pregnancy, and other conditions.

Irrigating solutions are used to remove foreign material and liquid from the external eye, to remove dyes, and to cleanse eyes of purulent drainage. Lubricants are used to treat dryness of the eye. Lubricants can be solutions, ointments, or artificial tear inserts or preparations.

AGENTS USED TO DIAGNOSE OCULAR DISORDERS

Drugs used to diagnose ocular disorders include local anesthetics, mydriatics, cycloplegics, and dyes. Anesthetics, mydriatics, and cycloplegics are used to relax eye structures and dilate the pupil for examination. Dyes are used to locate corneal foreign bodies, determine tear break-up time, assess potency of the nasolacrimal drainage system, and detect pathology in retinal blood vessels by angiography. Several preparations are available for staining ocular structures. Two commonly known and used dyes are fluorescein and rose bengal.

Fluorescein is a yellow acid of the xanthine group of dyes. It is available as a solution and as filter paper strips for topical instillation. Injectable preparations are also available for intravenous use.

Topical fluorescein instillation often is used before tonometry is used for measurement of IOP. One drop of solution or momentary placement of an impregnated strip into the conjunctival cul-de-sac causes a greenish discoloration around any area where the epithelial barrier is broken. When using a filter paper strip, wet the tip of the sterile strip in sterile saline solution before its introduction into the eye. Wetting the strip tip facilitates delivery of the dye into the eye and decreases the sensation of irritation. An occasional complaint of stinging is the only common side effect from topical instillation of fluorescein. Care should be taken to avoid facial staining by the tears after the use of the solution or paper strips.

Injectable fluorescein is used for fluorescein angiography to evaluate retinal blood vessels. After injection of 10 ml of a 5% solution in an antecubital vein, the dye usually is visualized in the central retinal artery within 13 seconds.[6] Before angiography, tell the client that fluorescein causes bright yellowish-orange urine for approximately 24 hours. In addition, the client's skin may have a yellowish cast for 6 to 12 hours after injection of the dye. Adverse effects from fluorescein angiography include nausea and vomiting, pruritis and urticaria, and allergic reaction of the immediate hypersensitivity type.

Rose bengal is an iodine derivative of fluorescein that can be applied topically as a 1% solution or with a moistened paper filter strip that contains 1.3 mg of rose bengal. Rose bengal, like fluorescein, does not stain normal cells. However, it does stain dead cells, degenerated cells, and mucus. Rose bengal is used most frequently to evaluate epithelial lesions associated with keratoconjunctivitis sicca. Eye discomfort and irritation are greater with rose bengal use than with fluorescein. A topical anesthetic may be applied before instillation to decrease uncomfortable eye sensations. Thorough irrigation of the eye after examination is recommended to remove excess dye since rose bengal stains eyelids, cheeks, fingers, and clothes.

Before instillation of either fluorescein or rose bengal, question clients about personal and family history of hypersensitivity to dye. Known hypersensitivity is a contraindication to usage.

CONCEPT REVIEW

Dyes used as diagnostic agents help in locating corneal foreign bodies, determining tear break-up time, monitoring potency of the nasolacrimal drainage system, and detecting pathology by angiography.

The two dyes most commonly used for the eye are fluorescein and rose bengal.

SUMMARY

The structures of the eye exist within a delicate balance that preserves and maintains vision. Glaucoma, inflammation, and infection are pathologic processes that often can be controlled or eliminated by pharmacologic treatment.

Some of the major effects of ophthalmic drugs are to relax select muscles of the eye, to alter the pressure within the eye, to reduce the reaction to antigens or irritants affecting the surface of the eye, and to eliminate infection. Ophthalmic dyes can be used to assess the eye mechanically or for pathology and to find foreign bodies.

Drugs used to treat the eye, although administered topically, can have widespread systemic effects. Many are self-administered. The nurse plays an important role as teacher in the treatment of ophthalmic conditions.

REFERENCES

1. Hole, J. (1993). *Human anatomy and physiology* (6th ed.). Dubuque, IA: Wm. C. Brown.
2. Guyton, A.C. (1992). *Human physiology and mechanisms of disease* (5th ed.). Philadelphia: W.B. Saunders.
3. Tortora, G., & Grabowski, S. (1993). *Principles of anatomy and physiology* (7th ed.). New York: Harper Collins College Publishers.
4. Seeley, R., Stephens, T., & Tate, P. (1992). *Anatomy and physiology* (2nd ed.). St. Louis: Mosby–Year Book.
5. Pavan-Lanston, D., & Dunkel, E.C. (1991). *Handbook of ocular drug therapy and ocular side effects of systemic drugs.* Boston: Little, Brown.
6. Barlett, J.D., & Jaanus, S.D. (Eds.). (1989). *Clinical ocular pharmacology* (2nd ed.). Boston: Butterworth.
7. U.S.P. - DI, 1994.
8. Hodgson, B., Kizior, R., & Kingdom, R. (1995). *1995 nurse's drug handbook.* Philadelphia: W.B. Saunders.
9. Gurwitz, J.H., Glynn, R.J., Monane, M., Everitte, D.E., Avorn, J., et al. (1993). Treatment for glaucoma: Adherence by the elderly. *American Journal of Public Health, 83,* 711–716.
10. Data Pharmaceutica, Inc. (1993). *1993 physician's genRx.* Smithtown, NY: Author.
11. U.S. Pharmacopeia Convention. (1990). *The United States pharmacopeia* (22nd rev.). Rockville, MD: Author.
12. Lehne, R. (1994). *Pharmacology for nursing care* (2nd ed.). Philadelphia: W.B. Saunders.
13. Fraunfelder, F.T., & Meyers, S.M. (1989). *Drug induced ocular side effects and drug interactions* (3rd ed.). Philadelphia: Lea & Febiger.
14. Smith, C.M., & Reynard, A.M. (Eds.). (1992). *Textbook of pharmacology.* Philadelphia: W.B. Saunders.
15. McEvoy, G.K., & Litvak, K. (Eds.). (1992). *AHFS drug information—92.* Bethesda, MD: American Society of Hospital Pharmacists.
16. American Pharmaceutical Association. (1990). *Handbook of nonprescription drugs* (9th ed.). Washington, DC: Author.

BIBLIOGRAPHY

Abramowicz, M. (Ed.). (1994). Oral pilocarpine for xerostomia. *Medical Letter on Drugs and Therapeutics, 36*(929), 76.

Kopecky, J. (1992). Ophthalmic drugs and anesthesia interactions. *CRNA: The Clinical Forum for Nurse Anesthetists, 3*(1), 16–21.

CHAPTER 65

Ear Preparations

JUDY MALKIEWICZ • JAN HOOT MARTIN

⊛ **Overview of Anatomy and Physiology**

LEARNING OBJECTIVES:

Describe the general structure of the ear.

Discuss the physiologic functions of the ear.

Explain how sound is transmitted and interpreted.

KEY TERMS:

External ear, middle ear, inner ear, tragus, tympanic membrane, eustachian tube, cochlea, pinna

⊛ **Nursing Considerations**

LEARNING OBJECTIVES:

Discuss the assessment of the ear.

List the most common nursing diagnoses for clients requiring otic medication.

Describe the proper administration of otic preparations.

KEY TERM: Furuncles

⊛ **Ear Preparations**

LEARNING OBJECTIVES:

Discuss the therapeutic uses of ear preparations.

Identify the most common undesired responses to otic preparations.

Explain the purpose and action of otic anesthetics.

Describe the desired actions of antibacterial otic preparations.

Discuss precautionary measures in using ceruminolytics.

Identify symptoms of ototoxicity.

Identify two highly ototoxic agents.

KEY TERMS:

Cerumen, ototoxicity

CONCEPTS AND TERMS TO REVIEW

Review the structure and function of the ear in a medical-surgical nursing text.

Review the use of antibiotics (Chapter 55) and corticosteroids (Chapter 42).

---

*T*his chapter reviews the basic anatomy and physiology of the ear, therapeutic uses of ear preparations, and nursing considerations for clients using ear preparations. Otically administered drugs are reviewed pharmacologically, including potential complications associated with their use. Drugs used systemically for the treatment of middle and inner ear disorders (antibiotics, analgesics, and corticosteroids) are discussed in other chapters of this text.

Topical ear preparations administered in the external ear canal are used most often for the prevention or treatment of external ear disorders. These preparations are instilled directly into the external meatus of the ear. Drugs used for otic administration include antibiotics, antiinfectives, antiinflamma-

tories, analgesics, anesthetics, drying agents, and cerumen solvents (ceruminolytics). For pathologies of the middle and inner ear, systemic drugs are generally required.

OVERVIEW OF ANATOMY AND PHYSIOLOGY

The ear is a sensory organ whose functions include hearing and the sense of balance. The ear consists of three structural parts: external, middle, and inner (Fig. 65–1). The structures and functions of these three parts are significant and integral to the process of hearing.

External Ear

The external ear is embedded in the temporal bone bilaterally at the level of the eyes. The ear is attached at approximately a 10-degree angle with the head. The **external ear** extends from the visible **pinna,** through the external canal to the lateral side of the **tympanic membrane,** or eardrum. The external canal is slightly S shaped and lined with cerum (wax)-producing glands, sebaceous glands, and hair follicles. The hair follicles and cerumen protect the tympanic membrane and the middle ear. The length of the external canal varies with age. In the adult the distance from the opening of the external canal to the tympanic membrane is approximately 1 to 1½ inches. In the infant and child the distance is ¼ to ½ inch. The **tragus** is a three-dimensional projection of skin-covered cartilage on the anterior portion of the external ear (Fig. 65–1). The external ear also includes the mastoid process, the bony ridge located over the temporal bone behind the pinna that covers the mastoid air cells. The mastoid air cells aid in the transmission of sound.[1]

Middle Ear

The **middle ear** consists of the medial side of the tympanic membrane and a compartment called the *epitympanum,* or *attic,* which contains the three bony ossicles: malleus, incus, and stapes. The tympanic membrane is embedded in the temporal bone and is surrounded by the mastoid air cells. The membrane is a thick, transparent sheet of tissue 9 mm in diameter. It provides a barrier between the external ear and the middle ear. The tympanic membrane is attached to the first bony ossicle, the malleus. The bony ossicles behind the tympanic membrane are joined together, although not rigidly, thus allowing vibratory movement. The middle ear is protected from the inner ear by the round and the oval window membranes. The **eustachian tube** originates from the floor of the middle ear at the proximal end and opens at the distal end in the nasopharynx. The distal opening in the nasopharynx is surrounded by adenoid lymphatic tissue. The eustachian tube allows equalization of pressure on both sides of the tympanic membrane. The eustachian tube is shorter, wider, and more horizontal in children than adults.

Inner Ear

The **inner ear,** lying on the other side of the oval window, contains the semicircular canals, the cochlea, and the distal end of the eighth cranial nerve (vestibulocochlear nerve). The **cochlea** is the spiral-shaped organ of hearing filled with endolymph and perilymph fluids. These fluids are important in the protection of the cochlea and the semicircular canals. These structures literally float in the fluids, which cushion

FIGURE 65–1   Anatomic features of the external ear, **A,** and internal ear, **B.** (From Ignatavicius, D.D., Workman, L.M., & Mishler, M.M. (1995). *Medical-surgical nursing: A nursing process approach* (2nd ed.). Philadelphia: W.B. Saunders, pp. 1352, 1353.)

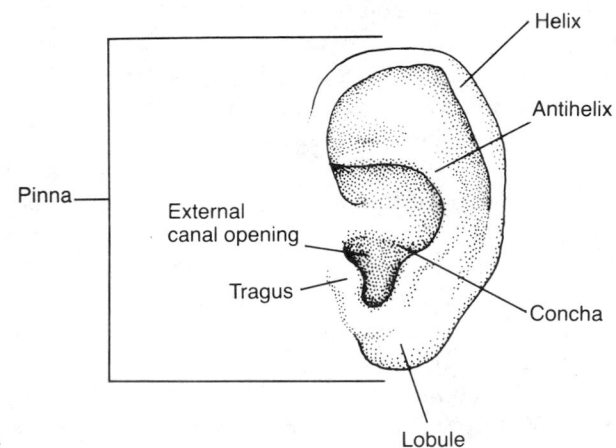

A

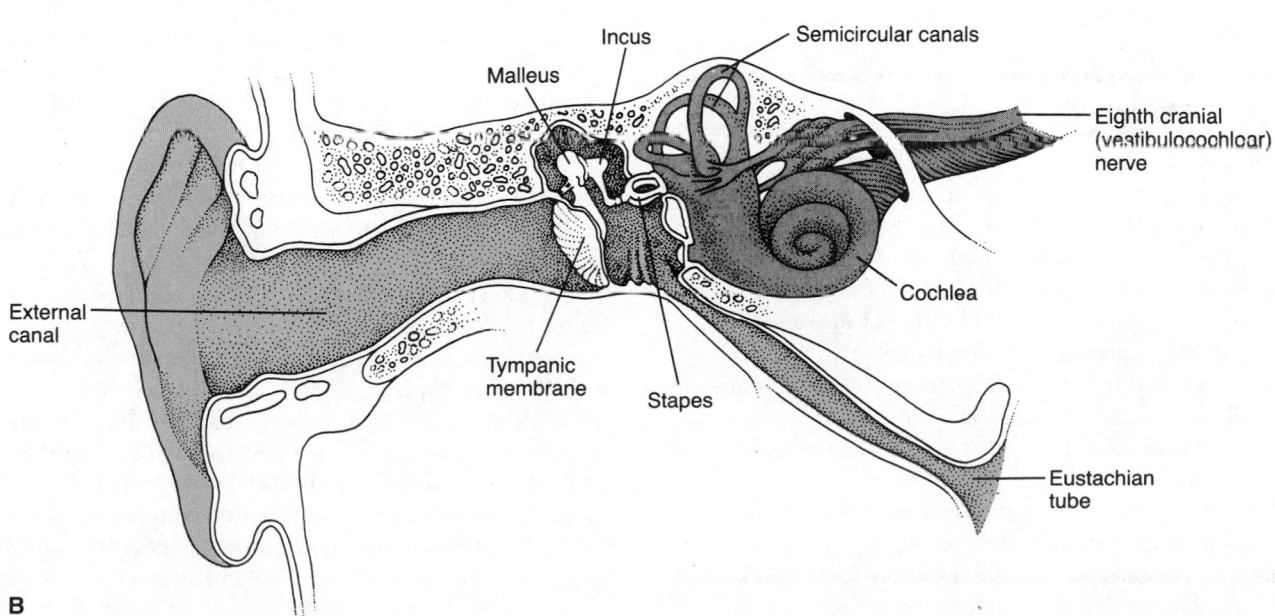

B

them against abrupt movements of the head. The cochlea's basilar membrane is approximately 30 mm long and is composed of thousands of fibers. The organ of Corti, the receptor end organ of hearing, is on the upper surface of the basilar membrane. The organ of Corti contains hair cells that rest on the fibers of the basilar membrane surrounded by the cochlear division of the eighth cranial nerve.

The eighth cranial nerve has two branches—the cochlear and the vestibular. The cochlear branch transmits neural impulses from the cochlea to the brain where they are interpreted as sound. Helping to maintain a person's sense of balance, the semicircular canals are structures that contain fluid and hair cells connected to the sensory nerve fibers of the vestibular portion of the eighth cranial nerve.

Physiology

Important physiologic functions of the ear are hearing and maintenance of balance. Hearing is accomplished when sound is delivered through the air to the external ear canal and the temporal bone covering the mastoid air cells. The sound waves strike the mastoid and the movable tympanic membrane, which is connected to the first bony ossicle, the malleus. The sound wave vibrations are transferred from the tympanic membrane to the malleus, the incus, and the stapes. From the stapes, the vibrations are transmitted to the cochlea. Receptors there transduce the vibrations into action potentials, which are conducted to the brain as neural impulses by the cochlear portion of the eighth cranial nerve. Thus sound is processed and interpreted by the brain.

The semicircular canals are part of the vestibular apparatus. As previously noted, they are filled with fluid and are composed of hair cells connected to the sensory nerve fibers of the vestibular portion of the eighth cranial nerve. When the client's head position changes, the hair cells are bent by the flow of fluid in the semicircular canals, which apprises the central nervous system of the client's relative position.

CONCEPT REVIEW

The ear's primary functions include hearing and providing a sense of balance. The ear has three distinct parts: external, middle, and inner. Use of external ear preparations is not indicated for otitis media and infections or inflammation of the inner ear. No external ear preparation should be used in the presence of a perforated tympanic membrane.

Antibiotic and antiinflammatory drugs are used for middle and inner ear problems and are often used in combination with external ear preparations to prevent inflammation.

Drying agents and ceruminolytics are used to prevent external ear pathologies.

NURSING CONSIDERATIONS

Assessing   Obtaining a **nursing history** is essential for all clients with ear disorders requiring drug therapy. The history includes a review of the present illness and possible causes of the ear disorder. Ask the client about bathing and swimming behaviors, recent trauma, any changes in hygiene activities, and products used in or around the ears. In addition, elicit information about any known allergies to drugs, foods, or preservatives and sensitivity of the skin to other products. Obtain a past medical history summarizing the client's overall health along with a list of current prescribed drugs. Determine if the female client is pregnant or lactating; this is always important when considering ear preparation therapy.

Clients requiring ear preparations should have a thorough **physical assessment** of the ear and possibly a hearing test before initiation of drug therapy to determine the extent of the pathology and the most appropriate treatment regimen. The assessment should include inspection and palpation of the ear, including an otoscopic examination. Inspect the mastoid process for redness and swelling, which are indications of inflammation. Gently tap one finger over the mastoid process, compress the tragus with one finger, and gently manipulate the pinna to assess for tenderness. Any resulting tenderness suggests an inflammatory process in either the external canal or the mastoid.

Assess the skin of the ear and surrounding structures for color, temperature, swelling, nodules, and lesions. The normal external canal is free from lesions and is dry, clean, and not reddened. Abnormalities of the external canal include **furuncles** (circumscribed inflammation of single hair follicles), large or hard accumulations of cerumen, scaliness, redness, swelling, and the presence of any foreign object. Ear pathologies can result in drainage or lymphatic involvement. Blood, cerebrospinal fluid, pus, or serous fluid may drain from the external ear. Document the color, odor, and consistency of any drainage from the external canal. Rarely discharge from the external ear is cultured, and antibiotic sensitivities are determined to guide the appropriate antibiotic treatment. Assess for enlargement and tenderness of preauricular and postauricular lymph nodes. Finally, note signs of systemic infection such as fever, malaise, anorexia, and fatigue.

When inflammation and extensive edema of the external canal exist, a temporary conductive hearing loss might be experienced. Assess hearing acuity to determine how any loss affects the client.

Any pain elicited during examination of the external ear requires *cautious* otoscopic examination because the speculum causes extreme pain when it contacts the inflamed tissue of the external canal. To accommodate the otoscopic speculum and allow clearer visualization of the canal and tympanic membrane, manipulate the external pinna up and backward for the adult, down and backward for the child. The tympanic membrane should be visualized to determine intactness, retraction, or bulging. At times the external ear canal edema prevents visualization of the tympanic membrane. Ear preparations should be used only when the tympanic membrane is intact to prevent complications such as ototoxicity and systemic absorption.

Diagnosing   Data gathered from the nursing history and physical examination are used to establish nursing diagnoses. The most common nursing diagnoses for clients requiring otic drugs follow:

- Pain related to inflammatory process and accumulation of fluid in the middle ear.
- Sensory or perceptual alterations (auditory) related to obstruction, infection, damage to the middle ear, or damage to the auditory nerve.
- Knowledge deficit regarding treatment plan.

Planning   Pain is a significant problem for clients with external otitis. Thus a primary client goal is to experience alleviation of ear pain. Other expected outcomes of otic drug therapy include the following:

- The client experiences an increase in auditory sensory perception to a functional level.
- The client demonstrates proper techniques when using ear preparations.
- The client demonstrates understanding of ototoxic effects of ear preparations.

Implementing   The treatment procedures for external ear disorders are generally performed at home or on an outpatient basis. Self-administration of ear preparations can be difficult at times. Suggesting that family or friends be instructed to help the client is useful. Therefore teach the client and significant others irrigation techniques (see box and illustration), when to use specific drugs (Table 65–1), and how to instill ear drops (see box and illustration on p. 896).

Tell the client to store ear preparations in a tightly closed container at room temperature. Otic preparations are warmed before administration for client comfort and to prevent vestibular stimulation (e.g., nausea, dizziness, ataxia). Warming is achieved best by holding the bottle of medication in the hand for 5 to 10 minutes or placing it in a pocket, allowing the drug to come to body temperature. To prevent destruction of the drug or burning of the skin, it should not be warmed in a microwave oven or boiling water. To avoid contamination of the entire bottle of medication, the dropper should *not* come in contact with the external ear. In addition, the client should be advised *not* to rinse the dropper after each use.

To achieve adequate distribution of otic preparations, teach the client to position the head with the involved ear facing upward. The pinna should be gently manipulated up and backward for the adult and down and backward for the child during instillation of the drug. After the prescribed numbers of drops are instilled, insert a cotton pledget into the external canal to prevent leakage of the medication. After the medication has been in place for the prescribed period of time, the soiled pledget is carefully removed and disposed. Thorough handwashing completes the procedure to prevent recurrent infection, spread of infection to the opposite ear, or contamination of another person.

Instruct the client to use the drug only for the prescribed number of days. Indiscriminate, prolonged use may result in

HOW TO IRRIGATE AN EAR

▶ Gather proper equipment: basin, appropriate syringe (soft rubber otic syringe or Toomey syringe), otoscope, and towel.

▶ Warm tap water to body temperature.

▶ Fill syringe with warm water.

▶ Place basin under the ear to be irrigated. Place a towel around the client's neck to avoid getting the client's clothing wet.

▶ Use otoscope to check the location of the impacted cerumen.

▶ Place the tip of the syringe at an angle so the fluid pushes at one side of the impaction and not directly on the impaction. This helps loosen the cerumen and avoids pushing cerumen further back in the canal. Avoid excessive pressure (see illustration).

▶ Watch fluid return for signs of cerumen plug removal and reexamine with otoscope.

▶ Continue to irrigate the ear with approximately 70 ml of warm water. If the cerumen does not drain out, wait approximately 10 min and repeat the procedure.

▶ Monitor the client for signs of nausea during the procedure. If the client becomes nauseated, stop the procedure.

▶ If the cerumen cannot be completely removed by irrigation, the client may place several drops of mineral oil into the ear three times a day for 2 d, after which irrigation may be repeated.

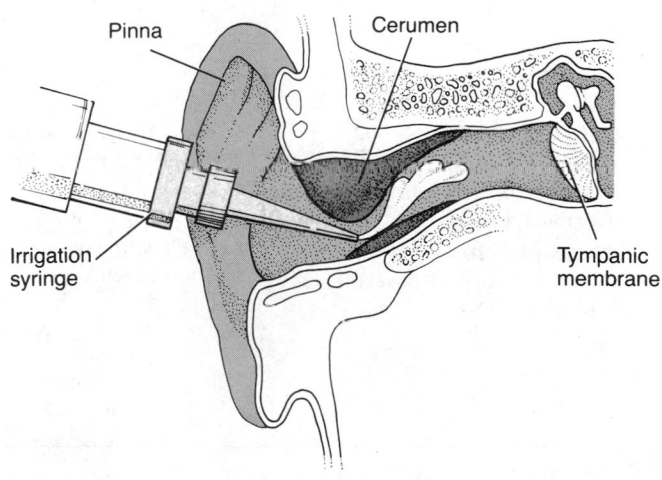

From Ignatavicius, D.D., Workman, L.M., & Mishler, M.M. (Eds.). (1995). *Medical-surgical nursing: A nursing process approach* (2nd ed., p. 1370). Philadelphia: W.B. Saunders.

TABLE 65–1
Major Drugs

Drugs	Dosage and Route of Administration	Nursing Considerations
ANTIBIOTICS **Chloramphenicol** (Chloromycetin Otic)	**Superficial Bacterial Infections of External Auditory Canal** 2–3 gtt tid to each ear Keep ear facing up for 1–2 min and use a cotton pledget to prevent medication leakage If necessary, a cotton wick or gauze may be inserted in the canal, kept moist by adding medication to wick	**Assess** Cerumen and debris should be removed before therapy. Drops should not be given to client with ruptured tympanic membrane. **Implement** Teach client how to administer to self. **Monitor** Discontinue if symptoms worsen. **Evaluate** Observe for decreased signs and symptoms of infection.
ANTIBIOTIC AND STEROID COMBINATIONS **Colistin Sulfate–Neomycin Sulfate–Thonsonium Bromide–Hydrocortisone Acetate Otic Suspension** (Coly-Mycin S Otic Drops) **Polymyxin B Sulfate–Neomycin Sulfate–Hydrocortisone** (Cortisporin Otic, Lazersporin-C, Pediotic, AK-Spore H.C., Cortatrigen, Cortisporin,* Drotic,* Otic-Care, Otocort,* Otomycin-HPN*)	**Superficial Infections of External Auditory Canal, Relief of Inflammation and Pain** 2–3 gtt tid or qid to each ear Keep ear facing up for 1–2 min and use a cotton pledget to prevent medication leakage If necessary, a cotton wick or gauze may be inserted in the canal, kept moist by adding medication to wick	**Assess** Cerumen and debris should be removed before therapy. Drug should not be given to client with ruptured tympanic membrane. **Implement** Teach client how to administer. **Monitor** Discontinue if symptoms worsen. Prolonged use can lead to overgrowth of other organisms. **Evaluate** Assess external auditory canal for decrease in symptoms.
STEROIDS **Desonide-Acetic Acid** (Tridesilon) **Hydrocortisone-Acetic Acid-Propylene Glycol** (V̄oSol-HC Otic, Acetasol HC)	**Inflammation of External Auditory Canal** 3–4 gtt to ear tid or qid Keep ear facing up for 1–2 min to prevent medication leakage	**Assess** Cerumen and debris should be removed before therapy. **Implement** Teach client how to administer to self. Teach client hazards of steroid use. **Monitor** Discontinue if symptoms worsen. Prolonged use can lead to overgrowth of other organisms. **Evaluate** Observe for decreased inflammation.
CERUMINOLYTICS **Triethanolamine Polypeptide Oleate-Condensate** (Cerumenex Drops) **Carbamide Peroxide** (Auro Ear Drops, Debrox, E-R-O, Murine Ear Drops)	**Emulsify or Disperse Cerumen; Protect Against Contamination** Fill ear canal with drug while client's head tilted at 45-degree angle Insert cotton pledget Allow to remain 15–30 min only Flush gently with lukewarm water using soft rubber syringe and avoiding excessive pressure For unusually hard impactions, repeat procedure	**Assess** Drug should not be used in presence of perforated tympanic membrane or otitis media. **Implement** Teach client to administer to self. **Evaluate** Assess for relief of symptoms.

*Contains potassium metabisulfite.

TABLE 65–1 *Continued*
Major Drugs

Drugs	Dosage and Route of Administration	Nursing Considerations
LOCAL ANESTHETICS AND TOPICAL DECONGESTANTS ***Benzocaine*** (Americaine-Otic) ***Benzocaine-Antipyrine*** (Allergen Ear Drops, Aurafair, Auralgan, Aurodex, Auroto) ***Benzocaine-Antipyrine-Phenylephrine*** (Tympagesic)	**Acute Otitis Media** Instill solution to run along the wall of external canal until it is filled Moisten a cotton pledget with drug and insert into ear Repeat q1–2h until pain and congestion relieved **Cerumen Removal** Fill ear canal three times daily for 2–3 d to help detach cerumen from wall of canal and to facilitate removal A cotton pledget moistened with drug should be inserted into the ear after instillation and after cerumen removal	**Assess** Do not use if tympanic membrane is perforated. Ask if client is taking any sulfonamides. Benzocaine antagonizes antibacterial activity of sulfonamides, and the two drugs should not be administered together. **Implement** Protect solution from light and heat. If solution is brown or contains a precipitate, do not use. Discard product 6 mo after opening. Avoid touching the ear with the dropper. Do not rinse dropper after use. Replace dropper in bottle after use and close tightly. Teach client how to administer to self. Drug can cause staining of clothes. **Evaluate** Observe for decreased pressure, congestion, or pain.
ANTIBACTERIALS, ANTIFUNGAL, ASTRINGENTS ***Acetic Acid–Burrow's Solution*** (Otic Domeboro) ***Boric Acid–Isopropyl Alcohol*** (Dri/Ear Drops, Ear-Dry) ***Acetic Acid*** (VōSol) ***Acetic Acid–Hydrocortisone*** (VōSol HC)	**Superficial Infections of External Ear Canal Caused by Organisms Susceptible to Action of Antimicrobial; Prevention of Infection by Drying of Canal After Exposure to Water** To promote continuous contact, insert wick saturated with drug into ear canal (wick may also be saturated after insertion) Keep wick in place for at least 24 h; keep moist by adding 3–5 gtt q4–6h	**Assess** Cerumen and debris should be removed before therapy. Do not use drug in presence of perforated tympanic membrane. **Implement** Store at room temperature. Keep container tightly closed. Teach client to administer to self. **Monitor** Discontinue use if sensitization or irritation occurs. **Evaluate** Observe for decreased signs and symptoms of infection or swelling.

systemic absorption and undesired clinical responses (Table 65–2). For the duration of use, advise the client to keep the ear dry by avoiding swimming and showering. Advise the client of potential undesired responses for the specific otic preparation in use. Warn the client it may be necessary to stop therapy if the symptoms worsen or if undesired responses occur.

Evaluating   Evaluation involves determining the efficacy of the otic preparation. When the drugs are effective, the client no longer complains of pain, edema, itching, or sensorial or perceptual alterations. Review the expected outcomes with the client to determine possible revisions of the initial plan of care.

Audiologic testing with tympanometry is done to assess hearing and to determine movement potential of the tympanic membrane. Decreased movement of the tympanic membrane indicates conductive hearing loss. These medical therapies are usually done only in cases failing to respond to initial treatment.

EAR PREPARATIONS

Therapeutic uses of external ear preparations include the treatment of external ear infection, inflammation, and pain and the removal of excessive or impacted cerumen. External ear preparations are not indicated for treatment of otitis media and infections or inflammation of the inner ear structures.[2] Because of the diverse symptomatology of external ear disorders, many ear preparations are combinations of drugs. For example, anti-inflammatory drugs are often given in combination with antibiotics to decrease symptoms of inflammation associated with the infection.

Otically administered drugs are used almost exclusively for their local actions. Direct otic administration allows better distribution of the drug to all surface areas of the external canal. Unless the infection is extensive, use of topical antibiotics is preferred in the treatment of external otitis. *No ear preparations*

HOW TO ADMINISTER EAR DROPS

▶ Remove old cotton pledget or ear wick if applicable. Be careful to dispose of this highly contaminated material properly. Wash hands thoroughly to prevent the spread of contamination to the other ear or to another person.

▶ Carefully irrigate external ear as needed to remove debris and cerumen.

▶ Gently warm medication by holding in hands. The drug may be placed in warm water, but care should be taken not to put it in hot water and not to wash off the label. Some drugs lose their potency if heated above body temperature. Mix drug by shaking thoroughly before instillation.

▶ Instill prescribed amount of drug (usually 2–6 gtt for adults and 3 gtt for infants and children) into external canal, pulling the pinna in the proper direction for the age of the client.

▶ Place a small cotton pledget into the canal to prevent loss of drug from the external ear. Tight occlusion with the pledget should be avoided, especially when instilling corticosteroids.

▶ If the external meatus is edematous and does not allow drugs to flow freely, an ear wick should be used. An ear wick is a small piece of fine mesh gauze placed through the swollen area of the external meatus (see illustration). Drugs are placed on the outside of the gauze and are allowed to be absorbed into the canal via the wick. The ear wick should be changed every 24 h.

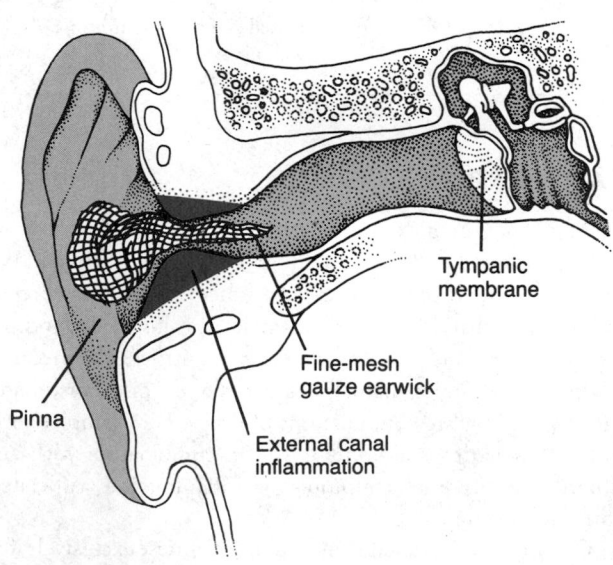

Illustration from Ignatavicius, D.D., Workman, L.M., & Mishler, M.M. (Eds.). (1995). *Medical-surgical nursing: A nursing process approach* (2nd ed., p. 1369). Philadelphia: W.B. Saunders.

are recommended by the Federal Drug Administration (FDA) for clients with perforated tympanic membrane.[3]

Other therapeutic uses of ear preparations include the prevention of external ear pathologies. Drugs used for prevention include drying agents and ceruminolytic preparations. Drying agents suppress the growth of organisms, and ceruminolytics help with the softening and removal of excessive or impacted cerumen.

Antibiotics

Similar to other **topical** antibiotics, otic antibiotics are used to treat superficial infections. Otic antibiotics act through direct contact with the surface area of the skin and are not designed for systemic absorption.

Chloramphenicol otic (Chloromycetin Otic) is a broad-spectrum antibiotic used for the treatment of external otitis.[4] The drug's mechanism of action is primarily bacteriostatic through inhibition of protein synthesis. Both gram-positive and gram-negative organisms are susceptible to chloramphenicol otic, including *Staphylococcus aureus, Escherichia coli, Haemophilus influenzae, Pseudomonas aeruginosa, Aerobacter aerogenes, Klebsiella pneumoniae,* and *Proteus* species.[3]

Relief of symptoms should occur within a week of the initial onset of therapy; treatment should last no longer than 10 days. Prolonged use should be avoided to prevent complications (e.g., contact dermatitis, bacterial resistance).[5] If pressure equalization tubes are in place, the tympanic membrane is perforated, or the middle or inner ear structures are involved, topical antibiotics are used only with extreme caution. Use of systemic antibiotics is preferred for the treatment of these conditions.

Contact dermatitis is the most common undesired response to any otic preparation. Signs and symptoms of dermatitis may include any or all of the following: itching, burning, angioneurotic edema (e.g., local wheals accompanied by swelling of subcutaneous tissue), urticaria, vesicular lesions, and maculopapular dermatitis.[5] Known hypersensitivity to this drug is a contraindication for the use of chloramphenicol otic. Additionally, clients known as allergic to kanamycin, paromomycin, streptomycin, or gentamicin should use this drug with caution.

Steroids and Combination Antibiotic and Steroid Drugs

Often antibiotics are given in combination with corticosteroids to treat otic infection and inflammation. Hydrocortisone is the most common corticosteroid combined with antibiotics for this purpose. The broad-spectrum antibiotic neomycin sulfate is included in each of the combination drugs because of its bactericidal effect.[6]

Corticosteroids are given to reduce dermal reactions to infections (e.g., inflammation, edema, pruritus, and pain). The mechanism of action for otic corticosteroids, as for other topical corticosteroids, remains unclear.

The amount of corticosteroid absorbed systemically is determined by the dosage instilled, the length of the treatment,

TABLE 65–2
Major Undesired Clinical Responses

Major Drugs	Undesired Clinical Responses and Contraindications	Nursing Considerations
ANTIBIOTICS	**Contraindications** Perforated tympanic membrane Hypersensitivity **Undesired Responses** Bone marrow hypoplasia and death have been reported after local application of chloramphenicol Prolonged use can lead to an overgrowth of nonsusceptible organisms, including fungi Ototoxic if product enters middle ear Local irritation; contact dermatitis (burning, stinging, pruritus, tenderness, erythema, rash, urticaria, edema)	Watch closely for signs and symptoms of local irritation or worsening of pretreatment symptoms. Discontinue use if irritation occurs.
STEROIDS	**Contraindications** Perforated tympanic membrane Hypersensitivity Presence of herpes simplex in external canal Vaccinia and varicella **Undesired Responses** Local irritation; contact dermatitis (burning, stinging, pruritus, tenderness, erythema, rash, urticaria, edema) Failure to heal Hypersensitive reaction to drug or preservatives; contains potassium metabisulfite Drying, folliculitis, hypertrichosis (excessive growth of hair), acneiform eruptions, hypopigmentation Overgrowth of secondary infection Systemic absorption leading to manifestations of Cushing's syndrome	Watch closely for signs and symptoms of local irritation or worsening of pretreatment symptoms. Discontinue use if irritation occurs. Systemic absorption is greater when an occlusive dressing is used. Systemic absorption is related to contact surface area and is greater with small children and infants.
ANTIBACTERIALS	**Contraindications** Perforated tympanic membrane Hypersensitivity **Undesired Responses** Local irritation; contact dermatitis (burning, stinging, pruritus, tenderness, erythema, rash, urticaria, edema)	Watch closely for signs and symptoms of local irritation or worsening of pretreatment symptoms. Discontinue use if irritation occurs.
LOCAL ANESTHETICS	**Contraindications** Perforated tympanic membrane Hypersensitivity **Undesired Responses** Local irritation; contact dermatitis (burning, stinging, pruritus, tenderness, erythema, rash, urticaria, edema) Rarer side effects: blurred or double vision, seizures, dizziness, diaphoresis, ringing or buzzing in ears, shivering or trembling, slow or irregular heartbeat, and unusual anxiety, excitement, nervousness, or restlessness	Watch closely for signs and symptoms of local irritation or worsening of pretreatment symptoms. Discontinue use if irritation occurs. Local anesthetics should not be used in children <1 y of age because of the threat of absorption through the skin. Rarely benzocaine induces methemoglobinemia, causing respiratory distress and cyanosis (IV methylene blue is the specific therapy for this condition).
CERUMINOLYTICS	**Contraindications** Perforated tympanic membrane Hypersensitivity **Undesired Responses** Local irritation; contact dermatitis (burning, stinging, pruritus, tenderness, erythema, rash, urticaria, edema)	Follow ceruminolytics with gentle irrigation of the external canal with warm water. If irritation occurs, plain anhydrous glycerin may be used as a substitute.

the integrity of the skin, and the use of a cotton pledget or other occlusive dressing. Greater potential for systemic absorption occurs when the external ear canal tissue integrity is compromised by infection or inflammation.[7] Once absorbed, the pharmacokinetics of topical corticosteroids are similar to those of systemic corticosteroids and can lead to comparable undesired responses. For more information on the side effects of systemic corticosteroids see Chapter 42.

Use of both topical and systemic corticosteroids is contraindicated in cases in which the client has herpes simplex, vaccinia, or varicella. If the tympanic membrane is not intact, topical corticosteroids are not used. Overgrowth of organisms, delayed healing, and contact dermatitis are the most common undesired responses to otic corticosteroid-antibiotic therapy.

Anesthetics

Otic anesthetics are used to alleviate pain and discomfort by relieving pressure and reducing inflammation. In addition, otic anesthetics facilitate the removal of excessive or impacted cerumen by decreasing the pain associated with irrigating procedures.[8]

The physiologic response of otic anesthetics on the ear includes reversible stabilization of the neuronal membrane, decreasing its permeability to sodium ions. This inhibition of the depolarization of the neuronal membrane thereby blocks the initiation and conduction of nerve impulses.[9]

Since otic anesthetic drugs do not tend to blanch the tympanic membrane or mask landmarks, the otoscopic examination is not distorted. However, indiscriminate use of anesthetic ear drops may mask symptoms of fulminating infection of the middle ear.

The desired actions of otic anesthetics are reduction of pain and pruritus in acute serous otitis media and acute external otitis. The use of otic anesthetics alone is often inadequate to relieve moderate to severe pain, and the use of oral analgesics may be necessary. Although otic anesthetics may provide symptomatic relief, appropriate antiinfective therapy is necessary when the pain is secondary to infection. Application of otic anesthetics may be repeated every 1 to 2 hours if necessary. Clients with no significant improvement after 48 hours of treatment should be reevaluated. The client should be cautioned not to use otic anesthetics if pregnant or lactating or is an infant less than 1 year of age.[10]

Antibacterials and Drying Agents

Antibacterial otic preparations contain either acetic or boric acid, astringents, and weak antimicrobials (antibacterial and antifungal). In addition, these preparations contain the drying agent isopropyl alcohol. The therapeutic use of otic antibacterial agents include the treatment of superficial infections of the external ear caused by organisms susceptible to the action of the antimicrobial and the acidification of the external ear.[10] Furthermore, the drying agent helps prevent recurrent external ear canal irritation.

The desired action of otic antibacterial agents is to eliminate susceptible organisms from the external auditory canal. After the use of antibacterial ear drops, the ear canal should be carefully dried with compressed air or a hair dryer. The client should be cautioned not to use cotton swabs to dry the canal.

Cerumen Solvents

Ceruminolytics soften, emulsify, and loosen excessive or impacted **cerumen** for removal. These agents act through both the cerumen-softening action of glycerin and the effervescence of the oxygen released from the carbamide peroxide to loosen debris.[10] However, because of the actions of these agents, cerumen solvents are irritating and may cause a severe eczematoid allergic reaction, especially with prolonged exposure. Cerumen removal is necessary for otoscopic examination, audiometry, and when the client experiences discomfort or hearing loss from excessive or dry cerumen.

Specific nursing considerations for cerumen solvents include careful instruction on the importance of limiting exposure to 15 to 30 minutes, flushing the ear canal with lukewarm water, and repeating the procedure for 2 to 10 days until the external ear canal is free of cerumen. In addition, the client should be cautioned to avoid contacting the periaural skin with the ceruminolytic. If contact does occur, the area should be washed immediately with soap and water. If the client experiences excessive irritation from the use of ceruminolytics, adequate softening of the cerumen can often be achieved with plain anhydrous glycerin. Once softened, the cerumen can be flushed out of the external canal with warm water irrigations.

CONCEPT REVIEW

Otic antibiotics treat superficial infections; they act through direct contact with the skin surface. Corticosteroids reduce skin reactions to infections. They are generally used in combination with antibiotic drugs to treat otic infection and inflammation. Systemic absorption of either otic antibiotics or corticosteroids is not desirable.

Otic anesthetics are helpful in relieving pressure and pain and reducing inflammation. They are used in irrigating procedures and in ear examination. They may provide symptomatic relief but often do not resolve the underlying process.

Antibacterials, drying agents, and cerumen solvents aid in preventing infection or impaction in the outer ear.

Life-Span Considerations

Since otic medications have not been systemically researched for safety in pregnant or lactating women, caution should be exercised in their use. Although no specific information about the use of otic preparations in infants or elderly versus younger adults exists, the friability of younger and older skin must be considered. Friability may contribute to a greater incidence of contact dermatitis and systemic absorption. Careful assessment for undesired responses is especially critical in the very young and the elderly. Otic anesthetics should not be given to clients less than 1 year of age because of the potential danger of systemic absorption. In addition, caution should be used when giving otic corticosteroids to infants because the potential for systemic absorption is greater.

Drug-Drug, Drug-Diet, and Drug-Environment Interactions

Benzocaine may antagonize the antibacterial activity of sulfonamides. To avoid any potential drug interaction, benzocaine preparations should be instilled in the ear first. After anesthesia has been achieved, the pool of benzocaine should be removed before the administration of any sulfonamide.

No known drug-diet interactions exist. However, clients allergic to sulfites should be cautioned that some steroidal otic preparations contain this substance (see Table 65–1).

Drug-environment interactions can occur. Clients should be instructed when using any ear preparation to avoid showering, swimming, or any activity that might dilute or wash out the medications.

OTC Otic Preparations

The FDA has approved some over-the-counter (OTC) preparations. However, these products should not be used indiscriminately. The client should consult a primary care provider or discuss his or her problem with the pharmacist be-

TABLE 65–3
OTC Otic Preparations

Preparation	Use
Acetic acid solutions	Mild forms of external otitis and swimmer's ear
Aluminum acetate solution (Burow's solution)	Local itching of the external ear caused by ear dermatitis
Carbamide peroxide	Ceruminolytic
Glycerin	Ceruminolytic

fore self-medicating. Listed in Table 65–3 are some of the types of the OTC otic preparations available.[11]

Ototoxicity

Many drugs damage inner ear structures and are termed *ototoxic*. Any route of administration can result in ototoxicity if a high concentration of the substance accumulates in the inner ear. Symptoms of ototoxic damage often occur even after completion of ototoxic drug therapy. This sometimes makes it difficult to adjust drugs as a means of preventing toxic effects.

Symptoms of **ototoxicity** depend on the area of the inner ear most affected by the drug. When the cochlea is damaged,

TABLE 65–4
Impact of Ototoxic Substances on Auditory and Vestibular Function

Drug	Auditory Problems*	Vestibular Problems*
ANTIBIOTICS	+ +	+
Amikacin (Amikin)	+–+ +	+
Chloramphenicol (Chloromycetin)	+–+ +	+
Erythromycin (E-Mycin)	+ +	+
Gentamicin (Garamycin)	+ +	+
Kanamycin	+ +	+
Neomycin	+ +	+
Streptomycin	+ +	+
Tobramycin (Nebcin)	+ +	+
Vancomycin (Vancocin)		
DIURETICS		
Acetazolamide (Diamox)	+ +	+
Furosemide (Lasix)	+ +	+
Ethacrynic acid (Edecrin)	+ +	+
NONSTEROIDAL ANTIINFLAMMATORY AGENTS		
Salicylates	+ +	
Ibuprofen	+	
Naproxen	+	
Indomethacin	+	+
OTHER DRUGS		
Cisplatin (Platinol)	+	+
Nitrogen mustard	+	+
Quinine (Quinamm)	+	+ +
Quinidine gluconate (Quinaglute)	+	+ +
Alcohol		+ +

Adapted from Ignatavicius, D.D., Workman, M.L., & Mishler, M.M. (Eds.). (1995). *Medical-surgical nursing: A nursing process approach* (2nd ed.). Philadelphia: W.B. Saunders.
*Symbols: +, slight; + +, significant.

the result is tinnitus and sensorineural hearing loss. Damage to the vestibular apparatus can produce vertigo, ataxia, lightheadedness, headache, giddiness, inability to focus or fixate on images, nausea, vomiting, and cold sweats. Vestibular or cochlear symptoms can be experienced unilaterally or bilaterally or can occur simultaneously. Symptoms vary in intensity from mild to severe and can be either reversible or permanent.

Many factors affect ototoxic drugs' effect on individual clients. Factors include dosage, renal function, concomitant use of other ototoxic chemicals, inherent susceptibility, age, and exposure to high-intensity noise.[1,12] Renal function plays an interesting part in the degree of ototoxicity resulting from many drugs. For example, aminoglycoside antibiotic therapy is both highly ototoxic and nephrotoxic. Nephrotoxicity leads to decreased clearing of the antibiotic and an increase in the toxic potential to the inner ear structures.[1]

Categories of ototoxic drugs include aminoglycosides and other antibiotics, loop diuretics, antimalarials, nonsteroidal antiinflammatory agents, and some chemotherapeutic agents.[1,12,13] A list of specific ototoxic substances along with the area affected is in Table 65–4. Aminoglycoside antibiotics are the most highly ototoxic drugs currently used. The half-life of the aminoglycoside in the perilymph of the inner ear is 8 to 15 hours versus the 2- to 3-hour half-life in the serum.

Another highly ototoxic drug is neomycin, a substance commonly found in topical otic preparations. Neomycin causes ototoxicity when given both systemically and topically. Because of the problems associated with the possible application of this toxic substance to middle ear structures, extreme caution must be used if neomycin is indicated for clients whose tympanic membrane is not intact.

Thorough client assessment and teaching are necessary to prevent extensive and permanent damage of the ear by potentially ototoxic preparations. Obtaining a drug history is necessary to detect clients who are taking numerous ototoxic drugs. Laboratory work to assess renal function and serum drug levels is also useful in determining the potential damage a drug may have. Clients should be taught to report immediately symptoms such as tinnitus, dizziness, fullness in the ears, changes in sound discrimination, or hearing loss to their health care provider.

CONCEPT REVIEW

Caution should always be used in administering otic drugs to pregnant or lactating women since the effects of these drugs have not been studied.

Clients must be informed of symptoms of ototoxicity. Damage to the inner ear structures is possible from a variety of drugs. The client must report symptoms promptly to prevent permanent damage.

SUMMARY

This chapter reviews the basic anatomy and physiology of the ear, therapeutic uses of ear preparations, and nursing considerations for clients when using ear preparations. Ear preparations are administered externally for the purposes of infection control, pain and inflammation reduction, and general hygiene of the ear. Efficacy of these drugs is best assured through careful client teaching. Teaching primarily includes reasons for administration, how to administer otic drugs, length of treatment, and potential undesired clinical responses. Indiscriminate and inaccurate use of otic preparations can result in sensory disturbances and emotional and physical pain.

REFERENCES

1. Ignatavicius, D.D., Workman, L.M., Mishler, M.M. (1995). *Medical-surgical nursing: A nursing process approach* (2nd ed.). Philadelphia: W.B. Saunders.
2. Facione, N. (1990). Otitis media: An overview of acute and chronic disease. *Nurse Practitioner, 15*(10), 11–21.
3. E. Neumann, Wallace Laboratories (personal communication, December 1987).
4. Ruddy, J., & Bickerton, R. (1992). Optimum management of the discharging ear. *Drugs, 43*(2), 219–235.
5. Smith, I., Keay, D., & Buxton, P. (1990). Contact hypersensitivity in patients with chronic otitis externa. *Clinical Otolaryngology, 15,* 155–158.
6. Leach, J., Wright, C., Edwards, L., & Meyerhoff, W. (1990). Effect of topical fosfomycin on polymyxin B ototoxicity. *Archives of Otolaryngology, Head and Neck Surgery, 116,* 49–53.
7. DiPiro, J., Talbert, R., Hayes, P., Yee, G., & Posey, M. (Eds.). (1989). *Pharmacotherapy: A pathophysiologic approach.* New York: Elsevier.
8. Woodcock, R.D. (1987). Pharmacologic principles for optimal sensory function. In M.K. Riley (Ed.), *Nursing care of clients with ear, nose, and throat disorders* (pp. 315–337). New York: Springer.
9. McEvoy, G.K. (Ed.). (1992). *AHFS drug information 92.* Bethesda, MD: American Society of Hospital Pharmacists.
10. *USP DI: Advice for the patient: Drug information in lay language* (11th ed.) (1991). Rockville, MD: United States Pharmacopeial Convention.
11. American Pharmaceutical Association. (1990). *Handbook of Nonprescription Drugs* (9th ed.). Washington, DC: Author.
12. Haybach, P.J. (1993). Ototoxicity: The inside story. *Nursing, 6,* 33–41.
13. Norris, C. (1988). Drugs affecting the inner ear. *Drugs, 36,* 754–772.

BIBLIOGRAPHY

Barnes, L., & Pell, R. (1992). *Head and neck pathology: A text atlas of differential diagnosis.* New York: Igaku-Shoin.
Katzung, B. (Ed.). (1992). *Basic and clinical pharmacology.* Norwalk, CT: Appleton & Lange.
Melmon, K.L., Morrelli, H., Hoffman, B., & Nierenberg, D. (Eds.). (1992). *Clinical pharmacology: Basic principles in therapeutics* (3rd ed.). NY: McGraw-Hill.
Pender, D. (1992). *Practical otology.* Philadelphia: JB Lippincott.

CHAPTER 66

Local Anesthesia

CAROL M. VIAMONTES • WILLIAM R. GERBER

⊛ Historical Background

LEARNING OBJECTIVE: Provide a brief history of local anesthesia.

KEY TERM: Local anesthesia

⊛ General Characteristics of Local Anesthetics

LEARNING OBJECTIVES:

Describe the function of local anesthetics.
Describe the types of local anesthetics.
Identify the general characteristics of each type of local anesthetic.

⊛ Therapeutic Uses of Local Anesthetics

LEARNING OBJECTIVES:

Explain how the most appropriate type of local anesthetic is determined.
Discuss the therapeutic uses and common representative drugs for each type of local anesthetic.
List the common types of peripheral nerve blocks.
Describe the administration of an intravenous nerve block.

KEY TERMS:

Topical (surface) anesthetic, surface coolant, local infiltration, peripheral nerve block, intravenous regional block, spinal block, saddle block, epidural (caudal) block

⊛ Nursing Considerations

LEARNING OBJECTIVES:

Review the assessment for local anesthetic administration.
Discuss nursing management for each type of local anesthetic.

KEY TERM: Eutectic mixture

⊛ Local Anesthetic Drugs

LEARNING OBJECTIVES:

List the usual routes of administration and contraindications for use of lidocaine.
Describe the adverse reactions to lidocaine.
Describe potential drug interactions using lidocaine.

⊛ Life-span Considerations

LEARNING OBJECTIVE: Describe the use of local anesthetic drugs throughout the life span.

⊛ Drug-Drug Interactions

LEARNING OBJECTIVE: Discuss potential drug-drug interactions involving local anesthetic drugs.

CONCEPTS AND TERMS TO REVIEW

Review techniques for intravenous administration.
Review anatomy and physiology of the spinal cord.
Reexamine Chapters 3 and 4 for information on dosage forms and routes of administration.
Read in Chapter 32 about lidocaine's use as an antiarrhythmic drug.

---

*A*nesthesia may be general, regional, or local; it may be administered by inhalation, intravenously, or locally by regional block, spinal, epidural, topical, or infiltrative methods. In Chapter 24 drugs administered by intravenous (IV) or inhalation methods were discussed; the focus of that chapter was general anesthetic drugs. The focus of this chapter is drugs used as local anesthetics.

HISTORICAL BACKGROUND

Local anesthesia is a process whereby sensory and motor innervation of a body part is interrupted by means of a chemical. The client experiences loss of sensation to a specific body part without accompanying loss of consciousness or loss of control of other vital functions. The anesthetic effect is usually transient and reversible.

The first local anesthetic discovered was cocaine, which was found in the leaves of the *Erythroxylon coca* plant. Peruvians chewed these leaves to achieve a mood-elevating effect. A secondary effect of chewing the leaves was a numbness of the oral cavity.

In 1884 Sigmund Freud used cocaine to wean a colleague from morphine addiction; this resulted in the individual's developing a cocaine addiction. In the same year Karl Koller, a Viennese ophthalmologist, discovered that cocaine could be used as a corneal anesthetic. The popularity of cocaine quickly spread; by the end of 1885 it was used in general, otolaryngology, obstetric, and gynecologic surgeries. Scientists discovered that diluting cocaine allowed infiltration of large body areas. By 1908 other routes of administration were used. However, because cocaine was addictive and somewhat toxic, other types of local anesthetic agents were developed. In 1948 lidocaine was synthesized. It had a superior ability to infiltrate body parts and not cause drug dependence. In addition, allergic reactions were rare.[1-3]

GENERAL CHARACTERISTICS OF LOCAL ANESTHETICS

Normally conduction of nerve impulses occurs as follows: a stimulus causes rapid depolarization of the nerve cell membrane. Depolarization occurs because sodium ions move from the extracellular to the intracellular space through sodium channels in the membrane. A gate mechanism in the channel controls the flow of the sodium ions. This depolarization is transmitted along the length of the nerve fiber. Potassium ions also move from the intracellular to the extracellular space through the same channels, causing depolarization and bringing the nerve cells back to a resting state.[1,2]

Local anesthetics prevent depolarization by diffusing across the nerve cell membrane. The anesthetic agent binds with certain receptors in the gate mechanism to block the sodium channels and inhibit the flow of sodium ions intracellularly. The result is a conduction blockade.

Local anesthetics act on both sensory and motor nerves. However, small, nonmyelinated pain fibers are most sensitive and are depressed first. Subsequent loss of function of other types of nerves occurs in the following order: temperature, touch, proprioception, and skeletal muscle tone.[1,2,4]

Local anesthetics are classified according to their chemistry and on the basis of clinical application. Chemically, local anesthetics are considered either esters or amides. Both types are comprised of aromatic, intermediate, and amine portions, which have lipophilic and hydrophilic properties. The ester or amide portion determines if the drug will be inactivated by hydrolysis in the plasma or metabolized in the liver.

Absorption of local anesthetics varies, depending on the site of injection, dose and concentration of the drug, degree of vasodilation caused by the drug, and presence or absence of a vasoconstrictor. Generally a more concentrated, higher dose shortens the onset and lengthens the duration of the effect. Vasodilation is caused by a direct effect on the blood vessels and anesthesia of sympathetic vasoconstrictor fibers. It results in more rapid absorption and occurrence of toxic side effects. To delay rate of absorption, vasoconstrictors can be mixed with local anesthetics.

CONCEPT REVIEW

Local anesthetics act on sensory and motor nerves, affecting loss of function in this order: temperature, touch, proprioception, and skeletal muscle tone. Local anesthetics are esters or amides, depending on whether the drug is inactivated by hydrolysis in the plasma or is metabolized in the liver.

Absorption depends on the site of injection, dose and concentration of the drug, degree of vasodilation caused by the drug, and presence or absence of a vasoconstrictor. To delay absorption, vasoconstrictors can be mixed with the anesthetics.

THERAPEUTIC USES OF LOCAL ANESTHETICS

As mentioned previously, local anesthetics are classified according to their chemical properties. In addition, they are classified according to clinical use, including topical use, local infiltration, peripheral nerve block techniques, and regional techniques such as epidural, caudal, and spinal blocks. The decision made by the primary care provider about the most appropriate local anesthetic is determined by the following criteria: (1) type of surgery; (2) desired speed of onset of anesthesia; and (3) site of injection of anesthetic.

Topical Use

Topical, or surface, anesthetics are used in producing anesthesia of the mucous membranes, wounds, burns, and various skin irritations. Topical anesthetics penetrate intact skin poorly but are more rapidly absorbed through mucous membranes and broken skin. They are used most commonly in minor surgical procedures to anesthetize the mucous membranes of the nose, mouth, tracheobronchial tree, esophagus, eye, rectum, genitalia, and urethra. They can also be used to alleviate the pain and itching associated with some types of dermatitis. Commonly used topical agents include cocaine, benzocaine, dibucaine hydrochloride, and tetracaine.

In certain minor surgical procedures such as arthrocentesis, local anesthesia can be achieved by freezing the skin surface with a **surface coolant.** The anesthetic effect is of relatively short duration, usually less than 60 seconds. Ethyl chloride is an example of a surface coolant. To apply ethyl chloride, the operative site should be prepared with an appropriate antiseptic. Petrolatum can be applied around the prepared site to protect the adjacent skin surface. Ethyl chloride is sprayed from a distance of 2 to 4 inches for a few seconds until the skin surface is white (usually 2 to 3 seconds). The injection or incision must be made quickly while the skin is still white. Caution should be used in spraying the skin surface for too long, for doing so can cause permanent tissue damage.[1,5]

Local Infiltration

Local infiltration anesthesia is produced by directly injecting the subcutaneous tissue of the area to be anesthetized. Only nerve endings are blocked; no attempt is made to identify individual nerves. A relatively dilute, somewhat large volume of solution is needed to anesthetize the operative site.

Certain drugs can be added to the anesthetic solution to enhance its effect. Vasoconstrictors such as epinephrine or phenylephrine delay absorption and prolong anesthesia. The vasoconstrictive effect also limits bleeding in the operative field. Sodium bicarbonate added to the anesthetic solution just before injection raises the solution's pH and speeds the onset of anesthesia. Adding sodium bicarbonate (1 ml of 8.4% solution) to 10 ml of lidocaine or mepivacaine may lessen the pain experienced by the client during the injection.[6–8]

Infiltration anesthesia is indicated for dental and minor surgical procedures such as excision of skin lesions or wound debridement. It is less effective in infected areas because the high acidity of the infected tissue decreases the drug's ability to infiltrate. In obstetrics local infiltration of perineal tissues is done to alleviate the pain associated with vaginal delivery and for repair of torn perineal tissues (episiotomy). Infiltration of subcutaneous tissues can also be used to treat chronic pain conditions arising from acute herpes zoster, post-herpatic neuralgias, subcutaneous fibrotic nodules, and neuromas. Commonly used anesthetic agents include lidocaine hydrochloride and bupivacaine hydrochloride.

Peripheral Nerve Blocks

A **peripheral nerve block** is injected into or around a specific nerve, a nerve trunk, or several nerve trunks emerging from the spinal column (paravertebral block). The effect is control of pain in an area supplied by that specific nerve or nerve trunk(s). A smaller volume of more concentrated solution is used rather than the larger, more dilute solution used in local infiltration. Lidocaine, bupivacaine, and chloroprocaine hydrochloride are used for this type of local anesthesia.[1]

Peripheral nerve blocks are used most commonly for surgical procedures.[4,9] They can also be used to diagnose and treat chronic pain conditions such as myofascial or idiopathic myalgias, phantom limb pain, vasospasm disorders, visceral pain, upper abdominal pain, burning pain of upper extremities and head, acute herpes zoster, and causalgias. Some of the more common types of peripheral nerve blocks and affected anatomic areas are listed below:

- **Cervical plexus block** above neck and supraclavicular fossa
- **Brachial plexus block** upper extremity from shoulder to hand

- **Intercostobrachial nerve block** medial aspect of upper arm
- **Median, ulnar, radial nerve blocks** hand
- **Intercostal nerve block** ribs, intercostal and subcostal spaces
- **Lumbar plexus block** lower extremity
- **Ankle block** foot

In obstetrics pudendal and paracervical blocks are commonly used.[10] The pudendal block involves injecting the anesthetic solution into the point where the pudendal nerve emerges from the sacrospinous ligament to innervate the perineum. In the paracervical block local anesthetic is injected at the 4 o'clock and 8 o'clock positions in the vaginal fornices. This block is effective in relieving pain associated with uterine contraction but can cause fetal bradycardia. The use of fetal heart monitoring is necessary when using the paracervical block.

Intravenous Regional Block

Intravenous (IV) regional block (Bier's block) is used for surgeries of short duration (40 to 60 minutes) of the arm or leg. A double pneumatic tourniquet is applied to the extremity, which then is elevated to drain it of venous blood. The distal tourniquet is inflated first to 300 mm Hg, followed by inflation of the proximal tourniquet. The distal tourniquet then is released, and the extremity assumes a mottled appearance. An anesthetic, usually lidocaine, is injected intravenously into the limb. The anesthetic diffuses across the peripheral circulation to the nerves. Onset of anesthesia is immediate, and duration continues until the proximal tourniquet is deflated.

When the tourniquet is released, the client is observed carefully for possible systemic toxic effects of the anesthesia. The tourniquet should not be deflated any sooner than 30 minutes after injection to ensure the anesthetic has become "fixed" in the tissue and to reduce the incidence of rapid systemic absorption.[9,11–13]

Spinal Block

Spinal, or intradural, block involves the injection of a local anesthetic into the cerebrospinal fluid in the subarachnoid space. A small volume of the anesthetic agent is mixed with a dextrose solution to make it hyperbaric (specific gravity heavier than cerebrospinal fluid). The solution is injected, and the client's position is adjusted to direct the flow either up, down, or to one side of the spinal cord. Once the desired dermatomes (skin regions) are anesthetized, the client is repositioned for surgery.[1]

Spinal anesthesia is used most commonly in clients having surgery in the lower abdomen below the umbilicus, the groin, or the lower extremities. A specific type of spinal anesthesia used in obstetrics is the saddle block.[10] The client is positioned so that she is sitting upright as the anesthetic is injected. This position is maintained until the anesthetic has diffused downward to anesthetize the perineal area. The body parts anesthetized are those areas that would have contact with a saddle when riding, hence the name **saddle block.** Local anesthetics used for spinal blocks include bupivacaine with dextrose, lidocaine with glucose, procaine, and tetracaine.

Epidural Block

Epidural (caudal) block is achieved by injecting the local anesthetic into the epidural space surrounding the dura mater at either the lumbar or sacral (caudal) level (Fig. 66–1). The anesthetic acts on the dorsal root ganglia and the nerve roots as they exit the spinal cord through the intervertebral foramina. Larger volumes of the anesthetic are needed than with a spinal block, and the onset of action is slower. The advantage of epidural over spinal anesthesia is that clients are less likely to experience untoward side effects because the anesthetic is not injected directly into the spinal cord. Clients are also less likely to experience spinal (postdural puncture) headaches since there is no leakage of spinal fluid.[10]

Epidural block is used commonly in obstetrics to control labor pain. It can also be used in other types of surgery involving the lower abdomen and lower extremities. In the treatment of chronic pain epidural anesthesia can be provided through a single injection for short-term treatment.[10] For long-term therapy an epidural catheter is inserted and is connected to an infusion pump.[4] Commonly used local anesthetics for epidural or caudal blocks include mepivacaine, bupivacaine, chloroprocaine, etidocaine, and lidocaine.

Specific information about individual local anesthetics is summarized in Table 66–1.

CONCEPT REVIEW

Topical anesthetics have a short duration of action. They are absorbed best through mucous membranes and broken skin and are used most commonly in minor surgical procedures.

Local anesthetics are injected into the subcutaneous tissue of the area to be anesthetized where they block nerve endings. The solution is fairly dilute and is used in relatively large volume. Local anesthetics can be mixed with drugs to delay or speed up the onset of anesthesia.

Peripheral nerve blocks involve injection of an anesthetic into or around a specific nerve, nerve trunk, or several nerve trunks emerging from the spinal col-

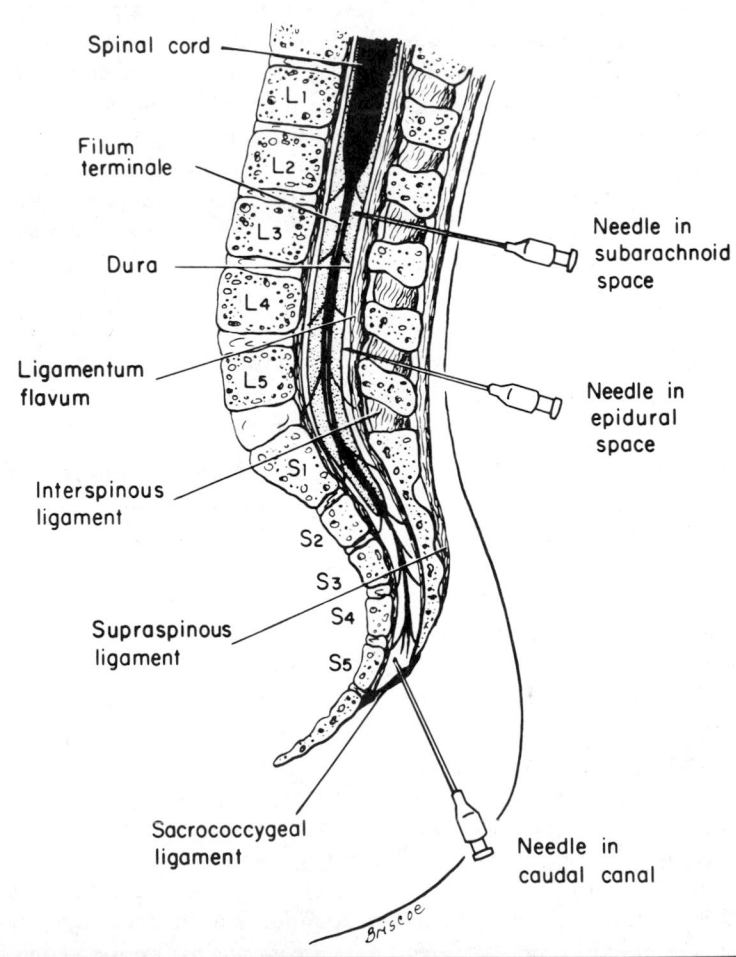

FIGURE 66–1   Schematic diagram of lumbosacral anatomy. Illustration shows needle placement for subarachnoid, lumbar epidural, and caudal blocks. (From Shnider, S.M., & Levinson, G. (1993). Anesthesia for obstetrics [3rd ed.]. Baltimore: Williams & Wilkins.)

umn to achieve control of pain in the area supplied by those nerves. The anesthetic is usually small in volume and is more concentrated than those used as a local anesthetic.

- IV regional block is used for short-duration surgeries of the arm or leg. A tourniquet must be maintained for at least 30 minutes after the injection to ensure the anesthetic is fixed in the tissue and will not create untoward systemic effects.
- Spinal block and epidural block are used primarily for surgeries below the umbilicus or during childbirth. In a spinal block the anesthetic agent is injected into the cerebrospinal fluid in the subarachnoid space. In an epidural block the drug is injected into the epidural space surrounding the dura mater at the lumbar or sacral level. Epidural block requires the use of larger volumes of anesthetic than does a spinal block and has a later onset of action, but it usually has fewer undesired clinical responses.

⊞ NURSING CONSIDERATIONS

The use of local anesthetics is gaining popularity for a variety of reasons. These anesthetics are used increasingly in high-risk populations such as the elderly and clients with cardiopulmonary diseases because these clients are not usually candidates for general anesthesia. In addition, more operative procedures have been identified that can be done in an ambulatory care setting with the use of local anesthetics. Various chronic pain conditions are also being managed with local anesthetics. Nurses currently see more of these types of clients and have more responsibility in their management.

Assessing   The purpose of a preanesthetic assessment is to gather enough information to determine a safe plan of care for the client undergoing any type of surgery with anesthesia. The first step is a **preanesthetic history.** The types of questions to ask are determined by the type of surgery and the local anesthetic but should include the following: age, drug history, past medical history (list of previous illnesses and surgeries), drug allergies and adverse reactions to drugs, and previous experiences with anesthesias. When asking the client about past experiences with anesthetics, include questions about complications and satisfaction with the anesthetic. Also determine if other family members have had complications from local anesthetics. A review of the medical record may yield additional information.

A review of systems can be used as a guide for a brief **physical assessment.** For cardiovascular status, obtain blood pressure and pulse. Determine if the client has active coronary artery or cardiac disease that may contradict the use of a vasoconstrictor as an additive to the local anesthetic. Respiratory assessment should include type and rate of respirations and smoking history. Neurologic assessment should include level of consciousness and orientation and preexisting neurologic symptoms (e.g., numbness or weakness of extremities).

Determine bowel and bladder status of clients receiving epidural or spinal anesthetics. For oropharyngeal or nasopharyngeal surgeries, determine if the client has a dental prosthesis or loose teeth.

In most ambulatory care settings time for a thorough preanesthetic assessment is limited. Many facilities make use of a health history or survey, which the client can complete during registration. The nurse can quickly review this information and ask questions about particular problem areas.

In addition to gathering information and doing a physical assessment, establish a bond with the client to allay fears about the anesthetic. Projecting a calm, unhurried appearance and answering all questions will reassure the client that he or she will receive optimal care.

Diagnosing   Many nursing diagnoses can be derived from the preanesthetic assessment. Some of them follow:
- Anxiety related to perceived loss of sensation from effects of anesthesia.
- Anxiety related to insufficient knowledge of perioperative and postoperative routines.
- High risk for aspiration related to depressive effect of anesthetic on gag reflex.
- High risk for injury to anesthetized body part related to freezing effects of surface coolant.
- High risk for injury to anesthetized body part(s) related to depressive effect of anesthetic on normal body defense mechanisms.
- High risk for alteration in tissue perfusion related to vasoconstrictive effects of epinephrine.
- High risk for altered respiratory function related to effects of local anesthetic.
- High risk for altered cardiovascular function related to effects of anesthesia.
- Alteration in comfort related to spinal headache.

Other nursing diagnoses may be identified based on the individual needs of the client.

Planning   As noted, preoperative contact with the client is limited. For this reason, standardized teaching plans developed for each population can be adapted for individual use. General goals should include (1) providing preoperative instruction to allay anxieties and to assist the client in coping with the anesthetic experience and (2) maintaining client safety during the administration of the anesthetic agent and throughout the duration of its effect.

Expected outcomes for the plan of care might include the following:
- Client identifies the source of anxiety and uses effective coping mechanisms.
- Client demonstrates understanding of basic perioperative and postoperative routines.
- Client does not experience aspiration.
- Client's skin surface and underlying tissues are protected from permanent damage.
- Client remains free of injury.
- Client's respiratory function is maintained.
- Client's cardiovascular functions are maintained.
- Client verbalizes pain relief.

TABLE 66–1
Local Anesthetics

Drug Name	Dosage and Route of Administration	Nursing Considerations
LIDOCAINE HYDROCHLORIDE (Xylocaine)	**Injection** LOCAL INFILTRATION, PERIPHERAL NERVE BLOCK, IV REGIONAL BLOCK, CERVICAL OR LUMBAR SYMPATHETIC BLOCK, EPIDURAL BLOCK, CAUDAL BLOCK Usual dose: 0.5%–4.0%, depending on site and length of procedure; duration, 1–1½ h but can be prolonged with epinephrine SADDLE BLOCK IN CESAREAN SECTION, SPINAL BLOCK IN LOWER ABDOMINAL SURGERY Usual dose: 1.5%–5%; onset of action, 3–20 min; duration, 1–1½ h	**Assess** Inquire about known cardiovascular disease; combination of lidocaine with epinephrine is used only with caution in client with this condition. Ask about history of hepatic disease; drug must be used with caution in such clients. Assess whether procedure involves surgery of fingers, toes, nose, or ear; use of epinephrine combination is contraindicated in such cases. Determine how solution with preservative will be used; it may not be used for epidural, caudal, or spinal block. Assess cardiovascular status (pulse, blood pressure). Assess respiratory function. Assess injection site for skin color and temperature. **Implement** Use small-gauge needle (No. 25–27). Check label carefully since solution is available both with and without epinephrine (see above). Discard cloudy, discolored, or crystallized solutions. Keep resuscitative equipment and emergency drugs available during anesthesia. Explain to client which body parts will be anesthetized, how long anesthesia will last, and the order in which sensation will return—proprioception, pressure, temperature, pain. Reassure client that effects are temporary. Instruct client not to chew gum, eat, or drink until ability to swallow returns. Do not exceed recommended dosage. Position client so that areas over bony prominences do not become reddened. Protect anesthetized extremities. For epidural block, give a test dose first to determine correct placement of catheter. **Monitor** For epidural and spinal blocks, monitor pulse, blood pressure, level of sensory loss, level of consciousness, urinary and bowel functions. Monitor respiratory function every hour, noting skin color, temperature, level of consciousness. If respiratory depression occurs, maintain open airway, administer oxygen, and contact primary care provider. Monitor pulse and blood pressure. If changes in pulse rate or BP occur, attach cardiac monitor to client and contact primary care provider. **Evaluate** Observe for desired anesthetic effect. As anesthetic effect wears off, note return of circulation.
	Topical SKIN PROBLEMS (CUTS, SCRATCHES, SUNBURN, INSECT BITES, BURNS, CONTACT DERMATITIS) Usual dose: up to 5 g (6-in length of 5% ointment), not to exceed 17 g in 24 h; onset of action, 3–5 min; duration, 1–1½ h MUCOUS MEMBRANE ANESTHESIA FOR ENDOTRACHEAL INTUBATION AND EXAMINATION OF THE URETHRA Usual dose of 2% jelly: depends on type of procedure but no more than 300 mg in 12 h; onset of action, 3–5 min; duration, 1–1½ h MUCOUS MEMBRANE ANESTHESIA OF MOUTH, NOSE, AND THROAT Usual dose of 4% solution: depends on procedure; onset of action, 3–5 min; duration, 1–1½ h	Apply ointment with cotton-tipped applicator. Instruct client to refrain from eating and drinking for 1 h after oral administration.

TABLE 66–1 *Continued*
Local Anesthetics

907

Drug Name	Dosage and Route of Administration	Nursing Considerations
LIDOCAINE HYDROCHLORIDE —CONT'D	ANESTHESIA OF MOUTH AND OROPHARYNX Usual dose of 10% oral topical spray: 1–2 metered sprays q1-2 h; onset of action, 3–5 min; duration, 1–1½ h	See above.
	INFLAMMATION AND PAIN OF MOUTH AND OROPHARYNX Usual dose of 2% viscous solution: 15 ml q3h not to exceed eight doses in 24 h; onset of action, 3–5 min; duration, 2–3 h	See above. Instruct client to swish solution in mouth; client may gargle solution for pharyngeal pain.
Bupivacaine Hydrochloride (Marcaine, Sensorcaine)	LOCAL INFILTRATION, PERIPHERAL NERVE BLOCK, RETROBULBAR BLOCK, SYMPATHETIC BLOCK, EPIDURAL, CAUDAL BLOCKS Usual dose: 0.25%–0.75%, depending on type of procedure; onset of action, immediate; duration, 3 h	Use is contraindicated with paracervical block and with topical anesthesia. See lidocaine.
	DENTAL SURGERY: LOCAL INFILTRATION, MAXILLARY AND MANDIBULAR BLOCKS Usual dose: 0.5% with 1:200,000 epinephrine; onset of action, 2–10 min; duration, up to 7 h	
	SPINAL ANESTHESIA FOR LOWER ABDOMINAL, PERINEAL SURGERIES AND CESAREAN SECTIONS Usual dose: 0.5%–0.75%; onset of action, immediate; duration, 3 h	
Mepivacaine Hydrochloride (Carbocaine)	LOCAL INFILTRATION, PERIPHERAL NERVE BLOCK, EPIDURAL AND CAUDAL BLOCKS, TRANSVAGINAL (PARACERVICAL PLUS PUDENDAL) BLOCK, THERAPEUTIC BLOCK FOR PAIN MANAGEMENT Usual dose: 0.5%–3%, depending on type of procedure; onset of action, 15 min; duration, 3 h; may be prolonged when mixed with levonordefrin	Use is contraindicated in clients with known hypersensitivity to methylparaben or in clients needing spinal anesthesia. Use caution in administering solutions with levonordefrin to clients with known cardiovascular disease. Monitor fetal heart rate when used as a paracervical block.
Procaine Hydrochloride (Novocain)	LOCAL INFILTRATION, PERIPHERAL NERVE BLOCKS, EPIDURAL BLOCKS, SPINAL BLOCK Usual dose: 10% for spinal anesthesia; 0.25%–0.5% for other blocks and local infiltration; onset of action, 2–5 min; duration, 1 h; may be prolonged when mixed with epinephrine	Use is contraindicated in clients with known hypersensitivity to para-aminobenzoic acid (PABA) derivatives. See lidocaine.
Chloroprocaine Hydrochloride (Nesacaine)	LOCAL INFILTRATION, PERIPHERAL NERVE BLOCK, RETROBULBAR BLOCK, EPIDURAL AND CAUDAL BLOCKS Usual dose: 1%–3%, depending on type of procedure; onset of action, 6–12 min; duration, 1 h; may be prolonged with epinephrine	Use is contraindicated in clients with known hypersensitivity to PABA derivatives. Use is contraindicated with spinal anesthesia. Monitor fetal heart rate when drug is used as a paracervical block. See lidocaine.
Tetracaine Hydrochloride (Pontocaine)	**Injection** SADDLE BLOCK Usual dose: 2–5 mg for vaginal delivery	Use is contraindicated in clients with known hypersensitivity to PABA derivatives. Tetracaine may be mixed with cerebrospinal fluid for prolonged spinal anesthesia. Solution may be cloudy. Store in refrigerator; protect from light.
	SPINAL ANESTHESIA TO PERINEUM 5 mg	
	SPINAL ANESTHESIA TO PERINEUM AND LOWER EXTREMITIES 10 mg	
	SPINAL ANESTHESIA UP TO COSTAL MARGIN 15–20 mg; onset of action, 15 min; duration, 3 h	See lidocaine.
	Injection with Glucose SADDLE BLOCK, SPINAL ANESTHESIA Usual dose: 2–5 mg in 10% glucose solution; onset of action, 15 min; duration, 3 h	

Table continued on following page.

TABLE 66–1 *Continued*
Local Anesthetics

Drug Name	Dosage and Route of Administration	Nursing Considerations
Tetracaine hydrochloride *Continued*	**Ophthalmic** CORNEAL AND CONJUNCTIVAL IRRITATION, ANESTHESIA FOR TONOMETRY, GONIOSCOPY, SUTURE REMOVAL FROM CORNEA, REMOVAL OF CORNEAL FOREIGN BODY Usual dose: 0.5% solution: 1–2 drops in eye before procedure; onset of action, 5 min; duration, 1–2 h	Recommend that client use eye patch after procedure. Inform client that transient eye stinging may be experienced for 30 sec after instillation. Systemic absorption is unlikely. Repeat use is not recommended because epithelial damage may occur.
	Topical HEMORRHOIDAL PAIN, PRURITUS, SUNBURN, CONTACT DERMATITIS, INSECT BITES Usual dose 5% ointment or 1% cream: no more than 1 oz daily	Clean and dry area thoroughly before application. Discontinue use if rash appears.
Benzocaine (Anbesol, Orajel, Americaine, Hurricaine, Auralgan)	**Topical Solution (Otic)** PAIN OF OTITIS MEDIA AND CERUMEN REMOVAL Usual dose: one dropper in affected ear canal; frequency determined by condition; duration, 1–2 h	Use is contraindicated in client with perforated eardrum. Keep drug in tightly capped, dark container. Do not use for more than 2 d. Benzocaine is used with an antibiotic for otitis media.
	5% Cream, 5% or 20% Ointment, 20% Aerosol Spray (Cutaneous) PAIN, BURNING, ITCHING FROM CONTACT DERMATITIS, SUNBURN, INSECT BITES Usual dose determined by condition	Use is contraindicated in clients with hypersensitivity to PABA derivatives (usually found in sun-blocking agents). Avoid contact with eyes. Avoid inhalation of aerosol spray. Observe affected area for allergic reactions (redness, swelling). Use is contraindicated if affected area is infected.
	20% Gel, Aerosol, Solution (Diagnostic) LOCAL ANESTHESIA BEFORE LARYNGOSCOPY, SIGMOIDOSCOPY, PROCTOSCOPY, AND INSERTION OF URINARY CATHETERS Usual dose: determined by procedure; duration, 1–2 h	Tell client to avoid eating or drinking for 1 h after application to oropharyngeal area.
	20% Ointment (Rectal) PAIN FROM HEMORRHOIDS AND RECTAL IRRITATION Usual dose: one applicator in rectum bid	Cleanse and dry rectal area before application. Discontinue if rectal bleeding or rash occurs.
	10% to 20% Jelly, 5- to 10-mg Lozenge, 20% Paste (Dental) PAIN FROM CANKER SORES, COLD SORES, GUM IRRITATION; PHARYNGEAL PAIN Usual dose: apply to affected area as needed	
Benzocaine, Butamben, Tetracaine (Cetacaine)	**Topical Solution or Spray, Gel, Ointment (Contains Benzocaine (14%), Tetracaine Hydrochloride (2%), Butamben (2%))** Usual dose as determined by procedure	Tell client to apply spray for 1–2 sec only. Apply ointment or solution with a cotton pledget. Hold the pledget in place until anesthesia is achieved. Do not apply to inflamed or ulcerated areas.

Implementing   Nursing interventions for clients receiving local anesthetics vary, depending on the type of local anesthetic, route of administration, and the operative procedure. In this section each major category of local anesthetic is presented with a brief discussion of nursing management.

Topical anesthetics   Topical anesthetics are administered to the oral cavity in the form of a jelly, paste, spray, lozenge, or solution for swishing and gargling. Instruct the client not to swallow the anesthetic solution unless specific instructions are given to do so. There is a potential for aspiration related to the depressive effect of the anesthetic on the gag reflex. Instruct the client not to eat or drink until he or she is able to swallow, usually 1 hour after administration. Duration of anesthesia may be slightly longer if epinephrine is used.

Local anesthetic preparations for skin problems usually come in a cream, ointment, or topical spray. Before application, cleanse the area thoroughly, dry it, and inspect it for changes in skin integrity. Report signs of wound infection to the primary care provider. If pruritus is present, instruct the client not to scratch affected areas. Keep client's nails trimmed short to avoid injury. Cotton mitts can be worn by small children or disoriented adults.

Apply creams or ointments sparingly to the affected area with a cotton ball or cotton-tipped applicator. Place a dressing or plastic wrap over the site to enhance the effectiveness of the medication. When using a topical spray, hold the container 3 to 4 inches from the site; spray sparingly.

A topical local anesthetic agent of interest is eutectic mixture of local anesthetics (EMLA). It comes as either a cream or ointment and is a formulation of two local anesthetics, lidocaine and prilocaine. A **eutectic mixture** consists of two or more chemical substances with different properties that can be dissolved together and remain compatible. The two anesthetics are present in greater concentrations than would be possible if they were formulated in individual preparations. EMLA is used in pediatric patients as a dermal anesthetic for relieving the pain associated with venipunctures.[13] It is applied to the selected venipuncture site 30 to 60 minutes before needle insertion. Duration of anesthetic effect varies with the length of time the cream is in contact with skin, but it usually lasts 1 to 2 hours.[14,15]

Rectal preparations come in the form of a suppository, ointment, cream, or aerosol foam. Suppositories are kept refrigerated until used. They can be lubricated with water or a water-soluble jelly to facilitate insertion. An applicator is usually provided with creams, ointments, and aerosol foams. The applicator should be cleaned with mild soap and water between uses. If bleeding occurs, the client should stop using the preparation and contact the primary care provider.

Topical eye anesthetics come in the form of a solution and are instilled in the eye with a dropper. Instruct the client to use the exact number of drops prescribed and not to allow the dropper to come in contact with the tissue surrounding the eye or the eyelid. Protect the anesthetized eye from injury; the anesthetic effect results in temporary absence of the blink reflex. Instruct the client to avoid rubbing the eye. An eye patch can be worn to prevent the introduction of foreign bodies.

Local anesthesia by injection   Before preparing any local anesthetic for injection, examine the solution for discoloration, cloudiness, and crystalline formation. If these conditions exist, discard the solution. Note the presence of additives such as epinephrine or preservatives. Anesthetics with preservatives are not used for spinal blocks. Discard bottles of anesthetic agents without preservatives after each use.

Before the procedure be sure resuscitative equipment and emergency drugs are present in case of an anaphylactic reaction. Place a blood pressure cuff on the client, and prepare a cardiac monitor for possible use. Short and ultrashort barbiturates (e.g., phenobarbital) must be available in the event of confusion. Access to short-acting muscle relaxants is necessary in case the client experiences respiratory or cardiac depression.

The client receiving local anesthetics by injection experiences a loss of sensation to the anesthetized part of the body, resulting in a potential for injury to the affected body part and anxiety to the client. The anesthetized area should be protected from injury since normal body defense mechanisms are absent. Anxiety can result because the client is unfamiliar with the changes in perception (i.e., absence of pain, loss of temperature and pressure sensations). Instruct the client that the anesthesia is temporary and sensation will return in a certain period of time.[14,16]

The client may also experience anxiety because he or she is awake during the procedure, especially if he or she lacks sufficient knowledge about perioperative and postoperative routines. Provide detailed explanations during and after the procedure to allay anxiety. Also use touch to provide reassurance to a frightened client.

There are also specific nursing considerations for the client receiving epidural, caudal, and spinal blocks.[10,17,18] With **epidural** and **caudal anesthesia,** the client usually is placed in a lateral decubitus position. The area for catheter insertion is identified and the skin cleansed with a disinfectant and draped. Using strict aseptic technique, the primary care provider inserts a large-gauge needle followed by the catheter. The needle is then removed. A test dose of the local anesthetic with epinephrine (usually 3 ml) is injected to rule out accidental placement of the catheter intravenously or in the subarachnoid or subdural spaces. Significant heart rate increase or seizures occurring within 60 seconds indicate IV injection. Respiratory depression, hypotension, generalized sensory anesthesia, and motor paralysis occurring within 3 to 5 minutes indicate subarachnoid and subdural injection.

Once correct placement of the epidural catheter is assured, tape the catheter securely to the client's back and monitor it for kinking, breaking, or slippage out of place during the procedure. Any movement by the client necessitates rechecking the position of the catheter. For the duration of the anesthesia, monitor pulse, blood pressure, skin color, and respirations. Vasodilation and cessation of sweating in the lower extremities are signs of effective anesthesia.

In the event of hypotension, stop the anesthesia, elevate the client's legs, increase IV fluid infusion, administer oxygen, and notify the primary care provider. Signs of impending confusion are increasing anxiety, restlessness, and twitching or trembling of the extremities.

Urinary retention sometimes occurs as a complication of epidural or caudal anesthesia.[19] The anesthetic can block motor and sensory inervation of the bladder. If the client voids in small amounts or has difficulty voiding, palpate the lower abdomen for urinary retention. Insert a urinary catheter if indicated.

In obstetrics an epidural or a caudal block is commonly used. During anesthetic administration, contractions are monitored. Epidural anesthesia diminishes contraction sensation and decreases the client's urge to push; thus labor can be delayed. After epidural catheter insertion, the client is maintained in a left lateral decubitus position to relieve pressure of the uterus on the inferior vena cava. Monitor the fetal heart rate because the anesthetic may cross the placental barrier and cause fetal bradycardia.

Monitor clients receiving **spinal anesthesia** for changes in cardiovascular, respiratory, urinary tract, and gastrointestinal (GI) status. A small percentage of clients may experience a spinal or postdural puncture headache, which is due to leakage of cerebrospinal fluid through the needle hole. A spinal headache usually disappears spontaneously in 2 to 3 days but can be treated with analgesics and large volumes of either IV or oral fluids to increase cerebrospinal fluid volume. If these conservative measures fail, the treatment of choice is an epidural blood patch. In this procedure 5 to 10 ml of the client's blood is placed in the epidural space to form a clot. The client is kept supine for 20 to 30 minutes after the procedure.

Other nursing measures for the client receiving spinal anesthesia include protecting the anesthetized area from injury and monitoring return of sensation. In some clients a transient nerve palsy occurs within 2 weeks after anesthesia. If this occurs, the client should immediately contact the primary care provider.

Evaluating To determine the effectiveness of the plan of care, review the expected outcomes with the client. If the outcomes were met, the nursing diagnosis is resolved. If outcomes have not been met, alter the plan of care by including additional nursing interventions or by rewriting the diagnosis.

LOCAL ANESTHETIC DRUGS
LOCAL ANESTHETIC PROTOTYPE
LIDOCAINE HYDROCHLORIDE

Lidocaine hydrochloride (Xylocaine) is one of the most frequently used local anesthetics.

Pharmacokinetics After its topical application, the onset of action of lidocaine is 3 to 5 minutes. For injection, the onset of action for a sensory block ranges from 3 to 20 minutes. Motor block is more complete with higher concentrations, ranging from a minimal block with 0.5% solution to a complete sensory and motor block with 2% solution. The duration of the block varies, depending on the technique, type of block, and drug concentration;

usually with lidocaine there is adequate anesthesia for 1½ to 2 hours.

Lidocaine is completely absorbed after administration. It is carried in the bloodstream in both free and protein-bound forms. Metabolism occurs in the liver where approximately 90% of it is rapidly metabolized into less active breakdown products. These metabolites plus the unchanged drug are excreted by the kidneys. Impaired renal function results in increased accumulation of metabolites in the bloodstream.

With normal hepatic and renal functioning, half of any given dose is eliminated within the first 1½ to 2 hours. This half-life may be doubled in the presence of liver disease.

Pharmacodynamics Epinephrine combined with lidocaine produces local vasoconstriction, which reduces local perfusion and thereby slows the systemic absorption of the agent. Its use also reduces blood loss through incisions.

Pharmaceutics Lidocaine is available in various preparations, including topical ointment, jelly, solution, and spray. For injection, it is prepared in sterile isotonic solutions in concentrations of 0.5%, 1%, 1.5%, and 2%. It is also available with or without the addition of dilute epinephrine (1:100,000 or 1:200,000).

Physiologic Responses to Lidocaine The desired response to lidocaine is local anesthesia through blockage of sensory or motor nerves. Thus the primary organ system affected is the nervous system. There are no desired effects on other organ systems, although undesired side effects and adverse reactions can occur.

Undesired Clinical Responses In general, adverse reactions occur more commonly when either high blood levels are present (e.g., excessive dosage or intravascular injection) or when there is hypersensitivity (allergic reaction).

Central nervous system (CNS) reactions can be related to CNS stimulation, CNS depression, or some combination of both. Excitatory symptoms include apprehension, nervousness, tinnitus, twitching, tremors, and in the extreme, convulsions. CNS depression includes confusion and drowsiness, which can progress in severe reactions to unconsciousness and respiratory arrest. Reactions that are a hybrid of stimulation and depression include blurred vision, diplopia, vomiting, or sensations of heat or cold. CNS reactions are rare with topical and local infiltration administration.

Adverse effects on the cardiovascular system are essentially cardiac depression. Such manifestations include bradycardia or hypotension. In the extreme, cardiac arrest occurs (Fig. 66–2).

Allergic reactions can occur as a result of hypersensitivity to either the lidocaine itself (very rarely) or to the preservative (methylparaben) in multidose vials. This latter risk is not present in single-dose vials because they do not contain the preservative. Allergic manifestations include skin lesions (urticaria, hives), edema (swelling), or respiratory compromise (wheezing or bronchospasms).

Contraindications and Precautions Lidocaine use is contraindicated for surgical procedures to the fingers, toes, or nose since circulation can be compromised. It is also used with caution in clients with known cardiovascular problems.[1,15,16] Resuscitative equipment and oxygen should always be available when this drug is used.

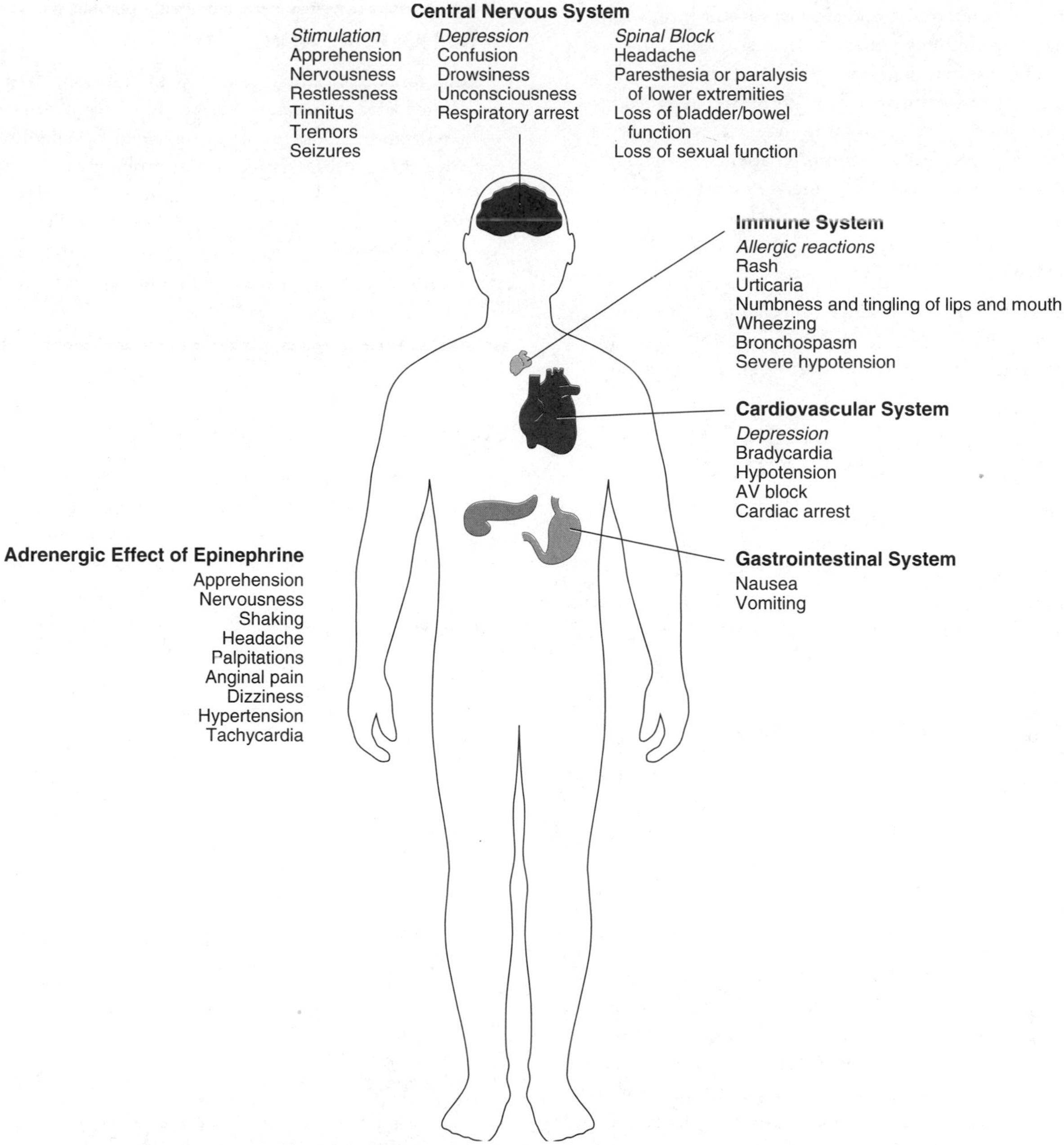

Central Nervous System

Stimulation	*Depression*	*Spinal Block*
Apprehension	Confusion	Headache
Nervousness	Drowsiness	Paresthesia or paralysis
Restlessness	Unconsciousness	of lower extremities
Tinnitus	Respiratory arrest	Loss of bladder/bowel
Tremors		function
Seizures		Loss of sexual function

Immune System

Allergic reactions
Rash
Urticaria
Numbness and tingling of lips and mouth
Wheezing
Bronchospasm
Severe hypotension

Cardiovascular System

Depression
Bradycardia
Hypotension
AV block
Cardiac arrest

Gastrointestinal System

Nausea
Vomiting

Adrenergic Effect of Epinephrine

Apprehension
Nervousness
Shaking
Headache
Palpitations
Anginal pain
Dizziness
Hypertension
Tachycardia

FIGURE 66–2   Common undesired clinical responses associated with local anesthetic drugs.

Drug-Drug and Drug-Environment Interactions Lidocaine with no antimicrobial preservatives (e.g., methylparaben) should be used for epidural or spinal anesthesia because the safety of preservatives in this setting has not been established.

Intramuscular (IM) lidocaine use may increase the creatine phosphokinase level and interfere with testing.

Store lidocaine at a controlled room temperature (15° to 30° C).

Life-Span Considerations Lidocaine is a Pregnancy Category B drug. It crosses the placenta and is distributed in breast milk.

🎋 NURSING RESEARCH

Brucia, J.J., Owen, D.C., & Rudy, E.V. (1992). The effects of lidocaine on intracranial hypertension. *Journal of Neuroscience Nursing, 24,* 205–214.

Endotracheal suctioning can temporarily increase intracranial pressure in patients who have suffered head injuries. Temporary increases in intracranial pressure have been harmful to such patients.

This article reviewed studies on the efficacy of lidocaine in decreasing the intracranial pressure response to endotracheal suctioning and similar stimuli in head-injury patients. Although there have been conflicting results in the research literature, current literature appears to indicate that the intratracheal administration of lidocaine before endotracheal suction may reduce the rise in intracranial pressure in head-injury patients, particularly when used with muscle relaxants or other anesthetic agents.

STUDENT ACTIVITIES

• Interview the clinical nurse specialist on the neurology unit. Determine if lidocaine is used to decrease intracranial pressure during endotracheal suctioning.

LIFE-SPAN CONSIDERATIONS

Because of potentially toxic effects of local anesthetics, dosages are determined by the client's age, weight, and preexisting health problems. Generally, smaller dosages are administered to children, adults of small stature, and elderly individuals. Compromised liver function also necessitates adjustments in dosages.

DRUG-DRUG INTERACTIONS

Interactions of local anesthetics with other drugs are relatively few, but careful observation of the client during administration is necessary. The interactions are summarized below.[14]

If other CNS depressants have been or are being administered with local anesthetics, the client may experience an additive CNS depressive effect. If this occurs, the dose of local anesthetic is reduced, and respiratory function is monitored.[8]

Interactions can also occur with local anesthetics containing vasoconstrictors such as epinephrine. If the client is also taking a monoamine oxidase (MAO) inhibitor, tricyclic antidepressant, phenothiazine, or oxytocic drug, then severe, sustained hypotension or hypertension can occur. The combined administration of these drugs should be done with caution and the client's blood pressure monitored.[8]

The general anesthetic drugs ethrane (Enflurane), fluothane (Halothane), chloroform, and cyclopropane, when given to a client receiving epinephrine in a local anesthetic, can precipitate cardiac arrhythmias. These combinations should be used with caution.

The two local anesthetics, chloroprocaine and bupivacaine, should not be mixed together. When these two drugs are combined, the action of bupivacaine is lessened.

Echothiophate iodide, a miotic agent used to treat glaucoma, can reduce the hydrolysis of procaine. This combination should be used with caution.

CONCEPT REVIEW

Duration of anesthetic block with lidocaine is determined by technique, types of block, and drug concentration. Dosages are determined by client's age, weight, and preexisting health problems.

Caution should be used in combining lidocaine with any other drug. Its use is contraindicated for surgical procedures to fingers, toes, or nose, and it is used with caution in clients with known cardiovascular problems.

SUMMARY

Local anesthetics are being used more frequently in today's health care management. Nurses have increased responsibility in assessing the client before and during administration of these drugs. Knowledge of allergies, past experiences with local anesthetics, and underlying health problems helps determine appropriate nursing management. Maintaining client safety is a priority because of loss of protective mechanisms. With the increased popularity of ambulatory surgery centers, comprehensive client teaching facilitates early discharge and return to routine activities.

REFERENCES

1. Ritchie, J.M., & Greene, N.M. (1990). Local anesthetics. In A. Gilman & L. Goodman, *The pharmacological basis of therapeutics* (8th ed.). New York: MacMillan.
2. Clark, W.G., Braeter, D.C., & Johnson, A.R. (1992). *Goth's medical pharmacology.* St. Louis: C.V. Mosby.
3. Penfield, A.J. (1986). *Gynecologic surgery under local anesthesia.* Baltimore: Urban & Schwarzenberg.
4. Citera, J. (1992). The use of local anesthetics in treatment of chronic pain. *Orthopaedic Nursing, 11*(1), 27–33.
5. Houghton, K. (1988). Local anesthesia. *Nursing Times, 84*(41), 63–66.
6. Covino, B.G., & Lambert, D.M. (1992). Pharmacology of local anesthetics. In D.E. Longnecker & F.L. Murphy (Eds.), *Introduction to anesthesia* (8th ed.) (pp. 195–212). Philadelphia: W.B. Saunders.
7. Berk, W.A., Welch, R.D., & Brooks, F.B. (1992). Controversial issues in clinical management of the simple wound. *Annals of Emergency Medicine, 21*(1), 72–80.
8. Smith, I., & White, P.F. (1992). Use of intravenous adjuvants during local and regional anesthesia. *Current Reviews in Nursing Anesthesia, 14*(23), 185–192.
9. Riegler, F.X. (1992). Nerve blocks. In D.E. Longnecker & F.L. Murphy (Eds.), *Introduction to anesthesia* (8th ed.) (pp. 229–245). Philadelphia: W.B. Saunders.
10. Shnider, S.M., Levinson, G., & Ralston, D.H. (1993). Regional anesthesia for labor and delivery. In S.M. Shnider & G. Levinson

(Eds.), *Anesthesia for obstetrics* (3rd ed.) (pp. 135–153). Baltimore: Williams & Wilkins.

11. Meeker, M.H., & Rothrock, J.C. (1991). *Alexander's care of the patient in surgery.* St. Louis: C.V. Mosby.

12. Spitzer, L.E. (1992). Sedation and analgesia techniques for regional anesthesia. *CRNA: The Clinical Forum for Nurse Anesthetists 3*(4), 190–194.

13. Snyder, B.A. (1990). Regional anesthesia in the pediatric patient. *Nurse Anesthesia 1*(1), 16–20.

14. Collins, V.J. (1993). *Principles of anesthesiology* (3rd ed.). Philadelphia: Lea & Febiger.

15. Wood, M. (1990). Local anesthetic agents. In M. Wood & A. Wood (Eds.), *Drugs and anesthesia: Pharmacology for anesthesiologists* (2nd ed.) (pp. 319–343). Baltimore: Williams & Wilkins.

16. Norris, R.L. (1992). Local anesthetics. *Emergency Medicine Clinics of North America, 10*(4), 707–718.

17. Wild, L., & Coyne, C. (1992). The basics and beyond: Epidural analgesia. *American Journal of Nursing, 92*(4), 26–34.

18. Haghenbeck, K. (1989). Nursing care following spinal anesthesia. *Critical Care Nurse, 9*(4), 22–25.

19. Bromage, P.R. (1993). Neurologic complications of regional anesthesia for obstetrics. In S.M. Shnider & G. Levinson (Eds.), *Anesthesia for obstetrics* (3rd ed.) (pp. 433–454). Baltimore: Williams & Wilkins.

BIBLIOGRAPHY

Arbey, C.J., & Lynch, W.S. (1992). Advances in local anesthesia. *Clinics in Dermatology, 10*(3), 275–283.

Dunnihoo, D.R. (1990). *Fundamentals of gynecology and obstetrics.* Philadelphia: J.B. Lippincott.

Grant, S., & Hoffman, R. (1992). Use of tetracaine, epinephrine and cocaine as a topical anesthetic in the emergency department. *Annals of Emergency Medicine, 21*(8), 987–997.

Guidelines for obstetrical anesthesia and conduction analgesia for the certified registered nurse anesthetist (1992). *Journal of the American Association of Nurse Anesthetists, 60*(2), 134–136.

Henrikson, M., & Wild, L. (1988). A nursing process approach to epidural analgesia. *Journal of Obstetric, Gynecological and Neonatal Nursing, 17*(5), 316–319.

Malamed, S.F., Sykes, P., Kubota, Y., Matsuura, H., & Lipp, M. (1992). Local anesthesia: A review. *Anesthesia and Pain Control in Dentistry, 1*(1), 11–24.

Miller, R.D. (1990). *Anesthesia* (3rd ed.). New York: Churchill Livingstone.

Petrone, S. (1989). Perioperative nurses must prepare themselves to monitor patients receiving local anesthesia. *Association of Operating Room Nurses Journal, 50*(2), 442–446.

Post anesthesia care standards for the certified registered nurse anesthetist (1992). *Journal of the American Association of Nurse Anesthetists, 60*(2), 132–133.

Drugs Affecting the Integumentary System

CHAPTER 67
Drugs Used to Treat Dermatologic Conditions

DRUGS USED TO TREAT
Dermatologic Conditions

V. LYNN HORNING • ROBERT J. KIZIOR

- **Anatomy and Physiology of the Skin**
  LEARNING OBJECTIVES:
  Discuss the function of the skin.
  Describe the general characteristics of the three layers of the skin.
  KEY TERMS:
  Dermis, epidermis, keratinocyte, melanocyte

- **Nursing Considerations**
  LEARNING OBJECTIVE: Develop a plan of care for the client requiring treatment for a dermatologic disease.

- **Acne Preparations**
  LEARNING OBJECTIVES:
  Discuss the pharmacodynamic properties of drugs used in acne treatment.
  Describe common undesired responses associated with drug therapy for acne.
  Identify several over-the-counter (OTC) acne preparations.
  KEY TERM: Acne vulgaris

- **Drugs Used to Treat Superficial Mycotic Infections**
  LEARNING OBJECTIVES:
  Describe the pharmacodynamics of major systemic drugs used to treat fungal infections (e.g., ketoconazole, griseofulvin).
  Describe the proper technique for applying topical drug preparations.
  Identify several OTC topical antifungal preparations.

- **Drugs Used to Treat Psoriasis**
  LEARNING OBJECTIVES:
  Explain the use of etretinate in the treatment of psoriasis.
  Discuss the pharmacodynamic properties of at least two other drugs used to treat psoriasis (e.g., coal tar, anthralin).
  Describe the use of phototherapy in the treatment of psoriasis.
  Explain the pharmacodynamic properties of topical corticosteroids.
  KEY TERM: Psoriasis

- **Drugs Used to Treat Vitiligo**
  LEARNING OBJECTIVE: Describe the use of phototherapy in the treatment of vitiligo.
  KEY TERM: Vitiligo

- **Enzymatic Agents**
  LEARNING OBJECTIVE: Discuss therapeutic agents (e.g., collagenase, sutilains, fibrinolysin) used in chemical debridement.

- **Drugs Used to Treat Scabies**
  LEARNING OBJECTIVE: Discuss drugs used to treat scabies.
  KEY TERM: Scabies

CONCEPTS AND TERMS TO REVIEW

Review the section in a medical-surgical textbook on skin disorders.

Review Chapter 3 for information about dosage forms of drugs applied topically.

Reviews Chapters 4 and 6 for information about factors influencing drug absorption and routes of percutaneous absorption.

Read appropriate sections in Chapter 58 for information on topical mycotic (fungal) infections and related drug therapy.

*T*he skin, or integument, is the largest organ in the body. It is exposed to the external environment and provides the first line of defense for the body. Skin disorders can result from various causes such as fungal, bacterial, or viral infections, parasitic infestations, reactions to substances encountered externally, reactions to internal changes, or new growth. This chapter provides an overview of the anatomy and physiology of the skin, common dermatologic disorders, and drug therapy for these disorders.

ANATOMY AND PHYSIOLOGY OF THE SKIN[1,2]

The skin or integumentary system covers the surface of the body, protecting it from environmental influences. It also protects deeper tissues from injury, from invasion by foreign organisms, and from drying. The skin contains the peripheral nerve endings of many sensory nerves; it is involved with temperature regulation, excretion, and absorption of materials.

Basic Structure of the Skin

The basic structure of the skin consists of an outer layer (the epidermis), the dermis, and a layer of subcutaneous tissue. The **epidermis** acts as a semipermeable membrane barrier, preventing substances from entering the body and also pre-venting body fluids from establishing equilibrium with the environment. The epidermis consists of five layers. The outermost layer, the stratum corneum, is composed of cells arranged in vertical stacks. These cells contain keratin and are regularly sloughed off. This layer is hygroscopic or water absorbing; it can swell in depth and width to form ridges over tight surfaces such as fingers.

Next to the stratum corneum is the stratum lucidum. The stratum lucidum is best seen in the palms of the hand and the soles of the feet where the stratum corneum (or horny layer) is thickest. The next layers are the stratum granulosum (or granular layer) and the stratum spinosum and the innermost layer, the stratum germinativum (Fig. 67–1).

The stratum germinativum consists of two types of cells, keratinocytes and melanocytes. **Keratinocytes** are capable of cell division, a process that occurs approximately every 19 days. Cell division produces daughter cells, which migrate to the skin surface, a process that requires an additional 28 to 60 days. Keratinocytes also produce several substances involved with inflammatory processes. **Melanocytes** produce melanin, which protects the skin from ultraviolet (UV) radiation. In Caucasians, melanin is found principally in the basal cell layer; in African-Americans it is distributed throughout the epidermis.

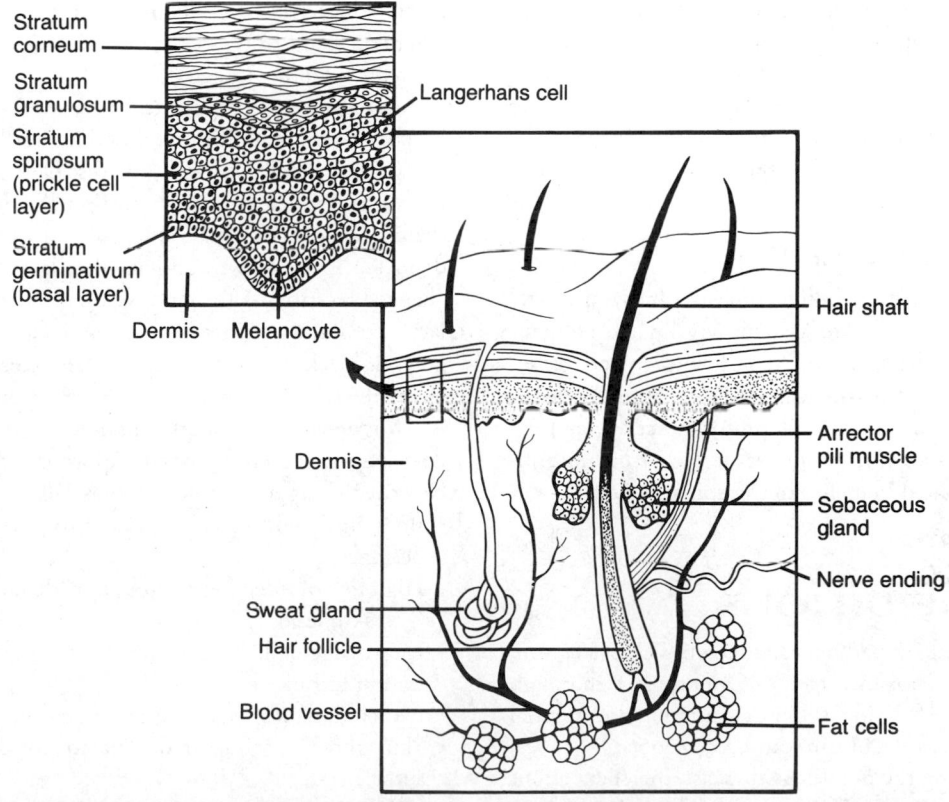

Stratum corneum

Stratum granulosum

Stratum spinosum (prickle cell layer)

Stratum germinativum (basal layer)

Langerhans cell

Dermis   Melanocyte

Hair shaft

Dermis

Arrector pili muscle

Sebaceous gland

Nerve ending

Sweat gland

Hair follicle

Blood vessel

Fat cells

FIGURE 67–1   Layers of the epidermis. (From Monahan, F.D., Drake, T., & Neighbors, M. (1994). *Nursing Care of Adults* (p. 156). Philadelphia: W.B. Saunders.

An additional cellular constituent of the epidermis is the Langerhans' cell. Langerhans' cells are probably manufactured in the bone marrow and have surface receptors active in the immune response.

The **dermis** protects deeper structures from mechanical injury. It is tough and resilient and consists of connective tissue, blood vessels, lymphatics, and nerve and elastic fibers (see Fig. 67–1). The dermis is composed of two layers, a papillary layer and a reticular layer. The papillary layer, which is located directly below the epidermis, is composed of coarsely arranged collagen fibers. Four types of collagen fibers account for 77% of the skin's dry weight.

Two main types of cells are found in the dermis, fibroblasts and mast cells. Fibroblasts synthesize collagen, elastic fibers, and ground substance, a gel-like substance composed of connective tissue cells and fibers. Mast cells are important because they contain an element called the *metachromatic granule,* which contains the anticoagulant heparin. Mast cells are also important because they manufacture histamine. Histamine through the formation and inactivation of kinins and prostaglandins, increases capillary permeability and vasodilation in the inflammatory process.

Subcutaneous tissue supports the dermis and the epidermis, serving as an area for fat storage. This layer of skin helps with temperature regulation of the body, provides nutritional support, and provides cushioning to the outer layers of the skin.

Blood Supply to Skin

The blood supply to the skin is derived from cutaneous branches of the subcutaneous musculocutaneous arteries. A small vessel plexus deep in the dermis progressively microbranches to the dermal papillary layer where arterioles interphase with capillary loops. The capillary loops drain into progressively larger vessels of the subcutaneous venous system.

Innervation of Skin

Motor innervation of the skin comes from sympathetic fibers of the autonomic nervous system. Myelinated postganglionic sympathetic fibers follow the course of blood vessels into and throughout the dermis where their terminals are involved with vasomotor control, pilomotor function, and eccrine secretion. Sensory innervation is derived from myelinated and nonmyelinated branches of the spinal nerves.

▨ NURSING CONSIDERATIONS

The skin is assaulted by pathogens, allergens, UV radiation, and a host of other noxious agents. Obtaining a thorough health history and performing a skin examination are essential before an appropriate plan of care can be developed.

Assessing During the **health history** ask the client about recent skin lesions or rashes. Have the client describe the time of onset and the duration of the lesions or rashes. Determine if the client is able to link his or her appearance to heat, cold, stress, exposure to toxic material, recent travel, new clothing, or change in detergents or skin care products. Document any history of drug allergies that have caused skin lesions or rashes.

Ask the client about a family or personal history of asthma, hay fever, or atopic dermatitis. Explore all complaints of pain, itching, burning, or tingling. Determine if the client has noticed any change in skin color. Ask how much time is spent outdoors and if sunscreen is used. Ascertain if there is a family or personal history of skin cancer or malignant melanoma.

Before starting the **physical assessment,** make certain the overhead lighting is adequate. Ask the client to undress so that the entire epithelial surface can be inspected. Wear gloves when examining lesions, mucous membranes, and any area that is itching or draining.

Begin by assessing the color of the skin. You are looking for changes in the client's normal skin color. Note if any of the skin is unusually pale or dark. Note details of the skin appearance. Record location of oily, dry, thick, or flaky skin areas. Use the dorsum (back) of your hand to assess skin temperature. Lightly palpate the skin to check tenderness, firmness, and depth of surface lesions. Assess skin turgor by lifting a fold of skin on the forearm and seeing how quickly it falls back into place.

The hair, nails, and mucous membranes are part of the integumentary system and must be included in the examination. Note whether the client has lost any hair on any part of the body. Determine if the alopecia is diffuse or patchy. Check the scalp and pubic hair for nits. To assess the fingernails, check the angle between the nail and the nail base. If the angle is greater than 160°, the client may have clubbing. Check the color and shape of the nails. Do the nails look discolored? Are the nails smooth? Ridged? Concave? Spoon shaped? Assess the toenails. Are the toenails thick? Ridged? Grooved? Inspect the mucous membranes for discoloration, lesions, or ulcerations.

Watch carefully for any growths. Determine if the growth is symmetric or asymmetric. Inspect the area to determine if the borders of the growth are regular or irregular. Measure the diameter of the growth and ask the client if the diameter has changed recently. Is the color of the growth uneven or irregular? Determine whether it contains shades of red, white, blue, gray, or black. Palpate the growth to determine if it is flat or elevated.

Diagnosing Nursing diagnoses are formulated after the data base has been analyzed. Appropriate diagnoses for the client requiring dermatologic drugs follow:

- Body image, disturbance, related to physical changes in appearance.
- High risk of infection related to inadequate primary defense (i.e., skin lesions).
- Knowledge deficit regarding treatment plan, drug administration technique.
- Noncompliance related to fear or anxiety.
- Skin integrity, impaired, related to disruption of skin surface.

Planning As with any client, teaching is an important concept. However, most of these individuals are treated on an outpatient basis; thus time spent with the client is brief.

Therefore you must develop comprehensive and easy-to-understand teaching plans. Provide written instructions or diagrams when possible. Perform a follow-up visit on or make a telephone call to ambulatory clients to determine the effectiveness of teaching and the efficacy of the drug therapy.

Develop expected outcomes to help evaluate effectiveness of the teaching plan. Appropriate outcomes include the following:

- Client verbalizes acceptance of self in situation.
- Client identifies interventions to reduce risk of infection.
- Client participates in learning process.
- Client performs necessary procedures correctly.
- Client verbalizes accurate knowledge of disease and understanding of treatment plan.
- Client displays healing of skin lesions without complications.

Implementing Familiarize yourself with the various dermatologic conditions. Learn the proper techniques for administering dermatologic drugs. You must understand this information so you can properly teach the client.

Evaluating Discuss the plan of care with the client. Determine if the expected outcomes have been met or if changes are needed in the plan.

CONCEPT REVIEW

Skin covers the surface of the body, protecting the body from environmental influences.

The skin consists of three layers: epidermis, dermis, subcutaneous tissue.

ACNE PREPARATIONS

Acne vulgaris affects approximately 80% of the teenage and young adult population and may be present into the middle years. In clients with acne vulgaris there is increased production of sebum from the sebaceous glands and the formation of comedones (blackheads and whiteheads) that plug the pores. Noninflammatory acne produces plugged follicles and a few pimples. Inflammatory acne is characterized by many pimples, pustules, nodules, and inflamed cysts. These lesions are found on the face, neck, chest, and shoulders. Current medical treatment is aimed toward prevention and suppression of lesions. Table 67–1 summarizes information about drugs used in the treatment of acne.

Isotretinoin

Pharmacotherapeutics Isotretinoin (Accutane) is a vitamin A derivative used to treat severe acne.[3-5]

Pharmacokinetics Peak levels of isotretinoin are reached in approximately 3 hours. The drug is excreted in the urine and bile and has a half-life of 10 to 20 hours.

Pharmacodynamics Isotretinoin exerts its action by decreasing sebum production and composition, inhibiting *Propionibacterium acnes* bacterial growth, inhibiting inflammation, and altering patterns of keratinization.

Pharmaceutics Isotretinoin is available in capsules of 10 to 40 mg. The initial dose is 0.5 to 1.0 mg/kg in divided doses, increasing to 2 mg/kg/d for 15 to 20 weeks.

Undesired clinical responses Isotretinoin has numerous undesired clinical responses. For example, conjunctivitis and cheilitis occur in a large number of clients. Other common responses include gastrointestinal (GI) upset, headache, pruritus, alopecia, epistaxis, lethargy, thirst, and bone and joint pain. Abnormal laboratory data include increased levels of serum glucose, triglycerides, cholesterol, alanine aminotransferase (ALT), aspartate aminotransferase (AST), and alkaline phosphatase. Increased photosensitivity and an increase in pseudotumor cerebri have also occurred.

Contraindications and precautions Isotretinoin therapy is contraindicated in clients receiving tetracycline or vitamin A supplements. Concomitant administration of tetracycline and isotretinoin has produced pseudotumor cerebri. Clients receiving both vitamin A and isotretinoin may develop avitaminosis.

Life-span considerations Isotretinoin must not be used by women who are pregnant or who may become pregnant. Reported teratogenic effects include severe central nervous system (CNS) abnormalities: hydrocephalus, microcephalus, cranial nerve deficits, skull abnormalities, and intelligence scores below 85. Abnormalities are attributed to interference with migration of neural crest cells early in embryonic development. Because of the potential for birth defects when taking isotretinoin while pregnant, female clients should have negative results from a pregnancy test within 2 weeks of start of therapy. In addition, therapy should begin on the second or third day of the next normal menstrual cycle. Clients should use contraception while receiving drug therapy and for up to 6 months after therapy is discontinued.

Specific drug-related nursing considerations Determine if the client has a history of or is currently taking vitamin preparations. Check the result of a serum pregnancy test. Instruct the client about undesired clinical responses. Provide information about correct dose administration of isotretinoin. Tell the client that if a dose is missed, the next dose should be taken as soon as possible. However, double dosing is inappropriate. Teach the client to avoid or restrict alcohol ingestion to minimize changes in triglyceride levels.

Support and encouragement should be provided the client because acne often gets worse before it improves. Family members should be included in client education efforts if the client is an adolescent. Reinforcing self-esteem by complimenting the client on improvement cannot be underestimated.

Tretinoin

Pharmacotherapeutics Tretinoin (Retin-A) is used to treat acne vulgaris grades I to III.[5]

Pharmacodynamics Tretinoin is a topically applied form of vitamin A. The drug increases cell turnover of the epidermis and decreases cohesiveness of keratinized cells. This action decreases the formation of existing comedones and inhibits the formation of new ones. Microcomedones are frag-

TABLE 67–1
Drugs Used in the Treatment of Acne

Drug Name	Dosage and Route of Administration	Nursing Considerations
Isotretinoin (Accutane) **HOW SUPPLIED** Capsules: 10, 20, 40 mg	**Severe Recalcitrant Cystic Acne** Initial dose: 0.5–1 mg/kg/d in two divided doses for 15–20 wk	**Assess** Assess the skin before therapy for severity of cysts, skin dryness, erythema. Ask whether the client is pregnant; use of this drug is contraindicated in pregnancy. Determine if the client is taking vitamins or vitamin A supplement; they are contraindicated with isotretinoin. Obtain triglyceride levels, liver function test results (AST, ALT, alkaline phosphatase), glucose value. **Implement** Capsules must be taken whole; do not crush. Give isotretinoin with meals. **Monitor** Monitor triglyceride levels and results of liver function tests. Assess the status of the skin. Teach the client to report any adverse clinical reactions (e.g., visual disturbances [with nausea, vomiting, or headache] or abdominal pain). **Evaluate** Evaluate the skin for decreased erythema, oiliness of the skin, comedones, noncystic lesions.
Tretinoin (Retin-A) **HOW SUPPLIED** Cream: 0.025%, 0.05%, 0.1% Gel: 0.025%, 0.01% Liquid: 0.05%	**Acne Vulgaris** Cream or gel: apply once daily before bedtime Liquid: apply once daily before bedtime; apply with fingertip, gauze pad, or cotton swab	**Assess** Assess the skin before therapy for severity of crysts, skin dryness, erythema. **Implement** Teach client to apply at night (alternate days to reduce excessive dryness and irritation). Teach client to wash area with mild soap 20–30 min before application. Client should allow the skin to dry completely before applying the medication. Teach client to avoid applying over sunburn or windburn. Encourage the use of sunscreens and protective clothing to minimize photosensitivity reactions. **Monitor** Assess the status of the skin. **Evaluate** Look for decreased erythema, oiliness, presence of comedones, or noncystic lesions.

mented, and plugs are expelled; closed comedones are converted to open comedones.

Pharmaceutics   Tretinoin is available in cream form in 0.025%, 0.05%, and 0.1% strengths; as a gel in 0.025% and 0.01% strengths; and as a solution in 0.05% strength. Tretinoin cream is more suitable for use in clients with dry skin; gel and solution forms are more suitable for clients with oily skins. The drug is applied nightly.

Undesired clinical responses   Potential undesired responses include excessive dryness and irritation of the skin. This response may be reduced by applying the drug on alternate days only.

Contraindications and precautions   Tretinoin use is contraindicated in clients hypersensitive to the drug.

Specific drug-related nursing considerations   Teach the client to cleanse the affected area with a mild soap 20 to 30

TABLE 67–1 *Continued*
Drugs Used in the Treatment of Acne

Drug Name	Dosage and Route of Administration	Nursing Considerations
Benzoyl Peroxide (Benzac-AC Wash, Desquam-X, Dryox, Fostex, Oxy-10) **HOW SUPPLIED** Liquid: 2.5%, 5%, 10% Bar: 5%, 10% Mask: 5% Lotion: 5%, 5.5%, 10% Cream: 5%, 10% Gel: 2.5%, 4%, 5%	**Acne Vulgaris, Oily Skin** Cleansers: wash once or twice daily Other dose forms: apply once daily for initial use; may increase to two or three times daily	**Assess** Assess the skin before use. Avoid use on inflamed, denuded, or highly sensitive skin. **Implement** Teach client to apply 30 min after washing to minimize irritation. Instruct the client to avoid contact with eyes, lips, inside of the nose, and sensitive areas of the neck. Initially client should keep peroxide on for 15 min a night; increase gradually until drug can be left on overnight. **Monitor** Monitor the status of the skin. **Evaluate** Inspect the skin for decreased evidence of acne.

minutes before the application of tretinoin and to let the skin dry completely. Instruct the client not to apply the drug over sunburn or windburn.

Many clients who take the drug experience increased sensitivity to sunlight. Teach the clients to use a sunscreen of SPF 15 or higher if direct sun exposure is unavoidable. Inform the client that increased sensitivity to wind and cold may also occur. Tell the client that dryness and peeling of the skin may occur in affected areas. Instruct male clients to avoid the use of shaving lotions or other products containing alcohol. Although drying and peeling may be expected, signs and symptoms such as severe burning, inflammation, blistering, and crusting are adverse reactions and should be reported.

Benzoyl Peroxide

Topical benzoyl peroxide is a bacteriostatic and comedolytic drug. It is one of the most effective nonprescription drugs available for acne.

Pharmacotherapeutics Mild to moderate forms of acne may respond to topical applications of benzoyl peroxide.

Pharmacodynamics Its exact mechanism of action is unknown, although benzoyl peroxide does increase the rate of sloughing of epithelial cells and destroy comedones. No benzoyl peroxide is absorbed systemically, regardless of the concentration applied.

Pharmaceutics Benzoyl peroxide is available in 2.5%, 5%, and 10% strengths and in a variety of dosage forms, including gels, lotions, creams, pads, sticks, and liquid cleansers.

Benzoyl peroxide has been combined with various drugs in attempts to improve the overall drug efficacy. Its combination with the antibiotic erythromcyin has proved more effective than either drug alone. Other combinations include miconazole and metronidazole.

Undesired clinical responses Primary undesired responses are irritation and excessive drying, which may be avoided by beginning treatment with a milder strength preparation. Clients with fair complexions are usually more sensitive to irritation.

Specific drug-related nursing considerations To minimize irritation, teach the client to apply benzoyl peroxide 30 minutes after washing. Warn the client to expect dryness and peeling of the skin. Cosmetics may be worn over the drug to conceal the skin changes.[6,7]

Topical Antibiotics

Topical antibiotics are useful in the treatment of mild to moderate inflammatory acne vulgaris. These drugs probably have no role in treating the comedo phase of the disease.

Topical antibiotics reduce the population of *P. acnes*, inhibit chemotaxis, and decrease the percentage of free fatty acids in the skin. Topical dosage forms of **erythromycin** and **clindamycin** are available and are of equal efficacy. Topical clindamycin is as effective or superior to oral tetracycline for treatment of mild to moderate acne. **Tetracycline** reduces the amount of keratin in sebaceous follicles and inhibits chemotaxis, phagocytosis, complement activation, and cell-mediated immunity. Tetracycline apparently is more concentrated in cells of inflamed skin.[6]

Topical antibiotics are usually applied to the affected area twice daily, in the morning and evening. The affected areas should be washed, rinsed, and dried before application of the drug. Most topical antibiotics produce occasional skin irritation and stinging upon application. Information about dosage forms, dosages, and nursing considerations is summarized in Table 67–2.

TABLE 67–2
Drugs Used in the Treatment of Acne: Antibiotics

Drug Name	Dosage and Route of Administration	Nursing Considerations
Clindamycin (Cleocin, Cleocin T, Clinda-Derm) HOW SUPPLIED Capsules: 75, 150, 300 mg Gel: 10 mg/ml Lotion: 10 mg/ml Topical solution: 10 mg/ml	**Acne Vulgaris** ADULTS Oral: 150 mg two times a day Topical: apply thin film to affected area two times a day	**Assess** Determine whether client has previous allergy to clindamycin. Assess skin before therapy for severity of cysts, skin dryness, erythema. **Implement** Instruct client to wash area 20–30 min before application, allow skin to dry completely, and then apply medication to the affected area. Administer oral form on empty stomach. If GI upset or nausea occurs, drug may be given with food. **Monitor** Assess for efficacy in relieving clinical manifestations of acne. Instruct client to report undesired clinical responses (e.g., diarrhea containing blood and mucus, abdominal pain, or fever). **Evaluate** Look for decreased erythema, oiliness of skin, decreased comedones, noncystic lesions.
Erythromycin (E-Mycin, Ery-Tab, E-Base, Staticin, Akne-mycin, A/T/S, T-Stat, Erygel) HOW SUPPLIED Tablets: 250, 333, 500 mg Capsules: 250 mg Solution: 1.5%, 2% Gel: 2% Ointment: 2%	**Acne Vulgaris** ADULTS Oral: initial dose up to 1 g/d Maintenance: 250–500 mg/d Topical: apply thin film to affected area two times a day	**Assess** Ask about previous allergic reaction to medication. Assess skin before therapy for severity of cysts, skin dryness, erythema. **Implement** Tell client to wash area 20–30 min before application, allow skin to dry completely, and apply to affected area. Administer on empty stomach; if GI upset or nausea occurs, give with food. **Monitor** Assess efficacy in relieving clinical manifestations of acne. **Evaluate** Examine the skin for decreased erythema, oiliness of skin, comedones, noncystic lesions.
Tetracycline (Achromycin, Sumycin, Topicycline) HOW SUPPLIED Capsules: 250, 500 mg Tablets: 250, 500 mg Topical solution: 2.2 mg/ml	**Acne Vulgaris** ADULTS Oral: initially 1 g/d in divided doses Maintenance: 125–500 mg/d Topical: apply thin film to affected area two times a day	**Implement** Same as for erythromycin except that client should also avoid antacids, dairy products, iron supplements for 2 h after administration.
Minocycline (Minocyn) HOW SUPPLIED Capsules: 50, 100 mg Tablets: 50, 100 mg	**Acne Vulgaris** ADULTS 50–200 mg/d	**Implement** Same as for erythromycin except that drug should be administered with a full glass of water and not at bedtime. Drug is in Pregnancy Category D; use should be avoided in women during last half of pregnancy.

Systemic Antibiotics

Acne that is resistant to topical antibiotics, covers large areas of the body, or has several large inflammatory nodules can be treated with oral antibiotics. Oral antibiotics have two modes of action. The primary mechanism is suppression of the *P. acnes* growth; the secondary mechanism is suppression of inflammation.

Tetracyclines are the most commonly used antibiotics for treating acne vulgaris. In the United States tetracycline hydrochloride, doxycycline, and minocycline are most commonly prescribed. **Erythromycin** is roughly as effective as tetracycline in the treatment of acne. Sulfanilamide drugs are often effective in treating acne resistant to tetracyclines or erythromycin.[6] These various groups of oral antibiotics are presented in more depth in Chapter 55.

CONCEPT REVIEW

Acne vulgaris affects 80% of the teenage and young adult population. This disease is caused by increased sebum production, proliferation of *P. acnes* bacteria, and changes in keratinization.

Several acne preparations are available, including isotretinoin, tretinoin, and benzoyl peroxide. In addition, topical and oral antibiotics are frequently prescribed.

OTC Preparations

Currently many OTC preparations are available for the treatment of acne. These products come in a variety of dosage forms: creams, cleansing bars, lotions, ointments, gels, pastes, medicated pads, and aerosol foams.

DRUGS USED TO TREAT SUPERFICIAL MYCOTIC INFECTIONS

Mycotic diseases of the skin such as tinea capitis, tinea corporis, or tinea pedis are caused by dermatophytes. These diseases are acquired by contact between a susceptible individual and an infected individual or animal. Transmission frequently occurs in surroundings such as dormitories, barracks, or locker rooms. Other environmental contributors to transmission are heat and humidity. In addition, perspiration and tight clothing can predispose skin to maceration, irritation, and infection. Chapter 58 provides a comprehensive description of superficial mycotic infections. In addition, the nursing process portion of that chapter summarizes important information about the nursing care of the client with a superficial mycotic infection. A review of appropriate sections of Chapter 58 provides a knowledge basis for caring for clients with topical mycotic infections.

Most superficial mycotic infections are treated with topical drug preparations. Compresses of Burow's solution, normal saline solution, or acetic acid may also be applied to relieve inflammation. Many topical antifungal drug preparations are available OTC (see Table 58–2, p. 791, and Table 67–3). Consultation with a primary care provider before using these preparations is recommended. Topical preparations of azoles or polyene antifungal drugs are prescribed for severe fungal infections. If the infection does not respond to topical drug therapy, systemic antifungal drugs (e.g., griseofulvin, miconazole, ketoconazole) may be prescribed. (Chapter 58 provides information on both topical and systemic antifungal drugs. Refer to that chapter for additional information.)

DRUGS USED TO TREAT PSORIASIS

Psoriasis is a skin disorder of unknown cause. It is characterized by erythematous papules and plaques, which are covered by silver-white scales. The epidermal cells affected by psoriasis proliferate seven times faster than normal and demonstrate increased metabolic activity and increased levels of DNA, RNA, and arachidonic acid. Psoriasis affects all racial groups and men and women equally. Predisposing factors to psoriasis includes stress, trauma, and infection.

Psoriasis may involve any area of the body. However, the part of the body affected influences the appearance of the lesions. For example, psoriasis of the scalp is usually characterized by erythema and diffuse scaling of thick plaques with exudate, fissures, and abscesses. Lesions on the legs, arms, and trunk are usually discreet or large plaques.[8]

Numerous dermatologic preparations are available for the treatment of psoriasis. For example, keratolytics such as salicylic acid are used to remove scales and to smooth the skin. Coal tar preparations are used to produce epidermal hyperplasia. Topical steroids such as fluocinonide (Lidex, Synalar) have an antiinflammatory and antimitotic action on psoriatic skin.

Etretinate

One of the most recent drugs to treat severe psoriasis is etretinate (Tegison). It is a retinoid derivative.

Pharmacotherapeutics   Because of the significant undesired responses associated with etretinate, it should be prescribed only by individuals knowledgeable in the systemic use of retinoids. Etretinate is recommended for individuals unresponsive to or intolerant of standard therapies (e.g., topical tar, ultraviolet A [UVA] light, psoralens plus UV light, systemic corticosteroids, and methotrexate).[9]

Pharmacokinetics   Etretinate is extensively metabolized after oral administration. It has a more significant first-pass metabolism to the acid form. The drug is more than 99% protein bound, predominantly to lipoprotein. Its active metabolite is bound to albumin. Metabolites of the drug are excreted in the bile and urine.[9]

Pharmacodynamics   The exact mechanism of action for etretinate is unknown. It appears to inhibit keratinization, proliferation, and differentiation of epithelial cells. It also has an antiinflammatory action.

Pharmaceutics   Etretinate is available in capsule form for oral administration. Table 67–4 summarizes information about dosage forms and dosages.

TABLE 67–3

Topical and Systemic Antifungal Preparations Used to Treat Superficial Fungal Infections

Drug Name	Dosage and Route of Administration	Nursing Considerations
Undecylenic Acid (Caldesene, Cruex, Desenex) HOW SUPPLIED Powder Cream Ointment	**Tinea Pedis (Athlete's Foot), Diaper Rash, Itching, Burning, Chafing, Prickly Heat, Tinea Cruris (Jock Itch)** Apply as needed or directed	**Assess** Assess skin and involved mucous membranes for open wounds. Make sure cultures have been taken. **Implement** Apply a small amount to cover affected area. Avoid use of occlusive dressings. **Monitor** Monitor skin and mucous membranes involved. Discontinue medication if skin irritation increases. **Evaluate** Assess the skin for decreased skin irritation and resolution of infection.
Econazole (Spectazole) HOW SUPPLIED Cream: 1%	**Tinea Pedis, Tinea Cruris, Tinea Corporis** Apply to affected area once daily **Cutaneous Candidiasis** Apply to affected area twice daily	Same as undecylenic acid.
Ciclopirox (Loprox) HOW SUPPLIED Cream: 1% Lotion: 1%	**Tinea Pedis, Tinea Cruris, Tinea Corporis, Cutaneous Candidiasis, Tinea Versicolor** Apply to affected area twice daily	Same as undecylenic acid.
Triacetin (Ony-Clear) HOW SUPPLIED Solution Cream Aerosol spray	**Treatment of Onychomycosis (Nail Fungus), Tinea Pedis, Tinea Cruris, Tinea Corporis, Monilial Impetigo, Dermatitis** Cream or solution: apply three times daily Tincture and spray—only for onychomycosis: apply two times daily	Same as undecylenic acid.
Oxiconazole (Oxistat) HOW SUPPLIED Cream: 1% Lotion: 1%	**Tinea Pedis, Tinea Cruris, Tinea Corporis** Apply to affected area one or two times daily	Same as undecylenic acid.
Sulconazole (Exelderm) HOW SUPPLIED Cream: 1% Solution: 1%	**Tinea Cruris, Tinea Corporis, Tinea Versicolor** Apply to affected area one or two times daily **Tinea Pedis** Apply two times daily to affected area	Same as undecylenic acid.
Nystatin (Mycostatin, Nilstat, Nystex) HOW SUPPLIED Cream: 100,000 U/g Ointment: 100,000 U/g Powder: 100,000 U/g	**Mycotic Infection Caused by Candida Species** Apply to affected area two to three times daily	Same as undecylenic acid.
Amphotericin (Fungizone) HOW SUPPLIED Cream: 3% Ointment: 3% Lotion: 3%	**Mycotic Infections Caused by Candida Species** Apply to affected area two to four times daily	Same as undecylenic acid.

TABLE 67–3 *Continued*

Topical and Systemic Antifungal Preparations Used to Treat Superficial Fungal Infections

Drug Name	Dosage and Route of Administration	Nursing Considerations
Haloprogin (Halotex) HOW SUPPLIED Cream: 1% Solution: 1%	**Tinea Cruris, Tinea Corporis, Tinea Versicolor** Apply to affected area two times daily	Same as undecylenic acid.
Naftifine (Naftin) HOW SUPPLIED Cream: 1% Gel: 1%	**Tinea Pedis, Tinea Cruris, Tinea Corporis** Apply to affected area once daily for cream and twice daily for gel	Same as undecylenic acid.
Terbinafine (Lamisil) HOW SUPPLIED Cream: 1%	**Tinea Pedis, Tinea Cruris, Tinea Corporis** Apply to affected area two times daily for tinea pedis and one or two times daily for tinea cruris and tinea corporis	Same as undecylenic acid.
Ketoconazole (Nizoral) HOW SUPPLIED Cream: 2% Tablets: 200 mg	**Tinea Pedis, Tinea Cruris, Tinea Corporis, Cutaneous Candidiasis** Topical: apply to affected area once daily Oral: 200 mg once daily (NOTE: Oral dose is for severe cutaneous dermatophyte infections not responding to topical therapy or griseofulvin.)	**Assess** Assess for the topical antifungals. Determine liver function as evidenced by AST, ALT, alkaline phosphatase, and bilirubin test results. **Implement** Give the oral form with meals to decrease nausea and vomiting. **Monitor** Monitor condition of the skin and liver function. **Evaluate** Observe the skin for resolution of signs and symptoms of fungal infections.
Griseofulvin (Fulvicin, Grifulvin, Grisactin, Gris-Peg) HOW SUPPLIED Microsize tablets: 250, 500 mg Microsize capsules: 125, 250 mg Microsize suspension: 125 mg/5 ml Ultramicrosize tablets: 125, 165, 250, 330 mg	For treatment of ringworm infections of the skin, hair, and nails, namely tinea corporis, pedis cruris, barbae, capitis, unguium (onychomycosis) **Tinea Corporis, Tinea Cruris, Tinea Capitis** ADULTS 500 mg (microsize), 330–375 (ultramicrosize) daily as single or divided dose **Tinea Pedis, Tinea Unguium** ADULTS 0.75–1 g (microsize); 660–750 mg (ultramicrosize) in divided doses CHILDREN (ALL USES) 11 mg (microsize)/kg/d or 7.3 mg (ultramicrosize)/kg/d	**Assess** Ask client if there is a history of allergy to penicillin (cross-sensitivity exists). Assess liver, renal function. **Implement** Give with or after meals. High-fat meals minimize GI upset and increase absorption. Teach client to avoid alcohol and ultraviolet light. **Monitor** Monitor condition of the skin and liver, renal function. Obtain complete blood count to monitor for blood dyscrasias. **Evaluate** Evaluate the skin for resolution of signs and symptoms of fungal infection.
Clioquinol (Vioform) HOW SUPPLIED Cream: 3% Ointment: 3%	**Eczema, Athlete's Foot, Other Fungal Infections** Apply two to three times daily for no longer than 1 wk	Same as undecylenic acid.
Miconazole (Micatin, Monistat-Derm, Micatin Liquid) HOW SUPPLIED Cream: 2% Powder: 2% Spray: 2%	**Tinea Pedis, Tinea Cruris, Tinea Corporis (Ringworm), Cutaneous Candidiasis (Moniliasis)** Apply to affected area two times daily **Tinea Versicolor** Apply to affected area once daily	Same as undecylenic acid.

Table continued on following page.

TABLE 67–3 *Continued*
Topical and Systemic Antifungal Preparations Used to Treat Superficial Fungal Infections

Drug Name	Dosage and Route of Administration	Nursing Considerations
Clotrimazole (Lotrimin, Mycelex) HOW SUPPLIED Cream: 1% Solution: 1% Lotion: 1%	**Tinea Pedis, Tinea Cruris, Tinea Corporis, Cutaneous Candidiasis, Tinea Versicolor** Apply to affected area two times daily	Same as undecylenic acid.
Tolnaftate (Genaspor, NP-27, Tinactin, Aftate) HOW SUPPLIED Cream: 1% Solution: 1% Gel: 1% Powder: 1% Spray powder: 1% Spray liquid: 1%	**Tinea Pedis, Tinea Cruris, Tinea Corporis, Tinea Versicolor, Onychomycosis** Apply two times daily	Same as undecylenic acid.

Undesired clinical responses Undesired clinical responses are related to vitamin A overdose. These responses include dried, cracked lips (cheilitis), epistaxis, pruritus, eye irritation, hair loss, palm, sole, and fingertip peeling, bone and joint pain, fatigue, and hyperlipidemia.

Contraindications and precautions Etretinate use is absolutely contraindicated in pregnant women or women contemplating pregnancy. It also is not recommended in nursing mothers.

Drug-drug, drug-nutrient, and drug-environment interactions Concurrent administration of vitamin A supplements and etretinate may cause symptoms of vitamin A hypervitaminosis. Etretinate should be administered with food. The capsules should be protected from light and stored at 15° to 30° C.[9]

Life-span considerations In the United States studies have not been conducted using etretinate in children. Therefore this drug should be used in this age group only if other treatment measures have failed.

Specific drug-related nursing considerations Administer etretinate with food.

Methotrexate Sodium

Methotrexate sodium is used primarily as an antiinflammatory or antineoplastic drug. However, it is prescribed for symptomatic control of severe psoriasis that has not responded to other forms of treatment. Methotrexate, which is specific for cells in the S phase, is effective for psoriasis therapy because a large number of psoriatic cells are in S phase. The drug acts directly on rapidly proliferating epidermal cells by inhibiting the synthesis of thymidylate, a DNA precursor. Methotrexate is discussed in detail in Chapter 69. See Table 67–5 for information on dosage forms, dosages, and nursing considerations associated with methotrexate use in psoriasis.

Coal Tar

Coal tar (e.g., Zetar) is a topical treatment for psoriasis. When applied to the skin, it causes transient epidermal hyperplasia that lasts 1 to 2 weeks. The hyperplasia is followed by cytostasis and epidermal thinning. Use with UVA light activates the coal tar, causing the drug to cross-link with DNA. This action prevents further epidermal cell replication and increases prostaglandin synthesis in the skin.

Application of coal tar can produce superficial folliculitis. Instruct the client to keep the coal tar away from the eyes. In addition, tell the client that coal tar stains skin and clothing and discolors hair and jewelry. Inform the client to avoid exposure to direct sunlight or sunlamps for 72 hours after treatment with coal tar.[9] See Table 67–5 for information about dosage forms, dosages, and nursing considerations.

Anthralin

Anthralin (Anthra-Derm, Anthra-Tex, Lasan) is an antipsoriatic drug with cytostatic, irritant, and weak antimicrobial properties. Anthralin is an anthrone derivative that inhibits DNA synthesis by binding with DNA. The drug also decreases epidermal proliferation by inhibiting mitochondrial activity. See Table 67–5 for information about dosage forms, dosages, and nursing considerations.

Calcipotriene

Calcipotriene (Dovonex) ointment, a synthetic vitamin D_3 analog, is used to treat moderate-plaque psoriasis. Its mechanism of action is unclear. Calcipotriene inhibits proliferation and enhances differentiation of human keratinocytes. Approximately 6% of a dose of the drug applied to psoriasis plaques is absorbed systemically. Calcipotriene is rapidly metabolized to inactive compound by the liver, and only traces of the drug are detectable in urine and feces after topical application.

A thin layer of calcipotriene ointment is applied twice daily to affected areas. Calcipotriene may be used in conjunction with anthralin cream. Undesired clinical responses include local burning, itching, and skin irritation. Dermatitis, dry skin, erythema, peeling, rash, or worsening of the psoriasis occasionally occurs.[10] See Table 67–5 for information about dosage forms, dosages, and nursing considerations.

Topical Corticosteroids

Topical corticosteroids are extremely useful in the treatment of various dermatologic conditions.

Pharmacotherapeutics In addition to the treatment of psoriasis, topical corticosteroids are used to relieve inflammation associated with contact dermatitis, eczema, localized burns, and insect bite reactions.[11]

Pharmacodynamics Topical corticosteroids modify the functions of epidermal and dermal cells and of leukocytes participating in proliferative and inflammatory skin diseases. After passage through the cell membranes, corticosteroids react with receptor proteins in the cytoplasm to form a steroid-receptor complex. This complex moves into the nucleus where it binds to DNA. The binding process changes the transcription of messenger RNA.[12,13]

Pharmaceutics Topical corticosteroids are classified according to potency. The most potent preparations are those that are fluorinated. These preparations should not be used on the face, on intertriginous areas, or for prolonged periods of time. Table 67–4 summarizes information about commonly prescribed topical corticosteroids.

Undesired clinical responses Common undesired clinical responses to topical corticosteroid therapy include burning and itching of skin and thinning of skin with easy bruising. In addition, dryness of the skin, skin rash, or irritation and skin redness or scaling of skin lesions may occur. Prolonged use of topical corticosteroids may cause glaucoma or cataracts.

Contraindications and precautions Topical corticosteroid use is contraindicated in clients with hypersensitivity to the drugs and in clients with conditions that include existing skin atrophy, infection at treatment site, herpes simplex, rosacea, perioral dermatitis, or acne.

Life-span considerations Topical corticosteroids are used in the pediatric population for a variety of skin disorders. The major undesired clinical response associated with this age group is skin atrophy. Low-potency preparations should be used for children.

Specific drug-related nursing considerations During assessment question the client about hypersensitivity to corticosteroids. Assess the skin carefully to establish a baseline description of the skin disorder.

Teach the client or a family member to apply the preparation after a shower or tub bath for best absorption. Instruct the client not to apply drug to weepy, denuded areas. Advise him or her that treated areas should not be exposed to sunlight.[14]

Phototherapy

The use of phototherapy or the combination of light and drugs is not new. UVA is the longest wave length in the UV light spectrum, measuring 320 to 400 nm. It is also the lowest form of light energy. UVA must be combined with a psoralen (photosensitizing agent) to be beneficial. The combination of a psoralen plus UVA wavelength equals psoralen ultraviolet A–range (PUVA).

PUVA acts to inhibit DNA synthesis and stimulate melanin pigmentation. This is accomplished by increasing the number of melanocytes and melanosomes and increasing the enzyme activity that stimulates melanin synthesis. The repigmentation of human skin that can be achieved with PUVA is believed to result from the migration of melanocytes in the hair follicles into the epidermis. PUVA is used in clients with severe psoriasis or that which has not responded to conventional or standard therapy. PUVA is effective in almost 90% of clients treated.

TABLE 67–4

Potency and Dosage Forms of Commonly Prescribed Topical Corticosteroids

Generic Name	Brand Name(s)	Potency	Dosage Forms
Alclometasone	Aclovate	Low	Cream, ointment
Amcinonide	Cyclocort	High	Cream, ointment, lotion
Betamethasone dipropionate (augmented)	Diprolene	Very high	Ointment, cream, gel, lotion
Betamethasone benzoate	Uticort	Medium	Cream, lotion, gel
Betamethasone dipropionate	Diprosone, Maxivate	High	Ointment, cream, lotion, aerosol
Betamethasone valerate	Valisone	High	Ointment, cream, lotion
Clobetasol	Temovate	Very high	Ointment, cream
Desonide	Tridesilon	Low	Ointment, cream, lotion
Desoximetasone	Topicort	High	Ointment, cream, gel
Dexamethasone	Decadron	Medium	Cream
Fluocinolone	Synalar	High	Ointment, cream, solution
Fluocinonide	Lidex	High	Cream, ointment, solution, gel
Flurandrenolide	Cordran	Medium	Ointment, cream, lotion
Fluticasone	Cutivate	Medium	Ointment, cream
Halcinonide	Halog	High	Ointment, cream, solution
Halobetasol	Ultravate	Very high	Ointment, cream
Hydrocortisone	Cort-Dome, Hytone	Medium	Ointment, cream, lotion, gel
Mometasone	Elocon	Medium	Ointment, cream, lotion
Triamcinolone	Aristocort, Kenalog	Medium	Ointment, cream, lotion

TABLE 67–5
Drugs Used in the Treatment of Psoriasis

Drug Name	Dosage and Route of Administration	Nursing Considerations
Etretinate (Tegison) **HOW SUPPLIED** Capsules: 10, 25 mg	Initial dose: 0.75–1 mg/kg/d in divided doses, not to exceed 1.5 mg/kg/d Maintenance dose: 0.5–0.75 mg/kg/d	**Assess** Take a history of liver function and blood lipid levels. Ask if client is pregnant. Etretinate is classified as Pregnancy Category X drug. Determine if client is nursing; nursing mothers should not receive drug. Assess the status of the skin. **Implement** Administer with milk or fatty food to increase absorption. Protect drug from light. Store drug at 15° to 30° C. Advise client against taking vitamin A during therapy. **Monitor** Monitor liver function and blood lipid test results. Observe for any changes in skin. **Evaluate** Assess the skin for improvement or resolution of skin lesions of psoriasis.
Methotrexate (Rheumatrex) **HOW SUPPLIED** Tablets: 2.5 mg Powder for injection: 20 mg/vial Injection: 25 mg/ml	**ADULTS** Oral: 10–25 mg/wk as single dose *or* 2.5 mg q12h in three divided doses Parenteral: 10–25 mg/wk as single dose	**Assess** Assess the skin before initiating therapy. Obtain a CBC with differential, renal and liver function tests. **Implement** Administer oral doses 1 h before or 2 h after meals. Administer IV at rate of 10 mg/min or less. **Monitor** Note any changes in skin. Obtain CBC, differential, and platelet count. **Evaluate** Observe the skin for improvement or resolution of skin lesions.
Methoxsalen (Oxsoralen) **HOW SUPPLIED** Capsules: 10 mg Lotion: 1% lesions of psoriasis	**Psoriasis** **ADULTS** Oral: Dosage based on patient weight; do not give more than once qod	**Assess** Assess skin for sunburn, diseases with photosensitivity (e.g., melanoma), squamous cell carcinoma. Ask about history of liver, GI, or cardiovascular disease or immunosuppression. Determine if client is pregnant; methoxsalen is classified in Pregnancy Category C. **Implement** Administer capsules with food or milk to decrease GI upset. Advise client not to sunbathe during 24 h before therapy. Advise that client must wear fully protective sunglasses during and 24 h after UVA treatment. Instruct client to avoid sun exposure for at least 8 h after drug ingestion. **Monitor** Observe the skin for effectiveness of treatment.

TABLE *67–5 Continued*
Drugs Used in the Treatment of Psoriasis

Drug Name	Dosage and Route of Administration	Nursing Considerations
Methoxsalen Continued		**Monitor—Continued** Obtain results of liver function, renal function, CBC, and ophthalmic examinations for cataracts. **Evaluate** Observe the skin for improvement or resolution of psoriatic lesions.
Coal Tar Preparations (Medotar, MG217 Medicated, Fototar, Tegrin for Psoriasis, Estar, Polytar, Zetar) HOW SUPPLIED Cream Ointment Lotion Gel Soap	Apply as directed (see individual products) Usually applied to affected area one to four times daily	**Assess** Assess the skin for acute eruptions or inflammation. Ask if client has a history of hypersensitivity. Ask if client is pregnant; coal tar is classified in Pregnancy Category C. Obtain information about renal function. **Implement** Apply thin coating on skin (avoid face and intertriginous areas). Protect adjacent skin with zinc oxide or petrolatum jelly. Cover with a loose, well-ventilated dressing to protect clothes and bedding. **Monitor** Inspect the skin for erythema, number or size of lesions, and appearance of skin irritation. Monitor renal function. **Evaluate** Observe the skin for suppression of disease (i.e., dry, scaling skin).
Calcipotriene (Dovonex) HOW SUPPLIED Ointment: 0.05%	Apply to affected area two times daily; rub in gently and completely	**Assess** Assess skin before initiating therapy. Obtain serum calcium levels. **Implement** Apply thin layer to affected area. **Monitor** Monitor for burning, itching, skin irritation, erythema. Obtain repeat serum calcium levels. **Evaluate** Observe the skin for improvement or resolution of psoriatic lesions.
Anthralin (Anthra-Derm, Lasan, Drithocreme) HOW SUPPLIED Cream: 0.1%, 0.2%, 0.25%, 0.4%, 0.5%, 1% Ointment: 0.1%, 0.25%, 0.4%, 0.5%	Apply to affected area once daily; apply sparingly only to psoriatic lesion; rub gently into skin until absorbed	**Assess** Ask if client is pregnant; anthralin is in Pregnancy Category C. **Implement** Use disposable gloves when applying drug. Apply sparingly only to psoriatic lesion. Rub gently into skin until absorbed. Wash affected areas with soap and water after 15–30 min of drug therapy. **Monitor** Inspect skin for signs of local irritation. **Evaluate** Observe skin for resolution of psoriatic lesions.

Methoxsalen

Methoxsalen (Oxsoralen) is a naturally occurring photoactive substance found in the seeds of the *Ammi majus* plant.

Pharmacotherapeutics   Use of oral methoxsalen with long-wave UVA (photochemotherapy) is indicated for symptomatic control of severe psoriasis.

Pharmacokinetics   Drug absorption and peak drug levels vary according to the dosage form administered. Methoxsalen is reversibly bound to serum albumin and is also taken up by epidermal cells. The drug is rapidly metabolized. Approximately 95% of the drug is excreted as metabolites in the urine within 24 hours.[9]

Pharmacodynamics   The mechanism of action for methoxsalen is not known. Methoxsalen, upon photoactivation, probably conjugates and forms covalent bonds with DNA.[9]

Pharmaceutics   Methoxsalen is available in capsule and lotion dosage forms. For the treatment of psoriasis, oral administration of the drug is used. See Table 67–5 for information on dosage forms and dosages.

Undesired clinical responses   The most common undesired response to methoxsalen is nausea. Other responses include insomnia, nervousness, and depression. When methoxsalen is combined with UVA, pruritus commonly occurs. Other responses from PUVA therapy include edema, dizziness, headache, malaise, hypopigmentation, skin rash, and urticaria.

Contraindications and precautions   Methoxsalen therapy is contraindicated in clients with a history of light-sensitive disease, invasive squamous cell carcinoma, or aphakia.

Drug-drug, drug-nutrient, and drug-environment interactions   Drugs such as griseofulvin, phenothiazines, nalidixic acid, thiazide diuretics, hypoglycemic agents, and some antibiotics produce photosensitivity. When administered concurrently with methoxsalen, an additive reaction to UVA may occur. Methoxsalen should be administered with milk or food to avoid gastric upset. In addition, a low-fat meal increases the blood level of the drug. Before, during, and after therapy, the client must be protected from the effects of the sun.

Life-span considerations   Methoxsalen is classified as a Pregnancy Category C drug. The drug should be administered to a pregnant woman only if clearly needed. It is not known if methoxsalen is excreted in human milk. Safety in children has not been established.

Specific drug-related nursing considerations   Nausea produced by methoxsalen can be minimized or avoided by administering the drug with food or milk or by dividing the dosage into two portions taken approximately 30 minutes apart.[9] After ingestion of methoxsalen, UVA-absorbing wraparound sunglasses should be worn during daylight hours for 24 hours. The protective eyewear is used to prevent irreversible binding of methoxsalen to the proteins and DNA of the lens. Cataracts form when enough binding occurs.

Instruct the client to avoid sun exposure for at least 8 hours after drug ingestion. If avoiding sun exposure is impossible, the client should wear protective clothing (i.e., gloves, long sleeves, hats) and sunscreens that filter out UVA. After PUVA therapy, protective sunglasses should be worn for 24 hours. Instruct the client not to sunbathe for 48 hours after therapy. Mild, transient erythema at 24 to 48 hours after PUVA therapy is an expected reaction and indicates that a therapeutic interaction between the drug and UVA occurred. See Table 67–5 for information about dosage forms, dosages, and nursing considerations.

CONCEPT REVIEW

Psoriasis is a chronic genetic disease that affects 1% to 3% of the population in the United States. It is characterized by recurring exacerbations and remission of thick scaly lesions.

A variety of measures, including systemic and topical drug therapy and UVA treatment, is used to reduce the symptoms of psoriasis.

DRUGS USED TO TREAT VITILIGO

Vitiligo is a condition in which pigment disappears from a patch of skin. The onset is sudden and may be associated with pernicious anemia, hyperthyroidism, and diabetes mellitus. Vitiligo is a concern of darkly pigmented individuals of all races. It also affects light-skinned individuals but not as often. Vitiligo appears at any age in men and women alike. Although the cause is unknown, inheritance and autoimmune factors have been implicated.

The lesion is a depigmented macular patch with definite borders that appears on the face, axillae, neck, or extremities. Lesion size varies from small to large macules involving large skin-surface areas. Depigmented areas, which burn in sunlight, appear bone colored or sometimes grayish blue.

Phototherapy   Treatment consists of psoralen administration in conjunction with UV radiation. (See section on PUVA under discussion of psoriasis.) **Methoxsalen ointment** (Oxsoralen) is used in the PUVA treatment instead of oral methoxsalen. A thin layer is applied within the margins of the vitiligo patch. (When applying methoxsalen, rubber gloves should be worn.) After 30 minutes, the treated area is exposed to UVA. With succeeding treatments, the intensity of UVA is increased. Repigmentation occurs gradually, with the repigmented patches blending in with surrounding skin. Therapy can be of long duration, covering a period of 4 to 12 months.

Phototoxic side effects include itching, blistering, hyperkeratosis, and pruritus. In particular, blistering may result if excess methoxsalen is applied, excessive UVA exposure occurs, or methoxsalen is not washed off after therapy.

Nursing care of the client receiving PUVA therapy for vitiligo involves the same elements as for the client receiving PUVA therapy for psoriasis. During therapy focus your nursing care on prevention of undesired clinical responses. After PUVA exposure, clients must be aware of the importance of avoiding direct sunlight on treated areas.[16,17]

Monobenzone Monobenzone is used to treat vitiligo clients with depigmentation too excessive to repigment. Monobenzone is available in a 20% topical cream (Benoquin).

ENZYMATIC DEBRIDING AGENTS

Enzymatic agents are used to cleanse and debride areas of necrotic tissue found in pressure ulcers, incisional, traumatic, or pyogenic wounds, and ulcers secondary to peripheral vascular disease. Commonly used debriding agents are collagenase, sutilains, and fibrinolysin-deoxyribonuclease. Table 67–6 summarizes information about these three agents.

Collagenase

Collagenase (Santyl) is available as a topical ointment. It dissolves undenatured collagen fibers that anchor necrotic tissue to the wound. Collagenase does not damage granulation tissue. The drug is effective in the environmental pH range of 6 to 8. Therefore use of sodium hypochlorite solution (Dakin's solution), buffered normal saline solution, or acidic cleansing solutions should be avoided. Collagenase usually is applied once daily.

Sutilains

Sutilains (Travase) is a proteolytic enzyme that digests necrotic tissue. It is optimally effective in a pH range of 6.0 to 6.8. Before applying the ointment, the affected area must be cleansed and irrigated with a sodium chloride or water solution. The area must be cleansed of antiseptics or heavy-metal antibacterials, which may denature the enzyme. The ointment is applied to a thin layer that extends beyond the area to be debrided by $\frac{1}{4}$ or $\frac{1}{2}$ inch. Once the ointment is administered, a loose, wet dressing is applied. The wound dressing should be changed three or four times daily. Undesired clinical responses include burning pain, paresthesias, transient dermatitis, and occasional bleeding.[9]

Fibrinolysin-Deoxyribonuclease

Elase is a combination of fibrinolysin and deoxyribonuclease. Fibrinolysin attacks primarily the fibrin of blood clots and fibrinous exudates, whereas deoxyribonuclease attacks deoxyribonucleic acid. The drug is applied one to three times daily with dressing changes.

DRUGS USED TO TREAT SCABIES

Scabies, a common skin disease, is caused by a mite *(Sarcoptes scabiei)*. The mite burrows into the cracked and folded regions of the skin and forms tunnels in the stratum corneum. Within the burrows, copulation occurs, and eggs are laid and hatched within 3 to 4 days. Resulting larvae form their own burrows and grow into adulthood within 2 months. Scabies is usually contracted after close personal contact with an infested individual.

Scabies lesions are small (1 to 4 mm) erythematous papules; some lesions have overlying dry scale or crust. Areas of the body commonly affected include hands, elbows, axillae, nipples, genitalia, feet, and web areas of the fingers. Scabies treatment consists of topical gamma benzene hexachloride (lindane) or crotamiton.[15] Table 67–7 summarizes information about these drugs.

Lindane

Lindane (Kwell, Scabene) is an ovicide and ectoparasiticide that affects *S. scabiei*. It is available as a topical cream or lotion. The drug is directly absorbed into the parasites and ova. Since lindane penetrates human skin and can produce CNS toxicity, the drug must be used according to recommended doses. The cream or lotion is applied to a dry skin surface. The drug should be left in place for 8 to 12 hours and removed by thorough washing. One application is usually sufficient.

Lindane is classified as a Pregnancy Category B drug and is secreted in human milk. Undesired clinical responses include eczematous irritation, and CNS reactions (i.e., dizziness, seizures) have been reported.[9]

Crotamiton

Crotamiton (Crotan, Eurax) is an effective scabicide and antipruritic drug. It is available as a cream or lotion. After a shower or bath, the cream or lotion is massaged into the skin from the chin to the toes, including folds and creases. A second application is recommended 24 hours later. A cleansing bath should be taken 48 hours after the last application.

Crotamiton is classified as a Pregnancy Category C drug. In addition, safety and effectiveness in children have not been established. Undesired responses include allergic sensitivity and skin irritation.[9]

CONCEPT REVIEW

Enzymatic debriding agents are used to cleanse areas of necrotic tissue found in pressure ulcers, incisional, traumatic, or pyogenic wounds, and ulcers secondary to peripheral vascular disease.

Commonly used debriding agents are collagenase, sutilains, and fibrinolysin-deoxyribonuclease.

Scabies, a skin disease produced by *Sarcoptes scabiei*, causes itching and erythema.

Scabicides such as lindane and crotamiton are used to treat scabies. Both drugs are available in lotion and cream dosage forms.

SUMMARY

Since dermatologic disorders are usually treated on an outpatient basis, nurses do not always have contact with the drugs used to treat these conditions. The nurse must routinely familiarize himself or herself with these drugs and their method of administration.

TABLE 67–6
Enzymatic Debriding Agents

Drug Name	Dosage and Route of Administration	Nursing Considerations
Collagenase (Santyl) HOW SUPPLIED Ointment	Apply once daily (more often if dressing becomes soiled)	**Assess** Check the area to be debrided; assess for evidence of infection. **Implement** Cleanse area with gauze pad saturated in 0.9% sodium chloride solution or hydrogen peroxide to remove necrotic material. Apply directly to deep wounds or to sterile gauze pad for shallow wound. Cover wound with gauze pad. Avoid application to healthy surrounding skin. **Monitor** Observe for evidence of infection. **Evaluate** Assess the treatment area for dissolution or sloughing and for development of granulation tissue.
Sutilaines (Travase) HOW SUPPLIED Ointment	Apply three to four times daily (after thoroughly cleansing and moistening wound); apply moist dressing after ointment	**Assess** Assess the area to be debrided; drug is most effective when applied while eschar is soft and moist. Ask if client is pregnant; drug should not be used during pregnancy. Inspect for presence of infection. **Implement** Necrotic tissue must be cleansed, irrigated before application. The area must be well moistened. After application, use loose, wet dressings. **Monitor** Monitor for a moist wound environment. Check for evidence of infection. **Evaluate** Evaluate the treatment area for dissolution or sloughing and development of granulation tissue.
Fibronolysin-desoxyribonuclease (Elase) HOW SUPPLIED Ointment Powder for solution	Apply thin layer and cover with nonadhering gauze two to three times daily	**Assess** Assess area to be debrided; dense, dry eschar must be removed surgically. Assess for presence of infection. **Implement** Before application, cleanse wound with water, peroxide, or 0.9% sodium chloride solution and dry gently. Apply thin layer of ointment, covering area with a nonadhering dressing (e.g., petrolatum gauze). Solution is applied topically as a liquid, spray, or wet dressing. If using wet dressing, ulcerated area is packed with gauze and allowed to dry, causing necrotic tissue slough to become enmeshed in the gauze. **Monitor** Monitor for evidence of infection. **Evaluate** Observe treatment area for dissolution or sloughing and development of granulation tissue.

TABLE 67–7
Scabicides

Drug Name	Dosage and Route of Administration	Nursing Considerations
Lindane (Kwell, G-well, Scabene) HOW SUPPLIED Cream: 1% Lotion: 1%	Apply thin layer to dry skin, rub thoroughly, and leave on for 8–12 h; remove by thorough washing; one application is usually sufficient	**Assess** Assess the skin and hair for signs of infestation, inflammation, abrasions. Assess family members and close friends for infestation. **Implement** Apply to body areas and scalp. Do not apply to face or eyes. Wear gloves to prevent systemic absorption. Wash recently worn clothing, bed linens, towels in very hot water to prevent spread of scabies. **Monitor** Monitor skin and hair for infestation. **Evaluate** Assess skin for resolution of signs of infestation with scabies.
Crotamiton (Eurax) HOW SUPPLIED Cream Lotion	Thoroughly massage into skin from neck down; repeat in 24 h	Same as for lindane.

REFERENCES

1. Hole, J. (1993). *Human anatomy and physiology* (6th ed.). Dubuque, IA: Wm. C. Brown.
2. Tortora, G., & Grabowski, S. (1993). *Principles of anatomy and physiology* (7th ed.). New York: Harper Collins College Publishers.
3. Flory, C. (1992). Skin assessment. *RN, 55*(6), 22–27.
4. Hanno, D. (1989). Accutane: An update for dermatology nurses. *Dermatology Nursing, 1*(1), 27–29.
5. Laudano, J., Leach, E., & Armstrong, R. (1990). Acne: Therapeutic perspectives with an emphasis on the role of isotretinoin. *Dermatology Nursing, 2*, 323–336.
6. Sykes, N., & Webster, G. (1994). Acne: A review of optimum treatment. *Drugs, 48*(1), 59–70.
7. Pochi, P. (1992). Treatment of teenage acne. *Physician Assistant, 16*(3), 147–150, 152, 162–164.
8. Grizzard, D. (1991). Understanding the pathophysiology of psoriasis: A nursing perspective. *Dermatology Nursing, 3*, 305–313.
9. Data Pharmaceutica, Inc. (1993). *1993 physicians' genRx.* Smithtown, NY: Author.
10. Abramowicz, M. (Ed.). (1994). Calcipotriene for psoriasis. *Medical Letter, 36*(928), 70–71.
11. Meola, T., Soter, N.A., Lim, H.W. (1991). Are topical corticosteroids useful adjunctive therapy for the treatment of psoriasis with ultraviolet radiation? A review of the literature. *Archives of Dermatology, 127*, 1708–1713.
12. Degreef, H., & Dooms-Goossens, A. (1993). The new corticosteroids: Are they effective and safe? *Dermatologic Clinics, 11*, 155–160.
13. Kragballe, K. (1989). Topical corticosteroids: Mechanisms of action. *Acta Dermato-Venereologica 69*(Suppl. 151), 7–10.
14. McPherson, M.L. (1993). The use of topical corticosteroids. *Journal of Home Health Care Practice, 5*(3), 50–55.
15. Copstead, L.C. (1995). *Perspectives on pathophysiology.* Philadelphia: W.B. Saunders.
16. Halder, R. (1991). Topical PUVA therapy for vitiligo . . . psoralen and ultraviolet A light. *Dermatology Nursing, 3*(3), 178–180.
17. Moore, S.M., & Lambert, V. (1991). Vitiligo: Care and treatment. *Dermatology Nursing, 3*(1), 15–20.
18. Madden, S., & Ho, V. (1990). Dermatologic therapy and management of special acquired conditions. In A. Goodman, T. Rall, A. Nies, and P. Taylor (Eds.), *The pharmacologic basic of therapeutics.* New York: Pergamon Press.

BIBLIOGRAPHY

Dicken, C., Edwards, L., Ellis, C., & Shalita, A. (1992). Retinoids: What role in your practice? *Patient Care, 26*(10), 18–21, 25–28, 31–32.
Farrington, E. (1993). Lidocaine 2.5%/prilocaine 2.5%: EMLA cream. *Pediatric Nursing, 19*, 484–486.
Marrs, R. (1991). Motivation—The key to control: Nurses' role in treatment of psoriasis. *Professional Nurse, 7*, 103–104, 106, 108.
Marrs, R. (1990). Vitiligo—The loss of pigmentation in skin patches. *Professional Nurse, 5*, 470–471.
Pershing, L.K., Lambert, L., Wright, E., Shah, V., & Williams, R. (1994). Topical 0.050% betamethasone dipropionate. Pharmacokinetic and pharmacodynamic dose response studies in humans. *Archives of Dermatology, 130*, 740–747.
Stone, L., & Garibaldinos, T. (1992). Apply daily . . . psoriasis. *Nursing: The Journal of Clinical Practice, Education, and Management, 5*(4), 8–19.
Stoukides, C. (1993). Topical medications and breastfeeding. *Journal of Human Lactation, 9*(3), 185–187.
Taylor, M. (1991). Treatment of acne vulgaris: Guidelines for primary care physicians. *Postgraduate Medicine, 89*(8), 40–42, 45–47.

Drugs Used to Treat Neoplastic Diseases

CHAPTER 68

OVERVIEW OF
Normal and Neoplastic Cell Growth

ELIZABETH ANN COLEMAN

⊛ **Physical Structure of the Cell**

LEARNING OBJECTIVES:

List five principal structures of the cell.
Describe the function of designated cellular structures.

KEY TERMS:

Cell membrane, centrioles, cytoplasm, endoplasmic
reticulum, Golgi apparatus, lysosomes,
mitochondria, nuclear membrane, nucleus,
organelles, ribosomes

⊛ **Normal Cell Division**

LEARNING OBJECTIVES:

Describe the role of DNA in normal cell division.
Summarize the major events that occur in mitosis.
Describe the events that occur during interphase.
Identify one factor that controls cell growth and
reproduction.

KEY TERMS:

Anaphase, interphase, metaphase, mitosis, prophase,
telophase

⊛ **Cell Differentiation**

LEARNING OBJECTIVE: Define the term *cell differentiation.*

⊛ **Abnormal Cell Division**

LEARNING OBJECTIVES:

Discuss the growth and spread of malignant tumors.
Identify four causes of malignancies.
Summarize the process of carcinogenesis.

KEY TERMS:

Anaplastic, benign, carcinogenesis, doubling time,
malignant, metastasis, oncogenes, proto-oncogenes,
undifferentiated

⊛ **Pharmacologic Therapy for Malignant
Neoplasms**

LEARNING OBJECTIVES:

Discuss the basis for drug selection.
Define the term *tumor kill.*
Explain five general principles of chemotherapy
administration.

KEY TERMS:

Cell-cycle specificity, tumor cell kill

CONCEPTS AND TERMS TO REVIEW

Review in an anatomy and physiology textbook the
functions of the various cell structures or organelles.
Study the process of normal cell division.
Reexamine the difference between mitosis and meiosis.

---

*T*his chapter presents an overview of normal and neoplastic cell growth. To understand how chemotherapy
works, knowledge of the following aspects of cell growth is
needed: role of deoxyribonucleic acid (DNA), the cell cycle,

control of cell growth, cell differentiation, abnormal cell division, and carcinogenesis. In addition to these topics, the chapter includes a discussion of the general effects of chemotherapy
agents on cells, factors that direct the selection of chemotherapy agents, and general principles of chemotherapy administration.

PHYSICAL STRUCTURE OF THE CELL

Cells vary greatly in size, shape, content, and function.
Commonly a cell consists of two major parts—a nucleus and
the cytoplasm. Activities of the cell are controlled by the **nu-**

cleus. This structure, the innermost part of the cell, is enclosed by a thin, double-layered **nuclear membrane.** A mass of fluid, the **cytoplasm,** surrounds the nucleus. It is enclosed by a **cell membrane** or cytoplasmic membrane.

Within the cytoplasm are highly organized structures, many of them called **organelles.** Some principal structures or organelles are **Golgi apparatus, mitochondria, endoplasmic reticulum, ribosomes, lysosomes,** and **centrioles.** Each organelle or structure performs specific metabolic functions for the cell.

NORMAL CELL DIVISION

Certain cells in the body divide almost continuously. For example, millions of blood cells are normally produced every second. Other cells never divide at all after birth (e.g., specialized muscle and nerve cells). Regulatory mechanisms within genes determine when cell division will occur and the growth characteristics of cells.

Role of DNA

Cellular function and activity are controlled by an essential nucleic acid—DNA. **DNA** is the self-reproducing component of chromosomes that carries genes. It is found in every cell in the body. DNA controls the production of protein enzymes capable of starting, stopping, and altering the rate of any cellular function. Since DNA is in the cell's nucleus and protein synthesis occurs outside the nucleus within the cytoplasm, **ribonucleic acid (RNA)** transfers the DNA genetic code to the area of protein synthesis.[1]

Cell Cycle

The cell's life cycle, usually referred to as the **cell cycle,** is the same for all dividing cells. This life cycle represents the period of time from cell reproduction to cell reproduction and lasts 10 to 30 hours. The cell cycle is ended by **mitosis,** the process of cell division that results in the formation of two new daughter cells. Mitosis lasts approximately 30 minutes. Therefore most of the cell cycle is represented by the interval between cell division called **interphase.** During interphase there are three distinct phases: S, G_1, and G_2. In the **G_1 (gap or growth) phase,** cells are engaged in growth, metabolism, and production of material needed for division. During the **S (synthesis) phase,** chromosomes are replicated. This phase is followed by a second growth phase, the **G_2 (gap or growth) phase.** Since no chromosomal replication occurs during the G phases, they are considered gaps or interruptions in DNA synthesis.[1-3]

In Figure 68–1, a fifth phase, G_0, is depicted lying outside the cell-cycle loop; it is the phase of noncycling cells. Cells in G_0 do not respond to signals prompting DNA synthesis as do the cells in G_1. These cells are in a resting phase. However, they continue to synthesize RNA and protein and to perform differentiation functions. Eventually some of the cells return to the cell-cycle loop.[1,2]

Mitosis consists of four subphases: prophase, metaphase, anaphase, and telophase (Fig. 68–2). During the first phase, **prophase,** the chromosomes coil tightly or contract, and the nuclear membrane dissolves. In addition, the mitotic spindle begins to form. During **metaphase,** the chromosomes separate or segregate. During **anaphase,** the chromatids of each chromosome separate and become daughter chromosomes. These

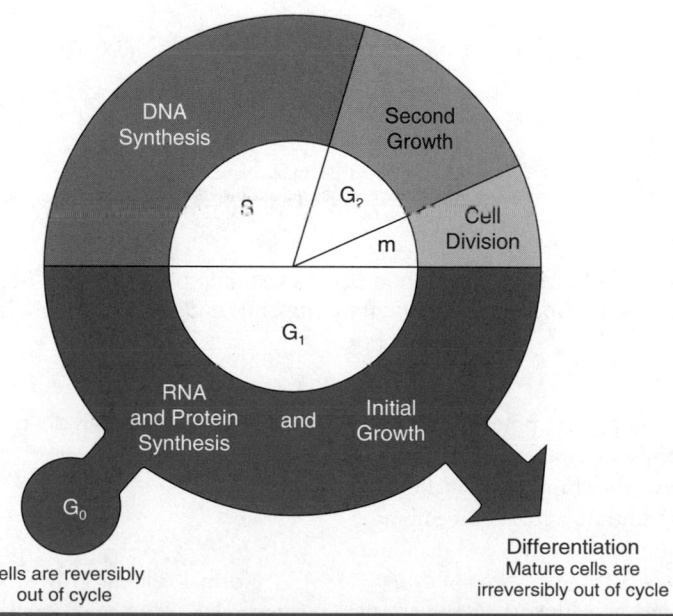

RNA and Protein Synthesis

Cells are reversibly out of cycle

Differentiation
Mature cells are irreversibly out of cycle

FIGURE 68–1   Phases of cell cycle. Relative length of each phase is reflected by the size of the compartments.

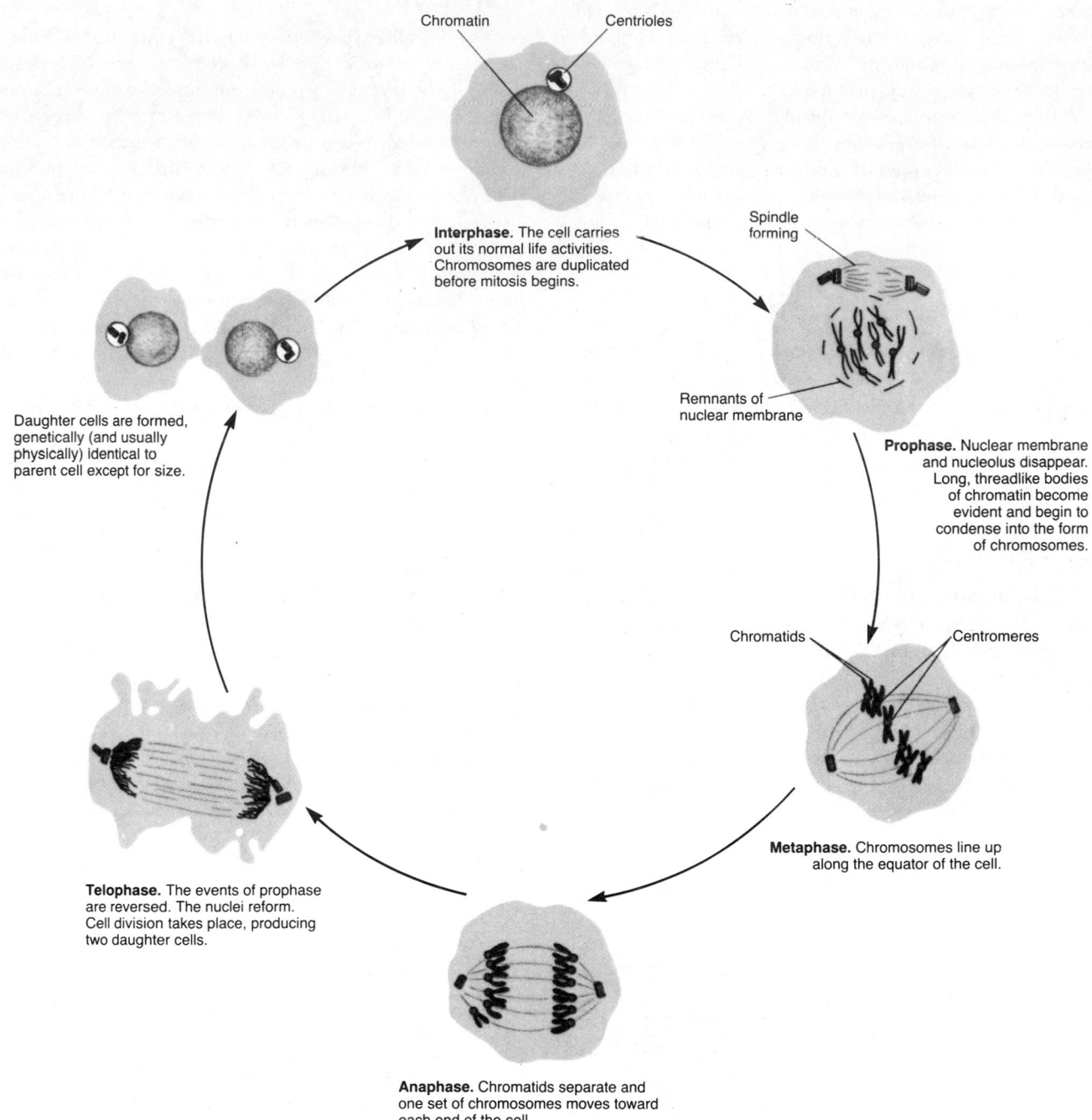

Chromatin   Centrioles

Interphase. The cell carries out its normal life activities. Chromosomes are duplicated before mitosis begins.

Spindle forming

Remnants of nuclear membrane

Prophase. Nuclear membrane and nucleolus disappear. Long, threadlike bodies of chromatin become evident and begin to condense into the form of chromosomes.

Daughter cells are formed, genetically (and usually physically) identical to parent cell except for size.

Chromatids   Centromeres

Metaphase. Chromosomes line up along the equator of the cell.

Telophase. The events of prophase are reversed. The nuclei reform. Cell division takes place, producing two daughter cells.

Anaphase. Chromatids separate and one set of chromosomes moves toward each end of the cell.

FIGURE 68–2   Cell division. Sequence begins with interphase. (From Solomon. E.P., & Phillips, G.A. [1991]. *Understanding human anatomy and physiology.* Philadelphia: W.B. Saunders.)

daughter chromosomes migrate to opposite poles of the cells. The final stage of mitosis, **telophase,** begins when the migration is complete. During telophase, the chromosomes elongate and form chromatin threads. In addition, a nuclear membrane appears around each chromosome set, forming two daughter cells.[1,3,4]

The intervals for the S, G_2, and M (mitosis) phases of cell division are similar for all types of cells, both normal and malignant. The longest and most varied phase is the G_1 phase, which extends from a few hours to several days. This variabil-

ity makes the cell-cycle time different for various types of cells.[2]

Normal cellular growth and reproduction are orderly and controlled. Thus the overall number of cells is held fairly constant. What regulates cell growth and reproduction? Why do some cells grow and reproduce to compensate for cellular insufficiency? Currently very little is known about the exact biologic mechanisms that direct cellular growth and replication. However, studies have suggested the involvement of several factors. For example, growth factors, polypeptides secreted by cells, exert specific and potent growth regulatory actions on cells. A substance, *maturation promoting factor* (MPF), may also be a key factor in the regulation of cell division. When this substance is activated, it induces cell division. In addition, most normal cells stop growing when they run out of space for growth.[5-7]

CELL DIFFERENTIATION

A special characteristic of cell growth and cell division is **cell differentiation.** This term describes the changes in physical and functional properties of cells as they proliferate in the embryo to form the different body structures. These changes involve transforming an unspecialized cell to a specialized cell. Thus these specialized cells differ from their ancestor cells. At present, the exact mechanism involved in producing cell differentiation is not known.[1,8]

CONCEPT REVIEW

The cell is considered the basic unit of life because it is the smallest self-sufficient unit in the body.

Most cells are bound by a cell membrane and have a nucleus and various organelles dispersed within the cytoplasm.

The stages in the life cycle of a cell include interphase, prophase, metaphase, anaphase, and telophase.

ABNORMAL CELL DIVISION

When cells of the body grow and divide without control, the excess tissue that develops is called a *tumor* or *neoplasm.* In tumors or neoplasms cell growth is progressive, and the rate of cell loss lags behind the rate of cell production. Tumors or neoplasms can be cancerous (**malignant**) or noncancerous (**benign**). Benign tumors usually are associated with a favorable prognosis. These tumors are well differentiated and do not invade surrounding tissue or break away and spread from the primary site to other locations in the body. However, malignant tumors are not well differentiated. They often invade surrounding tissues and/or spread to other body parts.

Growth and Spread of Malignant Cells

Malignant tumor growth cannot be explained adequately by cell-cycle kinetics. Different malignancies have similar cell *generation times* (time needed for a cell to complete the cycle from the end of mitosis until the beginning of the next mitosis) but have distinctly different growth rates. In addition, malignant tumors do not double in volume every 2 days, even when the cell-cycle time is approximately 2 days. Therefore tumor growth must be described in the context of tissue-growth kinetics, not cell-cycle kinetics.[2]

When tissues from malignant tumors are examined, it is clear that not all tumor cells are proliferating. In fact, most of the tumor cells are in the G_0 phase. They are either dead or have differentiated and no longer have the ability to replicate. These tumor cells in the G_0 phase just add to the tumor bulk. As the number of dead tumor cells increases, large areas of ischemic necrosis within the tumor develop as the tumor outstrips its blood supply.

Tumors grow much more rapidly early in their life spans. By the time a tumor is clinically detectable, it may have undergone 30 **doubling times,** the time required for a tumor to double in size. Additional doubling of the tumor's size occurs much more slowly and represents a small percentage of the tumor's growth.[2]

As the size of the tumor increases, it usually becomes too large for its environment. Initially the cells invade surrounding tissues and compete with normal tissue for space and nutrients. Eventually the normal tissue decreases in size and dies. As mentioned previously, the growth of a normal cell is inhibited by contact on all sides with other cells. This is called *contact inhibition.* Malignant cells do not respond in the same manner; they invade healthy tissues to make space for their growth.

After invasion of surrounding tissues, some malignant cells may detach from the initial or primary tumor and invade a body cavity or enter the blood or lymph. If these cells survive, they invade adjacent body tissues and establish secondary tumors. This is known as **metastasis.**

Malignant cells also lose the ability to differentiate like normal cells, with the degree of loss varying among tumors. Malignant cells that closely resemble normal cells from the tissue of origin are called **well differentiated.** Cells that have no similarity to the tissue of origin are **undifferentiated** and are called **anaplastic.** The degree of differentiation affects prognosis, with poorly differentiated cells indicating a poor prognosis.[3,9]

Causes of Malignancies

Why does a normal cell lose control and become malignant? Environmental agents, genetics, and viruses are known contributing factors. Studies have shown that some viruses cause malignancies in humans. These agents infect cells and convert them to virus producers. Numerous environmental factors, including inhaled substances (e.g., hydrocarbons, cigarette smoke, radon gas from the earth, and asbestos) and ingested substances (e.g., cytotoxic drugs, food high in saturated fats, and ultraviolet and ionizing radiation) produce cancer. Any environmental agent that is capable of producing cancer is called a *carcinogen.*[5,10-13]

Genetic factors that cause malignancies include specific chromosomal abnormalities, oncogenes, and mutated antioncogenes. **Oncogenes** are genes with the ability to transform a normal cell into a malignant cell when inappropriately activated. Oncogenes develop from normal genes that regulate growth and development called **proto-oncogenes.**[5,9,14]

Carcinogenesis

A normal cell undergoes malignant transformation through a process called **carcinogenesis.** The first stage of carcinogenesis is **initiation.** During this stage, exposure to a known producer of cancer occurs. However, malignancy may not develop. The second stage of carcinogenesis, **promotion,** increases the chance for malignancy. During this stage, the dose and duration of exposure to the promoting agent are important, but the effects still are reversible if the promoting agent is removed. In the third stage, **progression,** development of the malignant tumor occurs. The period of time between exposure to the promoting agent and the development of a malignant tumor is called the *latency period.*[9]

CONCEPT REVIEW

Abnormal cell division results in either a benign or malignant tumor or neoplasm.

Maligant cells divide continuously, invading and spreading to adjacent tissues and other portions of the body.

Viruses, genetic factors, chemicals, and environmental factors are linked to the development of malignant cells.

PHARMACOLOGIC THERAPY FOR MALIGNANT NEOPLASMS

Stage of tumor development, cell-cycle specificity, tumor location, drug resistance, and drug toxicity must be considered when determining which chemotherapeutic agent to use. Since most chemotherapeutic agents interfere with the synthesis or function of DNA, chemotherapy kills those tumor cells that are growing or replicating. As indicated previously, chemotherapy is most effective against tumors with high growth fractions. The **growth fraction** (ratio of dividing cells to total cells) is highest when the tumor is small. Thus early diagnosis and early treatment are important. If they are not possible, surgical debulking or radiation therapy can reduce the size of the tumor so that chemotherapy can be more effective.[2,15]

Cell-Cycle Specificity

Tumor cell kill, or killing effect, for most chemotherapeutic drugs is related to the cell cycle. **Cycle-specific drugs** are effective only if cells go through the cell cycle and if the drug makes contact with the cells while they are in a particular phase of the cell cycle. For example, methotrexate (Mexate) and fluorouracil (Adrucil) are most effective during S (synthesis) phase. Vincristine (Oncovin) and vinblastine (Velban) only work during the metaphase stage of mitosis.

Cycle-nonspecific drugs are effective only if cells go through the cell cycle, but tumor cells are killed during any phase of the cell cycle. Cisplatin (Platinol), cyclophosphamide (Cytoxan), and doxorubicin (Adriamycin) are examples of cycle-nonspecific drugs. There are a few chemotherapeutic drugs for which tumor cell kill is not related to the cell cycle. These drugs kill nondividing cells.[16,17]

Tumor Location and Route of Administration

Some tumors may not respond to chemotherapy because of their location and the drug's inability to reach the area. For example, chemotherapy given intravenously make not reach a tumor in the central nervous system because of the blood-brain barrier. Researchers are currently developing alternate drug delivery mechanisms to alleviate this problem.[17]

Drug Resistance

Tumor cell kill is also influenced by tumor cells' resistance to a specific chemotherapeutic agent. Resistance arises as tumor cells mutate spontaneously. Resistance to one chemotherapy drug often results in resistance to other chemotherapeutic agents, even those that are structurally unrelated.

Multidrug resistance is associated with the expression of a cell-surface glycoprotein, P-170, that repels certain chemotherapeutic drugs. Nonchemotherapeutic drugs that interfere with calcium entry into cells and thus stabilize cell membranes (e.g., the antiarrhythmic drug verapamil [Calan]) have been used to circumvent P-170 multidrug resistance. These drugs restore sensitivity to the chemotherapeutic drug, allowing the drug to make contact with the cells and destroy them.[2]

In the early stages of growth tumor cells differ only slightly from the tissue of origin, which means the tumor cells are well differentiated. As the tumor increases in size, its cells become less differentiated, or more anaplastic, and more difficult to kill. These anaplastic cells have a higher mutation rate, which results in drug resistance. In addition, chemotherapeutic drugs can act as mutagens, causing a higher mutation rate and thus drug resistance. Cancer researchers are attempting to find agents that would cause cancer cells to "grow up" or become differentiated (i.e., more like the normal cell of the tissue of origin) rather than trying to kill undifferentiated cells.[2]

Drug Toxicity

Drug toxicity is another major problem during drug selection. Both the drug dose and the duration of therapy are limited by the level of toxicity to normal body tissues. While chemotherapeutic agents are destroying tumor cells, they are also destroying normal cells. Whether malignant or normal, the cellular destruction is greatest for those cells that are the fastest growing. For example, since the intermitotic or generation time is most rapid for normal cells in the bone marrow, most chemotherapeutic drugs rapidly destroy these cells as they kill tumor cells.[17]

CONCEPT REVIEW

Chemotherapeutic drugs interrupt cellular division or damage the cell's DNA.

Tumor cell kill is influenced by cell-cycle specificity, tumor location, drug resistance, and drug toxicity.

SUMMARY

A review of normal and neoplastic cell growth facilitates an understanding of how chemotherapy affects cellular function. Neoplastic cells, unlike normal cells, are not held in check by homeostatic mechanisms that maintain a predetermined number of cells in normal tissues. As normal cells undergo malignant transformation through a process known as *carcinogenesis,* the transformed anaplastic cells acquire the ability to metastasize. Since surgery and radiotherapy are limited to local treatment of a malignant tumor, chemotherapy is necessary treatment for metastatic disease.

Most chemotherapy drugs work by interrupting or altering DNA synthesis or function, but the mechanism of activity for the major categories of chemotherapy drugs varies within the cell cycle. Chemotherapy works best during the early stages of the disease when the tumor's doubling time is rapid. It is most important that all courses of the drug therapy regimen, which usually consists of multiple drugs, be given.

REFERENCES

1. Guyton, A. (1991). *Textbook of medical physiology* (8th ed.). Philadelphia: W.B. Saunders.
2. Cooper, M.R., & Cooper, M.R. (1991). Principles of medical oncology. In A.I. Holleb, D.J. Fink, & G.P. Murphy, (Eds.). *American Cancer Society textbook of clinical oncology.* Atlanta: American Cancer Society.
3. Hole, J. (1993). *Human anatomy and physiology* (6th ed.). Dubuque, IA: Wm. C. Brown.
4. Solomon, E., & Phillips, G. (1987). *Understanding human anatomy and physiology.* Philadelphia: W.B. Saunders.
5. Park, M., & Woude, G.F. (1989). Principles of molecular cell biology of cancer: Oncogenes. In V.T. De Vita, S. Hellman, & S. Rosenberg, (Eds.). *Cancer: Principles and practice of oncology,* (3rd ed.) (Vol. 2). Philadelphia: J.B. Lippincott.
6. Roberts, A.B., & Sporn, M.B. (1989). Principles of molecular cell biology of cancer: Growth factors related to transformation. In V.T. De Vita, S. Hellman, & S. Rosenberg, (Eds.). *Cancer: Principles and practice of oncology* (3rd ed.). (Vol. 2). Philadelphia: J.B. Lippincott.
7. Woude, S.V., & Woude, G.F. (1989). Principles of molecular cell biology of cancer: General aspects of gene regulation. In V.T. De Vita, S. Hellman, & S. Rosenberg, (Eds.). *Cancer: Principles and practice of oncology* (3rd ed.). (Vol. 2). Philadelphia: J.B. Lippincott.
8. Tortora, G., & Grabowski, S. (1993). *Principles of anatomy and physiology* (7th ed.). New York: Harper Collins.
9. Vincent, B., & Mirand, A. (1991). The nature of cancer. In S.B. Baird, M.G. Donehower, V.L. Stalsbroten, & T.B. Ades, (Eds.). *A cancer source book for nurses* (6th ed.). Atlanta: American Cancer Society.
10. Greenwald, P. (1989). Principles of cancer prevention: Diet and nutrition. In V.T. De Vita, S. Hellman, & S. Rosenberg, (Eds.). *Cancer: Principles and practice of oncology* (3rd ed.) (Vol. 2). Philadelphia: J.B. Lippincott.
11. Rowley, J.D. (1989). Principles of molecular cell biology of cancer: Chromosomal abnormalities. In V.T. De Vita, S. Hellman, & S. Rosenberg, (Eds.). *Cancer: Principles and practice of oncology* (3rd ed.). (Vol. 2). Philadelphia: J.B. Lippincott.
12. Shields, P.G., & Harris, C.C. (1991). Molecular epidemiology and the genetics of environmental cancer. *JAMA, 266,* 681-768.
13. Trichopoulos, D., Mollo, F., Tomatis, L., Agapitos, E., et al. (1992). Active and passive smoking and pathological indicators of lung cancer risk in an autopsy study. *JAMA, 268,* 1697-1701.
14. Cooper, G.M. (1990). *Oncogenes.* Boston: Jones & Bartlett.
15. V.T. De Vita, (1989). Principles of chemotherapy. In V.T. De Vita, S. Hellman, & S. Rosenberg, (Eds.). *Cancer: Principles and practice of oncology,* (3rd ed.). (Vol. 2). Philadelphia: J.B. Lippincott.
16. Lobert, S., & Correla, J.J. (1992). Antimitotics in cancer chemotherapy. *Cancer Nursing, 13*(1), 22-33.
17. Petersen, J. (1991). Chemotherapy. In S.B. Baird, M.G. Donehower, V.L. Stalsbroten, & T.B. Ades, (Eds.). *A cancer source book for nurses* (6th ed.). Atlanta: American Cancer Society.

BIBLIOGRAPHY

Alberts, B., Bray, D., Lewis, J., Raff, M., Roberts, K., & Watson, J.D. (1989). *Molecular biology of the cell.* New York: Garland Publishing.

Cassidy, J., & Macfarlane, D.K. (1991). The role of the nurse in clinical cancer research. *Cancer Nursing, 14,* 124-131.

Collins-Hattery, A.M., & Blumberg, B.D. (1991). S phase index and ploidy prognostic markers in node negative breast cancer: Information for nurses. *Oncology Nursing Forum, 18*(1), 59-62.

Cullen, J.W. (1989). Principles of cancer prevention: Tobacco. In V.T. De Vita, S. Hellman, & S. Rosenberg, (Eds.). *Cancer: Principles and practice of oncology* (3rd ed.). (Vol. 2). Philadelphia: J.B. Lippincott.

Dudjak, L.A., & Fleck, A.E. (1991). BRMs: New drug therapy comes of age. *RN, 54*(10), 42-48.

Ersek, M. (1991). Biological response modifiers. In S.B. Baird, M.G. Donehower, V.L. Stalsbroten, & T.B. Ades (Eds.). *A cancer source book for nurses* (6th ed.). Atlanta: American Cancer Society.

Fry, R.J. (1989). Principles of carcinogenesis: Physical. In V.T. De Vita, S. Hellman, & S. Rosenberg, (Eds.). *Cancer: Principles and practice of oncology* (3rd ed.). (Vol. 2). Philadelphia: J.B. Lippincott.

Howley, P.M. (1989). Principles of carcinogenesis: Viral. In V.T. De Vita, S. Hellman, & S. Rosenberg, (Eds.). *Cancer: Principles and practice of oncology* (3rd ed.). (Vol. 2). Philadelphia: J.B. Lippincott.

Malloy, J. (1991). Administering intraperitoneal chemotherapy: A new approach. *Nursing '91, 21*(1), 58-62.

Mayer, D.K. (1990). Biotherapy: Recent advances and nursing implications. *Advances in Oncology Nursing, 25,* 291-305.

Walters, P. (1990). Chemo: A nurses' guide to action, administration, and side effects. *RN Magazine, 53*(2), 53-67.

CHAPTER 69

Antineoplastic Drugs

NORMA L. PINNELL • ROBERT J. KIZIOR

⊛ **Classification of Antineoplastic Drugs and Nursing Considerations**
LEARNING OBJECTIVES:
List the five main classes of antineoplastic drugs, determined by their mechanism of action.
Describe special precautions to take in administering antineoplastic agents.
Explain why these precautions are needed.
Name the three primary modes of intravenous administration of antineoplastic drugs.
List the most universal undesired clinical responses to chemotherapy.
Develop a plan of care for a client undergoing combination chemotherapy.
KEY TERMS:
Mucositis, alopecia, myelosuppression

⊛ **Alkylating Agents**
LEARNING OBJECTIVES:
Describe the mechanism of action of alkylating agents.
Name the major undesired clinical responses to these drugs.

⊛ **Antimetabolites**
LEARNING OBJECTIVES:
Explain the cell cycle specificity of cytarabine.
List the routes by which cytarabine can be administered.
Describe the mechanism of action of antimetabolic drugs.

⊛ **Antineoplastic Antibiotics**
LEARNING OBJECTIVES:
Describe the major adverse reaction to bleomycin.
List three common indications for antineoplastic antibiotics.

⊛ **Plant Alkaloids**
LEARNING OBJECTIVES:
Explain the meaning of the term *mitotic inhibitor*.
Name three commonly used plant alkaloids.
KEY TERM: Mitotic inhibitor

⊛ **Hormones**
LEARNING OBJECTIVES:
Discuss the possible mechanism of action of hormonal agents.
Describe possible undesired clinical responses to hormonal therapy.
Give two reasons why diethylstilbestrol use is contraindicated during pregnancy.

⊛ **Miscellaneous Agents**
LEARNING OBJECTIVES:
Explain the mechanism of action of asparaginase.
Discuss the major adverse reaction to asparaginase's use.
Describe the necessary precautions to take in case this reaction should occur.

⊛ **Investigational Drugs**
LEARNING OBJECTIVE: Discuss the use of investigational drugs in the treatment of cancer.
KEY TERM: Investigational agent

*T*he use of chemotherapeutic drugs to fight cancer dates
back to World War I when mustard gases, used as
weapons because of their vesicant action on the skin and mucous membranes, were observed to have toxic effects on other
tissues, especially the hematopoietic system. Research eventually supported the hypothesis that these systemic effects might
reduce the number of malignant cells in individuals with certain cancers.

Although chemotherapy was once used only as a last resort
in cancer treatment, it now is used as adjuvant therapy after
surgery or radiation therapy. Primary chemotherapy commonly is used for many neoplasms. Chemotherapeutic drugs
may be administered as a single agent; however, they are administered more often in combinations to increase therapeutic
results and decrease toxic effects.

Antineoplastic drugs affect both normal and malignant cells
by altering cellular activity during one or more phases of the
cell cycle. Although normal cells die along with tumor cells,
normal cells have a greater ability to repair themselves than do
tumor cells.

Chemotherapeutic drugs kill a percentage of cells, and that
percentage is governed by the dosage administered. Thus
multiple doses of a drug or drugs are necessary to reduce the
number of tumor cells to the point that the body's immune
system can eliminate the remainder.[1] Antineoplastic drugs are
most effective on rapidly dividing cancer cells in the early
stages of tumor growth. Thus early detection and treatment
are important.

CLASSIFICATION OF ANTINEOPLASTIC DRUGS

There are several different ways to classify antineoplastic drugs.
For example, the drugs may be categorized into general types
based on the stage of the cell cycle at which they exert their effect. (See Chapter 68 and Tables 69–4 through 69–9.)
Antineoplastic drugs are also divided into classes determined
by their mechanism of action: alkylating agents, antimetabolites, antineoplastic antibiotics, plant alkaloids, and hormones.
This classification system is used in Chapter 69. In addition,
miscellaneous agents and investigational drugs are considered
in this chapter.

▦ NURSING CONSIDERATIONS

Nursing care of the client with cancer involves careful attention to the physical and psychologic status of the client. It also
involves the use of many precautions to protect the client and
nurse from the adverse effects of the potent agents used. The
nursing process provides a framework to organize this complex
area of nursing care.

Assessing   A general health history and physical assessment are required before therapy. Obtain baseline laboratory
values for red blood count (RBC), white blood count (WBC),
and platelets. Assess the intravenous (IV) site selections and
the condition of oral mucosa before initiating therapy.

Determine the client's level of readiness to learn and his or
her ability to understand the information needed for his or her
self-care. Assess the client's and family's readiness to cope with
the ramifications of the disease. Observe the client for potential impediments to learning such as excessive fatigue and increased anxiety. Find out what the client knows about cancer
in general and about his or her own condition specifically.
Determine whether the client or a family member has had any
previous experience with the disease.

Identify potential contraindications for specific chemotherapeutic agents or situations requiring dosage adjustments.
Inquire whether the client has allergies and list any medications (over-the-counter [OTC] or prescribed) the client is
taking.

Diagnosing   Analyze the assessment data to determine
the relevant nursing diagnoses. Some of the more frequent
nursing diagnoses related to cancer chemotherapy follow:

- High risk for injury related to side effects of therapy.
- High risk for infection related to decreased WBCs or venous
  access devices.
- Altered oral mucous membranes related to decreased saliva-
  tion or inflammation (stomatitis, mucositis).
- Altered nutrition: less than body requirements, related to
  anorexia, nausea, and vomiting.
- Colonic constipation related to decreased activity or drug
  side effects.
- Fatigue related to anemia or effects of cancer.
- Anxiety related to effects and outcomes of treatment.
- Ineffective individual coping related to multiple stressors or
  overwhelming threat to self.
- Knowledge deficit of therapy, effects, and precautions.
- Body image disturbance related to alopecia.
- Dysfunctional grieving related to loss of body part or altered
  appearance or function.
- Altered family processes related to illness and therapy.[2]

Planning   Given the potential for adverse reactions and
the potential for psychosocial disturbance, planning for care
during chemotherapy should involve ongoing monitoring of
client status and client and family counseling and education.
Planning should also take into account whether the chemotherapy is administered in a hospital or in an ambulatory care
setting. The following expected outcomes are applicable:

- The client experiences no infection or inflammation.
- The client exhibits no bleeding.
- The client maintains adequate tissue integrity.
- The client maintains adequate nutritional status.
- The client achieves relief of pain and discomfort.

- The client demonstrates increased activity tolerance and decreased fatigue.
- The client progresses through the grieving process.
- The client exhibits improved body image and self-esteem.[3]

Implementing Implementation of nursing care in the client undergoing chemotherapy involves (1) administering the medication; (2) assisting the client to cope with undesired clinical responses to chemotherapeutic agents; and (3) educating and supporting the client and family in the period after the chemotherapy.

Administering the medication When dealing with chemotherapeutic drugs, take special precautions to protect yourself and others from unnecessary exposure to the agents. (These drugs are highly toxic whether they are inhaled or absorbed through the skin.) Always wear gloves, and follow National Institutes of Health (NIH) guidelines concerning gowns, masks, and eye protectors. Avoid contaminating anything with the agents. Dispose of all contaminated materials in specially identified containers. Administer the agents precisely according to schedule, using strict asepsis to prevent client infection. When the client's platelet count drops, avoid the use of all trauma (e.g., rectal temperature or injection).[4, 5]

The goal of chemotherapy administration is to optimize drug availability. Many diverse routes have been developed to deliver drugs in high concentrations to areas of greatest need and to improve the antitumor effects. The current routes of administration include intrathecal (IT), intraarterial (IA), intracavity (IC), subcutaneous (SC), intramuscular (IM), topical, oral, and IV.

The most common routes of chemotherapy administration are oral and IV. The oral route is usually preferred, but absorption can be unpredictable. In addition, there may be obstacles to this route (e.g., the condition of the gastrointestinal [GI] tract, the client's state of consciousness or willingness to comply with the treatment schedule, and the availability of oral forms of the drug).

The IV route is the most common method of delivering chemotherapy. It allows absorption of the drug, which in turn provides predictable blood levels. IV drugs are administered through a peripheral access, a vein in the client's arm or hand, through a central venous access device (e.g., a silicone, Silastic catheter), or through an implanted infusion port. See Table 69–1 for the routine maintenance of two of the more frequently used types of venous access devices. Standing orders and antidote kits must be available before administration of IV antineoplastic drugs. Extravasation is an emergency and must be dealt with at once.

Three methods of IV administration are commonly used to provide chemotherapeutic agents:

- **IV push:** direct administration of the drug into the IV cannula through either a butterfly needle or an angiocatheter
- **Piggyback IV administration:** introduction of drug

TABLE 69–1

Maintenance of Silastic Catheters and Implanted Infusion Ports

Type of Infusion Device	Routine Maintenance
SILASTIC CATHETERS	
Hickman Broviac	Irrigate qod with 3 ml heparin and saline solution (10–100 U heparin/ml).
Chemocath Silastic	Brisk irrigations prevent outflow obstruction.
Hemed Silicone Quinton Silastic	Routine clamping is not recommended. (However, when clamping catheter, clamp over protective covering.)
Raaf Catheter	Change dressing qod for 2–3 wk after insertion. (Thereafter, apply adhesive bandage to access site.) Prevent undue tension on catheter. Tape catheter to person at all times. Change cap(s) q7d. Showering and bathing are permitted.
Groshong Catheter	Never clamp the catheter. Catheter requires no heparinization. Pressure-sensitive valve remains closed when not in use. Irrigate briskly with 5 ml of normal saline solution (NSS) once q7d or after use. Irrigate with 20 ml saline solution after blood aspiration or transfusion of blood product. Do not use needle through injection cap.
INFUSION PORTS	
Mediport Infuse-A-Port Port-a-Cath S.E.A.-Port Groshong Port* Q-Port Hickman Port	Puncture with Huber point needle only for Mediport and Q-Port; Infusaid needles only for Infuse-A-Port; Huber needles for Port-A-Cath, Groshong and Hickman Ports; S.E.A.-Port infusion needles with a 90-degree angle only for S.E.A.-Port. Irrigate q4wk with heparin and saline solution (3–5 ml 100 U heparin/ml). Give 20 ml NSS flush after blood drawing. For arterial ports, irrigate once per week with 3–5 ml 100 U heparin/ml. Flush catheter after each use. Place no restrictions on client activity.

*Exceptions for Groshong Port: (1) in between usage flush with 10 ml NSS q4wk; (2) irrigate with 20 ml NSS flush after medications, total parenteral nutrition, and blood drawing.

through an injection port (usually the port closest to the client) in the tubing of continuous IV infusion

- **Sidearm administration:** as in piggybacking, administration of drug into a port connected to the main infusion cannula; the drug may run as a brief infusion for several minutes (a bolus infusion) or up to several days, 24 hours each day (a continuous infusion); again as in piggyback administration, permits dilution of the chemotherapeutic agent with the main infusion fluid

When high concentrations of an antineoplastic drug are needed and systemic concentrations must be minimized, the IT, IA, and IC routes can be used.

Assisting the client The client's acceptance of his or her cancer and the subsequent psychologic coping with the disease are complicated by the side effects of the agents administered. The nurse's role in decreasing these effects can have a significant impact on the client's sense of well being and potentially on the client's response to treatment. Response to chemother-

apy is very individual. Some tolerate the regimen well, whereas others become very ill. The most common undesired clinical responses to chemotherapeutic agents are nausea and vomiting, mucositis, alopecia, and bone marrow suppression (Fig. 69–1). They are discussed briefly here because they are common to most of the antineoplastic drugs and they have a profound effect on the client.

A number of measures can be taken to decrease nausea, vomiting, and other GI complaints resulting from many chemotherapeutic agents. Administer antiemetics the night before the initiation of chemotherapy and regularly (e.g., at 6-hour intervals) while the nausea continues. For many of the drugs this period is predictable. Administer the chemotherapeutic agents at night or during the late afternoon if possible, and instruct the client to experiment with different eating patterns while receiving the medication. The client can assess his or her tolerance to the drug by avoiding meals before, during, or immediately after the initial administration. Discourage intake of

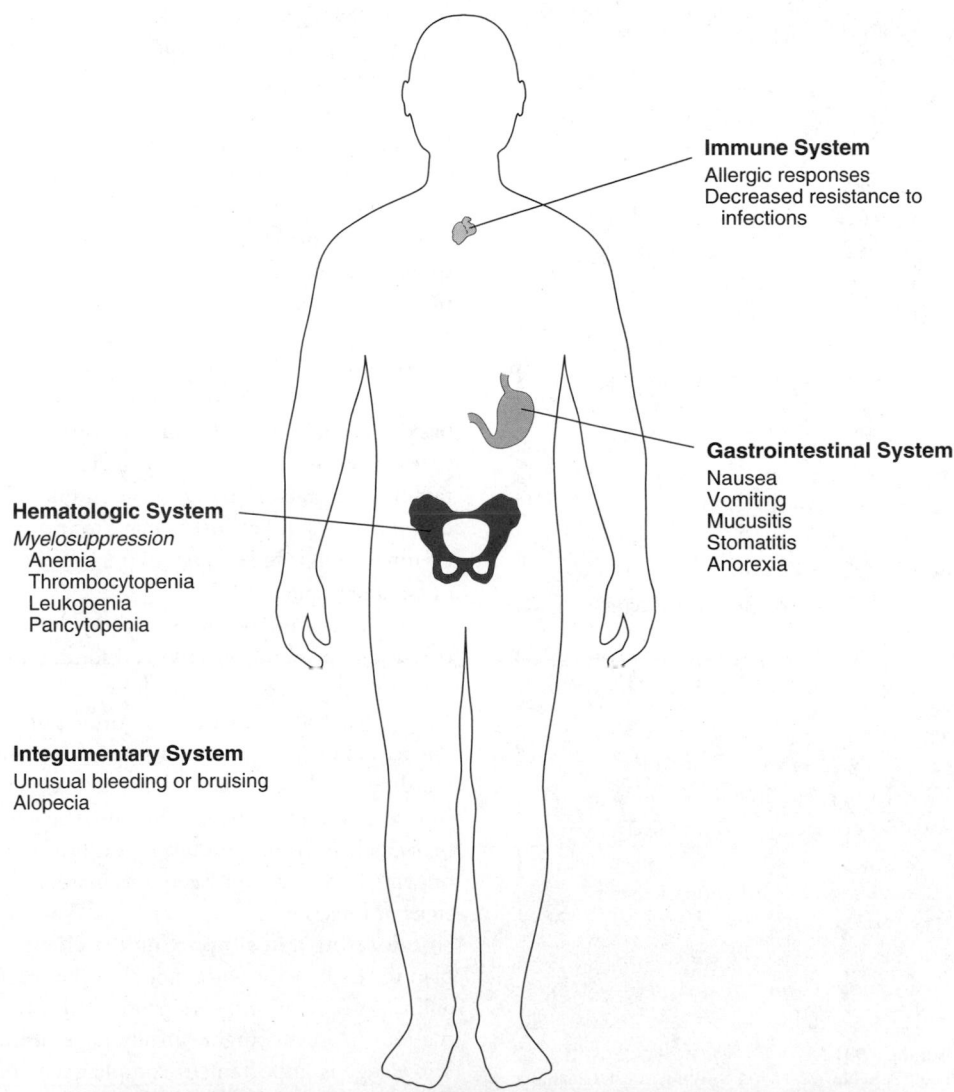

Immune System
Allergic responses
Decreased resistance to
  infections

Gastrointestinal System
Nausea
Vomiting
Mucusitis
Stomatitis
Anorexia

Hematologic System
Myelosuppression
  Anemia
  Thrombocytopenia
  Leukopenia
  Pancytopenia

Integumentary System
Unusual bleeding or bruising
Alopecia

FIGURE 69–1   Common adverse reactions to prototype antineoplastic drugs.

foods that are heavy, greasy, fatty, sweet, or spicy. If the client is able to tolerate foods on the day of therapy, recommend small, frequent meals with a bland diet consisting of, for example, cottage cheese, applesauce, and vanilla ice cream. Urge the client to increase fluid intake to 3 quarts per day. (See box.)

Provide an environment that is relatively free from odors. Immediate surroundings should be clean, quiet, and subdued. The client should keep weight and diet diaries to monitor how much is being consumed and retained. If the client's weight proves unstable, refer the client to a dietician for counseling. If a home caregiver is preparing meals for the client, he or she should also be encouraged to attend the dietary counseling sessions.[2,6,7]

CLIENT TEACHING ABOUT NAUSEA AND VOMITING

▶ Avoid big meals so your stomach won't feel too full. Eat small meals throughout the day.

▶ Drink liquids at least an hour before or after mealtime instead of with your meals.

▶ Eat and drink slowly.

▶ Stay away from sweet, fried, or fatty foods.

▶ Eat foods cold or at room temperature so you won't be bothered by strong smells.

▶ Chew your food well for easier digestion.

▶ If nausea is a problem in the morning, try eating dry foods like cereal, toast, or crackers before getting up. (Don't try this if you have mouth or throat sores or if you are troubled by a lack of saliva.)

▶ Drink cool, clear, unsweetened fruit juices such as apple or grape juice or light-colored sodas such as ginger ale that have lost their fizz.

▶ Suck on ice cubes, mints, or tart candies. (Don't use tart candies if you have mouth or throat sores.)

▶ Try to avoid odors that bother you such as cooking smells, smoke, or perfume.

▶ Prepare and freeze meals in advance for days when you don't feel like cooking.

▶ Rest in a chair after eating, but don't lie flat for at least 2 hours.

▶ Wear loose-fitting clothes.

▶ Breathe deeply and slowly when you feel nauseated.

▶ Distract yourself by chatting with friends or family members, listening to music, or watching a movie or TV show.

▶ Use relaxation techniques to help prevent anticipatory nausea.

▶ Avoid eating for at least a few hours before treatment if nausea usually occurs during chemotherapy.

From National Cancer Institute. (1991 Dec.). *Chemotherapy and you: A guide to self-help treatment.* (3rd ed., Pub. No. 92-1136). Washington, DC: United States Department of Health and Human Services.

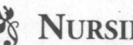 ## NURSING RESEARCH

Edwards, J.N., Herman, J., Wallace, B., Pavy, M., & Harrison-Pavy, J. (1991). Comparison of patient-controlled and nurse-controlled antiemetic therapy in patients receiving chemotherapy. *Research in Nursing and Health, 14,* 249–257.

The purpose of this quasiexperimental pilot study was to compare the effect of patient-controlled (PCAE) and nurse administered (NCAE) antiemetic therapy for controlling chemotherapy-induced nausea and vomiting. Twenty subjects were randomly assigned to either the PCAE group, who received IV antiemetic medication through a patient-controlled pump, or the NCAE group, who received antiemetic drugs from the nurse. Nausea, vomiting, sedation, and drug consumption were measured. There was no difference in nausea scores between the two groups. However, subjects in the PCAE group used significantly less medication than subjects in the NCAE group.

STUDENT ACTIVITIES

• In your agency determine the usual method of administering antiemetic drugs to clients receiving antineoplastic drugs.

• Compare chart data from clients receiving antineoplastic drugs and determine route and frequency of administration of antiemetic drugs.

Mucositis is the presence of sores on mucous membranes; this condition primarily affects the mouth (stomatitis). The sores can be painful and can interfere with eating. The box on p. 947 contains client teaching points about the care of these sores.

Alopecia, or hair loss, is a common complication arising from therapy with antineoplastic drugs. Hair usually grows back, although the color and texture may be different after therapy. Turbans, scarves, and hairpieces are helpful in maintaining a satisfactory body image through this period. Instruct clients to use soft hairbrushes and to use low heat when drying their hair. Advise clients *not* to use brush rollers, dye their hair, or get a permanent.

Bone marrow suppression (**myelosuppression,** the decrease of bone marrow activity, resulting in decreased numbers of circulating leukocytes, erythrocytes, and platelets) is a common effect of antineoplastic drug administration. Consequences such as immunosuppression, hypoxia, increased bleeding tendency, and fatigue are associated with this response. Take extra precautions in keeping the immunosuppressed client from unnecessary exposure to those who are sick or who have recently been vaccinated, and watch for early signs of infection.

Educating and supporting the client   Gear the teaching plan for each client with cancer to that particular individual's ability to take in and retain new information. Review information the client might already have heard, especially if this knowledge is important to compliance with the medical regimen. Provide written materials as follow-up.

CLIENT TEACHING ABOUT STOMATITIS

▶ If possible, see your dentist before you start chemotherapy to have your teeth cleaned and to take care of any problems such as cavities, abscesses, gum disease, or poorly fitting dentures. Ask your dentist to show you the best ways to brush and floss your teeth during chemotherapy. Chemotherapy can make you more likely to get cavities, so your dentist may suggest using a fluoride rinse or gel each day to help prevent decay.

▶ Brush your teeth after every meal. Use a soft toothbrush and a gentle touch; brushing too hard can damage soft mouth tissues. If your gums are too sensitive for even a soft toothbrush, use a cotton swab or gauze. Use a nonabrasive toothpaste or a paste of baking soda and water.

▶ Rinse your toothbrush well after each use and store it in a dry place.

▶ Avoid commercial mouthwashes that contain a large amount of salt or alcohol. Ask your doctor or nurse about a mild mouthwash that you might use.

▶ If you develop sores in your mouth, be sure to contact your doctor or nurse because you may need medical treatment for the sores.

From National Cancer Institute. (1991 Dec.). *Chemotherapy and you: A guide to self-help treatment* (3rd ed., Pub. No. 92-1136). Washington, DC: United States Department of Health and Human Services.

Tell the client what to expect in terms of how the drug will be administered, how often, and for how long. Explain that the interval between doses allows the normal cells to recover. Explain as much as possible about how the drug or drugs act, when the client can expect to experience any undesired reactions, what they might be, and how long they might last. Reassure the client about changes that are usually reversible. Make sure the client knows which reactions require an immediate call to the primary care provider. Give the client oral and written information about the many cancer support groups and community resources that are available.

Evaluating Review client goals in terms of compliance with the medical regimen, physical responses to chemotherapy, and resolution of emotional issues that have arisen as a result of the disease. Make any adjustments that are necessary in treatment goals and expected outcomes. Encourage expression of feelings throughout the process of dealing with cancer. Monitor test results and evaluate the client's response to medical treatment.

CONCEPT REVIEW

Drugs used in the treatment of cancer can be categorized according to their cell cycle specificity or according to their mechanism of action. Most operate by interfering with the supply of nutrients to or the genetic components of the cell. Antineoplastic drugs kill normal cells also, but normal cells are better equipped for self-repair.

Dosing schedule is a balance between the time needed for the body to repair itself and the need to kill rapidly dividing tumor cells.

There are many modes of administering antineoplastic agents, with IV push, piggyback, and sidearm the most common.

Meticulous nursing technique must be maintained at all times for the protection of the client and of others who come in contact with him or her.

ALKYLATING AGENTS
ALKYLATING AGENT PROTOTYPE
BUSULFAN

Pharmacotherapeutics Busulfan is the drug of choice in treatment of chronic myelogenous leukemia. Alkylating agents also are used for treating other conditions such as brain tumors, metastatic malignant melanoma, and Hodgkin's disease.

Pharmacokinetics Alkylating agents are rapidly cleared from the plasma and are inactivated. The inactivated products are excreted in the urine. Consequently, it may not be necessary to reduce the usual effective dose in clients with decreased renal function.

Pharmacodynamics Alkylating agents are highly reactive compounds that interact chemically with cellular DNA. The alkyl groups form strong bonds, usually intermittently (not continuously) down the DNA strand. They may bond two separate DNA strands, nucleic bases on the same DNA molecule, or DNA to RNA. This tight binding prevents replication, thereby inhibiting cell growth. The nitrosoureas, which are lipid soluble, are also in the alkylating group.[4,10]

Pharmaceutics Busulfan is available in tablets for oral administration. (Dosages for antineoplastic agents are often determined by nomogram according to client weight or body surface area.) Common dosages and nursing considerations for alkylating agents are provided in Table 69–2.

Undesired Clinical Responses The primary undesired clinical response to busulfan is bone marrow suppression. See Table 69–3 for other undesired clinical responses specific to this compound.

Contraindications and Precautions Alkylating agents should not be used in clients with known sensitivity to the agent; with severe leukopenia, thrombocytopenia, or anemia; or who are pregnant or breast-feeding. They should be used with caution in clients receiving radiation therapy or other antineoplastics.

Drug-Drug Interactions Busulfan may cause additive myelosuppression when used with other myelosuppressive drugs. Alkylating agents and all antineoplastics may interact with a number of OTC or prescription drugs. Check information specific to each drug against client's chart.

TABLE 69–2

Prototype Antineoplastic Drugs: Dosage and Nursing Considerations

Drug Name	Nursing Considerations
BUSULFAN Dosage: 2–8 mg daily PO	**Assess** Assess for disease resistance to previous therapy with drug. Use drug with extreme caution in client with compromised bone marrow reserve. Avoid use, if possible, during pregnancy, especially first trimester; use is not recommended while breast-feeding. Drug is in Pregnancy Category D. Ask about concurrent medications (e.g., antigout drugs). Obtain results of baseline hemoglobin, hematocrit, white blood count (WBC), differential, platelet count, hepatic and renal function tests. **Implement** Give drug at same time each day. Give drug on empty stomach if nausea and vomiting occur. Drug may be carcinogenic, mutagenic, or teratogenic. Handle with extreme caution. Encourage adequate daily fluid intake. Teach client not to have immunizations without consulting primary care provider and to avoid people who have just received live virus vaccine. Teach client to report persistent nausea and vomiting, consistent cough, congestion, difficulty breathing, fever, signs of local infection, bruising or unusual bleeding. Encourage client to use contraception during therapy. **Monitor** Obtain repeat laboratory test results weekly. Drug may increase blood and urinary uric acid levels and interfere with test results. Look for undesired clinical responses (hyperpigmentation of the skin, gastrointestinal [GI] distress, weight loss). Monitor for toxic effects (fever, sore throat, bruising or unusual bleeding, dizziness, muscle twitching or weakness, dyspnea, tonic-clonic seizures).
CYTARABINE (CYTOSINE ARABINOSIDE) Dosage (varies): 60–100 mg/m² IV 1 h qd for 10 d	**Assess** Inquire whether client is pregnant. If possible, do not use during pregnancy, especially first trimester. Drug is not recommended while breast-feeding. Drug is in Pregnancy Category D. Ask if client is taking other medications (antigout medication, bone marrow depressants, cyclophosphamide). Obtain baseline WBC and platelet count results. **Implement** Drug may be carcinogenic, mutagenic, or teratogenic. Handle with extreme care during preparation and administration. Check solution; discard if hazy. Reconstituted solution is stable for 48 h at room temperature. IV infusion solutions at concentrations up to 0.5 mg/ml are stable for 7 d at room temperature. Encourage increased fluid intake. Teach client not to have vaccinations and to avoid persons who have just been vaccinated with live virus vaccine. Teach client to report any fever, sore throat, signs of local infection, bruising or unusual bleeding, excessive weakness, numbness or neuropathy, or persistent nausea or vomiting. Encourage client to use contraceptives during therapy. **Monitor** Cytarabine may interfere with laboratory values for aspartate aminotransferase (AST), bilirubin, alkaline phosphatase, uric acid tests. Obtain repeat WBC and platelet count results. Monitor for undesired clinical reactions (GI problems, motor and sensory neuropathy, fever). Assess for toxicity: hematologic toxicity, cytarabine syndrome (fever, myalgia, rash, conjunctivitis, malaise, chest pain), hyperuricemia, central nervous system (CNS), GI, or pulmonary toxicity.
BLEOMYCIN SULFATE Dosage: 10–20 U/m² IM, IV, SC weekly or twice weekly	**Assess** Ask about previous allergic reaction to drug. Ask if client is pregnant. Avoid use of drug if possible during pregnancy, especially first trimester. Breast-feeding is not recommended during therapy. Bleomycin is a Pregnancy Category C drug. Ask if client is receiving other antineoplastics (e.g., cisplatin). Obtain baseline chest x-ray results.

TABLE 69–2 *Continued*

Prototype Antineoplastic Drugs: Dosage and Nursing Considerations

Drug Name	Nursing Considerations
BLEOMYCIN SULFATE—CONT'D	**Implement** Drug may be carcinogenic, mutagenic, or teratogenic. Handle with extreme care during preparation and administration. Refrigerate powder. Reconstitute with 5% dextrose or 0.9% NaCl solution for injection. Solution is stable at room temperature for 24 h. Teach client that fever and chills occur less frequently with continued therapy. Tell client not to have or be near a person who has had live virus immunization without consulting primary care provider. Tell client to report nausea and vomiting that persist at home. **Monitor** Obtain results of repeat chest x-ray studies q1-2wk. Monitor for common undesired clinical responses: anorexia, weight loss, rash, hyperpigmentation, blistering. Observe client for indications of toxicity: interstitial pneumonitis, bone marrow depression, renal or hepatic effects. If present, discontinue therapy and report at once.
ETOPOSIDE Dosage (varies): diluted in 100–250 ml 0.9% NaCl solution slowly over 30–60 min Also given orally.	**Assess** Inquire about history of impaired hepatic function. Ask if client is pregnant. Drug use is not recommended during pregnancy or while client is breast-feeding. Etoposide is a Pregnancy Category D drug. Inquire about use of concurrent medications. Etoposide may increase bone marrow depression if bone marrow depressants are being used. Obtain baseline hematology test results. **Implement** Drug may be carcinogenic, mutagenic, or teratogenic. Handle with extreme care during preparation and administration. Refrigerate gelatin capsules. Concentrate for the injection is clear yellow. Diluted solutions of 0.2–0.4 mg/ml are stable for at least 48 h at room temperature. Discard if crystallization occurs. Administer by slow IV infusion (over 30–60 min). Use syringes with Luer-lok fittings for handling concentrate to prevent displacement of needle from syringe. Monitor for anaphylactic reaction during IV administration. Teach client to avoid immunization (or individuals vaccinated) with live virus vaccines. Teach client to report fever, sore throat, signs of local infection, bruising, unusual bleeding, or persistent vomiting. Teach client signs of peripheral neuropathy. **Monitor** Monitor results of hemoglobin, hematocrit, WBC, differential, platelet count studies. Assess daily bowel activity and consistency. Observe for undesired clinical responses (mild nausea and vomiting, anorexia, alopecia). Provide antiemetics if necessary. Monitor for signs of toxicity: leukopenia, thrombocytopenia, anemia, pancytopenia, hepatotoxicity. Assess for paresthesias.
DIETHYLSTILBESTROL Dosage (oral): Breast: 10 mg/m²/d in divided doses Prostate: 0.5–1.5 mg/m²/d	**Assess** Obtain vital signs, weight, and blood glucose level. Ask whether client is pregnant or plans to be pregnant. Ask about hypersensitivity to estrogen, previous jaundice, or thromboembolic disorders. **Implement** Advise client of possible breast and libido changes. Instruct client about potential fluid retention and the need to maintain decreased sodium intake. Tell client not to take other drugs without consulting primary care provider. Teach female client to perform self-breast examination and to use a nonhormonal form of contraception. Tell client to avoid sun and ultraviolet light. **Monitor** Take weight daily. Report a gain of 5 lb/wk. Instruct client to report warmth and tenderness in calf region and other indications of thrombotic disorders such as sudden severe headache, shortness of breath, or loss of coordination. Take blood pressure at least daily. Monitor blood glucose level four times/d in diabetic clients.

Table continued on following page.

TABLE 69–2 *Continued*
Prototype Antineoplastic Drugs: Dosage and Nursing Considerations

Drug Name	Nursing Considerations
ASPARAGINASE (L-ASPARAGINASE) Dosage (varies greatly): follow protocol and administer IV or IM	**Assess** Obtain baseline temperature. Inquire about any history of use of this agent and any adverse reactions to it. Inquire about history of pancreatitis. Perform skin test and hepatic, renal, pancreatic, blood glucose, complete blood count, differential, and central nervous system function tests before therapy begins and when 1 wk or more has elapsed between doses. **Implement** Administer acetaminophen ½–1 h before infusion is ordered. Have equipment ready for handling possible allergic reaction. Teach client to increase fluid intake to protect renal function. Instruct client not to have immunizations without approval of primary care provider and to avoid exposure to anyone who has recently been immunized. Administer drug IV over 30–45 min. Observe for temperature elevation and signs of anaphylaxis (wheezing, facial flushing, hives). **Monitor** Obtain repeat hepatic function test results. Discontinue medication at first sign of renal failure or pancreatitis (abdominal pain, vomiting, nausea) and notify primary care provider. Monitor for hematologic toxicity (fever, sore throat, easy bruising) and anemia (excessive tiredness or weakness).

TABLE 69–3
Undesired Clinical Responses to Prototype Antineoplastic Drugs

Drug Name	Response
Alkylating Agent: busulfan	More common Anemia Leukopenia: usually begins 10–15 d after starting therapy, with nadir at 11–30 d; after withdrawal, recovery usually occurs within 12–20 wk Pancytopenia possible; recovery takes up to 2 y after drug withdrawal Missed or irregular menstrual periods Hyperpigmentation of skin, especially in clients with dark skin Less common Bronchopulmonary dysplasia with pulmonary fibrosis (busulfan syndrome); occurs within 8 mo–10 y after starting therapy (average, 4 y); symptoms—low-grade fever, cough, dyspnea; treatment unsatisfactory; condition usually fatal within 6 mo of diagnosis Rare Cataracts (symptoms—blurred vision): may occur after prolonged therapy
Antimetabolite: cytarabine	More common Leukopenia or infection: initially leukocytes fall within first 24 h, reaching nadir at 7–9 d following a brief rise; a second, deeper fall reaches nadir at d 15–24; rapid recovery within the next 10 d Stomatitis, anorexia, nausea, vomiting Thrombocytopenia: platelets fall by d 5, reaching nadir at 12–15 d, with a rise to baseline over the next 10 d Less common Central nervous system toxicity, including numbness; unusual tiredness at high doses Hyperuricemia, especially in patients with leukemia or lymphoma Diarrhea, headache, dizziness, itching, loss of hair Rare Pain at injection site Bone or muscle pain, skin rash Difficulty swallowing, heartburn Gastrointestinal hemorrhage Liver toxicity Megaloblastic anemia Difficulty urinating

TABLE 69–3 *Continued*
951

Undesired Clinical Responses to Prototype Antineoplastic Drugs

Drug Name	Response

Antibiotic: bleomycin	More common
	  Fever, chills: occur in up to 60% of clients; begin within 3–6 h, last 4–12 h; with contin-
	    ued use, fevers less frequent
	  Pneumonitis: occurs in up to 40% of clients, usually within 4–10 wk; occurrence higher in
	    elderly and in those receiving >400 U total dose; may be irreversible and fatal; pul-
	    monary function returns to normal in approximately 2 y.
	Less common
	  Idiosyncratic reaction consisting of hypotension, confusion, fever, chills, wheezing; occurs
	    in 1% to 60% of lymphoma clients; may occur immediately or several hours after the
	    first or second dose; if not treated, may progress to sweating, dehydration, hypotension,
	    and renal failure or cardiopulmonary collapse
	  Weight loss
	Rare
	  Liver or renal toxicity; vascular toxicity (including cerebrovascular accident), myocardial in-
	    farction

Plant Alkaloids: etoposide (VP-16)	More common
	  Anemia
	  Leukopenia: nadir of granulocyte count at 7–14 d, with complete recovery by d 20
	  Thombocytopenia: nadir of platelet count by 9–16 d, with complete recovery by d 20
	  Loss of appetite, nausea, vomiting
	  Loss of hair; may progress to complete baldness; is reversible
	Less common
	  Stomatitis
	  Unusual tiredness, diarrhea
	Rare
	  Anaphylaxis: fast heartbeat, fever, chills, wheezing, shortness of breath, hypotension; blood
	    pressure returns to normal several hours after discontinuing IV infusion
	  Pain at injection site
	  Difficulty walking, numbness or tingling in fingers, toes

Hormones: diethylstilbestrol (estrogen)	More common
	  Breast pain, tenderness
	  Enlargement of breasts (females)
	  Gynecomastia (males) in treatment of prostate cancer
	  Swelling of feet, lower legs, rapid gain in weight (sodium and fluid retention)
	  Abdominal cramping
	  Loss of appetite
	  Nausea
	Less common
	  Amenorrhea
	  Breakthrough bleeding
	  Prolonged or heavier menses
	  Breast tumors
	  Involuntary jerky muscular movement
	  Hepatitis
	  Gallbladder obstruction (pain in stomach, side, or abdomen)
	  Thromboembolic complications (may lead to increased risk of myocardial infarction, pul-
	    monary embolism, thrombophlebitis)
	  Mild diarrhea
	  Dizziness, headaches, decreased libido in males, increased libido in females
	  Vomiting (with high dosages)

Miscellaneous: asparaginase	More common
	  Allergic reactions: difficulty in breathing, joint pain, skin rash or itching; may be severe or
	    fatal
	  Decrease in blood clotting factors, especially factors V and VIII; symptoms—unusual
	    bleeding or bruising
	  Liver toxicity: within 2 wk of treatment
	  Pancreatitis (severe stomach pain, nausea, vomiting)
	Less common
	  Central nervous system effects: confusion, hallucinations, mental depression, unusual tired-
	    ness
	  Hyperglycemia
	  Hyperuricemia (especially in clients with leukemia and lymphoma)
	  Hypoalbuminemia, renal failure
	  Stomatitis
	Rare
	  Immunosuppression, leukopenia, leg vein thrombosis, hyperthermia, seizures

TABLE 69–4

Alkylating Agents: Cell Cycle Specificity and Indications for Use

Drug Name	Cell Cycle Specific	Indications for Use
Busulfan (Myleran)	No	Chronic myelogenous leukemia
Carboplatin (Paraplatin)	No	Ovarian carcinoma
Carmustine (BiCNU)	No	Brain tumors, multiple myeloma, Hodgkin's and non-Hodgkin's lymphomas
Chlorambucil (Leukeran)	No	Chronic lymphocytic leukemia, malignant lymphomas
Cisplatin (Cis-Platinum, CDDP, Platinol)	No	Metastatic testicular or ovarian tumors, advanced bladder cancer
Cyclophosphamide (Cytoxan)	No	Adenocarcinoma of ovary, breast cancer, malignant lymphomas, retinoblastoma, multiple myeloma, leukemias, mycosis fungoides, neuroblastoma
Estramustine (Emcyt, Estracyt)	No	Prostatic carcinoma
Ifosfamide (IFEX, IFX, Isophosphamide)	No	Germ cell testicular cancer
Lomustine (CeeNU, CCNU)	No	Brain tumors, Hodgkin's disease
Mechlorethamine (Mustargen, HN2, nitrogen mustard)	No	Polycythemia vera, mycosis fungoides, Hodgkin's disease, lymphosarcoma, chronic myelocytic or lymphocytic leukemia, bronchogenic cancer
Melphalan (Alkeran, L-phenylalanine mustard, L-sarcolysin)	No	Multiple myeloma, ovarian carcinoma
Streptozocin (Zanosar, Streptoozotocin)	No	Metastatic islet cell cancer of pancreas
Thiotcpa (TSPA, TESPA, Thiotepa)	No	Adenocarcinoma of breast or ovary, papillary cancer of urinary bladder

Data from Hodgson, B.B., Kizior, R.J., & Kingdon, R.T. (1995). *Nurse's drug handbook* (pp. 1088–1091). Philadelphia: W.B. Saunders.

Life-Span Considerations Always use antineoplastics with caution in the elderly or the very young. Busulfan may cause fetal harm when administered to pregnant women. It is not known whether busulfan is excreted in human milk.

MISCELLANEOUS DRUGS IN CATEGORY

Other drugs in the alkylating group and their cell specificity and indications are listed in Table 69–4.

CONCEPT REVIEW

Alkylating agents bind different parts of the tumor DNA (the strands, the bases, or DNA to RNA) to prevent tumor cell replication.

They have a strong bone marrow suppressive effect that can be compounded when they are used in combination with other antineoplastics.

ANTIMETABOLITES

ANTIMETABOLITE PROTOTYPE

CYTARABINE

Pharmacotherapeutics Cytarabine is prescribed for treatment of acute or chronic myelocytic leukemia and of acute lymphocytic leukemia.

Pharmacokinetics Antimetabolites function in ways similar to those of normal essential metabolites. Anti-metabolites are minimally metabolized, and most of each dose is excreted intact in the urine.

Pharmacodynamics Cytarabine is cell cycle specific to the S phase of the cell cycle. Antimetabolites may "trick" cells into incorporating them along metabolic pathways essential for synthesizing RNA and DNA, thus causing transmission of a false message; or they may block the enzymes necessary for synthesizing essential compounds. In either case they prevent DNA synthesis.

Pharmaceutics Cytarabine is available as a powder for IV, IT, or SC administration. Common dosages for antimetabolic agents are provided in Table 69–2.

Undesired Clinical Responses Undesired clinical responses to cytarabine administration include stomatitis, bone marrow depression, diarrhea, and other GI symptoms. See Table 69–3 for responses specific to this agent.

Contraindications and Precautions Cytarabine use is contraindicated in clients who have shown sensitivity to the drug. General precautions for antineoplastic agents should be observed.

Drug-Drug Interactions Cytarabine in combination therapy can cause reversible decreases in steady-state plasma digoxin concentration. It may also antagonize the effects of gentamicin.

Life-Span Considerations Cytarabine can cause fetal harm when administered to pregnant women. It is not known whether cytarabine is excreted in human milk.

MISCELLANEOUS DRUGS IN CATEGORY

Other drugs in the alkylating group, their cell specificity, and indications for their use are listed in Table 69–5.[13,14]

TABLE 69–5
Antimetabolites: Cell Cycle Specificity and Indications for Use

Drug Name	Cell Cycle Specific	Indications for Use
Cytarabine (Cytosar, cytosine arabinoside, ARA-C)	Yes	Acute, chronic myelocytic leukemia, acute lymphocytic leukemia
Floxuridine (FUDR, 5-FUDR)	No	Gastrointestinal adenocarcinoma metastatic to the liver
5-Fluorouracil (Adrucil, Efudex, fluorouracil, 5-FU)	No	Cancer of colon, rectum, breast, stomach, pancreas
Hydroxyurea (Hydrea)	No	Melanoma, chronic myelocytic leukemia, carcinoma of ovary
6-Mercaptopurine (Purinethol, 6-MP)	Yes	Acute lymphatic myelogenous leukemia
Methotrexate (Folex, Amethopterin, Mexate)	Yes	Gestational choriocarcinoma, choriocarcinoma destruens, hydatidiform mole, acute lymphocytic leukemia
6-Thioguanine (Thioguanine)	Yes	Acute nonlymphocytic leukemia

Data from Hodgson, B.B., Kizior, R.J., & Kingdon, R.T. (1995). *Nurse's drug handbook* (pp. 1088–1091). Philadelphia: W.B. Saunders.

CONCEPT REVIEW

Antimetabolites "starve" cancer cells by one of two methods: either they trick the cells into incorporating them instead of essential metabolites, or they block the cells from absorbing the metabolites they need to reproduce.

Some antimetabolites operate at a specific point in the cell cycle.

ANTINEOPLASTIC ANTIBIOTICS
ANTINEOPLASTIC ANTIBIOTIC PROTOTYPE
BLEOMYCIN

Pharmacotherapeutics Bleomycin is used to treat conditions such as Hodgkin's disease and non-Hodgkin's lymphomas, testicular carcinoma, and squamous cell carcinoma of the head, neck, and uterine cervix.

Pharmacokinetics Bleomycin achieves high concentrations in the skin and lungs but does not enter the central nervous system (CNS). Most of the drug is excreted unchanged in the urine.

Pharmacodynamics The exact mechanism of action of bleomycin is unknown. Evidence suggests that the drug inhibits DNA synthesis. It may also inhibit RNA and protein synthesis.

Pharmaceutics Bleomycin is supplied as a sterile powder and is administered IV, IM, or SC. Dosage information for bleomycin is provided in Table 69–2.

Undesired Clinical Responses Bleomycin is associated with pneumonitis leading to fibrosis.[1,10] It is unusual in that it causes minimal bone marrow toxicity. Undesired responses to bleomycin are listed in Table 69–3.

Contraindications and Precautions Bleomycin use is contraindicated in clients with a demonstrated hypersensitivity to it. It should be used with extreme caution in clients with impaired renal function or compromised pulmonary function.

Drug-Drug Interactions When used in combination with other antineoplastic agents, bleomycin may cause pulmonary toxicity at lower doses.

MISCELLANEOUS DRUGS IN CATEGORY

Other drugs in the antineoplastic antibiotics group, their cell specificity, and indications for their use are listed in Table 69–6.

TABLE 69–6
Antineoplastic Antibiotics: Cell Cycle Specificity and Indications for Use

Drug Name	Cell Cycle Specific	Indications for Use
Bleomycin (Blenoxane)	Yes	Squamous cell carcinoma, lymphomas, testicular carcinoma
Dactinomycin (Cosmegen)	No	Wilms' tumor, rhabdomyosarcoma, choriocarcinoma, testicular carcinoma, Ewing's sarcoma
Daunorubicin (Cerubidine, Daunomycin, Rubidomycin)	No	Acute lymphocytic, nonlymphocytic leukemia
Doxorubicin (Adriamycin, Rubex)	No	Acute lymphoblastic leukemia, acute myeloblastic leukemia, Wilms' tumor, neuroblastoma, soft-tissue and bone sarcomas, breast and ovarian carcinoma, transitional cell bladder carcinoma, thyroid carcinoma, Hodgkin's or non-Hodgkin's lymphoma, bronchogenic carcinoma, gastric carcinoma
Idarubicin (Idamycin)	No	Acute myeloid leukemia
Mitomycin (Mutamycin)	No	Disseminated adenocarcinoma of stomach and pancreas

Data from Hodgson, B.B., Kizior, R.J., & Kingdon, R.T. (1995). *Nurse's drug handbook* (pp. 1088–1091). Philadelphia: W.B. Saunders.

CONCEPT REVIEW

Antineoplastic antibiotics operate by an unidentified mechanism. They appear to inhibit DNA synthesis and DNA-dependent RNA synthesis and to delay or inhibit mitosis.

Their wide absorption in the lungs may lead to pulmonary toxicity, but they cause little bone marrow toxicity.

PLANT ALKALOIDS

PLANT ALKALOID PROTOTYPE
ETOPOSIDE

Pharmacotherapeutics Etoposide is approved for use in the treatment of refractory testicular cancer and small cell cancer of the lung. Other plant alkaloids are indicated for conditions such as small cell and non-small cell lung cancer, ovarian cancer, breast tumor and metastatic breast tumor, and mycosis fungoides.

Pharmacokinetics Etoposide has low penetration to the CNS. It is eliminated intact in the urine.

Pharmacodynamics Etoposide works by preventing DNA strand breaks from resealing. The resulting damage arrests the cell cycle in the G_2 phase, preventing the cell's entering the metaphase (M phase). The plant alkaloids are called **mitotic inhibitors.** Many crystallize the mitotic spindle proteins during metaphase, arresting mitosis and causing cell death.[15]

Pharmaceutics Etoposide is administered orally or intravenously. Dosage information for etoposide is supplied in Table 69–2.

Undesired Clinical Responses Bone marrow suppression is the major toxicity associated with use of etoposide. Other undesired clinical responses are listed in Table 69–3.

Contraindications and Precautions Etoposide use is contraindicated in clients who have shown a hypersensitivity to the compound or to any of its components. It should be used with caution in the presence of bone marrow suppression.

Life-Span Considerations Etoposide is categorized as a Pregnancy Category D drug. It is not known whether this drug is excreted in human milk. Safe and effectiveness in children have not been established.

MISCELLANEOUS DRUGS IN CATEGORY

Vinblastine and vincristine are perhaps the most commonly used plant alkaloids.[1] Some plant alkaloids, their phase specificity, and indications for use are listed in Table 69–7.[16,17]

CONCEPT REVIEW

Plant alkaloids are called *mitotic inhibitors* because they act on the cell during or before mitosis to prevent cell division; thus they are cell cycle specific to the M phase. Myelosuppression is the most common toxicity associated with their use.

HORMONES

HORMONE PROTOTYPE
DIETHYLSTILBESTROL

Pharmacotherapeutics Diethylstilbestrol (DES) is an estrogen used in treating carcinomas of the breast in postmenopausal women and selected men and in treating carcinomas of the prostate.

Pharmacokinetics DES is well absorbed from the GI tract and is widely distributed throughout the body. It is 50% to 80% bound to protein. It is metabolized in the liver and is excreted primarily in the urine.[18,19]

Pharmacodynamics The exact mechanism of action of most hormones on cancer cells is not understood. Hormones are not cytotoxic. However, evidence shows that hormonal agents can alter the tumor's environment and so inhibit its growth.

Pharmaceutics DES is supplied in oral tablet form and in ampules for IV administration. Dosages for DES are provided in Table 69–2.

Undesired Clinical Responses Use of DES in men is associated with changes in secondary sexual characteristics. Other common and less common undesired clinical responses to DES are listed in Table 69–3.

Contraindications and Precautions DES use is contraindicated during pregnancy. It carries many precautions to use. The nurse should check the package insert before administering the drug.

Drug-Drug Interactions DES can interfere with several endocrine and liver function tests.

TABLE 69–7

Common Plant Alkaloids: Cell Cycle Specificity and Indications for Use

Drug Name	Cell Cycle Specific	Indications for Use
Etoposide (VePesid, VP 16-213)	Yes	Refractory testicular tumor, small cell lung cancer
Vinblastine (Velban)	Yes	Hodgkin's disease, lymphocytic lymphoma, histiocytic lymphoma, mycosis fungoides, advanced testicular carcinoma, Kaposi's sarcoma, breast cancer
Vincristine (Oncovin)	Yes	Acute leukemia, Hodgkin's disease, non-Hodgkin's malignant lymphoma, rhabdomyosarcoma, neuroblastoma, Wilms' tumor
Vinorelbine (Navelbine)	Yes	Metastatic breast cancer, non-small cell lung cancer, ovarian cancer, Hodgkin's disease

Data from Hodgson, B.B., Kizior, R.J., & Kingdon, R.T. (1995). *Nurse's drug handbook* (pp. 1088–1091). Philadelphia: W.B. Saunders.

TABLE 69–8
Selected Hormones: Cell Cycle Specificity and Indications for Use

Drug Name	Cell Cycle Specific	Indications for Use
Diethylstilbestrol diphosphate (Stilphostrol)	No	Breast cancer, prostatic carcinoma
Estramustine (Emcyt)	No	Prostatic carcinoma
Flutamide (Eulexin)	No	Metastatic prostatic carcinoma
Goserelin (Zoladex)	No	Prostatic carcinoma
Leuprolide (Lupron)	No	Advanced prostatic cancer, endometriosis
Medroxyprogesterone (Depo-Provera)	No	Endometrial and renal carcinoma
Megestrol (Megace)	No	Breast and endometrial carcinoma
Tamoxifen Citrate (Nolvadex)	No	Metastatic breast cancer
Testolactone (Teslac)	No	Breast carcinoma

Data from Hodgson, B.B., Kizior, R.J., & Kingdon, R.T. (1995). *Nurse's drug handbook* (pp. 1088–1091). Philadelphia: W.B. Saunders.

Life-Span Considerations DES is categorized as a Pregnancy Category X drug. It is associated with limb-reducing effects in the fetus and is reported to encourage a rare form of vaginal or cervical cancer in females repeatedly exposed to the drugs in utero.

MISCELLANEOUS DRUGS IN CATEGORY

Besides the estrogens and antiestrogens, the other categories of hormones used in treatment of cancer are (1) androgens, (2) progestins, (3) gonadotropin-releasing hormone analogs, and (4) glucocorticoids. Some of these hormones, their cell specificity, and uses are listed in Table 69–8. (See Chapters 42, 62, and 63 for additional information on hormones.)

CONCEPT REVIEW

Hormones are not cytotoxic. They appear to prevent tumor growth by altering the environment in which the tumor exists. They may affect secondary sexual characteristics when administered to men.

Their use is contraindicated during pregnancy because of the severe effects they can have on the fetus and on grown females who were exposed to it in utero.

MISCELLANEOUS AGENTS
MISCELLANEOUS AGENT PROTOTYPE
ASPARAGINASE

Pharmacotherapeutics Asparaginase is used in the treatment of acute lymphocytic leukemia. It is most effective when used in combination with other drugs.

Pharmacokinetics Distribution of asparaginase is restricted to the vascular system. It does not cross the blood-brain barrier. It is inactivated by serum proteases.

Pharmacodynamics Asparaginase is an enzyme. It deprives cells of asparagine, an amino acid needed to synthesize protein. Because normal cells can produce their own asparagine, its action is mostly limited to neoplastic cells lacking asparagine synthetase.

Pharmaceutics Asparaginase is supplied as a lyophilized drug or powder for reconstitution. It is administered intravenously or intramuscularly and must be closely monitored at each administration. Dosages for asparaginase are listed in Table 69–2.

Undesired Clinical Responses Asparaginase is a foreign protein and as such may cause a severe allergic reaction. Preparations for treatment of anaphylaxis should be made before the administration of each does.[1,4] Other undesired responses to asparagines are listed in Table 69–3.

Contraindications and Precautions Asparaginase use is contraindicated in clients with pancreatitis or a history

TABLE 69–9
Miscellaneous Agents: Cell Cycle Specificity and Indications for Use

Drug Name	Cell Cycle Specific	Indications for Use
Asparaginase (Elspar)	No	Acute lymphocytic leukemia
Interferon alfa-2a (Roferon-A)	No	Hairy cell leukemia, AIDS-related Kaposi's sarcoma
Interferon alfa-2b (Intron A)	No	Hairy cell leukemia, condyloma acuminatum, AIDS-related Kaposi's sarcoma
Interferon alfa-n3 (Alferon N)	No	Condyloma acuminatum
Levamisole (Ergamisol)	No	Duke's stage C colon cancer
Mitotane (Lysodren)	No	Adrenal cortical carcinoma
Procarbazine (Matulane)	No	Hodgkin's disease
Pegaspargase (Oncaspar)	Yes	Acute lymphoblastic leukemia

Data from Hodgson, B.B., Kizior, R.J., & Kingdon, R.T. (1995). *Nurse's drug handbook* (pp. 1088–1091). Philadelphia: W.B. Saunders.

of pancreatitis and in clients who have had a previous anaphylactic reaction to it. It must be handled and administered carefully. Inhalation of dust or vapors and contact with skin or eyes must be avoided.

Drug-Drug Interactions Asparaginase interferes with interpretation of thyroid function test results.

Life-Span Considerations Asparaginase is a Pregnancy Category C drug and is not recommended for use in pregnant women. It is not known whether asparaginase is excreted in breast milk. Asparaginase toxicity is reported as greater in adults than in children.

OTHER DRUGS IN CATEGORY

Other miscellaneous drugs, their cell cycle specificity, and indications for their use are listed in Table 69–9.

CONCEPT REVIEW

Asparaginase is an enzyme that deprives cells of asparagine, an amino acid essential to protein synthesis. Normal cells produce their own asparagine, so asparaginase is more specifically active against neoplastic cells, which lack aspragine synthetase.

As a foreign substance, asparaginase can cause anaphylaxis. Precautions must be in place to handle such an emergency each time this agent is given.

INVESTIGATIONAL DRUGS

Anticancer drugs undergoing clinical trials and not yet approved by the Food and Drug Administration (FDA) are called **investigational agents.** The term *investigational* also includes drugs already approved by the FDA if a new use for the drug is being tested. Drugs in clinical trials are sometimes provided to clients by the National Cancer Institute, through cooperative group protocols and cancer centers, or directly from pharmaceutical companies.[18]

The introduction of new pharmacologic agents to treat neoplastic disease challenges the nurse to understand their uses, administration, and side effects and to establish new protocols for managing those side effects. The nurse will continue as a primary educator and provider of information to the client and the client's family.

SUMMARY

Care of the client with cancer provides some of the most complex challenges in nursing. To fulfill the requirements of oncologic nursing, the nurse must understand the basic mechanisms and effects of the antineoplastic agents, must administer many of those agents with a wide variety of sophisticated equipment, and must provide primary emotional and educational support in one of the most frightening of medical diagnoses. Furthermore, the nurse must take extreme care in performing physical tasks with these clients, both because of the

clients' compromised status and because of the toxicity of the compounds administered. As new developments and treatment are approved, nursing care of the client with cancer will remain a demanding and stimulating area to pursue.

REFERENCES

1. Tenenbaum, L. (1994). *Cancer chemotherapy and biotherapy* (2nd ed.). Philadelphia: W.B. Saunders.
2. Linton, A.D., Matteson, M.A., & Maebius, N.K. (1995). *Introductory nursing care of adults.* Philadelphia: W.B. Saunders.
3. Smeltzer, S.C., & Bare, B.G. (1992). *Brunner and Suddarth's textbook of medical-surgical nursing* (7th ed.). Philadelphia: J.B. Lippincott.
4. Hodgson, B.B., Kizior, R.J., & Kingdon, R. (1995). *Nurse's drug handbook.* Philadelphia: W.B. Saunders.
5. Valanis, B., Vollmer, W., Labuhn, K., & Glass, A. (1993). Acute symptoms associated with antineoplastic drug handling among nurses. *Cancer Nursing, 16,* 288–295.
6. Davis, J.R., & Sherer, K. (1994). *Applied nutrition and diet therapy for nurses* (2nd ed.). Philadelphia: W.B. Saunders.
7. Health Science Communications. (1991). *Coping with the side effects of chemotherapy.* Philadelphia: Wyeth-Ayerst Laboratories.
8. Edwards, J.N., Herman, J., Wallace, B., Pavy, M., & Harrison-Pavy, J. (1991). Comparison of patient-controlled and nurse-controlled antiemetic therapy in patients receiving chemotherapy. *Research in Nursing and Health, 14,* 249–257.
9. U.S. Department of Health and Human Services. (1991). *Chemotherapy and you: A guide to self-help during treatment.* Washington, D.C.: National Cancer Institute.
10. Lehne, R.A., Moore, L., Crosby, L., & Hamilton, D. (1994). *Pharmacology for nursing care* (2nd ed.). Philadelphia: W.B. Saunders.
11. Abramowicz, M. (Ed.). (1993). Drugs of choice for cancer chemotherapy. *Medical Letter on Drugs and Therapeutics, 35*(897), 43–50.
12. Boddy, A., Yule, S., Wyllie, R., Price, L., Pearson, A., & Idle, J. (1993). Pharmacokinetics and metabolism of ifosfamide administered as a continuous infusion in children. *Cancer Research, 53,* 3758–3764.
13. Bostrom, B., & Erdmann, G. (1993). Cellular pharmacology of 6-mercaptopurine in acute lymphoblastic leukemia. *American Journal of Pediatric Hematology/Oncology, 15*(1), 80–86.
14. Holtzclaw, B., & Rutledge, D. (1990). Use of amphotericin B in immunosuppressed patients with cancer. *Oncology Nursing Forum, 17,* 737–742.
15. Lobert, S., & Correla, J. (1992). Antimitotics in cancer chemotherapy. *Cancer Nursing, 15*(1), 22–23.
16. Lilley, L., & Scott, H. (1993). What you need to know about taxol. *American Journal of Nursing, 93*(12), 46–50.
17. U.S. Pharmacopeial Convention. (1990). *United States pharmacopeia* (22nd rev.). Rockville, MD: Author.
18. Data Pharmaceutica, Inc. (1993). *1993 physicians' genRx.* Smithtown, NY: Author.
19. Ignatavicious, D., & Bayne, M. (Eds.). (1995). *Medical-surgical nursing: a nursing process approach.* Philadelphia: W.B. Saunders.

BIBLIOGRAPHY

Baird, S.B., McCorkle, R., & Grant, M. (1991). *Cancer nursing: A comprehensive textbook.* Philadelphia: W.B. Saunders.
Cassidy, J., Macfarlane, D.K. (1991). The role of the nurse in clinical cancer research. *Cancer Nursing, 14*(3), 124–131.
Furlong, T.O. (1993). Neurologic complications of immunosuppressive cancer therapy. *Oncology Nursing Forum, 20*(9), 1337–1354.
Groenwald, S.L., Frogge, M.H., Goodman, M., & Yarbro, C.H.

(1993). *Cancer nursing: Principles and practice* (3rd ed.). Boston: Jones & Bartlett.

Nail, L.M., Jones, L.S., Greene, D., Schipper, D.L., & Jansen, R. (1991). Use and perceived efficacy of self-care activities in patients receiving chemotherapy. *Oncology Nursing Forum, 19*(5), 993–997.

Palmer, P., & Meyers, F.J. (1990). An outpatient approach to the delivery of intensive consolidation chemotherapy to adults with acute lymphoblastic leukemia. *Oncology Nursing Forum, 17*(4), 553–558.

Parker, G.G. (1992). Chemotherapy administration in the home. *Home Healthcare Nurse, 10*(1), 30–36.

Pinkel, D. (1993). Intravenous mercaptopurine: Life begins at 40. *Journal of Clinical Oncology, 11*(9), 1826–1831.

Rodman, J.H., Relling, M.V., Stewart, C.F., Synold, T.W., McLeod, H., Kearns, C., Stute, N., Crom, W.R., & Evans, W.E. (1993). Clinical pharmacokinetics and pharmacodynamics of anticancer drugs in children. *Seminars in Oncology, 20*(1), 18–29.

Schulmeister, L. (1992). An overview of continuous infusion chemotherapy. *Journal of Intravenous Nursing, 15*(6), 315–321.

Smith, D.B., & Babaian, R.J. (1992). The effects of treatment for cancer on male fertility and sexuality. *Cancer Nursing, 15*(4), 271–275.

Drugs for Fluid, Electrolyte, and Nutritional Balance

CHAPTER 70

Fluid, Electrolyte and Nutritional Balance

NORMA L. PINNELL • MARTHA A. SPIES

⊛ **Principles of Nutrition**
    LEARNING OBJECTIVES:
        Discuss the role of nutrition in health maintenance.
        Explain the importance of a balance between energy
            intake in foods and energy output.
    KEY TERMS:
        Basal metabolic rate, calorie, kilocalorie

⊛ **Nutrients**
    LEARNING OBJECTIVE: Describe the function of each
        major nutrient.
    KEY TERMS:
        Anabolism, catabolism

⊛ **Recommended Daily Allowances**
    LEARNING OBJECTIVE: Explain recommended daily
        allowances.

CONCEPTS AND TERMS TO REVIEW

Read about major nutrients in a nutrition textbook.

Nutrition is the sum of the processes of ingestion, digestion, absorption, transportation, and use of nutrients. With proper nutrition, the organism can grow, function, and reproduce.

PRINCIPLES OF NUTRITION

All foods supply a source of energy to the body in the form of calories. (A **calorie** is the amount of heat needed to raise the temperature of 1 g of water 1 degree Celsius.) Nutritional requirements are generally expressed in **kilocalories** (kcal). Caloric needs vary with age, sex, rate of growth, body size, activity level, and other factors.[1]

Energy is produced as carbon atoms are split from glucose, fatty acids, and amino acids. This energy can be used to maintain body heat or can be stored as adenosine triphosphate (ATP), which provides the energy required for all the work performed by body cells. Carbohydrates comprise the major energy source used by the body, followed by lipids and then proteins. **Basal metabolic rate** (BMR) represents the energy required to maintain necessary physiologic processes at rest. The BMR and level of physical activity are major determinants of total energy requirements.[2,3]

NUTRIENTS

Nutrients are foods that contain the elements necessary for body function. Six categories of nutrients have been identified: water, carbohydrates, proteins, lipids, vitamins, and minerals.

Water

Water is necessary for life and is present in all body tissues. Water is involved in all biochemical processes and the transport of nutrients and waste products. Water helps regulate body temperature, acts as a lubricant, and is part of cell structure. It is contained in two major compartments: the intracellular and extracellular. Most body water is in the intracellular compartment. The extracellular compartment includes the intravascular and interstitial spaces. The thirst center in the hypothalamus, antidiuretic hormone (ADH), and aldosterone act as regulators of water intake.[2-3]

Carbohydrates

Carbohydrates provide the chief source of energy in most diets, yielding 4 kcal/g. The simplest carbohydrates are the monosaccharides and include glucose, fructose, and galactose. Disaccharides are composed of two monosaccharides and include sucrose, maltose, and lactose. Starch, glycogen, and cellulose are the major polysaccharides and consist of multiple monosaccharides. All carbohydrates must be broken down to monosaccharides for absorption by the gastrointestinal (GI) tract. Glucose is the form in which carbohydrates circulate in the bloodstream and is the only source of energy for the central nervous system. Excess carbohydrate intake is converted to glycogen and is stored in the liver or converted to fat when glycogen stores are filled. It is released when the body needs energy. Daily intake of carbohydrates is necessary to avoid using proteins as a source of energy.

Proteins

Foods containing proteins are necessary for growth and repair of all tissues and provide 4 kcal/g when used for energy. Proteins are used by the body in the manufacture of substances such as hormones, enzymes, and antibodies and are involved in normal fluid and acid-base balances. The end products of the digestion of proteins are amino acids. Essential amino acids are those that humans cannot synthesize from other amino acids. Food sources of essential amino acids are called *complete proteins* and include dairy products, meat, and eggs. Examples of incomplete protein sources are cereals, legumes, and vegetables. Nonessential amino acids can be synthesized in the liver from other amino acids.

One of the waste products of protein metabolism is nitrogen, and the body's nitrogen balance is a good indicator of the client's protein status. In positive nitrogen balance, body tissues are adequately replaced and repaired, and new tissue growth, or **anabolism,** can take place. In negative nitrogen balance, break down, or **catabolism,** of body tissues takes place faster than replacement. This can occur when protein is used to meet the body's need for energy.

Lipids

Lipids provide a concentrated source of energy that spares protein as an energy source. Lipids allow proper absorption of fat-soluble vitamins, contribute to satisfaction with food intake at meals, and when stored, provide the body's main source of energy storage, cushioning, and insulation. Lipids furnish 9 kcal/g of calories. The smallest lipid units are fatty acids, which can be short, medium, or long chain. Long-chain fatty acids are less easily absorbed from the GI tract. Essential fatty acids (linoleic acid, linolenic acid, and arachidonic acid) cannot be synthesized by the body and must be ingested in the diet.

Vitamins

Vitamins are organic compounds necessary to regulate metabolic processes and to serve as catalysts in biochemical reactions. Many vitamins are not single chemicals but groups of chemically and functionally related compounds.

Vitamins can act as enzymes or hormones. They must be supplied through the diet or dietary supplements because they are not produced by the body. The fat-soluble vitamins are A, D, E, and K, and fat is required for their absorption from the GI tract. Fat-soluble vitamins can be stored by the body. Water-soluble vitamins are C and the B vitamins—folic acid, niacin, biotin, and pantothenic acid. These vitamins are not stored by the body, and intake must be provided daily.

Minerals

Minerals are important in the regulation of body processes and the production of body tissues. Minerals must be ionized (electrolytes) to be absorbed and transported throughout the body. **Macrominerals** are required in daily amounts greater than 100 mg and include calcium, chloride, magnesium, potassium, sodium, and phosphorus. **Microminerals** are needed in daily amounts less than 100 mg and include chromium, cobalt, copper, fluorine, iodine, iron, manganese, molybdenum, selenium, and zinc.[2-4]

RECOMMENDED DAILY ALLOWANCES

A list of recommended daily allowances (RDAs) has been available since the early 1940s. The RDAs are the levels of intake of essential nutrients considered adequate to meet the needs of healthy individuals. RDAs do not represent minimal or average nutritional requirements. Instead, they designate the minimal need plus a margin of safety sufficient to accommodate variations in nutritional needs. RDAs are not meant to assist individuals in making sensible food choices but are a means of assessing dietary adequacy.[1]

SUMMARY

To meet the nutritional needs of an individual, all major nutrients—water, carbohydrates, proteins, lipids, vitamins, and minerals—must be considered. To ensure proper nutrition, the individual's energy intake must meet, and not greatly exceed, the energy output.

REFERENCES

1. Bolander, V.B. (1994). *Sorensen and Luckmann's basic nursing: A psychophysiologic approach* (3rd ed.). Philadelphia: W.B. Saunders.
2. Williams, S. (1991). *Nutrition: Essentials and diet therapy* (9th ed.). St. Louis: Mosby–Year Book.
3. Davis, J., & Sherer, K. (1993). *Applied nutrition and diet therapy for nurses.* Philadelphia: W.B. Saunders.
4. Poleman, C.M., & Peckenpaugh, N.J. (1991). *Nutrition Essentials and diet therapy* (6th ed.). Philadelphia: W.B. Saunders.

CHAPTER 71

Fat-Soluble Vitamins

PATRICIA UGO • PAMELA MOHLER PICKENS

⊛ **Nursing Considerations**

LEARNING OBJECTIVE: Conduct a nutritional assessment on a client.

⊛ **Fat-Soluble Vitamins**

LEARNING OBJECTIVES:

Explain the physiologic roles of each fat-soluble vitamin.

Describe the signs of deficiency for each fat-soluble vitamin.

List clients at risk for deficiency of each fat-soluble vitamin.

Discuss administrative and toxicity issues for each fat-soluble vitamin.

Identify the three active forms of vitamin A.

Discuss the difference between vitamin D_2 and vitamin D_3.

Describe the influence of selenium on vitamin E requirement.

KEY TERMS:

Calcitriol, carotenoids, cholecalciferol, ergocalciferol, osteomalacia, retinal, retinoids, retinoic acid, retinol, retinol-binding protein, rickets, tretinoin

---

CONCEPTS AND TERMS TO REVIEW

Read overview provided in Chapter 70.

Review ingestion and digestion processes in an anatomy and physiology textbook.

Review nutrition textbook for sources of exogenous fat-soluble vitamins.

Consumers in the United States, convinced that they need more and better nutrients, spend millions of dollars each year on vitamin and nutritional products. In most cases the average individual does not need supplementation. In fact, some vitamins and minerals can be toxic if consumed in amounts greater than the recommended dietary allowance (RDA).

This chapter focuses on fat-soluble vitamins and emphasizes the indications of vitamin deficiency, drugs and diseases that contribute to deficiency states, and the function of the vitamins in the body.

▨ NURSING CONSIDERATIONS

Proper nutrition promotes growth, maintains health, and helps the body resist infection and other disease states.

Assessing During the **health history** include a dietary history and intake record. These data can confirm adequate nutrition or detect altered nutritional status.

Ask the client if there has been a recent change in diet. If so, have the client describe the duration and specific changes. Question the client about significant weight gain or loss or change in appetite. Determine if the client takes any over-the-counter (OTC) preparations or prescription drugs. Inquire specifically about vitamin and mineral supplements and appetite suppressants. Analyze the drug history for drugs that might contribute to vitamin deficiency or toxicity. Ask if the client uses "health" foods. If so, determine which ones and how much of each is consumed.

As you continue to gather data, consider the following aspects:

• Daily intake of alcoholic beverages
• Daily intake of beverages containing caffeine
• Food allergies
• History of an eating disorder
• Developmental needs of the individual
• Bowel habits
• Relationship between food intake and stress
• Economic status

Collect a history of health problems. Some diseases (e.g., alcoholism, hypoparathyroidism, malabsorption syndromes, and diarrhea) contribute to vitamin deficiencies or toxicities.

During the **physical assessment** inspect the client's overall appearance, particularly the skin, hair, mouth membranes, eyes, and nails. These structures frequently reflect altered nutrition. If possible, weigh the patient and obtain an accurate height measurement. Compare these findings with standard measurements. Review appropriate laboratory studies (e.g., hemoglobin, hematocrit, serum iron, total protein).[1]

Diagnosing Based on analysis of your findings, identify appropriate nursing diagnoses. Listed below are diagnostic labels developed through the North American Nursing Diagnosis Association (NANDA) that are appropriate for nutritional problems. Under each diagnostic label are examples of defining characteristics for that label.

- Nutrition, altered, less than body requirements.
  Lack of interest in food
  Reported inadequate food intake
  Body weight 20% or more under ideal weight
  Sore, inflamed buccal cavity
  Excessive loss of hair
- Nutrition, altered, more than body requirements.
  Weight 10% over ideal for height and frame
  Eating in response to internal cues other than hunger
  Eating in response to external cues (e.g., time of day)
  Observed dysfunctional eating patterns
- Nutrition, altered, high risk for more than body requirements.
  Reported or observed obesity in one or both parents
  Observed use of food as reward or comfort measure
  Dysfunctional eating patterns
  Reported or observed higher baseline weight at beginning of each pregnancy

Planning Most of the interventions associated with nutritional problems involve client teaching. Teaching must take into consideration the cultural needs of the client and the client's food preferences and dislikes. Stress the importance of eating well-balanced, nutritious meals. Provide the client a list of the major food groups and appropriate servings per group. In addition, plan to show the client sample meal plans.

With the client, develop appropriate expected outcomes. Examples of outcomes follow:

- Client demonstrates progressive weight gain or loss toward goal.
- Client demonstrates lifestyle changes to maintain appropriate weight.
- Client maintains optimal individual diet and exercise program.
- Client maintains weight at a satisfactory level for height and body build.

Implementing If the client is consuming less than the body requirement, several nursing interventions are appropriate:

- Alter diet as indicated (e.g., mechanical soft, small feedings, snacks).
- Offer flavoring agents if sodium is restricted.
- Limit fiber, which may lead to early satiety.
- Minimize unpleasant odors.
- Provide oral hygiene before and after meals.
- Assist client to obtain resources such as food stamps.

For the client consuming more than body requirements, consider the following interventions:

- Discuss client's view of self.
- Review eating behaviors with client.
- Determine client's motivation for weight loss.
- Assist client to choose nutritious foods that are within financial budget.

Evaluating Weigh the client at least weekly. Review laboratory studies. Discuss expected outcomes with the client and determine if they were met. In addition, determine what changes in the plan of care are needed.

VITAMIN A

Retinoids are a group of structurally and functionally related chemicals derived from animal tissues and collectively referred to as *vitamin A*. **Retinol** is the form of vitamin A found in mammals. **Carotenoids** are a related group of chemicals derived from plant tissues. More than 400 different carotenoids have been identified in human foodstuffs; only β-carotene can be bioconverted to vitamin A in significant amounts. Thus retinol from animal tissue foods and β-carotene from plant tissue foods constitute the primary dietary sources of vitamin A.

Pharmacotherapeutics Dietary vitamin A occurs as a fat-soluble molecule. Vitamin A used in the preparation of oral vitamin supplements may be present as the fat-soluble molecule or as a water-soluble salt. Vitamin A is used systemically to prevent or treat vitamin A deficiencies and is used topically to treat dermatologic disorders.

Deficiency states are associated with fasting blood retinol levels below 20 μg/dl in children less than 11 years and below 30 μg/dl in adults. During vitamin A deficiency, epithelial cells become dry, flattened, and keratinized. Respiratory, gastrointestinal (GI), and genitourinary cells are also affected. Cilia dry and break off, and secretory functions of mucous membranes decrease, leading to tissue sloughing. The risk for infection increases, especially in the elderly client. Common indications of vitamin A deficiency are listed in the box on p. 964.[2]

Deficiencies most often occur in children under the age of 5 years who have poor dietary intake. Individuals with diseases that alter fat digestion and absorption or impair liver storage may also develop vitamin A deficiencies. Vitamin A deficiency is commonly encountered in clients with fat malabsorption syndromes, chronic diarrhea, pancreatic insufficiency, biliary cirrhosis, and sprue. Alcoholism has been associated with decreased liver storage of vitamin A.

Drug-induced deficiencies are generally associated with decreased storage or decreased absorption of vitamin A. Drugs that induce increased microsomal activity in the liver may lead to markedly diminished liver stores of vitamin A. In these situations serum levels of vitamin A and retinol-binding protein (RBP) are generally normal or only slightly lowered if normal recommended intake of vitamin A is maintained. Decreased vitamin A intake in these clients leads to rapid development of a deficiency state. Drugs implicated in lowering hepatic vitamin A stores include phenytoin, methadone, caffeine, benzodiazepines, heroin, α-methyldopa, phenobarbital, phenothiazines, phenelzine sulfate, hydrocortisone, and pred-

COMMON INDICATIONS OF VITAMIN A DEFICIENCY

Skin
Follicular hyperkeratosis ("goose flesh")

Eyes
Impaired visual adaptation in the dark (night blindness)
Corneal, conjunctival, fundic dryness
Corneal ulceration
Bitot's spots (gray triangular deposits on the conjunctiva near the cornea)
Keratomalacia (dryness, ulceration, perforation of cornea)

Central Nervous System
Raised cerebral spinal fluid pressure
Decreased taste and smell sensation
Altered vestibular functions

Others
Decreased corticosteroid production
Growth failure
Faulty bone and tooth development
Fetal malformations
Impaired resistance to infections

---

nisone. Corticosteroids also cause decreased levels of cellular retinoic acid–binding protein and may contribute to localized tissue deficiencies. Consumption of aluminum salts such as aluminum hydroxide and aluminum sucralfate has been associated with decreased absorption of vitamin A from the gut. Cholestyramine, mineral oil, and broad-spectrum antibiotics also interfere with absorption of vitamin A.[3] Table 71–1 summarizes diseases and drugs that contribute to vitamin A deficiency.

Pharmacokinetics   Dietary vitamin A is absorbed from the small intestine, especially from the jejunum. Absorption varies, with 7% to 67% of oral doses absorbed. When in the fat-soluble state, vitamin A absorption depends on the presence of bile salts, pancreatic lipase, and dietary fats and proteins. Absorption of water-soluble salts of vitamin A such as vitamin A acetate depends less on these factors.[2,4]

Approximately 90% of the total body vitamin A content is found in the liver. Studies using radiolabeled vitamin A have indicated that vitamin A storage is complex, involving three distinct levels or pools of storage. A given dose of vitamin A remains in circulation, combined to its carrier proteins, for 24 hours after consumption. The body attempts to excrete any vitamin in excess of the required amounts from this pool. Transfer of vitamin A to the second, metabolically active pool occurs over days 2 through 9. Short-term storage of vitamin A for use in functional metabolism continues over days 9 through 43. By day 43, 30% to 60% of the dose has been transferred into the third, long-term storage pool. Based on

this information, treatment of vitamin A deficiency is more effective if smaller doses are administered over a long period of time instead of larger doses for a short period of time.[2,5]

Once delivered to the liver, retinyl esters are hydrolyzed to free retinol. Free retinol is then bound to a special carrier protein, **retinol-binding protein,** and is released into the bloodstream. In the bloodstream the retinol-RBP combination further combines with transthyretin (prealbumin) for transport to target tissues throughout the body. Cells that require vitamin A for proper functioning have RBP-specific binding sites. Target cells for vitamin A activity include the rod cells of the eyes, epithelial cells of the genitourinary, integumentary, and respiratory tracts, mucosal cells of the GI tract, and tooth germ cells. When the RBP portion of the retinol-RBP-transthyretin complex binds to the receptor site, the retinol is released into the cell. The RBP-transthyretin complex then leaves the cell and is transported to the kidney, where RBP is metabolized and transthyretin returned to circulation. Once within the target cell, retinol is metabolized into one of three active forms (i.e., chromoform, retinyl phosphate, retinoic acid), depending on the functional needs of the cell.

Under normal circumstances 1900 to 2400 IU of retinol are metabolically deactivated each day by hepatic glucuronidation. Retinol-glucuronide is excreted from the body in the bile. Increased levels of vitamin A in the body stores stimulate increased glucuronidation. Metabolism of vitamin A to retinol-glucuronide continues regardless of dietary intake. Eventually this action leads to the development of a deficiency state if intake of vitamin A is insufficient to replace losses.

Mechanism of action   Vitamin A is active within the human body in three forms: retinol, retinal, and retinoic acid. Although vitamin A is necessary for several physiologic functions, only the role of **retinal** in vision is clearly understood. Visual adaptation to dim light requires the presence of rhodopsin, or visual purple, in the rods of the retina. As 11-*cis* retinal, vitamin A provides a key portion of the rhodopsin molecule. Deficient production of 11-*cis* retinal is linked with night blindness (nyctalopia).

Retinoic acid appears to act at the gene level to affect growth and cell differentiation. It is key to the synthesis of glycoproteins and functions to help maintain epithelial tissue integrity. Along with retinol and retinal, retinoic acid supports female hormone production, oogenesis, fertilization, and implantation. Retinol or retinal is necessary to support placental and fetal development. Both retinol and retinoic acid are necessary for complete testicular function in males. In fetal gum tissue vitamin A is necessary for proper function of the ameloblasts, epithelial cells responsible for depositing enamel on the newly forming teeth. Recent clinical research supports the theory that vitamin A plays a critical role in cell-mediated immunity and in the complement system.[6]

Pharmaceutics   Vitamin A is available in capsules for oral administration and in parenteral solution for intramuscular (IM) injections and intravenous (IV) infusions. Table 71–2 provides RDA dosage information about vitamin A.

Undesired clinical responses   Vitamin A toxicity is generally associated with fasting blood retinyl ester levels greater

TABLE 71–1

Drugs and Diseases That Contribute to Vitamin Deficiencies and Toxicities

Vitamin	Disease States Contributing to:		Drugs and Drug Groups Contributing to:	
	Vitamin Deficiency	**Vitamin Toxicity**	**Vitamin Deficiency**	**Vitamin Toxicity**
A	Alcoholism Fat malabsorption syndromes, including cystic fibrosis, sprue, pancreatic insufficiency, biliary cirrhosis, chronic diarrhea Prematurity Proximal small bowel resection	Protein calorie malnutrition Cirrhosis Viral hepatitis Renal failure	Aluminum hydroxide Benzodiazepines Broad-spectrum antibiotics Cholestyramine Methadone α-Methyldopa Mineral oil Neomycin Phenelzine sulfate Phenobarbital Phenothiazines Phenytoin Steroids Sucralfate	Tetracycline
D	Osteolytic cancer Hypoparathryoidism Hyperthyroidism Malabsorption Short bowel syndrome Chronic renal disease	Sarcoidosis Hyperparathyroidism Hypophosphatemia	Bisacodyl (chronic) Cholestyramine Colestipol Corticosteroids (?) Glutethimide Isotretinoin Mineral oil Phenobarbital Phenytoin Primidone	Thiazide diuretics
E	β-Thalassemia major Prematurity Selenium deficiency Malabsorption syndromes Cholestasis		Antacids Broad-spectrum antibiotics Cholestyramine Mineral oil Phenobarbital Phenothiazines Phenytoin Primidone Polyunsaturated fatty acid (PUFA)–rich fat supplements	
K	Hemorrhagic disease of the newborn Biliary obstruction Malabsorption syndromes such as cystic fibrosis, sprue, inflammatory bowel disease, short bowel syndrome		Antibiotics Clofibrate Coumarin Mineral oil Phenobarbital Phenytoin Primidone Salicylates Vitamin A megadose Vitamin E megadose	

than 5 μg/dl. Toxicity occurs when liver storage is overwhelmed or there is insufficient RBP to bind and transport retinol. In these situations excess retinol and retinyl esters bind to very-low-density lipoproteins (VLDL) and are transported to cells throughout the body. The VLDL assists the vitamin to penetrate cell walls, leading to cell wall disruption and cellular swelling and rupture. Maintenance of adequate vitamin E intake diminishes but does not eliminate the risk of toxic effects from vitamin A.[7]

Although it is possible to obtain a toxic dose of vitamin A from dietary intake, most instances of toxicity are associated with the use of vitamin supplements. Acute toxicity is associated with single doses greater than 300,000 IU or 25,000 IU/kg of body weight. Chronic toxicity can occur with doses of 25,000 IU or more daily for a month or more. Indications of acute and chronic toxicity are illustrated in Figure 71–1.[3,5,8]

Contraindications and precautions Viral hepatitis, protein-energy malnutrition (PEM), cirrhosis, and other liver diseases increase the risk of toxicity by lowering the amount of vitamin A necessary to cause adverse effects. Although alcohol increases the risk of vitamin A toxicity in animal models, data in humans are unclear. Low-protein diets have been implicated in increased risk of liver damage and general toxicity by aggravating the stimulation of gluconeogenesis and the increased protein turnover associated with high vitamin A intake. For this reason, alcoholic clients requiring vitamin A supplementation should be treated with small doses and monitored carefully for signs of liver toxicity.[8]

Clients with renal failure have decreased renal clearance of RBP and are at increased risk of toxicity. Chronic doses as low as 5000 IU daily may lead to signs and symptoms of toxicity in a renal failure client.[8]

Clients with eating disorders have elevated plasma vitamin A levels. These elevations are probably related to hemoconcentration or diminished kidney clearance of retinol-binding protein. Chronic vitamin A supplementation in these individuals may be contraindicated.[4,9]

Life-span considerations The appropriate daily dose of vitamin A is age and sex dependent. Recommended oral and intravenous (IV) doses of vitamin A are listed in Table 71–2. Vitamin A activity is expressed in microgram retinol equivalents (μg RE) or in international units (IU). One μg RE is equivalent to 3.33 IU of retinol. Because of the risks associated with vitamin A toxicity, recommended amounts should not be routinely exceeded, especially in children and pregnant or lactating women.[10,11] Normal fasting blood retinol levels are 20 to 90 μg/dl for a child (<11 years) and 30 to 90 μg/dl for an adult.[12]

Vitamin A is teratogenic. Doses of 18,000 to 25,000 IU and above per day before and during pregnancy have been linked to an increased risk of fetal deformities of the head, face, and genitourinary system.

Specific nursing considerations Because of increased risks of toxicity, care should be taken in administering vitamin A supplements in clients with renal or liver dysfunction. Do not administer vitamin A supplements to clients with renal dysfunction severe enough to require chronic dialysis unless and until a deficiency state begins to develop. In addition, because several indications of vitamin A toxicity are similar to those of uremia (scaly skin, pruritus, headache, double vision, nausea, hypercalcemia), assess clients with renal failure carefully. Pregnant clients should not receive vitamin A supple-

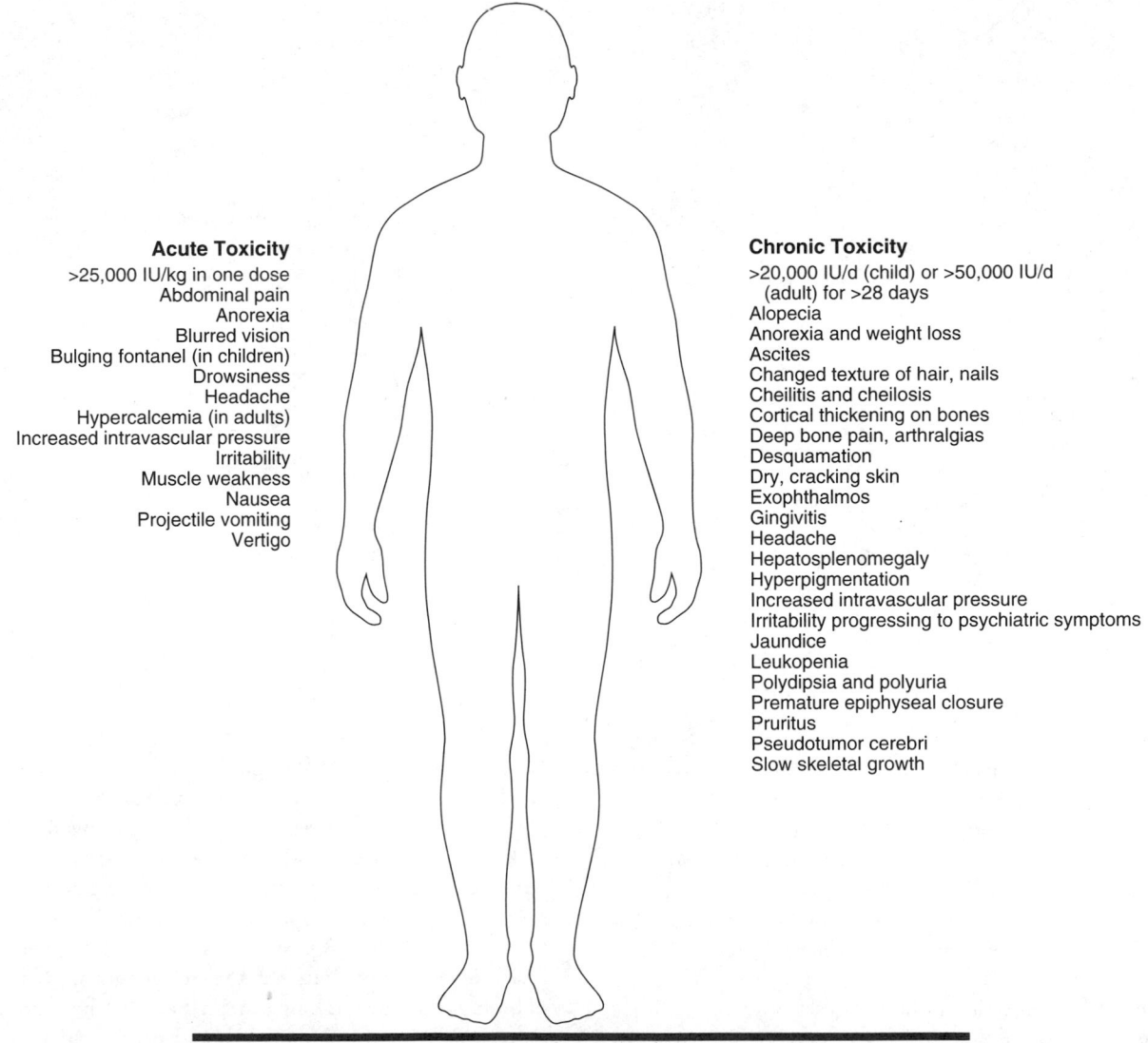

Acute Toxicity

>25,000 IU/kg in one dose
Abdominal pain
Anorexia
Blurred vision
Bulging fontanel (in children)
Drowsiness
Headache
Hypercalcemia (in adults)
Increased intravascular pressure
Irritability
Muscle weakness
Nausea
Projectile vomiting
Vertigo

Chronic Toxicity

>20,000 IU/d (child) or >50,000 IU/d
    (adult) for >28 days
Alopecia
Anorexia and weight loss
Ascites
Changed texture of hair, nails
Cheilitis and cheilosis
Cortical thickening on bones
Deep bone pain, arthralgias
Desquamation
Dry, cracking skin
Exophthalmos
Gingivitis
Headache
Hepatosplenomegaly
Hyperpigmentation
Increased intravascular pressure
Irritability progressing to psychiatric symptoms
Jaundice
Leukopenia
Polydipsia and polyuria
Premature epiphyseal closure
Pruritus
Pseudotumor cerebri
Slow skeletal growth

FIGURE 71–1   Common indications of acute and chronic vitamin A toxicity.

TABLE 71–2
Recommended Dosages of Vitamin A*

Client	Oral Dose	Intravenous Dose
Child		
<11 y	70 μg/kg/d	70 μg/kg/d
	Maximum: 700 μg/d	Maximum: 700 μg/d
Male		
>10 y	1000 μg/d	1000 μg/d
Female		
>10 y	800 μg/d	1000 μg/d
Pregnant	800–1000 μg/d	
Lactating	1200 μg/d	

*1 μg = 3.3 IU.

ments in excess of 800 μg RE (3000 IU)/d unless need is clearly established. Because of the extended half-life of vitamin A in the body, all sexually active, fertile women should be taught about the fetal risks associated with intake in excess of the RDA.[3]

Exposure of IV nutrient solutions to fluorescent lighting or sunlight can lead to photodegradation of vitamin A. Avoid placement of the solution in direct sunlight or near high-intensity lamps. Vitamin A binds to the plastic of IV administration sets over time. Prolonged exposure of vitamin A–containing solution to the administration bag or tubing can lead to significantly decreased availability of vitamin A to the client. To minimize the combined risks of photodegradation and binding, add the vitamin to the IV solution close to the scheduled infusion time.[5,13]

Avoid the use of daily doses of >25,000 IU unless a clear need has been established. Counsel parents that administration of large doses of vitamin A to children for long periods of time may lead to premature epiphyseal closure and bone malformations. If administration of vitamin A is deemed medically necessary, coadministration of vitamin E or zinc and taurine supplements may improve response to vitamin A and permit the use of smaller doses.[5,14]

Review with the client the risks of vitamin A toxicity. Instruct clients with small children in the house to keep vitamin A supplements out of reach of children. Advise them of the indications of acute overdose in children. Educate clients with high alcohol use or liver disease of the risks of high vitamin A supplementation.

Educate clients on sources of dietary vitamin A. Vitamin A can be obtained from many food products such as cream, egg yolk, and unwashed butter, which are natural sources of vitamin A. Counsel clients with biliary or fat malabsorption disorders about the risks of vitamin A deficiency. Instruct them about the use of water-soluble salts and vitamin A precursors as possible supplements.

MISCELLANEOUS DRUG PREPARATIONS

Vitamin A has beneficial effects in the treatment of several skin disorders, including acne. However, the use of systemic vitamin A for the treatment of skin disorders has proved too toxic. Therefore topical preparations containing vitamin A or synthetic retinoids are used.

When prepared in an appropriate solvent, both retinol and retinoic acid (**tretinoin**, or all-*trans*-retinoic acid) are absorbed through the stratum corneum and into the epithelial cells. Studies using radiolabeled tretinoin indicate that 9% to 50% of the drug preparation is absorbed into the skin within 16 hours of application when an occlusive dressing is used. These studies also indicate that 0.1% to 6% of the dose is excreted into the urine within 56 hours. Once vitamin A is absorbed into the cell, it is used, metabolized, and excreted in a manner identical to that of systemically obtained vitamin A. Extensive use of highly concentrated topical vitamin A preparations, combined with occlusive dressings, can lead to localized toxicity.[3,15]

Initial studies indicate that retinoic acid may work at the genetic level to affect cell differentiation. In clients with acne this may mean a reversal of hyperkeratosis of the sebaceous follicle, preventing the occlusion of the follicle and the formation of acne lesions. Topical tretinoin stimulates the synthesis of gap junctions. These intercellular membrane structures are found between epithelial cells and are implicated in the organization, coordination, and growth of new epithelial tissue. This mechanism may contribute to the clearing of fine wrinkles, reduction in skin coarseness and freckling, and increased pinkness seen during the experimental treatment of photo-damaged (sun-aged) skin with topical tretinoin.

Since topical tretinoin therapy requires up to 12 weeks of therapy to achieve results, counsel the client on the need to continue therapy until adequate results are achieved.[3] Instruct the client to use mild soaps and a gentle scrubbing and drying action on affected areas. Teach him or her to clean and completely dry the skin before each application to minimize irritation. Tretinoin may increase skin sensitivity to sun, wind, and cold; instruct clients about the importance of using sunblocks and, if necessary, noncomedogenic moisturizers. Some clients develop a blush, slight irritation, or peeling or have mild aggravation of their acne during the early stages of therapy. These problems should resolve as the skin becomes accustomed to the drug. Emphasize the importance of using only the prescribed amount of preparation since excessive use of the preparation increases the incidence of irritation, peeling, and other side effects.

CONCEPT REVIEW

In oral supplements vitamin A is present as a fat-soluble molecule or a water-soluble salt. It is used systemically to treat or prevent deficiency states. A topical preparation is available for the treatment of skin conditions.

Oral vitamin A is absorbed from the small intestine and primarily stored in the liver. It is most effective when administered in small doses over a long period of time.

Vitamin A is used with caution in individuals with impaired liver or kidney function. In high doses it is teratogenic.

Vitamin A can be degraded by sunlight or fluorescent lighting. It also binds to the plastic of IV administration sets.

VITAMIN D

Vitamin D comprises a group of chemicals that exhibit hormonal characteristics. Vitamin D is derived endogenously or exogenously. **Endogenous vitamin D** is formed by the action of ultraviolet light on 7-dehydrocholesterol in the skin. This action produces D_3 **(cholecalciferol).** Formation of vitamin D_3 is influenced by the intensity and length of ultraviolet light exposure and by the melanin content of the skin. Once formed, vitamin D_3 is transported from skin cells to the liver on specialized vitamin D carrier sites on globulin proteins.

Exogenous vitamin D comes from foods or vitamin supplements as vitamin D_2 **(ergocalciferol)** or vitamin D_3. Natural and fortified food sources such as cereals, milk, margarine, and chocolate beverage mixes provide limited amounts of both vitamin D_2 and vitamin D_3. These vitamin forms are also available through vitamin supplements and synthetic analogs of vitamin D. Absorbed in the small intestines in the presence of bile salts, dietary vitamin D and oral supplements are incorporated into chylomicrons for transport through the sympathetic system to the liver.[2,4] In this text the focus is on exogenous vitamin D.

Pharmacotherapeutics Deficiency states are consistently associated with serum 25-hydroxycholecalciferol levels below 5 ng/ml of blood; low blood levels are present before clinical indications of bone demineralization are identified. Poor bone demineralization is characterized as **rickets** in children and **osteomalacia** in adults. Complaints of bone pain or tenderness and proximal muscle weakness may accompany vitamin D deficiency. In addition, secondary hyperparathyroidism may develop as the body attempts to compensate for the vitamin deficiency. Hypocalcemia or hypophosphatemia may be present in some clients. These conditions may be accompanied by hypocalcemic tetany.

Disease states that decrease the production or excretion of biliary salts or pancreatic enzymes or that interfere with the absorption of fats (e.g., sprue) may lead to a vitamin D deficiency. Laxatives such as bisacodyl and mineral oil and bile acid sequestrates, including colestipol and cholestyramine, decrease absorption of vitamin D from the gut lumen. Phenytoin, phenobarbital, and primidone cause increased enzyme activity in the liver, leading to enhanced metabolism of vitamin D to inactive compounds. Deficiencies caused by these drugs apparently are dose related. Additionally, use of a ketogenic diet with anticonvulsant therapy in epileptic children causes bone loss in excess of that seen with use of the drugs alone.[3]

Glucocorticoid steroids such as hydrocortisone decrease the rate of renal hydroxylation of vitamin D. Because the development of osteopenia appears directly related to the dose of

steroid, this interference with vitamin D activity is postulated as the major mechanism of this adverse effect. Use of vitamin D supplementation to inhibit or reverse the process is under investigation.[3] Table 71–1 contains a summary of diseases and drugs that contribute to vitamin D deficiency.

Pharmacokinetics Ergocalciferol and cholecalciferol, both of which are chemically inert, are stored in the liver until needed. They are then metabolized to 25-hydroxycholecalciferol (calcidiol). Calcidiol is transported by the carrier globulin to the kidneys, where it is metabolized in the proximal convoluted tubules to 1,25-dihydroxycholecalciferol **(calcitriol),** the active form of the vitamin. The hydroxylation and release of calcitriol from the kidneys are stimulated by parathyroid hormone (PTH), low serum phosphate levels, estrogen, prolactin, and growth hormone. Calcitriol is degraded in the liver by dehydroxylation; most metabolites are excreted as calcitroic acid in bile. Two to 5% of vitamin D excretion is in urine.[2,4,16]

Mechanism of action Vitamin D works with PTH and calcitonin to maintain calcium and phosphorus homeostasis. It stimulates active absorption of calcium and phosphorus from the small intestines and stimulates release and mineralization of calcium and phosphorus from and to bone. It enhances kidney resorption of calcium and phosphorus. Calcitriol receptors have been located in cells of the stomach, parathyroid glands, gonads, pancreas, skeletal and cardiac muscles, brain, monocytes, lymphocytes, dermis, and hair roots.[2]

Pharmaceutics Vitamin D is administered most frequently in combination with other vitamins and minerals. Table 71–3 summarizes RDA IV and oral dosages for different age groups.

Undesired clinical responses Vitamin D toxicity is associated with oral doses greater than 50 μg/d (2000 IU) of cholecalciferol in children and oral doses greater than 125 μg/d (5000 IU) in adults. Toxic IV doses have not been clearly established. Many of the acute and chronic signs and symptoms of vitamin D toxicity are related to hypercalcemia secondary to elevated vitamin activity; therefore vitamin D

TABLE 71–3
Recommended Dosages of Vitamin D*

Client	Oral Dose	Intravenous Dose
Infant		
<6 mo	7.5 μg/d	4 μg/kg/d if <3 kg
<11 y		1 μg/kg/d
		Maximum: 10 μg/d
Male		
6 mo–25 y	10 μg/d	
>10 y		5 μg/d
>25 y	5 μg/d	
Female		
6 mo–25 y	10 μg/d	
>10 y		5 μg/d
>25 y	5 μg/d	
Pregnant	10 μg/d	5 μg/d
Lactating	10 μg/d	5 μg/d

*1 μg = 40 IU.

toxicity must be differentiated from primary hypercalcemia. Common signs and symptoms of toxicity are illustrated in Figure 71–2.

Contraindications and precautions   Newborn infants delivered to hypercalcemic mothers, including mothers who are vitamin D toxic, may have suppressed parathyroid gland function, which may lead to hypocalcemia, tetany, and seizure activity in the infant. Some infants born to hypercalcemic mothers have had supravalvular aortic stenosis.

Drug-drug interactions   Because vitamin D therapy leads to increased serum calcium levels, clients receiving digoxin therapy should be monitored closely for signs and symptoms of digoxin toxicity. Concurrent use of cholecalciferol and magnesium-containing antacids in chronic renal dialysis clients may lead to hypermagnesemia.[8]

Life-span considerations   The normal serum level of vitamin D_3 1,25-dihydroxycholecalciferol is 24 to 45 pg/ml. Plasma vitamin D_3 25-hydroxycholecalciferol levels range from 15 to 80 ng/ml in the summer to 14 to 42 ng/ml in the winter.[17]

Specific nursing considerations   Monitor the client with renal failure carefully for signs and symptoms of osteomalacia. The decreased ability to hydroxylate cholecalciferol to its active form may develop at any time during the course of renal disease. Some individuals require supplementation with 1,25-dihydrocholecalciferol or with dihydrotachysterol from the onset of renal failure, whereas others may not require supplementation until the disease process has been long established. Monitor the client receiving these supplements closely for signs and symptoms of vitamin D toxicity.

Assess clients receiving vitamin D as part of their parenteral nutrition regimen for changes in serum calcium and phosphorus levels. Those wholly dependent on parenteral nutrition therapy can easily develop hypocalcemia if vitamin D supplementation is inadequate; hypercalcemia may be a sign of vitamin D excess. Serum calcium levels greater than 10 mg/dl are

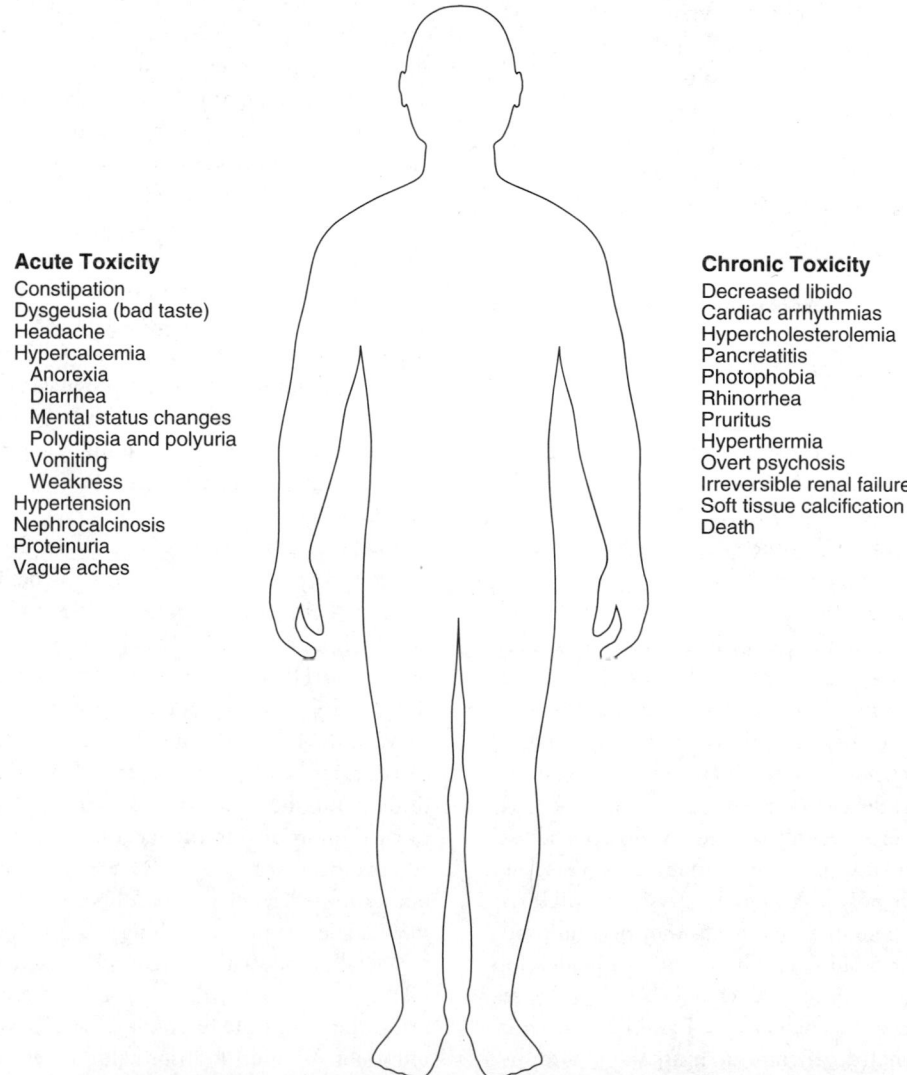

Acute Toxicity
Constipation
Dysgeusia (bad taste)
Headache
Hypercalcemia
  Anorexia
  Diarrhea
  Mental status changes
  Polydipsia and polyuria
  Vomiting
  Weakness
Hypertension
Nephrocalcinosis
Proteinuria
Vague aches

Chronic Toxicity
Decreased libido
Cardiac arrhythmias
Hypercholesterolemia
Pancreatitis
Photophobia
Rhinorrhea
Pruritus
Hyperthermia
Overt psychosis
Irreversible renal failure
Soft tissue calcification
Death

FIGURE 71–2   Common indications of acute and chronic vitamin D toxicity.

dangerous. Determine serum calcium levels twice weekly for clients receiving activated vitamin D_3 supplementation until the dosage and response to therapy have stabilized.

Vitamin D may bind to plastic tubing and bags used in IV administration sets. To minimize the loss of vitamin D, add the vitamin preparation to the IV solution close to the time of administration.[5]

Discourage clients from consuming more than the RDA of vitamin D unless the need for higher doses is clearly established. Caution nursing mothers that oral supplementation of vitamin D causes excretion dihydrocholecalciferol into the breast milk.

CONCEPT REVIEW

Endogenous vitamin D_3 is derived from cholesterol that is converted by ultraviolet light to cholecalciferol. Cholecalciferol is stored in the liver and is converted in the kidneys to the active hormone calcitriol. Calcitriol is degraded in the liver and excreted as calcitroic acid in the bile. Exogenous vitamin D_2 (ergocalciferol) is absorbed in the small intestines in the presence of bile salts. It is metabolized in the liver and is excreted like natural vitamin D.

Vitamin D works to maintain calcium and phosphorus balance. Deficiency of vitamin D produces rickets in children and osteomalacia in adults. Phenytoin, primidone, phenobarbital, and corticosteroids may decrease levels of active vitamin D.

VITAMIN E

Eight tocopherols constitute the group of chemicals generically classified as *vitamin E*. Of the eight, α-tocopherol has the highest biologic activity and is used as the standard of vitamin E activity. β-Tocopherols and γ-tocopherols also contribute significantly to dietary vitamin E activity.

Pharmacotherapeutics Vitamin E supplements are used to prevent or treat vitamin E deficiency in humans. Mild deficiency states are characterized by depressed serum levels, with no clinical sequelae. Because of the large storage pool of vitamin E and the slow depletion of adipose and muscle stores, moderate to severe deficiency states may require 5 years or more to develop. As the deficiency of vitamin E progresses, cell membranes become more permeable and in vitro hemolysis occurs. Infants, particularly premature infants and those fed formula enriched with polyunsaturated fatty acids (PUFAs) and iron, may develop hemolytic anemia as they become moderately depleted. Older infants, children, and adults develop neurologic abnormalities as the deficiency state progresses from moderate to severe; less frequently, vitamin E deficiency is associated with retinal degeneration, muscular dystrophy, myopathies, and reproductive failure. A study of cholestatic, cirrhotic clients linked vitamin E deficiency with decreases in hand-eye coordination, fine motor speed, vasomotor activity, and the ability to accomplish written connect-the-dots activities.[18]

Other individuals at risk of developing vitamin E deficiency include those with deficient dietary intake or high intake of PUFAs. Clients with steatorrhea from postgastrectomy syndrome, biliary atresia, cirrhosis, cystic fibrosis, sprue, inflammatory bowel disease, or pancreatic disorders may also develop vitamin E deficiency.

Vitamin E deficiency may develop as a result of concurrent drug therapy. Evidence exists that anticonvulsant drugs such as phenobarbital and phenytoin may decrease hepatic storage of vitamin E. Phenothiazines may also decrease available vitamin E. Use of drugs that decrease the absorption of fats or sequester bile salts in the gut (e.g., cholestyramine and mineral oil) leads to decreased absorption of vitamin E from the gut. In addition, antacids and broad-spectrum antibiotics may decrease vitamin E absorption. Clients receiving long-term therapy with any of these drugs may require vitamin E supplementation.[3,8,19] Table 71–1 contains a summary of diseases and drugs that contribute to vitamin E deficiency.

Also under investigation is the use of vitamin E in platelet aggregation and atherosclerotic disease and ischemia and reperfusion injuries.[20] Recent studies have suggested a role for vitamin E in the prevention of long-term diabetic complications.[21] Studies in animal models have demonstrated a role for vitamin E in delaying or minimizing the development of induced cataracts; its role in the development of cataracts in humans is under investigation.[20]

Pharmacokinetics Vitamin E is absorbed from the small intestine with variable efficacy. Absorption is best in the jejunum, with lesser absorption in the duodenum and ileum. In most individuals 25% to 80% of a dose is absorbed. Absorption requires the presence of bile salts and pancreatic lipase and is improved in the presence of mixed dietary fats. Administration of vitamin E with PUFAs may lead to decreased absorption of the vitamin. Vitamin E is collected into chylomicrons and is delivered to the liver through the lacteal lymphatics.[4,19]

In the liver vitamin E is liberated from the chylomicrons and is incorporated into VLDLs for delivery into the blood. Vitamin E is released from VLDLs and transported in low-density lipoproteins (LDLs) in men, with high-density lipoproteins (HDLs) as secondary transports. Women use HDL as the primary transport lipoprotein for vitamin E.[19,20]

Vitamin E–specific binding sites have been identified on hepatocytes and erythrocytes. Vitamin E is distributed throughout the body tissues, with tissue concentrations directly proportional to the fat content of the tissue. The plasma and liver stores of vitamin E are very labile and are rapidly mobilized in deficiency states. Adipose and muscle stores are less mobile and are preserved longer during deficiency states.[18]

Metabolically active vitamin E is excreted unchanged in the bile. It is unknown whether any of the excreted vitamin E is reabsorbed from the fecal matter as it passes through the small intestines. Vitamin E absorbed in excess of needs is converted by the liver to lactone. The lactone is further esterified to glucuronic acid, which is excreted in the urine.[19]

Mechanism of action Vitamin E is a very potent antioxidant and free radical scavenger. It prevents peroxidizing reactions and inhibits fats, including the phospholipid components of cell membranes, from becoming rancid. Because of its effects on such widely distributed cellular components, vitamin E has been implicated in efficient drug detoxification by hepatic microsomes, in the functioning of mitochondria, in the synthesis of heme proteins, and in neuromuscular function.

Vitamin E is used in the prevention or control of bronchopulmonary hyperplasia and retrolental fibroplasia in premature infants who require high concentrations of oxygen. The hyperoxemia present in these infants is damaging to retinal and pulmonary tissues, possibly through increased production of peroxide free radicals. Vitamin E binds to the peroxides, preventing tissue damage.[2,3,19] At very high doses, vitamin E inhibits synthesis of some prostaglandins (PGEs) such as PGE_2.

Pharmaceutics Vitamin E is available in oral, parenteral, and topical dosage forms. Table 71–4 provides RDA dosage information.

Selenium and vitamin E perform complementary roles. The amount of selenium present in the diet influences the amount of vitamin E necessary to prevent the occurrence of deficiency symptoms. Clients who maintain recommended selenium intake require lower vitamin E intake, with improved responsiveness to the lower vitamin doses.[12,19]

Undesired clinical responses Although vitamin E is considered fairly innocuous, high doses are not without risk. Toxicity related to ingestion of oral vitamin E capsules and tablets is relatively uncommon and is associated with doses in excess of the RDA. Toxic reactions to vitamin E are more common when it is administered by injection. However, this result may be due to nonvitamin components of the injection preparations.[3,19]

Vitamin E depresses vitamin K–dependent clotting factor activity, leading to prolonged clotting times. This effect may be compounded by decreased platelet aggregation secondary to suppression of prostaglandin metabolism. High doses of vitamin E have been linked to incidents of pulmonary embolism, hypertension, hypertriglyceridemia, fatigue, gynecomastia, breast tenderness, breast tumors, myopathy, intestinal cramps, and urticaria and to aggravation of diabetes mellitus.[3,8] There also have been reports of necrotizing enterocolitis in premature infants receiving vitamin E supplements.

Contraindications and precautions In clients with β-thalassemia major, an inborn error of metabolism frequently accompanied by vitamin E deficiency, supplementation of vitamin E has led to an unexpected toxic response. These clients develop increased tissue accumulation of iron, culminating in heart and liver failure.[2]

Life-span considerations Daily vitamin E needs are determined by the age and sex of the client. For example, infants up to the age of 6 months require 3 mg of d-α-tocopherol daily; this dosage increases to 4 mg/d for their second 6 months. Pregnant clients should consume 10 mg of d-α-tocopherol daily to ensure that adequate supplies are available for the developing fetus. Likewise, lactating clients should consume 12 mg/d for the first 6 months of breast-feeding and 11 mg/d for the second 6 months of breast-feeding.[3,12,19]

Clients receiving long-term birth control pill therapy may benefit from maintaining good vitamin E nutriture. Preliminary data suggest that maintaining vitamin E status decreases the platelet aggregation that can occur with extended use of birth control pills.[20]

Specific nursing considerations Vitamin E deficiencies and toxicities are very uncommon. The greatest risk for both occurs in premature newborns, particularly those dependent on parenteral feedings. Because IV fat emulsions are high in polyunsaturated fatty acids, which increase vitamin E requirements, monitor clients receiving these solutions for signs of hemolytic anemia or neurologic abnormalities.[12]

Vitamin E, like the other fat-soluble vitamins, adheres to plastic bags and infusion devices used for preparing and administering IV solutions. To minimize loss of the vitamin from the solution, add it to the solution close to the infusion time.[19]

TABLE 71–4
Recommended Dosages of Vitamin E*

Client	Oral Dose	Intravenous Dose
Infant		
<6 mo	3 mg/d	0.7 mg/kg/d Maximum: 7 mg/d
6–12 mo	4 mg/d	
Child		7 mg/d
1–3 y	6 mg/d	
3–10 y	7 mg/d	
Male		
>10 y	10 mg/d	10 mg/d
Female		
>10 y	8 mg/d	10 mg/d
Pregnant	10 mg/d	
Lactating	12 mg/d	

*1 mg = 1 IU.

CONCEPT REVIEW

Vitamin E comprises eight tocopherols; the most active is α-tocopherol. Vitamin E is absorbed best from the jejunum; absorption requires the presence of bile salts and pancreatic lipase. The vitamin is distributed throughout body tissue, with highest concentrations in the most fatty tissue. Metabolically active vitamin E is excreted unchanged in the bile; excess vitamin E is converted by the liver and excreted in the urine.

Vitamin E is a potent antioxidant and free radical scavenger. It assists in drug detoxification and in prevention and control of bronchopulmonary hyperplasia and retrolental fibroplasia in premature infants receiving oxygen. Vitamin E may be useful in improving immune function.

Deficiencies and toxicities are both uncommon. Severe vitamin E deficiency may take 5 years or more to develop.

VITAMIN K

The generic term *vitamin K* is used to refer to several compounds, the most important of which are two naturally occurring chemicals, K_1 (phytonadione or phylloquinone) and K_2 (farnoquinone or menaquinone), and one synthetic chemical, K_3 (menandiol or menadione).[12]

Vitamin K₁

Pharmacotherapeutics Because newborns are at increased risk for hemorrhagic complications as a result of hypoprothrombinemia, vitamin K_1 is administered at birth. Newborns should receive a prophylatic dose of 0.5 to 1 mg of K_1 intramuscularly if the mother did not receive a 1- to 5-mg supplement of K_1 during the 24 hours before delivery. If hypoprothrombinemic hemorrhage occurs, the newborn can be treated with 1 to 2 mg, either subcutaneously or intramuscularly, daily until the problem is corrected.[3]

An adult with severe bleeding complicated by hypoprothrombinemia may require transfusions and IV administration of 5 to 50 mg of vitamin K_1 to stabilize the individual and reverse the hypoprothrombinemia. If blood loss is particularly severe and rapid or if the hypoprothrombinemia is profound, a second IV dose may be necessary in 6 to 8 hours.[3]

Deficiency of vitamin K is associated with hypoprothrombinemia and decreased production of clotting factors II, VII, IX, and X. Individuals with a deficiency bruise easily and exhibit prolonged bleeding and clotting times. GI bleeding, epistaxis, and hematuria may also occur. Use of injectable drugs in these individuals is associated with an increased risk of hemorrhage or hematoma at the injection site.

Coumarin and other warfarin derivatives function by inhibiting the production of vitamin K–dependent clotting factors. The amount of vitamin K in the body influences the effectiveness of warfarin in preventing clot formation. Changes in the dietary intake of K_1 can increase or decrease the response to warfarin.[22]

Both clofibrate and mineral oil bind vitamin K_1, trapping it in the gut and preventing its absorption. Large doses of vitamin A or vitamin E may also interfere with absorption of K. Clients taking these drugs on a regular basis may need vitamin K supplementation. Primidone, phenobarbital, and phenytoin have been implicated in increased metabolic inactivation of vitamin K.[3,8] Diseases associated with altered fat absorption such as sprue, biliary obstruction, short bowel syndrome, liver parenchyma disease, inflammatory bowel disease, and pancreatic disease have been linked to decreased absorption of vitamin K from the small bowel. Table 71–1 summarizes diseases and drugs that contribute to vitamin K deficiency.

Pharmacokinetics Vitamin K_1 is absorbed from the proximal small intestines in the presence of bile salts. Passing directly from the intestinal cells to the bloodstream, vitamin K_1 is delivered to the liver, where it is stored briefly as the 2,3-epoxide. The liver uses vitamin K_1 in the formation of clotting factors II, VII, IX, and X. Vitamin K_1 is distributed throughout the body by the bloodstream, although little tissue storage occurs. Vitamin K_1 crosses the placenta and into breast milk.

Concentrations in breast milk are usually low but do increase with maternal supplementation.[2,21,23]

Mechanism of action Vitamin K plays a vital role in the carboxylation of several precursor chemicals necessary for the production of four clotting factors. When vitamin K is present in insufficient amounts, production of prothrombin and other chemicals necessary for the formation of blood clots drops. In this state the ability to form blood clots is diminished, and significant blood loss can occur from otherwise minor wounds.

Vitamin K may play a role in the production of a matrix protein found in the bone by influencing key carboxylation enzymes. Similar proteins have been identified in the kidney, placenta, spleen, lung, and blood. The significance of this activity is not yet known.[24]

Pharmaceutics Vitamin K_1 is available in oral and parenteral dosage forms. The parenteral solutions are for IV, IM, or SC administration. Table 71–5 provides information on dosages and routes of administration for vitamin K treatment.

Undesired clinical responses Normal blood and tissue levels have not been defined for vitamin K. Vitamin K is monitored indirectly through assessment of the prothrombin time. Use of the prothrombin time must be combined with clinical assessment to reach valid conclusions about vitamin K status.[24]

Adverse reactions are uncommon but may occur, especially if the vitamin is administered by injection. Anaphylactic and allergic reactions have been reported, occurring most frequently with IV dosing. These reactions may be related to components of the diluent rather than the vitamin itself. Because these reactions are independent of the size or dilution of the dose or the rate of administration, IV administration should be reserved for emergencies, and support equipment should be readily available if needed. Hypersensitive reactions to oral doses are usually manifested as urticaria; urticaria may also occur at injection sites. Continued dosing after cutaneous reactions may lead to the development of scleroderma-like plaques at the injection sites.[3,24]

On rare occasions the use of large doses of K_1 have been associated with hemolytic anemia and hyperbilirubinemia in premature or low-birth-weight neonates. Despite these occurrences, K_1 is considered the safest of the vitamin K supplements and is the supplement of choice for neonates requiring vitamin K.[2,24]

Life-span considerations Recommended intakes of K_1 are based on the assumption that 50% of an individual's vitamin K needs are met by absorption of bacterially produced K_2. Infants and children require 4 to 5 μg of K_1 per kilogram of body weight per day; adults require 70 μg of K_1 daily.[12]

CONCEPT REVIEW

Vitamin K_1 (phytonadione or phylloquinone) and K_2 (farnoquinone or menaquinone) are naturally occurring chemicals. Vitamin K_3 (menandiol or menadione) is synthetically produced.

Vitamin K is vital to the clotting process. Deficiency of vitamin K produces ease of bruising and prolonged

TABLE 71–5
Vitamin K: Forms and Dosages

Dosage Form	Dosage Recommendation
PHYTONADIONE (Aquamephyton) HOW SUPPLIED Oral: 5-mg tablets	***Anticoagulant-Induced Prothrombin Deficiency*** 10–20 mg
IV	***Serious or Life-Threatening Prothrombin Deficiency*** Usual dose: 5–10 mg; up to 50 mg can be used
Oral, IV, IM, or SC	***Hypoprothrombinemia Due to Other Causes*** Usual dose: 2.5–25 mg; up to 50 mg can be used
IM	***Prophylaxis, Hemorrhagic Disease of the Newborn*** 0.5–1 mg within 1 h of birth
IM or SC	***Treatment, Hemorrhagic Disease of the Newborn*** Initial dose: 1 mg; may be repeated daily
MENADIOL SODIUM DIPHOSPHATE (Synkayvite) HOW SUPPLIED Oral IM, SC, IV	Adults: 5–10 mg/d Adults: 5–15 mg one to two times/d Children: 5–10 mg one to two times/d

bleeding and clotting times, which may lead to GI bleeding, epistaxis, and hematuria.

IV administration of vitamin K_1 should be used only in emergencies since allergic reactions and anaphylaxis have been reported.

Vitamin K₂

Pharmacotherapeutics Newborn infants have sterile guts and little, if any, K_2 production perinatally. Breast milk contains only 2 µg/L; therefore a breast-fed newborn may obtain very little dietary K during the first few weeks of life. Many infant formulas are supplemented to provide 5 µg of vitamin K in as little as 125 ml of formula to decrease this risk.[12,24]

Deficient production or absorption of K_2 in the small bowel produces a deficiency state clinically indistinguishable from a K_1 deficiency. Since the production of K_2 depends on the health of intestinal bacteria, drugs and therapies that weaken or destroy gut flora lead to loss of vitamin K_2 production, with a resultant deficiency in absorbed K. Broad-spectrum antibiotics, especially cefamandole and other cephalosporins, have been linked to the development of vitamin K-responsive coagulopathies. Absorption of vitamin K_2, as K_1, is inhibited by administration of fat-trapping drugs such as mineral oil and cholestyramine. Clients receiving chronic therapy with these drugs may require vitamin K supplementation. Similarly, diseases associated with fat malabsorption decrease the absorption of K_2.

Pharmacokinetics In humans vitamin K_2 is produced by intestinal flora, released into the gut lumen, and absorbed into the bloodstream from the distal small bowel with the assistance of bile salts and pancreatic juices. The human body has no capacity to produce vitamin K_2 on its own. It is believed the vitamin K present in fecal matter represents unabsorbed or excess K_2.[12]

Gut flora may produce as much as 2 µg of vitamin K_2 per kilogram of body weight per day. Absorption of vitamin K_2 is estimated to provide up to 50% of the total daily vitamin K needs. Once absorbed, vitamin K_2 is transported to the liver where, like K_1, it is metabolized to the active hydroquinone. Metabolism, activity, and excretion of vitamin K_2 does not differ significantly from that of K_1.

CONCEPT REVIEW

Vitamin K_2 is produced by intestinal flora, released into the gut lumen, and absorbed into the bloodstream from the small bowel. Drug therapies that alter gut flora, especially some cephalosporins, can alter availability of vitamin K_2 and lead to clotting disorders. Extended periods of parenteral feeding can produce the same effect.

Metabolism, action, excretion, and signs of deficiency are similar to those of vitamin K_1.

Vitamin K₃

Two forms of vitamin K_3 exist, menadione and menadiol. Although vitamin K_3 (Synkavite) has recently been withdrawn from the U.S. market, it continues to be used in other countries.

Pharmacotherapeutics Vitamin K_3 is useful in treating hypoprothrombinemia caused by many drugs, including salicylates and antibiotics. It is *not* effective in treating hypoprothrombinemia and bleeding associated with warfarin therapy or hepatic failure. Vitamin K_3 does not provide a benefit in the treatment of hereditary hypoprothrombinemia.

Menadiol is useful as a vitamin K supplement in clients with obstructive cholestasis who have impaired absorption of fat-soluble forms of vitamin K. When given intramuscularly or subcutaneously, vitamin K_3 can control hypoprothrombinemic bleeding within 2 hours and return prothrombin levels to normal within 24 hours. Because of the delayed onset on action, transfusion of blood products may be necessary until the bleeding is controlled. If a single dose provides no response, alternate therapy should be used. Large doses of K_3 can cause prolonged prothrombin times, especially in clients with hepatic dysfunction.[3,24]

Mechanism of action Menadione is fat soluble and requires the presence of bile salts for absorption. Menadiol is water soluble and is absorbed in the small intestines without the need for bile salts. Both menadione and menadiol pass directly into the bloodstream.

Although vitamin K_3 is more potent than either K_1 or K_2 on a weight basis, it is slower to act. Based on animal models, it appears menadione and menadiol must be converted to menaquinone to act on the formation of clotting factors. Once converted, vitamin K_3 acts on and is acted on by the body in a manner identical to that for K_1 and K_2.[3,24]

Pharmaceutics Menadiol is a manmade chemical. Determining usual doses of menadiol depends on the severity of the deficiency, the route of administration, and the age of the client. Children usually require 50 to 100 μg/d orally for minor deficient states or 5 to 20 mg/d parenterally for more severe deficiencies. Adult doses range from 5 to 10 mg/d orally to 5 to 30 mg/d by injection.[3] Table 71–5 provides additional information on dosage forms, dosages, and routes of administration.

Undesired clinical responses Vitamin K_3 is associated with a high incidence of severe adverse effects in neonates and premature infants and is not recommended for use in these clients. Sequelae of vitamin K_3 use in neonates include brain damage, hemolytic anemia, kernicterus, hyperbilirubinemia, hemoglobinuria, and death. Because vitamin K_3 can cross the placenta, its administration to pregnant women can lead to adverse effects on the fetus and is contraindicated.[3]

Adverse effects in older children and adults are less severe but deserve consideration. Orally administered vitamin K_3 may cause GI upset and headache. Some clients have hypersensitivity reactions or allergic reactions to K_3. Injectable forms of menadiol contain metabisulfite, which may induce anaphylaxis or asthmatic reactions in clients sensitive to sulfites.[3]

Nursing Considerations for Vitamin K

Vitamin K is monitored indirectly by assessing prothrombin activity and identifying signs and symptoms of deficiency or toxicity. Assess clients regularly for signs of abnormal bleeding; check individuals receiving IV vitamin K frequently for anaphylactic or hypersensitive responses to therapy. Reassess frequently any client with a history of hepatic, biliary, or pancreatic disease who is receiving broad-spectrum antibiotic therapy or who is solely dependent on parenteral nutrition.

Stability of vitamin K in IV solutions has not been determined. Published guidelines have recommended the use of normal saline solution, 5% dextrose in water, or 5% dextrose in normal saline solutions free from preservatives. In the event IV administration of vitamin K is required for a client, consult the most recently published guidelines available or the institutional guidelines for administration to determine the most appropriate method for this client.

Controversy exists about the safety and efficacy of adding vitamins K_1 and K_3 to parenteral nutrition solutions. Although many institutions have guidelines for regular administration of K_1 or K_3 in parenteral nutritional solutions, consistent guidelines are not universal.

Vitamin K–rich foods include green leafy vegetables such as cabbage and spinach. Other food sources include cow's milk, vegetable oils, margarine, egg yolks, tomatoes, muscle meats, and liver. Changes in the diet can profoundly alter the anticoagulant response in clients stabilized by coumarin. Counsel individuals receiving oral anticoagulant therapy about the importance of maintaining stable dietary habits. Tobacco is also high in vitamin K. Advise individuals who wish to start or stop chewing tobacco or using snuff to contact their primary care provider to assess possible changes in their anticoagulant needs.

CONCEPT REVIEW

Menadione is fat soluble, needing bile salts for its absorption. Menadiol is water soluble and is absorbed in the small intestines. Both pass directly into the bloodstream.

Menadiol is a useful treatment agent. It is administered orally or by injection. Menadiol is contraindicated for use in pregnant women, neonates, or premature infants because of severe risk of undesired clinical response. It should be used with caution, especially in injectable form, and cardiac support equipment should be kept in readiness. The latest published guidelines should be consulted before administering the vitamin intravenously.

SUMMARY

Fat-soluble vitamins, A, D, E, and K, are stored in the body; therefore their daily intake is not necessary. Toxicity to some fat-soluble vitamins has been recognized for years. It usually results from megadoses of synthetic vitamins but has been reported in individuals whose diet includes large amounts of fish liver. Processing, storage, and preparation of foods have fewer effects on fat-soluble vitamins than on water-soluble vitamins. In addition, many foods are fortified by the addition of vitamins A and D.

REFERENCES

1. Morton, P.G. (1993). *Health assessment in nursing* (2nd ed.). Springhouse, PA: Springhouse.
2. Doenges, M.E., & Moorhouse, M.F. (1991). *Nurses' pocket guide: Nursing diagnoses with interventions* (3rd ed.). Philadelphia: F.A. Davis.
3. Williams, S.R. (Ed.). (1991). *Nutrition and diet therapy* (9th ed.). St. Louis: Mosby–Year Book.
4. American Hospital Formulary Service (1992). In G.K. McEvoy (Ed.), AHFS Drug Information 92. Bethesda, MD: American Society of Hospital Pharmacists.
5. Linder, M.C. (Ed.). (1991). *Nutritional biochemistry and metabolism: With clinical applications* (2nd ed.). East Norwalk, CT: Appleton & Lange.
6. Sitren, H.S. (1991). Vitamin A. In T.G. Baumgartner (Ed.), *Clinical guide to parenteral micronutrition* (2nd ed.). (pp. 343–368). Available from Lyphomed, Division of Fujisawa, USA.
7. Krinsky, N.I. (1991). Effects of carotenoids in cellular and animal systems. *American Journal of Clinical Nutrition, 53,* 238S–246S.
8. Hathcock, J.N., Hattan, D.G., Jenkins, M.Y., McDonald, J.T., Sundaresan, P.R., & Wilkening, V.L. (1990). Evaluation of vitamin A toxicity. *American Journal of Clinical Nutrition, 52,* 183–202.
9. Flodin, N.W. (1990). Micronutrient supplements: Toxicity and drug interactions. *Progress in Food and Nutrition Science, 14,* 277–331.
10. Mira, M., Stewart, P.M., & Abraham, S.F. (1989). Vitamin and trace element status of women with disordered eating. *American Journal of Clinical Nutrition, 50,* 940–944.
11. Robbins, S.T., & Fletcher, A.B. (1993). Early vs delayed vitamin A supplementation in very-low-birth-weight infants. *Journal of Parenteral and Enteral Nutrition, 17,* 220–225.
12. Underwood, B.A. (1994). Maternal vitamin A status and its importance in infancy and early childhood. *American Journal of Clinical Nutrition, 59* (Suppl.), 5175–5245.
13. Food and Nutrition Board of the National Research Council. (1989). *Recommended dietary allowances* (10th ed.). Washington, D.C.: National Academy Press.
14. Billion-Rey, F., Guillaumont, M., Frederich, A., & Aulagner, G. (1993). Stability of fat-soluble vitamins A (retinol palmitate), E (tocopherol acetate), and K_1 (phylloquinone) in total parenteral nutrition at home. *Journal of Parenteral and Enteral Nutrition, 17,* 56–60.
15. Fawzi, W.W., Herera, M.G., Willett, W.C., Nestal, P., et al. (1994). Dietary vitamin A intake and the risk of mortality among children. *American Journal of Clinical Nutrition, 59,* 401–408.
16. Hirschel-Scholz, S., Siegenthaler, G., & Saurat, J.H. (1989). Ligand-specific and non-specific in vivo modulation of human epidermal cellular retinoic acid binding protein (CRABP). *European Journal of Clinical Investigation, 19,* 220–227.
17. Catado, C., et al. (1992). *Nutrition and diet therapy: Principles and practice* (3rd ed.). St. Paul, MN: West.
18. Chernecky, C.C., Krech, R., & Berger, B. (1993). *Laboratory tests and diagnostic procedures.* Philadelphia: W.B. Saunders.
19. Arria, A.M., Tarter, R.E., Warty, V., & VanThiel, D.H. (1990). Vitamin E deficiency and psychomotor dysfunction in adults with primary biliary cirrhosis. *American Journal of Clinical Nutrition, 52,* 383–390.
20. Sitren, H.S. (1991). Vitamin E. In T.G. Baumgartner (Ed.), *Clinical guide to parenteral micronutrition* (2nd ed.) (pp. 389–408). Available from Lyphomed, Division of Fujisawa, USA.
21. Packer, L. (1991). Protective role of vitamin E in biological systems. *American Journal of Clinical Nutrition, 53,* 1050S–1055S.
22. Sitren, H.S. (1991). Vitamin K. In T.G. Baumgartner (Ed.), *Clinical guide to parenteral micronutrition* (2nd ed.) (pp. 411–427). Available from Lyphomed, Division of Fujisawa, USA.
23. Davis, J., & Sherer, K. (1993). *Applied nutrition and diet therapy for nurses* (2nd ed.). Philadelphia: W.B Saunders.
24. Poleman, C.M., & Peckenpaugh, N.L. (1991). *Nutrition: Essentials and diet therapy* (6th ed.). Philadelphia: W.B. Saunders.

BIBLIOGRAPHY

Baker, D.E., & Campbell, R.K. (1992). Vitamin and mineral supplementation in patients with diabetes mellitus. *Diabetes Educator, 18*(5), 420–427.

Brunier, G. (1994). Calcium/phosphate imbalances, aluminum toxicity, and renal osteodystrophy. *ANNA Journal, 21,* 171–179.

Hunter, D. et al. (1993). A prospective study of the intake of vitamins C, E, and A and the risk of breast cancer. *New England Journal of Medicine, 329,* 234–240.

Specker, B.L. (1994). Do North American women need supplemental vitamin D during pregnancy or lactation? *American Journal of Clinical Nutrition, 59,* 4849–4915.

CHAPTER 72

Water-Soluble Vitamins

PATRICIA UGO • PAMELA MOHLER PICKENS

⊛ **Water-Soluble Vitamins**

LEARNING OBJECTIVES:

Describe the physiologic role of each water-soluble vitamin.

List the signs of deficiency for each water-soluble vitamin.

Identify clients at risk for deficiency of each water-soluble vitamin.

Discuss administrative and toxicity issues for each water-soluble vitamin.

List dietary sources for each water-soluble vitamin.

⊛ **Vitamin C**

LEARNING OBJECTIVES:

List the signs of scurvy.

Discuss the administration of injectable ascorbic acid.

KEY TERM: Scurvy

⊛ **Vitamin B₁: Thiamin**

LEARNING OBJECTIVE: Differentiate between the two forms of thiamin deficiency.

KEY TERM: Beriberi

⊛ **Vitamin B₂: Riboflavin**

LEARNING OBJECTIVE: Discuss therapeutic uses for riboflavin.

KEY TERMS:

Angular stomatitis, cheilosis

⊛ **Vitamin B₃: Niacin, Niacinamide**

LEARNING OBJECTIVES:

Differentiate between nicotinic acid and nicotinamide.

Discuss therapeutic uses for nicotinic acid.

Describe niacin glossitis.

Explain the "three Ds" that characterize pellagra.

KEY TERM: Pellagra

⊛ **Vitamin B₅: Pantothenic acid**

LEARNING OBJECTIVE: Name six common dietary sources of vitamin B₅.

⊛ **Vitamin B₆: Pyridoxine**

LEARNING OBJECTIVES:

List the three naturally existing forms of pyridoxine.

Explain what is meant by *pyridoxine-dependent infant*.

⊛ **Vitamin B₁₂: Cobalamin**

LEARNING OBJECTIVES:

Describe the cause of pernicious anemia.

Clarify what is meant by "tobacco amblyopia."

Explain how differentiating between primary and secondary folate deficiency is relevant to cobalamin deficiency.

KEY TERM: Pernicious anemia

⊛ **Folic Acid**

LEARNING OBJECTIVES:

Discuss the complications that may arise from folate deficiency during pregnancy.

Explain the relationship between zinc and folate and its implications in pregnancy.

List three folate antagonists.

⊛ **Biotin**

LEARNING OBJECTIVES:

Identify diseases that contribute to biotin deficiency.

List four drugs that contribute to biotin deficiency.

⊛ **Bioflavonoids and Other Vitamin-like Substances**

LEARNING OBJECTIVE: Identify vitamin-like substances found in the human body.

KEY TERMS:

Bioflavonoids, carnitine, choline, inositol, *para-aminobenzoic acid*

Water-soluble vitamins (C, B, folic acid, biotin) have relatively small body stores and usually require daily supplementation to maintain adequate body levels. Nevertheless, months or years of deficient intake may occur before the development of deficiency states for some water-soluble vitamins. Because many water-soluble vitamins are heat sensitive, they deteriorate rapidly when exposed to the heat of cooking. Toxic events are less common with water-soluble vitamins because of the body's ease in disposing of excess vitamins through the urine, but overdoses can occur.

VITAMIN C

Vitamin C (ascorbic acid) has a long history of use. The name *ascorbic acid* is derived from the vitamin's ability to reverse the scorbutic symptoms associated with scurvy.

Pharmacotherapeutics Vitamin C is used to treat vitamin deficiency states. Clinical deficiency occurs when plasma levels are less than 0.2 mg/L of plasma. Classic ascorbic acid deficiency is known as **scurvy.** Descriptions of scurvy first appeared in the literature when extended sea journeys became common. The discovery that eating citrus fruits could protect sailors from scurvy inspired the British fleet to carry barrels of limes for its crew and led to the use of the slang term *limey* when referring to a British sailor.

Although fullblown scurvy may take up to 6 months to manifest, early symptoms appear in otherwise healthy individuals after approximately 1 month of deficient intake. Early changes include physical fatigue, weakness, and loss of appetite. As collagen production fails, collagen-dependent structures, including blood vessels and skin, show signs of disruption. Petechial (spot) hemorrhages appear on the extremities, followed by the development of follicular hyperkeratosis ("goose flesh"), especially on the buttocks, thighs, and calves. With continued deficient intake, the gums swell and bleed easily, and bleeding occurs around hair roots. Clients classically are initially seen with Sjögren's, or sicca, syndrome, which includes loose teeth and fillings, hair loss, itchy skin, and dry eyes and mucous membranes. Tissues bruise easily, and minor stresses on joints may lead to bleeding into the joint space. Vasomotor instability, accompanied by pitting edema and psychologic disorders, may develop.[1,2]

Individuals with subclinical ascorbate deficiency have decreased resistance to infection. Ascorbic acid has been implicated in the proper functioning of both cellular and humoral immunity.[3,4] During ascorbic acid deficiency, neutrophil chemotaxis is inhibited, and modulation of cyclic nucleotide levels in B and T cells is altered. Ascorbic acid may also play a role in moderating histamine and prostaglandin release and prostacyclin production. Administration of ascorbic acid in vitamin-deficient clients decreases the incidence of infections, including respiratory tract infections such as colds. There is no definite evidence that administration of ascorbic acid to individuals who are not deficient provides any additional protection from infection.

Ascorbic acid administration improves wound healing in clients who are scorbutic or subclinically deficient. Although many clinicians administer ascorbic acid to nondeficient individuals to improve traumatic and surgical wound healing, there is no scientific evidence that ascorbate in excess of physiologic doses provides any extra benefit in healing.[5]

Deficiency states are more common among individuals with alcoholic or nonalcoholic liver disease, rheumatoid disease, or malignant diseases and among those who smoke. In addition, clients with diabetes mellitus have decreased serum and leukocyte concentrations of ascorbic acid.[6] Individuals with renal failure that requires hemodialysis frequently need ascorbic acid supplements to replace the vitamin removed by the dialysis procedure.[7,8] Table 72–1 summarizes diseases and drugs that contribute to vitamin C deficiency.

Pharmacokinetics Vitamin C exists as either L-ascorbic acid or dehydroascorbic acid; both forms are water soluble. Absorption after oral intake of vitamin C occurs by either passive diffusion or through a sodium-dependent carrier. The percent of absorption decreases with increasing intake and ranges from 20% to 90%. Vitamin C is stored in all tissues, with the highest concentrations in the adrenal and pituitary glands and lower concentrations in the liver, spleen, and brain. Humans have approximately 100 days of storage. After metabolism of vitamin C, it is excreted in the urine. Vitamin C can also be excreted from the kidneys without being metabolized.[9]

Mechanism of action Precise mechanisms of action for ascorbic acid are still under investigation. Ascorbic acid does play a role in several oxidation-reduction pathways in the body. Ascorbic acid or dehydroascorbic acid is necessary for collagen formation, tissue repair, activation of folic acid, cellular respiration, immune function, synthesis of carnitine, fats, and proteins, and metabolism of iron, tyrosine, and carbohydrates.[5]

Ascorbic acid is postulated to play several roles in heme production, including the facilitation of iron absorption from the gut and oxidation of copper and iron for incorporation into heme and heme-producing enzymes. Doses of 200 mg or more of ascorbic acid have been suggested for every 30 mg of elemental iron to be absorbed. The effectiveness of ascorbic acid in this role apparently is improved when the two nutrients are consumed with food.[8]

Pharmaceutics The recommended dietary allowance (RDA) of ascorbic acid for adults is 60 mg. Ascorbic acid is supplied in a variety of oral dosage forms; tablets, timed-release capsules, and syrups. It is also available as sodium ascorbate, a soluble salt, for parenteral use. Parenteral forms are available for intramuscular (IM), intravenous (IV), and subcutaneous (SC) usage. The usual adult dosage for scurvy is 0.3 to 1 g/d.

Undesired clinical responses   Toxic reactions to ascorbic acid are rare, but they have been reported. Doses of 1000 mg or more may cause nausea, vomiting, or heartburn. Some patients report an increased incidence of diarrhea and abdominal cramps. Headaches, sleepiness, fatigue, flushing, and insomnia have also been reported.[8–10]

Contraindications and precautions   Anemia is common in scorbutic patients, probably as a result of decreased iron absorption. Paradoxically, ascorbic acid may interfere with the absorption of copper, which is also important for heme production.

Drug-drug and drug-environment interactions   Ethanol interferes with the absorption of ascorbate from the gut. Vitamin C is sensitive to heat, with metals such as iron and copper acting as catalysts. It is unstable in total parenteral nutritional (TPN) solutions because of the cupric ion and oxygen. Heat increases the rate of oxidative degradation of ascorbic acid, and the inhalation of heated air while smoking is associated with increased breakdown of ascorbate in the blood of the pulmonary capillaries.[9]

Interference with laboratory tests   Ascorbic acid interferes with the results of several clinical tests for the abnormal presence of blood or glucose. Tests that use oxidase enzymes are particularly prone to interference from ascorbic acid, often providing false-negative results. Recent ascorbic acid intake may cause false-negative results from blood and urine glucose tests and urine occult blood tests. Doses greater than 1 g have caused false-negative results in stool occult blood tests.

Life-span considerations   Most healthy individuals have whole blood ascorbic acid levels of 10 to 20 μg/dl. Because the blood level is highly affected by recent intakes of ascorbic acid, measurement of leukocyte vitamin content has been proposed as a more sensitive marker of total body status. Unfortunately, facilities to measure leukocyte levels are not widely available, so whole blood levels are used most commonly.[8,11]

Vitamin requirements are increased during growth and in response to physiologic stress or smoking. Pregnancy and lactation increase the need for ascorbic acid and may precipitate a deficiency state in an individual with marginal intake of the vitamin.[7]

Nursing considerations   Scurvy is uncommon in the United States today, but subclinical or subtle deficiencies may be seen in clients receiving chronic dialysis, cancer clients, smokers, alcoholics, and individuals with chronically poor diets. Monitor clients who have recently stopped consuming high doses of ascorbic acid and newly delivered infants of mothers who consumed high doses during pregnancy closely for signs and symptoms of rebound scurvy, including easy bruising, increased bleeding times, and painful joints. Be certain that the daily dosage of clients who have been taking large doses of ascorbic acid before admission is not suddenly discontinued unless continuing the ascorbic acid is contraindicated during the client's current health crisis.

Oral ascorbic acid is more beneficial when administered in several small doses each day. Oral doses greater than 500 mg are associated with stomach upset when taken on an empty stomach. Doses greater than 1000 mg are associated with nau-

sea and diarrhea. Administering the daily dose in several small doses throughout the day or administering it with meals may alleviate these problems. Administration of ascorbic acid with meals also decreases ascorbate's interference with copper absorption while still assisting in iron absorption. Ascorbic acid for injection can be very irritating to the tissues. Dilute it before its administration as an extended infusion to diminish the incidence of tissue damage.

Elderly individuals are often marginally depleted, possibly because of decreased intake of ascorbic acid–rich fruits and vegetables. Encourage intake of fresh fruits and vegetables (e.g., citrus fruits, strawberries, tomatoes, potatoes, red and green peppers, and dark green leafy vegetables). Fruits in the apple family, including rose hips, provide a good but less concentrated source of ascorbic acid, whereas meats, breads, and dairy products contain much lower amounts.[1,2]

CONCEPT REVIEW

Ascorbic acid (vitamin C) plays a role in oxidation-reduction pathways. It is necessary for activities such as collagen formation, tissue repair, immune function, and heme production.

Severe ascorbic acid deficiency is called *scurvy*. Its symptoms can appear within a month of deficient vitamin C intake. Subclinical deficiency can decrease resistance to infection.

Vitamin C may interfere with absorption of copper (less so when administered with food). It interferes with some clinical tests for the abnormal presence of blood or glucose and with tests using oxidase enzymes. When administered intravenously, it is diluted to prevent tissue damage.

VITAMIN B$_1$: THIAMIN

Vitamin B$_1$, thiamin, is a critical cofactor in energy use in the body. When thiamin is absent, it is impossible for the body to use glucose or the gluconeogenic amino acids as energy sources.

Pharmacotherapeutics   Thiamin is used to treat deficiency states, which may develop rapidly or slowly, depending on the dietary intake of and physiologic demands for thiamin. If thiamin intake is stopped completely, fatal deficiency states can develop in as few as 3 weeks.

Thiamin deficiency is commonly known as beriberi, which means "I can't, I can't." Individuals with chronic beriberi experience profound muscle weakness, which leaves them unable to perform even simple tasks. There are two types of beriberi; the types reflect differences in diet, lifestyle, and speed of onset. *Dry beriberi* is the chronic form of thiamin deficiency. It develops when insufficient thiamin intake is accompanied by decreased caloric intake and decreased physical activity. Dry beriberi is characterized by decreased muscular strength and the onset of peripheral and central neuropathies. The second form of thiamin deficiency, *wet beriberi,* occurs acutely when high intake of alcohol or carbohydrates is associated with low thiamin intake. Wet beriberi is characterized by high-output heart failure with peripheral venous dilation, sodium and water retention leading to edema, and biventricular myocardial failure. It may mimic congestive heart failure (CHF) in some clients. Chronic intake of alcohol with a thiamin-poor diet may manifest as an encephalopathic state known as *Wernicke's syndrome,* which is characterized by loss of memory, disorientation, and confabulation (creating improbable stories to cover losses of memory). Thus alcoholic patients with thiamin deficiency may be seen initially with dry or wet beriberi, with Wernicke's encephalopathy, or with the combined amnesiac and hallucinatory effects of Wernicke-Korsakoff's syndrome. Chronic thiamin undernutrition may also lead to irreversible central nervous system (CNS) lesions.[1,12]

Precipitating factors involved in thiamin deficiency include long-term dialysis, chronic febrile infections, and intake of diets high in raw fish, which contain antithiamin compounds, or nonenriched grain. Other less common precipitating factors include pregnancy, hyperthyroidism, infection, and hepatic disease. These conditions require the intake of increased levels of thiamin. (Table 72–1 summarizes diseases and drugs that contribute to the development of vitamin B_1 deficiency.)

Treatment of thiamin deficiency with thiamin injections can lead to reversal of many of the signs and symptoms within hours. Cardiac function, edema, and peripheral neuropathies respond quickly; CNS symptoms such as psychoses and confusion respond more slowly. CNS involvement may not resolve completely if long-standing deficiency has led to nerve damage.[8]

Pharmacokinetics Thiamin can be absorbed passively in the small intestine at high levels and by an active carrier in the jejunum. The large intestine may also absorb thiamin by passive diffusion. In the intestine thiamin is phosphorylated to thiamin pyrophosphate (TPP) and secreted into the portal blood. Most of the thiamin is stored as TPP; half of the thiamin is stored in muscle. Many thiamin metabolites are excreted in the urine.[9]

Mechanism of action TPP, in combination with magnesium, is a required cofactor for the oxidative decarboxylation of α-keto acids and for transketolase activity in the pentose-phosphate pathway of glucose use. Thus thiamin is required for the use of glucose, fructose, valine, isoleucine, and leucine as energy sources. Thiamin is *not* required for entry of fatty acids into the Krebs' (citric acid) cycle. TPP is the primary active form of thiamin, although thymidine triphosphate (TTP) is required for maintenance of nervous conduction.[9]

Pharmaceutics Thiamin is available in tablets (5 to 500 mg) for oral administration and in parenteral solution (100 to 200 mg/ml) for IM or IV administration. Oral doses ranging from 5 to 30 mg daily, in divided doses, are recommended for 1 month in deficient-nonemergent situations. Emergency treatment requires parenteral doses, with doses up to 100 mg recommended for adults and up to 25 mg for children.[8]

Treatment of metabolic disorders requires client-specific dosage determinations. Although many individuals respond well to daily doses of 10 to 20 mg, some clients may require up to 4 g of thiamin daily in divided doses.[8]

Undesired clinical responses Oral and parenteral doses of up to 500 mg of thiamin have been administered with no untoward effects. Toxic reactions to thiamin are very rare, but they are possible. The most common type is hypersensitivity reactions, including anaphylaxis and circulatory collapse, which usually occur in clients who have received multiple IV doses of the vitamin. Some individuals report gastric upset after receiving large oral doses of thiamin.[8,10]

Contraindications and precautions The only contraindication to thiamin use is a history of sensitivity to it or any ingredient in the oral or parenteral dosage forms.

Drug-drug and drug-environment interactions Drugs that decrease the residency time of food in the gut may decrease thiamin absorption. Diuretic therapy can enhance excretion of thiamin. Chronic phenytoin therapy has also been associated with decreased blood thiamin levels, but the nature and significance of this interaction are unclear.[10]

Thiamin is light sensitive. It should be stored at controlled room temperature. All forms of thiamin are stable at a pH of less than 5.5.

Life-span considerations The amount of thiamin needed daily is related to the activity level and caloric intake of the individual. To ensure adequate thiamin intake to meet metabolic needs plus replace daily urinary losses, most individuals require approximately 0.5 mg of thiamin per 1000 kcal consumed or used. The RDA is a minimum intake of 1 mg/d for all nonpregnant, nonlactating individuals above the age of 7 years and a minimum of 1.5 mg daily during pregnancy and lactation.

Nursing considerations Closely assess individuals, especially if they are alcoholic, who have inadequate nutritional intake for extended periods for signs and symptoms of thiamin deficiency. Monitor carefully new or worsening neurologic symptoms if IV dextrose solutions are used because the administration of calories without thiamin aggravates or brings to the surface preexisting thiamin deficiency.

Elderly individuals have a higher incidence of mildly deficient intake and subclinical deficiency of thiamin. Assess these clients for possible thiamin deficiency when investigating a new onset of mental status changes, edema, or CHF.

Because thiamin is light sensitive and deteriorates if left exposed to light, add it to large-volume IV solution containers immediately before administration to ensure as much of the dose gets to the client as possible. Avoid hanging thiamin-containing solutions in direct sunlight or near bright lights such as phototherapy lamps.

If a client is suspected of being hypersensitive to thiamin, precede IV dosing by a small intradermal test dose. If the intradermal dose elicits a significant local or systemic response, do not institute IV dosing.

Instruct pregnant individuals about the importance of eating a balanced diet, including thiamin-source foods. Good sources of thiamin are enriched or unrefined grain products, nuts, brewer's yeast, organ meats, legumes, and lean cuts of pork. Most pregnant women do not need an oral supplement if they consume adequate calories from a balanced diet.

CONCEPT REVIEW

Thiamin is critical to the body's use of glucose or gluconeogenic amino acids as energy sources. Treatment of deficiencies is usually oral but may require IM or IV doses in life-threatening situations.

The two forms of thiamin deficiency are dry beriberi and wet beriberi. The two forms reflect speed of onset, differences in diet and lifestyle, and signs and symptoms.

Causes of thiamin deficiency vary from excessive alcohol intake to a diet high in raw fish. Although many symptoms may reverse dramatically within hours, CNS effects are slower to resolve and may not resolve completely. Elderly clients should be assessed for thiamin deficiency when there is a new onset of mental status changes, edema, or CHF.

VITAMIN B₂: RIBOFLAVIN

Riboflavin (lactoflavin, vitamin G) is a required component in flavin enzymes in the body. Dietary riboflavin intake is derived from the release of riboflavin from flavin enzymes within the food stuffs.

Pharmacotherapeutics Riboflavin is used primarily to treat or prevent deficient states. Because riboflavin is key in maintaining adequate niacin and pyridoxine activity, deficiency of riboflavin is usually combined with niacin or pyridoxine deficiency, making it difficult to identify signs and symptoms specific to riboflavin deficiency. A common sign of riboflavin deficiency is the development of **angular stomatitis** or **cheilosis**.[7] This breakdown at the corners of the mouth is associated with repeated cracking and healing and may lead to the development of scar tissue. Individuals may also be seen initially with sore throat, hyperemic oral mucosa, glossitis (magenta tongue), normochromic normocytic anemia, or seborrheic dermatitis, usually at the nasolabial folds, scrotum, or vulva. Some clients report itching or burning of the eyes, excessive blinking, tearing, difficulty focusing, visual distortions, and eyestrain; corneal neovascularization, pinkeye, and pupil dilation are sometimes identified on examination.[8,9]

Deficiency states are usually associated with deficient dietary intake, often due to restricted milk intake or diminished absorption from the gut. Metabolic disorders leading to decreased conversion of riboflavin to the flavin enzymes have been reported. Decreased absorption may occur in clients with celiac sprue (gluten-sensitive enteropathy), lactose intolerance, chronic diarrhea, malignancy and resection of the bowel, and hypermotility disorders. Alcoholics are also at increased risk of riboflavin deficiency as part of a general B-vitamin complex deficiency.

Absorption of riboflavin may be decreased by the presence of copper, iron, zinc, nicotinamide, tryptophan, ascorbic acid, caffeine, or sodium saccharin. These food components may form chelates or complexes with riboflavin, decreasing the amount of riboflavin available for absorption. Nevertheless, riboflavin absorption generally is improved when it is taken with food.[11] Table 72–1 summarizes diseases and drugs that contribute to riboflavin deficiency.

Riboflavin has been used with variable success to treat a wide variety of syndromes, including burning feet syndrome, muscle cramps, migraine headaches, acne, and congenital methemoglobinemia. The precise mechanisms for its usefulness in these disorders is unclear and may be derived from the interrelationship of riboflavin with niacin and pyridoxine activity.[8] Riboflavin activity antagonizes and is antagonized by boric acid activity. Riboflavin has been used successfully as adjunctive therapy in the treatment of accidental boric acid ingestion and overdose.

Pharmacokinetics Before absorption, riboflavin must be released from dietary protein by acidic gastric conditions. Once released, it is absorbed by passive and active mechanism; only 25 mg is absorbed daily. There is minimal storage of riboflavin; storage is mainly in the plasma complexed with proteins and intracellularly with flavoprotein complexes. The amount of riboflavin excreted in the urine provides a fairly accurate measure of riboflavin intake.[9]

Mechanism of action As a component of flavin adenine dinucleotide (FAD), riboflavin is a necessary cofactor for the conversion of tryptophan to niacin. As a component of flavin mononucleotide (FMN), riboflavin is a necessary cofactor for the conversion of pyridoxine to its functional form. The FAD and FMN enzymes are also key in oxidative phosphorylation reactions, oxidation of fatty acids and amino acids, and purine degradation. Flavin adenosine dinucleotide is a requisite cofactor for erythrocyte glutathione reductase (E-GR) activity in red blood cells.[9]

Pharmaceutics Riboflavin is available in oral and IV dosage forms. Daily doses for deficiency states range from 5 to 10 mg.

Undesired clinical responses Riboflavin is a relatively nontoxic substance. No known oral overdoses have been identifed, even when it has been taken in large amounts. IV administration of high doses of riboflavin has been linked to photohemolysis in neonates. Other than pain at the injection site, no other adverse effects have been linked to IV riboflavin therapy.[11]

Drug-drug and drug-environment interactions Theophylline and caffeine decrease absorption of riboflavin; other methylxanthines such as theobromine in chocolate may also decrease absorption. Penicillin inhibits the renal excretion of riboflavin; the clinical significance of this interaction is minimal. Probenecid also decreases renal secretion of riboflavin and decreases absorption from the gut. Chlorpromazine decreases conversion of riboflavin to FAD and FMN. The tricyclic antidepressants amitriptyline and imipramine also inhibit metabolism of riboflavin.[11]

Use of oral contraceptive drugs has been associated with increased use of riboflavin. Women with marginal or poor diets are at increased risk for riboflavin deficiency during oral contraceptive therapy and may require supplementation.[8]

Riboflavin is light sensitive; increased exposure to ultraviolet light can cause increased loss of the vitamin. Individuals receiving phototherapy, especially neonates being treated for hyperbilirubinemia, are at increased risk for development of riboflavin deficiency.[11]

Life-span considerations   Normal serum riboflavin levels are poorly defined. Serum levels are greatly influenced by recent riboflavin intake and do not correlate strongly with total body stores. Erythrocyte riboflavin content correlates well with total body stores, with a normal level of 20 µg/dl.[7,11]

Because flavin enzymes play an important role in energy use, recommendations for riboflavin intake are linked to caloric intake. In general, clients require approximately 0.6 mg of riboflavin per 1000 kcal consumed. Increased needs in pregnancy and lactation are related to the increased metabolism of the mother and to the needs of the growing fetus and infant.[7]

Nursing considerations   Riboflavin deficiency as a single entity is rare; most riboflavin-deficient individuals are initially seen with multiple B vitamin deficiencies. Assess clients with lactase deficiency who restrict milk intake for adequacy of riboflavin intake from other dietary sources. Likewise assess individuals with hypermotile GI tracts or diarrhea and counsel them on the need for adequate riboflavin intake. Foods rich in riboflavin include dairy products, meats, including poultry and fish, enriched and fortified grains and bakery products, broccoli, asparagus, turnip greens, and spinach.

Encourage clients requiring oral riboflavin supplements to take them with food to maximize absorption. Supplements should not be taken with coffee, tea, or other caffeinated beverages or with beverages containing saccharin. Because riboflavin is sensitive to light, avoid hanging IV solutions containing riboflavin in direct sunlight or near phototherapy lamps.

CONCEPT REVIEW

Riboflavin is a required element in flavin enzymes in the body. It is necessary for the conversion of tryptophan to niacin and of pyridoxine to its functional form. Riboflavin plays an important role in energy use and may also provide a protective service to the eye.

Deficiency of riboflavin is usually combined with niacin or pyridoxine deficiency or multiple B vitamin deficiencies. Signs of riboflavin deficiency are angular stomatitis and cheilosis. Substances such as theophylline, caffeine, and the theobromine in chocolate can decrease absorption of riboflavin. Malabsorption syndromes and phototherapy may also create deficiencies.

VITAMIN B₃: NIACIN, NICOTINAMIDE

Niacin, also known as *nicotinic acid,* is the chemical precursor of niacinamide, which is also known as *nicotinamide.* These chemicals are not identical in activity. Nicotinic acid has no direct vitamin activity but alters serum cholesterol levels when administered in high doses. Nicotinamide is the active vitamin and has no effect on serum cholesterol levels at any dose.[8]

Nicotinic acid is produced endogenously by metabolism of tryptophan. Approximately 60 mg of tryptophan produces 1 mg of nicotinic acid (one niacin equivalent). This endogenous supply is not sufficient to meet daily needs and must be supplemented with an exogenous (dietary) source.[7]

Pharmacotherapeutics   The primary therapeutic use for niacin is the treatment or prevention of deficient states. Niacin deficiency rarely occurs as a single entity disease. It usually occurs in combination with thiamin, riboflavin, or pyridoxine deficiency. It can be caused by poor intake of niacin or by deficient conversion of tryptophan to niacin. Hartnup disease and carcinoid tumors are associated with decreased conversion of tryptophan to niacin and may be complicated by niacin deficiency.[8]

In rare instances deficiency due to increased niacin use occurs in clients with hyperthyroidism, diabetes mellitus, cirrhosis, pregnancy, or lactation. Individuals with cancer who are under considerable stress may also have increased niacin needs.[8,13]

Birth control pills stimulate conversion of tryptophan to niacin, which may lead to more rapid depletion of endogenous stores. Isoniazid has niacin antagonist activity, and clients should receive a niacin supplement during long-term isoniazid therapy to prevent encephalopathic changes and psychosis due to pellagra.[10] Table 72–1 summarizes some of the diseases and drugs that contribute to niacin deficiency.

Pellagra refers to the complex of niacin deficiency symptoms. Pellagra was originally identified in individuals subsisting on diets dependent primarily on corn. The term *pellagra* (Italian for "skin dry") refers to the skin roughness that occurs during niacin deficiency. Early literature describing this deficiency sometimes referred to it as *"mal de la rosa"* in reference to the rosy hue of the photosensitive skin rash seen with the syndrome. Classic pellagra affects the skin, gastrointestinal (GI) mucosa, and the CNS. It is typified by the three Ds: *d*ermatitis, *d*iarrhea (due to intestinal mucositis), and *d*ementia. If left untreated, pellagra can cause death.[9]

Glossitis is an early sign of niacin deficiency. Classic niacin glossitis is described as a "beefy red," swollen, raw-looking tongue. The tongue may have a scalloped edge, caused by edema pressing the tissues of the tongue against the inner aspects of the teeth.[14]

Nicotinic acid is used to treat other medical problems. Large doses of nicotinic acid have been suggested for use as adjunctive therapy for clients with vertigo, peripheral vascular disease, vascular spasm, Meniere's syndrome, and migraine headaches (when associated with vascular insufficiency). No clear scientific data confirm the usefulness of nicotinic acid in these cases. A wide variety of other uses for nicotinic

TABLE 72–1

Diseases and Drugs That Contribute to Vitamin Deficiencies and Toxicities of Water-Soluble Vitamins

	Diseases		Drugs and Drug Groups	
Vitamin	**Deficiencies**	**Toxicities**	**Deficiencies**	**Toxicities**
C (ascorbic acid)	Alcoholism Cancer Rheumatoid disease Smoking Rebound scurvy Large wounds, burns Achlorhydria Gastrointestinal bleeds Diarrhea Hemodialysis Liver disease		Copper (in total parenteral nutrition [TPN] solutions)	
B₁ (thiamin)	Alcoholism Chronic fever Hyperthyroidism Liver cirrhosis Malabsorption syndrome, including sprue Hemodialysis		Apomorphine Diuretics Laxatives Phenytoin (?)	Penicillin
B₂ (riboflavin)	Alcoholism Hypothyroidism Phototherapy Hypermotility disorders Chronic diarrhea Malabsorption syndromes Celiac sprue Lactose intolerance Stomach or bowel resection		Amitriptyline Boric acid Broad-spectrum antibiotics Caffeine Chloramphenicol Chlorpromazine Imipramine Oral contraceptives Saccharin Theophylline Urea	
B₃ (niacin)	Riboflavin deficiency Thiamin deficiency Pyridoxine deficiency Alcoholism Diabetes mellitus Malignancies Hyperthyroidism Chronic diarrhea Cirrhosis		Isoniazid 5-Fluorouracil 6-Mercaptopurine Oral contraceptives	
B₅ (pantothenic acid)	Alcoholism Ulcerative colitis Granulomatous colitis Liver disease		Estrogen and progesterone combinations	
B₆ (pyridoxine)	Riboflavin deficiency Alcoholism Pregnancy Hypermetabolic states Cancer Asthma Sickle cell anemia Uremia		Cycloserine Hydralazine Isoniazid Levodopa (high dose) Oral contraceptives Penicillamine Phenelzine	
B₁₂ (cobalamin)	Vegetarianism Alcoholism Pregnancy Hyperthyroidism Thyrotoxicosis Increased hematopoiesis Hemolytic anemia Resection of gastric fundus Parietal cell disorders Gastric atrophy Zollinger-Ellison syndrome		Aminoglycosides Anticonvulsants Chloramphenicol Colchicine Ethanol Metformin Neomycin Oral contraceptives *Para*-aminosalicylic acid Potassium chloride (extended release) Vitamin C (high dose)	Prednisone (?)

TABLE 72–1 *Continued*

Diseases and Drugs That Contribute to Vitamin Deficiencies and Toxicities of Water-Soluble Vitamins

Vitamin	Diseases		Drugs and Drug Groups	
	Deficiencies	Toxicities	Deficiencies	Toxicities
B$_{12}$ (cobalamin) *Continued*	Celiac sprue			
	Tropical sprue			
	Crohn's disease			
	Bowel strictures			
	Intestinal resections			
	Bowel cancers			
	Intestinal parasites			
	Liver disease			
	Renal disease			
	Pancreatic disease			
Folic acid	Vitamin C deficiency		Anticonvulsants	
	Vitamin B$_{12}$ deficiency		Arabinoside	
	Alcoholism		L-Asparginase	
	Pregnancy		Azulfidine	
	Chronic exfoliative dermatitis		6-Azauridine	
	Chronic fever		Azathioprine	
	Hyperthyroidism		Barbiturates	
	Increased hematopoiesis		Cholestyramine	
	Chronic hemolytic anemia		Cycloserine	
	Sickle cell anemia		Cytosine	
	Thalassemia		5-Fluorouracil	
	Lymphoproliferative cancers		Glutethimide	
	Intestinal strictures, resection		Hydroxyurea	
	Sprue		6-Mercaptopurine	
	Hemodialysis		Metformin	
	Liver disease		Methotrexate	
			Nitrofurantoin	
			Pentamidine	
			Procarbazine	
			Pyrimethamine	
			Thioguanine	
			Trimethoprim	
			Triamterene	
Biotin	Egg white injury		Carbamazepine	
	TPN therapy		Phenytoin	
	Alcoholism		Primidone	
	Alcoholic fatty liver			
	Cirrhosis			
	Achlorhydria			

acid is under investigation, including as treatment for drug-induced hallucinations, chronic brain syndrome, unipolar depression, hyperkinesis, motion sickness, acne, leprosy, and alcohol dependence.[8]

Pharmacokinetics Nicotinic acid is absorbed passively in the intestine; nicotinamide is not readily absorbed. Storage of niacin occurs in all tissues, but total storage is low. The liver is the primary site of nicotinic acid formation from tryptophan. With a normal intake of niacin, most of the metabolites are excreted in the urine.[9]

Mechanism of action Niacin provides its vitamin activity through the functioning of the nicotinamide-containing cofactors, nicotinamide adenine dinucleotide (NAD) and nicotinamide adenine dinucleotide phosphate (NADP). As NAD, nicotinamide acts with riboflavin-based cofactors in several oxidative enzyme systems. Both NAD and NADP act

as hydrogen carriers for glycogenolysis, tissue respiration, and lipid metabolism.[9]

As previously indicated, the action of nicotinic acid to lower blood cholesterol is independent from the vitamin activity. Similarly, nicotinic acid acts as a vasodilator at pharmacologic doses (>250 mg/d), whereas nicotinamide has no effect on vasodilation. The mechanism by which nicotinic acid affects vascular dilation and cholesterol levels is unknown at this time.[8]

Pharmaceutics Niacin is available as tablets and sustained-release capsules for oral administration. Parenteral solution for IM, IV, and SC administration is also available. Nicotinamide is dispensed in tablets for oral administration and as a parenteral solution. Table 72–2 provides information on dosage forms, dosages, and routes of administration.

When initiating therapy with nicotinic acid, increase the

TABLE 72–2
Niacin: Dosage Forms, Dosages, and Routes of Administration

Dosage Form	Dosage and Route of Administration
NICOTINIC ACID (Nicobid, Nicolar)	*Mild Deficiency* 10–20 mg/d
HOW SUPPLIED Timed-release capsules: 125, 250, 500 mg Scored tablets: 500 mg Elixir: 10 mg/ml SC, IM, or IV injection: 100 mg/ml	*Pellagra* Oral: 125 or 250 mg bid morning and evening or 500 mg once a day, not to exceed 500 mg/d without consulting primary care provider *Hypercholesterolemia* Initial dose: 250 mg after the evening meal; increase q4-7d to 1.5–2 g/d; after 2 mo may increase to 3–4 g/d; do not exceed 6 g/d
NICOTINAMIDE HOW SUPPLIED Tablets: 50–1000 mg Injection: 100 mg/ml	*Pellagra* 150–500 mg/d Not of use in clients with hypercholesterolemia

dosage slowly. For example, increasing the dose on a weekly basis decreases the incidence of undesired responses and allows the body to adapt to the increasing dose.

Undesired clinical responses Although no deaths have been reported from nicotinic acid or nicotinamide overdose, both can cause undesired clinical responses, with nicotinic acid more toxic than nicotinamide. As happens in the deficiency state, adverse reactions to niacin frequently involve the skin, GI tract, and CNS.

Flushing from peripheral vasodilation in face, neck, and chest is the most common undesired response reported. This response is probably mediated by histamine and prostacyclin. Dermatologic reactions include pruritus, dry skin, rash, dry mouth, keratosis nigricans, increased sebaceous gland activity, and burning, stinging, or tingling skin.[8] Figure 72–1 lists common undesired clinical responses associated with niacin.

GI complaints such as nausea, vomiting, heartburn, hunger pains, bloating, flatulence, activation of peptic ulcer disease, and diarrhea also occur. These problems are due, at least in part, to increased GI motility and gastric acid secretion stimulated by the histamine released by the nicotinic acid administration. Effects on the CNS include dizziness, syncope, blurred vision, transient headache, toxic amblyopia, proptosis, nervousness, and panic. Other effects include loss of central vision as a result of macular edema, hypotension, decreased glucose tolerance, glycosuria, increased uric acid levels, and increased liver function test results.[10]

Adverse effects from nicotinic acid are generally dose related and subside with a decrease in the dose. Most clients develop a tolerance as therapy continues. Tolerance may develop in a few days to 2 weeks. Some individuals remain intolerant at any dose or develop intolerance only after extended therapy. Use of 325 mg of aspirin concurrently with nicotinic acid controls the flushing, probably through inhibition of prostaglandin synthesis.[8]

Contraindications and precautions Niacin use is contraindicated in individuals with known idiosyncrasy to niacin, hepatic dysfunction, or active peptic ulcer.

Drug-drug and drug-environment interactions Antihypertensive drugs may have an additive vasodilating effect to

that of niacin and produce postural hypotension. Diabetic or potential diabetic clients should be observed for decreased glucose tolerance.[15]

Niacin is heat stable and is not significantly lost during the cooking process.

Life-span considerations Use of therapeutic niacin during pregnancy and lactation or in women of child-bearing age requires that the benefits be weighed against the potential hazards to mother and child. Insufficient data are available about usage in children.[15]

Nursing considerations Nicotinic acid doses greater than 2 g are associated with peripheral vasodilation, which may be very uncomfortable for the client. Counsel clients that their body will adjust within the first 2 weeks of therapy. Discourage clients from increasing the dose of nicotinic acid above 3 g unless directed to do so by their primary care provider. Monitor individuals receiving doses greater than 3 g daily for signs and symptoms of arrhythmias and GI problems.

Dietary niacin is available from yeast, meats, cereals, milk, eggs, and green vegetables. Note that most of the natural niacin in grain products is bound into nonabsorbable molecules. Most processed grain products in the United States are enriched with absorbable synthetic niacin.

CONCEPT REVIEW

Niacin, or nicotinic acid, has no direct vitamin activity but alters serum cholesterol levels and acts as a vasodilator when administered in high doses. Niacin provides its vitamin activity through the nicotinamide-containing NAD and NADP.

The complex of niacin deficiency symptoms is called *pellagra* and is typified by dermatitis, diarrhea, and dementia. Glossitis is an early sign of niacin deficiency. Toxic doses affect the skin, GI tract, and CNS. In correcting the deficiency, start with a low dose and titrate the dose upward on a weekly basis.

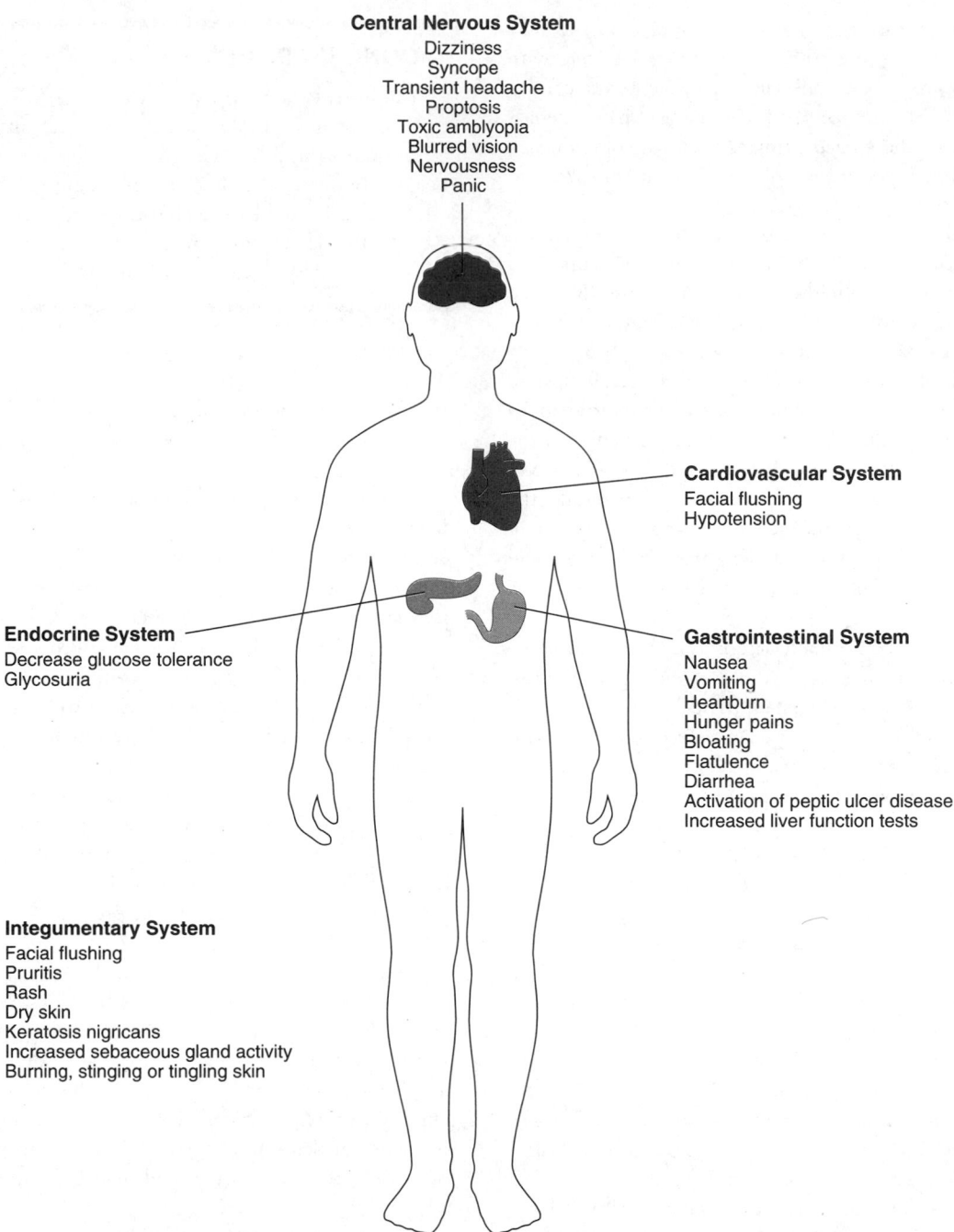

Central Nervous System
Dizziness
Syncope
Transient headache
Proptosis
Toxic amblyopia
Blurred vision
Nervousness
Panic

Cardiovascular System
Facial flushing
Hypotension

Endocrine System
Decrease glucose tolerance
Glycosuria

Gastrointestinal System
Nausea
Vomiting
Heartburn
Hunger pains
Bloating
Flatulence
Diarrhea
Activation of peptic ulcer disease
Increased liver function tests

Integumentary System
Facial flushing
Pruritis
Rash
Dry skin
Keratosis nigricans
Increased sebaceous gland activity
Burning, stinging or tingling skin

FIGURE 72–1   Common undesired clinical responses associated with niacin.

VITAMIN B₅: PANTOTHENIC ACID

Vitamin B₅, pantothenic acid, is present in plant and animal tissues as a component of coenzyme A (CoA). It is primarily as CoA that pantothenate is absorbed, with a bioavailability of approximately 50%. The gut microflora does produce some pantothenate, but it is unknown if any of this pantothenate is absorbed or whether it plays a significant role in pantothenate homeostasis.[11]

Pharmacotherapeutics   Therapeutic pantothenic acid is used to treat vitamin B₅ deficiencies. Pantothenate deficiency is associated with urinary excretion of less than 1 mg of pan-

tothenate per day. It is extremely uncommon as a single-entity deficiency and usually occurs in combination with other B vitamin deficiencies. Pantothenate deficiency is characterized by the "burning feet" syndrome, which features numbness, tingling, and burning of the feet and hands. Other signs and symptoms of the syndrome include vomiting, malaise, fatigue, insomnia, abdominal distress, burning cramps, very rapid heartbeat on exertion, anorexia, constipation, hyperactive deep tendon reflexes, somnolence, increased susceptibility to infections, and glossitis.[11]

Individuals with ulcerative or granulomatous colitis may

have decreased pantothenate absorption, and diabetics may have increased urinary excretion.[11] Few drugs interfere with pantothenate homeostasis. Estrogen and progesterone combinations such as oral contraceptives may increase pantothenate requirements, but the data on this subject are controversial. Table 71–1 summarizes diseases and drugs that contribute to pantothenate deficiency.

Pharmacokinetics Absorption of pantothenate is almost complete at normal intakes. After absorption, it is transported from the intestine through the portal vein. Most (80%) of pantothenic acid is stored as CoA, with the highest levels in the liver. Pantothenate is excreted in the urine.[9]

Mechanism of action As CoA or acyl carrier protein (ACP), pantothenate is a necessary cofactor for more than 70 different enzymes in the body. As CoA, pantothenate is the ACP for energy extraction from glucose and fats, cholesterol synthesis, heme synthesis, amine acetylation (including the synthesis of acetylcholine from choline), and acetylation of some drugs. As ACP, pantothenate is a part of the fatty acid synthase enzyme complex, which synthesizes fatty acids in the cytosol.[9,11]

Pharmaceutics Pantothenic acid is available in single-ingredient tablets and in many multivitamin preparations. Therapeutic dosages range from 10 to 100 mg/d.

Undesired clinical responses Adverse reactions to pantothenate are very rare. Some cases of diarrhea and water retention have been reported by individuals taking large doses. Intake of more than 250 mg/d has been associated with increased risk of generalized dermatitis, itching, tingling, difficulty breathing, urticaria, and erythema. The precise mechanism of these toxic effects has not been explained.[10,11]

Drug-drug and drug-environment interactions Pantothenate may prolong the effects of succinylcholine when given in large doses.[8] It is water soluble and labile to acid, alkali, and heat.

Life-span considerations Typical daily intake of pantothenate in the American adult diet is 10 to 20 mg. The recommended safe and effective dose for infants is 2 to 3 mg/d. For children the recommended dose is 3 to 5 mg/d; individuals more than 10 years old require 4 to 7 mg/d.[7]

Nursing considerations Assess all clients with a documented B vitamin deficiency for pantothenate status. Assess all individuals with pantothenate deficiency for deficiencies in other B vitamins. Although many of the signs and symptoms of pantothenate deficiency are nonspecific, complaints of tingling or burning feet unrelieved by elevation of extremities and rest provide a specific indication of a probable need for pantothenate supplementation.

Pantothenate is found in a wide variety of foodstuffs. Egg yolk, kidney, liver, and yeast are excellent pantothenate sources. Broccoli, lean beef, skimmed milk, sweet potatoes, and molasses are also good sources, although they are not as rich in CoA content.

VITAMIN B₆: PYRIDOXINE

Another of the B vitamins, vitamin B_6, exists naturally in three chemical forms: pyridoxine phosphate, pyridoxal phosphate

CONCEPT REVIEW

Pantothenic acid, a component of CoA, is a necessary cofactor for more than 70 different enzymes in the body. Pantothenate deficiency, usually occurring in combination with other B vitamin deficiencies, is characterized by the "burning feet" syndrome, along with GI symptoms, rapid heart-beat during exertion, hyperactive deep tendon reflexes, and glossitis.

(PLP), and pyridoxamine phosphate. All three forms are equally potent and function via the same mechanisms within the body.

Pharmacotherapeutics Because pyridoxine is intricately involved with the metabolism and use of so many other nutrients, its deficiency rarely occurs as a single entity. Clients in mild deficiency states may be seen initially with irritability, depression, or nervousness. Peripheral neuropathies may also develop in the early stages of deficiency. Progression of the deficiency may lead to the development of seizures as γ-aminobutyric acid (GABA) neurotransmitter production in the brain falls. Pyridoxine deficiency is also accompanied by a seborrheic skin rash and anemia.[8]

Genetic pyridoxine deficiency, causing rapid urinary excretion of pyridoxic acid, leads to epileptiform seizure activity in some newborn infants. Although the exact cause is unclear, many of these infants are delivered to mothers who received high doses of pyridoxine during pregnancy. The infants are termed *pyridoxine-dependent infants*.[16]

Certain disease states can contribute to pyridoxine deficiency. For example, hypermetabolic states, high fat intake, and high protein intake temporarily increase pyridoxine use. Cancers, asthma, sickle cell anemia, and some liver disorders also cause pyridoxine deficiency. Clients with uremia or chronic alcoholism are frequently deficient in body stores. The incidence of deficiency increases with age, in part because of decreased plasma binding and increased urinary losses of PLP.[16]

The drugs isoniazid, penicillamine, hydralazine, cycloserine, and phenelzine inhibit pyridoxine activity. Therapy with most of these drugs invariably leads to the development of pyridoxine deficiency, and vitamin supplementation during therapy is recommended.[8] Estrogen therapy decreases serum pyridoxine levels and may contribute to the development of deficiency states. Bowel-sterilizing antibiotic therapy may trigger a deficiency state in a client with borderline intake because of the loss of pyridoxine production by gut microflora and decreased pyridoxine absorption. Table 72–1 summarizes diseases and drugs that contribute to pyridoxine deficiency.

Pyridoxine has been used in the treatment of emesis of pregnancy to decrease nausea and vomiting. Similarly, pyridoxine is undergoing study as a possible treatment for premenstrual syndrome, postpartum depression, and depression associated with estrogen therapy.[8] Pyridoxine administration is also a useful adjunct in treating isoniazid, hydralazine, and cycloserine toxicities, especially in overdose situations. Although no scientific data exist to verify its effectiveness, pyridoxine use has been recommended for the treatment of such diverse health problems as acne, radiation sickness, motion sickness, vertigo, hyperkinesis, absence seizures, and tardive dyskinesia.[8]

Pharmacokinetics   After oral administration, pyridoxine is absorbed via passive diffusion. Pyridoxine is transported as a free vitamin bound to albumin. It is converted to pyridoxal in the liver. After pyridoxal is formed, it is phosphorylated by pyridoxal kinase to PLP. Most of the body's store of vitamin B_6 is as PLP. Excretion of the vitamin occurs through the urine as pyridoxic acid.[9]

Mechanism of action   Pyridoxine is a cofactor in more than 50 different enzyme systems in the body. It is a key cofactor in the production of all known CNS neurotransmitters and is necessary for the formation of nicotinic acid from tryptophan. Vitamin B_6 plays a role in the decarboxylation and transanimation of amino acids and in the transfer of sulfur to serine from methionine to form cysteine. It is necessary for the production of porphyrin, a necessary component of heme. In addition to contributing to the metabolism of amino acids, pyridoxine helps transport amino acids from the intestines into the bloodstream.[9,16] Pyridoxine is a cofactor for lipid metabolism and for glycogen phosphorylase activity. It plays an active role in maintaining immune function and in endocrine metabolism and is necessary for the formation of sphingolipid, a component of nerve myelin sheaths.

Pregnancy is associated with increased excretion of tryptophan metabolites, reflecting increased or altered tryptophan use. Supplemental pyridoxine returns the excretion pattern to normal, suggesting increased pyridoxine activity during pregnancy.

Pharmaceutics   The drug preparation pyridoxine hydrochloride is available in solution for IM or IV administration and in tablets for oral administration.

In cases of dietary deficiency, the dosage is 10 to 20 mg/d for 3 weeks. To prevent drug-induced pyridoxine deficiency and decrease the risk of drug toxicity, daily doses of 10 to 50 mg of pyridoxine are recommended for individuals receiving isoniazid or penicillamine. Clients receiving cycloserine therapy benefit from daily pyridoxine intake of 100 to 300 mg administered in divided doses.[8,16]

Therapeutic dosages of 2 to 60 mg/d may be useful for clients with carpal tunnel syndrome and preeclampsia. Daily doses of 100 mg or more are used to control emesis associated with pregnancy.[9] If pyridoxine-dependent infants are unresponsive to traditional anticonvulsant therapy, the seizures are often effectively controlled with daily administration of 2 to 30 mg of pyridoxine.[8,16]

Undesired clinical responses   Pyridoxine toxicity is associated with widespread nonspecific axonal degeneration. Doses greater than 2 g/d may lead to neurotoxicities, particularly of peripheral sensory neurons. Difficulty walking, decreased vibratory sense, and decreased proprioception (ability to locate one's extremities in space) frequently develop. The senses of temperature, touch, and pain are usually less affected. Deep tendon reflexes may be diminished without altered CNS function. Although the CNS is well protected from excessive levels

of pyridoxine by the blood-brain barrier, some cases of convulsions after high pyridoxine doses have been reported.[8]

Contraindications and precautions   Therapeutic pyridoxine use is contraindicated in an individual with a history of sensitivity to pyridoxine.

Drug-drug and drug-environment interactions   Pyridoxine supplements should not be administered to clients receiving levodopa because pyridoxine antagonizes the action of levodopa. Pyridoxine may be administered concurrently in clients receiving preparations containing both levodopa and carbidopa.[15] Pyridoxine hydrochloride should be protected from exposure to light.

Life-span considerations   Total body stores of pyridoxine in adults range from 16 to 25 mg. Plasma PLP levels are considered the best indicator of pyridoxine status. Reported mean plasma PLP levels are 38 to 68 pmol/ml for nonpregnant women and 50 to 60 pmol/ml for men. In general, plasma PLP levels of 50 pmol/ml or above are considered normal.

Because pyridoxine use rises and falls in parallel to amino acid intake and use, many clinicians recommend administering 0.02 mg of pyridoxine for each gram of protein consumed. If the client is pregnant or lactating, an additional 0.5 to 0.6 mg should be consumed daily.

The long-term effects of high-dose pyridoxine (>100 mg/d) use in pregnancy are not known, although short-term therapy appears safe. Some clinicians have suggested a link between fetal exposure to high pyridoxine levels and the development of pyridoxine dependency. High blood pyridoxine levels inhibit lactation in breast-feeding women.[8]

Nursing considerations   Closely monitor clients receiving drug therapies that inhibit pyridoxine activity. Since pyridoxine is toxic at high doses, monitor individuals with high daily intakes carefully for neurotoxicity, especially ataxia and decreased proprioception.

CONCEPT REVIEW

Vitamin B_6 (pyridoxine) is a cofactor in more than 50 enzyme systems in the body and is key in the production of all known CNS neurotransmitters. This vitamin is necessary for formation of nicotinic acid from tryptophan and for the production of porphyrin. Pyridoxine also transports amino acids from the intestines into the bloodstream. It is active in maintaining immune function and in endocrine metabolism.

No specific deficiency state for pyridoxine has been identified. Mild deficiency may be evidenced by seborrheic skin rash, irritability, depression, nervousness, and, in the early stages, peripheral neuropathies. Toxicity is associated with widespread axonal degeneration. Deficiency may exist in infants whose mothers took high doses of pyridoxine prenatally.

Pyridoxine hydrochloride is the drug preparation. It is used in treating emesis of pregnancy, premenstrual syndrome, postpartum depression, and depression associated with estrogen therapy. It is also a useful adjunct with isoniazid, penicillamine, or cycloserine therapy, which deplete the vitamin.

VITAMIN B₁₂: COBALAMIN

Vitamin B_{12}, cobalamin, belongs to a group of related chemicals known as **corroids,** which must contain the trace element cobalt to be active. Cyanocobalamin and hydroxocobalamin are synthetic forms of natural cobalamin.

Pharmacotherapeutics Vitamin B_{12} preparations are used to prevent or treat deficiency states. Individuals at risk of deficiency are those with poor intake, altered gut pH, decreased production of salivary R binder, and decreased production of the intrinsic factor (IF). In addition, pathologies that increase metabolism or excretion of cobalamin or alter use of the vitamin can contribute to a deficiency state. Several drugs cause or contribute to cobalamin deficiency. Chloramphenicol, which suppresses the bone marrow, interferes with cobalamin-induced hematopoiesis. Colchicine, neomycin, aminoglycosides, extended-release potassium chloride products, aminosalicylic acid, anticonvulsants, and possibly oral contraceptives interfere with binding or absorption of cobalamin. In addition, excessive and extended alcohol consumption interferes with intrinsic factor production. Cobalt irradiation of the small bowel decreases the absorptive capability of the tissue.[8] Table 71–1 summarizes diseases and drugs that contribute to cobalamin deficiency.

The classic cobalamin deficiency state is known as **pernicious anemia.** Pernicious anemia is characterized by a megaloblastic, macrocytic anemia; it is due to impaired DNA synthesis in the erythrocyte. Pernicious anemia often is accompanied by GI lesions, which often manifest as constipation. In the mild state of deficiency, bilateral paresthesia of the fingers and feet develops. Caused by demyelination of neurons, this paresthesia is associated with disturbances in proprioception and vibratory sense. As the deficiency progresses, spastic ataxia develops, caused by subacute combined degeneration of the spinal cord. In rare cases cobalamin-deficient heavy smokers may suffer "tobacco amblyopia" as the optic nerve becomes involved, impairing vision and causing scotomata and occasionally blindness.[8,16]

Treatment of cobalamin deficiency leads to a rapid reversal of the anemia and GI lesions, but any neurologic damage resolves slowly. In cases of chronic deficiency, the client may not fully recover from neurologic damage. Repeated incidents of deficiency increase the risk of permanent neurologic damage. If the cause of the deficiency is not corrected, a relapse may occur as rapidly as 2 years and as long as 10 years after resolution of the original insult. For this reason, most clinicians recommend regular monthly injections for the balance of the client's life span.[8]

A secondary functional folate deficiency may develop during cobalamin deficiency. Primary versus secondary folate deficiency must be differentiated since the administration of folic acid to a client with secondary folate deficiency masks cobalamin-deficient pernicious anemia but allows neurologic toxicity to progress.[8]

Cobalamin also has limited use in nondeficient states. Cobalamin-containing cofactors convert methylmalonate to succinate and homocystine to methionine. Because of this role in methylmalonate metabolism, large doses of cobalamin sometimes are used in the treatment of methylmalonic aciduria, an inborn error of metabolism.[8,16]

Pharmacokinetics Nutritional vitamin B_{12} is absorbed passively from the GI tract. In the GI tract it binds with IF. This complex of vitamin and IF binds to receptors in the ileum and is taken into the cell. From the intestinal cells, vitamin B_{12} is transported to other tissues bound to a protein. Storage of vitamin B_{12} occurs mostly in the liver. The storage of vitamin B_{12} is sufficient to last for 3 to 6 years. Unmetabolized vitamin B_{12} is excreted primarily via the bile.[9]

Mechanism of action Cobalamin is a required cofactor in fat and carbohydrate metabolism and in protein synthesis, including the synthesis of myelin and nucleoproteins. It plays an important role in cell reproduction and must be present to support cell division in rapid-turnover tissues such as the gut mucosa. Cobalamin is necessary for the activation of folic acid and plays a role in controlling hematopoiesis. As adenosylcobalamin, the vitamin is active in propionic acid metabolism. As methylcobalamin, it is necessary for the synthesis of succinyl-CoA.[15,16]

Pharmaceutics Vitamin B_{12} is available in oral and parenteral dosage forms. For a nutritional deficiency, 0.05 mg IM weekly for 2 weeks followed by 1 μg/d orally is recommended. For deficiency caused by impaired absorption, 100 μg IM monthly or at least every 3 months is recommended. For many clients with pernicious anemia, oral doses of vitamin B_{12} of 1000 μg/d eliminate the need for IM injections and are effective.[9,17,18]

Undesired clinical responses Cobalamin toxicity is very rare, but it can occur. At high doses, cobalamin can cause mild transient diarrhea, peripheral vascular thrombosis after injection, itching, transitory exanthema, urticaria, feeling of swelling of the entire body, anaphylaxis, and death. Allergic reactions, especially anaphylaxis, are extremely rare. Allergenic responses are most likely to occur with injection of the synthetic cobalamins, **cyanocobalamin** and **hydroxocobalamin.**[8,9]

Adverse responses to physiologic doses may also occur. Increased blood volume resulting from stimulation of hematopoiesis has contributed to pulmonary edema and CHF in a few clients. Clients with megaloblastic anemia who are treated with cobalamin may manifest depletion of serum potassium content because hematopoiesis incorporates the potassium into new erythrocytes. Cobalamin administration has unmasked previously undiagnosed polycythemia vera in some individuals. Additionally, cobalamin therapy may trigger gout attacks in susceptible individuals because of increased nucleic acid turnover.[8]

Contraindications and precautions Synthetic cobalamin should not be used in individuals with known hypersensitivity to the preparations.

Drug-drug and drug-environment interactions Parenteral solutions of cyanocobalamin and hydroxocobalamin should be protected from light and stored at a controlled room temperature. Clients who have intact gastric fundi may have increased absorption of cobalamin when taking prednisone. This result is believed due to steroid-induced increases in intrinsic factor release.[8,15]

Life-span considerations Because of the efficiency of the biliary cycling of cobalamin, very little daily intake is needed. Most individuals easily meet their cobalamin needs with their diet.

Nursing considerations Evaluate both folic acid status and cobalamin status when assessing an individual. Monitor hematologic parameters, including reticulocyte count and hemoglobin and hematocrit levels, to confirm appropriate response to therapy. Monitor individuals with megaloblastic anemia who have a poor dietary intake or a history of CHF carefully for the first week of replacement therapy. Return of hematopoiesis may trigger fatal hypokalemia or CHF. Because the risk of neurologic damage increases with each return to the deficiency state, counsel clients who are receiving treatment for pernicious anemia about the importance of regular monthly maintenance injections for the balance of their life span.

Liver, kidney, fish, and shellfish, muscle meat, and dairy foods are the best dietary sources of cobalamin. Only very minute amounts are found in plants. Cobalamin from a purely vegetarian diet is insufficient to maintain body cobalamin stores. Strongly encourage vegetarians to obtain cobalamin supplementation.

CONCEPT REVIEW

Vitamin B_{12} (cobalamin) is a required cofactor in fat and carbohydrate metabolism and in protein synthesis. It is important in cell reproduction and division and for activation of folic acid.

Vitamin B_{12} requirements are easily met except in alcoholics or clients following strict vegetarian diets lacking in milk, eggs, fish, and poultry. Supplementation is recommended for these clients. Vitamin B_{12} is administered orally and IM.

The classic cobalamin deficiency state is pernicious anemia, which may be accompanied by GI lesions and CNS symptoms. The anemia and GI symptoms resolve quickly with treatment, but the CNS symptoms may resolve slowly or incompletely. Relapse may occur, so lifelong therapy is recommended.

Secondary functional folate deficiency may develop during cobalamin deficiency and must be correctly identified. Treatment of secondary folate deficiency may mask cobalamin deficient pernicious anemia and allow CNS toxicity to progress. Conversely, cobalamin administration may partially mask folate-deficient anemia.

FOLIC ACID

Most of the folic acid found in foods is in the form of folate polyglutamates. Folic acid is heat sensitive and light sensitive when dissolved in water.

Total body stores of folate are 5 to 12 mg. Concentrations in various body tissues range widely. Normal serum concentrations are 0.005 to 0.015 µg/ml of blood serum. Concentrations within erythrocytes normally range from 0.175 to 0.316 µg/ml of cells. Cerebral spinal fluid concentrations normally range from 0.016 to 0.021 µg/ml of fluid. This concentration is higher than serum concentrations but lower than erythrocyte concentrations.[7,8,16]

Pharmacotherapeutics Therapeutic folic acid is used to treat or prevent deficiency states. Deficiency states are commonly associated with serum concentrations of less than 0.002 µg/ml. Lack of folate intake for 4 to 5 months generally is required before deficiency symptoms present. Deficiency may occur because of decreased intake, decreased absorption, increased metabolism, or increased excretion. In the case of chronic alcoholism, the combination of poor intake and decreased absorption with altered metabolism produces deficiency. Anticonvulsant drugs such as phenytoin, barbiturates, and phenobarbital have been implicated in decreased folate absorption. Primidone, oral contraceptives, nitrofurantoin, and sulfasalazine have been identified as agents that increase metabolic inactivation of folate in the liver.[8]

Zinc deficiency may also lead to decreased absorption of folic acid. Conversely, alternate coadministration of high doses of folic acid and zinc may lead to decreased absorption of zinc.[10] Some researchers, noting a relationship between folic acid supplementation and low serum zinc levels with increased incidence of fetal distress in pregnancy, suggest that pregnant women taking folate supplements should consider zinc supplementation.

Folate deficiency can manifest as a secondary complication of cobalamin deficiency because of the lack of cobalamin cofactor for tetrahydrofolic acid synthesis. Folate deficiency frequently appears as a complicating factor in clients with scurvy because ascorbic acid deficiency decreases the body's ability to retain folates.[10]

Increased use without concomitant increases in intake can lead to deficiency states. Common causes of increased use include periods of rapid cell division such as during pregnancy, with cancers, during rapid growth, and with increased hematopoiesis and in clients with chronic hemolytic anemia. Hypermetabolic states such as chronic fever and hyperparathyroidism have also been linked with increased folate use.[16]

Deficiency states due to increased loss have been associated with renal dialysis, liver disease, and chronic exfoliative dermatitis. Poisons such as arsenic and benzene also can contribute to folate deficiency. Riboflavin increases the rate of degradation of folic acid in IV solutions, especially when exposed to ultraviolet light.

Many drugs act as folate antagonists. Methotrexate, pyrimethamine, and trimethoprim are folate antagonists that prevent the formation of tetrahydrofolate within the cell. When these drugs are used in high doses or for prolonged periods of time, folate deficiency may develop. Purine antagonists (e.g., 6-mercaptopurine, thioguanine, and azathioprine) and pyrimidine antagonists (e.g., 5-fluorouracil and 6-azidouridine) may also precipitate folate deficiency symptoms by interfering with folate-mediated DNA synthesis. Metformin, cytosine arabinoside, hydroxyurea, procarbazine, L-asparginase, triamterene, pentamidine, glutethimide, cholestyramine, and sulfasalazine also have been implicated in interfering with folate activity. Isoniazid and cycloserine impair folate activity through the same pathways, and the combined use of these two drugs leads to the rapid development of folate deficiency.[1,8] Table 72–1 summarizes drugs and diseases that contribute to folic acid deficiency.

In some individuals large doses of folate reverse the mucosal deficit caused by tropical sprue. The precise mechanism of this mucosa-sparing response is unclear but may reflect a reversal of disease-induced inhibition of cell division or a repair of disease-altered host DNA.[8]

Pharmacokinetics   The ileum is the primary site of passive and facilitated absorption of oral folic acid. The amount of folic acid stored by humans is 2 to 10 mg, lasting from 3 to 6 months with no intake. Approximately half of the stored amount is in the liver as polyglutamates. Folic acid is excreted mainly in the bile, with 0.1 mg/d reabsorbed. The amount excreted is increased in clients with liver disease. It is also excreted in the urine as a metabolite.[9]

Mechanism of action   Folate is metabolically active as tetrahydrofolic acid. In this form folate is a cofactor for 1-carbon transfers in the synthesis of amino acids, purines, and thymidylates and for the methylation of transfer RNA. It is necessary for nucleic acid synthesis and cell division. Tetrahydrofolic acid is a cofactor in amino acid transamination (e.g., in the conversion of histidine to glutamic acid) and in the interconversion of serine and glycine and the conversion of homocystine to methionine. Folate is also required for the generation of formate.[7,8,16]

Pharmaceutics   Daily dose requirements vary with age and metabolic activity. Recommended oral and parenteral doses are listed in Table 72–3. Clients receiving anticonvulsant therapy who have chronic hemolytic anemia, chronic infections, or chronic alcohol consumption may require additional folic acid supplementation to prevent the occurrence of deficiency.[7,8]

Undesired clinical responses   Allergic responses to folate administration are rare but have been documented. The most common manifestations of folate allergy are erythema, rash, itching, and general malaise. Less commonly, bronchospasms occur.[8]

In rare cases folate doses greater than 15 mg/d for longer than 1 month are associated with GI and CNS changes. Complaints include anorexia, nausea, abdominal distention, flatulence, bad or bitter taste, altered sleep patterns, difficulty concentrating, irritability, overactivity, excitement, mental depression, confusion, and impaired judgment. Prolonged folic acid supplementation may lead to decreased serum cobalamin levels and may mask the hematologic manifestations of cobalamin deficiency.[8,10]

TABLE 72–3
Recommended Dosages of Folic Acid

Client	Oral Dose	Intravenous Dose
Infant		14 μg/kg/d
<6 mo	25 μg/d	Maximum: 140 μg/d
6–12 mo	35 μg/d	
Child		140 μg/d
1–3 y	50 μg/d	
4–10 y	75–100 μg/d	
Male		400 μg/d
11–14 y	150 μg/d	
>15 y	200 μg/d	
Female		400 μg/d
11–14 y	150 μg/d	
>15 y	180 μg/d	
Pregnant	400 μg/d	
Lactating	280 μg/d	

Contraindications and precautions   Therapeutic use of folic acid is contraindicated in individuals with known hypersensitivity to the vitamin or drug preparation.

Drug-drug and drug-environment interactions   Antibiotics, particularly tetracyclines, may cause falsely low serum folate levels when a microbiologic assay technique is used.

Large doses of folate stimulate seizure activity in some individuals whose seizure disorders are under control by phenytoin. This is due to a decrease in serum phenytoin levels caused by a folate-induced increase in phenytoin metabolism.[7,8]

Life-span considerations   Folate deficiency during pregnancy, particularly at the time of conception, is linked to an increased risk of fetal neural tube defects, particularly spina bifida and anencephaly. The Center for Disease Control and Prevention (CDC) has estimated that the incidence of neural tube defects in the United States would decrease by 99% if all fertile women maintained daily intakes of folic acid of 0.8 to 1 mg. Paternal folic acid levels at the time of conception may also contribute to the risk for defects, but sufficient epidemiologic evidence is not yet available to allow the CDC to develop similar recommendations for men.[1]

Nursing considerations   Because of the long-term neurologic damage that can occur when cobalamin deficiency is inadvertently masked by the use of a folate supplement, all individuals suspected of being folate deficient must be assessed for cobalamin deficiency also. Similarly, regularly assess anyone receiving long-term folate supplementation for a new onset of cobalamin deficiency. This is particularly important in pregnant women since cobalamin deficiency can result in both fetal and maternal complications.

Closely monitor clients with seizures who are stabilized by use of phenytoin therapy if folate supplementation is begun. Monitor serum phenytoin levels and adjust doses to maintain a seizure-free state.

Counsel all fertile women, regardless of sexual activity or contraceptive use, about the risks for fetal defects associated with folate deficiency. Encourage women who do not have adequate dietary intake to supplement their folate up to 1 mg daily. Dietary folate intake can be increased by consuming a diet rich in liver, kidneys, yeast, mushrooms, green leafy vegetables, whole grains, legumes, oranges, and bananas.

CONCEPT REVIEW

Folate is metabolically active as tetrahydrofolic acid. It is necessary for nucleic acid synthesis, cell division, and generation of formate.

Folate deficiency is associated with megaloblastic, macrocytic anemias and malabsorption syndromes. Deficiency at conception is connected to spina bifida and anencephaly in the neonate.

Zinc and folic acid may interfere with each other's absorption. Low zinc levels in pregnancy may lead to fetal distress; consequently, zinc intake should be supplemented if the client is taking folic acid supplements while pregnant.

Many drugs act as folate antagonists. Folate may stimulate seizure activity in some individuals whose disorders are controlled by phenytoin therapy.

BIOTIN

Biotin is a chemical that is present in virtually every food substance. Although its role has been recognized since the 1930s, the essential nature of biotin intake was not fully recognized until the use of IV nutrition became common. IV nutrient solutions do not contain biotin unless it is intentionally added to the solution. Thus the institution of IV feedings led to the confirmation of the thirteenth essential vitamin.

Pharmacotherapeutics   The main therapeutic use of biotin is the treatment and prevention of a vitamin deficiency. Biotin deficiency rarely occurs in individuals taking oral foods. When deficiency does occur, it is most often associated with the *egg-white syndrome*. In this syndrome avidin, a glycoprotein found in raw egg whites, binds biotin in the gut, preventing its absorption and leading to biotin deficiency.[8]

Since biotin is not a natural component of IV nutrient sources, clients totally dependent on IV nutrition for an extended period of time constitute a high-risk group for biotin deficiency. Infants are at the greatest risk and develop the deficiency relatively quickly, often within the first half year.[16] Adults can continue several years before signs and symptoms of deficiency develop. Indications of biotin deficiency are generally associated with urinary biotin excretion levels below 6 µg in 24 hours.

Symptoms of biotin deficiency include anorexia, nausea, vomiting, glossitis, mental depression, alopecia, and a dry scaly or seborrheic dermatitis. Pallor, increased serum cholesterol levels, and increased serum bile pigment content may also be noted.[1,2]

Serum biotin levels drop progressively throughout pregnancy, but no known adverse effects to mother or fetus have been linked to this phenomenon. Decreased biotin levels have also occurred in alcoholics, persons with achlorhydria, the el-

derly, and some athletes.[1,2] Individuals with liver cirrhosis usually have a 20% drop in biotin levels, whereas clients with fatty liver disease have an 80% or more drop in biotin levels.[16]

Saccharin inhibits biotin activity. Long-term therapy with phenytoin, primidone, phenobarbital, or carbamazepine sometimes leads to depressed biotin levels, probably through altered hepatic metabolism.[16] Antibiotic therapy may decrease biotin absorption by killing biotin-producing bacteria in the gut. The clinical significance of these interactions is minimal except in individuals who undergo extended periods without enteral food intake or parenteral biotin supplementation.[7,16] Table 72–1 summarizes drugs and diseases that contribute to biotin deficiency.

Pharmacokinetics   Biotin as an acid is only slightly soluble in water, but as a salt it is water soluble. The proteolytic product of biotin digestion is biocytin. Absorption is rapid and active in the upper small intestine and passive in the large intestine. There is little storage of biotin, probably 1 mg total. Most storage occurs in the liver as cytoplasm and mitochondrial carboxylases. Biotin is excreted in the urine.[9]

Mechanism of action   Although as many as eight biotin-dependent coenzyme systems have been identified in the animal kingdom, only four coenzyme systems have been identified in humans. All known biotin coenzymes act to move carboxyl groups from one molecule to another or to fix CO_2. The biotin coenzyme pyruvate carboxylase is essential for gluconeogenesis, and the coenzyme acetyl-CoA carboxylase is essential for fatty acid synthesis. Propionyl-CoA carboxylase plays an essential role in maintaining neuronal function by supporting propionate metabolism. Catabolism of branched chain amino acids requires the presence of 3-methylcrotonyl CoA carboxylase; failure of this enzyme system yields organic acids toxic to human beings and can cause metabolic acidosis.[1,2,9]

Pharmaceutics   Therapy for biotin deficiency requires 150 to 300 µg/d for 3 to 5 days. Larger doses of 5 mg/d for 2 to 3 weeks may be useful for treatment of seborrheic dermatitis and Leiner's disease.[9]

Undesired clinical responses   No indications of biotin toxicity have been reported. Doses as high as 10 mg/d appear safe. No hypersensitivity reactions to either enteral or parenteral biotin have been reported.[10,16]

Drug-drug interactions   As previously indicated, saccharin inhibits biotin activity. In addition, long-term therapy with phenytoin, primidone, phenobarbital, or carbamazepine can lead to depressed biotin levels, and antibiotic therapy may decrease biotin absorption.

Life-span considerations   Although serum and urinary biotin levels are fairly well correlated with dietary intake, insufficient data are available to determine normal biotin levels. The daily biotin requirement is probably related to age and growth rate. Recommended oral and parenteral doses of biotin are listed in Table 72–4.

Nursing considerations   Biotin in solution is light sensitive; therefore protect all IV solutions containing biotin from unnecessary exposure to light.

Food sources of biotin are difficult to avoid. The richest sources are liver, egg yolk, soy flour, cereals, and yeast. Plant

TABLE 72–4
Recommended Dosages of Biotin

Client	Oral Dose (Safe and Adequate)	Intravenous Dose
Infant		2 μg/kg/d
<6 mo	10 μg/d	Maximum: 20 μg/d
6–12 mo	15 μg/d	
Child		20 μg/d
1–3 y	20 μg/d	
4–6 y	25 μg/d	
7–10 y	30 μg/d	
Male		60 μg/d
>11 y	30–100 μg/d	
Female		60 μg/d
>11 y	30–100 μg/d	
Pregnant	—	
Lactating	—	

sources generally have higher levels of free biotin, although much of the biotin found in wheat is bound into an nonabsorbable form. Fruits and muscle meats are relatively poor sources of biotin.

CONCEPT REVIEW

Biotin coenzymes move carboxyl groups from one molecule to another or fix CO_2. Biotin is available in almost all food, and its deficiency is rare in individuals consuming an oral diet. The exception occurs in individuals who eat raw egg whites, which bind biotin in the gut.

BIOFLAVONOIDS AND OTHER VITAMIN-LIKE SUBSTANCES

Many chemicals are frequently found in association with vitamins in food. Some are structurally related to recognized vitamins. As yet, none of these chemicals has clearly demonstrated any vitamin-like activity in man.

Bioflavonoids are similar in structure to vitamin C, and some clinicians have suggested that they might act as substitutes for ascorbate in some of its activities. Bioflavonoids commonly occur in fruits and are especially rich in the rinds of citrus fruits.[1,2]

Inositol and **choline,** as components of lecithin, have developed a reputation as key players in maintaining adequate liver function, but their specific roles are unclear. These chemicals are widely available in food, and no specific deficiency states have been defined.[1,7] Choline is an important precursor molecule for the neurotransmitter acetylcholine. Clients completely dependent on TPN to meet their needs receive choline as part of the fat emulsion; it is unclear whether the amount supplied is sufficient to meet patient needs. Large oral doses of choline are generally well tolerated, although they may be associated with a fishy body odor, salivation, sweating, and GI distress.[19]

Para-**aminobenzoic acid (PABA)** is a component of the folic acid molecule and is widely distributed throughout food, both as part of folic acid and as free PABA. It is involved in a wide variety of functions throughout the body, but a deficiency state has never been identified for PABA. The most common nonnutritive use of PABA is as a topical sunscreen.[1]

Carnitine is an important cofactor in fatty acid synthesis and storage. Carnitine is found in both plant and animal foods, with the highest concentrations in muscle meats. Carnitine deficiency is almost unheard of in humans, who usually can manufacture needed amounts. It has been identified in some premature infants receiving TPN. In these infants insufficient carnitine was produced in utero to allow the newborn to process IV fats adequately. The fact that a specific deficiency state associated with carnitine has been identified in a few individuals with limited dietary carnitine intake has led some practitioners to classify it as a conditionally essential nutrient.[20,21]

CONCEPT REVIEW

Vitamin-like substances have not been proved to produce specific effects in humans, although they are frequently found in association with vitamins in food. No specific deficiency state has been associated with any of these substances except carnitine.

SUMMARY

Water-soluble vitamins include the B vitamins, vitamin C, biotin, and folic acid. These vitamins are stored in small quantities in the body and therefore require daily supplementation. However, some deficiency states may take months or a year to develop. Water-soluble vitamins are sensitive to light and heat.

Toxicities are less common with water-soluble than with fat-soluble vitamins because the body can easily excrete excess amounts in the urine. Periods of altered metabolism or rapid cell division (e.g., pregnancy, cancer, or hypermetabolic states) may lead to deficiency states.

REFERENCES

1. Williams, S. (1991). *Basic nutrition and diet therapy* (9th ed.). St. Louis: Mosby–Year Book.
2. Davis, J., & Sherer, K. (1993). *Applied nutrition and diet therapy for nurses* (2nd ed.). Philadelphia: W.B. Saunders.
3. Chandra, R.K. (1991). Collum Award Lecture: Nutrition and immunity: From the past and new insights into the future. *American Journal of Clinical Nutrition, 53,* 1087–1101.
4. Delafuente, J.C. (1991). Nutrients and immune responses. *Rheumatic Disease Clinics of North America, 17*(2), 203–212.
5. Nelson, J.L., Alexander, J.W., Jacobs, P.A., Ing, R.D., & Ogle, C.K. (1992). Metabolic and immune effects of enteral ascorbic acid after burn trauma. *Burns, 18*(2), 92–97.
6. Baker, D.E., & Campbell, R.K. (1992). Vitamin and mineral supplementation in patients with diabetes mellitus. *Diabetes Educator, 18*(5), 420–427.
7. Food and Nutrition Board of the National Research Council. (1989). *Recommended Dietary Allowances* (10th ed.). Washington, DC: National Academy Press.

8. American Hospital Formulary Service. (1992). In G.K. McEvoy (Ed.), *AHFS Drug Information 92* (pp. 2158–2159). Bethesda, MD: American Society of Hospital Pharmacists.

9. Horvath, P. (1992). Vitamins as therapeutic agents. In C.M. Smith & A.M. Reynard (Eds.), *Textbook of pharmacology* (pp. 1067–1089). Philadelphia: W.B. Saunders.

10. Flodin, N.W. (1990). Micronutrient supplements: Toxicity and drug interactions. *Progress in Food and Nutrition Science, 14,* 277–331.

11. Sitren, H.S., Baily, L.B., Cerda, J.J., & Anderson, C.R. (1991). Ascorbic acid (vitamin C). In T.G. Baumgartner (Ed.), *Clinical guide to parenteral micronutrition* (2nd ed.) (pp. 487–503). Available from Lyphomed, Division of Fujisawa, USA.

12. Zak, J., III, Burns, D., Lingenfelser, T., Steyn, E., & Marks, I.N. (1991). Dry beriberi: Unusual complication of prolonged parenteral nutrition. *Journal of Parenteral and Enteral Nutrition, 15*(2), 200–201.

13. Weisburger, J.H. (1991). Nutritional approach to cancer prevention with emphasis on vitamins, antioxidants, and carotenoids. *American Journal of Clinical Nutrition, 53,* 226S–237S.

14. Whitney, E.N., Cataldo, C.B., & Rolfes, S.R. (Eds.). (1991). *Understanding clinical nutrition* (3rd ed.) Saint Paul, MN: West Publishing.

15. Data Pharmaceutics, Inc. (1993). *1993 physicians' genRx.* Smithtown, NY: Author.

16. Bailey, L.B. (1991). Pyridoxine (vitamin B6). In T.G. Baumgartner (Ed.), *Clinical guide to parenteral micronutrition* (2nd ed.) (pp. 521–537). Available from Lyphomed, Division of Fujisawa, USA.

17. Hathcock, J., & Trowndle, G. (1991). Oral cobalamin for treatment of pernicious anemia. *Journal of American Medical Association, 265,* 96–97.

18. Lederle, F.A. (1991). Oral cobalamin for pernicious anemia—Medicine's best kept secret. *Journal of American Medical Association, 265,* 94–95.

19. Canty, D.J., & Zeisel, S.H. (1994). Lecithin and choline in human health and disease. *Nutrition Reviews, 52,* 327–339.

20. A role for carnitine in medium-chain fatty acid metabolism. (1991). *Nutrition Reviews, 49,* 243–245.

21. Metabolic effects of carnitine supplementation in subjects with low plasma carnitine levels. (1990). *Nutrition Reviews, 48,* 159–161.

BIBLIOGRAPHY

Cerrato, P.L. (1993). OTC interactions: Vitamins and minerals. *RN Magazine, 56,* 28–33.

Dickerson, J.W. (1993). Ascorbic acid, zinc, and wound healing. *Journal of Wound Care, 2,* 350–353.

Trujillo, E.B. (1993). Effects of nutritional status on wound healing. *Journal of Vascular Nursing, 11*(1), 12–18.

Wells, L. (1994). At the front line of care: The importance of nutrition in wound management. *Professional Nurse, 9,* 525–526, 528–530.

CHAPTER 73

 # Minerals

PATRICIA UGO • PAMELA MOHLER PICKENS

⊛ **Minerals**

LEARNING OBJECTIVES:
List the physiologic roles of each mineral.
Describe the signs of deficiency for each mineral.
List clients at risk for deficiency for each mineral.
Discuss administrative and toxicity issues for each mineral.
List dietary sources for each mineral.

⊛ **Iron**

LEARNING OBJECTIVES:
Describe the role of transferrin in iron metabolism.
Discuss the impact of iron deficiency on the developing fetus.

KEY TERMS:
Apotransferrin, heme, hemochromatosis, hemoglobin, myoglobin, pica, transferrin

⊛ **Chromium**

LEARNING OBJECTIVE: Discuss the primary therapeutic value of chromium.
KEY TERM: Glucose tolerance factor

⊛ **Zinc**

LEARNING OBJECTIVES:
Discuss the primary therapeutic use of zinc.
Describe the relationship between zinc deficiency and gastrointestinal fluid loss.

⊛ **Copper**

LEARNING OBJECTIVE: Discuss the use of a complete blood count to confirm the presence of copper deficiency.
KEY TERMS:
Ceruloplasmin, Wilson's disease

⊛ **Selenium**

LEARNING OBJECTIVE: Discuss the similarity between selenium and vitamin E.

⊛ **Manganese**

LEARNING OBJECTIVE: Identify the population group most at risk of developing manganese toxicity.

⊛ **Fluorine**

LEARNING OBJECTIVE: Explain the benefits and problems involving fluorine and teeth care.
KEY TERMS:
Fluorosis, fluoritosis

⊛ **Iodine**

LEARNING OBJECTIVE: Describe the paradox that occurs with the Wolff-Chaikoff effect.
KEY TERMS:
Colloid, cretinism, goiter, goitrogenic

⊛ **Molybdenum**

LEARNING OBJECTIVE: Describe the effect of high doses of molybdenum on copper absorption.

CONCEPTS AND TERMS TO REVIEW

Read the section on nursing considerations in Chapter 71.
Review the content in Chapter 70 on minerals.
Read the section on a nutrition textbook on minerals.
Read the sections in Chapter 74 on major minerals in the body (e.g., potassium, calcium, magnesium).

*B*ody minerals are inorganic elements that are involved in a variety of processes. These minerals are generally classified as *macrominerals* and *trace minerals* or *microminerals*. Information on macrominerals is included in Chapter 74. Trace minerals, or microminerals, are the focus of this chapter.

Many trace minerals have been identified within the human body. Fewer than a dozen are known as essential; the remaining trace minerals are probably environmental contaminants. Like vitamins, trace minerals have no intrinsic caloric value, although they may assist in the effective production or use of energy within the cells. In the modern world trace mineral deficiencies commonly are associated with poor dietary intake or with the routine intake of highly refined, unfortified grain foods.[1]

IRON

Although iron is the most abundant metal in the universe and is one of the most abundant minerals in the body, the amount needed on a daily basis is very small, qualifying it as a trace mineral.

Pharmacotherapeutics   Most iron preparations are prescribed to prevent or treat iron deficiency states. Iron deficiency is the most common nutritional disease in man. Signs and symptoms of deficiency may appear before a measurable drop in hemoglobin concentration is noted. Iron deficiency anemia is associated with decreases in mean corpuscular volume (MCV), mean corpuscular hemoglobin (MCH), serum iron, serum iron-binding capacity (transferrin saturation), and serum ferritin. Concurrently, increases occur in serum transferrin levels and intracellular protoporphyrin concentrations.

Iron deficiency anemia is usually secondary to rapid growth when needs are increased in excess of intake. It may also be due to or complicated by decreased dietary intake of iron, decreased absorption of iron, increased loss of iron, multiple pregnancies, or copper deficiency (sideroblastic anemia).

The severity of the signs and symptoms of iron deficiency are not directly related to the severity of the anemia. Iron deficiency can manifest in every organ system. Decreased oxygen-carrying capacity during anemia produces tachycardia, dependent edema, decreased exercise tolerance, and altered mental status. Anemia is also associated with impaired leukocyte function and increased risk of infection. Iron deficiency is associated with koilonychia, which is characterized by lusterless, thin, brittle, and flattened fingernails that progress to a spoon or bowl shape. Anemic individuals may complain of paresthesia, cold extremities, weakness, fatigue, listlessness, headache, burning tongue, or dysphagia. Appetite may become capricious, and **pica** (consumption of nonnutritive substances) may develop, for pica of wood products, starches, earth, and ice is frequently associated with iron deficiency. Angular stomatitis develops, and glossitis may also occur. Vague gastrointestinal (GI) complaints, including nausea, vomiting, diarrhea, constipation, eructation, and flatulence, are frequently reported. Some patients develop achlorhydria, which further impairs digestion and nutrient absorption.[2-4]

Pharmacokinetics   The absorption rate is influenced by total body iron stores, the form of dietary iron consumed, and the concentration of dietary iron present in the gut. Iron availability is best in the form of hemoglobin and myoglobin in meats. (**Myoglobin** is an iron-containing globulin within muscle tissue.) Iron in human milk, lactoferrin, is the next best source. Iron in cow's milk and most inorganic salts (nonheme iron) is relatively poorly absorbed.

Absorption of heme and nonheme iron occurs in the duodenum and jejunum. **Heme,** which is the iron-containing component of hemoglobin, is split from the globulin in the intestinal lumen and is assimilated intact. Intramucosal heme-splitting enzymes then release the ionic iron for transfer from the cells into the blood. Absorption of nonheme iron is mediated by **transferrin. Apotransferrin** (noniron-containing transferrin) is secreted by the mucosal cells into the gut lumen, where it binds to the dietary iron. The transferrin is then reabsorbed into the mucosal cells. Passage of the transferrin into the bloodstream is inversely proportional to total body iron stores. In iron deficiency states larger quantities of transferrin pass from the mucosal cells into the bloodstream. In iron-replete states the predominance of the transferrin remains within the mucosal cells. Much of this iron is lost from the body into the feces through the normal turnover (desquamation) of the mucosal cells. Iron from shed cells can be reabsorbed as it passes further through the intestines.

In the target tissues transferrin binds to specific cell receptors, which allow transport of the transferrin into the cell. The iron is removed from the transferrin, and the apotransferrin is returned to circulation.[2,5]

Mechanism of action   Iron is well recognized for its role in oxygen transport. Incorporated into the core of the **hemoglobin** molecule, iron binds to oxygen in the pulmonary circulation and releases it as the blood passes through other body tissues. After releasing an oxygen molecule, the hemoglobin binds to CO_2 produced by the tissues and delivers it to the pulmonary circulation where it is released into expired breath. The myoglobin molecule maintains a small store of oxygen within the muscle that can be used for aerobic metabolism during muscle use.

Iron also plays a role in several enzyme systems. Iron is key to the function of cytochrome oxidase. Some of the peroxidase and catylase enzymes also depend on iron for proper functioning.[2,3,5]

Pharmaceutics   Ferrous sulfate is the most common oral iron preparation. It is available in a variety of dosage forms. The usual therapeutic dosage is 2 to 3 mg/kg of body weight. In actual practice 300 mg three times a day is a widely prescribed dosage regardless of the adult's size.[5] As the dosage of iron is increased, the percent that is absorbed decreases. Table 73–1 provides additional information about dosage forms, dosages, and routes of administration.

Undesired clinical responses   The classic iron toxicity syndrome is known as **hemochromatosis.** Hemochromatosis can be caused by idiopathic or iatrogenic causes. *Idiopathic hemochromatosis* is caused by an autosomal-recessive inborn error of metabolism, which leads to excessive iron absorption. The iron is deposited in organs and soft tissues, causing fibrotic and cirrhotic destruction of the liver, heart, pancreas, and other organs. Age, sex, and alcohol ingestion can influence expression of the disease. It is usually diagnosed in adults, but the damage can begin in childhood.

The most common of the *iatrogenic,* or *acquired, causes* is the administration of multiple blood transfusions in a client

TABLE 73–1
Iron: Dosage Forms, Dosages, and Routes of Administration

Drug Name	Dosage and Route of Administration
FERROUS SULFATE: 20% ELEMENTAL IRON (Mol-Iron, Feratab, Fer-In-Sol, Feosol, Fer-Iron, Slow-Fe) HOW SUPPLIED Tablets: 195, 300, 324 mg Capsules: 250 mg Tablets, time-release: 525 mg Syrup: 90 mg/5 ml Elixir: 220 mg/5 ml Drops: 150 mg/ml	**Iron Deficiency (expressed as elemental iron)** Adults 100–200 mg/d CHILDREN 2–12 y: 3 mg/kg/d in 3–4 divided doses 6 mo–2 y: Up to 6 mg/kg/d in 3–4 divided doses INFANTS 10–25 mg/d in 3–4 divided doses
Iron Dextran (InFe D) HOW SUPPLIED Injection: 50 mg/ml	**Iron Deficiency Anemia** See package insert for amount specific to client weight (lb) and laboratory-observed hemoglobin level; drug is given undiluted and slowly (1 ml or less/min)

receiving renal dialysis. Aggressive treatment of thalassemia or sideroblastic anemia can also lead to iron overload syndromes.

Acute iron toxicity is a significant problem in children; a lethal dose of iron sulfate for a 2-year-old child can be as little as 3 g. Lethal doses of iron sulfate in adults range from 200 to 250 mg/kg of body weight. Signs and symptoms of acute toxicity include vomiting, abdominal pain, lethargy, dyspnea, and bloody diarrhea. In children necrotizing gastroenteritis may occur. The acute symptoms may be followed by brief improvement and sudden deterioration, leading to severe metabolic acidosis, coma, and death.[5,6]

When iron is administered intravenously, anaphylaxis may occur, although the incidence is rare. Headache, urticaria, fever, malaise, lymphadenopathy, and arthralgia are more commonly reported. Epinephrine, aminophylline, and support equipment should be available when the first dose is administered.[5,7] See box for emergency treatment for iron poisoning.

Contraindications and precautions Care should be used when administering iron to infants with concurrent vitamin E deficiency; this may lead to hemolysis. The presence of benzyl alcohol in the injectable iron products has been linked to a gasping syndrome in neonates.

Drug-drug and drug-nutrient interactions Iron is best absorbed from an acidic media. Antacids, which raise gastric pH, decrease iron absorption, whereas gastric acidifiers such as ascorbic acid improve absorption. High-dose zinc supplements interfere with copper absorption, which in turn leads to secondary iron deficiency anemia.

Several dietary components decrease nonheme iron absorption, including tannins in teas, phosphates, polyphenols in vegetables, oxalates, and cereal brans. Nonheme iron absorption can be improved by the consumption of lactic acid, citric acid, meat, fish, or poultry. Solid foods decrease absorption of milk iron in infants; absorption of heme iron is relatively unaffected by the presence or absence of food.

EMERGENCY TREATMENT FOR IRON POISONING

▶ **Deferoxamine mesylate,** an iron-chelating agent, is used to treat iron poisoning. Deferoxamine is available in 500-mg vials. It can be administered IM or IV.

▶ Usual initial dose: 1 g, followed by 500 mg 4 h and 8 h after initial dose. It is recommended that dosage not exceed 6 g/d.

▶ If IV route is needed, infusion rate should not exceed 15 mg/kg/h.

Data from Bettigole, R. (1992). Drugs acting on the blood and blood-forming organs. In C.M. Smith & A.M. Reynard (Eds.; pp. 784–789). *Textbook of pharmacology.* Philadelphia: W.B. Saunders; and from Data Pharmaceutics, Inc. (1993). *1993 physicians' genRx.* Smithtown, NY: Author.

Life-span considerations Men and postmenopausal women typically require 14 μg of iron/kg/d to maintain their body stores. A dose of 10 mg/d is generally adequate to meet the needs of these populations. Premenopausal women require up to 22 μg/kg or approximately 15 mg of iron daily to maintain their iron stores.[8]

During the second and third trimesters of pregnancy women should consume an additional 15 mg/d or a total of 30 mg/d to provide adequate iron for both the growing fetus and the maternal support tissues. During lactation no additional iron is needed above the basic 15 mg/d until menstruation resumes. When menstruation resumes, an additional 1 to 5 mg/d should be consumed until the child is weaned.[2,7,9]

Premature infants may need as much as 0.7 mg/kg/d to make up for lack of iron accumulation in utero. In general, this dose is continued until the infant has reached delivery age or the iron stores have reached normal levels. Total body stores in full-term infants are usually well maintained by daily iron doses of 6 mg until they are 6 months old. From age 6 months to 10 years, the daily requirement is 10 mg. A male teenager should consume 11 to 14 mg/d until full maturity is reached. A female teen, like her adult counterpart, should consume 15 mg/d once menarche is reached.

Specific drug-related nursing considerations   Counsel clients that taking iron supplements may cause reversible tooth staining. This staining is diminished if the iron is placed on the back of the tongue for swallowing. Iron supplements may cause the stools to darken. This darkening must be differentiated from the black, tarry stools of GI bleeding, preferably by stool guaiac testing. Iron supplements do *not* cause false-positive guaiac test results in properly performed tests.

Teach the client that compliance with therapy is most critical during the first month of therapy since that is when the majority of the deficiency correction occurs. Because the percent of the dose absorbed decreases as the deficiency corrects, encourage compliance for a full 12 months to ensure complete reversal of the deficiency state.

Store oral iron products in properly fastened childproof containers out of reach of children. Iron tablets are approximately the same size and colors of a popular candy treat and offer a tempting sight to young children. Poisoning may occur when a child is taken to visit a home in which no children live and the iron preparations have been left in easy reach by the unsuspecting homeowner.

MISCELLANEOUS DRUG PREPARATIONS

Iron dextran injection has been available in the United States for many years. It is available in 2-ml ampules and 10 ml vials containing 50 mg/ml for IM or intravenous (IV) use. Both sizes contain 0.9% sodium chloride. When administering iron dextran IM, use the Z-track method. Pull the tissues tautly away from the injection site, drawing tissues diagonally. After the drug is administered into the muscle, release the tissues, allowing them to return to their normal position while displacing the needle track. This method prevents the drug's leaking back along the needle track and causing tissue staining around the injection site.

When administering IV iron dextran, administer a small test dose first and monitor for anaphylaxis or gasping syndrome. If the test dose is tolerated, administer the balance of the dose. Have emergency assistance for anaphylaxis available during administration against the unlikely occurrence of a reaction.

CONCEPT REVIEW

Heme is the iron-containing component of hemoglobin, which is split from the globulin in the intestinal lumen and is assimilated intact. Apotransferrin is secreted by the mucosal cells into the gut lumen; it binds to nonheme (dietary) iron and, as transferrin, carries the iron with it into the mucosa. Most transferrin remains within the mucosal cells if the body has enough iron; if iron is depleted, more transferrin passes into the bloodstream.

Iron plays an important role in oxygen transport, releasing oxygen as the blood passes through body tissues. In muscle tissue the iron-containing globulin is called *myoglobin*.

Iron deficiency is a common disease. Complete reversal of the deficiency may take 12 months. Iron toxicity is known as *idiopathic* or *iatrogenic hemochromatosis*. Iron can be fatal to children in fairly small amounts; prompt treatment of accidental ingestion is critical.

CHROMIUM

Also known as **glucose tolerance factor (GTF),** chromium is a necessary cofactor for insulin activity. The trivalent ionic form of chromium is the only biologically active form in humans.

Pharmacotherapeutics   Chromic chloride is the pharmacologic preparation of chromium. It is used as a supplement to IV solutions administered for total parenteral nutrition (TPN). Its administration helps maintain chromium serum levels and prevent depletion of endogenous stores.

Relative insulin resistance, glucose intolerance, weight loss, peripheral neuropathy, elevated circulating insulin, glycosuria, fasting hyperglycemia, elevated serum cholesterol and triglyceride levels, and encephalopathy have all occurred in individuals with induced chromium deficiencies. Chromium deficiency may also impair growth, decrease sperm count and fertility, and decrease longevity, although these sequelae have not been clearly demonstrated in humans. An increased risk for atherosclerosis has been linked with chromium deficiency.[2,7,10]

Pharmacokinetics   Serum chromium is bound to transferrin in the β-globulin fraction. Typical blood levels from chromium range from 1 to 5 μg/L. However, blood levels are not a meaningful indicator of tissue stores. Excretion of chromium is through the kidneys, ranging from 3 to 50 μg/d. Biliary excretion through the small intestine may be an ancillary route for small amounts of chromium.[7]

Mechanism of action   As a part of the GTF, chromium potentiates the action of insulin, affecting carbohydrate and lipid metabolism. The precise mechanism of this potentiation has not been clarified. The GTF does bind to insulin in vitro, and it is presumed that it also binds in vivo.[2,7]

Pharmaceutics   Chromic chloride is available in parenteral preparations for IV administration. The additive should be administered in not less than 1 dl of fluid. For the adult receiving TPN, the recommended dosage is 10 to 15 μg of chromium/d. For the pediatric client a dosage of 0.14 to 0.20 μg/kg/d is recommended.

Undesired clinical responses   Trivalent chromium is nontoxic to humans. However, dermatitis has been reported in some clients after exposure to either the trivalent or hexavalent chromium.[10]

Contraindications and precautions   Direct IM or IV injection of chromic chloride is contraindicated since the acidic pH of the solution can cause extensive tissue irritation. The presence of severe renal disease may make it necessary to reduce or omit chromium doses.[7]

Drug-nutrient interactions   Exposure of chromic chloride to heat should be minimized. The product should be protected from freezing. Storage at room temperature is recommended.

Life-span considerations   Chromic chloride is classified as a Pregnancy Category C drug. It is not known if it is excreted in human milk. Safety and effectiveness in children have not been established.[7]

Specific drug-related nursing considerations   Brewer's yeast is the richest known dietary source of chromium. Mushrooms, prunes, nuts, asparagus, wine, and beer are all good sources. Meat, especially liver and other organ meats, whole grains and wheat germ, and American cheese are also valuable dietary sources of chromium. Chromium is leached from stainless steel during the preparation of acidic foods and may provide an additional chromium source. Raw sugar cane contains a significant amount of chromium, which is lost during the refining process.

CONCEPT REVIEW

Chromium, or glucose tolerance factor, is biologically active in humans only in the trivalent ionic form. It potentiates the action of insulin.

Deficiencies are rare except in clients receiving long-term parenteral nutrient therapy. The mineral is virtually nontoxic to humans.

Chromic chloride is the drug preparation of chromium. It is available in parenteral preparations for IV administration.

ZINC

Zinc plays a vital role in the function of a wide variety of enzyme systems. Much of zinc's activity is aimed at stabilizing cell membranes and assisting polysomes during protein synthesis.

Pharmacotherapeutics   The primary therapeutic use of zinc is to prevent or treat zinc deficiency. Zinc deficiency in humans manifests as perinasal, periorbital, or perioral dermatitis that spreads rapidly to the upper and lower extremities and the perianal area. The dermatitis may be seen initially as an eczematoid, seborrheic, acneiform, pustular, or papular rash. Glucose intolerance, mental depression, alopecia, diarrhea, sore throat, stomatitis, and loss of or change in sense of taste have been reported in clients receiving parenteral nutrition deficient in zinc content.[1-3]

Zinc deficiency is associated with diets highly dependent on cereal proteins, with minimal intake of animal proteins. Clients with anorexia nervosa, cancer anorexia, protein-energy malnutrition, pancreatic insufficiency, cystic fibrosis, inflammatory bowel disease (IBD), nephrotic syndrome, short-bowel syndrome, thalassemia, and thermal burns are prone to zinc deficiency. Other specific groups at risk are premature infants, the elderly, pregnant or lactating women, alcoholics, and individuals who practice pica.[2,3,11]

Zinc is also lost in exudative fluids in wounds. This exudative loss, combined with increased metabolic needs, places burn patients at risk for zinc deficiency.[12] Individuals with chronic renal failure have decreased zinc levels in their plasma, hair, and leukocytes. These decreased levels are associated with the presence of uremia and occur regardless of the type of dialysis used.

Mechanism of action   More than 80 metalloenzymes require zinc for proper functioning. Many of these enzymes such as DNA-RNA polymerase and thymidine kinase are involved in the processes of cell division and growth by contributing to protein synthesis. Zinc metalloenzymes are also necessary for the function of thymulin and other thymic hormones involved in the stimulation of T-cell differentiation.[2,3]

Pharmaceutics   Zinc is available as a mineral supplement in the pharmacologic preparations of zinc, zinc chloride, and zinc sulfate. Zinc and zinc chloride are available only for IV administration. Zinc sulfate is available in a capsule for oral administration and in a parenteral solution for IV administration.[7]

Some sources recommend that 70 to 80 μg/kg/d be administered to tumor-bearing clients. Similarly, an additional 2 mg daily is recommended during acute catabolic states and 12 to 17 mg for each liter of intestinal fluid lost from diarrhea or ileostomies. Premature infants should receive 300 μg/kg/d to replace zinc accumulation that normally occurs during the third trimester of fetal growth.

Undesired clinical responses   Chronic consumption of oral zinc can cause toxic effects. Gastric erosions, impaired iron and copper absorption, and anemia have been reported in individuals consuming more than 5 mg/d from nonfood sources. Consumption of 23 mg/d can result in asymptomatic hyperamylasemia.[13]

Acute zinc toxicity is primarily associated with GI symptoms. Acute doses greater than 25 mg cause nausea and epigastric distress and lead to a metallic taste in the mouth. Doses of 225 to 450 mg are emetic. Rapid administration of IV zinc may cause signs of acute zinc toxicity. Other signs of IV toxicity include flushing, sweating, and blurred vision.

Drug-drug and drug-nutrient interactions   Use of chelating agents, antimetabolites, anabolic agents, and diuretics has been associated with low zinc levels. For example, penicillamine therapy for Wilson's disease (hypercupremia) frequently causes zinc deficiency. Diuretics that accelerate potassium and magnesium losses are more likely to cause increased urinary excretion of zinc than are potassium-sparing diuretics.

Although administration of zinc with food decreases the gastric upset that may occur with therapeutic supplementation doses, absorption of zinc is best when administered on an empty stomach.

Life-span considerations Adults require 12 to 15 mg of dietary zinc daily. Children should consume 10 to 15 mg daily, but infants require only 5 mg daily from their diets. Lactating women should consume sufficient dietary zinc to ensure absorption of 5.5 mg/d.

Specific drug-related nursing considerations Individuals with chronic intestinal losses such as from intestinal fistulas or diarrhea should be monitored for clinical signs of zinc deficiency. A rash on the face around the nose, cheeks, and chin is often the first indication of zinc deficiency. Delayed wound healing after a large burn or traumatic or surgical injury may also indicate a deficiency in zinc stores.

Encourage clients to meet their zinc needs from dietary sources to diminish the risk of chronic toxicity. Also discourage clients from preparing acidic foods such as tomato-based sauces in galvanized steel vessels.

Seventy percent of dietary zinc typically comes from animal protein sources. Muscle meats, liver, eggs, and seafoods (especially oysters) are rich zinc sources. The balance is primarily from cereals. Although some cereals contain zinc concentrations comparable to those from animal sources, absorption from plant sources is less complete.

CONCEPT REVIEW

Zinc is vital to the functioning of many enzyme systems, stabilizing cell membranes and assisting in protein synthesis. Zinc deficiency is associated with low intake of animal protein and a variety of disorders. The classic symptom of zinc deficiency is dermatitis that occurs around the nose, eye, mouth, and anus.

High doses of zinc can interfere with copper metabolism. Chronic zinc consumption can cause toxic effects.

Zinc is available as a mineral supplement in the pharmacologic preparations of zinc, zinc chloride, and zinc sulfate.

COPPER

Copper plays an important role in the formation of red and white blood cells in the bone marrow.

Pharmacotherapeutics Therapeutic copper is used to prevent or treat deficiency states. Copper deficiency can be acquired or inborn. **Menkes' kinky-hair syndrome** is an X-linked, **inborn** copper deficiency syndrome. Menkes' syndrome occurs in male infants, with onset in early infancy. The syndrome is named for the brittle, steel-wool, kinky hair (or pili torti) that characterizes the disease. Absorption of copper is decreased, and poor use of available copper occurs. The hypochromic iron deficiency anemia of Menkes' syndrome can be microcytic, normocytic, macrocytic, or multicytic. Neutropenia is a common occurrence, as are subperiosteal hemor-

rhages. Some infants' legs swell as the hemorrhages spread periosteally. Skeletal modifications occur, including demineralization, microfractures, and metaphyseal changes, resulting in growth retardation. Cerebral and cerebellar degeneration leads to lethargy, mental retardation, and uncontrollable seizures. Defective elastin and connective tissue formation produces diffuse arterial aneurysms, hypotonia, and retinal dystrophy. Depigmentation of the hair and skin and hypothermia are also common problems. Eventually, Menkes' syndrome leads to death.[2,3]

Acquired copper deficiency in an infant or child can occur in either sex. It is identical in presentation to Menkes' syndrome with the exception of the hair changes, hypothermia, hypotonia, lethargy, mental retardation, and retinal dystrophy. Acquired deficiency is usually secondary to increased copper use in this age group.

An adult with acquired deficiency is initially seen with sideroblastic anemia and neutropenia. The bone marrow shows cavity formation, development of sideroblastic and megaloblastic cells, reduced numbers of maturing neutrophils, and granulocyte stem cells that contain vacuoles or cavities in the protoplasm. Skeletal defects, demyelination and degeneration of nervous system, defects of pigmentation and structure of hair, reproductive failure, myocardial degeneration, decreased arterial elasticity, soft-tissue calcification, metaphalangeal spurring, and osteoporosis have also been linked to acquired deficiency.[8,13] Deficiency states in adults can occur in individuals receiving long-term TPN therapy.

Pharmacokinetics Dietary copper is primarily bound into insoluble molecules and must be freed through digestion before absorption. Once released from the bound state, most dietary copper is absorbed in the jejunum or ileum. The presence of bile may improve the solubility and absorption of copper. The amino acid histidine probably acts as a carrier molecule during copper absorption. Two absorptive mechanisms, one active and one passive, have been described.[13]

Once absorbed, copper binds to albumin and free amino acids in the mesenteric blood flow for delivery to the liver. Approximately 5% of the copper in the bloodstream is bound. **Ceruloplasmin** is the primary transport protein for copper. Each ceruplasmin molecule can transport up to six copper ions. Ceruloplasmin levels are increased during pregnancy and in clients with tuberculosis, schistosomiasis, advanced cystic fibrosis, and several oncologic states. Although most copper transport involves ceruloplasmin, individuals with low ceruloplasmin levels can still have adequate and even toxic delivery of copper to peripheral tissues.

Copper excretion is primarily biliary. The amount excreted daily in the bile ranges from 0.9 to 2.5 mg. Enterohepatic recirculation is possible, although not clearly defined. Thirty to 50 μg is lost daily in the urine. During biliary obstruction the capacity for urinary excretion increases slightly. Insignificant amounts of copper are lost in skin, sweat, and hair.[14]

Mechanism of action Several copper-containing enzymes are essential for the proper use of iron. Cuproenzymes are key for erythropoiesis, leukopoiesis, skeletal mineralization, connective tissue synthesis, myelin formation, thermoregulation, melanin pigment synthesis, catecholamine metabolism, oxidative phosphorylation, antioxidant protection, immune function, and cardiac function. Copper is also believed to play a role in glucose metabolic regulation by affecting insulin receptor sites and in cholesterol metabolism.[2,8]

Pharmaceutics The amount of dietary copper deemed safe for daily intake varies with age and weight. Most adults do well with oral intakes of 1.5 to 3 mg daily. Premature infants require 100 μg/kg/d; term infants require 75 μg/kg/d or 60 μg/100 kcal consumed in the diet. Children and adolescents between the ages of 1 and 15 years require 35 to 45 μg/kg/d.

The main pharmacologic preparation of copper is **cupric sulfate.** Cupric sulfate is available as a parenteral solution for IV administration. This preparation provides 0.4 mg of copper/ml in multiple-dose and single-dose vials. For the metabolically stable adult receiving TPN, 0.5 to 1.5 mg/d should be added to the TPN solution. For full-term infants and children, 20 μg/kg/d should be added to the TPN solution. Limited data are available for premature infants, who may require larger doses.[7]

Daily dosages (0.1 mg/kg) of copper sulfate have been administered by mouth to some clients and have resulted in clinical responses.[5]

Undesired clinical responses Oral copper acts as an emetic, with 10 mg producing nausea and 250 mg causing vomiting. The irritant effects of copper on the gastric mucosa may lead to gastric hemorrhage. The liver is the organ most susceptible to toxic accumulation of copper, and acute copper toxicity is associated with hepatic necrosis and intravascular hemolysis, leading to jaundice. In severe cases fatal hemolytic anemia may occur. The probable lethal dose of copper is between 3.5 and 35 g as a single dose.

Chronic copper toxicity is associated with oral doses of more than 200 mg daily or IV doses greater than 0.5 mg/d. With chronic overdose, hepatic cellular damage results.

Wilson's disease, or hepatolenticular degeneration, is a spontaneous, toxic accumulation of copper in the liver, the basal ganglia of the brain, the kidneys, and the corneas. The clinical signs of Wilson's disease include low ceruloplasmin concentrations, hepatic cirrhosis, ataxia, and characteristic yellow Kayser-Fleischer rings around the corneas.[15]

Contraindications and precautions The multiple-dose cupric sulfate preparation should not be administered to clients with known sensitivity to benzyl alcohol. In addition, this solution is hypotonic and must not be administered by direct IM or IV route. It must be diluted for IV administration.[7]

Drug-drug and drug-environment interactions Several drugs alter serum copper levels, usually by affecting ceruloplasmin levels. Acute administration of high-dose corticosteroid therapy increases serum copper levels, whereas chronic corticosteroid use decreases serum copper levels. Oral contraceptives increase ceruloplasmin levels by 100% to 200%. Cigarette smoking and anticonvulsant drug therapy are also linked with elevated ceruloplasmin levels.

A few drugs interfere with copper absorption. Alkalinization of the GI tract with antacids decreases copper absorption; the use of antiulcer drugs that block acid secretion in the stomach may have a similar effect. Oral intake of high doses of zinc decreases copper absorption by competing for binding sites. Iron taken in large amounts may decrease copper absorption. The presence of calcium may reverse zinc's inhibition of copper absorption.[14]

Syringes equipped with aluminum needles or hubs must not be used with cupric sulfate since the solution is acidic. Cupric sulfate is physically compatible with the electrolytes and vitamins present in TPN solutions. However, it degrades ascorbic acid in the solutions; thus it should be added to the TPN solution immediately before infusion. Store the drug preparation at controlled room temperatures.[7]

Life-span considerations During the third trimester the fetus requires approximately 100 μg of copper/kg/d. Thus pregnant women may require supplementation to prevent maternal and fetal deficiency. Premature infants require supplementation to allow adequate accumulation of body stores. Breast-feeding mothers may also require supplementation to provide adequate copper for neonatal growth.

Cupric sulfate is classified as a Pregnancy Category C drug.

Specific drug-related nursing considerations The current standard for monitoring copper status is the plasma ceruloplasmin level. However, a simple complete blood count (CBC) can provide a rapid, relatively inexpensive screening tool for detecting copper deficiency. The combined presence of neutropenia, low reticulocyte count, and microcytic hypochromic anemia in the presence of adequate iron strongly suggests the presence of copper deficiency.

The best dietary sources of copper are shellfish (especially oysters) and legumes. Muscle meats, liver, and brains are also relatively good copper sources. Rice and milk are low in copper; thus encourage individuals with diets heavy in rice or milk products to incorporate some copper-rich foods into their diet.

CONCEPT REVIEW

Copper is important in the formation of red and white blood cells in bone marrow. Ceruloplasmin, the primary transport protein for copper, can transport up to six copper ions per molecule. Copper-containing enzymes (cuproenzymes) enable the proper use of iron and perhaps aid in regulation of glucose metabolism.

Copper deficiency can be acquired or inborn. Inborn deficiency is called *Menkes' kinky-hair syndrome.* The acquired form is often associated with protein-calorie malnutrition, GI dysfunction, and long-term TPN therapy.

Cupric sulfate is the pharmacologic preparation. It is usually added to TPN solutions to prevent or treat deficiency states.

SELENIUM

Selenium plays an important role in scavenging and destroying peroxides and free radicals in the mitochondria and cytoplasm.

This role is closely linked to the free radical scavenging activity of vitamin E.[16]

Pharmacotherapeutics The therapeutic value of the drug preparation is in the treatment or prevention of selenium deficiency. The classic selenium deficiency state is known as *Keshan disease.* This syndrome was originally identified in Chinese children whose diets consisted of foods grown in selenium-deficient soil. A similar syndrome has been seen in individuals receiving long-term, selenium-poor parenteral nutrition.

Acute onset of selenium deficiency is characterized by the sudden onset of cardiac failure. Clients with chronic deficiency states are initially seen with moderate to severe cardiomegaly and varying degrees of diminished cardiac function. The heart becomes enlarged and flabby.[17] Other signs and symptoms of selenium deficiency include decreased immune and inflammatory responses, hemolysis, altered response to toxic chemicals, cataract formation, muscle pain, liver necrosis, and pancreatic degeneration.[18,19]

Aside from eating diets poor in selenium content, the highest risk of deficiency occurs in persons with poor general dietary intake or decreased absorption or increased losses of selenium. Premature infants, clients with cancer, the elderly, alcoholic individuals, and other clients with poor oral intake are at risk. Increased selenium losses from the GI tract such as occur during nasogastric suctioning, with high-output enterocutaneous fistulas, and with IBD are also linked with the development of selenium deficiency.[18,19]

Pharmacokinetics Absorption of dietary selenium depends on the solubility of the compound. Selenium is mainly excreted by the kidneys.

Mechanism of action Selenium activity is linked to its place in the glutathione peroxidase enzyme. With assistance from manganese and copper, this selanoenzyme plays an important role in removing free radicals from body tissues by converting the free radicals to water and other, less harmful, waste products. It acts as a synergistic antioxidant with vitamin E.[2,19]

Pharmaceutics Selenium is available as a parenteral drug preparation for IV administration. The IV solution contains 40 µg/ml.

Undesired clinical responses Dietary intake of more than 5 to 10 parts per million on a chronic basis is associated with toxicity. Intake of 1.5 mg daily is classiifed as a chronically toxic dose. Daily intake of 1 mg, taken for a 2-year period, causes thickened fingernails and garliclike body odor. Daily intake of 5 mg is linked to fingernail changes and hair loss.[8] Intake of 27.3 mg daily causes nausea, vomiting, diarrhea, hair and nail changes, fatigue, and peripheral neuropathies.

Life-span considerations Based on the assumption of 80% bioavailability, an adult male should consume 70 µg of dietary selenium per day. A nonpregnant woman should consume 55 µg/d, and pregnant women require a total of 65 µg/d. Infants less than 6 months of age require 10 µg/d, whereas 6- to 12-month-old infants should receive 15 µg/d.

Because little is known about the effects of selenium supplementation on fetuses and infants, use of selenium supplements in pregnant women and infants require extreme caution.

Specific drug-related nursing considerations The food content of selenium varies with the amount of selenium in the soil. Seafood, legumes, whole grains, low-fat meats and dairy products, and vegetables are sources of selenium.

CONCEPT REVIEW

Selenium is similar to and is linked to the free radical scavenging activity of vitamin E, which converts free radicals to water and other waste products.

Classic selenium deficiency is called *Keshan disease.* Deficiency is rare and is found most often in clients receiving TPN. Both acute and chronic forms of deficiency affect the heart.

Selenium toxicity can be evidenced by a garliclike body odor and changes in hair and nails.

MANGANESE

The essential nature of manganese is not as clearly established as that of other trace minerals. However, because of the key metabolic roles of manganese-containing metalloenzymes, few clinicians argue the importance of maintaining adequate manganese stores.

Pharmacotherapeutics Manganese supplements are used to prevent or treat deficiency states. Manganese deficiency, as a single entity, is unlikely to occur except in individuals intentionally excluding manganese from the diet or receiving manganese-poor TPN. Usually manganese deficiency is encountered in a chronically malnourished individual who has multiple nutrient deficiencies.

Although manganese deficiency has been documented in several animal models, only a few diagnosed cases have been seen in humans. Manganese depletion is associated with mild dermatitis, reddening of the hair and beard, slow nail, hair, and beard growth, intermittent nausea and vomiting, decreased serum phospholipid and triglyceride levels, and moderate weight loss. Neonates with low manganese levels accumulated in utero are at increased risk of developing ataxia and of poor development of inner ear structures.[16]

Pharmacokinetics Manganese is bound to a specific transport protein, transmanganin. It is widely distributed but concentrates in the mitochondria-rich tissues such as the brain, kidney, pancreas, and liver. Excretion of manganese occurs mainly through the bile. In the event of obstruction, ancillary excretion routes include pancreatic juice.[7]

Mechanism of action Manganese serves as an activator for enzymes such as polysaccharide polymerase, cholinesterase, and pyruvate carboxylase.

Pharmaceutics Drug preparations of manganese, manganese chloride, and manganese sulfate are available. All three preparations are parenteral solutions of 0.1 or 0.5 mg/ml for IV administration. IV doses of manganese to meet daily needs are 2 to 10 μg/kg for children less than 15 years old and 0.15 to 0.8 mg/d for adults.[14]

Undesired clinical responses Manganese toxicity is an uncommon event. It is most likely to occur in workers exposed to airborne manganese in dust or fumes. It has been proposed that manganese toxicity may also occur in clients with severe biliary disease. The signs and symptoms of manganese toxicity are probably due to a manganese-induced potentiation of dopamine autooxidation. Manganese toxicity is characterized by parkinsonian symptoms, including excitement, tremors, irritation, compulsive behavior, mask facies, discoordinate gaze, and paralysis agitans.[14,16]

Contraindications and precautions Direct IM or IV injection of manganese parenteral solution is contraindicated since the acid of the solution may cause tissue irritation.[7]

Drug-environment interactions Parenteral solutions should be stored at a controlled room temperature. Manganese sulfate should not be prepared with syringes equipped with aluminum needles or hubs.

Life-span considerations Manganese sulfate is classified as a Pregnancy Category C drug. To maintain manganese homeostasis, most individuals must consume 0.035 to 0.070 mg/kg/d. This translates into a 2- to 5-mg oral daily dietary intake for adults and a 0.3- to 1-mg oral daily intake for infants.[8]

Specific drug-related nursing considerations Clinically efficient monitoring and assessment tools for manganese status are under development. Assessment of deficiency or toxicity must be made based on the clinical presentation of the individual or on a stated history of dietary deficiency or environment exposure. Dietary manganese is supplied best by grains and cereals, tea, fruits, and vegetables. Animal source foods are relatively poor sources of manganese.

CONCEPT REVIEW

Manganese deficiency has been documented in only a few humans. Although the nature of its action is not clearly understood, it is recognized as an essential trace mineral.

Although manganese deficiency is unlikely, toxicity can occur from exposure to airborne manganese in some work environments.

FLUORINE

Metabolically active as fluoride, most individuals in the United States know of fluorine for its role in preventing dental caries. Fluoridation of drinking water is common in areas of the United States where natural fluoride content is low. In most communities the target level of fluoride in the water is one part per million. In several countries, including the United States, the use of fluoridated table salt has been considered; as yet its use in the United States is very limited. Most of the fluoride consumed from treated water, dentifrices, and supple-

ments is as the sodium salt. Each gram of sodium fluoride provides 0.425 g of fluoride ion.

Pharmacotherapeutics Topical fluoride application and dietary intake are useful in the prophylaxis of dental caries. The greatest benefits occur in children during times of tooth development.

A specific fluoride deficiency state has not been defined. Epidemiologic studies link decreased fluoride intake with increased risk of dental caries in youth and of osteoporosis during old age. Several epidemiologic studies have suggested an increased incidence of decreased bone density and increased mineralization of the aorta in individuals chronically consuming low-fluoride water.

Pharmacokinetics Ninety percent of fluoride excretion is in the urine. Most of the balance is excreted in the feces, with a small amount lost in perspiration.

Fluoride typically is present in the blood at levels of 0.04 to 0.4 μg/g of whole blood. The fluoride ion is present in concentrations of 0.01 to 0.2 μg/ml of plasma and 0.2 to 1.1 μg/ml of urine.

Mechanism of action Fluoride is easily and rapidly incorporated into **apatite,** the calcium phosphate salt that provides the basic mineral structure of bone and tooth tissues. When fluoride replaces hydroxide in the apatite molecule, the structure becomes more stable and less vulnerable to demineralization. Tooth enamel has a high affinity for fluoride, which provides the enamel with improved resistance to acid attack. The incorporation of fluoride into bone tissues increases bone stability and tensile strength. This is believed to provide some measure of prophylaxis against osteoporosis.

Pharmaceutics A dose of 5 to 10 g of sodium fluoride is lethal in an adult male. The doses recommended for use in the treatment of osteoporosis, 50 mg/d, may lead to toxic effects with chronic use.

Undesired clinical responses Fluoride toxicity is known as **fluorosis** or **fluoritosis.** Fluorosis affects the permanent teeth in children consuming high levels of fluoride in drinking water or from excessive oral supplements. Paradoxically, fluorosis leads to weak, chalky enamel, which pits and stains, leading to the characteristic dark, mottled appearance. In adults prolonged intake of high doses of fluoride is associated with bone changes in the spine and the knees (genu valgum). Deterioration of kidney function, nerve function, and muscle function also occurs. Epidemiologic studies suggest there is no increase in cancer risk from the chronic consumption of fluoridated water.[8]

Life-span considerations Safe and effective intake for adults ranges from 1.5 to 4.0 mg. Dietary intake is usually adequate, and intake of a supplement is rarely necessary. Fluoride intake for children aged 7 years to adulthood should be 1.5 to 2.5 mg/d. Four- to 6-year-old children should take in 1.0 to 2.5 mg/d, and 1- to 3-year-old children require 0.5 to 1.5 mg/d. The safe and effective intake for infants up to 5 months of age is 0.1 to 0.5 mg/d, and 0.2 to 1.0 mg/d is recommended for infants 6 to 12 months old.

Specific drug-related nursing considerations Monitor children regularly for signs of fluorosis. If fluorosis is suspected, advise the parent to withhold supplements and seek a full dental examination. Also, monitor women receiving chronic fluoride therapy for fluorosis, especially for decreases in kidney function.

Encourage individuals taking oral fluoride supplements to avoid consuming antacids within 1 hour before or after the fluoride dose to decrease the risk of interaction.

Instruct individuals using topical applications of fluoride for the prevention of dental caries to maintain the application for at least 5 minutes to achieve the desired effects. In other words, a session of brushing the teeth with a fluoridated dentifrice should last at least 5 minutes, or the mouth should not be rinsed for at least 5 minutes after brushing. Similarly, use of a fluoride mouthwash requires a 5-minute rinsing session or a delay of at least 5 minutes after using the mouthwash before rinsing the mouth, eating, or drinking. Some fluoride mouthwashes are formulated so they can be swallowed after swishing; teach the patient to confirm with the child's dental care provider whether it is appropriate to swallow the mouthwash.

Instruct parents of young children never to administer more than the prescribed dose of a fluoride supplement to a child. Tell the parent to reassess fluoride supplementation needs if the family moves or if a change in water supply (e.g., from well to municipal water) occurs.

The primary dietary source of fluoride is drinking water. Although most foods contain small amounts of flouride, seafood, fish, fish products, and tea leaves are the highest food sources.

CONCEPT REVIEW

Fluorine is metabolically active as fluoride, which is commonly used to prevent dental caries. It is used in topical and oral dosage forms. The usual source of fluoride is drinking water, and the target level is one part per million.

A decrease in fluoride intake is linked to tooth decay, especially in children. Toxicity (fluorosis, fluoritosis) in children leads to weak, chalky enamel with a mottled appearance. In adults toxicity can cause bone changes in the spine and knees.

IODINE

The heaviest element known as essential for human life, iodine plays a role only in the thyroid hormone system.

Pharmacotherapeutics Iodide deficiency is classically associated with the formation of a **goiter,** or an enlarged thyroid gland. As the iodine deficiency decreases iodide stores, less thyroxine (T_4) is produced. This leads to decreased serum T_4 levels. This decrease stimulates increased production of thyroid-stimulating hormone (TSH). The increased serum levels of TSH stimulate hypertrophy of the thyroid gland. With its increased size, the gland attempts to improve capture of iodide ions from the blood. The size of the goiter reflects the amount

of tissue necessary to achieve a new level of homeostasis and adequate T_4 production.

Foods and drugs that stimulate the formation of goiters are known as **goitrogenics.** Bromide and thiocyanate compete with iodide for entrance into the gland. Cassava contains cyanogen glucosides, which are metabolized to thiocyanates and can cause goiter formation. Lithium inhibits thyroid hormone release, decreasing serum T_4 levels and stimulating goiter development. Cabbage, kale, cauliflower, broccoli, rutabaga, turnip, brussel sprouts, and mustard greens contain the chemical goitrin, and individuals highly dependent on these vegetables in their diets are prone to goiter formation.

In addition to goiter formation, several other signs and symptoms are common to iodide deficiency. Complaints of cold intolerance, weight gain, somnolence, dry skin, and constipation are common. The clients frequently are seen with bradycardia, hyporeflexia, increased serum cholesterol levels, decreased glucose absorption, or anemia. If the deficiency occurs during the prenatal period or childhood years, a syndrome known as **cretinism** may occur. Children with cretinism are likely to suffer from mental deficiency, spasticity, goiter, deafmutism, and dysarthralgia. With the squat, shortened stature common to cretinism, these children often walk with a shuffling gait. The longer a child lives with an iodide-deficient intake, the more profound these problems become and the less likely they can be reversed. For this reason, newborns in the United States are routinely screened for hypothyroidism.[2,3,15]

Clients who depend on IV nutrition generally do not require active iodine supplementation. In these individuals iodide needs are met incidentally from two sources: iodide as a trace contaminant in several IV nutrient solutions and iodine absorbed through the skin from topical germicides used to maintain IV catheter sites. The precise amounts of iodine obtained from these sources are not known.

Pharmacokinetics Dietary iodines are converted to iodide for absorption. (Iodide is a two-part compound of iodine.) Although iodide ions can be absorbed throughout the GI tract, most of the absorption occurs in upper bowel. Iodide selectively concentrates in salivary glands, thyroid glands, and gastric glands. Lesser amounts are found in the mammaries, ovaries, placenta, and skin. The iodide concentration in the thyroid gland may reach 40 to 50 times the plasma iodide concentrations.

Iodide intake in the form of the thyroid hormones, T_4 and triiodothyronine (T_3), does not require digestion of the hormone before absorption. Thyroid hormones are absorbed from the GI tract intact.

Iodide ions are taken up by the thyroid follicular cells, which contain thyroglobulin and thyroid peroxidase enzyme. The iodide binds to the tyrosyl residues within the thyroglobulin, forming monoiodothyroglobulin (MIT) and diiodothyroglobulin (DIT). Thyroid peroxidase acts on MIT and DIT, coupling the phenolic side chains to form T_3 (MIT plus DIT) and T_4 (DIT plus DIT). They are stored in the thyroid storage fluid, known as **colloid,** until needed.

Mechanism of action Although T_3 is far more potent, T_4 is more abundant and is believed the workhorse of the thyroid hormones. The thyroid hormones play a key role in energy metabolism and contribute to normal growth and development.

Pharmaceutics Radioactive iodines are used to treat hyperthyroidism. Information on these drugs is presented in Chapter 41.

Undesired clinical responses Persistent plasma iodine levels greater than 20 μg/ml are associated with the Wolff-Chaikoff effect. Paradoxically, rather than causing an increase in T$_4$ levels, organification of iodine is blocked, and goiter formation may occur. Iodine overload is a relatively recent phenomenon seen in developed countries. Incidental iodine administration due to widespread use of iodized salt for human and feed animal consumption, the addition of iodine-containing compounds to food products, and the use of iodine-containing germicides in the sterilization of food preparation equipment has led to significant increases in the amounts of iodine consumed. Iodine overload can lead to, or exacerbate, acne in adolescents and young adults.

Iodine toxicity, in the form of elevated thyroid hormone levels, occurs in persons with Graves' disease. The general signs and symptoms of hyperthyroidism include weight loss, hyperactivity, heat intolerance, tachycardia, excessive sweating, diarrhea, tremors, decreased serum cholesterol levels, increased glucose absorption, and negative nitrogen balance. Extremely elevated serum levels of thyroid hormones are associated with the development of thyrotoxicosis or thyroid storms.

Drug-drug interactions Clients requiring lithium therapy should receive regular assessment of their thyroid status. Because of the goitrogenic properties of thiocyanate, individuals who require prolonged therapy with nitroprusside may develop mild thyroid deficiencies.

Prolonged use of iodinated glycerol or potassium iodide solutions causes depression of thyroid hormone release in some individuals. Elderly clients appear to carry a higher risk for this interaction.

Life-span considerations The daily iodide requirement for adults is 150 μg, which is easily met in the United States through the use of iodized salt. This requirement is increased during growth phases such as pregnancy, lactation, and adolescence. Clients with iodine-deficiency goiter require a higher dose until the deficiency state has been reversed.

Specific drug-related nursing considerations When assessing an individual with a goiter, enlarged thyroid gland, or signs and symptoms of hypothyroidism, obtain a complete dietary and drug history. The intake of goitrogenic substances and the intake of excess iodine must be ruled out.

Seafood is the best natural source of iodine, with oceanic seafood providing more than freshwater fish. Vegetables, meats, eggs, dairy products, breads, and cereals contain fair amounts. Fruits are very low in iodine content. The primary dietary source of iodine in the United States is iodized salt, which contains 1 mg of iodide in every 10 g of salt.[2] Drinking water and homegrown vegetables provide variable amounts of iodide, depending on the soil content in the area. Encourage individuals who use no table salt and those who use nontraditional salt sources (e.g., "sea salt") to review their diet with a

qualified nutritionist to determine whether they are consuming adequate iodine.

CONCEPT REVIEW

Iodine, the heaviest element essential for human life, is important in the thyroid hormone system. T$_3$ and especially T$_4$ play key roles in energy metabolism, growth, and development.

Goiter is the classic sign of thyroid deficiency. Deficiency in the prenatal period or childhood can lead to cretinism.

Toxic levels of iodine are associated with Wolff-Chaikoff effect. Elevated thyroid hormone levels may lead to thyrotoxicosis or thyroid storm.

MOLYBDENUM

The first human molybdenoenzyme, xanthine oxidase, was recognized as requiring molybdenum in 1953.

Pharmacotherapeutics Molybdenum deficiency has never been reported in humans consuming oral diets. It does occur in clients receiving long-term molybdenum-poor TPN. Epidemiologic data associate low molybdenum intake with an increased incidence of esophageal cancer. Animal model studies suggest that molybdate-deficient diets can lead to impaired urate clearance, growth retardation, shortened life expectancy, renal xanthine calculi, and decreased flavoenzyme activity. Reports on children receiving molybdenum-poor diets link a deficient intake with intolerance to sulfur-containing amino acids, dislocated ocular lenses, seizures, and mental retardation.[2,18,19]

Mechanism of action Molybopterin acts as a cofactor in several oxidation-reduction reactions. As a cofactor to aldehyde oxidase, molybopterin plays a role in the detoxification of pyrimidines, purines, and pteridines. Working with sulfite oxidase, molybopterin participates in methionine and cystine metabolism. As a component of the xanthine oxidase system, molybopterin is necessary to metabolize xanthine and hypoxanthine to uric acid.

Pharmaceutics Molybdenum is available as a parenteral solution for IV administration. The solution contains 25 μg/ml molybdenum as 46 μg/ml ammonium molybdate tetrahydrate.

Molybdenum needs in clients receiving parenteral nutrition are not clearly established. Not all clinicians agree that molybdenum should be included in any but the longest term parenteral nutrition therapies. The Committee on Clinical Issues in Health and Disease of the American Society of Clinical Nutrition recommends that adults receiving parenteral nutrition receive 100 to 200 μg of molybdenum. The pediatric subcommittee further recommends that pediatric clients receiving parenteral nutrition therapy receive 0.25 μg/kg/d. No differentiation is made between term and premature infants.

Undesired clinical responses Molybdenum does not appear to have any direct toxic effects in humans. It may, however, contribute to secondary copper deficiency through competition for absorption sites, and most of the indications of molybdenum toxicity can be traced to secondary copper deficiency. The presence of increased serum molybdenum levels and normal copper levels has been linked to high serum uric acid levels and the development of gout. Increased plasma molybdenum levels occur during liver disease. The significance of this increase in unclear.

Drug-drug interactions Tungsten is a molybdenum antagonist. In addition, because of its relationship with xanthine oxidase function, it is possible that molybdenum levels affect the clearance of the methylxanthine drugs such as theophylline. As yet, however, no reports of such an interaction have surfaced in the literature.

Life-span considerations The safe and effective dietary intake of molybdenum for an adult is 75 to 250 μg/d. Infants up to 12 months of age should consume 15 to 40 μg/d. The safe and effective dietary intake for children is 25 to 150 μg/d.

Specific drug-related nursing considerations Assess clients receiving long-term parenteral nutrition therapy regularly for molybdenum deficiency and consider them as candidates for molybdenum supplementation. Assess individuals who have an apparent copper deficiency despite adequate oral intake for excessive molybdenum intake. Do not add molybdenum to parenteral nutrition formulas unless copper is also present in the solution. Because molybdenum excretion is closely linked to renal function, monitor clients with renal failure closely.

Meats are the best source of dietary molybdenum. Grains and legumes are good alternate sources. Supplementation of molybdenum is probably not necessary in individuals consuming an oral diet.

CONCEPT REVIEW

Molybdenum is important in several oxidation-reduction reactions in the body. Molybdenum deficiency has been reported primarily in association with administration of tungsten, a molybdenum antagonist. Molybdenum may not have any direct toxic effects. However, it can contribute to secondary copper deficiency.

SUMMARY

Trace minerals, or microminerals, are important in the functions of the human body. In most instances these elements are ingested in an oral diet. However, clients receiving long-term TPN are at risk for deficiencies. Many of the trace minerals are so closely related that a deficiency or excess in one affects others.

REFERENCES

1. Baumgartner, T.G. (1993). Trace elements in clinical nutrition. *Nutrition in Clinical Practice, 8,* 251–263.
2. Williams, S. (1991). *Basic nutrition and diet therapy* (9th ed.). St. Louis: Mosby–Year Book.
3. Davis, J., & Sherer, K. (1993). *Applied nutrition and diet therapy for nurses* (2nd ed.). Philadelphia: W.B. Saunders.
4. Beard, J.L. (1994). Iron deficiency: Assessment during pregnancy and its importance in pregnant adolescents. *American Journal of Clinical Nutrition, 59,* 5025–5105.
5. Bettigole, R. (1992). Drugs acting on the blood and blood-forming organs. In C.M. Smith & A.M. Reynard (Eds.), *Textbook of pharmacology* (pp. 784–789). Philadelphia: W.B. Saunders.
6. Roberts, J.R. (1993). Assessing iron poisoning. *Emergency Medicine, 25*(10), 6.
7. Data Pharmaceutics, Inc. (1993). *1993 physicians' genRx.* Smithtown, NY: Author.
8. Food and Nutrition Board of the National Research Council. (1989). *Recommended dietary allowances* (10th ed.). Washington, D.C.: National Academy Press.
9. Engstrom, J.L., & Sittler, C.P. (1994). Nurse-midwifery management of iron-deficiency anemia during pregnancy. *Journal of Nurse Midwifery, 39*(Suppl.), 20S–34S.
10. Anderson, R. (1988). Selenium, chromium, and manganese. In M. Shils & V. Young (Eds.), *Modern nutrition in health and disease* (7th ed.; pp. 268–277). Philadelphia: Lea & Febiger.
11. Keenan, J.M., & Morris, D.H. (1993). How to make sure your older patients are getting enough zinc. *Geriatrics, 48*(10), 57–58, 63–65.
12. Dickerson, J.W. (1993). Ascorbic acid, zinc, and wound healing. *Journal of Wound Care, 2,* 350–353.
13. Solomon, N. (1988). Zinc and copper. In M. Shils and V. Young (Eds.), *Modern nutrition in health and disease* (7th ed.; pp. 238–262). Philadelphia: Lea & Febiger.
14. Solomons, N.W. (1991). Zinc. In T.G. Baumgartner (Ed.), *Clinical guide to parenteral micronutrition* (2nd ed.; pp. 215–234). (Available from Lyphomed, Division of Fujisawa, USA.)
15. Copstead, L.C. (1995). *Perspectives on pathophysiology.* Philadelphia: W.B. Saunders.
16. Levander, O. (1988). Selenium, chromium, and manganese. In M. Shils and V. Young (Eds.), *Modern nutrition in health and disease* (7th ed.; pp. 263–267). Philadelphia: Lea & Febiger.
17. Lockitch, G., Wong, L.T.K., Davidson, P., Riddell, D., & Massing, B. (1990). Cardiomyopathy associated with non-endemic selenium deficiency in a caucasian adolescent. *American Journal for Clinical Nutrition, 5*(2), 72–77.
18. Escott-Stump, S. (1992). *Nutrition and diagnosis—Related care* (3rd ed.). Baltimore: Williams & Wilkins.
19. Linder, M.C. (Ed.). (1991). *Nutritional biochemistry and metabolism: With clinical applications* (2nd ed.). East Norwalk, CT: Appleton & Lange.

BIBLIOGRAPHY

Cerrato, P.L. (1993). OTC interactions: Vitamins and minerals. *RN Magazine, 56,* 28–33.
Drown, D.J. (1993). Serum iron: A new cardiovascular risk factor? *Progress in Cardiovascular Nursing, 8*(1), 46–47.
Nurses' Drug Alert. (1994). Iron overload and the CNS. *Nurses' Drug Alert, 18*(5), 34–35.
Scholl, T.O., & Hediger, M.L. (1994). Anemia and iron deficiency anemia: Compilation of data on pregnancy outcome. *American Journal of Clinical Nutrition, 59,* 4925–5015.
Shenkin, A. (1993). Trace elements and acute illness. *Care of the Critically Ill, 9*(2), 60–63.
Trujillo, E.B. (1993). Effects of nutritional status on wound healing. *Journal of Vascular Nursing, 11,* 12–18.
Wells, J. (1994). At the front line of care: The importance of nutrition in wound management. *Professional Nurse, 9,* 525–526, 528–530.

Agents Affecting the Volume and Ion Content of Body Fluids

MARTHA A. SPIES

⊛ **Alterations in Fluid Volume and Osmolality**

LEARNING OBJECTIVES:

Discuss the way fluids move into and out of cells and between vascular and interstitial spaces.

Describe isotonic fluid imbalances and how they occur.

Describe osmolar fluid imbalances and how they occur.

Explain the body's response to blood loss.

KEY TERMS:

Active transport, filtration pressure, osmosis, osmolality, isotonic, hypertonic, hypotonic, fluid volume excess, fluid volume deficit, hyperosmolar imbalance, hypoosmolar imbalance, diffusion, extracellular fluid, intracellular fluid, hydrostatic pressure, oncotic pressure

⊛ **Alterations in Electrolyte Balance**

LEARNING OBJECTIVES:

Describe briefly the regulation of electrolyte balance.

Identify the characteristics and causes of major electrolyte imbalances.

⊛ **Alterations in Acid-Base Balance**

LEARNING OBJECTIVES:

Describe how the body regulates acid-base balance.

Identify the characteristics and causes of respiratory acidosis and respiratory alkalosis.

Identify the characteristics and causes of metabolic acidosis and metabolic alkalosis.

⊛ **Nursing Considerations**

LEARNING OBJECTIVES:

Explain the importance of assessment of fluid, electrolyte, and acid-base balance.

Identify some common nursing diagnoses associated with fluid, electrolyte, and acid-base balance.

Discuss nursing interventions involved in fluid, electrolyte, and acid-base balance disturbances.

Describe the administration of blood or blood components.

KEY TERMS:

Infiltration, phlebitis, fluid volume overload

⊛ **Fluid Replacement**

LEARNING OBJECTIVES:

List the functions of crystalloid, colloid, and blood products.

Identify and discuss the characteristics of and nursing considerations for prototype crystalloid solutions.

Discuss the characteristics and functions of plasma expanders.

Discuss the characteristics and functions of protein products.

Describe potential complications of blood product administration.

Develop a plan of care for a client requiring fluid replacement.

KEY TERMS:

Plasmapheresis, neutropenia

⊛ **Agents Used With Alterations in Electrolyte Balance**

LEARNING OBJECTIVES:

Discuss the purpose and nursing considerations associated with potassium supplementation.

Discuss nursing considerations for agents used for hyperkalemia.

Describe nursing considerations associated with magnesium supplementation.

⊛ **Agents Used With Alterations in Acid-Base Balance**

LEARNING OBJECTIVES:

Discuss the purpose of agents used with alterations in acid-base balance.

Develop a plan of care for a client requiring treatment for acid-base imbalance.

CONCEPTS AND TERMS TO REVIEW

Review the following terms: osmosis, osmolality, hypertonic, hypotonic, hyperosmolar imbalance, and hypoosmolar imbalance.

Review Chapter 35 for an overview of the renal system.

Read the section on blood composition and fluid and electrolyte physiology in an anatomy-physiology textbook.

Read the section on acid-base balance in a medical-surgical textbook.

Review Chapter 34 for information on blood components.

The general pharmacologic effects of products discussed in this chapter are to replace the deficient elements and thus to restore normal physiologic function. Therapeutically, these products are used when the client cannot adapt to sudden or excessive losses of fluids, electrolytes, acids, bases, blood, or blood components. Fluid replacement products (e.g., intravenous [IV] fluids and blood products) increase the circulating blood volume. Electrolyte replacements reverse the adverse effects of any electrolyte deficits. The administration of acidifying or alkalinizing agents restores the serum pH to normal and fosters normal cellular mechanisms. When a client experiences an excess serum level of an electrolyte, pharmacologic measures to reduce the elevated serum level can be administered.

ALTERATIONS IN FLUID VOLUME AND OSMOLALITY

Regulation of Body Fluids

In the human body fluid is contained in two major fluid portions: **extracellular fluid (ECF)** and the **intracellular fluid (ICF).** ECF is divided between the intravascular and the interstitial spaces. The fluid in the interstitial space bathes the cells; and the cell membrane determines the movement of fluid into and out of each cell. Fluids move freely between the ECF and the ICF to transport necessary nutrients to cells and to carry waste products away from cells. Most fluid is obtained from the intake of water and other beverages and food. The kidneys provide the primary route of excretion of water; aldosterone and antidiuretic hormone (ADH) regulate fluid and electrolyte balance.

Capillaries comprise the site of water movement between the vascular and interstitial spaces. Fluid movement into and out of capillaries is determined by a balance between two opposing pressures.[1] The first of these pressures is **hydrostatic pressure,** which is determined by arterial and venous pressures. Hydrostatic pressure tends to push water, electrolytes, and other solutes out of the capillary. The other pressure is **oncotic pressure,** which is largely determined by serum proteins, especially albumin. Because protein molecules are large and cannot move out of the capillary, they hold water in the capillary. Hydrostatic pressure is higher on the arterial than the

venous side of the capillary bed; oncotic pressure stays constant throughout the capillary bed. The net effect of these forces is called **filtration pressure.** Filtration pressure causes fluids and solutes to move. Because of net filtration pressure, fluid and electrolytes tend to leave the vascular space on the arterial side and return to the vascular space on the venous side of the capillary bed.

Fluids and solutes can move into and out of cells by the processes of diffusion, active transport, and osmosis. **Diffusion** is the passive movement of solutes across a semipermeable membrane from a site of greater concentration of the solute to a site of lesser concentration. **Active transport** is the movement of solutes across a membrane against a concentration gradient (i.e., from an area of lesser concentration of the solute to an area of greater concentration). Active transport requires the use of energy. **Osmosis** is the movement of water across a semipermeable membrane. The water moves from an area of lesser concentration of solutes to an area of greater concentration.

The concentration of intravascular fluids is referred to as serum **osmolality.** Normal serum osmolality is 275 to 295 mOsm/kg. The principal solutes that contribute to serum osmolality are sodium, glucose, and urea. Serum sodium accounts for 97% to 98% of the serum osmolality.[2] The concentration of fluids, or tonicity, on two sides of a semipermeable membrane can be the same **(isotonic),** resulting in no net movement of fluid from one side to the other as a result of osmosis. In contrast, the concentration of fluids on one side can be more concentrated than on the other; the more concentrated side is referred to as **hypertonic.** For example, the intracellular concentration of fluids may be greater than the interstitial concentration. The osmotic pressure on the more concentrated intercellular side draws water from the interstitial side. This results in an increase in volume in the first compartment, which in this example results in cellular swelling.[3] In the previous example the lesser concentrated interstitial space is described as **hypotonic.** A hypotonic fluid is pulled into more concentrated sites, resulting in shrinkage or contraction of the hypotonic space. Once the concentration of fluids on the two sides of the semipermeable membrane becomes isotonic, the movement of water by osmosis stops.

Isotonic Fluid Imbalances

An isotonic fluid imbalance occurs when fluid and electrolytes or other solutes are gained or lost from the body in equal or isotonic proportions. The gain of isotonic fluids is called **fluid volume excess.** Examples of causes of fluid volume excess are heart failure and renal failure.[4] The excess fluid escapes from the vascular space and becomes trapped in the interstitial space as edema. Diuretics are often given to reduce this edema (see Chapter 36).

The imbalance resulting from the loss of isotonic fluids is called **fluid volume deficit.** The most common causes of fluid volume deficit are gastrointestinal (GI) losses, especially vomiting and diarrhea. Fluid is lost from the vascular space, and this loss results in decreased circulating blood volume. The client may experience hypotension, tachycardia, and decreased urinary output. The usual treatment is fluid and electrolyte replacement by the oral or IV administration of isotonic fluids.

Osmolar Fluid Imbalances

Fluid and electrolytes are not always lost in isotonic proportions. This results in alterations in the client's serum osmolality. When the client experiences an alteration that results in decreased fluids in proportion to electrolytes and solutes, the fluid in the vascular space becomes more concentrated, a **hyperosmolar imbalance.** This imbalance occurs when fluids are lost in excess of electrolyte loss or when the client gains electrolytes or other solutes. An example of fluid loss in excess of electrolyte loss occurs with a deficiency of ADH hormone. This produces an alteration called *diabetes insipidus.* The treatment of diabetes insipidus usually includes the administration of ADH. The administration of hyperosmolar tube feeding or total parenteral nutrition (TPN) formulas can produce a gain of solutes (see Chapter 75).

Assessment data associated with a hyperosmolar imbalance include increases in serum osmolality (>295 mOsm/kg), hematocrit (>54% males, >47% females), blood urea nitrogen (BUN; >20 mg/dl), and serum sodium (>145 mEq/L). These increases occur because the fluid in the vascular space becomes more concentrated. The client may experience thirst and dry mucous membranes. The common treatment for hyperosmolar imbalance (with hypernatremia) includes the IV administration of hypotonic fluids.[1]

When the client experiences an alteration in which fluid is retained in excess of electrolytes or when solutes are lost more rapidly than fluids, a **hypo-osmolar imbalance** occurs. In these situations the fluid in the vascular space becomes less concentrated. Causes of hypo-osmolar imbalance include excess secretion of ADH syndrome (of inappropriate antidiuretic hormone [SIADH], compulsive water drinking, and the loss of sodium in excess of fluids as a result of diuretic therapy.

Assessment data associated with hypo-osmolar imbalance include decreases in serum osmolality (<275 mOsm/kg), hematocrit (<40% males, <37% females), BUN (<10 mg/dl), and serum sodium (<135 mEq/L). If the serum sodium level becomes extremely low (<125 mEq/L) or suddenly decreases, the client may experience nausea, malaise, seizures, or coma.[1] Treatment includes restriction of electrolyte-free water intake for mild imbalances and the administration of hypertonic saline solutions for more severe imbalances.[3]

Alterations in Blood and Blood Components

Any blood loss results in a decreased hemoglobin count (<13.5 g/dl males, <12 g/dl females), hematocrit, and red blood cells count (RBCs), $<4.2 \times 10^6$ μl males, $<3.6 \times 10^6$ μl females). Clients may experience fatigue and pallor. If the loss of blood is severe or sudden, the client may experience hypotension, tachycardia, and postural hypotension because of decreased circulating blood volume. Treatment includes the administration of iron products when the blood loss is chronic

and the client is hemodynamically stable. See Chapter 73 for discussion of iron-containing products. If the degree of blood loss is severe, RBCs or plasma expanders can be administered.[5]

Clients who are malnourished or who have an abnormal loss of protein such as those with burns or nephrotic syndrome may require products containing protein, especially albumin. Decreased levels of serum protein (<6 g/dl) and albumin (<3.8 g/dl) can indicate both the need for administration of a protein product and the client's response to the product.

Clotting is altered with many conditions (e.g., hemophilia or liver disease). Diagnostic tests used to determine alterations in the clotting process include prothrombin time (PT; normal, 10 to 14 seconds, or 100%), partial thromboplastin time (PTT; normal, 30 to 45 seconds), platelets (150,000 to 350,000/mm³), and measurement of specific clotting factors. Disorders of clotting are treated by the administration of products containing components needed for clotting (e.g., platelets and specific clotting factors).

CONCEPT REVIEW

Fluids and solutes move in and out of cells by diffusion, active transport, and osmosis.

The principal solutes that contribute to serum osmolality are sodium, glucose, and urea.

Isotonic fluid imbalance occurs when fluid or solutes are gained or lost in equal proportions.

Osmolar fluid imbalance occurs when the concentration of vascular fluid becomes abnormal.

Fluid and solute imbalance can also involve blood and blood components, including serum protein and clotting factors.

ALTERATIONS IN ELECTROLYTE BALANCE

Regulation of Electrolyte Balance

Electrolytes are substances that break into ions when placed in solution. Ions are positively or negatively charged. The most abundant electrolytes in the ECF are sodium, chloride, and bicarbonate. The most abundant electrolytes in the ICF are potassium, phosphate, and magnesium. In healthy individuals the primary sources for electrolytes are food and liquids. The kidney is involved in precise regulation of serum levels of electrolytes through the processes of diffusion, filtration, and active transport. The effect of aldosterone in the kidney is to regulate the reabsorption of sodium and the excretion of potassium.[2] Aldosterone stimulation causes renal retention of sodium, resulting in passive retention of water. Another role of the kidney in electrolyte balance is to act as the only normal route of loss for potassium and magnesium. Other substances can be involved in the regulation of electrolyes (e.g., parathormone and vitamin D regulate phosphorus and calcium balances).

Sodium

The normal serum sodium level is 135 to 145 mEq/L. Because sodium is the major cation in the ECF, one of its major functions is maintenance of normal serum osmolality and volume. Changes in serum osmolality can affect ICF volume, which may result in alterations in cell function, especially in the nervous system. Sodium contributes to normal neuromuscular irritability by participating, along with potassium and calcium in the conduction of nerve impulses.[6] Sodium also contributes to acid-base balance by exchanging with hydrogen ions in the kidneys, allowing the excretion of hydrogen ions.[7]

Hypernatremia can result from the loss of water from the extracellular compartment or from the retention of sodium (e.g., water deprivation or in a client with diabetes insipidus). Both of these situations result in a serum sodium levels greater than 145 mEq/L. Because of increased serum osmolality, water is pulled from the ICF by osmosis, and cellular shrinkage occurs. The result of cellular shrinkage is most evident in altered neurologic function (i.e., lethargy, irritability, and disorientation).

Hyponatremia can result from the gain of water into the extracellular compartment or from the loss of sodium. Conditions associated with the occurrence of hyponatremia include SIADH, use of thiazide diuretics in combination with low-salt diet, and GI losses of sodium in excess of water (vomiting, diarrhea, suction). The serum level is less than 135 mEq/L. Changes in serum sodium levels should be monitored closely. Symptoms of hyponatremia such as nausea and malaise appear at 125 mEq/L. When the serum sodium level reaches 110 to 115 mEq/L, seizures and coma may occur.[1] Treatment includes the administration of sodium-containing products such as IV fluids.

Potassium

Potassium is the major cation of the ICF; the normal serum level is 3.5 to 5.3 mEq/L. The major route of excretion for potassium is the kidney, so any decrease in renal function results in an elevated serum potassium level. The body has no strong conservation mechanism for potassium, so polyuria can result in hypokalemia. Potassium is involved in the muscle contraction and electric conduction in the heart. Potassium participates in the transmission of nerve impulses and the contraction of skeletal muscles by participating in provoking an action potential in excitable tissues.[8] Potassium has a role in acid-base balance and is exchanged for hydrogen ions in the kidneys and between the ICF and ECF.

Hyperkalemia is caused by any condition that decreases renal excretion of potassium, causes potassium to move out of the ICF, or increases the intake or availability of potassium. Acute or chronic renal failure is an important cause of hyperkalemia. Other causes include excessive administration of potassium supplements or use of salt substitutes that contain potassium and the use of potassium-sparing diuretics (see Chapter 36). In clients with hyperkalemia the serum level is greater than 5.3 mEq/L. A serum potassium level greater than 6 mEq/L is associated with cardiac effects such as peaked narrow T waves and shortened QT interval. Higher levels of 7 to 8 mEq/L are associated with ventricular arrhythmias and cardiac arrest.[1] Weakness, paresthesias, nausea, abdominal cramping, and diarrhea also may occur. Treatment includes dietary restriction of potassium. In addition, dialysis and sodium polystyrene sulfonate (Kayexalate) can be used to remove potassium from the body.

Hypokalemia can be caused by the administration of potassium-losing diuretics; loss of GI contents by vomiting, suction, or diarrhea; lack of dietary intake; or steroid administration. In clients with hypokalemia the serum level is less than 3.5 mEq/L. With hypokalemia, the client may experience increased sensitivity to digitalis products, cardiac arrhythmias such as atrial or ventricular premature contractions, paresthesias, or decreased bowel motility. The treatment includes oral or IV potassium replacement.

Magnesium

Magnesium is found primarily in bone and in the intracellular space. The normal serum magnesium level is 1.5 to 2.5 mEq/L. Magnesium is eliminated by the kidneys and the intestines. It participates in metabolic functions, acting as an intracellular enzyme and contributing to carbohydrate and protein metabolism. It also affects neuromuscular and smooth muscle function.

Hypermagnesemia can be caused by any condition that results in decreased excretion of magnesium or excessive intake of magnesium. Common causes are renal failure and administration of antacids containing magnesium. In this alteration the magnesium level is greater than 2.5 mEq/L. The client may experience hypotension, flushed skin, hypoactive deep tendon reflexes, respiratory depression, or cardiac arrhythmias. Treatment includes restriction of magnesium intake, so sources present in food and drugs must be identified and limited. Adequate renal function must be verified before the administration of any oral or IV drug containing magnesium.[1] Dialysis may be used to lower the serum magnesium level.

Hypomagnesemia can be caused by any situation that reduces intake of magnesium or results in increased loss of magnesium. Common causes include malnutrition, especially that associated with chronic alcoholism, and GI losses of magnesium with vomiting, suction, or diarrhea. The serum level in clients with hypomagnesemia decreases below 1.5 mEq/L. The client may experience hyperactive deep tendon reflexes, tetany with positive Chvostek's and Trousseau's signs, and cardiac arrhythmias. Treatment includes magnesium replacement through increased dietary sources or through administration of supplements.

Calcium

Most calcium in the body is found in bones and teeth. The normal serum calcium level is 4.0 to 5.5 mg/dl (2.1 to 2.6 mEq/L) of ionized calcium (i.e., the calcium that is not bound to elements such as albumin or anions in the serum. The normal total serum calcium level is 8.5 to 10.5 mg/dl (4.3 to 5.3 mEq/L). Calcium and phosphorus have an inverse relationship so that changes in the serum phosphorus level causes reciprocal changes in the serum calcium level.[1] For example, when the serum phophorus concentration increases as a result of decreased renal secretion in a client with renal failure, the serum calcium level decreases. Calcium contributes to bone structure and strength and participates in the coagulation process. It is important to the transmission of nerve impulses and the contraction of muscles.[6]

Hypercalcemia can occur when there is increased absorption of calcium from the GI tract or from the bone or when there is decreased renal excretion of calcium. Conditions that cause hypercalcemia include excessive intake of products containing calcium such as antacids; prolonged bed rest, which promotes the movement of calcium out of bones into the bloodstream; decreased serum phosphorus; malignant conditions that result in bone destruction (e.g., multiple myeloma); and therapy with thiazide diuretics, which potentiate the action of parathormone on the kidneys.[1] With hypercalcemia, the client's serum calcium level is greater than 5.5 mg/dl. The client can experience muscle weakness, decreased memory, confusion, cardiac arrhythmias, and renal stones. If the hypercalcemia is prolonged and is caused by elevated parathormone effect, calcium moves out of the bones, placing the client at increased risk for spontaneous fractures. Treatment includes administration of normal saline solution IV and loop diuretics to increase the urinary excretion of calcium.

Hypocalcemia can be caused by conditions in which there is an excessive loss of calcium or in which there is a decreased intake of calcium. Causes include hyperphosphatemia associated with renal failure and hypoparathyroidism. With hypocalcemia, the client's serum calcium level is less than 4 mg/dl. The client can experience paresthesias, hyperactive deep tendon reflexes, and tetany with positive Chvostek's and Trousseau's signs. If the hypocalcemia is prolonged, calcium moves out of the bones, placing the client at increased risk for spontaneous fractures. Calcium products are administered to elevate the serum level of calcium.

Phosphorus

Phosphorus is found primarily in the bone combined with calcium and within cells. Phosphorus found in the vascular compartment is primarily in the form of phosphates. The normal serum phosphate level is 2.5 to 4.5 mg/dl. Phosphorus is an important component of bones and teeth. It participates in metabolic processes and acid-base balance; contributes to the function of muscle, RBCs, and the nervous system; and facilitates energy storage and transfer.

Hyperphosphatemia can be caused by any condition that increases the intake of phosphorus or decreases the elimination of phosphorus. The major cause of hyperphosphatemia is renal failure because the kidneys provide the major route of excretion for phosphorus. In clients with hyperphosphatemia the serum level is greater than 4.5 mg/dl. In addition, tetany may be present because of the associated hypocalcemia. Treatment focuses on restricting dietary intake of phosphorus and administering phosphorus-binding antacids (e.g., aluminum hydroxide).

Hypophosphatemia can be caused by a shift of phosphorus from the ECF into the ICF. One situation that causes such a shift occurs when enteral or parenteral nutrition is started in the client after a period of malnutrition (refeeding syndrome). In clients with this syndrome, as anabolic processes begin, serum phosphorus moves into muscle cells, and the serum level decreases. Additional causes of hypophosphatemia include decreased absorption of phosphorus from the GI tract and increased renal losses. The serum phosphate level is less than 2.5 mg/dl in clients with hypophophatemia. The client can experience neurologic alterations such as irritability, weakness, and paresthesias, which can progress to seizures and coma. Treatment focuses on providing dietary sources and providing phosphorus supplements.

CONCEPT REVIEW

Electrolytes are substances that dissolve into ions in solutions. The most abundant electrolytes in ECF are sodium, chloride, and bicarbonate; the most abundant in ICF are potassium, phosphate, and magnesium. The kidneys help regulate electrolyte levels through diffusion, filtration, and active transport.

Sodium is the major cation in ECF and helps maintain normal serum osmolality and volume. Changes in serum osmolality can affect ICF volume, causing alterations in cell functions, particularly in the nervous system.

Potassium is the major cation in ICF. Potassium is involved in muscle contraction and electric conduction in the heart. The body has no strong conservation mechanism for potassium, so changes in renal function affect the serum potassium level.

Magnesium, found in bone and intracellular space, acts as an intracellular enzyme and contributes to carbohydrate and protein metabolism. It also affects neuromuscular and smooth muscle function. Common causes of hypermagnesemia are renal failure and ingestion of antacids containing magnesium.

Calcium contributes to bone and teeth structure and participates in the coagulation process. In both hypercalcemia and hypocalcemia, calcium moves out of bones, placing the client at risk for spontaneous fractures. Phosphorus is also an important component of bones and teeth. It is involved in metabolic processes and contributes to the function of muscle, RBCs, and the nervous system. Calcium and phosporus have an inverse relationship: changes in the serum phosphorus level cause reciprocal changes in the serum calcium level.

ALTERATIONS IN ACID-BASE BALANCE

Regulation of Acid-Base Balance

Chemical buffers take up or release hydrogen ions so that the serum pH is maintained in a narrow range of normal (normal arterial pH, 7.35 to 7.45) despite the constant addition of acid metabolites from cells and food. The bicarbonate–carbonic acid system, organic phosphates, proteins (e.g., hemoglobin), and bone are examples of chemical buffers.[4] Although these buffers react quickly to changes in serum pH, they provide only short-term regulation. The bicarbonate–carbonic acid system is an extracellular buffering system, and the other buffers are intracellular.

The lungs regulate the hydrogen ion level by eliminating CO_2. CO_2 is formed as hydrogen ions combine with bicarbonate to form carbonic acid, which then dissociates into water and CO_2 in the extracellular buffering system. Respiratory compensation is stimulated by metabolic acidosis or alkalosis. The lungs respond immediately to changes in CO_2 in the blood by altering the rate and depth of respirations, but the respiratory changes decline over a 1- to 2-day period.[1] The respiratory compensation is lessened if the client has a primary respiratory disease (e.g., chronic obstructive pulmonary disease [COPD]) because it may interfere with the changes in respiratory rate and depth necessary to restore normal pH.

The kidneys perform the slowest but most powerful of the processes involved in acid-base regulation. The kidneys reabsorb and regenerate bicarbonate.[1] The kidneys also secrete hydrogen ions. The renal compensation occurs over a period of days, but the kidneys demonstrate long-term maintenance of the compensatory changes. When renal function is impaired (e.g., with renal failure), the compensatory mechanisms are weakened or absent.

Alterations in Acid-Base Balance

Respiratory acidosis Respiratory acidosis results from any condition that decreases alevolar ventilation, leading to CO_2 retention.[4] Common conditions associated with respiratory acidosis are COPD and neuromuscular diseases that interfere with respiratory rate and depth. The client with respiratory acidosis can have a decreased arterial pH of less than 7.35 and an arterial CO_2 level greater than 45 mmHg. In addition, the client may experience confusion and dizziness if the changes are acute. The acidotic state stimulates chemical buffers and renal mechanisms. Compensatory mechanisms include an increase in the amount of systemic bicarbonate. Treatment focuses on supporting the client's respiratory efforts to increase the elimination of CO_2.

Respiratory alkalosis Respiratory alkalosis occurs when alveolar hyperventilation causes the excessive loss of CO_2.[6] Hyperventilation can occur when a client is anxious, when ventilator settings result in overbreathing, during periods of hypoxemia (e.g., in high altitudes), or during periods of hypermetabolism (e.g., during a fever or with anemia). With respiratory alkalosis, the client's arterial pH increases above 7.45, and the arterial CO_2 decreases below 35 mmHg. The client may experience dizziness and paresthesias and may develop tetany caused by a decreased serum calcium level. Respiratory alkalosis often is short-lived and can be reversed when the client's hyperventilation is resolved. Treatment focuses on removing the cause of the hyperventilation.

Metabolic acidosis Metabolic acidosis occurs when the serum bicarbonate level is decreased because of loss of base, increased hydrogen ion levels, or the inability of kidneys to eliminate hydrogen ions.[4] Conditions that can cause metabolic acidosis include the abnormal loss of GI secretions containing bicarbonate (e.g., with diarrhea); diabetic ketoacidosis; lactic acidosis; poisoning with salicylates or methanol; and renal failure.[1] A decreased arterial pH level below 7.35 and a decreased serum bicarbonate level below 22 mEq/L are present with metabolic acidosis. The client may experience rapid, deep respirations as the lungs compensate for the decreased bicarbonate by blowing off CO_2. A reduction of CO_2 restores the normal relationship between bicarbonate and hydrogen ion levels. However, the body's ability to adapt to any further acid-base alterations is limited. If the acidosis continues, the client may become lethargic, confused, and even comatose. Treatment includes reversal of the initial cause of the acidosis (e.g., insulin is administered to the client with diabetic ketoacidosis). In some situations sodium bicarbonate is administered intravenously.

Metabolic alkalosis Metabolic alkalosis results from the accumulation of base or from loss of acid. Conditions that can cause metabolic alkalosis include loss of gastric secretions containing hydrochloric acid through vomiting or suction or hypokalemia caused by the administration of diuretics, especially loop and thiazide diuretics, or excessive mineralocorticoids.[1] (Hypokalemia causes excretion of hydrogen ions by the kidneys in exchange for potassium ions. The potassium ions are reabsorbed. Hydrogen ions move from the ECF to the ICF in exchange for potassium, which is moving to the vascular space to maintain the serum level.) In metabolic alkalosis, the client has an increased arterial pH greater than 7.45 and an increased bicarbonate level greater than 26 mEq/L. The client may experience depressed respiratory rate and depth, dizziness, paresthesias, and neuromuscular irritability. Treatment focuses on treating the underlying cause and replacing fluid volume, potassium, and chloride.

CONCEPT REVIEW

Chemical buffers act as short-term regulators of serum pH. The bicarbonate–carbonic acid system is an extracellular buffing system, whereas the other buffers are intracellular. The lungs also regulate the hydrogen ion level through elimination of CO_2. The kidneys are powerful, long-term regulators of acid-base balance, acting through reabsorption and regeneration of bicarbonate and through secretion of hydrogen ions. Acid-base regulation can be severely affected by pulmonary or kidney disorders.

Respiratory acidosis results from decreased alveolar ventilation leading to CO_2 retention. Respiratory alkalosis occurs when alveolar hyperventilation results in excessive loss of CO_2. Metabolic acidosis results from a decrease of serum bicarbonate or other base or through increased hydrogen ion levels. Metabolic alkalosis results from the loss of hydrogen irons or the accumulations of bicarbonate or other base.

⊞ NURSING CONSIDERATIONS

When administering drugs that affect fluid, electrolyte, or acid-base balance, perform a systematic assessment and formulate relevant nursing diagnoses, focusing on alterations in these areas to determine the continued need for the drug and whether it is safe to administer it. Planning, intervention, and evaluation complete the use of the nursing process so that appropriate care is given to prevent or intervene in clients with alterations in fluid, electrolyte, or acid-base balance.

Assessing A basic component of the nursing **health history** in the areas of fluid, electrolyte, and acid-base balance is to obtain information about medical conditions that place the client at risk for alterations. For example, vomiting or diarrhea, heart or renal failure, cirrhosis of the liver, major burns, or hemorrhage places clients at risk of fluid balance alterations. Certain drugs and treatments (e.g., diuretics and glucocorticoids, surgery, or GI suction or tube feedings) also place the client at risk. Changes in dietary intake, metabolic and endocrine function, or excretion place the client at risk for alterations in electrolyte balance. Conditions such as renal failure, COPD, and diabetes mellitus place the client at risk for alterations in acid-base balance (see box).

ASSESSMENT OF RISK FACTORS AND SUBJECTIVE CHANGES RELATED TO FLUID, ELECTROLYTE, AND ACID-BASE BALANCE

Risk Factors

1. Determine if the client has a history of heart or renal failure, cirrhosis of the liver, diabetes mellitus, chronic obstructive lung disease, or recent surgery.

2. Assess the quantity of alcohol consumed daily, weekly, monthly.

3. Ask if client is currently taking diuretics or glucocorticoids.

4. Determine if the client has any of the following: major burn, severe infection, vomiting, diarrhea, blood loss, gastrointestinal suction, or tube feeding.

Signs and Symptoms
Assess for the following:
• Recent, unexplained weight loss or weight gain
• Recent increase in thirst
• Change in amount or color of urine
• Swelling of feet and ankles
• Difficulty breathing
• Weakness, fatigue, or loss of coordination
• Dizziness when initially standing up
• Numbness or tingling in hands or feet
• Hand tremors or muscle cramps
• Heart palpitations
• Headaches
• Abdominal cramps
• Confusion
• Change in level of alertness
• Irritability or mood swings

Another important component of the nursing history is the presence of symptoms that indicate alterations in these areas (see box). For example, the client may relate a history of the loss of body fluids or a change in body weight. The family should be used as a source of data because some alterations can lead to changes in the client's cognitive function or emotional status. For any change, determine the onset, the severity, and the presence of any associated symptoms. All of these data help determine the extent of the imbalance.

The data relevant to fluid, electrolyte, and acid-base balance are found in every body system, so the **physical assessment** must be comprehensive (see on p. 1013). One isolated piece of information (e.g., a change in intake and output) is not sufficient to identify the presence of an alteration; you must look for patterns in the data. Monitor the client frequently. Early recognition of alterations facilitates treatment and prevents complications. To determine if a fluid imbalance exists, assess fluid intake and output, body weight, skin turgor, condition of mucous membranes, presence of thirst or edema, vital signs, and hand and neck vein filling. To determine if an alteration in electrolyte levels or acid-base balance exists, assess the client's level of consciousness and behavior, deep tendon reflexes, muscle strength, and activity tolerance.

Infants and children are at greater risk than adults for the development of fluid volume deficit. This age group has a larger percentage of total body water and of fluid in the extracellular compartment.[9] In addition, infants and children have a relatively larger body surface area than adults. Fluid losses occur more rapidly and produce fluid imbalances quickly. The volume of intake and output of an infant is approximately half that of the adult. Infants and children cannot concentrate urine as efficiently as adults, predisposing them to fluid volume deficit. Acid-base buffering mechanisms are less well deveoped at this age than in the adult, and infants and children tend to develop metabolic acidosis more easily.[9] Common medical conditions that predispose infants and children to fluid, electrolyte, and acid-base alterations include fevers, upper respiratory infections, and vomiting and diarrhea. Infants and small children are less able than adults to describe symptoms such as thirst or changes in sensation such as paresthesias. Therefore you must carefully monitor them for early changes indicating an imbalance such as listlessness, irritability, or changes in skin turgor, body weight, or urinary output.

Changes in physiologic function that accompany aging decrease the elderly adult's ability to avoid alterations in fluid, electrolyte, and acid-base balances. In addition, these changes lengthen the time it takes for the elderly individual to adapt. The elderly person is more at risk than younger adults for fluid volume deficit because of a decrease in total body water and a relatively larger extracellular volume than intracellular volume. In addition, the aging kidneys do not concentrate urine nor eliminate metabolic wastes as efficiently; as a result, the elderly individual is at greater risk for fluid volume deficit and metabolic acidosis. Because of decreased chest wall compliance, lung tissue elasticity, number of alevoli, and respiratory muscle strength, the elderly individual cannot eliminate CO_2 as efficiently. This limits the elderly person's ability to compen-

PHYSICAL ASSESSMENT FINDINGS ASSOCIATED WITH FLUID, ELECTROLYTE, AND ACID-BASE ALTERATIONS

Neuromuscular Findings
Muscle weakness
Flaccid paralysis
Hypoactive deep tendon reflexes
Hyperactive deep tendon reflexes
Positive Chvostek's and Trousseau's signs
Tetany
Seizures
Depression
Irritability
Lethargy
Confusion
Coma

Cardiovascular Findings
Distended neck veins
Irregular heart rhythm
Bradycardia
Tachycardia
Hypertension
Hypotension
Slow capillary refill
Slow capillary emptying

Respiratory Findings
Crackles in the lungs
Bradypnea
Tachypnea
Hyperventilation
Hypoventilation

Skin and Mucous Membrane and Extremity Findings
Edema (note location and severity)
Dry mucous membrane
Inelastic skin turgor

Gastrointestinal Findings
Diminished bowel sounds
Hyperactive bowel sounds
Vomiting
Diarrhea

Renal Findings
Oliguria
Polyuria
Dark urine

Body Temperature
Hyperthermia
Hypothermia

Body Weight
Weight loss >2% of total body weight
Weight gain >2% of total body weight

---

sate for metabolic alterations and predisposes him or her to respiratory acidosis. The aging skin becomes less able to accomplish body cooling. Because of decreased skin elasticity, skin turgor is not a reliable indicator of fluid balance.[10] The elderly individual does not recognize thirst easily. The drive to ingest fluids in the presence of fluid volume deficit or hyperosmolar fluid imbalance may be decreased, and the risk for hypernatremia is increased.[10]

Fluid, electrolyte, and acid-base balance affects many laboratory tests, so you must monitor test results. Correlate these results with the client's current status to help verify the presence of an alteration. Laboratory tests related to fluid balance include tests that depend on the vascular volume such as serum osmolality, hematocrit, sodium, and BUN. A complete blood count (CBC) and clotting studies such as PT and PTT help identify the need for the administration of blood or a blood component in the client with decreased circulating blood volume related to hemorrhage. Serum creatinine and BUN levels reflect renal function; increases in these levels may indicate an inability of the kidneys to excrete fluid, electrolytes, and elements involved in acid-base balance. Serum electrolyte levels are used to determine the presence of alterations in electrolyte balance. Tests on the urine (e.g., specific gravity, pH, osmolality, and electrolytes) are also important indicators of fluid,

electrolyte, and acid-base alterations. Arterial blood gas determinations measure the acid-base balance.

Diagnosing To formulate accurate nursing diagnoses in the areas of fluid, electrolyte, and acid-base alterations, you must identify patterns among the data obtained during the assessment phase. Nursing diagnoses common for clients with fluid, electrolyte, or acid-base alterations follow:

- Fluid volume deficit related to hyponatremia or decreased fluid intake.
- Fluid volume excess related to hypernatremia or excessive fluid intake.
- Decreased cardiac output related to decreased fluid volume.
- High risk for injury related to muscle weakness, dizziness.
- Knowledge deficit regarding treatment plan.

Planning Care of the client with fluid, electrolyte, or acid-base imbalances occurs on two levels. During the acute episode you must assist with the medical plan of care. Once the acute episode is stabilized, you must focus on preparing the client for self-care.

The pharmacologic management of alterations in fluid, electrolyte, and acid-base balances focuses on the replacement or supplementation of deficient fluids or electrolytes or correction of acid-base imbalances. In some instances drugs are used to lower abnormally elevated levels of electrolytes. To assist with this therapy, you must know why the product is prescribed and how to evaluate its effectiveness. In addition, you must monitor the client for the development of excessive levels of the product being given. For example, the range of normal serum potassium and magnesium levels is very narrow so that the client can quickly develop an elevated serum level during replacement therapy. When blood or blood products are administered, care must be exercised to prevent complications such as incompatibility reactions.

When the client has a condition that predisposes to fluid, electrolyte, and acid-base alteration, teach the client and family to identify situations that place the client at risk of further alterations. For example, the client with renal failure who develops vomiting or diarrhea can quickly develop electrolyte deficiencies or acid-base alterations. The client and family must be aware of how to prevent the development of such alterations and must know the assessment data that indicate an alteration has developed and must be reported. For example, the client with fluid alterations must know how to obtain an accurate daily weight.

Many clients have special dietary needs to provide deficient elements or to decrease excessive levels of elements. Clients must be taught the sources of the nutrients and the amounts to take. A dietician can be a valuable resource for dietary instruction.

The client receiving long-term drug therapy must understand how to take the drug safely and effectively. If IV fluids or infusion with blood or blood products is required, home health nursing care will be needed. The client or a caregiver may need instruction in the care of the IV site and measures to maintain patency of the IV device. The client or a caregiver also must be taught the indications and care of local complications at the IV site.

Outcomes identified during the planning phase reflect maintenance or improvement of the client's fluid, electrolyte, or acid-base balance and prevention of complications. Outcome statements must be individualized for each client. General outcomes include the following:

- The client's intake and output are balanced.
- The client's body weight is within 2 pounds of normal body weight.
- The client has elastic skin turgor, moist mucous membranes.
- The client is free of injury.
- The client's blood pressure is greater than 100/60, heart rate is less than 100 bpm, and the respiratory rate is less than 20 per minute.
- The client has normal laboratory test results (serum and urinary electrolytes, arterial blood gases, serum and urinary osmolality, hematocrit, and BUN).

Implementing Nursing interventions for the client receiving **IV fluids** focus on detecting and preventing complications. The most common local complications of IV therapy are infiltration and phlebitis. **Infiltration** is the inadvertent administration of IV fluids into the subcutaneous tissue around the vein. The client experiences pain proximal to the insertion site; swelling, pallor, and coolness of the skin are usually noted proximal to the insertion site. The flow of IV fluids usually slows down or stops from increased pressure in the interstitial space. A preventive measure for infiltration is providing secure taping to prevent movement of the IV catheter. When infiltration occurs, discontinue the IV infusion and restart it in another site.

Phlebitis is inflammation of the vein often caused by the contamination of the insertion site or the equipment or the administration of irritating substances such as potassium or antibiotics. The client experiences pain at the insertion site and along the course of the vein proximal to the insertion site. Redness, warmth, and swelling along the course of the vein can be noted. A preventive measure for phlebitis is the use of sterile technique during the insertion of the IV catheter and whenever any part of the system is disconnected or changed. Rotate the IV site at 48- to 72-hour intervals. Do not allow IV solutions to hang for longer than 24 hours. Select a vein of sufficient size and blood flow to dilute irritating IV solutions or additives. A filter can be used to remove bacteria or particulate matter. As with an infiltration, when phlebitis occurs, discontinue the infusion of the fluids and restart it in another site.

Systemic complications of IV therapy are not as common as the local complications. However, they are potentially more serious. **Fluid volume overload** is the most common systemic complication. It occurs when the IV fluids are given at a rate that exceeds the client's cardiac and renal adaptive capacity. The overload results in a rapid increase in the vascular volume, which can cause acute failure of the left side of the heart and pulmonary edema. When they occur, acute dyspnea, orthopnea, tachycardia, and tachypnea develop. To prevent fluid volume overload, monitor the rate of infusion of the IV fluids at least every hour to detect an inadvertent increase in the rate. An IV pump or controller may be used to regulate the rate more precisely, but its use does not eliminate the need for regular monitoring. If the rate of IV fluid administration falls behind schedule, increase the flow to the rate ordered. Do not exceed the ordered rate in an attempt to catch the fluids up to schedule.

Administration of blood or blood components is also an important function of the nurse. To prevent complications, exercise care in obtaining the correct blood product, identifying the correct client, using appropriate equipment to administer the product, infusing the product correctly, and monitoring for the appearance of complications. Before a transfusion is administered, obtain a sample of the client's blood to identify his or her blood type and to crossmatch the donor blood with that of the client. Note any history of prior blood transfusion reactions. Obtain vital signs in your pretransfusion assessment. They are used as a basis of comparison with results during the transfusion to identify the appearance of complications. Administer the transfusion through a catheter no smaller than No. 18 gauge to prevent hemolysis of RBCs and to allow larger cells to infuse freely. Use special tubing to provide adequate filtration of the blood and to allow the administration of normal saline solution before, during, or after the transfusion. (Only normal saline solution is used with a blood transfusion because other solutions cause hemolysis of RBCs when mixed with blood.)

In most cases a nurse must obtain the blood from the blood

bank. The nurse must check the requisition and blood bag label with laboratory personnel. In addition, he or she must verify the client's name, agency identification number, ABO blood type, and Rh group, the number of the donor, and the expiration date of the blood. This same information is checked by two nurses on the floor. Any discrepancy must be clarified before the blood is administered. The blood transfusion must be started within 30 minutes of the unit of blood's removal from refrigeration and must be finished within 4 hours to prevent bacterial growth and the deterioration of the cellular components.

During the transfusion monitor the client and the transfusion frequently. For the first 15 minutes administer the blood slowly, take the client's vital signs, and assess the client for the appearance of symptoms of a transfusion reaction. An **acute hemolytic reaction** occurs when ABO-incompatible blood is infused. The client may experience chills, back pain, and hypotension. Also possible is an **anaphylactic reaction** caused by infusion of immunoglobulin A (IgA) proteins to a client who has developed IgA antibodies. With an anaphylactic reaction, the client may experience anxiety, urticaria, wheezing, and tightness and pain in the chest. If these reactions occur, immediately stop the infusion because these are potentially fatal reactions. A **febrile, nonhemolytic reaction** is the most common transfusion reaction. It occurs when the client is sensitized to the donor's white blood cells (WBCs), platelets, or plasma proteins. Prevent this reaction by administering leukocyte-poor products, by using a leukocyte filter, or by administering acetaminophen, antihistamines, and steroids. If these measures fail, the client may experience chills and fever. A **mild allergic reacton** can also be experienced when the client is sensitive to the donor's plasma proteins. The client may experience flushing, itching, and urticaria. Administer antihistamines and steroids before the transfusion to moderate this reaction. Other reactions include circulatory overload and sepsis (Fig. 74–1).

Evaluating   To determine the effect of the administration of products used to treat fluid, electrolyte, or acid-base alterations, obtain data relevant to each of the identified outcomes. Assess the client's intake and output, body weight, skin turgor,

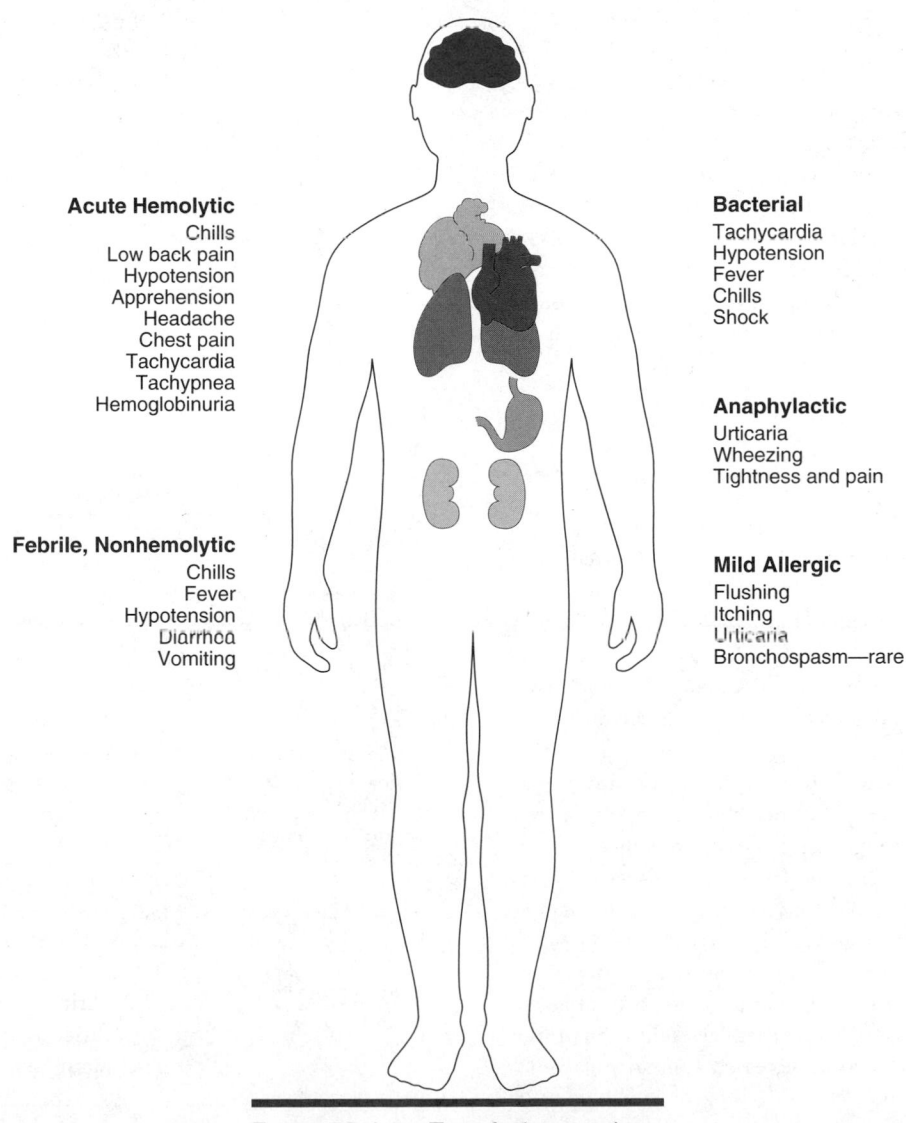

Acute Hemolytic
Chills
Low back pain
Hypotension
Apprehension
Headache
Chest pain
Tachycardia
Tachypnea
Hemoglobinuria

Febrile, Nonhemolytic
Chills
Fever
Hypotension
Diarrhea
Vomiting

Bacterial
Tachycardia
Hypotension
Fever
Chills
Shock

Anaphylactic
Urticaria
Wheezing
Tightness and pain

Mild Allergic
Flushing
Itching
Urticaria
Bronchospasm—rare

FIGURE 74–1   Transfusion reactions.

mucous membrane moistness, and vital signs regularly. Measure the client's intake and output; it should be balanced at approximately 2500 ml/24 h. Take care to include all routes of intake (oral or IV) and output (urinary, GI losses, or drains and tubes). It is expected that the client will maintain body weight without signs of fluid retention or loss. The vital signs will be maintained at a normal range or return to normal. If the client has been hypotensive because of fluid losses, the administration of IV fluids or blood products results in the return of the blood pressure to a normal level. The skin turgor will be elastic, and the mucous membranes will be moist. Trends in the serum and urinary levels of electrolytes and osmolality, arterial blood gases, CBC, and BUN help determine the effectiveness of therapy.

Changes in neuromuscular function predispose the client to injury because of changes in level of consciousness and changes in strength and coordination. Therefore monitor the client for the occurrence of injury.

The client and caregiver should be able to verbalize the complications of therapy and how to detect them. If the client is receiving an IV infusion of fluids or blood products, the client or caregiver must demonstrate care of the infusion site and how to manage complications or emergencies.

The primary medical therapy focuses on ordering and monitoring laboratory tests. The frequency of performing the laboratory tests varies, depending on the severity of the client's condition (e.g., the client being treated for diabetic ketoacidosis requires frequent determinations of arterial blood gas levels to evaluate the effectiveness of treatment on the pH and bicarbonate). The frequency of monitoring laboratory tests also depends on how actively fluids and electrolytes are being gained or lost. For example, when the client is experiencing profound vomiting, the body's ability to adapt to the fluid and electrolyte loss may not be successful; thus a rapid response is required to prevent vascular collapse (Table 74–1).

CONCEPT REVIEW

Assessment is crucial in obtaining information that may identify risk factors for fluid, electrolyte, and acid-base alterations. Changes in dietary intake, metabolic and endocrine function, or excretion place client at risk for electrolyte balance disturbances. Renal failure, COPD, and diabetes mellitus place clients at risk for alterations in acid-base balance. Assessment should be frequent and comprehensive, involving level of consciousness and behavior, deep tendon reflexes, muscle strength, and activity tolerance.

Because of their relatively larger body surface area and less well-developed buffering mechanism, infants and children are at greater risk than adults for fluid and acid-base disturbances. Similarly, the elderly are at greater risk because of their decrease in total body water, relatively larger extracellular volume than intracellular volume, and decreased function of compensatory systems.

Pharmacologic management of alterations in fluid, electrolyte, and acid-base balances focuses on the replacement or supplementation of deficient fluids, electrolytes, or blood components; the correction of acid-base imbalances; and the detection and prevention of complications. The client and family must be made aware of how to prevent and identify alterations and of sources and necessary quantities of important nutrients.

 ## NURSING RESEARCH

Metheny, N., Merritt, S., & Myers, J. (1991). Testing of alteration in potassium balance: Hypo- and hyperkalemia as nursing diagnoses. In *Classification of nursing diagnoses: Proceedings of the Ninth Conference held in Orlando, FL, 1990*. Philadelphia: J.B. Lippincott.

The purpose of the study was to assess two proposed nursing diagnoses: alteration in potassium balance: hypokalemia; and alteration in potassium balance: hyperkalemia. A review of 210 potential clients was done; of them, 48 individuals with hypokalemia and nine clients with hyperkalemia were identified. Common factors in assessment and interventions were identified. Refinement of the data collection tools is required before more testing of these diagnoses can be done.

STUDENT ACTIVITIES

• Review the charts of 10 clients, each with hypokalemia or hyperkalemia. List all the common ele-

TABLE 74–1
Major Medical Therapies

Test	Indication
Serum electrolytes	Monitor for excesses or deficiencies in serum level of electrolytes
Complete blood count (CBC)	Monitor for blood loss, decreased platelets and white blood cells
Prothrombin time (PT), partial thromboplastin time (PTT)	Monitor clotting ability of the blood
Serum osmolality, blood urea nitrogen (BUN), hematocrit	Monitor serum concentration, which reflects vascular volume
Serum creatinine (and BUN)	Monitor renal function; decreased renal function results in inability to maintain fluid, electrolyte, or acid-base balance
Arterial blood gases	Monitor acid-base balance
Urinary pH	Monitor renal response to acid-base processes
Urinary osmolality, specific gravity	Monitor concentration of urine
Urinary electrolytes	Monitor ability of kidney to eliminate electrolytes

ments defining the history of clients with these conditions. List common treatments and undesired clinical responses associated with those treatments.

- Write out a nursing diagnosis for either hypokalemia or hyperkalemia; list the pertinent assessment questions, a plan of care, implementation considerations, and important items to evaluate.

FLUID REPLACEMENT

IV replacement of fluids is given when the client has been losing isotonic fluids, hypertonic or hypotonic fluids, or blood. IV fluids that do not contain proteins are called *crystalloids.* Crystalloid products are used to replace fluid and electrolytes, treat acid-base disorders, and provide a small number of calories. Products that contain protein or starch molecules are called *colloids.*[5] Colloid solutions are used to increase capillary oncotic pressure so that intravascular volume is increased. These solutions can be used to expand vascular volume quickly when the client has experienced a rapid loss of blood. Whole blood or a component of whole blood is used to replace vascular volume, RBCs, or another element present in plasma that is decreased because of bleeding or the inability of the body to manufacture the substance in the amount needed for adaptation.

Crystalloid Solutions

DEXTROSE IN WATER

Pharmacotherapeutics A basic crystalloid solution is dextrose in water (Table 74–2). This solution is used to maintain or replace ECF or ICF fluid. Solutions with a concentration of 50% are given intravenously in small volumes (e.g., 50 ml) to reverse the effects of severe, insulin-induced hypoglycemia. Small volumes (2 to 12 ml) of dextrose in water solutions are given to infants and children to control acute hypoglycemia. The more concentrated solutions (e.g., 25%) can be given as part of the formula used for TPN (see Chapter 75).

Pharmacokinetics The dextrose in these solutions is rapidly metabolized to CO_2 and water.[1] As a result, hypotonic water is provided for ECF and ICF volume maintenance and replacement. Any excess water is excreted by the kidneys. When hypotonic dextrose solutions are given as the only fluid replacement, a hypotonic fluid imbalance can result. Solutions with a concentration of dextrose equal to or greater than 20% are hypertonic. Dextrose in water solutions contain no electrolytes.

Pharmacodynamics Dextrose in water solutions provides fluid and calories in clients with inadequate oral intake. The number of calories provided by these solutions depends on the volume given and the percentage of dextrose in the solution. Dextrose concentrations of 2.5%, 5%, and 10% do not provide sufficient calories (85 cal/L, 170 cal/L, and 340 cal/L, respectively) to maintain normal nutrition (Table 74–3). More concentrated solutions are available, ranging from 20% to 70%.[11]

Life-span considerations IV dextrose in water solutions are given cautiously in the very young and the very old because of the clients' immature or diminished renal function. Too-rapid infusion of fluids increases the risk of acute fluid volume excess, possibly resulting in pulmonary edema.

Drug-drug and drug-environment interactions Solutions containing dextrose may be physically incompatible with drugs given simultaneously through the IV line (Table 74–4). Consult compatibility charts for this information. If an incompatible drug is ordered, use of a second IV line is necessary. Blood and blood components are physically incompatible with dextrose and must be given through a separate line. Solutions containing dextrose increases serum blood glucose levels, interfering with the effectivness of hypoglycemic agents such as insulin and the oral hypoglycemic agents. Solutions containing dextrose are given cautiously to clients receiving corticosteroids because of the danger of hyperglycemia.[11]

Dextrose in water solutions should be protected from freezing and extreme heat.

Undesired clinical responses The administration of dextrose solutions can cause local IV site complications such as phlebitis and tissue necrosis if the fluid escapes into the subcutaneous space. These solutions can cause fluid volume excess, confusion, or unconsciousness.

Dextrose solutions can cause a transient elevation in blood glucose levels, which can cause a spurious rise in the serum blood glucose level (see box).

Contraindications IV solutions containing dextrose should not be given to clients with severe hyperglycemia. Use of hypertonic solutions ($\geq$10%) is contraindicated in the presence of a hyperosmolar fluid imbalance.

Specific drug-related nursing considerations Administer dextrose in water solutions with a concentration greater than 10% through a central vein because their use is associated with a higher incidence of phlebitis. When concentrated dextrose solutions (i.e., 25%) are given, monitor the client for hyperglycemia and glycosuria. Observe for confusion or decreased level of consciousness; these signs may indicate that a hyperglycemic, hyperosmolar imbalance is present. Observe for fluid volume excess.

UNDESIRED CLINICAL RESPONSES ASSOCIATED WITH CRYSTALLOID INTRAVENOUS SOLUTIONS

Saline Solution
Fluid volume excess with pulmonary edema and congestive heart failure
Hyperchloremic metabolic acidosis

Dextrose in Water Solution
Transient elevation in serum glucose level

Multiple Electrolyte Solutions
Hyperkalemia
Hypermagnesemia
Hypercalcemia

TABLE 74–2

Selected Crystalloid Intravenous Solutions

Solution	Desired Action, Dosage	Nursing Considerations
Dextrose in water (D₅W; D₁₀W)	Maintenance or replacement of ECF and ICF Dosage: usually given in 250-, 500-, or 1000-ml volumes over 8–24 h	Solution contains insufficient nutrients for tissue growth and repair; provides calories. Solution contains no electrolytes. Rate of infusion varies. Solutions ≥10% can cause phlebitis: administer in a large vein. Do not use as diluent for blood or administer simultaneously through same infusion set.
Saline (0.9% normal saline; 0.45% normal saline)	Replacement of serum sodium Expansion of vascular volume Maintenance or replacement of ECF and ICF Dosage: usually given in 250-, 500-, or 1000-ml volume over 8–24 h; 250 ml of 0.9% normal saline solution can be given over 1 h as a fluid challenge to assess renal function	Change IV tubing at least every 24–48 h. Maintain accurate intake and output. Monitor major electrolyte and acid-base balance. Solution classified in pregnancy category C. Incidence of adverse reactions increases in elderly. Incompatible with amphotericin B, levarterenol, mannitol.
Multiple electrolyte solutions (Isolyte, Normosol, Plasma-Lyte, Ionosol, lactated Ringer's, Ringer's)	Maintenance and replacement of ECF and electrolytes Maintenance of acid-base balance Dosage: usually given in 250-, 500-, or 1000-ml volume over 8–24 h	Solutions provide selected electrolytes in concentrations similar to normal serum levels.

SALINE SOLUTIONS

Pharmacotherapeutics A second category of crystalloid solutions consists of saline products (see Table 74–2). Saline solutions (0.9%) are given to replace serum sodium and to expand the vascular volume. They are also used in other ways (e.g., flushing IV lines, diluting drugs, and as part of the blood transfusion process).

Another common saline solution consists of 0.45% saline. This solution is hypotonic and is used to provide free water to replace fluid lost from the ECF and the ICF. Provided is 77 mEq/L of both sodium and chloride, which is enough to prevent sudden drops in the serum level of these electrolytes.

Hypertonic saline solutions (3% and 5% sodium chloride) can be given to correct severe sodium depletion. Because these solutions are extremely hypertonic, they must be administered carefully.[1]

Pharmacokinetics Sodium and chloride ions and water reach the plasma and elevate the serum levels of sodium and chloride. The water increases circulating blood volume. Excess sodium, chloride, and water are eliminated by the kidneys.

Pharmacodynamics Normal serum osmolality ranges from 275 to 295 mOsm/L, with sodium, chloride, and bicarbonate ions contributing most to the serum concentration. Saline solutions contain sodium and chloride ions in percentages reflecting the ratio of serum sodium to the total cations in the serum. The usual concentration of sodium is 0.9%/L. Solutions of 0.9% sodium chloride are called *normal saline solutions*. Although the total concentration of these two electrolytes is normal, the actual number of electrolytes is greater than normal serum levels (154 mEq sodium, 154 mEq chloride) because only two electrolytes are contributing to the concentration of the solution.[1] For this reason, normal saline solutions must be given with caution to clients not able to adjust to increased serum levels of sodium (e.g., clients with heart or renal failure).

Life-span considerations Saline solutions must be given with caution to elderly clients. The diminished renal function and limited cardiac reserve of these clients interfere with the excretion of the sodium and chloride ions so that excess water may not be excreted, resulting in fluid volume excess. Overdose is possible in newborn or very small infants.[11]

Drug-drug and drug-environment interactions Use of saline solutions may increase the excretion of lithium (see Table 74–4). Glucocorticoid use increases the retention of sodium and water. Solutions containing saline may be physically incompatible with drugs given simultaneously through the IV line (see Table 74–4).

Saline products should be protected from freezing and excessive heat. They should be stored at 25° C. Brief exposure to heat less than or equal to 40° C does not harm these solutions.[11]

Undesired clinical responses The administration of saline solutions can cause local IV site complications such as phlebitis and tissue necrosis if the fluid escapes into the subcutaneous space.

The administration of sodium and chloride ions may cause hypernatremia and hyperchloremia. These conditions can result in the loss of bicarbonate ions and development of meta-

TABLE 74–3
Crystalloid Solutions

How Supplied	Desired Action
DEXTROSE 5% IN WATER (D₅W)	
Volumes: 10, 25, 50, 100, 130, 150, 250, 400, 500, 1000 ml	Maintenance or replacement of fluid; is isotonic when administered, becomes hypotonic after dextrose is metabolized, and can replace ECF or ICF losses as necessary
SALINE SOLUTIONS	Replacement of serum sodium; expansion of vascular volume
0.9% sodium chloride (normal saline; 0.9% NaCl; 0.9% NS; NS) Volumes: 1, 2, 2.5, 3, 4, 5, 10, 20, 25, 30, 50, 100, 130, 150, 250, 500, 1000 ml	
0.45% sodium chloride (half normal saline; 0.45% NaCl; 0.45% NS; ½ NS) Volumes: 3, 5, 500, 1000 ml	Maintenance or replacement of ECF and ICF
DEXTROSE IN SALINE SOLUTIONS	
Dextrose 5% in 0.9% sodium chloride (D₅–0.9% NaCl; D₅–0.9% NS; D₅NS) Volumes: 250, 500, 1000 ml	Provides calories, sodium, and chloride
MULTIPLE ELECTROLYTE SOLUTIONS	
Lactated Ringer's (LR) Volumes: 250, 500, 1000 ml	Provides sodium, potassium, calcium, chloride, lactate

TABLE 74–4
Interactions With Crystalloid Intravenous Solutions

Solution	Interaction
Dextrose in water	Physical incompatibility with other drugs
	Physical incompatibility with blood products
	Decreased effectiveness of insulin and oral hypoglycemic agents
Saline	Increased lithium excretion
	Retention of sodium and water increased by glucocorticoids
Multiple electrolyte solutions	Physical incompatibility with drugs
	Development of arrhythmias when products containing calcium are administered to clients receiving digitalis products
	Action of verapamil (Calan, Isoptin) antagonized by calcium

bolic acidosis.[11] The administration of sodium chloride can cause hyperchloremic metabolic acidosis by diluting bicarbonate ions.[12] The elevated serum sodium level can cause hypokalemia. Solutions that contain sodium in concentrations of 0.9% or greater can cause fluid volume excess by increasing serum osmolality that stimulates the kidneys to retain water resulting in increased vascular volume and possibly pulmonary edema.

Contraindications Use of saline solutions is contraindicated in the client with severe hypernatremia or fluid retention. Use of very concentrated saline solutions (3% and 5%) is contraindicated with elevated, normal, or only slightly decreased plasma sodium and chloride concentrations.[11]

Specific drug-related nursing considerations Administer saline solutions with extreme caution to clients at risk of sodium retention (e.g., clients with heart and renal failure, cirrhosis of the liver, or hyperaldosteronism or who have just had surgery). Observe clients for changes indicating fluid retention (e.g., edema, shortness of breath). Monitor the client's serum electrolyte, serum osmolality, and arterial blood gas values. Report any increase in serum sodium or osmolality level to the primary health care provider.

DEXTROSE IN SALINE SOLUTIONS

Dextrose in 5% and 10% solutions is combined with saline in 0.2% to 0.9% concentrations (see Table 74–3). These solutions can be used to provide hydration, sodium, chloride, and limited calories. The solutions are hypertonic.

MULTIPLE ELECTROLYTE SOLUTIONS

Pharmacotherapeutics These solutions contain multiple electrolytes in various concentrations (see Table 74–2). Multiple electrolyte solutions are used to replace balanced losses of fluid and electrolytes (e.g., from vomiting) or to maintain postoperative fluid and electrolyte balance. Multiple electrolyte solutions may also contain dextrose, 5% or 10%, which provides a limited number of calories. These solutions also are used to treat mild metabolic acidosis.

Pharmacokinetics A commonly given multiple electrolyte solution is lactated Ringer's. The osmolality of this solution is 272 mOsm/L, which is isotonic in relation to the vascular space.[11] The concentration of the electrolytes in lactated Ringer's solution (sodium, potassium, calcium, and chloride) is similar to that of the normal serum levels. Lactate is metabolized by the liver to bicarbonate. Lactated Ringer's solution does not contain magnesium or phosphorous. Other solutions such as Plasma-Lyte 56 and Isolyte S contain magnesium but do not contain calcium.

Drug-drug interactions   The individual components of multiple electrolyte solutions affect compatibility with drugs administered through the same IV line (see Table 74–4). Calcium must be administered cautiously to the client receiving digitalis because calcium can precipitate arrhythmias. Calcium also can antagonize the effects of verapamil. Other interactions may occur with individual electrolytes present in the solution.

Undesired clinical responses   Undesired responses related to use of multiple electrolyte solutions reflect the effects of the dextrose and electrolytes contained in the solutions. Dextrose in 5% and 10% concentrations has few side effects other than a transient elevation of the blood glucose level while the solution is infusing. The administration of solutions containing potassium, magnesium, and calcium can result in increased serum levels of these electrolytes, especially in the presence of renal insufficiency.

Contraindications   Lactated Ringer's solution must be given cautiously to clients with lactic acidosis because failure to convert lactate to bicarbonate can worsen the acidosis.[1]

Specific drug-related nursing consideration   Before a solution containing potassium or magnesium is administered, establish the adequacy of urinary output because these electrolytes normally are excreted only by the kidneys.

Colloid Solutions

PLASMA EXPANDERS

Pharmacotherapeutics   Plasma expanders are used in life-threatening situations in which there is a rapid, severe loss of vascular volume (e.g., with hemorrhage, burns, or surgery). Hetastarch and dextran are two examples of plasma expanders. Blood products provide the preferred solution for replacement of blood loss because plasma expanders do not have oxygen-carrying capacity. However, plasma expanders can be administered to replace vascular volume without the need for blood typing and crossmatching.[13] Dextran is used to prevent deep-vein thrombosis and pulmonary embolisms in clients undergoing procedures with high risk of these conditions (e.g., orthopedic surgery).[11] Dextran also is used to prime the pumps used in extracorporeal circulation.

Pharmacokinetics   Small hetastarch molecules are eliminated by the kidneys. Hetastarch is effective for up to 36 hours.[14] The mean half-life of hetastarch is 17 days.[11]

Dextran is a synthetic polysaccharide that can have a low molecular weight of 40,000 or a high molecular weight of 70,000 or 75,000. Dextran is eliminated by renal excretion, with 75% of low-molecular-weight and 50% of high-molecular-weight dextran eliminated within 24 hours.[11] The remaining dextran is degraded to glucose.

Pharmacodynamics   Plasma expanders are synthetic solutions that contain large molecules that cannot diffuse out of the capillaries (Table 74–5). These solutions exert an oncotic pressure in the capillaries that draws fluid by osmotic pressure into the vascular space from the interstitial space. These solutions usually increase the vascular volume to an extent equal to or slightly greater than the volume infused. Low-molecular-weight dextran decreases platelet adhesiveness.[14]

Life-span considerations   Total dosage of plasma expanders in children should not exceed 20 ml/kg. Safey of these products for use during pregnancy and lactation is not known. Plasma expanders should be given cautiously to the elderly because the increased plasma volume may exceed the elderly per-

TABLE 74–5
Colloid Intravenous Solutions

Product	Desired Action, Dosage	Nursing Considerations
Plasma expanders	Expand vascular volume	Expanders can be used without blood typing
Hetastarch	Dosage: 20 ml/kg/h	and cross-matching.
Dextran 40	Dosage: 20 ml/kg/h for first 24 h; 10 ml/kg/h on days 2–5	Monitor for fluid volume excess.
		Monitor hemodynamic parameters (e.g., vital
Dextran 70	Dosage: 20–40 ml/min for emergency situations	signs) to evaluate the client's response.
Proteins	Maintenance of serum oncotic pressure Restoration of vascular volume Maintenance of blood pressure	
Plasma protein fraction (Plasmanate, Plasma-Plex, Plasmatein, Protenate)	Dosage: 5–8 ml/min	Administration faster than 10 ml/min can result in hypotension.
Albumin (Albuminar, 5% and 25%; Albutein, 5% and 25%; Buminate, 5% and 25%; Normal Serum Albumin (Human), 5% and 25%; Plasbumin, 5% and 25%)	Can be given rapidly if blood volume is greatly reduced If client is normotensive, usual rate is 2–4 ml/min	Albumin can expand vascular volume, which can result in fluid volume excess. Monitor blood pressure and laboratory test results to determine response.
5%	Available as 50, 250, 500, 1000 ml	
25%	Available as 10, 20, 50, 100 ml	

son's capacity to adjust because of diminished renal function and impaired cardiac function.

Drug-drug and drug-environment interactions Hydrolysis of dextran can cause a falsely elevated blood glucose level result. Serum bilirubin, total protein, blood typing and crossmatching results, and tests of renal and hepatic function may also be affected.

Hetastarch should be stored at room temperature equal to or less than 40° C and should not be frozen.

Low-molecular-weight dextan should be stored between 15° and 30° C and should be protected from freezing. High-molecular-weight dextran should be stored at a constant temperature equal to or less than 25° C. High-molecular-weight dextran contains no bacteriostatic agent, so any solution remaining after administration should be discarded.

Undesired clinical responses Plasma expanders can cause allergic reactions, and their use may result in fluid volume excess and pulmonary edema.

Hetastarch can cause the following adverse reactions: vomiting, mild temperature elevation, chills, itching, submaxillary and parotid gland enlargement, influenza-like symptoms, headache, muscle pain, and peripheral edema.

Dextran can cause hypernatremia, sudden hypotension, nausea and vomiting, fever, or joint pains. Dextran is also associated with complications such as phlebitis, thrombosis, and extravasation at the IV insertion site.

Contraindications Plasma expander use is contraindicated in clients with severe bleeding disorders or severe cardiac or renal failure. Dextran use is contraindicated for the individual with a known allergy to it.

Specific drug-related nursing considerations Monitor laboratory studies to detect adverse reactions such as decreased hematocrit levels; decreased serum osmolality; prolonged bleeding time, PT, and PTT; and thrombocytopenia.

Monitor for the development of hypersensitivity reactions, especially immediately after the initiation of therapy. Hypersensitivity can occur as urticaria, flushing, wheezing, or a feeling of chest tightness. Monitor the urinary output and specific gravity. The urinary output should increase in response to the increased vascular volume. The specific gravity increases as the large molecules are eliminated. If the urinary output does not increase, discontinue the infusion

Ensure that the client's blood has been typed and crossmatched before administering dextran because it can interfere with these procedures.

PROTEINS

Pharmacotherapeutics Serum proteins are administered to maintain plasma oncotic pressure, to restore circulating blood volume, and to maintain blood pressure in situations such as hypovolemic shock, burns, and hypoproteinemia. Protein products are given to reduce peripheral and interstitial edema. The most common products are albumin, 5% and 25% solutions, and plasma protein fraction, a variable combination of albumin with globulin and gamma globulin.

Pharmacokinetics Plasma protein fraction and albumin contain 130 to 160 mEq of sodium.[11] These products are heat treated to prevent their carrying the risk of viral transmission. They may be given without typing or crossmatching.

Pharmacodynamics Protein molecules are large, naturally occurring substances that exert an osmotic pressure within the vascular space to keep fluid from leaking into the interstitial space and becoming trapped as edema fluid. In some situations albumin and a loop diuretic such as furosemide are given to draw edema fluid from the interstitial space into the vascular space from which it is excreted by the kidneys into the urine under the influence of the diuretic. This process may result in fluid volume excess and pulmonary edema.

Life-span considerations Administration of protein products can cause fluid volume excess in elderly clients with diminished renal and cardiac function.

Drug-drug and drug-environment interactions Administration of protein products with protein hydrolysates, amino acid solutions, or alcohol can cause protein precipitation.

Protein products should be stored at room temperature less than or equal to 30° C and should not be frozen. Plasma protein fraction contains no preservative, and any solution remaining after administration should be discarded.

Undesired clinical responses Rapid administration of protein products may cause fluid volume excess; the client will experience shortness of breath and pulmonary edema. Hypotension can occur with rapid infusion or while cardiopulmonary bypass is being used. Protein products can cause an allergic reaction; the client may experience fever and chills, flushing, urticaria, back pain, headache, rash, nausea, vomiting, increased salivation, hyperthermia, tachycardia, and hypotension.

Contraindications Use of protein products is contraindicated for the client with a history of allergic reaction to plasma proteins. Other contraindications are severe anemia, cardiac failure, renal insufficiency, and the presence of normal or increased vascular volume.[11]

Specific drug-related nursing considerations Monitor the client for fluid volume excess by observing for shortness of breath, crackles in the lungs, and changes in vital signs and urinary output.

Blood and Blood Components

Because of possible hemolysis of the donor cells, no medications or IV fluids should be infused at the same time as blood or blood products.

RED BLOOD CELLS

Whole blood and packed RBCs are given to replace losses of circulating blood volume and RBCs. Whole blood and packed RBCs increase the volume and oxygen-carrying capacity of blood (Table 74–6). The volume of whole blood products is approximately 500 ml, and that of packed RBCs is approximately 250 ml. Both products provide the same number of RBCs, but packed RBCs are given more safely to clients with impaired cardiac or renal function because of the smaller volume delivered.[15] Leukocyte-poor RBCs, irradiated RBCs, and washed RBCs are used to prevent hypersensitivity reactions to blood components. All blood products may be sources of hepatitis B virus (HBV) and human immunodeficiency virus (HIV) despite careful screening of blood donors and testing of blood products. Universal precaution techniques must be used when administering blood or blood components. In addition, all blood products must be typed and crossmatched before administration, RBC products must be stored under refrigeration. The infusion should be initiated within 30 minutes of the blood unit's removal from refrigeration and must be complete within 4 hours.

BLOOD COMPONENTS AFFECTING CLOTTING

Fresh frozen plasma Fresh frozen plasma, the fluid portion of whole blood, is used to replace clotting factors when the client has multiple factor deficiencies or other coagulopathies. It contains the components of the coagulation system, other proteins, fats, carbohydrates, and minerals found in whole blood. Fresh frozen plasma is obtained from a single donor, prepared from whole blood, and frozen within 6 hours of collection.[16] Fresh frozen plasma can also be obtained by **plasmapheresis,** a process in which whole blood is withdrawn from a donor, the blood component is removed, and the remaining blood volume is returned to the donor. This product can be the source of viral infections (HBV and HIV) and must be ABO compatible with the recipient's blood. The product takes 20 minutes to thaw and must be administered within 24 hours of thawing.

Specific clotting factors Specific clotting factors can be derived from plasma and administered in a concentrated form. Clotting factors available include factor VIII, used to treat hemophilia, factor IX, and von Willebrand's factor. Some factor VIII products are treated with heat or chemicals to reduce the transmission of viruses.

Platelets Platelets are given to prevent or treat bleeding resulting from inadequate numbers of platelets or platelets that do not function normally. Platelets are obtained from pooled,

TABLE 74–6
Blood and Blood Components

Product Name	Dosage and Route of Administration	Nursing Considerations
Red Blood Cells (packed red blood cells) HOW SUPPLIED 250, 500 ml	**Replace Blood Loss** **Expand Vascular Volume** **Increase Oxygen-Carrying Capacity of Blood** 250–500 ml over 4 h	Carefully identify client and blood product. Monitor for development of transfusion reactions. Monitor hemodynamic parameters (e.g., vital signs) and CBC to evaluate client's response.
BLOOD COMPONENTS AFFECTING CLOTTING ***Fresh Frozen Plasma (FFP)*** HOW SUPPLIED 200 ml	**Prevention of Abnormal Bleeding** 200 ml infused over 15–20 min up to 1–2 h	Allow 20 min for FFP to thaw. Infuse plasma within 24 h.
Factor VIII—Antihemophilic Factor (Hemofil M, Humate-P, Koate-HS, Koate-HT, Monoclate-P, Profilate HP) HOW SUPPLIED Freeze-dried; requires reconstitution; single-dose vials; single-dose bottles with number of units labeled	**Acute Bleeding** 8–30 U/kg q8–12h **Prevention of Bleeding** Client >50 kg: 500 U/d Client <50 kg: 250 U/d	Store and reconstitute as directed by manufacturer. Administer promptly to prevent microbial growth.
Platelets HOW SUPPLIED 200–300 ml	Volume varies with number of units ordered; usual order, 6–10 U with total volume, 200–300 ml Rate: 150–200 ml/h	Rapid rate of infusion may result in fluid volume excess. Complete infusion within 4 h.
BLOOD COMPONENTS AFFECTING IMMUNE FUNCTION ***Granulocytes*** HOW SUPPLIED 300–400 ml	**Prevention of Infection** 300–400 ml Rate: slowly over 2–4 h	Monitor vital signs and client's response because transfusion reactions are common. Transfuse within 24 h of collection.
Immunoglobulins (Venoglobulin-I, Gammar-IV, Gamimune N, Gammagard, Iveegam, Sandoglobulin) HOW SUPPLIED 10–250 ml after reconstitution	Rate varies with product Can be given IM	Give slowly for first 15–30 min to detect anaphylaxis.

random donors or from single donors. The advantage of using a single-donor source is the ability to match the human leukocyte antigen from the donor precisely to minimize sensitization to the donor platelets.[15] Plateletpheresis is used to remove approximately 500 ml of platelet-rich plasma. Platelets are usually stored no longer than 5 days. Platelets can be the source of HIV and HBV infections; each unit should be tested. Generally platelets are not ABO and Rh matched.[17]

BLOOD COMPONENTS AFFECTING IMMUNE FUNCTION

Granulocytes Granulocytes are given to treat **neutropenia**, which is a decrease in the number of white blood cells (WBCs). Granulocytes are not given until the leukocyte count is less than 500. Granulocytes are obtained by leukapheresis. In this process the WBCs are removed from the donor's blood, and the remaining plasma and RBCs are returned to the donor. The donor may develop hypocalcemia, resulting in circumoral and digital tingling. The use of granulocytes has decreased because of the use of newer, more effective antibiotics and chemotherapy regimens that minimize the occurrence of neutropenia.

Immunoglobulins Intravenous immunoglobulin (IVIG), a concentrated form of immunoglobulin G (IgG),[18] is also known as *gamma globulin*. IVIG is obtained from the pooled serum of many donors, so it contains multiple antibodies to a wide range of bacteria and viruses. It can be used in the treatment of immune thrombocytopenia purpura, bone marrow suppression, and chronic lymphocytic leukemia and in clients infected with HIV and those who have had a bone marrow transplant. Side effects do not occur often, but the administration of IVIG is associated with the possibility of HBV and HIV transmission and the occurrence of anaphylaxis.[19] The infusion is given slowly for the first 15 to 30 minutes to allow the early detection of an anaphylactic response.

CONCEPT REVIEW

Crystalloid products (e.g., dextrose in water, saline solutions, dextrose in saline solution) are used to replace fluid and electrolytes, treat acid-base disorders, and provide a small number of calories.

Colloid solutions (e.g., plasma expanders, proteins) are used to increase capillary oncotic pressure so that intravascular volume is increased.

Whole blood or its components are used to replace vascular volume, RBC, or other elements of plasma.

AGENTS USED WITH ALTERATIONS IN ELECTROLYTE BALANCE

Deficiencies in serum electrolytes can be caused by many illnesses and treatments. These deficiencies can occur singly or in combination. When they occur, the effects are experienced in many body systems so that the client's level of health can be profoundly affected. Electrolyte supplements are used to prevent or treat serum electrolyte deficiencies. Excessive levels of serum electrolytes, particularly hyperkalemia, can also occur.

Potassium Supplements and Replacements

Pharmacotherapeutics Hypokalemia is one of the most commonly occurring electrolyte alterations; therefore potassium preparations are given frequently, either for prevention of hypokalemia or for maintenance of the normal serum potassium level. Clinical situations that require potassium administration include decreased intake of potassium; administration of potassium-losing diuretics; the treatment of diabetic ketoacidosis, prolonged vomiting or diarrhea; and hyperaldosteronism.

Pharmacokinetics Potassium is administered orally or intravenously. Hyperkalemia is more likely to occur during potassium replacement therapy if dietary intake of potassium increases suddenly, renal function decreases, or the client is elderly. The major route for excretion of potassium is the kidneys. The urinary output must be monitored whenever a potassium product is given. If urinary output falls below 10 to 20 ml/h, potassium excretion decreases, and dangerous elevation of serum potassium can quickly occur. The client's serum potassium level must be monitored to verify the adequacy of the potassium replacement and to detect hyperkalemia.

Pharmacodynamics Potassium is the principal intracellular cation of most body tissues. Potassium ions participate in a number of essential physiologic processes, including the maintenance of intracellular tonicity; transmission of nerve impulses; contraction of cardiac, skeletal, and smooth muscles; and maintenance of normal renal function.

Pharmaceutics The prototype potassium product is potassium chloride. The usual dosage is individualized to the client's situation and can range from 16 to 24 mEq/d in divided doses to prevent hypokalemia and 40 to 100 mEq/d for treatment of hypokalemia.[11] Liquid preparations of potassium chloride are often given as 10% and 20% solutions, which provide 20 and 40 mEq of potassium per 15 ml, respectively. Potassium chloride is particularly helpful in treating hypokalemia associated with metabolic alkalosis since chloride depletion commonly occurs in clients with this disorder. Other potassium salts such as potassium bicarbonate, potassium citrate, potassium acetate, and potassium gluconate are useful in treating the hypokalemia associated with the metabolic acidosis caused by renal tubular acidosis (Table 74–7).

Life-span considerations Potassium is classified as a Pregnancy Category C drug. Normal potassium ion content in human milk is approximately 13 mEq/L. Potassium replacement should have little or no effect on this level. Safety and effectiveness in children have not been established.

Drug-drug interactions Simultaneous use of potassium-sparing diuretics or salt substitutes with products containing potassium can produce an elevated serum potassium level.[11] Administration of angiotensin-converting enzyme (ACE) inhibitors such as captopril (Capoten) and enalapril (Vasotec) can cause potassium retention due to decreased aldosterone levels.[11] Cholinergic blocking drugs that slow GI motility may increase the risk of GI ulceration when tablets or enteric-coated capsules are given orally.[11] Potassium replacement therapy is not given to digitalized clients with complete heart block.[1]

Undesired clinical responses Orally administered potassium salts are irritating to the stomach and can cause nausea, vomiting, diarrhea, or abdominal pain. Rarely the client may experience a skin rash. Enteric preparations can cause GI ulceration and are rarely given. The most serious side effect is hyperkalemia.

Contraindications Use of potassium replacement products is contraindicated in clients with severe renal impairment, untreated adrenocortical insufficiency, and hyperkalemia. Client's urinary output must be at least 25 ml/h.

Specific drug-related nursing considerations Oral preparations of potassium are supplied as liquids, powders, effervescent tablets, capsules, tablets, and salt substitutes. Clients often complain that these preparations have a strong, unpleasant taste. This taste can interfere with clients' willingness to continue potassium replacement for long-term therapy. Oral preparations can be given with food or fluids to decrease gastric irritation. Liquid potassium preparations can be diluted in a small amount of juice or milk and followed by a larger volume of juice or milk. Dilute each 20 mEq of potassium in at least 90 ml of beverage. Mix or dissolve powders and effervescent preparations completely in 3 to 8 ounces of cold beverage. Tablets should not be chewed or crushed. Review the client's drug history for drugs that may cause potassium retention or contain potassium.

Always dilute IV preparations of potassium before their administration. A concentration of 40 to 80 mEq in 1000 ml is generally a safe concentration to administer intravenously over an 8-hour period.[11] For situations requiring a more rapid correction of hypokalemia administer concentrations of 40 mEq/dl at a rate no faster than 10 to 40 mEq/h. When a concentrated potassium solution is being administered, monitor the client's cardiac rhythm constantly to detect changes associated with hyperkalemia such as peaked T waves, prolonged PR intervals, or absent P waves.[1] Never give potassium products IV push because of the danger of cardiac arrest.[1] Do not add potassium to an infusing bag of IV fluids that has less than 500 ml remaining, for the resulting concentration will be too great. When potassium is added to an infusing bag of IV fluids, take care to disperse the potassium uniformly throughout the bag by inverting the bag several times.[1] If this is not done, the potassium may be concentrated at the bottom of the bag and be given too rapidly. Giving concentrated solutions of potassium can cause phlebitis when peripheral veins are used; therefore administration through a central vein is preferred.

Agents Used for Hyperkalemia

Hyperkalemia can be a life-threatening electrolyte imbalance, and its presence may require emergency measures to ensure prompt reduction of the serum levels, to move potassium into body cells, or to protect the heart from the cardiotoxic effects of hyperkalemia. One treatment is hemodialysis, which is used to remove excess serum potassium quickly. Another therapy is the infusion of glucose and insulin or the administration of sodium bicarbonate to foster the movement of potassium into cells.

HYPERKALEMIA AGENT PROTOTYPE

SODIUM POLYSTYRENE SULFONATE

Sodium polystyrene sulfonate (Kayexalate) is a cation exchange resin used to reduce elevated serum potassium levels.

Pharmacokinetics and Pharmacodynamics The resin is given orally through a feeding tube or by enema into the GI tract. Sodium ions are released from the resin and exchanged for potassium ions in the intestine, particularly the colon. The resin is excreted in the stool along with the retained potassium. The potassium-lowering effect of this product is slow and variable. After oral administration the onset of action varies from 2 to 12 hours; the onset is even longer after rectal administration.[11] The resin should remain in the GI tract for a minimum of 30 to 60 minutes (see Table 74–7).

Life-Span Considerations Sodium polystyrene sulfonate is classified as a Pregnancy Category C drug. It is not known if the drug is excreted in human milk.

Drug-Drug and Drug-Environment Interactions Systemic alkalosis can occur when nonabsorbable cation-donating antacids and laxatives such as magnesium hydroxide or aluminum carbonate are given with sodium polystyrene sulfonate. Compounds containing cations (e.g., antacids or laxatives containing calcium or magnesium) elevate the GI levels of these cations, which then compete with potassium for exchange with sodium. This effect decreases the effectiveness of the exchange process.

The drug should be stored in a refrigerator and used within 14 days of repackaging. Suspensions should be freshly prepared and stored no longer than 24 hours.

Undesired Clinical Responses Gastric irritation with nausea and vomiting can occur with sodium polystyrene sulfonate use. The occurrence of this side effect may result in the need to give the resin by enema. Constipation and impaction present a problem, especially in the elderly. Administering the product in a hypertonic vehicle such as sorbitol may prevent constipation. Rarely diarrhea occurs. Hypocalcemia and hypomagnesemia may result because these cations may also exchange for sodium in the GI tract. Hypernatremia may occur and not be tolerated well in the client with heart or renal failure or hypertension.

Specific Drug-Related Nursing Considerations Mix the oral preparation of sodium polystyrene sulfonate with sorbitol to produce fecal moistness by osmotic action. Monitor serum electrolyte values.

Magnesium Supplements and Replacements

Magnesium sulfate is administered as replacement therapy in clients with hypomagnesemia and to prevent and control convulsions associated with severe toxemia of pregnancy,

TABLE 74–7

Selected Electrolyte Therapy Products

Product	Desired Action, Route and Dosage	Nursing Considerations

POTASSIUM PRODUCTS
Potassium chloride
    Liquids (Kaochlor, Kay Ciel, K-Lor)
    Powders (K-Lyte/CL)
    Capsules and tablets (Kaon-CL, Slow-K, K-Tab, K-Dur, Micro-K Extencap)
Potassium gluconate (Kaon)
Potassium citrate (Bi-K)
Potassium gluconate, potassium citrate (Twin-K)
Potassium acetate, potassium bicarbonate, potassium citrate (Tri-K)
Potassium bicarbonate, potassium chloride, potassium citrate (Kaochlor-eff [effervescent tablets])
Potassium bicarbonate, potassium citrate (Effer-K [effervescent tablets])
Salt substitutes (Adolph's Salt Substitute, Morton Salt Substitute, NoSalt, Nu-Salt)
	Maintenance or replacement of serum potassium
	Route: oral or IV
	Dosage: for prevention of hypokalemia, 16–24 mEq/d; for maintenance of normal potassium level, 40–100 mEq/d
		Ensure client has adequate urinary output before administration of any product containing potassium.
		Administer oral products with food and fluid (20 mEq: 90 ml).
		Dilute IV products (e.g., 40 mEq/L) and administer over 8 h.
		Use caution when administering a solution with a higher concentration or at a more rapid rate because these changes may cause cardiac arrhythmias.
		Monitor peripheral IV sites for phlebitis.
		Completely mix or dissolve powders and effervescent preparations in 3–8 oz of water before administration.

SODIUM POLYSTYRENE SULFONATE (Kayexalate) **HOW SUPPLIED** Powder in 1-lb jars	Decrease in serum potassium Routes: oral, rectal Dosage: oral, 15–60 g/24 h; give 15 g one to four times/d; enema, 30–50 g q6h	Have client retain enema at least 30–60 min. Follow enema administration with one or two tap-water enemas to flush out the resin.
MAGNESIUM SULFATE (Vicon Forte, Eldertonic) **HOW SUPPLIED** Capsules: multivitamin with 70 mg magnesium sulfate Elixir: 2 mg with other vitamins and minerals in sherry wine base	Maintenance or replacement of serum magnesium Prevention of convulsions Routes: IM, IV Dosage: IM, 1–5 g q4-6h; IV, varies but total amount not to exceed 30–40 g/d Can be given in concentrations up to 20% (200 mg/ml) at 150 mg/min	Give IM injections in a large muscle.

epilepsy, and nephritis.[20–22] (See Table 74–7.) Magnesium products should be given cautiously in the presence of renal insufficiency because the kidneys are the primary route of excretion for magnesium. Their use also is contraindicated in clients with heart block or myocardial damage.

Administration of magnesium with neuromuscular-blocking agents, central nervous system (CNS) depressants, or general anesthetics can result in respiratory depression or enhancement of CNS depression.

Oral preparations of magnesium can cause diarrhea. Vasodilation, resulting in flushing and sweating, can occur during replacement therapy, even when the serum level remains within the therapeutic range of 1.5 to 2.5 mEq/L. However, the flushing and sweating can also indicate hypermagnesemia, so serum levels of magnesium must be carefully monitored. Hypotension, depressed or absent deep tendon reflexes, complete heart block, and respiratory paralysis all indicate the development of severe hypermagnesemia. Before IM

administration and every 15 to 60 minutes during initial IV administration, vital signs, deep tendon reflexes, and the client's mental status must be checked.

CONCEPT REVIEW

Hypokalemia is a commonly occurring electrolyte disturbance, and it can be treated by administering potassium orally or intravenously.

Hyperkalemia can be life threatening, requiring emergency measures such as hemodialysis to remove excess serum potassium.

Hypomagnesemia is corrected by administration of magnesium sulfate, which prevents or controls convulsions associated with severe toxemia of pregnancy, epilepsy, and nephritis.

AGENTS USED WITH ALTERATIONS IN ACID-BASE BALANCE

The treatment of acid-base imbalances involves the use of drugs that are acids or bases. These drugs provide the acidifying or alkalinizing substances necessary for maintenance of normal pH.

Treatment of Acidosis

SODIUM BICARBONATE

Sodium bicarbonate is given to buffer excess hydrogen ions (i.e., metabolic acidosis) or to increase the serum bicarbonate level associated with diarrhea. Sodium bicarbonate is also used to alkalinize the urine of clients with barbiturate, lithium, or salicylate toxicities in an attempt to enhance renal excretion of these substances. Sodium citrate, sodium acetate, and sodium lactate, which are metabolized into bicarbonate by the liver, are used for the same purposes.

Sodium bicarbonate is never the only treatment for metabolic acidosis. Specific therapies to reverse or treat the underlying cause must also be implemented (e.g., insulin should be used to correct diabetic ketoacidosis). Correction of metabolic acidosis should be accomplished gradually so that sudden alkalosis does not develop. Sodium bicarbonate is given orally as a tablet or powder or intravenously (Table 74–8).

Sodium bicarbonate is classified as a Pregnancy Category C drug. It should be protected from excessive heat and freezing and should be stored at room temperature.

Administration of glucocorticoids together with products containing sodium may result in excessive sodium retention and edema. Administration of sodium bicarbonate may decrease the effectiveness of chlorpropamide, lithium, salicylates, and tetracyclines because of increased renal clearance of the drugs.[11] Administration of sodium bicarbonate may prolong the effect of amphetamines, ephedrine, flecainide, mecamylamine, pseudoephedrine, quinidine, and quinine because of increased half-life and duration of action. Physical compatibility of sodium bicarbonate with other medications in IV solutions and tubings must be checked.

Sodium bicarbonate contains a high concentration of sodium, so it must be given cautiously to clients with heart or renal failure to prevent fluid volume excess and possible pulmonary edema. Its use is contraindicated in clients with chloride losses or hypocalcemia. The development of metabolic alkalosis as a consequence of sodium bicarbonate administration is associated with hyperirritability or tetany.[11]

Infiltration of intravenously administered sodium bicarbonate must be avoided because cellulitis and tissue necrosis can occur at the insertion site; thus administration of an IV solution containing sodium bicarbonate must be discontinued immediately if infiltration is suspected. The arm with the insertion site should be elevated and local warmth applied. Do not use a sodium bicarbonate solution unless it is clear. The unused portion should be discarded.

TROMETHAMINE

Tromethamine (Tham) is a highly alkaline product used to prevent or correct acidosis. It is used primarily on a short-term basis to correct the acidosis associated with cardiac bypass surgery and cardiac arrest (see Table 74–8). Tromethamine is sodium free. It is given intravenously and combines with hydrogen ions to form bicarbonate.

Respiratory depression can occur with tromethamine administration, especially in clients with chronic hypoventilation or in those receiving medications that depress respirations. Short-term hypoglycemia also can occur. Overdosage with tromethamine can result in alkalosis, fluid volume excess, or hyperosmolar fluid imbalance. Tromethamine use is contraindicated for the client with severe renal dysfunction.[11] Its use is contraindicated also in clients with hyperphosphatemia and hypocalcemia.

Since tromethamine is strongly alkaline, it can cause phlebitis, so it should be administered into a large vein with a high blood flow. If the drug infiltrates, it can cause inflammation, vascular spasms, and tissue damage; therefore the infusion site should be inspected frequently and the infusion discontinued immediately to prevent tissue necrosis and sloughing if signs of an infiltration develop. Correction of metabolic acidosis should be accomplished cautiously so that alkalosis does not develop.

Treatment of Alkalosis

SODIUM CHLORIDE

As normal saline, sodium chloride is given intravenously to clients experiencing metabolic alkalosis (see Table 74–6). Sodium chloride is also given to replace serum chloride lost through the chronic administration of loop or thiazide diuretics. The administration of sodium chloride provides chloride ions and increases the vascular volume, which allows the kidneys to excrete excess bicarbonate to correct the alkalosis.[22]

The administration of sodium chloride can result in hypernatremia and fluid volume excess. Sodium chloride use is contraindicated for the client with hypernatremia and fluid volume excess. It is also contraindicated in clients with hyperchloremia.

The client receiving sodium chloride should be monitored carefully for the development of hypertension and pulmonary edema. Serum chemistry levels should be reviewed regularly.

AMMONIUM CHLORIDE

Ammonium chloride is administered to correct metabolic alkalosis when the client cannot tolerate sodium or large volumes of fluid administration (see Table 74–8). Use of ammonium chloride can also correct hypochloremia.

Ammonium chloride is administered orally or intravenously. Ammonium is converted into urea in the liver, releasing hydrogen ions that buffer excessive bicarbonate ions and correct alkalosis.

Ammonium chloride use is contraidicated for clients with hepatic insufficiency who cannot tolerate increased ammonium levels and may develop encephalopathy. It is also contraindicated for clients with severe renal dysfunction. The effects of ammonia toxicity include muscular twitching, headache, confusion, decreasing level of consciousness, brady-

TABLE 74–8
Drugs Affecting Acid-Base Balance

Product	Desired Action, Route and Dosage	Nursing Considerations
ALKINALIZERS		
Sodium Bicarbonate	Treatment of metabolic acidosis	If infiltration is suspected, stop the IV infusion immediately.
HOW SUPPLIED	Increase serum bicarbonate level	Check for physical incompatibility with other IV additives.
IV solution: multiple dilutions available	Route: IV	
	Dosage: for routine administration, 2–5 mEq/kg over 4–8 h; for severe imbalances, 90–180 mEq/L over 1–1½ h	
Tromethamine	Prevention or control of acidosis after cardiac surgery or cardiac arrest	Administer through a large vein.
HOW SUPPLIED	Route: IV	If infiltration is suspected, stop the infusion immediately.
IV solution: 36 mg/ml	Dosage: 3.5–9 ml/kg, up to 500–1000 ml	
ACIDIFIERS		
Sodium Chloride	Replacement of fluid volume	
HOW SUPPLIED	Replacement of serum chloride	
Parenteral solution for IM, IV, SC use	To lower serum pH	
	Route: IV	
	Dosage: 250, 500, 1000 ml over 8–24 h	
Ammonium Chloride	To lower serum pH	Monitor arterial blood gas results.
HOW SUPPLIED	Route: IV	Do not give more rapidly than 5 ml/min.
IV solution: 5.35 g/20 ml	Dosage: 100–200 mEq in 500–1000 ml	

cardia, and vomiting.[11] Other effects are hyperventilation, pallor, diaphoresis, and thirst.

The IV infusion of ammonium chloride should go into a large vein to prevent phlebitis. Correction of alkalosis should be accomplished cautiously so that acidosis does not develop.

CONCEPT REVIEW

Sodium bicarbonate frequently is used to treat metabolic acidosis.

Tromethamine is used on a short-term basis to correct the acidosis associated with cardiac surgery and cardiac arrest.

Sodium chloride (as normal saline solution) is administered intravenously to clients experiencing metabolic alkalosis.

Ammonium chloride is used to treat metabolic alkalosis and to correct hypochloremia.

SUMMARY

The body contains fluids in two compartments: within the cells (intracellular fluid [ICF]) and outside the cells in intravascular or interstitial spaces (extracellular fluid [ECF]). Capillaries provide the site of fluid movement between vascular and interstitial spaces. Fluid movement is governed by hydrostatic and oncotic pressure; the net effect is called *filtration pressure,* which moves fluid and electrolytes out of the vascular space on the arterial side and into the vascular space on the venous side of the capillary bed. Diffusion, active transport, and osmosis move fluids and solutes into and out of cells. Fluids may be gained or lost from the body in equal proportions (isotonic imbalance) or in abnormal proportions (hypo-osmolar or hyperosmolar imbalance).

The primary electrolytes in the ECF are sodium, chloride, and bicarbonate. The most abundant electrolytes in the ICF are potassium, phosphate, and magnesium. An imbalance can be caused by loss of an electrolyte from the body or by movement of the electrolyte from one basic compartment to another (e.g., from ICF to ECF).

Arterial pH is maintained in healthy individuals between 7.35 and 7.45. Chemical buffers support this balance within the cells; the bicarbonate-carbonic acid system maintains it in extracellular space. The lungs assist by releasing CO_2. The kidneys provide long-term maintenance by reasbsorbing and regenerating bicarbonate; they are the slowest but most powerful regulators of acid-base balance. Acid-base imbalances are categorized as respiratory or metabolic.

All fluid replacement products must be used with care, especially in children and the elderly. Crystalloid products include solutions of dextrose in water, saline, and dextrose in saline. They replace fluid and electrolytes and provide a small number of calories. Colloid solutions increase intravascular volume by increasing capillary oncotic pressure; colloid solutions include plasma expanders and proteins. Whole blood or components of whole blood also are used in replacement therapy.

One of the most common alterations in electrolyte balance is hypokalemia; potassium preparations are given orally or intravenously for prevention of hypokalemia or for potassium maintenance. Hyperkalemia can be life threatening; in such cases hemodialysis is performed to remove the excess potassium quickly. Hyperkalemia can also be corrected by infusion of glucose and insulin, by administration of sodium bicarbonate, or by administration of sodium polystyrene sulfonate orally, by feeding tube, or by enema. Another less common alteration in electrolyte balance is hypomagnesemia; replacement magnesium is provided.

Alterations in acid-base balance are treated to restore the normal pH. Acidosis is corrected with sodium bicarbonate or an alkaline product such as tromethamine. The underlying cause of acidosis must always be treated. Alkalosis can be corrected with NaCl or ammonium chloride. When correcting either imbalance, care must be taken not to overtreat and produce the opposite imbalance.

REFERENCES

1. Metheny, N. (1992). *Fluid and electrolyte balance: Nursing considerations* (2nd ed.). Philadelphia: J.B. Lippincott.
2. Cogan, M. (1991). *Fluid and electrolytes: Physiology and pathophysiology.* East Norwalk, CT: Appleton & Lange.
3. Sterns, R., & Spital, A. (1990). Disorders of water balance. In J. Kokko & R. Tannen (Eds.), *Fluids and electrolytes* (2nd ed.; pp. 139–194). Philadelphia: W.B. Saunders.
4. Horne, M., Heitz, U., & Swearingen, P. (1991). *Fluid, electrolyte, and acid-base balance: A case study approach.* St. Louis: Mosby–Year Book.
5. Sommers, M. (1990). Fluid resuscitation following multiple trauma. *Critical Care Nurse, 10*(10), 74–83.
6. McCance, K., & Huether, S. (1990). *Pathophysiology: The biologic basis for disease in adults and children.* St. Louis: Mosby–Year Book.
7. Toto, R. (1990). Metabolic acid-base disorders. In J. Kokko & R. Tannen (Eds.), *Fluids and electrolytes* (2nd ed.; pp. 301–390). Philadelphia: W.B. Saunders.
8. Kokko, J., & Tannen, R. (1990). *Fluids and electrolytes* (2nd ed.). Philadelphia: W.B. Saunders.
9. Mollahan, J., & Riddle, I. (1992). Fluid balance in infants and children. In N. Metheny (Ed.), *Fluid and electrolyte balance: Nursing considerations* (2nd ed.; pp. 337–350). New York: J.B. Lippincott.
10. Robinson, S. (1992). Fluid balance in the elderly patient. In N. Metheny (Ed.), *Fluid and electrolyte balance: Nursing considerations* (2nd ed.; pp. 351–361). New York: J.B. Lippincott.
11. Olin, B. (1992). *Drug facts and comparisons.* St. Louis: J.B. Lippincott.
12. Wesson, D. (1991). Hyperchloremic metabolic acidosis. In H. Adrogue (Ed.), *Acid-base and electrolyte disorders* (pp. 97–115). New York: Churchill Livingstone.
13. Kuhn, M. (1991). Colloids vs crystalloids. *Critical Care Nurse, 11*(5), 37–51.
14. Rice, V. (1990). Parenteral fluids: Part two—Specifics of replacement therapy. *Canadian Intravenous Nurses Association Journal, 6*(3), 6–7.
15. Phillips, L. (1993). *Manual of IV Therapeutics.* Philadelphia: F.A. Davis.
16. Perez, W., & Viets, J. (1990). Transfusion and coagulation: An overview and recent advances in practice modalities: Part I: Blood banking and transfusion practices. *Nurse Anesthesia, 1,* 149–161.
17. Murphy, S. (1990). Preservation and clinical use of platelets. In W. Williams, E. Beutler, A. Erslev, & M. Lichtman (Eds.), *Hematology* (4th ed.; pp. 1654–1658).
18. Timmerman, P. (1993). Intravenous immunoglobulin in oncology nursing practice. *Oncology Nursing Forum, 20,* 69–75.
19. Frey, A. (1991). The immune system, Part II: Intravenous administration of immune globulin. *Journal of Intravenous Nursing, 14,* 396–405.
20. Yarnell, R. P., & Craig, M. (1991). Detecting hypomagnesemia: The most overlooked electrolyte imbalance. *Nursing '91, 21*(7), 55–57.
21. Owens, M.W. (1993). Keeping an eye on magnesium. *American Journal of Nursing, 93*(1), 66–67.
22. Graves, L. (1990). Disorders of calcium, phosphorus, and magnesium. *Critical Care Nursing Quarterly, 13* (3), 3–13.

BIBLIOGRAPHY

Baranowski, L. (1992). Current trends in blood component therapy: The evolution of a safer, more effective product. *Journal of Intravenous Nursing, 15,* 136–151.

Baranowski, L. (1991). Filtering out the confusion about leukocyte-poor blood components. *Journal of Intravenous Nursing, 14,* 295–306.

Cullen, L. (1992). Interventions related to fluid and electrolyte balance. *Nursing Clinics of North America, 27,* 569–597.

Korzets, A., et al. (1992). Electrolyte complications associated with fleet enemas. *Journal of the American Geriatric Society, 40,* 620–621.

Metheny, N. (1990). Why worry about IV fluids? *American Journal of Nursing, 90*(6), 50–57.

Millam, D.A. (1993). How to teach good venipuncture technique. *American Journal of Nursing, 93*(7), 38–41.

National Blood Resource Education Program's Nursing Education Working Group. (1991). Transfusion nursing: Trends and practices for the '90's. *American Journal of Nursing, 91*(6), 42–56.

Sachter, J. (1992). Magnesium in the 1990s: Implications for acute care. *Topics in Emergency Medicine, 14*(1), 23–50.

Schrier, R. (1992). *Renal and electrolyte disorders* (4th ed.). Boston: Little, Brown.

U.S. Food and Drug Administration. (1993). *Physician's genRx.* Smithtown, NY: Author.

CHAPTER 75

Enteral and Parenteral Nutritional Therapy

MARTHA A. SPIES

✹ Nursing Considerations

LEARNING OBJECTIVES:

Use the nursing process to develop a plan of care for the client with the diagnosis, "Alteration in nutrition: less than body requirements."

Identify nursing interventions appropriate for the implementation of enteral and parenteral nutrition.

KEY TERM: Anthropometric measurements

✹ Enteral Nutritional Therapy

LEARNING OBJECTIVES:

Describe the components of enteral nutrition solutions.

Identify possible complications and side effects of enteral nutrition administration.

KEY TERMS:

Hypertonic, isotonic, osmolality

✹ Parenteral Nutritional Therapy

LEARNING OBJECTIVES:

Describe the components of parenteral nutrition solutions.

Identify possible complications and side effects of parenteral nutrition administration.

CONCEPTS AND TERMS TO REVIEW

Read the section on nursing considerations in Chapter 71.

Review the content in Chapter 70 on fluid, electrolyte, and nutrition balance.

Read the section in a nutrition textbook on enteral and parenteral nutritional therapy.

Review the section of a medical-surgical textbook on enteral and parenteral nutrition.

---

*T*he intake of nutrients in optimal amounts and combinations is necessary to maintain health and to allow healing in times of illness. When healthy, the individual normally obtains the recommended amounts and kinds of nutrients through the oral ingestion of food and fluids. The gastrointestinal (GI) tract provides a pathway for digestion and absorption of nutrients and elimination of waste. Malnutrition is a serious problem in the individual experiencing either acute or chronic illness. Malnutrition can occur when an individual is unable to ingest sufficient nutrients to maintain optimal

health or experiences an injury that results in an increased need for nutrients.

When a client cannot ingest food and fluid orally but the GI tract is intact and functioning, **enteral nutrition** (the provision of nutrients to the GI tract) is the preferred method to deliver nutrients; it maintains normal GI mucosal structure and function and reduces costs.[1] When the GI tract is not able to perform the processes involved in supporting normal nutrition, nutrients can be given intravenously (**parenteral nutrition**).

▨ NURSING CONSIDERATIONS

Assessing During the **health history** obtain a nutritional history. This information identifies risk factors and provides information regarding indicators of nutritional alterations. Ask the client about a recent change in body weight; a 10% decrease in the absence of a planned dietary change is a major indicator that the client is experiencing a nutritional deficiency. The presence of chronic health conditions, especially ones that affect the body's metabolism or processes such as diabetes mellitus, malabsorption, renal or liver disease, provides evidence of the need for special dietary strategies. In addition, alterations of the mouth, pharynx, or esophagus indicate the client requires either enteral or parenteral nutrition. Recent surgery, injury, infection, or other acute illness may increase the body's need for nutrients, especially protein, to aid healing. Individuals with cancer may have alterations such as anorexia, nausea, and vomiting, which interfere with normal nutrition. Rapidly dividing tumors can produce special nutritional demands on the client because the tumor itself can use a large amount of amino acid (especially glutamine) and ketone bodies. These alterations may be due to the malignant process or to chemotherapy or radiation therapy. Ask the client to provide a food diary of all foods and fluids ingested in the last 24 hours.

Anthropometric measurements are noninvasive methods used to measure nutrition indirectly as reflected in changes in growth, development, body fat, and muscle tissue. Specialized knowledge and skills are required to obtain and interpret anthropometric measurements accurately, so they should always be made by trained individuals. Body weight is determined by using a calibrated beam balance scale. Body weight measurement is the most common assessment of nutritional status and reflects total weight of lean body mass and fat. A decrease in body weight 10% to 20% below recommended body weight is associated with malnutrition. The client's height is measured to detect growth failure in the infant or child. The client's weight in relation to height is compared to standards for the total population to detect obesity or malnutrition.

Other anthropometric measurements include midarm circumference and triceps skin-fold thickness. Together these measurements indirectly determine the arm muscle area and arm fat area, which can be used to estimate lean body mass and protein reserves.[2-4]

Laboratory tests provide more objective data than the history or anthropometric data. A combination of test results is more meaningful than any single test result. A standard protocol for laboratory tests may be determined by the nutritional support team, or the laboratory tests may be ordered by the primary care provider as indicated by the client's condition. A decreased level of serum proteins, especially serum albumin, reflects malnutrition and can result in edema because of decreased serum oncotic pressure. Prealbumin has a serum half-life of 2 to 3 days, so a change in nutrient intake can be detected within 7 days, allowing a more rapid detection of malnutrition.[5] A serum level of prealbumin less than 15 mg/dl indicates serum protein depletion. The normal serum protein level is 6.3 to 7.9 g/L, and the normal serum albumin level is 3.8 to 5 g/dl. Transferrin is a protein that regulates iron absorption and transport. A serum transferrin level less than 240 mg/dl is associated with loss of protein stores in body tissues. A decreased total lymphocyte count (in the absence of bone marrow suppression) evaluates the status of the immune system and the adequacy of tissue protein stores. A serum level less than 1000/mm³ suggests significant protein depletion.

The formula for determining nitrogen balance is based on the difference between nitrogen intake (all routes) and nitrogen loss through the urine plus the unmeasured losses through the skin and GI tract:

Nitrogen intake − (Urinary nitrogen + Change in BUN + 4)
where change in BUN (g) = (0.6 × weight [kg]) (BUNf − BUNi)

Note: i and f refer to initial and final levels of BUN

This calculation must be done carefully. There is a tendency to overestimate intake and underestimate loss, which can result in an inaccurate assumption that the client will experience anabolism.[5]

To improve the specificity and sensitivity of nutritional assessment, the Prognostic Nutritional Index (PNI) was developed as a multiparameter index to use to predict nutritional need.[5] The formula for the PNI is:

PNI (%risk) =
158 − 16.6 (albumin [g]) − 0.78 (triceps skinfold [mm]) −
0.2 (transferrin [mg/dl]) − 5.8 (skin test reactivity [0–2])

During the **physical assessment,** systematic inspection can reveal changes associated with malnutrition. Examination of the face and head of the malnourished client will reveal thinning hair that lacks the shine of healthy hair. The skin and conjunctiva may be pale if iron deficiency is present. The lips and tongue may be dry if the client is experiencing a fluid deficit. The angle of the lips and the tongue may be inflamed, and the gums may bleed easily.

Muscle mass and strength may be diminished when the person is experiencing protein or calorie deficiency. Deep tendon reflexes may be hyperactive or hypoactive with imbalances in calcium and magnesium levels. Generalized edema can occur with hypoalbuminemia because serum proteins exert oncotic pressure, which keeps fluid in the vascular space. A decreased serum albumin level allows fluid to leak into the interstitial space where it becomes trapped.

Indirect calorimetry is a method used to determine a client's energy expenditure and caloric needs. This test measures the resting energy expenditure (REE) based on oxygen consumption and CO_2 production.[5] The REE is measured 2 hours after eating, with the client lying down and resting for 30 minutes. The total daily energy expenditure is usually 130% of the REE.

The client's age and physical condition affect nutritional needs. Children of all ages need sufficient quantities of all nutrients to sustain the intense periods of growth they experience. Infants' percentage of body weight as water is larger, so any condition that increases loss of fluids (e.g., vomiting or diarrhea) can quickly lead to dehydration. Women who are pregnant or nursing children need increased levels of all nutrients to maintain maternal health and to provide adequate nutrition for the fetus or infant. Nutritional requirements remain stable during adulthood and are decreased from the levels needed to maintain health in childhood and adolescence. With aging, the caloric need decreases because of decreased BMR.

Diagnosing The nursing diagnosis "Alteration in nutrition: less than body requirements" is defined as a state in which an individual who may consume food orally experiences (or is at risk of experiencing) reduced weight related to an inadequate intake or metabolism of nutrients.[6] This diagnosis refers to an inability to ingest, digest, or absorb nutrients in quantities sufficient to fulfill nutritional requirements.[7] One of the most objective defining characteristics is weight 20% or more under that recommended for height and body frame. Other important supporting assessment data include a caloric intake less than the minimum daily requirement for the client's current metabolic need. Anthropometric and laboratory measurements and physical examination findings support the presence of malnutrition.

Planning Teach the client who will receive enteral or parenteral nutrition in the hospital to focus on the reason the nutritional support will be given and what the client will experience. For the client who requires enteral or parenteral nutrition at home, give the client or caregiver more extensive information so that the procedure can be done safely, comfortably, and effectively. It is often necessary for a caregiver to be available because the malnourished client may not have the energy to perform the necessary procedures. Begin the teaching in the hospital and expect that it will be reinforced or completed by home health nurses after the client is discharged.

An appropriate level of cleanliness must be established in the home to prevent infection. The client or caregiver must be able to prepare the tube feeding formula. Teach the client that all of the equipment used in formula preparation must be carefully cleaned because of the danger of bacterial contamination. Parenteral nutrition solutions will be delivered already prepared to the client's home. Total nutrient admixtures often are used to decrease the number of bags or bottles that must be hung. When insulin is needed, teach the client to add it to the bag because it is not stable in the solutions for long periods. Give the client or caregiver information on safe storage of the tube feeding or parenteral nutrition formula, especially if the tube feeding formula is prepared from a powder. An appropriate source of power must be available for one or more pumps. The client or caregiver must be able to demonstrate proper care of the feeding tube or vascular access device and equipment such as pumps. This care may include performing dressing changes for gastrostomy tubes or retaping nasally placed tubes and periodic flushing of all enteral tubes. The client or caregiver must know how to test placement of the tube and how to check gastric residual volumes. The client or caregiver also needs to know appropriate actions to implement if the tube becomes dislodged or if there is a large residual volume. For parenteral nutrition, teach the client or caregiver how to use careful sterile technique when attaching parenteral solutions and irrigating vascular access devices. Clients often prefer receiving intermittent feedings at night so that they are not connected to a pump for prolonged periods of time and can participate in more normal activities.

Teach the client to obtain his or her body weight at least weekly, to monitor intake and output daily; and to report immediately any temperature elevation. Urine or blood sugar values also must be monitored, especially during parenteral nu-

trition. Teach the client to have telephone numbers of resource persons available if complications develop or equipment malfunctions. Clients or caregivers must know how to obtain supplies and equipment and to arrange for reimbursement. The client will have weekly medical follow-up examinations until he or she is stable; when he or she is stable, the frequency of follow-up examinations can be every other month.

The identified outcomes reflect maintenance or improvement of the client's level of nutrition through the provision of enteral or parenteral nutrition. Outcome statements must be individualized for each client. General outcomes include the following:

- Client gains 0.5 to 1.0 pound per week.
- Client receives sufficient calories to meet metabolic needs.
- Serum albumin, transferrin, and total lymphocyte levels are normal.
- Client or caregiver demonstrates appropriate care for tube-feeding or parenteral nutrition equipment.

ENTERAL NUTRITIONAL THERAPY Basic considerations when planning nursing care for a client receiving enteral nutrition include the route that will be used and the placement of the feeding tube in the GI tract. Tubes can be orogastric, nasogastric, or nasoduodenal. The nasoduodenal route is used because of its association with a lower incidence of pulmonary aspiration. When the tube feeding is given over a long period, the tube can be inserted surgically or with fluoroscopy as an esophagostomy, a gastrostomy, or a jejunostomy. These insertions are used to avoid the discomfort of the oral or nasal insertion of a feeding tube. Know the tube type and size used. Small-bore pliable tubes are more comfortable for the client but are associated with a higher incidence of pulmonary aspiration and tube clogging. In addition, traditional methods for checking the placement of the tube are not reliable.[8]

To administer tube feedings accurately and safely, you must know the type of formula to give and the strength and rate to use. To obtain the necessary number of calories and nutrients, the client usually needs to receive 1000 to 2000 ml each 24 hours. Check the formula container for an expiration date, or when the formula is prepared by the agency's dietary department, check the time of expiration. Also be familiar with the characteristics of the formula (e.g., whether it contains lactose or fiber). Most formulas have a caloric density of 1.0 to 1.5 kcal/ml and contain 55% carbohydrate, 30% fat, and 15% protein.[1] Note the **osmolality** of the formula (i.e., its concentration expressed in milliosmoles per kilogram of solution). Many formulas are **isotonic,** having the same concentration as another solution (280 to 300 mOsm/kg), but some formulas are **hypertonic,** or more concentrated (400 to 1100 mOsm/kg).

Tube feedings are usually given as bolus, intermittent, or continuous feedings. **Bolus feedings** indicate the administration of 100 to 400 ml of formula over 1 to 5 minutes every 3 to 4 hours. Bolus feedings are not tolerated well because of the sudden increase in GI volume and osmolality. **Intermittent feedings** indicate the administration of 100 to 400 ml of formula over 15 to 30 minutes or longer four to six times each day. This schedule more closely resembles a normal meal pattern in which there is alternate filling and emptying of the stomach and intestines, and it allows the client to take part in normal activities between the feeding times. Intermittent feedings are tolerated better when given into the stomach because gastric secretions dilute the hypertonic solution before it is released into the duodenum.[1] **Continuous feedings** are given over 24 hours using a pump to regulate the rate. Continuous feedings are generally associated with increased absorption of nutrients, achievement of a positive nitrogen balance, and decreased incidence of diarrhea when compared with bolus feedings. Continuous feedings are used when the feedings are given into the duodenum or the jejunum because they are better tolerated there.

When tube feedings are begun, anticipate diluting the formula or giving it more slowly to decrease the incidence of GI complications such as cramping, nausea, or diarrhea. Initiate isotonic formulas at full strength but at a slower rate such as 50 ml/h. The rate can be increased 25 ml/h every 8 to 12 hours until the client is receiving the volume necessary to deliver the required calories and nutrients. When hypertonic tube feedings are given or tube feedings are given into the duodenum or jejunum, dilute the formula to half strength and start at 50 ml/h or slower. Generally first increase the rate to the level needed to deliver the necessary volume each hour and then increase the dilution of the formula until the client is receiving the necessary volume of full-strength formula.[9] The rate and strength of the formula should not be changed simultaneously because it will then be impossible to determine whether an adverse reaction is related to the change in volume or the change in osmolality.

PARENTERAL NUTRITIONAL THERAPY   Since parenteral nutrition is given into a vein, planning nursing interventions includes all of the factors involved in administering general IV therapy and those specific to administering a comprehensive nutritional product. Parenteral nutrition usually is administered into the superior vena cava to prevent phlebitis by diluting the hypertonic parenteral nutrition solutions with high-volume blood flow. Usual insertion sites are the subclavian or internal jugular veins, which allow threading the catheter into the superior vena cava. The vascular access device can be percutaneously placed or surgically implanted. All elements of nutrition, including sufficient calories for long-term support of growth and tissue maintenance and repair, can be administered through this route. A peripheral site may be used on a short-term basis to administer amino acids, 5% or 10% carbohydrate solutions, lipids, and other nutrients to provide 1400 to 2000 kcal/d for clients who can meet some nutritional needs through oral intake.[10]

Knowledge of the composition of the parenteral fluid enables the nurse to plan comprehensive nursing care. Crystalline amino acids are given to increase anabolism, decrease catabolism, and promote wound healing.[11] Formulas for infants and children differ from those for adults because some amino acids that are nonessential for adults are essential for infants and children.[12] Strongly hypertonic amino acid solutions cannot be given through a peripheral vein. Amino acid solutions have been developed to meet the special needs of clients with alterations in hepatic and renal function.

Calories are provided by a combination of carbohydrate and fat or lipid administration. These nonprotein sources of calories spare protein for use in anabolic processes. Carbohydrates should not be the only source of nonprotein calories because carbohydrate metabolism produces CO_2, which increases minute ventilation and can precipitate respiratory failure in the client with an already existing alteration in respiratory function.[13] The calories provided by lipid products should not exceed 60% of the total calories. Lipids are given to provide calories and to prevent deficiencies of essential fatty acids. Amino acids and dextrose often are administered together in the same bag with the majority of other necessary nutrients, but the lipids are administered in a separate container. The lipid container should be hung higher than the amino acid–dextrose line to prevent backflow of the lipids into the other line (lipids have a lower specific gravity).

A newer process that may decrease infection rates and costs is available in which amino acids, dextrose, lipids, and other nutrients are mixed in the same bag (3-in-1 mixtures, or total nutrient admixture [TNA]). These solutions have a higher pH and lower osmolality than traditional solutions and possibly may be given through a peripheral vein.[14] Disadvantages of these solutions include decreased stability in the bag, more difficulty with incompatibilities, decreased flexibility in composition, and inability to inspect for particulate matter or to use filters.[15]

The TPN formula usually provides 3000 ml of fluid per 24 hours. This volume may not be tolerated by a client with cardiac and renal alterations. The caloric concentration can be increased so the total volume of fluid administered is tolerated better by the client.

Implementing

ENTERAL NUTRITION   Nursing interventions for the client receiving tube feedings focus on detecting and preventing complications.

One of the most serious complications with tube feedings is aspiration of stomach contents into the lungs, especially when the client has an impaired gag reflex. To prevent aspiration, elevate the head of the client's bed at least 30 degrees to prevent upward migration of the tube. As the client receives tube feedings, monitor tube placement. The position of the small-bore, pliable tube in the GI tract should be verified by x-ray film before tube feedings are begun. Aspiration of stomach contents into a syringe can be done with many of the tubes to verify position. When stomach contents are aspirated, measure the gastric residual volume. If the volume is greater than 100 to 150 ml or 50% of the volume infused in an hour, stop the tube feeding and notify the primary care provider because this indicates that gastric emptying is delayed, which can increase the risk of vomiting and aspiration. Return the aspirated material to the GI tract to prevent the removal of fluid and electrolytes. If the client vomits, stop the tube feeding.

🌿 NURSING RESEARCH

Metheny, N., Reed, L., Berglund, B., & Wehrle, M.A. (1994). Visual characteristics of aspirates from feeding tubes as a method for predicting tube location. *Nursing Research, 43*(5), 282–287.

The purpose of this research was to determine whether the location of a tube used in enteral feeding could be predicted by the visual characteristics of tube aspirates. A sample of 880 feeding tube aspirates was classified by clarity and color. Gastric aspirates were most often cloudy and green, tan or off-white, or bloody or brown. Intestinal fluids were mostly clear and yellow to bile colored. Pleural fluid without blood was usually pale yellow and serous, and tracheobronchial secretions were generally tan or off-white mucus. However, blood in respiratory aspirates altered expected characteristics of that fluid.

Staff nurses were told about these characteristics and then were shown 106 photographs of aspirates. Their ability to identify gastric and intestinal aspirates improved after reading the list of criteria for each category. However, their accuracy in predicting respiratory aspirates decreased.

The study concluded that criteria lists are helpful in distinguishing between gastric and intestinal placement but are of little value in assessing respiratory samples.

STUDENT ACTIVITIES

- Assist in aspiration of tube feedings and assess the color and clarity of the aspirate (clear or cloudy) against the guidelines above.
- Obtain input from several nurses working in respiratory care areas about their criteria for identifying respiratory secretions. Inquire how they assess sputum with blood admixture. Compare their remarks with the results of this study. 🌿

Assess the GI tract to determine the response to the tube feeding. Monitor bowel sounds to ensure that neither a mechanical obstruction nor a paralytic ileus is present; tube feedings cannot be given safely in the presence of an obstruction. An indirect indicator of gastric retention is an increasing abdominal girth.

One of the most frequent complications of tube feedings is diarrhea. Possible causes of diarrhea include lactose, high fat content (>20 g of fat/L), or low fiber content in the formula; decreased serum albumin level, which makes the tube feeding formula relatively hypertonic; drugs such as H_2-blockers or antibiotics; or use of hypertonic formulas.[16] If the use of hypertonic liquid drugs probably caused the diarrhea, dilute them before administration. Another possible cause of diarrhea is bacterial contamination of the equipment or formula. To prevent this, change the bag and tubing every 24 hours, and do not hang the formula for longer than 4 to 6 hours. Use careful technique in handling the equipment and formula (e.g., clean the tops of cans before opening). If diarrhea occurs, antidiar-

rheal medications, a formula with fiber, a bulk-forming product, or *Lactobacillus acidophilus* (Lactinex), which restores normal flora, can be used (see Chapter 48). The rate and strength of the formula can be decreased, especially if the formula is hypertonic. However, decreasing the rate and strength may reduce the number of calories and the nutrients provided to levels less than necessary to maintain positive nitrogen balance.

A mechanical complication that can occur is clogging of the tube. This can occur with a small tube diameter, viscous formula, or improper administration of medications through the tube. Use of polyurethane tubes and flushing with warm water or Coca-Cola periodically and with medication administration can help to prevent clogging.[17]

PARENTERAL NUTRITION   Store total parenteral nutrition (TPN) solutions in the refrigerator and administer them completely within 24 hours of hanging the bag. TPN may be initiated slowly at 40 ml/h and advanced gradually by 20 ml/h to allow the client's metabolism to adapt to the increase in glucose and osmolality.[18] Discard TPN solutions if they are cloudy, are an inappropriate color, or show particulate matter. Discard total nutrient admixtures if they look like cream that has separated.

Dextrose, protein, and lipids are sources of calories in the TPN. Dextrose concentrations generally range from 25% to 35%, with an osmolality of 1200 to 1700 mOsm/L. These hypertonic solutions must be administered through a central vein.[11] Crystalline amino acid products are manufactured in concentrations ranging from 3.5% to 15%. Lipid solutions are isotonic and can be given through a peripheral vein but are often given with the TPN solution. The lipid-TPN mixture is unstable; thus the lipid insertion site must be close to the vascular access device, minimizing the time that the solutions are mixed. Start lipid administration slowly (0.5 to 1.0 ml/min for 15 to 30 minutes). Monitor the client for nausea, chills, muscle aches, pain in the chest or back, and urticaria.[12] Too rapid administration can result in dilution of serum electrolytes, overhydration, pulmonary edema, impaired pulmonary diffusion, or metabolic acidosis. Chronic adverse reactions include hepatomegaly and splenomegaly, thrombocytopenia and leukopenia, focal seizures, and fever. If no adverse reaction is noted during the first 15 to 30 minutes, increase the rate to no greater than 125 ml/h. The lipid molecules are large, so these solutions cannot be infused through a filter. Use special tubing to administer lipids because lipids can pull a toxic substance from plastic tubing.

One of the most serious complications associated with the use of TPN is sepsis. The most common causative organisms are *Staphylococcus aureus* and *Candida albicans*.[19] Gram-positive bacteria can colonize the catheter by migrating from the skin to the catheter on a fibrin sleeve that forms along the surface of the catheter. Fungi usually enter the bloodstream from the GI tract.[9] Nursing interventions aimed at prevention of sepsis include careful use of sterile technique during all manipulation of the TPN solutions, tubing, and dressings. Use one bag of solution sufficient to meet the client's needs for 24 hours to minimize the number of times the system is opened for bag changes. Use filters that can remove bacteria for any solution not containing lipids. Reserve use of the IV line for the TPN solution to minimize the number of entries into the system. Change tubing and filters daily with the bag change. Change dressings every 24 to 72 hours using sterile technique. Inspect the dressing to detect loss of occlusiveness and any wetness that could increase the access of organisms to the insertion site. Check the client's temperature for elevation every 4 hours. Note other signs that may indicate sepsis such as the appearance of glucose intolerance or mental status changes. When temperature elevation is noted, use measures to detect the source of the fever, especially blood cultures. If no other source of infection (e.g., urinary or respiratory tract infection) is found, remove the TPN catheter, culture the tip of the catheter, and initiate antibiotic treatment.

Evaluating To determine the effect of the nutritional therapy, obtain the client's body weight daily. After the nutritional therapy is established, obtain the body weight three times a week or weekly. The expected result is a gain of 2 to 3 pounds each week. Measure the client's weight using standard conditions (i.e., same scale, same time of day, same or similar clothing). This standard approach ensures that any change in weight is actually due to a change in body mass. If a sudden change in weight occurs out of proportion to the nutritional therapy, investigate other causes for the change (e.g., loss or retention of fluids because of a complication).

Calculate the client's intake of nutrients from the volume and composition of nutrients administered. Do this twice weekly as nutritional therapy is initiated; it can then be done weekly after the client's intake is stabilized at a sufficient level. The client's caloric intake should be 28 (range, 25 to 30) kcal/kg/24 h, or approximately 3000 kcal/24 h unless the client is very hypermetabolic; for example, an extensively burned client's caloric need can increase to 50 kcal/kg/24 h.[20] Include any oral intake in the calculations along with the enteral or parenteral solutions. Determine the number of calories and the intake of proteins, carbohydrates, fats, minerals, and vitamins. Use the volume of tube-feeding formula that is actually infused rather than the ordered volume. Many factors can decrease the infused volume (e.g., the rate or strength of the formula is decreased when the client experiences diarrhea, the tube becomes clogged or is pulled out, or the tube feeding is turned off for periods of time while the client is placed flat for therapy).

Monitor laboratory test results at least weekly initially to evaluate the effect of nutritional therapy. Later the frequency

TABLE 75–1
Major Medical Tests

Test	Initial Frequency	Later Frequency
Blood glucose: fingerstick (detects glucose intolerance and determines need for insulin)	Four times/24 h	Four times/24 h
or		
Urinary glucose: used for clients with normal glucose tolerance to screen for changes in blood glucose	Four times/24 h	Four times/24 h
Serum electrolytes: evaluates adequacy of nutritional formulas; detects complications Sodium Potassium Magnesium Chloride Calcium Phosphorus Bicarbonate	Daily	Twice weekly
Serum osmolality: monitors adequacy of fluid replacement and detects hyperosmolar imbalance	Daily	Weekly
Protein metabolism: determines adequacy of amino acid and caloric replacement Total protein Albumin Blood urea nitrogen (verifies kidney's ability to excrete increased urea) Creatinine Hemoglobin Transferrin Total lymphocyte count Prothrombin time	Twice weekly	Weekly
Serum triglycerides: monitors for hyperlipidemia, which can occur when lipids do not clear within 6–8 h of administration	Weekly	Weekly
Serum transaminases: monitors for liver inflammation and fatty liver infiltration, especially during first 2 wk of therapy	Twice weekly	Weekly
Trace minerals: monitors for adequate replacement Zinc Copper Chromium Selenium	Weekly	Weekly or less frequently

for doing the tests may be monthly or longer. Serum albumin levels should increase but may return to normal gradually over 2 to 3 weeks.[5] Nitrogen balance is a sensitive indicator of nutritional adequacy and can become positive within 2 to 3 days.[5] Serum transferrin levels are expected to increase to 240 to 489 mg/dl within 7 days. Total lymphocyte count will increase to 1000 to 4000/mm[3]. Certain assessment factors (e.g., upper arm circumference) are not sensitive enough to detect the immediate effect of nutritional support, and repeating them is not necessary until nutritional support has been used for 1 month or longer.[5,21]

Evaluate the client's and caregiver's ability to implement all of the care necessary for administration of enteral or parenteral nutrition before discharging the client to home. Do this by having the client or caregiver assume total responsibility for the nutritional therapy and perform all of the necessary steps independently while you observe for correct technique. In this way you can detect any errors and correct them immediately. In addition, have the client or caregiver verbalize major complications, how to prevent or detect them, and what steps to take if a complication develops. A home health nurse needs to make similar evaluations when the client returns home because anxiety can cause forgetfulness, and modifying procedures to fit the actual home environment may be necessary.

The primary care provider monitors laboratory test results during the administration of nutritional therapy to evaluate its effectiveness. The frequency of testing changes from the early period of nutritional therapy (i.e., first 3 to 5 days while the client is adapting to increasing glucose intake) to later periods when the client has adapted to the administration of concentrated nutrient solutions. Laboratory testing also is done to detect the presence of complications when clinical assessment data change (Table 75–1).

CONCEPT REVIEW

Enteral and parenteral nutrition is used when a client is unable to ingest nutrients by the normal oral route in amounts sufficient to maintain health and allow healing. It is necessary in these circumstances to prevent malnutrition and to provide the essential components of normal nutrition: proteins, carbohydrates, lipids, vitamins, minerals, and water. A guideline for nutritional deficit is body weight 20% or more under that recommended for height and body frame.

Enteral nutrition delivers food into the GI tract; it is less expensive than parenteral nutrition, and it maintains normal GI mucosal structure and function. Short-term enteral feeding can be by orogastric, nasogastric, or nasoduodenal tube. Long-term feeding tubes can be inserted surgically (esophagostomy, gastrostomy, or jejunostomy). A tube feeding is given as a bolus, intermittently, or continuously. The rate and strength of the formula given are increased gradually but separately so that client response to rate or strength can be gauged accurately. Volume and color

of gastric contents are important indicators of tube placement and gastric emptying. Clogging of tubes and aspiration of the feedings are two serious complications.

Parenteral nutrition is used when the GI tract cannot perform the processes involved in supporting normal nutrition. It is usually administered into the superior vena cava through subclavian or internal jugular veins. Differences in formula can affect placement of the inserting needle. With parenteral nutrition, calories are provided by a combination of carbohydrate and fat or lipid administration, which spares protein for use in anabolic processes; such formulas can be administered separately or in combination with amino acids. The most serious complication associated with the use of TPN is sepsis.

The effect of nutritional therapy is determined by weighing the client daily at first, then three times a week or weekly. The expected result is a gain of 2 to 3 pounds per week. The client's actual intake of nutrients is calculated twice a week initially and weekly after the intake is stabilized. Laboratory test results are also monitored to evaluate the effectiveness of therapy.

ENTERAL NUTRITIONAL THERAPY

Prototype Formulas

MODULAR FORMULAS

A modular formula consists of a single nutrient that can be combined with other single nutrients to produce an individually tailored formula for use in situations in which existing formulas do not meet a client's needs. Modular nutrients include sources of carbohydrates, fats, proteins, water, vitamins, and minerals. They can be given by tube, added to food or nutrient formulas, or given as an oral liquid (Table 75–2). The use of modular formulas is more expensive than using complete formulas because of manufacturing and preparation costs.

Carbohydrate modules are inexpensive and easily digested and combine readily with most liquid formulas. Carbohydrates differ in their osmolality, and some are more concentrated, increasing the risk of side effects such as diarrhea or hyperosmolar fluid imbalance. The prototype carbohydrate module is Polycose, which is derived from cornstarch by hydrolysis and contains 50 or 94 g of carbohydrate in each 100 ml. It supplies calories in situations in which the client's usual food sources do not meet caloric needs (Table 75–3).

Fat modules can contain long-chain (e.g., corn oil or safflower oil) or medium-chain triglycerides and are used to supplement caloric intake. The prototype medium-chain triglyceride product is MCT Oil, which is a liquid and provides 115 kcal/15 ml. MCT Oil is more expensive than products containing long-chain triglycerides, but it is digested and absorbed more easily. Medium-chain triglycerides do not contain all of the essential fatty acids, so deficiencies can develop (Table 75–3).

Protein modules contain intact protein (e.g., pureed beef, egg white solids); hydrolyzed protein, which are peptides and free amino acids; or crystalline amino acids, which require no further digestion before intestinal absorption. Crystalline proteins have the least pleasant taste and have an increased osmolality. Protein modules are more expensive than carbohydrate or fat modules. The prototype amino acid protein module is Nutrisource Protein, which is a powder. It has a higher ratio of branched chain–enriched amino acids (BCAAs) to aromatic amino acids, which makes it useful for clients with alterations in hepatic function because BCAAs can be metabolized as an energy source independent of liver function.[22] Only small amounts of BCAAs are metabolized by the liver, so BCAAs that flow to the liver after a meal are transferred intact into the

TABLE 75–2
Selected Tube Feeding Formulas

Formula	Clinical Uses	Nursing Considerations
MODULAR Polycose MCT Oil Nutrisource Protein	Provides single nutrient to supplement other intake or to compound a complete formula specific to client's individualized needs	Most formulas are supplied as a powder, so preparation can be complex and expensive; carefully store prepared formula to prevent contamination. Small, frequent feedings are tolerated better than larger, less frequent feedings. When used individually, these formulas do not provide complete nutrition.
BLENDERIZED Compleat-Regular Vitaneed	Provides complete nutrition when GI tract is functioning	Most formulas contain lactose and may cause diarrhea. Use large-bore tube.
POLYMERIC: MILK BASED Meritene Sustagen	Provides complete nutrition when GI tract is functioning	Formulas contain lactose and may cause diarrhea.

POLYMERIC: LACTOSE FREE
Ensure
  Ensure HN
  Ensure Plus
  Ensure Plus HN
Isocal
  Isocal HCN
Jevity
Magnacal
Osmolite
  Osmolite HN
Sustacal
  Sustacal HC
	Provides complete nutrition when GI tract is functioning	Polymeric formulas can be isotonic or hyperosmolar; hyperosmolar formulas may cause more GI effects such as cramping and diarrhea; hyperosmolar formulas are started at a slower rate and are diluted.

MONOMERIC
Criticare HN
Precision Isotonic
  Precision HN
  Precision LR
Vital HN
Vivonex HN
  Vivonex T.E.N.
	Provides complete nutrition when GI tract function is altered (e.g., impaired pancreatic or gallbladder function, impaired absorption in the small intestine)	Formulas are hypertonic and must be started slowly and diluted. They can be given through a needle jejunostomy.

SPECIAL FORMULAS Amin-Aid Glucerna Hepatic-Aid II Pulmocare Stresstein	Provides nutritional formulas specific to client's alterations (e.g., client with renal and hepatic failure, diabetes mellitus, respiratory failure, trauma and stress)	Formulas may not provide all necessary nutrients, so careful monitoring is important.

Abbreviations: GI, gastrointestinal; HC, high calorie; HN, high nitrogen; HCN, high calorie, high nitrogen; LR, low residue; TEN, total enteral nutrition. Data from Fischer, J. (1991). Metabolism in surgical patients. In D. Sabiston (Ed.), Textook of surgery: The biological basis of modern surgical practice (pp. 103–140). Philadelphia: W.B. Saunders; Feucht, S. (1992). Appendix 33: Enteral nutrition products. In L. Mahan & M. Arlin (Eds.), Krause's food, nutrition, and diet therapy (8th ed; pp. 843–857). Philadelphia: W.B. Saunders; and Olin, B. (1992). Drug facts and comparisons. St. Louis: Facts and Comparisons Division, J.B. Lippincott.

TABLE 75–3
Prototype Enteral Formulas

Formula	Caloric Density (kcal/ml)	Volume Needed to Meet 100% RDA (ml/24h)	Osmolality (mOsm/kg)
Polycose	2.0	Incomplete	Same as that of added liquid
MCT Oil	7.67	Incomplete	Unknown
Nutrisource Protein	400 (powder)	Incomplete	Unknown
Compleat-Regular	1.0	1500	450
Sustagen	1.8	1030	1100
Ensure	1.0	1897	470
Vivonex HN	1.0	3000	810
Amin-Aid	2.0	Incomplete	700

Data from Fischer, J. (1991). Metabolism in surgical patients. In D. Sabiston (Ed.), *Textbook of surgery: The biological basis of modern surgical practice* (pp. 103–140). Philadelphia: W.B. Saunders; and Mahan, L., & Arlin, M. (1992). Methods of nutritional support. In L. Mahan & M. Arlin (Eds.), *Krause's food, nutrition, and diet therapy* (8th ed; pp. 507–526). Philadelphia: W.B. Saunders.

systemic circulation.[23] Skeletal muscle is the primary organ of metabolism for BCAAs (see Table 75–3).

COMPLETE FORMULAS

Blenderized formulas Blenderized formulas contain intact foods blended into a liquid consistency. These formulas are nutritionally complete, contain fiber, and promote normal GI function and bowel movements. They are used for clients with functioning GI tracts who have an altered ability to ingest and swallow food (see Table 75–2). Blenderized formulas have a high viscosity, so use of a large-bore tube is necessary.[24] The prototype blenderized formula is Compleat-Regular (see Table 75–3). The blenderized formulas usually contain lactose, which may cause diarrhea.

Polymeric formulas Polymeric formulas contain all the essential nutrients in complex forms that require a normally functioning GI tract for digestion and absorption (see Table 75–2). These formulas have a caloric density of 1, 1.5, or 2 kcal/ml. The higher density formula can be used (2 kcal/ml) to provide nutritional needs for clients with fluid restrictions, but hyperosmolar imbalance can occur. Polymeric formulas are generally well tolerated. When fiber is in the formula, it can clog small tubes and should not be used.[24] When these formulas are milk based, they contain lactose, which may cause diarrhea. The prototype milk-based formula is Sustagen, and the lactose-free formula is Ensure (see Table 75–3).

Monomeric formulas Monomeric formulas contain nutrients in more simple or basic forms (e.g., peptides or amino acids as protein, simple glucose molecules, and vegetable oils or medium-chain triglycerides as fat). These formulas do not require digestion and are easily absorbed so that clients with GI alterations can receive them (see Table 75–2). These formulas are hypertonic and are associated with diarrhea. The prototype formula is Vivonex HN (see Table 75–3).

Special formulas Special formulas are designed for use in clients with specific disease states in which the type of nutrients administered is important (see Table 75–2). Clients with hepatic failure benefit from a formula with a higher level of BCAAs and smaller amounts of aromatic amino acids. Formulas for use in clients with renal failure include only essential amino acids as the source of protein along with low levels of sodium and potassium. Clients with respiratory failure benefit from a formula in which a higher percentage of calories is provided by fats rather than carbohydrates so that CO_2 levels are kept lower. A formula for use in clients with diabetes mellitus has a lower percentage of calories derived from carbohydrates and a higher percentage of calories from fats and proteins than other formulas. BCAAs are metabolized by muscle cells into glutamate and alanine. The glutamate is converted into glutamine, which is used for energy production. Glutamine is important in the immune response and wound healing because it is the major source of energy for lymphocytes and fibroblasts.[23] Therefore formulas available for clients with trauma or stress have higher levels of BCAAs and unrestricted amounts of aromatic amino acids. The prototype special formula is Amin-Aid (see Table 75–3).

Undesired Clinical Responses

Because of the constant infusion of solutes, especially carbohydrates in the tube-feeding formula, the client is at risk for hyperglycemia, hypernatremia, and hyperosmolar fluid imbalance (Table 75–4). The very young and the elderly are at particular risk because they cannot efficiently excrete excess solutes, particularly with hypertonic formulas. Bowman et al.[25] did a retrospective review of 55 charts and found that 50% of clients over age 60 years developed elevated serum sodium levels while receiving hyperosmolar tube-feeding formulas in contrast to 10.3% receiving hypoosmolar formulas and 12.7% receiving isoosmolar formulas. When these elevated levels occur, the client's serum osmolality increases. To detect this increase, measure all routes of intake and output, noting a decreased urinary output in relation to intake. Assess the client's mucous membranes to note drying, and test skin turgor periodically. Monitor serum blood sugar and sodium levels, note any increases, and report them to the primary care provider. To prevent hyperosmolar fluid imbalance, administer free water (e.g., 100 ml of water every 4 to 6 hours) at intervals to most clients. The water is used by the body to dilute the concentrated vascular and cellular spaces, thus preventing increased serum osmolality.

TABLE 75–4
Undesired Clinical Responses Associated With Enteral Nutrition

Undesired Response	Mechanism	Nursing Considerations
Hyperglycemia, hypernatremia, hyperosmolar fluid imbalance	Constant administration of solutes leads to osmotic diuresis and decreased intravascular volume; substances in the serum become more concentrated (hyperosmolar fluid imbalance).	Measure intake and output. Assess moistness of mucous membranes. Assess skin turgor. Monitor for and report elevations in serum sodium, glucose, and osmolality levels. Administer plain water as ordered.
Hypokalemia, hypophosphatemia	Potassium and phosphorus move from intravascular space to intracellular space during the anabolism that occurs with refeeding.	Monitor serum levels of potassium and phosphorus and report decreases; undesired response usually occurs in first week of nutritional therapy.

Hyponatremia can result from water retention (excess ADH) or from sodium loss through diarrhea or diuresis.[26] Hypokalemia and hypophosphatemia can occur, especially when the client has experienced prior poor nutrition. Potassium and phosphorus are needed during the periods of anabolism experienced during early refeeding. These electrolytes move from the intravascular space to the intracellular space. A study of 25 clients revealed that the serum phosphorous level decreased from a range of 2.4 to 4.8 mg/dl at the start of tube feedings to 0.5 to 1.2 mg/dl after 2 to 5 days of isotonic enteral feedings.[27]

Interactions

When liquid drugs are mixed with enteral feeding formulas, physical incompatibilities can cause the mixture to thicken, which can clog the tube. Hypertonic drugs can increase the osmolality of the resulting fluid. Both of these effects can be lessened by flushing the tube with water and diluting the drug with water. The absorption or effect of some drugs can be altered by the tube-feeding formula (Table 75–5). To avoid this alteration, delivery of the tube feeding must be stopped for as long as 2 hours before and after the administration of the drug. This action decreases the total volume of nutrients delivered, so use of another route may be necessary.

CONCEPT REVIEW

Modular enteral formulas combine single nutrients to tailor nutrition to the needs of a particular client. They provide separate carbohydrates, fats, proteins, vitamins, and minerals.

Complete formulas can be blenderized intact foods, polymeric formulas, monomeric formulas with simple or basic nutrient elements, or special formulas designed for use with specific disease states.

With enteral feeding, client risks include hyperglycemia, hypernatremia, and hyperosmolar fluid imbalance. Hypokalemia and hypophosphatemia can also occur. Monitoring intake and output is especially important.

PARENTERAL NUTRITIONAL THERAPY

Prototype Formulas

PERIPHERAL PARENTERAL NUTRITION

ProcalAmine uses glycerol as a calorie source. This product contains 3% amino acids and 3% glycerin, providing 130 nonprotein calories per liter.[18] In addition, each liter contains electrolytes. ProcalAmine is designed for administration through a peripheral vein to preserve body protein and improve nitrogen balance in well-nourished, mildly catabolic clients who require only short-term parenteral nutrition. Other peripheral parenteral nutrition solutions include crystalline amino acids, 3% or 4%, dextrose in water solutions, 5% or 10%, and fat emulsions, 10% or 20% (Table 75–6).

CENTRAL PARENTERAL NUTRITION

Crystalline amino acid products are manufactured in concentrations ranging from 3.5% to 15%, with varying concentrations of dextrose and electrolytes (see Table 75–6). This allows the choice of a formula to meet the client's precise nutritional needs. A prototype crystalline amino acid product is Aminosyn (Table 75–7). Other brand names include Travasol, FreAmine, TrophAmine, and Novamine.

Carbohydrates are provided in solutions of dextrose in water ranging in concentration from 2.5% to 70%. Concentrations ranging from 25% to 38.5% are used most commonly for TPN. Solutions with a concentration greater than 50% rarely are used because of extreme hypertonicity (e.g., dextrose 70% has an osmolarity of 3535 mOsm/L).[28]

Lipid products are available as 10% (providing 1.1 kcal/ml) or 20% (providing 2 kcal/ml) solutions. These fat emulsions are composed of soybean or safflower sources of triglycerides. Fat emulsions are low osmolality and can be given safely through a peripheral vein. Intralipid 10% and Intralipid 20% are prototypes of the fat emulsions (see Table 75–7).

OTHER COMPONENTS

Electrolytes, trace minerals, and vitamins are added to the TPN solution. They are added separately when the client has

TABLE 75–5
Interactions of Drugs With Formulas

Effect	Drug
INTERACTIONS WITH ENTERAL FORMULAS*	
Physical incompatibility	Dimetane elixir
	Dimetapp elixir
	Robitussin expectorant
	Sudafed syrup
	Mellaril oral solution
	Thorazine concentrate
	Feosol Elixir
	KCL Liquid
	Klorvess syrup
	MCT Oil
	Amphojel
	Bentyl
	Kaon liquid
	Mylanta-II
	Paregoric
	Riopan
	Tagamet
Increased osmolality	Digoxin
	Theophylline
	Phenytoin
	Methyldopa
	Furosemide
Decreased drug effect	Warfarin
	Phenytoin
	Ampicillin
	Aspirin
	Cephalosporins
	Oxacillin
	Tetracycline
	Digoxin
	Levodopa
	Metoprolol
	Propranolol
INTERACTIONS WITH PARENTERAL FORMULAS†	
Physical incompatibility	Ampicillin
	Tetracycline
	Amphotericin B
Decreased drug effect	Ampicillin
	Kanamycin

*Data from Melnik, G. (1989). Pharmacologic aspects of enteral nutrition. In J. Rombeau & M. Caldwell (Eds.), *Clinical nutrition: Enteral and tube feeding* (pp. 472–509). Philadelphia: W.B. Saunders.
†Data from LaFrance, R., & Miyagawa, C. (1991). Pharmaceutical considerations in total parenteral nutrition. In J. Fischer (Ed.), *Total parenteral nutrition* (pp. 57–98). Boston: Little, Brown.

individualized needs or when products are available that contain the most commonly needed items. For example, Tracelyte contains zinc, copper, manganese, chromium, sodium, potassium, calcium, magnesium, acetate, chloride, and gluconate. Hyperlyte contains sodium, potassium, calcium, magnesium, acetate, and gluconate. Lypholyte and TPN Electrolytes contain all of the electrolytes in Hyperlyte except for gluconate.[28] Vitamin preparations are also given. Vitamins B_{12} and K often are excluded from the TPN formula and are given by subcutaneous injection once weekly.

Because each client has unique metabolic needs, TPN prescriptions are formulated to provide precise nutritional support. The volume of fluid, the osmolality, and the concentration of each nutrient can be varied to meet the needs of clients with renal or hepatic disease, high energy needs, or diabetes mellitus (Table 75–8).

Undesired Clinical Responses

One of the side effects of TPN is glucose intolerance. When it develops, the client experiences hyperglycemia, glucosuria, and osmotic diuresis (Table 75–9). Glucose intolerance often occurs during the first 2 to 3 days of parenteral nutrition because the client's body does not adapt to the amount of glucose in the TPN solution by increasing insulin production. However, if the client's blood glucose level suddenly rises after being stable, suspect the development of sepsis. To prevent hyperglycemia during the initiation of TPN, start a 25% glucose solution slowly (e.g., 60 ml/h) and increase the rate gradually (e.g., 20 ml/h every 24 to 48 hours) until the desired volume is established.[9] Always use a volume-control pump for TPN administration to prevent errors in the rate of infusion of the solution. Perform urine or finger-stick blood glucose determinations every 6 hours around the clock to detect hyperglycemia. Add regular insulin to the TPN solution or give it subcutaneously to lower elevated blood sugar levels. Decrease the percent of nonprotein calories that come from glucose by administering more lipids.

Another side effect of TPN administration is hyperosmolar hyperglycemic nonketotic coma. With this imbalance, the client loses fluid from the vascular space as the elevated blood glucose level causes osmotic diuresis. The client experiences a blood sugar level greater than 500 mg/dl, glucosuria, and elevated serum osmolality greater than 350 mOsm/L. The client is thirsty and has poor skin turgor. Give insulin to decrease the hyperglycemia and administer hypotonic intravenous fluids (e.g., 0.45% sodium chloride).[13] Stop administration of the TPN solution.

Hypoglycemia theoretically can occur when administration of the TPN solution is abruptly discontinued after the client's insulin production has become adapted to the constant infusion of the concentrated glucose source. However, research findings indicate that initiating the TPN solution at the full rate resulted in a mean increase in plasma glucose of 60 mg/dl (79 plus or minus 14 in diabetic clients).[29] In this same study, during the discontinuation phase the mean plasma glucose level decreased 40 plus or minus 20 mg/dl and returned to baseline within 60 minutes. If hypoglycemia does occur, it can result in diaphoresis and confusion, especially in pediatric clients. Preventive interventions include use of a pump to prevent undetected decreases in the rate of infusion, tapering solutions over a 1- to 2-hour period when TPN is discontinued, and replacing the TPN solution with a 10% dextrose solution infusion if the TPN solution must be discontinued abruptly.

Interactions

The stability of the solution and the compatibility of the components in the solution are difficult to establish because of

TABLE 75-6
Selected Total Parenteral Nutrition Solutions

Formula	Clinical Uses	Nursing Considerations
PERIPHERAL ProcalAmine Crystalline amino acids Dextrose, 5% or 10% Fat emulsions	Provide amino acids with dextrose, glycerol, or fats for calories to prevent protein catabolism for short periods; can also provide electrolytes and vitamins	Formula can be used for 2–3 wk for maintenance of nutrition. It may not provide sufficient nutrients for the client with increased metabolism or severe nutritional deficits.
CENTRAL	Provide long-term nutrition for clients with increased metabolic needs or decreased nutrition	Anticipate use of TPN when the GI tract cannot be used.

Crystalline amino acids
   Aminosyn
   FreAmine
   Novamine
   Travasol
	Promote anabolism, reduce catabolism, promote wound healing, and maintain intravascular fluid volume	Solutions with a concentration greater than 4% are hypertonic and cannot be given peripherally.
		Formulas for infants and children differ from formulas for adults because of differing needs for growth.

Dextrose in water solutions	Provide nonprotein calories to spare protein for anabolism	Solutions greater than 10% are hyperosmolar and must be given through a central vein.

Fat emulsions
   Intralipid
   Nutrilipid
   Soyacal
   Liposyn
	Provide nonprotein calories to spare protein for anabolism
	Provide essential fatty acids
		Sources are safflower and soybean oils.

FLUID, ELECTROLYTES, TRACE METALS Tracelyte Hyperlyte Lypholyte TPN Electrolytes Multivitamin additive Berocca Parenteral Nutrition	Provide replacement for normal and altered losses	Periodic monitoring is necessary to verify adequate maintenance therapy.

Data from Olin, B. (1992). *Drug facts and comparisons.* St. Louis: Facts and Comparisons Division, J.B. Lippincott.

TABLE 75-7
Prototype Parenteral Formulas

Formula	Nutrient	Osmolarity (mOsm/L)
Aminosyn 3.5%	Nitrogen: 0.55 g/dl	357
Aminosyn 8.5%	Nitrogen 1.34 g/dl	850
Dextrose 25%	Carbohydrate: 250 g/L, 850 cal/L	1330
Intralipid 10%	1.1 cal/ml	260
Intralipid 20%	2 cal/ml	260

Data from Olin, B. (1992). *Drug facts and comparisons.* St. Louis: Facts and Comparisons Division, J.B. Lippincott.

TABLE 75-8
Example of TPN Formula

Nutrient	Amount
Calories (kcal/L)	1020
Carbohydrates (g/L)	250
Amino acids (g/L)	28.5–42.5
Calories to nitrogen ratio	127:1
Osmolality (mOsm/kg)	1825
Electrolytes	
Sodium (mEq/L)	30–55
Potassium (mEq/d)	60–90
Chloride (mEq/L)	30–55
Calcium (mEq/d)	6–12
Magnesium (mEq/d)	16–20
Acetate (mEq/L)	46–70
Phosphorus (mM/d)	18–28
Trace elements	
Zinc (mg/d)	2.5–4
Copper (μg)	300–500
Chromium (μg)	10–20
Molybdenum (μg)	100–200
Selenium (μg)	40–80
Vitamins	Added daily

Data from Berger, R., & Adams, L. (1989). Nutritional support in the critical care setting (Part 2). *Chest, 96,* 372–380; and Inadomi, D., & Kipple, J. (1994). Fluid and electrolyte disorders in total parenteral nutrition. In M. Maxwell, C. Kleeman, & R. Narins (Eds.), *Maxwell and Kleeman's clinical disorders of fluid and electrolyte metabolism* (5th ed.; pp. 1437–1462). New York: McGraw-Hill.

TABLE 75–9
Undesired Clinical Responses Associated with Total Parenteral Nutrition

Undesired Response	Mechanism	Nursing Considerations
Hyperglycemia, glucosuria, osmotic diuresis	When insulin production does not match the increased intake of carbohydrates, blood sugar level increases, and excess glucose is excreted by the kidneys along with increased loss of fluid.	Initiate TPN gradually as ordered. Use a pump to regulate the TPN rate. Monitor blood sugar levels by performing finger-stick blood sugar checks q6h. Administer insulin as ordered. Decrease amount of calories obtained from dextrose by increasing the amount of fat.
Hyperosmolar, hyperglycemic, non-ketotic coma	Elevated blood glucose level causes an osmotic diuresis. Blood sugar and serum osmolality are increased.	Monitor for complaints of thirst. Monitor skin turgor. Administer insulin and hypotonic IV fluids. Stop administration of TPN solution.
Hypoglycemia	When administration of TPN solution is discontinued abruptly, endogenous insulin production continues and may cause blood sugar level to decrease rapidly.	Use a pump to regulate the rate. Replace TPN solution with 10% dextrose solution if TPN solution must be abruptly discontinued. Taper delivery of TPN solutions over 1–2 h.

the complex nature of TPN solutions. Because of this difficulty and to prevent infection, drugs are not given piggyback into the TPN line. It helps to add certain drugs (e.g., H_2-blockers) to the TPN solution for constant administration. Careful verification of compatibility must be done before any drug is added to the solution (see Table 75–5).

CONCEPT REVIEW

Parenteral formulas range from peripheral products designed for short-term use in preserving body protein and improving nitrogen balance to central parenteral products designed to fulfill long-term, more complex needs. Electrolytes, minerals, and vitamins are added to the TPN solution to prevent or correct deficiencies.

Some undesired clinical responses to TPN therapy are glucose intolerance, sepsis, hyperosmolar hyperglycemic nonketotic coma, and (with abrupt discontinuation) hypoglycemia. Drugs can be administered piggyback into the TPN line only after their compatibility has been verified.

SUMMARY

The incidence of malnutrition among hospitalized clients is high. The nurse's role is to identify clients at risk for malnutrition or clients actually experiencing malnutrition. General categories of risk factors include the inability to ingest sufficient nutrients to maintain optimal health and conditions such as infection or injury that cause an increased metabolic rate. Nutrition can be provided to the client through the enteral route as an oral diet or as tube feedings. If use of enteral feeding is contraindicated for a client, parenteral nutrition is ad-

ministered. Both routes for nutrition necessitate using careful nursing care to maintain the prescribed nutrient intake and to prevent complications.

REFERENCES

1. Rombeau, J., & Kripke, S. (1991). Enteral nutrition. In J. Fischer (Ed.), *Total parenteral nutrition* (pp. 423–446). Boston: Little, Brown.
2. Davis, J.R. & Sherer K. (1994). *Applied nutrition and diet therapy for nurses.* Philadelphia: W.B. Saunders.
3. Peckenpaugh, N.J., & Poleman, C.M. (1995). *Nutrition: essentials and diet therapy.* Philadelphia: W.B. Saunders.
4. Ignatavicius, D.D., & Bayne, M.V. (1995). *Medical-surgical nursing: A nursing process approach.* Philadelphia: W.B. Saunders.
5. Smith, L., & Mullen, J. (1991). Nutritional assessment and indications for nutritional support. *Surgical Clinics of North America, 71,* 449–457.
6. Carpenito, L. (1992). *Nursing diagnosis: Application to clinical practice* (4th ed.). Philadelphia: J.B. Lippincott.
7. Gettrust, K., & Brabec, P. (1992). *Nursing diagnosis in clinical practice: Guides for care planning.* Albany, NY: Delmar.
8. Metheny, N., Spies, M., & Eisenberg, P. (1988). Measures to test placement of nasoenteral feeding tubes. *Western Journal of Nursing Research, 10,* 367–383.
9. Fischer, J. (1991). Metabolism in surgical patients. In D. Sabiston (Ed.), *Textbook of surgery: The biological basis of modern surgical practice* (pp. 103–140). Philadelphia: W.B. Saunders.
10. Weinstein, S. (1992). Administering P.P.N. *Nursing 92, 22*(1), 32H–32J.
11. Torosian, M., & Daly, J. (1991). Solutions available. In J. Fischer (Ed.), *Total parenteral nutrition* (pp. 13–24). Boston: Little, Brown.
12. Worthington, P., & Wagner, B. (1989). Total parenteral nutrition. *Nursing Clinics of North America, 24,* 355–372.
13. von Allmen, D., & Fischer, J. (1991). Metabolic complications. In J. Fischer (Ed.), *Total parenteral nutrition* (pp. 47–56). Boston: Little, Brown.
14. Hoheim, D., O'Callaghan, T., Joswiak, B., Boysen, D., & Bommarito, A. (1990). Clinical experience with three-in-one admixtures administered peripherally. *Nutrition in Clinical Practice, 5,* 118–122.
15. Mahan, L., & Arlin, M. (1992). Methods of nutritional support.

In L. Mahan & M. Arlin (Eds.), *Krause's food, nutrition, and diet therapy* (8th ed.; pp. 507–526). Philadelphia: W.B. Saunders.

16. Kohn, C., & Keithley, J. (1989). Enteral nutrition: Potential complications and patient monitoring. *Nursing Clinics of North America, 24,* 339–353.

17. Metheny, N., Eisenberg, P., & McSweeney, M. (1988). Effect of feeding tube properties and three irrigants on clogging rates. *Nursing Research, 37,* 165–169.

18. LaFrance, R., & Miyagawa, C. (1991). Pharmaceutical considerations in total parenteral nutrition. In J. Fischer (Ed.), *Total parenteral nutrition* (pp. 57–98). Boston: Little, Brown.

19. Berger, R., & Adams, L. (1989). Nutritional support in the critical care setting (Part 2). *Chest, 96,* 372–380.

20. Gottschlich, M., Alexander, J., & Bower, R. (1990). Enteral nutrition in patients with burns or trauma. In J. Rombeau & M. Caldwell (Eds.), *Clinical nutrition: Enteral and tube feeding* (pp. 306–324). Philadelphia: W.B. Saunders.

21. McMahon, M., & Bistrian, B. (1990). The physiology of nutritional assessment and therapy in protein-calorie malnutrition. *Disease-a-Month, 36,* 373–417.

22. Sax, H., & Hasselgren, P. (1991). Indications. In J. Fischer (Ed.), *Total parenteral nutrition* (pp. 3–11). Boston: Little, Brown.

23. Dudrick, P., & Souba, W. (1991). Amino acids in surgical nutrition. *Surgical Clinics of North America, 71,* 459–476.

24. Martyn-Nemeth, P., & Fitzgerald, K. (1992). Clinical considerations: Tube feeding in the elderly. *Journal of Gerontological Nursing, 18*(2), 30–36.

25. Bowman, M, Eisenberg, P., Katz, B., & Metheny, N. (1989). Effect of tube feeding osmolality on serum sodium levels. *Critical Care Nurse 9,* 22–28.

26. Metheny, N. (1992). *Fluid and electrolyte balance: Nursing considerations.* Philadelphia: J.B. Lippincott.

27. Hayek, M., & Eisenberg, P. (1989). Severe hypophosphatemia following the institution of enteral feedings. *Archives of Surgery, 124,* 1325–1328.

28. Olin, B. (1992). *Drug facts and comparisons.* St. Louis: Facts and Comparisons Division, J.B. Lippincott.

29. Krzyda, E., Andris, D., Whyiple, J., Street, C., Ausman, R., Schulte, W., & Quebbeman, E. (1993). Glucose response to abrupt initiation and discontinuation of total parenteral nutrition. *Journal of Parenteral and Enteral Nutrition 17,* 64-67.

BIBLIOGRAPHY

Baumgartner, T., & Cerda, J. (1991). Total parenteral nutrition. In J. Kassirer (Ed.), *Current therapy in internal medicine* (3rd ed.; pp. 65–75). Philadelphia: B.C. Decker.

Bliss, D., Guenter, P., & Settle, R. (1992). Defining and reporting diarrhea in tube-fed patients—What a mess! *American Journal of Clinical Nutrition, 55,* 753–759.

Bockus, S. (1991). Troubleshooting your tube feedings. *American Journal of Nursing, 91*(5), 24–30.

Bodkin, N., & Hansen, B. (1991). Nutritional studies in nursing. In J. Fitzpatrick, R., Taunton, & A. Jacox (Eds.), *Annual review of nursing research* (Vol. 9; pp. 203–220). New York: Springer.

Buckner, M. (1990). Perioperative nutrition problems: Nursing management. *Critical Care Nursing Clinics of North America, 2,* 559–566.

Campbell, I., Morton, R., Macdonald, I., Judd, S., Shapiro, L., & Stell, P. (1990). Comparison of the metabolic effects of continuous postoperative enteral feeding and feeding at night only. *American Journal of Clinical Nutrition, 52,* 1107–1112.

Campos, A., & Meguid, M. (1992). A critical appraisal of perioperative nutritional support. *American Journal of Clinical Nutrition, 55,* 117–130.

Carlson, D., & Jordan, B. (1991). Implementing nutritional therapy in the thermally injured patient. *Critical Care Clinics of North America, 3,* 221–235.

Eisenberg, P. (1991). Pulmonary complications from enteral nutrition. *Critical Care Clinics of North America, 3,* 641–649.

Eschleman, M. (1991). *Introductory nutrition and diet therapy* (2nd ed.). Philadelphia: J.B. Lippincott.

Grant, M., & Ropka, M. (1991). Alterations in nutrition. In S. Baird, R. McCorkle, & M. Grant (Eds.), *Cancer nursing: A comprehensive textbook* (pp. 717–741). Philadelphia: W.B. Saunders.

Heather, D., Howell, L., Montana, M., Howell, M., & Hill, R. (1991). Effect of a bulk-forming cathartic on diarrhea in tube-fed patients. *Heart and Lung, 20,* 409–413.

Heimburger, D. (1990). Diarrhea with enteral feeding: Will the real cause please stand up? *Heart and Lung, 88,* 89–90.

Kuhn, M. (1990). Nutritional support for the shock patient. *Critical Care Clinics of North America, 2,* 201–220.

Laquatra, I. *Nutrition in clinical nursing.* Albany, NY: Delmar Publishers.

Mickschl, D., Davidson, L., Flournoy, D., & Parker, D. (1990). Contamination of enteral feedings and diarrhea in patients in intensive care units. *Heart and Lung, 19,* 362–370.

Orr, M. (1992). Hyperglycemia during nutrition support. *Critical Care Nurse, 12,* 64–70.

Quillman, S. (1990). *Nutrition and diet therapy.* Springhouse, PA: Springhouse.

Payne-James, J., & Silk, D. (1991). Enteral nutrition: Liquid formula diets. In J. Kassirer (Ed.), *Current therapy in internal medicine* (3rd ed.; pp. 58–64). Philadelphia: B.C. Decker.

Pesola G., Hogg, J., Eissa, N., Matthews, D., & Carlon, G. (1990). Hypertonic nasogastric tube feedings: Do they cause diarrhea? *Critical Care Medicine, 18,* 1378–1382.

Smith, C., Marien, L., Brogdon, C., Faust-Wilson, P., Lohr, G., Gerald, K., & Pingleton, S. (1990). Diarrhea associated with tube feeding in mechanically ventilated critically ill patients. *Nursing Research, 39,* 148–152.

Miscellaneous Drug Categories

CHAPTER 76

Antiseptics, Disinfectants, and Sterilants

GAIL ESTOCK HALLER • NORMA L. PINNELL

⊛ Medical and Surgical Asepsis

LEARNING OBJECTIVES:

Define *asepsis*.
Differentiate between medical and surgical asepsis.
Provide examples of sterile and clean techniques.
Explain the infectious process.

KEY TERMS:

Asepsis, medical asepsis, surgical asepsis, sterilization, sterile technique, clean technique

⊛ Nursing Considerations

LEARNING OBJECTIVES:

Identify nursing measures for a client at risk of developing an infection.
List appropriate nursing diagnoses for a client at risk of developing an infection.

⊛ Antiseptics and Disinfectants

LEARNING OBJECTIVES:

Discriminate between antiseptics and disinfectants.
Define classifications of antiseptics and disinfectants.
Discuss the pharmacologic actions of antiseptics and disinfectants.
Identify specific groups of antiseptics and disinfectants.

KEY TERMS:

Antiseptic, disinfectant, bactericide, bacteriostatic, germicide

⊛ Sterilants

LEARNING OBJECTIVES:

Summarize the pharmacologic actions of sterilant agents.
Describe undesired clinical responses of sterilant agents.

CONCEPTS AND TERMS TO REVIEW

Read section on infectious process in Chapter 54.
Read section on inflammatory process in Chapter 49.
Review definitions for sterilization, asepsis, disinfectant and antiseptic.

---

*P*ractices that prevent the spread of infection have changed over the years. As more knowledge has been gained about infections, precautions have become more and more specific. The current emphasis is to recognize that all moist body sites and substances from humans are potentially infectious.

Some individuals enter the health care system specifically for treatment of known infections; others develop infections—nosocomial infections—after entering the system. Whatever the source, once an infection develops, nursing measures are needed to control its spread. This chapter discusses medical and surgical asepsis; differentiates between antiseptics and disinfectants; and describes specific groups of antiseptics and disinfectants.

MEDICAL AND SURGICAL ASEPSIS

Asepsis means the absence of pathogenic bacteria. In the health care delivery system, medical asepsis and surgical asepsis are used to reduce the number and spread of pathogens. **Surgical asepsis** is the preparation and handling of material in a manner that prevents the client's exposure to any living microorganisms. **Sterilization,** destroying all forms of microbial life, is the goal of surgical asepsis. **Medical asepsis** refers to the practices that inhibit or reduce the transfer of microorganisms from one place to another. The practices used in surgical asepsis are called *sterile* techniques; practices used in medical asepsis are called *medical* aseptic technique.[1]

Clean technique involves the use of chemicals, thermal energy (e.g., radiation), pasteurization, and mechanical energy (e.g., dishwashers, hand washing). **Sterile technique** includes the use of thermal energy (e.g., steam autoclave) and liquid chemicals or ethylene oxide. Some of the factors affecting any sterilization process are time, type of microorganism, and number of microorganisms.[1]

☒ NURSING CONSIDERATIONS

Infection control is so important that infection control measures must be applied in every aspect of client care.

Assessing During the **health history** assess for factors that contribute to infection. For example, collect a 24-hour nutritional history to determine if the client's food and fluid intake is adequate. Ask about the presence of chronic illness. Determine if the client lives in a home environment with small children. Question the client about routine hygiene practices (e.g., how frequently does the client bathe? How frequently does the client brush his or her teeth?).

During the **physical assessment** assess for classic indications of inflammation (i.e., redness, warmth, swelling, and pain in a specific location). Assess the client for wounds, and note if the wound has a purulent discharge. Determine if the client's urine is cloudy or if malaise or fever is present. Review the laboratory data. Check for hematologic changes (e.g., leukocytosis) or abnormal urinalysis results. Determine the results of specific serologic tests; these tests are used to determine antigen-antibody reactions.

Diagnosing A frequently used nursing diagnosis for clients with the potential for infection is "High risk for infection." According to the North American Nursing Diagnosis Association (NANDA) this diagnosis means "the state in which an individual is at increased risk for being invaded by pathogenic organisms."[2] Numerous causative factors include interrupted skin integrity, decreased ciliary action, stasis of body fluids, inadequate white blood cells, and chronic disease or malnutrition.

Other appropriate nursing diagnoses follow:
- Fear related to decreased protective mechanisms.
- Impaired social interaction related to fear of infection.

Planning If the client is at risk of an infection, plan how to break at least one link in the infectious process to prevent the infection (see Fig. 54–1). If infection is present, plan how to prevent the spread of the infection.

As with any plan of care, expected outcomes must be identified. Appropriate outcomes include the following:
- Client remains free of infection.
- Client identifies measures to cope with fears.
- Client verbalizes measures to decrease threat of infection.

Implementing One of the most important nursing interventions associated with infection prevention is hand washing. Nurses' hands are frequently the vectors of hospital-acquired infection. The main causative agents for nosocomial infections are *Staphylococcus aureus* and gram-negative bacilli. These organisms are spread via contact rather than through the airborne route.[3,4]

Some nursing interventions have been designed specifically to prevent the spread of infection. They are usually called *isolation precautions*. These precautions are established by the agency but must follow the Centers for Disease Control and Prevention (CDC) recommendations. The CDC has also established universal precautions that should be followed by all health care workers (see box). Refer to agency policy and pro-

---

UNIVERSAL PRECAUTIONS

Universal precautions are intended to prevent parenteral, mucous membrane, and nonintact skin exposures of health care workers to blood-borne pathogens. Universal precautions apply to blood and to other body fluids containing visible blood, semen, vaginal secretions, cerebrospinal fluid, synovial fluid, pleural fluid, peritoneal fluid, pericardial fluid, and amniotic fluid. Universal precautions do not apply to feces, nasal secretions, sputum, sweat, tears, urine, and vomitus unless they contain visible blood.

Barrier Guidelines
1. Disposable gloves (vinyl, latex) should be worn when in contact or when there is potential for contact with blood, body fluids, or other fluids that may contain human immunodeficiency virus (HIV). Gloves should be removed after each client contact. Rubber gloves can be used for equipment cleaning.
2. Hands should be washed between clients, after any exposure, and after removal of gloves.
3. Protective eyewear, face shields, and/or masks should be worn during procedures that may aerosolize blood.
4. Impervious gowns should be worn when there is potential for exposure to large quantities of blood, such as in the labor and delivery area or emergency room.

Needle Precautions
1. Needles should never be recapped after use; keep in mind that most needlesticks are the result of missed needle recapping.
2. Do not cut, break, or bend needles after use; this may release aerosolized blood from the needle shaft.
3. Do not leave used needles lying around.
4. Do not dispose of needles in ordinary receptacles; instead, use appropriately labeled, impermeable needle containers.

Data from the Centers for Disease Control (1988). Update: Universal precautions for prevention of transmission of human immunodeficiency virus, hepatitis B virus, and other bloodborne pathogens in health-care setting. *Morbidity and Mortality Weekly Report, 37*(3), 377–388.

cedure manuals and other resources for specific information on isolation precautions.

Evaluating During the evaluation phase determine if the expected outcomes were achieved and if the client remained free of infection. Review the current physical assessment and laboratory data and compare the findings to the baseline data.

CONCEPT REVIEW

Agents used to kill or inhibit microbial growth are antiseptics and disinfectants.

Medical asepsis involves practices that inhibit or reduce the transfer of microbes from one individual to another.

Surgical asepsis uses practices that destroy all microorganisms.

Illness caused by microorganisms can be prevented with interruption of the infectious process. Use of careful medical aseptic technique by health care providers, including appropriate hand washing, is essential.

ANTISEPTICS AND DISINFECTANTS

Agents used to kill or inhibit microbial growth are classified as antiseptics or disinfectants. Since these terms describe different actions, they should not be used interchangeably. An **antiseptic** is a chemical agent applied to living tissue; it inhibits the growth and development of microorganisms but does not necessarily kill them. A **disinfectant** is a chemical agent applied to inanimate objects; it destroys pathogens. Some agents, in different strengths or concentrations, are used for both purposes.[5,6]

Classifications

Antiseptics and disinfectants are categorized as bactericidal or bacteriostatic in nature. **Bacteriostatic** means that the agent inhibits the growth and development of the microorganism but does not kill the entire microorganism population. **Bactericides** kill microorganisms; however, they may not kill fungi, spores, or viruses. **Germicide** is a solution that affects many types of microorganisms, including bacteria, spores, viruses, and fungi. Many germicides can be used on both inanimate objects and living tissue.[5]

General Pharmacologic Actions

The use of antiseptics and disinfectants kills or inhibits microbial growth in one of three ways: protein denaturation, surface tension reduction, and biochemical interference. Agents that act by **protein denaturation** produce a change in the structure of the cell protein of the microorganism. This results in coagulation and destruction of the microorganism. If the agents act by **surface tension reduction,** they alter the permeability of the microorganism's cell membrane, leading to lysis and destruction of the cell. Those agents acting by

biochemical interference interfere with the metabolic processes of the microorganisms to survive and multiply. Table 76–1 summarizes action and indications for some antiseptics and disinfectants.

CONCEPT REVIEW

Both antiseptics and disinfectants are categorized as bactericidal or bacteriostatic.

Inhibition or destruction of microbial growth is achieved by one of three actions: biochemical interference, surface tension reduction, and protein denaturation.

Phenolic Compounds

Solutions of phenol are antiseptic or bactericidal, depending on the strength of the concentration.

PHENOL

Phenol in its pure state (i.e., carbolic acid) is not used. However, it is the parent compound of substituted phenols, which are used to formulate various phenolic disinfectants such as cresol. Substituted phenols include halogenated phenols (hexachlorophene) and the alkyl-substituted phenols (cresol and resorcinol).

Phenol denatures microbial protein structures; in high concentrations it can precipitate cellular proteins. In aqueous solutions of 1% to 2% phenol kills all but the hepatitis virus and bacterial or fungal spores within 20 minutes. It destroys spores after 12 hours of contact. Gram-positive and gram-negative bacteria are highly susceptible to phenol compounds.[5,6]

Phenol compounds are used to disinfect inanimate objects and surfaces when bactericidal action is needed in the presence of organic soils. As general purpose disinfectants, these compounds are effective for use on floors, walls, and furniture in high-risk areas such as operating rooms, nurseries, delivery rooms, intensive care units, and dialysis units.[5,6]

Phenol and phenol compounds are available in several over-the-counter (OTC) products, including Campho-Phenique, Castaderm, Funginail, and Osti-Derm.

Nursing considerations Solutions of phenol are poisonous if ingested or applied to abraded skin.

CRESOL

Cresol is effective in disinfecting excreta, bedpans, toilets, sinks, and equipment. Because it irritates the skin, its use is limited to disinfection of inanimate objects and surfaces. Lysol, a 50% solution of cresol in vegetable oil in a 2% to 5% strength, is also useful for disinfecting inanimate objects.[5–7]

Nursing considerations Cresol is highly toxic if ingested. It is easily absorbed through intact skin. After accidental skin contact, wash the area with large amounts of water. Avoid contact with the eyes.

TABLE 76–1
Antiseptics and Disinfectants: Actions and Applications

Agent	Action	Application Method
PHENOLS AND RELATED COMPOUNDS		
Cresol (Lysol)	Disinfectant	Topical
Carbolic acid	Disinfectant	Topical
Hexachlorphene	Antiseptic	Topical
DYES		
Gentian violet	Antiseptic	Topical
Crystal violet	Antiseptic	Topical
HEAVY METALS		
Mercury compounds		
Mercurochrome (merbromin 2%)	Antiseptic	Topical
Thimerosol (Merthiolate)	Antiseptic	Topical
Silver compounds		
Silver nitrate	Antiseptic, disinfectant	Topical
Silver nitrate (solid form)	Cauterization and removal of granulation tissue	Topical
Silver sulfadiazine	Antiseptic	Topical
HALOGENS		
Chlorine compounds	Antiseptic, disinfectant	Topical
Sodium hypochlorite	Disinfectant	Topical
Halazone		
Iodine Compounds and Iodophors	Antiseptic, disinfectant	Topical
Iodine tincture	Antiseptic, disinfectant	Topical
Iodine solution	Antiseptic	Topical spray, gargle, shampoo, scrub, vaginal douche
Povidone-iodine		
OXIDIZING AGENTS	Antiseptic	Topical
Hydrogen peroxide		
BIGUANIDES	Antiseptic	Tincture (4%) for surgical scrub, skin wound cleansing, and hand-washing agent
Chlorhexidine (Hibiclens)		
SURFACE-ACTING AGENTS	Antiseptic	Topically for superficial injuries and as a skin preparation; for sterilizing instruments with addition of antirust agent
Benzalkonium chloride (Zephiran, Bactine, Germicin)		
ALCOHOLS	Antiseptic, disinfectant	Topical (70%)
Isopropanol	Antiseptic, disinfectant	Topical (70%)
Ethanol		
ACIDS	Antiseptic, disinfectant	Topical for surgical dressings, burn therapy solution, dermatologic lotion, bladder irrigation, douching
Acetic		
Boric	Antiseptic	Topical for eyewash solution and ointment
MISCELLANEOUS	Antiseptic	Topical
Nitrofurazone		
STERILANT AGENTS		
Aldehydes	Disinfectant, sterilant	With isopropanol alcohol, disinfection of instruments
Formaldehyde	Disinfectant, sterilant	Disinfection and sterilization of instruments
Glutaraldehyde	Alkylating agent acting as a disinfectant	Gaseous sterilization of optical instruments, pacemakers, and plastic machinery parts
Ethylene oxide		

HEXACHLOROPHENE

Hexachlorophene is a white solid with low solubility in water. It is more soluble at alkaline pH and forms emulsions with soaps and detergents. Hexachlorophene is bacteriostatic against staphylococci and other gram-positive bacteria. It has a cumulative antibacterial effect.

Hexachlorophene is used as a 3% cleansing emulsion. It is used to disinfect hands and as a preliminary skin cleanser before surgery. Initial action on skin bacteria is slow, but adsorption of hexachlorophene to the skin can provide sustained and cumulative action. This compound can be absorbed through intact skin, but absorption usually occurs through abraded skin.[5,6]

Nursing considerations Hexachlorophene is not recommended for use on infants less than 6 months old because of its neurotoxic potential. For individuals with sensitive skin, it may cause erythema, dryness, and scaling. Clients with prolonged exposure to hexachlorophene must be observed for indications of central nervous system (CNS) toxicity (e.g., double vision, lethargy, changes in sensorium, and seizures. Do not leave these agents in contact with skin or mucous membranes; avoid their contact with the eyes.[5,6]

Rosaniline Dyes

Rosaniline dyes comprise a group of basic dyes used occasionally for antiseptic or antifungal purposes. Included in this group are gentian violet, crystal violet, methyl violet, brilliant green, and fuchsin.

Gentian violet is derived from coal tar; it has an antibacterial and antifungal effect. Gentian violet is used as a topical antiinfective agent for intravaginal *Candida* and vulvitis. It also is used as a stain in the laboratory for histology, bacteriology, and cytology studies. In addition, gentian violet is used to treat thrush.[8,9] Gentian violet in a 1% or 2% solution is available as an OTC antifungal product.[10]

Nursing considerations Advise parents or caregivers that children can be attracted to rosaniline solutions because of their color. These preparations must be stored out of reach of children. Counsel the client that treated areas of the skin and clothing that comes in contact with dye may become permanently discolored.

Heavy Metals

Since ions of heavy metal have a strong affinity for protein, salts of heavy metals have been used as antimicrobial and antiseptic agents. However, many of these preparations have been replaced with safer, more effective products.

MERCURY COMPOUNDS

Although mercurial antiseptics have been widely used, their effectiveness is limited. They are primarily bacteriostatic and probably act by inhibiting bacterial sulfhydryl enzymes. However, they also inhibit tissue enzymes.

Organic mercurial salts are more effective than inorganic salts. Although slow acting, organic salts are also less irritating and less toxic than inorganic agents. The effectiveness of inorganic salts is enhanced by vehicles that prolong the duration of action of the metal.

Merbromin (Mercurochrome) was the first organic mercurial agent used in medicine. It is less effective as a skin antiseptic than other organic mercurials. In addition, serous fluids reduce its antimicrobial potency. It is available in a 2% solution as an OTC product.[10]

Thimerosal (Merthiolate) has antibacterial and antifungal properties but is less effective than ethanol. It is found in several types of topical products, including aqueous solutions, tinctures, ointments, creams, and aerosols. Systemic toxicity occurs less frequently with thimerosal than with other mercurials because the mercury in thimerosal is tightly bound to the organic configurations. The usual concentration is 0.1%. It is available OTC as a Merthiolate solution and tincture.[10]

Nursing considerations If mercury compounds are used extensively or on large areas of abraded skin, mercury may be absorbed and systemic poisoning produced. These products can cause hypersensitivity reactions. Tincture of thimerosal should not be used on infants or young children.

SILVER COMPOUNDS

Silver compounds (e.g., silver nitrate and silver sulfadiazine) have been used as antimicrobial agents since ancient times. The first medicinal use of a silver compound was the instillation of silver nitrate 1% solution into the eyes of newborn infants to prevent gonorrheal ophthalmia neonatorum.

Silver nitrate is available as a topical solution, topical applicator, ophthalmic solution, and crystals. These preparations act as astringents. Topical solutions (10%) are used for treating pruritis and impetigo; 25% to 50% solutions are used to treat plantar warts and papillomatous growths. The solid dosage form of silver nitrate is used to cauterize wounds or mucous membranes; it can be used to remove granulation tissue. Treatment with silver nitrate applicator can result in permanent skin discoloration.

Silver sulfadiazine (Silvadene, Thermazene) is available in a 10% topical cream. The cream is easy to apply and washes off easily. It has broad antimicrobial activity against a variety of gram-negative and gram-positive bacteria and yeast. Silver sulfadiazine is used topically for the prevention and treatment of infections in second- and third-degree burn sites. Silver sulfadiazine is not recommended for use in an at-term pregnancy; it is classified as a Pregnancy Category B drug. It is also not recommended for use on newborns during the first 2 months of life.[5,6,11]

Nursing considerations Solutions of silver nitrate should be stored at 15° to 30° C and should be protected from light. Since allergic skin reactions have been reported, question the client about allergy to silver; monitor for a possible reaction. Silver nitrate 1% ophthalmic solution can cause eye redness or irritation; other preparations can cause skin irritation. With long-term therapy, permanent skin discoloration occurs.

Halogens

Halogen-based disinfectants are oxidizing agents. Important halogens are iodine compounds, iodophors, and chlorine compounds; chlorine compounds are the strongest of the groups.[5,6]

IODINE COMPOUNDS

Free iodine is a bluish-black solid that normally is premixed with water or alcohol to make a solution or tincture. It is slightly soluble in water; aqueous solutions are made by adding sodium or potassium iodine. Free iodine is more active at acid than alkaline pH, and the presence of organic matter interferes with drug potency. Iodine is effective against bacteria, viruses, fungi, and protozoa. It is less effective against spores.

Iodine compounds are used in a variety of situations (e.g., to treat abrasions, minor wounds, and infected wounds; to prepare the skin before surgery or venipuncture; as a part of indwelling catheter care). Some of the antiseptic or disinfectant compounds include tincture of iodine containing 2% iodine in alcohol, strong tincutre of iodine containing 7% iodine in alcohol, iodine solution containing 2% iodine in water, and strong iodine solution containing 5% iodine in water. Of the two dosage forms, solution and tincture, use of solutions is preferred since they have fewer irritating properties.[5,6,11]

IODOPHORS

Iodophors are organic complexes of iodine combined with a carrier or surface-active agent. The carriers increase the solubility of the iodine and provide prolonged release of iodine. Povidone-iodine is an example of an iodophor.

Povidone-iodine (Betadine) combines the water-soluble iodine with povidone; approximately 10% of the free iodine is released. Povidone-iodine is sporicidal. Povidone-iodine is available in tincture and aqueous solution forms. OTC preparations are available as 2% spray, shampoo, foam skin cleanser, ointment, 0.05% to 1% vaginal douche preparations, and 5% creams. (Use of povidone-iodine vaginal douches is contraindicated during pregnancy.) Povidone-iodine is also a component of mouthwashes and gargles.

Nursing considerations Before using iodine compounds and iodophors, assess for a history of allergy to iodine. Discontinue use of these preparations if irritation, erythema, or edema develops. After topical application, povidone-iodine can be absorbed; use it with caution in clients with abnormal renal or thyroid function.[12] Educate clients to purchase products in small quantities because evaporation of the vehicle increases the concentration of the drug.

CHLORINE COMPOUNDS

Chlorine compounds are oxidizing agents; the end products of their reaction with microorganisms and organic material are inactive chlorides. The following types of chlorine compounds are commonly used as disinfectants: sodium hypochlorite, calcium hypochlorite, and lithium hypochlorite. These compounds act by slowly yielding hypochlorous acid when combined with water.[5,6]

Hypochlorites have a wide antibacterial spectrum, although they are less active against spores than against nonsporing bacteria. Gram-positive and gram-negative bacteria are highly susceptible to hypochlorites. In addition, the hypochlorites show activity against lipid and nonlipid viruses. Chlorine disinfectants have a wide range of uses, ranging from the treatment of water supplies to inactivation of hepatitis B virus in blood. Sodium hypochlorite, 5% solution, is used for disin-fecting walls, floor, and instruments and as a household bleach. A 0.5% solution (Dakin's Solution) is used as an antiseptic for fungal infections or as a wound disinfectant. When properly diluted, it can be used as an irrigation for treatment of bladder and vaginal infections.[6]

Chloramines are compounds in which chlorine in water is linked chemically with nitrogen to release hypochlorous acid. The action of chloramines is slower and more prolonged than that of hypochlorite solutions.

Nursing considerations Chlorine compounds are irritating to delicate tissue and mucous membranes; they are extremely toxic if ingested. Keep these compounds away from light and out of reach of children. Since the diluted solutions are not stable, prepare the solutions fresh daily.

Oxidizing Agents

Chlorine dioxide, peracetic acid, and hydrogen peroxide—oxidizing agents—are used mainly for their sporicidal activity. Each has a broad spectrum of biocidal action. **Chlorine dioxide** is used to treat water; it removes tastes and odors by breaking down phenolic compounds. The bacterial activity of chlorine dioxide is similar to that of other chlorine disinfectants, and the sporicidal action occurs independently of pH over the range of 6 to 10.[6]

Hydrogen peroxide (3% solution) is the most widely used antimicrobial oxidizing agent. Enzymatic release of oxygen from hydrogen peroxide occurs when it comes into contact with blood or tissue fluid. The mechanical release of the oxygen has a cleansing effect on a wound, but organic matter reduces its effectiveness. The duration of action is only as long as the period of active oxygen release. Dilute solutions are unstable, especially in the presence of tissue that contains the enzyme catalase. This compound must be used only in areas where the released gas can escape. Hydrogen peroxide is active against most types of microorganisms, but enteric viruses and bacterial spores require a high concentration for lethal action.[6,10] Hydrogen peroxide is available as an OTC product.

Nursing considerations To delay decomposition of oxidizing agents, store them in tightly capped amber containers; protect the solutions from light and air. Ingestion of small amounts of the solution is not harmful, but if large amounts are ingested, the solution may harm the stomach.

🌿 NURSING RESEARCH

Tombes, M., & Gallucci, B. (1993). The effects of hydrogen peroxide rinses on normal oral mucosa. *Nursing Research, 42,* 332–336.

The purpose of this study was to provide a controlled setting in which to assess the usefulness of hydrogen peroxide as an oral rinsing agent. Three groups were established: group one used normal saline solution; group two used one-quarter strength hydrogen peroxide solution; and group three used one-half strength hydrogen peroxide. The study involved subjective and objective observations on daily use of the rinsing agents, weekly examinations for 5 weeks, and a follow-up examination 1 week after the study had concluded.

Results of the study showed that highly significant differences were found between pretreatment and treatment oral scores. These results suggest that hydrogen peroxide rinses are associated with mucosal abnormalities and that their use may alter the microflora of the mouth in a detrimental way. Use of alternatives such as normal saline solution, tap water, and sodium bicarbonate solution should be explored.

STUDENT ACTIVITIES

- Interview 10 clients receiving hydrogen peroxide rinses as part of their oral care. Inquire about subjective responses to the rinse (e.g., tingling, dryness). Ask if there have been any observable changes in the oral mucosa since using the hydrogen peroxide. Check the clients' charts for any recorded mucosal changes.
- Interview 10 clients receiving an alternative rinsing agent for oral care. Ask if there have been any undesired subjective responses to the agent. Check clients' charts for any objective mucosal changes.

Biguanides

Chlorhexidine is a cationic biguanide; it is a basic substance that forms salts with inorganic and organic acids. Chlorhexidine is active in the pH range of 5.5 to 8. The compound is effective against gram-positive and, to a lesser extent, gram-negative bacteria. Its antibacterial activity is cumulative with regular use. Soaps and other anionic detergents react with chlorhexidine and inactivate it.

Chlorhexidine is available in several formulations commercially. As 4% sudsing scrub (Hibiclens), it is used as a wound cleanser, surgical scrub, and hand-washing agent. Other preparations include mouth rinses and gels, obstetric lubricant creams, and aqueous solutions.[6,10]

Nursing considerations Local reactions to chlorhexidine are rare, but contact with eyes and ears is to be avoided. Chlorhexidine can be toxic to the cornea and should not be used for preoperative cleansing of the face and neck. In addition, if it reaches the middle ear, it may cause hearing loss.[14]

Surface-Acting Agents

Surface-active agents possess antiseptic properties but are not effective as disinfectants. Although the mechanism of action of these agents is unknown, the action is probably related to their ability to alter bacterial cell membrane permeability. These compounds are bacteriostatic in high concentrations and are not extremely irritating or toxic.

The **quaternary ammonium compound,** benzalkonium chloride, is a cationic surface-acting detergent. Benzalkonium chloride is used topically as a skin antiseptic, as a treatment for superficial injuries, and for preoperative skin preparation and scrubs. It also is used to sterilize surgical instruments.

Other quaternary ammonium compounds include benzethonium chloride and methylbenzethonium chloride. These compounds are available OTC in formulations such as creams, dusting powders, and aqueous or alcoholic solutions. For application to diseased or abraded skin, use of concentrations of 1:5000 to 1:20,000 is recommended. For use on intact skin and minor abrasions, use of a concentration of 1:750 is recommended.[10]

Nursing considerations Aqueous solutions of quaternary ammonium compounds can become contaminated and become a source of nosocomial infections. Concentrated solutions can injure delicate tissue and cause chemical burns if contact with tissues is allowed. These compounds are also irritating to the eyes. Benzalkonium chloride is inactivated by soap and can form a film under which bacteria can survive.

Alcohols

Ethyl alcohol and isopropyl alcohol are colorless liquids that evaporate at room temperature. They act by denaturation of proteins. Ethyl alcohol is less effective as a fat solvent than isopropyl alcohol. Water must be added to alcohols to obtain the maximum rate of biocidal action. (Usually use of a 70% ethyl alcohol solution and a 60% to 70% isopropyl alcohol solution is recommended.) The low surface tension of the alcohol-water mixtures gives these solutions a wetting ability and allows them to penetrate into crevices of the human skin or inanimate objects. Alcohols coagulate or precipitate proteins in serum, pus, sputum, and other biologic materials. This action may protect microorganisms from effective contact with the alcohol.[6]

Gram-positive and gram-negative bacteria are highly susceptible to both forms of alcohol solution. These solutions are effective as topical skin antiseptics. Ethyl alcohol may be used as a surface disinfectant. It is the agent of choice if contamination with *Mycobacterium tuberculosis* or other pathogenic acid-fast bacteria is likely.[6]

Nursing considerations Alcohols are irritants and toxic to tissue cells. They are toxic when ingested and must be kept out of the reach of children. Apply alcohol to the skin surface with friction, leave it on the skin for 2 minutes, and do not fan the area to hasten drying.

NURSING RESEARCH

Butz, A., Laughton, B., Gullet, D., & Larson, E. (1991). Alcohol-impregnated wipes as an alternative in hand hygiene. *American Journal of Infection Control, 18*(2), 70–76.

In this study four hand-wash products were assessed to determine their efficacy in reducing bacterial counts on hands. The products were ethyl alcohol–impregnated wipes, a liquid detergent containing 1% triclosan, a liquid detergent base containing 4% chlorhexidine gluconate, and a liquid, nonmedicated soap (control).

The study found that repeated washing with alcohol-impregnated wipes resulted in reductions in colony counts comparable to those with nonmedicated soap. The wipes were perceived by study subjects as milder than the two antiseptic products. The study concluded that in nonacute situations, use of alcohol-impregnated wipes could be a good alternative to use of medicated soap solutions and that their use might encourage compliance, especially when hand-washing facilities were in inconvenient locations.

STUDENT ACTIVITIES

- Make a chart of the hand-washing locations in your facility. Note how they are stocked (solutions, hand-drying equipment). Approximate the distance from these locations to six work stations. Assess the convenience of the hand-washing locations.
- Interview 10 nurses about hand-washing techniques and frequency. What is their preferred method of hand cleaning? How often in a shift do they accomplish it? Obtain their response to the idea of using alcohol-impregnated wipes (with emollients) as an alternative to their current method of hand washing.

Acids

A large family of organic acids and a few inorganic acids are found as preservatives in food products. Some are also used as preservatives in pharmaceutical products, antifungal preparations, and disinfectants. Available acid compounds include acetic acid, lactic acid, benzoic acid, and sulphuric acid.

Acetic acid (ethanoic acid) is the most commonly used drug in this group. It can be used as a diluted compound or as the natural product, vinegar. Acetic acid is germicidal to many microorganisms in a 5% solution; it is bacteriostatic at lower concentrations. Vinegar is frequently used by home health nurses because it is available and economic.[5,16,17]

Weak acetic acid solutions are used as a vaginal douche in the prevention or suppression of *Trichomonas, Candida,* and *Gardnerella vaginalis* microorganisms and to treat mild forms of external otitis.[10] Acetic acid, 1% solution, has also been used for surgical dressings.

Nursing considerations Hypersensitive reactions can result from the preservatives in the vinegar. Strong concentrations may cause irritation of mucosal tissues.

CONCEPT REVIEW

A variety of antiseptics and disinfectants are available.
Selection is based, in part, on the type of microorganism involved, area being treated (i.e., animate or inanimate object), source of contamination, and extent of contamination.

STERILANTS

Agents used as sterilants destroy all forms of microbial life. These agents are used to provide surgical asepsis.

Aldehydes

Two aldehydes are currently important as disinfectants, glutaraldehyde and formaldehyde. Gram-positive and gram-negative bacteria are highly susceptible to both.

FORMALDEHYDE

Formaldehyde is used as a disinfectant as a liquid or vapor. Liquid preparations are diluted with water or alcohol. Formaldehyde is a microbicidal agent with lethal action against bacteria and their spores, fungi, and many viruses. Formaldehyde combines readily with proteins but is less effective in the presence of protein organic matter. It is active at acid or alkaline pH.

Formaldehyde is combined with isopropyl alcohol or hexachlorophene to produce a potent germicide. Preparations with isopropyl alcohol are used for disinfection of instruments; formaldehyde is also used as a preservative agent in some vaccines. As a vapor, formaldehyde is used as a disinfectant of closed rooms, heat-sensitive medical materials, and hospital bedding.

GLUTARALDEHYDE

Glutaraldehyde has powerful microbicidal action against bacteria, fungi, spores, mycelia, and viruses. Although glutaraldehyde is less volatile than formaldehyde, fumes may irritate the respiratory tract, skin, mucous membranes, and eyes. Glutaraldehyde is used for disinfection of surgical and dental instruments, lensed instruments, and some plastic equipment.

Nursing considerations In common with other alkylating agents, aldehydes are potentially carcinogenic, and precautions against inhalation of vapors are needed. When working with aldehydes, provide adequate ventilation and wear gloves, goggles, and masks to prevent respiratory and eye irritation.

Ethylene Oxide

Ethylene oxide is a colorless, flammable, toxic gas used for sterilization of heat- and moisture-sensitive items. Given the proper conditions of time, temperature, concentration, and humidity, ethylene oxide is a highly reactive alkylating agent that can produce microbial death.

Excessive exposure to ethylene oxide can result in reproductive abnormalities, including genetic damage, neurologic damage, and cancer. It also irritates skin and mucous membranes. After sterilization, aeration time must be allowed to permit diffusion of residual ethylene oxide, thus reducing exposure levels for clients and personnel. The Occupational Safety and Health Administration (OSHA) has issued standards for permissible exposure to ethylene oxide; monitoring hospital personnel can reduce the risk of exposure.[18–20]

CONCEPT REVIEW

Sterilant agents are used to destroy all forms of microbial life; thus they are included in the practices of surgical asepsis.
The aldehydes, formaldehyde and glutaraldehyde, and ethylene oxide are commonly used as sterilants.
Ethylene oxide toxicity is an occupation hazard for hospital personnel.

SUMMARY

In a health care setting medical and surgical asepsis is used to reduce the number and spread of microorganisms. Although proper hand washing is still the most efficient method for accomplishing the reduction of microorganisms, the use of antiseptics, disinfectants, and sterilants is also important. Antiseptics are applied to living tissue, and disinfectants are used on inanimate objects. These agents may be bacteriostatic, bactericidal, or both.

REFERENCES

1. Bolander, V.B. (1994). *Sorensen and Luckmann's basic nursing: A psychophysiologic approach* (3rd ed.). Philadelphia: W.B. Saunders.
2. Doenges, M., & Moorhouse, M.F. (1991). *Nurse's pocket guide: Nursing diagnoses with interventions* (3rd ed.). Philadelphia: F.A. Davis.
3. Gould, D. (1991). Nurses' hands as vectors of hospital-acquired infection: A review. *Journal of Advanced Nursing, 16,* 1216–1225.
4. Goldmann, D., & Larson, E. (1992). Handwashing and nosocomial infection. *New England Journal of Medicine, 327,* 120–122.
5. Russell, A., Hugo, W., & Ayliffe, G. (Eds.). (1992). *Principles and practice of disinfection, preservation, and sterilization* (2nd ed.). Boston: Blackwell Scientific Publications.
6. Gardner, J., & Peel, M. (1991). *Introduction to sterilization, disinfection and infection control* (2nd ed.). New York: Churchill Livingston.
7. Melker, M., & Rothrock, J. (1991). *Alexander's care of the patient in surgery* (9th ed.). St. Louis: C.V. Mosby.
8. Utter, A.R. (1990). Gentian violet treatment for thrush: Can its use cause breastfeeding problems? *Journal of Human Lactation, 6*(4), 178–180.
9. Wilson-Clay, B. (1991). More on thrush and the use of gentian violet. *Journal of Human Lactation, 7*(2), 58.
10. American Pharmaceutical Association. (1990). *Handbook of nonprescription drugs* (9th ed.). Washington, DC: Author.
11. Data Pharmaceutica, Inc. (1993). *1993 physician's genRx.* Smithtown, NY: Author.
12. Welch, J. (1992). Efficacy and safety of povidone-iodine underscored. *Journal of Emergency Nursing, 18*(3), 191–192.
13. Tombes, M., & Gallucci, B. (1993). The effects of hydrogen peroxide rinses on normal oral mucosa. *Nursing Reserach, 42,* 332–336.
14. Hibiclens and eye damage. (1992). *Nurses' Drug Alert, 16*(4), 25–26.
15. Butz, A., Laughton, B., Gullet, D., & Larson, E. (1991). Alcohol-impregnated wipes as an alternative in hand hygiene. *American Journal of Infection Control, 18*(2), 70–76.
16. Kirkis, J. (1991). Home healthcare. *Infection Control and Hospital Epidemiology, 12,* 140, 142.
17. Simmons, B., Trusler, M., Roccaforte, J., Smith, P., & Scott, R. (1992). Infection control for home health. *Infection Control and Hospital Epidemiology, 11,* 363–370.
18. Recommended Practice Coordinating Committee, AORN, Inc. (1992). Proposed recommended practices: Steam and ethylene oxide (EO) sterilization. *AORN Journal, 55,* 228–237.
19. Rogers, B., & Travers, P. (1991). Overview of work-related hazards in nursing: Health and safety issues. *Heart and Lung, 20,* 486–497.
20. Haney, P., Raymond, B., & Lewis, L. (1990). Ethylene oxide: An occupational hazard for hospital workers. *AORN Journal, 51,* 480–486.

BIBLIOGRAPHY

Ansari, S., Springthorpe, V., Sattar, S., Tostowaryk, W., & Wells, G. (1991). Comparison of cloth, paper, and warm air drying in eliminating viruses and bacteria from washed hands. *American Journal of Infection Control, 19*(5), 243–249.

Bakker, P., Van Doorne, H., Gooskens, V., & Wieringa, N. (1992). Activity of gentian violet and brillant green against some microorganisms associated with skin infections. *International Journal of Dermatology, 31*(3), 210–213.

Belkin, N. (1992). Barrier materials: Their influence on surgical wound infections. *AORN Journal, 55*(6), 1521–1528.

Bennett, J., & Brachman, P. (1992). *Hospital infections* (3rd. ed.). Boston: Little, Brown.

Bhargave, K., Shirali, G., & Abhyankar, K. (1992). Treatment of allergic and vasomotor rhinitis by the local application of different concentrations of silver nitrate. *Journal of Laryngology and Otology, 106*(8), 699–701.

Bruch, M., & Larson, E. (1989). Regulation of topical antimicrobials: History, status and future perspective. *Infection Control and Hospital Epidemiology, 10*(11), 505–508.

Chevalier, J., & Cremieux, A. (1992). Comparative study on the antimicrobial effects of hexomedine and betadine on the human skin flora. *Journal of Applied Bacteriology, 73*(4), 342–348.

Collins, E. (1990). Protective isolation vs. handwashing in the prevention of infection in the cardiac transplant recipient, *Chart, 87*(3), 9.

deToledo, A., & Chandler, J. (1992). Conjunctivitis of the newborn. *Infectious Disease Clinics of North America, 6*(4), 807–813.

Dick, M., Dick, R., & Mundell, D. (1991). Contacts between two compounds should be avoided. *ANNA Journal, 18*(4), 410.

Goldman, D., & Larson. (1992). Hand-washing and nosocomial infection. *New England Journal of Medicine, 327,* 120–122.

Gould, D. (1991). Nurses' hands as vectors of hospital-acquired infection: A review. *Journal of Advanced Nursing, 16*(10), 1216–1225.

Gruendemann, B. (1990). Surgical asepsis revisited. *Journal of Ophthalmic Nursing and Technology, 9*(6), 250–253.

Haney, P., Raymond, B., & Lewis, L. (1990). Ethylene oxide: An occupational health hazard for hospital workers. *AORN Journal, 51*(2), 480–481, 483, 485–486.

McDowell, S. (1991). Are we using too much betadine? *RN, 54*(7), 43–45.

Miner, N., & Ross, C. (1991). Clinical evaluation of coldspor, a glutaraldehyde-phenolic disinfectant. *Respiratory Care, 36*(2), 104–109.

Nurses' Drug Alert. (1990). Eosinophilia caused by food dye. *Nurses' Drug Alert, 14*(8), 64.

Restucco, A., Mortensen, M., & Kelley, M. (1992). Fatal ingestion of boric acid in an adult. *American Journal of Emergency Medicine, 10*(6), 545–547.

Saydak, S. (1990). A pilot test of two methods for the treatment of pressure ulcers. *Journal of Enterostomal Therapy, 17*(3), 139–142.

Snelling, C., Inman, R., Germann, E., Boyle, J., Foley, B., Kester, D., Fitzpatrick, D., Warren, R., & Courtemanche, A. (1991). Comparison of silver sulfadiazine 1% with chlorhexidine digluconate 0.2% to silver sulfadiazine 1% alone in the prophylactic topical antibacterial treatment of burns. *Journal of Burn Care and Rehabilitation, 12*(1), 13–18.

Watanakunakorn, C., Brandt, J., Durkin, P., Santore, S., Bota, B., & Stahl, C. (1992). The efficacy of mupirocin ointment and chlorhexidine body scrubs in the eradication of nasal carriage of staphylococcus aureus among patients undergoing long-term hemodialysis. *American Journal of Infection Control, 20*(3), 138–141.

Williams, D., Elder, E., & Worley, S. (1988). Is free halogen necessary for disinfection? *Applied and Environmental Microbiology, 54*(10), 2583–2585.

CHAPTER 77

Drugs Used to Manage Poisoning

ELLEN J. BURGE • ROBERT J. KIZIOR • NORMA L. PINNELL

⊛ **Nursing Considerations**
LEARNING OBJECTIVE: Develop a plan of care for the client requiring treatment for poisoning.

⊛ **Prevention of Poisoning**
LEARNING OBJECTIVE: Discuss four specific preventive measures to reduce the risk of poisoning in the home.

⊛ **Management of Poisoning Victim at Home**
LEARNING OBJECTIVE: Describe therapeutic measures for treating the poisoning victim at home.
KEY TERM: Ipecac

⊛ **Management of Poisoning Victim in Hospital**
LEARNING OBJECTIVES:
Describe measures used to stabilize the poisoning victim.
Discuss contraindications for the use of emetics and gastric lavage.
Discuss the use of antidotes and antagonists in the treatment of poisoning.
KEY TERMS:
Emetics, gastric lavage

CONCEPTS AND TERMS TO REVIEW

Read about the nursing care of clients with medical emergencies in a medical-surgical nursing textbook. Review sections of this textbook that provide information on antidotes.

---

*P*oisoning, either unintentional or deliberate, remains a major cause of death. More than one half of accidental poisoning involves children less than 6 years of age. Although accidental poisoning is common in the United States, many cases go unreported. In the latest data available from poison control centers, there were more than 1.8 million exposures to poison. However, this figure represents only approximately 10% of the estimated cases of poison exposures.[1,2] In addition to accidental poisoning, poison exposures include suicide attempts, industrial poisoning, and criminal poisoning. Criminal tampering with over-the-counter (OTC) drugs, baby formulas, and other materials is also a form of poisoning.

✎ NURSING CONSIDERATIONS

The nurse's role in preventing and treating poisoning follows the steps in the nursing process.

Assessing   When the client is initially seen, obtain an accurate **health history** from the client or the individual accompanying the client. Include in the history the following questions:
• Was the substance inhaled, injected, ingested, or confined to skin surfaces?
• When did the exposure occur?
• What amount of exposure occurred (e.g., number of tablets, quantity of liquid, amount of skin contact)?
• Is there a history of allergies?
• Is there a history of medical problems?
• Is there a history of prescribed, OTC, or illicit drug use?
    Perform a rapid **physical assessment** of the individual. (A complete assessment is not possible until after the client is stabilized.) If poisoning is suspected, examine the lips and mouth for signs of burns, excess salivation, or difficulty swallowing. Note the odor of the breath. Is the odor of petroleum products

or cleaning compounds present? Note the client's respiratory and pulse rate and blood pressure.[3]

Diagnosing   Nursing diagnoses depend on the condition of the client and type of poison. For example, physical signs associated with poisoning from heavy metals (e.g., lead, arsenic, alcohols, and salicylates) include nausea, vomiting, and diarrhea. Physical signs seen with poisoning from phenothiazines, amphetamines, carbon monoxide, and strychnine include convulsions. In addition, nursing diagnoses may reflect the risk for poisoning:

• High risk for poisoning related to reduced vision.
• High risk for poisoning related to lack of drug education.
• High risk for poisoning related to drugs being stored in unlocked cabinets accessible to children.
• High risk for poisoning related to flaking and peeling paint.
• High risk for injury related to seizure activity.
• High risk for aspiration related to vomiting.

Planning   During the immediate care of a poisoning victim, there is not time to develop a written plan of care. However, expected outcomes that reflect immediate and long-term needs include the following:

• Client maintains airway patency.
• Client remains free of injury.
• Client corrects environmental hazards.
• Client lifestyle changes are needed to promote safe environment.

Implementing   All nurses, especially those in emergency departments, must have a working knowledge of drugs commonly used or abused. In addition, the nurse must be knowledgeable about the management and complications of poisoning and overdoses. The immediate care of the poisoning victim in the home and hospital is discussed in a later section of this chapter.

Evaluating   The goal of medical and nursing therapy is effective reversal of the effects of the poison. Vital signs should be stabilized, and the client should be free from injury.

PREVENTION OF POISONING

Preventing accidental poisoning is cost effective, decreases hospital stays, and decreases stress on the caregiver(s) and client. Prevention frequently starts with the actions of the nurse at the time of discharge. Before any client is discharged with prescription drugs, the nurse must furnish the client information about drug action, undesired clinical responses, and indications of drug overdose. In addition, he or she must determine if the client is prepared for accidental poisoning in the home.

🌿 NURSING RESEARCH

Brannan, J.E. (1992). Accidental poisoning of children: Barriers to resource use in a black, low-income community. *Public Health Nursing, 9*(2), 81–86.

This descriptive study examined factors that influence use of poison prevention measures and poison control center resources in a black, low-income, innercity community. A convenience sampling was used to recruit 32 mothers of children less than age 10 years at two federally funded health centers and two community food pantries.

Subjects were interviewed using a semistructured interview form. Analysis of the data indicated that the majority of subjects had a considerable degree of awareness of poisoning susceptibility, severity, and prevention. However, few had access to or had used the poison control center's telephone number. Only 56% of the subjects had received direct information about poisoning, with recall usually more accurate when information was obtained outside of the prenatal and postpartum settings.

STUDENT ACTIVITIES

• Determine resources for poison prevention and treatment within your community.
• Determine education programs available at your assigned agency.   🌿

Questions that should be addressed during discharge planning include the following:
• Are emergency numbers available at each phone?
• Is the poison control number available?
• Is there syrup of ipecac available for use in the home?

Advise clients to keep emergency numbers and their name, address, and a list of all prescription and OTC drugs used at each phone. In addition, many poison control centers have stickers that can be used to denote harmful substances. With proper teaching, children can learn that items marked with the special poison control stickers are harmful. However, advise the parents or caregivers not to rely only on the stickers; harmful substances must be kept out of the reach of children. Instruct caregiver(s) to check with the poison control center or primary care provider before administering the syrup.

Ask elderly clients about the members of their household. Do small children reside with them? If not, do they have small children that come to visit? Do they plan on using child-resistant caps for their drugs? If clients are not using child-resistant caps, remind them to take extra precautions and to store drugs out of reach of children. In some instances clients may need to install locks on cabinets to ensure safe drug storage.

Advise clients using transdermal delivery systems to store and dispose of them in a safe manner. Studies have shown that poisoning has occurred when young children reapply or chew on new or discarded patches.[5,6] Remind parents and caregivers not to treat medicine as candy, a practice frequently followed in an attempt to gain the cooperation of the child. Advise the parent that the administration of drugs should never be made into a game.

Another important role of the nurse is assessment of the home environment for hazards. Proper storage of drugs should be confirmed. Are the drugs actually stored in a child-resistant container? Remind the client how easy it is for small children to climb and reach places that adults consider safe. Is paint peeling from walls or ceilings? Has the home been checked for lead levels? Have children living in the home been checked for lead levels?

Although most families with small children are aware that detergents and cleaning materials are potential hazards, they may overlook less obvious poisons. For example, many common house and garden plants are dangerous, especially to children. They range from the white flowers and leaves of lily of the valley, to iris roots, poisonous mushrooms, green tubers of a potato, leaves of rhubarb, and philodendron. Many commonly used Christmas decorations such as poinsettias and the white berries of mistletoe are also poisonous.[7–10] Other hazardous materials include pesticides and plant fertilizers that are stored improperly.

CONCEPT REVIEW

Nurses play an important role in preventing accidental poisoning. This role includes client education and assurance that emergency and poison control center telephone numbers are available.

MANAGEMENT OF POISONING VICTIM AT HOME

When poisoning is discovered in the home, act immediately. Do *not* waste time waiting for symptoms to develop. Also do *not* rely on the client for accurate information about the amount or type of substance ingested. The first thing to do is to contact the poison control center. The poison control center can provide the most current data on nontoxic and poisonous material. The center needs to know the name of the substance, age of the client, time lapsed since contact, size of the container, estimate of the amount ingested, obvious signs and symptoms, existing illness, and current prescribed or OTC drugs. Provide the center information about the level of consciousness of the individual and if the client has vomited.

Instructions from the poison control center will vary. The center may instruct the caregiver to follow first aid information included on the label of the product. When the ingested material is caustic, the caller may be instructed to dilute the poison. For children, 100 ml of melted ice cream, milk, or plain water may be used. For adults, the dose is 200 ml. Ingestion of larger amounts of diluents is not recommended because the poison may be forced out of the stomach into the small intestine, thus producing faster absorption. When petroleum distillates such as gasoline are ingested, only milk should be used as a diluent. Only water is used if oil-soluble substances are involved.

If the poison is noncaustic, the poison control center may suggest use of an emetic. The most frequently recommended emetic is ipecac. If ipecac is not available, emesis can be initiated by stimulating the gag reflex.

Ipecac

Ipecac contains two alkaloids, emetine and cephaeline. The drug irritates the gastric mucosa and stimulates the vomiting center located in the medullary center. (See Table 77–1 for information on dosage and nursing considerations.) Vomiting usually occurs with 5 to 30 minutes in 90% of the clients. The original dose of ipecac can be repeated once if vomiting does not occur within 30 minutes. (It should not be repeated in infants.)

Abuse of ipecac is possible. Reports of parents administering ipecac to children to produce chronic vomiting and diarrhea have been documented. In addition, individuals with eating disorders (i.e., binge and purge eating, or bulimia) may use ipecac. Serious, potentially fatal, chronic toxicity can result from abuse of ipecac. Initial indications of abuse include generalized weakness and aching, especially in the neck and extremities. Stiffness, hyperreflexia, and difficulty performing tasks that requires muscular activity (e.g., climbing stairs) may follow. Speech is usually affected (i.e., slurred speech or dysphagia). Cardiotoxicity with flattened or inverted T waves, supraventricular tachycardia, atrial premature contraction, prolonged QT or PR intervals, decreased contractility, ventricular tachycardia and fibrillation, and cardiac arrest may occur. Emetine is eliminated slowly from the body, and recovery from excessive use may be prolonged.[11,12]

CONCEPT REVIEW

Management of poisoning victims in the home involves contacting the poison control center and proving first aid treatment, including the administration of syrup of ipecac.

Ipecac is safe and effective when administered to properly selected clients. It produces vomiting by a local irritant effect on the gastric mucosa and by a central medullary effect. The central medullary effect is produced by emetine and cephaeline, two alkaloids present in ipecac.

MANAGEMENT OF POISONING VICTIM IN HOSPITAL

Essential care of the poisoned client at the hospital includes the following:
- Stabilize the client.
- Identify the toxic substance.
- Eliminate the substance from the body.
- Support the client and significant other both physically and psychologically.[3]

Stabilize Client

The primary concerns in caring for a poisoned client are maintaining a patent airway and adequate cardiac output to maintain peripheral and renal perfusion. Usually an airway is inserted and oxygen administered. In some situations the use of mechanical ventilation is necessary. An intravenous line should be started. If fluid replacement is needed, normal saline or lactated Ringer's solution is administered intravenously.

TABLE 77–1
Drugs Used in the Management of Poisoning

Drug Name	Dosage and Route of Administration	Nursing Considerations
Charcoal, Activated (Superchar, Actidose, Liqui-Char) **HOW SUPPLIED** Powder: 15, 30, 40 g Liquid: 25 g in 120 ml, 30 g in 150 ml, 50 g in 240 ml	30–100 g (or 1 g/kg or approximately 5 to 10 times the amount of poison ingested) as a suspension	**Assess** Assess client's level of consciousness and determine material ingested. Ensure that emesis is complete; do not give if emesis is not complete. Obtain vital signs, blood pressure, and respiratory status. **Implement** Administer dose by mixing powder with tap water, forming thick syrup or slurry. Flavoring or fruit juice may be used; avoid milk or milk products, which reduce charcoal's absorptive capacity. Dose may be repeated if client vomits. Rapid ingestion may cause vomiting. **Monitor** Monitor vital signs, blood pressure, respiratory status. **Evaluate** Observe for therapeutic effect (absorption of poison is ended when charcoal is no longer in stool).
Ipecac Syrup (Ipecac) **HOW SUPPLIED** Syrup: 1.5%, 2%	**ADULTS** 15–30 ml followed by three to four glasses of water **CHILDREN** 1–12 y of age: 15 ml followed by one to two glasses of water <1 y: 5–10 ml followed by one half to one glass of water	**Assess** Do not administer if client has lost consciousness, if client is having seizures (convulsions), or if client is already vomiting profusely or has lost gag reflex. Determine the amount ingested. Do not induce emesis if petroleum distillates, volatile oils, or caustic substances were ingested. Obtain vital signs, blood pressure, and respiratory status. **Implement** Administer dose, followed by several ounces of warm water (do not give with milk or a carbonated beverage). Keep client active or jostled to enhance the emetic effect. **Monitor** Expect client to vomit within 5–30 min. Dose may be repeated once if there is no vomiting in this time. Monitor vital signs, blood pressure, and respiratory status. **Evaluate** Observe for vomiting within 30 min of administration.

Monitoring serum glucose levels is important since hypoglycemia can mask a variety of neurologic symptoms. In addition, use of a urinary catheter and a cardiac monitor may be necessary.

Identify Toxic Substance

If the client is transported to the hospital, take the suspected poisoning agent with the client. In addition, transport any empty bottles or containers found near the client since the labels may help identify ingredients in mixtures. Once in the hospital, appropriate laboratory studies (e.g., serum acetaminophen, cyanide, heavy metals, and toxicology screens such as heavy metal screen, serum toxicology drug screen) are ordered.

Eliminate Substance from Body

Since most poisoning results from oral ingestion, efforts to decrease gastrointestinal absorption are commonly used. This is accomplished by evacuation of gastric contents by (1) induc-

tion of emesis or gastric lavage, (2) use of activated charcoal, or (3) use of saline solution cathartics.

Emetics   The drug of choice for inducing emesis is syrup of ipecac. Its use is indicated after ingestion of almost all poisons. (See discussion of ipecac in earlier section.)

Induced emesis is contraindicated in the following situations:

- CNS depression: Clients who are lethargic or unresponsive, who lack a gag reflex, or who are unable to protect their airway effectively are at increased risk of pulmonary aspiration.
- Caustic material: Caustic material may further damage mucosal membranes when vomiting occurs. It may also cause gastric or esophageal perforations.
- Seizures: Postictal clients may aspirate gastric contents.
- Petroleum distillates ingestion: The risk of aspiration increases with compounds of very high viscosity (e.g., motor oil, mineral oil).

Gastric lavage   Gastric lavage (irrigation of the stomach) is used when induction of emesis cannot be performed. Lavage is accomplished by using a large-bore gastric tube (36 to 42 French for adults, 26 to 28 French for children). Use of smaller tubes should be avoided since they may not allow return of large tablet or capsule fragments and are easily occluded by food.

With the client in a left Sims' position and the head down, normal saline solution, half-normal saline solution, or tap water is instilled into the stomach. The amount of fluid instilled varies, depending on the age and tolerance of the client. Usually 250 to 500 ml is used in adults. Volumes in excess of 500 ml should be avoided because large volumes may foster passage of the substance into the duodenum. Lavage is carried out until fluid return is clear. The normal total lavage volume rarely exceeds 10 L. Approximately 10 to 12 washings with a total volume of 2 L are recommended for children.[3]

Gastric lavage is not without dangers. Inadvertent pulmonary placement of the tube and subsequent instillation of lavage fluids may occur. In addition, there is a risk of emesis or of esophageal or gastric perforation when passing the lavage tube.

Absorptive agents   Absorptive agents such as activated charcoal are also used. **Activated charcoal** may be prescribed after emesis or lavage. (Syrup of ipecac is inactivated and is absorbed by activated charcoal; therefore if ipecac has been administered, activated charcoal should be administered only when emesis is complete.) Activated charcoal absorbs and inactivates simple and complex poisons.

The powder form of the drug is prescribed most frequently. The recommended dose for children is 5 to 10 times the amount of poison ingested, with a minimum of 30 g mixed with 250 ml of water. If administered on a full stomach, larger doses may be necessary. The adult dose is 1 g/kg of body weight mixed as a suspension in 180 to 250 ml of water. Flavoring or fruit juice may be added to increase the palatability of the mixture. However, ice cream, sherbet, and milk ingestion should be avoided since they reduce the drug's absorptive capacity. The client drinks the mixture, or it is instilled through a nasogastric tube.[13-15] (See Table 77–1 for information on dosages and nursing considerations associated with activated charcoal.)

Antidotes and antagonists   Specific antidotes or antagonists are available for several drugs (Table 77–2). These products are used to reverse the action of the drug or to counteract drug overdose.[16,17] For example, **flumazenil** (Romazicon) acts as a benzodiazepine antagonist. (See Chapter 18 for information on flumazenil and benzodiazepines.) **Naloxone** (Narcan) is an antidote for narcotics and narcotic derivatives, and **physostigmine** (Antilirium) is used as an antidote for atropine, scopolamine, and tricyclic antidepressants. (See Chapter 19 for information on naloxone and Chapter 26 for information on physostigmine.)

TABLE 77–2

Antidotes Commonly Used in Managing Poisoned or Overdosed Clients

Substance	Antidote
Cholinesterase inhibitors (e.g., organophosphate insecticides, nerve gases, carbamates)	Atropine
Iron	Deferoxamine
Insulin	Dextrose 50%
Mercury, arsenic, lead, heavy metals	Dimercaprol, disodium edetate, penicillamine
Methanol, ethylene glycol	Ethanol
Lead	EDTA (ethylenediamine tetraacetic acid)
Acetaminophen	*N*-Acetylcysteine (Mucomyst)
Narcotics and narcotic derivatives, opiates	Naloxone (Narcan)
Cyanide	Amyl nitrite, sodium nitrite, sodium thiosulfate
Carbon monoxide	Oxygen
Cholinesterase inhibitors	2-PAM (Protopam)
Atropine, scopolamine, tricyclic antidepressants	Physostigmine (Antilirium)
Anticoagulants (e.g., warfarin [Coumadin])	Vitamin K

From Black, J.M., & Matassarin-Jacobs, E. (1993). *Luckmann and Sorensen's medical-surgical nursing* (4th ed., p. 2251). Philadelphia: W.B. Saunders.

CONCEPT REVIEW

General management of acute poisoning consists of supportive and symptomatic care. Focus is on maintaining a patent airway and sufficient cardiac output to assure adequate tissue perfusion.

Evacuation of gastric contents is accomplished by induction of emesis or gastric lavage. In some situations an adsorptive agent such as activated charcoal or a saline solution cathartic is used.

SUMMARY

The primary role of the nurse concerning poisoning is prevention. Careful assessment of the client's home and community environment is essential. Client education must focus on risks of poisoning found in these areas and first aid treatment in the case of poisoning.

REFERENCES

1. Litovitz, T.L., Holm, K.C., Bailey, K.M., & Schmitz, B.F. (1992). 1991 Annual report of the American Association of Poison Control Centers national data collection system. *American Journal of Emergency Medicine, 10,* 452–505.
2. Litovitz, T., & Manoguerra, A. (1992). Comparison of pediatric poisoning hazards: An analysis of 3.8 million exposure incidents. *Pediatrics, 89,* 999–1006.
3. Black, J., & Matassarin-Jacobs, E. (1993). *Luckmann and Sorensen's medical-surgical nursing: A psychophysiologic approach.* Philadelphia: W.B. Saunders.
4. Brannan, J.E. (1992). Accidental poisoning of children: Barriers to resource use in a black, low-income community. *Public Health Nursing, 9*(2), 81–86.

5. Morelli, J. (1993). Pediatric poisonings: The 10 most toxic prescription drugs. *American Journal of Nursing, 93*(7), 26–29.

6. Wiley, J.F., Wiley, C.C., Torrey, S.B., & Henretig, F.M. (1990). Clonidine poisoning in young children. *Journal of Pediatrics, 116,* 654–658.

7. Arena, J.M. (1989). Plants that poison. *Emergency Medicine, 21*(11), 20–24, 31–32, 34–35, 37–38, 48–51, 58–64.

8. Yew leaf ingestion can be cardiotonic. (1994). *Nurses' Drug Alert, 18*(10), 76.

9. Manoguerra, A.S. (1991). Poisonous plants, part 2. *Emergency, 23*(7), 23–26.

10. Manoguerra, A.S. (1991). Poisonous plants, part 1. *Emergency, 23*(6), 26, 28–29.

11. Ipecac misuse. (1994). *Nurses' Drug Alert, 18*(7), 52.

12. American Pharmaceutical Association. (1990). *Handbook of nonprescription drugs* (9th ed.). Washington, DC: Author.

13. Bayer, M.J., Klatzko, M., & Julig, K. (1990). The poisoned patient. *Patient Care, 24*(11), 176–180, 185, 188.

14. Davis, J.E. (1991). A consideration not to be overlooked: Activated charcoal in acute drug overdoses. *Professional Nurse, 6,* 710–712, 714.

15. Burkhart, K., et al. (1992). The adsorption of isopropanol and acetone by activated charcoal. *Journal of Toxicology, 30,* 371–375.

16. Brogden, R.N., & Coa, K.L. (1991). Flumazenil: A reappraisal of its pharmacologic properties and therapeutic efficacy as a benzodiazepine antagonist. *Drugs, 42,* 1061–1089.

17. Watson, D.S. (1993). The use of the benzodiazepine antagonist flumazenil. *AORN Journal, 57,* 497, 499–502.

BIBLIOGRAPHY

Everson, G.W., Bertaccini, E.J., & O'Leary, J. (1991). Use of whole bowel irrigation in an infant following iron overdose. *American Journal of Emergency Medicine, 9,* 366–369.

Fiser, D.H., Moss, M.M., & Walker, W. (1990). Critical care for clonidine poisoning in toddlers. *Critical Care Medicine, 18,* 1124–1128.

Foltin, G.L., & Goldfrank, L. (1993). Emergency care of the poisoning victim. *Hospital Medicine, 29*(12), 33–34, 41–43, 47–48.

Heidelman, S.M., & Sarnaik, A.P. (1990). Clonidine poisoning in children. *Critical Care Medicine, 18,* 618–620.

Hsu, J., & Williams, S. (1991). Injury prevention awareness in an urban Native American population. *American Journal of Public Health, 81,* 1466–1468.

Jacobson, B.J., Rock, A.R., Cohn, M.S., & Litovitz, T. (1989). Accidental ingestions of oral prescription drugs: A multicenter survey. *American Journal of Public Health, 79,* 853–856.

Mofenson, H.C. (1992). Is activated charcoal useful for acetaminophen overdose beyond two hours after ingestion? *Annals of Emergency Medicine, 21,* 894.

Olson, D.K., Sax, L., Gunderson, P., & Sioris, L. (1991). Pesticide poisoning surveillance through regional poison control centers. *American Journal of Public Health, 81,* 750–753.

Tenenbein, M. (1991). Multiple doses of activated charcoal: Time for reappraisal? *Annals of Emergency Medicine, 20,* 529–531.

Voltey, S.R., Bossee, G.M., Bayer, M.J., & Hoffman, J.R. (1991). Flumazenil: A new benzodiazepine antagonist. *Annals of Emergency Medicine, 20,* 181–188.

Weinman, S.A. (1993). Emergency management of drug overdose. *Critical Care Nurse, 13*(6), 45–51.

CHAPTER 78

DRUGS USED FOR
Diagnostic Procedures

SHARON JONES LAYTON • NORMA L. PINNELL

⊛ **General Characteristics**
LEARNING OBJECTIVE: Describe the function of diagnostic agents.

⊛ **Nursing Considerations**
LEARNING OBJECTIVE: Develop a plan of care for a client receiving diagnostic agents.

⊛ **Skin Testing Agents**
LEARNING OBJECTIVES:
   Describe the therapeutic uses of skin testing agents.
   Identify the major skin testing agents and their benefits and drawbacks.
   Discuss primary nursing activities related to skin testing agents.
   Discuss modified clonal selection theory.
   Discuss methods of introducing immunogens into the body.
   Provide rationale for the preferred method of skin testing.
   Compare and contrast old tuberculin and tuberculin, purified protein derivative, testing.
   Discuss the interpretation of the response to tuberculin injection.
   Discuss the objectives and procedure for the two-step method.
KEY TERMS:
   Immunogen, delayed (cell-mediated) hypersensitivity, T lymphocytes, patch test, scratch test, intradermal test, tuberculin anergy

⊛ **Imaging Agents**
LEARNING OBJECTIVES:
   Describe the therapeutic uses of imaging agents.
   Identify the major imaging agents and their benefits and drawbacks.
   Discuss primary nursing activities related to imaging agents.
   Identify factors to consider in evaluating the toxicity of a contrast medium.
KEY TERMS:
   Opacity, thrombogenic, barium sulfate, radiopaque agents

⊛ **Provocative Agents**
LEARNING OBJECTIVES:
   Describe the therapeutic uses of provocative agents.
   Identify the major provocative agents and their benefits and drawbacks.
   Discuss primary nursing activities related to provocative agents.
KEY TERM: Provocative

⊛ **In Vivo Markers and Tracers**
LEARNING OBJECTIVES:
   Describe the therapeutic uses of in vivo markers and tracers.
   Identify the major in vivo markers and tracers and their benefits and drawbacks.
   Discuss primary nursing activities related to in vivo markers and tracers.
KEY TERMS:
   Isotope, radioisotope, radiopharmaceutical

The nurse must know about the drugs used in conjunction with the wide range of diagnostic procedures available to assist in the evaluation of a client's disease or condition. Although not actually administering the diagnostic drugs, the nurse often provides care before and after the testing occurs. The correct preparation of the client physically and the education of the client and his or her significant others usually are considered nursing responsibilities. When the examination is finished, the nurse must provide the correct medication or treatment for that particular examination, be alert for possible complications, and provide information and support while awaiting the examination results. In recent years the explosion in the field of imaging techniques has brought a host of new drugs used to provide or enhance the contrast of one part of the body in comparison to another. The nurse's responsibility is not only to know what tests his or her client is undergoing but also to know about the drugs involved in the testing procedures.

GENERAL CHARACTERISTICS

Drugs used for diagnostic procedures display a variety of characteristics. Some are relatively innocuous (e.g., barium sulfate); others are active agents and as such, can have far reaching effects on the body. Highly iodinated compounds can cause iodism—irritation of the eye, nose, and throat, symptoms resembling a bad cold, and an unpleasant taste in the mouth. Although many of these drugs are used only as a diagnostic aid, some also have therapeutic applications. In general, these drugs provide a means to assess the allergic or immune status, to get a picture of a cavity or organ, or to measure the function of an organ or body system. The actual process used to achieve these outcomes in part defines the needed characteristics of that type of drug. For example, drugs involved in the imaging of some part of the body must have opacity as a characteristic. Radioisotopes used as tracers must be able to incorporate into a particular molecule. They must also emit enough radiation to be picked up by the scanning device without causing harm to the client. Another type of drug is used for skin testing; these drugs must elicit a specific reaction that can be easily identified without being severe enough to put the individual at risk for anaphylactic reaction. See chapter 49 for more information on the immune response. Specific characteristics of the diagnostic drugs are addressed later in this chapter.

These drugs are not measured according to their therapeutic use because they are used for testing purposes. The criteria used to assess the efficacy of a drug used for diagnostic testing are different from those for drugs used prophylactically or therapeutically. Some of the parameters used to evaluate diagnostic drugs are sensitivity, specificity, accuracy, and reproducibility. Identification of anything that might interfere with the drug's use for testing is important to prevent skewing the test results in some fashion.

▨ NURSING CONSIDERATIONS

Assessing Assess each testing procedure to determine what type of preparation is required, necessary postprocedure interventions, effects of the drug used for the procedure, and possible interactions with therapeutic drugs currently in use or with drugs recently used in other testing procedures. For example, a client scheduled for a thyroid function evaluation and for a procedure that involves the use of an iodinated contrast media must have the thyroid function procedure done first because the iodinated contrast media skews thyroid function test results for months. Pertinent individual client assessment includes any history of allergy or reaction to the drug(s) involved in the testing procedure(s), an assessment of the client's ability to understand and follow directions, and the physical status of the client in regard to ability to tolerate the procedure. Be alert for the less obvious possibilities for an allergic reaction (e.g., corticotropin use is contraindicated in clients with a sensitivity to porcine proteins).

Diagnosing Analysis of the data obtained during the nursing history and physical assessment constitutes the basis for the formulation of the appropriate nursing diagnoses and the development of the plan of care.

Nursing diagnoses appropriate for the client undergoing diagnostic testing stem from the process of preparing the client for the test procedure, the test itself, posttest procedures, and the process of waiting for the outcome of the test. Possible nursing diagnoses follow:

- Anxiety related to the process of the test procedure.
- Bowel elimination, alteration in: constipation related to barium ingestion.
- Bowel elimination, alteration in: diarrhea related to test preparation.
- Fear related to possible test outcome.
- Fluid volume deficit, high risk related to test preparation.
- Knowledge deficit regarding test procedure(s).
- Nutrition, alteration in: less than body requirements related to test preparation.
- Oral mucous membrane, alteration in, related to test preparation or procedure.
- Self-concept, disturbance: body image related to testing process.
- Skin integrity, impairment of: high risk related to positioning during the testing process.
- Sleep pattern disturbance related to test preparation or procedure.
- Urinary elimination, alteration in patterns, related to test procedure.

Planning Once the needs of the client have been identified, a plan of care can be initiated. Much of the nursing care for the client undergoing diagnostic testing involves the following areas: education about all the phases of the testing process; procedures indicated for the preparation of the client for the test; any posttest nursing interventions dictated by the individual test; and nursing interventions related to any nursing diagnoses identified as a consequence of the results of the tests. The test results may trigger a whole new group of needs. For example, if a hiatal hernia is identified on x-ray film, the client probably will need education about dietary changes, positioning after meals, and medications.

Possible expected outcomes for the plan of care include the following:

- Client verbalizes understanding of possible bowel and urinary changes related to testing and names ways to cope with them.
- Client expresses feeling about possible test outcomes.
- Client describes ways to maintain fluid volume and adequate nutrition.
- Client expresses understanding that testing produces temporary changes in oral mucous membranes or skin integrity.
- Client identifies altered self-concept or inability to sleep related to upcoming procedures.

Implementing   In general, interventions include providing needed education, monitoring fluid balance, and assessing for possible untoward reactions to drugs administered or intolerance to the testing procedure.

The education process should start from the first interaction with the client and continue throughout the entire process. Often people do not remember what information has been given to them verbally, so reinforce any teaching done with written information to which the client may refer at a later time. If more than one diagnostic test will be done, consider the prevention of conflicts in preparation and diagnostic drugs used. Also consider client tolerance and convenience, especially if the tests will be done on an outpatient basis.

Evaluating   There are various approaches to determining how effective the education process was. They include getting the client to list possible interventions for a particular situation, eliciting a description of the disease or condition in the client's own words, and asking what information has been given about the outcome of the test(s). Evaluation of the preparation process is primarily based on accomplishing the correct procedures in the correct time frames before the test. If the preparation involves a series of enemas to cleanse the bowel, the outcome criteria should reflect both this purpose and the maintenance of the fluid balance during and after the preparation or testing process.

CONCEPT REVIEW

If a drug is a good diagnostic agent, it must be sensitive, specific, and accurate and must provide reproducible results. Anything (e.g., food, another drug, environmental factors) that interferes with the drug must be identified.

Nursing intervention for diagnostic testing involves preparing the client physically, mentally, and emotionally for the testing itself and for learning the results of testing; it also may involve further client education and planning, depending on test results.

Use of written materials is always useful, especially if more than one procedure is planned.

SKIN TESTING AGENTS

Skin testing is used for determining the allergy status of a person, to assess the immune status, or to test for the presence of specific antibodies to a past or present infection with a particular organism. Skin testing for a present or previous exposure to a particular microorganism takes advantage of a known immune system mechanism. At some point, the individual exposed to an **immunogen** (any cell or molecule that produces an immune response). This exposure sets in motion a process called the *modified clonal selection theory*, which results in the production of antibodies specific for that particular immunogen.[2] When a second exposure (the skin test) occurs, the observed response is called **delayed hypersensitivity** or **cell-mediated hypersensitivity**. This response involves the migration of **T lymphocytes** (specific to the immunogen) to the site of the immunogen exposure. The reaction of the T lymphocytes and the immunogen cause the release of a series of mediators. These mediators cause the development of an inflammation at the site. The delay in the response is caused by the time required for the migration of the T lymphocytes, which usually takes approximately 36–48 hours.[3] The cell containing the immunogen eventually is destroyed.

Three methods are used to introduce the immunogen into the body: the patch test, scratch test, and intradermal test. With the **patch test**, an adhesive patch impregnated with the immunogenic substance is placed on the skin. With the **scratch test**, the skin is abraded and the immunogenic substance applied to that area. With the **intradermal test**, the immunogenic substance is injected intradermally. The preferred method is the intradermal test because the dosage of the immunogen can be controlled much more precisely than with the other methods, thus increasing the accuracy of the testing process.

Major Skin Testing Agents

The number of skin testing agents used for the purpose of detecting the presence of specific antibodies in relation to a past or present infection by a specific organism is small. Table 78–1 lists the skin testing agents found in this category. Some of these agents are used for **anergy** testing (anergy is the loss of ability to mount cutaneous delayed hypersensitivity reactions) in addition to testing for a past or present infection. Of note is the use of the mumps skin test antigen at the same time as the tuberculin skin testing on human immunodeficiency virus (HIV) seropositive individuals. This practice provides information in about both the reaction to the tuberculosis testing and the presence of cutaneous anergy and helps predict the oc-

TABLE 78-1
Major Skin Testing Agents

Agent	Action, Dosage, Route of Administration, Interpretation Timing	Nursing Considerations
Tuberculin	**Clinical use:** Assist in the diagnosis of tuberculosis and in the differentiation from other mycotic and bacterial infections; assist in the evaluation of cell-mediated immune status. **Desired action:** Area of induration at the injection site; erythema not considered a positive reaction **Dosage:** 0.1 ml of 5 TU/0.1 ml solution **Route of administration:** Intradermal route—most accurate and preferred **Interpretation timing:** 48–72 h after injection NOTE: *Never administer 250 TU/0.1 ml strength tuberculin as an initial test* because of the risk of necrosis at the site.	**Assess** Obtain history; look for any history of hypersensitivity or positive response to the test and for any family history or clinical manifestations of tuberculosis. Assess ability to follow directions and understand information about test interpretation. **Implement** Administer test, being careful to use correct technique. Make sure a bleb forms, indicating the test was done correctly; if not, repeat the test in another site at least 5 cm away. Provide instructions about interpretation of the test in 48–72 h. Observe for any untoward reactions to the test; although anaphylactoid reactions are rare, be prepared for such a reaction. Interpret the test using CDC guidelines. Provide appropriate education and counseling in response to the test outcome. **Evaluate** Client identifies the purpose of the test, describes the testing process, and describes his or her role in that process. Untoward reactions to the test are recognized and properly treated. Positive test outcomes are reported to all appropriate agencies.
Coccidioidin	**Clinical uses:** Assist in diagnosis of coccidioimycosis and in differentiation from other mycotic and bacterial infections; assist in the evaluation of cell-mediated immune status **Desired action:** Area of induration at the injection site; erythema not considered a positive reaction **Dosage:** usual dose, 0.1 ml of 1:100 solution; for individuals with disseminated coccidioimycosis or thin-walled coccidioidal pulmonary cavities—recommended dosage, 0.1 ml of 1:10 solution; presence of potential or confirmed diagnosis of coccicioidal erythema nodosum—strength of the solution, 1:10,000 **Route of administration:** Intradermal **Interpretation timing:** First reading at 24 h after injection, with a second reading after 48 h **Contraindications:** Use is contraindicated for individuals with allergy or sensitivity to mercury. In presence of potential or confirmed diagnosis of coccidioidal erythema, a 1:10,000 strength must be used for testing.	**Assess** Obtain history; look for any history of hypersensitivity or positive response to the test, presence of a potential or confirmed diagnosis of coccidioidal erythema nodosum, and any family history or clinical manifestations of coccidioimycosis. Since the preparation contains thimerosal, look for any history of allergy to mercury. Assess ability to follow directions and understand information about test interpretation. **Implement** Administer test, being careful to use correct technique and dosage. Make sure a bleb forms, indicating the test was done correctly; if not, the test must be repeated in another site at least 5 cm away. Provide instructions about interpretation of the test after 24 h to avoid false-negative reports after 48 h. Observe for any untoward reactions to the test for at least 15 min; be prepared for immediate systemic reaction. Interpret the test appropriately. Provide appropriate education and counseling in response to the test outcome. **Evaluate** Client identifies the purpose of test, describes the testing process, and describes his or her role in that process.

Table 78–1 *Continued*
Major Skin Testing Agents

Agent	Action, Dosage, Route of Administration, Interpretation Timing	Nursing Considerations
Coccidioidin *Continued*		***Evaluate—Continued*** Untoward reactions to the test are recognized and properly treated. Positive test outcomes are reported to all appropriate agencies.
Histoplasmin	**Clinical use:** Assist in the diagnosis of histoplasmosis and in the differentiation from other mycotic and bacterial infections; assist in the evaluation of cell-mediated immune status **Desired action:** Area of induration at injection site **Dosage:** 0.1 ml **Route of administration:** Intradermally **Interpretation timing:** 48–72 h after injection	***Assess*** Obtain history; look for any history of hypersensitivity or positive response to the test and any family or clinical manifestations of histoplasmosis. Assess ability to follow directions and understand information about test interpretation. ***Implement*** Administer test, being careful to use correct technique and dosage. Too large a dose may cause severe erythema and induration followed by necrosis and ulceration. Make sure a bleb forms, indicating the test was done correctly; if not, the test must be repeated in another site at least 5 cm away. Be prepared for a hypersensitive or anaphylactic reaction by having epinephrine available. ***Monitor*** Monitor for the development of vesiculation, ulceration, and necrosis at the test site in the histoplasmin-sensitive person. ***Evaluate*** A client identifies the purpose of the test, describes the testing process, and describes his or her role in that process. Untoward reactions to the test are recognized and properly treated. Positive test outcomes are reported to all appropriate agencies.
Penicilloylpolylysine (PPL)	**Clinical use:** Assist in evaluation of risk of hypersensitive reaction to administration of penicillin G **Desired action:** Scratch test—pale wheal ≥5–15 mm in diameter; intradermal test—itching and marked increase in size of bleb caused by injection, especially when compared to control site **Dosage:** Scratch test—small drop of PPL smoothed on 3–5 mm long scratch made by sterile 20-gauge needle; intradermal test—0.01–0.02 ml of PPL preparation **Route of administration:** Either as a scratch test or intradermally **Interpretation timing:** Reaction visible within 15 min of test administration **Contraindications:** PPL skin test should not be administered with other skin testing agents or penicillin-type drugs.	***Assess*** Obtain personal and family history about any previous treatment with a penicillin or cephalosporin. If such a history is elicited, probe for any untoward effects or allergic reactions noted during treatment. Assess client's ability to follow directions and understand information about test interpretation. ***Implement*** If there is any history of allergic reactions, do *NOT* administer the test. *Always* administer the scratch test first. If there is no reaction or a questionable reaction to the scratch test, administer the intradermal test. Observe for and be prepared for a hypersensitive or anaphylactic reaction to the test.

Table continued on following page.

TABLE 78–1 *Continued*
Major Skin Testing Agents

Agent	Action, Dosage, Route of Administration, Interpretation Timing	Nursing Considerations
Penicilloylpolylysine (PPL) *Continued*		**Implement—Continued** If the client has a reaction to the control site done in conjunction with the intradermal test, it may be difficult to interpret the response to the testing process correctly. Such a reaction should be reported to the primary care provider for further evaluation. Provide education about the testing process and potential outcomes. **Evaluate** Client identifies purpose of the test, describes the testing process, and describes his or her role in that process. Untoward reactions to the test are recognized and properly treated. Positive test outcomes are reported to the primary care provider.
Mumps skin test allergen	**Clinical use:** Assessment of cell-mediated immunity; *Not* used for the immunization, diagnosis, or treatment of mumps virus infection **Desired action:** Area of induration at injection site $\geq$ 5 mm; exception—HIV-seropositive individual in whom any indurated area is considered positive; erythema not considered a positive reaction **Dosage:** 0.1 ml **Route of administration:** Intradermal injection only **Interpretation timing:** Check injection site in 48–72 h NOTE: Mumps skin test allergen should be administered with other antigens to which the person has probably been exposed. **Contraindications:** Agent should not be used in persons with a hypersensitivity to avian protein or thimerosal.	**Assess** Obtain history; look for any history of hypersensitivity to the test. Investigate a history of hypersensitivity to avian protein or to thiomerosal since this compound has the potential to precipitate an anaphylactic reaction to either one. Assess client's ability to follow directions and understand information about test interpretation. **Implement** Administer the test carefully, using the correct technique and dosage. Observe for the appearance of a bleb, indicating correct adminstration of the test. Provide instructions about interpretation of test after 48–72 h. Observe for any untoward reactions to the test for at least 15 min; be prepared for immediate systemic reaction. Interpret the test appropriately. Provide appropriate education and counseling in response to the test outcome. **Evaluate** Client identifies the purpose of the test, describes the testing process, and describes his or her role in that process. Untoward reactions to the test are recognized and properly treated. Positive test outcomes are reported to all appropriate agencies.

currence of the initial opportunistic infection.[4] Included in this category is the agent used to test for the risk of a hypersensitive reaction to the administration of penicillin G because this agent is not only a diagnostic agent but also works using the delayed reaction hypersensitivity process. Response to testing with penicilloyl-polylysine possibly indicates a hypersensitivity to other penicillins and to the cephalosporins. However, at this time labeling does not include this indication as approved by the Food and Drug Administration (FDA).

If the individual being tested is *anergic,* or abnormally inactive, there will be a false-negative test result. If the history and clinical presentation point to diagnosis of the infection, other methods of making a positive diagnosis should be used. This situation also identifies the need for anergy testing and, if appropriate, further exploration into the cause of an identified anergic state. In some cases the individual was selectively anergic to a skin testing agent.[4]

Undesired clinical responses Undesired responses are

---

similar for skin testing agents. These responses are listed in the box.

Life-span considerations   No studies have been with any of the skin testing agents to find out if they could cause fetal harm. Each situation must be evaluated to see if the diagnostic process can be completed without this portion of the process. If the skin test must be included to make the diagnosis, another question should be asked and answered: Which is greater—the risk of teratogenic effects or the risk of an undiagnosed and thus untreated infection? In the case of testing for hypersensitivity to penicillin G, the question should be: Can another drug be administered? If not, the risk of giving penicillin therapy without skin testing versus the risk of using skin testing with antigen in a pregnant woman should be evaluated. The geriatric client's immune sensitivity may wane, creating a need to administer the Mantoux test a second time to take advantage of the booster effect. The booster effect is a positive reaction to a second testing after an insignificant reaction to the initial test. This effect is seen in persons with waning sensitivity (e.g., those with recent viral infection). This second testing should be done 1 week after the initial testing.[4] This testing process is known as the *two-step-method* and should be used not only in this situation but also for the initial testing process of groups on whom periodic testing will be done (e.g., direct health care providers). By initial use of the two-step-method, two objectives are met: (1) prevention of false-negative results and (2) prevention of incorrect identification of seroconversion at a later date.

Drug-drug, drug-nutrient, drug-environment interactions   Interactions between the testing agent and other drugs, diet, and environmental factors can cause either a false-positive or false-negative test result. Table 78–2 lists specific interactions for each testing agent.

Intradermal Tuberculin Testing

Determining exposure to tuberculosis is a common use of intradermal testing. Since dosage regulation is a problem with multiple-puncture devices, the American Thoracic Society (ATS) and the U.S. Centers for Disease Control (CDC) both recommend the use of the intradermal injection (Mantoux) test to evaluate the status of individuals exposed to a case of clinical tuberculosis, individuals in the position of a likely exposure, or those suspected of having tuberculosis.

Therapeutic uses and clinical indications   tuberculin skin testing is used to identify those infected with *Mycobacterium tuberculosis*. The approach is from two aspects: (1) to test individuals identified as probably infected and (2) to help in the confirmation of the diagnosis when symptoms are present. Another use for tuberculin is in conjunction with other immunogens to evaluate an individual's delayed hypersensitivity status. Table 78–3 provides further details in these areas.

Physiologic response   Response to the introduction of tuberculin may be seen as quickly as 6 hours after administration. Maximal reaction occurs in 48 to 72 hours. In most individuals the reaction remains visible for approximately 4 days before gradually going away. The usual physiologic responses are erythema and induration, frequently accompanied by pruritis.

Undesired clinical responses   Other responses to tuberculin are vesiculation, ulceration, necrosis, and pain. In a few cases severe scarring has occurred at the injection site. Severe response to tuberculin is infrequent; when it does occur, it occurs usually in an individual with a high level of sensitivity. On rare occasions a hypersensitive response to tuberculin or to the agents added to the preparation occurs immediately after injection. This response usually consists of a wheal, with or without accompanying erythema and induration, which peaks in approximately 6 hours and leaves within 24 hours. Because of the time frames involved, this hypersensitive response should not interfere with the evaluation of the testing site. Systemic response usually does not occur unless the tuberculin is accidentally injected subcutaneously instead of intradermally. In the individual highly sensitive to tuberculin, systemic effects include a febrile reaction or acute inflammation around old tuberculosis lesions. Reports of anaphylactoid reactions to tuberculin have been very rare.[4] Since this testing process is based on the immune system's response to an immunogen, the potential for an anaphylactic reaction always exist. Therefore always have equipment for the proper treatment of such a reaction readily available.

Test interpretation   Both old tuberculin (OT) and tuberculin, purified protein derivative (PPD), may be used with the multiple-puncture device; however, only PPD is used for the Mantoux test procedure. PPD is available in three strengths. Both the CDC and the ATS recommend the use of the intermediate strength solution: 5 tuberculin units (TU)/0.1 ml.[4] The standard Mantoux test is 0.1 ml of this solution. This test is the most accurate and reliable tuberculin skin test presently available. Interpretation of the Mantoux test is based on duration only, and reading should be done 48 to 72 hours after the injection of the tuberculin. To promote objective reading of the response, the outer perimeters of the induration are identified by applying steady pressure from normal skin toward the indurated area, using a pen to mark the area, and repeating the procedure on the other side of the indurated area. These lines should be parallel to the long axis of the forearm to allow measurement between the lines, which is easy and objective. Interpretation of the response to the injection is di-

TABLE 78–2
Interactions Associated With Major Skin Testing Agents

Agent	Drug Name	Diet	Laboratory Tests and Environment
Tuberculin	**Viral vaccines:** May suppress any reaction for 4–6 wk after immunization **Bacille Calmette-Guérin (BCG) Vaccination:** usually causes a positive reaction; however, varies with time, age, and exposure to active tuberculosis; should investigate any positive reaction in individual known to have received BCG vaccination for presence of active tuberculosis **Systemic corticosteroids or amniocaproic acid:** Suppress reactivity to tuberculin test	Malnourishment suppresses a positive reaction.	Positive reaction may be caused by an infection due to another mycobacterium; other diagnostic procedures are needed when a positive reaction occurs. False-negative reactions have occurred in client with HIV, AIDS, Hodgkin's disease, lymphoma, chronic lymphocytic anemia, sarcoidosis, or any condition that affects the lymph system. Suppression of a positive reaction may also occur in presence of dehydration, chronic renal failure, or situations causing high levels of stress (e.g., burns, surgery, mental illness). Administration of the test in an area of atopic dermatitis, sun damaged skin, or ultraviolet treatment produces a false-negative reaction. PPD solutions should be stored at 2° to 8° C, should be protected from light, and should not be frozen. PPD solutions may be stored for 30 d in prefilled syringes at 2° to 8° C, but this practice is not recommended.
Coccidioidin	Does not interfere with serologic tests for coccidioidomycosis	Malnourishment suppresses a positive reaction.	Positive reaction may be caused by an infection due to another mycobacterium; other diagnostic procedures may be needed when a positive reaction occurs. Commercially prepared dilutions should be stored at 2° to 8° C. Further dilutions should be stored at 2° to 8° C and used within 24 h.
Histoplasmin	**Serologic test for histoplasmosis:** draw before administration of histoplasmin **Viral vaccines:** May suppress any reaction for 3 wk after immunization **Corticosteroids or immunosuppressants:** Suppress reactivity to the test	—	A positive reaction may be caused by an infection caused by another mycobacterium, necessitating other diagnostic procedures when a positive reaction occurs. Preparation should be stored at 2° to 8° C.
Penicilloylpolylysine (PPL)	**Skin tests using penicillin or other penicillin-derived reagents:** may potentiate any reaction	—	Store at 2° to 10° C. If agent is left at room temperature for more than 1 d, discard it.
Mumps skin test antigen		Malnourishment may suppress a positive reaction.	Mumps skin test antigen should be stored at 2° to 8° C; avoid freezing.

vided into three groups based on the degree of exposure or likelihood of the presence of tuberculosis or HIV infection. Group 1 includes those individuals who have had close contact with someone with clinical tuberculosis, those known or strongly suspected to have HIV infection, intravenous (IV) drug users, and those strongly suspected to have tuberculosis. An area of induration of 5 mm or more is considered positive. Group 2 includes individuals at greater risk to acquire tuberculosis than the general public: clients with medical conditions that predispose them to tuberculosis, individuals from countries with a high prevalence of the disease, individuals who work or reside in long-term care facilities, and individuals with low socioeconomic backgrounds. For this group an area of in-

duration of 10 mm or greater is considered positive. Group 3 consists of individuals with no risk factors and therefore at low risk of exposure to tuberculosis. An indurated area of 15 mm or greater is considered a positive response for this group. Erythema is *not* considered in the process of interpreting the test. However, if there is an area of erythema greater than 10 mm without any induration, the injection may have been made too deeply and the test should be repeated to clarify the situation.

Nursing considerations   Since skin testing usually is done by nursing personnel, nursing implications are found throughout the testing process. Administer the test correctly to avoid a systemic distribution of the tuberculin and to promote

TABLE 78–3
Therapeutic Uses and Clinical Indications for Tuberculin

Uses	Clinical Indications
Screening well individuals	Identification of clients with asymptomatic infections with Mycobacterium tuberculosis
	Identification of individuals who would benefit from preventive therapy
	Periodic surveillance of individuals at risk for exposure to tuberculosis (e.g., personnel and long-term residents in hospitals, nursing homes, mental institutions, prisons)
	Periodic surveillance of children not identified as being in some risk category: well-child screening done at 12–15 mo of age, before entry into school system, and at 14–16 y of age
	Abnormal chest x-ray film compatible with past tuberculosis
	Individuals at high risk for recent exposure: immigrants from Asia, Africa, Latin America, low socioeconomic background
	Children at high risk: living in areas of high prevalence; black, Hispanic, Asian, native Americans, and native Alaskans: socioeconomically deprived; immigrants from Asia, Africa, the Middle East, Latin American, or the Caribbean with medical risk factors for tuberculosis
	Epidemiologic studies used to identify areas of high incidence of the disease
Testing individuals with other diseases	Any client with HIV infection or at risk for HIV infection
	Any client with a medical condition that increases the risk to contract tuberculosis (e.g., silicosis, diabetes, immunosuppressive therapy, lymphoma)
	New enrollees in a drug treatment program or enrollees not yet tested
Testing symptomatic individuals	To aid in the diagnosis of the disease; important to note that an individual's positive test result by itself does *not* make the diagnosis of a case of clinical tuberculosis
Anergy testing	Any individual considered at risk for either HIV or tuberculosis infection

a clear response to the test. Inject the dosage intradermally, usually on the flexor surface of the forearm approximately 4 inches (10 cm) below the elbow, using a tuberculin syringe and short 26- or 27-gauge needle. Interpret the test in a timely manner, using the guidelines previously identified. Be precise in the measurement of any indurated area to ensure correct interpretation of the test response. Be prompt in reporting the test results to the primary care provider, thus promoting the proper treatment of the disease. In addition, notify the proper state and federal agencies so that other contacts can be identified and tested.

The nurse plays a major role in the education of the client and any significant others about the meaning of the test results, modes of transmission of the disease, required reporting, and the need for and probable content of medical management. A positive diagnosis of tuberculosis cannot be made on the basis of the skin test alone. Referral for medical management triggers additional testing to confirm or deny any diagnosis suggested by the positive skin test result. After a positive diagnosis of tuberculosis has been made, the nursing role is one of support in acceptance of the diagnosis, reinforcement of the need to take prescribed medicine faithfully, and education about follow-up visits. The importance of taking the prescribed medication cannot be emphasized too strongly since it is believed that the appearance of strains of tuberculosis resistant to standard treatment is due in large part to the noncompliance of those individuals treated for the disease.

CONCEPT REVIEW

Skin testing agents can identify allergies, immune status, or antibodies caused by a particular immunogen.
Methods used to determine delayed hypersensitivity are the patch test, scratch test, and intradermal test.

One of the most common and important tests performed intradermally is the tuberculin test. A positive test result requires notification of the primary care provider and state and federal authorities.
Other drugs, diet, and testing or environmental factors may interact with skin testing agents.

IMAGING AGENTS

Imaging agents are used to promote the visualization of some part of the body. The mechanism used varies according to the part of the body studied. The first imaging agents were the bismuth salts, used to enhance visualization of the gastrointestinal (GI) tract.[5] Since then, the number of drugs and the methods used for visualization of some part of the body have changed markedly. Imaging agents are subdivided into groups for easier classification and better understanding of them. The most common subdivisions are drugs used as radiographic contrast agents, diagnostic radiopharmaceuticals used for nuclear medicine procedures, and contrast agents used for magnetic resonance imaging (MRI).

Major Imaging Agents

Drugs used to provide contrast during conventional radiographic procedures are selected primarily because of their **opacity** to x-rays. X-rays cannot pass through such agents, thus leaving a distinct impression on the radiographic film. This property allows the outlining of a cavity or tissue space. In addition, in some cases this testing procedure also gives information about the level of function of a particular organ—if it is not visualized, it is not functioning (e.g., the gallbladder). Although opacity on x-ray film is the desired action of radiographic contrast agents, a balance must be struck between obtaining as high a concentration as possible in the cavity or tissue space for the study without causing harm. This requires study of the pharmacokinetics and pharmacodynamics of any agent used. The two agents used to confer opacity are barium and iodine.

Barium sulfate is particularly suited for evaluation of the GI tract because of its insolubility, which precludes systemic absorption.[6] The agent used to suspend the barium depends on which area of the GI tract will be studied. Some compounds combine barium and a gas-producing agent to use the double-contrast method (barium for opacity and gas to distend, thus improving the outlining of the area) for better visualization.

Since barium is *not* used systemically because of the toxicity of barium ions, intravascular administration of a **radiopaque** iodine is used to visualize the blood vessels and organs or spaces of the body. As with barium, the agent used to suspend the iodine varies with the area studied. If an iodized compound must be introduced into a body cavity today, the newer water-soluble iodine compounds are used.[6] (Table 78–4).

Undesired clinical responses and contraindications Undesired clinical responses and contraindications for major imaging agents are summarized in Table 78–5. Nursing considerations associated with these concerns are also provided.

Factors to consider when evaluating the toxicity of a contrast medium include the cation in the preparation; the osmolarity, volume concentration, and viscosity of the solution; and the rate and route of administration. In general, the lower the compound in each category, the less toxic it is.

Drug-drug, drug-nutrient, drug-environment interactions The interaction of imaging agents and other drugs, nutrients, laboratory tests, and the environment are summarized in Table 78–6.

BARIUM SULFATE

Barium is not absorbed systemically when introduced orally or rectally. It is eliminated from the body in the feces. The length of time barium remains in the GI tract and the rate of elimination in the feces depend on the specific preparation used and the motility status of the GI tract at the time of testing. This transit time is also the time available for radiologic studies. In an individual with a normal GI tract, barium administered orally usually is excreted in 24 hours. When administered rectally, the barium usually is expelled with the enema; however, some may remain in the colon for several weeks in the presence of decreased motility. Aspiration of barium when administered orally seldom occurs, and when it does, it is usually not harmful. Aspiration of large amounts of barium may cause pneumonitis or nodular gramulomas of interstitial lung tissues.[4] A weakness in the bowel wall may predispose the client to bowel perforation after rectal administration of barium. The perforation probably is caused by hydrostatic pressure of the instilled barium sulfate or trauma to the colon by the enema tip. Partial perforation can lead to dissection of the intestinal wall layers. If complete intestinal perforation occurs, barium spills into the peritoneal cavity, accompanied by a large fluid loss.

IODIZED COMPOUNDS

Iodized compounds are used to provide visualization of body cavities, angiography, urography, and visualization of the gallbladder. The degree of opacity is directly proportional to the iodine content of the compound. Although drugs that contain organic iodine are effective radiographic contrast agents, they also can cause significant undesired clinical responses. In general, the adverse reactions that occur after the administration of iodized compounds can range from discomfort to severe anaphylactoid reactions. Therefore competent personnel and appropriate facilities to treat such reactions should always be available when these drugs are used. Specific undesired clinical responses provided in Table 78–5. Since all iodized compounds interfere with thyroid function testing, this type of testing should be done before the use of iodized contrast agents.

Iodized fatty acid and oils Iodized fatty acid and oils were used for myelography, sialography, bronchography, and hysterosalpingography before computed tomography (CT), water-soluble contrast agents, and (MRI) became available.[5] After iodized fatty acids and oils (e.g., ethiodized oil) are instilled into the lymph vessel, they are readily distributed throughout the lymphatic system. In addition, they can enter the vascular system via lymphatic-venous anastomoses, particularly in the presence of lymph node tumors and obstruction of lymph flow. After reaching the vascular system, as much as 65% of the dose may be obtained in the pulmonary circulation as microemboli. Visualization of the lymph nodes and lymph vessels occurs immediately after instillation of the drug. Elimination from the body is slow (6 to 18 months).

When used for intrauterine instillation to visualize the uterine plus fallopian tube anatomy, there is sufficient contrast to visualize the uterus and fallopian tube cavities immediately. Elimination of the drug from this area of the body is also slow. If the drug leaks into the peritoneal cavity, it is absorbed into the vascular system over 3 to 6 months. If an obstruction is present in the fallopian tubes, incomplete absorption of the drug may occur, leaving the drug in the body for years. In general, the metabolization of iodized fatty acids and oils to fatty acid and inorganic iodine is a slow process.[4]

Oral iodized agents Oral iodized agents are used to visualize the gallbladder and never achieve a high concentration in the blood since they are absorbed from the intestine, circulated bound to albumin, and concentrated in the gallbladder. Excretion occurs in the same manner as bilirubin. Oral iodine compounds can promote the sickling of cells in individuals homozygous for sickle cell disease. However, these oral agents are seldom used since ultrasound and scintigraphy are available. The ultrasound process is used to detect gallstones, whereas scintigraphy is used to detect cholecystitis.[6]

Water-soluble ionic iodized agents Water-soluble ionic iodized agents are used as the contrast in a wide variety of radiographic diagnostic procedures. **Diatrizoate** and **iothalamate salts** in various preparations are effective contrast agents with relatively low toxicity. These drugs are rapidly absorbed into the extracellular compartment after intramuscular or intraarticular injection or after injection into an intervertebral

Text continued on p. 1077.

TABLE 78–4
Major Imaging Agents

1069

Drug Name	Uses, Action, Dosage and Route of Administration, Interpretation Timing	Nursing Considerations
BARIUM Barium sulfate	**Clinical use:** Contrast medium to detect and evaluate abnormalities of the gastrointestinal (GI) tract; in computed tomography (CT) to provide increased radiodensity of GI tract, thus permitting better study of structures outside that system **Desired actions:** Opacification and visualization of GI tract **Dosage:** Concentration, dosage, and suspending agents, colors, flavors, and preservatives based on study being done **Route of administration:** Orally, rectally, or via nasogastric tube, depending on area studied **Interpretation timing:** Serial radiographs taken from time of administration until all of study area of GI tract visualized	***Assess*** Assess for signs of pyloric stenosis and obstruction or perforation of GI tract. All phases (preparation, test, posttest treatment) of the test can be very exhausting; therefore assess client's ability to tolerate test, including fluid balance status. ***Implement*** Provide education about the purpose of the test, testing procedure, and any posttest treatments (e.g., enema, laxative) involved. If client cannot eat and drink before the test, provide mouth care and monitor fluid balance status. Since barium can cause constipation or impaction, administer a cathartic or enema after the test. If the test is done on an outpatient basis, provide proper instructions for administration of cathartic or enema. Teach client to report untoward signs and symptoms to primary care provider. Assess for status of GI tract function after the test is completed; document any passage of stool completely. Evaluate how well the procedure was tolerated and institute any other interventions that may be needed (e.g., bed rest, hydration). Provide emotional support during the posttest period as needed.
IONIC IODINATED COMPOUNDS Diatrizoate meglumine	**Clinical use:** Radiographic contrast medium for excretion urography, retrograde urography, retrograde cystourethrography; contrast enhancement of CT of brain; peripheral venography, peripheral arteriography, cerebral angiography, aortography, angiocardiography, operative or postoperative T-tube cholangiography, percutaneous transhepatic cholangiography, splenoportography, arthrography, discography; contrast enhancement of CT of body **Desired actions:** Visualization of a body cavity, including regions of the vascular system (veins, arteries, heart, and major blood vessels), site of an obstruction, lesions, or abnormal structures or pathways **Dosage:** Form, dosage, and concentration individualized according to test, technique, and the physical status of the individual being tested **Route of administration:** Varies according to the test **Interpretation timing:** Serial radiographs taken from time of administration until all of study	***Assess*** Obtain a thorough history. Since specific testing for iodine sensitivity is not possible, look for history of any previous sensitivity to iodine, iodine compounds, or foods that contain iodine. Assess for bronchial asthma, allergy, or family history of allergy and for a history of renal, hepatic, or thyroid disease and sickle cell disease. All phases (preparation, test, posttest treatment) of the test can be very exhausting; therefore assess client's ability to tolerate the test, including fluid balance status. ***Implement*** Since this compound can cause some type of allergic reaction, equipment and staff should be prepared and available to treat any reaction. Provide education about the purpose of the test, testing procedure, and any posttest treatments (e.g., enema, laxative) involved. Since this drug can be used for a variety of radiographic tests, be familiar with potential side effects (see Table 78–5). Intravascular administration of any drug carries the risk of extravasation and resultant tissue necrosis. Be alert for complaints of stinging, burning at the injection site.

Table continued on following page.

TABLE 78–4 *Continued*
Major Imaging Agents

Drug Name	Uses, Action, Dosage and Route of Administration, Interpretation Timing	Nursing Considerations
Diatrizoate meglumine *Continued*		**Implement—Continued** If test is done on an outpatient basis, provide instructions for any posttest interventions that may be needed and indicate any untoward developments that should be reported. Assess status or function of the organ or system visualized after the test is completed. Assess the fluid balance status before and after the test. Promote complete fluid balance before testing to prevent renal failure. Evaluate how well the procedure was tolerated and institute any other interventions that may be needed (e.g., bed rest, hydration). Provide emotional support during the posttest period.
Diatrizoate sodium	**Clinical uses:** Radiographic contrast medium for excretion urography, retrograde urography, retrograde cystourethrography; contrast enhancement of CT of the brain; peripheral venography, intraosseous venography, peripheral arteriography, aortography, selective renal arteriography, operative and postoperative T-tube cholangiography, splenoportography, and hysterosalpingography; the use of this contrast medium not recommended for cerebral angiography; may be used for visualization of GI tract after administration orally or rectally **Desired actions, dosage, route of administration, and interpretation timing:** same as for diatrizoate meglumine	Nursing assessment and interventions are the same as for diatrizoate meglumine.
Iothalamate meglumine	**Clinical uses:** Same procedures as diatrizoate meglumine **Desired actions, dosage, route of administration, and interpretation timing:** Same as for diatrizoate meglumine	Nursing assessment and interventions are the same as for diatrizoate meglumine.
Iothalamate sodium	**Clinical uses:** Excretion urography, contrast enhancement of CT of the brain, aortography, and angiocardiography **Desired actions, dosage, route of administration, and interpretation timing:** Same as for diatrizoate meglumine	Nursing assessment and interventions are the same as for diatrizoate meglumine.
Iodamide meglumine	**Clinical uses:** Radiographic contrast medium for excretion urography and contrast enhancement of CT of the brain **Desired actions:** Visualization of urinary tract, maximum contrast enhancement of CT of brain **Dosage:** Excretion urography—according to client's size and age; CT enhancement—4.5 ml/kg of 24% solution for adults **Route of administration:** IV **Interpretation timing:** Serial radiographs taken from time of administration until all of study area visualized	Nursing assessment and interventions are the same as for diatrizoate meglumine.
Iodipamide meglumine	**Clinical uses:** Radiographic contrast medium for cholecystography and cholangiography **Desired actions:** Visualization of hepatic and common bile ducts and gallbladder **Dosage:** According to size and age	Nursing assessment and interventions are the same as for diatrizoate meglumine.

TABLE 78–4 *Continued*
Major Imaging Agents

Drug Name	Uses, Action, Dosage and Route of Administration, Interpretation Timing	Nursing Considerations
Iodipamide meglumine *Continued*	**Route of administration:** IV **Interpretation timing:** Serial radiographs taken from time of administration until all of study area visualized	
Iophendylate	**Clinical uses:** Radiographic contrast medium for conventional lumbar, cervical, thoracic, and total columnar myelograply **Desired actions:** Visualization of tumors or herniation of the intervertebral disc or other lesion compressions of the spinal cord **Dosage:** According to size and age **Route of administration:** Lumbar subarachnoid injection **Interpretation timing:** Serial radiographs taken from time of administration until all study area visualized	Nursing assessment and interventions are the same as for diatrizoate meglumine except for the intravascular concerns. In addition, since this compound is injected into the subarachnoid space, the client must remain horizontal for 24 h after completion of the examination. Observe for signs of meningeal irritation, chronic adhesive arachnoiditis, aseptic techniques, and signs of a subarachnoid bleeding. Rare instances of parethesias, paraplegia, and focal seizures have been reported; be alert for such occurrences.
Ethiodized oil	**Clinical uses:** Radiographic contrast medium for lymphography and hysterosalpinography **Desired actions:** Visualization of lymph vessels, lymph nodes, uterus, and fallopian tubes **Dosage:** Varies according to test performed **Route of administration:** Varies according to the test performed **Interpretation timing:** Serial radiographs taken from time of administration until all of study area visualized	Nursing assessment and interventions are the same as for diatrizoate meglumine except for the intravascular concerns. In addition, when the compound is injected into the lymph vessels(s), observe for the development of symptoms of compromised pulmonary function, infection of the cutdown site, delayed wound healing, and lymphadenitis. When the compound is used for hysterosalpingography, observe for symptoms of leakage into the peritoneal cavity.
COMBINATION IONIC IODINATED COMPOUNDS Diatrizoate meglumine and diatrizoate sodium; diatrizoate meglumine and iodipamide meglumine; iothalamate meglumine and iothalamate sodium	**Clinical uses, desired actions, dosage protocols, route of administration, and interpretation timing:** Same as diatrizoate meglumine	Nursing assessment and interventions are the same as for diatrizoate meglumine.
NONIONIZED IODINATED COMPOUNDS Metrizamide	**Clinical uses:** Contrast medium for conventional and CT lumbar, thoracic, cervical, and total columnar myelography and for CT cisternography; may also be used for conventional cisternography and ventriculography in children **Desired actions:** Opacification of subarachnoid space of the spinal column, thus delineating the nerve anatomy by contrast; in children, opacification of the ventricles and cisterns of the brain **Dosage:** Varies according to age, condition of client, nature of pathology, degree and extent of contrast needed, and equipment and technique used **Route of administration:** Injection into the subarachnoid space; for cisternography or ventriculography in children, direct injection into the cistern or ventricle	*Assess* Obtain a complete history, including any iodine sensitivity, epilepsy, the presence of any local or systemic infection, severe cardiovascular disease, impaired hepatic chronic alcoholism, multiple sclerosis, pheochromocytoma, or sickle cell anemia. Assess for history of anticonvulsant therapy. Assess client's ability to follow directions and understand information provided. *Implement* Be alert for any allergic reaction and have the appropriate medications and equipment available. Since this drug may cause seizures if inadvertent intracranial entry occurs, be prepared to intervene if seizures ensue.

Table continued on following page.

TABLE 78–4 *Continued*
Major Imaging Agents

Drug Name	Uses, Action, Dosage and Route of Administration, Interpretation Timing	Nursing Considerations
Metrizamide *Continued*	**Interpretation timing:** Contrast for conventional or CT myelography achieved for the lumbar area within minutes after injection; opacification of other areas varies according to distance from injection area and positioning techniques used; opacification for CT studies available much longer than for conventional studies	***Implement—Continued*** If there is a history of seizures, premedication with anticonvulsant drugs may be considered. Include assessment for abnormal central nervous system signs and symptoms after testing is done. Assess the fluid balance status before testing and monitor throughout the testing process. Provide education about the purpose of the test, testing procedure, and when the test results will be known. Assess how well the procedure was tolerated. Provide psychosocial support during the posttest period. Nursing assessment and interventions are the same as for metrizamide.
Iopamidol	**Clinical uses:** Radiographic contrast media for contrast enhancement of CT cisternography, angiography, and myelography using intrathecal administration **Desired actions:** Opacification of a body cavity, allowing visualization of the cavity and in some instances, by inference, delineation of a body organ or tissue **Dosage:** Concentration and amount adjusted for the test performed and for age **Route of administration:** Intrathecal or IV **Interpretation timing:** Rapid absorption, allowing visualization within 1 h	
Iohexol	**Clinical uses:** Opacification of a body cavity providing visualization for lumbar, thoracic, cervical, and total columnar myelography; angiocardiography, including ventriculography and selective coronary arteriography; hysterosalpingography; visualization of the joint spaces, peritoneal herniations, pancreatic and bile ducts and bladder, GI tract **Desired actions:** Opacification of a body cavity, allowing visualization of the cavity and in some instances, by inference, delineation of a body organ or tissue **Dosage:** Varies according to test performed **Route of administration:** Intrathecal, intravascular **Interpretation timing:** Varies with route of administration; in general, visualization achieved in a matter of minutes with intrathecal and intravascular administration	***Assess*** Obtain a complete history, including any iodine sensitivity, epilepsy, the presence of any local or systemic infection, severe cardiovascular disease, impaired hepatic function due to chronic alcoholism, multiple sclerosis, pheochromocytoma, or sickle cell anemia. Assess for use of neuroleptic or anticonvulsant drugs. Evaluate the current fluid balance status. Assess ability to follow directions and understand information provided. ***Implement*** Be alert for any allergic reaction and have the appropriate medications and equipment available. Since this drug may cause seizures if inadvertent intracranial entry occurs, be prepared to intervene if seizures ensue. If there is risk of seizure, premedication with anticonvulsant drugs may be considered. Include assessment for abnormal central nervous system signs and symptoms after testing is done. Promote complete hydration before the testing procedure. After intrathecal administration, keep the head of the bed elevated 45 degrees and move the client passively for several hours after the procedure.

TABLE 78–4 *Continued*
Major Imaging Agents

1073

Drug Name	Uses, Action, Dosage and Route of Administration, Interpretation Timing	Nursing Considerations
Iohexol *Continued*		**Implement—Continued** Provide education about the purpose of the test, testing procedure, and when the test results will be known. Assess how well the procedure was tolerated. Provide psychosocial support during the posttest period. Nursing assessment and interventions are similar to those for iohexol.
Ioversol	**Clinical uses:** Angiography, including cerebral, coronary, peripheral, visceral, renal arteriography, and left ventriculography; contrast-enhanced CT head and body imaging, IV excretory urography, IV digital subtraction angiography and venography **Desired actions:** Visualization of a body cavity or enhancement of CT imaging **Dosage:** Varies according to procedure performed **Route of administration:** Intravascular **Interpretation timing:** Visualization possible within 15–20 min after injection	
Ioxaglate meglumine and ioxaglate sodium	**Clinical uses:** Urography, arthrography, angiography, angiocardiography, arteriography, aortography, venography, hysterosalpinography, and CT **Desired actions, dosage, route of administration and interpretation timing:** Same as for other contrast media in section NOTE: Although this contrast medium is ionic, since it has the same advantages as nonionic contrast media, it is placed in the same section.	Nursing assessment and interventions are similar to those of the other agents in this section.
ORAL CHOLECYSTOGRAPHIC COMPOUNDS		
Iocetamic acid, iopanoic acid, ipodate calcium, ipodate sodium	**Clinical uses:** Radiographic contrast medium in oral cholecystography, cholangiography **Desired actions:** Radiographic opacification of gallbladder **Route of administration:** Oral; ipodate salts—oral, rectal **Interpretation timing:** 10–20 h after oral administration; ipodate salts—1–5 h after ingestion	**Assess** Obtain a thorough history, including any history of previous sensitivity to iodine, iodine compounds, foods that contain iodine, bronchial asthma, or allergy or family history of allergy. Elicit any history of hyperuricemia, renal, hepatic, or severe GI absorption disorders or cardiovascular disease. The thyroid gland is affected by iodine, so note any history of thyroid disease. Since ipodate sodium capsules contain the FD & C yellow No. 5, which may cause an allergic reaction, assess for history of allergic reaction. **Implement** Provide a diet containing fat for 1 or more days before the examination. Administer the contrast medium as directed by the radiologist. Administer a laxative or enema as ordered by the radiologist. Make sure the client receives nothing by mouth except water after administration of the contrast medium. Promote complete hydration to prevent uric acid nephropathy in the hyperuricemic person. Provide education about the purpose of the test, testing procedure, and when the test results will be known. Assess how well the procedure was tolerated. Provide psychosocial support during the posttest period.

TABLE 78–5

Undesired Clinical Responses and Contraindications Associated With Major Imaging Agents

Undesired Clinical Responses	Contraindications	Nursing Considerations
BARIUM		
Cramping secondary to distention of the intestine, constipation, intestinal obstruction, retention of barium in the appendix, perforation of the colon	Presence of obstructing lesions, known obstruction(s) of the colon, known or suspected gastrointestinal (GI) tract perforation Cautions: suspected tracheoesophageal fistula, presence of acute ulcerative colitis or acute diverticulitis, <24 h after rectal or colonic biopsy, <24 h after cessation of GI bleeding, pregnancy	Obtain a thorough history and physical assessment before test to assist in forming nursing diagnoses and to detect any conditions that would preclude use of a particular contrast medium. After the test, monitor bowel sounds and bowel movements to detect possible bowel obstruction and to evaluate evacuation of barium.
IONIC IODINATED COMPOUNDS		

Most common side effects: nausea, vomiting, flushing, hypotension, hypertension, tachycardia, bradycardia, cardiac arrhythmias
Other side effects:
  Anaphylactoid reactions—urticaria, angioedema, hypotension, cardiac or respiratory arrest, acute renal failure
  Respiratory system effects—coughing, spasm, wheezing, pulmonary or laryngeal edema
  Nervous system effects—restlessness, confusion, anxiety, headache, dizziness, tremors, seizures, paresis, neurotoxicity (lethargy, disorientation, agitation, severe headache, seizures, loss of vision)
Direct toxic effects—acute renal failure, nephropathy
  Transient anticoagulant effect: altered thyroid function test results
	Any known hypersensitivity to iodine or other component of the contrast media
	Presence of multiple myeloma, advanced renal disease, severe concomitant hepatic and renal impairment, severe cardiovascular disease, severe hypertension, severe debilitation, anuric states, endotoxemia or fever, severe thyrotoxicosis, client with diabetes with a serum creatinine level >3 mg/dl, and individuals homozygous for sickle cell disease
	Intrathecal administration contraindicated in the presence of significant local or systemic infection
	Safe use during pregnancy not established
	Caution: in presence of hyperthyroidism, known or suspected pheochromocytoma
		Since there is a degree of risk involved, obtain consent for the test.
		As with the barium contrast media, obtain a thorough history and physical assessment.
		Monitor client for the occurrence of the possible side effects.
		Keep equipment and personnel available in the event an anaphylactoid reaction occurs.
		Assess the fluid balance status and promote complete hydration before the test; monitor intake and output closely after the test.
		Closely observe the injection site for signs and symptoms of extravasation.

NONIONIC IODINATED COMPOUNDS		
See ionic iodinated compounds	See ionic iodinated compounds	See ionic iodinated compounds
ORAL IMAGING AGENTS		
Mild transient symptoms: restlessness, sensations of warmth, sneezing, perspiration, salivation, flushing, pressure in the upper abdomen, dizziness, nausea, vomiting, diarrhea, chills, fever, headache, pallor and tremors Hypersensitive reactions and (rare) anaphylactoid reactions Altered renal function tests and possibly acute renal failure Altered thyroid function test results Promotion of the sickling phenomenon in individuals homozygous for sickle cell disease **Ipodate salts:** bitter taste, precordial pain and palpitation	Any individual with a history or previously demonstrated hypersensitivity to iodine, severe renal impairment or advanced hepatorenal disease Clients with known or suspected hepatic or biliary disorders who have recently received an oral cholecystographic agent Safe use during pregnancy not established Caution: any individual with history of allergies, asthma, hay fever, or urticaria, renal or hepatic disease, hyperuricemia or cardiovascular disease **Iopanoic acid:** use contraindicated in presence of severe GI disorders that prevent absorption **Ipodate salts:** known hypersensitivity to FD & C yellow No. 5	Nursing considerations are the same as for the other imaging agents. This method of visualizing the gallbladder and bile ducts is not the method of choice with the current availability of ultrasonic and scintigraphic procedures.

TABLE 78–6

Interactions Associated With Major Imaging Agents

Imaging Agent	Drug Effects	Laboratory Tests, Environment
Barium sulfate	—	Client is required to fast before testing with any of the imaging agents.
Diatrizoate meglumine	Anticoagulant drug effects: may be enhanced General anesthesia: may increase incidence of adverse reactions Hypotension-causing agents (e.g., morphine sulfate, meperidine hydrochloride): may exacerbate hemodynamic effects Physically incompatible with diphenhydramine hydrochloride or promethazine hydrochloride	Contact of blood and this drug in a syringe has produced clots. Agent interferes with thyroid function test results based on a measurement of iodine for up to 16 d and with urinary chemical testing for up to 2 d. Radiographic visualization may not be adequate if GI tract is filled with feces or air. Protect agent from light.
Diatrizoate sodium	Anticoagulant drug effects: may be enhanced General anesthesia: may increase incidence of adverse reactions Physically incompatible with diphenhydramine hydrochloride	Contact of blood and this drug in a syringe has produced clots. Agent interferes with thyroid test results based on a measurement of iodine for up to 16 d and with urinary chemical testing for up to 2 d. Erythrocyte sludging, agglutination, and crenation and transient changes in coagulation may occur. Protect agent from strong light.
Iothalamate meglumine	May enhance anticoagulant drug effects General anesthesia: may increase incidence of adverse reactions Physically incompatible with promethazine hydrochloride	Contact of blood and this drug in a syringe has produced clots. Agent interferes with thyroid test results based on measurement of iodine. Agent may produce falsely decreased results in urinary total hydroxyproline determinations. Agent may interfere with urinary chemical testing for up to 2 d. Erythrocyte sludging, agglutination, and crenation and transient changes in coagulation may occur. Protect agent from strong light.
Iothalamate sodium	May enhance anticoagulant drug effects General anesthesia: may increase incidence of adverse reactions Physically incompatible with promethazine hydrochloride	See iothalamate meglumine.
Iodamide meglumine	Physically incompatible with diphenhydramine hydrochloride	Agent interferes with thyroid function test results based on a measurement of iodine for up to 16 d and with urinary chemical testing for up to 2 d. Protect agent from strong light.
Iodipamide meglumine	Oral ipodate calcium: may partially inhibit biliary excretion IV administration of iodipamide meglumine after oral administration of ipodate calcium: may increase incidence and severity of adverse effects Insufficient visualization of the biliary ducts possible in clients receiving methyltestosterone Probenecid: may decrease biliary concentration of iodipamide meglumine Incidence of a syndrome resembling myocardial infarction seen when meperidine hydrochloride was administered concurrently with iodipamide meglumine Physically incompatible with brompheniramine maleate, chlorpheniramine maleate, diphenhydramine hydrochloride, genatmicin sulfate, and promethazine hydrochloride	Agent interferes with thyroid function test results based on a measurement of iodine for 3–4 mo and with urinary chemical testing for up to 2 d. Protect agent from light and excessive heat.

Table continued on following page.

TABLE 78–6 *Continued*
Interactions Associated With Major Imaging Agents

Imaging Agent	Drug Effects	Laboratory Tests, Environment
Iophendylate		Agent interferes with thyroid function test results based on a measurement of iodine for a few months to several years. Protect agent from light.
Ethiodized oil		Agent is physically incompatible with rubber. Agent interferes with thyroid function test results based on a measurement of iodine for several months to 1 y. Protect agent from light; do not use if the color has darkened.
Metrizamide	Increased risk of seizures if administered concurrently with drugs that lower the seizure threshold (e.g., phenothiazines, antipsychotic drugs, monamine oxidase inhibitors, tricyclic antidepressants, central nervous system [CNS] stimulants)	Agent interferes with urinary chemical testing for up to 2 d and possibly with thyroid function test results based on a measurement of iodine. Agent contains no preservatives and should be used immediately. Protect agent from excessive heat and light.
Iopamidol	—	Agent interferes with thyroid function test results based on a measurement of iodine. Agent contains no preservatives and should be used immediately. Protect agent from excessive heat and light.
Iohexol	General anesthesia: may increase incidence of adverse reactions Hypotension-causing agents (e.g., morphine sulfate, meperidine hydrochloride): may exacerbate hemodynamic effects Increased risk of seizures if administered concurrently with drugs that lower the seizure threshold (e.g., phenothiazines, antipsychotic drugs, monamine oxidase inhibitors, tricyclic antidepressants, CNS stimulants) Incompatible with antihistamines	Agent reduces the iodine-binding capacity of the thyroid for up to 2 wk, rendering tests using iodine-containing isotopes inaccurate during that time. Contact of blood and this drug in a syringe has produced clots.
Ioversol	Interacts with oral cholecystographic agents to promote renal toxicity in individuals with liver dysfunction General anesthesia: may increase incidence of adverse reactions Hypotension-causing agents (e.g., morphine sulfates, meperidine hydrochloride): may exacerbate hemodynamic effects	Contact of blood and this drug in a syringe has produced clots. Agent interferes with thyroid function test results based on a measurement of iodine for up to 16 d and with urinary chemical testing for up to 2 d. Protect agent from light. Store below 30° C.
Ioxaglate meglumine	Interactions similar to those of other iodine-containing imaging agents	
Ioxaglate sodium	Interactions similar to those of other iodine-containing imaging agents	
Iocetamic acid	Aspirin: may counteract uricosuric effect when dose of 600 mg given concomitantly with the imaging agent and then repeated in 2 h	Sulfobromophthalein retention and total serum bilirubin concentrations may be increased for a few days after administration. Agent interferes with urine testing for at least 2 d. Agent interferes with thyroid function test results based on a measurement of iodine for several months.
Iopanoic acid	Cross-reactions with other iodinated imaging agents possible Aspirin: may counteract uricosuric effect when dose of 600 mg given concomitantly with the imaging agent and then repeated in 2 h	Sulfobromophthalein retention and total serum bilirubin concentrations may be increased for a few days after administration. Agent interferes with urine testing for at least 3 d. Agent interferes with thyroid function test results based on a measurement of iodine for several months. Agent may cause false low values in tests for metanephrine.

TABLE 78–6 *Continued*

Interactions Associated With Major Imaging Agents

Imaging Agent	Drug Effects	Laboratory Tests, Environment
Ipodate calcium; ipodate sodium	May partially inhibit biliary excretion of iodipamide meglumine Incidence and severity of adverse effects possibly increased if iodipamide meglumine is administered within 24 h of this imaging agent	Sulfobromophthalein retention and total serum bilirubin concentrations may be increased for a few days after administration. Agent interferes with urine testing for at least 3 d. Agent interferes with thyroid function test results based on a measurement of iodine for several months. Store agent in tightly closed containers and protect from light.

disc or into the spleen. When these agents are instilled into the GI tract or the urinary bladder, little absorption occurs into the blood. Intravascular injection not only provides visualization of the arteries and veins, but since the drug is excreted in the urine with little absorption or secretion in the renal tubules, it also is effective in excretion urography. In clients with normal renal function these drugs are almost completely excreted, unchanged, in the urine within 24 hours. A small percentage of the drugs are excreted in the feces. In those with impaired renal function a much greater percentage is excreted in the feces by way of biliary elimination. Peritoneal dialysis or hemodialysis removes diatrizoates and iothalamates. Since the diatrizoates and iothalamates are ionic, they function as osmotic diuretics and as such interfere to some degree with the tubular reabsorption of water.

Iodamide meglumine is used for excretion urography and contrast enhancement of CT of the brain. **Iodipamide** differs from the diatrizoates, iothalamates, and iodamide meglumine. It is rapidly distributed throughout the extracellular fluid and appears in the bile within 10 to 15 minutes. In the individual with normal renal and hepatic function, iodipamide meglumine is excreted primarily in the feces via the biliary pathway, and approximately 5% to 20% is excreted renally. If hepatic function is compromised, an increase in elimination occurs through the renal route.

Nonionized compounds, recently developed as radiopaque contrast media, have proved superior in that they are good contrast media but do not have the undesired clinical responses of the ionized compounds. Both the diatrizoates and iothalamates are fully substituted triiodinated compounds and as such become ionized in aqueous solutions. The nonionic compounds have a lower osmolality, making them safer to use in cardiac studies.[6] Both the ionic and nonionic contrast media have transient anticoagulant effects. Conversely, when these contrast media come in contact with blood in a syringe, clotting occurs. There is concern that they may have a **thrombogenic** effect. At this time the nonionic compounds are significantly more expensive, making the decision to use them economically difficult for the radiology department personnel.

The choice of contrast media to use for a particular radiographic study is dictated by the area and the administration route that will be used and by the characteristic body distribution and elimination. Although iothalamate meglumine, iothalamate sodium, diatrizoate meglumine, and diatrizoate sodium are considered good choices for intravascular injection, iothalamate meglumine is selected for certain procedures because it is less toxic to the neural tissue and to the vascular endothelium.

• • •

Life-span considerations When considering the life-span aspects of imaging agents, the first consideration is the exposure to radiation. In most instances the benefits of the examination must outweigh the risks before proceeding with the examination, especially if the client is pregnant. Use of iodinated contrast media has not been studied in human models. No teratogenic effect have been noted in studies of metrizamide, iohexol, and iopamidol in laboratory animals. Many of the iodinated contrast media cross the placental barrier, and the rest are assumed to do so; therefore use of these compounds is not recommended during pregnancy. Precautions must also be taken in the case of nursing mothers. Iodamide meglumine, metrizamide, ioversol, and iohexol are distributed in milk. The manufacturers of the last two recommend discontinuing nursing for at least 24 hours after administration of the contrast media. Both ioversol and iohexol may be used in children, but the risk of adverse events is greater than in adults. The long-term effects of iodine administration and exposure to radiation are not fully known. The thyroid gland may be permanently affected after a myelography and bronchography using iodinated contrast media. Radiation exposure is cumulative, and certain probable adverse effects can be projected. They include infertility, birth defects, and the potential for changes in normal cell structure, with concomitant impact on the occurrence of malignancy and growth and development.

Nursing considerations Obtain a thorough history, especially about any history of allergy to iodine, contrast media, shellfish, and iodine-containing compounds. Determine if kidney, thyroid, or liver disease exists. Discuss a positive history with the primary care provider ordering the test and with the radiologist. Administering a test dose of the compound has not proved a reliable predictor of a reaction, and skin testing in this situation has no value. Although pretreatment with prednisone, diphenhydramine, or ephedrine has not always proved successful in preventing anaphylactoid reaction, its use should be considered. Since neither testing for a reaction nor pretreatment with corticosteroids or antihistamines has proved reliable, the best action is to avoid the use of iodinated contrast media in those individuals who appear at risk. If testing must be done using an iodinated compound, a nonionic compound should be used. If the client is hyperthyroid, the use of iodinated contrast media may precipitate thyroid storm.

Another aspect of the testing procedure to consider is the exposure to radiation. Determine during history taking whether the female client is pregnant. If she is or may be pregnant, notify the primary care provider and radiologist. Care should be taken to prepare the client properly to prevent any delay or needless repetition of the test. Since preparation and posttest treatment vary from one facility to another and from one type of test to another, consult the policies and procedures of the facility for precise information.

In general, if the client is not able to eat and drink before the test, mouth care should be provided and the fluid balance status monitored. If you assist with the radiologic procedure in some manner, consider the possibility of radiation exposure. Obtain a lead shield before your participation in the testing procedure. Since the reaction to the testing compound could include nausea and vomiting, prepare by bringing an emesis basin and tissues. Radiology rooms are often cold. Make the individual as physically comfortable as possible, (e.g., provide a blanket, pillow); provide psychologic support. Client education should include the reason for the test, expected outcomes, when the test results will be available, and who will tell the client of the test results.

Osmotic diuresis can occur, particularly when ionic iodinated compounds are used. Maintenance of a balanced fluid status helps prevent acute renal failure secondary to pretesting dehydration. Observe for any signs of a fluid volume deficit, including monitoring the intake and output both before and after the test. Table 78–4 lists the major imaging agents, their desired actions, dosage, route of administration, and nursing implications. Table 78–5 provides information about major undesired clinical responses, contraindication, and nursing considerations.

CONCEPT REVIEW

Imaging agents can be categorized as radiographic contrast agents, diagnostic radiopharmaceutical agents used for nuclear medicine procedures, and contrast agents used for magnetic resonance imaging.

The main radiographic contrast agents are barium (best for the GI tract) and iodine (used for blood vessels, organs, and body spaces). Iodized fatty acids and oils also are sometimes used for visualization of lymph nodes and vessels or of the uterus and fallopian tubes, but their elimination is very slow.

Water-soluble ionic iodized agents are effective contrast agents with relative low toxicity. They are used for visualization of arteries and veins and in excretion

urography. In clients with normal renal function, they are excreted almost completely and unchanged in the urine within 24 hours.

Nonionized radiopaque contrast media provide good contrast and do not have the adverse reactions of ionized compounds. They are safer for use in cardiac studies. Both ionic and nonionic contrast media have transient anticoagulant effects.

PROVOCATIVE AGENTS

Provocative agents are used to provoke a predictable response used to diagnose a specific condition or disease state. Although skin testing for systemic allergy is a type of provocative testing, the response from such testing is milder than from provocative testing because the dose is controlled to limit the overall systemic effect. Provocative testing, however, stimulates or inhibits a gland or system and may be both uncomfortable and dangerous because of the widespread effect on the body. All of the agents are administered in a parenteral form providing a quick response. They are rapidly removed from the plasma by the body and distributed in the tissues. Excretion routes vary from agent to agent and include the urine or bile; in many cases the excretion route is unknown.

Major Provocative Agents

Sometimes an agent (e.g., edrophonium chloride) can be used for both diagnosis of a disease and for evaluation of treatment of the disease. **Edrophonium chloride** is administered intravenously, provoking a response (improvement in muscle strength) within 1 to 3 minutes. If the response is positive, myasthenia gravis is the diagnosis. If the diagnosis has already been made, an evaluation of the treatment may be needed to determine if the client has been given too low or too high a dose of cholinesterase inhibitors. If the dosage is too low, the response is an increase in muscle strength; however, if the dose is too high, an increase in muscle weakness is not seen.

Histamine phosphate is an example of an agent that can be used to test for two different problems: achlorhydria and pheochromocytoma. When evaluating the gastric ability to produce hydrochloric acid, the gastric contents are analyzed for an increase in the secretion of hydrochloric acid. Absence of a gastric response demonstrates achlorhydria. The loss of the stomach's ability to produce hydrochloric acid is a characteristic of pernicious anemia, so in effect, two diagnoses are aided by one test. Testing for pheochromocytoma involves evaluating blood pressure response and urinary catecholamine levels. A rise within specific parameters in both the blood pressure and urinary catecholamines is considered positive for pheochromocytoma.

Provocative agents can be divided into two groups: naturally occurring and synthetically produced agents. In some cases synthetically produced agents caused significantly fewer adverse reactions than the naturally occurring agents. Many of these agents also have therapeutic uses (Table 78–7).

Text continued on p. 1084.

TABLE 78-7
Major Provocative Agents

Drug Name	Uses, Action, Dosage, and Route of Administration, Interpretation Timing*	Nursing Considerations
NATURALLY OCCURRING DRUGS Corticotropin	**Clinical uses:** Aids in the diagnosis of a adreno-cortical insufficiency. **Desired action:** To elicit a response by the adrenal cortex (i.e., increased cortisol secretion) **Dosage:** For 8 h infusion—10–25 U diluted in compatible infusion fluid; method may be repeated on each of 4 or 5 successive days if no initial response is obtained; rapid screening–25 U intramuscularly or rapid IV administration **Route of administration:** IV, IM **Interpretation timing:** 8-h infusion method—comparison of baseline serum cortisol levels before testing with levels obtained, at a minimum, 1 h after starting IV infusion and at the completion of the infusion; determination of 24-h urinary 17-oxyhydrocorticosteroid and 17-ketosteroid levels should be obtained before beginning the test and another 24-h collection done starting with onset of infusion; rapid screening method—timing of the serum level draws after the injection occur over a longer period of time	***Assess*** While obtaining a complete nursing history, include evaluation for any hypersensitivity to corticotropin or porcine proteins. Note if client has been or is receiving cortisone, hydrocortisone, estrogens, spironolactone because they interfere with test results. Assess client's ability to follow directions and comprehend information provided in the teaching process. ***Implement*** Provide teaching about the test purpose and the procedure itself. Closely observe for any hypersensitivity reaction. Have equipment, supplies and staff available if a reaction occurs. If client has a suspected sensitivity to porcine proteins, perform hypersensitivity testing before the test is done. Observe for any local induration, pain, or development of an abscess when the IM route is used. ***Evaluate*** Evaluate tolerance of testing procedure. Assess the client's understanding of the test purpose and procedure and his or her knowledge about how the test results will be provided.
Histamine	**Clinical uses:** Test for achlorhydria, pheochromocytoma **Desired action:** Achlorhydria—production of hydrochloric acid; pheochromocytoma—increase in systolic blood pressure >20 mmHg and diastolic blood pressure >10 mmHg and increase urinary catecholamine levels **Dosage:** Achlorhydria—0.01 mg/kg; pheochromocytoma—0.01 mg initially; if no response after 5 min, 0.05 mg **Route of administration:** Achlorhydria—SC; pheochromocytoma—IV **Interpretation timing:** Achlorhydria—gastric contents show increase in hydrochloric acid in four samples obtained q15 min after injection; pheochromocytoma—rise in blood pressure within 5 min after injection; a 2-h urine sample collected before and after the injection	***Assess*** Obtain history of allergies, asthma, gastric ulcer, bronchial disease, cardiovascular disease, urticaria, hypertension, hypotension, vasomotor instability, and renal disease. (If client has a diagnosis of pheochromocytoma, using this drug to test for achlorhydria may cause a severe adverse reaction.) Assess the client's ability to follow directions and comprehend information provided in the teaching process. ***Implement*** This testing agent may precipitate severe allergic reactions and marked hypertension or hypotension. Be alert for both systemic and, if administered subcutaneously, local reactions. Have equipment, supplies, and staff available if a reaction occurs. If the blood pressure is >150 mmHg systolic and >100 mmHg diastolic, notify primary care provider before testing. Teach the client and significant other(s) about the test's purpose and procedure. Discuss how the test results will be provided and by whom. ***Evaluate*** Evaluate tolerance of testing procedure.

*Many of the drugs mentioned have other applications that are not mentioned in this chapter.

Table continued on following page.

TABLE 78–7 *Continued*
Major Provocative Agents

Drug Name	Uses, Action, Dosage, and Route of Administration, Interpretation Timing*	Nursing Considerations
Histamine *Continued*		**Evaluate—Continued** Assess the client's understanding of the test purpose and procedure and his or her knowledge about how the test results will be provided.
Secretin	**Clinical uses:** Diagnosis of pancreatic exocrine disorders, gastrinoma **Desired action:** Pancreatic disorders—increase in volume and bicarbonate content of pancreatic secretions; gastrinoma—increased serum gastrin levels **Dosage:** pancreatic disorders—1 CU/kg; gastrinoma—2 CU/kg **Route of administration:** IV over 1 min **Interpretation timing:** Pancreatic disorders—gastric and duodenal secretion samples taken during the first hour after injection; gastrinoma—serum samples obtained during the first 30 min after injection	**Assess** Obtain history of any allergy, asthma, vagotomy, anticholinergic therapy, and inflammatory bowel disease. This test involves the insertion of a double-lumen, Dreiling-type tube. Evaluate client's ability to cooperate and tolerate such a procedure. Assess the client's ability to follow directions and comprehend information provided in the teaching process. **Implement** If there is a history of hypersensitivity, allergy, or asthma, administer a test dose before injection of the agent for testing purposes. If there are no allergic reactions 1 min after the test dose is administered, injection of the agent for testing purpose may be done. Have facilities available to intervene if an allergic reaction does occur. Support the client during the tube insertion procedure and throughout the remainder of the test. Teach the client and significant others about the test's purpose and procedure. Discuss how test results are provided and by whom. **Evaluate** Evaluate tolerance of testing procedure. Assess client's understanding of the test purpose and procedure and his or her knowledge about how the test results will be provided.
Thyrotropin	**Clinical uses:** Diagnosis of subclinical hypothyroidism, low thyroid reserve; differentiation between primary and secondary hypothyroidism; detection of thyroid cancer remnant; evaluation of treatment efficacy **Desired action:** Increased thyroid hormone production **Dosage:** Differential diagnosis of subclinical hypothyroidism or low thyroid reserve—10 IU; differential diagnosis primary and secondary hypothyroidism or treatment evaluation—10 IU/d for 1–3 d; diagnosis of thyroid cancer remnant—10 IU daily for 3–7 d **Route of administration:** IM or SC **Interpretation timing:** After the administration cycle is completed	**Assess** Include in the nursing history any history of angina pectoris, cardiac failure, hypopituitarism, adrenal cortical suppression, corticosteroid therapy, coronary thrombosis, untreated Addison's disease, and hypersensitivity to thyrotropin. Assess the client's ability to follow directions and comprehend information provided in the teaching process. **Implement** Observe for nausea, vomiting, headache, fever, tachycardia, ventricular fibrillation, and menstrual irregularities. This testing agent may cause allergic reactions; be alert for signs and symptom of such a reaction. Have facilities available for intervening should an allergic reaction occur. Teach the client and significant others about the test purpose and procedure.

TABLE 78–7 *Continued*
Major Provocative Agents

Drug Name	Uses, Action, Dosage, and Route of Administration, Interpretation Timing*	Nursing Considerations
Thyrotropin *Continued*		**Implement—Continued** Discuss how test results are provided and by whom. **Evaluate** Evaluate tolerance of testing procedure. Assess client's understanding of the test purpose and procedure plus his or her knowledge about how the test results will be provided.
SYNTHETIC DRUGS Arginine	**Clinical uses:** Evaluation of pituitary growth hormone reserve **Desired action:** Increase in the plasma growth hormone **Route of administration:** IV **Interpretation timing:** Plasma sampling done 30 min before and immediately before injection for baseline and then at time of initiation of injection and at 30-min intervals for $2\frac{1}{2}$ h	**Assess** Obtain history of allergy or hypersensitivity reactions, sickle cell anemia, renal disease, and a complete drug history. Assess the client's ability to follow directions and comprehend information provided in the teaching process. **Implement** Evaluate the drug history and current drug regimen for any possible drug interactions. Since this testing agent is hypertonic and is a vesicant, administer it through an indwelling catheter; be careful to prevent extravasation. Be alert for any allergic type reactions. Provide client a diet with at least 150–300 g carbohydrate for 3 d immediately before the test. Provide teaching to the client and significant other(s) about the purpose of the test and the test procedure. **Evaluate** Evaluate tolerance of testing procedure. Assess client's understanding of the test purpose and procedure and his or her knowledge about how the test results will be provided.
Cosyntropin	**Clinical uses:** Diagnosis of adrenocortical insufficiency **Desired action:** Increase in serum cortisol level **Dosage:** 0.25 mg **Route of administration:** IM or IV **Interpretation timing:** Rapid screening method—30 min or possibly 60 min after administration; serial administration, which involves administration of testing on successive days by either IV infusion or IM injection followed by the rapid screening—30–60 min after rapid screening injection	**Assess** Include in the nursing history all current medications, especially cortisone, hydrocortisone, estrogens, and spironolactone since they interfere with test results. Although this testing agent is much less likely to cause an allergic reaction than corticotropin, obtain a history of allergic reaction or hypersensitivity to corticotropin or cosyntropin. **Implement** Be alert for any allergic type reactions. Provide teaching to the client and significant other(s) about the purpose of the test and the test procedure. **Evaluate** Evaluate tolerance of testing procedure. Assess client's understanding of the test purpose and procedure plus his or her knowledge about how the test results will be provided.

Table continued on following page.

TABLE 78–7 Continued
Major Provocative Agents

Drug Name	Uses, Action, Dosage, and Route of Administration, Interpretation Timing	Nursing Considerations
Edrophonium	**Clinical uses:** Differential diagnosis of myasthenia gravis; differentiation between cholinergic crisis and myasthenic crisis; evaluation of treatment therapy **Desired action:** Myasthenia gravis diagnosis—increase in muscle strength; differentiation between cholinergic crisis and myasthenic crisis—increased oropharyngeal secretion and muscle weakness with cholinergic crisis, improved respirations and muscle strength with myasthenic crisis; evaluation of treatment—improvement in undertreated clients and increased muscle weakness in overtreated clients **Dosage:** Myasthenia gravis diagnosis—2 mg initially; if no response, give 8 mg; differentiation between cholinergic crisis and myasthenic crisis—1 mg initially followed by 1 mg after 1 min if no increased impairment occurs; evaluation of treatment—1–2 mg 1 h after oral intake of drug used to treat myasthenia gravis **Route of administration:** 1V **Interpretation timing:** Myasthenia gravis diagnosis—45 sec after injection; differentiation between cholinergic crisis and myasthenic crisis—1 min; evaluation of treatment—1 min	***Assess*** Obtain history of allergy or hypersensitivity reactions, myocardial infarction, complete drug history, including current anticholinesterase treatment, sulfite sensitivity (sodium sulfite is in commercial preparations), bronchial asthma. Assess client's ability to follow directions and comprehend information provided in the teaching process. ***Implement*** Respiratory arrest, increased salivation, and muscle weakness may occur. Have facilities available for respiratory support and for intervention should an allergic or hypersensitive reaction occur. Teach the client and significant others about the test's purpose and procedure. Provide psychologic support during testing process. Discuss how test results are provided and by whom. ***Evaluate*** Evaluate tolerance of testing procedure. Assess the client's understanding of the test purpose and procedure plus his or her knowledge about how the test results will be provided.
Gonadorelin	**Clinical uses:** Evaluation of hypothalamic-pituitary gonadotropic function **Desired action:** Increase in serum luteinizing hormone **Dosage:** 100 μ **Route of administration:** SC or IV **Interpretation timing:** Serum sampling: done at 15, 30, 45, 60, and 120 min after administration	***Assess*** Obtain history of allergy or hypersensitivity and a complete drug history to assist in identification of any potential drug interactions with the testing agent. Assess client's ability to follow directions and comprehend information provided in the teaching process. ***Implement*** Teach the client and significant others about the test's purpose and procedure. Discuss how test results will be provided and by whom. ***Evaluate*** Evaluate tolerance of testing procedure. Assess the client's understanding of the test purpose and procedure plus his or her knowledge about how the test results will be provided.
Metyrapone	**Clinical uses:** Evaluation of hypothalamic-pituitary function, particularly hypopituitarism and Cushing's syndrome **Desired action:** Increase in urinary 17-hydroxy-corticosteroids and 17-ketogenic steroids **Dosage:** 750 mg q4h for six doses or single dose of 30 mg/kg **Route of administration:** Oral **Interpretation timing:** After a control urine collection and a corticotropin test to rule out adrenal insufficiency, metyrapone administration followed by urine collection	See gonadorelin.

TABLE 78–7 *Continued*
Major Provocative Agents

Drug Name	Uses, Action, Dosage, and Route of Administration, Interpretation Timing	Nursing Considerations
Pentagastrin	**Clinical uses:** Evaluation of gastric acid secretion; helpful in testing for acidity associated with pernicious anemia, atrophic gastritis, or gastric carcinoma; hypersecretion in clients with possible duodenal ulcer or postoperative stomal ulcer; diagnosis of Zollinger-Ellison syndrome **Desired action:** Increase in gastric acid secretions **Dosage and route of administration:** Usual—SC 6 μg/kg **Interpretation timing:** First 60 min after administration	**Assess** Include any history of allergy or hypersensitivity and of pancreatic, hepatic, or biliary tract disease in the nursing history. Assess for presence of acute, penetrating, or bleeding peptic ulcers since the use of this testing agent is contraindicated if they are present. Assess client's ability to follow directions and comprehend information provided in the teaching process. **Implement** Observe for any adverse reactions. Since the testing procedure involves the insertion of a nasogastric tube, provide support and teaching in this area. Teach the client and significant others about the test's purpose and procedure. Discuss how test results will be provided and by whom. **Evaluate** Evaluate tolerance of testing procedure. Assess the client's understanding of the test purpose and procedure plus his or her knowledge about how the test results will be provided.
Tolbutamide sodium	**Clinical uses:** To help in the diagnosis of insulinomas, pancreatic carcinoma, acute pancreatitis, and mild diabetes mellitus **Desired action:** Decrease in the true serum glucose level **Dosage:** 1 g **Route of administration:** IV **Interpretation timing:** Baseline serum sample drawn before administering the drug; frequency and number of serum samples obtained after administration of the testing agent depend on suspected disease state	**Assess** Include in the nursing history a drug history and known hypersensitivity to this testing agent or other sulfonylurea drugs. Identify drugs that might potentiate the hypoglycemic effect of this drug. Obtain fasting blood glucose levels. **Implement** Most of the interventions are based on the fact that action of the testing agent is to lower the serum glucose level. If the fasting level of serum glucose is low, it may fall dangerously low after administration of the drug. Have both carbohydrate and 25% to 50% glucose for IV injection readily accessible in case severe hypoglycemia occurs. Although the likelihood of hypersensitivity reaction is low in comparison to other testing agents, have facilities to handle such an emergency available. Observe for hypoglycemic signs and symptoms not only at the immediate time of testing but also, for several hours afterward. Teach the client and significant others about the test's purpose and procedure, including the need for adrenal insufficiency testing. Discuss how test results will be provided and by whom. **Evaluate** Evaluate tolerance of testing procedure. Assess the client's understanding of the test's purpose and procedure plus his or her knowledge about how the test results will be provided.

Table continued on following page.

TABLE 78–7 *Continued*
Major Provocative Agents

Drug Name	Uses, Action, Dosage, and Route of Administration, Interpretation Timing	Nursing Considerations
Xylose	**Clinical uses:** Diagnosis of malabsorptive conditions **Desired action:** Normal level of urinary or serum xylose; actual results vary according to particular testing method used **Route of administration:** Oral **Interpretation timing:** Varies according to test method used NOTE: Normal test results vary with age.	**Assess** Collect a thorough nursing history, including any history of renal disease or impaired renal function, thyroid dysfunction, pernicious anemia, iron deficiency anemia. Assess for the presence of vomiting or diarrhea, dehydration, overgrowth of bacteria, gastric stasis, and any condition that affects cardiovascular function. All of these conditions can cause the inaccurate test results. Collect a drug history since certain drugs can also skew test results. Assess the ability of the client to tolerate the test which may occasionally cause GI cramping, bloating, abdominal discomfort, vomiting and diarrhea. Assess the client's ability to follow directions and comprehend information provided in the teaching process. **Implement** Encourage adequate fluid intake both before and during testing. Be sure that all of the test dose has been ingested; fill the glass with water after the test dose has been taken. Have client drink the water. Assess tolerance of the test. Be alert for the occurrence of any adverse effects. Teach the client and significant others about the test's purpose and procedure. Discuss how test results will be provided and by whom. **Evaluate** Evaluate tolerance of testing procedure. Assess the client's understanding of the test's purpose and procedure plus his or her knowledge about how the test results will be provided.

Undesired clinical responses and contraindications
Table 78–8 summarizes undesired clinical responses and contraindications associated with major provocative agents.

Life-span considerations No provocative testing agents except tolbutamide have been sufficiently tested for use during pregnancy or in children. Since provocative testing agents are used over a short length of time, in many instances there is only one injection of the testing agent, and the long-term effect of the drug is not a consideration. The effect of these testing agents on elderly individuals is primarily related to the procedure itself rather than the testing agent. For example, some agents require the insertion of a nasogastric tube for recovery of GI secretions. Others require serial sampling of serum urine, which may make the testing procedure painful or complex and thus difficult to understand.

Drug-drug, drug-nutrient, drug-environment interactions Interactions between the provocative testing agents

and other drugs and the environment do occur; however, the occurrence is less frequent since provocative testing agents are used over a short time and in some cases are naturally occurring compounds. See Table 78–9 for more information on the individual provocative testing agents.

CORTICOTROPIN TEST

Corticotropin (ACTH) is used to present the concept behind the use of provocative agents.

Therapeutic use Corticotropin is used to test the function of the adrenal gland and to diagnose adrenocortical insufficiency.

Physiologic response Corticotropin is produced by the anterior pituitary to maintain and control the function of the adrenal cortex. Exogenous and endogenous corticotropin stimulate the adrenal cortex to secrete cortisol (hydrocortisone) and numerous weakly androgenic substances. The corticotropins

Table 78–8

Undesired Clinical Responses and Contraindications Associated With Provocative Agents

Major Undesired Clinical Responses	Contraindications	Nursing Considerations
NATURALLY OCCURRING AGENTS		
Corticotropin		
Hypersensitivity reaction: urticaria, dizziness, nausea, vomiting, and mild fever; anaphylactic shock, wheezing, circulatory failure, death	Porcine protein sensitivity or history of hypersensitivity	Identify any history of allergies or hypersensitivity history that would preclude the use of this testing agent.
Transient local pain, induration, or abscess: may occur if injected subcutaneously or intramuscularly		Closely observe client during the testing process to identify any reaction.
Histamine		
Headache, tachycardia, nervousness, marked hypertension or hypotension, bronchial constriction, dyspnea, flushing, dizziness, visual symptoms, syncope, abdominal cramps, nausea and vomiting, diarrhea, metallic taste, urticaria, and asthma	Geriatric clients or clients with severe hypertension as defined as a blood pressure with a systolic reading >150 mmHg and diastolic reading >100 mmHg	Monitor both the blood pressure and pulse closely.
Local or systemic allergic reactions	This testing agent not specifically contraindicated for those clients with a history of asthma, bronchial disease, bronchospasm, or serious allergic conditions, but risk of a severe adverse reaction is much higher than in other individuals	If the client does have pheochromocytoma, the blood pressure may rise dangerously high; if not, it may fall transiently but quickly. Observe client for the onset of respiratory problems and any allergic reactions.
Secretin		
Potential for a hypersensitive reaction; in addition, client may develop hypersensitivity and be at risk if test is repeated	History of hypersensitivity to secretin, acute pancreatitis, apprehensive or very nervous individuals since testing procedure requires insertion of double-lumen tube into stomach and duodenum	Assess for contraindications; if present, notify primary care provider. During the testing procedure monitor for signs and symptoms of adverse or allergic reaction.
	History of vagotomy or inflammatory bowel disease	
Thyrotropin		
Nausea, vomiting, headache, fever, tachycardia, atrial fibrillation, postinjection flare, urticaria, and menstrual irregularities	History of angina pectoris, cardiac failure, hypopituitarism, coronary thrombosis, untreated Addison's disease, and hypersensitivity to thyrotropin	See secretin.
Hypotension associated with anaphylactic reaction	Caution advised if the client is receiving treatment with corticosteroids	
SYNTHETIC AGENTS		
Arginine		
Rapid IV administration: flushing, nausea, vomiting, numbness, headache, and local venous irritation	History of allergies Presence of uremia	See secretin.
Extravasation of the testing agent: tissue necrosis		
Oral administration: bloating and abdominal pain		
Potential for an allergic reaction exists		
High chloride content may pose a threat to individuals with an electrolyte imbalance		
Cosyntropin		
Hypersensitivity reactions	History of hypersensitivity to cosyntropin	See secretin.

Table continued on following page.

TABLE 78–8 *Continued*

Undesired Clinical Responses and Contraindications Associated With Provocative Agents

Major Undesired Clinical Responses	Contraindications	Nursing Considerations
Edrophonium		
Anticholinesterase agents: nausea, vomiting, diarrhea, abdominal cramps, dysphagia, excessive salivation and sweating, arrhythmias, laryngospasm, increased tracheobronchial secretions, and bronchospasm; weakness, muscle cramps, or fasiculations also possible, as is a brief period of refractoriness to anticholinesterase medications Clients with a history of myocardial infarction: more likely to experience hypotension and bradycardia Clients with myasthenia gravis who are receiving anticholinesterase medication: at risk for cholinergic crisis Respiratory paralysis possible Hypersensitive reaction possible, including allergic reactions to sulfite	Mechanical obstruction of the intestinal or urinary tracts Allergy to sulfite sodium, history of hyperreaction to edrophonium, bronchial asthma Individuals currently taking a cardiac glycoside Caution used when administering this testing agent in client with cardiac arrhythmias	Since there is a risk of cholinergic crisis, have atropine available to counteract the muscarinic effects of the drug. Have facilities available in the event of a respiratory or cardiac arrest. Closely observe client for the onset of any adverse reactions.
Gonadorelin		
Headache, nausea, light-headedness, abdominal discomfort, and flushing If administered subcutaneously, possibility of local reactions: swelling, pain, and pruritus at site Hypersensitivity: rare	Hypersensitivity to gonadorelin or any of its components	Obtain a thorough allergy and drug history. Observe for the onset of any adverse reactions, including a hypersensitivity reaction.
Metyrapone		
Nausea, abdominal discomfort, dizziness, vertigo, headache, sedation and allergic rash Less frequently: a fall in arterial blood pressure and a moderate increase in heart rate	Individuals with adrenocortical insufficiency or a known hypersensitivity to metyrapone	See gonadorelin.
Pentagastrin		
Abdominal pain or cramps, borborygmi, urge to defecate, nausea, vomiting, blood-tinged mucus, flushing, tachycardia, palpitation, hypotension, sensation of tightness in chest, dizziness, faintness, drowsiness, transient blurring of vision, tiredness, headache, tremulousness, shortness of breath, chills, sweating, paresthesia (numbness, tingling, and pain at injection site)	Presence of acute, penetrating, or bleeding peptic ulcers or a history of hypersensitivity Caution used with clients with pancreatic, hepatic, or biliary tract disease	See gonadorelin.
Tolbutamide sodium		
Venospasm or thrombophlebitis with thrombosis of the vein used for injection Severe hypoglycemia Hypersensitivity reaction	Clients with known hypersensitivity to the testing agent or other sulfonylurea drugs	See gonadorelin.
Xylose		
Nausea, intestinal bleeding, borborygmi, vomiting, cramping, abdominal discomfort, diarrhea	No known contraindications	See gonadorelin.

TABLE 78–9

Interactions Associated With Major Provocative Agents

Agent	Drug	Diet	Laboratory Tests/Enivornment
NATURALLY OCCURRING AGENTS			
Corticotropin	Cortisone, hydrocortisone: skew baseline reading upward and the test results downward Estrogens: raise both the baseline and test results Spironolactone: erroneously raises the test results Prednisone, dexamethasone, and betamethasone: not detected by the testing method and do not affect the testing outcomes	—	Agent is stable after reconstitution at room temperature for 24 h and at 2° to 8° C.
Histamine	Antihypertensive agents, sympathomimetic agents, sedatives and opiates: should not be given for 24 h before the test; if possible, expand the time to 72 h	—	Agent is stable in air and unstable in light.
Secretin	Acetazolamide, anticholinergics, mepenzolate bromide, atropine, methantheline bromide, and propantheline bromide: decrease secretin-stimulated pancreatic secretion	Fast for 12–15 h before test; nothing by mouth during test	For long-term stability, store agent at −20° C; for short-term storage, store at 25° C. Once reconstituted, use immediately.
Thyrotropin	Caution advised if receiving current therapy with corticosteroids		Agent is stable for 2 wk after reconstitution at 2° to 8° C.
SYNTHETIC AGENTS			
Arginine	Estrogens and estrogen-progestin combination oral contraceptives: may elevate the growth hormone response and paradoxically reduce glucagon and insulin response Medroxyprogesterone acetate: skews the growth hormone response downward Norethindrone: may reduce the insulin response Potassium-sparing diuretics: may cause hyperkalemia Spironolactone: may cause severe hyperkalemia, especially in clients with severe hepatic disease Plasma glucagon response: may be suppressed by use of long-term sulfonylurea oral antidiabetic agents	Fast overnight before and during test	Agent is stable at room temperature. Protect from heat. If agent is frozen, discard it. Do not use agent if discolored or if the container has no vacuum.
Cosyntropin	Cortisone and hydrocortisone: skew the baseline upward and the test results downward Estrogens: raise both the baseline and the test results upward, but the relationships not affected Prednisone, dexamethasone, and betamethasone: do not affect the testing procedure Enzymes: inactive drug	—	After reconstitution, agent is stable for 24 h at room temperature and for 21 d at 2° to 8° C.
Edrophonium	Anticholinesterase drugs: interfere with test results and should be discontinued at least 8 h before testing Edrophonium: may prolong the phase I block of depolarizing muscle relaxants (e.g., succinylcholine, decamethonium) Effects of nondepolarizing muscle relaxants (e.g., atacurium, gallamine, metocurine, pancuronium, tubocurarine, vecuronium): antagonized by edrophonium Muscarinic effects of this drug: antagonized by atropine Digitalis: may increase sensitivity of cardiac muscle to edrophonium, causing atrioventricular block and possibly prolonged ventricular asystole	—	Agent is stable at 25° C.

Table continued on following page.

TABLE 78–9 *Continued*
Interactions Associated With Major Provocative Agents

Agent	Drug	Diet	Laboratory Tests/Enivornment
Gonadorelin	Test results: inaccurate if drugs used that affect pituitary secretion of gonadotropins (preparations that contain androgens, estrogens, progestins, or glucosteroids) Spironolactone and levodopa: elevate the test response Oral contraceptives and digoxin: suppress the test response	—	Agent is stable at room temperature. Use within 24 h after reconstitution.
Metyrapone	Phenytoin: may invalidate test results; discontinue any therapy with phenytoin at least 2 wk before testing Estrogens, progestins, corticosteroids, phenothiazines chlordiazepoxide, chlorpromazine, amitriptyline, phenobarbital, and methysergide: may produce subnormal response Estrogen-progestin oral contraceptives: may either raise or lower the test response	—	Store agent in tight, light-resistant container. Protect from excessive heat. Metyrapone darkens with exposure to light.
Pentagastrin	None	—	Agent is stable in air and unstable in light.
Tolbutamide sodium	Salicylates, sulfonamides, phenylbutazone, probenecid, monamine oxidase inhibitors, chloramphenicol and any drug that would potentiate the hypoglycemic effect: should not be taken for at least 3 d before test	Diet should contain 150–300 g of carbohydrates for at least 3 d before test	Store agent at 15° to 30° C. Agent must be used within 1 h after reconstitution.
Xylose	Indomethacin, neomycin, colchicine, aspirin, metoclopramide, phenobarbital, or large doses of aminosalicylic acid: cause inaccurate test results	Fast overnight and throughout the test procedure	Store agent at 15° to 30° C in tight containers. Agent must be used within 4 y of manufacture.

also slightly increase aldosterone production. In the normal individual the rate of corticotropin release is regulated by the negative corticosteroid feedback system and nervous system stimulation.

Pharmacokinetics   Corticotropin is transported in the plasma bound to corticosteroid-binding globulin. Corticotropin is absorbed by the tissues over 8 to 16 hours after IM injection and very rapidly after IV injection. The exact mechanism of elimination is not known.

Pharmaceutics   When corticotropin is used for testing purposes, the dose is small both in the amount and the time over which it is administered, thus avoiding many of the undesired clinical responses. Its usual dose to test for adrenocortical insufficiency is 10 to 25 U given intravenously over 8 hours.

Test interpretation   Cortisol levels should peak after 1 hour and drop off in 2 to 4 hours after IV administration of corticotropin. When the repository method is used, the agent is administered subcutaneously; peak levels occur 3 to 12 hours after administration. The adrenal cortex has been "provoked" into responding by releasing cortisol; this response allows the diagnostician to add to the data about that client, thus aiding the diagnostic process. By itself, this test cannot be used to make the diagnosis of adrenocortical insufficiency. Additional tests are needed to complete the diagnosis and to determine the cause of the insufficiency.

Nursing considerations   Obtain a thorough drug history since the use of cortisone, hydrocortisone, estrogen, spironolactone, prednisone, dexamethasone, and betamethasone changes test outcomes. The primary problem encountered with the use of corticotropin as a testing agent is hypersensitivity to it. Therefore assess previous exposure to the agent and history of sensitivity to porcine proteins (corticotropin is extracted from the pituitaries of pigs). Whenever it is suspected that the client is sensitive to porcine proteins, perform hypersensitivity skin testing. Explain the procedure to the client before testing. Include an explanation of the purpose of the test and information about the number and frequency of serum and urine sample collections in the teaching. Give the client information about when to expect the test results and who will provide such information.

CONCEPT REVIEW

Provocative testing stimulates or inhibits a gland or system and has a widespread effect on the body.

Provocative agents usually are administered parenterally to provide a quick response.

These agents are used to test conditions such as adrenocortical insufficiency, poor production of hydrochloric acid (signpost of pernicious anemia), and myasthenia gravis.

Provocative agents are naturally occurring or synthetic; in some cases the synthetic drugs are more easily tolerated by the body.

Drug-drug or drug-environment interactions are not a major consideration because of the short-term use of the agents.

IN VIVO MARKERS AND TRACERS

In vivo markers and tracers are used to evaluate the functioning ability of an organ or tissue. To accomplish this, specific types of tissue or compounds within the body must be identified. Dyes, radioactive material, and miscellaneous compounds are used to "tag" the tissue or compound for identification by a chemical, color assay, or imaging technique. Nonradioactive substances that provide information through chemical analysis or evaluation of color change and radioactive substances that provide information by identification of their distribution in the body are used for tags.

Mode of Action

The **nonradioactive agents** are relatively inert and are passed through the body unchanged. This passage through the body does not cause changes in function, and the agents are used to evaluate organ function, identify structure better,

---

RADIOPHARMACEUTICAL TERMINOLOGY

Alpha particles characterized by decrease in activity as the thickness of tissue (absorber) increases; penetrate only approximately 100 μm into tissue

Beta radiation has two particles—beta+ and beta− ; penetrates 1 mm into tissue

Gamma radiation is electromagnetic, whereas alpha and beta radiation is particulate; is the most penetrating radiation of all; penetrates more than 25 cm into tissue

Half-life time required for the nuclide to decay by one half

Ionizing radiation impact of radiation on tissue, resulting in changed or disrupted bonds between atoms, thus changing how and if the cell will survive

Isotope type of nuclide that has the same number of protons but a different number of neutrons

Nuclide an atom identified by the number of protons and neutrons in the nucleus

Rad unit of measurement of absorbed ionizing radiation energy; 1 rad equals 100 ergs of radiation energy per gram of tissue

Radioactive element one that undergoes spontaneous reaction (decay)

Radiopharmaceutical combination of a radionuclide and another compound; used to "tag" a tissue or component thereof

Roentgen unit of exposure dose to χ or gamma radiation; quantity of χ or gamma radiation that produces one electrostatic unit of charge in 1 cc of air

---

trace flow, and measure compartment volumes. They are administered parenterally and are both rapidly distributed and excreted.

The **radioactive agents** are used for a wide variety of evaluation techniques. An **isotope** is a form of an nuclide (type of atom) that has the same number of protons as other forms of the nuclide but has a different number of neutrons. When an element undergoes spontaneous decay (change in the ratio of neutrons to protons), it is radioactive, a **radioisotope**. During the process of spontaneous decay, particles are lost, creating a "radiation" of energy. The range of *alpha and beta particles* is not very far in tissue (100 μm to 1 mm) and therefore not readily detectable from outside the body. **Gamma particles**, on the other hand, have an acceptable range (25 cm) and are detectable through the use of gamma radiation detection devices. A desirable radioisotope for diagnostic purposes should have an effective range in tissue, be detectable, and have as low a level of radiation as possible. Radioisotopes for diagnostic purposes are chosen based on half-life, quantity required, and body retention time. Radioisotopes that have a short half-life, are detectable using only a small quantity, and are rapidly excreted are used. **Radiopharmaceuticals** are radioactive compounds composed of a radionuclide and a chemical pharmaceutical. Clinically useful radiopharmaceuticals are those that use one or more localization mechanisms (e.g., technetium Tc 99m aggregated albumin injection—the macroaggregate becomes lodged in the small pulmonary capillaries, providing pulmonary information; as the macroaggregates disintegrate, they are taken to the liver and phagocytosed, providing information about that organ). Detection of the radiopharmaceuticals in the body is carried out using different techniques, depending on the agent used and information desired. A large number of radiopharmaceuticals currently are in use.

Therapeutic Uses and Clinical Indications

In vivo markers and tracers have a wide variety of diagnostic uses (see box on page 1090). The test interpretation and standards generally are predicated on the mechanism of location and the half-life.

RADIOPHARMACEUTICS

Indocyanine green   Indocyanine green has a half-life of 2.2 to 3 minutes and is highly bound to plasma proteins. It is eliminated by active uptake into hepatic parenchymal cells for transport to bile for excretion in the stool. A serum sample is obtained 20 minutes after injection and prepared for a photometric reading. Since indocyanine green is transported through the body but does not become a part of it, the results should be a dye retention in the body of less than 4%. Any amount greater than 4% indicates liver dysfunction.

Sodium pertechnetate Tc 99m   Sodium pertechnetate Tc 99m has been used for the detection and location of cranial lesions, thyroid and salivary gland imaging, placental localization, and blood-pool imaging. Currently it is combined with other compounds in radiopharmaceuticals used to evaluate a

need further education about any disease or condition identified by the test.

CONCEPT REVIEW

In vivo markers and tracers assist in evaluating an organ or tissue, fluid volume, flow rate, or diffusion and concentration ability. They "tag" a tissue or compound for identification by a chemical, color assay, or imaging technique.

In vivo markers and tracers can be nonradioactive or radioactive. Nonradioactive agents are relatively inert, do not cause changes in body function, and pass through the body unchanged.

Radioisotopes must have a level of radioactivity that can be detected outside the body, a short half-life, and a rapid excretion time and must be able to tag the body part using only a small quantity of the radioisotope.

The most useful radiopharmaceuticals localize to specific body parts.

Some uses of in vivo markers are testing heart or liver function, locating cranial lesions or position of the placenta, and imaging the thyroid, the salivary glands, and the lung.

SUMMARY

Drugs used for diagnostic procedures provide a means to assess the allergic or immune status, to obtain a picture of a cavity or organ, and to measure the function of an organ or body system. Drugs used for skin testing must elicit a specific, identifiable reaction without putting the client at risk for anaphylactic reaction. Drugs used for imaging must be opaque to the scanning device used whereas those used as provocative agents must cause a systemic reaction and must be monitored very carefully. Drugs used as tracers must be incorporated in particular molecules and must emit enough radiation to be seen on a scan without hurting the client. Even if the agents have therapeutic uses, the dosages of diagnostic agents for testing are much smaller (i.e., the smallest amount needed to obtain the desired reaction). The nurse's role in helping clients undergoing testing involves careful preparation for the tests themselves and providing education and support in light of possible test results.

REFERENCES

1. Chase, G.D. (1990). Medical applications of radioisotopes. In A.R. Gennaro (Ed.), *Remington's pharmaceutical sciences* (pp. 624–652). Easton, PA: Mack.
2. Zink, G.L. (1990). Principles of immunology. In A.R. Gennaro (Ed.), *Remington's pharmaceutical sciences* (pp. 1379–1388). Easton, PA: Mack.
3. Cunningham, R.K., & Smith, C.M. (1992). Interactions: Drug allergy; drug-drug; drug-food. In C.M. Smith & A.M. Reynaud (Eds.), *Textbook of pharmacology* (pp. 1090–1103). Philadelphia: W.B. Saunders.
4. McEvoy, G.K. (Ed.) (1992). Diagnostic agents. *American Hospital Formulary Service drug information* (pp. 1389–1481). Bethesda, MD: American Society of Hospital Pharmacists.
5. Swinyard, E.A. (1990). Diagnostic drugs. In A.R. Gennaro (Ed.), *Remington's pharmaceutical sciences* (pp. 1272–1285). Easton, PA: Mack.
6. Carr, E.A. (1992). Diagnostic drugs. In C.M. Smith & A.M. Reynaud (Eds.), *Textbook of pharmacology* (pp. 1027–1049). Philadelphia: W.B. Saunders.

BIBLIOGRAPHY

Radwin, L.E. (1990). Research on diagnostic reasoning in nursing. *Nursing Diagnosis, 1,* 70–77.

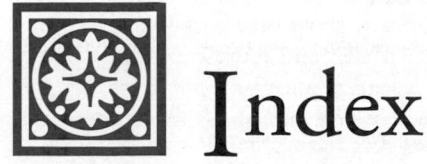

Index

Note: Page numbers in *italics* refer to illustrations; page numbers followed by t refer to tables.

GUIDE TO NURSING RESEARCH